Krause's

FOOD, NUTRITION, & DIET THERAPY

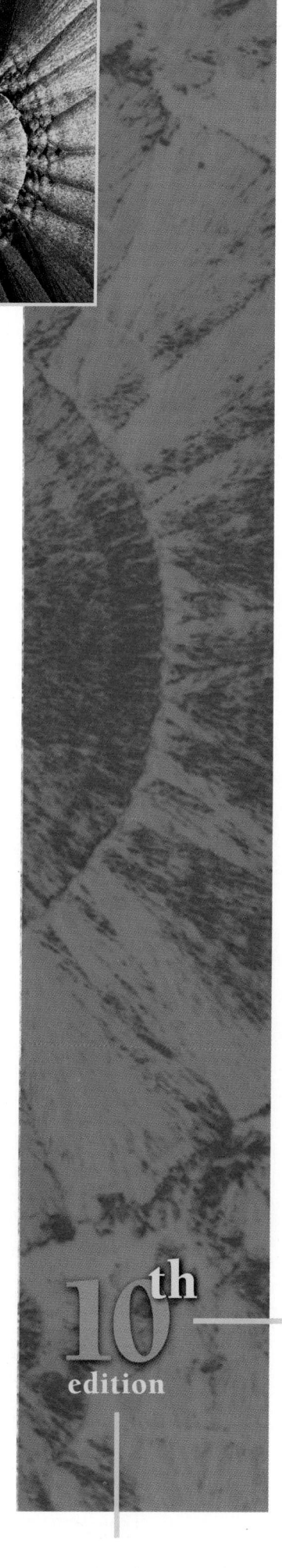

Krause's

FOOD, NUTRITION, & DIET THERAPY

edited by

L. Kathleen Mahan, MS, RD, CDE
Clinical Associate
Department of Pediatrics
School of Medicine
University of Washington
Seattle, Washington
and
Nutrition Consultant
Nutrition by Design
Seattle, Washington

Sylvia Escott-Stump, MA, RD, LDN
Dietetic Programs Director
East Carolina University
Greenville, North Carolina
and
Consulting Nutritionist
Nutritional Balance
Greenville, North Carolina

W.B. Saunders Company
A Division of Harcourt Brace & Company
Philadelphia London Toronto Montreal Sydney Tokyo

W.B. SAUNDERS COMPANY
A Division of Harcourt Brace & Company

The Curtis Center
Independence Square West
Philadelphia, Pennsylvania 19106

Cover illustration: Crystallized Vitamin C

Library of Congress Cataloging-in-Publication Data

Krause's food, nutrition, and diet therapy / edited by L. Kathleen Mahan, Sylvia Escott-Stump. — 10th ed.
p. cm.
Includes bibliographical references and index.
ISBN 0–7216–7904–8
1. Diet therapy. 2. Nutrition. 3. Food. I. Mahan, L. Kathleen. II. Escott-Stump, Sylvia.
RM216.M285 2000
615.8′54—dc21 99–16752

KRAUSE'S FOOD, NUTRITION, AND DIET THERAPY ISBN 0–7216–7904–8

Printed in the United States of America

Last digit is the print number: 9 8 7 6 5 4 3 2 1

This edition is dedicated to the memory of Marie Krause Mendelson (1906–1994) whose idea led to a universally recognized, authoritative, and popular textbook. During her lifetime Marie wrote the first five editions and gave encouragement for subsequent editions.

It is our wish that students and practitioners acknowledge the dedication with which this work was begun in 1952 by Marie Krause Mendelson.

—The Authors, 10th Edition

Preface

The tenth edition of this classic text continues to recognize the increasing importance of nutrition in achieving and maintaining optimal health and fitness and as a component of complete and effective health care. Its purpose is to furnish theoretical knowledge and clinical information in a form that will be useful to students in nursing, dietetics, and other allied health professions, many of whom are receiving education and training in an interdisciplinary clinical setting. It is valuable as an ancillary text for use in other disciplines such as medicine, dentistry, child development, and health education. As always, with its extensive appendices, tables, illustrations, figures, and clinical insight boxes providing practical hands-on procedures and clinical tools, it continues to be the textbook that can accompany the graduating student into clinical practice as a treasured reference source. All of the popular features have been retained in this edition, and all material has been updated and referenced extensively to reflect the most current information available.

Authors

This edition introduces new guest authors who join those who have participated in previous editions. There has also been the addition of many new reviewers. The contributions of these reputable authors and reviewers, all of whom are experts in their fields, reflect the effort of this text to cover the increasing sophistication of nutritional care and education.

Organization and Content

This edition is organized into five parts. Two of these, **Nutrition Basics** and **Nutrition in the Life Cycle,** are appropriate for use as the text for a basic nutrition course. Although Parts 3, 4, and 5 are progressively more clinical in content, sections of Part 4—**Nutrition for Health and Fitness**—fit very well into a basic nutrition course. The third part **Nutrition Care,** and the fifth part **Medical Nutrition Therapy,** provide the basis for training in diet therapy and add the background information and hands-on tools necessary for successful clinical practice.

Part 1—Nutrition Basics—continues to furnish material appropriate for teaching basic nutrition. A new chapter—**Macronutrients**—synthesizes the content of the previous three chapters on carbohydrates, lipids, and proteins into one chapter. The chapter is more useful because the content is more integrated, and the student can refer to one place. Practical information is provided by many tables with useful clinical applications such as calculation of energy requirements and expenditure, and the best food sources for each vitamin and mineral.

In **Part 2—Nutrition in the Life Cycle**—an expert group of guest authors presents in-depth information on the importance of nutrition from pregnancy throughout the aging process. These chapters discuss the nutrition issues in each life stage. A new chapter on **Nutrition in the Adult Years** presents knowledge relating the beginning of chronic disease seen in the elderly to the nutrition habits and intakes in adulthood. The role of phytonutrients, antioxidants, and fiber of a plant-based diet in delaying or preventing chronic disease and optimizing health, are highlighted.

Part 3—Nutrition Care—covers the concepts of the individual's nutritional status as a reflection of eating habits, pharmacological and nutritional treatment, and the nutrition resources in the community. There are three new chapters in this section—Chapters 17, 19, and 21. **Chapter 17—Laboratory Data in Nutrition Assessment**—discusses a patient's biochemical data and how they are interpreted and integrated into the complete assessment. It is complemented by the extensive Appendix 32, which gives the details of every laboratory test. **Chapter 19—Integrative Medicine and Herbal Therapy**—discusses alternative therapies and the role of botanicals in nutritional care. **Chapter 21—Counseling for Change**—presents the transtheoretical model for counseling the client who needs to make changes in eating habits. All of these chapters are much needed, practical chapters that students and clinicians will find very useful.

Part 4—Nutrition for Health and Fitness—continues to bring together nutrition concepts that have particular meaning in the achievement and maintenance of health and fitness, and the prevention of chronic disease. Chapters on dental health and bone health, atherosclerotic heart disease, hypertension, and athletic training and sports focus on the role of nutrition in the prevention of problems in these areas. The previous chapter on weight control has been replaced with two chapters: **Nutrition for Weight Management** and **Nutrition in Eating Disorders.** We felt that the now extensive material on eating disorders warranted its own chapter. Although theories of cancer prevention would also be appropriate to this section, these are discussed in the chapter on **Medical Nutrition Therapy for Neoplastic Disease** that appears in Part 5.

Part 5—Medical Nutrition Therapy—continues to reflect the current knowledge and trends in nutrition therapy. All 15 of the chapters are written by specialists in the nutritional aspects of conditions such as diabetes, renal disease, and pulmonary disease. And most of these chapters have been reviewed by additional specialists, making the content extremely up-to-date and useful.

Features New to the Tenth Edition

One of the most significant changes made to this edition is the increased emphasis on pathophysiology. Responding to the needs of our readers, we highlighted pathophysiology content throughout the **Medical Nutrition Therapy** chapters. Additionally, we have included new algorithms that illustrate pathophysiology and signs of disease, and present appropriate medical and nutritional management. We feel this new emphasis will better equip students to understand the illness process and provide optimum nutritional care.

Throughout the text we have incorporated the new **Dietary Reference Intakes (DRIs)** that were available. They are designated as Recommended Dietary Allowances (RDA), Adequate Intakes (AI) or Tolerable Upper Levels of Intake (UL). Those RDAs that were not changed at the time of printing are designated as such.

We have also added **itnernet website addresses** to most chapters to give the student additional resources for study. These website references continue to make this text current and practical.

In the extensive Appendices the reader will still find, all in one place, the clinical references and tools that have always been a valued feature of this text. There are two new appendices. **Appendix 3, the ICD-9 Codes** for nutritional therapy diagnoses, will be very useful to the clinician and administrator for documenting the effectiveness of medical nutritional therapy. **Appendix 54—Glycemic Indices of Foods—**contains the most comprehensive table available and will be very useful to the clinician or student working with athletes, people with diabetes, or others in whom maintenance of optimal blood glucose or insulin levels is a challenge.

The large **Appendix 41—Nutritive Values of the Edible Parts of Foods—** has been condensed and the previous tables on **folic acid** and **zinc content of foods** have been incorporated into it. **Clinical Insight, New Directions,** and **Focus On** boxes have been expanded and continue to provide the student and teacher with "nice to know" information and suggest areas for further discussion, study, or research.

Ancillary

New to this edition is the **Instructor's Electronic Resource** CD-ROM. The Instructor's Electronic Resource CD-ROM consists of an Instructor's Manual, Lecture View and ExaMaster.

The **Instructor's Manual** presents for each text chapter an overview of the chapter, learning objectives, and teaching strategies to enhance teaching and learning. **LectureView** is a PowerPoint presentation utilizing 200 images from the text and 220 prepared word slides showcasing important content. With this tool instructors can custom build exciting, visual classroom presentations. The **ExaMaster** computerized test bank offers the instructor a variety of testing options using the 800 available test questions.

L. Kathleen Mahan, M.S., R.D., C.D.E.
Sylvia Escott-Stump, M.A., R.D., L.D.N.

Acknowledgments

We wish to acknowledge the hard work and support of Maura Connor, Senior Acquisitions Editor, Terri Ward, Senior Developmental Editor, and Sharon Iwanczuk, Artist, at W.B. Saunders Company; Mary McDonald, Production Editor; Elizabeth Summers, who prepared some of the vitamin tables; Susan Casey, Sarah Eitelbach, Renee Willett, and Toi Borthwick, who helped with the procuring some of the new photographs; and reviewers for the tenth edition. We would also like to thank the authors of the ancillary materials to accompany the tenth edition. Most important is the loyal support from our families, without whom this work could not be completed: Robert, Carly, and Ana Raab; Elsa and Jim Mahan; Clara Escott; Russ, Matthew, and Lindsay Stump; Florianne Stump; and Joyce Stanley and family.

Reviewers

Leila T. Beker, PhD, RD, LD
Assistant Clinical Professor of Pediatrics
College of Medicine & Health Sciences
George Washington University
Attending Nutritionist
Children's National Medical Center
Washington, DC

Peter L. Beyer, MS, RD
Associate Professor
Dietetics and Nutrition
University of Kansas Medical Center
Kansas City, KS

Carmen Boyd, MS, RD, LPC
Southwest Missouri State University
Springfield, MO

Tracey L. Carlyle, MS, RD
Loyola University Chicago
Chicago, IL

Joseph Y. Chang, PhD
Vice President
Research and Development
Pharmanex, Inc.
Simi Valley, CA

Judith L. Dodd, MS, RD, CFCS, FADA
Clinical Dietetics and Nutrition
School of Health and Rehabilitation Services
University of Pittsburgh
Pittsburgh, PA

Robert Earl, MPH, RD
Director of Public Health
International Food Information Council
Washington, DC

Barbara Eldridge, RD
Clinical Research Associate
University of Colorado Health Sciences Center and Cancer Center
Denver, CO

Miriam Erick, MS, RD, CDE
Department of Nutrition
Brigham and Women's Hospital
Boston, MA

Rachel M. Fournet, PhD, RD, LDN
University of Southwestern Louisiana
Lafayette, LA

Barbara Gollman, MS, RD, LD
The Good Food Group
Dallas, TX

Cynthia Hamilton, MS, RD, LD, CNSD
Cleveland Clinic Foundation
Cleveland, OH

Karen S. Kubena, PhD, RD
Associate Dean for Academic Affairs
College of Agriculture & Life Sciences
Professor of Nutrition
Texas A&M University
College Station, TX

Edith Lerner, PhD, LD
Case Western Reserve University
Cleveland, OH

Tara Prather Liskov, MS, RD, CD-N
Yale-New Haven Hospital
New Haven, CT

Dan Lukaczer, ND
HealthComm International
Gig Harbor, WA

Suzanne Martin, PhD, RD
College of the Ozarks
Point Lookout, MO

Sarah L. Morgan, MD, MS, RD, FADA, FACP
The University of Alabama at Birmingham
Birmingham, AL

Renee Piazza-Barnett, MEd, RD, LD, CNSD
Nutrition Support & Vascular Access Department
The Cleveland Clinic Foundation
Cleveland, OH

Nancy F. Sheard, ScD, RD
University of Vermont
Burlington, VT

Linda R. Shoaf, PhD, LDN, RD
Private Practice
Rutherford, TN

Kay S. Soltesz, PhD, RD, LD
Bluffton College
Bluffton, OH

Arleen Banks Tate, MS, RD, LD
Johns Hopkins Bayview Medical Center
Baltimore, MD

Stella L. Volpe, PhD, RD, FACSM
University of Massachusetts
Amherst, MA

Kerri Wiggins, MS, RD
Renal Dietitian
Skagit Valley Kidney Center
Mt. Vernon, WA

Contributors

Chapter Contributors

Diane M. Anderson, PhD, RD, CSP, FADA
Associate Professor of Pediatrics
Neonatal Nutritionist
Medical University of South Carolina
Charleston, South Carolina
Chapter 9, Nutrition for the Low–Birth-Weight Infant

John J. B. Anderson, PhD
Professor of Nutrition
Schools of Public Health and Medicine
University of North Carolina
Chapel Hill, North Carolina
Chapter 5, Minerals
Chapter 28, Nutrition for Bone Health

Cynthia Taft Bayerl, MS, RD
Director, Perinatal and Pediatric Nutrition Programs
Massachusetts Department of Public Health
Boston, Massachusetts
Chapter 14, Nutrition in the Community

Jacqueline R. Berning, PhD, RD
Assistant Professor, Department of Biology
University of Colorado
Colorado Springs, Colorado
Nutrition Consultant
Denver Broncos Football Club, Denver Nuggets Basketball Club, University of Colorado–Boulder Athletic Department, and Cleveland Indians Minor League Baseball Teams
Chapter 25, Nutrition for Exercise and Sports Performance

Peter L. Beyer, MS, RD
Associate Professor, Department of Dietetics and Nutrition
University of Kansas Medical Center
Kansas City, Kansas
Chapter 1, Digestion, Absorption, Transport, and Excretion of Nutrients
Chapter 30, Medical Nutrition Therapy for Upper Gastrointestinal Tract Disorders
Chapter 31, Medical Nutrition Therapy Therapy for Lower Gastrointestinal Tract Disorders

Abby S. Bloch, PhD, RD, FADA
Associate Professor
New York University Graduate School of Education
Nutrition and Food Studies
New York, New York
Formerly Coordinator (30 years)
Clinical Nutrition Research
GI/Nutrition Service
Department of Medicine
Memorial Sloan-Kettering Cancer Center
New York, New York
Chapter 22, Enteral and Parenteral Nutrition Support

Susan T. Borra, RD
Senior Vice President, Director of Nutrition
International Food Information Council
Washington, DC
Chapter 15, Guidelines for Dietary Planning

Cynthia M. Brylinsky, MS, RD
Director, Guest Services
North Central and Eastern Regions
Penn State Geisinger Health System
Geisinger Medical Center
Danville, Pennsylvania
Chapter 20, The Nutritional Care Process

Timothy H. Carlson, PhD, RD
Senior Scientist
Pacific Biometrics, Inc.
Seattle, Washington
Chapter 17, Laboratory Data in Nutrition Assessment

Gerald F. Combs, Jr., PhD
Professor of Nutrition
Division of Nutrition Science
Cornell University
Ithaca, New York
Chapter 4, Vitamins

Patrick J. Connolly, MD
Resident, Section of Neurosurgery
Indiana University School of Medicine
Indianapolis, Indiana
Chaper 42, Medical Nutrition Therapy for Neurologic Disorders

Robert Earl, MPH, RD
Director of Public Health
International Food Information Council
Washington, DC
Chapter 15, Guidelines for Dietary Planning

Susan Ettinger, PhD, RD
Chair and Associate Professor
Department of Clinical Nutrition
New York Institute of Technology
Old Westbury, New York
Chapter 3, Macronutrients: Carbohydrates, Proteins, and Lipids

Cathy Fagen, MA, RD
Perinatal Nutritionist
Long Beach Memorial Medical Center
Long Beach, California
Chapter 7, Nutrition During Pregnancy and Lactation

Marcy Fenton, MS, RD
HIV Nutrition Advocate
AIDS Project Los Angeles
Los Angeles, California
Chapter 40, Medical Nutrition Therapy for Human Immunodeficiency Virus (HIV) Infection and Acquired Immonodeficiency Syndrome (AIDS)

Carol B. Frankmann, MS, RD, LD, CNSD
Director
Department of Clinical Nutrition
University of Texas
M. D. Anderson Cancer Center
Houston, Texas
Chapter 39, Medical Nutrition Therapy for Neoplastic Disease

Marion J. Franz, MS, RD, LD, CDE
Director, Nutrition and Professional Education
International Diabetes Center
Minneopolis, Minnesota
Teaching Specialist
Department of Food Services and Nutrition
University of Minnesota
St. Paul University
St. Paul, Minnesota
Chapter 34, Medical Nutrition Therapy for Diabetes Mellitus and Hypoglycemia of Nondiabetic Origin

Therese Ann Franzese, MS, RD, CD-N
Director, Clinical Dietetic Internship
Assistant Professor
New York Institute of Technology
School of Allied Health Sciences
Department of Clinical Nutrition
Old Westbury, New York
Director of Nutrition Counseling
Club Sports International
New York, New York
Chapter 43, Medical Nutrition Therapy for Rheumatic Disorders

Victoria A. Haken, MS, RD, CNSD
Adjunct Professor
New York University
New York, New York
Associate Director
Food and Nutrition Services
New York Methodist Hospital
Brooklyn, New York
Chapter 18, Interactions Between Drugs and Nutrients

Kathleen A. Hammond, MS, RD, LD, CNSD, BSN, RN
Clinical Instructor, Nutrition Support
University of Georgia
Athens, Georgia
Coordinator, Continuing Education
Clinical Nutrition Specialist
NHC/Nations Healthcare, Inc.
Department of Professional Practice
Alpharetta, Georgia
Chapter 16, Dietary and Clinical Assessment

Nancy G. Harris, MS, RD, LDN
Lecturer
Department of Nutrition and Hospitality Management
School of Human Environmental Services
East Carolina University
Consultant
Cypress Glen Retirement Community
Greenville, North Carolina
Chapter 13, Nutrition in Aging

Jeanette M. Hasse, PhD, RD, FADA, CNSD
Transplant Nutrition Specialist
Baylor University Medical Center
Dallas, Texas
Chapter 32, Medical Nutrition Therapy for Liver, Biliary System, and Exocrine Pancreas Disorders

Rachel K. Johnson, PhD, RD
Associate Dean and Associate Professor
Department of Nutrition and Food Sciences
University of Vermont
Burlington, Vermont
Chapter 2, Energy

Tracy Stopler Kasdan, MS, RD
President
Nutrition Etc., Inc.
Plainview, New York
Professor
Aldephia University
Garden City, New York
Chapter 35, Medical Nutrition Therapy for Anemia

Debra A. Krummel, PhD, RD
West Virginia University School of Medicine
Morgantown, West Virginia
Chapter 26, Nutrition in Cardiovascular Disease
Chapter 27, Nutrition in Hypertension
Chapter 36, Medical Nutrition Therapy for Heart Failure and Transplant

Ida Laquatra, PhD, RD
Nutrition Consultant
Shape Up America
Heinz Institute of Nutritional Sciences, Inc.
Pittsburgh, Pennsylvania
Chapter 23, Nutrition for Weight Management

Betty Lucas, MPH, RD, CD
Lecturer, Family and Child Nursing
Nutritionist
Center on Human Development and Disability
University of Washington
Seattle, Washington
Chapter 10, Nutrition in Childhood

Susan G. Manchester, RD, LDN, CNSD
Clinical Dietitian
Rhode Island Hospital
Providence, Rhode Island
Chapter 33, Medical Nutrition Therapy for Metabolic Stress: Sepsis, Trauma, Burns, and Surgery

Laura E. Matarese, MS, RD, FADA, CNSD
Manager, Nutrition Support Dietetics
Cleveland Clinic Foundation
Cleveland, Ohio
Chapter 32, Medical Nutrition Therapy for Liver, Biliary System, and Exocrine Pancreas Disorders

Kimberly Mathai, MS, RD, CN
Nutrition Consultant
Nutrition by Design
Adjunct Faculty, Nutrition Department
John Bastyr University
Seattle, Washington
Chapter 12, Nutrition in the Adult Years
Chapter 19, Integrative Medicine and Herbal Therapy

Charles Mueller, MS, RD, CNSD
Adjunct Clinical Assistant Professor
Department of Food and Nutrition Studies
New York University
Nutrition Research Manager
General Clinical Research Center
Cornell University Medical Center
New York, New York
Chapter 22, Enteral and Parenteral Nutrition Support

Donna H. Mueller, PhD, RD, FADA
Associate Professor, Nutrition and Food Sciences
Department of Bioscience and Biotechnology
Drexel University
Adjunct Staff, Department of Pathology and Laboratory Medicine
St. Christopher's Hospital for Children
Philadelphia, Pennsylvania
Chapter 37, Medical Nutrition Therapy for Pulmonary Disease

Pamela Reichert-Anderson, MA, RD
Registered Dietitian
Long Island Jewish Hospital/Schneider Children's Hospital
New Hyde Park, New York
Chapter 24, Nutrition in Eating Disorders

Janet Schebendach, MA, RD
Nutritionist-in-Charge
Center for Eating Disorders
Division of Adolescent Medicine
Schneider Children's Hospital
New Hyde Park, New York
Chapter 24, Nutrition in Eating Disorders

Leeann R. Shiveley, MPH, RD
Study Manager
Epidemiology and Medical Studies Program
Research Triangle Institute
Rockville, Maryland
Formerly Senior Clinical Dietitian
John Hopkins Hospital
Baltimore, Maryland
Chaper 42, Medical Nutrition Therapy for Neurologic Disorders

Ellyn Silverman, MPH, RD, CHES
President
ECS Nutrition Services
Long Beach, California
Chapter 40, Medical Nutrition Therapy for Human Immunodeficiency Virus (HIV) Infection and Acquired Immonodeficiency Syndrome (AIDS)

Linda G. Snetselaar, PhD, RD
Associate Professor
Department of Preventive Medicine and Environmental Health
University of Iowa
Iowa City, Iowa
Chapter 21, Counseling for Change

Bonnie A. Spear, PhD, RD
Assistant Professor
Department of Pediatrics
Division of General Pediatrics and Adolescent Medicine
University of Alabama at Birmingham
Birmingham, Alabama
Chapter 11, Nutrition in Adolescence

Riva Touger-Decker, PhD, RD, FADA
Assistant Professor
University of Medicine and Dentistry of New Jersey
Newark, New Jersey
Chapter 29, Nutrition for Oral and Dental Health

Cristine M. Trahms, MS, RD, FADA
Lecturer, Department of Pediatrics
Head, Nutrition Center on Human Development and Disabilities
University of Washington
Seattle, Washington
Chapter 8, Nutrition in Infancy
Chapter 44, Medical Nutrition Therapy for Metabolic Disorders

Susan J. Whitmire, RD, CNSD
Clinical Dietitian
Adult Critical Care Medicine/Nutrition Support Service
Penn State Geisinger Health System
Danville, Pennsylvania
Chapter 6, Water, Electrolytes, and Acid-Base Balance

Katy G. Wilkens, MS, RD
Manager, Nutrition Services
Northwest Kidney Centers
Seattle, Washington
Chapter 38, Medical Nutrition Therapy for Renal Disorders

Sherry Hubbard Wilson, RD, LD
Liason
American Dietetic Associatioon
American Academy of Allergy, Asthma, and Immunology
Oklahoma City, Oklahoma
Chapter 41, Medical Nutrition Therapy for Food Allergy and Food Intolerance

Marion F. Winkler, MS, RD, CNSD
Clinical Teaching Associate of Surgery
Brown University School of Medicine
Surgical Nutrition Specialist
Rhode Island Hospital
Providence, Rhode Island
Chapter 33, Medical Nutrition Therapy for Metabolic Stress: Sepsis, Trauma, Burns, and Surgery

Pathology Algorithm Contributors

John J. B. Anderson, PhD
Department of Nutrition
Schools of Public Health and Medicine
University of North Carolina
Chapel Hill, North Carolina

Sanford C. Garner, PhD
Duke University Medical Center
Durham, North Carolina

Contents in Brief

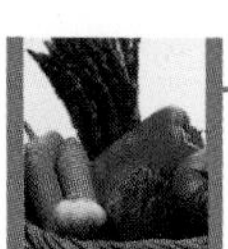

PART 1 • Nutrition Basics

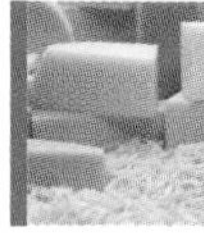

PART 2 • Nutrition in the Life Cycle

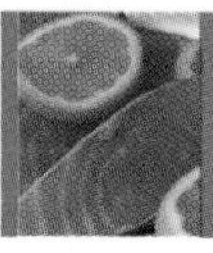

PART 3 • Nutrition Care

NOTICE

Contents

PART 1 • Nutrition Basics

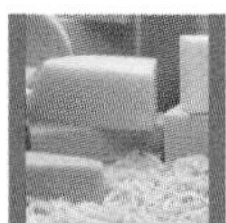

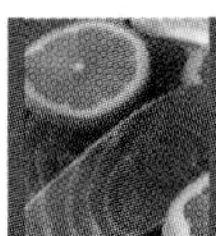

PART 3 • NUTRITION CARE

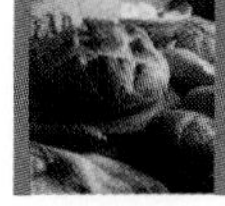

PART 4 • NUTRITION FOR HEALTH AND FITNESS

Krause's

FOOD, NUTRITION, & DIET THERAPY

PART 1

Nutrition Basics

Food and nutrients provide the energy and building materials for the countless substances that are essential to the growth and survival of living things. The manner in which nutrients become integral parts of the body and contribute to its function depends on the physiologic and biochemical processes that govern their actions.

This section opens with an overview of the processes of digestion, absorption, transportation, and excretion because these functions determine the fate of the food after it enters the body. Foods invite consumption for a variety of reasons, including form, texture, and flavor, as well as a host of psychosocial factors. Once inside the alimentary tract, however, their relative attractiveness is no longer an issue, as processes of digestion reduce them all to the same common denominators and make them available in a size and form capable of absorption and transportation to individual cells.

Proteins, fats, and carbohydrates all contribute to the total energy pool, but the energy that they yield is all in the same form. Utilization and conservation of this energy to build and maintain the body requires the involvement of vitamins and minerals. They function as coenzymes, catalysts, and buffers in the miraculous watery arena of metabolism.

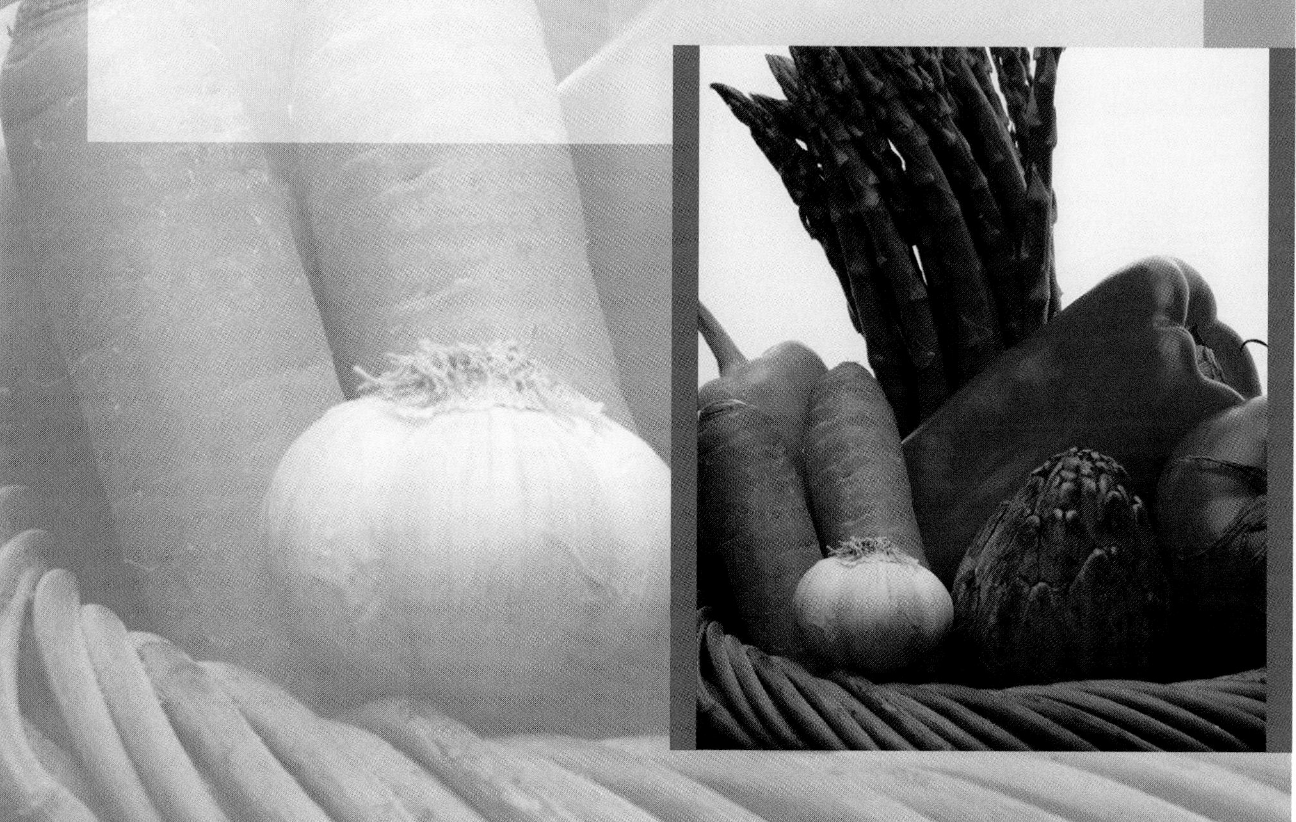

CHAPTER 1

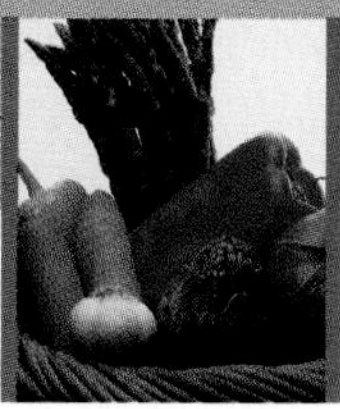

Digestion, Absorption, Transport, and Excretion of Nutrients

PETER L. BEYER, MS, RD

Chapter Outline

- The Gastrointestinal Tract
- Overview of Digestive and Absorptive Processes
- The Small Intestine—Primary Site for Nutrient Absorption
- Role of the Large Intestine

Key Terms

ACTIVE TRANSPORT—the movement of particles, in combination with a carrier protein, across cell membranes and epithelial layers, a process requiring expenditure of energy

AMYLASE (PTYALIN)—an enzyme, secreted in saliva and from the pancreas, that catalyzes the hydrolysis of starch

BRUSH BORDER—the microvilli that greatly increase the surface area of the intestinal mucosal cell

CHELATION—the process by which a mineral is bound to a ligand—usually an acid, organic acid, or sugar—so that it is in a form capable of being absorbed into the intestinal cell

CHOLECYSTOKININ (CCK)—a hormone secreted by the proximal small bowel that stimulates the pancreas to secrete enzymes (and, to a lesser extent, bicarbonate and water), stimulates gallbladder contraction, slows gastric emptying, and may possibly regulate appetite

CHYME—the semi-fluid, gruel-like material produced by the gastric digestion of food

COLONIC SALVAGE—the process of fermenting and absorbing dietary carbohydrates, fiber, and amino acids from the large intestine

ENTEROGASTRONE—a hormone, secreted by the duodenal mucosa in response to the presence of fat in the duodenum, that inhibits gastric secretion and motility, thus slowing the delivery of further lipid into the duodenum

FACILITATED DIFFUSION—movement of particles across a membrane via a carrier protein

GASTRIC INHIBITORY POLYPEPTIDE (GIP)—a hormone released from the intestinal mucosa in the presence of fat and glucose that inhibits gastric acid secretion and stimulates insulin release

GASTRIN—a hormone produced by the antral mucosa of the stomach that stimulates gastric secretions and motility

GLUCAGON-LIKE PEPTIDE 1 (GLP-1)—a hormone released from the intestinal mucosa that slows gastric emptying, lowers glucagon concentration, stimulates proinsulin synthesis, and increases insulin sensitivity

LACTASE—the intestinal enzyme that hydrolyzes lactose to glucose and galactose

MALTASE—the intestinal enzyme that hydrolyzes maltose into glucose units

MICELLE—a complex of free fatty acids, monoglycerides, and bile salts that allows for the absorption of lipid products into the intestinal mucosal cell

MICROVILLI—minute cylindrical processes on the surface of the intestinal cells that greatly increase the absorptive surface area of the cells

PANCREATIC LIPASE—an enzyme in pancreatic juice that hydrolyzes the ester linkages between fatty acids and glycerol

PARIETAL CELLS—large cells scattered along the walls of the stomach that secrete the hydrochloric acid in gastric juice

PASSIVE DIFFUSION—the random movement of particles through openings in cellular membranes depending on electrochemical and concentration gradients

PERISTALSIS—the movement by which the alimentary canal propels its contents

PROTEOLYTIC ENZYMES—trypsin, chymotrypsin, and carboxypolypeptidase, which break down protein into proteoses, peptones, peptides, and amino acids

SECRETIN—a hormone released from the duodenal wall into the bloodstream, which stimulates the pancreas to secrete water and bicarbonate and inhibits gastrin secretion

SUCRASE—the intestinal enzyme that hydrolyzes sucrose to glucose and fructose

VILLI—the numerous, finger-like projections that cover the surface of the mucosa of the small intestine

Most of the major nutrients in foods are bound in large molecules that cannot be absorbed from the intestine because of their size or because they are not soluble. The digestive system is responsible for reducing these large molecules into smaller, readily absorbed units and for converting the insoluble molecules into soluble forms. Proper function of the absorptive and transport mechanisms is crucial to delivering the products of digestion to individual cells. Derangements of any of these systems can result in malnutrition, even in the presence of an adequate diet.

THE GASTROINTESTINAL TRACT

The primary roles of the gastrointestinal (GI) tract are to (1) extract macronutrients, protein, carbohydrate, lipid, water, and ethanol from ingested foods and beverages, (2) absorb necessary micronutrients and trace elements, and (3) serve as a physical and immunologic barrier to microorganisms, foreign material, and potential antigens consumed with foods or formed during the passage of foods through the GI tract. In addition to its primary roles, the GI tract also participates in many other regulatory and metabolic functions that affect the entire body.

The human GI tract is well suited for digesting and absorbing nutrients from a tremendous variety of foodstuffs, including meats, dairy products, fruits, vegetables, grains, complex starches, sugars, fats, and oils. With few exceptions, the human GI tract is remarkably efficient. Humans can consume a wide variety of foods, ranging in chemical composition from simple to complex, and can consume the foods in random combinations without significant loss of digestive effectiveness. Depending on the nature of the diet consumed, about 92% to 97% of it is digested and absorbed. The primary exception to this rule is that the human GI tract is unable to digest most plant fibers. Compared to ruminants and animals with very large cecums, humans are considerably less efficient at extracting energy from grasses, stems, seeds, and other coarse fibrous materials. Humans lack the enzymes to hydrolyze the chemical bonds that link the molecules of sugars forming plant fibers. Fibrous foods are fermented by bacteria in the human colon, but only 5% to 10% of the energy needed by humans can be derived from this process.

The GI tract, which extends from the mouth to the anus, is one of the largest organs in the body (Fig. 1–1). It is configured in a pattern of folds, pits, and finger-like projections, called **villi,** which are lined with epithelial cells and even smaller, cylindrical extensions called **microvilli.** The result is a tremendous increase in surface area compared to that expected from a smooth, hollow cylinder. In ad-

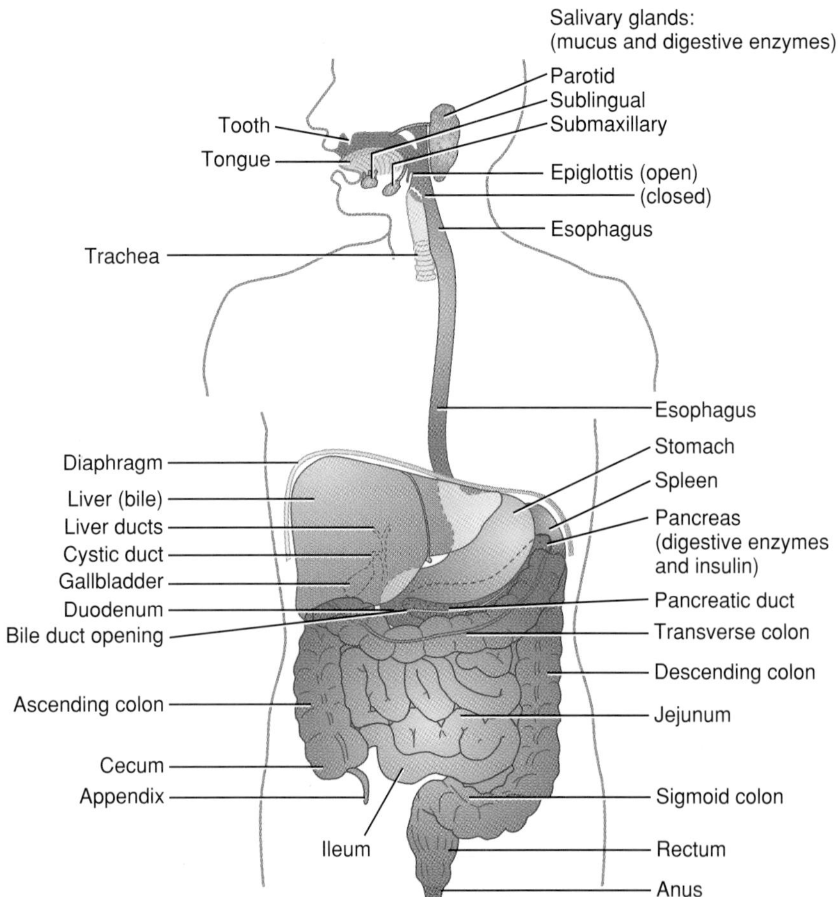

FIGURE 1–1 The digestive system.

dition to having a large surface area, the GI tract is extremely active in carrying out the physiologic and metabolic functions of secretion, absorption, nutrient processing, and cellular reproduction. The cells lining the gastrointestinal tract have a life span of approximately 3 to 5 days before they are sloughed into the lumen and "recycled." They are fully functional only for the last 2 to 3 days as they migrate from the crypts to the distal one third of the villi.

It is becoming increasingly apparent that the health of the host is dependent on appropriate health and function of the GI tract (see Chapter 12). Because of the unusually high metabolic activity and requirements of the GI tract, it is more susceptible than most tissues to micronutrient deficiencies, protein calorie malnutrition, and damage resulting from toxins, drugs, irradiation, or interruption of its energy blood supply. Approximately 45% of the energy requirement of the small intestine and 70% of the energy requirement of cells lining the colon are supplied by nutrients passing through its lumen. After several days of starvation, the GI tract atrophies; that is, the surface area declines markedly and secretions, synthetic functions, and absorptive capacity are reduced. Refeeding, even with less than adequate calories, results in cellular proliferation and return of normal GI function after only a few days. Maximum function of the human gastrointestinal tract appears to depend on frequent consumption of a healthy diet rather than feedings interspersed with prolonged fasts (Bengmark and Jeppsson, 1995; Spiller, 1994).

OVERVIEW OF DIGESTIVE AND ABSORPTIVE PROCESSES

In the mouth, the particle size of foods is reduced by chewing, and foods are mixed with salivary secretions that prepare foods for swallowing. The esophagus transports foods and beverages from the oral cavity and the pharynx to the stomach. In the stomach, foods are diluted with more fluids and mixed with proteolytic enzymes. Up to this point, only small amounts of starch and lipid digestion have taken place, and protein digestion has only begun. When foods are the appropriate consistency and concentration, the stomach allows passage of its contents into the small intestine, where most digestion takes place. In the first 100 cm of small intestine, a flurry of activity occurs, resulting in the digestion and absorption of most of the foodstuffs ingested. Starches are exposed to powerful enzymes from the pancreas and are reduced to simple sugars. Enzymes from the pancreas and brush border of the small intestine complete the digestion of proteins, converting them into small peptides and amino acids. Fats are reduced from visible droplets to microscopic emulsions where the lipases from the pancreas can attack and reduce the fats to mixtures of smaller molecules, primarily fatty acids and monoglycerides. In addition to secretions from the mouth and stomach, the secretions from the pancreas, small intestine, and gallbladder also contribute a considerable amount of fluid. In all, about three times more fluid is secreted from the alimentary tract than is consumed orally.

Along the remaining length of the small intestine, macronutrients, minerals, vitamins, trace elements, and most of the remaining water are absorbed before reaching the colon.

The large intestine or *colon* and *rectum* absorb most of the remaining liter or so of fluid delivered from the small intestine, and the colon absorbs electrolytes and, to some extent, some of the final products of digestion. The intestinal flora play an essential role in fermentation of ingested fiber and remaining carbohydrates and amino acids. Fermentation of carbohydrate results in the production of *short chain fatty acids (SCFA)* and gases. SCFAs help maintain normal mucosal function, "salvage" some of the residual energy substrates, and facilitate the absorption of remaining salts and water (Mortensen and Clausen, 1996). The large intestine also provides temporary storage for waste products which serve as a medium for bacterial synthesis of some vitamins. The rectum and *anus* control defecation.

Role of Enzymes in Digestion

Digestion of foodstuffs is accomplished by hydrolysis under the direction of enzymes. Cofactors, such as hydrochloric acid, bile, and sodium bicarbonate support the digestive and absorptive processes. The digestive enzymes, which are primarily *exoenzymes*, are synthesized within specialized cells in the mouth, stomach, pancreas, and small intestine and are released to catalyze hydrolysis of nutrients in areas external to the cell. *Endoenzymes* are localized in the lipoprotein membranes of the mucosal cells and attach to their substrates as they enter the cell. Table 1–1 summarizes the gastrointestinal enzymes and their functions.

Normally, 92% to 97% of the mixed American diet is digested and absorbed. Water, monosaccharides, vitamins, minerals, and alcohol are usually absorbed in their original form. The disaccharides and polysaccharides, lipids, and proteins must, for the most part, be converted to their simple constituents before they are absorbed.

Regulators of Gastrointestinal Activity

Neural Mechanisms

The neural control of gastrointestinal contractile and secretory activity consists of a local system located in the gut wall—the *enteric nervous system*—and an external system of nerve fibers from the autonomic nervous system (Furness and Costa, 1987). Mucosal receptors sensitive to the composition of chyme (e.g., acidity) and lumen stretch (e.g., full-

TABLE 1–1 SUMMARY OF ENZYMATIC DIGESTION AND ABSORPTION*

SECRETION AND SOURCE OF SECRETION	ENZYME	SUBSTRATE	ACTION AND PRODUCTS OF ACTION	ABSORPTION
Saliva from salivary glands in mouth	Ptyalin (salivary amylase)	Starch	Hydrolysis to form disaccharides (dextrins and maltose) and branched oligosaccharides	
Gastric juice from gastric glands in stomach mucosa	Renin	Casein (milk protein)	Curdling of casein to prepare it for pepsin action	
	Pepsin	Protein (presence of HCl)	Hydrolysis of peptide bonds to form polypeptides and amino acids	
	Lipase (tributyrinase)	Fat (tributyrin)	Hydrolysis to form free fatty acids	
Exocrine secretion from pancreas	Trypsin (activated trypsinogen)	Protein and polypeptides	Hydrolysis of interior peptide bonds to form polypeptides	
	Chymotrypsin (activated chymotrypsinogen)	Proteins and peptides	Hydrolysis of interior peptide bonds to form polypeptides	Pinocytosis of small peptides
	Carboxypolypeptidase	Polypeptides	Hydrolysis of terminal peptide bonds (carboxyl end) to form amino acids	Amino acids absorbed into blood
	Ribonuclease Deoxyribonuclease	Ribonucleic acids Deoxyribonucleic acids	Hydrolysis to form mononucleotides	
	Elastase	Fibrous protein	Hydrolysis to form peptides and amino acids	
	Lipase	Fat (presence of bile salts)	Hydrolysis to form monoglycerides, fatty acids	
	Cholesterol esterase	Cholesterol	Hydrolysis to form esters of cholesterol and fatty acids	Micelles → mucosal cells → chylomicrons → lymph
	α-Amylase	Starch and dextrins	Hydrolysis to form dextrins and maltose	
Small intestine enzymes, most of which are located in the brush border	Carboxypeptidase Aminopeptidase Dipeptidase Nucleosidase	Polypeptides	Hydrolysis of peptide bonds to form amino acids	Amino acids absorbed into blood
	Nucleosidase	Nucleotides	Hydrolysis to form nucleosides and H_3PO_4	
	Nucleosidase	Nucleosides	Hydrolysis to form purines, pyrimidines, and pentose	
	Enterokinase	Trypsinogen	Activates to trypsin	
	Lipase (enteric)	Monoglycerides	Hydrolysis to fatty acids and glycerol	Micelles → mucosal cells → chylomicrons → lymph
	Sucrase	Sucrose	Hydrolysis to glucose and fructose	Glucose, galactose, and fructose absorbed into blood
	α-Dextrinase (isomaltase)	Dextrin (isomaltose)	Hydrolysis to glucose	Glucose, galactose, and fructose absorbed into blood
	Maltase	Maltose	Hydrolysis to glucose	Glucose, galactose, and fructose absorbed into blood
	Lactase	Lactose	Hydrolysis to glucose and galactose	Glucose, galactose, and fructose absorbed into blood

*There are no digestive enzymes in the large intestine. Digestion and absorption are completed by the time the colon is reached. Only water, salt, vitamins, and minerals are absorbed thereafter.

ness) send impulses to muscle and secretory cells of the intestinal tract via transmitters of the submucosal and myenteric plexuses. These neurotransmitters include enkephalin, somatostatin, serotonin, bombesin, substance P, vasoactive intestinal polypeptide (VIP), and neurotensin. Table 1–2 summarizes the site and primary action of each of these neurotransmitters.

Autonomic innervation is supplied by the sympathetic fibers that run along blood vessels and by the parasympathetic fibers in the vagus nerve. In general, the *parasympathetic* nerves innervate specific areas of the alimentary tract, whereas the *sympathetic* system inhibits activity. Acid secretion from parietal cells in the stomach is stimulated by vagal activity in response to the sight or smell of food.

Hormonal Mechanisms

Regulation of the gastrointestinal system involves the action of a large number of hormones, several of which have complex actions that extend beyond the GI tract. More than 80 hormones and hormone-like growth factors secreted by more than 20 different types of neuroendocrine cells have been identified (Holst et al., 1996; Modlin and Basson, 1993). The functions of several GI hormones have been well described, but the actions of several other hormones are still not completely understood, and newer peptides with hormonal or growth-enhancing properties are still being evaluated. Only a few of the primary hormones are reviewed here and in Table 1–3. Knowledge of major hormone functions becomes especially important when the sites for their secretion or action are diseased or removed in surgical procedures or when hormones and their analogues are used therapeutically.

Gastrin, a hormone that stimulates gastric secretions and motility, is secreted from cells in the antral mucosa of the stomach. Secretion is initiated by (1) distention of the antrum, such as after a meal; (2) impulses from the vagus nerve, such as may be triggered by the thought of food; and (3) the presence in the antrum of secretagogues, such as partially digested proteins, fermented spirits (e.g., wine), caffeine, and food extracts (e.g., bouillon). When the lumen pH gets too acidic, a feedback mechanism reduces acid secretion by inhibiting gastrin release.

Secretin, a hormone released from the duodenal wall into the bloodstream, opposes both the action and secretion of gastrin. Secreted in response to acidic chyme emptied into the duodenum, it stimulates the pancreas to secrete water and bicarbonate into the duodenum. Neutralization of the acidity protects the duodenal mucosa from prolonged exposure to acid and provides the appropriate environment for the activity of intestinal and pancreatic enzymes.

Other cells of the small bowel mucosa secrete **cholecystokinin (CCK),** an important multifunctional hormone whose release is stimulated by the amino acids and fatty acids produced in protein and fat digestion (Liddle, 1997). The functions of this hormone are (1) stimulation of the pancreas to secrete enzymes and, to a lesser extent, bicarbonate and water; (2) stimulation of gallbladder contraction as well as contraction of the colon and rectum; (3) slowing of gastric emptying; and (4) possibly, a role in limiting food intake (see Chapter 23).

Gastric inhibitory polypeptide (GIP), which is released from the intestinal mucosa in the presence of fat and glucose, inhibits gastric acid secretion and stimulates insulin release. **Glucagon-like peptide 1 (GLP-1)** slows gastric emptying, lowers glucagon concentrations, stimulates (pro)insulin synthesis, increases insulin sensitivity, and may help to control food intake. As a result of GIP and GLP-1, an enteral glucose load results in less of an increase in blood glucose than an equal amount of glucose administered intravenously (Nauck et al., 1997).

Motilin, released by the cells of the upper small intestine in response to alkalinity of the duodenum, increases the rate of gastric emptying and stimulates gut motility. Erythromycin, an antibiotic, has been shown to serve as an agonist (stimulator) of motilin receptors, and both erythromycin and analogues of motilin are being used therapeutically to treat delayed gastric emptying (Minami et al., 1996).

TABLE 1–2 GASTROINTESTINAL NEUROTRANSMITTERS

NEUROTRANSMITTER	SITE OF RELEASE	MAIN ACTION
Bombesin	Gut, CNS, lung	Stimulates release of gut hormone
Enkephalin	Gut, CNS	Exerts opiate-like effect (endorphin system)
Neurotensin	Ileum, CNS	Inhibits release of gastric emptying and acid secretion
Somatostatin	Gut, CNS	Inhibits release of gastric and pancreatic hormones; decreases pancreatic enzyme production; inhibits gallbladder contraction
Substance P	Gut, CNS, skin	Sensory (mainly pain)
Vasoactive inhibitory polypeptide (VIP)	All tissues	Stimulates secretions of pancreas and small intestine; stimulates liver glycogenolysis; inhibits gastric acid output; vasodilates; relaxes smooth muscle

CNS, central nervous system.

TABLE 1–3 IMPORTANT FUNCTIONS OF GASTROINTESTINAL HORMONES

HORMONE	SITE OF RELEASE	STIMULANTS OF RELEASE	ORGAN AFFECTED	EFFECT ON ORGAN
Gastrin	Antral mucosa of stomach	Polypeptides	Esophagus	Increases resting pressure of lower esophageal sphincter
		Amino acids		
	Duodenum	Caffeine	Stomach	Stimulates secretion of HCl and pepsinogen by parietal and chief cells, respectively
	Jejunum	Alcohol		Increases gastric antral motility
		Food extracts		
		Distention of stomach antrum	Gallbladder	Weakly stimulates contraction of gallbladder
		Vagal nerve	Pancreas	Weakly stimulates pancreatic secretion of bicarbonate
Secretin	Duodenal mucosa	Gut acidity (pH <4–5)	Esophagus	Reduces resting pressure of lower esophageal sphincter
			Stomach	Reduces gastric and duodenal motility
				Stimulates pepsinogen secretion
				Inhibits gastrin-stimulated gastric acid secretion
			Duodenum	Decreases motility
				Increases mucus output of Brunner's glands
			Pancreas	Increases ouput of H_2O and bicarbonate
				Increases some enzyme secretion as well as insulin release
			Liver	Increases volume and electrolyte output of bile
Cholecystokinin-pancreozymin (CCK-PZ)	Proximal small bowel	Amino acids (especially tryptophan)	Small bowel	Increases motility
			Gallbladder	Causes contraction
		HCl	Pancreas	Stimulates enzyme secretion
		Fat		Potentiates effect of secretin on pancreas
		Protein		Slows gastric emptying
				May mediate feeding behavior
Gastric inhibitory polypeptide (GIP)	Small intestine	Glucose	Stomach	Inhibits gastrin-stimulated gastric acid secretion
		Fat	Pancreas	Stimulates insulin secretion
Enteroglucagon and glucagon	Duodenum	Carbohydrate	Liver	Stimulates glycogenolysis
	Jejunum	Long-chain triglycerides	Pancreas	Inhibits enzyme secretion
			Small intestine	Inhibits motility
Motilin	Duodenum	Alkalinity in the duodenum	Stomach	Decreases gastric emptying
	Jejunum			Regulates gut motility (?)
Somatostatin	Antrum of stomach	Gastric and duodenal acidity	Pancreas	Inhibits release of insulin and glucagon
	Upper small intestine			Decreases enzyme production
	Hypothalamus (primarily)	Amino acids		
		Fat (?)	Stomach	Inhibits gastrin release
			Gallbladder	Inhibits contraction
			Other	Suppresses secretion of growth hormone
				Suppresses secretion of thyroid-stimulating hormone

Somatostatin is a hormone with far-reaching actions. Its general actions appear to be inhibitory and antisecretory, but it also regulates a number of other hormones. Somatostatin and its analogue octreotide are being used to treat certain malignant diseases (Bajetta et al., 1996; Farthing, 1996), as well as a number of GI disorders, such as diarrhea, short bowel syndrome, pancreatitis, dumping syndrome, and gastric hypersecretion. Table 1–3 summarizes the functions of these hormones.

Digestive Process (see Fig. 1–2)

Digestion in the Mouth

In the mouth, the teeth function to grind and crush food into small particles. The food mass is simultaneously moistened and lubricated by saliva, about 1.5 L of which is produced daily by three pairs of salivary glands: the parotid, submaxillary, and sublingual glands. A serous secretion containing **amylase (ptyalin)** begins the digestion of starch. The amount of starch digestion is minimal, and the

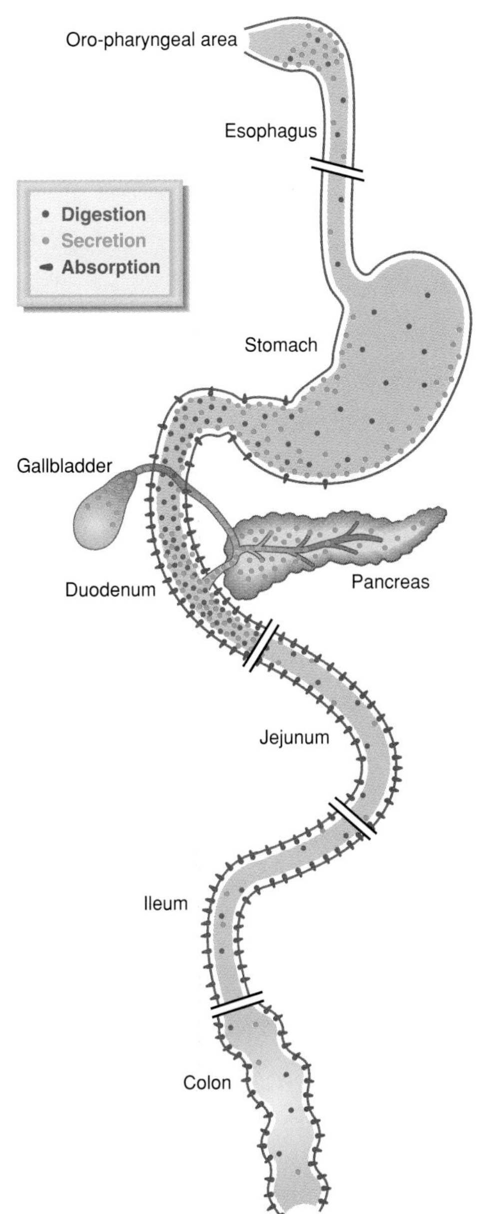

FIGURE 1–2 Sites of secretion, digestion, and absorption.

amylase becomes inactive when it reaches the acid contents of the stomach. Another type of saliva contains mucus, a protein that causes particles of food to stick together and lubricates the mass for ease of swallowing. The oropharyngeal secretions also contain a lipase which is capable of digesting some fats. Because fatty materials are still mixed with whole foods, are not adequately processed, and are not retained in the mouth or esophagus for any length of time, the contribution of this lipase to overall fat digestion is usually minimal.

The masticated food mass, called a *bolus,* is passed back to the pharynx under voluntary control, but throughout the esophagus, the process of swallowing (*deglutition*) is involuntary. **Peristalsis** then moves the food rapidly into the stomach. (Swallowing is discussed further in Chapter 42, Neurologic Disease.)

Digestion in the Stomach

Food particles are propelled forward and mixed with gastric secretions by wave-like contractions that progress forward from the upper portion of the stomach, the fundus, to the antrum and pylorus. In the stomach, gastric secretions are mixed with foods and beverages. An average of 2000 to 2500 mL of gastric juice is secreted daily. The gastric secretions contain hydrochloric acid (secreted by the parietal cells scattered along the walls of the stomach), a protease, gastric lipase, mucus, intrinsic factor, and the gastrointestinal hormone gastrin. In the process of gastric digestion, most of the foods become semiliquid (**chyme**), containing approximately 50% water. Digestion of protein begins in the stomach, primarily by the action of *pepsin.* Pepsin is secreted in an inactive form (pepsinogen), which is converted by hydrochloric acid to its active form. Pepsin is active only in the acid environment of the stomach and serves primarily to change the shape and size of some of the proteins in a normal mixed meal.

Lipases secreted into the stomach are not usually the primary agents for the digestion of the usual long chain fatty acids (LCFAs) in dietary lipids. Varying amounts of triglycerides composed of medium chain fatty acids (MCFAs) and SCFAs may be digested in the stomach, but the normal adult diet contains few of these fats. Lipases secreted in the upper portions of the GI tract may have increased importance in infant diets and may have significance in pancreatic insufficiency or short bowel syndrome when MCFAs may be included in the diet.

When foods are consumed, significant numbers of microorganisms are also consumed. The acid in the stomach is quite strong, with a pH ranging from about 1 to 4. The combination of the acid pH and the proteolytic enzymes results in the killing of most of the microorganisms ingested. Achlorhydria, gastrectomy, GI disease, or poor nutrition may increase the risk of bacterial overgrowth in the intestine.

The stomach continually mixes and churns food and normally releases the mixture in small quantities into the small intestine. The amount emptied with each contraction of the antrum and pylorus varies with the volume and type of food consumed, but is only a few milliliters at a time. The stomach normally empties within 1 to 4 hours. When eaten alone, carbohydrates leave the stomach most rapidly, followed by protein, fat, and fibrous foods. In a mixed meal, emptying of the stomach depends on the overall volume and characteristics of the foods. Liquids empty more rapidly than solids, large particles empty more slowly than small particles, and concentrated foods tend to empty more slowly than meals of low caloric concentration (Collins et al., 1996). These factors play an important role for the practitioner who counsels patients with nausea, vomiting, diabetic gastroparesis, or partial obstruction, or who advises patients during refeeding after gastrointestinal surgery or malnutrition.

The sphincters guarding the entrance to and the exit from the stomach prevent backflow of the mixture from the stomach into the esophagus and pharynx and from the duodenum into the stomach. These sphincters can become excessively stimulated during emotional upsets; when the exit pyloric valve tightens or goes into spasms, the pain can be excruciating. Irritation from nearby ulcers may also alter the performance of this structure. Certain foods and beverages may alter the lower esophageal sphincter (LES) pressure, permitting backflow or reflux of the GI contents into the esophagus. See Chapter 30 for further discussion of these factors.

Digestion in the Small Intestine

The small intestine is the primary site for digestion of foods and nutrients. The small intestine is divided into the duodenum, the jejunum, and the ileum, as shown in Figure 1–2. Most of the digestive process is completed in the duodenum and upper jejunum, and the absorption of nutrients is largely complete by the middle of the jejunum. The acidic chyme from the stomach enters the duodenum, where it is mixed with duodenal juices and the secretions from the pancreas and biliary tract. The dilution from secreted fluids, and especially bicarbonate ions in pancreatic fluid, helps to neutralize acid chyme and allows the enzymes of the small intestine and pancreas to operate at a more neutral pH.

CCK is secreted from the small intestine in response to the presence of fats and protein. CCK stimulates the secretion and release of bile from the liver and gallbladder. Bile is a mixture consisting predominantly of water and bile salts and small amounts of pigments and cholesterol. Through their emulsifying properties, the bile salts facilitate the digestion and absorption of lipids. The pancreas secretes enzymes capable of digesting all of the major nutrients. **Proteolytic enzymes** include *trypsin* and *chymotrypsin,* carboxypolypeptidase, ribonuclease, and deoxyribonuclease. Trypsin and chymotrypsin are secreted in their inactive forms and are activated by *enterokinase,* which is secreted in response to contact of chyme with the intestinal mucosa. Pancreatic amylase is secreted to hydrolyze starch. Most of the ingested starches are digested to oligosaccharides and disaccharides. Enzymes lining the brush border of the villi further reduce the molecules to monosaccharides prior to absorption. Varying amounts of "resistant" starches and almost all dietary fiber escape digestion in the small intestine (Cummings and Englyst, 1995; Levin, 1994).

Fluids containing large amounts of bicarbonate ion, secreted under the influence of secretin, neutralize the highly acidic chyme. Intestinal contents move along the small intestine at a rate of 1 cm/min, taking from 3 to 8 hours to travel the entire length to the ileocecal valve (Guyton and Hall, 1996). The ileocecal valve, like the pyloric valve, serves as a "brake" to regulate the movement of intestinal material passed into the colon.

THE SMALL INTESTINE—PRIMARY SITE FOR NUTRIENT ABSORPTION

The primary organ of absorption is the small intestine, which is characterized by its enormous absorptive area. This is attributable to its extensive length—10 to 12 ft (3 to 4 m)—as well as to the ordering of the mucosal lining into convolutions (*valvulae conniventes*). These folds are covered with finger-like projections called villi, which in turn are covered by microvilli, or the **brush border.** (See "*Focus On:* Unstirred Water Layer.") The combination of folds, villous projections, and microvillous border results in an enormous absorptive surface of about 250 m^2 (Chang et al., 1996; Guyton and Hall, 1996; Caspary, 1992). The villi rest on a supporting structure called the *lamina propria,* composed of connective tissue, in which the blood and lymph vessels receive the products of digestion (Fig. 1–3). Each day, the small intestine absorbs 200 to 300 g of monosaccharides, 60 to 100 g of fatty acids, 50 to 100 g of amino acids and peptides, and 50 to 100 g of ions. The capacity for absorption in the healthy in-

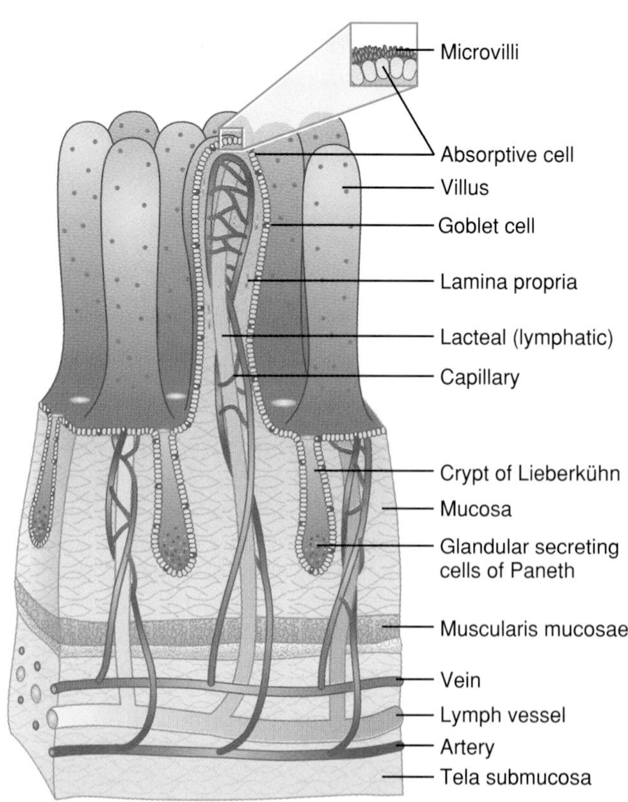

FIGURE 1–3 Diagram of villi of the human intestine showing their structure and blood and lymph vessels.

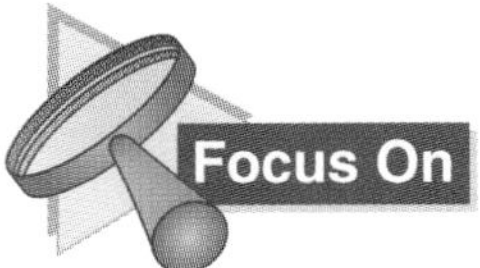

Unstirred Water Layer

The unstirred water layer (UWL) is a collection of watery plates that form a boundary between the intestinal lumen and the brush border membranes. Emulsification of fats in the small intestine is followed by digestion, primarily by pancreatic lipase, into beta-monoglycerides (one fatty acid attached to the middle glycerol carbon) and free fatty acids. When the concentration of bile salts reaches a certain level, they combine to form micelles that are organized with the polar ends of the molecules oriented toward the watery lumen of the intestine. The lipid breakdown products of the fat digestion are rapidly solubilized in the central portion of the micelles and carried to the area of the brush border (see Fig. 1–7).

At the surface of the UWL, the micelles detach from their lipid passengers and return to the lumen for further transport. The monoglycerides and fatty acids are thus left to make their way across the lipophobic UWL to the more lipid-friendly membrane cells of the brush border. Upon arrival, they are rapidly taken up for processing and entry into the transport system.

Because the UWL slows the progress of lipids from the lumen into the mucosal cell, it may be the major rate-limiting factor in the speed of lipid absorption (Thompson, 1989).

dividual far exceeds the normal macronutrient and caloric requirements. All but 1 to 1.5 L of the 7 L of fluids secreted from the upper portions of the GI tract is reabsorbed. The 1.5 to 3 L of fluid ingested daily is also absorbed in the small intestine. About 95% of the secreted bile salts are absorbed as bile acids in the distal ileum. Without this "recycling" of bile acids from the GI tract, de novo synthesis of bile acids in the liver would not keep pace with needs for adequate lipid digestion. Bile salt insufficiency becomes clinically important in patients who have resections of the small bowel and diseases affecting the small intestine, such as Crohn's disease, celiac sprue, and cystic fibrosis. The distal ileum is also the site for vitamin B_{12}/intrinsic factor absorption.

Absorptive Mechanisms

Diffusion and Active Transport

Absorption is an extremely complex process, combining the relatively simple process of **passive diffusion,** in which nutrients pass through the intestinal mucosal cells (enterocytes or colonocytes) into the bloodstream, with the more intricate process of *active transport*.

Diffusion involves random movement through openings in the membranes of the mucosal cell walls using channel proteins (*simple diffusion*) or in combination with a carrier protein (**facilitated diffusion**) (Fig. 1–4).

Active transport requires the input of energy to move ions or other substances, in combination with a carrier protein, across a membrane against an energy gradient. Some nutrients may share the same carrier and thus compete for absorption. Carrier systems can also become saturated, and the absorption of the nutrient is thus slowed. The best-known carrier is the *intrinsic factor* responsible for the absorption of vitamin B_{12}.

Some molecules are moved from the intestinal lumen into the mucosal cell by means of *pumps,* which require energy derived from adenosine triphosphate (ATP), and a carrier. The absorption of glucose, sodium, galactose, potassium, magnesium, phosphate, iodide, calcium, iron, and amino acids is thought to occur in this manner.

Pinocytosis has been described as a "drinking in" or engulfing of a small drop of intestinal contents by the epithelial cell membrane. In this manner, large particles, such as whole proteins, may be absorbed in a small quantity. The movement of for-

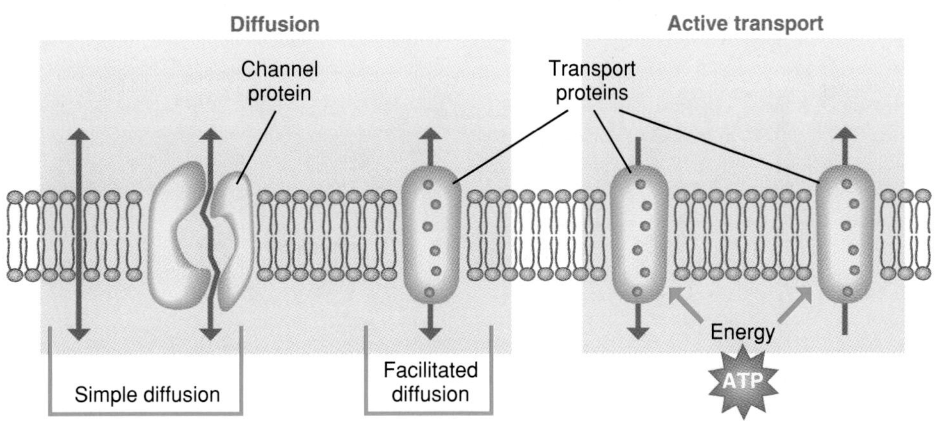

FIGURE 1–4 Diagram illustrating transport pathways through the cell membrane, as well as the basic mechanisms of transport.

eign proteins across the gastrointestinal tract into the bloodstream, where they cause allergic reactions, may be the result of pinocytosis. The immunoglobulins from breast milk are probably absorbed in this manner.

Digestion and Absorption of Nutrients

Carbohydrates and Fiber

Most dietary carbohydrates are consumed in the form of starches, disaccharides, and monosaccharides. Starches usually make up the greatest proportion of carbohydrates, and they exist as two major types of polysaccharides. Polysaccharides (including those of most plant fibers) are large molecules composed of straight or branched chains of sugar molecules joined together, primarily in alpha 1–4 and 1–6 linkages. Most of the dietary starches are amylopectins, the branching polysaccharides, and amylose, the straight-chain–type polymers (Levin, 1994; Chang, 1996).

In the mouth, the enzyme salivary **amylase** (ptyalin), which operates at a neutral or slightly alkaline pH, starts the digestive action on starch, hydrolyzing it into smaller molecules (Fig. 1–5). The activity of amylase is halted by contact with hydrochloric acid. If the digestible carbohydrate were to remain in the stomach long enough, the acid hydrolysis would eventually reduce much of it to the monosaccharides. However, the stomach usually empties itself before significant digestion can take place, and carbohydrate digestion occurs almost entirely in the proximal small intestine.

Pancreatic **amylase** breaks the large starch molecules at alpha 1–4 linkages to create maltose, maltotriose, and "alpha-limit" dextrins remaining from the amylopectin branches. Enzymes from the brush border of the enterocytes further break the disaccharides and oligosaccharides into monosaccharides. **Maltase** from the mucosal cells, for example, reduces the disaccharide maltose to two molecules of glucose. These outer-cell membranes also contain the enzymes **sucrase, lactase,** and *isomaltase* (or *alpha-dextrinase*), which act on sucrose, lactose, and isomaltose, respectively (Fig. 1–6).

The resultant monosaccharides—glucose, galactose, and fructose—pass through the mucosal cell and, via the capillary of the villus, into the bloodstream, where they are carried by the portal vein to the liver. Glucose and galactose are absorbed by active transport, primarily by a carrier that is sodium-dependent; fructose is more slowly absorbed by facilitated diffusion that is probably also sodium-dependent (Levin, 1994). This understanding of monosaccharide absorption is the reason for the use of sodium-glucose drinks for rehydrating athletes and for rehydration fluids for infants with diarrhea. Glucose is transported from the liver to the tissues, although some glucose is stored in the liver and muscles as glycogen. A small amount of fructose may be converted to glucose before it passes from the intestinal cell into the blood, but most is transported as fructose to the liver where, like galactose, it is converted to glucose. Consumption of large amounts of lactose (especially in lactase-deficient individuals), fructose, stachyose, raffinose, and alcohol sugars (sorbitol, mannitol, or xylitol) can result in considerable amounts of these sugars passing unabsorbed into the colon (Levin, 1994; Rumessen and Gudmand-Hoyer, 1988) and may cause gas and diarrhea. Some forms of carbohydrate cannot be digested by humans. Cellulose, hemicelluloses, pectins, gums, and other forms of fiber pass relatively unchanged to

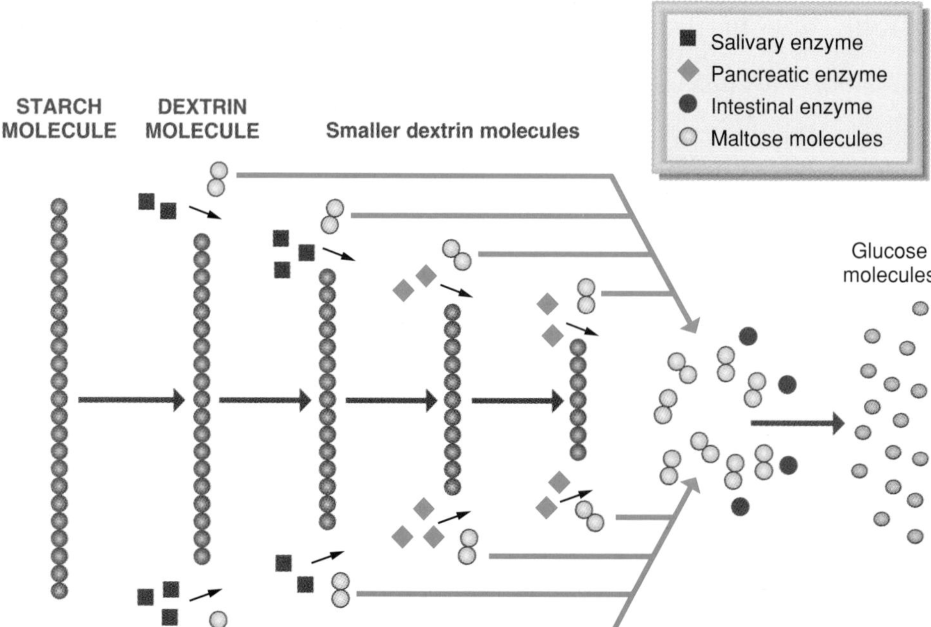

FIGURE 1–5 The gradual breakdown of large starch molecules to glucose by enzymes in digestion.

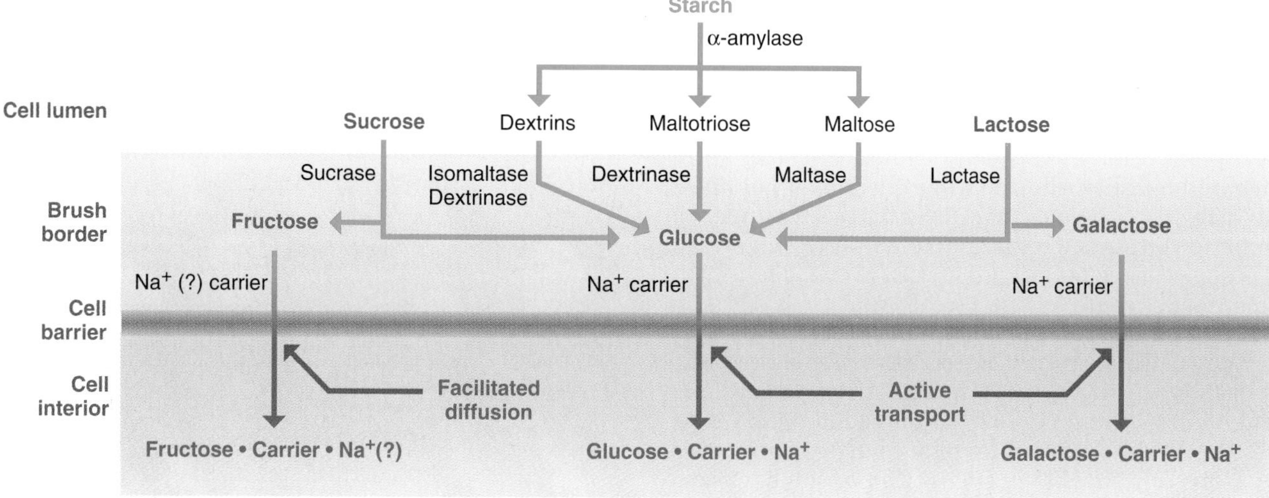

FIGURE 1–6 The process of digestion and absorption of carbohydrates. Sodium, along with either glucose or galactose, combines with the carrier. The sugar-carrier-sodium ion complex is transported across the cell membrane into the interior of the cell. Once inside the cell, the glucose diffuses passively across the serosal membrane, and the sodium is actively pumped back out of the cell. The driving force for glucose transport against a concentration gradient is the gradient of sodium ion across the membrane that contains the glucose carrier.

the colon, where they are partially fermented by bacteria in the colon. Neither salivary nor pancreatic amylase have the ability to split the cellulose bond. Cows and other ruminants, however, can subsist on high-fiber feeds because of the bacterial digestion that takes place in the rumen. Some "resistant" starches and sugars are less well digested or absorbed than others, and consumption of large amounts may result in the passage of significant amounts of these into the colon where they, like fiber, are fermented to SCFAs and gases. Starches resistant to digestion tend to include uncooked starchy foods and plant foods with high protein and fiber content, such as legumes and whole grains (Bjorck et al., 1994; Cummings and Englyst, 1995).

Proteins

Protein digestion begins in the stomach, where proteins are split into proteoses, peptones, and large polypeptides. Inactive *pepsinogen* is converted to the enzyme pepsin when it comes in contact with hydrochloric acid and other pepsin molecules. Unlike any of the other proteolytic enzymes, pepsin digests collagen, the major protein of connective tissue. Most protein digestion takes place in the duodenum, however, and the contribution of the stomach to the total process is small (Caspary, 1992; Chang et al., 1996; Murray et al., 1996).

Contact of chyme with the intestinal mucosa stimulates release of *enterokinase,* an enzyme that transforms inactive pancreatic *trypsinogen* into active *trypsin,* which in turn activates the other pancreatic proteolytic enzymes. Pancreatic *trypsin, chymotrypsin,* and *carboxypolypeptidase* break down intact protein and continue the breakdown started in the stomach until small polypeptides and amino acids are formed.

Proteolytic *peptidases* located on the brush border also act on polypeptides, changing them to amino acids, dipeptides, and tripeptides. Usually, many small peptides are efficiently absorbed intact. The final phase of protein digestion takes place in the brush border, where dipeptides and tripeptides are hydrolyzed to their constituent amino acids by peptide hydrolases. The presence of antibodies to many food proteins in the circulation of healthy individuals indicates that immunologically significant amounts of large intact peptides escape hydrolysis and can enter the portal circulation (see Chapter 41).

Amino acids are absorbed through four distinct active transport systems: one each for neutral, basic, and acidic amino acids, and one for proline and hydroxyproline. Amino acid transport is controlled by the same type of sodium co-transport mechanism that has been identified for glucose. Absorbed peptides and amino acids are transported to the liver via the portal vein for release into the general circulation.

Almost all protein is absorbed by the time it reaches the end of the jejunum, and only 1% of ingested protein is found in the feces. Some amino acids may remain in the epithelial cells and are used in the synthesis of intestinal enzymes and new cells. Most of the endogenous protein from intestinal secretions and desquamated epithelial cells is also digested and "recycled" and absorbed from the small intestine.

Lipids

Small amounts of fat are digested in the mouth with lingual lipase, but greater amounts are digested in the stomach from the action of *gastric lipase (tributyrinase).* Gastric lipase hydrolyzes some or part of the triglycerides, especially short-chain triglycerides (as in butter), into fatty acids and glycerol. However, the major portion of fat digestion takes place in the small intestine as a result of pancreatic lipase. Entrance of fat stimulates the release of **enterogastrone,** which acts to inhibit gastric secretion and motility, thus slowing the delivery of lipids. As a result, a portion of a large fatty meal may remain in the stomach for up to 4 hours or longer.

The presence of fat and protein in the small intestine also stimulates the secretion of CCK. This, in turn, stimulates biliary and pancreatic secretions.

The peristaltic action of the small intestine breaks large fat globules into smaller particles, and the emulsifying action of the bile keeps them separated and thus more accessible to digestion by **pancreatic lipase.** Bile is a secretion of the liver composed of bile acids (primarily conjugates of cholic and chenodeoxycholic acids with glycine or taurine), bile pigments (which color the feces), inorganic salts, some protein, cholesterol, lecithin, and many compounds, such as detoxified drugs, that are metabolized and secreted by the liver. From its storage organ, the gallbladder, about 2 pt of bile are secreted daily in response to the stimulus of food in the duodenum and stomach.

The free fatty acids and monoglycerides produced by digestion form complexes with bile salts called **micelles.** The micelles facilitate passage of the lipids through the watery environment of the intestinal lumen to the brush border (see "*Focus On:* Unstirred Water Layer" and Fig. 1–7). The bile salts are then released from their lipid components and are returned to the lumen of the gut. Most of the bile salts are actively reabsorbed in the terminal ileum and are recycled back to the liver to enter the gut again via the gallbladder. This efficient recycling process is known as the *enterohepatic circulation.* The pool of bile acids may circulate anywhere from 3 to 15 times per day, depending on the amount of food ingested.

In the mucosal cell, the fatty acids and monoglycerides are reassembled into new triglycerides. A few are further digested into free fatty acids and glycerol and then reassembled to form triglycerides. These triglycerides, along with cholesterol and phospholipids, are surrounded by a beta-lipoprotein coat forming *chylomicrons,* as shown in Figure 1–7. The globules pass into the lacteals of the villi by a process of exocytosis. Chylomicrons are transported by the lymphatic vessels to the thoracic duct and are emptied into the bloodstream at the junction of the left internal jugular and left subclavian veins. The chylomicrons are then carried to the liver, where the triglycerides are repackaged into lipoproteins and transported primarily to the adipose tissue for metabolism and storage.

Cholesterol is absorbed in a similar manner after being hydrolyzed from the ester form by *pancreatic cholesterol esterase.* The fat-soluble vitamins A, D, E, and K are also absorbed in a micellar fashion, although water-soluble forms of vitamins A, E, and K and carotene can be absorbed in the absence of bile acids.

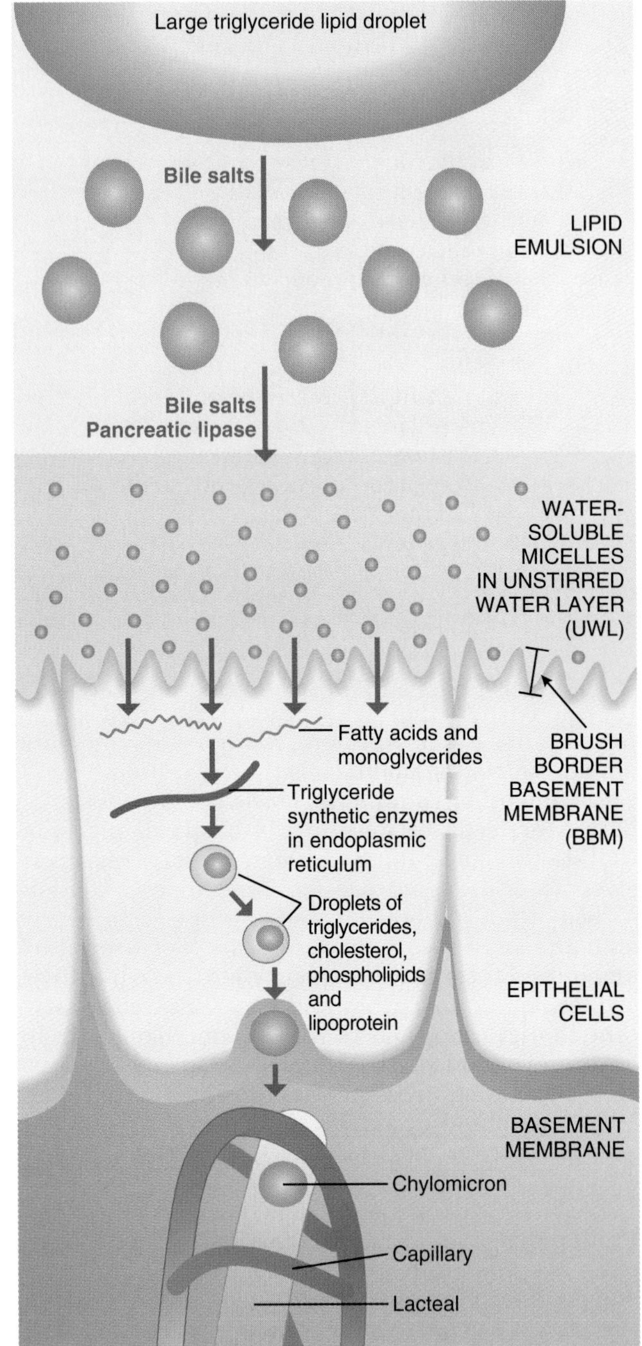

FIGURE 1–7 Summary of fat absorption.

Under normal conditions, about 95% to 97% of ingested fat is absorbed into lymph vessels. Because of their shorter length and thus increased solubility, fatty acids of 12 carbons or less can be absorbed directly into the mucosal cell without the presence of bile and micelle formation. After entering the mucosal cell, they are able to go directly without esterification into the portal vein, which carries them to the liver.

This capability of MCFAs is clinically useful. Some individuals cannot efficiently absorb the usual types of dietary fat (long-chain triglycerides) because they lack necessary bile salts for micellar formation or the means for transporting triglycerides out of the intestinal epithelial cells into the lymphatics, as occurs in abetalipoproteinemia. In these cases, medium-chain triglycerides, with fatty acid chain lengths of C8 and C10, are the principle sources of dietary fat. Medium-chain triglycerides do not require micellar and chylomicron formation and are able to enter the portal circulation (see Chapter 31).

Increased motility, intestinal mucosal changes, pancreatic insufficiency, or the absence of bile can decrease absorption of fat. When undigested fat appears in the feces, the condition is known as steatorrhea (see Chapter 31).

Other Nutrients

Vitamins, minerals, and fluids are absorbed simultaneously through the intestinal mucosa. Various factors affect bioavailability of vitamins and minerals in this process, including the presence or absence of other specific nutrients. Each day, about 8 to 9 L of fluid from the body pass back and forth across the membrane of the gut to keep the nutrients in solution. Figure 1–8 illustrates the present understanding of the sites and routes of absorption of nutrients.

Most vitamins and water pass unchanged from the small intestine into the blood by passive diffusion. Drugs are mostly absorbed by passive diffusion; those absorbed by active transport may compete with nutrients at the cell membrane. The result may decrease or increase actual absorption of either the medication or the nutrient.

Mineral absorption is more complex and proceeds in three stages. The *intraluminal* stage consists of the chemical reactions and interactions that take place in the stomach and intestines. These reactions, which are predominantly determined by the pH of the luminal contents and the composition of the food entering from the stomach, primarily affect the cations. The small anionic elements, such as fluoride, are not influenced by either pH or the composition of the diet and are absorbed quite freely. Cations, which are soluble in the acidic pH of the stomach, form insoluble hydroxides when the chyme passes into the higher-pH small intestine. These cations are kept available for absorption by ligands, such as amino acids and other organic acids and sugars, which form coordination or **chelation** compounds with the elements.

The *translocation stage* involves passage across the membrane into the intestinal mucosal cell. Transport of small anions may be by simple diffusion. For most cationic elements, the mechanism is either facilitated diffusion or active transport. For many minerals, more than one method of translocation may be operable, depending on the concentration of a particular trace element in the intestinal contents.

During the *mobilization stage,* minerals are either transported across the serosal surfaces of the intestinal cells into the bloodstream or are sequestered within the cell. Iron and zinc, for example, are either bound to proteins within the intestinal cell (chelated) or added to the intracellular pool. The ions in the pool are then mobilized and transported across the serosal surface, whereas the protein-bound ions are either released to become part of the pool or remain bound, in which case they are lost with the cell during desquamation.

The gastrointestinal tract is the site of important interactions between minerals. Medication with iron or zinc may depress the absorption of copper. Copper, in turn, may lower iron and molybdenum absorption. Cobalt absorption is increased in patients with iron deficiency, but cobalt and iron compete and inhibit each other's absorption. These interactions probably reflect a lack of complete specificity of the absorption mechanisms.

Metals are transported bound to protein carriers. The proteins are either specific, such as transferrin, which binds with iron, or general, such as albumin, which binds a variety of minerals. A fraction of each mineral is also carried in the serum in the form of amino acid or peptide complexes. Specific protein carriers are usually undersaturated, and the reserve capacity may be a buffer against excessive exposure. Toxicity from minerals usually results only after this buffering capacity is exceeded.

Factors Affecting Digestion

Psychologic Factors

The appearance, smell, and taste of food as it is served, along with the prevailing emotional climate, have an impact on digestion. Sight, smell, taste, and even the thought of food increase secretions of saliva and the stomach juices and increase muscular activity of the gastrointestinal tract. Emotions of fear, anger, and worry stimulate the hypothalamus to activate the autonomic nervous system, which in turn depresses secretions, inhibits peristalsis, and slows propulsion of food by increasing sphincter tone (Mattes, 1997).

Bacterial Action

The gut microflora make up a complex community in which about 100 species have been identified. At birth, the gastrointestinal tract is essentially sterile, but implantation of various microorganisms soon takes place. *Lactobacillus* is the chief component of the flora until the infant begins to eat solid foods. *Escherichia coli* then becomes predominant in the distal ileum, and the primary colonic flora appear to be anaerobic, with species of the genus *Bacteroides* occurring most frequently. Lactobacilli are also present in the stools of most persons ingesting an ordinary mixed diet.

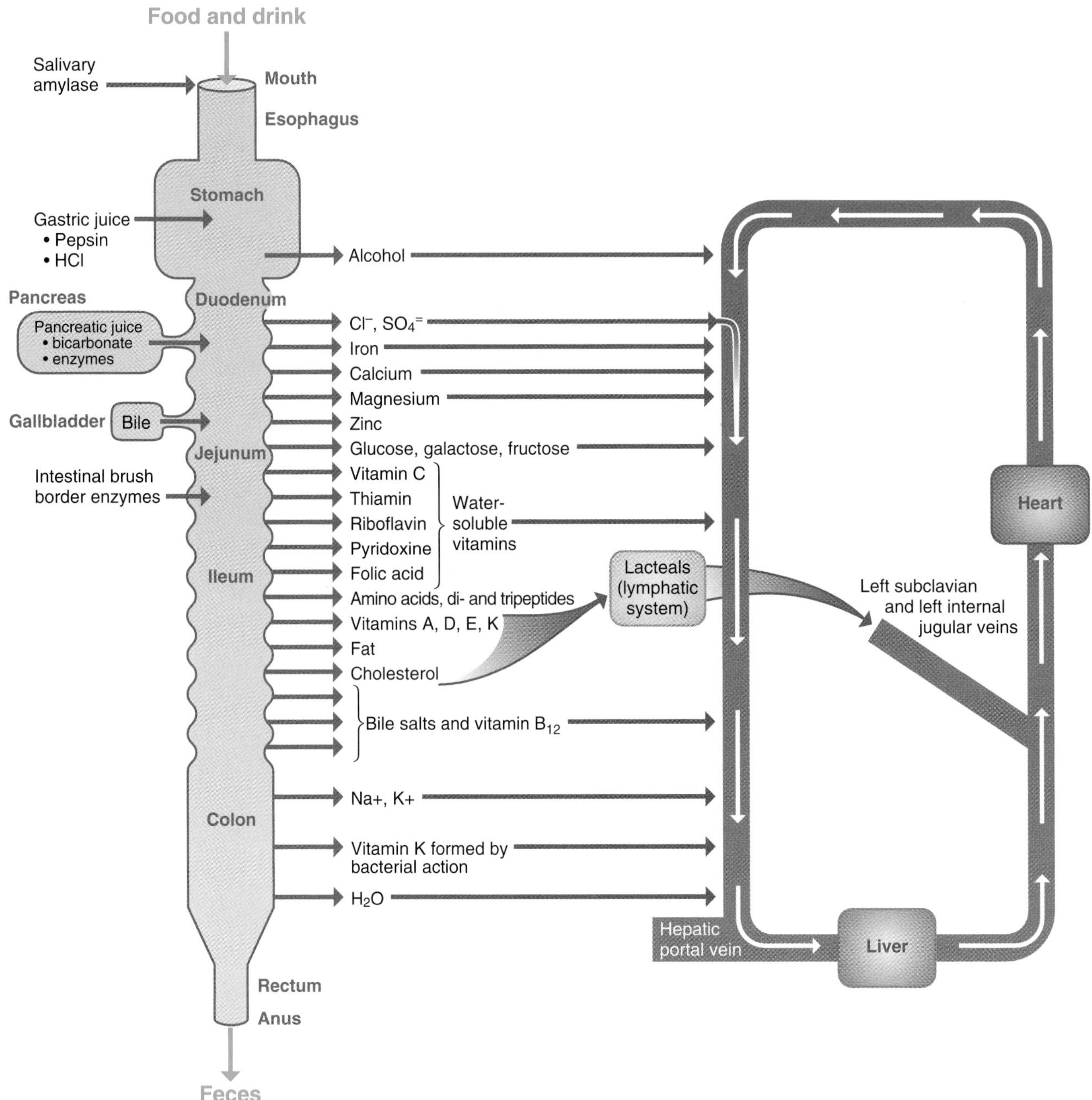

FIGURE 1–8 Sites of secretion and absorption in the gastrointestinal tract.

Normally, there is very little bacterial action in the stomach because the hydrochloric acid acts as a germicidal agent. However, conditions marked by decreased secretion of hydrochloric acid may lower resistance to bacterial action, occasionally leading to inflammation of the gastric mucosa (gastritis) or an increased risk of overgrowth in the small intestine, which is usually relatively sterile.

Bacterial action is most intense in the large intestine. Colonic bacteria contribute to the formation of gases (hydrogen, carbon dioxide, oxygen, ammonia, and, in some individuals, methane), acids (e.g., acetic, proprionic, butyric, and lactic), and various potentially toxic substances (e.g., indole, phenol), many of which contribute to the odor of feces.

Although dietary intake alters the fecal flora, the response is highly individualized and variable. The ingestion of increased carbohydrate and fiber, in general, leads to increased fermentation in the large intestine; protein yields increased putrefaction. If faulty absorption in the small intestine allows large amounts of carbohydrate or protein to reach the large intestine, bacterial action may lead to the formation of excessive gas or certain toxic substances. In patients who are significantly malnourished, have GI disease, or have not been fed via the GI tract, there may be increased risk of bacterial translocation. This is the movement of microorganisms across cells lining the bowel into the circulation, which can lead to serious consequences of infection and, possibly, to multi-stage organ failure (Bengmark and Jeppsson, 1995) (see Chapter 33).

Effects of Food Processing

In general, properly cooked foods are more digestible than raw foods. Cooking of meat, for example, loosens the connective tissue, aids chewing, and makes the meat more accessible to the digestive juices. Fiber is softened by cooking, and cooking may make the digestible nutrients attached to fibrous components more available. Raw fruits and vegetables, however, maintain the presence of their active enzymes, which also can facilitate the onset of their digestion in the mouth and stomach. Small, frequent meals are sometimes more completely digested than fewer, large meals.

In some circumstances, chemical reactions take place between food and the secretions of the digestive system. *Acrolein,* a decomposition product produced by frying foods at excessive temperatures, retards the flow of digestive juices. Meat extracts, on the other hand, stimulate secretion of digestive secretions, hormones, and enzymes.

ROLE OF THE LARGE INTESTINE

The large intestine is the site of the absorption of water, salts, and the vitamins synthesized in that organ by bacterial action. It is approximately 5 ft long and consists of the cecum, colon, and rectum. Most of the water contained in the 500 to 1000 mL of chyme entering the colon each day is absorbed, leaving 50 to 200 mL to be excreted in the feces. Normally, as the colonic contents move forward slowly at a rate of 5 cm/hr, almost everything remaining with nutritional value is absorbed.

Large amounts of mucus secreted by the mucosa of the large intestine protect the intestinal wall from excoriation and bacterial activity and provide the medium for binding the feces together. Bicarbonate ions secreted in exchange for absorbed chloride ions help to neutralize the acidic end products of bacterial action.

Colonic bacteria continue the digestion of some materials that have resisted previous digestive activity. In the process, several nutrients are formed by bacterial synthesis that are available for absorption and contribute to the nutrient intake. These nutrients include vitamin K, vitamin B_{12}, thiamin, and riboflavin. Vitamin K, in particular, contributes significantly to the available nutrient supply.

Intestinal flora help to ferment any carbohydrate that remains malabsorbed or resistant to digestion, and help convert dietary fiber into SCFAs and gases. Rapid absorption of SCFAs enhances absorption of sodium and water and helps reduce the osmotic load of accumulating carbohydrate. The process of fermenting and absorbing dietary carbohydrates is called **colonic salvage** (see Fig. 1–9). Fermentation of residual carbohydrate, fiber, and some amino acids salvages a small amount of residual energy substrate; increases the production of SCFAs, which provide fuel for the colonocytes; stimulates colonocyte proliferation and differentiation; reduces the osmotic load of malabsorbed sugars; and enhances the absorption of electrolytes and water (Bengmark and Jeppsson, 1995). The ability to salvage carbohydrates is limited in the human, and colonic fermentation normally disposes of about

SITUATIONS OF INCREASED CARBOHYDRATE MALABSORPTION WITH COLONIC FERMENTATION
In normal individuals, after consumption of:
• lactose when lactase deficiency is present
• dietary fiber
• resistant starch, olestra (sucrose polyester), acarbose (amylase inhibitor)
• small amounts of sorbitol, mannitol, xylitol, or lactulose
• significant amounts of fructose
• fairly large amounts of sucrose
In patients with malabsorption secondary to:
• gastric resection and modest ingestion of sugars, carbohydrates
• pancreatic insufficiency
• short bowel syndrome
• inflammatory bowel disease
• celiac sprue
• disaccharidase deficiencies
SMALL INTESTINE
Fermentation of malabsorbed carbohydrate and fiber by colonic microbes leads to:
• short chain fatty acids SCFAs (butyrate, propionate, acetate, and lactate)
• gases (H_2, CO_2, N, CH_4)
SCFAs:
serve as fuel and stimulate proliferation and differentiation of cells; reduce osmolality, enhance absorption of Na^+ and water
COLON
Significant malabsorption leads to bloating, abdominal distention, flatulence, acidification of stool, and, possibly, diarrhea.

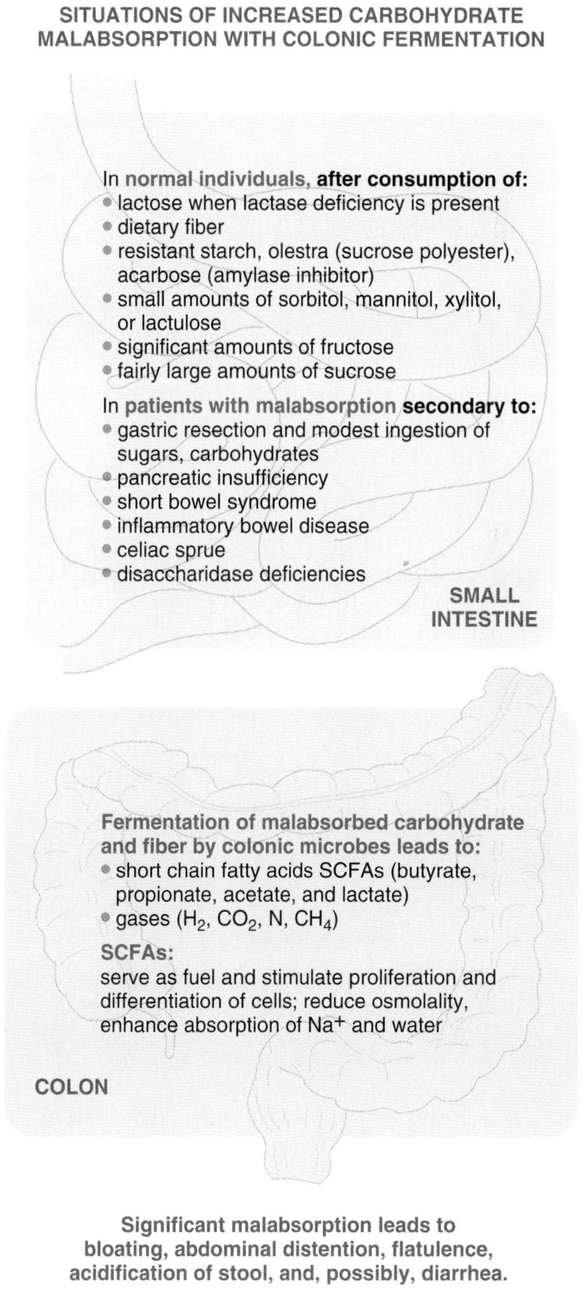

FIGURE 1–9 Colonic fermentation of malabsorbed carbohydrate/fiber.

CASE STUDY

After reading about the benefits of a powdered fiber supplement in a magazine, Mary J. consumed a 20-g dose of a soluble fiber source, in addition to increasing her dietary fiber intake from about 10 g per day to 25 g. Later that day, she suffered abdominal cramping and distention, increased flatulence, and loose stools.

1. What is the likely explanation for her symptoms?
2. How could she have accomplished her goal of increasing fiber without experiencing such severe symptoms?
3. Is the total amount of fiber intake reasonable?

20 to 25 g of carbohydrate over a 24-hour period. Excess amounts of carbohydrate and fermentable fiber in the colon can cause abdominal (colonic) distention, bloating, pain, increased flatulence, and sometimes, loose stools, especially if the individual consumes a large amount at once. Adaptation appears to occur in individuals consuming diets high in carbohydrates and fiber that are resistant to human digestive enzymes. Current research indicates that consumption of about 25 to 30 g of dietary fiber from fruits, vegetables, and whole grains is valuable for (1) maintaining the health of the cells lining the colon, (2) preventing excessive intracolonic pressure, and (3) preventing constipation and, perhaps, other colonic disorders without interfering with mineral balance.

The feces consist of 75% water and 25% solids, but these proportions vary greatly. About one third of the solid matter consists of dead bacteria. Inorganic materials and fats make up 20% to 40%, and protein constitutes approximately 2% to 3%. The remainder includes undigested dietary fiber, sloughed epithelial cells, and dried components of digestive juices, such as bile pigments.

Defecation, or expulsion of feces through the anus, occurs with varying frequency, ranging from three times daily to once every 3 days or more. Normal stool weight is in the range of 100 to 200 g, and mouth-to-anus transit time may vary from 18 to 72 hours. A diet that includes abundant amounts of fruits, vegetables, and whole grains typically results in shorter overall GI transit time, more frequent evacuations, and larger and softer stools.

CITED REFERENCES

Bajetta E, et al. The role of somatostatin analogues in the treatment of gastro-enteropancreatic endocrine tumors. Digestion 57:72S, 1996.

Bengmark S, Jeppsson B. Gastrointestinal surface protection and mucosal reconditioning. J Parent Ent Nutr 19:410, 1995.

Bjorck I, et al. Food properties affecting digestion and absorption of carbohydrates. Am J Clin Nutr 59(suppl):699S-705S, 1994.

Caspary WF. Physiology and pathophysiology of intestinal absorption. Am J Clin Nutr 55(suppl):299S, 1992.

Chang EB, et al. Gastrointestinal, Hepatobiliary, and Nutritional Physiology. Philadelphia: Lippincott-Raven, 1996.

Collins PJ, et al. Effects of increasing solid component size of a mixed solid/liquid meal on solid and liquid gastric emptying. Am J Physiol 271:G539, 1996.

Cummings JH, Englyst HN. Gastrointestinal effects of food carbohydrate. Am J Clin Nutr 61(suppl):938S, 1995.

Farthing MJ. The role of somatostatin analogues in the treatment of refractory diarrhoea. Digestion 57(suppl):107S, 1996.

Furness JB, Costa M. The Enteric Nervous System. Edinburgh: Churchill Livingstone, 1987.

Gardner MIG. Gastrointestinal absorption of intact proteins. Ann Rev Nutr 8:329, 1988.

Guyton AC, Hall JE. Textbook of Medical Physiology, 9th ed. Philadelphia: WB Saunders, 1996.

Holst JJ, et al. Gastrointestinal endocrinology. Scand J Gastroenterol 216(suppl):27S, 1996.

Levin RJ. Digestion and absorption of carbohydrates—from molecules and membranes to humans. Am J Clin Nutr 59(suppl):690S, 1994.

Liddle RA. Cholecystokinin cells. Annu Rev Physiol 59:221, 1997.

Mattes RD. Physiologic responses to sensory stimulation by food: Nutritional implications. J Am Diet Assoc 97:406, 1997.

Minami T, et al. Effects of erythromycin in chronic idiopathic intestinal pseudo-obstruction. J Gastroenterol 31:855, 1996.

Modlin IM, Basson MD. Clinical applications of gastrointestinal hormones. Endocrinol Metab Clin North Am 22:823, 1993.

Mortensen PB, Clausen MR. Short-chain fatty acids in the human colon: Relation to gastrointestinal health and disease. Scand J Gastroenterol 216:132, 1996.

Murray RK, et al. Harper's Biochemistry, 24th ed. Stamford, CT: Appleton and Lange, 1996.

Nauck MA, et al. Glucagon-like peptide 1 (GLP-1) as a new therapeutic approach for type 2 diabetes. Exp Clin Endocrinol Diabetes 105:187, 1997.

Rumessen JJ, Gudmand-Hoyer E. Functional bowel disease: Malabsorption and abdominal distress after ingestion of fructose, sorbitol and fructose-sorbitol mixtures. Gastroenterology 95:694, 1988.

Spiller RC. Intestinal absorptive function. Gut 31(suppl):5S, 1994.

Thompson ABR, et al. Lipid absorption: Passing through the unstirred layers, brush border membrane and beyond. Can J Physiol Pharmacol 71:531, 1989.

ADDITIONAL REFERENCES

Johnson LR, et al. Physiology of the Gastrointestinal Tract, 3rd ed., vols. 1 and 2. New York: Raven Press, 1994.

Minami H, McCallum RW. The physiology and pathophysiology of gastric emptying in humans. Gastroenterology 86:1592, 1984.

CHAPTER 2

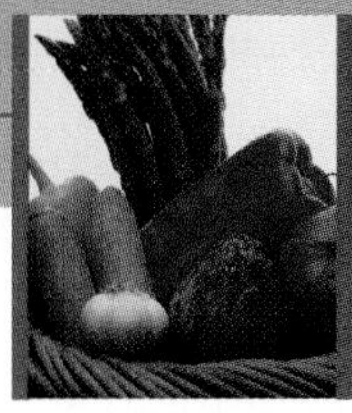

Energy

RACHEL K. JOHNSON, PhD, MPH, RD

CHAPTER OUTLINE

- Components of Energy Expenditure
- Measurement of Energy Expenditure
- Estimating Energy Requirements
- Calculating Food Energy
- Recommended Energy Allowances

Key Terms

BASAL ENERGY EXPENDITURE—the amount of energy used in 24 hours by a person who is lying quietly, 12 to 18 hours after the last meal, in a thermoneutral environment

BASAL METABOLIC RATE—measurement of the basal energy expenditure, usually expressed as kcal/kg body weight/hr or as kcal/24 hours

CALORIE—the amount of energy required to raise the temperature of 1 mL of water by 1° C at 15° C

DIRECT CALORIMETRY—measurement of the amount of energy expended by monitoring the rate at which a person loses heat from the body to the environment when placed inside a structure large enough to permit moderate amounts of activity.

DOUBLY LABELED WATER—a method of measuring total energy expenditure in free-living people using two stable isotopes of water (^2H_2O and $H_2{}^{18}O$); the difference in the turnover rates of the two isotopes measures CO_2 production rate, from which total energy expenditure can be calculated.

ENERGY EXPENDED IN PHYSICAL ACTIVITY—energy expended in voluntary exercise and involuntary activity, such as shivering and fidgeting; the most variable component of total energy expenditure

FACULTATIVE THERMOGENESIS—a portion of the thermic effect of food; "excess" energy expended above the obligatory thermogenesis, thought to be partially mediated by sympathetic nervous system activity

INDIRECT CALORIMETRY—a method for estimating energy production by measuring O_2 consumption and CO_2 production rather than by directly measuring heat transfer; measurements typically take 30 minutes to 1 hour to complete

JOULE—the measure of energy in terms of mechanical work; the amount of energy required to accelerate 1 N a distance of 1 m; 1 kcal is equal to 4.184 kJ

KILOCALORIE (KCAL OR CAL)—1000 calories; sometimes written as Calorie

OBLIGATORY THERMOGENESIS—a portion of the thermic effect of food; the energy required to digest, absorb, and metabolize nutrients

RESTING ENERGY EXPENDITURE—energy expended for the maintenance of normal body functions and homeostasis; represents the largest portion of total energy expenditure (60% to 75%)

RESTING METABOLIC RATE—measurement of the resting energy expenditure, usually expressed as kcal/kg body weight/hr or as kcal/24 hours

RESPIRATORY QUOTIENT—the ratio of moles of CO_2 produced to the moles of O_2 consumed

THERMIC EFFECT OF FOOD—the increase in energy expenditure associated with the processes of digestion, absorption, and metabolism of food; represents approximately 10% of a person's total energy expenditure and includes facultative thermogenesis and obligatory thermogenesis; often called diet-induced thermogenesis (DIT)

TOTAL ENERGY EXPENDITURE—the sum of the resting energy expenditure, energy expended in physical activity, and the thermic effect of food; the energy expended by an individual in 24 hours

Energy is defined as the capacity to do work. In the study of nutrition, it refers to the manner in which the body makes use of the energy locked in the chemical bonding within food.

The ultimate source of all energy in living organisms is the sun. Through the process of *photosynthesis*, green plants intercept a portion of the sunlight reaching their leaves and capture it within the chemical bonds of glucose. Proteins, fats, and other carbohydrates are synthesized from this basic carbohydrate to meet the needs of the plant. Animals and humans obtain these nutrients and the energy they contain by consuming plants and the flesh of other animals.

Energy is released by the metabolism of food, which must be supplied regularly to meet the energy needs for the body's survival. Although all energy eventually appears in the form of heat, which is dissipated into the atmosphere, the unique processes within the cells first make possible its use for all of the tasks required to maintain life. Among these processes are chemical reactions that accomplish synthesis and maintenance of body tissues, electrical conduction of nerve activity, the mechanical work of muscle effort, and heat production to maintain body temperature.

COMPONENTS OF ENERGY EXPENDITURE

Energy is expended by the human body in the form of resting energy expenditure (REE), the thermic effect of food (TEF), and energy expended in physical activity (EEPA) (Hildreth and Johnson, 1995). These three components make up a person's daily **total energy expenditure** (TEE) (Fig. 2–1). Except in extremely active subjects, the REE constitutes the largest portion (60% to 75%) of the TEE (Poehlman, 1993). The TEF represents approximately 10% of the total daily energy expenditure. The contribution of physical activity is the most variable component of TEE, which may be as low as 100 kcal per day in sedentary people or as high as 3000 kcal per day in very active people.

Resting Energy Expenditure

Resting energy expenditure (REE) is the energy expended in the activities necessary to sustain normal body functions and homeostasis. These activities include respiration and circulation, the synthesis of organic compounds, the pumping of ions across membranes, the energy consumed by the central nervous system, and maintenance of body temperature. Of the total, 29% is used by the liver, much of which is involved in synthesizing glucose and ketone bodies as fuels for the brain (Table 2–1).

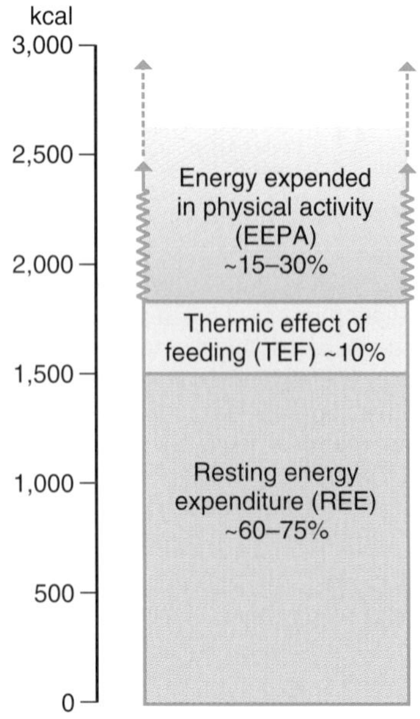

FIGURE 2–1 The components of total energy expenditure (TEE). (From Poehlman ET, Horton ES. Energy needs: Assessment and requirements in humans. In: Modern Nutrition in Health and Disease. Baltimore, MD: Williams & Wilkins, 1988.)

TABLE 2–1 APPROXIMATE ENERGY EXPENDITURE OF ORGANS IN HUMAN ADULTS

ORGAN	% OF REE
Liver	29
Brain	19
Heart	10
Kidney	7
Skeletal muscles (at rest)	18
Remainder	17
	100

(Adapted from Grande F. Energy expenditure of organs and tissues. *In:* Kinney JM (ed). Assessment of Energy Metabolism in Health and Disease. Columbus, OH: Ross Laboratories, 1980, pp. 88–92.)
REE, resting energy expenditure.

The term **basal energy expenditure** (BEE) is also used to describe this portion of daily energy expenditure. BEE can be simply defined as the minimal amount of energy expended that is compatible with life. BEE is the amount of energy used in 24 hours by a person who is lying at physical and mental rest, at least 12 hours after the last meal, in a thermoneutral environment that prevents the activation of heat-generating processes, such as shivering. **Basal metabolic rate** (BMR) measurements are made early in the morning, before the person has engaged in any physical activity, and with no ingestion of tea or coffee or inhalation of nicotine for at least 12 hours before the measurement. If any of the conditions for BMR are not met, the energy expenditure should be termed the **resting metabolic rate** (RMR). For practical reasons, the BMR is now rarely measured. In its place, RMR measurements are used, which in most cases, are higher than the BMR.

Factors Affecting Resting Energy Expenditure

A number of factors cause the REE to vary among individuals. Major determinants are body size and composition. In addition, age, sex, and hormonal status affect REE as well.

Body Size. Larger people have higher metabolic rates than do people of smaller size. A difference in weight of 10 kg would lead to a difference in RMR of approximately 120 kcal per day in adult men or women, or a difference in total daily energy expenditure of approximately 200 kcal per day in people with little physical activity.

Body Composition. The major single determinant of REE is fat-free mass (FFM) or lean body mass (LBM) (Poehlman and Horton, 1998). FFM is the metabolically active tissue in the body, and so most of the variation in REE between people can be accounted for by the variation in their FFM. FFM can be measured most accurately by using reference body composition methods. These include underwater weighing, measuring total body water using stable isotopes of deuterium or 18-oxygen, total body potassium counting, and dual-energy x-ray absorptiometry (DXA). DXA is a novel scanning technique that accurately estimates bone mineral, fat, and fat-free soft tissue. Radiation exposure is minimal, on the order of a single day's background radiation, for a whole body composition analysis (Fig. 2–2). However, owing to the expense and impractical nature of these reference methods, other, less accurate methods are often used in practice to estimate body composition. These include skinfold anthropometry, bioelectrical impedance, and near infrared interactance.

AGE. The loss of FFM with aging is associated with a decline in RMR, amounting to about a 2% to 3% decline per decade after early adulthood. These changes in body composition can be attenuated by exercise; exercise can help maintain a higher lean body mass and, thus, a higher RMR (Poehlman, 1993).

Because it is determined by the FFM, the REE is highest during periods of rapid growth, chiefly during the first and second years of life, and reaches a lesser peak through the ages of puberty and adolescence in both sexes. The additional energy required to cover the cost of synthesizing and depositing body tissue is about 5 kcal/g of tissue gained (Roberts and Young, 1988). Growing infants may store as much as 12% to 15% of the energy value of their food intake in the form of new tissue. As a child becomes older, the caloric requirement for growth is reduced to about 1% of the total energy requirement.

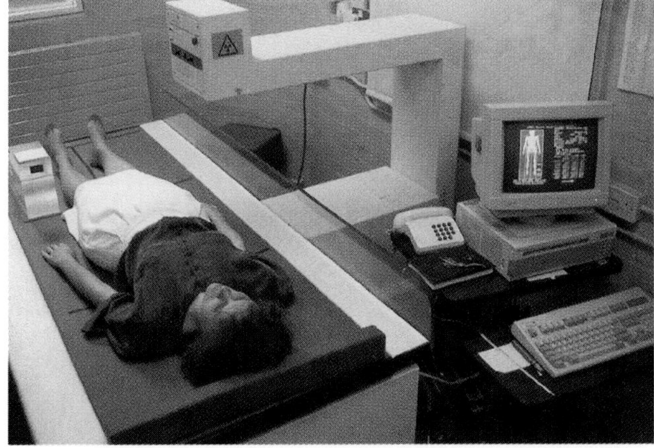

FIGURE 2–2 Dual-energy x-ray absorptiometry (DXA) is a scanning technique that accurately estimates bone mineral, fat, and fat-free soft tissue. Radiation exposure for a whole body analysis is minimal, being approximately equivalent to the x-ray associated with a dental x-ray. (From The Dunn Nutrition Centre, University of Cambridge, Cambridge, UK.)

SEX. Sex differences in metabolic rate are primarily attributable to differences in body size and composition. Women, who generally have more fat in proportion to muscle than men, have metabolic rates that are around 5% to 10% lower than men of the same weight and height.

HORMONAL STATUS. Hormonal status can impact metabolic rate, particularly in endocrine disorders, such as hyperthyroidism and hypothyroidism, when energy expenditure is increased or decreased, respectively. Stimulation of the sympathetic nervous system, such as occurs during emotional excitement or stress, increases cellular activity by the release of epinephrine, which acts directly to promote glycogenolysis. Other hormones, such as cortisol, growth hormone, and insulin, also influence metabolic rate.

The metabolic rate of adult females fluctuates with the menstrual cycle. An average of 359 kcal/day difference in the BMR has been measured between its low point, about 1 week before ovulation at day 14, and its high point, just before the onset of menstruation. The mean increase in energy expenditure is about 150 kcal/day during the second half of the menstrual cycle (Webb, 1986). During pregnancy, RMR seems to decrease in the early stages, whereas later in pregnancy, the metabolic rate is increased by the processes of uterine, placental, and fetal growth and by the mother's increased cardiac work (Goldberg et al., 1993).

OTHER FACTORS AFFECTING METABOLIC RATE. Fevers increase the metabolic rate by about 7% for each degree rise in body temperature above 98.6° F, or by 13% for each degree above 37° C.

RMR is also affected by extremes in environmental temperature. People living in tropical climates usually have RMRs that are 5% to 20% higher than those living in a temperate area. Exercise in temperatures greater than 86° F also imposes a small additional metabolic load of about 5% owing to increased sweat gland activity. The extent to which energy metabolism increases in extremely cold environments depends on the insulation available from body fat and protective clothing.

Athletes with greater muscular development show approximately a 5% increase in basal metabolism over that in nonathletic individuals owing to their greater FFM. Habitual exercise does not cause significantly prolonged stimulation of metabolic rate per unit of active tissue, but it does cause an 8% to 14% higher metabolic rate in men who are moderately and highly active, respectively, owing to increased LBM (Horton and Geissler, 1994). These differences appear to be related to the individual, not to the activity itself.

Thermic Effect of Food

The **thermic effect of food** (TEF) is the increase in energy expenditure associated with the consumption of food. It accounts for approximately 10% of TEE (Poehlman and Horton, 1998). TEF is also referred to as *diet-induced thermogenesis* (DIT). TEF can be separated into obligatory and facultative (or adaptive) subcomponents. **Obligatory thermogenesis** is the energy required to digest, absorb, and metabolize nutrients. This includes the synthesis and storage of protein, fat, and carbohydrate. Adaptive or **facultative thermogenesis** is the "excess" energy expended above the obligatory thermogenesis, thought to be attributable to the metabolic inefficiency of the system stimulated by sympathetic nervous activity.

Factors Affecting the Thermic Effect of Food

The TEF varies with the composition of the diet, being greater after carbohydrate and protein consumption than after fat. This is attributable to the metabolic inefficiency of metabolizing carbohydrate and protein in comparison with fat. Fat is stored very efficiently with only 4% wastage, compared with 25% wastage when carbohydrate is converted to fat for storage. These factors are thought to contribute to the obesity-promoting characteristics of fat (Prentice, 1995). The role of TEF in weight management is discussed further in Chapter 23.

Spicy foods both enhance and prolong the effect of the TEF. Meals with added chili and mustard increase the metabolic rate significantly more than unspiced meals, and this effect may be prolonged for more than 3 hours (McCrory et al., 1994) (Fig. 2–3). Cold, caffeine, and nicotine also stimulate the TEF. The amount of caffeine in one cup of coffee (100 mg), if ingested every 2 hours for 12 hours, has been shown to increase the TEF by 8% to 11% (Dulloo et al., 1989). Nicotine has a similar effect (Hofstetter, 1986).

Energy Expended in Physical Activity

The **energy expended in physical activity** (EEPA) is the most variable component of total energy expenditure. It may range from as little as 10% in the bedridden person to as much as 50% of total energy expenditure in the athlete. EEPA includes energy expended in voluntary exercise, as well as the energy expended involuntarily in activities like shivering, fidgeting, and postural control.

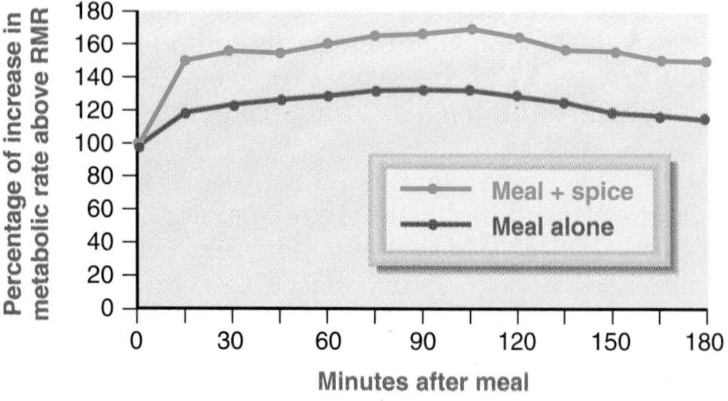

FIGURE 2–3 The effect of adding spices to a meal on the resting metabolic rate (RMR) of healthy subjects. (From McCrory P, et al. Energy balance, food intake and obesity. In: Hills AP, Wahlqvist ML [eds.]. Exercise and Obesity. London: Smith-Gordon and Co., Ltd., 1994, p. 117.)

TABLE 2–2 APPROXIMATE ENERGY EXPENDITURE FOR LEVELS OF ACTIVITY EXPRESSED AS MULTIPLES OF RESTING ENERGY EXPENDITURE (REE)

ACTIVITY CATEGORY	ENERGY AS MULTIPLE OF REE	KCAL/MIN
Resting Sleeping, reclining	REE × 1.0	1–1.2
Very light Seated and standing activities, painting trades, driving, laboratory work, typing, sewing, ironing, cooking, playing cards, playing a musical instrument	REE × 1.5	Up to 2.5
Light Walking on a level surface at 2.5 to 3 mph, garage work, electrical trades, carpentry, restaurant trades, house cleaning, child care, golf, sailing, table tennis	REE × 2.5	2.5–4.9
Moderate Walking 3.5 to 4 mph, weeding and hoeing, carrying a load, cycling, skiing, tennis, dancing	REE × 5.0	5.0–7.4
Heavy Walking with load uphill, tree felling, heavy manual digging, basketball, climbing, football, soccer	REE × 7.0	7.5–12.0

(From Food and Nutrition Board, National Research Council, National Academy of Sciences. Recommended Dietary Allowances, 10th ed. Washington, DC: National Academy Press, 1989, p. 27.)

Factors Affecting the Energy Expended in Physical Activity

EEPA varies considerably depending on *body size* and the efficiency of individual habits of motion. The level of *fitness* also affects the energy expenditure of voluntary activity, probably owing to increased muscle mass. Table 2–2 categorizes activity into five general levels as multiples of the REE and as energy expenditure expressed in kcal/min. The higher level of energy expenditure in each category represents male subjects with their relatively greater LBM.

EEPA tends to decrease with *age,* a trend that is associated with a decline in FFM and an increase in fat mass. Men generally have a higher EEPA than women, primarily because of their larger body size and greater FFM.

Mental activity does not appreciably affect the energy requirement.

MEASUREMENT OF ENERGY EXPENDITURE

Units of Measurement

The standard unit for measuring energy is the **calorie,** which is the amount of heat energy required to raise the temperature of 1 mL of water at 15° C by 1° C. Because the amounts of energy involved in the metabolism of foodstuffs are fairly large, the **kilocalorie,** equal to 1000 calories, is commonly used. A popular convention is to designate kilocalorie by "Calorie" (with a capital "C"). In this text, kilocalorie is abbreviated as kcal.

The **joule,** which measures energy in terms of mechanical work and is the amount of energy required to accelerate 1 Newton (n) over 1 m, is widely used in countries other than the United States. One kilocalorie is equivalent to 4.184 kJ (see "*Clinical Insight:* The Joule").

Measuring Human Energy Expenditure

There are a variety of methods available to measure human energy expenditure. It is important to gain an understanding of the differences in these methods and how they can be applied in both practical and research settings.

DIRECT CALORIMETRY. **Direct calorimetry** monitors the amount of heat produced by a subject placed inside a structure large enough to permit moderate amounts of activity. These structures are referred to as whole room calorimeters. Direct calorimetry provides a measure of energy expended in the form of heat, but provides no information on the kind of fuel being oxidized. The method is also limited by the confined nature of the testing conditions. Hence, the measurement of total energy expenditure using this method is not representative of a free-living environment because physical activity within the chamber is limited. The method is also limited by its high cost, complex engineering, and a scarcity of appropriate facilities around the world.

INDIRECT CALORIMETRY. **Indirect calorimetry** estimates energy expenditure by determining the oxygen consumption and carbon dioxide production of the body over a given period of time. The equipment varies, but the person commonly breathes into a mouthpiece or ventilated hood through which their expired gases are collected. Indirect calorimetry has the advantage of mobility and low equipment cost. The most widely used form of indirect calorimetry is the measurement of RMR through a respirator gas-exchange canopy (Fig. 2–4). These ventilated hoods are useful for both short- and long-term measurements, but are less advantageous in measuring EEPA. However, indirect calorimetry can be used to measure EEPA during various activities in a laboratory setting. Metabolic carts are often used at the hospital bedside to assess patients' energy requirements.

Data are obtained from indirect calorimetry in a form that permits calculation of the **respiratory quotient** (RQ):

$$RQ = \text{moles } CO_2 \text{ expired/moles } O_2 \text{ consumed}$$

This determination is converted into kilocalories of heat produced per square meter of body surface per hour and is extrapolated to energy expenditure in 24 hours.

The RQ depends on the fuel mixture being metabolized. The RQ for carbohydrate is 1.00, because the number of CO_2 molecules produced is equal to the number of O_2 molecules consumed.

RQ =		
	Carbohydrate	1.0
	Mixed diet	0.85
	Protein	0.82
	Fat	0.7

The energy value of 4.825 kcal/L of oxygen consumed (5 kcal/L for ease of calculation) is used as the factor for estimating the energy expenditure based on oxygen consumption. This unit is called a *metabolic equivalent* (MET).

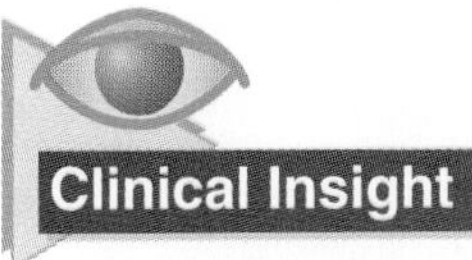

THE JOULE

The joule, a unit of energy based on mechanical energy, is defined as the work done by a force of 1 N acting through a distance of 1 m. The International Organization for Standardization has recommended the adoption of the joule (J) as the preferred unit for energy measurement in all branches of science. This recommendation was adopted by the U.S. National Bureau of Standards in 1964; in 1970, the Committee on Nomenclature of the American Institute of Nutrition recommended that replacement be effected as soon as the mechanics of the transition could be established. Although the joule has been in use internationally for a number of years, the United States and Canada have not made the change to date.

The multiplier recommended by the Committee on Nomenclature, International Union of Nutritional Sciences, to convert kilocalories to kilojoules (kJ) is 4.184 (although 4.2 may be used). Energy values per gram of each nutrient, expressed in kilojoules, are as follows: carbohydrate, 17 kJ; protein, 17 kJ; and fat, 38 kJ. Because the energy content of diets is usually greater than 1000 kJ, the megajoule (mJ), equivalent to 1000 kJ, is often used.

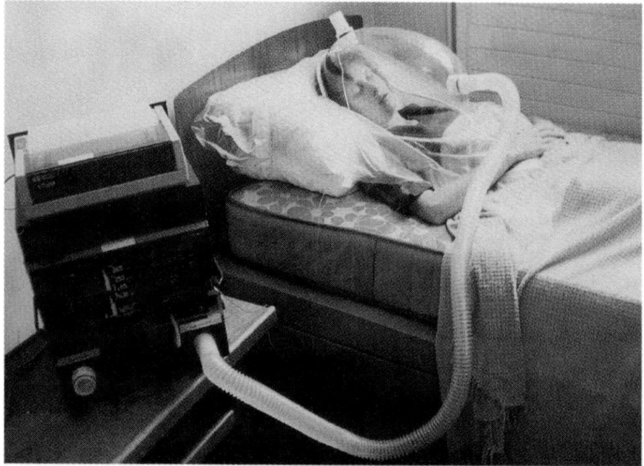

FIGURE 2–4 Measuring resting metabolic rate using a ventilated hood system. (From The Dunn Nutrition Centre, University of Cambridge, Cambridge, UK.)

Doubly Labeled Water

The **doubly labeled water** (DLW) technique for measuring TEE revolutionized our understanding of energy requirements and energy balance in humans. The method was first applied to humans in 1982; since that time, the number of studies using the technique has mushroomed. The method is based on the principle that carbon dioxide production can be estimated from the difference in the elimination rates of body hydrogen and oxygen. The principle of the method is that, after administering a loading dose of water labeled with deuterium oxide (^2H_2O) and oxygen-18 ($H_2{}^{18}O$) (hence the term "doubly labeled water"), the deuterium is eliminated from the body as water and the oxygen-18 is eliminated as water and carbon dioxide (Fig. 2–5). The elimination rates of the two isotopes are measured over a period of 10 to 14 days by periodic sampling of body water through urine, saliva, or plasma. The difference between the two elimination rates is a measure of carbon dioxide production. Carbon dioxide production can then be equated to total energy expenditure using standard indirect calorimetric techniques for the calculation of energy expenditure.

Advantages and Disadvantages of the Doubly Labeled Water Technique

There are a number of advantages to the DLW technique which make it the ideal method for measuring TEE in a variety of populations. First, it provides a measure of energy expenditure that incorporates all the components of TEE: REE, TEF, and EEPA. The technique is easily administered, and the subject is then able to engage in free-living activities throughout the measurement period, thus providing a measure of the person's usual and typical daily TEE. This is beneficial in individuals, such as infants, young children, the elderly, and the disabled, who cannot easily withstand the rigorous testing involved in the measurement of oxygen consumption during various activities. DLW also provides a method by which other, more subjective estimates of energy intakes (diet recalls and records) and energy expenditure (physical activity logs) can be validated (Schoeller, 1990). Most importantly, the method is accurate and has a precision of 2% to 8%.

There are also drawbacks to the DLW technique, however—namely, the expense of the stable isotopes and the expertise required to operate the highly sophisticated and costly mass spectrometer for analysis of the isotope enrichments (see "*Clinical Insight:* Estimating Energy Requirements").

Measuring the Thermic Effect of Food

Actual measurement of TEF is appropriate only for research purposes. For practical purposes, it is determined as 10% of the sum of the RMR and the EEPA.

Measuring Energy Expended in Physical Activity

In conjunction with indirect calorimetry, the DLW method can be used to obtain a caloric value of EEPA. A postprandial RMR is measured using indi-

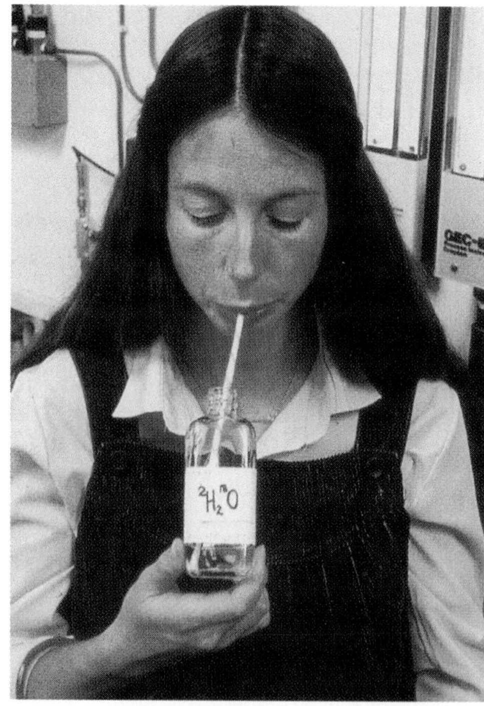

FIGURE 2–5 A woman consumes a loading dose of water labeled with deuterium oxide (^2H_2O) and oxygen-18 ($H_2{}^{18}O$) prior to undergoing a doubly labeled water (DLW) measurement of total energy expenditure. (From The Dunn Nutrition Centre, University of Cambridge, Cambridge, UK.)

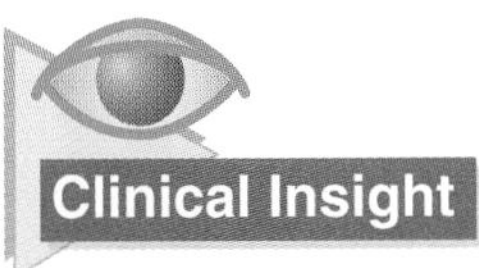

Estimating Energy Requirements

Scientists have had the capacity to measure total energy expenditure (TEE) in humans using the doubly labeled water (DLW) technique for the past decade. Unfortunately, due to its high cost and small number of laboratories worldwide with the required technical expertise, there have been a relatively small number of measurements of TEE across the age and sex groups and special conditions (pregnancy, lactation) for which RDAs for energy are established. Thus, clinicians still rely heavily on prediction equations to estimate energy requirements in their patients. As more measurements of TEE are conducted using DLW, increasingly accurate tools to estimate TEE should be available. In addition, the new Dietary Reference Intakes (DRIs) for energy should take into account TEE measurements conducted to date using DLW and be revised accordingly. In the meantime, clinicians can use the best formulas available to estimate energy requirements in their clients. However, these equations should be used only as a guide or starting point, after which the client must be monitored closely and interventions devised based on individual needs that promote the attainment of optimal nutritional status.

rect calorimetry, which incorporates a measure of the TEF. An estimate of EEPA can then be determined by subtracting the postprandial RMR from the TEE that is measured using DLW (Goran et al., 1995). This method is generally only used in research settings, but can be used to validate other, more practical and easily administered methods of measuring physical activity. These include activity diaries; motion sensor devices, such as pedometers or accelerometers; and heart rate monitoring. Because these methods are dependent on the accuracy of a person's record keeping, their memory of activity patterns, their enthusiasm for wearing a motion sensor device, and assumptions about the correlation between heart rate and oxygen consumption during exercise, the estimates of EEPA obtained while using them can often be inaccurate (Russ et al., 1997).

ESTIMATING ENERGY REQUIREMENTS

Knowledge of energy requirements throughout the life cycle; during various physiological conditions, like pregnancy and lactation; and in various disease states is essential to the promotion of optimal health. In the past, the measurement of energy intake served as an important tool from which recommendations for energy requirements for all age groups were derived (WHO, 1985). However, since the advent of the DLW technique, scientists have begun to establish accurate energy requirements based on the actual measurement of TEE in free-living subjects.

Measuring Energy Intake in Humans

Traditionally, recommendations for energy requirements have been based on self-recorded (diet record) or self-reported (24-hour recall) estimates of food intake. It is now well accepted, however, that these methods do not provide accurate or unbiased estimates of a person's energy intake, and that underreporting of food intake is pervasive in dietary surveys (Black, 1996). This conclusion is based on findings from studies using the DLW technique to measure TEE to assess the accuracy of estimates of energy intake. These studies are based on the principle of energy balance; that is, in groups of weight-stable individuals, energy intake must equal TEE. Thus, on a group basis, measurements of TEE using DLW can be used to validate estimates of energy intake (Schoeller, 1990).

It has been shown that the percentage of people who underreport their food intake ranges from 10% to 45%, depending on their ages, sex, and body compositions. Underreporting tends to increase as children age, is worse among women than men, and is more prevalent and severe among the obese in comparison with the lean (Johnson et al., 1998). Thus, until methods of determining energy intake are developed that minimize the problem of underreporting, it is no longer acceptable to base recommendations for energy requirements on estimates of energy intake (Livingstone, 1995). According to the World Health Organization (WHO), "As a matter of principle we believe the estimates of energy requirements should, as far as possible, be based on estimates of energy expenditure" (WHO, 1985).

Total Energy Requirements Estimated from DLW Studies

Values for energy requirements for various age and sex groups can be obtained from a meta-analysis of 574 free-living measurements of TEE using DLW (Black et al., 1996). The data shown in Table 2–3 are compiled from healthy, free-living people aged 2 to 95 years. Information is also presented on basal metabolic rate and physical activity levels. These data will be used in the establishment of future recommendations for energy intake and can be used to evaluate other estimates of energy requirements.

TABLE 2–3 TOTAL ENERGY EXPENDITURE (TEE) OF DIFFERENT AGE AND SEX GROUPS FROM A META-ANALYSIS OF 574 FREE-LIVING DLW MEASUREMENTS*

AGE GROUP (yr)	n	AGE (yr) Mean	TEE KCAl/d Mean	BMR KCAl/d Mean	PAL FACTOR
Females					
1–6	21	4.9	1316	861	1.57
7–12	24	9.2	1914	1148	1.68
13–17	26	14.8	2727	1603	1.73
18–29	89	24.4	2488	1483	1.70
30–39	76	33.8	2392	1435	1.68
40–64	47	51.6	2345	1388	1.69
65–74	24	69.1	2057	1268	1.62
>75	12	82.8	1459	981	1.48
Males					
1–6	29	4.7	1459	909	1.64
7–12	32	9.8	2345	1364	1.74
13–17	31	14.5	3373	1938	1.75
18–29	56	22.5	3301	1794	1.85
30–39	36	34.3	3421	1962	1.77
40–64	15	50.6	2751	1675	1.64
65–74	22	68.6	2637	1651	1.61
>75	34	80.8	2201	1435	1.54

(Reprinted with permission from Black AE. Physical activity levels from a meta-analysis of doubly labeled water studies for validating energy intake as measured by dietary assessment. Nutr Rev 54:172, 1996.)

DLW, doubly labeled water; *TEE*, total energy expenditure; *BMR*, basal metabolic rate; *PAL*, physical activity level factor; MJ = kcal (4.184) ÷ 1000. TEE = BMR × PAL × 1.1.

Estimating Resting Metabolic Rate

Because it is still not feasible to measure TEE, or even RMR, whenever information about the energy requirements of a person is needed, practitioners still rely heavily on formulas that estimate energy needs using multiples of RMR. The total daily energy requirement is commonly estimated by adding estimates of RMR, the EEPA, and the TEF. There are two major limitations to this approach: (1) the formulas do not take into account the amount of FFM that represents the metabolically active tissue and (2) the level of physical activity is highly variable in normal, healthy people, ranging from a low of 200 kcal/day to 1250 kcal/day (Poehlman and Horton, 1998).

More than 190 equations have been developed to predict RMR from people's physical characteristics (commonly, age, height, weight, and gender) (Green et al., 1994). The most widely used equation in the United States is probably the Harris-Benedict equation, which was developed in 1919 (Harris and Benedict, 1919). These equations, as well as other standard equations, are shown in Table 2–4.

The Harris-Benedict formulas have been found to overestimate REE by 7% to 24% (Daly et al., 1985; Owen et al., 1986 and 1987). The Mifflin–St. Jeor equations correct for this overestimation. However, their use results in an unexplained variability of 30% among individuals of the same sex, height, and weight, possibly owing to individual differences in metabolic efficiency (Mifflin et al., 1990). The WHO has adopted the equations that utilize body weight, as presented in Table 2–5.

Calculating REE in obese individuals involves the question of whether the increased surface area related to excessive fatness in fact increases the REE, as adipose tissue is not as metabolically active as FFM. Use of the actual body weight of a person who is more than 125% of ideal body weight (IBW) results in an REE that is too high. On the other hand, using IBW for the calculations does not allow for the increased LBM needed for structural support of the extra adipose tissue, or for the in-

TABLE 2–4 METHODS FOR PREDICTING RESTING ENERGY EXPENDITURE (REE)

Harris and Benedict (1919)

For children and adults, all ages

Women: REE (kcal) = 655. + 9.56 W + 1.85 H − 4.68 A

REE (kJ) = 2741 + 40 W + 7.74 H − 28.35 A

Men: REE (kcal) = 66.5 + 13.75 W + 5.0 H − 6.78 A

REE (kJ) = 278 + 57.5 W + 7.74 H − 19.56

(A = age; W = weight in kilograms; H = height in centimeters)

Mifflin–St. Jeor (Mifflin et al, 1990)

For adults 19 to 78 years of age

REE (female) = 10 W + 6.25 H − 5 A − 161

REE (male) = 10 W + 6.25 H − 5 A + 5

(A = age; W = weight in kilograms; H = height in centimeters)

REE Based on Age, Sex, and Body Weight Alone

See Table 2–5.

Abbreviated Version for Persons of Normal Height and Weight

REE (female) = weight (kg) × 0.95 kcal/kg × 24 hr

REE (male) = weight (kg) × 1 kcal/kg × 24 hr

TABLE 2–5 EQUATIONS FOR PREDICTING RESTING ENERGY EXPENDITURE (REE) FROM BODY WEIGHT ALONE

SEX AND AGE RANGE (yr)	EQUATION TO DERIVE REE IN KCAL/DAY	SD*
Males		
0–3	(60.9 × wt[†]) – 54	53
3–10	(22.7 × wt) + 495	62
10–18	(17.5 × wt) + 651	100
18–30	(15.3 × wt) + 679	151
30–60	(11.6 × wt) + 879	164
>60	(13.5 × wt) + 487	148
Females		
0–3	(61.0 × wt) – 51	61
3–10	(22.5 × wt) + 499	63
10–18	(12.2 × wt) + 746	117
18–30	(14.7 × wt) + 496	121
30–60	(8.7 × wt) + 829	108
>60	(10.5 × wt) + 596	108

(Adapted from Food and Nutrition Board, National Research Council, National Academy of Sciences. Recommended Dietary Allowances, 10th ed. Washington, DC: National Academy Press, 1989.)

*Standard deviation (SD) of the differences between actual and computed values.

[†]Weight of person in kilograms.

creased energy expenditure required to move the excess weight.

Ideally, REE of the obese should be based on LBM determined by underwater weighing or other methods (Cunningham, 1982; Webb, 1981) (see Chapter 23). However, when it is necessary to estimate energy requirements of the obese, the following formula has been recommended (Wilkens, 1986):

$$(\text{ABW} - \text{IBW}) \times 0.25 + \text{IBW} = \text{weight to be used for calculating REE}$$

In this formula, ABW is actual body weight; IBW is ideal body weight, and 0.25 is the percentage of excess body weight that is metabolically active.

Estimating Energy Expended in Physical Activity

Energy expended in physical activity can be estimated by using tables such as Appendix Table 31. The calculation should include a factor for body size or weight to allow for the extra energy expended by larger persons. Table 2–6 lists factors derived from DLW studies that can be used if the general level of activity of the person is known (Shetty et al., 1996).

Children's average daily EEPA is actually much less than previously believed. According to the 1989 Recommended Dietary Allowances (RDAs), children were thought to have daily energy expenditures of 1.7 to 2.0 times the REE (Food and Nutrition Board, 1989). Recently, however, studies using the

TABLE 2–6 FACTORS FOR PHYSICAL ACTIVITY LEVELS (PAL) BASED ON DOUBLY LABELED WATER (DLW) STUDIES

LIFE STYLE AND LEVEL OF ACTIVITY	FACTOR FOR PAL
Chair-bound or bed-bound	1.2
Seated work with no option of moving around and little or no strenuous leisure activity	1.4–1.5
Seated work with discretion and requirement to move around but little or no strenuous leisure activity	1.6–1.7
Standing work (e.g., housework, shop assistant)	1.8–1.9
Significant amounts of sport or strenuous leisure activity (30–60 minutes four to five times per week)	+0.3 (increment)
Strenuous work or highly active leisure	2.0–2.4

(Adapted from Shetty PS, et al. Energy requirements of adults: An update on basal metabolic rates (BMRs) and physical activity levels (PALs). Eur J Clin Nutr 50(suppl 1):S11, 1996.)

DLW technique have shown that children's TEE is actually only 1.3 to 1.4 times the REE (Goran et al., 1997). According to these findings and others based on the DLW method, and given the increasing prevalence of obesity in U.S. children (Troino et al., 1995), it is now believed that the RDAs for energy for infants and children are currently set too high (Cryan and Johnson, 1997) (see Chapter 15) (see www.cdc.gov/needphp/dnpa/).

Total Energy Expenditure

Table 2–7 presents calculations for estimating TEE in an individual. Stress and injury would increase the total energy requirements. These factors are discussed throughout the text.

TABLE 2–7 CALCULATION OF ESTIMATED TOTAL ENERGY EXPENDITURE (TEE)

1. Determine IBW in kilograms. This can be determined from (1) a record of the person's constant weight, (2) Appendix Table 19, or (3) a formula presented in Chapter 23.
2. Determine resting energy expenditure (REE)—see Table 2–4 or 2–5.
3. Add factor for physical activity level (PAL)—see Table 2–6.
4. Add thermic effect of food (TEF)—10% of REE plus PAL
5. Sum equals the approximate daily energy requirement

Sample calculation of total energy expenditure (TEE)

Example: 20-year-old woman, 165 cm tall and weighing 55 kg
Activity: standing work

a. determine IBW (55 kg is IBW for this woman)
b. REE = 655 + 9.56 (55) + 1.85 (165) – 4.68 (20) = 1392.5 kcal
c. multiply by a PAL factor of 1.8

$$1392.5 \times 1.8 = 2506.4 \text{ kcal}$$

d. add 10% TEF of 250.6

$$2506.4 + 250.6 = 2757 \text{ kcal/day}$$

Measuring the Energy in Food

The total energy available from a food is measured by means of a *bomb calorimeter*. This device consists of a closed container in which a weighed food sample, ignited with an electric spark, is burned in an oxygen atmosphere. The container is immersed in a known volume of water, and the rise in the temperature of the water after ignition of the food is used to calculate the heat energy generated.

Not all of the energy in foods and alcohol is available to the body's cells. The processes of digestion and absorption are not completely efficient, and the nitrogenous portion of amino acids is not oxidized, but is excreted in the form of urea. Therefore, the biologically available energy from foods and alcohol is expressed in values rounded off slightly below those obtained using the calorimeter. These values for protein, fat, carbohydrate, and alcohol, summarized in Figure 2–6, are 4, 9, 4, and 7 kcal/g, respectively. The kilocalorie content of various foods is shown in Appendix 41.

CALCULATING FOOD ENERGY

Although the energy value of each nutrient is known precisely, only a few foods, such as oils and sugars, are made up of a single nutrient. More commonly, foods contain a mixture of protein, fat, and carbohydrate. The energy value of one medium-sized egg (50 g), for example, calculated in terms of weight, is derived from protein (13%), fat (12%), and carbohydrate (1%) as follows:

$$\text{Protein: } 13\% \times 50 \text{ g} = 6.5 \text{ g} \times 4 \text{ kcal/g} = 26 \text{ kcal}$$
$$\text{Fat: } 12\% \times 50 \text{ g} = 6 \text{ g} \times 9 \text{ kcal/g} = 54 \text{ kcal}$$
$$\text{Carbohydrate: } 1\% \times 50 \text{ g} = 0.5 \text{ g} \times 4 \text{ kcal/g} = 2 \text{ kcal}$$
$$\text{Total} = 82 \text{ kcal}$$

Energy values of foods based on chemical analyses may be obtained from the U.S. Department of Agriculture's (USDA's) Nutrient Data Laboratory. To obtain information about USDA food composition publications, and to do simple nutrient analyses on-line, one may access the following Internet address: *http://www.nal.usda.gov/fnic/foodcomp.* Another source of nutrient values for common serving sizes of foods is: *Bowes and Church: Food Values of Portions Commonly Used*, 17th ed., 1998. Many computer software programs that use the USDA nutrient database as the standard reference are also available and have been reviewed extensively (Nieman et al., 1992). The approximate energy content of any diet can be estimated from Appendix 41.

Kilocalories in alcoholic beverages may be calculated as shown in the accompanying box (*"Clinical*

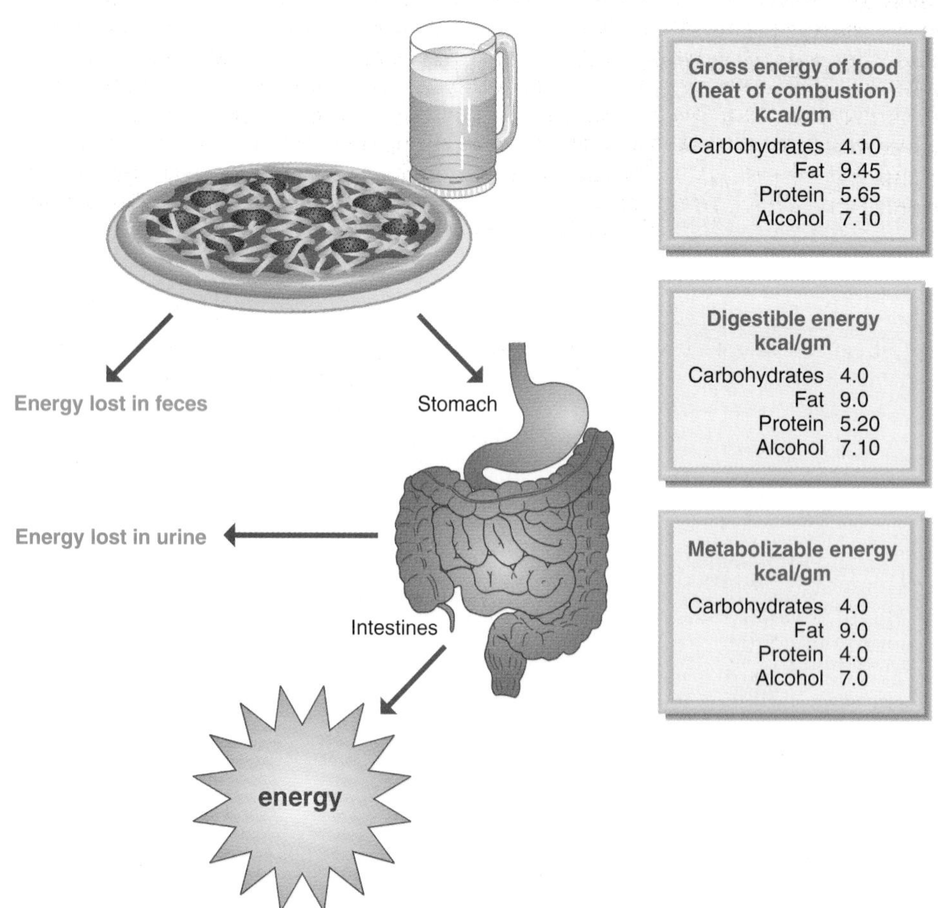

Gross energy of food (heat of combustion) kcal/gm	
Carbohydrates	4.10
Fat	9.45
Protein	5.65
Alcohol	7.10

Digestible energy kcal/gm	
Carbohydrates	4.0
Fat	9.0
Protein	5.20
Alcohol	7.10

Metabolizable energy kcal/gm	
Carbohydrates	4.0
Fat	9.0
Protein	4.0
Alcohol	7.0

FIGURE 2–6 Energy value of food.

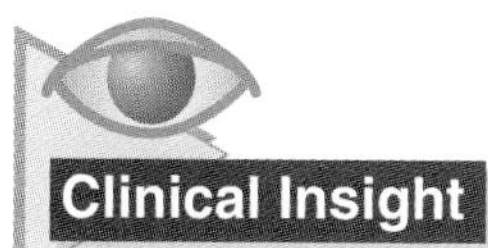

Calculation of Energy Content of Alcoholic Beverages and Mixes

The energy value of alcoholic beverages, expressed in kilocalories, can be determined by the following equation (Gastineau, 1976):

kcal = oz of beverage × proof × 0.8 kcal/proof/1 oz

Proof is defined as the proportion of alcohol to water or other liquids in an alcoholic beverage. The standard in the United States defines 100-proof as being equal to 50% of ethyl alcohol by volume.

To determine the percentage of ethyl alcohol in a beverage, divide the proof value by 2. For example, a volume of 86-proof whiskey contains 43% ethyl alcohol.

The latter part of the equation—0.8 kcal/proof/1 oz—refers to the factor necessary to account for the caloric density of alcohol (7 kcal/g) and the fact that not all of the alcohol in liquor is available for energy. For example, the number of kilocalories in 1½ oz of 86-proof whiskey would be determined as follows:

1½ oz × 86 proof × 0.8 kcal/proof/1 oz = 103 kcal

Insight: Calculation of Energy Content of Alcoholic Beverages and Mixes") and Appendix 44.

RECOMMENDED ENERGY ALLOWANCES

The recommendations for energy intake for adults, revised in 1989 by the Food and Nutrition Board, National Research Council, National Academy of Sciences, are presented in Table 2–8. The recommended allowances are based on a light-to-moderate activity level and are calculated by using the WHO equations for calculating REE. REEs are multiplied by an activity factor appropriate for the individual's age and sex. The activity factors for men aged 19 to 24, 25 to 50, and 51 to 75 are 1.67, 1.6, and 1.5, respectively. Factors for women of the same age groups are 1.6, 1.55, and 1.5. Allowances for persons with heavy activity patterns should be adjusted to 2.0 times the REE or higher. The average daily energy allowances for the reference man (79 kg) and woman (63 kg) are 2900 kcal and 2200 kcal, respectively.

It is anticipated that, as much as possible, future recommendations for energy intake will be based on

TABLE 2–8 RECOMMENDED DIETARY ALLOWANCES FOR ENERGY

		WEIGHT		HEIGHT			AVERAGE ENERGY ALLOWANCE (KCAL)*		
CATEGORY	AGE (yr) OR CONDITION	(kg)	(lb)	(cm)	(in)	REE† (KCAL/DAY)	Multiples of REE	Per kg	Per day‡
Infants	0.0–0.5	6	13	60	24	320		108	650
	0.5–1.0	9	20	71	28	500		98	850
Children	1–3	13	29	90	35	740		102	1300
	4–6	20	44	112	44	950		90	1800
	7–10	28	62	132	52	1130		70	2000
Males	11–14	45	99	157	62	1440	1.70	55	2500
	15–18	66	145	176	69	1760	1.67	45	3000
	19–24	72	160	177	70	1780	1.67	40	2900
	25–50	79	174	176	70	1800	1.60	37	2900
	51 +	77	170	173	68	1530	1.50	30	2300
Females	11–14	46	101	157	62	1310	1.67	47	2200
	15–18	55	120	163	64	1370	1.60	40	2200
	19–24	58	128	164	65	1350	1.60	38	2200
	25–50	63	138	163	64	1380	1.55	36	2200
	51 +	65	143	160	63	1280	1.50	30	1900
Pregnant	1st trimester								+0
	2nd trimester								+300
	3rd trimester								+300
Lactating	1st 6 months								+500
	2nd 6 months								+500

(From Food and Nutrition Board. National Research Council, National Academy of Sciences. Recommended Dietary Allowances, 10th ed. Washington, DC: National Academy Press, 1989.)

*In the range of light to moderate activity, the coefficient of variation is ± 20%.

†Calculation is based on FAO equations (see Table 2–5), then rounded.

‡Figure is rounded.

CASE STUDY

Allen Q. has been active all of his life due to his work. Now, at the age of 54, he wants to start a structured exercise program that includes walking three times a week, swimming twice a week, and occasional tennis. After obtaining his physician's approval for this general increase in activity, Allen Q. schedules an appointment to see you, the nutrition counselor. He is 5 ft 8 in tall, weighs 175 lb, and has no prior medical conditions that are a factor in his health care treatment. He is a landscape architect who engages in low to moderate activity levels during the workday.

1. What other information is needed to give Allen appropriate nutritional guidance?
2. What specific advice may be useful to Mr. Q. on days that he is more active than usual?
3. Allen thinks he can double his energy intake because of this increase in activity. Calculate his normal needs, and estimate for him the increases that will actually occur based on his planned activities.

actual measurements of energy expenditure using the DLW method (Black et al., 1996). The method has been adopted by many laboratories around the world and is now being applied to people of all ages, ranging from premature infants to the very elderly, and to people in a variety of circumstances, ranging from bedridden patients to elite athletes (Cryan and Johnson, 1997) (see Tables 2–3 and 2–6). As these data become available, it will become possible to establish more accurate recommendations for energy needs in different age and sex groups and during various physiological conditions and disease states.

CITED REFERENCES

Black AE. Physical activity levels from a meta-analysis of doubly labeled water studies for validating energy intake as measured by dietary assessment. Nutr Rev 54:170, 1996.

Black AE, et al. Human energy expenditure in affluent societies: An analysis of 574 doubly-labelled water measurements. Eur J Clin Nutr 50:72, 1996.

Cryan J, Johnson RK. Should the current recommendations for energy intake in infants and young children be lowered? Nutr Today 32:69, 1997.

Cunningham JJ. An individualization of dietary requirements for energy in adults. J Am Diet Assoc 80:335, 1982.

Daly JM, et al. Human energy requirements: Overestimation by widely used prediction equation. Am J Clin Nutr 42:1170, 1985.

Dulloo AG, et al. Normal caffeine consumption: Influence on thermogenesis and daily energy expenditure in lean and post-obese human volunteers. Am J Clin Nutr 49:44, 1989.

Food and Nutrition Board, National Research Council, National Academy of Sciences. Recommended Dietary Allowances, 10th ed. Washington, DC: National Academy Press, 1989.

Gastineau CF. Alcohol and calories. Mayo Clin Proc 51(2):88, 1976.

Goldberg GR, et al. Longitudinal assessment of energy expenditure in pregnancy by the doubly labeled water method. Am J Clin Nutr 57:494, 1993.

Goran MI, et al. Energy requirements across the life span: New findings based on measurement of total energy expenditure with doubly labeled water. Nutr Res 15:115, 1995.

Goran MI, et al. Physical activity related energy expenditure and fat mass in young children. Int J Obes 21:171, 1997.

Green JH. Assessment of energy requirements. In: Heatley RV, Green JH, Losowsky MS. Consensus in Clinical Nutrition. Cambridge, UK: Cambridge University Press, 1994.

Hildreth HG, Johnson RK. The doubly labeled water technique for the determination of human energy requirements. Nutr Today 30:254, 1995.

Hofstetter A. Increased 24-hour energy expenditure in cigarette smokers. N Engl J Med 314:79, 1986.

Horton T, Geissler C. Effect of habitual exercise on daily energy expenditure and metabolic rate during standardized activity. Am J Clin Nutr 59:13, 1994.

Johnson RK, et al. The multiple-pass 24-hour recall method underestimates energy intake in U.S. low-income women: A doubly labeled water study. J Amer Diet Assoc 98:1136, 1998.

Livingstone MBE. Assessment of food intake: Are we measuring what people eat? Br J Biomed Sci 52:58, 1995.

McCrory P, et al. Energy balance, food intake and obesity. In: Hills AP, Wahlqvist ML (eds). Exercise and Obesity. London: Smith-Gordon and Co., Ltd., 1994.

Mifflin MD, et al. A new predictive equation for resting energy expenditure in healthy individuals. Am J Clin Nutr 51:241, 1990.

Nieman DC, et al. Comparison of six microcomputer dietary analysis systems with the USDA nutrient database for standard reference. J Am Diet Assoc 92:48, 1992.

Owen OE, et al. A reappraisal of caloric requirements in healthy women. Am J Clin Nutr 44:1, 1986.

Owen OE, et al. A reappraisal of the caloric requirements of men. Am J Clin Nutr 46:875, 1987.

Poehlman ET. Regulation of energy expenditure in aging humans. Geriatr Biosci 41:552, 1993.

Poehlman ET, Horton ES. Energy needs: Assessment and requirements in humans. In: Bloch AS, Shils ME (eds.). Modern Nutrition in Health and Disease. Baltimore: Williams & Wilkins, 1998.

Prentice AM. All calories are not equal. International Dialogue on Carbohydrates 5(4):1, 1995.

Roberts SB, Young VR. Energy costs of fat and protein deposition in the human infant. Am J Clin Nutr 48:951, 1988.

Russ J, et al. Physical activity related energy expenditure in children by doubly labeled water as compared with the Caltrac accelerometer. J Am Diet Assoc 97:A73, 1997.

Schoeller DA. How accurate is self-reported dietary energy intake? Nutr Rev 48:373, 1990.

Shetty PS, et al. Energy requirements of adults: An update on basal metabolic rates (BMRs) and physical activity levels (PALs). Eur J Clin Nutr 50 (suppl 1): S11, 1996.

Troino R, et al. Overweight prevalence and trends for children and adolescents. Arch Pediatr Adolesc Med 149:1085, 1995.

Webb P. Energy expenditure and fat-free mass in men and women. Am J Clin Nutr 34:1816, 1981.

Webb P. 24-hour energy expenditure and the menstrual cycle. Am J Clin Nutr 44:614, 1986.

Wilkens K (ed.). Suggested Guidelines for Nutrition Care of Renal Patients. Chicago: American Dietetic Association, 1986, p. 34.

WHO. Energy and protein requirements. Report of a Joint FAO/WHO/UNU Expert Consultation. (Technical Report Series 724). Geneva: World Health Organization, 1985.

ADDITIONAL REFERENCES

Harris JA, Benedict FG. A Biometric Study of Basal Metabolism in Man (Publication No. 279). Washington, DC: Carnegie Institute of Washington, 1919.

Jebb SA, Elia M. Techniques for the measurement of body composition: A practical guide. Int J Obes 17:611, 1993.

Klesges LM, Klesges RC. The assessment of children's physical activity: A comparison of methods. Med Sci Sports Exerc 19:511, 1987.

McNeill G. Energy. In: Garrow JS, James WPT (eds.). Human Nutrition and Dietetics. New York: Churchill Livingstone, 1993.

Murgatroyd PR, et al. Techniques for the measurement of human energy expenditure: A practical guide. Int J Obes 17:549, 1993.

Schoeller DA. Measurement of energy expenditure in free-living humans by using doubly labeled water. J Nutr 118:1278, 1988.

CHAPTER 3

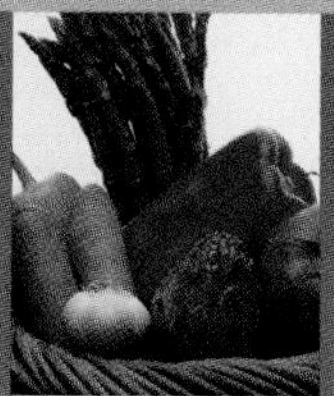

Macronutrients: Carbohydrates, Proteins, and Lipids

SUSAN ETTINGER, PHD, RD

Chapter Outline

- Development of Macronutrients
- Carbohydrates
- Fats and Lipids
- Amino Acids and Protein
- Macronutrient Utilization and Storage in the Fed State
- Macronutrient Catabolism from Body Stores in the Fasted State

Key Terms

AMINO ACID—an organic compound containing an amino (NH_2) group and a carboxyl (COOH) group, which functions as one of the building blocks of protein

AMINO ACID SCORE—a method of protein evaluation in which the milligrams of the limiting indispensable amino acid in the test protein are divided by the milligrams of the same indispensable amino acid in the reference protein

AMYLOSE—a form of starch; long straight chains of glucose units

CARNITINE—a required cofactor derived from the essential amino acids, methionine and lysine; carnitine facilitates transfer of long-chain fatty acids across the mitochondrial membranes for use as an energy source

CELLULOSE—a structural carbohydrate in plants that resists hydrolysis in the human digestive tract

CHITIN—a homopolymer of *N*-acetylglucosamine in the exoskeleton of invertebrates

CHOLESTEROL—a sterol found in cell membranes of all animal tissues that is also necessary for production of bile and steroid hormones

CHYLOMICRON—a lipoprotein particle formed after lipid absorption to transport dietary triglyceride and cholesterol in the blood

CONDITIONALLY ESSENTIAL AMINO ACIDS—amino acids that become essential under certain conditions

DENATURATION—"unraveling" or breaking down of the tertiary structure of proteins by mechanical agitation, heat, cold, acidity, or alkalinity

DEXTRIN—an intermediate product of starch hydrolysis

DEXTROSE—glucose produced by the hydrolysis of cornstarch

DIETARY FIBER—the amount of plant material remaining after treatment with digestive enzymes and reduction with acid and alkali

DIGLYCERIDE (DIACYLGLYCEROL)—a lipid with only two fatty acids attached to the glycerol molecule

DISACCHARIDE—a sugar capable of being hydrolyzed to two monosaccharide molecules

ESSENTIAL AMINO ACIDS—amino acids for which synthesis is inadequate to meet metabolic needs and that must be supplied in the diet; threonine, tryptophan, histidine, lysine, leucine, isoleucine, methionine, valine, and phenylalanine, formerly called "indispensable"

ESSENTIAL FATTY ACIDS (EFA)—fatty acids the body needs, but cannot synthesize; the two main EFAs are linoleic and α-linolenic acids

FATTY ACID—a straight carbon chain, usually with an even number of carbons and a carboxyl group at one end and a methyl group at the other end

FRUCTOOLIGOSACCHARIDE—a nonabsorbed polymer of fructose; supports the growth of colonic bacteria

FRUCTOSE—a monosaccharide occurring in fruit, honey, and some vegetables; the sweetest of the monosaccharides

GALACTOSE—a monosaccharide produced by the hydrolysis of lactose by digestive enzymes

GLUCOSE—the main monosaccharide in blood and an important source of energy for living organisms; plentiful in fruits, sweet corn, corn syrup, honey, and certain roots

GLYCOGEN—branched-chain glucose polymer used for glucose storage in animals

GLYCOLIPID—a compound that contains a long-chain fatty acid, one to seven monosaccharides, and varying side groups; high concentrations are found in the brain

HEMICELLULOSES (NONCELLULOSE POLYSACCHARIDES)—a group of nondigestible carbohydrate heteropolymers that contain fewer glucose units and a variety of other carbohydrate units

HYDROGENATION—the process of adding hydrogen to unsaturated fatty acids to increase saturation and stability

ISOPRENOID—a large group of lipids with alternating single- and double-bond structure (conjugated double bonds). As part of vitamin E and beta carotene, the structure acts as an antioxidant to quench free radicals. The structure is found in phytochemicals such as lycopene and limonine

KETONE BODIES—three compounds (acetoacetic acid, acetone, β-hydroxybutyric acid) formed during fatty acid oxidation

LACTOSE—a disaccharide composed of glucose and galactose; the principal sugar found in mammalian milk

LECITHIN (PHOSPHATIDYLCHOLINE)—a phospholipid substituted with choline. Found in the membranes of biologic organisms. As part of bile, it emulsifies fats; as part of lipoproteins, it transports triglyceride and cholesterol

LIPOPROTEINS—circulating particles that contain varying amounts of triglyceride, cholesterol, phospholipids, and protein, which solubilize lipids for blood transport

MACRONUTRIENTS—are defined as those macromolecules in plant (and animal) structures that can be digested, absorbed, and utilized by another organism as energy sources and as substrate for synthesis of the carbohydrates, fats, and proteins required to maintain cell and system integrity as illustrated in Figure 3–1

MANNITOL—a sugar alcohol that exists in fruit, is poorly digested, and yields about half as many calories as glucose

MONOGLYCERIDE (MONOACYLGLYCEROL)—a lipid with only one fatty acid attached to the glycerol molecule

MONOSACCHARIDE—sugar incapable of being hydrolyzed to a simpler form

MONOUNSATURATED FATTY ACID (MUFA)—a fatty acid containing one double bond

NONESSENTIAL AMINO ACIDS—amino acids the body that are able to synthesize to meet metabolic requirements

OMEGA-3 FATTY ACIDS—fatty acids with the first double bond located at the third carbon from the methyl end

PEPTIDE—any compound of low molecular weight that yields two or more amino acids on hydrolysis; constituent part of proteins

PHOSPHOLIPID—a lipid containing fatty acids, an alcohol, and a phosphorous compound; widely distributed in cell membranes

POLYPEPTIDE—a peptide that contains from a few to as many as 300 amino acids

POLYSACCHARIDE—a carbohydrate that on hydrolysis yields more than 10 monosaccharide units

POLYUNSATURATED FATTY ACID (PUFA)—a fatty acid containing at least two double bonds

PROTEIN—a complex nitrogenous compound make up of amino acids in peptide linkages

PROTEIN DIGESTIBILITY CORRECTED AMINO ACID SCORE—official assay for evaluating protein quality

RESISTANT STARCH—the fraction of starch modified by cooking or processing that still resists enzyme action unless pretreated with alkali

SATURATED FATTY ACID (SFA)—a fatty acid that has no double bonds, with a general formula $C_nH_{2n}O_2$

SORBITOL—a sugar alcohol occurring naturally in fruits; in mammals is found in some tissues such as the lens of the eye

STRUCTURED LIPID—synthetic triglyceride with medium-chain fatty acids and long-chain fatty acids interesterified to glycerol; used in parenteral nutrition formulas

SUCROSE—ordinary table sugar; a disaccharide composed of glucose and fructose found in sugar cane, sugar beets, molasses, maple syrup, maple sugar, fruit, vegetables, and honey

TRANSAMINATION—reversible transfer of an amino group from an amino acid to a keto acid, forming a new keto acid and a new amino acid without the appearance of ammonia

TRANS-FATTY ACIDS—stereoisomers of the naturally occurring cis-fatty acids; artifacts of the hydrogenation process

TRIGLYCERIDE (TRIACYLGLYCEROL)—a lipid consisting of three fatty acid chains esterified to a glycerol molecule

UREA—the chief nitrogenous end product of protein metabolism and the chief nitrogenous constituent of urine

XYLITOL—a noncariogenic sugar alcohol absorbed one fifth as rapidly as glucose and often used in sugarless chewing gum

DEVELOPMENT OF MACRONUTRIENTS

All living organisms obtain energy from the sun. *Photosynthesis* describes the sequential process through which green plants transduce light energy into chemical bonds. Chemical energy is stored within the newly formed molecule by linking energy-poor carbon dioxide to hydrogens and other carbons. The first **macronutrient** formed in this process is a carbohydrate. Two carbohydrates linked as the **disaccharide,** sucrose, are used for transporting energy to nonphotosynthesizing tissues, roots, tubers, and seeds, for use and storage as starch **polysaccharide** granules. Although plants use carbohydrates primarily for energy and as a basis for structural tissues, they also use carbohydrate precursors to synthesize specialized fats and amino acids for growth and reproduction. Thus, plants are the primary source for all macronutrients required for animals and humans. Depending on their position in the food chain, some animals and humans also consume other animals for their macronutrient content.

The early part of this chapter discusses the structure, properties, food sources, and clinical implications of the three classes of macronutrients—carbohydrate, lipids, and proteins. Digestion and transport have been discussed in Chapter 1. The last section briefly reviews the mechanisms through which the cell accesses stored nutrients during periods of fasting to maintain energy and structural substrates necessary for life. Figure 3–1 shows substrate utilization.

CARBOHYDRATES

Plant carbohydrates vary widely in sweetness, texture, rate of *digestion,* and degree to which they are absorbed after passage through the human gastrointestinal tract. The diversity, physiologic properties, and potential health benefits of carbohydrate sources in the food supply can best be appreciated by examining the chemical properties of each major carbohydrate type. Carbohydrates can be categorized as (1) monosaccharides, (2) di- and oligosac-

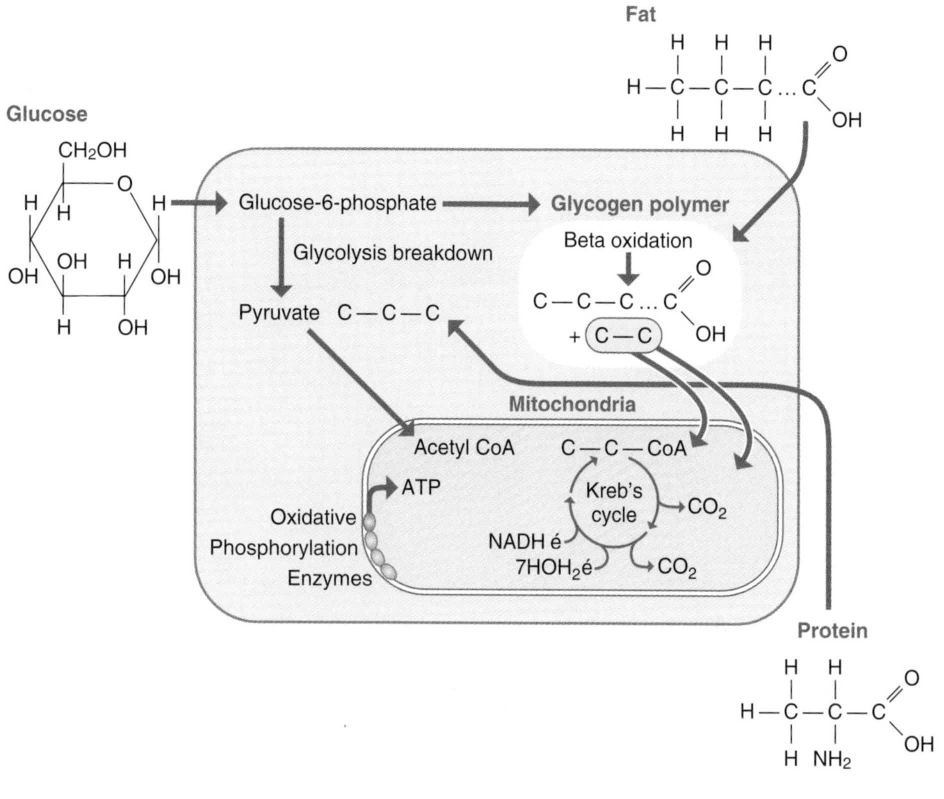

FIGURE 3–1 Typical cell use of macronutrients for energy.

charides, and (3) polysaccharides—starch and fibers (Table 3–1).

Monosaccharides

Monosaccharides are seldom found free in nature, but are linked into di- and polysaccharide forms. Only a fraction of the many monosaccharide structures formed in nature can be absorbed and utilized by humans. It is likely that the sweet taste of edible sugars, especially fructose and sucrose, was of great evolutionary advantage, because sweetness would have guided early humans to select plant foods of the greatest nutritional value. Table 3–2 indicates sweetness values of common sugars and artificial sweeteners.

The smallest carbohydrate unit has the formula, $(CH_2O)n$, where *n* can be any integer from 3 to 7. Although twelve hexose (6 carbons) and six pentose (5 carbons) isomers can be formed in nature, only three hexoses—glucose, galactose, and fructose—can be absorbed by humans (see below). The edible hexoses differ in chemical behavior, taste, sweetness, and dietary source. These differences result from slight, but significant, differences in their chemical structure. As illustrated in Figure 3–2, **glucose** and **galactose** contain an aldehyde group on carbon 1 (C-1) compared with the ketone at C-2 in **fructose.** The active aldehyde and ketone carbons perform two special functions: (1) they can react with the hydroxyl group of C-5 to form a ring structure as illustrated, and (2) once the ring is formed, the active carbons can link to other sugars by forming a glycosidic linkage with another hydroxyl group. Because the hydroxyl group on C-1 can "reduce" (donate hydrogen to) metals such as copper and iron, glucose and galactose are called "reducing sugars." Note that the active ketone at C-2 in fructose reacts with the hydroxyl at C-5 to form a five-membered, rather than a six-membered, ring formed by the aldoses, glucose and galactose.

Specific Monosaccharide Characteristics

Glucose is the most widely distributed sugar in nature, although it is seldom consumed in its monosaccharide form. In polymer form, glucose is present as starch and cellulose and is found in all edible disaccharides. Glucose, both as a monomer and linked with fructose as the disaccharide, sucrose, makes up a large fraction of the total solid content of fruits and vegetables.

Fructose (levulose, fruit sugar) is the sweetest of all monosaccharides, although its sweetness varies. When tasted in crystalline form, it is twice as sweet as sucrose. If it is dissolved in liquid, the sweetness rapidly declines, possibly because dissolved fructose is free to assume less sweet configurations (Shallenberger, 1976). Fruits contain from 1% to 7% fructose, with some fruits containing considerably greater concentrations. Fructose makes up about 3% of the dry weight in vegetables and about 40% in honey. As fruit ripens, it becomes sweeter be-

TABLE 3–1 TYPES, SOURCES, AND END PRODUCTS OF CARBOHYDRATES

CARBOHYDRATES	FOOD SOURCES	END PRODUCTS OF DIGESTION	REMARKS
Polysaccharides			
Indigestible			
1. Cellulose	Stalks and leaves of vegetables; outer covering of seeds	—	May be partially split to glucose by bacterial action in large bowel
2. Hemicelluloses			These substances have an affinity for water, form bulk, slow gastric emptying time, and may bind bile acids.
3. Pectins	Fruits	—	
4. Gums and mucilages	Plant secretions and seeds		
5. Algal substances	Seaweeds and algae	—	
Partially digestible			
1. Inulin	Jerusalem artichokes, onions, garlic, and mushrooms	Fructose	Digestion is incomplete; further splitting by bacteria may occur in the large bowel; may be production of flatus from raffinose and stachyose.
2. Galactogens	Snails	Galactose	
3. Mannosans	Legumes	Mannose	
4. Raffinose	Sugar beets, kidney beans, lentils, and navy beans	Glucose, fructose, and galactose	
5. Stachyose	Beans	Pentoses	
6. Pentosans	Fruits and gums		
Digestible			
1. Starch and dextrins	Grains; vegetables (especially tubers and legumes)	Glucose	The most important group quantitatively; usually accompanied by some maltose
2. Glycogen	Meat products and seafood	Glucose	
Disaccharides and Oligosaccharides			
1. Sucrose	Cane and beet sugars, molasses, and maple syrup	Glucose and fructose	
2. Lactose	Milk and milk products	Glucose and galactose	
3. Maltose and maltotriose	Malt products, some breakfast cereals	Glucose	
4. Lactulose	Synthetic products	Not metabolized	Does not appear in foods; is synthetic, not digested; and is used as a laxative
5. Trehalose	Mushrooms, insects, yeast	Glucose	
Monosaccharides			
Hexoses			
1. Glucose	Fruits, honey, corn syrup	Glucose	In fruits and vegetables the contents of glucose and fructose depend on species ripeness and state of preservation.
Sorbitol*	Fruits, vegetables, dietetic products		
2. Fructose	Fruits, honey	Fructose	
3. Galactose		Galactose	These monosaccharides do not occur in free form in foods.
4. Mannose		Mannose	
Mannitol*	Pineapples, olives, asparagus, sweet potatoes, carrots, and dietetic products		
Pentoses			
1. Ribose	—	Ribose	Ribose, xylose, and arabinose do not occur in free form in foods. They are derived from pentosans of fruits and from the nucleic acids of meat products and seafood.
2. Xylose	Fruits, vegetables, cereals, mushrooms, seaweed, dietetic chewing gum, and other dietetic products	Xylose	
Xylitol*			
3. Arabinose	—	Arabinose	
Carbohydrate Derivatives			
1. Ethyl alcohol	Fermented liquors		
2. Lactic acid	Milk and milk products	Absorbed as same	These substances are the products of natural or induced carbohydrate breakdown.
3. Malic acid	Fruits		

*Sugar alcohol forms of the designated sugars.

TABLE 3–2 SWEETNESS OF SUGARS AND ARTIFICIAL SWEETENERS

SUGAR OR SUGAR PRODUCT	SWEETNESS VALUE	ARTIFICAL SWEETENERS	SWEETNESS VALUE
Levulose, fructose	173	Cyclamate (banned in US)	30
Invert sugar	130	*Aspartame (Nutra-Sweet)	180
Sucrose	100	Acesulfame-K (Sunette)	200
Glucose	74	Saccharin (Sweet 'n Low)	300
Sorbitol	60	Sucralose	600
Mannitol	50	Alitame (approval pending)	2000
Galactose	32		
Maltose	32		
Lactose	16		

*Nutritive (has calories).

cause the sucrose it contains is enzymatically cleaved to glucose and fructose.

Honey is made from plant nectar (sucrose) harvested by the honeybee. The honeybee secretes an enzyme, invertase, which hydrolyzes sucrose to glucose and fructose, increasing the sweetness of the product. As indicated above, approximately 40% of the sugar in mature honey is free fructose. Because the molecular configuration of fructose determines its relative sweetness, the degree of crystallization influences the sweetness of honey. Honey is calorie dense; 1 tablespoon of honey contains 64 kcal, whereas an equal amount of sugar contains 46 kcal. It also contains vitamins and minerals, but in trace amounts inconsequential in terms of daily needs. Commercial honey has been heated to 150° to 160°F to prevent crystallization and yeast formation; "organic" or "raw" honey has not been heat treated. Although heat treatment is not sufficient to destroy spores of the ubiquitous *Clostridium botulinum,* the high sugar content of honey prevents germination of these spores and risk for deadly botulism. Normal adults are not at risk, but the immature gastrointestinal tracts of very young infants may promote spore germination. For this reason, it is recommended that honey not be used to sweeten pacifiers or fed to infants under 1 year of age.

High-fructose corn syrup is intensely sweet and inexpensive. It is manufactured by enzymatically changing the glucose in cornstarch to fructose. High-fructose corn syrup is added to canned and frozen fruits to preserve the structure of the fruit. It penetrates the fruit easily and preserves the natural form, flavor, and color. When added to soft drinks, it adds body without affecting or masking flavors.

Di- and Oligosaccharides

Monosaccharide units are joined by glycosidic linkage between the active aldehyde or ketone carbon and any hydroxyl on any other sugar. The hydroxyl group on the active carbon can rapidly change position from above (beta-β) to below (alpha-α) the ring. Once two sugars are linked, the position is frozen (Fig. 3–3) as in the edible disaccharide sugars, sucrose, lactose, and maltose. It should be noted that each hexose has six hydroxyl groups each in one of two possible orientations, above or below the ring. Random linkage between hydroxyl groups of different sugars creates a bewildering variety of di- and oligosaccharide configurations in nature. One glucose molecule, for example, can form glycosidic links between the six carbons on a second glucose, both in α and β positions to form 11 different configurations. The most common configurations are maltose in α linkage as starch and cellobiose in β linkage as cellulose. Only maltose can be cleaved and absorbed as glucose. The other linkages are found in the vast diversity of **dietary fibers.** The number of possible configurations formed by linking different isomers or more than two sugars is enormous.

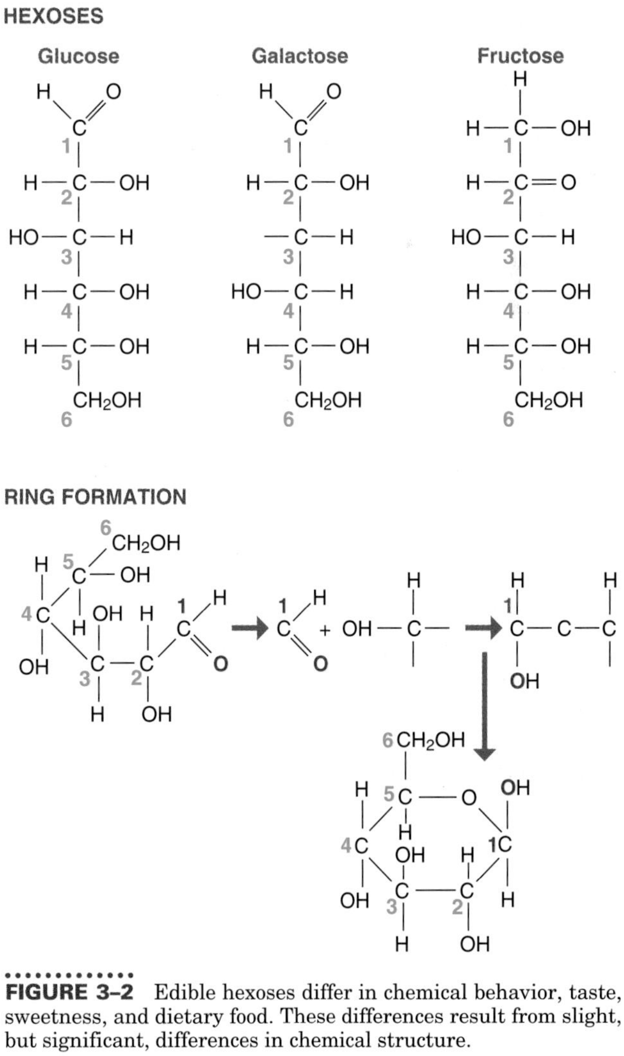

FIGURE 3–2 Edible hexoses differ in chemical behavior, taste, sweetness, and dietary food. These differences result from slight, but significant, differences in chemical structure.

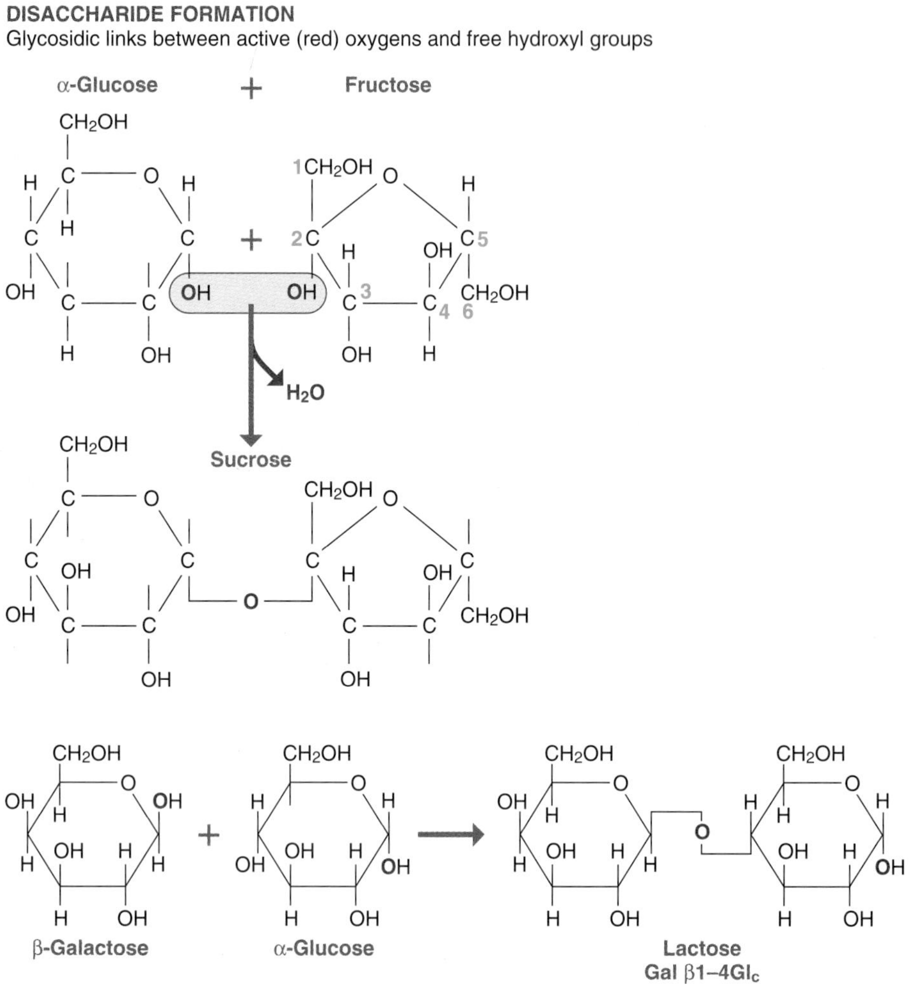

DISACCHARIDE FORMATION
Glycosidic links between active (red) oxygens and free hydroxyl groups

α-Glucose + Fructose

Sucrose

β-Galactose + α-Glucose → Lactose Gal β1–4Glc

FIGURE 3–3 Disaccharide formation. Glycosidic links between active (red) oxygens and free hydroxyl groups.

Human absorptive capacity for carbohydrate is limited. Despite the enormous variety of possible di- and oligosaccharide configurations in the food supply, humans utilize only a few. Amylase, secreted by the salivary glands and the pancreas, cleaves only the α bond between two glucose molecules. Enzymes in the brush border of the intestinal mucosal cell hydrolyze only the following four glycosidic bonds.

sucrase = α bond between glucose C-1 and fructose C-2 [Glcα1-2Fru]
maltase = α bond between glucose C-1 and glucose C-4 [Glcα1-4Glc]
isomaltase = α bond between glucose C-1 and glucose C-6 [Glcα1-6Glc]
lactase = β bond between galactose C-1 and glucose C-4 [Galβ1-4Glc]

Carbohydrates containing any other linkages cannot be digested and must be classified as dietary fiber as discussed below.

Oligosaccharides are low molecular weight polymers containing 2 to 20 sugar molecules. Because they are small, they are readily water soluble and often quite sweet (Roberfroid et al., 1993). Nondigestible oligosaccharides are resistant to stomach acid and the action of amylase and intestinal hydrolytic enzymes. They enter the large intestine intact and can be fermented by indigenous bacteria. *Raffinose,* found in sugar beets, is a trisaccharide made from galactose-glucose-fructose. *Strachyose,* a tetrasaccharide composed of two galactoses, one glucose, and one fructose, is found in vegetables such as legumes and squash. Because they are fermented by gut bacteria, oligosaccharide ingestion is often accompanied by complaints of gas and bloating.

Fructooligosaccharides (FOS) are naturally occurring polymers of fructose, usually attached to an initial glucose molecule. FOS can also be made commercially by an enzymatic action on sucrose. FOS are totally resistant to digestion in the upper gastrointestinal tract and utilized almost entirely by bifidobacteria in the colon (Hidaka et al., 1986). FOS are 0.4 to 0.6 times as sweet as sucrose, but because they are not absorbed proximally, they have been estimated to supply only 1 kcal/g (Roberfroid et al., 1993). When ingested chronically, they have been reported to enhance intestinal flora growth, relieve constipation, improve blood lipids, especially triglycerides, and suppress the production of putrefactive substances. Trautwein et al. (1998), using a Syrian hamster model, reported that inulin (FOS) exerts a hypocholesterolemic effect. Evidence on the effect of FOS on human blood lipids is conflicting. Some studies (Jenkins et al., 1991) reported raised low-density lipoprotein (LDL) concentrations, possibly due to production of acetate, a precursor to cholesterol and lipids, by gut fermentation. Lipid-lowering action of FOS appears to involve changes in hepatic triglyceride synthesis, very low-density lipoprotein (VLDL) secretion, or reabsorption of bile acids. Chronic consumption of dietary FOS also alters glucose metabolism. Luo et al. (1996) reported decreased basal hepatic glucose production on 20 g FOS/day compared with sucrose in healthy human subjects.

Specific Di- and Oligosaccharide Characteristics

Sucrose *(table sugar, cane sugar, beet sugar, grape sugar)* is formed by glucose and fructose linked together by their active carbons (Glcα1-2Fru). Dietary sucrose can be hydrolyzed to glucose and fructose monomers in dilute acid or in the presence of the enzyme invertase. When sucrose is used in preparation of acidic foods, for example, to sweeten fruit drinks, it becomes inverted within a few hours. Note that honey is also invert sugar.

Invert sugar is used commercially because it is sweeter than equal concentrations of sucrose. Glucose and fructose also make smaller crystals than sucrose; thus invert sugar is preferred to sucrose in preparation of delicate candies and icings.

Lactose *(milk sugar)* is made almost exclusively in the mammary glands of most lactating animals, however, not in whale or hippopotamus. It accounts for 7.5% and 4.5% of the composition of human and cow's milk, respectively. It is less soluble than the other disaccharides and is only about one sixth as sweet as glucose. The β linkage (Galcβ1-4Glc) in lactose is hydrolyzed by lactase in the intestinal cell. It should be noted that lactase is expressed late in the development of the intestinal cell toward the end of its migration to the tip of the intestinal villi, hence, the reason it is often the first enzyme lost in intestinal diseases.

Most mammals do not consume milk after weaning. It has been estimated that the vast majority of the world's human populations, as is true for nonhuman mammals, have limited ability to express the lactase enzyme after weaning. On the other hand, a small minority of human populations, largely from Northern European extraction, continue to express large amounts of the enzyme throughout life. Genetic modification is thought to have allowed these populations to express lactase throughout life and thus to absorb the lactose in milk from their herd animals during the severe winters of North Europe. Such a mutation would have allowed individuals to survive while others perished. Early humans who survived would have transmitted the altered gene to their offspring. As a result, their decendents are able to consume large amounts of lactose-containing milk without difficulty. Lactose intolerance in these adults thus appears to be the norm, rather than the exception. It should be noted that lactose intolerance, while uncomfortable, does not appear to damage the gastrointestinal tract or to be associated with long-term disease pathology (see Chapter 31).

Galactose is rarely free in nature. Most dietary galactose is produced from lactose (milk sugar) by hydrolysis during the digestive process.

Maltose (malt sugar) is formed by hydrolysis of starch polymers. Maltose is seldom found naturally in the food supply as the disaccharide but is consumed in a number of food products. The germinating seed produces *diastase,* an enzyme that hydrolyzes starch to maltose for use by the new plant, thus sprouted grains contain maltose. Diastase is also used commercially to hydrolyze starch to maltose (malt) used in beer making. Because maltose, the disaccharide, is sweeter than starch polymer, barely malt is also used as a sweetener. It is often found in commercial products marketed as "sucrose free," even though maltose and sucrose have the same caloric value.

Dextrose is glucose that is produced after hydrolysis of cornstarch. This form is commonly used in food production.

Dextran and *levan* are structural bacterial products derived from a variety of sugars, including sucrose and maltose. Some bacteria produce dextran, a linear polymer containing isomaltose (glucose with α 1–6 branch) as a repeating unit. Levan is a repeating polymer of fructose units in 2,6-fructoside linkage formed from sucrose. Dental plaque consists of levan-producing bacteria embedded in the sticky, adherent matrix they produce. Individuals whose mouth flora includes levan-producing bacteria are prone to dental plaque, especially when they consume high amounts of sucrose. This explains the utility of using a bactericidal mouth rinse to control dental plaque.

Inulin, an FOS found in artichokes, chicory, onions, and asparagus, is a polymer of fructose in β (2–1) linkage. It is readily fermented in the cecum and colon and has recently been shown to have a lipid-lowering effect, specifically decreasing plasma triglyceride concentrations (see FOS section, above). Other rich sources of FOS include tomatoes, bananas, barley, rye, garlic, onion, and Jerusalem artichoke. Extensive testing revealed that naturally occurring and commercially produced FOS (marketed under the brand name, Nutraflora ™) are safe, with no significant adverse effects at doses up to 2,170 mg/kg/day (Spiegel et al., 1994). The authors propose that the addition of FOS to yogurt containing *Bifidobacterium infantis* cultures is safe, improves product taste, and enhances gut flora growth.

Polysaccharides—Starch

Plants store carbohydrates as starch granules formed by linking α glucans (α glucans are glucose polymers in α-1,4 straight chains with α-1,6 branches) into a complex granular structure. The more carbohydrate the plant makes during photosynthesis, the greater the rate of starch formation. Starch is stored in plastids (storage vesicles) called *leukoplasts* (Gr. *leukos* = white) adapted for starch storage (amyloplasts). Some *amyloplasts* can grow quite large; for example, the amyloplasts in the potato can be as large as an average animal cell. Edible plants make two types of starch, amylopectin and amylose. **Amylose** is a smaller, linear molecule (10^5 to 10^6 daltons) with fewer than 1% branches. *Amylopectin* is highly branched, containing up to 5% α-1,6 branches, with a very high molecular weight (10^7 to 10^8 daltons). Because of its larger size, amylopectin is more abundant in the food supply and makes up a greater fraction of the starch in grains and starchy tubers.

Specific Starch Characteristics

Starch granules are encased by rigid cellulose walls in plants and are inaccessible to digestive enzymes. This accounts for the poor digestibility of raw potato and grains. Cooking causes the granules to swell, gelatinizes the starch, softens and ruptures the cell wall, and makes the starch more digestible. *Resistant starch* resists enzyme breakdown from cooking or processing and is poorly digested. Starches from different plant sources, such as corn, arrowroot, rice, potato, tapioca, and other plants, are all glucose polymers with the same chemical composition. Their unique characteristics are determined by the relative numbers of glucose units in straight and branched configuration.

Waxy starch is obtained from corn and rice strains bred to contain a greater percentage of branched amylopectin chains. When dissolved in water, waxy starch forms a smooth paste that does not gel unless in very high concentrations. The product remains thick during freezing and thawing, making it an ideal thickener for commercially frozen fruit pies, sauces, and gravies.

Modified food starch is chemically or physically modified to change its hot paste viscosity, ability to gel, and other texture properties. Pregelatinized starch, dried on hot rolls or drums and made into powder, is porous and rapidly rehydrated with cold liquid. The starch rapidly thickens, making it useful for instant puddings, salad dressings, pie fillings, gravies, and baby food. Because it is purified, smaller amounts of modified starch are required for thickening, in contrast to flour and other nonmodified starches that also contain protein, fibers, and other structural constituents.

Dextrins are large linear glucose polysaccharides of intermediate lengths cleaved from starch by α amylase. Amylase cleaves amylose and amylopectin at different rates depending on the starch structure and its integration into the individual foods. Amylose is a linear, tightly coiled macromolecule with limited sites for amylase action. In contrast, amylopectin is highly branched, more "open," and has many points at which amylase can act, yielding readily available maltose. Amylopectin branch points not cleaved by amylase are called *limit dextrins.* Limit dextrins can subsequently be digested to glucose by the mucosal enzyme, isomaltase. As a result, starch digestion and subsequent glucose availability vary with the amylose and amylopectin content of specific foods. Glucose in amylopectin-rich foods is more easily hydrolyzed, and consumption of these foods results in a higher postprandial blood glucose rise. The glycemic index, discussed below and in Chapters 12 and 25 and Appendix 54, describes the extent to which individual foods raise blood glucose.

Animal Carbohydrate—Glycogen

Plants use carbohydrates, especially cellulose, to make up their structural components. In contrast, animal structure is made predominately from the protein collagen. Carbohydrates are used primarily for energy and for minor, but essential, signaling and identification functions. Carbohydrate consumed in excess of immediate energy requirements is stored in all cells as the polymer, **glycogen.** Glycogen is a branched glucose polymer similar to amylopectin, but the branches in glycogen are shorter and more frequent (Fig. 3–4). Because it is a carbohydrate, glycogen contains water molecules [$(CH_2O)n$]. The additional water makes glycogen a large and cumbersome molecule, unsuitable for long-term energy storage. The 70-kg "reference man" stores only an 18-hour fuel supply as glycogen, compared to a 2-month supply as fat. If all human energy stores were glycogen, it has been estimated that humans would need to carry 60 additional pounds (Alberts et al., 1995). About 150 g of glycogen is stored in muscle; this amount can be increased fivefold with physical training (see Chapter 25). The glycogen store in human liver is about 90 g and is involved in the hormonal control of

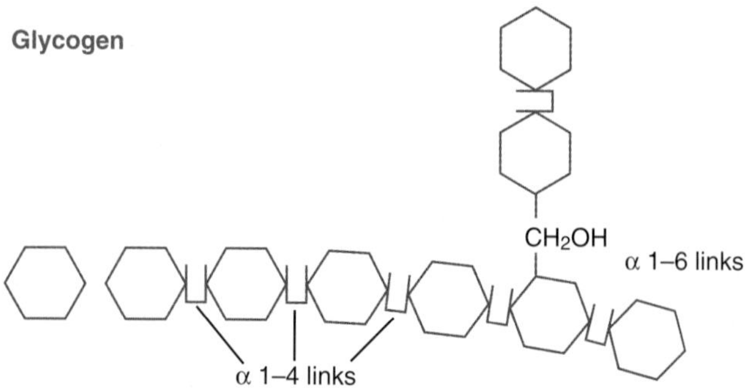

FIGURE 3–4 Glycogen is a branched glucose polymer similar to amylopectin, but the branches in glycogen are shorter and more frequent.

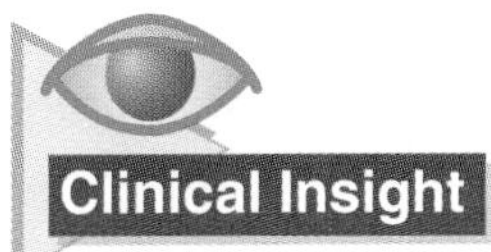

Hormonal Controls of Blood Sugar Levels

A number of mechanisms function to maintain blood glucose at a remarkably constant level (70 to 100 mg/100 mL) under fasting conditions. A battery of hormones is involved in regulating blood sugar levels. *Insulin* is produced by the beta cells of the islets of Langerhans in the pancreas. It has been called the "feasting hormone" because its liberation is enhanced by a high glucose level in the blood and to a lesser extent by the ingestion of protein or infusion of amino acids or **ketone bodies.** Insulin release is also stimulated by the action of glucagon and the gastrointestinal hormones, as well as by the vagus nerve and certain drugs (e.g., glucotrol, an oral hypoglycemic agent). The mechanism by which insulin lowers blood glucose involves an increase in the rate of glucose utilization for oxidation, glycogenesis, and lipogenesis. Facilitated diffusion of glucose into muscle and adipose cells is increased, glucose is stored as glycogen in the liver and muscle cells, and the uptake of glucose by adipose and liver cells for conversion into fat is enhanced.

Glucagon, produced by the alpha cells of the islets of Langerhans, has an effect exactly opposite to that of insulin. It causes a rise in the amount of sugar in the blood by increasing glycogenolysis and gluconeogenesis and stimulates the release of insulin from the pancreas. Insulin and glucagon may thus be considered antagonists, and their opposing effects at least in part maintain carbohydrate metabolism in a steady state.

Epinephrine, a hormone produced by the adrenal medulla, favors the breakdown of liver and muscle glycogen to yield blood glucose *(glycogenolysis)* and decreases the release of insulin from the pancreas, thus raising the blood sugar. Secretion of epinephrine is increased during anger or fear, and the subsequent glucose formation provides extra energy for crisis response.

Glucocorticoids, steroid hormones elaborated by the adrenal cortex, also influence blood glucose levels by stimulating gluconeogenesis. These hormones reduce glucose utilization and also increase the rate at which protein is converted into glucose, thus counteracting the action of insulin.

Severe lowering of blood glucose concentration increases *thyroxine* secretion. Hepatic glycogenolysis and gluconeogenesis are increased, leading to a rise in blood glucose concentration. Thyroxine also increases the rate of hexose absorption from the intestine.

Growth hormone, elaborated by the anterior pituitary gland, also raises the blood glucose level by increasing amino acid uptake and protein synthesis by all cells, diminishing cellular uptake of glucose, and increasing the mobilization of fat for energy.

---

blood sugar (see the accompanying box "*Clinical Insight:* Hormonal Controls of Blood Sugar Levels").

Despite its presence in animal tissue, meat and other animal products do not contain appreciable glycogen. In response to epinephrine and other stress hormones released at slaughter, glycogen stores are largely depleted. Glucose released is converted to lactic acid after death.

Nondigestible Carbohydrate Homopolymers: Cellulose

The structure of plants, from the giant redwood tree to the most delicate flower, is composed almost entirely of carbohydrate. Plant structural carbohydrate is formed largely from **cellulose,** a simple polymer of glucose in β (1–4) glycosidic linkage. Cellulose is the most abundant organic compound in the world, constituting 50% or more of all the carbon in vegetation. The enormously long molecule folds back on itself like a ribbon (Fig. 3–5) and is held in place by hydrogen bonds formed between the hydroxyls on adjacent loops. The ribbon structure gives cellulose fibrils great mechanical strength but limited extensibility; it is the strength of cellulose fibrils that allows trees to grow to great heights. The maximal size of cellulose fibrils has been estimated by hydrolyzing samples of cellulose to cellobiose, two glucose molecules joined in β-glycosidic linkage. Samples were found to contain from 150 to 1,250 cellobiose units per molecule, with molecular weights ranging from 50,000 to 400,000 daltons. It is likely that the original cellulose molecules were several fold larger, because these samples were taken from much larger, water-insoluble cellulose preparations (Smith et al., 1978).

Nondigestible Carbohydrate Heteropolymers: Hemicellulose and Gums

Plants contain multiple types of fibers. Plant cell wall construction consists of cellulose microfibrils embedded in a matrix of heteropolysaccharide. This construction is analogous to animal connective tissue structure with collagen, embedded in a proteo-

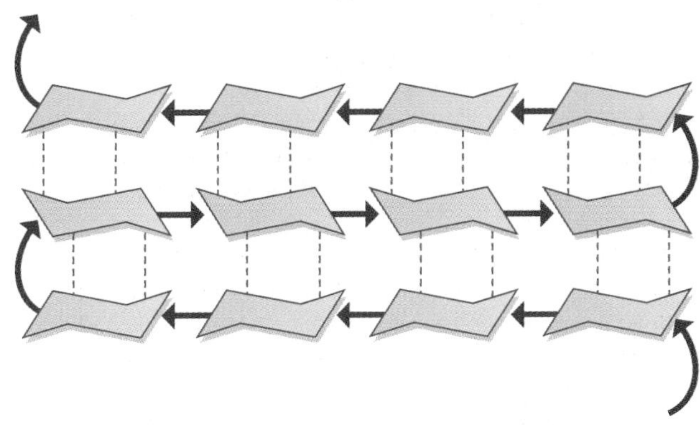

FIGURE 3–5 Schematic of the ribbon-like structure of cellulose. Note the cross-links between adjacent molecules.

TABLE 3–3 SOURCES OF FIBER COMPONENTS

INSOLUBLE		
CELLULOSE	**HEMICELLULOSE**	**LIGNIN**
Whole-wheat flour Bran Vegetables	Bran Whole grains	Mature vegetables Wheat Fruits and edible seeds, such as strawberries
SOLUBLE		
GUMS	**PECTIN**	
Oats Legumes Guar Barley	Apples Citrus fruits Strawberries Carrots	

glycan matrix. In plants, carbohydrate heteropolymers are made from two or more different types of sugar units. The basic cellulose polymer is substituted with other carbohydrates and with noncarbohydrate residues depending on the purpose for which the fiber will be used. For example, *β glucans* consist of β (1–4) cellulose bonds interspersed with β (1–3) bonds. This makes the molecule less linear and more soluble. Oats and barley are rich in β glucans and thus are classified as *soluble fibers* (see Table 3–3). **Hemicellulose** fibers contain cellulose molecules substituted with other sugars (see Table 3–4). Hemicelluloses are named for the predominant sugar in the backbone, xylan, galactan, or mannan, or in the side chain, arabinose or galactose. The hemicellulose class, glucomannans, includes arabinoxylans and xyloglucans (Schneeman and Tietyen, 1994). *Pectins* and *gums* are more water soluble than hemicelluloses. They are composed of a galacturonic acid backbone with rhamnose units inserted at intervals and with side chains of arabinose and galactose.

Specific Fiber Characteristics

Pectin is found in apples, citrus fruits, strawberries, and other fruits. The galacturonic acid structure absorbs water and forms a gel, making it widely used for making jams and jellies. Pectin gel cooked with sugar and fruit juice or pulp is stable for months at room temperature. Such jams and jellies are often sealed with wax to prevent bacterial or fungal growth. Pectin is added to fat-free yogurt and other products to provide texture and stability.

Gums and *mucilages* are similar in structure to pectin except that the galactose units are combined with other sugars (glucose) and polysaccharides. They are found in plant secretions or seeds, for example, guar gum. The specific textural qualities of these fibers are commercially useful when added to processed foods such as ice cream.

Lignin is a woody fiber found in the stems and seeds of fruits and vegetables and in the bran layer of cereals. It is actually not a carbohydrate but is a polymer composed of phenylopropyl alcohols and acids. Lignin may have properties that are useful in cancer prevention.

Algal polysaccharides are extracted from seaweed and algae and are used as thickening and stabiliz-

TABLE 3–4 DIETARY FIBER CONTENT OF FOODS IN COMMONLY SERVED PORTIONS*

FOOD GROUP	<1 g	1–1.9 g	2–2.9 g	3–3.9 g	4–4.9 g	5–5.9 g	>6 g
Breads (1 slice)	Bagel White French	Whole wheat	Bran muffin (1)	NA[†]	NA	NA	NA
Cereals (1 oz)	Rice Krispies Special K Cornflakes	Oatmeal Nutri-Grain Cheerios	Wheaties Shredded Wheat	Most Honey Bran	Bran Chex 40% Bran Flakes Raisin Bran	Corn Bran	All-Bran Bran Buds 100% Bran
Pasta (1 cup)	NA	Macaroni Spaghetti	NA	Whole-wheat spaghetti	NA	NA	NA
Rice (½ cup)	White	Brown	NA	NA	NA	NA	NA
Legumes (½ cup) cooked	NA	NA	NA	Lentils	Lima beans Dried peas	NA	Kidney beans Baked beans Navy beans
Vegetables (½ cup unless stated)	Cucumber Lettuce (1 cup) Green pepper	Asparagus Green beans Cabbage Cauliflower Potato w/out skin (1) Celery	Broccoli Brussels sprouts Carrots Corn Potato w/skin (1) Spinach	Peas	NA	NA	NA
Fruits (1 medium fruit unless stated)	Grapes (20) Watermelon (1 cup)	Apricots (3) Grapefruit (½) Peach w/skin Pineapple (½ cup)	Apple, w/out skin Banana Orange	Apple, w/skin Pear, w/skin Raspberries (½ cup)	NA	NA	NA

*From Slavin JL. Dietary fiber: Classification, chemical analyses, and food sources. J Am Diet Assoc 87:1164, 1987.
[†]Not applicable.

ing agents in many processed foods. One of this class, *carrageenan,* is a sulfated polygalactant algal polysaccharide extracted from macroalgae or seaweed (Evans, 1989). In nature, the mucilaginous polysaccharide confers structural integrity to the sea plants. As cell wall constituents, alginate, carrageenan, and agar prevent desiccation, provide for selective adsorption of ions, and facilitate bioadhesion of the plant to rocks and other anchors. Algal polysaccharides are used commercially because they form weak gels with proteins and stabilize a food mixture, preventing suspended ingredients from settling. Carrageenan is an ingredient in pudding and is used commercially to add body to infant formulas, ice cream, milk pudding, and sour cream products.

Carrageenan was initially assumed to be poorly absorbed and harmless at levels as high as 15% of the diet of rodents and other experimental animals. Early on, species differences were observed. Animal models such as guinea pigs and rabbits appeared highly sensitive to carrageenan and developed intestinal ulcers at levels less than 1% of the diet (Jacobson, 1972). Recently investigators have observed microscopic mucosal changes throughout the colon associated with carrageenan absorption into the mucosal cell. Because carrageenan is a highly active polyanionic electrolyte that can cause breakdown of mucosal integrity (Marcus et al., 1992), these changes have been linked to colonic ulceration in these animals. Carrageenan at high doses has been reported to induce mucosal thymidine kinase activity in rats (Calvert and Satchithanadam, 1992), resulting in proliferation of the colonic mucosa. In humans, it is both a T-cell mitogen and toxic to macrophages (Sugawara et al., 1982). Carrageenan damages human cells in culture and has caused filament disassembly and cell death in human mammary myoepithelial cells at concentrations as low as 0.00014% (Tobacman, 1997). In view of its wide use in commercial food preparation and uncertainty as to the extent of human sensitivity to carrageenan, further investigation is urgently needed.

Chitin, a homopolymer of *N*-acetyl-β-D-glucosamine, is a polysaccharide produced by lower animal forms for structural support. This polymer is folded like cellulose except that the hydroxyl on carbon 2 of each residue is replaced by acetylated amino groups. Chitosan is a polymer of glucosamine obtained by the deacetylation of chitin (Shiau and Yu, 1998). Chitin is widely distributed among organisms. Although found in algae, fungi, and yeasts, its best known use is in the exoskeleton of arthropod, mollusks, and marine invertebrates including lobster and shrimp. In many of these organisms, chitin forms a matrix on which minerals are deposited, much as collagen forms a matrix for vertebrate bone mineralization.

Chitin and chitosan have been studied for their hypocholesterolemic effect. The strong positive charge on chitosan binds negatively charged lipids, blocking their absorption. Hypercholesterolemic mice given chitosan for 20 weeks had significantly lower blood cholesterol levels (64% of controls) and highly significant inhibition of atherogenesis in the aorta (Ormrod et al., 1998). On the other hand, chitosan feeding resulted in severe malabsorption of fat-soluble vitamins and bone minerals in rats (Deuchi et al., 1995). Again, more research is needed to assess the safety of this substance for long-term human consumption.

The Impact of Carbohydrate and Fiber on Human Physiology

A growing body of evidence suggests that dietary carbohydrate, especially nonabsorbable oligosaccharides, and fiber exert significant impact on human physiology. It is now recognized that specific carbohydrates not only modulate whole body energy dynamics but also affect disease processes.

Impact on Nutrient Absorption and Utilization

Glucose regulation and the glycemic index. Digestion of dietary carbohydrate in the upper gastrointestinal tract provides glucose, fructose, and galactose for intestinal absorption. The presence of nonabsorbable oligosaccharides and viscous dietary fibers such as pectins, β glucans, and gums in fruits, vegetables, and cereals reduces the efficiency of enzyme hydrolysis and slows the rate at which glucose enters the bloodstream. Starch encased in its seed coat or coarsely ground is not efficiently hydrolyzed to glucose because digestive enzymes are prevented from reaching the starch. Starch granules subjected to moist heat and subsequent cooling become dense and less available to enzyme action. Thus, the physical form, as well as food processing and cooking methods, influence the energy availability of dietary carbohydrate.

The *glycemic index* is a ranking of foods based on the postprandial blood glucose response compared with a reference food (Jenkins, 1981). This index integrates multiple influences on glucose availability and is proposed as a means for prescribing diabetic and energy-controlled diets. Hundreds of studies have confirmed that the glycemic index concept is reproducible, predictable within the concept of mixed meals, and clinically useful in the dietary management of diabetes and hyperlipidemia (Brand Miller, 1994). Published data on the glycemic indices of individual foods has been consolidated for the convenience of users (Foster-Powell and Brand Miller, 1995). See Appendix 56.

Consumption of a diet low on the glycemic index influences multiple parameters of glucose and lipid metabolism. A low- compared with a high-glycemic index diet in healthy young volunteers reduced serum fructosamine, an indicator of protein glycosylation, reduced 24-hour urinary C peptide, an indicator of insulin secretion, and lowered the 12-hour glucose profile (Jenkins et al., 1987). Reaven (1995) postulated that a cluster of defects including non–insulin-dependent-diabetes mellitus (NIDDM), obesity, hyperlipidemia, high blood pressure, and risk for coronary heart disease, called *syndrome X,* occur together in a large subset of the population (see Chapter 12). A growing body of literature supports the concept that the insulin response to dietary glucose availability determines the clinical course of several important human diseases (Cohen et al., 1990; Kiens and Ricter, 1996). A subset of the population is especially susceptible to diet-induced abnormalities of glucose metabolism. This may reflect subtle changes in the genes that regulate glucose uptake or utilization and determine the extent to which an individual is able to tolerate dietary carbohydrate (Salas et al., 1998). Thus, the bioavailability and absorption rate of specific dietary carbohydrates can play a pivotal role in blood glucose utilization and disposal, especially in individuals with genetic patterns that increase their risk for carbohydrate intolerance.

Lipid absorption and regulation of blood lipids. Insoluble fibers such as wheat bran, lignin, and chitin bind bile acids and reduce fat and cholesterol absorption. Insoluble fibers do not always alter serum cholesterol levels, partly because hepatic cholesterol synthesis can compensate for cholesterol malabsorption. *Soluble fibers,* such as viscous pectin, guar gum, oat bran, psyllium husk, beans and legumes, and fruits and vegetables, appear to specifically lower the LDL cholesterol. The hypocholesterolemic effects vary with the type and amount of fiber.

Mechanisms proposed for the lipid-lowering effects of soluble fibers include: (1) fibers bind fecal bile acids and increase excretion of bile acid-derived cholesterol; (2) fibers prevent dietary fat and cholesterol absorption by binding bile acids or fat and lipids; (3) fermentable oligosaccharides and dietary fiber are converted to short-chain fatty acids by intestinal bacteria; and (4) fibers, especially the "soluble" fibers from oats and soy, lower blood lipids by mechanisms that are presently unclear.

Vitamin and mineral absorption. Nonnutrient components of plants, including tannins, saponins, lectins, and phytates, interact with dietary macronutrients, vitamins, and minerals and can reduce macro- and micronutrient absorption. Phytate, a six-carbon ring with phosphate bound to each carbon (myo-inositol 1,2,3,4,5,6 hexakis dihydrogen phosphate) is found in the seed coat of grains and legumes and has the ability to bind metal ions, especially calcium, copper, iron, and zinc (Couzy et al., 1998). Because calcium catalyzes the action of amylase, excess phytate also reduces starch hydrolysis. Phytate is hydrolyzed by the enzyme, phytase, produced by growing yeast; thus, the phytate content is lowered in leavened bread (Jenkins et al., 1994).

Other constituents of fiber also bind nutrients and prevent their absorption (e.g., dephytinized insoluble fiber from oat, wheat, or rice bran bound metals) (Bergman et al., 1997). In contrast, some fiber constituents increase nutrient absorption. Soluble fiber from inulin and sugar beet enhance calcium absorption without an adverse effect on other metals (Coudray et al., 1997). Thus, dietary carbohydrate can inhibit or enhance nutrient absorption, depending on its form and processing.

Impact on Stool Bulk, Colonic Motility, and Cancer

Stool bulk and colonic motility. Cellulose and other insoluble fibers increase stool bulk directly by adsorbing water molecules into their structure. The capacity to increase the volume of the intestinal contents accounts for the utility of bran and other cellulose-containing fibers as treatment for constipation and irritable bowel syndrome (see Chapter 31). Soluble fibers are largely metabolized during gut transit, and only a small fraction of the ingested fiber is excreted. Because they provide nutrients to the colonic bacteria, pectins, gums, and some hemicelluloses in fruits and vegetables increase stool bulk by increasing microbial growth (Schneeman and Tietyen, 1994). Over 50% of the stool bulk is bacteria, thus the influence of soluble fiber on microbial growth can be impressive. For example, cabbage increases stool weight by 70%, but very little cabbage fiber remains after colonic transit.

Prevention of cancer. Dietary fiber appears to exert an overall preventive effect on cancer risk. Insoluble fibers such as cellulose bind fat-soluble carcinogens and remove them from the intestinal tract. On the other hand, some soluble fibers may actually increase cancer risk. Soluble-fiber polysaccharides such as gum arabic and carrageenan, widely used as stabilizers and emulsifiers in the food industry, have been postulated to increase cancer risk. At least three mechanisms have been proposed: (1) soluble fibers reduce the ability of insoluble fibers to adsorb and excrete carcinogens; (2) if carcinogen-bound soluble fibers are digested by colonic bacteria, the carcinogen can be deposited on the mucosal cells; and (3) soluble-fiber polysaccharides may cross the intestinal epithelium and carry with them carcinogens in solution (Harris et al., 1993).

Impact on Short-Chain Fatty Acids Production

In a healthy person, 70% to 80% of dietary fiber is metabolized in the colon to carbon dioxide, hydrogen, methane, and *short-chain fatty acids (SCFA).* Acetate, butyrate, and proprionate account for about 85% of all SCFA produced in the human colon. SCFA are readily absorbed by the intestinal and colonic mucosa and have the following effects: (1) enhance sodium and water absorption; (2) increase colonocyte proliferation; (3) increase metabolic energy production; (4) enhance colonic blood flow; (5) stimulate the autonomic nervous system; and (6) increase gastrointestinal hormone production (Compher et al., 1997).

Over 70% of the fuel for colonocytes is the SCFA, *butyrate* (4C). The preference of colonocytes for butyrate was found even in the neonatal rat in the immediate postbirth period before butyrate is available from bacterial fermentation (Krishnan et al., 1998). Butyrate is under intensive study for its ability to inhibit colon carcinoma cell growth. Two mechanisms have been suggested, one involving hyperacetylation of histones and the other related to impaired responsiveness to epidermal growth factors (Meng et al., 1998). *Proprionate* (3C) is absorbed and cleared by the liver and may be important in hepatic lipid or glucose metabolism. *Acetate* (2C) is rapidly metabolized to carbon dioxide by peripheral tissues and can serve as substrate for lipid and cholesterol synthesis.

Protective Influences

Phytochemicals are nonnutrient constituents in plants that affect hormonal and enzymatic processes and reduce risk for cancer and chronic disease by mechanisms not yet understood (Messina, 1995; Persky and Van Horn, 1995). Many phytochemicals have isoflavone or isoprenoid structures (described below) that quench free radicals and confer antioxidant protection on the gastrointestinal tract (Molteni et al., 1995) (see Chapter 12).

In summary, carbohydrates have the general formula, $(CH_2O)n$ and provide the same energy (4 kcals) per gram. They are formed by plants in a bewildering array of possible single unit and polymer structures. Humans have the ability to digest only a few of the many possible bonds linking carbohydrate units with each other and with other types of organic molecules. Over 80% of edible carbohydrates are absorbed as single glucose units. Table 3–5 shows carbohydrates as a percentage of weight in foods. Depending on their structure, nondigestible carbohydrates pass to a greater or lesser degree through the intestine and are excreted (see Chapter 1). During this passage, some fibers hold water, are metabolized by gut bacteria, or act as antioxidants to protect the colonic mucosa.

FATS AND LIPIDS

Lipid Structures and Functions

Fats and lipids constitute approximately 34% of the energy in the human diet. Because fat is energy rich and provides 9 kcal of energy per gram, humans are able to obtain adequate energy within a reasonable daily consumption. Fat deficient diets cannot provide adequate calories and contribute to malnutrition in many parts of the world. Dietary fat is stored in adipose (fat) cells located in depots on the human frame. The ability to store and access large amounts of fat enables the human to go without food for weeks and sometimes months. This ability is thought to have contributed to survival of early humans in times of famine.

Some fat deposits are not accessed during a fast and are classified as *structural fat.* These fat pads hold the body organs and nerves in position and protect them against traumatic injury and shock. Fat pads on the palms and buttocks protect the bones from mechanical pressure. Humans also have a subcutaneous layer of fat that insulates the body, preserving body heat and maintaining body temperature. Dietary fat is also essential for the digestion, absorption, and transport of the fat-soluble vitamins. As described in Chapter 1, dietary fat depresses gastric secretions, slows gastric emptying, and stimulates biliary and pancreatic flow, thereby facilitating the digestive process.

Possibly because fat is essential for survival, humans and other animals appear to have a "hard

TABLE 3–5 CARBOHYDRATE CONTENT OF FOODS (% OF WEIGHT)

SUGAR	CARBOHYDRATE (%)	STARCH	CARBOHYDRATE (%)
Concentrated Sweets		**Grain Products**	
Sugar: Cane, beet, powdered,	99.5	Starches: Corn, tapioca, arrowroot	86–88
brown, maple	90–96	Cereals (dry): Corn, wheat, oat, bran	68–85
Candies	70–95	Flour: Corn, wheat (sifted)	70–80
Honey (extracted)	82	Popcorn (popped)	77
Syrup: Table blends, molasses	55–75	Cookies: Plain, assorted	71
Jams, jellies, marmalades	70	Crackers, saltines	72
Carbonated, sweetened beverages	10–12	Cakes: Plain, without icing	56
		Bread: White, rye, whole wheat	48–52
Fruits		Macaroni, spaghetti, noodles, rice (cooked)	23–30
Prunes, apricots, figs (cooked, unsweet)	12–31	Cereals (cooked): Oat, wheat, grits	10–16
Bananas, grapes, cherries, apples, pears	15–23		
Fresh: Pineapples, grapefruits, oranges,		**Vegetables**	
apricots, strawberries	8–14	Boiled: Corn, white and sweet potatoes, lima and	
Milk		dried beans, peas	15–26
Skim	6	Beets, carrots, onions, tomatoes	5–7
Whole	5	Leafy: Lettuce, asparagus, cabbage, greens, spinach	3–4

TABLE 3–6 FAT CONTENT OF SOME COMMON FOODS*

0 Grams of Fat	**7–10 Grams of Fat**
Most fruits and vegetables	Cheese, cheddar, 1 oz
Nonfat milk	Milk, whole, 1 cup
Nonfat yogurt	Bologna, beef, 1 slice
Plain pasta and rice	Sausage, 1 patty
Angel food cake	Steak, sirloin, broiled, 3 oz
Popcorn, air-popped, unbuttered	Potatoes, French fried, 10
Soft drinks	Chow mein, chicken, 1 cup
Jam, jelly	Chocolate candy bar, 1 oz
1–3 Grams of Fat	Corn chips, 1 oz
Popcorn, oil-popped, unbuttered, 1 cup	Doughnut, cake type, plain, 1
Low-calorie salad dressing, 1 T[†]	Mayonnaise, 1 T
Baked beans, ½ cup	**15 Grams of Fat**
Soup, chicken noodle, canned, 1 cup	Hot dog, beef, 2 oz
Whole-wheat bread, 1 slice	McDonald's Chicken McNuggets, 6 pieces
Dinner roll, 1	Peanut butter, 2 T
Waffle, frozen, 4″, 1	Pork chop, broiled, 3 oz
Coleslaw, ½ cup	Sunflower seeds, dry roasted, ¼ cup
Flounder or sole, baked, 3 oz	Avocado, ½ medium
Chicken, without skin, roasted, 3 oz	Chop suey, beef and pork, 1 cup
Tuna, canned in water, 3 oz	Cinnamon roll, 1
Cheese, cottage, 2% fat, ½ cup	**20 Grams of Fat**
Ice milk, soft serve, ½ cup	Cheesecake, 1⁄12 cake
4–6 Grams of Fat	Lasagna with meat, 1 medium piece
Low-fat yogurt, 1 cup	Macaroni and cheese, homemade, 1 cup
Cheese, mozarella, part-skim, 1 oz	Peanuts, dry roasted, ¼ cup
Chicken, roasted with skin, 3 oz	Ground beef, broiled, 3 oz
Egg, scrambled, 1	**25+ Grams of Fat**
Turkey, roasted, 3 oz	Polish sausage, 3 oz
Granola, 1 oz	Cheeseburger, large
Muffin, bran, 1 small	Pie, pecan, ⅛ 9″
Pizza, cheese, ¼ of 12″	Chicken pot pie, frozen, baked, 1 pie
Burrito, bean, 1	Quiche, bacon, ⅛ pie
Brownie, with nuts, 1 small	
Margarine or butter, 1 tsp	
Popcorn, oil-popped, buttered, 1 cup	
French dressing, regular, 1 T	

*Data from Healthy Dividends, Rosemont, IL, National Dairy Council, 1990.
[†]T, tablespoon.

wired" taste for fat. Consider the sensory properties of high-fat chocolate compared with the intense sweetness of fat-free chocolate. Food manufacturers use fat for its textural properties; fat in ice cream contributes to its smoothness, and fat in baked goods increases the tenderness of the product by "shortening" the strands of gluten in batters and doughs (Vail, 1978). Great chefs know that a judicious amount of fat adds to the palatability of the meal and produces a feeling of satiety after a meal. Table 3–6 shows the fat content of common foods.

Unlike carbohydrates, lipids are not polymers but rather small molecules extracted from animal and plant tissues. They are a heterogeneous group of compounds characterized by their insolubility in water and can be classified into six major groups:

1. **Fatty acids**—long hydrocarbon chains with carboxylic acid head groups
2. **Triglycerides**—neutral esters of glycerol and fatty acids
3. **Phospholipids**—ionic esters of glycerol, fatty acids, and phosphate
4. Lipids not containing glycerol—*sphingolipids, alcohols, waxes, terpenes,* and *steroids*
5. Lipids combined with other compounds—**glycolipids** and *glycoproteins,* usually found in the biomembrane
6. *Synthetic lipids.*

Table 3–7 shows lipid classification. Figure 3–6 shows some structures.

Fatty Acids

Fatty acids are rarely free in nature and almost always linked to other molecules by their hydrophilic (water-loving) carboxylic acid head group. They exist primarily as unbranched hydrocarbon chains with an even number of carbons variably saturated with hydrogen. Fatty acids are classified according to the number of carbons in the chain, the number of double bonds, and the position of the first double bond. Both chain length and saturation contribute to the melting temperature of a fat. In general, fats with shorter fatty acid chains or with more double bonds are liquid at room temperature. Saturated fats, especially those with long chains, as in beef tallow (18C), are solid at room temperature. Because triglycerides in natural foods are mixtures of fatty acids of different melting points, fatty acids

TABLE 3–7 CLASSIFICATION OF LIPIDS

SIMPLE LIPIDS

• Fatty acids
• Neutral fats: Esters of fatty acids with glycerol
  • monoglycerides, diglycerides, triglycerides
• Waxes: Esters of fatty acids with high molecular weight alcohols
  • Sterol esters (e.g., cholesterol ester)
  • Nonsterol ester (e.g., retinol palmitate [vitamin A esters])

COMPOUND LIPIDS

• Phospholipids: Compounds of phosphoric acid, fatty acids, and a nitrogenous base
  • Glycerophospholipids (e.g., lecithins, cephalins, plasmologens)
  • Glycosphingolipids (e.g., sphingomyelins)
• Glycolipids: Compounds of fatty acids, monosaccharides, and a nitrogenous base (e.g., cerebrosides, gangliosides, ceramide)
• Lipoproteins: Particles of lipid and protein

MISCELLANEOUS LIPIDS
• Sterols (e.g., cholesterol, vitamin D, bile salts) • Vitamins A, E, K

(From Examples of current and proposed ingredients for fats. J Am Diet Assoc 92:472, 1992.)

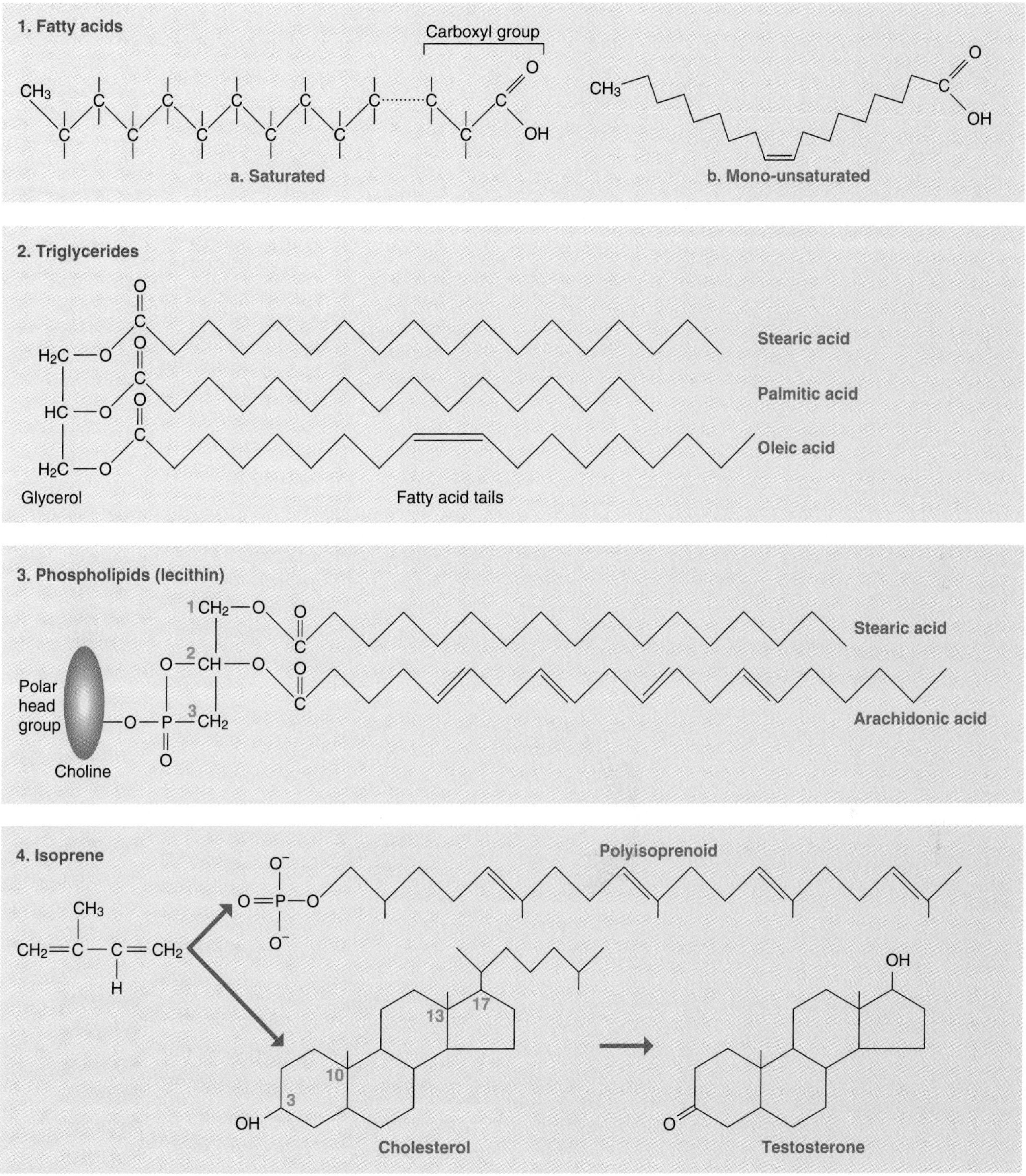

FIGURE 3–6 Structures of physiologically important fats and lipids.

solidify at a different rate during cooling. Some manufacturers cool the oil and filter out solidified particles before sale; the "winterized" oil will remain clear during refrigeration. Olive oil, about 75% monounsaturated fatty acid, becomes cloudy and viscous when cooled. In contrast, coconut oil is highly saturated but semiliquid at room temperature because of the predominance of SCFA (8–14C).

CHAIN LENGTH

Plants and animals require fatty acids of specific chain length and saturation for structural and metabolic needs. Each organism has evolved the capacity to synthesize and elongate its own fatty acids; thus, food sources will necessarily differ with respect to the composition of fatty acid chain lengths they contain. In general, butter and milk

TABLE 3–8 COMMON FATTY ACIDS*

COMMON NAME	SYSTEMATIC NAME	NO. OF CARBON ATOMS†	NO. OF DOUBLE BONDS	TYPICAL FAT SOURCE
Saturated Fatty Acids				
Butyric	Butanoic	4	0	Butterfat
Caproic	Hexanoic	6	0	Butterfat
Caprylic	Octanolic	8	0	Coconut oil
Capric	Decanoic	10	0	Coconut oil
Lauric	Dodecanoic	12	0	Coconut oil, palm kernel oil
Myristic	Tetradecanoic	14	0	Butterfat, coconut oil
Palmitic	Hexadecanoic	16	0	Palm oil, animal fat
Stearic	Octadecanoic	18	0	Cocoa butter, animal fat
Arachidic	Elcosanoic	20	0	Peanut oil
Behenic	Docosanoic	22	0	Peanut oil
Unsaturated Fatty Acids				
Caproleic	9-Decenoic	10	1	Butterfat
Lauroleic	9-Dodecenoic	12	1	Butterfat
Myristoleic	9-Tetradecenoic	14	1	Butterfat
Palmitoleic	9-Hexadecenoic	16	1	Some fish oils, beef fat
Oleic	9-Octadecenoic	18	1	Olive oil, canola oil
Elaidic	9-Octadecenoic	18	1	Butterfat
Vacceric	11-Octadecenoic	18	1	Butterfat
Linoleic	9, 12-Octadecadienoic	18	2	Most vegetable oils esp. safflower, corn, soybean, cottonseed
Linolenic	9, 12, 15-Octadecatrienoic	18	3	Soybean oil, canola oil, walnuts, wheat germ oil, flaxseed oil
Gadoleic	9-Eicosenoic	20	1	Some fish oils
Arachidonic	5, 8, 11, 14-Eicosatetraenoic	20	4	Lard, meats
—	5, 8, 11, 14, 17-Eicosapentaenoic (EPA)	20	5	Some fish oils, shellfish
Erucic	13-Docosenoic	22	1	Canola oil
—	4, 7, 10, 13, 16, 19-Docosahexaenoic (DHA)	22	6	Some fish oils, shellfish

*Adapted from Institute of Shortening and Edible Oils. Food fats and oils, 6th ed. Washington, DC: Author, 1988.
†All double bonds are in the *cis* configuration except for elaidic acid and vaccenic acid, which are *trans*.

fat contain predominately SCFA with 4 to 6 carbons, coconut oil contains fats with 12 to 14 carbons, and animals, **long-chain fatty acids** with 16 to 20 carbons (Table 3–8).

SATURATION

Each carbon in the fatty acid chain has four binding sites. In a **saturated fatty acid (SFA),** all binding sites not linked to carbon are "saturated" with hydrogen. **Monounsaturated fatty acid (MFA)** contains only one double bond; **polyunsaturated fatty acids (PUFA)** contain two or more double bonds. In MFA and PUFA, one or more pairs of hydrogens have been removed and double bonds are formed between adjacent carbons. As is the case with fatty acid chain length, each organism has evolved its own optimal fatty acid composition. Because fatty acids with double bonds are vulnerable to oxidative damage, humans and other warm-blooded organisms store fat predominantly as saturated *palmitic* ($C_{16}H_{32}O_2$ = C16:0) and *stearic* ($C_{18}H_{36}O_2$ = C18:0) *fatty acids.* On the other hand, the biomembrane must be both stable and flexible for optimal function. To achieve this requirement, biomembrane phospholipids contain one saturated and one highly polyunsaturated fatty acid, the most abundant of which is arachidonic acid (C20:4). The most abundant MFA in human blood is monounsaturated *oleic* ($C_{18}H_{34}O_2$ = C18:1) *acid.* Food sources of fatty acids are found in Table 3–9.

LOCATION OF DOUBLE BONDS

Fatty acids are also characterized by the location of the double bonds. Two conventions are used to describe the location of the double bonds. In the

TABLE 3–9 FOOD GROUP SOURCES OF FATTY ACIDS*

FATTY ACID GROUP†	MEATS, POULTRY, FISH (%)	FATS AND OILS (%)	DAIRY PRODUCT (%)	LEGUMES, NUTS (%)	EGGS (%)	OTHER (%)
SFA	39	34	20	2	2	3
MUFA	35	48	8	4	2	3
PUFA	18	68	2	6	2	6

*Data from Life Science Research Office, Federation of American Societies for Experimental Biology. Nutrition monitoring in the United States—An update report on nutrition monitoring. Prepared for the US Department of Agriculture and the US Department of Health and Human Services. Public Health Service. Washington, DC: US Government Printing Office, September 1989; DHHS publication no. (PHA) 89-1255.
†SFA, saturated fatty acids; MUFA, monounsaturated fatty acids; PUFA, polyunsaturated fatty acids.

first, the Greek capital letter delta (Δ) refers to the carbon preceding the double bond. For example, Δ9 refers to the double bond between carbons 9 and 10. In the second convention, lower case Greek letters are used to refer to the placement of the carbons within the fatty acid. Alpha (α) refers to the first carbon adjacent to the carboxyl group, beta (β) to the second carbon, and omega (ω) to the last carbon (omega number). Double bonds labeled with ω are counted from the terminal methyl carbon. Thus, *arachidonic acid* (20:4 ω-6), the major highly polyunsaturated fat in the membranes of land animals, is an *omega-6* fatty acid. It has four double bonds, the first is 6 carbons from the terminal methyl group. *Eicosapentaenoic acid (EPA)* (*eicosa* = 20; *pent* = 5; 20:5 ω-3) is found in marine organisms and is an **omega-3 fatty acid.** It has five double bonds, the first is 3 carbons from the terminal methyl group. Plants make oils of both omega-6 and omega-3 fatty acid types. *Linoleic acid* (C18:2 ω-6) has 18 carbons and two double bonds, and *alpha (α) linolenic acid (ALA)* (C18:3 ω-3) has 18 carbons and three double bonds and is of the omega-3 type. MFA, for example, oleic acid (C18:1 ω-9) found in olive and canola oil, has the double bond 9 carbons from the methyl group and is classed as *nonomega-9* fatty acids.

SOURCES OF FATTY ACIDS

Food group sources of saturated, monounsaturated, and polyunsaturated fatty acids are shown in Table 3–9. Sources of omega-3 fatty acids from selected marine sources are listed in Table 3–10. Note that values for omega-3 fatty acid content can differ in the food sources. For example, eggs from chickens fed fish meal are higher in omega-3 fatty acids (Farrell, 1998). Similarly, the omega-3 fatty acid content of fish differs by species (Atlantic versus Chinook salmon) and by their origin (farm raised or wild). Considerable variation has been identified in omega-3 fatty acid content of the same food analyzed using different nutrient data bases. For this reason, the values given in Table 3–10 and elsewhere should be used as a rough estimate, rather than a precise calculation of omega-3 fatty acid intake.

TABLE 3–10 SOURCES OF OMEGA-3 FATTY ACIDS

FOOD SOURCE (100 g edible portion—raw)	TOTAL FAT (g)	OMEGA-3 FAT DHA (22:6 ω-3) EPA (20:5 ω-3)
Anchovy	4.8	1.4
Bluefish	6.5	1.2
Catfish—channel	4.3	0.3
Flounder	1.0	0.2
Haddock	0.7	0.2
Herring—Atlantic	9.0	1.6
Lobster—northern	0.9	0.2
Mackerel—Atlantic	13.9	2.5
Pompano—Florida	9.5	0.6
Salmon—Atlantic	5.4	1.2
Salmon—Chinook	10.4	1.4
Salmon—pink	3.4	1.0
Sardines—in sardine oil	15.5	3.3
Shrimp	1.1	0.3
Trout—brook	2.7	0.4
Tuna	2.5	0.5

Adapted from Conner SL, Conner WE. Are fish oils beneficial in the prevention and treatment of coronary artery disease? Am J Clin Nutr (4 suppl):1020S–1031S, 1997.
DHA, docosahexenoic acid; EPA, eicosapentoic acid.

THE ω-6:ω-3 RATIO

It has been postulated that humans evolved on a diet lower in saturated fat and higher in ω-3 fatty acids than is consumed today (Crawford, 1992). Early humans either lived by the oceans and subsisted primarily on fish or, if they lived inland, consumed large quantities of green plants high in ALA (C18:3 ω-3). ALA is a precursor to EPA (C20:5 ω-3) and to the longer *docosahexaenoic acid* (DHA) (C22:6 ω-3). The Paleolithic diet is thought to have been richer in marine and plant sources of ω-3 fatty acids and lower in ω-6 fatty acid sources, resulting in a ratio of ω-6:ω-3 that approximated 1:1. In contrast, the modern diet is richer in ω-6 fatty acids from animal protein and vegetable oils and lower in ω-3 fats from vegetables and fish, with an estimated ω-6:ω-3 ratio of 8 to 12:1. Unofficial recommendations in the field and from the World Health Organization (WHO) suggest that the ratio should be lower, 5 to 10:1 (see Chapter 12).

The human brain and central nervous system, as well as membranes throughout the body, require ω-3 fatty acids, especially EPA and DHA for optimal function (Connor et al., 1992). It has been proposed that greater availability of long-chain ω-3 fatty acids allowed humans to develop their complex brain and neural system. Long-chain, highly polyunsaturated **essential fatty acids** must be obtained from the diet, either preformed or from dietary precursors. Precursors for the synthesis ω-3 and ω-6 fatty acids are made by the chloroplasts of marine phytoplankton and land plants, respectively. Animals higher on the evolutionary scale cannot introduce double bonds closer to the terminal than C-7 nor can mammalian cells interconvert ω-3 to ω-6. Humans can desaturate and elongate ALA (C18:3 ω-3) into EPA (C20:5 ω-3) and DHA (C22:6 ω-3). Linseed or flaxseed (57%), canola (8%), and soybean (7%) oils, as well as green leaves, are plant sources of ALA. Sources of long-chain ω-3 fatty acids are primarily marine: cod liver oil, mackerel, salmon, as well as crab, shrimp, and oyster. Egg yolk, especially from chickens fed ω-3-containing feed, is also a source of ω-3 fatty acids. See "*Clinical Insight:* Essential Fatty Acid Deficiency."

Triglycerides

Triglycerides (formally called triaglycerols) are formed by joining three fatty acids to a glycerol side chain. Because free fatty acids contain a carboxylic

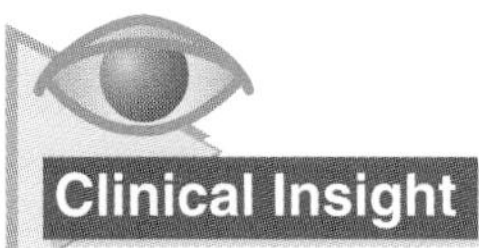

Essential Fatty Acid Deficiency

Deficiencies of both ω-3 and ω-6 essential fatty acids are seen clinically and can be differentiated by predominant symptoms. Common findings with ω-6 deficiency include growth retardation, skin lesions, reproductive failure, fatty liver, and polydipsia. In contrast, ω-3 fatty acid deficiency spares growth and reproduction, but is associated with reduced learning, impaired vision, and polydipsia. Evidence is accumulating linking ω-3 fatty acid deficiency to attention deficit hyperactivity disorder (Stevens et al., 1995). Abnormal ω-6:ω-3 ratios have been linked to changes in vascular membrane lipid composition and increased incidence of atherosclerosis and inflammatory disorders (Reaven, 1995).

(COOH) acid head group, fatty acids can react with other molecules and are potentially dangerous. To avoid tissue damage, biologic organisms bind three fatty acids to glycerol. The OH group on each fatty acid is bound to an OH group on glycerol. At each site, a molecule of water is released and an ester (-O-) linkage is formed. Fatty acids linked to glycerol are neutral and the triglyceride is water insoluble (hydrophobic). "Neutral fats" can be safely transported in the blood and stored in the fat cell (adipocyte) as an energy reserve. Over 95% of lipids in the food supply are in the triglyceride storage form.

The fatty acids that make up the triglyceride in a food source reflect the needs of the plant or animal. Milk fat and coconut and palm kernel oils have a high percentage of short- (4–6C) and medium- (6–12C) chain fatty acids. As mentioned above, SFAs are relatively inert and not susceptible to oxidative damage during storage. Thus land animals store fat in longer, largely saturated fatty acids (16C and 18C). Fish oils and marine-derived fats contain even longer, but highly unsaturated fatty acids (20C and 22C). Cold water creatures must maintain their fatty acids in liquid form even at low temperatures, and increased numbers of double bonds lower the temperature at which the fat is liquid and available for metabolic functions.

Phospholipids

Phospholipids are derivatives of phosphatidic acid, a triglyceride modified to contain a phosphate group at the third position as shown in Figure 3–6. Phosphatidic acid is esterified to a nitrogen-containing molecule, choline, serine, inositol, or ethanolamine. Phospholipids are named for the nitrogenous base: phosphatidylcholine, phosphatidylethanolamine, or phosphatidylserine. The resulting molecule is polar at physiologic pH. The phosphate-containing portion of the molecule is charged and forms hydrogen bonds with water while the two fatty acids form hydrophobic interactions with other fats. The hydrophilic head groups face outward to the extracellular media and inward to the cytoplasm, whereas the fatty acid tails form hydrophobic interactions in the membrane center and maintain optimal biomembrane fluidity. Phospholipids are called biologic *amphiphiles* (Gr. *ampho* = both) because their hydrophilic head group and hydrophobic fatty acid tail groups form an emulsification between water and oil at the phase interface and act as a detergent to "dissolve" the fat into the water.

Phospholipids make up more than 50% of the biomembrane lipid bilayer and provide a lipid barrier to unregulated transport of water-soluble molecules into the cell. Phospholipids usually contain one SFA (C16-C18) at C-1, and a highly PUFA (C16–C20) at C-2. The SFA is relatively inert; the PUFA is bent because of the double bonds (see Membrane Viscosity below). γ-Linolenic acid (C18:3 ω-3), arachidonic acid (C20:4 ω-6), and ω-3 substitutes can be cleaved from the lipid bilayer and provide substrate for synthesis of prostaglandins and other local mediators of cell activity as described below. The third position on the glycerol molecule is occupied by a phosphate esterified to a nitrogenous base such as choline, ethanolamine, or serine.

LECITHIN

Lecithin (phosphatidylcholine) and its derivative, *sphingomyelin,* are the two major phospholipids in the biomembrane outer leaflet and are essential to biomembrane structure and function. Lecithin is also a major component of the high-density phospholipid and protein disk (high-density lipoprotein, HDL) used to remove cholesterol from cell membranes. HDL uses its copper-dependent enzyme, lecithin-cholesterol acyltransferase, to transfer a fatty acid from lecithin to free cholesterol taken from the cell membrane. The resultant neutral cholesterol is stored in the HDL lipid center for safe transport to the liver.

Lecithin is made by the body, both de novo and in biomembranes, by adding three methyl groups to another phospholipid, phosphatidylethanolamine. It is also widely distributed in the food supply. Liver, egg yolk, soybeans, peanuts, legumes, spinach, and wheat germ are rich sources. Remember that all cells contain lecithin as a lipid bilayer component. Thus, animal products are a source of lecithin. Because of its emulsifying properties, lecithin is added to food products such as margarine, snack crackers, and confections. Although supplemental lecithin has been used empirically to reduce risk for hyperlipidemia, conclusive support for this hypothesis is meager. Note that lecithin is a fat and contains 9 kcal/g. At this time, it is recommended that healthy persons use dietary sources of lecithin that also contain ω-3 fatty acids and essential nutrients rather than purified lecithin supplements.

Trans-Fatty Acids: Membrane Viscosity

In natural unsaturated fatty acids, the two carbons participating in a double bond each bind a hydrogen on the same side of bond (cis-isomer form). Because the two remaining hydrogens take up space, the cis configuration causes the fatty acid to crimp or bend toward the empty side, as shown in Figure 3–6. The more double bonds per fatty acid, the more bends in the molecule. **Hydrogenation** of unsaturated fat can occur during anaerobic fermentation in the rumen of cows and sheep and by chemical methods that add hydrogen to liquid oils to form a stable and solid fat. Hydrogen can be added both in the natural cis position (two hydrogens on the same side of the double bond) and in the trans position (one hydrogen on opposite sides of the double bond). Depending on the process, the final product has a mixture of cis and trans double bonds with **trans-fatty acids** ranging from 0% to 50% (Katan and Mensink, 1992).

Membrane function depends on the three-dimensional configuration of membrane fatty acids. The cis double bonds in membrane PUFA form kinks and pack more loosely, making the membrane less stiff and rigid. Proteins embedded in a biomembrane float or sink, depending on membrane fluidity. Thus, the viscosity of a biomembrane is important for protein signaling, hormone responsiveness, and other membrane protein. Because trans-fatty acids do not kink, but pack as tightly as SFAs in biomembranes, dietary intake of trans-fatty acids can influence membrane fluidity and could be detrimental to cell function.

TRANS-FATTY ACIDS AND CHRONIC DISEASE

Clinical and epidemiologic studies suggest that higher intakes of trans-fatty acids are associated with increased risk for coronary heart disease, cancer, and other chronic diseases (Simopolus, 1994). Trans-fatty acids have been shown to inhibit the desaturation and elongation of linoleic and ALA to form long-chain essential fatty acids as indicated above. Major sources of trans-fatty acids in the U.S. diet are partially hydrogenated margarine, shortening, commercial frying fats, high-fat baked goods, and salty snacks containing these fats. Butter and animal fat can also contain trans-fatty acid from bacterial fermentation as indicated above.

Long-chain PUFA are critical for fetal brain and organ development. Until more is known about the extent of risk, it is recommended that dietary consumption of hydrogenated and saturated fatty acids be reduced (Lichtenstein, 1995). This modification will reduce trans-fatty acid intake as well. The role of trans-fatty acids in atherosclerosis is discussed in Chapter 26.

Eicosanoids and Paracrine Mediators

Arachidonic (C20:4 ω-6) and eicosapentenoic (C20:5 ω-3) acids bound to C-2 in the phospholipid bilayer (see Fig. 3–7) is cleaved by a phospholipase in response to inflammatory mediators. Cleaved fatty acids enter the pathways for *eicosanoid* (*eicosa* =

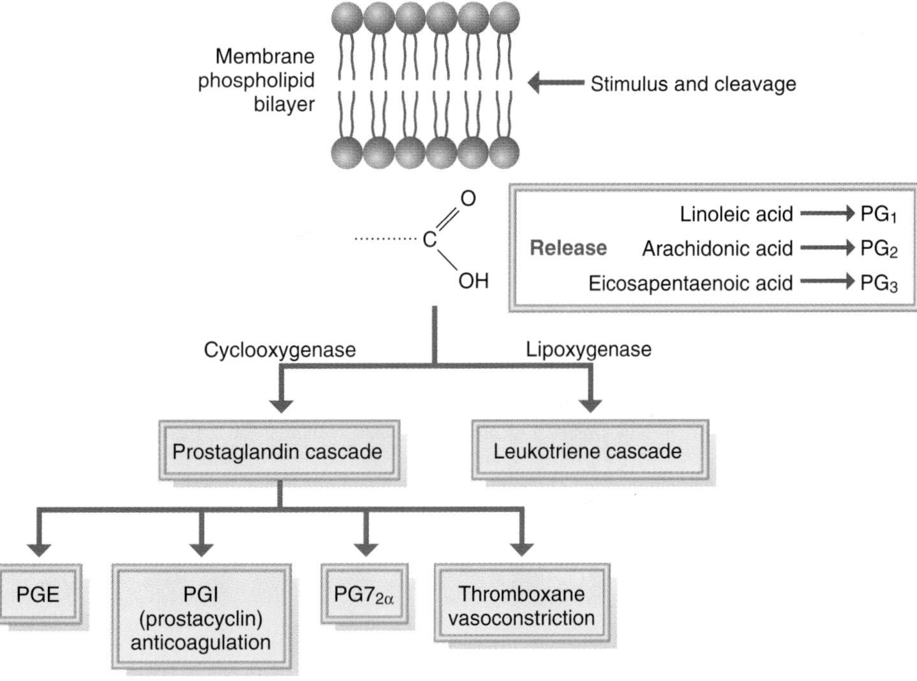

FIGURE 3–7 Eicosanoid synthesis following phospholipid cleavage in the biomembrane. Injury, inflammation, and other stimuli cleave the highly unsaturated fatty acid at the C-2 position of the membrane phospholipid. Arachidonic acid (AA) or eicosapentaenoic acid (EPA) are the major fatty acids released; the pathway entered depends on the degree to which the target tissue expresses the enzyme. The cyclooxygenase pathway leads to prostaglandin (PG), thromboxane, and prostacyclin synthesis. The lipoxygenase pathway expressed in large amounts in lung and bronchi leads to leukotriene synthesis and subsequent bronchoconstriction. Note the point at which steroidal and nonsteroidal anti-inflammatory drugs act.

20) synthesis in the production of local *(paracrine)* hormones. These hormones are made nearby (*para* = alongside) in contrast to endocrine hormones made by distant organs and transported in the blood. As indicated in Figure 3–7, injury or inflammation cleaves PUFA from the membrane. PUFA is processed by eicosanoid synthetic pathways to form any of a variety of paracrine hormones including prostaglandins, thromboxanes, prostacyclins, and leukotrienes. These paracrine hormones have multiple local functions. They can alter the size and permeability of the blood vessels, alter the activity of platelets and contribute to blood clotting, and modify the processes of inflammation. Eicosanoids can have markedly different functions. The eicosanoid product of a cleaved PUFA depends on the cell type (platelets or endothelial cells) and the type of PUFA (arachidonic ω-6 or eicosapentenoic ω-3 acids) in the membrane. Note that membrane cleavage is inhibited by cortisone and prostaglandin synthesis is inhibited by aspirin, hence, steroidal and nonsteroidal drugs are used as anti-inflammatory agents. See "*Clinical Insight:* Bleeding Tendency."

There are bewildering varieties and functions of inflammatory interleukins, cytokines, chemokines, clotting factors, growth factors, adhesion factors, and other molecules not yet identified that are influenced by dietary lipid consumption. Too little is known yet to make more than a few basic recommendations as to the amount and type of dietary lipids that provide optimal biomembrane substrate. The role of ω-3 fatty acids in cardiovascular disease is discussed in Chapter 26, and their role in the pathogenesis of arthritis and inflammatory conditions in Chapter 43.

Sphingolipids, Alcohols, Waxes, Isoprenoids, and Steroids

All organisms produce small amounts of complex lipids with specialized, critical functions. Many of these lipids do not contain glycerol and are built from two carbon acetyl coenzyme A (CoA) units.

Sphingolipids are lipid esters attached to a sphingosine base rather than a glycerol. They are widely distributed in the nervous systems of animals and in the membranes of plants and lower eukaryotes such as yeast. Sphingomyelin includes the nitrogenous base, choline, and makes up more than 25% of the myelin sheath, the lipid-rich structure that protects and insulates cells of the central nervous system. Sphingomyelin is found, along with phosphatidylcholine, in the outer leaflet of all biomembranes. Sphingolipids are constantly synthesized and degraded in the lysosome.

Sphingolipidoses refers to a group of genetic lipid storage diseases in which sphingolipid degradation through the lysosomal pathway is blocked. Tay-Sachs disease is an example of a lipid storage disease. In this disease, enzyme deficiency results in accumulation of the lipid metabolite, especially in the brain. Severe nervous system degeneration, mental retardation, and blindness are seen, and the patients die, usually by age 4.

Long-chain alcohols are metabolic by-products. The feces contains cetyl alcohol, a by-product of palmitic acid. Beeswax is rich in the alcohol, myricyl pamitate. *Waxes* consist of long-chain fatty acids bound to long-chain alcohols. These molecules are almost completely water insoluble and are often used as water repellants, as in the feathers of birds and on the leaves of plants.

Isoprenoids, activated derivatives of isoprene, are an extraordinarily large and diverse group of lipids built from one or more five-carbon units (see Fig. 3–6). Isoprene contains alternating single and double (conjugated) bonds; conjugated bond structures can quench free radicals by accepting or donating electrons. Terpene is a generic term for all compounds synthesized from isoprene precursors. As a group, isoprenoids include essential oils of plants: turpentine from trees and limonene from lemons. Plant pigments that transfer electrons in photosynthesis are also isoprenoids. This group contains lycopene (red pigment in tomatoes), carotenoid (yellow and orange pigments in squash and

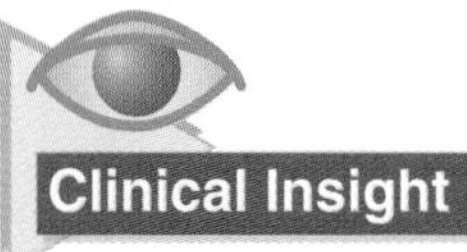

Clinical Insight

Bleeding Tendency

Arachidonic acid (C20:4 ω-6) is a precursor of the prostaglandin, thromboxane A_2 (TXA_2), a strong activator of platelet aggregation, vasoconstriction, and clot formation (Connor and Connor, 1997). Marine fish and oils in the diet increase the number of eicosapentaenoic acid (C20:5 ω-3) molecules in the platelet biomembrane. If EPA, rather than arachidonic acid, is cleaved from the membrane, the prostaglandin TXA_3 is formed. This hormone is much weaker than TXA_2, and platelets are less likely to aggregate. Fish oil also reduces fibrinogen and other clotting proteins, increases platelet survival, and decreases the risk to form a thrombus. At the same time, fish oil ingestion causes vascular endothelial cells to produce more prostacyclin (PGI_3) and to secrete more endothelial cell-derived relaxation factor. These mediators counter vasoconstriction and inhibit the tendency to clot. Omega-3 fatty acids inhibit the desaturase enzyme, thereby reducing the amount of arachidonic acid formed from γ-linolenic acid. Thus, eicosanoids made from EPA inhibit the tendency to clot, whereas eicosanoids from arachidonic acid increase clotting. The ratio of ω-6:ω-3 fatty acid in the membrane appears to be of utmost importance, and the ratio is largely determined by the type of dietary fatty acids ingested.

carrots), and the yellow/green chlorophyll group. Fat-soluble vitamins A, D, E, and K, and the electron transducer, coenzyme Q, have isoprenoid structures. Vitamin E, lycopene, and β carotene are effective antioxidants. Nonnutritive phytochemicals with antioxidant function usually have an isoprenoid structure (see Chapter 12).

Steroids constitute a class of lipids derived from a four-membered saturated ring as illustrated in Figure 3–6. Several important steroid derivatives are made in the body. Glucocorticoids (cortisone) and mineralocorticoids (aldosterone) are made in the adrenal gland, androgens (testosterone) and estrogens (estradiol) are made in the testes and ovaries, respectively, and bile acids are made in the liver. Vitamin D hormone is made when ultraviolet rays from the sun cleave cholesterol in subcutaneous fat to form cholecalciferol (D_3). Synthetic vitamin D is made by irradiating the plant steroid, ergosterol, to form ergocalciferol (D_2).

Cholesterol also plays an important role in membrane function. The rigid, four-ringed cholesterol molecule is bound into the hydrophobic membrane by its hydroxyl group (see Fig. 3–6). The stiff, planar rings spread apart and partially immobilize the fatty acid chains near the polar region. At the same time, the nonpolar hydrocarbon tail contributes to greater fluidity in the interior of the membrane. Plasma membranes contain large amounts of cholesterol, up to one molecule for every phospholipid molecule (Alberts et al., 1994). See "*New Directions:* Mevacor, Reductase Inhibitors, and Cholesterol-Reducing Drugs."

Glycolipids include the cerebrosides and gangliosides with their base sphingosine and very long-chain fatty acids (22C). Cerebrosides contain galactose; gangliosides also contain glucose and a complex compound containing an amino sugar. Structurally, both compounds are components of nerve tissue and certain cell membranes, where they play a role in lipid transport.

Synthetic lipids are commercially synthesized for specific purposes. Examples include medium-chain triglycerides (MCT), structured lipids, and fat replacers.

Medium-chain triglycerides (MCT) are SFAs with a chain length between 6 and 12 carbons. They are short enough to be water soluble, require less bile salts for solubilization, are not re-esterified in the enterocyte, and are transported as free fatty acid, bound to albumin, through the portal system. Because the portal blood flow rate is about 250 times faster than lymph flow, MCT are digested quickly and are not likely to be affected by intestinal factors that inhibit fat absorption (Linscheer and Vergroesen, 1994). They are not stored in adipose tissue but are oxidized to acetic acid. Natural MCT occur in milk fat, coconut oil, and palm kernel oil. Commercial MCT oil is a by-product of margarine production; it contains approximately 65% caprylic acid (C8:0) and 25% capric acid (C10:0), with the remaining fatty acids less than 6C and greater than 10C in length. MCT oils provide 8.25 kcal/g. Clinically, MCT oil is used for patients with fat malabsorption or in catabolic states such as acquired immunodeficiency syndrome and cancer. Specific uses of MCT oil are discussed in Chapter 22.

Structured lipids include MCT oil esterified with a desired fatty acid such as linoleic acid or ω-3 lipid. The combined product is absorbed faster than the long-chain triglyceride alone. Clinically, structured lipids are under investigation for parenteral and enteral formulas used in specific cases, for example, to enhance immune function or athletic performance.

Fat substitutes are structurally different from fats and do not provide readily absorbable nutrients. Their commercial importance is that they imitate the texture, mouth feel, and sensory effects of fat. Fat replacers differ in their macronutrient base and the extent to which they mimic the characteristics of fat. Caloric value of these substitutes varies between 5 kcal/g (caprenin) and 0 kcal/g (olestra, carrageenan). Table 3–11 gives examples of fat replacers and their properties.

The largest group of fat replacers is derived from plant polysaccharides such as gums, cellulose, dextrins, fiber, maltodextrins, starches, and polydextrose. Some products can be digested and provide 4 kcal/g. If the carbohydrate is hydrated (contains more water), the energy in the molecule can be as little as 1 to 2 kcal/g. Cellulose and nonabsorbable fibers provide no energy. Alcohols of carbohydrates (polyols such as sorbitol) are not fully absorbed and metabolized and provide less than 4 kcal/g.

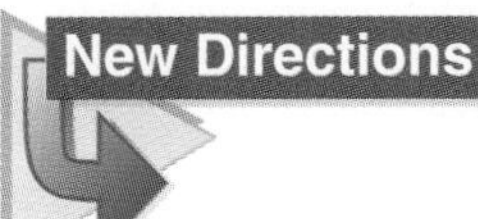

Mevacor, Reductase Inhibitors, and Cholesterol-Reducing Drugs

The first committed step in cholesterol biosynthesis is the formation of 6-carbon mevalonate using the enzyme, *3-hydroxy-3-methylglutaryl-CoA reductase (HMG CoA reductase).* By reducing the precursor for cholesterol synthesis, drugs such as Mevacor, reductase inhibitors, and statins lower serum cholesterol. By inhibiting cholesterol biosynthesis, especially in the liver, they are drugs of choice for high-risk hyperlipidemic patients. However, mevalonate is also used as precursor for complex lipids and their derivatives, including coenzyme Q. Conclusive evidence on risk versus benefit has not been demonstrated. The drugs do not reduce triglyceride synthesis and, thus, are not used for hypertriglyceridemia.

TABLE 3–11 EXAMPLES OF FAT REPLACERS AND THEIR FUNCTIONS AND PROPERTIES

CLASS OF FAT REPLACERS	TRADE NAMES	APPLICATIONS	FUNCTIONAL PROPERTIES
Carbohydrate-based			
Polydextrose	Litesse,[a] Sta-Lite[b]	Dairy products, sauces, frozen desserts, salad dressings, baked goods, confections, gelatins, puddings, meat products, chewing gum, dry cake and cookie mixes, frostings and icings	Moisture retention, bulking agent, texturizer
Starch (modified food starch)	Amalean I & II,[c] N-Lite,[d] Instant Stellar,[e] Sta-Slim,[b] OptaGrade,[e] Pure-gel[f]	Processed meats, salad dressings, baked goods, fillings and frostings, condiments, frozen desserts, dairy products	Gelling, thickening, stabilizing, texturizer
Maltodextrins	CrystaLean,[e] Maltrin,[f] Lycadex,[g] Star-Dri,[b] Paselli Excell,[h] Rice-Trim[i]	Baked goods, dairy products, salad dressings, spreads, sauces, fillings and frostings, processed meat, frozen desserts, extruded products	Gelling, thickening, stabilizing, texturizer
Grain-based (fiber)	Betatrim,[j] Opta,[e] Oat Fibere,[k] Snowite,[k] TrimChoice,[b] Fibrim[l]	Baked goods, meats, extruded products, spreads	Gelling, thickening, stabilizing, texturizer
Dextrins	N-Oil,[d] Stadex[b]	Salad dressings, puddings, spreads, dairy products, frozen desserts, chips, baked goods, meat products, frostings, soups	Gelling, thickening, stabilizing, texturizer
Gums (xanthan, guar, locust bean carrageenan, alginates)	Kelcogel,[m] Keltrol,[n] Viscarin,[o] Gelcarin,[o] Fibrex,[p] Novagel,[q] Rohodigel,[j] Jaguar[r]	Salad dressings, processed meats, formulated foods (eg, desserts and processed meats)	Water retention, texturizer, thickener, mouth feel, stabilizer
Pectin	Grindsted,[s] Slendid,[t] Splendid[t]	Baked goods, soups, sauces, dressings	Gelling, thickening, mouth feel
Cellulose (carboxy-methyl cellulose, microcrystalline cellulose)	Avicel,[q] cellulose gel, Methocel,[u] Solka-Floc,[v] Just Fiber[w]	Dairy products, sauces, frozen desserts, salad dressings	Water retention, texturizer, stabilizer, mouth feel
Fruit-based (fiber)	Prune paste, dried plum paste, Lighter Bake,[x] WonderSlim,[y] fruit powder	Baked goods, candy, dairy products	Moisturizer, mouth feel
Protein-based	Simplesse,[z] K-Blazer,[aa] Dairy-lo,[bb] Veri-lo,[bb] Ultra-Bake,[b] Powerpro,[cc] Proplus,[dd] Supro[dd]	Cheese, mayonnaise, butter, salad dressing, sour cream, spreads, bakery products	Mouth feel
Fat-based	Caprenin,[ee] Olean,[ee] Benefat,[bb] Dur-Em[w] Dur-Lo[w]	Chocolate, confections, bakery products, savory snacks	Mouth feel
Combinations	Prolestra,[ff] Nutrifat,[ff] Finesse[ff]	Ice cream, salad oils, mayonnaise, spreads, sauces, bakery products	Mouth feel

[a]Cultor Food Science, Inc, Ardsley, NY
[b]AE Staley Manufactuing Co, Decatur, IL
[c]Cerestar USA, Inc, Hammond, IN
[d]National Starch and Chemical Co., Bridgewater, NJ
[e]Opta Food Ingredients, Bedford, MA
[f]Grain Processing Corp, Muscatine, IA
[g]Roquette America, Inc, Keokuk, IA
[h]AVEBE America Inc, Princeton, NJ
[i]Zumbro, Inc, Hayfield, MN
[j]Rhone-Poulenc, Inc, Cranbury, NJ
[k]Canadian Harvest USA, Cambridge, MN
[l]Protein Technologies International, Pryor, OK
[m]Monsanto, Chicago, IL
[n]Kelco, Division of Merck, Clark, NJ
[o]FMC Corp, Rockland, ME
[p]Purity Foods, Okemos, MI
[q]FMC Corp, Philadelphia, PA
[r]Aston Chemicals, Aylesbury, Buckinghamshire, England
[s]Danisco, New Century, KN
[t]Hercules Inc, Wilmington, DE
[u]Dow Chemical, Midland, MI
[v]Fiber Sales and Development Corp, Green Brook, NJ
[w]Loders Croklaan, Glen Ellyn, IL
[x]Sunsweet Growers, Yuba City, CA
[y]The Heart Garden Corporation, Los Angeles, CA
[z]Nutrasweet, San Diego, CA
[aa]Kraft Food Ingredients, Memphis, IN
[bb]Cultor Food Science, Ardsley, NY
[cc]Land O'Lakes Food Division, Arden Hill, MN
[dd]Protein Technologies International, St. Louis, MO
[ee]Procter and Gamble, Cincinnati, OH
[ff]Reach Associates, South Orange, NJ

(From American Dietetic Association. Position of the American Dietetic Association: Fat replacers. J Am Diet Assoc 98:463, 1998.)

Protein fat replacers alter the texture of a product in a variety of ways. Microparticulated proteins can act like small ball-bearings to provide fatlike mouth feel. Protein replacers contribute between 1.3 and 4 kcal/g and augment the protein content of the food. Note that some proteins can stimulate an allergic or antigenic response in susceptible individuals.

Fat sources can be modified to reduce gastrointestinal absorption, thereby reducing caloric availability. Mono- and **diacylglycerols** are used as emulsifiers and contribute the sensory properties of fat with fewer calories (~5 kcal/g). Salatrim (short- and long-chain fatty acid triglyceride molecule) also contains about 5 kcal/g because of reduced absorbability.

The aim of reducing gastrointestinal fat absorption prompted creation of a new synthetic fat replacer, a sucrose polyester with the generic name, olestra. Sucrose is esterified with six to eight fatty acids to form hexa-, hepta-, and octa-esters. The fatty acid chains range in length from 12 to 24C and are dervied from edible oils such as soybean, cottonseed, and corn. The product has the physical properties of natural dietary fats. Because they are nonabsorbable, sucrose polyesters do not contribute calories to the diet.

Concern has been raised as to the long-term effects of fat substitutes. In particular, if fat substitutes are not absorbed, can they bind essential fatty acids and fat-soluble vitamins and contribute to their malabsorption (Gershoff, 1995)? On the other hand, sufficient research has been done for the Food and Drug Administration (FDA) to grant most fat substitute the status of generally recognized as safe. In the case of sucrose polyester, the FDA determined that it was not previously found in food, classified it as a food additive, and required extensive data on the ingredient's safety before allowing it to be added to food (Clydesdale, 1997). The American Dietetic Association (1998) has reviewed fat replacers and concluded that "fat replacers may offer a safe, feasible, and effective means to maintain the palatability of diets with controlled amounts of fat and/or energy."

Food Sources of Fat and Recommendations

The vast array of fat types in the diet, coupled with the growing realization that the type of dietary fat consumed may have important consequences in the body, suggests that recommendations about dietary fat consumption must consider fat type as well as fat amount. The following guidelines are suggested with the understanding that fat metabolism is a dynamic and ever-changing field.

Fat Sources

Animals maintain their storage fats as saturated as possible but still liquid at body temperature, thus storage fat depots in foods of land animal origin are primarily saturated (SFA). Marine animals, especially those from cold waters, must maintain their fat in liquid form as unsaturated oils (PUFA). Plants that grow in temperate climates, corn and soybeans, form PUFA oils, mainly linoleic acid (C18:2 ω-6) stored in their seeds. Some tropical plants, such as coconut, cocoa, and palm, store saturated fats, possibly because their growing temperature is higher. MFA is found in olive oil, canola oil, peanut oil, peanuts, pecans, almonds, and avocados. Omega-3 PUFA come primarily from marine sources (see Table 3–8) although vegetable precursors can be obtained from flaxseed and canola oils and green leafy sources.

Amount of Fat in the Diet

Reduced amounts of total fat, with low saturated fat and cholesterol, and increased intake of complex carbohydrates have been recommended to reduce serum cholesterol and risk for chronic disease, especially heart disease, blood pressure, stroke, and renal disease (Krauss et al., 1996; McCarron, 1997). On the other hand, evidence is accumulating that serum triglycerides may be an important risk factor. The Consensus Panel on Triglyceride, High-Density Lipoprotein and Coronary Heart Disease of the National Institutes of Health (NIH) has stated that raised triglyceride-rich lipoproteins (VLDL) and lowered HDL can increase risk for heart disease both by contributing to plaque formation and by increasing clotting tendency (NIH, 1993). Starch and sucrose, used to replace dietary fat, may actually increase risk in certain groups of individuals by raising triglyceride concentrations (Daly et al., 1997). Individuals with hypertriglyceridemia or hyperinsulinemia (or both) appear to be sensitive to the effects of dietary sucrose and fructose. Furthermore, several studies have suggested that low-fat, high-carbohydrate diets lower HDL concentrations, thereby increasing risk for heart disease. Diets high in MUFA can be advised as an alternative to high-carbohydrate diets in diabetic and carbohydrate-sensitive patients (Garg, 1994.) Until more is known it seems prudent to recommend a diet low in saturated fats, with high fiber and moderate amounts of ω3 and monounsaturated fat.

Type of Fat in the Diet

Saturated fatty acids are known to increase, and PUFA to decrease, plasma lipids. However, too much PUFA can be dangerous. Double bonds are highly reactive and bind oxygen to form peroxides when exposed to air or heat. Oxidized fats produce the off flavors and odors described as rancidity. Saturated fat and partially hydrogenated oils have fewer oxygen-binding sites and thereby have increased stability and longer shelf life. PUFA-rich oils are also reactive in cooking. When subjected to routine frying or cooking practices, PUFA can generate high levels of toxic aldehyde products that promote cardiovascular disease. To prevent toxic product formation, PUFA are often fortified with vitamin E or synthetic antioxidants such as butylated hydroxyanisole (BHA) and butylated hydroxytoluene (BHT). However, toxic products were seen during cooking, even in the presence of antioxidants such as vitamin E. Saturated and MFA, especially olive oil, similarly thermally stressed did not produce these toxic products (Grootvelt et al., 1998). These data suggest that monounsaturated fats, with only one reactive bond, may be safer than PUFA, and yet not increase risk for heart disease.

Risk from Dietary Cholesterol

Because high serum cholesterol concentrations have been associated with risk for heart disease, dietary restriction of cholesterol-rich foods such as eggs, has been recommended. However, serum cholesterol levels are homeostatically controlled, and individual response to dietary cholesterol is highly variable (Hegsted, 1986). Eggs, for example, contain approximately 250 mg cholesterol each. Bronsgeest-Schoute et al. (1979) removed all eggs from the diet of 44 selected subjects. Serum cholesterol concentrations rose in 16 subjects and remained the same or decreased in the remainder. Vorster et al. (1992) reported that 14 eggs per week did not raise serum cholesterol concentrations or contribute to heart disease risk in young healthy subjects. It should be remembered that eggs are an inexpensive source of high biologic value protein and also contain ω-3 fatty acids and lecithin, both substances associated with reduced risk for hyperlipidemia and heart disease.

In summary, lipids play a major role in cell biology. As energy stores in adipocytes they provide a concentrated source of fuel, especially in the fasting state. As structural fat pads, they protect organs and bones from injury. Phospholipids are integral to all biomembranes where they function as lipid barriers, insulators, and substrates for paracrine hormones and complex lipids. Fat-soluble vitamins A and D regulate metabolic functions in diverse ways. Vitamin E protects membranes from oxidative damage. Science is just beginning to understand the full extent of lipid action and the precise interactions between dietary and endogenous lipids at the molecular level.

At present, it is impossible to conclusively dictate optimal dietary lipid recommendations. In view of the well-described mammalian preference for fat, apparently "hard wired" into the human physiology, we can conclude that the human requires fat in the diet. Until more is known, the recommendation to consume a variety of SFA, PUFA, and MFA in the diet and to avoid harsh cooking practices appears justified. In short, moderation and diversity are the keys.

AMINO ACIDS AND PROTEIN

Protein: The Nitrogen Cycle and Dietary Protein Sources

In a never-ending "nitrogen cycle," plants use the nitrogen to form their own **amino acids** and **proteins.** Animals eat the plants and use the amino acids for their tissues. Humans eat animals and plants for their amino acids and rearrange the nitrogen to make the pattern of amino acids required. Finally, everybody dies; organic molecules are degraded by microorganisms, nitrogen goes back into the soil to be used by nitrogen-fixing bacteria, and the cycle starts again.

Nitrogen contained in all amino acids originates as nitrogen gas (N_2) in the biosphere. Certain microorganisms, *Rhizobium* bacteria in soil, cyanobacteria in fresh water, and blue-green algae in sea water have the capacity to utilize inorganic nitrogen and "fix" it into organic molecules such as ammonia. Soil bacteria attach to the roots of plants such as soybean, clover, and alfalfa. A symbiotic relationship is formed, in which the bacteria provide organic nitrogen in exchange for sugars and other nutrients from the plant. This accounts for the high nitrogen content in legumes such as soybeans and beans. Agricultural practices take advantage of this phenomenon; farmers "rotate" legume crops with corn and wheat to provide added nitrogen to the soil.

Whereas plant structure is primarily carbohydrate, the structure of humans and animals is built on protein. Protein also represents an energy source. Nitrogen can be removed from amino acids in a process called deamination, and the resulting carbohydrate can be used for energy at the rate of 4 kcal/g. Protein in muscles and body tissue is in constant turnover. Tissue protein is degraded and nitrogen excreted in the urine. New protein is required daily to maintain the body in steady state.

The Recommended Dietary Allowance for protein is 0.8 g/k body weight for a healthy adult. To obtain this quantity of protein, humans require that dietary protein make up approximately 10% to 15% of their total energy intake. Protein requirements are increased during hypermetabolic stress and in disease, as discussed in Chapter 33. Protein-rich foods are obtained primarily from animal flesh or from animal products such as eggs and milk. Most plant foods are relatively poor in protein, with the exception of legumes and beans.

Amino Acids, Protein Synthesis, and Protein Three-Dimensional Structure

Amino Acid Structure

Amino acids are carbohydrates with an amino (NH_2) group added to the α carbon (the carbon next to the carboxyl group), as indicated in Figure 3–8. Carbohydrate skeletons can be made in the body, for example, from intermediates in metabolic pathways. Because we can make these amino acids, they are called **nonessential amino acids.** For example, pyruvate formed during glycolysis can be aminated to alanine. **Essential amino acids,** indicated in Figure 3–8 with an asterisk, have carbon skeletons that we cannot make and can obtain only from the diet. We can transfer nitrogen between amino acids and carbohydrates through a process called **transamination.** This process requires vitamin B_6 and is done by multiple forms of

All amino acids have the same general structure $HO-C(=O)-C^{\alpha}(NH_2)(H)-R$ where R is different for each.

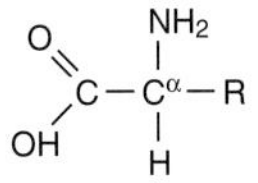

Amino acids are abbreviated using both a three letter and a single letter code as given below.
Amino acids marked with an asterisk* are essential; those with ** are essential in infants and in chronic diseases.

FUNCTIONAL TYPE	AMINO ACID (abbr.)	R GROUP	CHARACTERISTICS OF THE AMINO ACID
Aliphatic	Glycine (Gly) G	H	Tiny R group (H) allows hairpin bends in the peptide chains
	Alanine (Ala) A	CH_3	Can be deaminated to pyruvate and used for glucose synthesis
	Valine (Val) V*	$-CH(CH_3)_2$	Branched chain amino acids—metabolized in muscle
	Leucine (Leu) L*	$-CH_2-CH(CH_3)_2$	Branched chain more hydophobic—Muscle metabolism
	Isoleucine (Ile) I*	$-CH(CH_3)-CH_2-CH_3$	Branched chain most hydophobic—Muscle metabolism
Sulfur	Cysteine (Cys) C**	$-CH_2-SH$	Essential for glutatione synthesis—synthesis limited in chronic diseases
	Methionine (Met) M*	$-CH_2-CH_2-S-CH_2$	Converted to S-adenosylmethionine (SAM), the universal methyl donor, and cysteine
Hydroxyl	Serine (Ser) S	$-CH_2-OH$	The hydroxyl group is phosphorylated to activate/inactivate protein
	Threonine (Thr) T	$-CH_2-CH_2-S-CH_3$	Also site for regulatory phosphorylation
Aromatic	Phenylalanine (Phe) F*	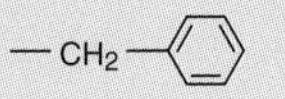 $-CH_2-$(benzene ring)	Converted to tyrosine for synthesis of norepinephrine, epinephrine and dopamine
	Tyrosine (Tyr) Y	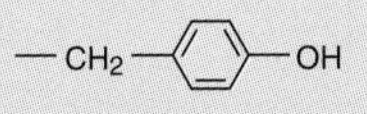 $-CH_2-$(benzene ring)$-OH$	Converted to neurotransmitters, norepinephrine, epinephrine and dopamine
	Tryptophan (Trp) W*	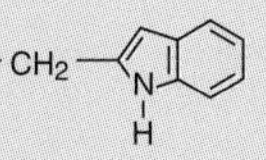 $-CH_2-$(indole ring, N–H)	Converted to neurotransmitter, serotonin and to niacin
Cyclic	Proline (Pro) P*	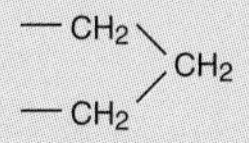 $-CH_2-CH_2-CH_2-$ (ring)	Allows triple helix; proline in collagen must be hydroxylated for crosslinkage
Basic	Lysine (Lys) K	$-CH_2-CH_2-CH_2-CH_2-\overset{+}{N}H_3$	Site for hydroxylation in proteins; hydrophylic, used in signalling
	Histidine (His) H**	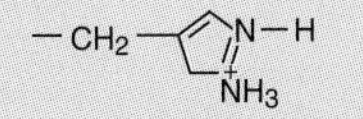 $-CH_2-$(imidazole ring, N–H, $\overset{+}{N}H_3$)	Hydrophilic, binds zinc in signalling proteins
	Arginine (Arg) R	$-CH_2-CH_2-CH_2-NH-C(=\overset{+}{N}H_2)-NH_2$	Formed in the urea cycle—essential for synthesis of nitric oxide signalling pathway
Acidic	Aspartic acid (Asp) D	$-CH_2-C(=O)O^-$	Takes a second nitrogen to form asparagine (Asn) N $-CH_2-C(=O)NH_2$
	Glutmic acid (Glu) E	$-CH_2-CH_2-C(=O)O^-$	Takes a second nitrogen to form glutamine (Gln) Q $-CH_2-CH_2-C(=O)NH_2$

FIGURE 3–8 Structures and functions of the 20 amino acids required by humans. All amino acids have the same general structure where R is different for each. Amino acids are abbreviated using both a three-letter and a single-letter code. Amino acids marked with an asterisk (*) are essential; those with double asterisks (**) are essential in infants and those with chronic diseases.

aminotransaminase enzymes using the following format:

carbohydrate + amino acid <==> amino acid + carbohydrate

The ability to transaminate carbohydrates increases the likelihood that all 20 amino acids will be available for protein synthesis (discussed below). Transamination also is used to remove nitrogen from amino acids degraded from tissue proteins. The nitrogen is bound to pyruvate to form alanine and transferred in the blood to the liver, where it is removed and enters the urea cycle for excretion in the urine.

As shown in Figure 3–8, the α carbon of the amino acid also binds a hydrogen atom and a side chain (R group). The carboxyl and α carbon on all amino acids are identical. It is the R group that dictates the identity of the amino acid. Figure 3–8 illustrates the general structure for an α amino acid. The R group for each amino acid is shown, together with the three-letter abbreviations commonly used and the single-letter abbreviations used when describing the amino acid sequence of a protein. Amino acids always essential are indicated with an asterisk, and those conditionally essential with double asterisks. A brief characterization of each amino acid is given, identifying the influence of R-group structure on amino acid function.

Protein Synthesis

Amino acids are important because they are used as substrates for protein synthesis. The patterns for all proteins are contained in the DNA of each organism. As illustrated in Figure 3–9, protein synthesis is a complex process through which the protein pattern is copied from the DNA onto RNA. The RNA message is taken to the cytoplasm where the amino acids are attached in linear precise sequence. Precise details of protein synthesis can be obtained in current biochemistry and cell biology texts. Figure 3–10 illustrates the end product of protein synthesis, the formation of the **peptide** bond. The peptide bond is formed between the carboxyl OH of the first amino acid and the nitrogen of the next. The pattern for protein synthesis is contained on messenger RNA (mRNA), directly copied from DNA. New proteins are built by attaching amino acids as dictated by the mRNA. When the protein has been built, it detaches from the message and is ready to be used. See "*Focus On:* DNA Transcription and RNA Translation."

Protein Folding: Three-Dimensional Structure

Proper folding of the completed linear amino acid chain is essential for a protein to perform its unique functions. The linear sequence of individual amino acids dictates the configuration of the ma-

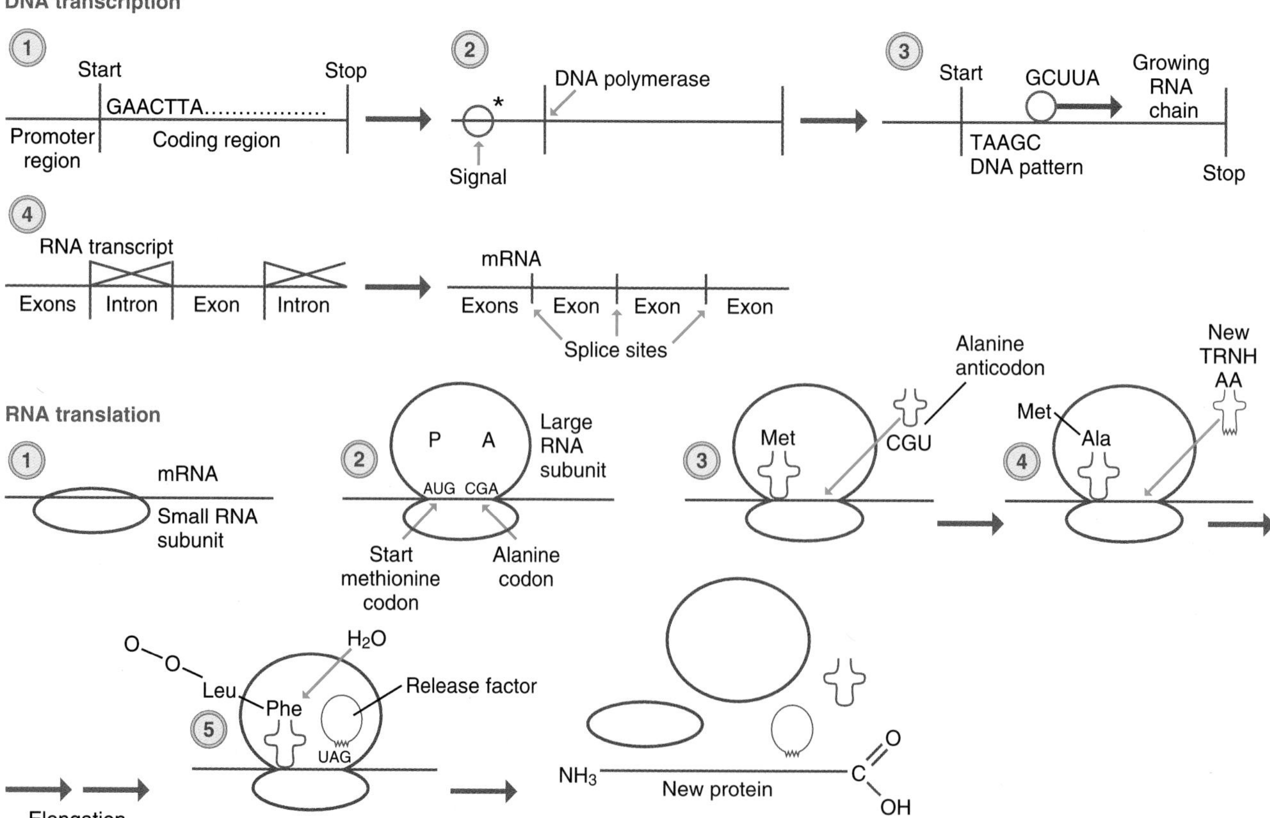

FIGURE 3–9 Summary of DNA transcription and RNA translation in the eukaryote cell.

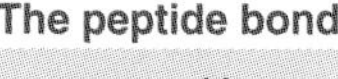

FIGURE 3–10 The peptide bond and protein folding.

ture protein. As indicated in Figure 3–10, R groups protrude from the newly synthesized peptide chain and are in position to react with each other. Folding is accomplished through hydrogen bonding, ionic bonding, and hydrophobic and other interactions between individual R groups on each amino acid. For example, a negative charge on one amino acid R group forms an attraction with a positive charge on another. This allows the protein to form a precise three-dimensional structure. Proteins assume four levels of structure as diagrammed in Figure 3–10.

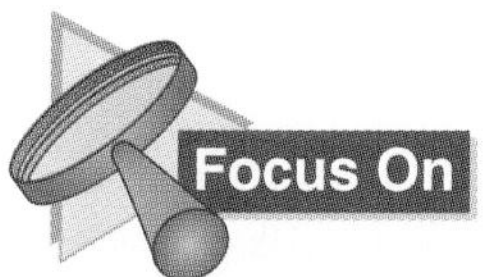

DNA Transcription and RNA Translation

DNA transcription occurs as follows:

1. All cells have the ability to make all proteins needed by the body. The linear sequence of each protein is dictated by the linear sequence of nucleotide bases, thymine, adenine, guanine, and cytosine. The linear sequence of three bases code for each of the 20 amino acids. Because four bases can be combined in 64 ways, more than one three-base codon can code for a single amino acid.
2. As they differentiate, cells inactivate codes for proteins. For example, only the red blood cell precursor makes hemoglobin.
3. In front of each coding region is a promoter region. The promoter region receives a signal that the protein is needed. Nutrients, including vitamins A and D, as well as minerals such as zinc, play major roles in regulating gene expression in the promoter region.
4. At the signal, RNA polymerase binds to the start code in the coding region, opens the double helix, and builds a new RNA chain the exact negative of the coding region.
5. When it reaches the end of the protein code, the stop code, the polymerase molecule detatches, releasing the completed RNA transcript. The DNA helix reforms and the RNA transcript is modified to remove introns (intervening sequences) not part of the protein coding pattern. The modified transcript is called messenger RNA (mRNA)
6. At the same time, in another region of the DNA, DNA polymerase molecules have made copies of ribosomal RNA (rRNA) and transfer RNA (tRNA).
7. mRNA, rRNA, and tRNA leave the nucleus and enter the cytoplasm.

RNA translation then follows these steps:

1. Small rRNA subunits are activated and bind mRNA.
2. Large rRNA subunits bind to hold the mRNA firmly. The mRNA is sandwiched between the two subunits with two three-base codons available for binding.
3. Each of 20 tRNA types binds the amino acid that matches its anti-codon region. The anti-codon recognizes and binds the mRNA codon. This ensures that linear amino acid sequence is an exact representation of the original DNA code.
4. The process continues. After each tRNA binds the A site, its amino acid is linked to the growing peptide chain by an enzyme, peptidyl transferase, which forms a peptide bond between the end carboxyl and the amino group of the incoming amino acid.
5. The ribosome moves forward; the tRNA now attached to the peptide chain is in the P site and another tRNA enters.
6. At the stop signal, UAG, a release factor, binds at the A site. It attaches a water molecule to the peptide chain, creating the carboxyl (COOH) terminus. The newly formed peptide chain detaches and the tRNA and rRNA units separate.

1. *Primary structure:* Peptide bonds are formed between sequential amino acids according to directions on mRNA. The completed protein is a linear chain of amino acids.
2. *Secondary structure:* Attractions between R groups of amino acids create helices and pleated sheet structures.
3. *Tertiary structure:* Helices and pleated sheets are folded into compact domains. Small proteins have one domain, large proteins have multiple domains.
4. *Quaternary structure:* Individual **polypeptides** can serve as subunits in the formation of larger assemblies or complexes. Subunits are bound together by a large number of weak noncovalent interactions; sometimes they are stabilized by disulfide bonds. For example, four hemoglobin monomers are joined to form the tetramer hemoglobin molecule.

Protein structure is critical for protein function. The active and catalytic sites at which protein action occurs are formed by juxtaposing functional groups from nearby and sometimes distant R groups. If the linear protein sequence is altered, as in certain genetic diseases, the protein is unable to form active sites and its activity is limited or eliminated entirely.

TABLE 3–12 ESTIMATES OF AMINO ACID REQUIREMENTS

	REQUIREMENTS (mg/kg/day) BY AGE GROUP			
AMINO ACID	Infants, Age 3–4 mo*	Children, Age ~2 yr†	Children, Age 10–12 yr‡	Adults§
Histidine	28	?	?	8–12
Isoleucine	70	31	28	10
Leucine	161	73	44	14
Lysine	103	64	44	12
Methionine plus cystine	58	27	22	13
Phenylalanine plus tyrosine	125	69	22	14
Threonine	87	37	28	7
Tryptophan	17	12.5	3.3	3.5
Valine	93	38	25	10
Total without histidine	714	352	216	84

Adapted, by permission from WHO. Energy and Protein Requirements Report of a Joint FAO/WHO/UNU Expert Consultation. Technical Report Series 724. Geneva: WHO, 1985, p. 65.

*Based on amounts of amino acids in human milk or cow's milk formulas fed at levels that supported good growth.

†Based on achievement of nitrogen balance sufficient to support adequate lean tissue gain (16 mg N/kg/day).

‡Based on upper range of requirement for positive nitrogen balance.

§Based on highest estimate of requirement to achieve nitrogen balance.

Dietary Protein Quality

As indicated above, proteins are formed on the basis of DNA instructions and use specific amino acids. Each organism makes only those proteins required to carry out the tasks required for its own uses. As a result, each source of dietary protein contains its own unique proportion of the 20 common amino acids (Table 3–12). Some organisms, especially plants, use uncommon amino acids that may cause trouble to human consumers (see below). Over 50 years ago, it was proposed that the nutritional quality of a protein depended on its amino acid profile and that the biologic value of a protein could be determined by the essential amino acid present in least concentration compared with human requirements (Block and Mitchel, 1946). This is the "most limiting amino acid" from which a "chemical score" of protein quality can be calculated.

Protein quality is also determined by measuring the amount of protein actually used by an organism. *Net protein utilization (NPU)* is the simplest method devised for this purpose. Dietary protein is equated with its metabolic products by measuring nitrogen (N) in the diet and biologic samples and converting it to the amount of protein on the basis of the formula [N (g) × 6.25 = protein (g)]. Nitrogen (N) content in the bodies of control animals is compared to N in the carcass of an experimental group fed a protein-free diet for the same length of time. The gain in N is compared with the N intake, and the proportion N retained in the body is computed to obtain the NPU. The NPU ranges from approximately 40 to 94, with protein from animal products near the top and that from vegetables near the lower end (Crim and Munro, 1994).

Soy protein originally received a low NPU until it was recognized that methionine, low in soy protein, is a limiting amino acid for the rat. Rats require approximately 50% more methionine than do humans (Sarwar et al., 1985). The WHO and the U.S. FDA adopted a corrected **protein digestibility corrected amino acid score** (PDCAAS) as the official assay for evaluating protein quality. The PDCAAS is based on amino acid requirements of children aged 2 to 5 years and represents the amino acid score after correcting for digestibility (Messina, 1995). Proteins that, after correcting for digestibility, provide amino acids equal to or in excess of requirements, receive a PDCAAS of 1.0. Soy protein has a PDCAAS of 1.0 and meets protein needs of human adults when consumed as a sole source of protein at the rate of 0.6 g/kg body weight (Young, 1991).

Protein Processing and Digestibility

The digestibility of protein sources is affected by multiple factors. Meat preparation procedures often use wine or vinegar marinade and moist heat to tenderize tough cuts of meat by the process of denaturation. Proteins are kept in proper configuration by hydrogen and ionic interactions; these bonds are loosened in the presence of acid, salt, and heat. By denaturing proteins these methods also soften gristle or connective tissue proteins and release muscle proteins from their attachments, thereby making all proteins more available to digestive enzymes.

Vegetable protein is less well digested than animal protein, partly because it is encased in carbohydrate cell walls and is less available. Some plants also contain enzymes that interfere with protein digestion. These enzymes must be heat inactivated before consumption. For example, soybeans contain a trypsinase that inactivates trypsin, the major protein digesting enzyme in the intestine.

Food processing can also damage amino acids and reduce their availability in the following ways (Crim, 1994). Mild heat treatment in the presence of reducing sugars (glucose and galactose), as in milk processing, causes loss of available lysine. Lactose reacts with lysine side chains and renders them unavailable. This reaction is called the "browning" or Maillard reaction and can cause significant lysine loss at high temperatures.

Under severe heating conditions in the presence of sugars or oxidized lipids, or even in their absence, all amino acids in food proteins become resistant to digestion. When protein is exposed to severe treatment with alkali, the amino acids lysine and cysteine can react together and form a potentially toxic lysinoalanine. Exposure to sulfur dioxide and other oxidative conditions can result in loss of methionine. Thermal processing and low-moisture storage of proteins can also result in reductive binding of vitamin B_6 to lysine residues, thereby inactivating the vitamin (Leklem, 1998).

Protein Complementarity

The chemical score for a plant protein is often very different from the needs of the human. Because certain amino acids are "limiting" in most plant foods, diets based on a single plant food staple do not foster optimal growth. Throughout history human cultures discovered traditional dishes that contain a mixture of vegetable proteins that compensated deficiencies with excesses and allowed the population to thrive. Protein complementarity was delineated by the book, *Diet for a Small Planet,* originally published by Lappe in 1971, and revised and republished in 1991. She describes a method to ensure that vegetable proteins with different chemical scores complement each other to provide complete proteins as indicated below:

EXCELLENT COMBINATIONS	EXAMPLES
Grains—legumes	rice/beans, pea soup/toast, lentil curry/rice
Grains—dairy	pasta/cheese, rice pudding, cheese sandwich
Legumes—seeds	garbanzo beans/sesame seeds as dip, falafel or soup

Other combinations, dairy—seeds, dairy—legumes, grains—seeds, are less effective because the chemical scores are similar and do not effectively complement.

In the 20th anniversary edition, Ms. Lappe has modified some of her concepts based on new information. Although it is not necessary to eat complementary proteins at the same meal, they should be eaten within 3 to 4 hours to ensure that all amino acids are available when needed. Most individuals, even those on a strict vegetarian diet, need not complement at all meals. Pregnant and nursing mothers should increase their protein intake more than energy intake.

As indicated above, the NPU of vegetable protein may not accurately reflect the available protein. If the diet is otherwise healthy and the overall protein intake above the minimal requirements, this is probably not of concern. Amino acid composition of some foods is found in Table 3–13.

Protein Utilization

Protein utilization in the body can best be understood as a black box. Dietary protein is digested and absorbed as discussed in Chapter 1. Products of protein digestion, di- and tripeptides and amino acids, as well as protein secreted into the gut lumen (enzymes, sloughed cells, etc.), are available for absorption and are transported in the portal vein to the liver. The liver can deaminate amino acids to carbohydrate or the amino acids can enter the amino acid pool. Homeostatic regulations control the concentrations of specific amino acids in the amino acid pool. Enzymes that destroy essential amino acids are inactive until concentration of their target reaches a specified "threshold." At that point, the activity of the catabolic enzyme rises, allowing the body to maintain essential amino acid concentrations at a constant level. Enzymes that destroy nonessential amino acids rise in direct proportion to the concentration of the specific amino acid. In this way the body carefully regulates the amino acid availability.

Body protein synthesis and breakdown (turnover) is regulated such that in health, the amount of protein taken in is exactly balanced by protein excreted in feces, urine, and skin. Protein balance studies have demonstrated the zero protein balance in health, the negative nitrogen balance in infection or trauma, and the positive balance in growth and pregnancy. Figure 3–11 shows the impact of a long-term high protein intake on children. Muscle mass is maintained in steady state with a fraction of muscle protein being destroyed and rebuilt daily using amino acids from the pool. Muscle mass can be measured as an index of somatic protein status.

Amino acids are also required for synthesis of visceral proteins by the liver and other tissues. Albumin, transferrin, retinol binding protein, and other serum proteins are measured to assess the capacity of the body to synthesize visceral proteins (see Chapter 17). Albumin and globulin are examples of *simple proteins* that yield only amino acids on hydrolysis.

TABLE 3–13 AMINO ACID COMPOSITION OF SOME FOODS

ESSENTIAL AMINO ACID	CHEESE, EGGS, MILK, AND MEAT	CORN	CEREAL	LEGUMES	WHOLE GRAINS (WITH GERM)	NUTS, SEED OILS, AND SOYBEANS	SESAME AND SUNFLOWER SEEDS	PEANUTS	GREEN LEAFY VEGETABLES	GELATIN	YEAST
Methionine			X	—	X	—	X	—	—	—	X
Isoleucine	X										
Leucine	X										
Lysine	X	—	—	X	X	X	—	—		—	
Phenylalanine											—
Threonine	X	—	—	X	—	X		—			X
Tryptophan		—		—			X			—	
Valine	X										

Adapted from Erhard D: Nutrition education for the "now" generation. J Nutr Educ 3:135, 1971.

X, high amount of amino acid present in that food; —, low amount of amino acid present in that food. Blank spaces indicate a general good balance of amino acids in the food.

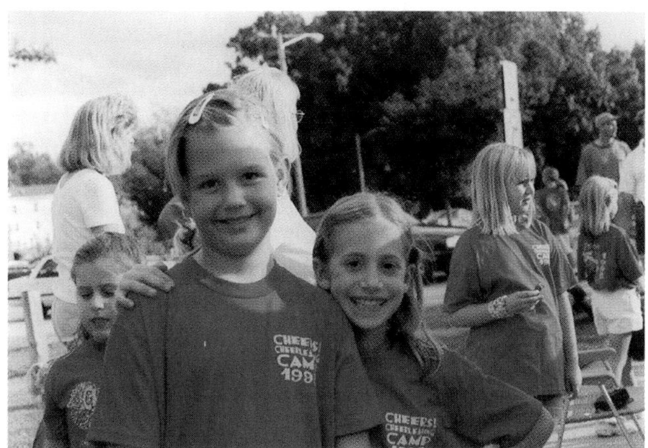

FIGURE 3–11 Both girls pictured are the same age. However, the child on the left consumed a high-protein diet over her lifetime. Genetics and protein consumption both impact overall height and growth rates.

Nitrogen Excretion: The Urea Cycle

Nitrogen in the form of ammonia (NH_3) is highly toxic, easily crosses biomembranes, and cannot be allowed to travel unbound throughout the body. In the fed state, pyruvate and other carbon skeletons take up nitrogen and transport it to the liver as nonessential amino acids, usually alanine and glutamic acid (from α-ketoglutarate). When the amino acids reach the liver, they are deaminated to carbohydrate. The ammonia ion is combined with carbon dioxide in the presence of high-energy phosphate and magnesium through action of the enzyme *carbamoyl phosphate synthase* to form the first intermediate of the **urea** cycle (see Chapter 44). Details of the urea cycle can be found in any biochemistry text.

Urea makes up 90% of urinary nitrogen in the fed state. Arginine, one of the basic amino acids pictured in Figure 3–8, is a by-product of the urea cycle. Recent research has found that arginine is required for formation of nitric oxide and other mediators of the inflammatory response (Abcouwer and Souba, 1998). Although classified as a nonessential amino acid, arginine may be essential for critically ill individuals, as discussed in Chapter 33.

Single Amino Acid Supplementation

Sulfur-containing amino acids, homocysteine, cysteine, methionine, and taurine concentrations are homeostatically regulated and are essential for growth and protein synthesis. Optimal regulatory pathways are dependent on adequate intake of micronutrients including folate, vitamin B_{12}, and vitamin B_6 (Stipanuk, 1998).

Conditionally essential nitrogen transporters include glutamine and arginine. Despite clear evidence that glutamine and arginine are nonessential amino acids and that their carbon skeletons are made in the body, evidence is accumulating that these nutrients are required in supraphysiologic amounts during the stress of exercise, surgery, trauma, sepsis, and other catabolic states. Abcouwer and Souba (1998) have reviewed current knowledge on metabolism and use of these amino acids in clinical patient management.

In summary, protein is essential for animal structure, routine housekeeping activities, fighting infections and other acute processes. Protein can also be used as an energy source, at 4 kcal/g, by removing the nitrogen and oxidizing the carbon skeleton. Protein consists of linear chains of amino acids linked precisely according to the dictates of protein coding regions in the DNA of all cells. Final protein configuration depends on interactions between the amino acid R groups. Genetic mutations that change the linear sequence of amino acids can change the final protein structure and drastically alter protein function, sometimes with lethal results. Dietary protein is digested and amino acids are absorbed and enter the circulating amino acid pool. This pool provides amino acids for synthesis of all body proteins. All body proteins are replaced at different rates; the net rate of protein turnover dictates the protein requirement for the individual. In the fed state, nitrogen is excreted from the body as urea.

MACRONUTRIENT UTILIZATION AND STORAGE IN THE FED STATE

Carbohydrate

As indicated in Chapter 1, absorbed carbohydrate is transported as plasma glucose in the portal vein. The cytoplasmic processes of glycolysis and mitochondrial oxidation of pyruvate to provide adenosine triphosphate (ATP) are described in detail in biochemistry texts. Briefly, glucose rise in the portal vein stimulates preformed insulin secretion from the pancreas. The liver is the first organ to receive portal blood glucose. The liver does not require insulin either to take up approximately 50% of absorbed glucose via receptors, or to phosphorylate glucose to glucose-6-phosphate, thereby retaining glucose in the cell. Insulin is required to enhance the oxidation of glucose in the cytosol through the glycolytic pathway. Insulin also stimulates *pyruvate dehydrogenase,* a thiamin-requiring mitochondrial enzyme that removes a carbon from pyruvate with the formation of acetate. Energy-rich bonds in the acetate molecule (bound to CoA) are broken, the energy transported to the oxidative phosphorylation enzymes on the inner mitochondrial membrane, and ATP is generated.

If carbohydrate intake is in excess of oxidative and storage capacity, the cell can convert carbohydrate to fat. Using a rat model of NIDDM, Kibir et al. (1998) studied the lipogenic effect of a diet with a high glycemic index (waxy starch, rich in amylopectin) compared with a diet with a low glycemic index (mung beans, high in amylose). Well-absorbed carbohydrate increased the synthesis of fatty acid synthase, an insulin-dependent enzyme that regulates fatty acid synthesis. The authors suggested that lipogenesis associated with diets of high glycemic index could eventually lead to hyperlipidemia and fat accumulation. Hirsch et al. (1996) also demonstrated lipogenesis on a low-fat diet in humans.

A high priority for cells is the storage of glucose for release into the blood in the fasting state. Glucose is stored as highly branched glycogen polymers. The cell adds glucose residues (as glucose-6-phosphate) to the growing end of preformed glycogen clusters. In the presence of insulin, glucose is added to the polymer in α 1–4 or α 1–6 linkage by the enzyme, *glycogen synthase.* Muscle glycogen is used within the muscle cell to provide ATP for muscle contraction. Its concentration within the muscle is dependent on the physical activity of the individual and can be greatly increased by physical training. Liver glycogen serves as a reservoir to provide a readily available supply of glucose to maintain blood glucose levels during the fasting state, as described below. A constant supply of blood glucose is especially important to maintain ATP production in the brain and central nervous system. Liver glycogen stores are dependent on food intake and are rapidly replenished with each meal.

Lipid Transport and Storage

Triglycerides from Gut to Adipocyte—Chylomicrons

Because they are fat soluble, lipids cannot be transported unbound through the aqueous media of the body. Lipid transport can best be understood as the conversion of water-insoluble lipids into water-soluble forms for transport and reversion to water-insoluble lipid esters once they have reached their cellular destination. Blood transport is accomplished by the formation of a variety of **lipoproteins,** fat encased in a coat of protein and phospholipid. Different lipoprotein types are characterized by their density, VLDL, LDL, and HDL, based on the relative proportions of fat, protein, and phospholipid they contain. Remember, fat floats on water because it is lighter (less dense) than water; thus, VLDL contains much more fat than HDL.

Absorbed fatty acids and **monoglycerides** are re-esterified into triglycerides within the mucosal cell and the fat-soluble center covered with a thin layer of protein. The protein component includes markers, apoproteins (apo) B, A, C, and E on the surface. The **chylomicron** contains only 2% protein, the rest is triglycerides (84%), cholesterol, and phospholipid. The lipid-rich particles leave the mucosal cell and travel through lymphatic channels to the thoracic duct that empties into the right side of the heart. Rapid blood flow in the heart prevents the large, lipid-rich chylomicrons from forming clumps and fat emboli. **Medium-chain fatty acids** are more water soluble and can be absorbed directly into the portal blood, thus bypassing the lymphatic system. Chylomicrons transport dietary fat and are usually found in serum only after meals. High concentrations of chylomicrons make the plasma appear milky after a high-fat meal.

Chylomicrons leave the heart through the aorta and are transported to the adipocyte (fat cell). An enzyme, *lipoprotein lipase* (LPL), is expressed on the membrane of endothelial cells lining capillaries in the region of the adipocytes and elsewhere. LPL is activated by membrane bound apo C to bind chylomicrons and cleave triglycerides, releasing fatty acids and monoglycerides that cross the fatty lipid membrane, enter the adipocyte, and become re-esterified to triglyceride for safe and hydrophobic storage. Note that insulin, the predominant hormone in the fed state, activates LDL and facilitates fat storage. The chylomicron remnant, relieved of some of its triglyceride content, is bound to liver receptors through its surface markers, apo B and apo E, and recycled. Chylomicrons also exchange cholesterol with other lipoproteins by means of apo A, and other markers.

Triglycerides from Liver to Adipocyte—Very Low-Density Lipoproteins

The liver receives fat from a number of sources: (1) from chylomicron remnants, (2) from circulating fatty acids (see below), (3) from uptake of intermediate lipoproteins (IDL) and other lipoproteins, and (4) from endogenous body synthesis. The liver re-esterifies fat from all sources and wraps it in a heavier coat of protein and phospholipid to form VLDL. This lipoprotein is relatively richer in cholesterol than the chylomicron, but still contains a large proportion of triglyceride. VLDL also contain apoproteins B, E, and C and pick up apo A as they circulate. In the fed state, large numbers of VLDL are formed and transported to the adipocyte where triglycerides are hydrolyzed, re-esterified, and stored. Even in the fasted state, VLDL are formed to carry endogenous lipids. It should be noted that insulin facilitates fat storage in many ways. It enhances fatty acid synthesis from carbohydrate in the liver and stimulates VLDL formation and secretion. Hyperinsulinemia, such as is found in the obese patient and the patient with NIDDM, is associated with hypertriglyceridemia (as VLDL) and excess fat storage (Reaven, 1995).

Cholesterol from Diet and Liver to All Cells—Low-Density Lipoproteins

All cells require cholesterol for their membranes. Cholesterol is substrate for steroid hormones including cortisone and estrogens; glands that produce steroid hormones require added cholesterol biosynthesis. The liver uses cholesterol for synthesis of bile acids. Dietary cholesterol is transported via chylomicrons and VLDL but is not removed by LPL activity. After LPL has cleaved additional triglyceride from VLDL, the "remnant" remaining is called an intermediate-density lipoprotein (IDL) if it is not entirely cleared of triglyceride. The LDL has been maximally cleaved of triglyceride. Although both can be taken up by the liver on receptors for apo B and apo E, all cells have LDL receptors that bind and take up these cholesterol-rich particles. The endocytic vesicle containing LDL is fused with a lysosome, thereby breaking it down to its component parts. The protein is recycled to the cellular amino acid pool and cholesterol is released for use by the cell. The extent to which each cell takes up LDL is regulated by the concentration of free cholesterol released from the LDL. Free cholesterol is inserted into the plasma membrane and stored as cholesterol ester for biosynthetic purposes. Free cholesterol regulates its own concentration by:

1. Downregulating cellular synthesis of the LDL receptor
2. Downregulating endogenous cholesterol synthesis

Cholesterol from Cells to the Liver and Excretion—High-Density Lipoproteins

The HDL facilitate cholesterol turnover by removing free cholesterol from cell membranes and scavenging cholesterol from other lipoproteins. HDL particles are formed in the liver as a protein–phospholipid disk. They circulate in the bloodstream, accumulating free cholesterol, which they esterify with fatty acid from their phosphatidylcholine (lecithin) phospholipid structure. The ability of HDL to function as a cholesterol transporter is dependent on the activity of its copper-dependent enzyme, *lecithin-cholesterol acyltransferase* to esterify cholesterol and store it in its hydrophobic center. When it has accumulated sufficient lipid to become spherical, HDL is taken up by the liver and recycled. Cholesterol is used for bile acid synthesis, stored in subcutaneous tissue where it can be formed into vitamin D, or secreted as VLDL.

Oxidized Lipid to Macrophages—Low-Density Lipoprotein Scavenger Pathway

Abundant evidence now supports the role of the macrophage (large cell that eats) in the pathogenesis of atherosclerosis (Chisolm and Penn, 1996) and discussed in subsequent chapters. Macrophages are distributed throughout the body and play a major role in immune defense. They also inhabit the subendothelial region of the arteries where they provide surveillance against foreign and microbial agents in the blood. Although macrophages do not recognize and ingest normal lipoproteins, they do recognize, possibly as foreign, lipoproteins in which the fat has been oxidized. Macrophages do ingest oxidized LDL and accumulate fat within their cytoplasm, giving them a foamy appearance, hence the name, foam cells. Ingestion activates the macrophage and triggers multiple cascades, some of which lead to atherosclerosis. Some macrophage signals include:

- Release of mediators to call more macrophages to the area—*chemotaxis*
- Release of growth factors that stimulate endothelial cells to proliferate—*mitogenesis*
- Stimulation of smooth muscle cells to proliferate and become fibroblast-like, releasing collagen and other connective tissue proteins

As a result, the vessel wall becomes thickened and fibrotic with raised plaques formed from proliferating smooth muscle cells and foam cells stuffed with lipid. When the thickened plaque prevents nutrient delivery, cells die and release their contents into the plaque, cholesterol crystallizes into sharp cholesterol shards, and the lumen of the vessel is compromised.

MACRONUTRIENT CATABOLISM FROM BODY STORES IN THE FASTED STATE

Starvation, meaning the absolute deprivation of food, leads to *marasmus.* It is at one end of the continuum of *protein-energy* (protein-calorie) *malnutrition.* At the opposite end is protein deprivation in the presence of carbohydrate intake. This condition is called *kwashiorkor,* from an African word meaning the disease that affects the first child after the second is born. The disease occurs when the first child is weaned from protein-rich mother's milk onto a protein-poor carbohydrate food source. Symptoms of protein-calorie malnutrition are observed at multiple points on the spectrum, hence the term, *marasmic kwashiorkor.*

The body has remarkable ability to withstand food deprivation. A series of adaptive changes allow access to stored macronutrients to provide for daily housekeeping activities of the body. Adaptation to starvation has evolutionary advantage because it allowed primitive peoples to undergo cycles of feast and famine.

Adapted Starvation—Marasmus

In the fasted state, and in the absence of insulin, catabolic hormones epinephrine, thyroxine, and glucagon suppress glycogen synthase and activate the enzyme, *glycogen phosphorylase.* The enzyme adds a phosphate to the last glycosidic linkage of glycogen, releasing one unit of glucose-1-phosphate. Glucose-1-phosphate is converted to glucose-6-phosphate and then to glucose by the liver enzyme, *glucose-6-phosphatase.* Note that only the liver expresses this enzyme and only the liver can release free glucose into the bloodstream. Muscles and other tissues do not express glucose-6-phosphatase and are unable to release free glucose. These tissues use glycogen to provide glucose for their own needs. Muscles can release pyruvate and lactate into the bloodstream. These metabolic products return to the liver and are resynthesized to glucose by the Cori cycle, discussed above. Note that glycogen is never totally depleted even with long-term starvation. A small amount of preformed glycogen is carefully guarded as a primer for glycogen resynthesis.

Because glucose is a required nutrient for the brain and nervous system, as well as red blood cells, white blood cells, and other glucose-requiring tissues, blood glucose must be maintained at all times. Because glycogen stores last only about 24 hours, glucose must be synthesized de novo using protein as a substrate. Muscle and other proteins are broken down. Released amino acids are transported to the liver for deamination and the carbon skeleton is used to remake glucose. This process is called *gluconeogenesis.* The most common amino acid substrate for this activity is alanine; deaminated alanine is pyruvate. Gluconeogenesis is not simply the reverse of glycolysis, but requires separate enzymes to reverse the irreversible enzymes of glycolysis, as detailed in any biochemistry text. It is important to note that fat is not a substrate for gluconeogenesis. Fat is released as an energy source during fasting and is used by muscles, including the heart muscle, to make ATP.

Protein from muscle breakdown and fat released from the adipocyte are both available as macronutrient energy sources during fasting. Release of these stored nutrients requires that insulin be kept low and that anti-insulin hormones, glucagon, cortisone, epinephrine and growth hormone, be increased. Anti-insulin hormones activate hormone-sensitive lipase enzyme on the adipocyte membrane; the enzyme cleaves stored triglycerides, releasing fatty acid and glycerol from the fat cell. Fatty acids travel to the liver bound to serum albumin and easily enter the liver cell. Fatty acids can not enter the liver mitochondria for use as an energy source unless they are bound to carnitine. Via the transport system, carnitine acyltransferase, fatty acid carnitine esters, can cross the mitochondrial membrane. Once inside the mitochondria, two carbon (acetate) segments are sequentially cleaved from long-chain fatty acids via the process of beta oxidation. Acetate is bound to coenzyme A to form acetyl CoA, and oxidized through the citric acid cycle. Excess acetyl CoA molecules not required for hepatocyte use are joined to form 4-carbon, energy-rich fragments called ketones.

Adaptation to starvation depends on ketone production. As the blood ketone level rises during fasting, the brain and nervous system, consumers of 80% of blood glucose, begin to use ketones as an energy source. Because the brain now has an alternative fuel to glucose, the demand on muscle protein for gluconeogenesis declines, thereby reducing the rate of muscle catabolism. Reduced muscle catabolism reduces the amount of ammonia received by the liver. Liver synthesis of urea falls precipitously, reflecting a slower rate of muscle protein deamination. As the fast extends through weeks, the rate of urea synthesis and excretion is minimized. In an adapted organism, urea is excreted at approximately the same rate as uric acid produced by the kidney.

Thus, in the individual "adapted" to starvation, protein losses are minimized and lean body mass spared. Although fat cannot be made into glucose, fat does provide fuel for the muscle and brain in the form of ketones. As long as water is available, the normal weight individual can fast for a month or two with no ill effects. Relatively normal nutritional indices, immune function, and other systems are maintained. When fat stores are exhausted, protein is used and the patient dies.

Nonadapted Starvation—Trauma and Sepsis

If the fasted individual develops an infection, inflammatory mediators such as interleukin-1 and tumor necrosis factor stimulate insulin secretion and prevent the development of mild ketosis. Without ketones, brain and other tissues require glucose, thereby limiting "adaption" to starvation. Muscle mass is eroded to provide glucose. The person with an infection rapidly develops negative nitrogen balance. When 50% of the protein stores are exhausted, the ability to recover is very poor and the patient dies because the respiratory muscles cannot support breathing.

Nonadapted Starvation—Kwashiorkor

Adaption to starvation is not possible in kwashiorkor because carbohydrate intake stimulates insulin production. Insulin is a storage hormone and prevents fat stores from being accessed for fuel. It also inhibits fat from being formed into ketones, thereby limiting adaption to starvation. In the presence of insulin, muscle breakdown is inhibited. Protein cannot be used to make albumin and other visceral proteins. Edema results because albumin exerts osmotic pressure in the vessels. If albumin concentration is low, fluid remains in the extracellular spaces and is clinically seen as edema. Compromised neural function and gastrointestinal absorption, decreased cardiac output, immune function, fatigue, and other symptoms of protein-calorie malnutrition result from inadequate protein synthesis, inadequate ATP production, and fluid accumulation in the tissues.

Nonadapted protein-calorie malnutrition is dangerous. Not only can unremitting protein loss become life threatening by compromising muscles of

CASE STUDY

Joe K. is a 38-year-old black man who recently began to increase his fiber intake at the recommendation of his physician because he has hyperlipidemia and is 50 lbs. overweight. From a diet history taken at your office, you have determined that Joe normally consumed 15 g of fiber per day prior to this change. He is now consuming 45 g on an average day. He is complaining about increased gas and flatulence from this change in his routine.

1. What changes would you suggest to Joe at this time about fiber intake? About fat intake?
2. What types and amounts of fiber would you recommend if Joe began to show signs of carbohydrate intolerance?
3. Calculate the fiber and protein content of your own diet for 3 days. How many grams of fiber did you eat? What foods would you add to your diet to change your intake to the recommended intake of 25 to 35 g daily? How much protein did you eat?
4. Joe's wife asks you about the benefits of a vegetarian diet. What suggestions will you make about proteins?

the heart and respiratory system, it can compromise the immune system. By limiting host defense, it makes the individual susceptible to a vicious cycle of infections, diarrhea, more nutrient loss, further compromised defense, and finally, opportunistic infections and death. Iatrogenic or "physician-induced" malnutrition was recognized early on as a danger in hospitalized patients (Butterworth, 1974). It remains so to this day (Souba and Wilmore, 1998).

In summary, macronutrients in the food supply are present in a vast variety of form and quality. Biologic organisms have a remarkable ability to utilize a wide diversity of plant and animal foods for growth and maintenance. If the organism is deprived of food, alternate adaptive mechanisms parcel stored macronutrients to maintain body integrity. When adaption mechanisms are compromised, serious disease and death can result.

REFERENCES

Abcouwer SF, Souba WW. Glutamine and arginine. In: Shils ME, et al. (eds.). Modern Nutrition in Health and Disease, 9th ed. Baltimore: Williams & Wilkins, 1998.

Alberts B, et al. Membrane structure (Chapter 11); Energy conversion, mitochondria and chloroplasts (Chapter 14). In: Molecular biology of the cell. New York: Garland, 1995.

American Dietetic Association. Position of the American Dietetic Association: Fat replacers. J Am Diet Assoc 98: 463, 1998.

Bergman CJ, et al. Mineral binding capacity of dephytinized insoluble fiber from extruded wheat, oat and rice brans. Plant Foods Hum Nutr 51:295, 1997.

Block RJ, Mitchel HH. Nutr Abstr Rev 16:249, 1946.

Brand Miller J. The importance of glycemic index in diabetes. Am J Clin Nutr 59:747S, 1994.

Bronsgeest-Schoute DC, et al. Dependence of the effects of dietary cholesterol and experimental conditions on serum lipids in man. III. The effects on serum cholesterol of removal of eggs from the diet of free-living, habitually egg-eating people. Am J Clin Nutr 32:2193, 1979.

Butterworth CE. The skeleton in the hospital closet. Nutrition 10:435, 1974.

Calvert RJ, Satchithanandam S. Effects of graded levels of high-molecular-weight carrageenan on colonic mucosal thymidine kinase activity. Nutrition 8:252, 1992.

Chisolm GM III, Penn MS, Oxidized lipoproteins and atherosclerosis. In: Fuster V, et al. (eds). Atherosclerosis and Coronary Artery Disease. Philadelphia: Lippincott-Raven, 1996.

Clydesdale FM. Olestra: The approval process in letter and spirit. Food Technol 51:104, 1997.

Cohen C, et al. Insulin response and glycemic effects of meals in non-insulin-dependent diabetes. Am J Clin Nutr 52:519, 1990.

Compher C, et al. Dietary fiber and its clinical applications to enteral nutrition. In: Rombeau JL, Rolandelli RH (eds). Enteral and Tube Feeding, 3rd ed. Philadelphia: Saunders, 1997.

Connor WE, et al. Essential fatty acids: The importance of n-3 fatty acids in the retinal and brain. Nutr Rev 50:21, 1992.

Connor SL, Connor WE. Are fish oils beneficial in the prevention and treatment of coronary artery disease? Am J Clin Nutr 66 (4suppl): 1020S, 1997.

Coudray C, et al. Effect of soluble or partly soluble dietary fibres supplementation on absorption and balance of calcium, magnesium, iron and zinc in healthy young men. Eur J Clin Nutr 51:375, 1997.

Couzy F, et al. Effect of dietary phytic acid on zinc absorption in the healthy elderly, as assessed by serum concentration curve tests. Br J Nutr 80:177, 1998.

Crawford MA. The role of dietary fatty acids in biology: Their place in the evolution of the human brain. Nutr Rev 50:3, 1992.

Crim MC, Munro HN. Proteins and amino acids. In: Shils ME, et al. (eds.). Modern Nutrition in Health and Disease. Philadelphia: Lea & Febiger, 1994.

Daly ME, et al. Dietary carbohydrates and insulin sensitivity: A review of the evidence and clinical implications. Am J Clin Nutr 66:1972, 1997.

Deuchi K, et al. Continuous and massive intake of chitosan affects mineral and fat-soluble vitamin status in rats fed on a high-fat diet. Biosci Biotechnol Biochem 59:1211, 1995.

Evans LV. Mucilaginous substances from macroalgae: An overview. Symp Soc Exp Biol 43:455, 1989.

Farrell DJ. Enrichment of hen eggs with n-3 long chain fatty acids and evaluation of enriched eggs in humans. Am J Clin Nutr 68:538, 1998.

Foster-Powell K, Brand Miller J. International tables of glycemic index. Am J Clin Nutr 62:871S, 1995.

Garg A. Efficacy of dietary fiber in lowering serum cholesterol. Am J Med 97:501, 1994.

Gershoff SN. Nutrition evaluation of dietary fat substitutes. Nutr Rev 53:305, 1995.

Grootveld M, et al. In vivo absorption, metabolism and urinary excretion of a,b-unsaturated aldehydes in experimental animals: Relevance to the development of cardiovascular diseases by the dietary ingestion of thermally stressed polyunsaturate-rich culinary oils. J Clin Invest 101:1210, 1998.

Harris PJ, et al. The effects of soluble-fiber polysaccharides on the adsorption of a hydrophobic carcinogen to an insoluble dietary fiber. Nutr Cancer 19:43, 1993.

Hegsted DM. Serum-cholesterol response to dietary cholesterol: A re-evaluation. Am J Clin Nutr 44:299, 1986.

Hidaka H, et al. Effects of fructooligosaccharides on intestinal flora and human health. Bifidobacteria Microflora 5:37, 1986.

Jacobson MF. Eater's Digest: The Consumer's Factbook of Food Additives. New York: Doubleday Anchor Books, 1972.

Jenkins DJA, et al. Glycemic index of foods: A physiological basis for carbohydrate exchange. Am J Clin Nutr 34:362, 1981.

Jenkens DJA, et al. Metabolic effects of a low glycemic index diet. Am J Clin Nutr 46:968, 1987.

Jenkins DJA, et al. Specific types of colonic fermentation may raise low-density lipoprotein cholesterol concentrations. Am J Clin Nutr 54:141, 1991.

Jenkins DJA, et al. Diet factors affecting nutrient absorption and metabolism. In: Shils ME, et al. (eds). Modern Nutrition in Health and Disease, 8th ed. Philadelphia: Lea & Febiger, 1994.

Katan MB, Mensink RP. Isomeric fatty acids and serum lipoproteins. Nutr Rev 50:46, 1992.

Kibir M, et al. A high glycemic index starch diet affects lipid storage-related enzymes in normal, and to a lesser extent in diabetic rats. J Nutr 128:1878, 1998.

Kiens B, Richter EA. Types of carbohydrate in an ordinary diet affect insulin action and muscle substrates in humans. Am J Clin Nutr 63:47, 1996.

Krauss RM, et al. Dietary guidelines for healthy American adults: A statement for health professionals from the Nutrition Committee, American Heart Association. Circulation 94:1795, 1996.

Krishnan S, et al. The ability of enteric diarrheal pathogens to ferment starch to short chain fatty acids in vitro. Scand J Gastroenterol 33:242, 1998.

Lappe FM. Diet for a Small Planet. New York: Ballantine Books, 1971 and 1991.

Leklem JE. Vitamin B_6. In: Shils ME, et al. (eds.). Modern Nutrition in Health and Disease, 9th ed. Baltimore: Williams & Wilkins, 1998.

Lichtenstein AH. Trans fatty acids and hydrogenated fat—What do we know? Nutrition Today 30:102, 1995.
Linscheer WG, Vergroesen AJ. Lipids. In: Shils ME, et al. (eds.). Modern Nutrition in Health and Disease, 8th ed. Philadelphia: Lea & Febiger, 1994.
Luo J, et al. Chronic consumption of short-chain fructooligosaccharides by healthy subjects decreased basal hepatic glucose production but had no effect on insulin-stimulated glucose metabolism. Am J Clin Nutr 63:939, 1996.
Marcus SN, et al. The pre-ulcerative phase of carrageenan-induced colonic ulceration in the guinea-pig. Int J Exp Pathol 73:515, 1992.
McCarron DA. Dietary patterns and blood pressure, N Engl J Med 337:637, 1997.
Meng AS, et al. Butyrate inhibits colon carcinoma cell growth through two distinct pathways. Surgery 124:248, 1998.
Messina M. Modern applications for an ancient bean: Soybeans and the prevention and treatment of chronic disease. J Nutr 125:567S, 1995.
Molteni A, et al. In vitro hormonal effects of soybean isoflavones. J Nutr 125:751S, 1995.
National Institutes of Health Concensus Conference. Coronary heart disease. JAMA 209:505, 1993.
Ormrod DJ, et al. Dietary chitosan inhibits hypercholesterolemia and atherogenesis in the apolipoprotein E-deficient mouse model of atherosclerosis. Atherosclerosis 138:329, 1998.
Persky V, Van Horn L. Epidemiology of soy and cancer: Perspectives and directions. J Nutr 125:709S, 1995.
Reaven GM. Pathophysiology of insulin resistance in human disease. Physiol Rev 75:473, 1995.
Roberfroid M, et al. The biochemistry of oligofructose, a nondigestible fiber: An approach to calculate its caloric value. Nutr Rev 51:137, 1993.
Salas J, et al. The SstI polymorphism of the apolipoprotein C-III gene determines the insulin response to an oral-glucose-tolerance test after consumption of a diet rich in saturated fats. Am J Clin Nutr 68:396, 1998.
Sarwar G, et al. Corrected relative net protein ratio (CRNPR) method based on differences in rats and human requirements for sulfur amino acids. J Am Oil Chem Soc 68:689, 1985.
Schneeman BO, Tietyen J. Dietary fiber. In: Shils ME, et al. (eds.). Modern Nutrition in Health and Disease, 8th ed. Philadelphia: Lea & Febiger, 1994, pp 89–100.
Shiau SY, Yu YP. Chitin but not chitosan supplementation enhances growth of grass shrimp, *Penaeus monodon.* J Nutr 128:908, 1998.
Simopoulos AP. Is insulin resistance influenced by dietary linoleic acid and trans fatty acids? Free Radic Biol Med 17:367, 1994.
Smith EL, et al. The carbohydrates. In: Principles of biochemistry. 7th ed. New York: McGraw-Hill, 1978.
Souba WW, Wilmore D. Diet and nutrition in the care of the patient with surgery, trauma and sepsis. In: Shils ME, et al. (eds.). Modern Nutrition in Health and Disease, 9th ed. Baltimore: Williams & Wilkins, 1998.
Spiegel S, et al. Safety and benefits of fructooligosaccharides as food ingredients. Food Technology, 48:85, 1994.
Stevens LJ, et al. Essential fatty acid metabolism in boys with attention-deficit hyperactivity disorder. Am J Clin Nutr 62:761, 1995.
Stipanuk MH. Homocysteine, cysteine and taurine. In: Shils ME, et al. (eds.). Modern Nutrition in Health and Disease, 9th ed. Baltimore: Williams & Wilkins, 1999.
Sugawara I, et al. Carrageenans, highly sulfated polysaccharides and macrophage-toxic agents: Newly found human T-lymphocyte mitogens. Immunobiology 163:527, 1982.
Tobacman JK: Filament disassembly and loss of mammary myoepithelial cells after exposure to lambda-carrageenan. Cancer Res 57:2823, 1997.
Trautwein EA, et al. Dietary inulin lowers plasma cholesterol and triacylglycerol and alters bile acid profile in hamsters. J Nutr 128:1937, 1998.
Vorster HH, et al. Egg intake does not change plasma lipoprotein and coagulation profiles. Am J Clin Nutr 55:400, 1992.
Young VR. Soy protein in relation to human protein and amino acid nutrition. J Am Diet Assoc 91:828, 1991.

ADDITIONAL REFERENCES

Asp N-G. Carbohydrates in human nutrition: The importance of food choice, especially the high carbohydrate diet. Am J Clin Nutr 59(S3): 679, 1994.
Bolton-Smith C, et al. Evidence for age-related differences in the fatty acid composition of human adipose tissue, independent of diet. Eur J Clin Nutr 51:619, 1997.
Canty DJ, Zeisel SH. Lecithin and choline in human health and disease. Nutr Rev 52:327, 1994,
Dudrick PS, Souba WW. Special fuels in parenteral nutrition. In: Rombeau JL, Caldwell MD (eds). Parenteral Nutrition, 2nd ed. Philadelphia: Saunders, 1993.
Gerrits P, Tsalikian E. Diabetes and fructose metabolism. Am J Clin Nutr 58(S):796S, 1993.
Hunt JR, et al. Zinc absorption, mineral balance, and blood lipids in women consuming controlled lactoovovegetarian and omnivorous diets for 8 wk. Am J Clin Nutr 67:421, 1998.
James MJ, et al. Simple relationships exist between dietary linoleate and the n-6 fatty acids of human neutrophils and plasma. Am J Clin Nutr 58:497, 1993.
Katan MB. Impact of low-fat diets on plasma high-density lipoprotein concentrations. Am J Clin Nutr 67(S):573S, 1998.
Mantzioris E, et al. Dietary substitution with α-linolenic acid-rich vegetable oil increases eicosapentaenoic acid concentrations in tissues. Am J Clin Nutr 59:1304, 1994.
O'Dell B. Fructose and mineral metabolism. Am J Clin Nutr 58(S):771S, 1993.
Potter J, et al. Colon cancer: A review of the epidemiology. Epidemiol Rev 15:499, 1993.
Sarkkinen ES, et al. Fatty acid composition of serum cholesterol esters, and erythrocyte and platelet membranes as indicators of long-term adherence to fat-modified diets. Am J Clin Nutr 59:364, 1994.
Torun B, Chew F. Protein-energy malnutrition. In Shils ME, et al. (eds.). Modern Nutrition in Health and Disease, 8th ed. Philadelphia: Lea & Febiger, 1994.
Warshaw HS, et al. Ingredients that replace fat: Their role in today's foods and challenges in educating people with diabetes. The Diabetes Educator 19:419, 1993.

CHAPTER 4

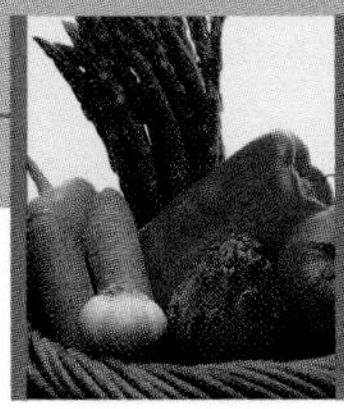

Vitamins

GERALD F. COMBS, JR., PHD

CHAPTER OUTLINE

- What Is a Vitamin?
- Chemical and Physical Properties of the Vitamins
- The Fat-Soluble Vitamins
- The Water-Soluble Vitamins
- Other Vitamin-Like Factors

Key Terms

ANTIOXIDANT—a substance that can inhibit reactions of free radicals such as reactive species of oxygen; used to describe vitamins C and E, some carotenoids, ubiquinones, and bioflavonoids

ASCORBIC ACID—a water-soluble vitamin, vitamin C, that plays essential roles in mineral metabolism and intracellular antioxidant functions; it is biosynthesized from glucose by most nonprimate species

BERIBERI—a neuropathy due to thiamin deficiency

BIOFLAVONOIDS—a group of vitamin-like substances found in plants and that have antioxidant activities

BIOTIN—a sulfur-containing vitamin synthesized by microorganisms in the lower gastrointestinal tract

CALCITRIOL—hormonally active form of vitamin D produced by the kidney; 1,25-dihydroxycholecalciferol (1,25-$[OH]_2D_3$)

CARNITINE—a vitamin-like factor that is essential for the oxidation of fatty acids; it can be biosynthesized from the amino acid lysine

CAROTENES—yellow or red pigments found in carrots, sweet potatoes, leafy vegetables, milk fat, and egg yolk, which can be converted into vitamin A (retinol) in the body

CHOLECALCIFEROL—the form of the fat-soluble vitamin D_3, produced when 7-dehydrocholesterol in the skin is photolysed by ultraviolet irradiation

CHOLINE—a metabolic precursor of the key structural element of membranes, phosphatidylcholine, and the neurotransmitter, acetylcholine; considered a B-complex vitamin for some species, but can be synthesized by humans

COBALAMIN—a B-complex vitamin, vitamin B_{12}, that has essential roles in the metabolism of single-carbon units and propionate

COENZYME Q_{10}—a ubiquinone that has redox properties, enabling it to function as a fat-soluble antioxidant

CYANOCOBALAMIN—the commercially available form of vitamin B_{12}

7-DEHYDROCHOLESTEROL—a precursor of vitamin D_3 found in the epidermal layer of the skin that on exposure to ultraviolet radiation becomes D_3

ERGOCALCIFEROL—a form of vitamin D (vitamin D_2) produced from the ultraviolet irradiation of the plant sterol ergosterol

FOLATE (FOLACIN)—a general term for those compounds with the metabolic activity of the B vitamin, folic acid

FOLIC ACID—a specific folic acid vitamer, pteroylglutamic acid

HYPERCAROTENODERMIA—accumulation of cartenoids in the skin with consequent yellowing

MENADIONE—a fat-soluble synthetic form of vitamin K

MENAQUINONE—a form of vitamin K produced by bacteria in the lower intestinal tract; a predominant form of vitamin K in animal tissue

***myo*-INOSITOL**—a vitamin-like factor that plays important metabolic roles as a constituent of phospholipids and a mediator of cellular responses to external stimuli; it is biosynthesized from glucose

NIACIN—vitamin B_3, the general term for the antipellagra vitamers, nicotinamide (also niacinamide) and nicotinic acid, that play essential roles as cofactors for numerous enzymes involved in the metabolism of carbohydrates, protein, and energy

NICOTINAMIDE—an amide of niacin lacking its vasodilatory activity

NIGHT BLINDNESS—impaired dark adaptation caused by loss of visual pigments due to vitamin A deficiency; also called nyctalopia

PANTOTHENIC ACID—a B-complex vitamin that plays essential roles in the synthesis and oxidation of fatty acids

PELLAGRA—a dermatitis caused by niacin deficiency in humans

PHYLLOQUINONE—the form of vitamin K produced by plants; a form of vitamin K found in animal tissue

PROVITAMIN—a dietary precursor to an active form of a vitamin

PYRIDOXINE—a B-complex vitamin, vitamin B_6, that plays essential roles in the metabolism of amino acids

PYRROLOQUINOLINE QUINONE—a vitamin-like factor that is thought to be involved in certain cellular oxidation-reduction reactions

RETINOL—a form of the antixerophthalmic vitamin, vitamin A, that is essential to the visual process as well as cell differentiation

RETINOL EQUIVALENT—a of measure of the vitamin A activity in foods

RIBOFLAVIN—a B-complex vitamin, vitamin B_2, that plays essential roles as cofactors of enzymes involved in many cell oxidation-reduction reactions
RICKETS—a disease of infants and young animals characterized by impaired mineralization of growing bone caused by deficiencies of vitamin D, calcium, or phosphorus
SCURVY—a disease characterized by impaired maturation of connective tissues caused by a deficiency of vitamin C
THIAMIN—a B-complex vitamin, vitamin B_1, that plays an essential role as a cofactor of enzymes involved in certain dehydrogenase and transketolase reactions
TOCOPHEROL—a form of the fat-soluble antioxidant vitamin, vitamin E
TRYPTOPHAN—an amino acid that serves as the metabolic precursor of niacin
UBIQUINONES—vitamin-like metabolites that play essential roles, as coenzyme Q_{10} in respiratory energy metabolism, and have antioxidant functions that may spare vitamin E in cells
VITAMER—one of multiple forms (all isomers and active analogues) of a vitamin
VITAMIN—an organic compound, essential in very small amounts in supporting normal physiologic function, that cannot generally be biosynthesized at rates equivalent to the needs of the body
VITAMIN K—a fat-soluble vitamin that plays essential roles in the biosynthesis of several proteins involved in blood clotting and bone mineralization
XEROPHTHALMIA—a disease, characterized by dryness leading to ulceration of the cornea, caused by deficiency of vitamin A

WHAT IS A VITAMIN?

The vitamin concept is relatively new compared to other nutrients such as protein or fat. Its emergence marked the birth of the field of nutrition as a science barely 100 years ago. For centuries it had been known that certain diseases were related to diet: scurvy could be prevented by eating green vegetables or fruits; night blindness could be treated with liver; beriberi was associated with the heavy dependence on polished rice as the major food; pellagra was associated with eating spoiled corn; and, with the industrial revolution in northern Europe, rickets came to be associated with low sunlight exposure and insufficient intakes of "good fats." Unfortunately, much of this knowledge was not appreciated by a medical community galvanized by the germ theory of disease that emerged in the 19th century. Therefore, by the turn of the last century, it was widely held that scurvy, beriberi, and rickets were each caused by a bacterium or bacterial toxin rather than by the simple absence of something required for good health.

Thus, the discovery by Christian Eijkman of a water-extractable factor in rice polishings that could prevent beriberi challenged the very dominance of the germ theory. Published in 1906, his was the first elaboration of the concept of an essential *micronutrient* at a time when good nutrition was thought to involve only protein, fats, carbohydrates, and minerals. Although Eijkman's discovery was associated with preventing certain clinical signs, it quickly became associated with the "accessory factors" that had emerged from bacteriology and that were used to describe the growth-promoting activities of certain foods for animals fed semipurified diets.

The new paradigm for nutrition was inaugurated by Funk who found Eijkman's antiberiberi factor to be an amine. In reference to its importance for life, Funk, in 1912 called it a "vital amine" "vitamine," proposing the existence of four (antiberiberi, antiscurvy, antirickets, antipellagra) such "vitamines." That not all of these subsequently proved to be amines (hence, the change to "vitamin") is less important than is the revolutionary concept that the term introduced. The new paradigm fostered research that, over the brief span of only five decades, produced fundamental understandings of the identities and functions of more than a dozen vitamins as well as many essential inorganic elements.

The term **vitamin** has come to describe a group of essential micronutrients that generally satisfy the following criteria.

- An organic *compound* distinct from fats, carbohydrates, and proteins
- A *natural component of foods* where it is usually present in minute amounts
- *Not synthesized by the host* in amounts adequate to meet normal physiologic needs
- Essential, also usually in minute amounts, for *normal physiologic function* (i.e., maintenance, growth, development, reproduction)
- By its absence or underutilization, causes a *specific deficiency syndrome*

This definition distinguishes this class of nutrients from proteins and amino acids, essential fatty acids, and essential inorganic elements. It points out the specificity of deficiency syndromes by which the vitamins were discovered. It places the vitamins in that portion of the chemical environment on which animals (including humans) must depend for survival, thus distinguishing them from hormones.

Despite its usefulness, this operating definition has limitations, as many species can, indeed, synthesize at least some of the vitamins. For example, most species (except those lacking the enzyme L-gulonolactone oxidase) can synthesize ascorbic acid; most species can synthesize choline and at least some niacin; and individuals exposed to modest amounts of sunlight can produce adequate amounts of vitamin D. Thus, the definition of a vitamin should be understood as having specific connotations to animal species, stage of development, diet or nutritional status, and physical environmental conditions.

The vitamins show few close chemical or functional similarities. Although several vitamins function as enzyme cofactors (vitamins A, K, and C, thiamin, niacin, riboflavin, vitamin B_6, biotin, pantothenic acid, folate, vitamin B_{12}), not all enzyme cofactors are vitamins. Some vitamins function as biologic antioxidants (vitamins E and C) and several function as cofactors in metabolic oxidation-reduction reactions (vitamins E, K, and C, niacin, riboflavin, pantothenic acid). Vitamins A and D are now recognized as functioning as hormones; vitamin A also serves as a photoreceptive cofactor in vision.

The nomenclature of the vitamins is in some cases rather complicated, reflecting both the terminology that evolved nonsystematically during the course of discovery, as well as more recent efforts to standardize vocabulary. The 13 families of vitamins comprise two to three times that number of important vitamers. **Vitamers** are the multiple forms (all isomers and active analogues) of vitamins. Vitamers function in metabolism in four general (and not mutually exclusive) ways: (1) as membrane stabilizers; (2) as hydrogen (H+) and electron (e-) donors and acceptors; (3) as hormones; and (4) as coenzymes. The type of metabolic function of a particular vitamer depends on its tissue/cellular distribution and its chemical activity, both of which are direct or indirect functions of its chemical structure (Combs, 1998) (Table 4–1).

CHEMICAL AND PHYSICAL PROPERTIES OF THE VITAMINS

The vitamins are usually classified into two groups, based on their solubilities. Some are soluble in nonpolar solvents: vitamins A, D, E, and K; others are soluble in polar solvents ("water soluble"): vitamin C, thiamin, riboflavin, niacin, vitamin B_6, biotin, pantothenic acid, folate, and vitamin B_{12}. Each of the former, "fat-soluble" vitamins, is comprised of five-carbon isopentyl units derived initially from acetyl coenzyme A (CoA). Vitamin functions are determined by their chemical and associated physical properties.

The enteric absorption of the fat-soluble vitamins depends on micellar dispersion in the intestinal lumen, whereas vitamins that are soluble in the intestinal lumen can be taken up by the absorptive surface of the gut more directly. For example, some of the water-soluble vitamins are absorbed by simple diffusion; others are absorbed via specific carriers; some (vitamins C, B_{12}, thiamin, and folate) are absorbed via carrier-dependent mechanisms at low doses and by simple diffusion at high doses.

The fat-soluble vitamins tend to be absorbed and transported with dietary lipids and tend to partition into the hydrophobic centers within cells (membranes and bulk lipid droplets). In contrast, the water-soluble vitamins are absorbed by passive and active processes, are transported bound to carriers

TABLE 4–1 VITAMINS, VITAMERS, AND THEIR FUNCTIONS

GROUP	VITAMERS	PROVITAMINS	PHYSIOLOGIC FUNCTIONS
Vitamin A	Retinol Retinal Retinoic acid	β-carotene Cryptoxanthin	Visual pigments; cell differentiation; gene regulation
Vitamin D	Cholecalciferol (D_3) Ergocalciferol (D_2)		Ca homeostasis; bone metabolism
Vitamin E	α-tocopherol γ-tocopherol		Membrane antioxidant
Vitamin K	Phylloquinones (K_1) Menaquinones (K_2) Menadione (K_3)		Blood clotting; Ca metabolism
Vitamin C	Ascorbic acid Dehydroascorbic acid		Reductant in hydroxylations in biosynthesis of collagen and carnitine and in the metabolism of drugs and steroids
Vitamin B_1	Thiamin		Coenzyme for decarboxylations of 2-keto acids and transketolations
Vitamin B_2	Riboflavin		Coenzyme in redox reactions of fatty acids and the TCA cycle
Niacin	Nicotinic acid Nicotinamide		Coenzymes for several dehydrogenases
Vitamin B_6	Pyridoxol Pyridoxal Pyridoxamine		Coenzymes in amino acid metabolism
Folic acid	Folic acid Polyglutamyl folacins		Coenzymes in single-carbon metabolism
Biotin	Biotin		Coenzyme for carboxylations
Pantothenic acid	Pantothenic acid		Coenzyme in fatty acid metabolism
Vitamin B_{12}	Cobalamin		Coenzyme in metabolism of propionate, amino acids, and single carbon fragments

TCA, tricarboxylic acid.

and in free solution, and may not be stored appreciably. In general, the fat-soluble vitamins are excreted with the feces via enterohepatic circulation; whereas, the water-soluble vitamins are excreted in the urine either intact (riboflavin, pantothenic acid) or as water-soluble metabolites as in the case of vitamin C, thiamin, niacin, riboflavin, pyridoxine, biotin, folate, and vitamin B_{12}.

THE FAT-SOLUBLE VITAMINS

Vitamin A

The first fat-soluble vitamin to be recognized was vitamin A. Two groups of research workers, McCollum and Davis at the University of Wisconsin, and Osborne and Mendel at Yale University, made the discovery almost simultaneously in 1913.

Vitamin A is the descriptor for compounds with the biologic activity of **retinol,** which was originally isolated from the retina where the vitamin functions in the visual pigments. Due to their similarities to retinol, the compounds are called *retinoids*. Vitamin A-active retinoids occur in nature in three forms: the alcohol (retinol); the aldehyde (retinal or retinaldehyde); the acid (retinoic acid). Plant pigments called carotenoids can yield retinoids on metabolism. Those that yield retinol are referred to as **provitamins** A; the most active of these is ß-carotene, which is a retinol dimer. Several hundred carotenoids occur in foods naturally; of these, some 50 are thought to have significant provitamin A activity.

Absorption, Transport, and Storage

The absorption of vitamers and provitamins A requires their initial digestion. First, preformed vitamin A and carotenoids from foods are released from proteins in the stomach. Then, *retinyl esters* are hydrolyzed in the small intestine to retinol, which is absorbed more efficiently than the esters. Carotenoids are cleaved within the intestinal mucosal cells into molecules of retinaldehyde, which are reduced to retinol and then esterified to retinyl esters, which are transported in the plasma.

The bioavailabilities of carotenoids depend on the efficiencies of both their absorption and their yield of retinol. This process appears to be one of fairly low efficiency, such that excess vitamin A is almost never obtained from carotenoids in foods. It is estimated that 80% to 95% of ingested retinyl esters are absorbed, but that this figure is only 40% to 60% for ingested ß-carotene. The absorption of carotenoids varies greatly and can be affected by other dietary factors such as the level and type of fat, the amount of protein, and the digestibility of proteins bound to carotenoids in foods.

Retinyl esters of both retinoid and carotenoid origin are transported via the lymphatic drainage of the intestine into the blood and then to the liver as constituents of chylomicra. They are deposited mostly in the liver but also in adipose tissue, the lungs, and the kidneys, as retinyl esters, mostly retinyl palmitate. That process involves hydrolysis to retinol followed by re-esterification. Some 50% to 80% of the vitamin A in the body is stored in the liver where it is bound to the *cellular retinol-binding protein (CRBP).* This storage capacity mitigates against the effects of highly variable patterns of vitamin A intake, particularly, against risks of deficiency during periods of low intake of the vitamin (Li and Norris, 1996).

Vitamin A can be mobilized from the liver for distribution to peripheral tissues. This process involves the de-esterification of retinyl esters, and the binding of retinol to a specific transporter, the *retinol-binding protein (RBP)* that travels in the plasma in a complex with transthyretin. In healthy individuals, plasma retinol is maintained within a narrow range of 40 to 50 μg/dL in adults and about half that in infants. Because hepatic RBP synthesis depends on the presence of both zinc and amino acids, both serum/plasma retinol and RBP levels can be affected by deficiencies of those nutrients as well as by chronic vitamin A deficiency severe enough to deplete hepatic retinyl ester stores. Thus, children with protein-calorie malnutrition typically show low circulating retinol levels that may not respond to vitamin A supplementation unless the protein deficiency is corrected.

The RBP-bound retinol is taken up by other tissues using a receptor-mediated process involving the transfer of retinol from RBP to CRBP after which apo-RBP is removed from the circulation by the kidney. Many tissues also contain other RBPs that are thought to be involved in the transport of specific retinoids within and between cells and to affect the presentation of their retinoid ligands to various receptors. These include two cellular retinoic acid-binding proteins (CRABPs), a retinal-binding protein (CRALBP), an interphotoreceptor retinol-binding protein (IRBP), and two families of nuclear retinoid receptors (RARs) (Mangelsdorf, 1994) (Fig. 4–1).

Metabolism

In addition to being esterified for storage, the transport form *retinol* can also be oxidized to *retinal* and then *retinoic acid* or conjugated as either *retinyl glucuronide* or *retinyl phosphate*. Once retinoic acid is formed, it is converted to forms that are readily excreted. Chain-shortened and oxidized forms of vitamin A are excreted in the urine; intact forms are excreted in the bile and lost with the feces. The intermediary metabolism of retinoids appears to be regulated by the CRBPs, which channel their ligands via protein-protein interactions among the various enzymes involved in their metabolism.

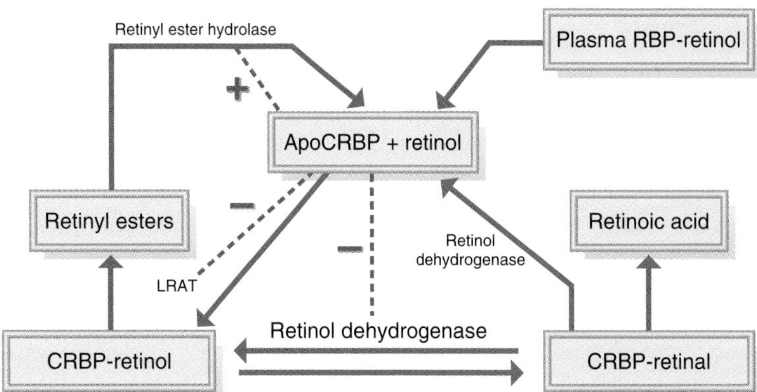

FIGURE 4–1 Roles of binding proteins in vitamin A metabolism. CRBP, cellular retinol-binding protein; RBP, retinol-binding protein. (From Combs GF. The Vitamins: Fundamental Aspects in Nutrition and Health, 2nd ed. Orlando, FL: Academic Press, 1998.)

Functions

Vitamin A has essential roles in vision, growth and development, the development and maintenance of epithelial tissue, immune functions, and reproduction. Each of these functions can be satisfied by ingesting provitamin A carotenoids, retinyl esters, retinol, or retinal, because each can be metabolized to yield the functional forms retinol, retinal, and retinoic acid. However, because retinoic acid cannot be reduced metabolically, it can only satisfy the so-called systemic functions of the vitamin (e.g., epithelial cell differentiation).

Retinal is a component of the visual pigments of the rod and cone cells of the retina and, as such, is essential to photoreception. The 11-*cis* isomer, 11-*cis*-retinal, constitutes the photosensitive group of the various proteins that comprise the visual pigments, collectively referred to as *opsins* (*rhodopsin* in the rods and *iodopsin* in the cones). Photoreception is effected by the light-induced isomerization of 11-*cis*-retinal to the all-*trans* form. This leads to the progression of the pigment through a series of unstable intermediates and, ultimately, to the dissociation of all-*trans*-retinal and opsin, which is coupled to nervous stimulation of the visual centers of the brain. This process is cyclic; 11-*cis*-retinal is regenerated enzymatically for subsequent binding to opsin.

The "systemic" functions of vitamin A are less well characterized but more important to health than are the visual functions. These include essential roles of the vitamin in the differentiation and growth of epithelial cells, in bone growth, and in tissue growth in general. In each of these roles, the function of vitamin A resembles that of a hormone because of the abilities of all-*trans*-retinoic acid to regulate gene expression at specific sites in the body (Maden, 1994). Retinoic acid-induced cell differentiation gives rise to many proteins that are presumed to be induced or activated by this system.

Measurement

To accommodate the various vitamers and provitamins A, a system of International Units (IU) was developed and continues to be in wide use. However, the newer designation, **retinol equivalents** (RE) is preferred in calculating the total vitamin A values of diets because this system accounts for both the differing biopotencies of preformed vitamin A and major provitamin A carotenoids that occur in foods. Retinol, ß-carotene, and other carotenoids can also be expressed directly in µg (Table 4–2).

Recommended Dietary Allowance (RDA)

The current RDA for vitamin A was established in 1989; it is expressed in µg RE. Dietary reference intakes (DRIs) have not yet been established for vitamin A. The current RDA for infants is based on the amount of retinol in human milk. Those for adults are based on levels that provide adequate blood levels and liver stores and are adjusted for differences in average body size. Increased amounts during pregnancy and lactation provide for fetal storage and the vitamin A in breast milk (Table 4–3).

Sources

Preformed vitamin A occurs only in foods of animal origin, either in storage areas such as the liver or associated with the fat of milk and eggs. Very high concentrations of vitamin A occur in cod and halibut liver oils. Nonfat milk, which by U.S. law can contain 0.1% fat, is routinely fortified with retinol in this country. Provitamin A carotenoids are found in dark green, leafy, and yellow-orange vegetables and fruit; deeper colors are associated with higher carotenoid levels. In much of the world, carotenoids supply most dietary vitamin A. The American food supply provides roughly equal amounts of preformed vitamin A and provitamin A carotenoids. Carrots, vegetable soups, greens, spinach, green

TABLE 4–2 RETINOL EQUIVALENTS (RE)

1 retinol equivalent	= 1 µg retinol
	= 6 µg β-carotene
	= 12 µg other provitamin A carotenoids
	= 3.33 IU vitamin A activity from retinol
	= 10 IU vitamin A activity from β-carotene

TABLE 4–3 RECOMMENDED DIETARY ALLOWANCES FOR VITAMIN A IN RETINOL EQUIVALENTS

AGE (y)	RDA (in μg RE/d)
Infants	
0.0–0.5	375
0.5–1.0	375
Children	
1–3	400
4–6	500
7–10	700
Males	
11–14	1000
15–18	1000
19–24	1000
25–50	1000
51+	1000
Females	
11–14	800
15–18	800
19–24	800
25–50	800
51+	800
Pregnant	800
Lactating	
1st 6 mo	1300
2nd 6 mo	1200

(From Food and Nutrition Board, National Research Council, NAS. Recommended Dietary Allowances, 10th ed. Washington, DC: National Academy Press, 1989.)
RDA, recommended dietary allowances; RE, retinol equivalents.

salad, orange juice, sweet potatoes, beef stew, mixed vegetables, and cantaloupe comprise the top 10 sources of provitamin A (Block, 1994). In many of these foods, vitamin A bioavailability is limited by binding of carotenoids to proteins; this can be overcome by cooking, which disrupts the protein association and frees the carotenoid. Table 4–4 lists the vitamin A content of selected foods.

Free retinol is relatively stable to heat and light; however, it can be destroyed by oxidation. Therefore, its biopotency can be reduced by the presence of transition elements (ferric iron, cupric copper) and protected by the use of vitamin E or synthetic antioxidants, or stabilized by esterification.

Deficiency

Globally, an estimated 250 million children are at risk for vitamin A deficiency. Vitamin A deficiency is the most important cause of blindness in the developing world. In 1991, nearly 14 million preschool children, most from south Asia, had clinical eye disease (xerophthalmia) due to vitamin A deficiency. Two-thirds of the new cases die within months of going blind, due to enhanced susceptibility to infections. Even subclinical vitamin A deficiency increases child morbidity and mortality (West et al., 1989). (See *"New Directions:* Vitamins and Immunity—The Antioxidant Story.")

One of the earliest signs of vitamin A deficiency is impaired vision due to the loss of visual pigments. This is manifest clinically as *night blindness* or *nyctalopia*. Subsequently, vitamin A deficiency leads to failures in its systemic functions characterized by impaired embryonic development, impaired spermatogenesis or spontaneous abortion, reduced osteoclast numbers resulting in excessive deposition of periosteal bone, anemia, and impaired immunocompetence (reduced numbers and mitogenic responsiveness of circulating T lymphocytes). Vitamin A deficiency also leads to the keratinization of the mucous membranes that line the respiratory tract, alimentary canal, urinary tract, skin, and epithelium of the eye. These changes hinder the roles that these membranes play in protecting the body against infections. Clinically, these conditions are manifest as poor growth, blindness due both to xerophthalmia and corneal ulceration, or to occlusion of the optic foramina as the result of periosteal overgrowth of the cranium, reproductive failure, or increased susceptibility to infections.

Primary deficiencies of vitamin A result from inadequate intakes of preformed vitamin A and provitamin A carotenoids. Secondary deficiencies can result from malabsorption due to insufficient dietary fat, biliary or pancreatic insufficiency, and impaired transport due to abetalipoproteinemia, liver disease, protein-energy malnutrition, or zinc deficiency.

TABLE 4–4 VITAMIN A CONTENT OF SELECTED FOODS

FOOD	RE
Liver, beef, 3.5 oz	10,602
Sweet potato, baked, 1 small	2,487
Carrots, raw, 1	2,025
Spinach, cooked, ½ cup	737
Squash, butternut, ½ cup	714
Cantaloupe, 1 cup	515
Apricots, dried, 10 large halves	253
Milk, 2%, 1 cup	139
Broccoli, cooked, ½ cup	108
Egg yolk, 1	99
Cheese, cheddar, 1 oz	86
Peach, 1 medium	47
Halibut, baked, 3 oz	46
Margarine, fortified, 1 tsp	41
Butter, 1 tsp	38
Orange, 1 medium	28
Apple, 1 medium	7
Crab, cooked, 3 oz	2

(From Pennington J. Bowe's and Church's Food Values of Portions Commonly Used, 17th ed. Philadelphia: Lippincott-Raven, 1998.)
RE, retinol equivalents.

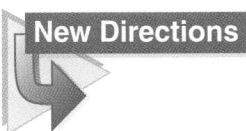

VITAMINS AND IMMUNITY—THE ANTIOXIDANT STORY

The body maintains a complex set of defenses against illness and infection. Skin, mucous membranes, and acidic secretions are among the first line of defense. Cellular immunity modified by the T cells of the thymus gland and antibodies are the next line of protection. Nutrients such as vitamin A (especially β-carotene and other carotenoids), vitamin E, vitamin C, vitamin B_6, and folacin protect the body by supporting antioxidant efforts. Iron, zinc, and selenium also have important roles. At least two long-term studies have shown a protective effect of vitamin E against the development of cardiovascular disease. (Rimm et al., 1993; Stamfer et al., 1993).

Damage from oxidation of cells can impair the body's defense against some cancers (American Council on Science and Health, 1993; Block, 1992; Blot et al., 1993; Hunter, 1993; International Life Sciences Institute, 1993). Chromosomal damage is directly related to cancer and cell mutation, and β-carotene is protective against x-ray damages (Umegaki et al., 1994). In an extensive vitamin/mineral supplementation trial in Linxian, China, 30,000 persons participated over a 5-year period. While results do not guarantee a reduction in esophageal and stomach cancers (Wang et al., 1994), the implications are that total mortality was decreased in the experimental group (American Council on Science and Health, 1993).

Longer trials with larger population groups are warranted. Several disturbing studies suggest that too large an intake of these nutrients may have a prooxidant effect. In one study, β-carotene has also been implicated as a contributor rather than a preventive agent in some types of lung cancer, especially in smokers (Caution, 1994). Finally, the Nurses Health Study, an ongoing investigative study of nutrient and food intakes of 89,494 U.S. women aged 34 to 59, found no specific correlation with vitamins C or E, but did find a protective correlation with dietary sources of vitamin A (Gerster, 1993; Hunter, 1993).

In the aging process, free radicals are thought to cause degenerative changes in the immune system, perhaps leading to cataract formation, atherosclerotic plaques, arthritis, and Parkinson's disease (Blumberg, 1992). A recent study of 88 healthy elderly (over age 65) who received placebo or vitamin E supplements showed that those receiving 200 mg or more of vitamin E daily had a statistically significant increase in delayed-type hypersensitivity response, an indicator of enhanced immune responsiveness (Meydani, 1977). Protection from DNA damage is believed to enhance the body's self-defense mechanisms. Vegetables, fruits, and their relationship to good health and wellness have been studied more extensively in the past decade than in previous years. The American Council on Science and Health has joined with the American Cancer Society and other agencies to recommend five servings daily of fruits and vegetables. The Food Pyramid also highlights the importance of both food categories. Since only about 9% of Americans consume enough antioxidants (vitamins A, C, and E) from their diet, nutrition counselors must make this recommendation a top priority in their practices (International Life Sciences Institute, 1993); School of Public Health, 1994). Substances in food such as phytochemicals may be as important as any single nutrient in supplemental form (American Council on Science and Health, 1993) (see Chapter 12). This area of research has generated much interest and will continue to stimulate new studies.

NIGHT BLINDNESS (NYCTALOPIA)

Impairment of dark adaptation—the ability to adapt from a bright light or glare to darkness, as encountered in night driving or entering a dark room from a brightly lighted one—is symptomatic of vitamin A deficiency. **Night blindness** results from the failure of the retina to regenerate rhodopsin. Individuals afflicted with night blindness have poor visual discriminatory ability and may not be able to see in dim light or at twilight.

XEROPHTHALMIA

Xerophthalmia involves atrophy of the periocular glands, hyperkeratosis of the conjunctiva, and, finally, involvement of the cornea, leading to softening or keratomalacia and blindness. Although the condition is now rare in the United States (where it is usually associated with malabsorption), it is more common in developing countries where it is a major source of blindness among children.

Loss of mucous membrane integrity due to vitamin A deficiency increases host susceptibility to bacterial, viral, or parasitic infections. The deficiency also leads to impairments in certain aspects of cell-mediated immunity, ultimately increasing the risk particularly for respiratory infections.

Vitamin A deficiency produces characteristic changes in skin texture. These involve *follicular hyperkeratosis (phrynoderma),* in which blockage of the hair follicles with plugs of keratin causes the "goose flesh" or "toad skin." The skin becomes dry, scaly, and rough. At first the forearms and thighs are involved, but in advanced stages, the whole body is affected (Fig. 4–2).

Acute vitamin A deficiency is treated with large oral doses of vitamin A. When it is part of concomitant protein-energy malnutrition, correction of this condition is also needed to realize benefits of vitamin A treatment. The signs and symptoms of deficiency respond to vitamin A supplementation in about the same order as they appear; night blindness responds very quickly, whereas the skin abnormalities may take several weeks to resolve. Massive intermittent dosing with large doses of vitamin A have been used in developing countries. Treatments with single doses of 200,000 IU (60,000

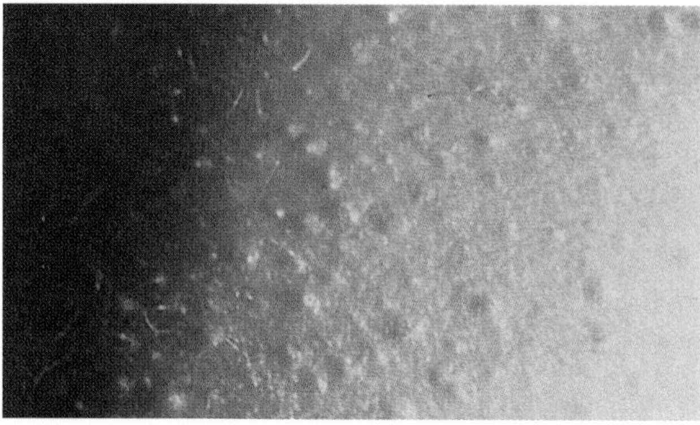

FIGURE 4–2 Follicular hyperkeratosis. Dry, bumpy skin associated with vitamin A or linoleic acid (essential fatty acid) deficiency. Linoleic acid deficiency may also result in eczematous skin, especially in infants. (From Taylor KB, Anthony LE. Clinical Nutrition. New York: McGraw-Hill, 1983, copyright by Harold H. Sandstead, MD.)

RE) of vitamin A have reduced child mortality by 35% to 70%. This approach is very costly, which has stimulated interest in increasing the vitamin A content of local food systems as a more sustainable approach to preventing the deficiency.

Toxicity

Persistent large doses of vitamin A (over 1000 times the required amount), which overcome the capacity of the liver to store the vitamin, can produce intoxication. This is marked by high plasma levels of retinyl esters associated with lipoproteins. Hypervitaminosis in humans is characterized by changes in the skin and mucous membranes. Dry lips (cheilitis) is a common early sign, followed by dryness of the nasal mucosa and eyes; later signs include dryness, erythema, scaling and peeling of the skin, hair loss, and nail fragility. Headache, nausea, and vomiting have also been reported. Very high intakes (exceeding 66,000 IU/day) can cause liver disease. Hypervitaminotic A animals frequently show bone abnormalities involving overgrowth of periosteal bone (Hathcock et al., 1990) (Table 4–5).

Hypervitaminosis A can be induced by single doses of retinol greater than 200 mg (660,000 IU) in adults or greater than 100 mg (330,000 IU) in children. Chronic hypervitaminosis A can result from chronic intakes (usually from misuse of supplements) greater than at least 10 times the RDA of 4.2 mg retinal (14,000 IU) for an infant or 10 mg retinal (33,000 IU) for an adult (Olson, 1996). Dramatic stories in the literature describe reddening and exfoliation of the skin in Arctic explorers and fishermen who feasted on polar bear liver (10 million IU/lb) or halibut liver.

Retinoids can be toxic to maternally exposed embryos (Maden, 1994). This is particularly true for 13-*cis*-retinoic acid (Accutane), a form that is very effective in treating severe cystic acne but which can cause craniofacial, central nervous system, cardiovascular, and thymic malformations of the fetus. Fetal malformations have also been linked to daily exposures of 20,000 to 25,000 IU of vitamin A from supplements, and pregnant women are advised against vitamin A intakes exceeding 10,000 IU/day.

The toxicities of carotenoids are low, and daily intakes of as much as 30 mg β-carotene are without side effects other than the accumulation of the carotenoid in the skin with consequent yellowing. **Hypercarotenodermia** can be differentiated from jaundice in that the former involves only the skin, leaving the sclera (white) of the eye clear. Hypercarotenodermia is reversible on cessation of excessive carotene intakes.

TABLE 4–5 SIGNS OF VITAMIN A TOXICITY

Serum vitamin A of 250–6600 IU/100 mL
Bone pain and fragility
Hydrocephalus and vomiting (infants and children)
Dry, fissured skin
Brittle nails
Hair loss (alopecia)
Gingivitis
Cheilosis
Anorexia
Irritability
Fatigue
Hepatomegaly and abnormal liver function
Ascites and portal hypertension

Vitamin D (Calciferol)

Vitamin D was first recognized by McCollum as the component of "good fats" that cured rickets. Now recognized as the "sunshine vitamin," it is really a hormone produced in the body by the photolytic action of ultraviolet light on the skin. Modest exposures to sunlight are sufficient for most people to produce their own vitamin D unless they spend most of their days indoors and, particularly, live in the northern latitudes. For such individuals, who must obtain the nutrient from their diets, it is a vitamin.

Two sterols found in the lipids of animals **(7-dehydrocholesterol)** or plants (*ergosterol*) can serve as precursors of vitamin D. Each of these can undergo photolytic ring-opening when exposed to ultraviolet irradiation to yield a provitamin form (7-dehydrocholesterol yields **cholecalciferol** or vitamin D_3; ergosterol yields **ergocalciferol** or vitamin D_2). Each provitamin requires further metabolism to yield the metabolically active forms, 1,25-dihydroxyvitamin D_3 and 1,25-dihydroxyvitamin D_2.

Vitamin D can thus be described as a *prohormone* because it does not need to be supplied from a source outside the body, and it serves as a precursor to the hormonal form 1,25-dihydoxyvitamin D_3 (also called **calcitriol**). In this manner, vitamin D plays an important role, along with calcium and phosphorus, in the maintenance of calcium homeostasis and in the maintenance of healthy bones and teeth. In these roles, it functions as part of a multihormone system also involving parathyroid hormone (PTH), calcitonin, and estrogen.

Absorption, Transport, and Storage

Ingested vitamin D is absorbed from the intestine along with lipids by micelle-dependent diffusion and is taken up by chylomicra in the lymphatic drainage of the intestine whereupon it is transferred in the plasma to a specific carrier, the *vitamin D-binding protein (DBP)* (also called *transcalciferin*). The efficiency of this absorption process appears to be about 50%. In contrast, vitamin D from the skin enters the capillary drainage of the skin where it is picked up by DBP.

Vitamin D is transported to peripheral tissues via DBP. Unlike the other fat-soluble vitamins, there is little hepatic storage of vitamin D; instead it partitions into the lipid phases of many tissues. Intracellularly, the active metabolite, 1,25-$(OH)_2$ vitamin D_3, is present exclusively bound to specific proteins referred to as *vitamin D receptors (VDRs)*; these are thought to mediate rapid, nongenomic actions of the vitamin. Nuclear vitamin D receptors (nVDRs) have also been identified; these are thought to mediate the transcription-dependent actions of the vitamin.

Metabolism

The prohormone form, vitamin D_3, is activated by two sequential hydroxylations. The first involves a side-chain reaction and occurs in the liver; it yields 25-hydroxyvitamin D_3 (25-hydroxycholecalciferol) whose biologic activity is some five times more potent than vitamin D_3. This metabolite is the predominant circulating form of the vitamin. It is further activated by ring hydroxylation, which occurs in the kidney and yields 1,25-dihydroxyvitamin D_3, which is some 10 times more active than vitamin D_3. The metabolic activation of vitamin D is regulated by PTH to maintain near-constant plasma calcium levels. A reduction in the plasma calcium level signals the secretion of PTH, which stimulates the production of 1,25-dihydroxyvitamin D_3. The side chains of both 25-hydroxyvitamin D_3 and 1,25-dihydroxyvitamin D_3 can be further metabolized to several other di-, tri-, and tetra-hydroxylated products. One (24,25-dihydroxyvitamin D_3) appears to be an alternative metabolite to 1,25-dihydroxyvitamin D_3; however, the metabolic roles of the others remain unclear (Fig. 4–3).

Functions

Vitamin D has essential metabolic roles in the maintenance of calcium and phosphorus homeostasis and cell differentiation. In each of these roles the functionally active form appears to be 1,25-dihydroxyvitamin D_3. However, only some of these roles fit the pattern of responses to a typical steroid hormone. Although birds can discriminate between vitamers D_3 and D_2, which differ only with respect to the methylation of their side chains, it is clear that mammals cannot.

The best characterized function of the vitamin is in the maintenance of calcium and phosphorus homeostasis in which 1,25-dihydroxyvitamin D_3 has different activities in several tissues. In the small intestine, it enhances the active transport of calcium across the gut, which involves stimulation of the synthesis of calcium-binding protein (*calbindin*) in the mucosal brush border. This also involves the stimulation of intestinal phosphate transport, perhaps involving acid phosphatase, which is also induced. In the bone, it functions in conjunction with PTH and estrogen to regulate the mobilization and deposition of calcium and phosphorus. In the kidney, it increases renal tubular reabsorption of both calcium and phosphate. These activities are coordinated with the purpose of maintaining plasma calcium within a narrow range of concentration. Under conditions that might otherwise lead to hypocalcemia, vitamin D activities restore plasma calcium by enhancing enteric absorption, renal retention, and mobilization from bone. Under conditions that tend to increase plasma calcium levels, these effects are reduced by inhibition of the production of the active metabolite. In addition, calcitonin secreted by the thyroid signals a suppression in bone mobilization and increases the renal excretion of calcium and phosphate.

These functions, as well as many others, involve both genomic and nongenomic pathways mediated by 1,25-dihydroxyvitamin D_3 interacting with a number of vitamin D receptors. More than 50 genes are known to be regulated by vitamin D (Whitfield, 1995). This number includes the gene for calbindin; however, most of the genes regulated by vitamin D are not involved in mineral metabolism. In addition, several biologic responses to 1,25-dihydroxyvitamin D_3 appear to be mediated by signal transduction mechanisms independent of the nuclear vitamin D receptors. This includes the rapid calcium transport response of intestinal mucosal cells (Wasserman, 1995).

Vitamin D appears to have metabolic roles in tissues not central to overall calcium homeostasis because 1,25-dihydroxyvitamin D_3 has been found in many soft tissues. Thus, it has been suggested that vitamin D may also be essential for cell differentiation, the functional maintenance of membranes, as well as the functions of several organs including skin, muscles, the pancreas, nerves, the parathyroid gland, and the immune system.

Measurement

Even though vitamin D is frequently expressed in terms of International Units (IU), the preferred terminology is micrograms (μg) of vitamin D_3. For nonavian species, vitamins D_2 and D_3 have equivalent biologic activities; hence, both are usually described as "vitamin D" or subsumed under the heading vita-

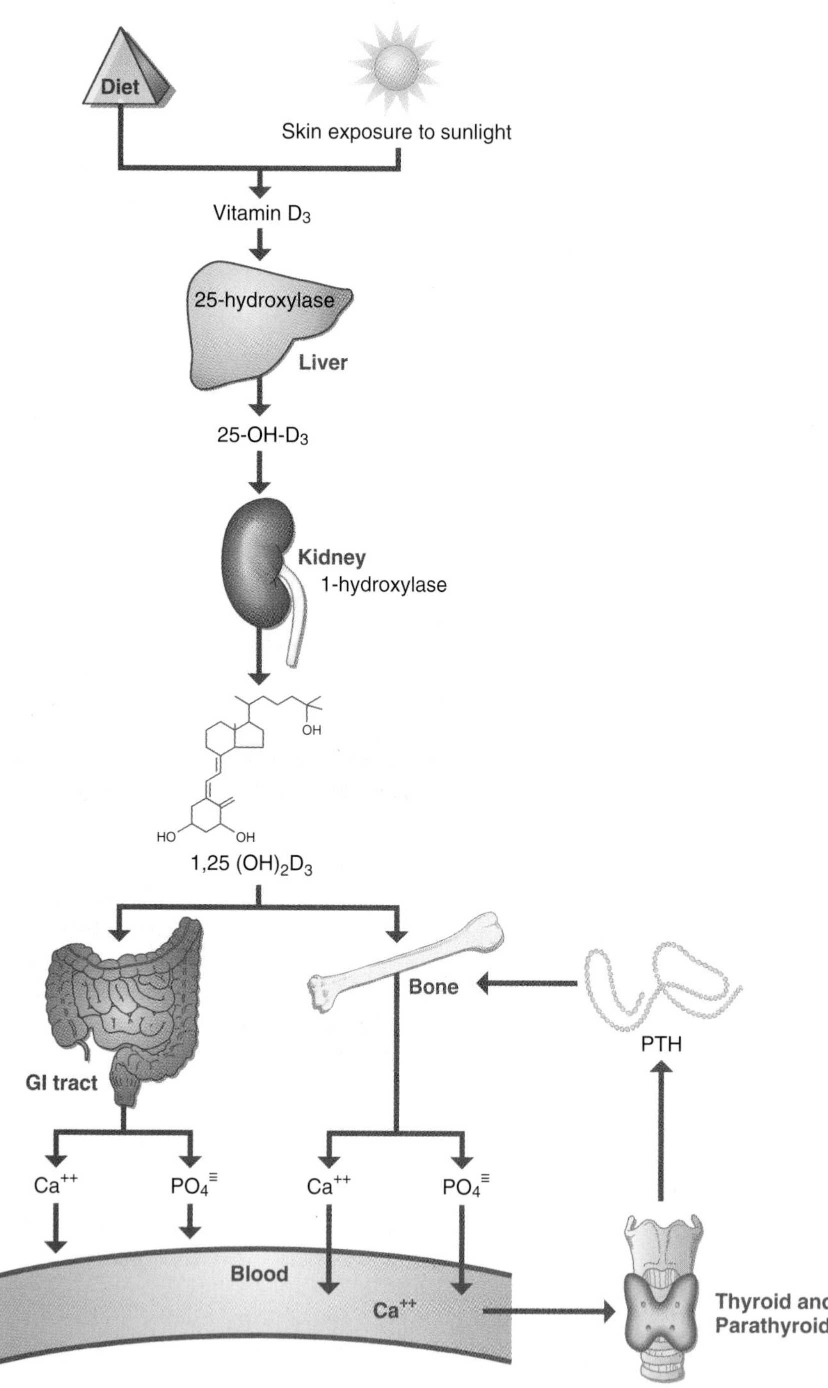

FIGURE 4–3 The metabolism and function of vitamin D. Vitamin D_3 (cholecalciferol) is changed to its biologically active forms, 25-$(OH)D_3$ and 1,25-$(OH)_2D_3$. 1,25-$(OH)_2D_3$ acts on the intestine to increase calcium and phosphate absorption, on the bones to increase calcium and phosphate resorption, and on the kidney to reduce calcium loss in the urine.

min D_3. In the feeding of poultry and other birds, however, it is important to use vitamin D_3, which has nearly 100 times the biopotency of vitamin D_2. One IU of vitamin D_3 is equal to 0.025 μg, and 1 μg of vitamin D_3 equals 40 IU of vitamin D_3 (Table 4–6).

Dietary Reference Intakes

In 1998, DRIs were established for vitamin D. These include the new adequate intakes (AIs) and tolerable upper intake levels (ULs), but not the estimated average requirement (EAR) or newly defined RDA.

Although 2.5 μg vitamin D daily is sufficient to prevent vitamin D-deficiency rickets, higher levels are recommended for infants and children throughout the period of their skeletal development. The AI is 5 μg/day for children. Continued intake of the vitamin at this level during adulthood is necessary to support the normal process of continual bone remodeling as well as adequate calcium and phosphorus homeostasis. The AI is increased to 10 μg/day for adults age 51 years and older and is increased even further to 15 μg/day (600 IU) for adults 71 years and older. The UL for vitamin D for infants is 25 μg/day (1000 IU) and for children and adults the UL is 50 μg/day (2000 IU) (Table 4–7).

TABLE 4–6 VITAMIN D TERMINOLOGY AND EQUIVALENTS

Terminology	
7-Dehydrocholesterol (vitamin D_3 precursor)	Ergosterol (vitamin D_2 precursor)
(Source: animal epidermis)	(Source: plant tissue)
Vitamin D_3	Vitamin D_2
25-hydroxycholecalciferol	25-hydroxyergocalciferol
Cholecalciferol	Ergocalciferol
$25\text{-(OH)}D_3$	$25\text{-(OH)}D_2$
(Source: precursor irradiation)	(Source: precursor irradiation)
Vitamin D_3 (active form)*	Vitamin D_2 (active form)*
1,25-dihydroxycholecalciferol	1,25-dihydroxyergocalciferol
Calcitrol	Ercalcitriol
$1,25\text{-(OH)}_2D_3$	$1,25\text{-(OH)}_2D_2$
(Source: kidney activation)	(Source: kidney activation)
Equivalents	
1 International Unit (IU) = 0.025 μg of cholecalciferol (vitamin D_3)	
1 μg cholecalciferol (vitamin D_3) = 40 IU vitamin D	

*Vitamin D_3 usually used to denote both active forms.

The normal adult is presumed to obtain sufficient vitamin D from exposure to sunlight and the incidental ingestion of small amounts in foods. Although the heavy pigment of dark-skinned people can block substantial amounts of ultraviolet radiation from reaching the deeper layers of the skin where vitamin D can be synthesized, this effect may be limiting only under conditions of routinely short periods of exposure.

Supplemental vitamin D is appropriate for individuals chronically shielded from sunlight, such as persons who are housebound, or living in northern latitudes or areas with high atmospheric pollution, wearing clothing that completely covers the body, and persons working at night, who stay indoors during the day.

TABLE 4–7 DIETARY REFERENCE INTAKES FOR VITAMIN D

LIFE-STAGE GROUP	ADEQUATE INTAKES (AI)*† μg/d	TOLERABLE UPPER INTAKE LEVELS (UL) (μg/d)
Infants		
0–6 mo	5	25
7–12 mo	5	25
Children		
1–3 y	5	50
4–8 y	5	50
Males		
9–13 y	5	50
14–18 y	5	50
19–30 y	5	50
31–50 y	5	50
51–70 y	10	50
>70 y	15	50
Females		
9–13 y	5	50
14–18 y	5	50
19–30 y	5	50
31–50 y	5	50
51–70 y	10	50
>70 y	15	50
Pregnancy and Lactation		
≤18 y	5	50
19–50 y	5	50

(From Institute of Medicine, Food and Nutrition Board. Dietary Reference Intakes for Calcium, Phosphorus, Magnesium, Vitamin D and Fluoride. Washington, DC: National Academy Press, 1997.)

*As cholecalciferol. 1 μg cholecalciferol = 40 IU vitamin D.

†In the absence of adequate exposure to sunlight.

Sources

Vitamin D_3 occurs naturally in animal products, the richest sources being fish liver oils. It is found in only small and highly variable amounts in butter, cream, egg yolk, and liver; both human and unfortified cow's milk tend to be poor sources of the vitamin, providing only 15 to 40 IU/L (0.4 to 1 μg/L). However, approximately 98% of all fluid milk sold in the United States is fortified with vitamin D_2 (usually at the level of 400 IU/qt), as is most dried whole milk and evaporated milk, as well as some margarines, butter, soy milks, certain cereals, and all infant formula products. Vitamin D is very stable and does not deteriorate when foods are heated or stored for long periods (Table 4–8).

Deficiency

Vitamin D deficiency is manifest as rickets in children and growing animals and as osteomalacia in adults.

RICKETS

Rickets is a disease involving impaired mineralization of growing bones. It can result from deprivation of vitamin D, but also from deficiencies of calcium and phosphorus. Rickets is characterized by

TABLE 4–8 VITAMIN D CONTENT OF SELECTED FOODS

FOOD	IU
Herring, fresh, raw, 1 oz	255
Salmon, 1 oz	142
Milk, cow's fortified, 1 cup	100
Sardines, canned, 1 oz	85
Liver, chicken, cooked, 3 oz	45
Shrimp, canned, 1 oz	30
Egg yolk	25
Milk, human, 1 cup	1–24
Liver, calf, cooked, 3 oz	12
Cream, light, 1 T	8
Cheese, cheddar, 1 oz	3
Oysters, 4	3
Butter, 1 tsp	1.4

(From USDA. Composition of Foods, Handbook No. 8 Series. Washington, DC: ARS, USDA, 1976–1986.)

structural abnormalities of the weight-bearing bones (e.g., tibia, ribs, humerus, radius, ulna) (Fig. 4–4) and is associated with accompanying bone pain, muscular tenderness, and hypocalcemic tetany. Soft, pliable, rachitic bones cannot withstand ordinary stresses and strains, resulting in the appearance of bowlegs, knock-knees, beaded ribs (the rachitic rosary), pigeon breast, and frontal bossing of the skull. Radiography reveals enlarged epiphyseal growth plates manifested as enlarged wrists and ankles resulting from their failure to mineralize and continue growth. Patients show increased plasma/serum levels of alkaline phosphatase, which is released by the affected osteoblasts.

Historically victims of rickets have been poor children in industrialized cities where exposure to sunlight is limited. Rickets continues to be a significant public health problem in China, and pockets have been identified in Nigeria and Bangladesh (Specker and Tsang, 1988). In North America, the vitamin D supplementation of foods has virtually eliminated the disease; however, prolonged breast-feeding without exposure to sunlight or vitamin D supplements can lead to rickets. Rickets can also occur in children with chronic problems of lipid malabsorption and in those receiving long-term anticonvulsant therapy (which reduces the circulating levels of 1,25-dihydroxyvitamin D_3).

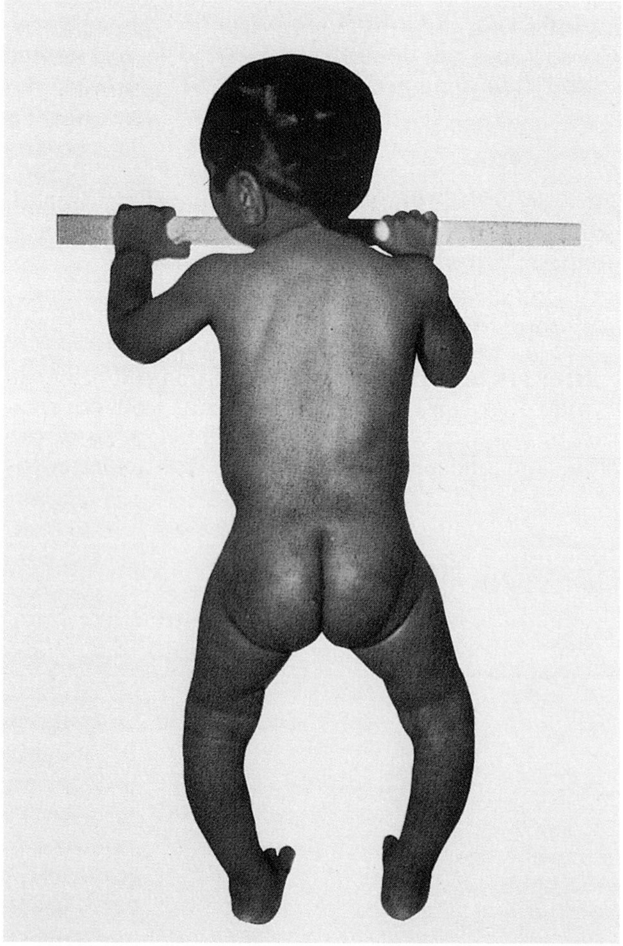

FIGURE 4–4 Rickets. Sign of vitamin D and calcium deficiencies in children (disorders of cartilage cell growth, enlargement of epiphyseal growth plates) and adults (osteomalacia). (From Latham MC, et al. Scope Manual on Nutrition. Kalamazoo, MI: The Upjohn Company, 1980, copyright by Rose Lee Nemir, MD.)

Rickets due strictly to vitamin D deprivation can be treated effectively with oral preparations of the vitamin or natural sources rich in the vitamin. For example, vitamin D concentrates of fish liver oil have been prescribed: 1 teaspoon (4 mL) of cod liver oil contains 360 IU of vitamin D. In cases of calcium-deficiency or hypophosphatemic vitamin D refractory rickets, vitamin D treatment alone may not be effective. Active vitamin D metabolites (25-(OH)D_3 or 1,25$(OH)_2D_3$) or a synthetic analogue are necessary.

OSTEOMALACIA

Osteomalacia occurs in adults with formed bones whose epiphyseal closures have made that region of the bone unaffected by vitamin D deficiency. The disease involves generalized reductions in bone density and the presence of pseudofractures especially of the spine, femur, and humerus. Patients experience muscular weakness and bone tenderness and have a greater risk of fracture particularly of the wrist and pelvis.

Prevention of osteomalacia is usually possible through the adequate supply of vitamin D, calcium, and phosphorus in the diet. It has been estimated that as little as 10 to 15 minutes of sun exposure on a clear summer day, two to three times a week, should be sufficient to prevent osteomalacia among most elderly people. (See *"Focus On:* Sunshine, Vitamin D, and Fortification.") Osteomalacia can be treated effectively with vitamin D_3 in doses of 1000 to 5000 IU/day; in cases complicated by lipid malabsorption daily doses as large as 50,000 IU have been used.

OSTEOPOROSIS

Osteoporosis is frequently confused with osteomalacia; however, it is a very different disease of the bone, one that involves diminished bone mass with the retention of normal histologic appearance (Heaney, 1993). Osteoporosis is associated with aging; it is thought to be a multifactorial disease involving impaired vitamin D metabolism and function associated with low or decreasing estrogen levels (see Chapter 28). It is the most common bone disease of postmenopausal women and also occurs in older men. A recent study of patients admitted to hospitals showed that an alarmingly high number had low levels of vitamin D (Thomas et al., 1998). Studies of the efficacies of various vitamers D in treating osteoporosis have been inconsistent; but two large studies involving the chronic use of 1,25-dihydroxyvitamin D_3 by women indicated significant retardation of the onset (and some reversal) of the signs and symptoms.

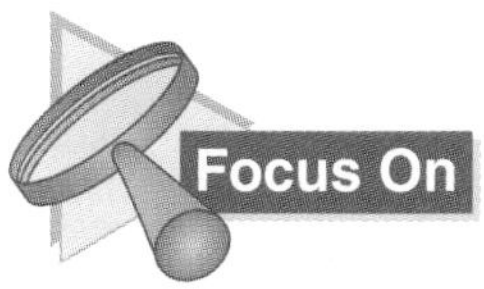

SUNSHINE, VITAMIN D, AND FORTIFICATION

Brief and casual exposure of the face, arms, and hands to sunlight is thought to equal about 200 IU vitamin D (5 mg), and prolonged exposure with erythema raises plasma 25-(OH)D_3 concentrations as much as long-term ingestion of vitamin D at a level of 10,000 IU (250 mg) daily (Haddad, 1992). Ultraviolet light penetration depends on the amount of melanin present, clothing type, blockage of effective rays by window glass, and the use of sunscreens. Casual exposure now appears to be sufficient to last through the winter months except in persons unable or unwilling to go outside. Fortification of foods with vitamin D appears to be adequate for these individuals, since vitamin D deficiency is now unusual in this country. Milk continues to be a food of choice for this type of fortification because of the presence of calcium. Soy milks are now also fortified with vitamin D and calcium to the same levels as cow's milk. However, milk and infant formulas rarely contain the amount of vitamin D stated on the label and may have an unknown level (Holick, 1992). Eight cases of hypervitaminosis D resulting from drinking milk fortified incorrectly and excessively were recently studied. Fortification must be carefully regulated by states and local dairies to prevent recurrence of this problem (Jacobus et al., 1992). Both over- and underfortification are dangerous and a unified monitoring program is needed (Chen et al., 1993).

Toxicity

Excessive intake of vitamin D can produce intoxication characterized by elevated serum calcium (hypercalcemia) and phosphorus (hyperphosphatemia) levels and, ultimately, the calcification of soft tissues (*calcinosis*) including the kidney, lungs, heart, and even the tympanic membrane of the ear, which can result in deafness. Patients often complain of headache and nausea (Table 4–9). Infants given excessive amounts of vitamin D may have gastrointestinal upsets, bone fragility, and retarded growth.

Hypervitaminosis D is a progressive intoxication, and individuals appear to vary in susceptibility. The tolerable upper intake level (UL) has been established at 1000 IU/day for infants and 2000 IU/day for children and adults. It is clear that infants and small children are most susceptible.

Vitamin E

Vitamin E was discovered in the 1920s as a fat-soluble factor required to prevent fetal death and resorption in rodents. When it was chemically identified in the subsequent decade, the vitamin was named tocopherol, from the Greek *tokos* (childbirth) and *pherein* (to bear).

Vitamin E is now recognized as having a fundamental role in the normal metabolism of all cells. Therefore, its deficiency can affect several different organ systems. Its function is related to several other nutrients and endogenous factors that, collectively, comprise a system that protects against the potentially damaging effects of reactive oxygen species that are formed metabolically or encountered in the environment.

Vitamin E is the descriptor for two families of biologically active substances: **tocopherols** and the related but much less biologically active compounds with saturated side chains, *tocotrienols*. The various vitamers of each series are named according to the position and number of methyl groups on their ring systems. Due to the stereoisomerism possible on the side chain, and the possibility for partial or multiple methylation of the nucleus, many tocopherol vitamers are possible. However, only a few occur naturally. The most important of these are α- and γ-tocopherol, each of which has an R,R,R-configured side chain (Fig. 4–5). Synthetic preparations of α-tocopherol are mixtures of eight possible stereoisomers; these are designated with the prefix "all-*rac*-" or "l" and they are about 25% less active metabolically than the natural forms ("d" forms).

TABLE 4–9 SIGNS OF VITAMIN D TOXICITY

Signs
Excessive calcification of bone
Kidney stones
Metastatic calcification of soft tissues (kidney, heart, lung, and tympanic membrane)
Hypercalcemia
Headache
Weakness
Nausea and vomiting
Constipation
Polyuria
Polydipsia

Absorption, Transport, and Storage

Vitamin E is absorbed in the upper small intestine by micelle-dependent diffusion and, like the other fat-soluble vitamins, its utilization depends on the presence of dietary fat and adequate biliary and pancreatic function. Esterified forms of the vitamin (e.g., tocopheryl acetate) are absorbed as the free alcohol after hydrolysis by nonspecific esterases at the duodenal mucosa. The absorption of vitamin E is highly variable, with efficiencies in the range of 20% to 70%. Absorbed vitamin E is taken up by chylomicra and intestinal very-low-density lipoproteins

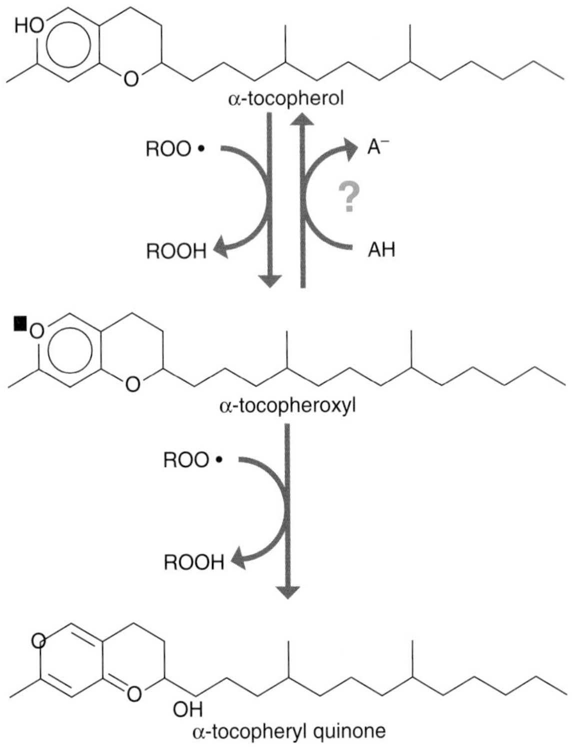

FIGURE 4–5 Mechanism of vitamin E scavenging oxygen-centered free radicals (ROO·). (From Combs GF. The Vitamins: Fundamental Aspects in Nutrition and Health, 2nd ed. Orlando, FL: Academic Press, 1998.)

(VLDL) in the lymphatic circulation. After they are taken to the liver they are incorporated into the triglyceride-rich VLDL and a portion is also partitioned into high-density lipoproteins (HDL).

The cellular uptake of vitamin E from VLDL and HDL in the plasma appears to involve both a receptor-mediated process as well as one mediated by lipoprotein lipase. These processes also appear to involve an intracellular *tocopherol-binding protein (TBP),* which facilitates the intracellular transport of the vitamin. In most nonadipose cells, vitamin E is located almost exclusively in membranes from which it can be mobilized; in adipose tissues, it is partitioned largely in the bulk lipid phase where it is not readily mobilized.

Metabolism

The metabolism of vitamin E is limited. The in vivo antioxidant function of the vitamin results in its oxidation primarily to the biologically inactive *tocopheryl quinone,* which can be reduced to *tocopheryl hydroquinone*. Glucuronic acid conjugates of the latter are secreted in the bile, making excretion with the feces the major route of elimination of the vitamin. With usual intakes of vitamin E, a very small portion is excreted in the urine as water-soluble, side-chain metabolites (*tocopheronic acid* and *tocopheronolactone*).

Functions

Vitamin E is the most important lipid-soluble **antioxidant** in the cell (Jacob, 1995). Localized in the hydrophobic environments of biologic membranes, it protects unsaturated membrane phospholipids from oxidative degradation due to highly reactive oxygen species and other free radicals (Burton, 1994). Vitamin E performs this function through its ability to reduce such radicals to harmless metabolites—a process referred to as *free radical "scavenging."*

As a membrane-resident free radical scavenger, vitamin E is now understood to be an important component of the cellular antioxidant defense system, which also involves other enzymatic (superoxide dismutases [SODs], glutathione peroxidases [GPXs], glutathione reductase [GR], catalase, thioredoxin reductase [TR]) and nonenzymatic factors (glutathione, uric acid) many of which are dependent on other essential nutrients. For example, the expressions of the GPXs and TR depend on adequate selenium status; the expressions of the SODs depend on adequate copper, zinc, and manganese status; the activity of GR depends on adequate riboflavin status. Therefore, the antioxidant function of vitamin E can be affected by the nutritional status with respect to one or more other nutrients. This is seen in several deficiency diseases of animals (e.g., myopathies, vascular disorders), where vitamin E can appear to be interchangeable with selenium—a phenomenon referred to as *nutritional sparing.*

This antioxidant function suggests that vitamin E and related nutrients may collectively be important in protecting against conditions related to oxidative stress, such as aging, air pollution, arthritis, cancer, cardiovascular disease, cataracts, diabetes, and infection. These areas are subjects of active research (Burning and Hennekeus, 1997; Halliwell, 1996).

Measurement

Because various E vitamers occur in different foods, they are generally quantified in terms that accommodate their differences in biologic activity. One system is that of International Units (IU) in which 1 mg of all-*rac*-α-tocopheryl acetate is defined as 1.0 IU, and 1 mg of the naturally occurring R,R,R-α-tocopherol (formerly called D-α-tocopherol) is defined as 1.49 IU. In recent years, this system has been largely replaced by the use of R,R,R-α-tocopherol equivalents (α-TE) in which 1 mg of the synthetic all-*rac*-α-tocopherol is defined as 0.74 α-TE, 1 mg R,R,R-α-tocopherol defined as 1 α-TE, and 1 mg γ-tocopherol defined as 0.1 mg α-TE. For most foods, the presence of non-α-tocopherols is such that the total α-TE value can be estimated at roughly 1.2 times the α-tocopherol content.

Recommended Dietary Allowance

The current RDA for vitamin E was established in 1989; DRIs have not yet been established although they are being worked on (Institute of Medicine,

1998) (Table 4–10). The need for vitamin E depends, in part, on the amounts of polyunsaturated fatty acids (PUFAs) consumed. For Americans, typical intakes are about 0.4 mg α-TE/mg PUFA; in the absence of evidence of significant vitamin E deficiency in this country, this ratio is thought to be adequate. Recent evidence, however, suggests that intakes greater than the now typical 7 to 9 mg α-TE per day, may be of particular benefit in reducing risk for a variety of disorders associated with oxidative stress.

Sources

The vitamers E are synthesized only by plants; therefore, they are found primarily in plant products, the richest sources being oils. Although vitamin E activity in foods is contributed by tocopherols (in leaves and other green parts) and tocotrienols (in bran and germ fractions), the predominant ones in common foods are α- and γ-tocopherols. Animal tissues tend to contain low amounts of vitamin E, the richest source being fatty tissues and tissues of animals fed large amounts of the vitamin. It has been estimated that nearly two thirds of the vitamin E in the typical American diet is supplied by salad oils, margarines, and shortenings, about 11% by fruits and vegetables, and about 7% by grains and grain products. Table 4–11 lists the vitamin E content of selected foods.

TABLE 4–10 RECOMMENDED DIETARY ALLOWANCES FOR VITAMIN E

AGE (y)	RDA (mg α-TOCOPHEROL EQUIVALENTS/d)
Infants	
0.0–0.5	3
0.5–1.0	4
Children	
1–3	6
4–6	7
7–10	7
Males	
11–14	10
15–18	10
19–24	10
25–50	10
51+	10
Females	
11–14	8
15–18	8
19–24	8
25–50	8
51+	8
Pregnant	10
Lactating	
1st 6 mo	12
2nd 6 mo	11

(From Food and Nutrition Board, National Research Council, NAS. Recommended Dietary Allowances, 10th ed. Washington, DC: National Academy Press, 1989.)
RDA, recommended dietary allowance.

TABLE 4–11 VITAMIN E CONTENT OF SELECTED FOODS

FOOD	VITAMIN E α-Tocopherol Equivalent (mg)
Wheat germ oil, 1 T	26.94
Sunflower oil, 1 T	7.14
Almonds, dried, 1 oz	6.72
Corn oil, 1 T	2.96
Soybean oil, 1 T	2.55
Avocado, Calif., 1	2.32
Olive oil, 1 T	1.74
Mayonnaise, 1 T	1.65
Margarine, 1 T	1.6
Baked beans, canned with pork, 1 cup	1.37
Apricots, frzn, sweetened, ½ cup	1.08
Salmon, raw, 3 oz	.85
Peas, canned, ½ cup	.64
Butter, 1 T	.24
Milk, nonfat or whole, 1 cup	nonfat—0.10, whole—0.24
Chicken, w/o skin, ½ breast	.23
Chocolate milk, plain, 2%, 1 oz	.13

(From Pennington T. Bowe's and Church's Food Values of Portions Commonly Used, 17th ed. Philadelphia: Lippincott-Raven, 1998.)

The free alcohol forms of vitamin E (e.g., tocopherols) are fairly stable, but they can be destroyed oxidatively when in contact with rancidifying fats and transition elements such as ferric iron. The corresponding esters (e.g., tocopheryl acetate) are very stable even to such oxidizing conditions. Because the vitamers E are insoluble in water, they are not lost by cooking in water, but can be lost by deep-fat frying.

Deficiency

The clinical manifestations of vitamin E deficiency vary considerably among species. In general, the targets are the neuromuscular, vascular, and reproductive systems. In the neuromuscular system vitamin E deficiency, which may take 5 to 10 years to develop, is manifested clinically as loss of deep tendon reflexes, impaired vibratory and position sensation, changes in balance and coordination, muscle weakness, and visual disturbances (Sokol, 1996). Symptoms in humans are uncommon and have occurred only in cases with lipid malabsorption (e.g., biliary atresia, exocrine pancreatic insufficiency) or lipid transport abnormalities (e.g., abetalipoproteinemia).

At the cellular level deficiency of vitamin E is accompanied by an increase in lipid peroxidation of the cell membrane. Because of this, vitamin E-deficient cells exposed to an oxidant stress will show more rapid injury and necrosis (Sokol, 1996).

The limited transplacental movement of vitamin E results in newborn infants having low tissue concentrations of vitamin E. Premature infants may, therefore, be at risk of vitamin E deficiency, because they typically have limited lipid absorptive capacity for some time.

Toxicity

Vitamin E is one of the least toxic of the vitamins. Both humans and animals appear to be able to tolerate relatively high intakes, at least 100 times the nutritional requirement. At very high doses, however, vitamin E can antagonize the utilization of other fat-soluble vitamins. Hypervitaminotic E animals have shown impaired bone mineralization, impaired hepatic vitamin A storage, and prolonged blood coagulation. The latter effect may be a concern for patients on anticoagulant therapy because a regular daily intake of 1200 IU vitamin E was found to exacerbate the effect of a coumarin drug.

Vitamin K

Vitamin K was discovered in 1935 by Dam in Copenhagen as a factor that prevented severe hemorrhagic disease in animals fed fat-free diets. The factor was named the *Koagulationsvitamin*, hence, vitamin K. It was isolated and synthesized in 1939. In addition to playing essential roles in blood clotting, vitamin K is now also recognized as functioning in bone formation (Heaney, 1993).

Vitamin K is the descriptor for 2-methyl-1,4-naphthoquinone and its derivatives exhibiting antihemorrhagic activity. Naturally occurring forms of the vitamin are **phylloquinones**. The phylloquinones (the vitamin K_1 series) have phytyl or further alkylated side chains with only one double bond on the proximal isoprene unit; they are synthesized by green plants. The **menaquinones** (the vitamin K_2 series) have side chains of varying numbers of isopentyl units each of which has a double bond; these are synthesized by bacteria. The synthetic compound with no side chain is called **menadione** (vitamin K_3) and humans and animals alkylate it to produce *menaquinones*. Menadione is the synthetic compound (vitamin K_3) and it is made in several forms. It is about twice as potent biologically as the naturally occurring forms—vitamins K_1 and K_2 (Suttie, 1995).

Absorption, Transport, and Storage

Like the other fat-soluble vitamins, most of the vitamers K are absorbed across the small intestine by micelle-dependent diffusion, which requires a minimum of dietary fat as well as adequate biliary and pancreatic function. The exceptions are the phylloquinones, which appear to be absorbed by an energy-dependent process. Due to the extreme difficulty in demonstrating signs of vitamin K deficiency in animals deprived of dietary sources of the vitamin, it can be inferred that menaquinones produced from the hind gut microflora can be absorbed across the colon. The absorbed vitamers K are incorporated into chylomicrons in the lymph and taken to the liver where they are transferred to VLDLs and low-density lipoproteins (LDLs) in which forms they are transported to peripheral tissues.

Vitamin K is found at low concentrations in many tissues in which it is localized in cellular membranes. Due to the metabolism of the vitamin, tissues show mixtures of vitamers K even when a sole form is fed. Most tissues contain phylloquinones as well as menaquinones.

Metabolism

Menadione can be alkylated in the liver; however, the side-chain metabolism of the phylloquinones and menaquinones appears only to be accomplished by enteric bacteria. The result of the latter phenomenon is that ingested phylloquinones can be converted to menaquinones by successive bacterial dealkylation and realkylation prior to absorption.

Both phylloquinones and menaquinones are catabolized by side-chain shortening and oxidation to produce metabolites that are excreted in the feces via the bile, frequently as glucuronic acid conjugates. Menadione is metabolized more rapidly; it is excreted primarily in the urine as a phosphate, sulfate, or glucuronide derivative.

The naphthoquinone ring system of the vitamers K can be altered by hepatic microsomal metabolism to yield *vitamin K epoxide*. This form, which normally constitutes some 10% of hepatic vitamin K, can be reduced back through a quinone form ultimately to the fully reduced dihydroxyvitamin K.

Functions

The basis of the metabolic role of vitamin K involves its oxidation to the epoxide form. This occurs as part of a system, the *vitamin K cycle,* that drives the γ-carboxylation of specific post-translational modification of protein-bound glutamyl residues (to produce *γ-carboxyglutamyl* [*GLA*] residues) on the vitamin K-dependent proteins (Ferland, 1998). The vitamin K cycle can be interrupted by certain inhibitors of the regeneration of reduced vitamin K; this includes the coumarin-type drugs warfarin and dicumarol and is the basis for their anticoagulant activities.

Several GLA-proteins have been identified: four plasma clotting factors including four coagulation-inhibiting factors, at least three proteins found in calcified tissues (including *osteocalcin;* see Chapter 28) and at least one protein found in calcified atherosclerotic tissue (*atherocalcin;* see Chapter 26). The vitamin K-dependent conversion of protein-GLA residues confers on those proteins the ability to bind ionic calcium (Vermeer et al., 1996). This is thought to be the basis of the various activities of the GLA proteins in blood clotting and calcified tissues because each reaction involves calcium.

TABLE 4–12 RECOMMENDED DIETARY ALLOWANCES FOR VITAMIN K

AGE (y)	RDA (μg/d)
Infants	
0.0–0.5	5
0.5–1.0	10
Children	
1–3	15
4–6	20
7–10	30
Males	
11–14	45
15–18	65
19–24	70
25–50	80
51+	80
Females	
11–14	45
15–18	55
19–24	60
25–50	65
51+	65
Pregnant	65
Lactating	
1st 6 mo	65
2nd 6 mo	65

(From Food and Nutrition Board, National Research Council, NAS. Recommended Dietary Allowances, 10th ed. Washington, DC: National Academy Press, 1989.)
RDA, recommended dietary allowance.

Measurement

Although the various vitamers K vary widely in their biopotencies, there has been no standardization of means for accommodating those differences when quantifying the amounts of the vitamin K in foods or diets. Each vitamer is expressed in terms of its mass in micrograms of vitamin K.

Recommended Dietary Allowance

An RDA for vitamin K was established for the first time in 1989; DRIs have not yet been established. The RDA, 1 μg/kg body weight, assumes half to be supplied by intestinal microbial synthesis and the remainder by the diet. Table 4–12 presents the RDA for age and sex categories.

Sources

Vitamin K is found in large amounts in green leafy vegetables, especially broccoli, cabbage, turnip greens, and dark lettuces, usually at levels greater than 100 μg/100g. The amounts of the vitamin in dairy products, meats, and eggs tend to be variable, 1 to 50 μg/g and fruits and cereals usually contain about 15 μg/g. Breast milk tends to be low in vitamin K content, providing insufficient amounts of the vitamin for infants less than 6 months of age (see Chapters 8 and 9). Table 4–13 shows the vitamin K content of some selected foods.

The analytical task of determining the vitamers K in foods is formidable; therefore, it is understandable that tabulated vitamin K values for food are often not accurate. Nevertheless, the absence of evidence of significant vitamin K deficiency in the general population would indicate that adequate amounts of the vitamin can normally be obtained by foods or enteric microflora.

Vitamin K is fairly stable; it is not destroyed by ordinary cooking methods nor is it lost in cooking water. It is, however, light and alkali sensitive.

Deficiency

The predominant sign of vitamin K deficiency is hemorrhage, which, in severe cases, can cause a fatal anemia. The underlying condition is *hypoprothrombinemia,* which is manifest as prolonged clotting time. Vitamin K deficiencies are rare among hu-

TABLE 4–13 AVERAGE VITAMIN K CONTENT OF SELECTED FOODS

FOOD		FOOD		FOOD		FOOD	
Milk and Milk Products (μg)		**Fats (μg)**		**Vegetables (μg)**		Green beans, cooked, ½ cup	22
Milk, cow's, 8 oz, whole	10	Corn oil, 1 T	8	Asparagus, raw, 4 spears	23	Chickpeas, 1 oz	74
Milk, human, 1 fl oz	0.6	Soybean oil, 1 T	76	Broccoli, frzn, ½ cup	63	Carrot, 1 med	9
Eggs (μg)		Safflower oil, 1 T	0	Cabbage, raw, ½ cup	52	**Fruits (μg)**	
Whole, 1 Lg	25	**Cereals and Grain Products (μg)**		Lettuce, iceberg, 1 leaf	22	Apple, 1 med	4
Meat and Meat Products (μg)		Oats, dry, 1 oz	18	Seaweed, dulse, dried, 3.5 oz	1700	Orange, 1 med	7
Beef, ground, 3.5 oz	4	Wheat bran, 1 oz	23	Potato, baked	6	Strawberries, 1 cup	21
Pork, 3.5 oz	88	Flour, whole wheat, 1 cup	36	Spinach, frzn, ½ cup	131	**Beverages (μg)**	
Beef, 3.5 oz	104	Wheat germ, 1 oz	10	Tomato, 1	28	Coffee, dry, 1t	0.7
Turkey, 3.5 oz	0			Turnip greens, cooked, ½ cup	82	Tea, green, dry, 1 oz	199
Veal, 3.5 oz	27						

(From Pennington J. Bowe's and Church's Food Values of Portions Commonly Used, 17th ed. Philadelphia: Lippincott-Raven, 1998.)

mans and have been associated with lipid malabsorption, destruction of intestinal flora as with chronic antibiotic therapy, and liver disease. Newborn infants, particularly those who are premature or are exclusively breast-fed, are susceptible to hypoprothrombinemia during the first few days of life as the result of poor placental transfer of vitamin K, and failure to establish a vitamin K-producing intestinal microflora. This is associated with *hemorrhagic disease of the newborn,* which is treated prophylactically by administering menadione intramuscularly on delivery. In animals, vitamin K deficiency can occur when access to feces is prevented; problems have been most frequently encountered in poultry raised on wire floors to prevent parasitic diseases.

Toxicity

Neither the phylloquinones or menaquinones have shown any adverse effects by any route of administration. Menadione, however, can be toxic; excessive doses (at least 1000 times the RDA) have produced hemolytic anemia in rats and severe jaundice in infants.

THE WATER-SOLUBLE VITAMINS

Thiamin, riboflavin, niacin, vitamin B_6, pantothenic acid, biotin, folic acid, vitamin B_{12}, and vitamin C are usually referred to as the water-soluble vitamins. In fact, their similar solubilities are about the only characteristic that they share. But, because of that general characteristic, these vitamins tend to be absorbed by both simple diffusion and carrier-mediated processes, and they tend to be distributed in the aqueous phases of the cell (cytoplasm, mitochrondrial matrix space). They function as essential cofactors or co-substrates of enzymes involved in various aspects of metabolism (Combs, 1998). Most tend to not be stored in appreciable amounts, making their regular consumption a necessity.

The discoveries of the water-soluble vitamins began at the turn of the last century with the recognition by Christian Eijkman, a Dutch physician in Java, that rice bran contained a factor that prevented a beriberi-like syndrome in the chicken. That discovery revolutionized the physiology of the day—giving birth to the field of nutrition and an intense period of investigation in the early decades of this century. When those studies revealed a fat-soluble factor that prevented xerophthalmia in the rat, the discoverers had called the new factor "fat-soluble A" thus distinguishing it from what would become "water-soluble B." Other fat-soluble factors (the fat-soluble vitamins A, D, E, and K) were quickly discovered, but the identification of "water-soluble B" was a bit slower. When another water-soluble factor, the antiscorbutic "vitamin C" was recognized, it became clear that "water-soluble B" had not been a single factor but, rather, a group of biologically active factors with similar physical properties and source distributions. Collectively, these factors became known as the "B complex." Ultimately, more than a half-dozen vitamins were teased out of that grouping.

Members of the B complex have an essential role in the metabolic processes of living cells, both plant and animal. They function as coenzymes or as prosthetic groups bound to apoenzymes. Four of these (thiamin, niacin, riboflavin, and pantothenic acid) are essential to the derivation of energy from glycolysis and the tricarboxylic acid (TCA) cycle (see Chapter 3).

Because of the close interrelationships among the B vitamins, an inadequate intake of one may impair utilization of others. Discrete deficiencies of single B vitamins are rarely seen clinically.

Thiamin

Thiamin (formerly, vitamin B_1) was the first of the B vitamins to be elucidated. It plays essential metabolic roles in carbohydrate metabolism and neural function. These involve the metabolic activation of the vitamin to *thiamin triphosphate (TTP),* also referred to as *cocarboxylase,* which serves as a coenzyme in energy metabolism and in the synthesis of pentoses. It has also been proposed that thiamin may have a nonmetabolic role in nerve transmission.

Absorption, Transport, and Storage

Thiamin is absorbed from the proximal small intestine both by active transport (at low doses) and passive diffusion (at high doses, e.g., >5 mg/day). The former process is inhibited by alcohol consumption, which interferes with active transport of the vitamin, and folate deficiency, which interferes with the replication of enterocytes. The mucosal uptake of thiamin is coupled to its phosphorylation to TPP in which form the vitamin is carried to the liver by the portal circulation.

In the plasma, thiamin occurs mostly as free thiamin and *thiamin monophosphate (TMP)* bound chiefly to albumin; but most (90%) of the circulating vitamin is carried as TPP by erythrocytes. Its uptake by cells of peripheral tissues appears to occur both by passive diffusion and active transport. Tissues retain thiamin as its phosphate esters, most of which are bound to proteins. Tissue levels of thiamin are variable, with no appreciable storage of the vitamin.

Metabolism

Thiamin is phosphorylated in many tissues to the di- and triphosphate esters by specific kinases. Each of these esters can be catabolized by a phosphorylase to yield TMP. Small amounts of some 20 other excretory metabolites (including thiochrome) are also produced.

Functions

The functional form of thiamin is TPP, also called cocarboxylase, which is a coenzyme for several enzymes involved in the metabolism of pyruvate and other α-keto acids. In this manner, thiamin is essential for the oxidative decarboxylation of α-keto acids including the oxidative conversion of pyruvate to acetyl CoA, which enters the TCA (Krebs) cycle to generate energy. It is similarly required for the conversion of α-ketoglutarate and the 2-ketocarboxylates derived metabolically from the amino acids methionine, threonine, leucine, isoleucine, and valine. Thiamin pyrophosphate also serves as the coenzyme for transketolase, which catalyzes 2-carbon fragment exchange reactions in the oxidation of glucose by the hexose monophosphate shunt.

Measurement

Thiamin is expressed quantitatively in terms of its mass, usually in milligrams.

Dietary Reference Intakes

In 1998, DRIs were established for thiamin; these include AIs for infants and the newly defined RDAs. In general, the EARs and RDAs are based on levels of energy intake, due to the direct role of thiamin in energy metabolism, whereas the AIs for infants are based on the thiamin levels typically found in human milk (Table 4–14).

TABLE 4–14 DIETARY REFERENCE INTAKES FOR THIAMIN

LIFE STAGE GROUP	RDA (mg/d)
Infants	
0–6 mo	0.2*
7–12 mo	0.3*
Children	
1–3 y	0.5
4–8 y	0.6
Males	
9–13 y	.9
14–18 y	1.2
19–30 y	1.2
31–50 y	1.2
51–70 y	1.2
>70 y	1.2
Females	
9–13 y	.9
14–18 y	1.0
19–30 y	1.1
31–50 y	1.1
51–70 y	1.1
>70 y	1.1
Pregnancy	
≤18 y	1.4
19–30 y	1.4
31–50 y	1.4
Lactation	
≤18 y	1.5
19–30 y	1.5
31–50 y	1.5

(From Institute of Medicine, Food and Nutrition Board. Dietary Reference Intakes for Thiamin, Riboflavin, Niacin, Vitamin B-6, Folate, Vitamin B-12, Pantothenic Acid, Biotin, and Choline. Washington, DC: National Academy Press, 1998.)
*AI, adequate intake; RDA, recommended dietary allowance.

Sources

Thiamin is widely distributed in many foods, most of which contain only low concentrations. The richest sources are yeasts and liver; however, cereal grains comprise the most important source of the vitamin in most human diets. Although whole grains are typically rich in thiamin, most of that is removed by milling and refining. Plant foods contain thiamin predominantly in the free form, whereas almost all of the thiamin in animal products exists in phosphorylated forms, mostly as TPP (Table 4–15).

Thiamin can be destroyed by heat, oxidation, and ionizing radiation, but it is stable during frozen storage. Cooking losses of the vitamin tend to be highly variable, depending on cooking time, pH, temperature, quantity of water used and discarded, and whether the water is chlorinated. Thiamin can be destroyed by several *sulfites* added in processing, by thiamin-degrading enzymes *(thiaminases)* present in fish, shellfish and some bacteria, and by certain heat-stable factors in several plants (e.g., ferns, tea, betel nut).

Deficiency

Thiamin deficiency is characterized by anorexia and weight loss as well as cardiac and neurologic signs. In humans, these are eventually manifest as **beriberi,** the symptoms of which include mental confusion, muscular wasting, edema (in "wet" beriberi), peripheral neuropathy, tachycardia, and cardiomegaly. The nonedematous ("dry") form of the disease is usually associated with energy deprivation and inactivity, whereas the "wet" form is usually associated with a high carbohydrate intake along with strenuous physical exertion. The latter is characterized by edema due to biventricular heart failure with pulmonary congestion. Without TPP, pyruvate cannot enter the TCA cycle and energy deprivation of the heart muscle results in heart failure. Beriberi has been reported in infants (infantile beriberi) fed formulated diets unsupplemented with thiamin; in these cases, deterioration was sudden and characterized by cardiac failure and cyanosis. Beriberi responds to thiamin treatment, particularly if neural damage and cardiac involvement are not great.

Historically, beriberi has been endemic among the poor in areas of the world where rice is the major staple food and, particularly, where people also consume raw fish or other sources of thiaminase. Such conditions will usually produce multiple

TABLE 4–15 THIAMIN CONTENT OF SELECTED FOODS

FOOD	mg
Yeast, brewer's, 1 oz	4.43
Pork chop, lean, 3.5 oz	0.82
Ham, lean, 3.5 oz	0.75
Sunflower seeds, shelled, 1 oz	0.59
Wheat germ, raw, ¼ cup	0.55
Milk, soy, 1 cup	0.39
Malt-o-meal, 1 cup	0.38
Beans, baked, 1 cup	0.34
Pasta, spaghetti, cooked, 1 cup	0.29
Rice, white, enriched, cooked, 1 cup	0.26
Doughnut, yeast, 1	0.22
Potato, baked, 1	0.22
Orange juice, from frzn conc., 1 cup	0.20
Squash, acorn, baked, ½ cup	0.17
Salmon, pink, baked, 3 oz	0.17
Bread, white, 1 slice	0.12
Peanuts, roasted, shelled, 1 oz	0.12
Milk, 2%, 1 cup	0.10
Tomato, 1	0.07
Chicken, breast, roasted, 3 oz, w/skin	0.06
Halibut, baked, 3 oz	0.06
Lettuce, romaine, 1 cup	0.06
Hamburger, lean, broiled med, 3.5 oz	0.05
Egg, 1	0.03

(From Pennington J. Bowe's and Church's Food Values of Portions Commonly Used, 17th ed. Philadelphia: Lippincott-Raven, 1998.)

nutritional deficiencies, making uncomplicated beriberi unlikely.

Frank thiamin deficiency is not common in the United States, due to the thiamin supplementation of rice. Subclinical thiamin deficiency occurs among alcoholics who tend to have inadequate intakes and impaired absorption of the vitamin. Affected individuals show an encephalopathy called *Wernicke-Korsakoff syndrome,* the signs of which range from mild confusion to coma. Many show an apparently inherited abnormal transketolase incapable of normal TPP binding. Table 4–16 summarizes symptoms of thiamin deficiency.

Toxicity

There is little information about the toxic potential of thiamin, although massive doses (1000 times nutritional needs) of the commercial form, thiamin hydrochloride, have suppressed the respiratory center with fatal results. Parenteral doses of thiamin at 100 times the recommended levels have produced headache, convulsions, muscular weakness, cardiac arrhythmia, and allergic reactions.

Riboflavin

The biologic significance of a yellow-green fluorescent pigment in milk, recognized in 1879, was first understood in 1932. The vitamin was synthesized and named **riboflavin** in 1935.

Riboflavin (formerly, vitamin B_2), is essential for the metabolism of carbohydrates, amino acids, and lipids and also supports antioxidant protection. It discharges these functions as the coenzymes *flavin adenine dinucleotide (FAD)* and *flavin adenine mononucleotide (FMN)*. Because of these fundamental roles in metabolism, riboflavin deficiencies are first manifest in tissues with rapid cellular turnover, such as the skin and epithelia.

Absorption, Transport, and Storage

Riboflavin is absorbed in the free form by a carrier-mediated process in the proximal small intestine. Because most foods contain the vitamin in its coenzyme forms, FMN and FAD, absorption follows the hydrolytic cleavage of free riboflavin from its various flavoprotein complexes. The mucosal uptake of free riboflavin is coupled to its phosphorylation to FMN.

Riboflavin is transported in the plasma both as free riboflavin and FMN, both of which are largely bound to plasma proteins, particularly *albumin*. A specific *riboflavin-binding protein (RfBP)* has also

TABLE 4–16 CLINICAL FEATURES OF THIAMIN DEFICIENCY

DEFICIENCY TYPE	FEATURES
Early stage of deficiency	Anorexia Indigestion Constipation Malaise Heaviness and weakness of legs Calf muscle tenderness "Pins and needles" and numbness in legs Anesthesia of skin, particularly at the tibia Increased pulse rate and palpitations
Wet beriberi	Edema of legs, face, trunk, and serous cavities Tense calf muscles Fast pulse Distended neck veins High blood pressure Decreased urine volume
Dry beriberi	Worsening of polyneuritis of early stage Difficulty walking Wernicke-Korsakoff syndrome; encephalopathy may occur —Loss of immediate memory —Disorientation —Nystagmus (jerky movements of eyes) —Ataxia (staggering gait)
Infantile beriberi (2–5 mo of age)	Acute —Decreased urine output —Excessive crying; thin and plaintive whining —Cardiac failure Chronic —Constipation and vomiting —Fretfulness —Soft, toneless muscles —Pallor of skin with cyanosis

been identified and is thought to function in the transplacental movement of the vitamin. Riboflavin is transported in its free form into cells that then convert it mostly to FMN but also to FAD, both of which are largely protein bound. Although small amounts of the vitamin are found in the liver and kidney, it is not stored to any appreciable degree and must, therefore, be supplied in the diet regularly.

Metabolism

Riboflavin is converted to its coenzyme forms by an adenosine triphosphate (ATP)-dependent phosphorylation to yield riboflavin-5′-phosphate, also called FMN, by the enzyme *flavokinase*. Most FMN is then converted to FAD by FAD-pyrophosphorylase. Both steps are regulated by thyroid hormones.

Most riboflavin in tissues occurs as non-covalently linked FAD in functional *flavoproteins,* but some enzymes contain covalently attached FAD. Protein-bound flavins are resistant to catabolism, which occurs to unbound forms of the vitamin. This involves the dephosphorylation of FAD to yield FMN and of FMN to yield free riboflavin by pyrophosphatases or alkaline phosphatase. Riboflavin can be glycosylated in the liver; the glycosylated metabolite is excreted, but it has been suggested that it may also have a direct metabolic function. Riboflavin can also be catabolized by oxidation, demethylation, and hydroxylation of its ring system to yield products that are lost in the urine along with free riboflavin, which constitutes the chief source of urinary excretion.

Functions

The flavin coenzymes FMN and FAD are versatile redox cofactors because they can participate in either one- or two-electron redox reactions, thus, serving as switching sites between obligate two-electron donors (e.g., nicotinamide adenine dinucleotide [NADH], succinate) and obligate one-electron acceptors (e.g., iron-sulfur proteins, heme proteins). Both FMN and FAD serve as prosthetic groups of several flavoprotein enzymes that catalyze oxidation-reduction reactions in the cells and function as hydrogen carriers in the mitochondrial electron transport system. In other cellular roles, riboflavin and nicotinamide adenine dinucleotide phosphate (NADPH)-dependent mechanisms appear to combat oxidative damage to the cell. In one study riboflavin was administered during experimental ischemia and appeared to lessen negative consequences (Christensen, 1993). The cataract study in Linxian, China suggests a beneficial effect of nutritional supplements on cataracts, at least in marginally nourished populations. Riboflavin was considered to be an important factor, but findings were not conclusive (Sperduto et al., 1993).

FMN and FAD are also coenzymes of dehydrogenases that catalyze the initial oxidations of fatty acids and of several intermediates in glucose metabolism. FMN is also required for the conversion of pyridoxine (vitamin B_6) to its functional form pyridoxal phosphate. FAD is also required for the biosynthesis of the vitamin niacin from the amino acid tryptophan (Decker, 1993).

Measurement

Riboflavin content of foods or requirements are expressed in milligrams.

Dietary Reference Intakes

In 1998, DRIs were established for riboflavin, which, like those for thiamin, include AIs for infants and the newly defined RDAs. In general, the RDAs were based on the amount required to maintain normal tissue reserves, based on urinary excretion, red blood cell riboflavin contents, and erythrocyte glutathione reductase activity. Riboflavin needs are increased during pregnancy and lactation to meet the needs of increased tissue synthesis and the losses of riboflavin secreted in breast milk (Table 4–17).

TABLE 4–17 DIETARY REFERENCE INTAKES FOR RIBOFLAVIN

LIFE STAGE GROUP	RDA (mg/d)
Infants	
0–6 mo	0.3*
7–12 mo	0.4*
Children	
1–3 y	0.5
4–8 y	0.6
Males	
9–13 y	.9
14–18 y	1.3
19–30 y	1.3
31–50 y	1.3
51–70 y	1.3
>70 y	1.3
Females	
9–13 y	.9
14–18 y	1.0
19–30 y	1.1
31–50 y	1.1
51–70 y	1.1
>70 y	1.1
Pregnancy	
≤18 y	1.4
19–30 y	1.4
31–50 y	1.4
Lactation	
≤18 y	1.6
19–30 y	1.6
31–50 y	1.6

(From Institute of Medicine, Food and Nutrition Board. Dietary Reference Intakes for Thiamin, Riboflavin, Niacin, Vitamin B-6, Folate, Vitamin B-12, Pantothenic Acid, Biotin, and Choline. Washington, DC: National Academy Press, 1998.)

*AI, adequate intake; RDA, recommended dietary allowance.

Sources

Riboflavin is widely distributed in foods bound to proteins as FMN and FAD. Rapidly growing, green leafy vegetables are rich in the vitamin; however, meats and dairy products are the most important contributors of the vitamin to the diets of Americans (Table 4–18). More than half of the vitamin is lost when flour is milled; however, most breads and cereals are enriched with riboflavin and contribute appreciably to the total daily intake.

Riboflavin is stable to heat, but it can be readily destroyed by alkali and exposure to ultraviolet irradiation. Very little of the vitamin is lost in the cooking and processing of foods; however, because of its sensitivity to alkali, the common practice of adding baking soda to soften dried peas or beans destroys much of their riboflavin content. Wax-lined paper containers protect milk against riboflavin loss from exposure to sunlight.

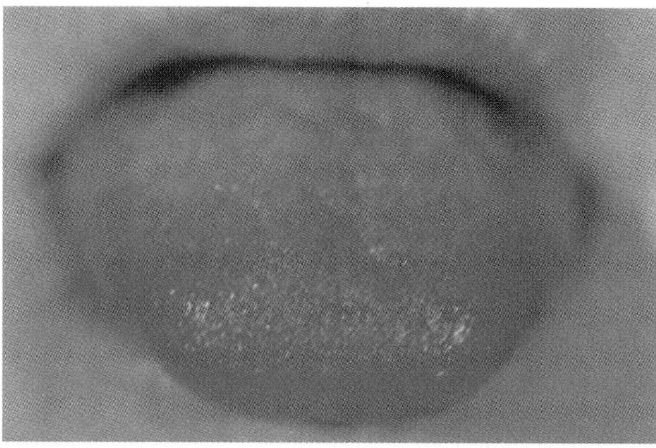

FIGURE 4–6 Magenta tongue is a sign of riboflavin deficiency. In contrast, a pale tongue is probably attributed to iron deficiency; a beefy red-colored tongue is caused by vitamin B-complex deficiency. (From McLaren DS. Color Atlas of Nutritional Disorders. England: Yearbook Medical Publishers, 1981.

Deficiency

Uncomplicated riboflavin deficiency becomes manifest after several months of deprivation of the vitamin. The early symptoms include photophobia, lacrimation, burning and itching of the eyes, loss of visual acuity, and soreness and burning of lips, mouth, and tongue. Subsequent symptoms include cheilosis (fissuring of the lips); angular stomatitis (cracks in the skin at the corners of the mouth); a greasy eruption of the skin in the nasolabial folds, scrotum, or vulva; a purple swollen tongue (Fig. 4–6); capillary overgrowth around the cornea of the eye; and peripheral neuropathy.

Phototherapy of infants with hyperbilirubinemia often leads to riboflavin deficiency (by photodestruction of the vitamin) if such therapy does not also include riboflavin administration. Otherwise, riboflavin deficiencies occur usually in combination with deficiencies of other water-soluble vitamins, such as thiamin and niacin. Table 4–19 summarizes signs of possible riboflavin deficiency.

TABLE 4–18 RIBOFLAVIN CONTENT OF SELECTED FOODS

FOOD	mg
Liver, beef, 3.5 oz	4.10
Yeast, brewer's, 1 oz	1.21
Milk, 2% fat, 1 cup	0.40
Yogurt, fruit flavored, low-fat, 1 cup	0.37
Clams, canned, 3 oz	0.36
Ice milk, soft serve, 1 oz	0.34
Egg, 1	0.25
Custard, bkd, ½ cup	0.25
Pork, roast loin, 3 oz	0.24
Cheese, feta, 1 oz	0.24
Bagel, plain, 1	0.22
Hamburger, lean, broiled med, 3.5 oz	0.21
Spinach, fresh, ckd, ½ cup	0.21
Cheese, cottage, 2% fat, ½ cup	0.21
Chicken, dark meat, 3 oz	0.19
Wheat germ, raw, ¼ cup	0.14
Cheese, colby, 1 oz	0.11
Milk, human, 1 oz	0.09
Trout, rainbow, farmed, bkd, 3 oz	0.07
Rice, brown, cooked, 1 cup	0.05
Orange, 1	0.05
Apple, 1	0.02

(From Pennington J. Bowe's and Church's Food Values of Portions Commonly Used, 17th ed. Philadelphia: Lippincott-Raven, 1998.)

Toxicity

There is no known toxicity for riboflavin; high oral doses are considered essentially nontoxic.

Niacin

Niacin is the generic term for **nicotinamide** (niacinamide) and nicotinic acid. It functions as a component of the pyridine nucleotide coenzymes *nicotinamide adenine dinucleotide (NAD)* and *nicotinamide adenine dinucleotide phosphate (NADP)*, which are present in all cells.

Niacin was identified as a result of the search for the cause and cure of **pellagra,** a disease common in Spain and Italy in the 18th century. The problem had reached sufficient proportions in the United States in the early 1900s that the Public Health Service enlisted Goldberger to investigate pellagra that was rampant in the southern states (Goldberger et al., 1918), where diets were based on cornmeal. He established that a nutrient deficiency was the cause of the disease and that it could be cured by a diet containing high-quality protein. Recognition of pellagra as a niacin deficiency disease followed the discovery in 1937 by Elvehjem that the pellagrous disease of black tongue in dogs was caused by lack of niacin. Since then it has been established that **tryptophan** is a precursor of niacin and tryptophan deficiency is also involved in pellagra.

TABLE 4–19 SIGNS OF POSSIBLE RIBOFLAVIN DEFICIENCY

Soreness and burning of lips, mouth, and tongue*
Cheilosis*
Angular stomatitis*
Glossitis*
Seborrheic dermatitis of nasolabial folds, vestibule of nose, and sometimes the ears and eyelids, scrotum, and vulva
Ocular pathology (sometimes)
—Inflammation of conjunctiva
—Superficial vascularization of cornea
—Ulcerations of cornea
—Photophobia
Anemia—normocytic and normochronic
Neuropathy
Purplish or magenta tongue*
Hypertrophy or atrophy of tongue papillae*

(Adapted from Goldsmith GA. Riboflavin deficiency. In: Rivlin RS (ed). Riboflavin. New York: Plenum Press, 1975.)

*Tongue and mouth changes are difficult to differentiate from those in niacin, folic acid, thiamin, vitamin B_6, or vitamin B_{12} deficiency.

Biosynthesis, Absorption, Transport, and Storage

Niacin can be synthesized from the amino acid tryptophan. Even though the efficiency of this process is low, dietary tryptophan intake is important to the overall niacin economy of the body.

Niacin in many foods, particularly those from animal sources, consists mostly of the coenzyme forms, NADH and NADPH, each of which must be digested to release the absorbed forms, nicotinamide (Nam) and nicotinic acid (NA). Many foods derived from plants, particularly grains, contain niacin in covalently bound complexes with small peptides and carbohydrates that are not released on digestion. These forms, collectively referred to as *niacytin,* are not biologically available, but can be rendered so by alkaline hydrolysis. Thus, the Central American tradition of soaking maize in lime water before preparing tortillas effectively increases the bioavailability of what otherwise is a low-niacin food.

Ultimately, Nam and NA are absorbed in the small intestine by carrier-mediated facilitated diffusion. Both are transported in the plasma in free solution, and each is taken up by most tissues by passive diffusion although some tissues (e.g., erythrocytes, kidney, brain) also have a transport system for NA. Niacin is retained in tissues by being converted mostly to NADH but also to NADPH.

Metabolism

The de novo synthesis of NADH and NADPH occurs from *quinolinic acid,* a metabolite of the indispensable amino acid tryptophan. This interconversion involves both FAD- and pyridoxal phosphate-dependent steps and therefore depends on adequate nutritional status with respect to riboflavin and, to a lesser extent, vitamin B_6. The rate-limiting enzymes in this pathway are *3-hydroxyanthranilic acid oxidase (3-HAAO)* and *picolinic acid carboxylase (PAC)*. Species with low 3-HAAO:PAC ratios (e.g., ducks, cats) are inefficient in converting tryptophan to niacin and, thus, have relatively high requirements for the preformed niacin. Humans appear to be moderately efficient at this conversion: about 60 mg tryptophan is required to produce 1 mg niacin. This aspect of tryptophan metabolism yields *nicotinic acid mononucleotide (NMN),* which is phosphoradenylated to form NAD.

Both NADH and NADPH can be produced from NA and Nam obtained from the diet. The latter is deamidated to yield NA, and NA is phosphoribosylated, adenylated, and then amidated to yield NADH which itself can be phosphorylated to yield NADPH.

The pyridine nucleotides NADH and NADPH are catabolized by hydrolysis to yield Nam, which can be deamidated to NA or methylated to yield *1-methylnicotinamide (mNAm)*. Urinary excretion of the vitamin consists of the NA, Nam, mNAm and oxidized metabolites of the latter such as 1-methyl-2-pyridone-5-carboxamide. The profile of urinary metabolites can be changed by deprivation of dietary protein.

Functions

The coenzymes NADH and NADPH are the most central electron carriers of cells, playing essential roles as co-substrates of more than 200 enzymes involved in the metabolism of carbohydrates, fatty acids, and amino acids. In general, NADH and NADPH facilitate stereospecific hydrogen transport by two-electron transfers, which using the hydride ion as the carrier, play very different roles in metabolism. The NADH-dependent reactions are involved in intracellular respiration, whereas most dependent on NADPH serve biosynthetic (e.g., fatty acids, sterols) functions.

Measurement

Niacin is expressed quantitatively in terms of its mass. Food values are often expressed in term of *niacin equivalents,* calculated from the preformed niacin content plus 1/60th of the tryptophan content.

Dietary Reference Intakes

In 1998, DRIs were established for niacin; these include AIs for infants, the newly defined RDAs, and the tolerable upper intake limits (ULs) (Table 4–20).

Sources

Significant amounts of niacin are found in many foods; lean meats, poultry, fish, peanuts, and yeasts are particulary rich sources. Niacin occurs predomi-

TABLE 4–20 DIETARY REFERENCE INTAKES FOR NIACIN

LIFE STAGE GROUP	RDA (mg NE/d)[†]	UL (mg NE/d)
Infants		
0–6 mo	2*	ND
7–12 mo	4*	ND
Children		
1–3 y	6	10
4–8 y	8	15
Males		
9–13 y	12	20
14–18 y	16	30
19–30 y	16	35
31–50 y	16	35
51–70 y	16	35
>70 y	16	35
Females		
9–13 y	12	20
14–18 y	14	30
19–30 y	14	35
31–50 y	14	35
51–70 y	14	35
>70 y	14	35
Pregnancy		
≤18 y	18	30
19–30 y	18	35
31–50 y	18	35
Lactation		
≤18 y	17	30
19–30 y	17	35
31–50 y	17	35

(From Institute of Medicine, Food and Nutrition Board. Dietary Reference Intakes for Thiamin, Riboflavin, Niacin, Vitamin B-6, Folate, Vitamin B-12, Pantothenic Acid, Biotin, and Choline. Washington, DC: National Academy Press, 1998.)

*AI, adequate intake; RDA, recommended dietary intake; UL, tolerable upper intake level; ND, not determinable due to lack of data.

[†]As niacin equivalents (NE). 1 mg niacin = 60 mg tryptophan; 0 to 6 mo = preformed niacin (not NE).

TABLE 4–21 NIACIN CONTENT OF SELECTED FOODS

FOOD	mg
Tuna, canned in water, 3 oz	11.8
Wheat flour, 1 cup	7.4
Corn grits, instant, 1 pkct	6.8
Cheerios, 1 cup	5.0
Beef, round choice, braised, 3.5 oz	4.1
Seaweed, spirulina, dried, 1 oz	3.7
Potato, baked with skin, 1 med	3.3
Bagel, plain, 1	3.2
Mushrooms, raw, ½ cup	1.4
Corn, yellow, ½ cup, boiled	1.3
Peach, raw, 1 med	0.9
Carrot, raw, 1 med	0.7
Salt pork, 1 oz	0.5
Cow's milk, 2%, 1 cup	0.2
Human milk, 1 fl oz	0.1
Whole egg, 1 large	0.0

(From Pennington J. Bowe's and Church's Food Values of Portions Commonly Used, 17th ed. Philadelphia: Lippincott-Raven, 1998.)

nantly as protein-bound NA in plant tissues, and as Nam, NADH and NADPH in animal tissues. Milk and eggs contain small amounts of niacin, but they are excellent sources of tryptophan, giving them significant niacin equivalent contents. Most tables of food nutrient composition list only preformed niacin, thus underestimating the total niacin equivalencies of many foods. Table 4–21 lists the niacin content of various foods.

Deficiency

Niacin deficiency in humans is first manifest as muscular weakness, anorexia, indigestion, and skin eruptions. Severe deficiency of niacin leads to pellagra, which is characterized by dermatitis, dementia, and diarrhea (the "3 Ds"); tremors; and sore tongue ("beef tongue"). The dermatologic changes are usually the most prominent: the skin develops a cracked, pigmented, scaly dermatitis in sun-exposed areas (Fig. 4–7). Central nervous system involvement is manifest as confusion, disorientation, and neuritis. Digestive abnormalities cause irritation and inflammation of the mucous membranes of the mouth and the gastrointestinal tract.

Patients with pellagra can also show clinical signs of riboflavin deficiency, evidencing the metabolic interrelationships of these vitamins. Patients are likely to have had very poor diets not only providing very little niacin but also lacking protein and other nutrients.

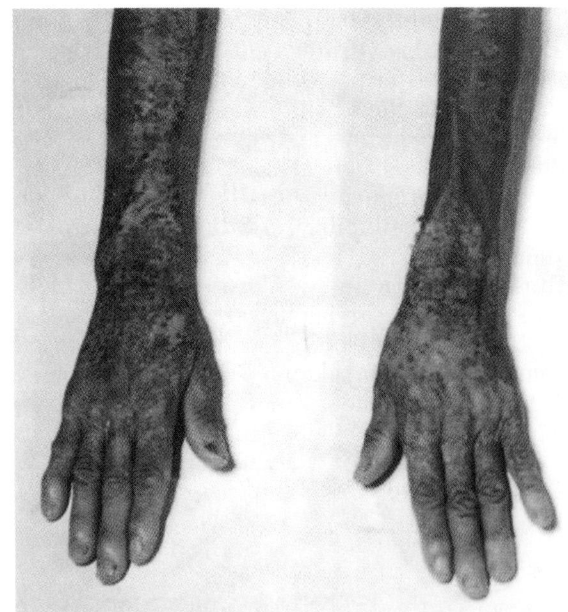

FIGURE 4–7 Pellagra. Pigmented keratotic scaling lesions resulting from deficiency of niacin. These lesions are especially prominent in areas exposed to the sun, such as hands, forearm, neck, and legs. (From Latham MC, et al. Scope Manual on Nutrition. Kalamazoo, MI: The Upjohn Company, 1980, copyright by Thomas Spies, MD.)

Toxicity

In general, the toxicity of niacin is low. There are, however, side effects of clinical uses of high doses of 1 to 2 g of NA three times per day, which have been used in attempts to lower blood cholesterol concentrations (see Chapter 26). The main side effect is a histamine release that causes flushing and that may be injurious to persons with asthma or peptic ulcer disease. Nam does not have this effect. High doses of niacin can also be toxic to the liver, and risks are greater with time-released forms of the vitamin (Reimund and Ramos, 1994). Megavitamin use should be monitored carefully because high doses are medication and not nutritional supplements.

Vitamin B_6

Vitamin B_6 is the descriptor for 2-methyl-3,5-dihydroxy methylpyridine derivatives exhibiting the biologic activity of **pyridoxine,** a compound that was formerly called pyridoxol. Pyridoxine was identified as another fraction of the vitamin B complex in 1938 and synthesized in 1939. The biologically active analogues of this alcohol form are the aldehyde pyridoxal and the amine pyridoxamine. The biologic activity of each depends on its metabolism to the coenzyme form *pyridoxal phosphate (PLP).*

Absorption, Transport, and Storage

The various forms of vitamin B_6 appear to be absorbed by passive diffusion primarily in the jejunum and ileum. Absorption is driven by phosphorylation to form PLP and *pyridoxamine phosphate* (PMP), and then by protein binding of each of these metabolites in the intestinal mucosa and blood.

The predominant form of the vitamin in the blood is PLP, most of which is derived from the liver after metabolism by hepatic flavoenzymes. Small amounts of free pyridoxine are also found in the circulation, but most is as PLP bound to albumin. Cells take up pyridoxal in preference to PLP; thus, the dephosphorylation of the latter is thought to occur as part of the cellular uptake process. On uptake, pyridoxal is again phosphorylated to PLP and PMP, the greatest levels being found in liver, brain, kidney, spleen, and muscle where they are bound to proteins. Muscle serves as the largest depot, containing 80% to 90% of the total body vitamin stores in the form of PLP bound to glycogen phosphorylase.

Metabolism

The vitamers B_6 are readily interconverted metabolically by phosphorylation/dephosphorylation, oxidation/reduction, and amination/deamination. The limiting step in this metabolism is catalyzed by the FMN-enzyme pyridoxal phosphate oxidase. Thus, deprivation of riboflavin can reduce the conversions of pyridoxine and pyridoxamine to the active coenzyme PLP.

In the liver, PLP is dephosphorylated and oxidized by FAD- and NAD-dependent enzymes to yield 4-pyridoxic acid and other inactive metabolites that are excreted in the urine.

Functions

The metabolically active form of vitamin B_6 is PLP, which serves as a coenzyme of numerous enzymes involved in practically all reactions in the metabolism of amino acids as well as several aspects of the metabolism of neurotransmitters, glycogen, sphingolipids, heme, and steroids. These roles relate to the ability of the PLP aldehyde group to react with primary amino groups and thus to stabilize the other bonds on the bound carbon. Thus, vitamin B_6 is essential for a variety of amino acid transaminases, decarboxylases, racemases, and isomerases. It is needed for the biosynthesis of the neurotransmitters serotonin, epinephrine, norepinephrine, and γ-aminobutyric acid, the vasodilator and gastric secretagogue histamine, and the porphyrin precursors of heme (Guilarte, 1993). The vitamin is also required for the metabolic conversion of tryptophan to niacin, the release of glucose from glycogen, the biosynthesis of sphingolipids in the myelin sheaths of nerve cells, and in the modulation of steroid hormone receptors.

Measurement

The vitamin B_6 content of foods is expressed in milligrams. However, this practice does not account for known differences in bioavailability of vitamin B_6 in different foods.

Dietary Reference Intakes

In 1998, DRIs were established for vitamin B_6, which include AIs for infants, and the newly defined RDAs, and ULs for children and adults. In general, needs for vitamin B_6 increase with increasing intakes of protein; adequate vitamin B_6 status appears to be maintained when the vitamin is consumed in an approximate ratio of 0.016 mg/g protein (Driskell, 1994) (Table 4–22).

Sources

Vitamin B_6 is widely distributed in foods, occurring in greatest concentrations in meats, whole-grain products (especially wheat), vegetables, and nuts (Table 4–23). Much of the vitamin B_6 in many foods is bound covalently to proteins or is glycosylated, the digestibilities of which result in much of the vitamin B_6 contents of foods having relatively low bioavailabilities. Because plants (e.g., potatoes, spinach, beans, and other legumes) generally contain more complexed forms of the vitamins than animal tissues, foods derived from animal sources

TABLE 4–22 DIETARY REFERENCE INTAKES FOR VITAMIN B_6

LIFE STAGE GROUP	RDA (mg/d)[†]	UL (mg/d)
Infants		
0–6 mo	.1*	ND
7–12 mo	.3*	ND
Children		
1–3 y	.5	30
4–8 y	.6	40
Males		
9–13 y	1.0	60
14–18 y	1.3	80
19–30 y	1.3	100
31–50 y	1.3	100
51–70 y	1.7	100
>70 y	1.7	100
Females		
9–13 y	1.0	60
14–18 y	1.2	80
19–30 y	1.3	100
31–50 y	1.3	100
51–70 y	1.5	100
>70 y	1.5	100
Pregnancy		
≤18 y	1.9	80
19–30 y	1.9	100
31–50 y	1.9	100
Lactation		
≤18 y	2.0	80
19–30 y	2.0	100
31–50 y	2.0	100

(From Institute of Medicine, Food and Nutrition Board. Dietary Reference Intakes for Thiamin, Riboflavin, Niacin, Vitamin B-6, Folate, Vitamin B-12, Pantothenic Acid, Biotin, and Choline. Washington, DC: National Academy Press, 1998.)

*AI, adequate intake; RDA, recommended dietary intake; UL, tolerable upper intake level; ND, not determinable due to lack of data.

tend to have superior vitamin B_6 bioavailabilities than those derived from plants.

Deficiency

Deprivation of vitamin B_6 leads to metabolic abnormalities resulting from insufficient production of PLP. These manifest clinically as dermatologic and neurologic changes in most species. Humans show symptoms of weakness, sleeplessness, peripheral neuropathies, cheilosis, glossitis, stomatitis, and impaired cell-mediated immunity. Due to the widespread distribution of the vitamin in foods, cases of vitamin B_6 deficiency are relatively rare. However, deficiency may be precipitated by medications (e.g., the antitubercular drug, isoniazid) that interfere with the metabolism of the vitamin (see Chapter 18). Infants fed a milk-based formula in which much of vitamin B_6 was unknowingly destroyed in processing developed irritability and convulsions, but recovered rapidly after an injection of the vitamin.

Toxicity

The toxicity of vitamin B_6 appears to be relatively low, although high, acute doses (several grams per day) have produced sensory neuropathy marked by changes in gait and peripheral sensation (Schaumberg et al., 1983). Many of the signs of vitamin B_6 toxicity appear to resemble those of vitamin B_6 deficiency.

Folate

Folate is the descriptor for a family of vitamers discovered in the course of investigations of the causes of nutritional anemias. It was chemically synthesized in the laboratory and established as a dietary nutrient in 1946. Named for their abundance in plant foliage, the term "folate" refers to pteroyl-

TABLE 4–23 PYRIDOXINE (VITAMIN B_6) CONTENT OF SELECTED FOODS

FOOD	mg	FOOD	mg
Liver, beef, 3.5 oz.	0.91	Peanut butter, 2 T	0.15
Oatmeal, 1 pkt	0.74	Brussel sprouts, cooked, ½ cup	0.14
Banana, 1	0.66	Cauliflower, cooked, ½ cup	0.11
Chicken, light meat, 3.5 oz	0.60	Orange juice, 1 cup	0.10
Potatoes, mashed, 1 cup	0.48	Milk, 2%, 1 cup	0.10
Avocado, California, 1	0.48	Tomato, raw, 1	0.10
Sunflower seeds, kernels, ¼ cup	0.45	Frankfurter, 1	0.07
Halibut, baked, 3 oz	0.34	Apple, 1 med	0.07
Chicken, dark meat, 3 oz	0.30	Egg, large, 1	0.07
Pork chop, baked, 3 oz	0.30	Apricots, dried halves, 10	0.05
Wheat germ, toasted, ¼ cup	0.28	Bread, whole-wheat, 1 slice	0.05
Rice, brown, cooked, 1 cup	0.28	Corn, canned, ½ cup	0.04
Prunes, dried, 10	0.22	Milk, human, 1 cup	0.03
Beef, hamburger, 3.5 oz	0.20	Cheese, cheddar, 1 oz	0.02
Rice, white, 1 cup	0.15	Bread, white, 1 slice	0.02

(From Pennington J. Bowe's and Church's Food Values of Portions Commonly Used, 17th ed. Philadelphia: Lippincott-Raven, 1998.)

monoglutamic acid and related compounds including those conjugated with one or more L-glutamic acid residues. The reduced compound, *tetrahydrofolic acid (FH_4)* functions metabolically as a carrier for several single-carbon derivatives, which are named according to the specific carbon moiety. Thus, the folates include a large number of chemically related species; an estimated 100 different folate vitamers are found in animals. Those from most natural sources usually have a single carbon unit at N-5 or N-10 or both; these forms participate in the metabolism of the *single carbon pool*.

Absorption, Transport, and Storage

Dietary folates are absorbed as the monoglutamate forms **folic acid,** 5-methyltetrahydrofolic acid, and 5-formyltetrahydrofolic acid in most species. This occurs by active transport mainly in the jejunum, but the vitamin can also be absorbed by passive diffusion.

Because most folate in foods is present in polyglutamate forms, absorption of the ingested vitamin depends on the ability to hydrolyze those forms to yield folyl monoglutamates. This step is accomplished by brush border and intracellular mucosal folyl conjugases. Because of inefficiencies in this step, the bioavailabilities of folate in food are typically about half those of the purified vitamin. This is the main reason for the recommendation for women intending to conceive that they supplement their diet with folic acid in addition to eating foods high in folate content.

Folate taken up by the intestinal mucosal cell is reduced to FH_4, which can either be transferred to the portal circulation or alkylated to 5-methyl-FH_4 before entering the circulation.

Because the folyl polyglutamates cannot cross biologic membranes, cellular uptake of folates involves exclusively the monoglutamate derivatives found in plasma. This occurs both by an energy-dependent process involving a specific folate-binding protein, as well as by a separate, carrier-mediated anion-exchange process. Within cells, FH_4 is methylated to 5-methyl-FH_4, which is retained intracellularly by binding to intracellular macromolecules and by further conversion to folyl polyglutamates (Wagner, 1996). The liver is the most important depot for folate, containing about half of the total body store as tetra-, penta-, hexa-, and heptaglutamates of 5-methyl-FH_4 and 10-formyl-FH_4. Tissues with high rates of cell division (e.g., intestinal mucosa) tend to show relatively low concentrations of 5-methyl-FH_4 and high concentrations of 10-formyl-FH_4; 5-methyl-FH_4 predominates in tissues with low rates of cell division.

Metabolism

Folates are metabolized in three ways: reduction of the pterin ring, reactions of the polyglutamyl side chain, and acquisition of single-carbon moieties at certain positions on the pterin ring. Ring reduction is catalyzed by the enzyme *7,8-dihydrofolate reductase,* high activities of which are found in liver, kidney, and rapidly dividing (e.g., tumor) cells. Side-chain reactions are accomplished by ATP-dependent *folyl polyglutamate synthetase,* which links glutamyl residues to the vitamin by peptide bonds involving the γ-carboxyl groups.

Folate is metabolically activated by conversion to one of several derivatives with single-carbon units substituted at the N-5 or N-10 (or both) positions of the pterin ring. The main source of the single-carbon fragments is *serine hydroxymethyltransferase,* which uses the dispensable amino acid serine and the single-carbon donor to produce 5,10-methylene-FH_4. Other enzymes similarly yield other single-carbon metabolites: 5-methyl-FH_4, 5,10-methenyl-FH_4, 5-formimino-FH_4, 5-formyl-FH_4, and 10-formyl-FH_4.

Tissue folates turn over by cleavage of their pteridine and para-aminoboenzoyl polyglutamate moieties. The latter is further degraded to a variety of water-soluble side-chain metabolites that are excreted in the urine and bile.

Functions

The folates function as enzyme co-substrates in many reactions of the metabolism of amino acids and nucleotides in which the fully reduced (tetrahydro-) form of each serves as an acceptor or donor of a single-carbon unit.

Folates serve several important roles in metabolism. They are necessary for the de novo synthesis of DNA by transferring formate (as 5,10-methenyl-FH_4) for purine synthesis and formaldehyde (as 5,10-methylene-FH_4) for thymidylate synthesis. It donates formate (as 10-formyl-FH_4) in purine synthesis. It is required for the conversion of histidine to glutamic acid, impairments of which result in accumulation of the intermediary product, *formiminoglutamic acid (FIGLU),* which is excreted in the urine. It provides labile methyl groups (as 5-methyl-FH_4) for the synthesis of methionine from homocysteine. This conversion also requires vitamin B_{12}, which passes the methyl group from 5-methyl-FH_4 to homocysteine; therefore, deficiencies of either folate or vitamin B_{12} can lead to homocysteinemia. Also because of this interrelationship, deprivation of vitamin B_{12} alone can produce a functional folate deficiency by interrupting the regeneration of FH_4, effectively trapping the vitamin as 5-methyl-FH_4—this is called the "methyl-folate trap." (See Fig. 35–7.)

Folate is essential for the formation of both red and white blood cells in the bone marrow and for their maturation. It serves as a single-carbon carrier in the formation of heme. Folate supplementation produces marked alleviation of pernicious anemia; however, the gastrointestinal symptoms and neurologic lesions of the anemia continue to progress. This "masking effect" is discussed in Chapter 35.

TABLE 4–24 DIETARY REFERENCE INTAKES FOR FOLATE*

LIFE STAGE GROUP	RDA (μg/d)	UL (μg/d)[c]
Infants		
0–6 mo	65[†]	ND
7–12 mo	80[†]	ND
Children		
1–3 y	150	300
4–8 y	200	400
Males		
9–13 y	300	600
14–18 y	400	800
19–30 y	400	1000
31–50 y	400	1000
51–70 y	400	1000
>70 y	400	1000
Females		
9–13 y	300	600
14–18 y	400[a]	800
19–30 y	400[a]	1000
31–50 y	400[a]	1000
51–70 y	400	1000
>70 y	400	1000
Pregnancy		
≤18 y	600[b]	800
19–30 y	600[b]	1000
31–50 y	600[b]	1000
Lactation		
≤18 y	500	800
19–30 y	500	1000
31–50 y	500	1000

(From Institute of Medicine, Food and Nutrition Board. Dietary Reference Intakes for Thiamin, Riboflavin, Niacin, Vitamin B-6, Folate, Vitamin B-12, Pantothenic Acid, Biotin, and Choline. Washington, DC: National Academy Press, 1998.)

*As dietary folate equivalent (DFE). 1 DFE = 1 μg food folate = 0.6 μg folic acid (from fortified food or supplement consumed with food = 0.5 μg synthetic (supplemental) folic acid taken on an empty stomach.

AI, adequate intake; RDA, recommended dietary intake; UL, tolerable upper intake level.

[a]In view of evidence linking folate intake with neural tube defects in the fetus, it is recommended that all women capable of becoming pregnant consume 400 μg synthetic folic acid from fortified foods and/or supplements in addition to intake of food folate from a varied diet.

[b]It is assumed that women will continue consuming 400 μg folic acid until their pregnancy is confirmed and they enter prenatal care, which ordinarily occurs after the end of the periconceptional period—the critical time for formation of the neural tube.

[c]The ULs for synthetic folic acid apply to forms obtained from supplements, fortified foods, or a combination of the two.

Measurement

Folates are expressed quantitatively, usually in micrograms. When applied to the quantitation of folate values of foods, this practice does not account for known differences in bioavailability of folates.

Dietary Reference Intakes

In 1998, DRIs were established for folate. The AIs were defined for infants, and the newly defined RDAs for children and adults are almost double the previous RDAs in most cases. Table 4–24 lists the new DRIs. These new DRIs for women include increased amounts for women who could become pregnant. Although low folate stores are found in approximately 10% of the population, this is not accompanied by signs of deficiency.

Sources

Folates occur, as reduced folyl polyglutamates (of mostly 5-methyl-FH_4 and 10-formyl-FH_4), in a variety of foods of both plant and animal origins. Liver, mushrooms, and green leafy vegetables (especially spinach, asparagus, and broccoli) are rich sources. Lean beef, potatoes, whole-wheat bread, and dried beans are good sources (Table 4–25). Methods for analyzing the concentration of folate in foods are difficult, and values in tables of food composition may be too low. Folate occurs in 150 different forms. The reduced forms in foods are easily oxidized and losses of 50% to 90% typically occur during storage, cooking, or processing at high temperatures.

The bioavailabilities of folates in foods also vary considerably. This relates to differences in the inherent biopotencies of the folate vitamers, the presence/absence of folyl conjugase inhibitors and folate binders, and the nutritional status of the host (e.g., deficiencies of iron and vitamin C can impair folate utilization). Thus, the relative bioavailabilities of folates in most foods are in the range of 25% to 50%.

Deficiency

Deficiencies of folate result in impaired biosynthesis of DNA and RNA, thus, reducing cell division, which is most apparent in cells with rapid multiplication rates, such as red blood cells, leukocytes, and epithelial cells of the stomach, intestine, vagina, and uterine cervix. This manifests as anemia, der-

TABLE 4–25 FOLIC ACID CONTENT OF SELECTED FOODS

FOOD	μg
Liver, beef, fried, 3.5 oz	220
Blackeyed peas, boiled, 1 cup	210
Yeast, active, dry, ¼ oz	164
Beans, white, boiled, ½ cup	144
Spinach, cooked, ½ cup	131
Wheat germ, raw, ¼ cup	81
Broccoli, cooked, 1 cup	78
Romaine lettuce, 1 cup	76
Fresh orange juice, 1 cup	75
Cabbage, raw, 1 cup	30
Egg, yolk, 1	25
Banana, 1	22
Almonds, dry roasted, 1 oz	18
Milk, 2%, 1 cup	15
Whole-wheat bread, 1 slice	14
Wheat bran, ¼ cup	12
White bread, 1 slice	9

(From Pennington J. Bowe's and Church's Food Values of Portions Commonly Used, 17th ed. Philadelphia: Lippincott-Raven, 1998.)

matologic lesions, and poor growth in most species. Early signs of deficiency in humans include nuclear hypersegmentation of circulating polymorphonuclear leukocytes followed by megaloblastic anemia and, then, general weakness, depression, and polyneuropathy (see Chapter 35).

Folate-responsive homocysteinemia, a condition associated with elevated risk for occlusive vascular disease, is prevalent among apparently healthy Americans, suggesting that subclinical folate deficiency may be common. The role of folate in normal cell division makes it particularly important in embryogenesis (Butterworth and Bendich, 1996). Thus, the finding that periconceptual folate supplementation can reduce the risk of serious birth defects (including neural tube defects) by as much as half stimulated the U.S. government to regulate the addition of folate to wheat flour (see Chapter 7).

Toxicity

No adverse effects of high oral doses of folate have been reported in animals, although parenteral administration of amounts some 1000 times the dietary requirement produce epileptiform seizures in the rat. It has been suggested that high levels of folate may render zinc unavailable through the formation of nonabsorbable complexes in the gut, and studies have shown that folate treatment can exacerbate the teratogenic effects of nutritional zinc deficiency in animals.

Vitamin B_{12}

Vitamin B_{12}, isolated in 1948 from liver extract, was the last vitamin to be identified; it was the extrinsic factor found to be effective in the treatment of pernicious anemia. The term vitamin B_{12} is now the descriptor for a family of compounds containing the porphyrin-like, cobalt-centered corrin nucleus. This family includes analogues containing cobalt-bound methyl-, 5′-deoxyadenosyl-, hydroxo- (OH^-), nitrito-, or aqua- (H_2O) groups; these are called methyl-, adenosyl-, hydroxo-, nitrito-, or aqua-cobalamin, respectively. Of the several **cobalamin** compounds that exhibit vitamin B_{12} activity, **cyanocobalamin** and *hydroxycobalamin* are the most active.

Absorption, Transport, and Storage

Vitamin B_{12} is absorbed by active transport and, at low efficiency (about 1%), by simple diffusion. The active process is mediated by a specific binding protein, the *intrinsic factor (IF),* which is present in gastric secretions. Intrinsic factor can bind any of the four cobalamins in a IF-vitamin B_{12} complex from which the vitamin is taken into the enterocyte by a process involving the binding to a specific membrane receptor on the ileal brush border.

After absorption, cobalamin is circulated to peripheral tissues bound to plasma proteins. In humans, some three fourths of the cobalamins in plasma are bound nonspecifically to glycoproteins referred to as *R proteins* of unknown physiologic importance (their vitamin B_{12} binding may be adventitious). Specific binding of the vitamers B_{12} occurs to two carrier proteins, *transcobalamins (TCs)* I and II.

Cellular uptake of vitamin B_{12} appears to be mediated by a specific TC-receptor that internalizes the TC-vitamin complex. After lysosomal degradation of TC, the free vitamin is released for binding to vitamin B_{12}-dependent enzymes.

In adequately nourished individuals, vitamin B_{12} is stored in appreciable amounts (~2000 μg), mainly in the liver, which typically accumulates a substantial store, some 5 to 7 years worth, most of which is in the form of adenosylcobalamin. An enterohepatic circulation of the vitamin also contributes to these stores.

Metabolism

Vitamin B_{12} is metabolically active only as derivatives that have either a 5′-deoxyadenosine or a methyl group attached covalently to the corrin ring cobalt atom. These conversions are accomplished by *vitamin B_{12} coenzyme synthetase* and *5-methyl-FH4:homocysteine methyltransferase,* respectively. Little, if any, metabolism of the corrinoid ring system occurs and the vitamin is excreted intact by both renal and biliary routes. Apparently, only the free cobalamins (not the adenosylated or methylated forms) in plasma are available for excretion.

Functions

Vitamin B_{12} functions in two coenzyme forms: *adenosylcobalamin* (for methylcalonyl-CoA mutase and leucine mutase) and *methylcobalamin* (for methionine synthetase). In these three reactions, these forms of the vitamin play important roles in the metabolism of propionate, amino acids, and single carbons, respectively. These steps are essential for normal function in the metabolism of all cells, especially for those of the gastrointestinal tract, bone marrow, and nervous tissue. Deprivation of the vitamin, therefore, is marked by increases in plasma and urinary levels of methylmalonic acid, aminoisocaproate, and homocysteine, and losses of FH_4 (via the methyl folate trap).

Measurement

Vitamin B_{12} is expressed in micrograms.

Recommended Dietary Allowance

The DRIs were established for vitamin B_{12}, which include AIs for infants, and the newly defined RDAs (Table 4–26). The adult RDA provides for substantial body stores in view of the prevalences of achlorhydria and atrophic gastritis associated with

TABLE 4–26 DIETARY REFERENCE INTAKES FOR VITAMIN B_{12}

LIFE STAGE GROUP	RDA (μg/d)
Infants	
0–6 mo	.4*
7–12 mo	.5*
Children	
1–3 y	0.9
4–8 y	1.2
Males	
9–13 y	1.8
14–18 y	2.4
19–30 y	2.4
31–50 y	2.4
51–70 y	2.4[a]
>70 y	2.4[a]
Females	
9–13 y	1.8
14–18 y	2.4
19–30 y	2.4
31–50 y	2.4
51–70 y	2.4[a]
>70 y	2.4[a]
Pregnancy	
≤18 y	2.6
19–30 y	2.6
31–50 y	2.6
Lactation	
≤18 y	2.8
19–30 y	2.8
31–50 y	2.8

(From Institute of Medicine, Food and Nutrition Board. Dietary Reference Intakes for Thiamin, Riboflavin, Niacin, Vitamin B-6, Folate, Vitamin B-12, Pantothenic Acid, Biotin, and Choline. Washington, DC: National Academy Press, 1998.)

*AI, adequate intake; RDA, recommended dietary allowance.

[a]Because 10% to 30% of older people may malabsorb food-bound vitamin B_{12}, it is advisable for those older than 50 years to meet their RDA mainly by consuming foods fortified with vitamin B_{12} or a supplement containing vitamin B_{12}.

cooked sea vegetables contained vitamin B_{12} in the same range as beef liver. Individuals consuming strictly vegetarian diets, particularly after 5 to 6 years, typically show lower circulating levels of the vitamin B_{12} unless they supplement with the vitamin. This is not true for ovolacto vegetarians whose diets include food sources of vitamin B_{12} (Thorogood, 1995).

Approximately 70% of the vitamin activity is retained during the cooking of most foods; however, appreciable amounts of the vitamin can be lost when milk is pasteurized or evaporated.

Deficiency

Vitamin B_{12} deficiency causes impaired cell division, particularly in the rapidly dividing cells of the bone marrow and intestinal mucosa, resulting from arrested synthesis of DNA. The ensuing reduction in mitotic rate results in abnormally large cells and a characteristic anemia (*megaloblastic anemia;* see Chapter 35). Cobalamin deficiency produces another clinical syndrome, a neurologic one. Neurologic abnormalities develop with much later onset in about one fourth of persons with megaloblastic anemia. These involve progressive neuropathy with nerve demyelination commencing peripherally and proceeding centrally. Symptoms include numbness, tingling and burning of the feet, and stiffness and generalized weakness of the legs.

Perhaps the most common cause of vitamin B_{12} deficiency is malabsorption of the vitamin due to inadequate production and secretion of IF. This results in the condition called *pernicious anemia,* which can result from atrophy of gastric parietal cells associated with aging, by hereditary deficiencies in IF synthesis, or by autoimmune incapacitation of IF. Although it is true that the chronic (sev-

losses of IF production, and of pernicious anemia in persons over 60 years of age.

Sources

Vitamin B_{12} is synthesized by bacteria, but the vitamin produced from the microflora in the colon is not absorbed. The vitamin is, however, found in the tissues of animals that require dietary sources of the vitamin to support critical functions in cell division and growth. The richest sources of the vitamin are liver and kidney, milk, eggs, fish, cheese, and muscle meats (Table 4–27).

Foods of plant origin contain the vitamin only through contamination or bacterial synthesis. Many people believe that fermented foods contain sufficient vitamin B_{12} to meet their needs; however, this theory is not supported by analysis (Specker et al., 1988). Six samples of tempeh (a fermented soybean product) were analyzed, and the vitamin B_{12} concentrations were negligible. In contrast, some

TABLE 4–27 VITAMIN B_{12} CONTENT OF SELECTED FOODS

FOOD	μg
Clams, canned, 3 oz	84.05
Liver, beef, 3.5 oz	71.00
Oysters, raw, Pacific, 3 oz	13.61
Crab, dungeness, raw, 3 oz	7.65
Tuna, light, canned, in water, 3 oz	2.54
Beef, hamburger, lean, broiled, 3.5 oz	2.35
Halibut, baked, 3 oz	1.16
Milk, 2%, 1 cup	0.89
Frankfurters, beef, 1	0.88
Pork chop, broiled, 3.5 oz	0.74
Egg, 1	0.50
Cheese, Edam, 1 oz	0.44
Chicken, white meat, 3.5 oz	0.32
Ice cream, vanilla, ½ cup	0.26
Yogurt, low fat, plain, 1 cup	0.24

(From Pennington J. Bowe's and Church's Food Values of Portions Commonly Used, 17th ed. Philadelphia: Lippincott-Raven, 1998.)

eral years) consumption of strict vegan diets without supplemental vitamin B_{12} typically leads to very low circulating levels of the vitamin, clinical signs among such individuals appear to be rare and may not be manifest for several years, except among breast-fed infants.

Many believe vitamin B_{12} deficiency to be a common disorder in the elderly (Carethers, 1988). It often presents with (1) a lemon-yellow tint resulting from concurrent anemia and jaundice from ineffective erythropoeisis; (2) a smooth, beefy red tongue; and (3) neurologic disorders. Psychiatric manifestations such as impaired mentation and depression may be present.

Toxicity

Vitamin B_{12} has no appreciable toxicity.

Pantothenic Acid

As its name suggests, **pantothenic acid** is widely distributed in foods; hence, cases of clinical deficiency are rare. The vitamin has critical roles in metabolism, being an integral part of two acylation factors: *coenzyme A (CoA)* in which the vitamin is linked via a phosphodiester group with adenosine-3′,5′-diphosphate, and *acyl-carrier protein (ACP)* in which it is similarly linked to a serine residue of the protein. In these forms, pantothenic acid is essential for the metabolism of fatty acids, amino acids, and carbohydrates and has important roles in the acylation of proteins.

Absorption, Transport, and Storage

Because pantothenic acid exists in most foods as CoA and ACP, the utilization of the vitamin depends on the hydrolytic digestion of these protein complexes to release the free vitamin as *4′-phosphopantetheine,* which is dephosphorylated to yield *pantetheine* and rapidly converted to pantothenic acid. Pantothenic acid is absorbed both by a process of active transport as well as by simple diffusion. It is then transported in the free acid form in solution in the plasma and is taken up by diffusion into erythrocytes, which carry most of the vitamin in the blood. Pantothenic acid is taken up by cells of peripheral tissues by an active transport process mediated by a specific carrier protein. Within the cell, the vitamin is converted to CoA, which is its predominant form in most tissues, particularly the liver, adrenals, kidney, brain, heart, and testes.

Metabolism

All tissues are capable of synthesizing CoA from pantothenic acid. This is a multienzyme process involving the phosphorylation of the vitamin to yield *4′-phosphopantothenic acid,* which is condensed with cysteine to yield *4′-phosphopantothenoylcysteine*. The latter product is decarboxylated to yield *4′-phosphopantetheine,* which is converted to CoA by a final phosphoadenosylation step that requires 4 moles ATP per mole CoA formed. The ACP contains 4′-phosphopantetheine that is transferred from CoA to bind to the apo-ACP by linkage to a specific serinyl residue.

Both CoA and ACP are degraded to yield free pantothenic acid and other metabolites. The vitamin is excreted mainly in the urine as free pantothenic acid as well as some 4′-phosphopantothenate. An appreciable amount (some 15% of daily intake) is oxidized completely and lost through the lungs as carbon dioxide.

Functions

Both CoA and ACP function metabolically as carriers of acyl groups. In each case the linkage with the transported group involves the reactive sulfhydryl of the 4′-phosphopantetheinyl prosthetic group. CoA forms high-energy thioester bonds with carboxylic acids, the most important of which is acetic acid, which can come from the metabolism of fatty acids, amino acids, or carbohydrates. As acetyl-CoA, that group can enter the TCA cycle to release energy from carbohydrate, or it can be used for the synthesis of fatty acids or cholesterol, or in acetylations of alcohols, amines, and amino acids. It also functions to activate fatty acids prior to their incorporation into triglycerides and as an acyl donor for proteins. The ACP is a component of the multienzyme complex fatty acid synthase in which it functions to transfer covalently bound intermediates between different active sites with successive cycles of condensation and reduction.

Measurement

Pantothenic acid is expressed in terms of its mass in milligrams.

Dietary Reference Intakes

For the first time, in 1998, AIs were established for pantothenic acid as part of the DRIs. No EARs or RDAs were established (Table 4–28).

Sources

Pantothenic acid is present in all plant and animal tissues. The most important sources in mixed diets are meats (particularly liver and heart); but mushrooms, avocados, broccoli, egg yolk, yeast, skimmed milk, and sweet potatoes are also good sources of the vitamin. Pantothenic acid is fairly stable to ordinary means of cooking and storage, although the vitamin can be lost from frozen meats during thawing. Because it is localized in the outer layers of grains, about half of the vitamin is lost in the

TABLE 4–28 DIETARY REFERENCE INTAKES FOR PANTOTHENIC ACID

LIFE-STAGE GROUP	AI (mg/d)
Infants	
0–6 mo	1.7
7–12 mo	1.8
Children	
1–3 y	2
4–8 y	3
Males	
9–13 y	4
14–18 y	5
19–30 y	5
31–50 y	5
51–70 y	5
>70 y	5
Females	
9–13 y	4
14–18 y	5
19–30 y	5
31–50 y	5
51–70 y	5
>70 y	5
Pregnancy	
≤18 y	6
19–30 y	6
31–50 y	6
Lactation	
≤18 y	7
19–30 y	7
31–50 y	7

(From Institute of Medicine, Food and Nutrition Board. Dietary Reference Intakes for Thiamin, Riboflavin, Niacin, Vitamin B-6, Folate, Vitamin B-12, Pantothenic Acid, Biotin, and Choline. Washington, DC: National Academy Press, 1998.)
AI, adequate intake.

milling of flour. Table 4–29 presents the pantothenic acid content of some foods.

Deficiency

Deprivation of pantothenic acid results in impairments in lipid synthesis and energy production. Clinical signs vary among different species; most frequently they involve the skin, liver, adrenals, and nervous system. Because the vitamin is so widely distributed in foods, deficiencies are rare; in humans, pantothenic acid deficiency has been observed only among severely malnourished patients, who experienced paresthesia in the toes and soles of the feet, and subjects treated with the antagonist ω-methylpantothenic acid (who developed burning sensations of the feet, depression, fatigue, insomnia, and weakness).

Toxicity

The toxicity of pantothenic acid is negligible; no adverse effects have been reported in any species following ingestion of large doses of the vitamin. Massive doses (e.g., 10 g/day) administered to humans have produced only mild intestinal distress and diarrhea.

Biotin

Biotin was first isolated in 1936 and synthesized in 1943. It had been previously observed that chicks and rats fed large amounts of raw egg whites developed eczema accompanied by alopecia around the eyes. The syndrome was cured by adding egg yolks to the diet of the affected animals, and the corrective factor in the yolk was named vitamin H. This proved to be the same as a potent growth factor in yeast called coenzyme r, and the factor was renamed biotin. Cases of biotin deficiency were identified in humans with the advent of total parenteral nutrition before the vitamin was added to tube-feeding solutions. Because the vitamin synthesized by the microflora in the colon can be absorbed, cases of deficiency are rare and there is a paucity of quantitative information about the biotin needs of humans.

Absorption, Transport, and Storage

Biotin in foods is largely protein bound. It is released by hydrolytic digestion to yield the biotinyllysine adduct *biocytin* from which free biotin is liberated by intestinal *biotinidase*. Free biotin is absorbed in the proximal small intestine by both facilitated and simple diffusion. Biotin can also be absorbed from the colon, which facilitates the utilization of the vitamin produced by hind gut microflora.

Biotin is transported in the plasma mostly as free biotin, but also as biotin metabolites including *bis-*

TABLE 4–29 PANTOTHENIC ACID CONTENT OF SELECTED FOODS

FOOD	mg
Liver, beef, braised, 3.5 oz	4.57
Chicken, white meat, w/o skin, baked, 3.5 oz	0.97
Ice milk, soft serve, 1 cup	0.78
Milk, 2% fat, 1 cup	0.78
Mushrooms, raw, ½ cup	0.77
Salmon, pink, baked, 3 oz	0.74
Corn, cooked, ½ cup	0.72
Dates, 10	0.65
Wheat germ, raw, ¼ cup	0.65
Liverwurst, 1 slice	0.53
Cheese, blue, 1 oz	0.49
Oatmeal, regular, cooked, 1 cup	0.47
Broccoli, boiled, ½ cup	0.40
Papaya, ½	0.33
Cheese, cottage, 2% fat, ½ cup	0.27
Peanut butter, creamy, 2 T	0.26
Strawberries, ½ cup	0.25
Orange juice, ½ cup	0.24
Yogurt, low fat, w/fruit, 1 cup	0.19
Bread, whole-wheat, 1 slice	0.15

(From Pennington J. Bowe's and Church's Food Values of Portions Commonly Used, 17th ed. Philadelphia: Lippincott-Raven, 1998.)

norbiotin and *biotin sulfoxide*. Some (12%) of this is bound to biotinidase, which also occurs in human milk. Biotin is taken into cells by a specific carrier-mediated process. Appreciable storage of the vitamin occurs in the liver; however, these stores appear to be poorly mobilized during periods of deprivation of the vitamin.

Metabolism

Free biotin is attached to each of its four apoenzymes by the formation of an amide linkage to the ε-amino group of a specific lysyl residue catalyzed by *biotin holoenzyme synthetase*. The biotin holocarboxylases normally turn over to yield biocytin from which free biotin is liberated by biotinidase. Little catabolism of biotin occurs; but some of the vitamin is oxidized to biotin sulfoxides. The vitamin is rapidly excreted in the urine (95% of an oral dose within 24 hours), half as free biotin and the balance as bisnorbiotin, biotin sulfoxides, and various side-chain metabolites.

Functions

Biotin functions as a mobile carboxyl carrier in four carboxylases of animals: pyruvate carboxylase, acetyl-CoA carboxylase, propionyl-CoA carboxylase, and 3-methylcrotonyl-CoA carboxylase. The catalytic action of each involves first the carboxylation of the vitamin followed by the transfer of the carboxyl group. *Pyruvate carboxylase* supports the formation of phosphoenolpyruvate in gluconeogenesis, replenishes the mitochondrial supply of oxaloacetate for the TCA cycle, and supports the formation of citrate for lipogenesis. *Acetyl-CoA carboxylase* catalyzes the first committed step in fatty acid synthesis. *Propionyl-CoA carboxylase* catalyzes the oxidation of odd-chain fatty acids and produces methylmalonyl-CoA for energy and glucose production. The enzyme *3-methylcrotonyl-CoA carboxylase* degrades the ketogenic amino acid leucine. These roles of biotin link it to the metabolic roles of folic acid, pantothenic acid, and vitamin B_{12}.

Measurement

When used to quantify the biotin in foods, the expression of biotin in terms of its mass fails to accommodate the known differences in bioavailability of biotin from various food sources.

Dietary Reference Intakes

In 1998, AIs were established for biotin as part of the DRIs; no EARs or RDAs have been established (Table 4–30).

TABLE 4–30 DIETARY REFERENCE INTAKES FOR BIOTIN

LIFE-STAGE GROUP	AI (μg/d)
Infants	
0–6 mo	5
7–12 mo	6
Children	
1–3 y	8
4–8 y	12
Males	
9–13 y	20
14–18 y	25
19–30 y	30
31–50 y	30
51–70 y	30
>70 y	30
Females	
9–13 y	20
14–18 y	25
19–30 y	30
31–50 y	30
51–70 y	30
>70 y	30
Pregnancy	
≤18 y	30
19–30 y	30
31–50 y	30
Lactation	
≤18 y	35
19–30 y	35
31–50 y	35

(From Institute of Medicine, Food and Nutrition Board. Dietary Reference Intakes for Thiamin, Riboflavin, Niacin, Vitamin B-6, Folate, Vitamin B-12, Pantothenic Acid, Biotin, and Choline. Washington, DC: National Academy Press, 1998.)
AI, adequate intake.

Sources

Biotin is widely distributed in foods, but few foods have high concentrations (Table 4–31). Milk, liver, egg yolk, and a few vegetables are the most important sources of the vitamin in human diets, and intestinal bacteria contribute appreciable amounts to human biotin nutrition. Fecal and urinary excretion considerably higher than dietary intake reflects the magnitude of microfloral synthesis.

The bioavailability of biotin varies considerably among different foods; this relates to differences in the digestibility of various biotin-protein complexes. Biotin is unstable to oxidizing conditions and is destroyed by heat, especially in the presence of lipid peroxidation.

Deficiency

Because biotin can be obtained from many foods as well as from gut microbial metabolism, simple biotin deficiencies in animals are rare. They can be induced, however, by feeding raw egg white or the active principle contained in that product, the heat-labile, biotin-binding protein *avidin*. Such treatments induce lesions in lipid metabolism and energy production that are characterized in most species as seborrheic dermatitis, alopecia, and paralysis. The few

TABLE 4–31 BIOTIN CONTENT OF SELECTED FOODS

FOOD	RANGE (μg/100 g)	FOOD	RANGE (μg/100 g)
Cereals		**Poultry**	10–11.3
Wheat germ	22–38	**Fish and Shellfish**	3–24
Oatmeal	22–31		
Wheat bran	22.4–25.5	**Vegetables**	0.2–4.1
Oatmeal, rolled oats	15.3–24.6	**Fruit**	0.2–2
Wheat bran	22.4–33.4		
Milk and Milk Products		**Nuts**	
Fresh whole, dried	2–16	Almonds, raw	18
Whole	1.6–2.4	Peanuts, roasted	34
Instant	16–24	Pecans	27
Eggs		Walnuts, peanut butter	37–39
Whole, cooked	20–25	**Miscellaneous**	
Yolk, raw	51.5–58	Chocolate	32
Meat and Meat Products		Molasses	9
Beef, liver	96	Yeast, brewer's	200
Beef, other	2.6–3.4	Yeast, Torula	100
Chicken, liver	170–210	**Human Milk**	18–22

(From Marshall MW. The nutritional importance of biotin—An update. Nutrition Today 22:26, 1987.)

cases of biotin deficiency that have been described in humans have involved patients receiving incomplete parenteral nutrition and nursing infants whose mothers' milk contained very low amounts of the vitamin. In each case, the signs included dermatitis, glossitis, anorexia, nausea, depression, hepatic steatosis, and hypercholesterolemia.

Inherited defects in all of the known biotin enzymes have been indentified in humans, but these are rare and usually have serious neurologic consequences.

Toxicity

There are no known toxic effects from biotin.

Ascorbic Acid

Vitamin C is the antiscorbutic factor, **ascorbic acid,** that was originally isolated from adrenal tissue, oranges, and cabbage. Although scurvy was first described during the Crusades and commonly plagued early explorers and voyagers, the specific relationship between scurvy, citrus foods, and ascorbic acid was not established until the 20th century. English sailors have been nicknamed "limeys" since the days when ships were required to carry citrus fruits (actually lemons) as a scurvy preventive.

The antiscorbutic factor was isolated and named *hexuronic acid* in 1928 by Szent-Gyorgyi, who found it in adrenal tissue, oranges, and cabbage. In 1932 both he and C. Glenn King demonstrated that hexuronic acid was vitamin C.

Vitamin C is a hexose derivative synthesized by plants and most animals from glucose and galactose. Humans, other primates, guinea pigs, some bats, and a few species of birds, however, lack an enzyme, *l-gulonolactone oxidase,* and thus cannot biosynthesize the factor, which for them is consequently a vitamin.

Absorption, Transport, and Storage

Species that cannot biosynthesize ascorbic acid absorb it by active transport as well as passive diffusion. The oxidized form of the vitamin, *dehydroascorbic acid,* is better absorbed than the reduced form, *ascorbate* or ascorbic acid. The former is not ionized at physiologic pH, is relatively hydrophobic, and is thus better able to penetrate membranes than the latter. Dehydroascorbic acid is reduced to ascorbate during this process. The efficiency of enteric absorption of the vitamin is high (80–90%) at low intakes but declines markedly at intakes greater than about 1 g/day.

Vitamin C is transported in the plasma in the reduced form (ascorbic acid) in free solution. It is taken up by cells both by the glucose transporter and by a specific active transport system. Each system moves *dehydroascorbic acid* into cells where it is readily reduced to *ascorbate*. The glucose transporter-based system of uptake is not as fast as the specific system, but it is stimulated by insulin and inhibited by glucose. Thus, diabetic patients with high glucose levels typically have high plasma levels of dehydroascorbic acid. The vitamin is concentrated mostly as dehydroascorbic acid in many vital organs, particularly the adrenals, brain, and eye.

Metabolism

Ascorbic acid is oxidized in vivo by two successive losses of single electrons. First the ascorbyl free radical (also called *monodehydroascorbic acid*) is formed. This intermediate can be further oxidized to dehydroascorbic acid (Fig. 4–8). Subsequently, the oxidized product undergoes irreversible hydrolysis to yield 2,3-diketo-L-gulonic acid, which can be decarboxylated to yield carbon dioxide and several five-carbon fragments (xylose, xylonic acid), or oxidized to yield oxalic acid and several four-carbon fragments (e.g., threonic acid). In addition, the vitamin can be converted to ascorbic acid 2-sulfate.

It has been suggested that ascorbic acid may also react with tocopheroxyl or urate radicals to regenerate the reduced species of each. Such reactions would extend the known antioxidant roles of vitamin C to the metabolic recycling of other antioxidants.

Functions

Vitamin C serves several metabolic functions as an enzyme cofactor, a protective agent, and as a reactant with transition metal ions. Each of these functions involves the reduction/oxidation properties of the vitamin. Because ascorbic acid easily loses electrons and because of its reversible monovalent oxidation to the ascorbyl radical, it can serve as a biochemical redox system involved in many electron transport reactions including those involved in the synthesis of collagen, the degradation of 4-hydroxyphenylpyruvate, the synthesis of norepinephrine, and the desaturation of fatty acids. That ascorbic acid can react with free radicals makes it an **antioxidant,** as it undergoes single-electron oxidation to the ascorbyl radical, which disproportionates to ascorbate and dehydroascorbate. By such reactions the vitamin can quench potentially toxic reactive oxygen species, such as superoxide or the hydroxyl radical, and regenerate tocopherol from the tocopheroxyl radical.

Ascorbate functions as a co-substrate for at least eight enzymes: three involved in lysine/proline hydroxylations, two required for carnitine biosynthesis, two functional in hormone biosynthesis, and one involved in the metabolism of the amino acid tyrosine. Of these, the best characterized is the role of vitamin C in the hydroxylation of proline to form hydroxyproline in the synthesis of *collagen*, the major protein on which the integrity of fibrous tissues (connective tissue, cartilage, bone matrix, tooth dentin, skin, and tendon) depends. Impairments of this function, in which the vitamin appears to maintain another cofactor, iron, in the reduced (Fe^{++}) state, are manifest as lesions in the healing of wounds and fractures, as well as in bruises, pinpoint hemorrhages, and bleeding gums.

Vitamin C is essential for the oxidation of phenylalanine and tyrosine, the conversion of folacin to tetrahydrofolic acid, the conversion of tryptophan to 5-hydroxytryptophan and the neurotransmitter serotonin, and the formation of norepinephrine from dopamine. It also reduces ferric to ferrous iron in the intestinal tract to facilitate absorption, and is involved in the transfer of iron from plasma transferrin to liver ferritin.

Ascorbic acid participates in the hydroxylation of certain steroids synthesized in adrenal tissue. Concentration is decreased under stress when adrenal cortical hormone activity is high. During periods of emotional, psychological, or physiologic stress, the urinary excretion of ascorbic acid is increased.

Vitamin C promotes resistance to infection through the immunologic activity of leukocytes, the production of interferon, the process of inflammatory reaction, or the integrity of the mucous membranes (Packer and Fuchs, 1997). The value of large amounts of ascorbic acid to prevent and cure the common cold has been reported, but these insights are controversial (see "*Clinical Insight:* Vitamin C and the Common Cold").

The role of vitamin C as an antioxidant is discussed in the earlier box, "*New Directions*: Vitamins and Immunity—The Antioxidant Story." Vitamin C intake protects lung function, as evaluated in 2256 adults in the first report of the National Health and Nutrition Examination Survey. After controlling for other risk factors and demographic factors, a positive significant correlation was found between pulmonary function and intake of this vitamin (Schwartz and Weiss, 1994). The relationship of vitamin C to cancer is discussed in Chapter 39.

Measurement

Vitamin C is expressed quantitatively as milligrams.

Recommended Dietary Allowances

The DRIs have not been formulated for vitamin C although they are being developed (Institute of Medicine, 1998). The current guidelines are the

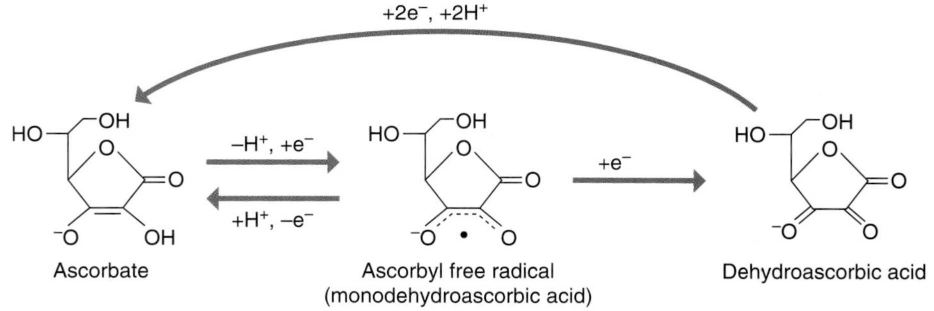

FIGURE 4–8 Oxidation-reduction reaction of vitamin C. (From Combs GF. The Vitamins: Fundamental Aspects in Nutrition and Health, 2nd ed. Orlando, FL: Academic Press, 1998.)

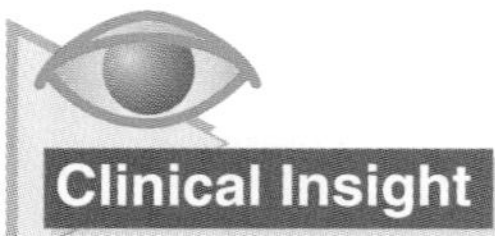

Vitamin C and the Common Cold

Interest in the use of vitamin C for treating the common cold dates from the 1940s, but the theory did not become popular until Linus Pauling wrote a book claiming that vitamin C in massive doses would protect against and cure the common cold. Sales of the vitamin skyrocketed despite considerable skepticism from the nutrition community. In subsequent years, several studies have modified or even discredited the original hypothesis.

1. Anderson and colleagues conducted a double-blind trial with 818 individuals in which a placebo group was compared with a treatment group that took 1 g/day of vitamin C and 4 g/day during the first 3 days of a cold. Although the vitamin C group experienced less illness, the differences were statistically insignificant. However, when those taking vitamin C did contract a cold it was less severe and resulted in 30% fewer days of disability (Anderson et al., 1972; Anderson, 1975).
2. In a study involving 641 children taking a placebo or 1 to 2 g vitamin C, Coulehan and colleagues found that although taking the vitamin did not prevent colds, those children who were taking vitamin C had 24% to 28% fewer days of sickness compared with a placebo group. However, a later study by the same investigator could not confirm the effectiveness of 1 g/day doses in reducing the severity of cold symptoms (Coulehan et al., 1974, 1976).
3. Wilson and Loh (1973) found that prophylactic doses of 200 to 500 mg/day reduced cold symptoms in girls but had no effect in boys.
4. Miller and co-workers conducted a double-blind study on co-twins ranging in age from 6 to 15 years in which subjects received either a placebo or 500 to 1000 mg of vitamin C per day depending on their size. They observed a 28% reduction in incidence of cold symptoms, a 17% reduction in total severity, and a 21% variation in total duration. The effect of the vitamin was more pronounced in younger girls. The authors concluded that even though large doses of vitamin C may have a detectable prophylactic effect in some age and sex groups, genetic, environmental, or subjective factors appear to account for a substantially greater fraction of the total morbidity (Miller et al., 1977).
5. Carr and colleagues studied a series of pairs of monozygotic twins aged 14 to 64 years who received either 1 g/day of vitamin C or placebo for 100 days. The perception of treatment was important, as those who thought they were on a "high dose" reported markedly fewer, shorter, and less severe colds than their co-twins who thought they were on a "low dose." In addition, there were significant correlations between cold symptoms reported and the personality trait of neuroticism (Carr et al., 1981).
6. One investigator concluded that ascorbic acid had an antihistaminic effect (Bouhuys, 1974). Other work has shown that persons with low plasma ascorbic acid levels have elevated blood histamine levels, which are lowered by supplementation with the vitamin.
7. Most people would suffer chronic diarrhea and possibly kidney stones if they were to take the 12,000 to 40,000 mg of vitamin C that Linus Pauling recommends (Marshall, 1992).

It has been concluded that benefits from ascorbic acid in fighting the common cold are not great enough to recommend routine large intakes. If there are benefits, they appear to be in reducing the severity of symptoms rather than preventing the cold.

RDAs of 1989. Although as little as 10 mg vitamin C is needed to prevent scurvy, that level does not provide acceptable reserves of the vitamin. The RDA of 60 mg for adults thus provides a margin of safety above that minimum value. Table 4–32 presents the RDAs for vitamin C.

Because of the lower concentrations of ascorbic acid in the serum of cigarette smokers, it is recommended that smokers increase their intake to at least 100 mg/day (Food and Nutrition Board, 1989).

Sources

Vitamin C is found in both plants and animal tissues as both ascorbic acid and dehydroascorbic acid. The best sources are fruits, vegetables, and organ meats, but the actual ascorbic acid contents of foods can vary with the conditions of growth and the degree of ripeness when harvested. Refrigeration and quick freezing help retain the vitamin. Most commercially frozen foods are processed so close to the source of supply that their ascorbic acid content is often higher than that of fresh foods that have been shipped across the country and spent time in storage and on supermarket shelves. Table 4–33 lists the vitamin C content of selected fruits and vegetables. Citrus fruits and juices are very important sources of the vitamin for many Americans who tend not to eat many servings of other fruits and vegetables.

Ascorbic acid is easily destroyed by oxidation and, because it is soluble in water, it is often extracted and discarded in cooking water. Sodium bicarbonate, added to preserve and improve the color of cooked vegetables, is highly destructive of vitamin C. The cumulative losses of the vitamin from prepared vegetables held 24 hours under refrigeration can be as high as 45% for fresh products and 52% for frozen products. As consumers eat out more frequently, and as more foods are supplied to restaurants or institutions partially prepared (e.g., shredded lettuce, peeled and diced vegetables) or served from open salad bars, this loss must be considered when evaluating dietary intake (Carlson and Tabacchi, 1988).

TABLE 4–32 RECOMMENDED DIETARY ALLOWANCES FOR VITAMIN C

AGE (y)	RDA (mg)
Infants	
0.0–0.5	30
0.5–1.0	35
Children	
1–3	40
4–6	45
7–10	45
Males	
11–14	50
15–18	60
19–24	60
25–50	60
51+	60
Females	
11–14	50
15–18	60
19–24	60
25–50	60
51+	60
Pregnant	70
Lactating	
1st 6 mo	95
2nd 6 mo	90

(From Food and Nutrition Board, National Research Council, NAS. Recommended Dietary Allowances, 10th ed. Washington, DC: National Academy Press, 1989.)
RDA, recommended dietary allowance.

Deficiency

Acute vitamin C deficiency results in **scurvy** in individuals unable to synthesize the vitamin. In human adults, signs are manifest after 45 to 80 days of vitamin C deprivation. In children, the syndrome is called Moeller-Barlow disease; it is seen in non–breast-fed infants who have no other source of vitamin C such as infant formulas at about 6 months of age when maternal vitamin C stores have been exhausted. In each case lesions occur in mesenchymal tissues and are seen as impaired wound healing, edema, hemorrhages, and weaknesses of bone, cartilage, teeth, and connective tissues (Fig. 4–9). Scorbutic adults may show swollen, bleeding gums and eventual tooth loss, lethargy, fatigue, rheumatic pains in the legs, muscular atrophy, skin lesions (Fig. 4–10), and various psychological changes (hysteria, hypochondria, depression).

Toxicity

The only consistent adverse effects of high doses of vitamin C in humans are gastrointestinal disturbances and diarrhea. This is fortunate because vitamin C is the most commonly used supplement in the United States, taken by 8% of young people and 44% of the elderly (Johnston and Luo, 1994). However, because the catabolism of vitamin C yields oxalate (among other metabolites), it is reasonable to be concerned about the possibility of high doses of

TABLE 4–33 VITAMIN C CONTENT OF SELECTED FOODS

FOOD	AMOUNT	mg	FOOD	AMOUNT	mg
Kiwi	1	74	Papaya	1 med	188
Broccoli			Lemon	1 (2½" diameter)	31
fresh, boiled	½ cup	158	Grapefruit	½	39
frozen, chopped, boiled	½ cup	37	Honeydew melon	1 cup	42
Brussel sprouts, frozen	½ cup	36	Cauliflower, from raw, cooked	½ cup	27
Cantaloupe	1 cup	68	Mustard greens, cooked	½ cup	18
Collards (cooked)	½ cup	7.5	Potato		
Pepper			baked, with skin	1 medium	20
sweet, yellow	1, large	341	baked, then peeled	1 medium	18
hot chili, raw	½ cup	109	peeled, then boiled	1 medium	10
Orange, navel	1 (2½" diameter)	75	mashed	½ cup	6
Orange juice			French fries	10	5
fresh	1 cup	124	chips	10 (1 oz)	9
frozen, diluted can	1 cup	97	Watermelon	1 cup	15
canned	1 cup	86	Sweet potato, baked	1 medium	28
Kale, from raw, cooked	½ cup	27	Spinach		
Turnip greens, from raw, cooked	½ cup	20	fresh	½ cup	8
Strawberries	½ cup	42	frozen, boiled	½ cup	12
Grapefruit juice			canned	½ cup	15
canned, unsweetened	½ cup	36	Cabbage		
Tomato			cooked	½ cup	15
fresh	1 (3" diameter)	23	raw	½ cup	11
canned, stewed	½ cup	15	Tangerine	1 (2¼" diameter)	26
juice	¾ cup	33	Okra, cooked	½ cup	10
Mango	1	57	Cranberry juice cocktail	¾ cup	67

(From Pennington J. Bowe's and Church's Food Values of Portions Commonly Used, 17th ed. Philadelphia: Lippincott-Raven, 1998.)

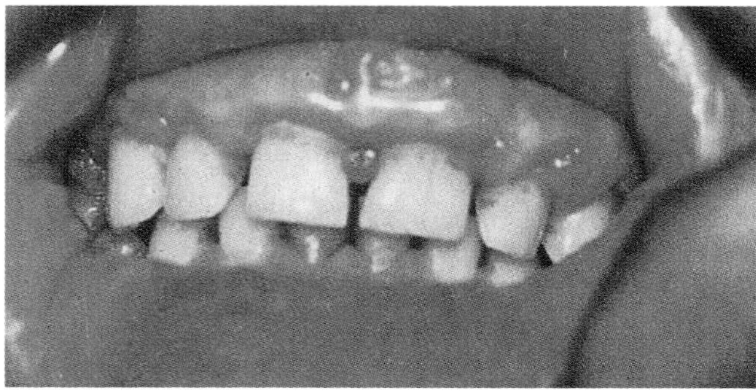

FIGURE 4–9 Scorbutic gums in vitamin C deficiency. Gums are swollen, ulcerated, and bleeding due to vitamin C-induced defects in oral epithelial basement membrane and periodontal collagen fiber synthesis. (From Taylor KB, Anthony LE. Clinical Nutrition. New York: McGraw-Hill, 1983, copyright by The Upjohn Company.)

the vitamin increasing the risk of forming renal oxalate stones. Clinical studies have shown, however, that subjects given multiple daily doses of the vitamin showed only slight oxaluria (Sauberlich, 1994). Nevertheless, prudence dictates avoiding such intakes for individuals with histories of forming renal stones. Excess ascorbic acid excreted in the urine can give a false-positive test for urinary glucose.

Table 4–34 summarizes information on the known vitamins.

OTHER VITAMIN-LIKE FACTORS

Other food factors have vitamin characteristics without meeting the criteria of vitamin status. These quasi-vitamins include some (e.g., choline, carnitine) that can be biosynthesized but may yield benefits on supplementation, some (e.g., choline, carnitine) that are required by nonhuman species, and some (e.g., choline, carnitine, *myo*-inositol, pyrroloquinoline quinone, the ubiquinones, the bioflavonoids) for which evidence of essentiality remains incomplete. Some, such as choline, may need to be provided in the diet only at certain stages of life.

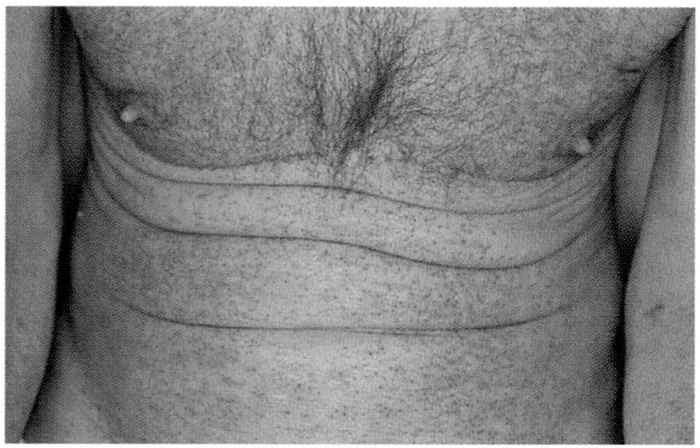

FIGURE 4–10 Scurvy. (From Callen WBS, et al. Color Atlas of Dermatology. Philadelphia: Saunders, 1993.)

Choline

Choline (2-hydroxy-*N,N,N*-trimethylenthanolamine), first discovered in 1862 and synthesized in 1866, is an essential component of animal tissues in which it has functional roles as *phosphatidylcholine (PC)* or *lecithin,* in membrane phospholipids, and as the neurotransmitter *acetylcholine (AC).* Choline can be biosynthesized from ethanolamine by sequential methylations using S-adenosylmethionine, but most humans obtain it from dietary phosphatides. Choline is widely distributed in food fats, occurring predominately in the form of PC in eggs, liver, soybeans, beef, milk, and peanuts. Free choline is present in liver, oatmeal, soybeans, iceberg lettuce, cauliflower, kale, and cabbage. Choline is released by the hydrolysis of PC by pancreatic and intestinal lipases and is absorbed by a carrier-mediated process as well as by passive diffusion. Absorbed choline is transported via chylomicra in the lymphatic circulation primarily in the form of PC; it is transferred to lipoproteins in that form for distribution to peripheral tissues.

Functions

Choline has several functions in metabolism (Zeisel and Blusztajn, 1994). As PC, it is a structural element of membranes, a precursor to the sphingolipids, and a promotor of lipid transport. As AC, it functions as a neurotransmitter and as a component of platelet-activating factor. Choline deficiency can occur in young poultry unable to synthesize it at rates equal to their needs. Deficient animals show fatty deposition in the liver, hemorrhagic kidney disease, and deformations of the bone organic matrix. Clear cases of choline deficiency have not been demonstrated in humans. However, supplemental choline has been used with some success to diminish short-term memory loss associated with Alzheimer's disease, and very high doses (up to 20 g/day) have been reported to alleviate symptoms of tardive dyskinesia and Huntington's disease (Canty and Zeisel, 1994).

Reference Dietary Intakes

The AIs were established for choline as part of the 1998 DRIs (Table 4–35).

Carnitine

Carnitine (β-hydroxy-γ-*N*-trimethylaminobutyrate) functions in the transport of long-chain fatty acids (as their acyl-CoA derivatives) into the mitochondria for oxidation as sources of energy; this process is called the *carnitine transport shuttle.* Preformed dietary carnitine is required by at least some insects, but mammals and birds can biosynthesize it

TABLE 4–34 SUMMARY OF VITAMINS

NAME	RDA FOR ADULTS*	SOURCES	STABILITY	COMMENTS
Fat-Soluble Vitamins				
Vitamin A (retinol; α-, β-, γ-carotene)	M: 1000 RE F: 800 RE	Liver, kidney, milk fat, fortified margarine, egg yolk, yellow and dark green leafy vegetables, apricots, cantaloupe, peaches.	Stable to light, heat, and usual cooking methods. Destroyed by oxidation, drying, very high temperature, ultraviolet light.	Essential for normal growth, development and maintenance of epithelial tissue. Essential to the integrity of night vision. Helps provide for normal bone development and influences normal tooth formation. Functions as antioxidant. Toxic in large quantities.
Vitamin D (calciferol)	M: 5–10 μg F: 5–10 μg Adequate Intake	Vitamin D fortified milk, irradiated foods, some in milk fat, liver, egg yolk, salmon, tuna fish, sardines. Sunlight converts 7-dehydrocholesterol to cholecalciferol.	Stable to heat and oxidation.	Really a prohormone. Essential for normal growth and development; important for formation and maintenance of normal bones and teeth. Influences absorption and metabolism of phosphorus and calcium. Toxic in large quantities.
Vitamin E (tocopherols and tocotrienols)	M: 10 α-TE F: 8 α-TE	Wheat germ, vegetable oils, green leafy vegetables, milk fat, egg yolks, nuts.	Stable to heat and acids. Destroyed by rancid fats, alkali, oxygen, lead, iron salts, and ultraviolet irradiation.	Is a strong antioxidant. May help prevent oxidation of unsaturated fatty acids and vitamin A in intestinal tract and body tissues. Protects red blood cells from hemolysis. Role in reproduction (in animals). Role in epithelial tissue maintenance and prostaglandin synthesis.
Vitamin K (phylloquinone and menaquinone)	M: 80 μg F: 65 μg	Liver, soybean oil, other vegetable oils, green leafy vegetables, wheat bran. Synthesized in intestinal tract.	Resistant to heat, oxygen, and moisture. Destroyed by alkali and ultraviolet light.	Aids in production of prothrombin, a compound required for normal clotting of blood. Involved in bone metabolism. Toxic in large amounts.
Water-Soluble Vitamins				
Thiamin	M: 1.2 mg F: 1.1 mg	Pork liver, organ meats, legumes, whole-grain and enriched cereals and breads, wheat germ, potatoes. Synthesized in intestinal tract.	Unstable in presence of heat, alkali, or oxygen. Heat stable in acid solution.	As part of cocarboxylase, aids in removal of CO_2 from alphaketo acids during oxidation of carbohydrates. Essential for growth, normal appetite, digestion, and healthy nerves.
Riboflavin	M: 1.3 mg F: 1.1 mg	Milk and dairy foods, organ meats, green leafy vegetables, enriched cereals and breads, eggs.	Stable to heat, oxygen, and acid. Unstable to light (especially ultraviolet) or alkali.	Essential for growth. Plays enzymatic role in tissue respiration and acts as a transporter of hydrogen ions. Coenzyme forms FMN and FAD.
Niacin (nicotinic acid and nicotinamide)	M: 16 mg NE F: 14 mg NE	Fish, liver, meat, poultry, many grains, eggs, peanuts, milk, legumes, enriched grains. Synthesized by intestinal bacteria.	Stable to heat, light, oxidation, acid and alkali.	As part of enzyme system, aids in transfer of hydrogen and acts in metabolism of carbohydrates and amino acids. Involved in glycolysis, fat synthesis, and tissue respiration.
Vitamin B_6 (pyridoxine, pyridoxal, and pyridoxamine)	M: 1.3–1.7 mg F: 1.3–1.5 mg	Pork, glandular meats, cereal bran and germ, milk, egg yolk, oatmeal, and legumes. Synthesized by intestinal bacteria.	Stable to heat, light, and oxidation.	As a coenzyme, aids in the synthesis and breakdown of amino acids and in the synthesis of unsaturated fatty acids from essential fatty acids. Essential for conversion of tryptophan to niacin. Essential for normal growth.
Folate (folic acid, folacin)	400 μg	Green leafy vegetables, organ meats (liver), lean beef, wheat, eggs, fish, dry beans, lentils, cowpeas, asparagus, broccoli, collards, yeast. Synthesized in intestinal tract.	Stable to sunlight when in solution; unstable to heat in acid media.	Essential for biosynthesis of nucleic acids, esp. important in early fetal development. Essential for normal maturation of red blood cells. Functions as a coenzyme: tetrahydrofolic acid.

(*continued*)

TABLE 4–34 SUMMARY OF VITAMINS (continued)

Vitamin B_{12} (cobalamin)	2.4 μg	Liver, kidney, milk and dairy foods, meat, eggs. Vegans require supplement.	Slowly destroyed by acid, alkali, light, and oxidation.	Involved in the metabolism of single-carbon fragments. Essential for biosynthesis of nucleic acids and nucleoproteins. Role in metabolism of nervous tissue. Involved with folate metabolism. Related to growth.
Pantothenic acid	5 mg Adequate Intake	Present in all plant and animal foods. Eggs, kidney, liver, salmon, and yeast are best sources. Possibly synthesized by intestinal bacteria.	Unstable to acid, alkali, heat, and certain salts.	As part of coenzyme A, functions in the synthesis and breakdown of many vital body compounds. Essential in the intermediary metabolism of carbohydrate, fat, and protein.
Biotin	30 μg Adequate Intake	Liver, mushrooms, peanuts, yeast, milk, meat, egg yolk, most vegetables, banana, grapefruit, tomato, watermelon, and strawberries. Synthesized in intestinal tract.	Stable.	Essential component of enzymes. Involved in synthesis and breakdown of fatty acids and amino acids through aiding the addition and removal of CO_2 to or from active compounds, and the removal of NH_2 from amino acids.
Vitamin C (ascorbic acid)	60 mg	Acerola (West Indian cherry-like fruit), citrus fruit, tomato, melon, peppers, greens, raw cabbage, guava, strawberries, pineapple, potato, kiwi.	Unstable to heat, alkali, and oxidation, except in acids. Destroyed by storage.	Maintains intracellular cement substance with preservation of capillary integrity. Co-substrate in hydroxylations requiring molecular oxygen. Important in immune responses, wound healing, and allergic reactions. Increases absorption of nonheme iron.

*M, male; F, female; RE, retinol equivalents; α-TE, alpha-tocopherol equivalents; NE, niacin equivalents; FMN, flavin adenine mononucleotide; FAD, flavin adenine dinucleotide.

from the amino acid lysine by a multistage process involving vitamin C. There are few data on the carnitine biosynthetic capacities of humans; but the low tissue levels typically seen in neonates fed diets low in carnitine (e.g., nonsupplemented soy-based formulas) suggest that they may have limited capacities for synthesizing the factor (Atkins and Clandinin, 1990). In some instances it may be a "conditionally essential nutrient" (Broquist, 1994).

Foods of plant origin are generally low in carnitine, but those from animals (particularly meats and dairy products) are good sources. Carnitine is absorbed across the gut with high efficiency by both active transport and simple diffusion (Li et al., 1992). About half of carnitine is acetylated during absorption; both free and acetylated forms are found in the circulation in plasma and erythrocytes. Carnitine is taken up mostly by skeletal peripheral tissues, which contain some 90% of body stores.

Tissue depletion of carnitine has been reported in adults undergoing hemodialysis, adults with liver disease, and in preterm infants. Supplemental carnitine has been found to correct the hypertriglyceridemia in such patients (Combs, 1998). Muscle weakness and hypoglycemia have also been described as clinical manifestations of carnitine deficiency (Metabolic, 1990).

myo-Inositol

***myo*-Inositol** (*cis*-1,2,3,5-*trans*-4,6-cyclohexanehexol) functions in metabolism as phosphatidylinositol (PI), which has a structural role in membranes, serves as a source of arachidonic acid for the biosynthesis of eicosanoids, and is itself a mediator of cellular responses to external stimuli. It is concentrated in the brain and cerebrospinal fluid, but also occurs in other tissues (Combs, 1998).

Mammals synthesize *myo*-inositol from glucose, but it is also obtained from fruits, grains, vegetables, nuts, legumes, and organ meats such as liver and heart. Dietary sources include various inositol phospholipids in animal products as well as *phytic acid* (inositol hexaphosphate) in plant materials. Because humans and most other mammals lack an intestinal phytase, phytic acid is not a useful source of *myo*-inositol, serving instead to interfere with the absorption of the divalent cations of calcium, iron, and zinc.

myo-Inositol is efficiently absorbed in free form by an active transport process. It is transported in the blood mostly in free form, with some as PI associated with lipoproteins. Free *myo*-inositol is converted in the tissue to PI, which is metabolized by sequential phosphorylations to the mono- (PIP) and

TABLE 4–35 DIETARY REFERENCE INTAKES FOR CHOLINE

LIFE-STAGE GROUP	AI* (mg/d)	UL (mg/d)
Infants		
0–6 mo	125	ND
7–12 mo	150	ND
Children		
1–3 y	200	1000
4–8 y	250	1000
Males		
9–13 y	375	2000
14–18 y	550	3000
19–30 y	550	3500
31–50 y	550	3500
51–70 y	550	3500
>70 y	550	3500
Females		
9–13 y	375	2000
14–18 y	400	3000
19–30 y	425	3500
31–50 y	425	3500
51–70 y	425	3500
>70 y	425	3500
Pregnancy		
≤18 y	450	3000
19–30 y	450	3500
31–50 y	450	3500
Lactation		
≤18 y	550	3000
19–30 y	550	3500
31–50 y	550	3500

(From Institute of Medicine, Food and Nutrition Board. Dietary Reference Intakes for Thiamin, Riboflavin, Niacin, Vitamin B-6, Folate, Vitamin B-12, Pantothenic Acid, Biotin, and Choline. Washington, DC: National Academy Press, 1998.)

AI, adequate intake; UL, tolerable upper intake level; ND, not determinable due to lack of data of adverse effects.

*Although AIs have been set for choline, there are few data to assess whether a dietary supply of choline is needed at all stages of the life cycle, and it may be that the choline requirement can be met by endogenous synthesis at some of these stages.

diphosphate (PIP_2) forms. Clear dietary needs for preformed *myo*-inositol have been demonstrated only for some fishes and the female gerbil. Deprivation of the factor produced anorexia, dermatologic lesions, and intestinal lipdystrophy.

Pyrroloquinoline Quinone

Pyrroloquinoline quinone (PQQ) (4,5-dihydro-4, 5-dioxo-1*H*-pyrrolo[2,3*f*]quinoline-2,7,9-tricarboxylic acid) was recently found to prevent mortality and skin lesions involving impaired collagen metabolism in mice fed a diet containing very low amounts of the factor. Although PQQ appears to function as a redox cofactor of some bacterial enzymes, its role in eukaryotes is not clear (Christensen, 1994; Combs, 1998). The factor appears to be present in egg yolk, glandular tissues, and many citrus fruits.

Ubiquinones

The **ubiquinones** are a group of substituted 1,4-benzoquinone derivatives with isopentyl side chains of variable length. The principle species has 10 such side-chain units and is referred to as **coenzyme Q_{10} (CoQ_{10})**; it was first isolated in 1957. The ubiquinones function as essential components of the mitochondrial electron transport chain in which they undergo reversible reduction/oxidation to pass electrons from flavoproteins (NADH or succinic dehydrogenases) to the cytochromes via cytochrome b_5. In addition, the redox properties of CoQ_{10} enable it to function as a fat-soluble antioxidant, much like α-tocopherol. Relatively high concentrations of the ubiquinones are maintained in tissues apparently by biosynthesis from endogenous precursors. It has been suggested that limited ubiquinone synthesis may play a role in the etiology of heart disease; indeed, supplemental CoQ_{10} has been found to be effective in cardiomyopathy and congestive heart failure (Folkers et al., 1993; Morisco et al., 1993; Permanetter, 1992). CoQ_{10} is concentrated in a variety of foods, notably fish oils, nuts, fish, and meats.

Bioflavonoids

The **bioflavonoids** (phenolic derivatives of 2-phenyl-1,4-benzopyrone) have no known immediate metabolic function; however, they have been shown to reduce capillary fragility and to potentiate the antiscorbutic activity of ascorbic acid both of which effects may involve their chelation of divalent metal ions (Cu^{++}, Fe^{++}) and their intrinsic antioxidant properties (Manach et al., 1996). Epidemiologic studies have demonstrated associations of diets high in bioflavonoids with reduced risks for cardiovascular disease and several cancers. The bioflavonoids are ubiquitous in foods of plant origin; more than 800 different bioflavonoids such as quercitin, rutin, and hesperidin have been isolated from plants in which they represent the major sources of noncarotenoid red, blue, and yellow pigments.

CASE STUDY

JoAnne T. is a 40-year-old African-American executive. She leads an active life and uses oral contraceptives. She works out regularly and eats a very-low-fat diet to manage her weight. She and her husband want to start a family. Her blood work indicates a low folacin level. She has a light breakfast of fruit, a sandwich and coffee for lunch, and a dinner of a green salad, pasta of some sort, and fruit and milk. She comes into your office for advice on how to improve her diet.

What recommendations do you have for her as her nutritional counselor?

1. What are your concerns about her diet?
2. What additional information do you need?
3. What would you recommend to her to improve her vitamin intake?
4. Would a supplement be useful for JoAnne?

CITED REFERENCES

American Council on Science and Health. Diet and Cancer, 2nd ed. New York, 1993.

Anderson TW, et al. Vitamin C and the common cold: A double-blind trial. Can Med Assoc J 107:503, 1972.

Anderson TW. Large scale trials of vitamin C. Ann N Y Acad Sci 258:498, 1975.

Atkins J, Clandinin MT. Nutritional significance of factors affecting carnitine dependent transport of fatty acids in neonates: A review. Nutr Res 10:117, 1990.

Block G. The data support a role for antioxidants in reducing cancer risk. Nutr Rev 50:207, 1992.

Block G. Nutrient sources of provitamin A carotenoids in the American diet. Am J Epidemiol 139:290, 1994.

Blot W, et al. Nutrition intervention trials in Linxian, China: Supplementation with specific vitamin/mineral combinations, cancer incidence, and disease-specific mortality in the general population. J Nat Cancer Inst 85:1483, 1993.

Blumberg J. Dietary antioxidants and aging. Contemp Nutr 17(3):1, 1992.

Bouhuys A. Colds and antihistamine effects of vitamin C. N Engl J Med 290:633, 1974.

Broquist HP. Carnitine. In: Shils ME, et al. (eds.). Modern Nutrition in Health and Disease, 8th ed. (vol. 1). Philadelphia: Lea & Febiger, 1994.

Buring JE, Hennekeus CH. Antioxidant vitamins and cardiovascular disease. Nutr Rev 55(2):S53, 1997.

Burton GW. Vitamin E: Molecular and biological function. Proc Nutr Soc 53:251, 1994.

Butterworth C Jr, Bendich A. Folic acid and the prevention of birth defects. Annu Rev Nutr 16:73, 1996.

Canty DJ, Zeisel SJ. Lecithin and choline in human health and disease. Nutr Rev 52:327, 1994.

Carethers M. Diagnosing vitamin B_{12} deficiency, a common geriatric disorder. Geriatrics 43:89, 1988.

Carlson BL, Tabacchi MH. Loss of vitamin C in vegetables during the food service cycle. J Am Diet Assoc 88:65, 1988.

Carr AB, et al. Vitamin C and the common cold: A second MZ cotwin control study. Acta Genet Med Cemellol 30:249, 1981.

Caution on use of antioxidants. Nutrition Today 29(2):4, 1994.

Chen T, et al. An update on the vitamin D content of fortified milk from the United States and Canada. (Letter). N Engl J Med 329:1507, 1993.

Christensen H. Riboflavin can protect tissues from oxidative injury. Nutr Rev 51:149, 1993.

Christensen HN. Is PQQ a significant nutrient in addition to its role as a therapeutic agent in the higher animal? Nutr Rev 52:24, 1994.

Combs GF Jr. The Vitamins: Fundamental Aspects in Nutrition and Health, 2nd ed. New York: Academic Press, 1998, p. 107.

Coulehan JL, et al. Vitamin C and acute illness in Navaho children. N Engl J Med 295:973, 1976.

Coulehan JL, et al. Vitamin C prophylaxis in a boarding school. N Engl J Med 290:6, 1974.

Decker KF. Biosynthesis and function of enzymes with covalently bound flavin. Annu Rev Nutr 13:17, 1993.

Driskell JA. Vitamin B-6 requirements of humans. Nutr Res 14:293, 1994.

Ferland G. The vitamin K-dependent proteins: An update. Nutr Rev 56:223, 1998.

Folkers K, et al. Nutrition and cardiac health. A deficiency of coenzyme Q_{10} is a dominant molecular cause of heart failure. J Optimal Nutrition 2:24, 1993.

Food and Nutrition Board (FNB), National Research Council, NAS. Recommended Dietary Allowances, 10th ed. Washington, DC: National Academy Press, 1989.

Gerster H. Anticarcinogenic effect of common carotenoids. Int J Vit Nutr Res 63:93, 1993.

Goldberger J, et al. A study of the diet of nonpellagrous and pellagrous households. JAMA 71:944, 1918.

Guilarte TR. Vitamin B_6 and cognitive development: Recent research findings from human and animal studies. Nutr Rev 51:193, 1993.

Haddad J. Vitamin D: Solar rays, the milky way or both? N Engl J Med 326:1213, 1992.

Halliwell B. Antioxidants in human health and disease. Annu Rev Nutr 16:33, 1996.

Hathcock JN, et al. Evaluation of vitamin A toxicity. Am J Clin Nutr 52:183, 1990.

Heaney RP. Nutritional factors in osteoporosis. Annu Rev Nutr 13:287, 1993.

Holick M, et al. The vitamin D content of fortified milk and infant formula. N Engl J Med 326:1178, 1992.

Hunter D. A prospective study of the intake of vitamins C, E and A and the risk of breast cancer. N Engl J Med 329:234, 1993.

Institute of Medicine, Food and Nutrition Board. Dietary Reference Intakes. Proposed Definition and Plan for Review of Dietary Antioxidants and Related Compounds. Washington, DC: National Academy Press, 1998.

International Life Sciences Institute. Disease prevention effects of antioxidants explored at ILSI meetings in Washington and Stockholm. ILSI News 11(5):1, 1993.

Jacob RA. The integrated antioxidant system. Nutr Res 15:755, 1995.

Jacobus C, et al. Hypervitaminosis D associated with drinking milk. N Engl J Med 326:1173, 1992.

Johnston C, Luo B. Comparison of the absorption and excretion of three commercially available sources of vitamin C. J Am Diet Assoc 94:779, 1994.

Li BUK, et al. The effect of enteral carnitine administration in humans. Am J Clin Nutr 55:838, 1992.

Li E, Norris AW. Structure/function of cytosolic vitamin A-binding proteins. Annu Rev Nutr 16:205, 1996.

Maden M. Vitamin A in embryonic development. Nutr Rev 52(suppl):S3, 1994.

Manach C, et al. Bioavailability, metabolism and physiological impact of 4-oxo-flavonoids. Nutr Res 16:517, 1996.

Mangelsdorf DJ. Vitamin A receptors. Annu Rev Nutr 52(suppl):S32, 1994.

Marshall C. Can megadoses of vitamin C help against colds? Nutr Forum 9(5):33, 1992.

Metabolic effects of carnitine supplementation in subjects with low plasma carnitine levels. Nutr Rev 48:159, 1990.

Meydani SN, et al. Vitamin E supplementation and in vivo immune response in healthy elderly subjects: A randomized controlled trial. JAMA 277: 1380, 1997.

Miller JZ, et al. Therapeutic effect of vitamin C. A co-twin control study. JAMA 237:248, 1977.

Morisco C, et al. Effect of coenzyme Q_{10} therapy in patients with congestive heart failure: A long-term multicenter randomized study. Clin Invest 71:S134, 1993.

Olson JA. Vitamin A. In: Zeigler EE, Filer LJ (eds.). Present Knowledge in Nutrition, 7th ed. Washington, DC: ILSI Press, 1996.

Packer L, Fuchs J (eds.). Vitamin C in Health and Disease. New York: Marcel Dekker, 1997.

Permanetter B. Ubiquinone (coenzyme Q_{10}) and the long term treatment of idiopathic dilated cardiomyopathy. Eur Heart J 13:1528, 1992.

Reimund E, Ramos A. Niacin-indused hepatitis and thrombocytopenia after 10 years of niacin use. J Clin Gastroenterol 18:270, 1994.

Rimm E, et al. Vitamin E consumption and the risk of coronary artery disease in men. N Engl J Med 328:1450, 1993.

Sauberlich HE. Pharmacology of vitamin C. Annu Rev Nutr 14:371, 1994.

Schaumberg HJ, et al. Sensory neuropathy from pyridoxine abuse. N Engl J Med 309:445, 1983.

School of Public Health. Our vitamin prescription: The big four. University of California at Berkeley Wellness Letter 10(4):1, 1994.

Schwartz J, Weiss S. Relationship between dietary vitamin C intake and pulmonary function in the first National Health and Nutrition Examination Survey (NHANES 1). Am J Clin Nutr 59:110, 1994.

Sokol RJ. Vitamin E. In: Zeigler EE, Filer LJ (eds.). Present Knowledge in Nutrition, 7th ed. Washington, DC: ILSI Press, 1996.

Specker BL, Tsang RC. Vitamin D in infancy. Cereal Foods World 33:788, 1988.

Specker BL, et al. Increased urinary methylmalonic acid excretion in breast-fed infants of vegetarian mothers and identification of and acceptable dietary source of vitamin B_{12}. Am J Clin Nutr 47:89, 1988.

Sperduto RD, et al. The Linxian cataract studies: Two nutrition intervention trials. Arch Ophthalmol 111:1246, 1993.

Stampfer MJ, et al. Vitamin E consumption and the risk of coronary artery disease in women. N Engl J Med 328:1444, 1993.

Suttie JW. The importance of menaquinones in human nutrition. Annu Rev Nutr 15:399, 1995.

Thomas MK, et al. Hypovitaminosis D in medical patients. N Engl J Med 338:777, 1998.

Thorogood M. The epidemiology of vegetarianism and health. Nutr Res Rev 8:179, 1995.

Umegaki S, et al. Beta-carotene prevents x-ray induction of micronuclei in human lymphocytes. Am J Clin Nutr 59:409, 1994.

Vermeer C, et al. Effects of vitamin K on bone mass and bone metabolism. J Nutr 126:1187S, 1996.

Wagner C. Symposium on the subcellular compartmentalization of folate metabolism. J Nutr 126:1228S, 1996.

Wang G, et al. Effects of vitamin/mineral supplementation on the prevalence of histological dysplasia and early cancer of the esophagus and stomach: Results from the general population trial in Linxian, China. Cancer Epidemiol Biomarkers Prevention 3(2):161, 1994.

Wasserman RH, Fullmer CS. Vitamin D and intestinal calcium transport: Facts, speculations and hypothesis. J Nutr 125:1971S, 1995.

West KP Jr, et al. Vitamin A and infection: Public health implications. Annu Rev Nutr 9:63, 1989.

Whitfield GK, et al. Genomic actions of 1,25-dihydroxyvitamin D_3. J Nutr 125:1690S, 1995.

Wilson CW, Loh HS. Common cold and vitamin C. Lancet 1:638, 1973.

Zeisel SH, Blusztajn JK. Choline and human nutrition. Annu Rev Nutr 14:269, 1994.

ADDITIONAL REFERENCES

Vitamin A

Goldberg J. Vitamin A and eyesight. Am J Epidemiol 128:700, 1988.
Krinsky NI. Carotenoids and cancer: Basic research studies. In: Frei B (ed.). Natural Antioxidants in Human Health and Disease. New York: Academic Press, 1994, p. 239.
Mangels A, et al. Carotenoid content of fruits and vegetables: An evaluation of analytic data. J Am Diet Assoc 93:284, 1993.
Mijewski S, et al. Decreased levels of vitamin A in serum of patients with psoriasis. Arch Dermatol Res 280:499, 1989.
Olson J. 1992 Atwater lecture: The irresistible fascination of carotenoids and vitamin A. Am J Clin Nutr 57:833, 1993.
Palozza P. Prooxidant actions of carotenoids in biologic systems. Nutr Rev 56:257, 1998.
Parker RS. Absorption, metabolism and transport of carotenoids. FASEB J 10:542, 1996.
Pfahl M, Chytil, F. Regulation of metabolism by retinoic acid and its nuclear receptors. Annu Rev Nutr 16:257, 1996.

Vitamin D

Bonner F, Stein W. Calcium homeostasis—An old problem revisited. J Nutr 125:1987S, 1995.
Hannah SS, Norman AW. 1,25$(OH)_2$Vitamin D_3-regulated expression of the eukaryotic genome. Nutr Rev 52:376, 1994.
Looker AC, Gunter EW. Hypovitaminosis D in medical patients. (Letter). N Engl J Med 339:344, 1998.
Season, latitude, and ability of sunlight to promote synthesis of vitamin D_3 in skin. Nutr Rev 47:252, 1989.
Vitamin D and psoriasis. Nutr MD 18(4):3, 1989.

Vitamin E

Allen RG. Oxygen-reactive species and antioxidant responses during development: The metabolic paradox of cellular differentiation. Proc Soc Exp Biol Med 196:117, 1991.
Cohn W, et al. Tocopherol transport and absorption. Proc Nutr Soc 51:179, 1992.
Maeda H, Akaike T. Oxygen free radicals as pathogenic molecules in viral diseases. Proc Soc Exp Biol Med 198:721, 1991.
Packer L, Fuchs J (eds.). Vitamin E in Health and Disease. New York: Marcel Dekker, 1993.

Vitamin K

Dowd P, et al. The mechanism of action of vitamin K. Annu Rev Nutr 15:419, 1995.
Furie B, Furie BC. Molecular basis of vitamin K-dependent carboxylation. Blood 75:1753, 1990.
Olson R. Vitamin K. In: Shils M, et al. (eds.). Modern nutrition in health and disease, 8th ed. Philadelphia: Lea & Febiger, 1994, p. 342.
Shearer MJ. Vitamin K. Lancet 345:229, 1995.

Thiamin

Rindi G. Thiamin. In: Ziegler EE, Filer LJ Jr (eds.). Present Knowledge in Nutrition, 7th ed. Washington, DC: ILSI Press, 1996, p. 160.
Tanphaichitr V. Thiamin. In: Shils M, et al. (eds.). Modern Nutrition in Health and Disease, 8th ed. Philadelphia: Lea & Febiger, 1994, p. 359.

Riboflavin

Bunce GE, Hess JL. Cataract—What is the role of nutrition in lens health? Nutrition Today 23(6):6, 1988.
Cimino JA, et al. Riboflavin metabolism in the hypothyroid human adult. Proc Soc Exp Biol Med 184:151, 1987.
McCormick D. Riboflavin. In: Shils M, et al. (eds.). Modern Nutrition in Health and Disease, 8th ed. Philadelphia: Lea & Febiger, 1994, p. 366.
Rivlin RS. Riboflavin. In: Ziegler EE, Filer LJ Jr (eds.). Present Knowledge in Nutrition, 7th ed. Washington, DC: ILSI Press, 1996, p. 167.

Niacin

Jacob RA, Swendseid ME. Niacin. In: Ziegler EE, Filer LJ Jr (eds.). Present Knowledge in Nutrition, 7th ed. Washington, DC: ILSI Press, 1996, p. 184.
van Eys J. Nicotinic acid. In: Machlin LJ (ed.). Handbook of Vitamins. New York: Marcel Dekker, 1991, p. 311.

Vitamin B_6

Driskell J. Vitamin B-6 requirements of humans. Nutr Res 14(2):293, 1994.
Lecklem J. Vitamin B6. In: Ziegler EE, Filer LJ (eds.). Present Knowledge in Nutrition, 7th ed. Washington, DC: ILSI Press, 1996, p. 174.
Pyridoxine and autism. Nutr MD 15(3):4, 1989.
Rall LC, Meydani SN. Vitamin B_6 and immune competence. Nutr Rev 51:217, 1993.

Folate

Antony AC. Folate receptors. Annu Rev Nutr 16:501, 1996.
Bailey LB. Dietary reference intakes for folate: The debut of dietary folate equivalents. Nutr Rev 56:294, 1998.
Henderson GB. Folate-binding proteins. Annu Rev Nutr 10:319, 1990.
Herbert V, Das K. Folic acid and vitamin B_{12}. In: Shils M, et al. (eds.). Modern Nutrition in Health and Disease, 8th ed. Philadelphia: Lea & Febiger, 1994, p. 402.

Vitamin B_{12}

Clementz GL. The spectrum of vitamin B_{12} deficiency. Am Fam Physician 41(1):150, 1990.
Herbert V. Vitamin B-12. In: Ziegler EE, Filer LJ Jr (eds.). Present Knowledge in Nutrition, 7th ed. Washington, DC: ILSI Press, 1996, p. 191.
Unrecognized cobalamin-responsive neuropsychiatric disorders. Nutr Rev 47:208, 1989.

Pantothenic Acid

Plesofsky-Vig N. Pantothenic acid. In: Ziegler EE, Filer LJ Jr (eds.). Present Knowledge in Nutrition, 7th ed. Washington, DC: ILSI Press, 1996, p. 236.
Plesofsky-Vig N. Pantothenic acid and coenzyme A. In: Shils M, et al. (eds.). Modern Nutrition in Health and Disease, 8th ed. Philadelphia: Lea & Febiger, 1994, p. 395.
Tahiliani AG, Benlich CJ. Pantothenic acid in health and disease. Vitam Horm 46:165, 1991.

Biotin

A role for biotin in bone growth. Nutr Rev 47:157, 1989.
Dakshinamurti K. Biotin. In: Shils M, et al. (eds.). Modern Nutrition in Health and Disease, 8th ed. Philadelphia: Lea & Febiger, 1994, p. 426.
Mock DM. Biotin. In: Ziegler EE, Filer LJ Jr (eds.). Present Knowledge in Nutrition, 7th ed. Washington, DC: ILSI Press, 1996, p. 220.

Vitamin C

Hemilä H. Vitamin C intake and susceptibility to the common cold. Br J Nutr 77:59, 1997.
Jacob R. Vitamin C. In: Shils M, et al. (eds.). Modern Nutrition in Health and Disease, 8th ed. Philadelphia: Lea & Febiger, 1994, p. 432.
Machlin LJ, Bendich A. Free radical tissue damage: Protective role of antioxidant nutrients. FASEB J 1:441, 1988.
Pauling L. Vitamin C and the Common Cold. San Francisco: Freeman, 1970.

Choline

McMahon KE. Choline, an essential nutrient? Nutrition Today 22(2):18, 1987.
Zeisel SH. Choline. In: Shils ME, et al. (eds.). Modern Nutrition in Health and Disease, 8th ed. (vol. 1). Philadelphia: Lea & Febiger, 1994, p. 449.

Carnitine

Metabolic effects of carnitine supplementation in subjects with low plasma carnitine levels. Nutr Rev 48:159, 1990.
Rebouche CJ, Paulson DJ. Carnitine metabolism and function in humans. Annu Rev Nutr 6:41, 1986.

myo-Inositol

Aukema HM, Holub BJ. Inositol. In: Shils ME, et al. (eds.). Modern Nutrition in Health and Disease, 8th ed. (vol. 1). Philadelphia: Lea & Febiger, 1994, p. 466.
Berdanier C. Is inositol an essential nutrient? Nutrition Today 22(2):18, 1987.

CHAPTER 5

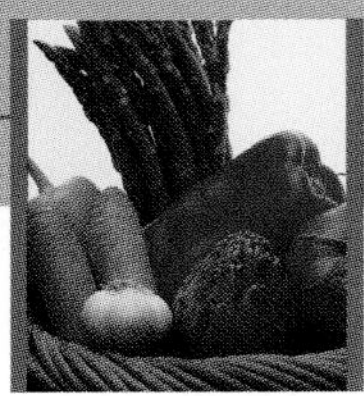

Minerals

JOHN J. B. ANDERSON, PhD

Chapter Outline

- Characteristics of Minerals
- Macrominerals
- Microminerals
- Ultratrace Elements
- Other Trace Elements

Key Terms

BIOAVAILABILITY—the availability of a mineral within the small intestine for absorption and the actual absorption (efficiency) of the mineral; implies retention of the mineral in the body and its utilization in cellular or tissue functions

CALBINDINS—calcium-binding proteins found in intestinal absorbing cells and other cells of the body

CERULOPLASMIN—a plasma protein that transports copper and acts as an oxidase (enzyme)

CRETINISM—a congenital condition, typically caused by severe iodine deficiency during gestation; characterized by arrested physical and mental development and subnormal intelligence

FERRITIN—an iron-apoferritin complex that is the major storage form of iron in the liver and other tissues

GLUCOSE TOLERANCE FACTOR—a biologically active chromium complex found in foods; its structure is unknown

GLUTATHIONE PEROXIDASE—a selenium-containing enzyme that is the major active form of selenium in cells

GOITER—a chronic enlargement of the thyroid gland, visible as a swelling at the front of the neck; commonly associated with iodine deficiency

GOITROGEN—a compound that blocks the uptake and utilization of iodine by thyroid cells and contributes to iodine deficiency and goiter

HEME IRON—the nonprotein, insoluble, iron-containing protoporphyrin that is a constituent of hemoglobin, myoglobin, and a few other proteins

HEMOGLOBIN—a conjugated protein containing four heme groups and globin with the property of reversible oxygenation

HEMOSIDERIN—a complex insoluble form of storage iron

HYDROXYAPATITE—a crystalline structure in bone, consisting of calcium phosphate and calcium carbonate

HYPERCALCIURIA—excessive urinary losses of calcium that may occur in individuals who have excessive intestinal absorption of calcium, or who have high-protein intakes, especially from animal protein

MACROMINERAL (BULK ELEMENT)—a mineral required by humans in amounts of 100 mg/day or more (i.e., in large quantities)

METALLOTHIONEIN—a nonenzymatic, zinc-binding protein found in intestinal absorbing cells and other tissues of the body, especially the liver

MICROMINERAL (TRACE ELEMENT)—a mineral required by humans in amounts of less than 100 mg/day (i.e., in quantities of a few milligrams or even micrograms)

MYOGLOBIN—an iron protoporphyrin-globin complex present in striated muscle that stores oxygen

NONHEME IRON—the form of iron found in plants, which is less well absorbed than heme iron

OXALIC ACID (OXALATE)—an organic acid, found in certain leafy vegetables, which binds with calcium and other divalent cations, thereby inhibiting their absorption from these foods

PHYTIC ACID (PHYTATE)—a phosphorus-containing compound, found in the outer husks of cereal grains, which binds with minerals and inhibits absorption

TETANY—muscle twitchings, spasms, and (eventually) convulsions caused by low blood levels of calcium or magnesium

THYROXINE (T_4)—an iodine-containing hormone secreted by the thyroid gland to regulate the rate of cell metabolism

TRANSFERRIN—a protein synthesized in the liver that transports iron in the blood to the erythroblasts for use in heme synthesis and to all other tissues; also carries chromium and a few other cations in blood, especially from the small intestine to tissues

TRIIODOTHYRONINE (T_3)—an iodine-containing thyroid hormone with several times the biologic activity of thyroxine

ULTRATRACE ELEMENTS—minerals found in the body, each of which occurs in small quantities and is typically measured in micrograms

The minerals represent a large class of micronutrients, most of which are considered essential. They are traditionally divided into macrominerals (bulk elements) and microminerals (trace elements). More recently, the term **ultratrace elements** has been used to describe elements that are consumed in microgram (μg) quantities each day. Macrominerals, such as calcium and phosphorus, are required in amounts of 100 mg/day or more, whereas the microminerals, such as iron and selenium, are required in much smaller amounts, typically less than 15 mg/day.

Knowledge about the trace elements has expanded over the past few decades because of greatly improved analytical techniques. Because there is still so little solid information about the essentiality of the ultratrace elements to human health, this group is covered only minimally in the final section of this chapter.

Except for the "other trace elements" and possibly boron, all minerals covered in this chapter are recognized as essential for human function, even though specific requirements have not been established for a few of them. Studies of patients receiving long-term total parenteral nutrition (TPN) have helped to determine the essentiality of and the required amounts for several trace elements.

CHARACTERISTICS OF MINERALS

Macrominerals occur in the body and food chiefly in the ionic state. For example, sodium, potassium, and calcium form positive ions (cations), whereas other minerals exist as negative ions (anions). The latter include chlorine (as chloride), sulfur (as sulfate), and phosphorus (as phosphates). Salts, such as sodium chloride and calcium phosphate, dissociate in solution, existing in body fluids and crystals as Na^+, Cl^-, Ca^{++}, and HPO_4^{--}. Minerals also occur as components of organic compounds, such as phosphoproteins, phospholipids, metalloenzymes, and other metalloproteins, such as hemoglobin.

Bioavailabilty of Minerals

Bioavailability has become a useful term in recent years to describe the chemical or physiochemical state of minerals within the lumen of the small intestine (Fairweather-Tait and Hurrel, 1996). With the exception of heme iron, practically all other elements are absorbed in the ionic state. Therefore, any elements that remain bound to organic molecules or other inorganic complexes after the digestive steps are completed will not be absorbed; that is, they are not bioavailable, and these unabsorbed minerals will be eliminated in the feces.

Once the ions are absorbed at the brush borders of the columnar intestinal epithelial cells or enterocytes, often referred to as the mucosal surface, they still must transfer through the cytosol of the absorbing cells before they are transported across the basolateral (serosal) membrane to the blood. This exit step of the absorptive process typically requires an active transport mechanism, at least for the mineral cations. If the cationic forms of the elements are not transported across the basolateral membrane, they remain in the absorbing cells, bound to proteins. For example, calcium ions bind to calbindins, iron to intestinal ferritin, and zinc to metallothionein, only to be excreted when the intestinal cells die and slough off into the intestinal lumen. (The low intestinal absorption efficiencies of these cations may have evolved to protect against potential toxicities that result from excessive absorption.) Low bioavailability may also result from the formation of soaps—for example, of calcium and magnesium—binding to free fatty acids in the lumen, in fat malabsorption, and from precipitation when one of a pair of ions (e.g., calcium, which combines with phosphates) is present in the lumen at a very high concentration. Mineral-mineral interactions also can result in depressed absorption of elements or low bioavailability (see the section that follows).

Many molecules in foods influence bioavailability, either by enhancing absorption or by interfering with or inhibiting absorption. Examples of inhibitors include the binding by phytates and oxalates of calcium and other divalent cations. Enhancers include ascorbate for nonheme iron, among others. Vegetarians tend to consume foods with increased quantities of many of the inhibiting factors, but they typically also ingest more ascorbic acid, an enhancer. In addition, the bioavailability of elements may be influenced by many physiologic factors, such as gastric acidity, homeostatic adaptations, and stress.

Bioavailability also is often used to refer to the absorption and utilization of the elements in tissue and cellular functions. This broader meaning of the term is not generally accepted because of the lack of quantification. Bioavailability cannot be quantified easily when its meaning is intended to include utilization in tissues; that is, beyond the chemical state of the elements within the gut lumen and absorption across the intestinal barrier to blood.

In general, certain elements typically have low bioavailability from foods (iron, chromium, manganese), whereas others have high bioavailability (sodium, potassium, chloride, iodide, fluoride). All other minerals, including calcium and magnesium, are of medium bioavailability.

Mineral-Mineral Interactions

Minerals can have negative interactions with other minerals, potentially affecting intestinal absorption, transport, utilization, and storage. For example, the absorption of zinc may be reduced by nonheme iron supplementation; excessive intake of zinc can reduce the absorption of copper; and excessive intakes of calcium may reduce the absorption of manganese, zinc, and iron (Deehr et al., 1990; Hallberg et al., 1991; Wood and Zheng, 1997). However, interaction studies are difficult to conduct, and definitive conclusions about these interactions await additional investigation. Other examples of interactions are covered in the sections on the individual elements.

Mineral Composition of the Body

Minerals represent about 4% to 5% of body weight, or 2.8 to 3.5 kg in adult women and men, respectively. Approximately 50% of this weight is calcium, and another 25% is phosphorus, existing as phosphates; almost all of the calcium and 70% of the phosphates are found in bones and teeth. The five other essential macrominerals (magnesium, sodium, potassium, chloride, and sulfur) and the eleven established microminerals (iron, zinc, iodide, selenium, manganese, fluoride, molybdenum, copper, chromium, cobalt, and boron) constitute the remaining 25%. The ultratrace elements, such as arsenic, aluminum, tin, nickel, vanadium, and silicon, provide a negligible amount of weight.

Functions of Minerals

Mineral elements have many essential roles, both as ions dissolved in body fluids and as constituents of essential molecules. The mineral ions in body fluids regulate the activities of many enzymes, maintain acid–base balance and osmotic pressure, facilitate the membrane transfer of essential nutrients and other molecules, and maintain nerve and muscular irritability. In some cases, mineral ions are structural constituents of extracellular body tissues, such as bones and teeth. Several minerals, such as zinc and iron, are involved in different ways in the growth process as well.

MACROMINERALS

Macrominerals, bulk elements, that are essential for adult humans in amounts of 100 mg/day or more are calcium, phosphorus (phosphates), magnesium, sulfur (sulfate), sodium, chloride, and potassium. Except for sulfur, these minerals typically exist in the ionic state in foods and in the body. Many organic molecules also contain phosphorus-containing groups, such as phospholipids, that are not in a free ionic form.

Calcium

Calcium, the most abundant mineral in the body, makes up about 1.5% to 2% of the body weight and 39% of the total body minerals. Approximately 99% of the calcium exists in the bones and teeth. (The calcium in teeth, however, is not mobilizable for return to the blood, as the minerals of erupted teeth are "fixed for life.") The remaining 1% of calcium is in the blood and extracellular fluids and within the cells of all tissues, where it regulates many important metabolic functions. Figure 5–1 illustrates the pathways of calcium metabolism.

The skeleton is not simply a store of calcium and other minerals; it is a dynamic tissue that returns calcium and other minerals to the blood and extracellular fluids upon demand. Bone also takes up calcium and other minerals from the blood when they are consumed (i.e., during the postprandial period). Late in life, however, bone retention of calcium derived from food and supplements is limited unless the calcium is consumed along with vitamin D or a bone-conserving drug. (The roles of calcium in bone metabolism are covered in Chapter 28.)

Food Sources and Intakes

Dark green leafy vegetables, such as kale, collards, turnip greens, mustard greens, and broccoli, and sardines, clams, oysters, and canned salmon are good sources of calcium. Soybeans also contain ample amounts of calcium. Oxalic acid limits the availability of calcium in rhubarb, spinach, chard, and beet greens. Fortified orange juice contains as much calcium as milk. Table 5–1 and Appendix 41 show the calcium content of selected foods.

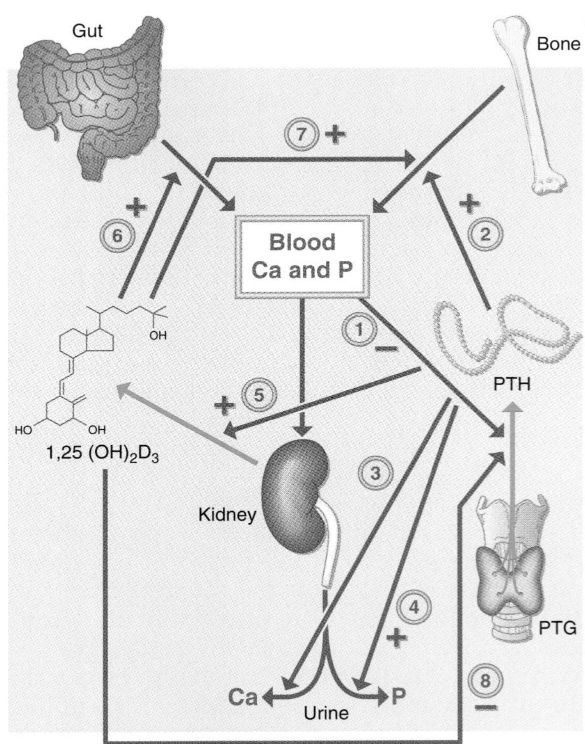

FIGURE 5–1 Schematic illustration of the pathways of calcium metabolism. The regulation of calcium metabolism involves intestinal absorption (gut), blood calcium (Ca) and phosphate (P) concentrations, bone, the kidneys, which produce the hormonal form of vitamin D (1,25[OH]$_2$D$_3$), and the parathyroid glands (PTG), which secrete parathyroid hormone (PTH). Steps 1 through 8 represent specific points of regulation.

TABLE 5–1 CALCIUM CONTENT OF SELECTED FOODS

FOOD	mg
Yogurt, low-fat, w/fruit, 1 cup	345
Milk, skim, 1 cup	302
Ice milk, soft-serve, 1 cup	274
Yogurt, frozen, 1 cup	240
Cheese, cheddar, 1 oz	204
Salmon, canned, w/bones, 3½ oz	185
Ice cream, vanilla, 1 cup	176
Rhubarb, cooked, ½ cup	174
Cheese, cottage, 2% fat, 1 cup	155
Spinach, frozen, cooked, ½ cup	138
Molasses, blackstrap, 1 T	137
Tofu, regular, ½ cup	130
Milk, dry, instant, nonfat, 2 T	104
Almonds, ¼ cup	92
Baked beans, white, ½ cup	64
Frankfurter, turkey, 1	58
Orange, 1 medium	52
Halibut, baked, 3 oz	51
Kale, fresh, cooked, ½ cup	47
Broccoli, cooked from fresh, ½ cup	36
Bread, whole-wheat, 1 slice	32
Waffle, frozen, 4" diameter, 1	29
Cheese, cream, 2 T	23
Oatmeal, cooked, 1 cup	19
Cream, half and half, 1 T	16
Chicken, breast, baked, 3 oz	13
Banana, 1 medium	7
Ground beef, lean, 3 oz	4

(From United States Department of Agriculture (USDA). Composition of Foods. USDA Handbook No. 8 Series. Washington, DC: ARS, USDA, 1976-1986.)

Calcium supplements are being used to increase calcium intake. The most common form is calcium carbonate, which is relatively insoluble, particularly at a neutral pH. Calcium citrate, although containing less calcium than calcium carbonate by weight, is much more soluble. Therefore, calcium citrate would be suitable for patients with achlorhydria (lack of hydrochloric acid in the stomach). The selection of the most appropriate calcium supplement depends on several factors, including physical and chemical properties, interactions with other medicines taken concurrently, and current medical conditions and age (Levenson and Bockman, 1994).

Beginning at the age of 11 years, median dietary calcium intakes in the United States are considerably less than the Adequate Intakes (AI) described in the next section (Fig. 5–2). Therefore, calcium intakes of Americans are insufficient for the critical ages of bone deposition in both genders, as well as being inadequate at other critical stages.

According to the Continuing Survey of Food Intakes of Individuals (CSFII) (U.S. Department of Agriculture, 1994), the top food sources of calcium in the U.S. diet are milk, cheese, bread, ice cream, sherbet, and frozen yogurt, along with cakes, cookies, quick breads, and doughnuts (Subar et al., 1998).

Dietary Reference Intakes (DRIs)

The AIs for calcium recommended by the Food and Nutrition Board (Institute of Medicine, 1998) are based on estimates of requirements of both genders throughout the life cycle. The tolerable upper intake levels (ULs) have also been established for this nutrient for the first time. These DRIs are given in Table 5–2. During several periods of the female life cycle, calcium intake is critical, namely, prepuberty and adolescence, postmenopause, and during pregnancy and lactation. In a study of adolescent girls, calcium intakes of 1300 mg or more each day were necessary for maximal calcium retention by the body (skeleton) (Yates et al., 1998). Men also need adequate amounts of calcium throughout the life cycle, but less is known about their requirements.

Absorption, Transport, Storage, and Excretion

Calcium is absorbed by all parts of the small intestine, but the most rapid absorption after a meal occurs in the duodenum where an acid medium (pH < 7) prevails. Absorption is slower in the remainder of the small bowel because of the alkaline pH, but the amount of calcium absorbed is actually greater in the lower segments of the small intestine, including the ileum. Usually, only 30% (or slightly less) of ingested calcium is absorbed by adults, but in a few individuals, as little as 10% may be absorbed. Although rare, some hyperabsorbing adults can absorb as much as 60% of ingested calcium.

Calcium is absorbed by two mechanisms: *active transport,* which operates predominantly at low luminal concentrations of calcium ions, and *passive transfer* or paracellular movement, which operates at high luminal concentrations of calcium ions. The active transport mechanism, mainly in the duodenum and proximal jejunum, is saturable, and it is controlled through the action of 1,25-dihydroxyvitamin D ($1,25[OH]_2D_3$), or vitamin D. This hormone

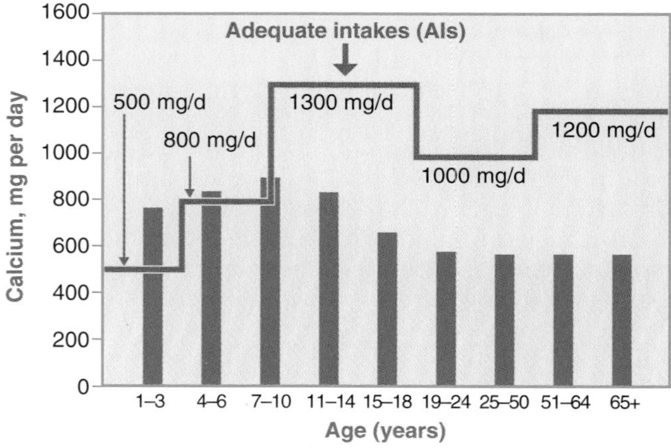

FIGURE 5–2 Median daily calcium intake for females in the United States compared to the adequate intakes established in 1998.

TABLE 5–2 DIETARY REFERENCE INTAKES FOR CALCIUM, PHOSPHORUS, MAGNESIUM, AND FLUORIDE

LIFE STAGE GROUP	CALCIUM (mg/day) AI	UL	PHOSPHORUS (mg/day) RDA	UL	MAGNESIUM (mg/day) RDA		UL[†]	FLUORIDE (mg/day) AI		UL
0–6 mo	210	ND	100*	ND	30*		ND		0.01	0.7
6–12 mo	270	ND	275*	ND	75*		ND		0.5	0.9
1–3 y	500	2500	460	3000	80		65		0.7	1.3
4–8 y	800	2500	500	3000	130		110		1.0	2.2
					Male	**Female**		**Male**	**Female**	
9–13 y	1300	2500	1250	4000	240	240	350	2.0	2.0	10
14–18 y	1300	2500	1250	4000	410	360	350	3.0	3.0	10
19–30 y	1000	2500	700	4000	400	310	350	4.0	3.0	10
31–50 y	1000	2500	700	4000	420	320	350	4.0	3.0	10
51–70 y	1200	2500	700	4000	420	320	350	4.0	3.0	10
> 70	1200	2500	700	3000	420	320	350	4.0	3.0	10
Pregnancy										
≤ 18 y	1300	2500	1250	3500		400	350		3.0	10
19–30 y	1000	2500	700	3500		350	350		3.0	10
31–50 y	1000	2500	700	3500		350	350		3.0	10
Lactation										
≤ 18 y	1300	2500	1250	4000		360	350		3.0	10
19–30 y	1000	2500	700	4000		310	350		3.0	10
31–50 y	1000	2500	700	4000		320	350		3.0	10

(Adapted from Institute of Medicine—National Academy of Sciences, Food and Nutrition Board. Dietary Reference Intakes: Recommended Levels for Individual Intake. The National Academy of Sciences, 1998.)

†, the UL for magnesium represents intake from a supplement or pharmacological agent only; not the intake from food and water.
ND, not determinable due to lack of data.
AI, adequate intake.
RDA, recommended dietary allowance.
UL, tolerable upper intake level.

increases calcium uptake at the brush border of the intestinal mucosal cell by an incompletely understood mechanism, and it also stimulates the production of calcium-binding proteins or **calbindins.** The second transfer mechanism, which is passive, nonsaturable, and independent of vitamin D, occurs along the entire length of the small intestine. When large amounts of calcium are consumed in a single meal, as from a dairy food or a supplement, much of the calcium that is absorbed occurs by this passive route. The active transport mechanism becomes much more important when calcium intakes are low and body requirements are not being met, that is, at levels typically well below recommended intakes at any stage of the life cycle.

The role of calbindins in the intestinal absorbing cells is to store calcium ions temporarily after a meal and to ferry them to the basolateral membrane for the final step of absorption. The calcium-binding proteins bind two or more calcium ions per protein molecule within the cytosol.

Most calcium is absorbed in the lower half of the small intestine, including the ileum, as shown by the devastating effect on calcium metabolism of surgical removal of the ileum (see Chapter 31). Calcium can also be absorbed in the colon, but only in small amounts.

Calcium is absorbed only if it is present in an ionic form. Calcium is not absorbed if it is precipitated by another dietary constituent, such as oxalate, or if it forms a soap with free fatty acids. These unabsorbed forms of calcium are excreted in the feces as calcium oxalates and calcium soaps.

A number of factors, both favorable and unfavorable, influence the bioavailability of calcium within the gut lumen, and hence, the absorption of calcium. In general, the greater the need and the smaller the dietary supply, the more efficient will be the absorption. Increased needs encountered in growth, pregnancy, lactation, and calcium deficiency, as well as levels of exercise resulting in high bone density, enhance calcium absorption.

As mentioned, vitamin D in its active hormonal form, $1,25(OH)_2D_3$, stimulates intestinal absorption through a complex series of steps, including transfer across the mucosal brush border to blood. Low vitamin D intakes or inadequate exposure to sunlight reduce calcium absorption, especially among the elderly (Gloth et al., 1995). An insufficient amount of vitamin D in its active form in blood reduces the absorption of calcium, if calcium is available in the diet. If dietary calcium intake is very low, however, an adequate circulating concentration of $1,25(OH)_2D_3$ may have little benefit in improving calcium status (Okonofua et al., 1991).

Calcium is best absorbed in an acid medium; thus, the hydrochloric acid secreted in the stomach favors calcium absorption by lowering the pH in the proximal duodenum. This also applies to calcium supplements. Taking calcium supplements with meals improves absorption, especially in the elderly (Heaney et al., 1989).

Lactose enhances calcium absorption in human infants. In adults, even those with lactose intolerance, lactose probably plays a role in absorption. The increased risk for osteoporosis in lactose intolerant individuals results from a low intake of calcium.

Oxalic acid in rhubarb, spinach, chard, and beet greens forms insoluble calcium oxalate in the digestive tract. For example, only 5% of the calcium in spinach is absorbed.

Phytic acid, a phosphorus-containing compound found principally in the outer husks of cereal grains, combines with calcium to form calcium phytate, which is also insoluble and cannot be absorbed.

Dietary fiber may decrease calcium absorption, but this may only be a problem in vegetarians who consume more than 30 g of fiber a day (Kelsey et al., 1979).

Medications can affect bioavailability or increase calcium excretion, both of which can contribute to bone loss.

Aging is characterized by a decreased efficiency of calcium absorption, probably due to achlorhydria and a blunted adaptive response of vitamin D to a decreased calcium intake (see Chapter 13).

In individuals with fat malabsorption, calcium absorption is decreased because of the formation of calcium–fatty acid soaps.

Calcium absorption does not appear to be affected by the amount of phosphate in the diet, unless phosphate is excessively high, or by the calcium: phosphorus ratio (see discussion on phosphorus).

RENAL EXCRETION

Normally, just over 50% of the ingested calcium is excreted in the urine each day, but an almost equivalent amount is also secreted into the intestine (and joins unabsorbed calcium in the feces). Calcium reabsorption from the renal tubules occurs by similar transport mechanisms as in the small intestine. Urinary calcium excretion varies throughout the life cycle, but it is typically low during periods of rapid skeletal growth. At menopause, calcium excretion is greatly increased, but in postmenopausal women treated with estrogen, less calcium is excreted. After approximately 65 years of age, calcium excretion declines, most likely because of decreased intestinal absorption of calcium. In general, urinary calcium correlates well with calcium intake.

A high urinary calcium excretion, that is, *protein-induced hypercalciuria,* has been reported to accompany a high-protein diet, especially from animal proteins, because of the generation of organic acids, like sulfate, from the sulfur-containing amino acids (Kerstetter and Allen, 1990). This hypercalciuric effect, however, has not been established in long-term studies of populations consuming diets high in meat. Consumption of large amounts of coffee, especially caffeinated coffee, may also increase urinary calcium losses. The presence of a high blood concentration of phosphate decreases renal calcium excretion.

SKIN LOSSES

Dermal losses occur in the form of sweat and exfoliation of the skin. The loss of calcium in sweat is about 15 mg/day. Strenuous physical activity with sweating will increase the loss, even in persons with a low calcium intake.

SERUM CALCIUM

Total serum calcium consists of three distinct fractions: free or ionized calcium (47.6%); complexes between calcium and anions, such as phosphate, citrate, or other organic anions (6.4%); and calcium that is protein-bound, primarily with albumin (46%). Serum albumin binds between 70% and 90% of the calcium that is protein-bound.

Ionized calcium (Ca^{++}), the regulated form, equilibrates rapidly with protein-bound calcium in blood. Serum ionized calcium concentration is controlled primarily by parathyroid hormone (PTH), the hormone secreted by the parathyroid glands, although other hormones have minor roles in its regulation. These other hormones include calcitonin, vitamin D, estrogens, and others (see the following section). Total serum calcium is maintained within a narrow range of 8.8 to 10.8 mg/dL, of which the ionized calcium concentrations range from 4.4 to 5.2 mg/dL. (Serum calcium values higher than the upper limit of normal are defined as hypercalcemic, whereas values below the lower limit are hypocalcemic; each abnormal status carries significant risk.) Serum levels of calcium are highest early in life, gradually declining throughout life, reaching the lowest levels during the elderly years (Anderson, 1991).

Several factors affect the relative distribution of calcium in blood serum or plasma. One of these is pH; the ionized fraction is increased in acidosis and decreased in alkalosis. Total calcium changes along with changes in plasma protein levels; however, the ionized fraction usually remains within normal limits. The strict regulation of ionized calcium makes it a useful diagnostic tool in assessing parathyroid gland function, monitoring kidney disease, and monitoring sick neonates for whom hypocalcemia could be life-threatening.

REGULATION OF SERUM CALCIUM

Calcium in bones is in equilibrium with calcium in the blood. PTH plays the major role in maintaining serum calcium at a normal concentration of about 10 mg/100 mL of blood serum (2.5 mmol/L). (The physiologic role of calcitonin in this regulation is not well established.) When the blood calcium concentration falls below this level, PTH stimulates the transfer of exchangeable calcium from the bone into the blood. At the same time, PTH promotes renal tubular resorption of calcium, and it indirectly stimulates increased intestinal absorption of calcium via the hormonal form of vitamin D-$1,25(OH)_2D_3$.

Other hormones, such as glucocorticoids, thyroid hormones, and sex hormones, also have important roles in calcium homeostasis. Glucocorticoids may impair calcium absorption via both active and passive mechanisms. Glucocorticoid excess leads to bone loss, particularly trabecular bone, a feature commonly found in patients receiving chronic glucocorticoid therapy at doses of 20 mg/day or higher. Thyroid hormones (T_4 and T_3) may stimulate bone resorption; chronic hyperthyroid conditions result in loss of both compact and trabecular bone.

In women, normal bone balance requires serum estrogen concentrations to be within normal limits. The rapid decline of serum estrogen concentration at menopause is a major factor contributing to bone resorption. Treating postmenopausal women with estrogen slows the rate of bone resorption (see Chapter 28). Bone resorption is also inhibited by testosterone.

Functions

Adequate dietary calcium is needed to permit optimal gains in bone mass and density in the prepubertal and adolescent years. These gains are especially critical for girls because the accumulated bone may provide additional protection against osteoporosis in the late years of life after menopause. Peak calcium retention by girls has been shown to occur in the prepubertal and early pubertal periods (Abrams and Stuff, 1994). Other studies also support the importance of obtaining sufficient calcium intakes by young girls for bone development (Jackman et al., 1997; Matkovic et al., 1995) (see Chapter 28).

Postmenopausal women need to obtain sufficient amounts of calcium to maintain bone health and to suppress PTH. The latter increases later in life in most individuals, perhaps as a result of inadequate calcium in the diet (see Chapters 28 and 13).

Additional amounts of calcium are recommended to meet the needs of pregnancy and lactation. Calcium requirements in pregnancy, infancy, childhood, and adolescence are discussed in detail in Chapters 7 through 11. In addition to its function in building and maintaining bones and teeth, calcium also has a number of metabolic roles in cells in all other tissues. Only small amounts of calcium, compared to the large needs of the skeleton, however, are required for all other cellular and extracellular functions.

The transport functions of cell membranes are influenced by calcium, which affects membrane stability in poorly understood ways. Calcium also influences the transmission of ions across membranes of cell organelles, the release of neurotransmitters at synaptic junctions, the function of protein hormones, and the release or activation of intracellular and extracellular enzymes.

Calcium is required for nerve transmission and regulation of heart muscle function. The proper balance of calcium, sodium, potassium, and magnesium ions maintains skeletal muscle tone and controls nerve irritability. A significant increase in serum calcium can cause cardiac or respiratory failure; a decrease results in **tetany** of skeletal muscles. In addition, calcium ions play a critical role in smooth muscle contractility.

Ionized calcium initiates the formation of a blood clot by stimulating the release of thromboplastin from blood platelets. Calcium ions also serve as required cofactors for several enzymatic reactions, including the conversion of prothrombin to thrombin, which aids in the polymerization of fibrinogen to fibrin and the final step in the formation of blood clots.

Deficiency

The development of peak bone mass requires adequate amounts of calcium as well as phosphorus, vitamin D, and other nutrients. Compared to adulthood, large amounts of calcium and phosphate are required for skeletal development; therefore, adequate intakes of these minerals and others exert significant impacts on peak bone mass development up to the time of puberty and through adolescence. After adolescence, bone gains may still occur, but the amounts of calcium required decline. Vitamin D status may or may not be a problem, depending on the intakes of calcium and phosphorus. Almost anytime during the life cycle when the calcium intake is well below the recommended amount, PTH concentrations in the blood increase. A persistent elevation may contribute to low bone mass (see the section on Phosphorus in this chapter and Chapter 28).

An inadequate intake of calcium, in addition to inadequate vitamin D, has also been demonstrated to contribute to osteomalacia (Marie et al., 1982) (see Chapters 4 and 28).

A low calcium intake may be an important factor in several chronic diseases, such as colon cancer (Chapter 39) and hypertension (Chapter 27), that commonly occur in Western societies.

Data from the Dietary Approaches to Stop Hypertension (DASH) show that adequate dietary intakes of calcium, magnesium, potassium, and other micronutrients from low-fat dairy foods, fruits, and vegetables can both substantially reduce blood pressure in those with hypertension and prevent the development of hypertension (Appel et al., 1997) (see Chapter 27). As a corollary to these studies, an analysis of intake patterns showed that low-calcium diets are also low in many other essential micronutrients needed for health (Barger-Lux et al., 1992).

PHYSICAL IMMOBILITY

Prolonged bed rest or periods of weightlessness during space travel promote significant calcium losses in response to a lack of tension or gravity on the bones. Older individuals with hip fractures or other illnesses who require prolonged recovery with limited activity also have increased calcium losses.

Toxicity

A very high intake of calcium (i.e., 2000 mg or more per day), especially in the presence of a high level of vitamin D, such as from excessive ingestion of combined supplements of calcium and vitamin D, is a potential cause of hypercalcemia. Such toxicity may lead to excessive calcification in soft tissues, especially the kidneys, which may be life-threatening. The tolerable upper intake levels (ULs) for calcium are shown in Table 5–2.

High intakes of calcium may also interfere with the absorption of other divalent cations, such as iron, zinc, and manganese (Argiratos and Samman, 1994; Copper deficiency . . . , 1985; Dawson-Hughes et al., 1986; Deehr et al., 1990; Hallberg et al., 1991; Wood and Zheng, 1997). Therefore, when a person needs to consume minerals as supplements, the iron supplement should be taken at a different time, that is, on an empty stomach if acceptable, whereas the calcium supplement should be taken with a meal. The same concerns have been expressed about the use of calcium supplements during pregnancy.

Other potential adverse effects of excessive calcium intakes, though not toxic effects per se, include constipation and the formation of renal stones. Constipation is common among elderly women who use calcium supplements, but the incidence of renal stones among users of calcium supplements is rare.

Phosphorus

Phosphorus, another essential element, ranks second to calcium in abundance in human tissues. About 80% is present in the skeleton and teeth as calcium phosphate crystals. The remaining 20% exists in the metabolically active pool in every cell in the body and in the extracellular fluid compartment. Serum inorganic phosphorus is closely maintained by PTH at levels of 3 to 4 mg/100 mL in adults, but it is not as closely regulated as serum calcium. Normal blood concentrations in infants are higher. Phosphorus balance is illustrated in Figure 5–3.

Most of the inorganic phosphate is present as $H_2PO_4^-$ and HPO_4^{--}. A small amount is bound to protein or complexed with calcium or magnesium. Almost 10% of the serum inorganic phosphorus is bound to protein.

Food Sources and Intakes

In general, good sources of protein are also good sources of phosphorus. Meat, poultry, fish, and eggs rank as excellent sources. Milk and milk products are good sources, as are nuts and legumes, cereals, and grains. However, in the outer coating of cereal grains, particularly wheat, phosphorus occurs in the form of phytic acid, which can complex with some minerals to form insoluble compounds. In conventional breads, phytic acid is converted to the soluble form of orthophosphate during the leavening process. However, in the unleavened breads commonly eaten in the Middle East, the availability of practically all minerals is reduced. Table 5–3 and Appendix 41 list the phosphorus content of selected foods.

The average intakes of phosphorus by adults in the United States are approximately 1300 mg/day for men and 1000 mg/day for women. Most phosphorus (about 60%) comes from milk, meat, poultry,

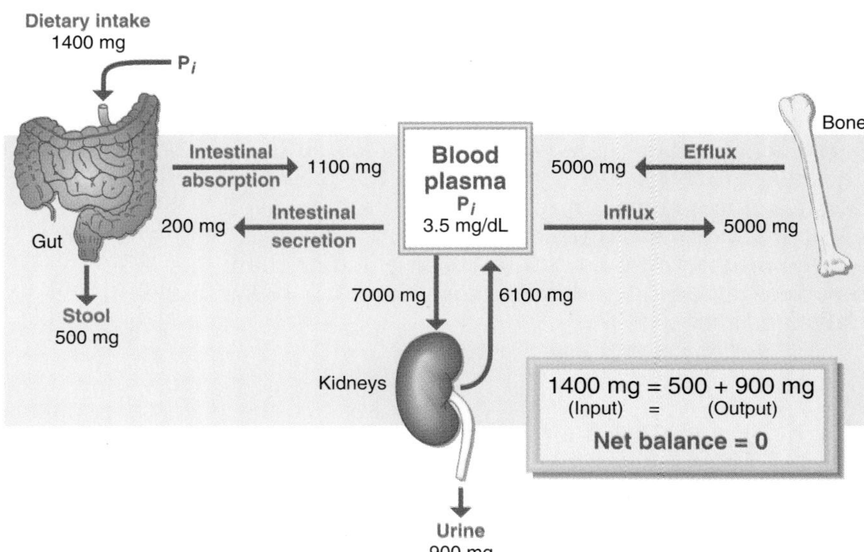

FIGURE 5–3 Phosphorus balance is maintained primarily by the amount of phosphate absorbed versus the amount excreted by the kidneys and intestine. Bone remains the major store of phosphate, as it does for calcium. The metabolic pathways have many similarities with those of calcium.

TABLE 5–3 PHOSPHORUS CONTENT OF SELECTED FOODS

FOOD	mg
Macaroni and cheese, 1 cup	322
Sole, baked, 3 oz.	248
Milk, 2% fat, 1 cup	232
Pizza, ⅛ of 15" diameter	216
Cheese, Swiss, processed, 1 oz	216
Split pea soup, 1 cup	213
Ham, 3 oz	210
Ice milk, soft-serve, 1 cup	202
Almonds, ¼ cup	184
Oatmeal, 1 cup	178
Lentils, cooked, ½ cup	178
Cheese, cottage, 2% fat, ½ cup	170
Cheese, cheddar, 1 oz	146
Yeast, brewer's, 1 T	140
Shrimp, boiled, 2 large	137
Baked beans (white), ½ cup	137
Ground beef, 3 oz	135
Tofu, regular, ½ cup	120
Potato, baked, with skin, 1	115
Garbanzo beans, canned, ½ cup	108
Egg, 1	86
Bread, whole-wheat, 1 slice	74
Peas, frozen, cooked, ½ cup	72
Cola beverage, 1 can (12 oz)	46
Potato chips, 14	43
Chocolate, dark, 1 oz	41
Bread, white, 1 slice	30
Lettuce, romaine, 1 cup	25
Cauliflower, fresh, ½ cup	23
Orange, 1	18

(From United States Department of Agriculture (USDA). Composition of Foods. USDA Handbook No. 8 Series. Washington, DC: ARS, USDA, 1976–1986.)

fish, and eggs. Another 20% is provided by cereals and legumes, and approximately 10% is derived from fruits and their juices. Other dietary sources, such as tea, coffee, and spices, supply approximately 3%. The estimated amount from food additives represents almost 10% (Calvo and Park, 1996).

The intakes of phosphorus in the United States are considerably higher than the 1998 recommended dietary allowances (RDAs), which have been reduced by the Food and Nutrition Board compared to the 1989 RDA values. A major shift in phosphorus intake has occurred over the past few decades since the widespread increase in the use of phosphate additives by the food industry; true phosphorus intakes may be 200 to 300 mg higher than reported intakes (Anderson and Barrett, 1994; Calvo and Park, 1996).

Dietary Reference Intakes

The Food and Nutrition Board in 1998 recommended DRIs for phosphorus that are somewhat lower than those for calcium for all age groups (see Table 5–2). Tolerable upper intake levels (ULs) were also established (Institute of Medicine, 1998).

Absorption, Transport, Storage, and Excretion

The relative amount of inorganic and organic phosphates in the diet varies with the type of phosphates consumed. Regardless of the form, most phosphates are absorbed in the inorganic state. Organically bound phosphate is hydrolyzed in the lumen of the intestine and released as inorganic phosphate, mainly through the action of alkaline phosphatase. Bioavailability depends on the form of the phosphate and the pH. The acidic milieu of the most proximal portion of the duodenum is important in maintaining phosphorus solubility and, therefore, bioavailability. In vegetarian diets, the major portion of the phosphorus occurs as phytate, which is poorly digested by humans. Humans do not have the enzyme phytase to cleave the phosphorus from the phytate; however, intestinal bacteria have the enzyme to hydrolyze some phosphate. The yeast used in making bread contains a phytase, which also releases some phosphate.

In general, the efficiency of absorption of phosphates approaches 60% in adults, almost twice as high as for calcium, and phosphate absorption is also much more rapid than that of calcium. For example, the peak of absorption of phosphates occurs approximately 1 hour after ingestion of a meal, whereas for calcium entry into the blood, the peak occurs 3 to 4 hours after a meal (Anderson, 1991).

RENAL AND INTESTINAL EXCRETION

The primary route of phosphorus excretion is renal. Major determinants of urinary phosphorus loss are an increased intake of phosphate, an increase in phosphate absorption, and the plasma phosphorus concentration. Other factors important in certain conditions are hyperparathyroidism, acute respiratory or metabolic acidosis, the intake of diuretics, and the expansion of extracellular volume. If PTH levels are high, additional phosphate is excreted by the urinary route. Reduced phosphate excretion is associated with dietary phosphorus restriction; increases in plasma insulin, thyroid hormone, growth hormone, or glucagon; metabolic or respiratory alkalosis; and extracellular volume contraction.

Regulation of urinary phosphate losses is not as precise as it is for calcium, but endogenous fecal phosphate excretion may be better regulated and serve as a way to eliminate some of the excessive phosphate when PTH levels are high. The latter route of excretion may be increased when the phosphate load in the blood and tissues is excessively high.

Functions

As phosphates, phosphorus participates in numerous essential functions of the body. DNA and RNA are based on phosphate. The major cellular form of energy, (adenosine triphosphate) (ATP), contains high-energy phosphate bonds, as does creatinine phosphate and phosphoenolpyruvate. Cyclic adenosine monophosphate (cAMP) acts as a secondary signal within cells following peptide hormone activation of many membrane receptors. As part of phospholipids, phosphorus is present in every cell membrane in the body. A number of phospholipid molecules also act as secondary messengers within the cytosol. Phosphorylation-dephosphorylation reactions control various steps in the activation or deactivation of cytosolic enzymes by kinases or phosphatases. Total intracellular concentrations of phosphate (but not ionic concentrations) are much higher than extracellular concentrations because phosphorylated compounds do not cross cell membranes easily and are trapped within the cell.

The *phosphate buffer system* is important in intracellular fluid and in the kidney tubules, where phosphate functions in the excretion of hydrogen ion. Filtered phosphate reacts with secreted hydrogen ions, releasing sodium in the process. The sodium, in turn, can be reabsorbed under the influence of aldosterone (see Chapter 6).

Finally, phosphates combine with calcium ions to form **hydroxyapatite,** the major inorganic molecule present in teeth and bones.

Deficiency

Phosphate deficiency is rare, but it could possibly develop in individuals who are taking drugs known as phosphate binders (see Chapter 38). The widespread and ultimately fatal consequences of severe phosphorus depletion reflect its ubiquitous role in body functions. Symptoms result primarily from decreased synthesis of ATP and other organic phosphate molecules. Neuromuscular, skeletal, hematologic, and renal abnormalities occur.

Because phosphorus is so widely available from foods, including processed foods, and soda type soft drinks, little likelihood of a dietary inadequacy exists. Clinical phosphate depletion and hypophosphatemia may result from long-term administration of glucose or TPN without sufficient phosphate, excessive use of phosphate-binding antacids, hyperparathyroidism, or treatment of diabetic acidosis, and it may occur in alcoholic patients with or without decompensated liver disease. Premature infants who are fed unfortified human milk may also develop hypophosphatemia.

Toxicity

A persistently elevated concentration of PTH may result because of the chronic consumption of a low calcium, high phosphorus diet. This condition has often previously been referred to as *nutritional secondary hyperparathyroidism*. In humans, the PTH levels in blood that result from a low Ca:P ratio typically remain within the normal range, but usually at the high end of the range. A persistently elevated PTH, even within the normal range, contributes to increased bone turnover that potentially can result in a reduction of bone mass and density (Calvo, et al., 1990). If this condition is chronic, it could contribute to fragility fractures because of excessive resorption and thinning of trabecular plates at bone sites throughout the skeleton. Individuals with a low Ca:P ratio would benefit from increasing their calcium intake from foods or supplements (Anderson, 1996). Adequate calcium intakes have been shown in several studies to reduce the serum PTH concentration, typically from the high end of the normal range to a lower level (Krall and Dawson-Hughes, 1994), but occasionally from a true hyperparathyroid level into the normal range. The mechanism by which a low dietary Ca:P ratio contributes to the development of a persistently elevated PTH concentration is illustrated in Figure 5–4. The persistently elevated PTH level contributes to both the limited bone mineralization during growth—that is, inadequate peak bone mass accumulation in adolescents and young adults—and the loss of bone mass in adults (Anderson, 1996).

Magnesium

Magnesium ranks second in content to potassium as an intracellular cation. The adult human body contains approximately 20 to 28 g, of which approximately 60% is found in bone, 26% in muscle, and the remainder in soft tissues and body fluids. Gen-

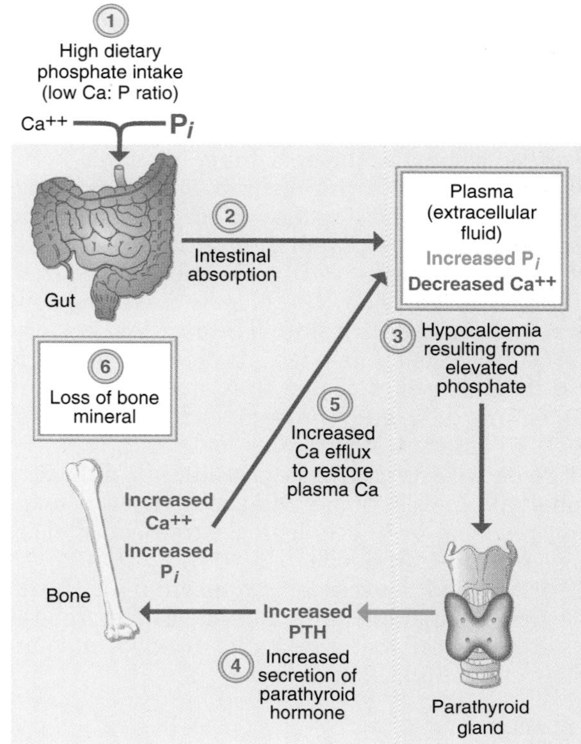

FIGURE 5–4 The mechanism through which a low dietary Ca:P ratio contributes to the development of a persistently elevated parathyroid hormone (PTH) concentration.

der differences in the body content of magnesium begin at prepuberty. Magnesium in bone is present in both exchangeable and nonexchangeable pools. Magnesium ions in the bone fluid compartment are much more exchangeable than magnesium ions that have become part of the crystal lattice. Normal serum levels are usually in the range of 1.5 to 2.1 mEq/L (0.75 to 1.1 mmol/L). About half the magnesium in plasma is free, approximately one third is bound to albumin, and the remainder is complexed with citrate, phosphate, or other anions.

Magnesium homeostasis is governed by intestinal absorption and renal excretion. No hormone is known to have a major role in the control of serum magnesium, although PTH has a minor role (Rude, 1998).

Food Sources and Intakes

Magnesium is abundant in many foods, and the ordinary diet should provide adequate amounts if the right foods are selected for consumption. Good sources are seeds, nuts, legumes, and unmilled cereal grains, as well as dark green vegetables, in which magnesium is an essential constituent of chlorophyll. Milk is a moderately good source of magnesium, especially because milk and other dairy products are so widely consumed; indeed, milk is the major contributor of magnesium (Pennington and Young, 1991). Fish, meat, and the most commonly eaten fruits (i.e., oranges, apples, and bananas) are poor sources of magnesium. Diets high in refined foods, meat, and dairy products are usually lower in magnesium than diets rich in vegetables and unrefined grains (Table 5–4). The mineral is lost during the refining of cereals, such as wheat flour and rice, and the processing of foods, such as sugar, and it is not added as part of the enrichment of cereals.

Figure 5–5 shows the median intakes of magnesium in males and females in the United States (Alaimo et al., 1994). Median intakes for both males and females subjects fall below the RDAs after 11 years of age; however, the elderly have the lowest intakes of any adult group. The low intakes of the elderly are consistent with studies of Norwegians older than 60 years of age that suggest subclinical magnesium deficiency among healthy elderly subjects (Gullestad et al., 1994).

High intakes of calcium, protein, vitamin D, and alcohol all increase the requirements for magnesium; physical or psychological stress may also increase magnesium needs.

The top food sources of magnesium in the U.S. diet (CSFII) include milk, bread, coffee, ready-to-eat cereals, beef, potatoes, and dried beans/lentils (Subar et al., 1998).

Dietary Reference Intakes

The RDAs for magnesium were increased in 1998 by the Food and Nutrition Board. For the first time, different recommendations were made for females and males beginning at puberty (see Table 5–2). ULs were also established as well as AIs for infants (Institute of Medicine, 1998).

TABLE 5–4 MAGNESIUM CONTENT OF SELECTED FOODS

FOOD	mg
Tofu, firm, ½ cup	118
Chili with beans, 1 cup	115
Wheat germ, toasted, ¼ cup	90
Cashews, roasted, ¼ cup	89
Halibut, baked, 3 oz	78
Swiss chard, cooked, ½ cup	75
Peanuts, roasted, ¼ cup	67
Chocolate chips, semisweet, ¼ cup	58
Baked potato with skin, 1	55
Cocoa powder, 2 T	52
Molasses, blackstrap, 1 T	52
Cereal, raisin bran, 1 oz	48
Spinach, fresh, 1 cup	44
Cheerios, 1 oz	39
Milk, 2% fat, 1 cup	33
Bread, whole-wheat, 1 slice	26
Chicken, breast, 3 oz	25
Green peas, frozen, cooked, ½ cup	23
Ground beef, lean, 3 oz	16
Fruits	10–25
Coffee, brewed, ¾ cup	9
Egg, 1	5

(From United States Department of Agriculture (USDA). Composition of Foods. USDA Handbook No. 8 Series. Washington, DC: ARS, USDA, 1976–1986.)

Absorption, Transport, Storage, and Excretion

The efficiency of absorption of magnesium varies widely, from 35% to 45%. Magnesium may be absorbed along the length of the small intestine, but most absorption occurs in the jejunum. As with other divalent cation minerals, the entry step of magnesium from the gut lumen occurs by two mechanisms: a carrier-facilitated process and simple diffusion. A saturable facilitated mechanism operates at low intraluminal concentrations, whereas paracellular movement across the mucosa predominates throughout the length of the small bowel when intraluminal concentrations are high. The efficiency of absorption varies with the magnesium status of the individual, the amount of magnesium in the diet, and the composition of the diet as a whole. Vitamin D has little or no effect on magnesium absorption.

No homeostatic system for serum magnesium regulation has been identified, but serum magnesium concentration is remarkably constant. Maintenance of these constant values depends on absorption, excretion, and transmembranous cation flux, rather than on hormonal regulation. Once in the cells, magnesium is bound mainly to protein and energy-rich phosphates. Magnesium balance is illustrated in Figure 5–6.

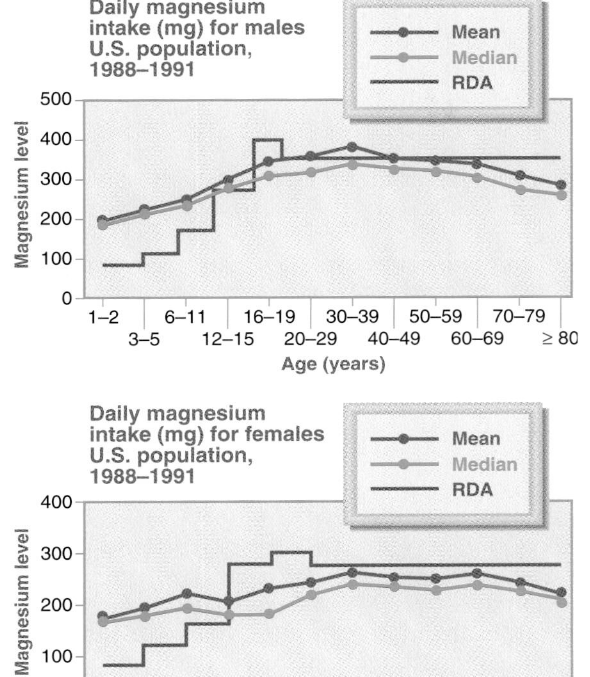

FIGURE 5–5 Median daily magnesium intake for males and females in the United States compared to the 1998 RDAs.

RENAL EXCRETION

The control of magnesium balance is governed primarily by the kidneys, which conserve magnesium efficiently, particularly when intake is low. Supplementing a normal intake increases urinary excretion, and the serum magnesium level remains normal. Diets low in magnesium reduce urinary excretion of magnesium. To meet the increased needs of lactating women, urinary excretion of magnesium tends to decrease (Dengel et al., 1994). Renal reabsorption varies inversely with that of calcium.

Functions

The major function of magnesium may be to stabilize the structure of ATP in ATP-dependent enzyme reactions. Magnesium is a cofactor for more than 300 enzymes involved in the metabolism of food components and in the synthesis of many products. Among the reactions requiring magnesium are the synthesis of fatty acids and proteins, phosphorylation of glucose and its derivatives in the glycolytic pathway, and transketolase reactions. Magnesium is important in the formation of cAMP, which was the first cytosolic "second messenger" to be identified as a mechanism for transmitting messages from outside the cells in response to either hormones, local hormone-like factors, or other molecules.

Magnesium plays a role in neuromuscular transmission and activity, working both in concert with and against the effects of calcium, depending on the system involved. In normal muscle contraction, calcium acts as a stimulator and magnesium acts as a relaxer. Magnesium acts as a physiologic calcium channel blocker, and it has been called "nature's blocker" (Iseri and French, 1994). The reactivity of vascular and other smooth muscle cells depends on the ratio of calcium to magnesium in blood. Large doses of magnesium can result in central nervous system (CNS) depression, anesthesia, and even paralysis, especially in patients with renal insufficiency. Thus, renal patients should not be given magnesium supplements. (See Chapter 38.)

Magnesium has been implicated in clinical problems that share an underlying pathophysiology of vasospasm and increased coagulation. Experimental studies have shown that low magnesium intakes affect the ratio of prostacyclin to thromboxane in

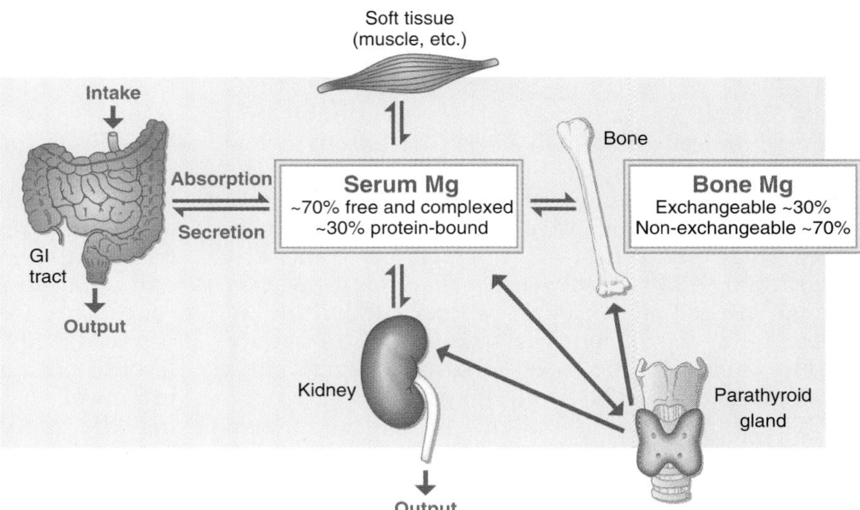

FIGURE 5–6 Magnesium balance is maintained largely by gastrointestinal (GI) absorption and renal excretion.

pregnancy-induced hypertension (see Chapter 7). The use of magnesium to inhibit atherogenesis or to prevent ischemic heart disease remains the subject of continuing study.

Deficiency

Although very rare, severe magnesium deficiency is manifested clinically by tremor, muscle spasm, personality changes, anorexia, nausea, and vomiting. Tetany, myoclonic jerks, athetoid movements, convulsions, and coma have also been reported in magnesium-deficient individuals. Hypocalcemia and hypokalemia typically occur early, together with impairment of the individual's responsiveness to PTH. Sodium retention may also occur.

The effects of severe magnesium depletion on bone metabolism include decreased PTH secretion by the parathyroid glands, very low concentrations of serum PTH, impaired responsiveness of bone and kidneys to PTH, decreased serum $1,25(OH)_2D_3$, vitamin D resistance, altered hydroxyapatite crystal formation, and impaired bone growth in the young or osteoporosis in the old (Rude, 1996). With continued depletion of magnesium, PTH concentrations decline even further. Intravenous administration of magnesium reverses the clinical signs and symptoms within a short time.

Moderate depletion of magnesium is apparently prevalent in elderly populations in Western nations (Gullestad et al., 1994). Such deficiencies are typically precipitated by chronic dietary intakes that are low in magnesium, especially in individuals who avoid dark green leafy vegetables, milk, and other goods sources of magnesium. Any other condition, such as an increased loss of magnesium, or a shift in electrolyte balance, especially a decline in potassium, will also trigger a moderate magnesium deficiency (Rude, 1998). Situations in which acute deficiencies may develop include renal disease, diuretic therapy, malabsorption, hyperthyroidism, pancreatitis, kwashiorkor, diabetes, parathyroid gland disorders, postsurgical stress, and vitamin D–resistant rickets.

Decreased magnesium status has been suggested as a factor contributing to the pathogenesis of several of the chronic diseases of Western nations (Shils, 1994). For example, both dysrhythmias and myocardial ischemia have been attributed to low magnesium intakes (Seelig and Heggtveit, 1974). Studies of magnesium use in patients with acute myocardial infarction (MI) suggest a reduced mortality with rapid post-MI magnesium treatment (Orlov et al., 1994). Moreover, oral supplementation in middle-aged and elderly women with mild to moderate hypertension has been found to reduce systolic and diastolic blood pressure significantly (Witteman et al., 1994). (See Chapter 27.)

Magnesium status is difficult to determine from serum measurements of magnesium because total serum magnesium remains constant over a wide range of intake levels. Leukocyte magnesium contents are much more sensitive to nutritional status, which makes them a superior marker. Urinary excretion of magnesium (and often, potassium) is less in magnesium-deficient individuals than in magnesium-replete subjects treated with magnesium, suggesting greater retention of magnesium and improved tissue magnesium status throughout the body in magnesium deficient individuals. Attention has been focused on the interrelationships of magnesium and other electrolytes, particularly potassium, and the effects of these interrelationships on the development of various tissue abnormalities. For example, low magnesium intake is now also considered to be a potential risk factor for hypertension, along with inadequate intakes of potassium, calcium, and other micronutrients (Appel et al., 1997).

Magnesium deficits may also be a factor in osteoporosis, although the mechanism has not been established. Researchers in Israel, who administered magnesium supplements for 2 years to postmenopausal women with established osteoporosis, demonstrated improved trabecular, but not cortical, bone mass (Stendig-Lindenberg et al., 1993). Further research on the linkage between magnesium and bone in postmenopausal women is needed.

Toxicity

Although excess magnesium can inhibit bone calcification, magnesium excesses from dietary sources, including supplements, are very unlikely to result in toxicity. However, ULs for magnesium from supplements or pharmacological agents were established for the first time in 1998. (See Table 5–2.) The only cases of toxicity have been reported in smelter workers who inhale or otherwise ingest so much magnesium dust that the body takes on a toxic load.

Sodium, Potassium, and Chloride

Three indispensable dietary constituents—sodium, potassium, and chloride—commonly known as the electrolytes, are related in the body. Sodium constitutes 2%, potassium 5%, and chloride 3% of the total mineral content of the body. These elements, which exist as ions in body fluids, are distributed throughout all body fluids (extracellular and intracellular). Sodium and chloride exist primarily in extracellular fluids, whereas potassium is mainly an intracellular element. These electrolytes are involved in maintaining at least four important physiologic functions of the body: water balance and distribution; osmotic equilibrium; acid–base balance; and intracellular/extracellular differentials in their concentrations, a result of functioning (living) membranes (see Chapter 6). The last role is responsible for the electrical potential gradients across membranes of all cells with nerve and muscle cells having the highest gradients. The Na/K/Ca/ATPase "pump" system is important in volume regulation, maintenance of membrane potential, and in the transport across membranes of sugars, amino acids, and other molecules.

All three elements are readily absorbed by the small intestine and are excreted primarily via the urine. Fecal and sweat losses are the other routes of elimination. Because these minerals are widely available in the diet, deficiencies do not usually occur in healthy individuals. Potassium, however, is underconsumed by large numbers of Americans, perhaps as many as 50% of adults. The reason for the poor potassium intakes is simply too little consumption of fruits and vegetables. Excessive consumption of sodium is common, and it contributes to the development of hypertension in a large percentage of the U.S. population.

Intakes and Sources

According to the National Health and Nutrition Examination Survey (NHANES) III, Phase 1 (1988–1991), median sodium intakes of individuals aged 20 years of age and older ranged from a low of 2172 mg for women 80 years and older to a high of 4126 mg for men 20 to 29 years of age (Alaimo et al., 1994). The electrolytes are discussed in detail in Chapter 6.

Major food sources of sodium in the U.S. diet (USDA, 1994) include foods to which salt is added during preparation or processing—cheese, ham, tomatoes, milk, salad dressings and mayonnaise, beef, ready-to-eat cereals, cakes, cookies, quick breads, and doughnuts (Subar et al., 1998).

The foods providing the highest levels of potassium in the U.S. diet (USDA, 1994) include milk, potatoes, beef, coffee, tomatoes, orange and grapefruit juice, and poultry (Subar et al., 1998). The Total Diet Study (Pennington and Young, 1991) also identified dairy food products as a primary source of potassium. See Appendix 41 for the sodium and potassium contents of various foods.

Recommended Intakes

Estimated minimal intakes for the electrolytes are included in the 1989 RDAs established by the Food and Nutrition Board (1989). Mean sodium intakes for adults should not exceed the maximum recommendation of 2400 mg/day. The Food and Nutrition Board has not released any new guidelines for these elements in their 1998 publications.

Deficiency

The major deficit in consumption of electrolytes involves potassium. This is because so many people avoid fruits and vegetables, which provide a good proportion of total potassium intake in healthy eaters. Insufficient intakes of potassium have been linked to both hypertension (Appel et al., 1997) and osteoporosis (New et al., 1997; Tucker et al., 1998) (see Chapters 27 and 28).

Toxicity

Excessive intakes of sodium, but not potassium, may contribute to the pathogenesis of several chronic diseases, including hypertension and osteoporosis, but by different mechanisms. High sodium intakes increase urinary calcium excretion because the kidneys reabsorb sodium preferentially over calcium. An increased loss of calcium secondary to high sodium intakes has been reported in both young girls (Matkovic et al., 1995) and postmenopausal women (Devine et al., 1995). Urinary sodium and calcium are negatively correlated (Nordin et al., 1993). In perimenopausal women, the restriction of salt reduces both sodium and calcium excretion; it may, thereby, improve calcium retention in the skeleton.

Sulfur

Sulfur occurs in the body as a constituent of three amino acids—cystine, cysteine, and methionine—and of many other organic molecules. As such, it is present in all cells and in extracelluar compartments, such as connective tissue. The tertiary structure of proteins is attributable, in part, to covalent bonding between cysteine residues where the -SH groups are oxidized to form disulfide (-S-S-) bridges. These bridges also provide the three-dimensional structural modifications necessary for the activity of some enzymes, insulin, and other proteins. Sulfhydryl groups of proteins also participate in diverse cellular reactions. For example, the poisonous effects of arsenic are due to its ability to bind sulfhydryl groups of enzymes. The sulfur of cysteine binds to iron-sulfur clusters that are present in electron transfer proteins involved in basic, life-sustaining processes, such as photosynthesis, nitrogen fixation, and oxidative phosphorylation.

Glutathione, a tripeptide-containing cysteine, acts as a donor of reducing equivalents for the reduction of hydrogen peroxide and organic peroxides by **glutathione peroxidase.** Sulfur may, therefore, be considered among the nutrients that serve as antioxidants.

Sulfur occurs as a component of heparin, an anticoagulant found in liver and some other tissues, and as chondroitin sulfate in bone and cartilage. Sulfur is also an essential component of three vitamins—thiamin, biotin, and pantothenic acid. Other important molecules, such as S-adenosyl methionine, also contain this element.

Excess inorganic sulfur is excreted in the urine as sulfates. The metabolism of sulfur-containing amino acids generates inorganic acids, especially sulfate anions in substantial amounts. The sulfates are thought to combine with calcium ions in the glomerular ultrafiltrate, thereby reducing the renal tubular reabsorption of calcium. This mechanism may explain as much as 50% of the calcium loss associated with protein-induced hypercalciuria, which is observed following consumption of meals rich in animal proteins.

Food sources of sulfur include meat, poultry, fish, eggs, dried beans, broccoli, and cauliflower.

In summary, according to established recommended intakes, calcium, magnesium, and potassium are underconsumed by a large percentage of the U.S. population. Indeed, all of the surveys conducted thus far have identified these nutrients as being consistently underconsumed by Americans. By contrast, the sodium and phosphorus (phosphate) intakes of large segments of the population have been found to exceed the recommended intake. The increasing use of mineral supplements has apparently not yet had a major impact in improving the intakes of calcium and magnesium.

MICROMINERALS (TRACE ELEMENTS)

A number of elements that are present in minute amounts in body tissues are essential to optimal growth, health, and development. **Microminerals** or **trace elements** are defined as those demonstrated, through appropriately designed and corroborated experiments, to be required for optimal performance of a particular function. Classically, each element exhibits a spectrum of action that depends on the element's dosage and the nutritional state of the recipient with respect to the element.

In the past, deficiency of a nutrient could easily be identified and defined. Increasing amounts of a nutrient evoked an increasing biologic response until a plateau was reached beyond which larger intakes could produce pharmacologic effects and, eventually, toxicity.

The spectrum of effects produced by trace element deficiencies is more subtle and difficult to identify today, in part because many of these effects occur at the cellular or subcellular level. For example, iron deficiency eventually results in a type of anemia that is easy to identify. Cellular effects cannot be identified as easily, but may actually be more harmful to the individual (see Chapter 35). Recent reports have indicated that a benign strain of virus became virulent while residing in a selenium-deficient host (Beck et al., 1994, 1995). This finding, discussed in greater detail in the section on selenium, illustrates the fact that current theories and knowledge about adequacy and deficiency are different from those of 10 years ago, and that the understanding of the various functions of trace and ultratrace minerals must continually be updated.

RDAs have been established for only four trace elements: iron, iodine, selenium, and zinc (Table 5–5). Ranges of estimated safe and adequate daily dietary intakes (ESADDIs) for four other trace elements—copper, manganese, chromium, and molybdenum—are presented in Table 5–6. Most recently, AIs and ULs have been designated for fluoride (see

TABLE 5–5 RDAs OF TRACE ELEMENTS ACROSS THE LIFE CYCLE

GROUP	AGE (yr)	IRON (mg/day)	ZINC (mg/day)	IODINE (μg/day)	SELENIUM (μg/day)
Infants	0.5–0.5	6	5	40	10
	0.5–1.0	10	5	50	15
Children	1–3	10	10	70	20
	4–6	10	10	90	20
	7–10	10	10	120	30
Males	11–14	12	15	150	40
	15–18	12	15	150	50
	19–24	10	15	150	70
	25–50	10	15	150	70
	51+	10	15	150	70
Females	11–14	15	12	150	45
	15–18	15	12	150	50
	19–24	15	12	150	55
	25–50	15	12	150	55
	51+	10	12	150	55
Pregnant		30	15	175	65
Lactating					
	1st 6 mo	15	19	200	75
	2nd 6 mo	15	16	200	75

(From Food and Nutrition Board, National Academy of Sciences—National Research Council. Recommended Dietary Allowances, 10th ed. Washington, DC: National Academy Press, 1989 [abridged].)

TABLE 5–6 ESADDIs FOR TRACE ELEMENTS ACROSS THE LIFE CYCLE

TRACE ELEMENT	GROUP	AGE (yr)	ESSADDI (μg)
Chromium			
	Infants	0–0.5	10–40
		0.5–1	20–60
	Children and Adolescents	1–3	20–80
		4–6	30–120
		7–10	50–200
		11+	50–200
	Adults		50–200
Copper			
	Infants	0–0.5	0.4–0.6
		0.5–1	0.6–0.7
	Children and Adolescents	1–3	0.7–1.0
		4–6	1.0–1.5
		7–10	1.0–2.0
		11+	1.5–2.5
	Adults		1.5–3.0
Manganese			
	Infants	0–0.5	0.3–0.6
		0.5–1	0.6–1.0
	Children and Adolescents	1–3	1.0–1.5
		4–6	1.5–2.0
		7–10	2.0–3.0
		11+	2.0–5.0
	Adults		2.0–5.0
Molybdenum			
	Infants	0–0.5	15–30
		0.5–1	20–40
	Children and Adolescents	1–3	25–50
		4–6	30–75
		7–10	50–150
		11+	75–250
	Adults		75–250

(Reprinted with permission from Food and Nutrition Board, National Academy of Sciences. Recommended dietary allowances, 10th ed. Washington, DC: National Academy Press, 1989.)

Table 5–2). Appropriate ranges for the remaining trace minerals cannot be established on the basis of present knowledge.

General Characteristics

Trace elements exist typically in two forms: as charged ions, or bound to proteins or complexed in molecules, such as metalloenzymes. Each element has different chemical properties that become critical in its functional role in cells or extracellular compartments. In blood and other tissue and cellular fluids, the trace elements do not exist in the free ionic state; rather, they are typically bound to transporting or holding proteins. In the case of fluoride ions, they become bound in the hydroxyapatite crystals of bones and teeth.

Food Sources

Compared to other sources, foods of animal origin are generally superior sources of trace elements because concentrations tend to be higher and the metals more available for absorption. Seafoods, in particular, are usually rich in nearly all micronutrients. One exception to the rule is manganese, which is readily available from plant sources. Trace elements are not distributed evenly in the wheat grain. The germ and outer layers that contain the most minerals are removed, to a large extent, by the milling process. The minerals that remain in white flour, however, are more readily available than some of those in whole-wheat flour, which are firmly complexed by molecules, such as phytate and fiber.

Functions

Many enzymes require small amounts of one or more trace metals for full activity. Metals function in enzyme systems by (1) direct participation in catalysis; (2) combination with substrate to form a complex on which the enzyme acts; (3) formation of a metalloenzyme that binds substrates; (4) combination with a reaction end product; or (5) maintenance of quaternary structure.

Minute concentrations of trace minerals affect the whole body through interaction with the enzymes or hormones that regulate masses of substrate. This ability is amplified if, in turn, the substrate has some regulatory function. Trace minerals may also interact with DNA to control the transcription of proteins important to the metabolism of that particular trace mineral.

Iron

Iron has been recognized as an essential nutrient for more than a century. Nutritional iron deficiency and iron deficiency anemia remain far too common in the year 2000, given the wide availability of iron-rich foods (see Chapter 35). Indeed, iron deficiency anemia is the world's most common nutritional deficiency disease. Many advances have been made in the study of iron metabolism and iron deficiency, but questions about the mechanisms regulating the intestinal absorption of iron and iron balance still persist.

The adult human body contains iron in two major pools: (1) functional iron in hemoglobin, myoglobin, and enzymes; and (2) storage iron in ferritin, hemosiderin, and **transferrin,** (a transport protein in blood (Fig. 5–7). Healthy adult men have about 3.6 g total body iron whereas the value in women is about 2.4 g. Table 5–7 lists the relative proportions of iron in the major pools in men and women. Adult women have much lower amounts of iron in storage than do men. Iron is highly conserved by the body; approximately 90% is recovered and reused every day. The rest is excreted, mainly in the bile. Dietary iron must be available to maintain iron balance—to meet this 10% gap—or else iron deficiency will result.

Two concerns about iron nutritional status predominate: the incidence of iron deficiency anemia and the role of excessive iron intakes in coronary heart disease and cancer. Because of food fortification and the use of iron supplements by so many individuals, high iron intakes by men and postmenopausal women may be contributing to the risk of these chronic diseases.

Food Sources and Intake

By far, the best source of dietary iron is liver, followed by oysters, seafoods, kidney, heart, lean meat, poultry, and fish. Dried beans and vegetables are the best plant sources. Some other foods that provide iron are egg yolks, dried fruits, dark molasses, whole-grain and enriched breads, wines, and cereals. Milk and milk products are practically devoid of iron. Corn is a notoriously poor source of iron, so it is not surprising that cultures consuming diets based primarily on corn have been found to have high rates of anemia. Iron skillets, and even

TABLE 5–7 RELATIVE PROPORTIONS OF IRON IN YOUNG, HEALTHY, ADULTS

	MEN		WOMEN	
IRON CONTENT	**mg**	**%**	**mg**	**%**
Functional				
Hemoglobin	2300	64	1700	73
Myoglobin	320	9	180	8
Heme enzymes	80	2	60	3
Nonheme enzymes	100	3	80	3+
Storage				
Ferritin	540	15	200	9
Hemosiderin	230	6	100	4
Transferrin	5	<1	4	<1
TOTAL	3575		2314	

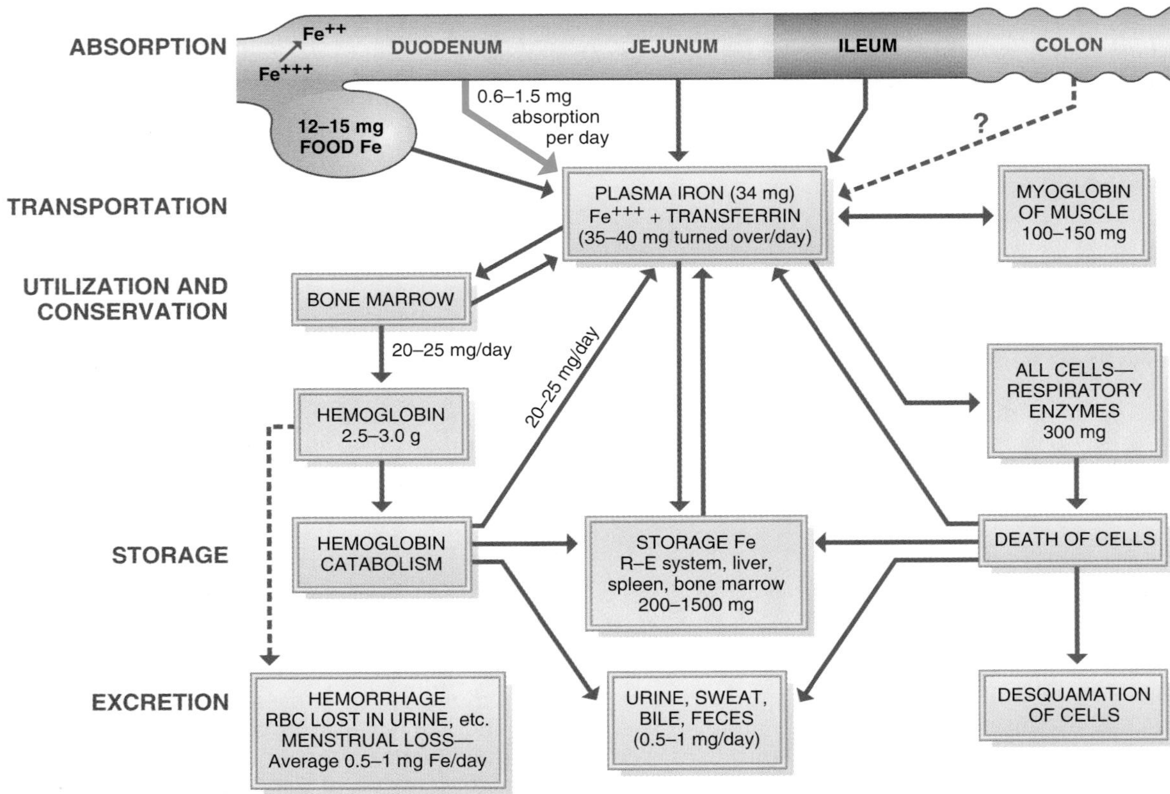

FIGURE 5–7 Schematic diagram of iron metabolism in adults. Most iron is absorbed from the duodenum and jejunum, after which it is transported as plasma iron or bound to transferrin. *R-E system*, reticuloendothelial system.

stainless steel pans, when used for cooking, add to the total iron intake.

The median iron intakes of most women are lower than the RDA, whereas the median intakes of men generally exceed the RDA, as reported in Phase I of NHANES III (Alaimo et al., 1994). An adequate diet containing meats and other animal sources typically has a high iron density, containing approximately 6 mg of iron per 1000 kcal. The average omnivorous woman consuming 2000 kcal, therefore, consumes 12 mg of iron, or approximately 80% of the RDA of 15 mg/day. This intake level appears to meet the needs of 86% of menstruating women. However, iron intakes totaling much less than 12 mg/day place women at risk—first for iron deficiency, and, then for iron deficiency anemia. However, iron consumption that meets the RDA of 15 mg/day should be sufficient to meet the needs of virtually all menstruating women. Women with high daily iron losses compensate with an increased rate of absorption, but even with this adaptation, insufficient stores of iron may exist.

The availability of iron derived from food is important in the consideration of dietary sources. For example, only 50% or less of the iron in whole-grain cereals and in some green vegetables is available in utilizable form. Table 5–8 and Appendix 41 present the iron content of selected foods. Vegetarian (vegan) women can obtain enough iron from their diet, but they must consume sufficient amounts of moderately iron-rich foods, such as legumes and dried fruits. Soy products are typically good sources of iron, as well as zinc.

Iron fortification of cereals, flours, and bread has added significantly to the total iron intake of the U.S. population. Fortified cereals have become a substantial source of iron for infants and children, as well as for adolescents and adults.

The foods that supply the greatest amount of iron in the U.S. diet (USDA, 1994) include ready-to-eat cereals fortified with iron; bread, cakes, cookies, doughnuts, and pasta (all fortified with iron); beef; dried beans/lentils; and poultry (Subar et al., 1998). Grain sources were also found to be primary foods providing iron in the Total Diet Study of the Food and Drug Administration (FDA) (Pennington and Young, 1991).

Recommended Dietary Allowance

The dietary allowances for iron established by the Food and Nutrition Board in 1989 remain the same. The RDA for iron is 10 mg for men and postmenopausal women and 15 mg for women of childbearing age (to replace the losses of menstruation and to provide for iron stores sufficient to support a pregnancy). The RDA for female adolescents is also set at 15 mg/day to provide for the iron needs of growth. For teenaged boys the RDA is 12 mg/day (see Table 5–5).

Full-term infants are born with a reserve supply of iron via placental transfer during fetal life. The RDA for a normal term infant is based on an average daily requirement of 1.5 mg/kg body weight during the first year of life (Taylor et al., 1988). The RDA is set at 10 mg/day beyond the first year of life, and it continues at that level until adolescence. Premature infants have limited iron stores because most of the iron and other trace minerals that are normally transferred during the last trimester of pregnancy are lacking. The need for iron to support rapid growth in premature infants becomes apparent at approximately 2 to 3 months of age (see Chapter 9).

Figure 5–8 shows the physiologic requirements of iron in relation to age. Requirements are highest during infancy and adolescence. Iron needs among males decrease after the adolescent growth spurt, whereas the iron needs of their female counterparts continue to be high until the menopausal transition. Iron allowances do increase during pregnancy (from 15 to 30 mg per day) but not during lactation, although supplements are frequently recommended by physicians for pregnant and lactating women.

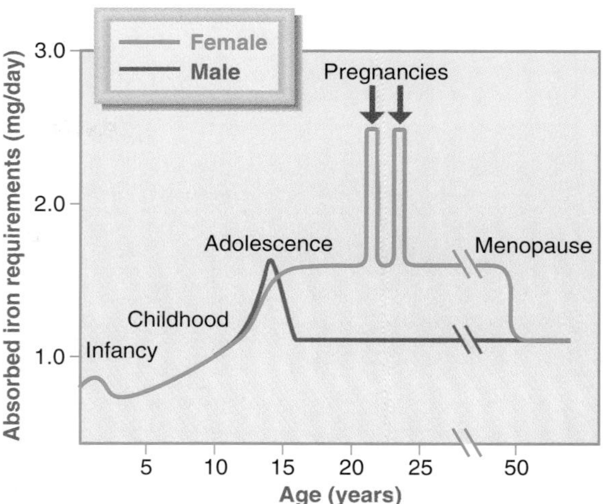

FIGURE 5–8 The absorbed iron requirement in males and females of various ages. The greatest requirements in relation to food intake occur during infancy. During childhood, requirements are the same for both sexes. During the adolescent growth spurt, there is an increase in iron needs, which is greater in male than in female adolescents. Because of menstruation, however, the requirement in women remains high, whereas in men, the requirement decreases after adolescence.

TABLE 5–8 IRON CONTENT OF SELECTED FOODS

FOOD	mg
Cereal, ready-to-eat, fortified, 1 cup	1–16
Clams, canned, ¼ cup	11.2
Beef liver, fried, 3 oz	5.3
Braunschweiger, 2 oz	5.3
Baked beans, 1 cup	5.0
Molasses, blackstrap, 1 T	5.0
Oysters, cooked, 1 oz	3.8
Venison, roasted, 3 oz	3.8
Baked potato, w/skin, 1	2.8
Soup, lentil and ham, 1 cup	2.6
Wheat germ, toasted, ¼ cup	2.5
Burrito, bean, 1	2.5
Soup, beef noodle, 1 cup	2.4
Rice, white, enriched, 1 cup	2.3
Spaghetti w/tomato sauce, 1 cup	2.3
Poptart, fortified, 1	2.2
Ground beef, lean, 3 oz	1.8
Apricots, dried halves, 10	1.7
Oatmeal, unfortified, 1 cup	1.6
Spinach, fresh, 1 cup	1.5
Cocoa powder, 2 T	1.5
Peas, frozen, cooked, ½ cup	1.3
Bread, whole-wheat, 1 slice	1.2
Chicken, breast, roasted, 1	0.9
Peanuts, dry roasted, ¼ cup	0.8
Pork chop, broiled, 1	0.7
Broccoli, fresh, cooked, ½ cup	0.7
Egg, 1	0.7
Blueberries, frozen, ½ cup	0.5
Wine, red, ½ cup	0.5
Raspberries, fresh, ½ cup	0.4
Cheese, cheddar, 1 oz	0.2
Milk, 2% fat, 1 cup	0.1

(From United States Department of Agriculture (USDA). Composition of Foods. USDA Handbook No. 8 Series. Washington, DC: ARS, USDA, 1976–1986.)

Absorption, Transport, Storage, and Excretion

Dietary iron exists in two chemical forms: **heme iron,** found in hemoglobin, myoglobin, and some enzymes; and **nonheme iron,** found predominantly in plant foods, but also in some animal foods, as in nonheme enzymes and ferritin. Heme iron (i.e., the intact ferroporphyrin ring) is absorbed across the brush border (mucosa) of intestinal absorbing cells (enterocytes) after it is digested from animal sources. Once heme enters the cytosol, the ferrous iron is enzymatically removed from the ferroporphyrin complex. The free iron ions combine immediately with *apoferritin* to form ferritin in the same way that free nonheme iron combines with apoferritin. **Ferritin** serves as both an intracellular store and a ferry that carries bound iron from the brush border to the basolateral membrane of the absorbing cell. The final step of absorption occurs at the basolateral membrane of the absorbing cell, the same as for nonheme iron, by an active transport mechanism by which iron ions are moved into the blood. A diagram of these steps is presented in Figure 5–9. The absorption of heme iron is affected only minimally by the composition of meals and gastrointestinal secretions. Heme iron represents only 5% to 10% of the dietary iron of individuals who consume a mixed diet, but absorption may be as high as 25%, compared with only 5% or so, for nonheme iron. Because vegans consume only plant

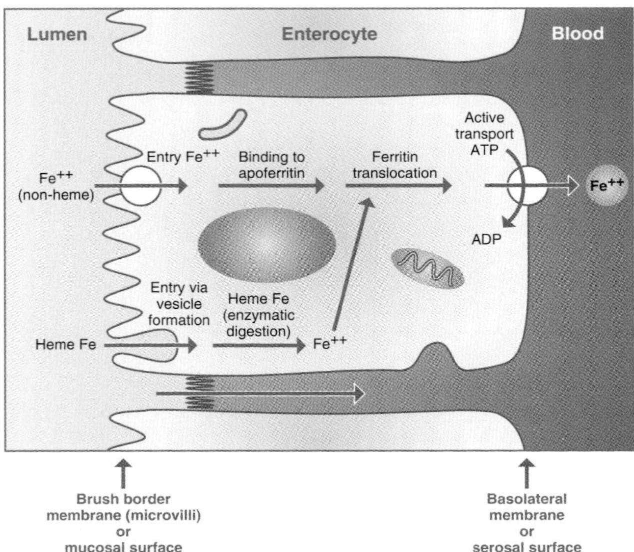

FIGURE 5–9 Schematic diagram of the intestinal absorption of iron from both heme and nonheme sources by an intestinal absorbing cell or enterocyte. Enterocytes contain two membranes—the brush border membrane and the basolateral membrane—as illustrated. The entry step of nonheme iron at the brush border membrane is different from that of heme iron. Heme iron enters by vesicle formation around the heme, whereas nonheme iron (ionic iron) enters by facilitated diffusion down a concentration gradient. Absorbed ions combine with apoferritin to form ferritin complexes that move across the cell by diffusion to the basolateral membrane for the exit step of absorption by active transport. The iron of heme iron is enzymatically removed and these ions exit at the basolateral membrane by an unknown mechanism. *ATP,* adenosine triphosphate; *ADP,* adenosine diphosphate.

foods, sufficient amounts of nonheme iron must be ingested and absorbed to meet body requirements.

Three steps of absorption also precede the entry of nonheme iron into the blood circulation (see Fig. 5–9). Nonheme iron must be digested free from plant sources and enter the duodenum and upper jejunum in a soluble (and ionized) form if it is to be transferred across the brush border (mucosa), the first step of absorption. The acid of gastric secretions enhances both the solubility and the change of iron to the ionic state—either as ferric (+3 oxidation state) or ferrous (+2 oxidation state) iron—within the gut luminal contents. Iron in the reduced or ferrous state is preferred for the entry step of absorption, but some ferric iron is also transferred across the brush border. Iron absorption is enhanced by the co-ingestion of vitamin C because ascorbic acid reduces ferric to ferrous iron, and it also binds or chelates the ferrous form, which allows the two entities to be absorbed together at the brush border (see below). Other food molecules, such as sugars and sulfur-containing amino acids, may also enhance iron entry by forming chelates with ionic iron. As chyme moves down the duodenum, the addition of pancreatic and duodenal secretions increases the pH of the contents to 7, at which point most ferric iron is precipitated unless it has been chelated. Ferrous iron, however, is significantly more soluble at a pH of 7, so these ions remain available for absorption in the remainder of the small intestine.

The efficiency of nonheme (but not heme) iron absorption appears to be controlled by the intestinal mucosa, which allows amounts of iron to enter the blood from the cytosolic ferritin pool according to the body's needs. The signal from the body to the absorbing cells may be *transferrin saturation,* that is, the percentage of iron bound to transferrin (see Fig. 5–9). Normally, transferrin saturation is 30% to 35% in healthy, iron-consuming individuals. The percentage can vary greatly, depending on both iron intake and bioavailability.

A low percentage, say 15%, of the *total iron-binding capacity* (TIBC) of transferrin would stimulate the absorbing cells to transport iron by the exit step at the basolateral membrane to the blood. Some researchers suggest that the amount of transferrin receptors on the basolateral membranes of the absorbing cells can be increased (i.e., upregulated) to permit more transport of iron to awaiting transferrin molecules, each of which has the capacity to bind two iron ions (atoms). At low saturation, increased numbers of vacancies are available on the transferrin molecules to take up iron and carry it to the bone marrow and other tissues to meet their needs. Conversely, if iron status in the body is excessive, TIBC may approach 40% to 50%, in which case the absorbing cells would be downregulated by this signal, and less iron would be allowed to be absorbed. The latter situation operates during iron overload to protect against toxicity.

The life span of the intestinal absorbing cells is approximately 5 to 6 days. During this time, they emerge from the crypts after cell division, pass up the villi to the tips, and eventually slough off as dead cells. It is during the life of the individual cell, signaled by the percent saturation of transferrin in the crypt or shortly thereafter, that the number of receptors for transferrin is set. Other cells formed before or after may have different numbers of receptors, depending on the nutritional supply of iron. In individuals with chronic underconsumption of iron, especially women in the childbearing years, the number of receptors may chronically be upregulated to maximize the efficiency of absorption of iron.

The efficiency of iron absorption (from gut lumen to blood) by adults with normal hemoglobin values averages between 5% to 15% of the iron (heme and nonheme combined) contained in food and supplements. Although absorption may be as high as 50% in those with iron deficiency anemia, this level of absorption is not common. Most women with iron deficiency, but not anemia, probably have absorption efficiencies of 20% to 30%. From 2% to 10% of nonheme iron in vegetables is absorbed, and from 10% to 30% of iron (both heme and nonheme) in animal sources is typically absorbed.

Several factors affect the intestinal absorption of iron, especially nonheme iron. The efficiency of iron absorption is determined, to some extent, by the foods from which it is derived. Some foods contain enhancing substances, such as ascorbic acid and the so-called meat factor explained in the next paragraph. Other foods contain complexing agents, such as phytates and oxalates, that inhibit absorption. Ascorbic acid, the most potent enhancer of iron absorption, forms a chelate with iron that remains soluble at the alkaline pH of the lower small intestine. Ascorbic acid enhances nonheme iron absorption especially well in women with low iron intakes (Hunt et al., 1994).

Animal proteins from beef, pork, veal, lamb, liver, fish, and chicken enhance absorption. The substance responsible for this improved absorption—termed the *meat factor*—is unknown. One theory is that the digestion products of both muscle and fat in beef interact to enhance iron absorption (Kapsokefalou and Miller, 1993).

Although the iron content of human milk is very low, it is highly bioavailable because of the presence of milk lactoferrin, which enhances iron absorption. Infants retain more iron from human milk than from cow's milk or infant formulas because of the presence of lactoferrin in breast milk. Whey protein (lactalbumin), which constitutes a greater percentage of the total protein in human milk than in cow's milk, may also improve iron absorption (Borch-Iohnsen et al., 1994).

The degree of gastric acidity enhances solubility and, therefore, the bioavailability of iron derived from foods. Therefore, achlorhydria (lack of gastric acid secretion), hypochlorhydria (inadequate acid secretion), or administration of alkaline substances, such as antacids, can interfere with nonheme iron absorption by not permitting the solubilization of iron in gastric and duodenal fluids. Gastric secretions also appear to increase the absorption of heme iron.

Physiologic states, such as pregnancy and growth, which demand increased blood formation, stimulate iron absorption. Also, more iron is absorbed in iron deficiency because of adaptive mechanisms that enhance nonheme iron absorption.

Foods with high phytate content have low iron bioavailability, but whether or not phytate is the cause is not clear. Tannins, which are polyphenols, in tea also reduce nonheme iron absorption. The presence of an adequate amount of calcium helps to remove phosphate, oxalate, and phytate that would otherwise combine with iron and inhibit its absorption.

The availability of iron from various compounds used for enrichment of foods or as supplements varies widely according to their chemical composition. Although iron in the ferrous form is most readily absorbed, not all ferrous compounds are equally available. Ferrous pyrophosphate is used frequently in products, such as breakfast cereals, because it does not add a gray color to the food. However, this compound and others, such as ferrous citrate and ferrous tartrate, are poorly absorbed. Iron is usually added to baby foods in an elemental form, the absorbability of which depends on the iron particle size.

Increased intestinal motility decreases iron absorption by decreasing contact time, and also by rapidly removing the chyme from the area of highest intestinal acidity. Poor fat digestion leading to steatorrhea also decreases iron absorption, as well as the absorption of other cations.

TRANSPORT

Iron (nonheme) is transported, bound to transferrin, to various tissues to meet their needs. It does not typically exist in the free ionic state in serum.

STORAGE

About 200 to 1500 mg of iron is stored in the body as ferritin and hemosiderin; 30% of the body's iron store is in the liver, 30% occurs in the bone marrow, and the rest is found in the spleen and muscles. Up to 50 mg/day can be mobilized from storage iron, 20 mg of which is used in hemoglobin synthesis. A schematic illustration of these events can be found in Figure 5–7. The amounts of circulating ferritin in blood correlate closely with total body iron stores, which makes this measurement an invaluable tool for clinical evaluation of iron status (see Chapters 17 and 35).

INTESTINAL EXCRETION

Iron is lost from the body only through bleeding and, in very small amounts, through fecal excretion, sweat, and the normal exfoliation of hair and skin. Most of the iron lost in the feces consists of that which could not be absorbed from food intake. The remainder comes from bile and the cells exfoliated from the gastrointestinal epithelium. Almost no iron is excreted in the urine.

Daily iron loss amounts to approximately 1 mg in the adult man and slightly less in the nonmenstruating woman. The loss of iron accompanying menstruation averages about 0.5 mg/day. Wide variations exist among individuals, however, and menstrual losses of more than 1.4 mg of iron daily have been reported in approximately 5% of normal women.

Functions

The functions of iron result from its ability to participate in oxidation and reduction reactions. Chemically, iron is a highly reactive element that can interact with oxygen to form intermediates that have the potential of damaging cell membranes or degrading DNA. Iron must be tightly bound to proteins to prevent these potentially destructive oxidant effects.

Iron metabolism is complex because this element is involved in so many aspects of life, including red blood cell function, myoglobin activity, and the roles of numerous heme and nonheme enzymes. Because of its oxidation-reduction (redox) properties, iron has a role in the respiratory transport of oxygen and carbon dioxide, and it is an active component of the cytochromes (enzymes) involved in the process of cellular respiration. Iron also appears to be involved in immune function and cognitive performance. Although these relationships have not been clearly identified, they underscore the importance of preventing iron deficiency anemia in the world population. Table 5–9 lists the major iron molecules in the body and their functions.

Hemoglobin, present in red blood cells, is synthesized in immature cells in bone marrow. Hemoglobin works in two ways: (1) the iron-containing heme combines with oxygen in the lungs, and (2) the heme releases the oxygen in tissues where it picks up carbon dioxide, only to release this gas in the lungs upon its return from the tissues. **Myoglobin,** also a heme-containing protein, serves as an oxygen reservoir within muscle.

Oxidative production of ATP within the mitochondria involves many iron-containing enzymes, both heme and nonheme. The *cytochromes,* present in cells, function in the respiratory chain in the transfer of electrons and the storage of energy through the alternate oxidation and reduction (redox) of iron ($Fe^{++} \leftarrow \rightarrow Fe^{+++}$). A number of water-insoluble drugs and endogenous organic molecules are transformed by the *cytochrome P-450 system* in the liver into water-soluble compounds that can be secreted in the bile and eliminated. Although these vital enzymes represent only a small portion of the total iron in the body (see Table 5–9) a decline in their cellular concentrations can have long-term consequences. Other enzymes, including several in the brain, also require iron to be active.

TABLE 5–9 IRON MOLECULES IN THE BODY

METABOLIC PROTEINS	
Heme Proteins	
Hemoglobin	Oxygen transport from lungs to tissues
Myoglobin	Transport and storage of oxygen in muscle
Enzymes-Heme	
Cytochromes	Electron transport
Cytochrome P-450	Oxidative degradation of drugs
Catalase	Conversion of hydrogen peroxide to oxygen and water
Enzymes-Nonheme	
Iron-sulfur and metalloproteins	Oxidative metabolism
Enzymes-Iron-Dependent	
Tryptophan pyrolase	Oxidation of tryptophan
TRANSPORT AND STORAGE PROTEINS	
Transferrin	Transport of iron and other minerals
Ferritin	Storage
Hemosiderin	Storage

An adequate iron intake is essential for the normal function of the immune system. Both iron overload and iron deficiency result in changes in the immune response. Iron is required by bacteria; therefore, iron overload (especially intravenously) may result in an increased risk of infection. Iron deficiency affects humoral and cellular immunity. Concentrations of circulating T lymphocytes are reduced in persons with iron deficiency, and mitogenic response is impaired. Natural killer (NK) cell activity is also reduced. Ribonucleotide reductase, the rate-limiting enzyme involved in DNA synthesis, is an iron enzyme. Production of interleukin-1 has been shown to be reduced in iron-deficient animals, and depressed interleukin-2 production has been reported in humans and animals. In one study, the immune response of apparently healthy elderly persons was improved when they were receiving iron supplements (Johnson et al., 1994) (see Chapter 13).

Two iron-binding proteins—transferrin (in blood) and lactoferrin (in breast milk)—appear to protect against infection by withholding iron from microorganisms that need it for proliferation.

Iron is used by brain cells for normal function at all ages (Beard et al., 1993). Iron is involved in the function and synthesis of neurotransmitters and, possibly, myelin. The detrimental effects of early iron deficiency anemia in children persist for many years (Lozoff, 1990; Walter, 1990).

Differences have been found between the scholastic performance, sensorimotor competence, attention, learning, and memory of anemic children and control subjects (Pollitt et al., 1976). Iron supplementation in children with iron deficiency anemia has been found to benefit their learning processes, as measured by school achievement test scores (Soemantri et al., 1985).

Changes occur in iron metabolism in certain disease states, such as Alzheimer's disease. Iron distribution in the brain has also been reported to change during normal aging (Johnson et al., 1994).

Deficiency

Iron deficiency, the precursor of iron deficiency anemia, is the most common of all nutritional deficiency diseases (see Chapter 35). In the United States and worldwide, iron deficiency anemia is the most common cause of anemia among both children and women of childbearing age. The groups considered to be at greatest risk for iron deficiency anemia are infants younger than 2 years of age, adolescent girls, pregnant women, and the elderly. Pregnant teenagers are frequently at high risk because of poor eating habits (see Chapters 7 and 11).

The final stage of the continuum of iron deficiency is manifested by a hypochromic, microcytic anemia. Anemia may be corrected by providing high-dose supplements in the form of ferrous sulfate or ferrous gluconate until blood parameters return to normal. To prevent further iron deficiency, individuals should be counseled regarding a diet that is appropriately rich in iron. See Figure 35–1 for the sequential changes in iron parameters that define normal conditions ranging from normal iron status to severe iron deficiency anemia. Figure 5–10 illustrates koilonychia, an iron-deficiency symptom.

Iron deficiency can be caused by injury, hemorrhage, or illness (e.g., blood loss secondary to hookworms or gastrointestinal diseases that interfere with iron absorption). Iron deficiency may also be aggravated by a poorly balanced diet containing insufficient iron, protein, folate, and vitamins B_{12}, B_6, and C. Anemia typically develops because of an inadequate amount of dietary iron or faulty iron absorption. Iron deficiency anemia is discussed in detail in Chapter 35.

Female athletes, especially cross-country runners and others involved in endurance sports, typically suffer from iron deficiency at some point in their training if they are not taking iron supplements or do not consume diets high in iron. The reason for the extra iron losses in these athletes has not been determined, but it is thought that iron losses through the gut are increased during the stressful conditions of training. One cross-country runner became so anemic that she developed hairline fractures of her proximal femur (hip), which illustrates the potential severity of the consequences of poor iron consumption (Anderson et al., 1998). It appears that the greater the intensity of training, the worse the iron parameters become in women (see Chapter 25).

Toxicity

The major cause of iron overload is *hereditary hemochromatosis;* transfusion overload is rare. The latter may be seen in individuals with sickle cell disease or thalassemia major who require transfusions for their anemia. Iron overload in Africans may be linked to dietary iron intake and a distinct gene, separate from any human leukocyte antigen–linked gene (Gordeuk et al., 1992). Genetic testing may eventually become a routine, readily available method for detecting this problem.

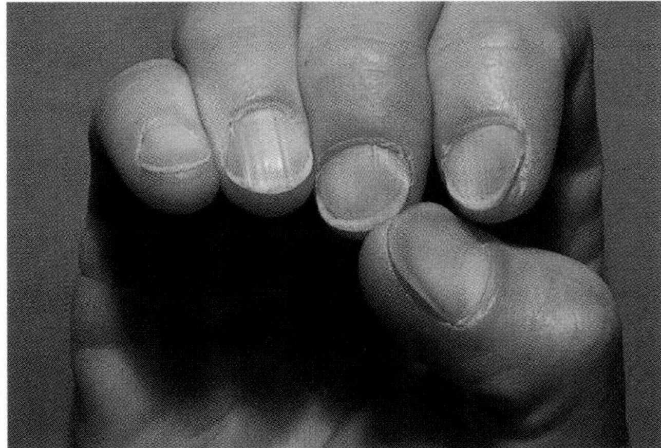

FIGURE 5–10 Koilonychia, thin, concave nails with raised edges, may be seen with iron deficiency anemia. (From Callen WBS, et al. Color Atlas of Dermatology. Philadelphia: WB Saunders, 1993.)

TABLE 5–10 THE CLINICAL MANIFESTATIONS OF IRON OVERLOAD (HEMOCHROMATOSIS)

Abnormal accumulation of iron in the liver
Excessive tissue ferritin levels
Elevated serum transferrin levels
Oxidation of low-density lipoprotein (LDL) cholesterol
Cardiovascular complications

The characteristic chemical parameters of iron overload are listed in Table 5–10 and are described further in Chapter 35.

Long-term ingestion of large amounts of iron or frequent blood transfusions can lead to abnormal accumulation of iron in the liver. Saturation of tissue apoferritin with iron is followed by the appearance of **hemosiderin,** which is similar to ferritin but contains more iron and is very insoluble. *Hemosiderosis* is an iron storage condition that develops in individuals who consume abnormally large amounts of iron or in those with a genetic defect resulting in excessive iron absorption. If the hemosiderosis is associated with tissue damage, it is called **hemochromatosis,** which is discussed further in Chapter 35.

Iron supplements may not be beneficial for either older (postmenopausal) women or older men because of the associated increased risks for heart disease and cancer. An intake of dietary iron in excess of the RDA by adult men and postmenopausal women may contribute to an enriched oxidative environment in the body that favors oxidation of low-density lipoprotein (LDL) cholesterol, arterial vessel damage, and other adverse effects involving the cardiovascular system. In addition, excessive iron may help generate excessive amounts of free radicals that attack cellular molecules, thereby increasing the number of potentially carcinogenic molecules within cells.

Zinc

The most readily available form of zinc occurs in animal flesh, particularly red meats and poultry. Meat intake is frequently low among preschoolers, perhaps because of personal preferences, possibly because of socioeconomic reasons, but usually because meats are displaced by cereal foods, milk, and milk products that children tend to prefer. In Hambidge's study, for example, some of the preschool children were found to eat as little as 1 oz of meat per day (Hambidge et al., 1976). This observation led to the fortification of infant and children's foods,

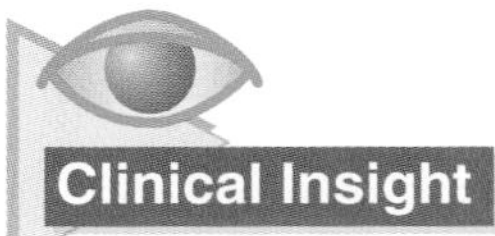

The Role of Zinc in Children's Health

The first studies linking zinc and growth were done in Iran and Egypt almost 3 decades ago. "Nutritionally dwarfed" boys, characterized by short stature, iron deficiency anemia, and delayed sexual maturity, showed remarkable improvement with zinc supplementation. Some grew as much as 5 inches in 1 year and showed parallel progression in gonadal development. The primary cause of zinc deficiency in these boys was identified as an impoverished diet consisting mainly of fibrous unleavened bread. Although the whole grains used to make the bread were relatively high in zinc, they also contained phytates, which are known to form insoluble complexes with both zinc and iron (Prasad, 1988).

At the time, the circumstances leading to growth impairment secondary to zinc deficiency were believed to be unique to less-developed countries. However, studies of preschool children from apparently well-nourished families in Denver demonstrated a correlation between short stature and low hair zinc levels (Hambidge et al., 1976). Other studies have supported these findings.

In addition to growth depression, mild zinc deficiency is probably associated with reduced resistance to infection in children, but it has been difficult to establish this linkage (Prentice, 1993). However, children with severe zinc-deficiency, as measured by plasma zinc concentrations, have been found to be at increased risk of both diarrhea and respiratory diseases (Bahl et al., 1998). Therefore, adequate zinc status plays a central role, not only in health promotion, but also in disease prevention.

especially cereals, with zinc. Milk is a good source of zinc, but high intakes of calcium from the milk can interfere with the absorption of both iron and zinc. Although the phytates from whole grains in unleavened breads may limit zinc absorption in Middle Eastern populations, this is less likely to be a problem in Western nations where breads, breakfast foods, and other cereal-based foods are made primarily from refined grains.

Nutritional assessment, including biochemical measurements, is necessary to detect the presence of a mild zinc deficiency in young children with suboptimal stature. However, a positive response of short children to zinc supplementation would provide some confirmatory evidence of zinc deficiency.

Zinc has only been known to be essential for humans since the now-classic studies of zinc deficiency in Iran and Egypt in the early 1960s (Halsted et al., 1972; Prasad et al., 1963). Severe zinc deficiency disease has been identified in undernourished populations, such as those in the Middle East, but a marginal form of deficiency has also been identified among low-income preschoolers in Denver and other cities in the United States (Hambidge et al., 1976). These marginal deficits have largely been corrected by food fortification over the last two decades (see the accompanying box, "*Clinical Insight:* The Role of Zinc in Children's Health").

Zinc is abundantly distributed throughout the human body and is second only to iron among trace elements. Zinc occurs in the human body in amounts of about 2 to 3 g, with the highest concentrations occurring in the liver, pancreas, kidney, bone, and muscles. Other tissues with high concentrations include various parts of the eye, prostate gland, spermatozoa, skin, hair, fingernails, and toenails. Zinc is primarily an intracellular ion, functioning in association with more than 100 different enzymes. Even though zinc is abundant in the cytosol, it is virtually all bound to proteins, but it is in equilibrium with a small ionic fraction.

Food Sources and Intakes

Meat, fish, poultry, and milk and milk products provide 80% of the total dietary zinc (Moser-Veillon, 1990). Oysters, other shellfish, meat, liver, cheese, whole grain cereals, dry beans, and nuts are also fairly good sources of zinc (Table 5–11 and Appendix 41). Soy products are also fairly good sources of zinc. In general, zinc intake correlates well with protein intake.

TABLE 5–11 ZINC CONTENT OF SELECTED FOODS

FOOD	mg
Oysters, Eastern, ½ cup	113.0
Oysters, Pacific, ½ cup	21.0
Wheat germ, toasted, ¼ cup	4.7
Ground beef, lean, 3 oz	4.6
Liver, beef, fried, 3 oz	4.6
Turkey, dark meat, baked, 3 oz	3.8
Beef enchilada, 1	2.3
Baked beans, with pork, ½ cup	1.9
Cheese, ricotta, part-skim, ½ cup	1.7
Pecans, ¼ cup	1.6
Tahini (sesame butter), 1 T	1.6
Peanuts, dry roasted, ¼ cup	1.4
Crab, canned, ¼ cup	1.3
Wild rice, cooked, ½ cup	1.1
Clams, canned, ¼ cup	1.1
Lobster, cooked, ½ cup	1.1
Cheese, Edam, 1 oz	1.1
Milk, 2% fat, 1 cup	1.0
Chicken, breast, baked, 1	1.0
Walnuts, English, ¼ cup	0.8
Gingerbread, 1 piece	0.6
Egg, 1	0.6
Salmon, baked, 3 oz	0.4

(From United States Department of Agriculture (USDA). Composition of Foods. USDA Handbook No. 8 Series. Washington, DC: ARS, USDA, 1976–1986.)

The zinc content of typical diets of adults in Western nations is between 10 and 15 mg/day (Food and Nutrition Board, 1989). Other researchers have suggested that the mean zinc intakes of adults are less than 10 mg/day for women and less than 15 mg/day for men (Moser-Veillon, 1990). The low intakes of women may be related to the lower total energy intake of women, rather than to the density of zinc in their diets. The zinc density of the American adult's diet is about 5.6 mg/1000 kcal.

The top foods supplying zinc in the U.S. diet (USDA, 1994) are beef, ready-to-eat cereals fortified with zinc, milk, poultry, bread, and cheese (Subar et al., 1998). Meats and other animal flesh foods were found to be the primary sources of zinc in the FDA's Total Diet Study (Pennington and Young, 1991).

Recommended Dietary Allowances

The 1989 RDA established 15 mg/day as the appropriate zinc intake for male adolescents and adults. Because of the lower body weight of adolescent and adult women, their RDA is 12 mg/day. The requirement for preadolescents is estimated at 6 mg/day, but because of greater dermal losses and more variation, the RDA has been set at 10 mg. The RDA for infants is 5 mg/day during the first year of life (see Table 5–5).

Oral contraceptive therapy may alter zinc distribution. However, there is no evidence that indicates these changes alter the dietary requirement (King, 1986).

Absorption, Transport, Storage, and Excretion

Both zinc absorption and excretion are controlled by poorly understood homeostatic mechanisms. The mechanism of absorption is by two pathways, similar to those of calcium: (1) a saturable carrier mechanism operating most efficiently at low zinc intakes which result in low luminal zinc concentrations and (2) a passive mechanism involving paracellular movement at high zinc intakes. Solubility of zinc in the gut lumen is critical, but zinc ions are generally bound to amino acids or short peptides in the lumen, and the ions are released at the brush border for absorption via the carrier mechanism. The entry step of absorption across the brush border is followed by the binding of zinc ions to **metallothionein** and other proteins within the cytosol of the absorbing cell. Metallothionein carries the zinc (via transcellular movement) to the basolateral border for the exit step from the absorbing cell to the blood. The exit step is by active transport because the blood concentration is significantly greater than the cytosolic ion concentration of zinc. The process of zinc absorption is illustrated in Figure 5–11.

Zinc absorption is affected by the level of zinc in the diet and the presence of interfering substances, especially phytates. Following the consumption of zinc in a meal, the serum zinc level rises and then declines in a dose-response pattern. A protein-rich diet promotes zinc absorption by forming zinc–amino acid chelates that present zinc in a more absorbable form. Zinc absorption is slightly increased during pregnancy and lactation (Fung et al., 1997). Absorbed zinc is taken up from the portal circulation initially by the liver, but most of the zinc is subsequently redistributed to other tissues. Impaired absorption is associated with a variety of intestinal diseases, such as Crohn's disease or pancreatic insufficiency.

Several dietary factors affect zinc absorption. Phytate decreases zinc absorption, but other complexing agents (e.g., tannins) do not. Copper and cadmium compete for the same carrier protein, so they reduce zinc absorption. Concern exists that high intakes of iron may reduce the amounts of zinc absorbed. High dietary calcium intakes reduce both zinc absorption and balance (Wood and Zheng, 1997). Folic acid may also reduce zinc absorption when zinc intake is low. On the other hand, high doses of zinc can impair absorption of iron from fer-

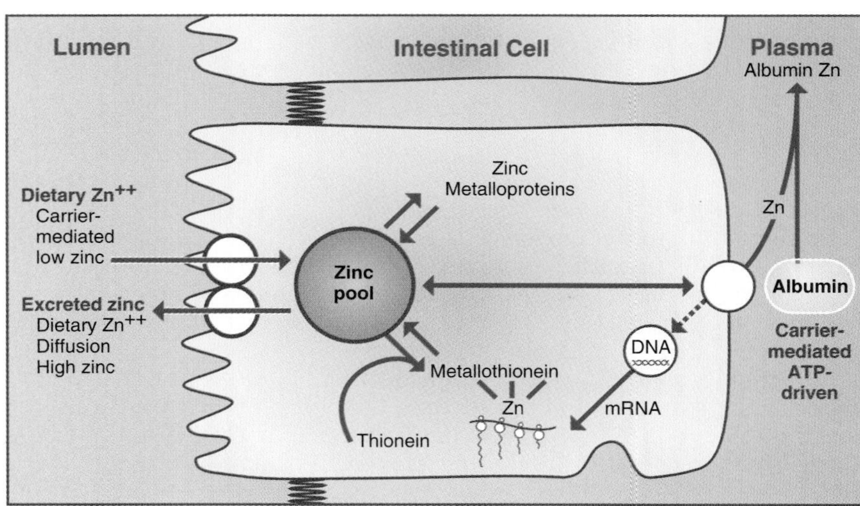

FIGURE 5–11 A model for zinc absorption showing the relationship between metallothionein and cysteine-rich intestinal protein.

rous sulfate, the form usually found in vitamin/mineral supplements (Crofton et al., 1989). Dietary fiber may also interfere with zinc absorption, but the significance of this interaction within the gut lumen is not clear.

Zinc absorption may be enhanced by either glucose or lactose and by soy protein fed alone or mixed with beef. Red table wine also increases zinc absorption, probably owing to the congeners present; white wine has not been studied. Just as with iron, zinc is better absorbed from human milk than from cow's milk.

TRANSPORT IN BLOOD

The amount of zinc transported in the blood depends on the availability not only of zinc, but also of albumin, a transport protein for many mineral cations. Albumin is the major plasma carrier, although some zinc is transported by transferrin and by alpha$_2$-macroglobulin. Most of the zinc in blood is localized in erythrocytes and leukocytes. Plasma zinc is metabolically active and fluctuates in response to dietary intake, as well as to physiologic factors, such as injury or inflammation. Plasma zinc levels drop by 50% in the acute-phase response to injury, probably from the sequestering of zinc by the liver, although transferrin may also increase its zinc content (King and Keen, 1994).

When zinc is administered intravenously, about 10% of the dose appears in the intestine within 30 minutes. Serum concentration declines after a zinc-free meal, possibly because the pancreas removes zinc from the circulation to produce and secrete zinc-metalloenzymes needed for digestion and absorption.

INTESTINAL EXCRETION

Excretion of zinc in normal individuals is almost entirely via the feces. However, increased urinary excretion has been reported in starvation and in patients with nephrosis, diabetes, alcoholism, hepatic cirrhosis, and porphyria. Plasma and urine concentrations of amino acids, specifically the zinc-binding cysteine and histidine, as well as other urinary metabolites, may have a role in increasing zinc losses in these patients.

Functions

Many questions regarding the biologic role of zinc in humans remain unanswered. Zinc participates in reactions involving either synthesis or degradation of major metabolites, such as carbohydrates, lipids, proteins, and nucleic acids. More than 200 zinc enzymes have been isolated from various species. Zinc is also involved in the stabilization of protein and nucleic acid structure and the integrity of subcellular organelles, as well as in transport processes, immune function, and expression of genetic information.

Metallothionein is the most abundant, nonenzymatic zinc-containing protein known at present. This low-molecular-weight protein is rich in cysteine and exceptionally high in metals, among which are zinc and lesser amounts of copper, iron, cadmium, and mercury. The biologic role of metallothionein has not been defined conclusively, but a function in zinc absorption has been postulated. It may have a role in the detoxification of metals as well as in their absorption.

Zinc is abundant in the nucleus, where it stabilizes RNA and DNA structure and is required for the activity of RNA polymerases important in cell division. Zinc also functions in chromatin proteins involved in transcription and replication.

A relationship between zinc intake and age-related macular degenerative (AMD) disease was suggested by early reports, but a recent publication by Stur et al. (1996) could not demonstrate a protective benefit of zinc supplementation (200 mg/day for 24 months) in the unaffected eye of patients with AMD in one eye.

Zinc gluconate lozenges, though widely touted to cure or prevent the common cold, have not been proved to be effective against this condition in a randomized, controlled trial of children and adolescents (Macknin et al., 1998).

Zinc appears in the crystalline structure of bone, in bone enzymes, and at the zone of demarcation. It is thought to be needed for adequate osteoblastic activity; formation of bone enzymes, such as alkaline phosphatase; and calcification. Unless bone resorption is occurring, the zinc in bone is not available (see Chapter 28).

Deficiency

The clinical signs of zinc deficiency in humans were first described in young boys in Iran and Egypt and included short stature, hypogonadism, mild anemia, and low plasma zinc levels (Prasad et al., 1963) (see previous box, "*Clinical Insight:* The Role of Zinc in Children's Health"). This deficiency is caused by a diet high in unrefined cereal and unleavened bread. These contain a high level of fiber and phytate, both of which chelate with zinc in the intestine and prevent absorption. The anemia seen in the youths may have reflected a coexisting iron deficiency from the same cause. Additional symptoms of zinc deficiency include hypogeusia (decreased taste acuity), delayed wound healing, alopecia, and diverse forms of skin lesions. A zinc-responsive night blindness has also been documented (Solomons and Cousins, 1984). Acquired zinc deficiency may occur as the result of malabsorption, starvation, or increased losses via urinary, pancreatic, or other exocrine secretions (Fig. 5–12).

Patients receiving TPN have developed signs of clinical zinc deficiency because of the underlying disease process. Patients with alcoholism may have altered zinc metabolism. Pregnant women and the elderly are also at increased risk of deficiency. In

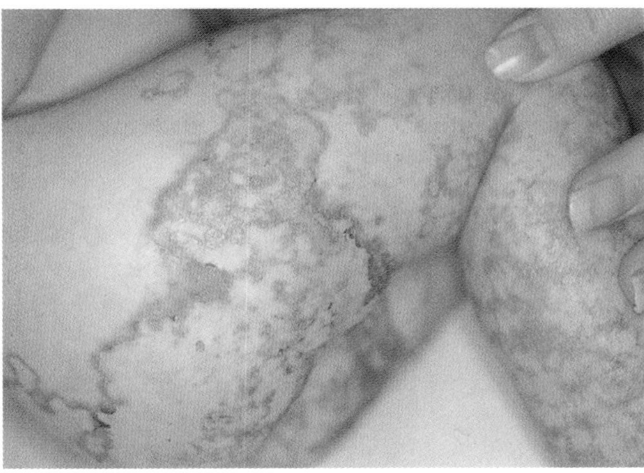

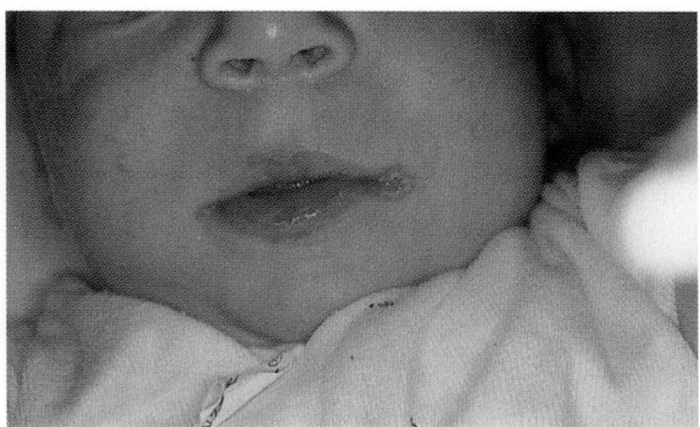

FIGURE 5–12 The two photos illustrate the cutaneous manifestations of zinc deficiency. (From Callen WBS, et al. Color Atlas of Dermatology. Philadelphia: WB Saunders, 1993.)

one study of institutionalized elderly, low-dose zinc supplementation partially reversed measures of poor zinc status (Boukaïba et al., 1993).

Acrodermatitis enteropathica, an autosomal recessive disease characterized by zinc malabsorption, results in eczematoid skin lesions, alopecia, diarrhea, intercurrent bacterial and yeast infections, and, eventually, death if left untreated. Symptoms are generally first observed at weaning from human milk to cow's milk.

Zinc deficiency results in a variety of immunologic defects. Severe deficiency is accompanied by thymic atrophy, lymphopenia, reduced lymphocyte proliferative response to mitogens, a selective decrease in T_4-helper cells, decreased NK cell activity, anergy, and deficient thymic hormone activity. Even mild zinc deficiency can reduce immune function, producing impaired interleukin-2 production, for example. In one study of such individuals, supplementation with zinc improved immune status (Prasad et al., 1993). Moderate zinc deficiency is associated with anergy and diminished NK cell activity, but not with thymic atrophy or lymphopenia. Table 5–12 summarizes the clinical manifestations of human zinc deficiency.

TABLE 5–12 CLINICAL MANIFESTATIONS OF ZINC DEFICIENCY IN HUMANS

Growth retardation
Delayed sexual maturation
Hypogonadism and hypospermia
Alopecia
Delayed wound healing
Skin lesions
Impaired appetite
Immune deficiencies
Behavioral disturbances
Eye lesions, including photophobia and night blindness
Impaired taste (hypogeusia)

Similarities between patients with sickle cell anemia and zinc deficiency suggest the possibility of a secondary zinc deficiency in that disease. (See Chapter 35.)

Low zinc intakes are associated with low concentrations of insulin-like growth factor 1 (IGF-1) in postmenopausal women, but the meaning of this finding is unclear (Devine et al., 1998). If calcium supplements are taken by postmenopausal women, it is possible that zinc absorption becomes suppressed, which in turn, reduces IGF-1, which normally supports tissue growth. Problems with low zinc intakes appear to be on the increase, in part because of the low bioavailability of zinc (Fairweather-Tait, 1998).

Athletes may also be at increased risk for zinc deficiency. Physical activity contributes to elevated mobilization of zinc from zinc stores for cellular needs (i.e., to supply zinc-metalloenzymes), even though the serum zinc concentration remains constant (Dolev et al., 1995) (see Chapter 25).

Toxicity

Excess oral ingestion of zinc to the point of toxicity (100 to 300 mg/day) is rare. Continued supplementation with zinc in excess of the RDA, however, will interfere with copper absorption (Fosmire, 1990). Zinc supplementation of 50 mg/day has been found to cause a decrease in high-density lipoprotein (HDL) cholesterol in adult men (Black et al., 1988). Zinc sulfate in amounts of 2 g/day or more can cause gastrointestinal irritation and vomiting. Inhalation of zinc fumes during welding can be toxic, but can be prevented with proper precautions.

The major type of zinc toxicity is seen in patients with renal failure treated with hemodialysis. Contamination of dialysis fluids from the adhesive plastic used on the dialysis coils or from galvanized pipes has been reported. The toxic syndrome in this case is characterized by anemia, fever, and CNS disturbances.

Fluoride

Fluoride is a natural element found in nearly all drinking waters and soil, although the fluoride content varies greatly (American Dietetic Association, 1994). For example, some well water may have much more fluoride than others, and those families who use well water need to monitor fluoride levels periodically to make sure that levels are not in the fluorotic range. Although fluoride is not considered to be an essential element, this anion is known to be important for the health of bones and teeth (see Chapter 29). The average skeleton contains 2.5 mg of fluoride.

Food Sources and Intakes

The major dietary sources of fluoride are drinking water and processed foods that have been prepared or reconstituted with fluoridated water. Seafoods also are high in fluoride, but the content of freshwater fish is lower than that in saltwater fish. The standard recommendation is 1 ppm in fluoridated community water supplies. An estimated difference in intake of almost 1 mg has been documented between children who consume 0.9 mg/day in an area with unfluoridated water and those who ingest approximately 1.7 mg/day in a fluoridated area (Singer et al., 1980). This difference is not so great, but intakes higher than 2 mg begin to raise concern about mild fluorosis.

Although fluorides exist in fruits and vegetables, the amounts in most foods, with the exception of seafood, are not significant. The amount in tea (from the leaves) can be quite substantial, depending on the brewing strength. One cup of tea may contain as much as 1.0 mg of fluoride. Soups and stews made with fish and meat bones also provide good amounts of fluoride. Mechanically deboned meat and fowl, as well as seafood and beef liver, are high in fluoride. Cooking foods in Teflon pans (a fluoride-containing polymer) may increase fluoride intake, although solid scientific data are not available.

Dietary Reference Intakes

The AIs for fluoride were established by the Food and Nutrition Board in 1998. AIs for adult men and women are 4 and 3 mg/day, respectively. Depending on age, the AIs range from 2.0 to 3.0 mg/day for children and adolescents and from 0.7 to 1.0 mg/day for young children between the ages of 1 and 8 years (see Table 5–2) (Institute of Medicine, 1998). For comparison, an 8-oz glass of fluoridated water (1 ppm or 1 mg/L) provides about 0.2 mg of fluoride. ULs were also established for fluoride.

Functions

Fluoride is considered to be important, if not essential, because of its beneficial effect on tooth enamel, conferring maximal resistance to dental caries, and on skeletal hydroxyapatite. The prevalence of dental caries has decreased by 50% in the last 15 to 20 years, owing mainly to the fluoridation of drinking water and the use of topical fluorides. The prevalence of dental caries has also declined in communities without fluoridated water. The cause is unknown, but probably includes the use of fluoridated toothpaste, topical fluoride application, and increased use of fluorides in the food chain, especially from fluoridated water used in food processing. Soft drinks typically are prepared with fluoridated waters at bottling plants in urban areas. See Chapter 29 for recommendations for fluoride supplementation.

Fluoride substitutes for the hydroxyl group on the lattice structure of calcium phosphate salts (i.e., hydroxyapatites) of the bones and teeth to form *fluoroapatite,* which is harder and less readily resorbed than hydroxyapatite. Recent placebo-controlled trials of supplementation in postmenopausal women with a slow-release fluoride preparation resulted in improved bone density and a reduction of hip fractures (Pak et al., 1995) (see Chapter 28).

Toxicity

A mild fluorosis can appear at daily doses of 0.1 mg/kg, that is, greater than about 2 to 3 ppm of fluoride in the drinking water (see Chapter 29). This type of discoloration of the teeth, or mottling, is not usually visible and has no adverse effect, except cosmetically. Higher intakes, however, lead to tooth flaking and more serious dental effects.

Some evidence suggests that fluoride intakes are increasing among toddlers and young children because of the proliferating sources of fluorides. When drinking water contained less fluoride, the average intake was less. Even the highest values did not exceed the recommendation of 0.08 mg/kg daily. Intakes of fluoride by young children may vary greatly because of the widespread availability of foods prepared with fluoridated water, the use of dentifrices, and other sources; therefore, some children are consuming total amounts of fluoride that exceed the optimal intake level (0.05 to 0.07 mg/kg daily) beyond which dental fluorosis may occur (Levy et al., 1995).

Copper

Copper, recognized for more than 100 years as a normal constituent of blood, has been established as an essential micronutrient only in recent years. Recent interest in copper, along with several other trace elements, has increased because of the many tissue functions of this trace element and the potential (though unlikely) risk of deficiency (Uauy et al., 1998). Concentrations of copper are highest in the liver, brain, heart, and kidney. Muscle contains a low concentration of copper, but because of its large mass, skeletal muscle contains almost 40% of all copper in the body. Recent investigations have greatly advanced knowledge of the physiologic roles of copper, copper homeostasis, and copper needs across the life cycle (Lönnerdal and Uauy, 1998).

Food Sources and Intakes

Copper is distributed widely in foods, especially animal products except for milk, and most diets provide between 0.6 and 2 mg/day. Foods high in copper are shellfish (oysters), organ meats (liver, kidney), muscle meats, chocolate, nuts, cereal grains, dried legumes, and dried fruits (Table 5–13). Animal flesh was found to be the primary source of copper in the Total Diet Study of the FDA (Pennington and Young, 1991). In general, fruits and vegetables contain little copper. Cow's milk, a poor source of copper, contains 0.015 to 0.18 mg/L, whereas the copper content of human milk, from which copper is well absorbed, ranges from 0.15 to 1.05 mg/L. Infants fed cow's milk may be at risk of copper deficiency because of the low copper content of this form of milk (Lönnerdal, 1996).

Copper intakes of individuals in several age categories in the United States have been consistently below recommended amounts, with adolescent girls consuming only approximately 50% of the ESADDI, according to estimated median intakes reported in the Total Diet Study of the FDA (Pennington and Schoen, 1996). Typically, the copper content of drinking water is not considered in diet surveys, but the amount of copper in water from copper pipes is considered to be very low, perhaps insignificant.

Copper intakes may be low in U.S. diets because ready-to-eat cereals typically were not fortified with copper, as they were for several other trace minerals, until recently (Johnson et al., 1998).

TABLE 5–13 COPPER CONTENT OF SELECTED FOODS

FOOD	mg
Beef liver, fried, 3 oz	2.4
Cashews, dry roasted, ¼ cup	0.8
Black-eyed peas, dried, cooked, ½ cup	0.7
Molasses, blackstrap, 2 T	0.6
Sunflower seeds, ¼ cup	0.6
Chocolate chips, semisweet, ¼ cup	0.5
V-8 juice, 1 cup	0.5
Tofu, firm, ½ cup	0.5
Beans, refried, ½ cup	0.5
Instant breakfast, fortified, 1 envelope	0.5
Cocoa powder, 2 T	0.4
Prunes, dried, 10	0.4
Salmon, baked, 3 oz	0.3
Tahini (sesame butter), 1 T	0.2
Pizza, cheese, ⅛ of 15"	0.2
Bread, whole-wheat, 1 slice	0.1
Milk chocolate, 1 oz	0.1
Milk, 2% fat, 1 cup	0.1

(From United States Department of Agriculture (USDA). Composition of Foods. USDA Handbook No. 8 Series. Washington, DC: ARS, USDA, 1976–1986.)

Estimated Safe and Adequate Daily Dietary Intakes

Although sufficient data are not available to establish an RDA, in 1989, ESADDIs of 1.5 to 3 mg/day for adolescents and adults were established for copper. The ESADDIs for children range between 0.7 and 2 mg/day; for infants, the ESADDIs are 0.4 to 0.6 mg during the first 6 months and 0.6 to 0.7 mg/day during the second 6 months (see Table 5–6). Premature infants, who are born with low copper reserves, may require increased dietary copper during their first few months of life (see Chapter 9). A review of the ESADDIs by the Food and Nutrition Board is to be undertaken in the near future.

Absorption, Transport, Storage, and Excretion

Copper absorption occurs in the small intestine. Entry at the mucosal surface is by facilitated diffusion. Exit at the basolateral membrane is primarily by active transport, but facilitated transfer may also occur at this membrane. Competition between copper ions and other divalent cations exists at each step. Within the intestinal absorbing cells, copper ions are bound to metallothionein with greater affinity than zinc or other ions. Some evidence suggests that the amount of copper absorbed is regulated by the amount of metallothionein in the mucosal cells. Net absorption of copper varies from 25% to 60%. Low absorption efficiencies help to regulate the retention of copper in the body; therefore, the percentage of absorption decreases with increased intake. Fiber and phytate, known to affect bioavailability of several minerals, do not appear to have an adverse effect on copper absorption.

TRANSPORT

Approximately 90% of the copper in serum is incorporated into ceruloplasmin; the rest is bound loosely to albumin, transcuprein, other proteins, and free amino acids, and possibly, to histidine. Copper is transported in the blood to other tissues, mainly bound to albumin. Copper is also present in blood as **ceruloplasmin,** a functional protein that acts as an enzyme at the blood-forming cells of the bone marrow. Both serum copper and immunoreactive ceruloplasmin levels tend to be higher in women than in men. The serum copper concentration is greatest in the neonate. It then decreases gradually during the first year of life.

Copper bound to albumin in blood may serve as a temporary storage site for copper. In the liver, copper binds to metallothionein, which serves as a storage form, and it is incorporated into ceruloplasmin and secreted into the plasma for the transport of copper to cells. Copper is also secreted from the liver as a component of bile, the major route of excretion of copper. Once in the gastrointestinal tract, copper becomes part of the pool that may be reabsorbed or excreted, depending on the body's need for copper. Biliary excretion increases in response to excessive intakes of copper, but not when intakes reach toxic levels.

Small amounts of copper are found in urine, sweat, and menstrual blood. Copper can be conserved by the kidney, if necessary, when substantial amounts are filtered through the glomeruli and reabsorbed in the tubules.

The interaction of copper with other nutrients illustrates the fallacy of taking excessive amounts of vitamin and mineral supplements above the recommended levels of consumption. In amounts of 150 mg/day, zinc has been shown to induce copper deficiency by overwhelming the capacity of metallothionein in intestinal absorbing cells to bind copper (Copper deficiency . . . , 1985), even though metallothionein has a greater affinity for copper than for zinc. High ascorbic acid intake (1500 mg/day) reduces blood concentrations of both copper and ceruloplasmin in human subjects and, therefore, decreases the functional properties of ceruloplasmin (Finley and Cerklewski, 1983). Combined high dietary iron and ascorbic acid intakes have essentially similar effects on copper status in rats (Johnson and Murphy, 1988).

Functions

Copper is a component of many enzymes, and clinical manifestations of copper deficiency are attributable to enzyme failures. Copper in ceruloplasmin has a well-documented role in oxidizing iron before it is transported in the plasma. Lysyl oxidase, a copper-containing enzyme, is essential in the lysine-derived cross-linking of both collagen and elastin, connective tissue proteins with great tensile strength (Rucker et al., 1998). Through the involvement of copper-containing electron transport proteins, copper also has roles in mitochondrial energy production. As part of copper-containing enzymes such as superoxide dismutase, copper protects against oxidants and free radicals and promotes the synthesis of melanin and catecholamines. Other functions of copper-containing enzymes have not yet been completely defined.

Deficiency

Copper deficiency has historically been assessed by a decrease in serum copper and ceruloplasmin levels, but more sensitive indicators of copper status—copper-containing enzymes in blood cells—have now been identified (Milne, 1998). Copper deficiency is characterized by anemia, neutropenia, and skeletal abnormalities, especially demineralization. Other changes may also follow, including subperiosteal hemorrhages, hair and skin depigmentation, and defective elastin formation. The failure of erythropoiesis, as well as cerebral and cerebellar degeneration, may lead to death. Neutropenia and leukopenia are the best early indications of copper deficiency in children. Copper deficiency anemia is discussed in Chapter 35.

Classical cases of copper deficiency were reported in the 1960s among Peruvian infants who were poorly nourished, had diarrhea, and who were fed diluted cow's milk (Cordano, 1998). Other cases of deficiency have been reported since then. Premature infants are likely to have copper deficiency unless given a copper supplement because most of the copper is normally transferred across the placenta during the last few months of a full-term pregnancy (see Chapter 9).

Copper is stored in the liver; therefore, deficiency develops slowly as copper stores become depleted. Deficiencies have not been reported in otherwise healthy humans consuming a varied diet. Low serum copper, ceruloplasmin, and superoxide dismutase levels provide supportive evidence of copper deficiency, but these markers are not sensitive to marginal copper status. Bone changes, including osteoporosis, metaphyseal spur formation, and soft-tissue calcification seen in infants receiving prolonged TPN, may resolve with copper supplementation. The only signs of copper deficiency found in adults are neutropenia and microcytic anemia, but deficiency is very rare in adults, probably because copper accumulates in the liver throughout life in most individuals.

Menkes' disease or kinky-hair syndrome is a sex-linked recessive defect that results in copper malabsorption, increased urinary copper loss, and abnormal intracellular copper transport, all of which cause an abnormal distribution of copper among organs and within cells. Affected infants have retarded growth, defective keratinization and pigmentation of the hair, hypothermia, degenerative changes in aortic elastin, abnormalities of the metaphyses of long bones, and progressive mental deterioration. These infants typically do not survive the first few months of life. Many of the features of this disorder result from interference with the cross-linking of collagen and elastin; these steps require one or more copper enzymes. Brain tissue is practically devoid of cytochrome C oxidase, and a marked accumulation of copper occurs in the intestinal mucosa, although serum copper and ceruloplasmin levels remain very low. Parenteral administration of copper results in transient improvement. Ataxia, mild learning difficulty, and connective tissue abnormalities are seen in patients with mild Menkes' disease (Procopis et al., 1981).

A new copper deficiency, only recently reported, manifests as a demyelinating neuropathy with chronic intestinal pseudo-obstruction, osteoporosis, testicular failure, retinal degeneration, and cardiomyopathy. The underlying problem appears to be a defect in hepatic processing of copper into ceruloplasmin (Buchman et al., 1994).

Decreased plasma copper is seen in patients with malabsorption diseases, such as celiac sprue, tropical sprue, protein-losing enteropathies, and nephrotic syndrome.

Low copper intakes may also contribute to reduced immune responses in otherwise healthy individuals (Kelley et al., 1995).

Toxicity

Copper toxicity from food consumption is considered to be impossible, but toxicity from excessive supplementation or from copper salts used in agriculture has been reported. Liver cirrhosis typically develops from toxic intakes, and abnormalities in red blood cell formation also occur.

Ceruloplasmin concentrations increase during pregnancy and with the use of oral contraceptives. Serum copper concentrations in pregnant women are approximately twice the values found in nonpregnant women. Serum copper concentrations are also elevated in patients with acute and chronic infections, liver disease, and pellagra. The physiologic significance of these elevations is not known, but bile also contains substantial amounts of copper under these conditions. Any chronic liver disease that interferes with the excretion of bile may contribute to the retention of copper. Primary biliary cirrhosis, as well as mechanical obstruction of the bile ducts, contributes to a progressive rise in liver copper content.

Wilson's disease (hepatolenticular degeneration) is a disease characterized by accumulation of copper to excessive levels in body tissues, including the eyes, as a result of a genetic deficiency in the liver synthesis of ceruloplasmin (see Chapter 32). A strict vegetarian diet may be beneficial in the treatment of patients with Wilson's disease because of the low copper content of fruits and vegetables (Brewer et al., 1993).

ULTRATRACE ELEMENTS

Iodine

Iodine deficiency in the United States and many Western nations has practically been eliminated with the iodinization of salt. People living in many mountainous areas of the world and a few low-lying delta regions, however, still have low iodine intakes because of low iodine content of the soil used in cultivating crops. Others living in lowlands may have high goitrogen consumption that reduces iodine utilization by the thyroid gland.

The body normally contains 20 to 30 mg of iodine, with more than 75% in the thyroid gland and the rest distributed throughout the body, particularly in the lactating mammary gland, gastric mucosa, and blood. The dietary requirement for iodine is for the synthesis of thyroid hormones; iodine becomes an integral part of the thyroid hormones.

Food Sources and Intakes

Iodine occurs in variable amounts in food and drinking water. Seafoods, such as clams, lobsters, oysters, sardines, and other saltwater fish, are the richest sources of iodine. Saltwater fish contain 300 to 3000 μg/kg of flesh; freshwater fish contain 20 to 40 μg/kg, but they are still good sources of this mineral. The iodine content of cow's milk and eggs is determined by the iodides available in the diet of the animal; the iodide content of vegetables varies according to the iodine content of the soil in which they grow.

Iodine also enters the food chain through the use of iodophors, which are used as disinfectants in dairy processing, coloring agents, and dough conditioners. These sources add significant amounts of iodine to the food supply. For example, cow's milk in the United States is high in iodine because of the use of iodofors. Table 5–14 lists the iodine content of various foods.

The use of iodized salt should still be advocated in certain areas to prevent goiter. The best way to obtain an adequate intake of iodine is to use iodized salt (76 μg of iodine per gram of salt for both United States and Canada) in preparing food. More than 50% of the table salt sold in the United States is iodized; however, iodized salt is not used in processed foods. Mandatory iodinization has been adopted by many nations, including Canada, but is not legally required in the United States, where iodine deficiency is now very rare.

The Total Diet Study of the FDA showed that median adult iodine intakes over the period 1982–1991 ranged from 130 to 140 μg/day for women and 182 to 204 μg/day for men. The median iodine intake for both male and female teenagers was even higher, with adolescent boys consuming almost twice the

TABLE 5–14 IODINE CONTENT OF SELECTED FOODS

FOOD	μg
Salt, iodized, 1 tsp	400
Bread, made with iodate dough conditioner and continuous mix process, 1 slice	142
Haddock, 3 oz	104–145
Bread, made with regular process, 1 slice	35
Cheese, cottage, 2% fat, ½ cup	26–71
Shrimp, 3 oz	21–37
Egg, 1	18–26
Cheese, cheddar, 1 oz	5–23
Ground beef, 3 oz	8

(From United States Department of Agriculture (USDA). Composition of Foods. USDA Handbook No. 8 Series. Washington, DC: ARS, USDA, 1976–1986.)

RDA (Pennington and Schoen, 1996). Intakes of iodine in the United States are clearly adequate because of both iodinization of salt and the use of iodofors.

A small subset of vegans who eat only uncooked, lactobacilli-rich food were tested for thyroid function and found to be within normal limits (Rauma et al., 1994). These vegans consume iodine in seaweed or in kelp tablets. Some of the individuals in this study had iodine intakes high enough to cause potential problems, but symptoms of toxicity were not observed.

Recommended Dietary Allowances

An iodine intake of 150 μg/day has been suggested as sufficient for all adults and adolescents. The RDA for pregnant and lactating women is increased to 25 μg and 50 μg, respectively. The RDA is 40 μg for infants up to 6 months of age, and 50 μg for older infants. The RDA for children is between 70 and 120 μg, increasing with age (or body size) (see Table 5–5).

Absorption, Transport, Storage, and Excretion

Iodine is absorbed easily in the form of iodide. In the circulation, iodine occurs both free and protein-bound, but the bound iodide predominates. Excretion is primarily via urine, but small amounts are found in the feces as a result of biliary secretion.

Functions

Iodine is stored in the thyroid gland, where it is used in the synthesis of **triiodothyronine (T_3)** and **thyroxine (T_4).** Uptake of iodide ions by the thyroid cells may be inhibited by goitrogens found in foods (see the following section). The hormone is degraded in target cells and in the liver, and the iodine is highly conserved under normal conditions. Selenium is important in iodine metabolism because of its presence in one enzyme responsible for forming active T_3 from thyroglobulin stored in the thyroid gland.

Deficiency

Millions of people worldwide living in less developed nations remain at risk for iodine deficiency (Tonglet et al., 1992). These individuals may suffer from moderate iodine deficiency, even when obvious goiter, a severe condition, is not evident. Iodine deficiency is a preventable cause of mental deficiency, including cretinism, especially during pregnancy (Hetzel, 1994). Use of iodized salt or the oral administration of a single dose of iodized oil would suffice to correct iodine deficiency for about 1 year. Weekly iodine supplements also are effective (Alnwick, 1998). Use of iodized salt should be encouraged in pregnancy, especially through the end of the second trimester (Xue-Yi et al., 1994).

Very low iodine intakes are associated with the development of endemic or simple **goiter,** which is an enlargement of the thyroid gland (Fig. 5–13). The deficiency may be nearly total, especially in mountainous areas and regions of high goitrogen intakes, or relative, subsequent to increased need for thyroid hormones, as occurs in women during adolescence, pregnancy, and lactation.

The World Health Organization (WHO) has estimated that the world incidence of goiter is approximately 200 million. In some countries, goiter is so common that it is regarded as a normal physical feature. In the United States, the prevalence rate of goiter for all ages is 1.9/1000 persons. The rate is higher in women than in men, and it is higher for older than younger age groups.

Goitrogens, substances occurring naturally in foods, can also cause goiter by blocking uptake of iodine from the blood by thyroid cells. Foods containing goitrogens include cabbage, turnips, rapeseeds, peanuts, cassava, and soybeans. Goitrogens are inactivated by heating or cooking. A fully satisfactory explanation for the development of goiter has not been established.

Severe iodine deficiency during gestation and early postnatal growth results in **cretinism** in infants, a syndrome characterized by mental deficiency, spastic diplegia or quadriplegia, deaf mutism, dysarthria, a characteristic shuffling gait, shortened stature, and hypothyroidism. Less severe variations of this syndrome may also exist, manifesting as moderate retardation in intellectual or neuromotor maturation.

Toxicity

Iodine intakes have a wide margin of safety. In some cases, however, goiter will develop slowly as a consequence of long-term excessive iodine intakes,

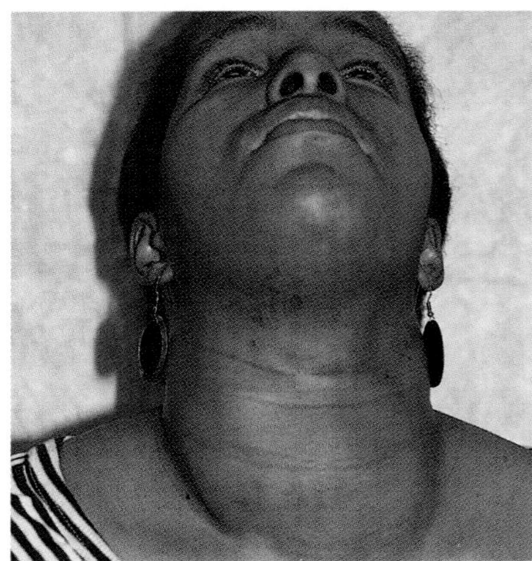

FIGURE 5–13 Goiter caused by iodine deficiency. (From Swartz MH. Textbook of Physical Diagnosis History and Examination, 3rd ed. Philadelphia: WB Saunders, 1998.)

well above physiologic requirements. The significance of excessive intakes of iodine in contributing to thyroid disease or disorder is not clear. At present, the level of iodine in foods is not considered to be a significant public health problem in the United States or Canada. However, two different studies—one in Canada and the other in the United States—reported intakes of iodine that were either greater than or approximately equal to recommended intake levels across the life cycle (Discher and Girous, 1987; Pennington and Schoen, 1996). These intakes are generally considered to be safe because adverse effects of high intakes have only been rarely reported in the United States and Canada.

Selenium

A rather narrow window of safety exists for selenium, below which deficiency occurs and above which toxicity develops. Only in China have these extremes been shown to relate to the soil content of selenium. A dietary intake of approximately 40 μg of selenium per day appears to be necessary to maintain *glutathione peroxidase (GSH-Px),* an enzyme containing selenium. The diets of practically all nations other than China supply selenium in sufficient amounts to maintain adequate levels of GSH-Px, so that selenium deficiency is extremely rare. GSH-Px, discovered to be a selenoenzyme in the early 1970s, is considered the major active form of selenium in tissues, although other selenium proteins have since been discovered.

Additional roles for selenium, not associated with GSH-Px, have recently been identified. Selenium, as selenomethionine or selenocysteine, exists in several proteins that have wide distribution in the body. *Cellular glutathione peroxidase (cGSH-Px)* has been found in almost all cells, as well as extracellularly, in serum and milk. This family of enzymes may help provide a reserve of selenium in proteins that can be drawn on when needed. *Phospholipid hydroperoxide glutathione peroxidase (phGSH-Px),* which has a distribution in lipid-soluble fractions of the cell, may have other roles in lipid and eicosanoid metabolism. *Type I iodothyronine 5′-diodinase,* an enzyme capable of converting T_4 to T_3, is a selenoprotein. *Selenoprotein P,* another selenium-containing molecule, may act as a free radical scavenger, or it may serve as a transporter of selenium. Selenium is used in the synthesis of these molecules in the anionic form, but in the molecules, selenium is covalently bound, as is sulfur, which it typically replaces in some of these molecules.

Tissue levels are influenced by dietary intake and reflect the geochemical environment. Regions of North America identified as low in selenium content are the Northeast, Pacific, Southwest, and the coastal plain of southeastern United States, as well as north central and eastern Canada. The lowest selenium content of soil exists in a few regions of China, especially in Keshan, where severe selenium deficiency was first reported in a human population in 1979. Other areas with low selenium content include parts of Finland and New Zealand.

Food Sources and Intakes

No comprehensive table of the selenium content of foods has been published. The selenium concentration in foods depends on the selenium content of the soil and water where the food was grown. Improvements in analytical techniques have resulted in changes being made to many earlier published data of the selenium content of foods over the last few decades. Table 5–15 and Appendix 41 list the selenium contents of some foods.

Major food sources of selenium are brazil nuts, seafoods, kidney, liver, meat, and poultry; fruits and vegetables are low in selenium content. The major food source of selenium identified by the FDA's Total Diet Study was animal flesh foods (Pennington and Young, 1991). Grains vary in selenium content depending on where they are grown.

Selenium content and GSH-Px activity in human breast milk are influenced directly by maternal selenium nutrition and by the form of selenium consumed (McGuire et al., 1993a). Plasma selenium concentrations of infants fed unsupplemented formula are lower than those of infants fed supplemented formula or human milk (McGuire et al., 1993b).

Data summarized for the FDA's Total Diet Study over the period 1982–1991 showed that the estimated median selenium intakes of both adults and children were greater than the age-specific RDAs (Pennington and Schoen, 1996). Mean intakes of 19 and 13 μg/day in men and women, respectively,

TABLE 5–15 SELENIUM CONTENT OF SELECTED FOODS

FOOD	μg
Brazil nuts, ¼ cup	380
Snapper, baked, 3 oz	148
Halibut, baked, 3 oz	113
Salmon, baked, 3 oz	70
Scallops, steamed, 3 oz	70
Clams, steamed, 20	52
Oysters, raw, ¼ cup	35
Lasagna, with meat, 1 piece	34
Wheat germ, toasted, ¼ cup	28
Molasses, blackstrap, 2 T	25
Sunflower seeds, ¼ cup	25
Granola, 1 cup	23
Ground beef, 3 oz	22
Chicken, breast, baked, 3 oz	17
Bread, whole wheat, 1 slice	16
Egg, 1	12
Milk, 2% fat, 1 cup	6
Cheese, cheddar, 1 oz	4

(From Hands ES. Food Finder: Food Sources of Vitamins and Minerals, 2nd ed. Salem, OR: ESHA Research, 1990.)

were reported in a low-selenium area of China where Keshan disease was prevalent (Yang et al., 1988). Typical diets consumed by Americans provide sufficient amounts of selenium daily both to prevent any deficiency of selenium and also to promote health (Levander et al., 1995). Selenium fortification of infant formulas with selenate has been shown to improve the selenium status of preterm infants (Tyrala et al., 1996).

Recommended Dietary Allowances

The RDAs for selenium were defined for the first time in the 1989 RDA as 55 and 70 μg for adult women and men, respectively, and 40 to 50 μg/day for adolescents. The RDA for children is 20 to 30 μg/day, whereas the RDA for infants is 10 to 15 μg/day. Pregnancy increases the RDA by 10 μg, and lactation increases it still further (see Table 5–5). Requirements may increase with the increased consumption of unsaturated fatty acids in the diet because of the need for the antioxidant activity of selenium.

Absorption, Transport, Storage, and Excretion

Absorption of selenium, which occurs in the upper segment of the small intestine, is more efficient under conditions of deficiency. Increased intake frequently results in increased excretion of selenium in the urine.

Selenium status is assessed by measuring selenium or GSH-Px in serum, platelets, and erythrocytes, or selenium in whole blood or urine. Erythrocyte selenium measurement is an indicator of long-term intake.

TRANSPORT IN BLOOD

Selenium is transported bound to albumin initially, and subsequently, bound to alpha$_2$-globulin.

Functions

Many, but not all, of the pathologic changes observed in selenium deficiency can be explained on the basis of inadequate levels of GSH-Px. Because GSH-Px acts together with other antioxidants and free radical scavengers, these molecules reduce cellular peroxides and free radicals, in general, to water and other harmless molecules.

In animal studies, selenium deficiency results in low plasma T_3 levels, but the mechanism of this interrelationship has not been described (Olin et al., 1994). The level of the selenium-containing enzyme, type I iodothyronine-5-iodinase, in thyroid cells may be too low to generate sufficient amounts of T_3.

The antioxidant effects of selenium and vitamin E may reinforce each other by the overlap of their protective actions against oxidative damage. These two antioxidant nutrients may participate in other cooperative activities that help maintain healthy cells. GSH-Px acts in both the cytosol and the mitochondrial matrix, whereas vitamin E exerts its antioxidative actions within cell membranes.

The GSH-Px reaction step is illustrated in Figure 5–14. Other selenium-dependent enzymes exist in mammalian systems, but less is known about the requirements of these enzymes for selenium.

Deficiency

Despite a wide range of selenium intakes from food, selenium deficiency is rare in humans. Based on information obtained from children receiving TPN, manifestations of selenium deficiency take years to develop, and repletion generally occurs within weeks or months (Litov and Combs, 1991).

Severe selenium deficiency in a population has only been reported for the Keshan region of China, but in another region of China, a severe selenium deficiency combined with a viral disease has also been reported. These two human diseases occur in areas where the content of selenium in the soil is very low. *Keshan disease,* a form of cardiomyopathy that mainly affects children and women, was first observed in the Keshan province of China. Since its discovery, supplementation programs in Keshan have totally eradicated the disease. In individuals with established disease, the response to supplementation is poor, probably because of other factors contributing to the myopathy.

The second selenium deficiency disease, discovered in Mongolia, is known as *Kashin-Beck disease* and is common in preadolescent and adolescent children. This disease has a viral component in which the virus flourishes in the absence (or low content) of selenium in the diet (Beck et al., 1994, 1995). Illness initially involves symmetrical stiffness, swelling, and, often, pain in the interphalangeal joints of the fingers, followed by a generalized osteoarthritis in which elbows, knees, and ankles are also involved (Sokoloff, 1988). Kashin-Beck disease may also have iodine deficiency as a risk factor. (Moreno-Reyes et al., 1998.)

Selenium deficiency has occasionally been reported in malnourished patients receiving long-term TPN (Brown et al., 1986). Children receiving TPN

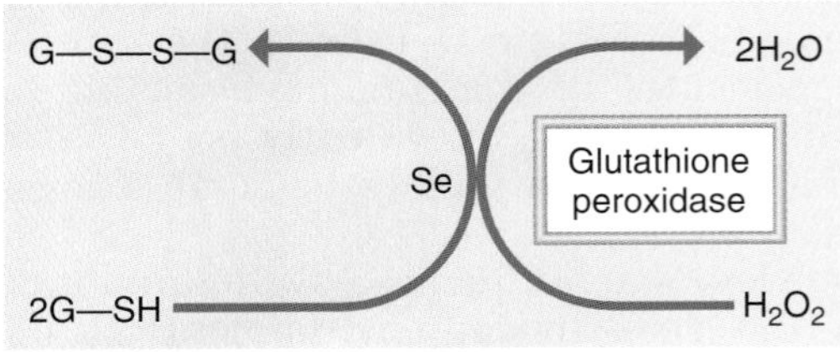

FIGURE 5–14 The enzymatic reaction catalyzed by the selenium-containing enzyme, glutathione peroxidase. Selenium is a prosthetic form of the enzyme that removes highly reactive hydrogen peroxide (H_2O_2) from within cells by converting it to water (H_2O), while at the same time converting two molecules of reduced glutathione (G-SH) to oxidized glutathione (G-S-S-G)

for up to 4 years have exhibited muscle weakness, pain, and tenderness, and elevated serum transaminase levels (Kien and Ganther, 1983; Vinton et al., 1987). Selenium supplementation resulted in improved serum selenium levels, and it also improved the clinical symptoms. Platelet GSH-Px activity was higher in patients receiving TPN when they were also receiving selenium supplementation than when the supplement was discontinued (Sando et al., 1992). Selenium deficiency should no longer be a problem in patients receiving long-term TPN or enteral nutrition because the preparation of these solutions now includes a trace element supplement. Insufficient intakes of selenium in patients with cystic fibrosis suggest that supplementation should be considered after any underlying malnutrition is assessed (Dworkin et al., 1987) (see Chapter 37).

Deficient selenium intakes may also contribute to carcinogenesis. Patients with some cancers have been shown to have low serum selenium levels, although the underlying mechanisms for this correlation have not been established. One possible mechanism is the failure of GSH-Px to scavenge free radicals efficiently in dividing cells. Epidemiologic analyses of population data to determine the relationship between low selenium intakes and cancer have been conflicting, and no conclusions can be drawn from these studies at this time.

Toxicity

Indicators of selenium toxicity and the level of dietary intake at which toxicity occurs have only been reported in China. Signs of toxicity, referred to as selenosis, include skin and nail changes, decay of teeth, and neurologic abnormalities.

Manganese

Manganese deficiency in humans was first reported in 1972, and the essentiality of this trace element in humans is well established. Symptoms of deficiency are weight loss; transient dermatitis; occasionally, nausea and vomiting; changes in hair color, and slow growth of hair and beard. Manganese deficiency in animals also affects reproductive capacity, pancreatic function, and several aspects of carbohydrate metabolism.

Food Sources and Intakes

The manganese content of foods varies greatly. The richest sources are whole grains, legumes, nuts, and tea. Fruits and vegetables are moderate sources. Animal tissues, seafood, and dairy products are poor sources. Relatively high amounts occur in instant coffee and tea. Human milk is relatively low in manganese.

The Total Diet Study of the FDA over the period 1962–1991 revealed that the median manganese intakes approximated the ESADDIs for adult men and women, but they were below the ESADDI for adolescent girls (Pennington and Schoen, 1996). Based on the apparent lack of manganese deficiency in the population, however, these intakes appear to be sufficient (Food and Nutrition Board, 1989).

Estimated Safe and Adequate Daily Dietary Intakes

In 1989, an ESADDI in the range of 2 to 5 mg/day was established for manganese for adults and children 11 years of age and older. For children, 1 to 3 mg/day is suggested depending on age (see Table 5–6).

Absorption, Transport, Storage, and Excretion

Manganese is absorbed throughout the small intestine. Iron and cobalt compete for common binding sites for absorption. Men absorb less manganese than women, a difference which may be related to iron status according to a study by Finley et al., (1994). In this study, manganese absorption was significantly associated with plasma ferritin; in another study, though (Greger et al., 1990) it was not found to correlate with serum iron concentrations in men. In young women, heme iron has no influence on manganese status, but diets high in nonheme iron were associated with lower serum manganese values, higher urinary manganese losses, and somewhat lower activity of a manganese-dependent enzyme, superoxide dismutase (Davis et al., 1992). Manganese is transported bound to a macroglobin, transferrin, and transmanganin. Excretion of manganese occurs mainly in the feces after secretion into the intestine via the bile.

Functions

The 10 to 20 mg of manganese contained in the adult human body tends to be concentrated predominantly in tissues rich in mitochondria. Manganese is a component of many enzymes, including glutamine synthetase, pyruvate carboxylase, and mitochondrial superoxide dismutase. In addition, manganese activates many other enzymes, most of which can also be activated by magnesium. Manganese is associated with the formation of connective and skeletal tissues, growth and reproduction, and carbohydrate and lipid metabolism.

Deficiency

The FDA Total Diet Study reported that manganese intakes were below recommended levels for adolescent girls (Pennington and Schoen, 1996), but no physiologic evidence of insufficiency has been reported. Data on the physiologic effects resulting from manganese deficiency are confined to the results of animal studies. These studies have established the essentiality of manganese for reproduction. Sterility occurs in both sexes; striking skeletal abnormalities and ataxia characterize the offspring of manganese-deficient mothers.

Toxicity

Manganese toxicity has occurred in miners as a result of absorption of manganese through the respiratory tract. The excess, which accumulates in the liver and CNS, produces Parkinson-like symptoms.

Chromium

A biologic role for chromium was first proposed in 1954. Chromium was not accepted as an essential nutrient until 1977, however, when patients receiving TPN exhibited abnormalities of glucose metabolism that were reversed by chromium supplementation. The low concentrations of chromium in food, body tissues, and body fluids have required careful and appropriate analytical techniques and new standard reference materials for accurate measurements.

Food Sources and Intakes

Precise assessment of chromium in foods is difficult; biologically available chromium and inorganic chromium cannot be distinguished from each other. Analyses done before 1980 must be viewed with caution because determinations were flawed by contamination and analytical problems.

Brewer's yeast, oysters, liver, and potatoes have high chromium concentrations; seafoods, whole grains, cheeses, chicken, meats, and bran are intermediate in chromium content. The refining of wheat removes chromium along with the germ and the bran; refining sugar fractionates the chromium into the molasses portion. Dairy products, fruits, and vegetables are low in chromium. Table 5–16 presents the chromium composition of selected foods.

TABLE 5–16 CHROMIUM CONTENT OF SELECTED FOODS

FOOD	(μg)
Broccoli, 1 cup	22.0
Turkey, leg, 3 oz	10.4
Juice, grape, 1 cup	7.5
Waffle, egg, 1	6.7
Ham, 3 oz	3.6
English muffin, 1	3.6
Cookies, chocolate chip, 1 large	3.4
Potatoes, mashed, 1 cup	2.7
Bagel, egg, 1	2.5
Juice, orange, 1 cup	2.2
Green beans, 1 cup	2.2
Beef cubes, 3 oz	2.0
Lettuce, 1 wedge	1.8
Barbecue sauce, 1 T	1.7
Ketchup, 1 T	1.0
American cheese, 1 oz	0.56
Maple syrup, 1 T	0.5

(From Anderson RA, Bryden NA, Polansky MM. Dietary chromium intake. Biol Trace Elem Res 32:117, 1992.)

Usual chromium intakes range between 25 and 35 μg/day for women and men, respectively. Chromium intakes are not assessed in the USDA, NHANES, or Total Diet Study surveys because of inadequate methodology.

Human breast milk, which has been analyzed according to carefully controlled conditions with appropriate standards, contains 3 to 8 nmol/L. According to Anderson et al. (1993), it is virtually impossible for exclusively breast-fed infants to obtain the current ESADDI for chromium. (The concentration of chromium in human breast milk is independent of the concentrations typically found in foods, serum, and urine.)

Estimated Safe and Adequate Daily Dietary Intake

The ESADDI for chromium is 50 to 200 μg/day for persons 7 years of age and older. Depending on the age of the child, an ESADDI of 10 to 120 μg/day has been established for younger children and infants (see Table 5–6).

Absorption, Transport, Storage, and Excretion

As with other minerals, organic and inorganic forms of chromium are absorbed differently. Organic chromium is readily absorbed, but quickly passes out of the body. Less than 2% of the trivalent chromium consumed is absorbed. Chromium absorption is increased by oxalate and is higher in iron-deficient animals than in animals with adequate iron status. The latter suggests a commonality with an iron absorption pathway. Chromium absorption reaches a plateau, where it remains at dietary intakes of 40 μg or more per day; at such high intakes, urinary excretion increases to maintain balance. Absorption from chromium chloride is modified by the type of dietary carbohydrate consumed; starch, rather than sugar, increases absorption. The absorption of chromium ions from chromium picolinate is greater than that from chromium chloride, whose absorption efficiency is 2% or less.

Both chromium and iron are carried by transferrin; however, albumin is also capable of assuming this role if iron transferrin saturation is high. Alpha- and beta-globulins and lipoproteins can also bind chromium.

Inorganic chromium is excreted primarily by the kidney, with small amounts being excreted through hair, sweat, and bile. Organic chromium is excreted through bile. Strenuous exercise, physical trauma, or an increased intake of simple sugar results in increased chromium excretion.

Functions

Chromium potentiates insulin action and, as such, influences carbohydrate, lipid, and protein metabolism. Although the chemical nature of the relationship between chromium and the activity of insulin has not been clearly identified, chromium may have a beneficial effect on serum triglyceride levels in patients with non–insulin-dependent diabetes mellitus (Lee and Reasner, 1994).

The proposed role of chromium in a so-called **glucose tolerance factor** is controversial. A possible chromium–nicotinic acid complex has been identified, but its structure has not been established by modern chemical techniques (Baumgartner, 1993). Chromium may regulate synthesis of a molecule that potentiates insulin action. Another possible role for chromium, similar to that of zinc, is in the regulation of gene expression.

Deficiency

Chromium deficiency results in insulin resistance and a few lipid abnormalities, which can be ameliorated by chromium supplementation. Insufficient chromium intakes may occur in the United States, but true deficiency is more likely to be significant in populations with very low chromium intakes, such as in some areas of China (Anderson et al., 1997a). Early in the development and use of TPN, some individuals receiving TPN showed impaired glucose tolerance or hyperglycemia with glycosuria and refractiveness to insulin (Freund et al., 1979; Jeejeebhoy et al., 1977). Deficiency of chromium in animals includes impaired growth, elevated serum cholesterol and triglyceride concentrations, increased incidence of aortic plaques, corneal lesions, and decreased fertility and sperm count.

Recent claims that the ingestion of high doses of chromium (as chromium picolinate) will improve strength, body composition, endurance, or other characteristics of physical fitness are controversial with some studies supporting these claims and others not (Anderson, 1998). Lukaski et al. (1996) found no benefits derived from chromium supplements in terms of body composition or strength in healthy men. However, both acute and chronic resistive exercise did increase urinary chromium losses in men who consumed the American Heart Association Phase I diet (with no supplements) (Rubin et al., 1998). The investigators concluded that these losses indicated increased absorption of chromium over the 16-week study.

Molybdenum

Molybdenum has been established as an essential micronutrient, particularly because of its requirement in the enzyme xanthine oxidase. Interrelationships between molybdenum, copper, and sulfate absorption in livestock, and between molybdenum intake and copper excretion in both humans and animals, have been demonstrated. Individuals receiving long-term TPN have displayed symptoms of molybdenum deficiency, including mental changes and abnormalities of sulfur and purine metabolism.

Food Sources and Intakes

Molybdenum is distributed widely in commonly used foods, such as legumes, whole-grain cereals, milk and milk products, and dark green leafy vegetables. Estimated intakes, as determined by the FDA's Total Diet Study, ranged from 50 μg/day in infants to 80 and 126 μg/day for 14- to 16-year-old girls and boys, respectively. These intakes were found to decrease slowly over the lifetime of the subjects to 74 and 101 μg/day for 60- to 65-year-old women and men, respectively (Pennington and Jones, 1987).

Estimated Safe and Adequate Daily Dietary Intakes

The daily requirements for molybdenum across the life cycle are not known. However, the 1989 ESADDIs range from 75 to 250 μg/day for adolescents and adults, and depending on age, from 25 to 150 μg/day for children (see Table 5–6).

Absorption, Transport, Storage, and Excretion

Molybdenum, which is found in minute amounts in the body, is readily absorbed from the stomach and small intestine, with the rate of absorption being higher in the proximal small intestine than in the distal small intestine. As with other minerals, molybdenum is absorbed by two mechanisms: carrier mediated and passive diffusion. Molybdenum is excreted primarily in the urine. Excretion, rather than absorption, is the homeostatic mechanism. Some molybdenum is also excreted in the bile.

Functions

Xanthine oxidase, aldehyde oxidase, and sulfite oxidase, all enzymes that catalyze oxidation-reduction reactions, require a prosthetic group containing molybdenum. Sulfite oxidase is important to the degradation of cysteine and methionine and also catalyzes the formation of sulfate from sulfite. Genetic sulfite oxidase deficiency is a fatal disorder of cysteine metabolism. Clinical symptoms include severe brain damage with mental retardation, dislocation of the lens, and increased urinary output of sulfate (Rajagopalan, 1987). Whether or not molybdenum is involved in the response of some asthmatics to sulfites is not known.

Deficiency

Molybdenum deficiency has not been established in humans except for patients treated with TPN. Symptoms of molybdenum deficiency include mental changes and abnormalities of sulfur and purine metabolism.

Toxicity

An excessive molybdenum intake of 10 to 15 mg/day is associated with a gout-like syndrome (Nielsen, 1996). However, there are no good biomarkers to accurately assess the presence of manganese excess (Greger, 1997).

Boron

The essentiality of boron for humans has not yet been established, but its essentiality for plants and animals is widely accepted. Boron, an ultratrace element, is obtained from foods as sodium borate, and it is rapidly and almost completely (90%) absorbed. The highest concentrations of boron are found in bone, spleen, and thyroid, although it is present in all other tissues of the body. The roles of boron in humans have not been well studied, and clinical entities of severe deficiency of boron have not been established (Nielsen, 1996). Additional studies of this ultratrace element, especially its relationship to bone metabolism, are being conducted.

Food Sources

Foods that are good sources of boron include plant foods, especially noncitrus fruits, leafy vegetables, nuts, and legumes. Wine, cider, and beer are other good sources.

Recommended Intakes

No recommended intakes have been established for boron.

Functions

Boron is associated with cell membranes and, in plants, is involved with the functional efficiency of cell membranes. Response to boron deprivation is enhanced when other nutrients that alter membrane functions are also deficient. Boron apparently binds to the active site of some enzymes, reducing their ability to function. Boron is also thought to compete with some enzymes for the coenzyme nicotinamide adenine dinucleotide.

Evidence from animal studies shows that boron deprivation affects two major organs: the brain and bone. With boron deficiency, brain composition and function are altered, and bone composition, structure, and strength are reduced. Because of the role of boron in bone, studies in humans have focused on its potential role in the development of osteoporosis. Some evidence suggests that boron may have actions similar to estrogens on bone (Nielsen, 1996) (see Chapter 28). One report involving a rodent model has suggested that boron may actually improve bone strength (Chapin et al., 1997).

Deficiency and Toxicity

Boron deficiency has not been reported in humans. No toxicity has been established either.

Cobalt

Most of the cobalt in the body appears with vitamin B_{12} stores in the liver. Blood plasma contains approximately 1 μg of cobalt per 100 mL.

Food Sources and Intakes

Cobalt occurs in foods; however, only microorganisms are able to synthesize vitamin B_{12}. Ruminant animals obtain cobalamin as the result of a symbiotic relationship with the microorganisms of their gastrointestinal tract. The microorganisms of monogastric species, such as humans, have an extremely limited capacity for synthesis in areas where the vitamin can be absorbed; therefore, humans must obtain vitamin B_{12}—and thus, cobalt—from animal foods, such as organ and muscle meats. In some circumstances, ordinary bacterial contamination of foods of vegetable origin may supply the minute amounts of this vitamin required for normal function. The 1984 Total Diet Survey estimated cobalt intakes of the American population to be in the range of 6.3 to 10.8 μg/day for adults and 7.6 to 11.6 μg/day for 14- to 16-year-olds (Pennington and Jones, 1987).

Strict vegetarians who avoid all animal products may become deficient in vitamin B_{12}. However, the deficiency may develop only after 3 to 6 years, or not at all.

Absorption, Transport, Storage, and Excretion

Cobalt may share at least part of the same intestinal transport mechanism as iron. Absorption is increased in patients with deficient iron intake, portal cirrhosis with iron overload, and idiopathic hemochromatosis. The major route of cobalt excretion is the urine; small amounts are excreted via feces, sweat, and hair.

Functions

The only known essential role of cobalt is as a component of *vitamin B_{12} (cobalamin)*. This vitamin is essential for the maturation of red blood cells and the normal function of all cells, not just red blood cells (see Chapters 4 and 35).

Dietary Reference Intakes

The dietary requirement for cobalt is expressed in terms of vitamin B_{12}. Approximately 2 to 3 μg of vitamin B_{12} is needed daily. (See Chapter 4 and Table 4–26 for the DRIs).

Deficiency

A deficiency of cobalt occurs only as it is related to a vitamin B_{12} deficiency. Insufficient vitamin B_{12} causes a macrocytic anemia. A genetic defect limit-

TABLE 5–17 MINERALS IN HUMAN NUTRITION

MINERAL	LOCATION IN BODY AND SELECTED BIOLOGIC FUNCTIONS	RDA, AI, OR ESADDI FOR ADULTS	FOOD SOURCES	LIKELIHOOD OF DEFICIENCY
Macronutrients Essential at Daily Levels of 100 mg or More				
Calcium	99% in bones and teeth Ionic calcium in body fluids is essential for ion transport across cell membranes. Calcium may also be bound to protein, citrate, or inorganic acids.	AI is 1000 mg for women and men 19–50 yrs 1200 mg for women and men 51+ yrs.	Milk and milk products, sardines, clams, oysters, kale, turnip greens, mustard greens, tofu	Dietary surveys indicate that many diets do not meet AIs for calcium. Because bone serves as a homeostatic mechanism to maintain calcium levels in the blood, many essential functions are maintained, regardless of dietary intake. Long-term dietary deficiency is probably one of the factors responsible for development of osteoporosis later in life.
Phosphorus	About 80% in inorganic portion of bones and teeth Phosphorus is a component of every cell, as well as of important metabolites, including DNA, RNA, ATP, and phospholipids. Phosphorus is also important to pH regulation.	RDA is 700 mg	Cheese, egg yolk, milk, meat, fish, poultry, whole-grain cereals, legumes, nuts	Dietary inadequacy is not likely if protein and calcium intake are adequate.
Magnesium	About 50% is located in bone; the remaining 50% is almost entirely inside body cells, with only about 1% located in extracellular fluid. Ionic Mg functions as an activator of many enzymes and so influences almost all body processes.	RDA is 400–420 mg for men, 310–320 mg for women, aged 14–70+ y	Whole-grain cereals, tofu, nuts, meat, milk, green vegetables, legumes, chocolate	Dietary inadequacy is considered unlikely, but conditioned deficiency is often seen in clinical medicine, usually associated with surgery, alcoholism, malabsorption, loss of body fluids, and certain hormonal and renal diseases.
Sodium	30%–45% in bone; major cation of extracellular fluid; only a small amount found inside cells Regulates body fluid osmolarity, pH, and body fluid volume	500–3000 mg	Common table salt, seafoods, animal foods, milk, eggs; abundant in most foods except fruit	Dietary inadequacy probably never occurs, although low blood sodium levels require treatment in certain clinical disorders. Sodium restriction may be necessary in certain cardiovascular and renal disorders.
Chloride	Mostly present in extracellular fluid; < 15% inside cells Major anion of extracellular fluid, functioning in combination with sodium Serves as a buffer and enzyme activator and is a component of gastric hydrochloric acid.	750–3000 mg	Common table salt, seafoods, milk, meat, eggs	In most cases, dietary intake has little significance except in the presence of vomiting, diarrhea, or profuse sweating, under which conditions a deficiency may develop.
Potassium	Major cation of intracellular fluid, with only small amounts in extracellular fluid Functions in regulating pH and osmolarity, and in cell membrane transfer. Ion is necessary for carbohydrate and protein metabolism.	2000 mg	Fruits, milk, meat, cereals, vegetables, legumes	Dietary inadequacy unlikely, but conditioned deficiency may be found in individuals with kidney disease, diabetic acidosis, excessive vomiting, diarrhea, or sweating. Potassium excess may be a problem in renal failure and severe acidosis.
Sulfur	Bulk of dietary sulfur is present in sulfur-containing amino acids needed for synthesis of essential metabolites. Functions in oxidation-reduction reactions. Sulfur also functions as part of thiamin and biotin, and as inorganic sulfur.	The need for sulfur is satisfied by essential sulfur-containing amino acids.	Protein foods, such as meat, fish, poultry, eggs, milk, cheese, legumes, nuts	Dietary intake is chiefly from sulfur-containing amino acids, and adequacy is related to protein intake.

(*continued*)

TABLE 5–17 MINERALS IN HUMAN NUTRITION (continued)

Macronutrients Essential at Daily Levels of a Few Milligrams				
Iron	About 70% in hemoglobin; about 25% stored in liver, spleen, and bone Iron is a component of hemoglobin and myoglobin, and is important in oxygen transfer. It is also present in serum transferrin and certain enzymes. Almost none occurs in ionic form.	10 mg for men, 15 mg for women	Liver, meat, egg yolk, legumes, whole or enriched grains, dark green vegetables, dark molasses, shrimp, oysters	Iron deficiency anemia occurs in women of reproductive age and in infants and preschool children. Deficiency may be associated in some cases, with unusual blood loss, parasites, or malabsorption. Anemia is the last effect of a deficient state.
Zinc	Present in most tissues, with greatest amounts occurring in the liver, voluntary muscle, and bone A constituent of many enzymes and of insulin, zinc is important in nucleic acid metabolism.	15 mg for men, 12 mg for women	Oysters, shellfish, herring, liver, legumes, milk, wheat bran	The extent of dietary zinc inadequacy in this country is not known. Conditioned deficiency may be seen in systemic childhood illnesses and in patients who are nutritionally depleted or who have been subjected to severe stress, such as surgery.
Copper	Found in all body tissues with the bulk located in the liver, brain, heart, and kidney Constituent of enzymes and of ceruloplasmin and erythrocuprein in blood. May be an integral part of DNA or RNA molecule	1.5–3 mg	Liver, shellfish, whole grains, cherries, legumes, kidney, poultry, oysters, chocolate, nuts	There is no evidence that specific deficiencies of copper occur in humans. Menkes' disease is a genetic disorder resulting in copper deficiency.
Iodine	Constituent of T_4 and related compounds synthesized by thyroid gland T_4 functions in the control of reactions involving cellular energy.	150 μg	Iodized table salt, seafoods, water and vegetables in non-goitrous regions	Iodization of table salt is recommended, especially in areas where food is low in iodine.
Manganese	Highest concentration in bone; also relatively high concentrations in pituitary, liver, pancreas, and gastrointestinal tissue Constituent of essential enzyme systems; rich in mitochondria of liver cells.	2.5–5.0 μg	Beet greens, blueberries, whole grains, nuts, legumes, fruit, tea	Deficiency unlikely to occur in humans
Fluoride	Present in bone and in teeth In optimal amounts in water and diet, flouride reduces dental caries and may minimize bone loss.	AI is 4 mg for men; 3 mg for women	Drinking water (1 ppm), tea, coffee, rice, soybeans, spinach, gelatin, onions, lettuce	In areas where fluoride content of water is low, fluoridation of water (1 ppm) has been beneficial in reducing the incidence of dental caries.
Molybdenum	Constituent of an essential enzyme (xanthine oxidase) and of flavoproteins	75–250 μg	Legumes, cereal grains, dark green leafy vegetables, organ meats	No available information
Cobalt	Constituent of cyanocobalamin (vitamin B_{12}), occurring bound to protein in foods of animal origin Essential to the normal function of all cells, particularly cells of bone marrow and nervous and gastrointestinal systems.	2.4 mg vitamin B_{12}	Liver, kidney, oysters, clams, poultry, milk	Primary dietary inadequacy is rare except when no animal products are consumed. Deficiency states may be found in association with lack of gastric intrinsic factor, gastrectomy, or malabsorption syndromes.
Selenium	Involved in fat metabolism, vitamin E, and antioxidant functions	70 μg in men, 55 μg in women	Grains, onions, meats, milk; vegetable content varies depending on selenium content of soil	Keshan disease is a selenium-deficient state. Deficiency has occurred in patients receiving long-term TPN without selenium supplementation.
Chromium	Associated with glucose metabolism	50–200 mcg	Corn oil, clams, whole-grain cereals, brewers' yeast, meats, drinking water, (variable)	Deficiency is found in severe malnutrition, states and may be factor in diabetes in the elderly and in cardiovascular diseases.

AI, adequate intake; *ATP*, adenosine triphosphate; *ESADDI*, estimated safe and adequate daily dietary intake; *RDA*, Recommended Dietary Allowance; *TPN*, total parenteral nutrition.

ing vitamin B_{12} absorption results in pernicious anemia, which is treated appropriately with massive doses of the vitamin. These forms of anemia are discussed in detail in Chapter 35.

Toxicity

A high intake of inorganic cobalt (free from cobalamin) in animal diets produces polycythemia (overproduction of red blood cells), hyperplasia of bone marrow, reticulocytosis, and increased blood volume.

The information on the microminerals (trace elements) known to be required by humans is summarized in Table 5–17. Fortification of ready-to-eat cereals has had a significant impact on the nutritional status of those living in the United States; preschool and school children who consume these cereals have improved health status according to standard indicators. The extent of the benefits of these nutritionally enhanced foods has not yet been evaluated fully.

Of the several trace elements, only a few—copper, zinc, and iron—have been found to be consistently deficient in the diets of those living in the United States. (In the United States, ready-to-eat cereals are now fortified with all three of these elements, so this situation may be remedied in the future.) Other trace elements, such as chromium and manganese, may also be consumed in inadequate amounts, but the evidence in support of the prevalence of these deficiencies is not sufficiently strong. The only micronutrient associated with concern about toxicity is fluoride. This concern is focused on the potential development of fluorosis in infants and children (see Chapter 29).

CASE STUDY

Miles P. is a 46-year-old Native American man with a history of high blood pressure (140/95), elevated serum cholesterol levels (240 mg/dL), and hypothyroidism. He currently takes a small dose of thyroid replacement hormone and a mild potassium-depleting diuretic. He has purchased an exercise bike for indoor use and has started a walking program. Other than increasing his activity levels, he plans to avoid all table salt and has become an avid label reader when he shops for groceries.

1. What concerns do you have about his intake of iodine, given his resolve to avoid table salt? From what other foods might he derive sufficient iodine?
2. His usual diet, which is low in fruits and vegetables, is likely to contain an insufficient amount of which minerals? What suggestions do you have for increasing the intake of these minerals?
3. He drinks very little milk. What would you recommend to increase his dietary calcium intake?
4. Fluoridated water is not available to Miles. Does this concern you?

OTHER TRACE ELEMENTS

Several other trace elements of uncertain essentiality exist in this class, including silicon, vanadium, aluminum, arsenic, tin, lithium, and nickel. A few other ultratrace elements may also be added to this list in the future. They are classified as ultratrace elements because of their very low quantities in human tissues. Requirements remain undefined for all of these elements because of their uncertain essentiality. The ultratrace elements remain enigmas because of their uncertain roles in human function. It has long been established that these elements exist in human tissues, especially in the skeleton, because of their abundance in the earth's surface, but the essentiality of any of these in humans remains questionable. These ultratrace elements have been reviewed by Nielsen (1996). The presence of several of these elements in various foods has been reported in the Total Diet Study of the FDA (Pennington and Jones, 1987).

CITED REFERENCES

Abrams SA, Stuff JE. Calcium metabolism in girls: Current dietary intakes lead to low rates of calcium absorption and retention during puberty. Am J Clin Nutr 60:739, 1994.

Alaimo K, et al. Dietary intake of vitamins, minerals and fiber of persons ages 2 months and over in the United States: Third National Health and Nutrition Examination Survey. Phase 1, 1988–91. Advance data from vital and health statistics; No 258. Hyattsville, MD: National Center for Health Statistics, 1994.

Alnwick D. Weekly iodine supplements work. Am J Clin Nutr 67:1103, 1998.

American Dietetic Association. Position of the American Dietetic Association: The impact of fluoride on dental health. J Am Diet Assoc 94:1428, 1994.

Anderson JJB. Calcium, phosphorus and human bone devlopment. J Nutr 126:1153S, 1996.

Anderson JJB. Nutritional biochemistry of calcium and phosphorus. J Nutr Biochem 2:300, 1991.

Anderson JJB, Barrett CJH. Dietary phosphorus: The benefits and the problems. Nutr Today 29(2):29, 1994.

Anderson JJB, Garner SC (eds.). Calcium and Phosphorus in Health and Disease. Boca Raton, FL: CRC Press, 1996.

Anderson JJB, et al. Nutrition and bone in physical activity and sport. In: Wolinsky I (ed.). Nutrition in Exercise and Sport, 3rd ed. Boca Raton, FL: CRC Press, 1998, p. 219.

Anderson RA. Chromium as an essential nutrient for humans. Reg Toxicol Pharmacol 26:S35, 1997a.

Anderson RA. Nutritional factors influencing the glucose/insulin system: Chromium. J Am Coll Nutr 16:404, 1997b.

Anderson RA. Effects of chromium on body composition and weight loss. Nutr Rev 56:266, 1998.

Anderson RA, et al. Breast milk chromium and its association with chromium intake, chromium excretion, and serum chromium. Am J Clin Nutr 57:519, 1993.

Anderson RA, et al. Elevated intakes of supplemental chromium improve glucose and insulin variables in individuals with type 2 diabetes. Diabetes 46:1786, 1997.

Appel IJ, et al. A clinical study of the effects of dietary patterns on blood pressure. N Engl J Med 336:1117, 1997.

Argiratos V, Samman S. The effect of calcium carbonate and calcium citrate on the absorption of zinc in healthy female subjects. Eur J Clin Nutr 48:198, 1994.

Bahl R, et al. Plasma zinc as a predictor of diarrheal and respiratory morbidity in children in an urban slum setting. Am J Clin Nutr 68:414S, 1998.

Barger-Lux MJ, et al. Nutritional correlates of low calcium intake. Clin Appl Nutr 2:39, 1992.

Baumgartner T. Trace elements in clinical nutrition. Nutr Clin Pract 8:251, 1993.

Beard JL, et al. Iron in the brain. Nutr Rev 51:157, 1993.

Beck M, et al. Increased virulence of human enterovirus (coxsackievirus B3) in selenium-deficient mice. J Infect Dis 170:351, 1994.

Beck M, et al. Rapid genomic evolution of a non-virulent coxsackievirus B3 in selenium-deficient mice results in selection of identical virulent isolates. Nature Med 1:433, 1995.
Black MR, et al. Zinc supplements and serum lipids in young adult white males. Am J Clin Nutr 47:970, 1988.
Borch-Iohnsen B, et al. High bioavailability to humans of supplemental iron in a whey concentrate product. Nutr Res 14:1643, 1994.
Boukaïba N, et al. A physiological amount of zinc supplementation: Effects on nutritional, lipid and thymus status of an elderly population. Am J Clin Nutr 57:566, 1993.
Brewer GJ, et al. Does a vegetarian diet control Wilson's disease? J Am Coll Nutr 12:527, 1993.
Brown MR, et al. Proximal muscle weakness and selenium deficiency associated with long-term parenteral nutrition. Am J Clin Nutr 43:549, 1986.
Buchman AL, et al. Copper deficiency secondary to a copper transport defect: A new copper metabolic disturbance. Metabolism 12:1462, 1994.
Calvo MS, et al. Persistently elevated parathyroid hormone secretion and action in young women after four weeks of ingesting high phosphorus, low calcium diets. J Clin Endocrinol Metab 70:1340, 1990.
Calvo MS, Park YM. Changing phosphorus content of the U.S. diet: Potential for adverse effects on bone. J Nutr 126:1168S, 1996.
Chapin RE, et al. Effects of dietary boron on bone strength in rats. Fund Appl Toxicol 35:205, 1997.
Copper deficiency induced by megadoses of zinc. Nutr Rev 43:148, 1985.
Cordano A. Clinical manifestations of nutritional copper deficiency in infants and children. Am J Clin Nutr 67(suppl):1012S, 1998.
Crofton RW, et al. Inorganic zinc and the intestinal absorption of ferrous iron. Am J Clin Nutr 50:141, 1989.
Davis CD, et al. Interactions among dietary manganese, heme iron, and non-heme iron in women. Am J Clin Nutr 56:926, 1992.
Deehr M, et al. Effects of different calcium sources on iron absorption in postmenopausal women. Am J Clin Nutr 51:95, 1990.
Dengel JL, et al. Magnesium homeostasis: Conversion mechanism in lactating women consuming a controlled-magnesium diet. Am J Clin Nutr 59:990, 1994.
Devine A, et al. Effects of zinc and other nutritional factors on insulin-like growth factor I and insulin-like growth factor binding proteins in postmenopausal women. Am J Clin Nutr 68:200, 1998.
Devine A, et al. A longitudinal study of the effect of sodium and calcium intakes on regional bone density in postmenopausal women. Am J Clin Nutr 62:740, 1995.
Discher PWF, Girous A. Iodine content of a representative Canadian diet. J Can Diet Assoc 48:24, 1987.
Dolev E, et al. Interpretation of zinc status indicators in a strenuously exercising population. J Am Diet Assoc 95:482, 1995.
Dworkin B, et al. Low blood selenium levels in patients with cystic fibrosis compared to controls and healthy adults. J Parenter Enteral Nutr 11:38, 1987.
Fairweather-Tait SJ. Zinc in human nutrition. Nutr Res Rev 1:23, 1998.
Fairweather-Tait SJ, Hurrell RF. Bioavailability of minerals and trace elements. Nutr Res Rev 9:295, 1996.
Finley EB, Cerklewski FL. Influence of ascorbic acid supplementation on copper status in young adult men. Am J Clin Nutr 37:553, 1983.
Finley JW, et al. Sex affects manganese absorption and retention by humans from a diet adequate in manganese. Am J Clin Nutr 60:949, 1994.
Food and Nutrition Board, National Research Council, National Academy of Sciences. Recommended Dietary Allowances, 10th ed. Washington, DC: National Academy Press, 1989.
Fosmire GJ. Zinc toxicity. Am J Clin Nutr 51:225, 1990.
Freund H, et al. Chromium deficiency during total parenteral nutrition. JAMA 241:496, 1979.
Fung EB, et al. Zinc absorption in women during pregnancy and lactation: A longitudinal study. Am J Clin Nutr 66:80, 1997.
Gloth FM III, et al. Vitamin D deficiency in homebound elderly persons. JAMA 274:1683, 1995.
Gordeuk V, et al. Iron overload in Africa. N Engl J Med 326:95, 1992.
Greger JL, et al. Intake, serum concentrations, and urinary excretion of manganese by adult males. Am J Clin Nutr 51:457, 1990.
Greger JL, Malecki EA. Manganese: How do we know our limits? Nutr Today 32:116, 1997.
Gullestad L, et al. Magnesium status in healthy free-living elderly Norwegians. J Am Coll Nutr 13:45, 1994.
Hallberg L, et al. Calcium: Effect on different amounts of nonheme and heme iron absorption in humans. Am J Clin Nutr 53:112, 1991.
Halsted JA, et al. Zinc deficiency in man—The Shiraz experiment. Am J Med 43:277, 1972.
Hambidge KM, et al. Zinc nutrition of preschool children in the Denver Head Start program. Am J Clin Nutr 29:734, 1976.
Heaney RP, et al. Meal effects on calcium absorption. Am J Clin Nutr 49:372, 1989.
Hetzel B. Iodine deficiency and fetal brain damage. N Engl J Med 331:1770, 1994.
Hunt J, et al. Effect of ascorbic acid on apparent iron absorption by women with low iron stores. Am J Clin Nutr 59:1381, 1994.
Institute of Medicine, Food and Nutrition Board, National Academy of Sciences. Dietary Reference Intakes. Washington, DC: National Academy Press, 1998.
Iseri LT, French JH. Magnesium: Nature's physiologic calcium blocker. Am Heart J 108:188, 1994.
Jackman LA, et al. Calcium retention in relation to calcium intake and postmenarcheal age in adolescent females. Am J Clin Nutr 66:327, 1997.
Jeejeebhoy KN, et al. Chromium deficiency, glucose intolerance and neuropathy reversed by chromium supplementation in a patient receiving long-term total parenteral nutrition. Am J Clin Nutr 30:531, 1977.
Johnson MA, et al. Iron nutriture in elderly individuals. FASEB J 8:609, 1994.
Johnson MA, Murphy CL. Adverse effects of high dietary iron and ascorbic acid on copper status in copper-deficient and copper-adequate rats. Am J Clin Nutr 47:96, 1988.
Johnson MA, et al. Copper, iron, zinc, and manganese in dietary supplements, infant formulas, and ready-to-eat cereals. Am J Clin Nutr 67(suppl):1035S, 1998.
Kapsokefalou M, Miller DD. Lean beef and beef fat interact to enhance nonheme iron absorption in rats. J Nutr 123:1429, 1993.
Kelley DS, et al. Effects of low-copper diets on human immune response. Am J Clin Nutr 62:412, 1995.
Kelsey J L, et al. Effect of fiber from fruits and vegetables on metabolic responses of human subjects. II. Calcium, magnesium, iron, and silicon balances. Am J Clin Nutr 32:1876, 1979.
Kerstetter JE, Allen LH. Dietary protein increases urinary calcium. J Nutr 120:134, 1990.
Kien CL, Ganther HE. Manifestations of chronic selenium deficiency in a child receiving total parenteral nutrition. Am J Clin Nutr 37:319, 1983.
King JC. Do women using oral contraceptive agents require extra zinc? J Nutr 117:217, 1986.
King JC, Keen CL. Zinc. In: Shils ME, Olson JA, Shike M (eds.). Modern Nutrition in Health and Disease, vol. 1, 8th ed. Philadelphia: Lea & Febiger, 1994.
Krall EA, Dawson-Hughes B. Osteoporosis. In: Shils M, Olson JA, Shike M (eds.). Modern Nutrition in Health and Disease, 8th ed. Philadelphia: Lea & Febiger, 1994, p. 1559.
Lee N, Reasner C. Beneficial effect of chromium supplementation on serum triglyceride levels in NIDDM. Diabetes Care 17:1449, 1994.
Levander OA, et al. Vitamin E and selenium. Proc Nutr Soc 54:475, 1995.
Levenson DI, Bockman RS. A review of calcium preparations. Nutr Rev 52:221, 1994.
Levy SM, et al. Sources of fluoride intake in children. J Public Health Dent 55:39, 1995.
Litov RE, Combs GF. Selenium in pediatric nutrition. Pediatrics 87:339, 1991.
Lönnerdal B. Bioavailability of copper. Am J Clin Nutr 63:821S, 1996.
Lönnerdal B, Uauy R (eds.). Genetic and environmental determinants of copper metabolism. Am J Clin Nutr 67(suppl):951S, 1998.
Lozoff B. Has iron deficiency been shown to cause altered behavior in infants? In: Dobbins J (ed.). Brain, Behavior and Iron in the Infant Diet. New York: Springer-Verlag, 1990.
Lukaski HC, et al. Chromium supplementation and resistance training: Effects on body composition, strength, and trace element status of men. Am J Clin Nutr 63:954, 1996.
Macknin ML, et al. Zinc gluconate lozenges for treating the common cold in children. JAMA 279:1962, 1998.
Marie PJ, et al. Histological osteomalacia due to dietary calcium deficiency in children. N Engl J Med 307:584, 1982.
Matkovic V, et al. Urinary calcium, sodium, and bone mass of young females. Am J Clin Nutr 62:417,1995.
McGuire MK, et al. Selenium status of infants is influenced by supplementation of formula or maternal diets. Am J Clin Nutr 58:643, 1993a.
McGuire MK, et al. Selenium status of lactating women is affected by the form of selenium consumed. Am J Clin Nutr 58:649, 1993b.
Milne DB. Copper intake and assessment of copper status. Am J Clin Nutr 67(suppl):1041S, 1998.
Moreno-Reyes R, et al. Kashin-Beck osteoarthropathy in rural Tibet in relation to selenium and iodine status. N Engl J Med 339:112, 1998.
Moser-Veillon PB. Zinc: Consumption patterns and dietary recommendations. J Am Diet Assoc 90:1089, 1990.
New SA, et al. Nutritional influences on bone density: A cross-sectional study in premenopausal women. Am J Clin Nutr 65:1831, 1997.
Nielsen FH. Other trace elements. In: Ziegler EE, Filer LJ Jr (eds.). Present Knowledge in Nutrition, 7th ed. Washington, DC: ILSI Press, 1996.
Nordin BEC, et al. The nature and significance of the relationship between urinary sodium and urinary calcium in women. J Nutr 123:1615, 1993.
Okonofua F, et al. Rickets in Nigerian children: A consequence of calcium malnutrition. Metabolism 40:209, 1991.
Olin KL, et al. Copper deficiency affects selenoglutathione peroxidase and selenodeiodinase activities and antioxidant defenses in weanling rats. Am J Clin Nutr 59:654, 1994.

Orlov MV, et al. A review of magnesium, acute myocardial infarction and arrhythmia. J Am Coll Nutr 13:127, 1994.
Pak CYC, et al. Treatment of postmenopausal osteoporosis with slow-release sodium fluoride: Final report of a randomized controlled trial. Ann Intern Med 123:401, 1995.
Pennington JAT, Jones JW. Molybdenum, nickel, cobalt, vanadium, and strontium in total diets. J Am Diet Assoc 87:1644, 1987.
Pennington JAT, Schoen SA. Total Diet Study: Estimated dietary intakes of nutritional elements, 1982–1991. Int J Vitam Nutr Res 66:350, 1996.
Pennington JAT, Young BE. Total Diet Study nutritional elements. J Am Diet Assoc 91:179, 1991.
Pollitt E, et al. Behavioral effects of iron deficiency among preschool children in Cambridge, MA. Fed Proc 37:487, 1976.
Prasad AS. Zinc and growth and development and spectrum of human zinc deficiency. J Am Coll Nutr 7:377, 1988.
Prasad A, et al. Zinc deficiency in elderly persons. Nutrition 9:218, 1993.
Prasad AS, et al. Zinc metabolism in patients with the syndrome of iron deficiency anemia, hepatosplenomegaly, dwarfism and hypogonadism. J Lab Clin Med 61:537, 1963.
Prentice A. Does mild zinc deficiency contribute to poor growth performance? Nutr Rev 51:268, 1993.
Procopis P, et al. A milk form of Menkes' syndrome. J Pediatr 98:97, 1981.
Rajagopalan KV. Molybdenum—An essential trace element. Nutr Rev 45:321, 1987.
Rauma AL, et al. Iodine status in vegans consuming a living food diet. Nutr Res 14:1789, 1994.
Rubin MA, et al. Acute and chronic resistive exercises increase urinary chromium excretion in men as measured with an enriched chromium stable isotope. J Nutr 128:73, 1998.
Rucker RB, et al. Copper, lysyl oxidase, and extracellular matrix protein cross-linking. Am J Clin Nutr 67(suppl):996S, 1998.
Rude RK. Magnesium deficiency: A cause of heterogeneous disease in humans. J Bone Miner Res 13:749, 1998.
Rude RK. Magnesium homeostasis. In: Bilezikian JP, Raisz LG, Rodan GA (eds.). Principles of Bone Biology. San Diego: Academic Press, 1996, p. 277.
Sando K, et al. Platelet glutathione peroxidase activity in long-term parenteral nutrition with and without selenium supplementation. J Parenter Enteral Nutr 16:54, 1992.
Seelig MS, Heggtveit HA. Magnesium interrelationships in ischemic heart disease: A review. Am J Clin Nutr 27:59, 1974.
Shils ME. Magnesium. In: Shils ME, Olson JA, Shike M (eds.). Modern Nutrition in Health and Disease, 8th ed., vol. 1. Philadelphia: Lea & Febiger, 1994, p. 164.
Singer L, et al. Fluoride intake of young male adults in the United States. Am J Clin Nutr 33:328, 1980.
Soemantri AG, et al. Iron deficiency anemia and educational achievement. Am J Clin Nutr 42:1221, 1985.
Sokoloff L. Kashin-Beck disease: Current status. Nutr Rev 46:113, 1988.
Solomons NW, Cousins RJ. Zinc. In: Solomons NW, Rosenberg IH (eds.). Absorption and Malabsorption of Mineral Nutrients. New York: Alan R. Liss, 1984, p. 125.
Stendig-Lindenberg G, et al. Trabecular bone density in a two year controlled trial of peroral magnesium in osteoporosis. Magnes Res 6:155, 1993.
Stur M, et al. Oral zinc and the second eye in age-related macular degeneration. Invest Ophthalmol Vis Sci 37:1225, 1996.
Subar AF, et al. Dietary sources of nutrients among US adults, 1989 to 1991. J Am Diet Assoc 98:537, 1998.
Taylor PG, et al. Daily physiological iron requirements in children. J Am Diet Assoc 88:454, 1988.
Tonglet R, et al. Efficacy of low oral doses of iodized oil in the control of iodine deficiency in Zaire. N Engl J Med 326:236, 1992.
Tucker KL, et al. Potassium, magnesium, and fruit and vegetable intakes are associated with greater bone mineral density in older men and women. Am J Clin Nutr 69:727, 1998.
Tyrala EE, et al. Selenate fortification of infant formulas improves the selenium status of preterm infants. Am J Clin Nutr 64:860, 1996.
Uauy R, et al. Essentiality of copper in humans. Am J Clin Nutr 67(suppl):952S, 1998.
US Department of Agriculture. Continuing Survey of Food Intakes of Individuals (CSFII): Diet and Knowledge Survey 1991. Springfield, VA: US Department of Commerce, National Technical Information Service, 1994.
Vinton NE, et al. Macrocytosis and pseudoalbinism: Manifestations of selenium deficiency. J Pediatr 111:711, 1987.
Walter T. Iron deficiency in infancy: A critical review. In: Dobbins J (ed.). Brain, Behavior and Iron in the Infant Diet. New York: Springer-Verlag, 1990.
Witteman JCM, et al. Reduction of blood pressure with oral magnesium supplementation in women with mild to moderate hypertension. Am J Clin Nutr 60:129, 1994.
Wood RJ, Zheng JJ. High dietary calcium intakes reduce zinc absorption and balance in humans. Am J Clin Nutr 65:1803, 1997.
Xue-Yi C, et al. Timing of vulnerability of the brain to iodine deficiency in endemic cretinism. N Engl J Med 331:1739, 1994.
Yang G, et al. Selenium-related endemic diseases and the daily selenium requirement of humans. World Rev Nutr Diet 55:98, 1988.
Yates AA, et al. Dietary reference intakes: The new basis for recommendations for calcium and related nutrients, B vitamins, and choline. J Am Diet Assoc 98:699, 1998.

ADDITIONAL REFERENCES

Allen LH, Wood RJ. Calcium and phosphorus. In: Shils M, Olson JA, Shike M (eds.). Modern Nutrition in Health and Disease, 8th ed. Philadelphia: Lea & Febiger, 1994, p. 144.
Anderson RA, et al. Chromium intake and excretion of patients receiving total parenteral nutrition: Effects of supplemental chromium. J Trace Elem Exp Med 1:9, 1988.
Andrews NC. Iron-transport across biologic membranes. Nutr Rev 57:114, 1999.
Beinert H, Kennedy MC. Aconitase: A two-faced protein: Enzyme and iron regulatory factor. FASEB J 7:1442, 1993.
Calvo MS. Dietary phosphorus, calcium metabolism, and bone. J Nutr 123:1627, 1993.
Chandra RK. Nutrition and immunity in the elderly. Nutr Rev 50:367, 1992.
Chesters JK, Arthur JR. Early biochemical defects caused by dietary trace element deficiencies. Nutr Res Rev 1:39, 1998.
Clarkson PM. Effects of exercise on chromium levels. Is supplementation required? Sports Med 23:341, 1997.
Conrad ME, et al. Alternate iron transport pathway. J Biol Chem 269:7169, 1994.
Cousins RJ. Metal elements and gene expression. Ann Rev Nutr 14:449, 1994.
Feler AG, et al. Subnormal concentrations of serum selenium and plasma carnitine in chronically tube-fed patients. Am J Clin Nutr 45:476, 1987.
Freund H, et al. Chromium deficiency during total parenteral nutrition. JAMA 241:496, 1979.
Gavin M, et al. Evidence that iron stores regulate iron absorption—A setpoint theory. Am J Clin Nutr 59:1376, 1994.
Goyer RA. Toxic and essential metal interactions. Ann Rev Nutr 17:37, 1997.
Hartz SC, et al (eds.). Nutrition in the Elderly: The Boston Nutritional Survey. London: Smith-Gordon, 1992.
Heaney RP, et al. Calcium absorbability from spinach. Am J Clin Nutr 47:707, 1988.
Heird WC, Gomez MR. Parenteral nutrition in low-birth-weight infants. Ann Rev Nutr 16:471, 1996.
Hempe JM, Cousins RJ. Cysteine-rich intestinal protein and intestinal metallothionein: An inverse relationship as a conceptual model for zinc absorption in rats. J Nutr 122:89, 1992.
Jackson JL, et al. A meta-analysis of zinc salt lozenges and the common cold. Arch Int Med 157:2373, 1997.
Johnson P, et al. Effects of age and sex on copper absorption, biological half-life and status in humans. Am J Clin Nutr 56:917, 1992.
Klimis-Tavantzis DJ. Manganese in Health and Disease. Boca Raton, FL: CRC Press, 1994.
Kok FJ, et al. Serum selenium, vitamin antioxidants and cardiovascular mortality: A 9-year follow up study in the Netherlands. Am J Clin Nutr 45:462, 1987.
Lloyd T, et al. Calcium supplementation and bone mineral density in adolescent girls. JAMA 270:841, 1993.
Massey LK, et al. Effect of dietary oxalate and calcium on urinary oxalate and risk of formation of oxalate kidney stones. J Am Diet Assoc 93:901, 1993.
Matkovic V, et al. Timing of peak bone mass in caucasian females and its implication for the prevention of osteoporosis. J Clin Invest 93:799, 1994.
Menendez C. Vitamin A and iron supplementation in pregnancy. Lancet 343:490, 1994.
Mertz W. Essential trace metals: New definitions based on new paradigms. Nutr Rev 51:2887, 1993.
Mertz W, et al (eds.). Risk Assessment of Essential Elements. Washington, DC: ILSI Press, 1994.
Mietzner TA, Morse SA. The role of iron-binding protein in the survival of pathogenic bacteria. Ann Rev Nutr 14:471, 1994.
Monsen ER. Iron nutrition and absorption: Dietary factors which impact iron bioavailability. J Am Diet Assoc 88:786, 1988.
Ophaug RH, et al. Dietary fluoride intake of 6-month and 2-year-old children in four regions of the United States. Am J Clin Nutr 42:701, 1985.
Repke JT, Villar J. Pregnancy-induced hypertension and low birth weight: The role of calcium. Am J Clin Nutr 54(suppl, pt. 1):237S, 1991.
Salonen J, et al. High stored iron levels are associated with excess risk of myocardial infarction in Eastern Finnish men. Circulation 86:803, 1992.

Seelig MS, Elin R. Is there a place for magnesium in the treatment of acute myocardial infarction? Am Heart J 132(2 pt., 2 suppl):472, 496, 1996.

Sempos C, et al. Body iron stores and the risk of coronary heart disease. N Engl J Med 330:1119, 1994.

Simon JA, et al. Calcium intake and blood pressure in elderly women. Am J Epidemiol 31:265, 1992.

Villar J, Repke JT. Calcium supplementation during pregnancy may reduce preterm delivery in high-risk populations. Am J Obstet Gynecol 163:1124, 1990.

Weaver CM, et al. Calcium absorption from foods. In: Burckhardt P, Heaney RP (eds.). Nutritional Aspects of Osteoporosis, vol. 85, Serono Symposium Series. New York: Raven Press, 1991, p. 133.

Winzerling JJ, Law JH. Comparative nutrition of iron and copper. Annu Rev Nutr 17:501, 1997.

Zarkadas M, et al. Sodium chloride supplementation and urinary calcium excretion in postmenopausal women. Am J Clin Nutr 50:1088, 1989.

Ziegler EE, Filer LJ Jr (eds.). Present Knowledge in Nutrition, 7th ed. Washington, DC: ILSI Press, 1996.

CHAPTER 6

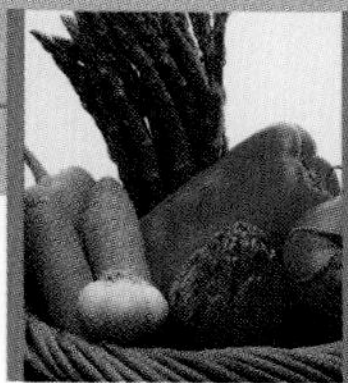

Water, Electrolytes, and Acid-Base Balance

SUSAN J. WHITMIRE, RD, CNSD

Chapter Outline

- Body Water
- Electrolytes
- Acid-Base Balance

Key Terms

ACID-BASE BALANCE—a dynamic state of equilibrium of hydrogen ion concentration in the body

ACIDOSIS—a state in which the pH of arterial blood decreases to below the normal range of 7.35 to 7.45 owing to an increase in circulating acids or a reduction in bicarbonate levels

ALKALOSIS—a state in which the pH of arterial blood exceeds the normal range of 7.35 to 7.45 owing to an increase in bicarbonate levels or a reduction in circulating acids

ANION GAP—the difference between measured cations and measured anions

BUFFER—a proton donor and acceptor system that helps preserve homeostasis of the hydrogen ion concentration

CONTRACTION ALKALOSIS—metabolic alkalosis resulting from hypovolemia; occurs when decreased blood flow to the kidneys stimulates reabsorption of water and sodium; bicarbonate is reabsorbed with the sodium, causing alkalosis

DEHYDRATION—excessive loss of body water

EDEMA—an abnormal accumulation of fluid in the intercellular tissue spaces or body cavities

ELECTROLYTE—a substance that dissociates into positively and negatively charged ions when dissolved in water

EXTRACELLULAR FLUID (ECF)—water and dissolved substances occupying spaces outside the cell

EXTRACELLULAR WATER (ECW)—water in the plasma, lymph, spinal fluid, and secretions

HYPERTONIC—a term describing a solution that, when bathing body cells, causes a net flow of water across the semipermeable cell membrane out of the cell

HYPOTONIC—a term describing a solution that, when bathing body cells, causes a net flow of water across the semipermeable cell membrane into the cell

INSENSIBLE WATER LOSS—water that is lost inperceptibly, such as when air is expired from the lungs or when water vapor escapes the skin's surface

INTERCELLULAR (INTERSTITIAL) WATER—water between and around the cells

INTRACELLULAR FLUID (ICF)—water and dissolved substances contained within the cell

INTRACELLULAR WATER (ICW)—water contained within the cell

METABOLIC ACIDOSIS—acidosis caused by an increase in circulating noncarbonic acids and/or an excessive loss of bicarbonate

METABOLIC ALKALOSIS—alkalosis caused by an increase in circulating bicarbonate and/or an excessive loss of acid

METABOLIC WATER—water derived from the metabolism of carbohydrate, protein, or fat

ONCOTIC PRESSURE (COLLOIDAL OSMOTIC PRESSURE)—the pressure at the capillary membrane that is caused by dissolved proteins in the plasma and interstitial fluids

OSMOLALITY—a measure of the osmotically active particles per kilogram of solvent in which the particles are dispersed

OSMOLARITY—a measure of the osmotically active particles per liter of solution

OSMOTIC PRESSURE—the pressure of a solution directly related to its solute osmolar concentration

RESPIRATORY ACIDOSIS—acidosis caused by acute or chronic retention of carbon dioxide by the lungs

RESPIRATORY ALKALOSIS—alkalosis caused by increased ventilation and elimination of carbon dioxide

SENSIBLE WATER LOSS—water that is lost with urine, feces, and sweat

"THIRD SPACE" FLUIDS—fluid that is both extracellular and extravascular (e.g., in tissues and cavities), the accumulation of which results in edema

WATER INTOXICATION—a state in which excess water increases intercellular volume and dilutes body fluids

Water is closer to being a universal solvent than any other material. It is, however, more than a passive solvent; it also participates actively in biochemical reactions and provides form and structure to the cells through turgor. It also provides a means of stabilizing body temperature.

Electrolytes are substances or compounds that, when dissolved in water, dissociate into positively and negatively charged ions. Electrolytes can be simple inorganic salts of sodium, potassium, or complex organic molecules.

Acid-base balance is the dynamic state of equilibrium of hydrogen ion concentration. Marked alterations in rates of chemical reactions can occur with only slight changes in hydrogen ion concentration. Protein-energy malnutrition, illness, trauma, and surgery can affect fluid, electrolyte, and acid-base balance, causing alterations in the composition and amount of tissue fluids. If these conditions are not corrected, dehydration, shock, and death can ensue.

BODY WATER

Water is the largest single component of the body. Metabolically active cells of the muscle and viscera have the highest concentration of water, whereas calcified tissue cells have the lowest. As a percentage of body weight, water varies among individuals, depending on the proportion of muscle to adipose tissue. Total body water is higher in athletes than in nonathletes, and it decreases significantly with age owing to diminished muscle mass (Fig. 6–1).

Functions of Water

Water is an essential component of all body tissues. As a solvent, it makes many solutes available for cell function and is the medium needed for all reactions. It also participates as a substrate in metabolic reactions and as a structural component providing form to cells. Water is essential to the physiologic processes of digestion, absorption, and excretion. It plays a key role in the structure and function of the circulatory system and acts as a transport medium for nutrients and all body substances. Water maintains the physical and chemical constancy of intracellular and extracellular fluids and has a direct role in maintaining body temperature. Evaporation of perspiration cools the body during warm weather; 600 kcal of body heat dissipates during the evaporation of 1 L of perspired water.

Loss of 20% of body water may cause death; loss of only 10% causes severe disorders (Fig. 6–2). In moderate weather, adults can live up to 10 days without water, and children can live up to 5 days. In contrast, it is possible to survive for several weeks without food.

Distribution of Body Water

Intracellular water (ICW) is the water contained within cells. **Extracellular water** (ECW), commonly estimated to account for 20% of body weight, includes the water in plasma, lymph, spinal fluid, and secretions, as well as the **intercellular (interstitial) water** between and around the cells. Most interstitial water is held in a gel in the intercellular

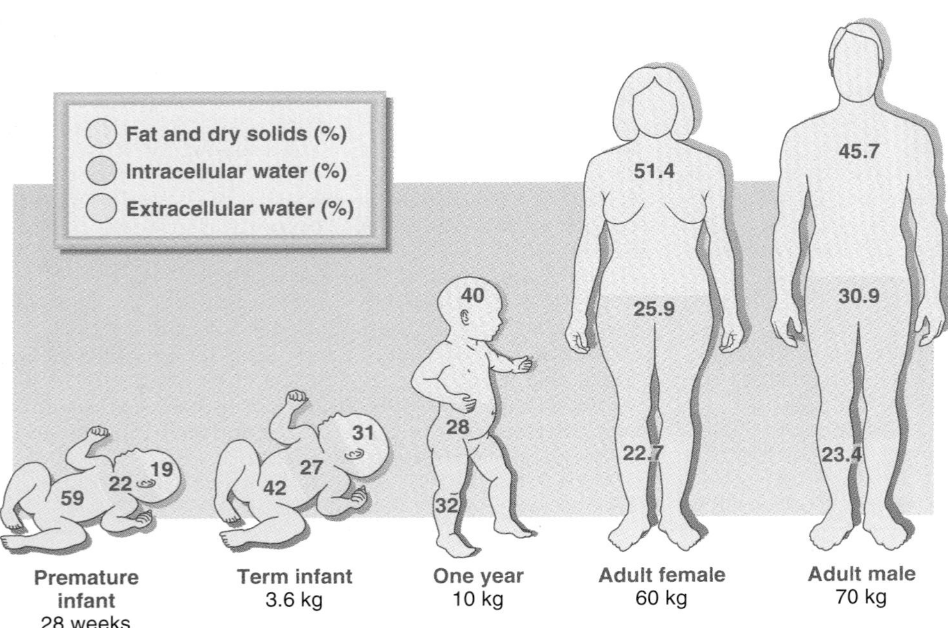

FIGURE 6–1 Distribution of body water as a percentage of body weight.

spaces and is continuous with the plasma through pores in the capillaries. Abnormal accumulation of fluid in the intercellular tissue spaces or body cavities is called **edema.**

The distribution of body water varies under different circumstances, but the total amount in the body remains relatively constant. Our understanding of body water in health and disease has improved through the use of bioelectrical impedance, a measurement of electrical conduction, to estimate body water (NIH Consensus Statement, 1996).

Water Balance

Homeostatic regulation by the gastrointestinal tract, kidneys, and brain keeps the water content of the fat-free body weight fairly constant. The amount of water taken in daily is approximately equivalent to the amount lost (Table 6–1).

Water Intake

In healthy individuals, water intake is controlled mainly by thirst. Thirst control centers are located in the ventromedial and anterior hypothalamus, close to the centers that regulate antidiuretic hormone (ADH). Thirst is stimulated when osmolality increases or extracellular volume decreases. The sensation of thirst serves as a signal to seek fluids.

Water is ingested as fluid and also as part of ingested food. The oxidation of foods in the body also produces **metabolic water** as an end product. The oxidation of 100 g of fat, carbohydrate, and protein yields 107, 55, and 41 g of water, respectively, for a total of approximately 200 to 300 mL/day.

Water is absorbed rapidly because it moves freely through membranes by diffusion. This movement is controlled mainly by osmotic forces generated by the inorganic ions in solution in the body (see "*Clinical Insight:* Osmotic Forces").

TABLE 6–1 WATER BALANCE (average figures in milliliters)

	WATER INTAKE
Fluids	1400
Water in food	700
Water from cellular oxidation of food	200
Total	2300

	WATER OUTPUT		
	Normal Temperature	Hot Weather	Prolonged Exercise
Urine	1400	1200	500
Water in feces	100	100	100
Skin (perspiration)	100	1400	5000
Insensible Loss			
Skin	350	350	350
Respiratory tract	350	250	650
Total	2300	3300	6600

(Modified from Guyton AC. Textbook of Medical Physiology, 9th ed. Philadelphia: WB Saunders, 1996.)

When water cannot be ingested orally, it may be administered intravenously in the form of salt (saline) solutions, which closely resemble body fluids; glucose solutions; or in blood, plasma, or protein hydrolysate mixtures. **Water intoxication** occurs as a result of an excess of water and **intracellular fluid** (ICF) volume, and is accompanied by osmolar dilution. If excessive water is given after surgery, trauma, or any condition that results in salt and water loss, and if ADH levels are not adjusted and the kidney cannot respond, water intoxication results. The increased volume of ICF causes the cells, particularly the brain cells, to swell, leading to symptoms of headache, nausea, vomiting, muscle twitching, convulsions with impending stupor, and possibly, death. Papilledema, blurring of vision, and blindness may also result.

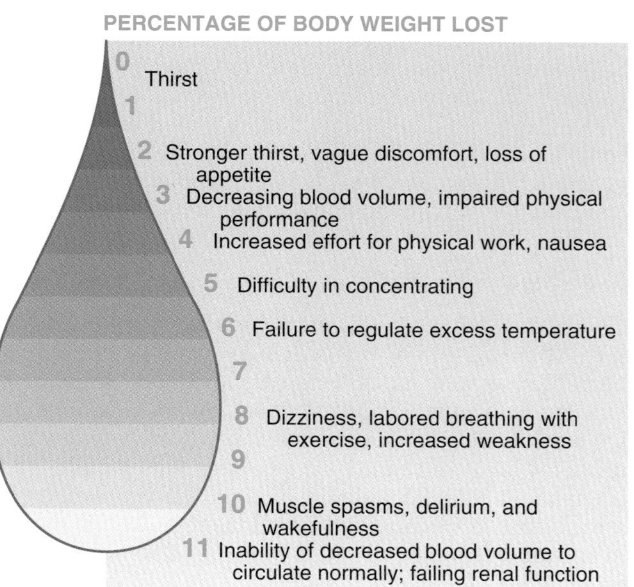

PERCENTAGE OF BODY WEIGHT LOST
0 Thirst
1
2 Stronger thirst, vague discomfort, loss of appetite
3 Decreasing blood volume, impaired physical performance
4 Increased effort for physical work, nausea
5 Difficulty in concentrating
6 Failure to regulate excess temperature
7
8 Dizziness, labored breathing with exercise, increased weakness
9
10 Muscle spasms, delirium, and wakefulness
11 Inability of decreased blood volume to circulate normally; failing renal function

FIGURE 6–2 Adverse effects of dehydration.

Water Elimination

Water loss normally occurs through the kidneys in the urine and through the gastrointestinal tract in the feces (termed **sensible water loss,** or measurable water loss), as well as through air expired from the lungs and water vapor lost through the skin (**insensible water loss,** or nonmeasurable water loss) (see Table 6–1). The kidney is the main regulator of sensible water loss. Insensible water loss is continuous and usually unconscious. Sweat, a detectable source of water loss, is distinct from insensible water loss through the skin. Perspiration losses vary greatly. Athletes can lose 3 to 4 lb during practice at 80° F and low humidity, and even more at higher temperatures (see Chapter 25).

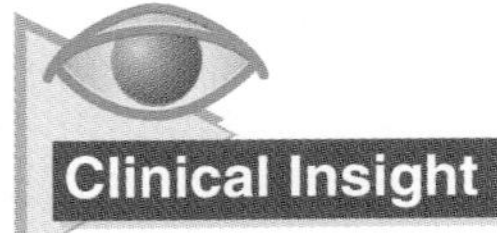

Osmotic Forces

Osmotic Pressure. **Osmotic pressure** is directly proportional to the number of particles in solution and usually refers to the pressure at the *cell membrane.* It is convenient (although not entirely accurate) to consider the osmotic pressure of the intracellular fluid as a function of its content of potassium, the predominant cation in the intracellular fluid. By contrast, the osmotic pressure of extracellular fluid may be considered relative to its content of sodium, the major cation present in extracellular fluid. Although variations in the distribution of sodium and potassium ions are the principal causes of water shifts between the various fluid compartments, chloride and phosphate also influence water balance. Proteins, which are nondiffusible because of their size, also play an important part in maintaining osmotic equilibrium.

Oncotic Pressure. **Oncotic pressure,** or **colloidal osmotic pressure,** is the pressure at the *capillary membrane* caused by dissolved proteins in the plasma and interstitial fluids. Oncotic pressure helps to retain water within blood vessels, thus preventing its leakage from plasma into the interstitial spaces. In stress and certain disease states in which the protein content of plasma is exceptionally low, water leaks into the interstitial spaces causing edema. This process is also referred to as *"third spacing."*

Osmole and Milliosmole. Concentrations of individual ionic constituents of extracellular or intracellular fluids are expressed in terms of *milliosmoles* per liter. One mole is equal to 1 gram molecular weight of a substance. Dissolved in 1 L of water, it becomes 1 osm. One milliosmole is equal to 1/1000th of an osmole. The number of milliosmoles per liter is equivalent to the number of millimoles per liter times the number of particles into which the dissolved substance dissociates. Thus, 1 mmo equals 1 mOsm for a nonelectrolyte (e.g., glucose). Similarly, 1 mmol equals 2 mOsm for an electrolyte containing only monovalent ions (e.g., NaCl). One milliosmole dissolved in 1 L of water has an osmotic pressure of 17 mm Hg.

Osmolality and Osmolarity. **Osmolality** is a measure of the osmotically active particles per kilogram of the solvent in which the particles are dispersed. It is expressed as milliosmoles of solute per kilogram of solvent (mOsm/kg). **Osmolarity** is the term formerly used to describe concentration, milliosmoles per liter of the entire solution; however, osmolality is now expressed in that form for most clinical work. In certain disease states, such as hyperlipidemia, it makes a difference whether it is stated as milliosmoles per kilogram of solvent or per liter of solution.

Serum Osmolality. Osmolality can be calculated for serum and extracellular fluids as follows:

$$\text{Serum osmolality} = (\text{serum Na [mEq/L]} \times 2) + \text{glucose (mg/dL)}/18 + \text{BUN (mg/dL)}/2.8$$

The average sum of the concentration of all the cations in serum is about 150 mEq/L. This is balanced by 150 mEq/L of anions to yield a total serum osmolality of about 300 mOsm/L. Osmolar imbalance is caused by a gain or loss of water relative to a solute, or a gain or loss of solute relative to water. An osmolality of less than 285 mOsm/L generally indicates water excess; an osmolality of greater than 295 mOsm/L indicates a water deficit.

Under normal conditions, the water contained in the 7 to 9 L of digestive juices and other extracellular fluids secreted daily into the gastrointestinal tract is almost entirely reabsorbed in the ileum and colon, except for about 100 mL that is excreted in the feces. Because this volume of reabsorbed fluid is about twice that of the blood plasma, excessive gastrointestinal fluid losses through diarrhea may have serious consequences, particularly for the very young and the very old.

Fluid loss secondary to diarrhea has been responsible for thousands of deaths of children in developing countries. Oral rehydration therapy with a simple mixture of water, sugar, and salts has been highly effective in reducing the number of deaths (see Chapter 31). Other abnormal fluid losses may occur as a result of emesis, hemorrhage, fistula drainage, burn and wound exudates, nasogastric and surgical tube drainage, and the use of diuretics.

When water intake is insufficient or water loss is excessive, the kidneys compensate by conserving water and excreting a more concentrated urine. The renal tubules increase water reabsorption in response to the hormonal action of ADH. During dehydration, the specific gravity of urine increases above the normal levels of 1.008 to 1.030, and the urine becomes remarkably darker in color.

Water balance is related directly to the homeostatic function of the internal environment. When excess water is lost, electrolyte balance is disrupted. Intentional dehydration as a result of excessive sweating or fluid restriction is a method of water loss that has frequently been used by young wrestlers trying to "make weight." It is a harmful practice that can adversely affect performance (see Chapter 25).

Requirement for Water

The body has no provision for water storage; therefore, the amount of water lost every 24 hours must be replaced to maintain health and body efficiency. Under ordinary circumstances, a reasonable allowance based on recommended caloric intake is 1 mL/kcal for adults and 1.5 mL/kcal for infants. This translates into 35 mL/kg of usual body weight in adults, 50 to 60 mL/kg in children, and 150 mL/kg in infants. In most cases, a suitable daily allowance for adults is 2.5 L, or approximately 2.5 to 3 quarts. Infants have an increased need for water because of the limited capacity of their kidneys to handle the renal solute load, their higher percentage of body water, and their large surface area per unit of body weight.

Thirst is usually an adequate guide for water intake, except in infants, heavily exercising athletes, the sick, and sometimes, the elderly, in whom thirst sensation may be diminished (see Chapter 13). Anyone sick enough to be hospitalized, regardless of diagnosis, is at risk for water and electrolyte imbalance. The elderly are particularly susceptible because of other causal factors, such as impaired renal concentrating ability, polypharmacy, fever, diarrhea, vomiting, and decreased ability for self-care. In cases of extreme heat or excessive sweating, thirst may not keep pace with the actual water requirement.

Signs of **dehydration** include poor skin turgor (although this may be present in well-hydrated older persons), skin tenting on the forehead, concentrated urine, decreased urine output, sunken eyes, dry mucous membranes of the mouth and nose, orthostatic blood pressure changes, and tachycardia (Sanservero, 1997).

During lactation, the need for water increases—theoretically, by an additional 600 to 700 mL/day—because of the high amounts required for milk production (see Chapter 7). Many successfully lactating women do not consume enough water to satisfy theoretical recommendations, but evidently meet their fluid needs with water contained in foods (Stumbo et al, 1985) (Table 6–2). Appendix 41 provides the amount of water contained in foods.

TABLE 6–2 PERCENTAGE OF WATER OF SOME COMMON FOODS

Food	%
Lettuce (iceberg)	96
Celery	95
Cucumbers	95
Cabbage (raw)	92
Watermelon	92
Broccoli (boiled)	91
Milk (nonfat)	91
Spinach	91
Green Beans (boiled)	89
Carrots (raw)	88
Oranges	87
Cereals (cooked)	85
Apples (raw, without skin)	84
Grapes	81
Potatoes (boiled)	77
Eggs	75
Bananas	74
Fish (baked haddock)	74
Chicken (roasted white meat)	70
Corn (boiled)	65
Beef (sirloin)	59
Cheese (Swiss)	38
Bread (white)	37
Cake (angel food)	34
Butter	16
Almonds (blanched)	5
Saltines	3
Sugar (white)	1
Oils	0

(From Pennington JA. Bowes and Church's Food Values of Portions Commonly Used, 17th ed. Philadelphia: JB Lippincott, 1994.)

Water Safety

Five of six Americans obtain their water from a public water supply. Safety issues related to drinking water stem from the increasing number of pathogens found in public drinking supplies. These pathogens, including Cryptosporidium, *Escherichia coli,* Giardia, and cyclospora, can cause widespread public health problems. Infants, the elderly, and those who are immunocompromised are the most susceptible and severely affected. Concern over the quality and safety of drinking water has prompted many consumers to rely on bottled water or to utilize home water filtration devices. Water-filtering devices that specify "one micron absolute," "NSF Standard 53 or 58" or "rated for cyst reduction," are the only ones capable of removing the organisms just mentioned. Interestingly, about 25% of all bottled water comes from the same municipal supplies that deliver water to people's homes. Until recently, consumers had no way of knowing whether the bottled water they were buying was actually tap water. In May of 1997, the U.S. Food and Drug Administration (FDA) issued a ruling on the labeling of bottled water that mandates the provision of information regarding the water's source. Water from public water supplies must be labeled as such, and bottled water terms now have legal definitions (Gershoff, 1996) (see "*Focus On:* U.S. FDA Definitions of Bottled Water Terms and Criteria for Labeling"). Information on public drinking supplies can be obtained from the municipal drinking contaminant and analysis reports that are required by the Environmental Protection Agency.

ELECTROLYTES

Electrolytes are substances or compounds that, when dissolved in water, dissociate into positively and negatively charged ions (cations and anions). Electrolytes can be simple inorganic salts of sodium, potassium, or magnesium, or complex organic molecules (Table 6–3).

Sodium

Sodium is the major cation of extracellular fluid. Various intestinal secretions, such as bile and pancreatic juice, contain substantial amounts of sodium. Thirty-five to 40% of the total body sodium is in the skeleton; however, most of this sodium is unexchangeable or only slowly exchangeable with that in body fluids. Contrary to common belief, sweat is hypotonic and contains a relatively small amount of sodium.

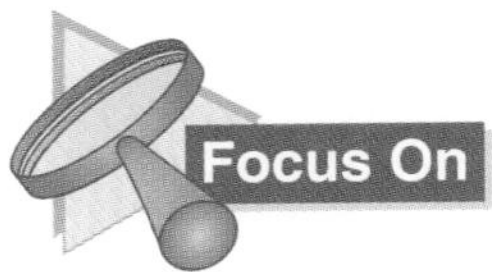

U.S. Food and Drug Administration (FDA) Definitions of Bottled Water Terms and Criteria for Labeling*

Artesian water or well water—water drawn from a well that taps into an underground, water-bearing layer of rock or sand

Ground water—water derived from an underground body of water that is not in contact with any surface water

Mineral water—water, drawn from an underground source, that must contain at least 250 ppm of dissolved solids. Minerals found in mineral water may include calcium, iron, and sodium. If the mineral content is 250 to 500 ppm, the statement "low mineral content" must appear on the bottle label. If the mineral content is greater than 1500 ppm, the statement "high mineral content" must appear. If the water contains greater than or equal to 20 mg calcium, 0.36 mg iron, or 5 mg sodium, the product must also carry a nutrition label (see Fig. 15–5).

Purified (demineralized) water—water from which all minerals and dissolved solids have been removed. It may be called distilled, deionized, or reverse osmosis, depending upon the removal method.

Sparkling water—naturally carbonated water that contains the same amount of carbon dioxide as it did when it left the source. This carbonation level may be maintained naturally or added during the bottling process.

Spring water—water derived from an underground formation from which water flows naturally to the surface. It may be collected at the spring or by tapping into the underground formation that feeds the spring.

Sterile (sterilized) water—water that meets the requirements of microorganism removal set by the U.S. Pharmacopeia.

Not sterile/Use as directed by physician or by labeling directions for use of infant formula—required wording when the label states or implies that the product is for use in feeding infants, but is not actually sterile

From a community water system or municipal source—required wording when the water comes from the same source as that which flows through the pipes of a city or town. The statement must appear "conspicuously."

*Note: Seltzer water, soda water, and tonic water fall under different regulations, as they may contain sugar and calories and would require nutritional labels.

Functions

As the predominant ion of extracellular fluid, sodium regulates the size of this compartment, as well as the plasma volume. Sodium also aids in the conduction of nerve impulses and the control of muscle contraction.

Absorption and Excretion

Sodium is readily absorbed from the intestine and carried to the kidneys, where it is filtered out and returned to the blood to maintain appropriate levels. The amount absorbed is proportional to intake.

About 90% to 95% of normal body sodium loss is through the urine; the rest is lost in feces and sweat. Normally, the quantity of sodium excreted daily is equal to the amount ingested. Sodium excretion is maintained by a mechanism involving the glomerular filtration rate, the cells of the juxtaglomerular apparatus of the kidneys, the renin-angiotensin-aldosterone system, the sympathetic nervous system, circulating catecholamines, and blood pressure (see Chapter 38).

Sodium balance is regulated by *aldosterone,* a mineralocorticoid secreted by the adrenal cortex (see Chapter 38). When blood sodium levels rise, the thirst receptors in the hypothalamus stimulate the thirst sensation. When blood levels are low, excretion of sodium through the urine decreases. Under certain circumstances, sodium and fluid regulation can be disrupted, resulting in abnormal blood sodium levels. The *syndrome of inappropriate antidiuretic hormone secretion* (SIADH) is characterized by concentrated low-volume urine and dilutional hyponatremia as water is retained. ADH secretion is inappropriate because it occurs in the absence of dehydration. SIADH can result from central nervous system disorders, pulmonary disorders, tumors, and certain medications.

Estrogen, which bears a slight resemblance to aldosterone, can also cause sodium and water retention. Changes in water and sodium balance during the menstrual cycle, pregnancy, and with oral contraceptive use are partially attributable to changes in progesterone and estrogen levels.

TABLE 6–3 NORMAL ELECTROLYTE CONCENTRATION OF SERUM

ELECTROLYTES	RANGE OF NORMAL
Cations	
Sodium	136–145 mEq/L
Potassium	3.5–5 mEq/L
Calcium	4.5–5.5 mEq/L (9.0–11 mg/dL)
Magnesium	1.5–2.5 mEq/L (1.8–3 mg/dL)
Anions	
Chloride	96–106 mEq/L
CO_2 (content) TCO_2	24–28.8 mEq/L
Phosphorus (inorganic)	3–4.5 mg/dL (1.9–2.85 mEq/L as HPO_4^{-2})
Sulfate (as S)	0.8–1.2 mg/dL (0.5–0.75 mEq/L as SO_2^{-2})
Lactate	0.7–1.8 mEq/L (6–16 mg/dL)
Protein	6–7.6 g/dL (14–18 mEq/L); depends on albumin level

Recommended Intake

Actual minimum requirements for sodium are not known. Estimates of such requirements are as low as 200 mg/day. The estimated minimum requirements for all ages, as cited in the 1989 Recommended Dietary Allowances (RDAs), are shown in Table 6–4. The low-salt syndrome is discussed in Chapter 36.

Acute and excessive intake of sodium leads to edema and hypertension; however, the kidneys are usually able to excrete the excess sodium. Of greater concern is chronic excessive sodium intake. An upper limit of 6 g/day of sodium chloride has been recommended, given the potential role of sodium in hypertension (see Chapter 27) (Food and Nutrition Board, 1989).

Sources

The major source of sodium is sodium chloride, or common table salt, of which sodium constitutes 40%. The mean daily salt intake in Western societies is about 10 to 12 g (4 to 5 g of sodium) per capita. Approximately 3 g of the daily salt intake occurs naturally in foods, 3 g is added during processing, and 4 g is added by the individual. Protein foods generally contain more sodium than do vegetables and grains, whereas fruits contain little or none. The sodium content of foods is discussed further in Chapter 36 and Appendix Table 41.

Chloride

Functions

Chloride is widely distributed throughout the body as the principal anion of extracellular fluids. Together with sodium, it helps to maintain water balance and osmotic pressure. The highest concentrations of chloride are in cerebrospinal fluid and gastric and pancreatic juices. Along with phosphate and sulfate, chloride helps to maintain acid-base balance in the body fluids. Chloride ions maintain osmotic equilibrium as bicarbonate levels in the plasma and red blood cells change. It has also been suggested that chloride plays a role in regulating the renin-angiotensin-aldosterone system (William and Dluhy, 1994). The reader is referred to Chapter 27 for a discussion of the possible role of chloride in hypertension.

Absorption and Excretion

Chloride is almost completely absorbed in the intestine and excreted in urine and sweat. Chloride loss parallels sodium loss. Excessive loss through sweat is minimized by aldosterone, which acts directly on the sweat glands. Extra chloride may be necessary to correct the metabolic alkalosis resulting from disease, the use of diuretics, or gastric losses from nasogastric suctioning or vomiting.

Sources

Most dietary chloride comes from sodium chloride or table salt, which is 60% chloride. The amount in food and added table salt provides approximately 3 to 9 g/day. Chloride in water contributes only a very small fraction of the chloride consumed in the diet.

Recommended Intake

The safe range of chloride intake for all ages, as determined by the Food and Nutrition Board, is shown in Table 6–4. A chloride deficiency syndrome has been described in infants receiving a chloride-deficient formula. The syndrome is characterized by loss of appetite, failure to thrive, muscle weakness, lethargy, and severe metabolic alkalosis with resultant hypokalemia (Grossman et al., 1980).

Potassium

Functions

Potassium, the major cation of intracellular fluid, is present in small amounts in extracellular fluid. Along with sodium, it is involved in maintaining

TABLE 6–4 ESTIMATED MINIMUM REQUIREMENTS FOR SODIUM, CHLORIDE, AND POTASSIUM IN HEALTHY PERSONS

AGE	WEIGHT (kg)	SODIUM (mg)*†	CHLORIDE (mg)*†	POTASSIUM (mg)‡
Months				
0–5	4.5	120	180	500
6–11	8.9	200	300	700
Years				
1	11.0	225	350	1000
2–5	16.0	300	500	1400
6–9	25.0	400	600	1600
10–18	50.0	500	750	2000
>18§	70.0	500	750	2000

(Reproduced with permission from Recommended Dietary Allowances, 10th ed., © 1989 by the National Academy of Sciences. Published by National Academy Press.)

*No allowance has been included for large, prolonged losses from the skin through sweat.

†There is no evidence that higher intakes of sodium or chloride confer any health benefit.

‡Desirable intakes of potassium may considerably exceed these values (e.g., 3500 mg for adults).

§No allowance is included for growth. Values for those younger than 18 years assume a growth rate at the 50th percentile reported by the National Center for Health Statistics and averaged for males and females. See Chapter 7 for information on pregnancy and lactation.

normal water balance, osmotic equilibrium, and acid-base balance. Along with calcium, it is important in the regulation of neuromuscular activity. Potassium also promotes cellular growth. The potassium content of muscle is related to muscle mass and glycogen storage; therefore, if muscle is being formed, an adequate supply of potassium is essential.

Absorption and Excretion

Potassium is readily absorbed from the small intestine. Eighty to 90% of ingested potassium is excreted in the urine; the remainder is lost in the feces. The kidneys maintain normal serum levels through their ability to filter, reabsorb, and excrete potassium under the influence of aldosterone. Ionized potassium is excreted in place of ionized sodium by means of the renal tubule exchange mechanism.

Sources

Dietary sources of potassium are listed in Chapter 38 and in Appendix Table 41. As a rule, fruits, vegetables, and fresh meat are good sources of potassium.

Recommended Intake

The minimum potassium requirement for adults is 1.6 to 2 g (40 to 50 mEq) per day, but higher levels are recommended because of the possible protective effect of potassium against hypertension. The safe range of recommended intakes for all ages is given in Table 6–4. Potassium deficiency arising from inadequate intake is not common in healthy individuals because potassium is widely distributed in foods. The average daily intake is estimated to be in the range of 0.8 to 1.5 g of potassium/1000 kcal. An adequate intake of milk, meats, cereals, vegetables, and fruits will provide ample potassium.

ACID-BASE BALANCE

Acid-base status is determined by pH, which is the negative of the hydrogen ion concentration logarithm. A low pH value represents an acidic state (acidosis), whereas a high pH value is indicative of an alkaline state (alkalosis). Maintaining the pH level within a normal range of 7.35 to 7.45 is crucial for many physiologic functions and biochemical reactions. The body is able to accomplish this despite the enormous acid load generated through diet and tissue metabolism. Disruption of acid-base balance may occur with certain diseases, with shifts in fluid status, as well as with certain medical and surgical treatment modalities (Table 6–5). If the condition remains uncorrected, a multitude of detrimental effects, ranging from electrolyte abnormalities to death, can ensue.

Acid Generation

Acids are generated exogenously through the ingestion of food, acid precursors, and toxins. They are generated endogenously through normal tissue metabolism. Fixed acids, such as phosphoric and sulfuric acid, are produced from the metabolism of phosphate-containing substrates and sulfur-containing amino acids, respectively. Organic acids, of which

TABLE 6–5 CLASSIFICATION OF THE FOUR MAJOR ACID-BASE IMBALANCES AND SOME OF THE CONDITIONS LEADING TO THESE IMBALANCES

TYPE AND ETIOLOGY OF IMBALANCE	RESPIRATORY IMBALANCE		METABOLIC IMBALANCE	
	Respiratory Acidosis	**Respiratory Alkalosis**	**Metabolic Acidosis**	**Metabolic Alkalosis**
Characteristics of failure	↑ H_2CO_3 level secondary to retention of CO_2	↓ H_2CO_3 level secondary to excessive expiration of CO_2 and H_2O	↑ H^+ (↓pH) concentration secondary to ↑ production or ↑ retention OR ↓ HCO_3^- secondary to excretion of large amounts of base from ECF	↓ H^+ (↑pH) concentration secondary to ↑ losses OR ↑ HCO_3^- secondary to abnormal retention of base in ECF
Associated diseases/conditions	Conditions involving ↓ lung surface area, such as emphysema Restrictive or obstructive lung diseases Certain neuromuscular disease in which respiratory function is impaired	Aftermath of severe exercise Anxiety reaction Early sepsis	Diarrhea Uremia Ketoacidosis secondary to uncontrolled diabetes mellitus Starvation ↑ fat, ↓ carbohydrate diet Drugs	Diuretics ↑ ingestion of alkali Loss of chloride Vomiting

ECF, extracellular fluid.

lactic acid and keto acids are examples, typically accumulate only in disease states. Carbon dioxide (CO_2), a volatile acid, is generated from the oxidation of carbohydrates, amino acids, and fat.

Regulation

A variety of regulatory mechanisms operate to maintain the pH level within very narrow physiologic limits. At the cellular level, **buffer** systems, composed of weak acids or bases and their corresponding salts, minimize the effect on pH caused by the addition of a strong acid or base. The buffering effect occurs through the formation of a weak acid or base, equivalent in amount to the strong acid or base that is added to the system (Fig. 6–3). Proteins and phosphates are the primary *intracellular buffers*, whereas the bicarbonate/carbonic acid system is the main *extracellular buffer*. Acid-base balance is also maintained through the actions of the kidneys and lungs. The kidneys regulate hydrogen ion secretion and bicarbonate (HCO_3^-) reabsorption. The lungs control alveolar ventilation, altering either the depth or rate of breathing. This, in turn, alters the amount of CO_2 expired.

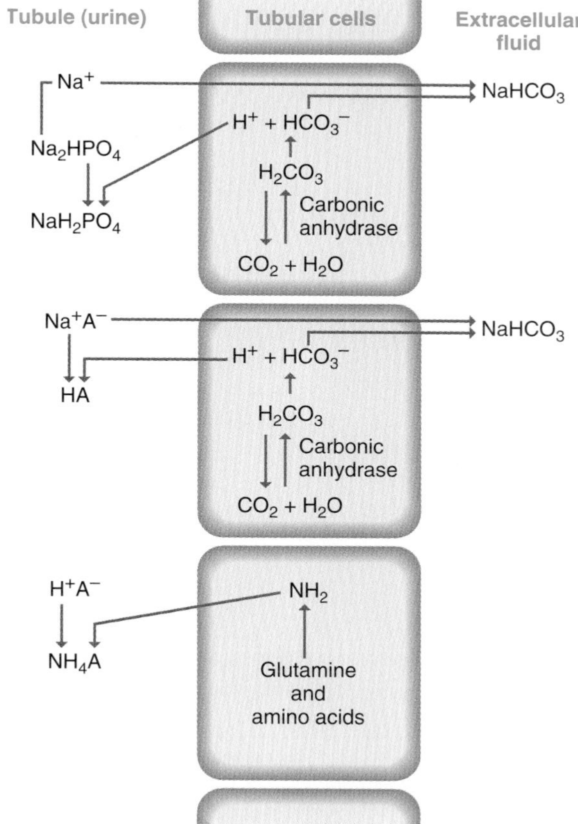

FIGURE 6–3 Generation of $NaHCO_3$ and clearance of H^+ by the three buffer systems that function in the kidney. *ECF,* extracellular fluid; *HA,* any acid in the body.

TABLE 6–6 NORMAL ARTERIAL BLOOD GAS (ABG) VALUES

pH	7.35–7.45
pCO_2	35–45 mm Hg
pO_2	80–100 mm Hg
HCO_3^-	22–26 mEq/L
O_2 Sat.	>95%

Acid-Base Disorders

Acid-base disorders can be differentiated based on metabolic and respiratory etiologies. The evaluation of acid-base status requires analysis of both serum electrolytes (see Table 6–3) and arterial blood gas (ABG) values (Table 6–6). *Metabolic* acid-base imbalances are manifested through changes in bicarbonate levels, which are reflected in the total CO_2 (TCO_2) portion of the electrolyte profile. TCO_2 includes HCO_3^-, H_2CO_3, and dissolved CO_2; however, all but 1 to 3 mEq/L is in the form of HCO_3^-. Thus, for ease of interpretation, TCO_2 should be equated with HCO_3^-. *Respiratory* acid-base imbalances are manifested through changes in pCO_2, the partial pressure of dissolved CO_2. This is reported in the ABG values, along with the pH, which reflects the overall acid-base status.

Metabolic Acidosis

Metabolic acidosis results from increased generation or accumulation of acids as in diabetic ketoacidosis, lactic acidosis, or uremia, or from excessive bicarbonate loss via the kidneys or intestinal tract. The **anion gap** is calculated to determine the etiology of the acidosis so that appropriate treatment can be instituted (see "*Clinical Insight:* Anion Gap," and Table 6–5).

Metabolic Alkalosis

Metabolic alkalosis results from the administration or accumulation of bicarbonate or its precursors, excessive acid loss (e.g., as may occur with nasogastric suctioning), or loss of extracellular fluid containing more chloride than bicarbonate (e.g., as may occur with villous adenoma or diuretic use). It may also result from volume depletion, whereby decreased blood flow to the kidneys stimulates reabsorption of sodium and water, which in turn increases bicarbonate reabsorption. This is known as **contraction alkalosis.** Alkalosis can also result from severe hypokalemia (serum K^+ <2.0 mEq/L). As potassium moves from the intracellular to the extracellular fluid, hydrogen ions move from the extracellular to the intracellular fluid to maintain electroneutrality. This produces an *intracellular acidosis,* which increases hydrogen ion excretion and bicarbonate reabsorption by the kidneys.

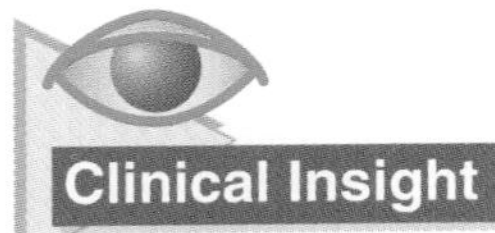

Clinical Insight

ANION GAP

The number of positively charged ions (cations) in the body equals the number of negatively charged ions (anions). However, not all cations and anions are routinely measured. Sodium is the principal measured cation, whereas chloride and bicarbonate are the principal measured anions. The term *anion gap* refers to the difference between measured cations and measured anions.

Anion gap (AG) = (serum Na^+) – (serum Cl^- + HCO_3^-)
Normal AG = 12–14 mEq/L

Nongap Metabolic Acidosis. *Nongap metabolic acidosis* occurs when the decrease in bicarbonate is balanced by an increase in chloride, resulting in a normal anion gap. This type of acidosis, also referred to as hyperchloremic metabolic acidosis, can occur in the following conditions, represented by the acronym, "USED CARP" (Wilson, 1992):

Ureterosigmoidostomy
Small bowel fistula
Extra chloride ingestion
Diarrhea
Carbonic anhydrase inhibitor
Adrenal insufficiency
Renal tubular acidosis
Pancreatic fistula

Anion Gap Metabolic Acidosis. *Anion gap metabolic acidosis* occurs when the decrease in bicarbonate is balanced not by increased chloride, but rather by other acid anions. This causes the calculated anion gap to exceed the normal range of 12 to 14 mEq/L. This type of acidosis, also referred to as normochloremic metabolic acidosis, can occur in the following conditions, represented by the acronym, "MUD PILES" (Wilson, 1992):

Methanol ingestion
Uremia
Diabetic ketoacidosis
Paraldehyde ingestion
Iatrogenic
Lactic acidosis
Ethylene glycol or ethanol ingestion
Salicylate ingestion

Respiratory Acidosis

Respiratory acidosis is caused by decreased ventilation and consequent carbon dioxide retention. Acute respiratory acidosis can occur as a result of sleep apnea, asthma, aspiration of a foreign object, or acute respiratory distress syndrome (ARDS), also known as adult respiratory distress syndrome. Chronic respiratory acidosis is associated with obesity hypoventilation syndrome, chronic obstructive pulmonary disease (COPD) or emphysema, certain neuromuscular diseases, and starvation cachexia.

Respiratory Alkalosis

Respiratory alkalosis results from increased ventilation and elimination of carbon dioxide. This can be mediated centrally (e.g., secondary to head injury, pain, anxiety, cerebrovascular accident, or tumors) or by peripheral stimulation (e.g., secondary to pneumonia, hypoxemia, high altitudes, pulmonary embolism, congestive heart failure, or interstitial lung disease).

Compensation

When a metabolic or respiratory acid-base imbalance develops, the body attempts to restore normal pH by developing a secondary or compensatory disorder to offset the effects of the first or primary disorder (Table 6–7). For example, in the presence of a primary respiratory acidosis, the kidneys compensate by increasing bicarbonate reabsorption, thereby creating a metabolic alkalosis to help increase pH. It should be noted that complete compensation does not occur. The pH level will still reflect the underlying disorder. In clinical practice, it is imperative to distinguish between primary and compensatory disturbances, as treatment is always directed toward the primary acid-base disturbance and its underlying cause.

TABLE 6–7 PRIMARY AND COMPENSATORY LABORATORY VALUE CHANGES IN ACID-BASE DISORDERS*

ACID-BASE DISORDER	pH	HCO_3^-	pCO_2
Metabolic acidosis	↓↓/↑ (net pH remains less than normal)	↓↓	↓ (compensatory respiratory alkalosis)
Metabolic alkalosis	↑↑/↓ (net pH remains greater than normal)	↑↑	↑ (compensatory respiratory acidosis)
Respiratory acidosis	↓↓/↑ (net pH remains less than normal)	↑ (compensatory metabolic alkalosis)	↑↑
Respiratory alkalosis	↑↑/↓ (net pH remains greater than normal)	↓ (compensatory metabolic acidosis)	↓↓

*↑↑/↓↓ denotes primary change, whereas ↑/↓ denotes compensatory change.

CASE STUDY

Phillip P. is a 6-ft-tall, 180-lb, 43-year-old man who was admitted to the intensive care unit following a motor vehicle accident in which he sustained a closed head injury, multiple facial and orthopedic fractures, and massive blood loss. Upon admission, he was hypotensive and in circulatory shock. Fluid resuscitation and blood transfusions were begun. Initial laboratory data revealed the following: pH, 7.10; pCO_2, 39; lactate, 9.3 mEq/L (elevated); sodium, 138 mEq/L; potassium, 4.9 mEq/L; chloride, 101 mEq/L; bicarbonate, 18 mEq/L. After the patient was hemodynamically stabilized, tube feedings were initiated using a high-nitrogen, 1 Kcal/mL enteral formula. Data obtained on the third day of hospitalization indicated the following: albumin, 2.1 g/dL; sodium, 129 mEq/L; serum osmolality, 273 mOsm/L; urine osmolality, 936 mOsm/L (high); cumulative intake/output (I/O), 14.6/4.0 L, and weight, 205 lbs.

1. Upon admission, an acid-base disorder was evident. What was it and what was its cause?
2. Marked hypoalbuminemia ensued as a result of what factors?
3. A review of weight and I/O records revealed a 25-lb weight gain and an intake that exceeded output by about 10 kg. The excess fluid had likely moved from the intravascular space to the __________ spaces due to the low __________ __________ resulting from the hypoalbuminemia.
4. On hospital day 3, a decrease in serum sodium level was noted, which prompted measurement of serum and urine osmolalities. Based on the results, the patient most likely had what syndrome? This condition was most likely caused by ___________.
5. The physician asked you to reevaluate the patient's tube feeding prescription based on the information just presented. You correctly recommended the following course:
   a. continue current tube feedings
   b. change to a more concentrated tube feeding formula
   c. add salt to the feedings
6. Phillip P. gradually improved, and after 3 weeks, was extubated and transferred out of the intensive care unit. His weight had decreased from 205 lb to 170 lb. Explain the cause(s) of his weight loss.

CITED REFERENCES

Food and Nutrition Board, National Research Council. Recommended Dietary Allowances, 10th ed. Washington, DC: National Academy Press, 1989.

Gershoff, SN (ed.). Making bottled water rules watertight. Tufts Univ Diet Nutr Lett, 13(11):2, 1996.

Grossman H, et al. The dietary chloride deficiency syndrome. Pediatrics 66:366, 1980.

NIH Consensus Statement. Bioelectrical impedance analysis in body composition measurement. National Institutes of Health Technology Assessment Conference Statement, December 12–14, 1994. Nutrition 12(11-2):749, 1996.

Pennington, JA. Bowes and Church's Food Value of Portions Commonly Used, 17th ed. Philadelphia: JB Lippincott, 1994.

Sanservero AC. Dehydration in the elderly: Strategies for prevention and management. Nurse Pract 22(4):41, 1997.

Stumbo PJ, et al. Water intakes of lactating women. Am J Clin Nutr 42:870, 1985.

William GH, Dluhy RG. Hypertensive states: Associated fluid and electrolyte disturbances. In: Narins RG (ed.). Maxwell and Kleeman's Clinical Disorders of Fluid and Electrolyte Metabolism, 5th ed. New York: McGraw-Hill, 1994, pp 1621–1622.

Wilson RF. Acid-base problems. In: Tintinalli JE, Krome RL, Ruiz E (eds.). Emergency Medicine: A Comprehensive Study Guide, 3rd ed. New York: McGraw-Hill, 1992.

ADDITIONAL REFERENCES

Adrogue HJ, Madias NE. Management of life-threatening acid-base disorders, Part I and Part II. N Engl J Med 338:26 and 107, 1998.

Avner ED. Clinical disorders of water metabolism: Hyponatremia and hypernatremia. Pediatr Ann 24:23, 1995.

Chernoff R. Thirst and fluid requirements. Nutr Rev 52(8, Pt. 2):S3, 1994.

Faber MD, et al. Common fluid and electrolyte acid-base problems in the intensive care unit: Selected issues. Semin Nephrol 14(1):8, 1994.

Gennari FJ. Hypokalemia. N Engl J Med 339:451, 1998.

Guyton AC. Textbook of Medical Physiology, 9th ed. Philadelphia: WB Saunders, 1996.

Hood VL, Tannen RL. Protection of acid base balance by pH regulation of acid production. N Engl J Med 12:819, 1998.

Horne MM, Swearingen PL. Pocket Guide to Fluids, Electrolytes, and Acid-Base Balance, 2nd ed. St. Louis: Mosby Year Book, 1993.

Humphreys MH. Fluid and electrolyte management. In: Way LW. Current Surgical Diagnosis and Treatment, 10th ed. Norwalk, CT: Appleton and Lange, 1994.

Koch SM, Taylor RW. Chloride ion in intensive care medicine. Crit Care Med 20:227, 1995.

Levine, BS. . . . About Water. Nutr Today 31(5):209, 1996.

McDonald RA. Disorders of potassium balance. Pediatr Ann 24:31, 1995.

Preuss HG. Fundamentals of clinical acid-base evaluation. Clin Lab Med 13:103, 1993.

Shires GT, et al. Fluid, electrolyte, and nutritional management of the surgical patient. In: Schwartz SI (ed.). Principles of Surgery, 6th ed. New York: McGraw-Hill, 1994.

PART 2

Nutrition in the Life Cycle

The importance of nutrition throughout the life cycle cannot be refuted. After all, we must eat to live. However, the significance of nutrition at specific times of growth, development, and aging is becoming increasingly appreciated.

The effect of proper nutrition during pregnancy on the health of the infant and mother in post-childbearing years has long been recognized. Maternal nutrition, and possibly even paternal nutrition, prior to conception affects the health of the newborn. It is now recognized that "fetal origin" has far more lifelong effects than originally thought.

Establishing good food habits during childhood lessens the possibility of inappropriate eating behavior (a phenomenon that occurs with disturbing frequency during adolescence) later in life. Although the influence of proper nutrition on one's own morbidity and mortality usually remains unacknowledged until adulthood, recent studies suggest that dietary practices aimed at preventing the degenerative diseases that appear later in life should be instituted in childhood.

It is clear that, during early adulthood, many changes begin that lead to the appearance of "diseases of aging" several years later. What is only beginning to become clear is that many of these changes can be accelerated or slowed over the years depending on the quality of the individual's nutritional intake, the health of the gut, and the function of the immune system.

With the rapid growth in the elderly population has evolved a need to expand the limited data currently available on nutrition in that population. Although it is known that energy needs decrease with aging, little is known about whether requirements for specific nutrients are increased or decreased. The identification of unique nutritional differences in the stages of aging assumes increasing significance as longevity increases.

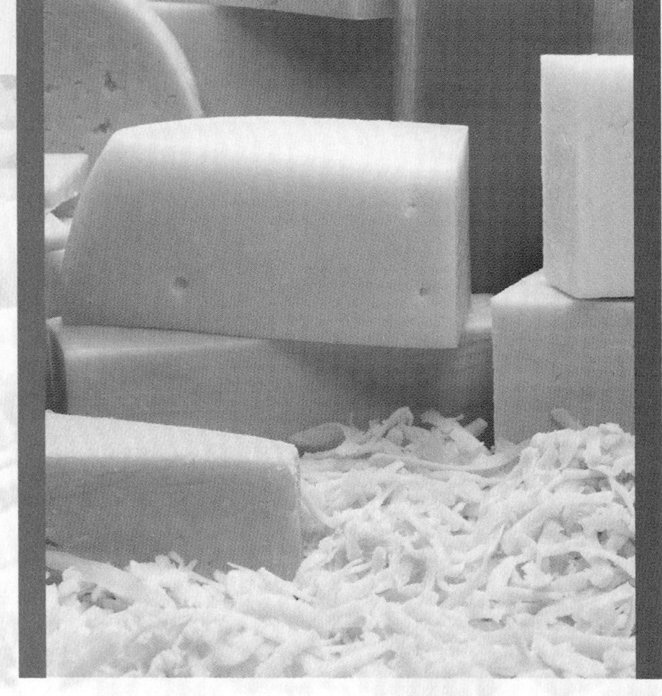

CHAPTER 7

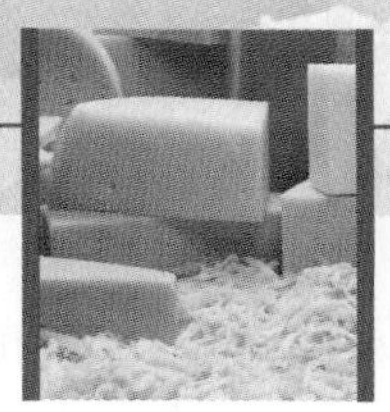

Nutrition During Pregnancy and Lactation*

CATHY FAGEN, RD, MA

Chapter Outline

- Pregnancy
- Lactation
- Nutrition, Fertility, and Conception

Key Terms

AMYLOPHAGIA—a form of pica involving consumption of excessive amounts of starch, such as laundry starch

COLOSTRUM—the thin, yellow, milky fluid secreted by the mammary gland a few days before and after birth, prior to secretion of mature milk

ECLAMPSIA—the late stage of pregnancy-induced hypertension characterized by proteinuria and, often, grand mal seizures occurring near the time of labor

FETAL ALCOHOL SYNDROME—a specific set of abnormal features resulting from exposure of the fetus to alcohol during gestation

GEOPHAGIA—a common pica of pregnancy involving the consumption of dirt or clay

GESTATIONAL DIABETES—diabetes that exists only during pregnancy

HYPEREMESIS GRAVIDARUM—prolonged and persistent vomiting during pregnancy

INFANT MORTALITY—infant deaths in the first year of life

LACTATION—the period of milk secretion

LET-DOWN—a distinct tingling sensation accompanying the movement of milk from the alveoli through the duct system and lactiferous sinuses to the nipple

NEURAL TUBE DEFECTS—developmental anomalies resulting in anencephaly or spina bifida; related to folic acid deficiency

OXYTOCIN—a hormone from the posterior pituitary that stimulates the movement of milk down to the nipple and the contraction of the uterine muscle

PERINATAL MORTALITY—the number of infant deaths occurring in the period that extends from 28 weeks' gestation to 4 weeks after birth

PICA—compulsive ingestion of unsuitable substances having little or no nutritional value

PREECLAMPSIA—the early stage of pregnancy-induced hypertension

PREGNANCY-INDUCED HYPERTENSION—a severe hypertension that may develop during pregnancy, usually after 20 weeks of gestation; accompanied by proteinuria, edema and, rarely, convulsions and coma

PROLACTIN—one of the hormones of the anterior pituitary gland that stimulates milk production by alveolar cells

TERATHANASIA—selective promotion of spontaneous abortion of defective fetuses

TERATOGEN—any agent (infectious, environmental, or nutritional) that causes a malformation in the fetus

PREGNANCY

Numerous factors interact to determine the progress and outcome of pregnancy. Although much remains to be learned about the role of nutrition in modifying this process, it is well accepted that the nutritional status of the pregnant woman affects the outcome of her pregnancy. This is especially true with respect to the birth weight of her infant, a factor closely related to **infant mortality,** and the infant's risk of long-term adverse health outcomes, such as hypertension, obesity, glucose intolerance, and cardiovascular disease (Barker, 1995).

*This chapter is a revision of a chapter, contributed by Bonnie S. Worthington-Roberts, PhD, and Marian Stone Neuhouser, PhD, RD, that appeared in the previous edition.

Sections of this chapter have been adapted, with permission, from Worthington-Roberts BS, Williams SR. Nutrition in Pregnancy and Lactation, 5th ed. St Louis: CV Mosby, 1993.

Effect of Nutritional Status on Pregnancy Outcome

Historical Perspective

The effects of undernutrition and the accompanying stress on previously well-nourished populations have been explored as a consequence of World War II, when severe food deprivation occurred in many parts of Europe. Retrospective studies in Germany, the Netherlands, and Russia indicate that the incidence of amenorrhea increased significantly, a protective phenomenon that reflects the nutritional unpreparedness of these energy-deprived women for pregnancy. In the Netherlands, 50% of the female population stopped menstruating. The smallest decline in fertility occurred among those living in rural areas and those who had priority access to food rations. The incidence of miscarriages and abortions, stillbirths, neonatal deaths, and neonatal malformations increased in women conceiving during famine. Surviving infants showed a significant reduction in mean birth weights and birth lengths (Hytton and Leitch, 1971; Susser and Smith, 1994). As living conditions improved, mean birth weight rose steadily, returning to normal by 1948.

Perinatal Mortality and Birth Weight

Low birth weight (LBW; <2500 g) is a major factor in infant deaths and certain long-term health problems, such as developmental disabilities and learning disorders in the United States. Infant mortality, whether due to intrauterine growth retardation or prematurity, is 40 times greater in LBW infants than in neonates of normal weight. Because **perinatal mortality** correlates better with birth weight than with length of gestation, it is widely believed that a substantial reduction in the rate of LBW would lead to a dramatic decline in infant mortality rates.

Although many inherited problems or perinatal insults cannot be prevented, poor gestational nutrition and low maternal weight gain, both of which are factors implicated in LBW, can be modified. In addition, it appears that poor nutritional status prior to conception and a low prepregnant weight of the mother negatively influence infant birth weight (Kramer, 1987).

Two indicators of maternal nutritional status have consistently been shown to correlate with infant birth weight: maternal size (height and prepregnancy weight) and the amount of weight gained during pregnancy.

Maternal Size. Big mothers tend to have big babies, and it has been proposed that maternal size is a conditioning factor on the ultimate size of the placenta. The size of the placenta determines the amount of nutrition available to the fetus, and eventually, the birth weight of the neonate. Mothers with low prepregnancy weights have much lighter-weight placentas than do heavier mothers (Naeye, 1979). There is a greater incidence of LBW and prematurity in babies born to underweight mothers than in those born to mothers of normal weight (Edwards et al., 1979). Adequate pregravid weight and satisfactory weight gain are particularly important for the offspring of short women (Luke et al., 1984). By reaching a higher prepregnancy weight or gaining extra weight during pregnancy, these women can improve their pregnancy outcome (Naeye, 1981).

Maternal Weight Gain During Pregnancy. The normal distribution of weight gain is illustrated in Figure 7–1. Less than half of the total weight gain resides in the fetus, placenta, and amniotic fluid; the remainder is found in maternal reproductive tissues, fluid, blood, and "maternal stores," a component composed largely of body fat. Gradually increasing subcutaneous fat in the abdomen, back, and upper thigh serves as an energy reserve for pregnancy and lactation.

Over the years, attitudes about the amount of weight gained during pregnancy have changed dramatically. In the early 1900s, a popular view held that large babies complicated the process of labor and delivery. As cesarean sections were rarely performed and maternal mortality was high at this time, restricting fetal size seemed justifiable. The philosophy of restricting maternal weight gain prevailed into the 1960s and is still espoused by a minority of clinicians. In 1915, however, poor maternal nutritional status was reported to have a profound influence on birth weight and outcome of pregnancy (Smith, 1916). Most subsequent studies have corroborated the observation that increased weight gain during pregnancy is associated with increased birth weight and a progressive decrease in the number of LBW infants. This relationship persists up to a weight gain of 26 to 35 lb, the range associated with optimal outcome. However, in very overweight mothers, increased weight gain is usually not associated with substantial increments in birth weight (Abrams and Laros, 1986). The Institute of Medicine (IOM) recommends a weight gain of 25 to 35 lb for women of normal weight, 28 to 40 lb for underweight women, and 15 to 25 lb for overweight women (IOM, 1990) (Table 7–1).

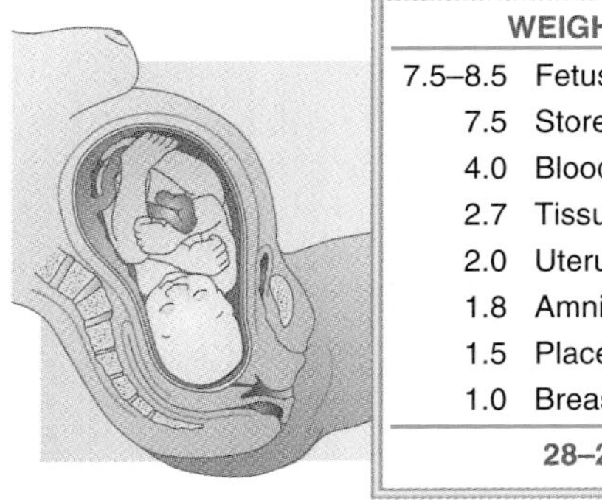

WEIGHT IN POUNDS	
7.5–8.5	Fetus
7.5	Stores of fat and protein
4.0	Blood
2.7	Tissue fluids
2.0	Uterus
1.8	Amniotic fluid
1.5	Placenta and umbilical cord
1.0	Breasts
28–29.0 pounds	

FIGURE 7–1 Distribution of weight gain during pregnancy.

TABLE 7–1 RECOMMENDED WEIGHT GAINS FOR PREGNANT WOMEN BASED ON BODY MASS INDEX (BMI)

WEIGHT CATEGORY BASED ON BMI*	TOTAL WEIGHT GAIN†		1ST TRIMESTER GAIN		2ND AND 3RD TRIMESTER WEEKLY GAIN	
	lb	kg	lb	kg	lb	kg
Underweight (BMI < 19.8)	28–40	12.5–18	5	2.3	1.07	0.49
Normal weight (BMI = 19.8–26)	25–35	11.5–16	3.5	1.6	0.97	0.44
Overweight (BMI > 26–29)	15–25	7–11.5	2	0.9	0.67	0.3
Obese (BMI > 29)	at least 15	6				

(Data from Subcommittee on Nutritional Status and Weight Gain During Pregnancy and Subcommittee on Dietary Intake and Nutrient Supplements During Pregnancy, Food and Nutrition Board, National Academy of Sciences. Nutrition During Pregnancy, Parts I and II. Washington, DC: National Academy Press, 1990.)

*Metric BMI = weight (kg)/height (m)^2. See Appendix 20.

†Young adolescents and black women should strive for gains at the upper end of the recommended range. Short women (< 62 in. or < 157 cm) should strive for gains at the lower end of the range.

Recommended weight gain goals are based on prepregnancy body mass index (BMI). The BMI calculation is explained in Chapter 16 and Appendix 20.

A BMI of between 20 and 26 is considered to be normal. A BMI of less than 20 represents underweight, a BMI greater than 26 indicates overweight, and a BMI exceeding 29 is indicative of obesity. A woman with a BMI of 22 would be considered normal weight and counseled to gain 25 to 35 lb during her pregnancy.

Weight gain curves now being used during pregnancy reflect the prepregnancy weight, height, and age of the mother. Figure 7–2 presents curves of desirable weight gain during pregnancy, as recommended by the Subcommittee on Nutritional Status and Weight Gain During Pregnancy (IOM, 1990).

Since the release of the 1990 Institute of Medicine report, few studies have dealt with the effects of biological factors on maternal weight gain (i.e., birth interval, parity, BMI, height, and physical activity). The composition of weight gain and rate of energy metabolism appear to affect infant birth weight (King, 1994). For example, water gain, which probably represents lean tissue gain, is a pre-

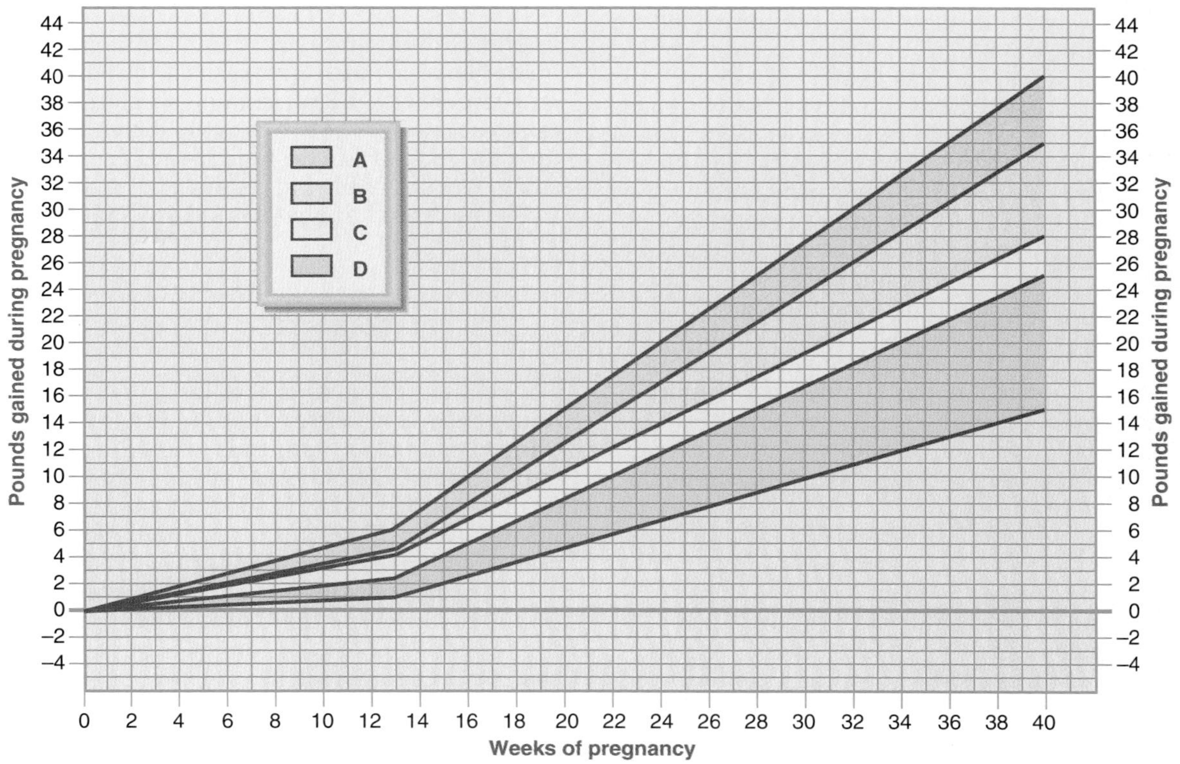

FIGURE 7–2 Women who are of normal weight prior to pregnancy should aim for a weight gain in the B–C range (25 to 35 lb) during the pregnancy. Underweight women should gain in the A–B range (28 to 40 lb). Women who are overweight prior to pregnancy should gain in the D range (15 to 25 lb).

dictor of birth weight, whereas fat tissue gain is not (Hickey, 1994; Lederman, 1996).

Obesity. Trends among U.S. women reveal an increasing prevalence of obesity. For example, the prevalence of overweight (BMI >27.8) among women aged 20 to 29 years increased from 12.6% in 1971 to 1974 to 20.2% in 1988 to 1991 (Kuczmarski et al., 1994).

When the obese woman (BMI of 29 or greater) becomes pregnant, there is an increased risk of very preterm (<32 weeks) delivery and early or late fetal death if this is her first pregnancy. In parous women who are obese and pregnant, there is an increased risk of late fetal death, with stillbirth occurring at 28 weeks or later (Cnattingius et al., 1998). The rate of preeclampsia also increases with increasing BMI (Eskenazi et al., 1991; Stone et al., 1994).

Another worrisome observation in obese pregnant women is the increased risk of delivering an infant with a neural tube defect, regardless of folic acid intake. Apparently adequate folate intake did not seem to provide protection in these women, as it does in normal-weight pregnant women (Werler et al., 1996; Shaw et al., 1996). It is possible that these women require even more folic acid.

Gestational weight gain is positively associated with postpartum weight retention. Indeed, many women with increased weight postpartum have gained more during their pregnancy than the upper limits recommended in the 1990 IOM report (Caulfield et al., 1996).

Gains of 15 to 25 lb have been recommended for the overweight woman to at least account for the weight of the fetus and the maternal support tissues. Lower gains are associated with an increased risk of intrauterine growth retardation (Edwards et al., 1996). Because obese women may be hesitant to gain any weight at all during pregnancy, they should be counseled that pregnancy is not a time for weight loss. Rather, an appropriate nutritional goal would be to emphasize choosing food of high nutritional quality and avoiding unnecessary, calorie-rich foods. Because obese women have an increased incidence of obstetric complications, including prolonged labor, pyelonephritis, diabetes, hypertension, and thromboembolism, the pattern of weight gain should be monitored carefully by the nutrition professional, and appropriate dietary recommendations made as needed.

Adolescence. About 1 million U.S. adolescents become pregnant every year. Teens have a higher rate of bearing LBW infants which is the greatest determinant of infant death and disability. Risk factors for poor outcome in pregnant adolescents are listed in Table 7–2 (Story, 1990). Teenage pregnancy continues to be viewed as one of the major public health problems in the United States, and is associated with significant medical and nutritional risks (Fig. 7–3). Dietary practices are one of the most important and controllable factors for both the teen and her baby. In counseling teen mothers, the nutrition professional must be aware of the teen's social, economic, and educational frameworks that influence her food choices (Konzelmann, 1996). It is recommended that adolescents, as a group, gain 28 to 40 lb during pregnancy; recommended weight gain is individualized depending on prepregnant weight and gynecologic age (years since menarche) (see Chapter 11). The benefits of prenatal counseling for teens are noted in Figure 7–4.

TABLE 7–2 RISK FACTORS FOR POOR OUTCOME OF PREGNANCY IN TEENS

Maternal age, especially 15 years or younger
Pregnancy less than 2 years after onset of menarche
Poor nutrition/low prepregnancy weight
Poor weight gain
Infection
Sexually transmitted diseases
Preexisting anemia
Substance abuse—smoking, drinking, drugs
Poverty
Lack of social support
Lack of education
Rapid repeat pregnancies
Lack of access to age-appropriate prenatal care
Late entry into the health care system
Unmarried status

(Story M (ed.). Nutrition Management of the Pregnant Adolescent. Washington, DC: U.S. Departments of Agriculture and Health and Human Services, March of Dimes Birth Defects Foundation, National Clearing House, 1990.)

Multiple Births. The incidence of multiple births in the United States is rising. Infants of multiple births have a much greater risk of being born premature, or with LBW, than do singletons. Adequate maternal weight gain has been shown to be particularly important in these high-risk pregnancies. Optimal weight gain and infant gestational ages for this population are presented in Table 7–3 (Luke, 1994, 1995, 1996).

Nutritional Supplementation During Pregnancy

Supplementation of a mother's diet during pregnancy may take the form of additional energy, protein, vitamins, or minerals exceeding her routine daily intake. Numerous studies have been performed, particularly in poverty-stricken, underdeveloped countries where prepregnancy nutritional status is likely to be inferior. The findings of many of these studies suggest that the worse the nutritional condition of the mother entering pregnancy, the more valuable an improved prenatal diet, nutritional supplementation, or both, are to her pregnancy course and outcome (Lechtig et al., 1975a).

In this country, the major food program for pregnant women, under the auspices of the U.S. Department of Agriculture (USDA), is the Special Supplemental Nutrition Program for Women, Infants and Children, better known as WIC. The WIC program,

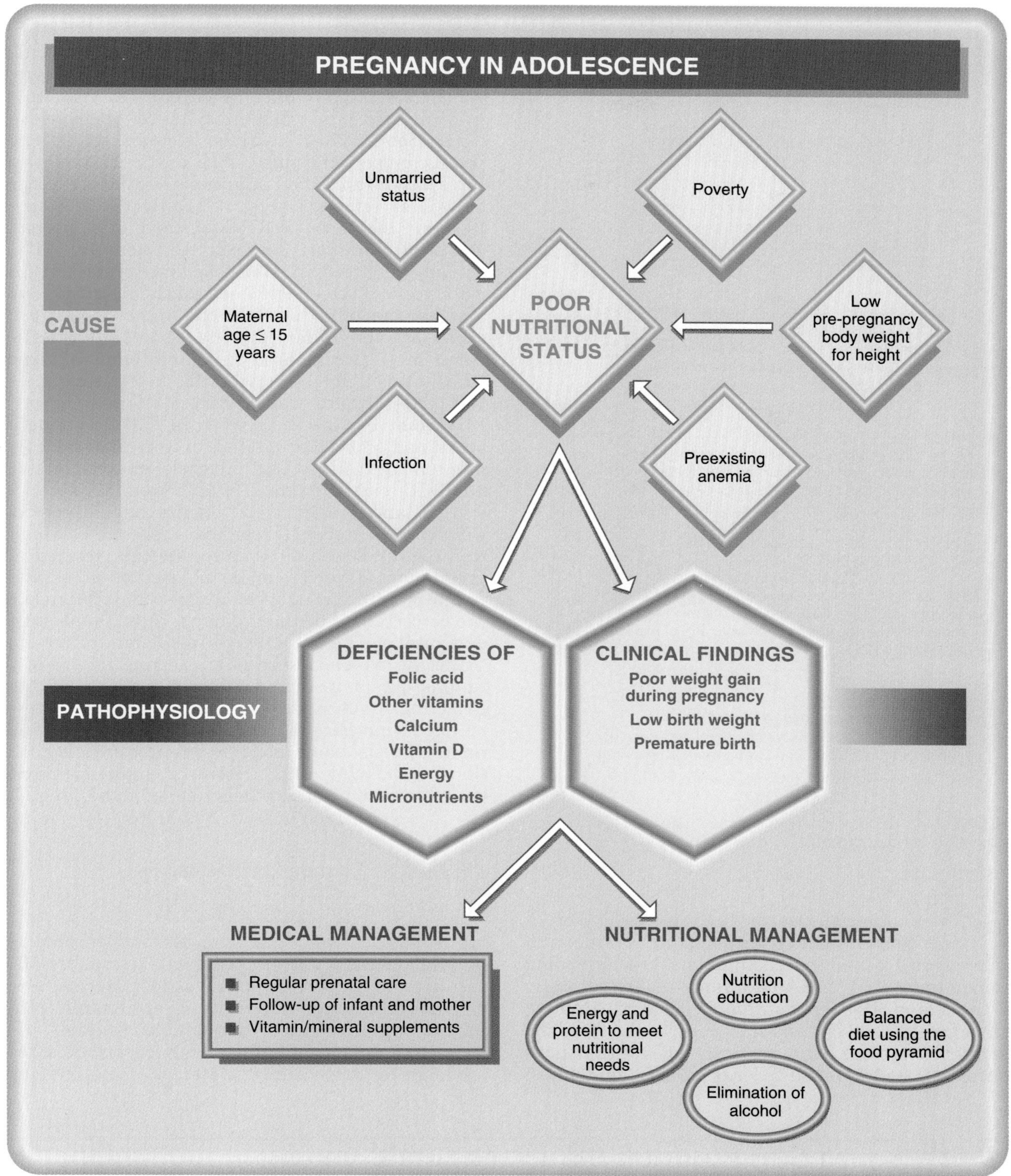

FIGURE 7–3 Pathophysiology algorithm—management of pregnancy in adolescence. (Algorithm content developed by John Anderson, Ph.D., and Sanford C. Garner, Ph.D., 2000.)

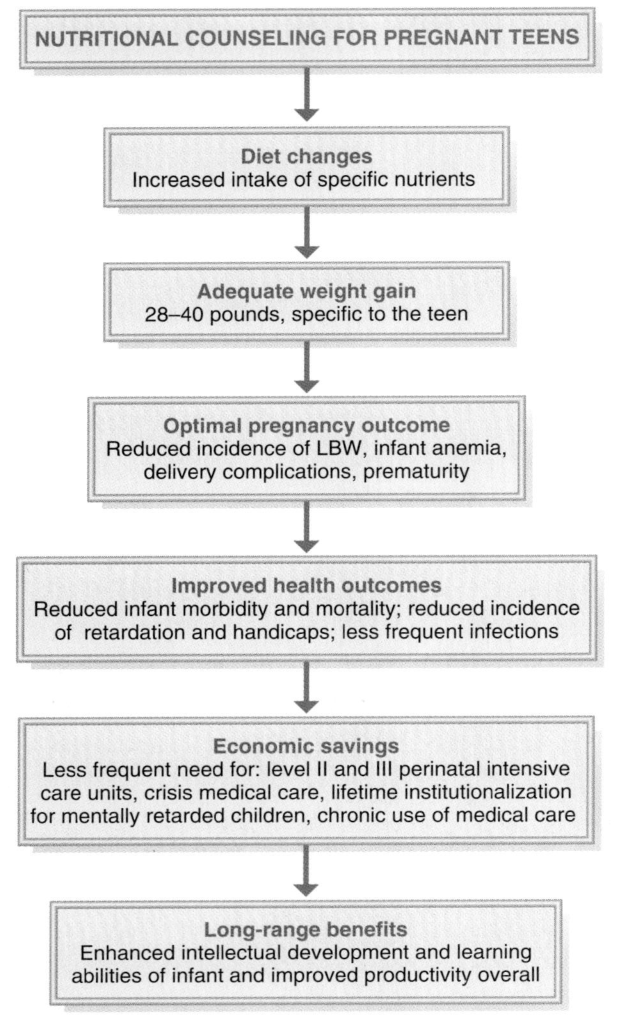
NUTRITIONAL COUNSELING FOR PREGNANT TEENS
Diet changes
Increased intake of specific nutrients
Adequate weight gain
28–40 pounds, specific to the teen
Optimal pregnancy outcome
Reduced incidence of LBW, infant anemia, delivery complications, prematurity
Improved health outcomes
Reduced infant morbidity and mortality; reduced incidence of retardation and handicaps; less frequent infections
Economic savings
Less frequent need for: level II and III perinatal intensive care units, crisis medical care, lifetime institutionalization for mentally retarded children, chronic use of medical care
Long-range benefits
Enhanced intellectual development and learning abilities of infant and improved productivity overall

FIGURE 7–4 Benefits of nutritional counseling in adolescent pregnancy. *LBW,* low birth weight.

which was originally authorized in 1972, serves pregnant women, non–breast-feeding postpartum women until 6 months postpartum, breast-feeding women up until 1 year, and infants and children up to the age of 5 years. To qualify for WIC services, participants must live in an area served by WIC, be at nutritional risk, and have an income that does not exceed 185% of the federal poverty guidelines. Criteria for "nutritional risk" vary from state to state but may include anemia, poor gestational weight gain, the infant failing to thrive, or a diet record showing an inadequate diet. WIC provides vouchers for foods high in vitamin A, vitamin C, iron, protein, and calcium. Some of the foods include iron-fortified breakfast cereals, milk, eggs, peanut butter, and juice. WIC participants also receive either individual or group nutrition education, as well as referrals to other health care resources. In many instances, WIC clinics also offer prenatal and well child care services. Additionally, WIC is actively involved in breast-feeding promotion. An evaluation of the effectiveness of the program found a higher mean birth weight and higher mean gestational age for infants born to women who participated in WIC compared to infants born to women who were eligible, but who did not participate in WIC. Also, there was a decreased prevalence of LBW and very low birth weight (VLBW) among infants, and a lower prevalence of iron deficiency anemia among toddlers and preschool children, associated with participation in WIC (Owen, 1997).

A balanced diet that results in appropriate weight gain during pregnancy generally supplies the required vitamins and minerals needed for pregnancy. However, many physicians prescribe a prenatal vitamin-mineral supplement because of the uncertainty of the woman's nutritional status and intake. The Institute of Medicine did not find sufficient evidence to recommend routine use of vitamins except in high-risk pregnancies (i.e., those involving undernourished, substance-abusing, or teenaged mothers, a short interval between pregnancies, a history of an LBW infant, multiple gestations, etc.) (IOM, 1990). However, supplementation with folate and iron is recommended in all pregnancies (see the section on Nutritional Requirements).

Physiologic Changes of Pregnancy

Blood Volume and Composition

Many physical and biochemical changes occur in normal pregnancy. Blood volume expands by 50%, resulting in a decrease in hemoglobin levels, blood glucose values, and serum levels of albumin, other serum proteins, and water-soluble vitamins. The decline in serum albumin levels contributes to a tendency for extracellular water to accumulate dur-

TABLE 7–3 WEIGHT GAINS OF MOTHERS AND MULTIPLE BIRTH BABIES*

PLURALITY	LIVEBORN INFANTS*	%LBW (<2500 g)	%VLBW (<1500 g)	MATERNAL WEIGHT BY 24 WKS.	WEIGHT GAIN TOTAL (lb)	WEEKS GESTATION	MEAN BIRTH WEIGHT (g)
Singletons	3,899,627	6	1	12	25–35	38–41	3700–4000
Twins	96,445	50	10	24	40–45	36–37	2500–2800
Triplets[+]	4168	90	32	36	50–60	34–35	1900–2200

(From Luke B. Managing maternal nutrition: Prenatal and postpartum. Perinat Nutr Rep 3: 2, 1997.)
LBW, low birth weight; *VLBW,* very low birth weight.
*Based on 1994 U.S. vital statistics.

ing pregnancy. The decrease in water-soluble vitamin concentrations makes determination of an inadequate intake or a deficient nutrient state difficult. By contrast, serum concentrations of fat-soluble vitamins and other lipid fractions, such as triglycerides, cholesterol, and free fatty acids, increase.

Cardiovascular and Pulmonary Function

To provide for the increased cardiac output that accompanies pregnancy, slight cardiac hypertrophy occurs, along with an increased pulse rate. In most women, blood pressure decreases during the first two trimesters because of peripheral vasodilation. It then returns to normal in the third trimester. Maternal oxygen requirements increase, and the threshold for CO_2 is lowered, making the pregnant woman feel dyspneic. Adding to this feeling of dyspnea is the fact that the growing uterus pushes the diaphragm upward, making breathing more difficult. Fortunately, more efficient gas exchange occurs in the lungs.

Gastrointestinal Function

During pregnancy, the function of the gastrointestinal system changes in several ways that affect nutritional status. Early on, nausea and vomiting may occur, followed by a return of appetite that, in some, may be ravenous. Cravings for and aversions to foods may be accompanied by a decreased ability to taste saltiness. This may, in fact, be a physiologic mechanism for increasing salt intake (Brown and Toma, 1986). At the same time that an increased progesterone level relaxes the uterine muscle to allow expansion with fetal growth, gastrointestinal motility also diminishes, to allow for increased absorption of nutrients. This often results in constipation. Additionally, a relaxed lower esophageal sphincter can cause regurgitation and heartburn (see the section on Heartburn that appears later in this chapter).

Renal Function

Increased blood volume produces a high glomerular filtration rate. It appears that the renal tubules are unable to adjust completely, and a percentage of nutrients that would have been reabsorbed in the nonpregnant woman are excreted in the urine. Increased amounts of amino acids, glucose, and water-soluble vitamins may appear in the urine. This may be a reason for the increased number of urinary tract infections seen in pregnant women.

The ability to excrete water is lowered, and edema in the legs and ankles is common and normal. This edema is not associated with perinatal mortality when the other symptoms of preeclampsia—hypertension and proteinuria—are absent. In fact, if it is not associated with other symptoms of preeclampsia, the presence of mild edema is associated with slightly larger babies and a lower rate of prematurity (Worthington-Roberts and Williams, 1993).

Placenta

Not only is the placenta the principal site of production for several hormones responsible for regulating fetal growth and development of maternal support tissues, but it is also the conduit for exchange of nutrients, oxygen, and waste products. Any damage to or inadequacy in the placenta compromises its ability to nourish the fetus, regardless of how well nourished the mother is, or how optimal her dietary intake. Placental size and the number of placental cells have been found to be 15% to 20% below normal in infants experiencing intrauterine growth failure. A small placenta has a relatively smaller surface area of placental peripheral villi, which are responsible for the transfer of nutrients to the fetus. The placental surface area may be the means by which maternal nutrition affects birth weight (Lechtig et al., 1975b).

Nutritional Requirements

Pregnancy is a time for growth and additional demand for nutrients. Subcommittees of the Institute of Medicine are currently reviewing and revising the 1989 Recommended Dietary Allowances (RDAs) for pregnancy and lactation in the United States and Canada. Some of the old RDAs have been replaced by Adequate Intakes (AIs) and others by new RDAs (see Chapter 15). Table 7–4 gives the most current RDAs and AIs.

Energy

Additional energy is required during pregnancy to support the metabolic demands of pregnancy and fetal growth.

RECOMMENDED INTAKE. The 1989 RDA for energy intake during pregnancy is an additional 300 kcal/day, with the qualification that unless body reserves are depleted at the onset of pregnancy, the extra 300 kcal should be added only in the second and third trimesters (Food and Nutrition Board, 1989). However, it should be recognized that, as long as the amount and rate of weight gain are within the desirable range, the range of acceptable energy intakes with good pregnancy outcomes is wide.

EXERCISE. Energy expended in voluntary physical activity is the largest variable in overall energy expenditure. Activities involving body movement require an increase in energy expenditure proportional to the increase in body weight. Most pregnant women compensate, however, by slowing their work pace as weight gain proceeds, so that total energy expenditure during a day may not be substantially greater than before.

For those women who become pregnant while

TABLE 7-4 DIETARY REFERENCE INTAKES: RECOMMENDED DIETARY ALLOWANCES AND ADEQUATE INTAKES FOR WOMEN

	14–18 YR OF AGE	19–30 YR OF AGE	31–50 YR OF AGE	PREGNANT	LACTATING
Energy (kcal)	2200	2200	2200	+0 1st tri. +300 2nd tri. +300 3rd tri.	+500
Protein (g)	44	46	50	60	65
Vitamin A (μg RE)	800	800	800	800	1300
Vitamin D (μg)* AI	5	5	5	5	5
Vitamin E (mg α-TE)	8	8	8	10	12
Vitamin K (μg)	55	60	65	65	65
Vitamin C (mg)	60	60	60	70	95
Thiamin (mg)	1.0	1.1	1.1	1.4	1.5
Riboflavin (mg)	1.0	1.1	1.1	1.4	1.6
Niacin (mg NE)	14	14	14	18	17
Vitamin B_6 (μg)	1.2	1.3	1.3	1.9	2.0
Folate (μg)**	400	400	400	600	500
Vitamin B_{12} (μg)	2.4	2.4	2.4	2.6	2.8
Biotin (μg)* AI	25	30	30	30	35
Pantothenic acid (mg)* AI	5	5	5	6	7
Choline (mg)* AI	400	425	425	450	550
Calcium (mg)* AI	1300	1000	1000	1000 (>18 yr old) 1300 (≤ 18 yr old)	1000 (>18 yr old) 1300 (≤ 18 yr old)
Phosphorus (mg)	1250	700	700	700 (> 18 yr old) 1250 (≤ 18 yr old)	700 (> 18 yr old) 1250 (≤ 18 yr old)
Magnesium (mg)	360	310	320	350 (> 18 yr old) 400 (≤ 18 yr old)	310 (> 18 yr old) 360 (≤ 18 yr old)
Fluoride (mg)* AI	3	3	3	3	3
Iron (mg)	15	15	15	30	15
Zinc (mg)	12	12	12	15	19
Iodine (μg)	150	150	150	175	200
Selenium (μg)	50	55	55	65	75

(Adapted from Food and Nutrition Board, National Academy of Sciences. Recommended Dietary Allowances, 10th ed., Washington, DC: National Academy Press, 1989 and Institute of Medicine; Food and Nutrition Board. Dietary Reference Intakes for Thiamin, Riboflavin, Niacin, Vitamin B_6, Folate, Vitamin B_{12}, Pantothenic Acid, Biotin and Choline. Washington, DC: National Academy Press, 1998; and Institute of Medicine, Food and Nutrition Board. Dietary Reference Intakes for Calcium, Phosphorus, Magnesium, Vitamin D and Fluoride. Washington, DC: National Academy Press, 1997.)

*Adequate Intake (AI).

tri., trimester; *RE*, retinol equivalents; α-*TE*, alpha-tocopherol; NE, niacin equivalents.

**This is synthetic folic acid from fortified foods or supplements.

maintaining an exercise program, it appears that continuing with the exercise does not affect the rate of weight gain or fat deposition during the first trimester. However, after the 15th week of gestation, regular exercise does reduce fat deposition and weight gain. The overall pregnancy weight gain, however, usually still remains appropriate (Clapp and Little, 1995). (See the accompanying box, "*Focus On:* Exercise in Pregnancy.")

Because individuals vary considerably in level and intensity of activity, it is best to advise women to eat enough to satisfy their physiologic appetite and support an appropriate rate of weight gain. Excessive exercise, combined with inadequate energy intake, may lead to suboptimal maternal weight gain and poor fetal growth. A pregnant woman should always discuss exercise with her doctor or health practitioner because pregnancy loosens ligaments, and excessive exercise can increase core temperatures.

Consequences of Energy Restriction. Optimal fetal growth occurs only when the mother is able to accumulate a critical amount of extra body stores during pregnancy. The effect of maternal malnutrition on the development of the fetus is a matter of concern, not only with respect to nutritionally deprived populations, but also with respect to the deliberate practice of restricting food intake to lose weight or prevent weight gain.

A once popular concept held that the fetus can protect itself by parasitizing the mother when nutritional status is less than optimal. However, evidence from famines in Holland and Germany during World War II clearly contradict this assumption. The deprived mothers appeared to be proportionately less affected than their infants, an observation that is consistent with animal data.

One recognized consequence of energy restriction is the increased production of ketone bodies and their ultimate spillage into the urine. Although it is known that the fetus can metabolize ketone bodies to some degree, the short- and long-term effects of maternal ketonemia are unclear. Both animal and human data indicate that ketone bodies are probably normally presented to the fetal brain at various times during pregnancy. After an overnight fast, maternal ketone body concentrations in the blood are greater in pregnant than in nonpregnant

EXERCISE IN PREGNANCY

Exercise programs have become increasingly popular with the heightened concern about weight control, particularly during the reproductive years when some women have a tendency to gain weight. Health care providers need sound scientific information on the benefits and risks of exercise during pregnancy to provide appropriate advice to such women.

Research shows that continuing a regular exercise regimen throughout pregnancy reduces subcutaneous fat deposition in mid-pregnancy and subcutaneous fat retention in late pregnancy. Rate of weight gain is limited after the 15th week, and the overall weight gain is reduced, but remains well within the normal range (Clapp & Little, 1995). Additional outcome data confirm that the incidence of obstetric complications in women who continue a regular exercise regimen throughout pregnancy is either unchanged or reduced (Clapp, 1993; Dewey and McCrory, 1994).

The potential benefits of prenatal exercise include improved fitness, prevention of gestational diabetes, facilitation of labor, and reduced stress. A healthy fetus is generally able to compensate for periods of transitory stress that occur during maternal exercise. However, pregnant women should follow particular guidelines to avoid extreme stress to either herself or the fetus. Guidelines for exercise during pregnancy have been developed by the American College of Obstetricians and Gynecologists (ACOG, 1998).

A woman who is just beginning an exercise program during pregnancy should exercise at a level that keeps her heart rate below 140 beats per minute. A good fitness program would be 1 hour of physical activity 3 days per week, with an intensity that keeps the maternal heart rate under 120 to 130 beats per minute (Revelli et al., 1992). The types of exercise that provide the best cardiovascular and psychological benefits with the least pregnancy risks are walking, jogging, stationary cycling, and swimming.

women, and ketonuria sometimes is seen. Extreme levels of ketonemia, however, may be an indicator of maternal malnutrition, with maternal-fetal competition for nutrients and the associated increased fetal risk.

Protein

Although the need for additional protein to support the synthesis of maternal and fetal tissues is well recognized, the required magnitude of the increase is uncertain. Efficiency of protein utilization in pregnant women appears to be about 70%, the same as that observed in infants. Needs are also variable, increasing as pregnancy proceeds, with greater demands occurring during the second and third trimesters. The current RDA of 60 g of protein for pregnant women represents an additional 10 to 16 g per day over nonpregnant protein requirements (Food and Nutrition Board, 1989).

Protein deficiency during pregnancy has adverse consequences, but limited intakes of protein and energy usually occur together, making it hard to separate the effects of energy deficiency from those of protein deficiency. Studies have shown that providing extra energy to mothers influences pregnancy outcome as much as providing energy and protein together (Lechtig, 1975a; Zlatnick and Burmeister, 1983). Thus, it appears that it is usually the energy deficit and not the protein deficit that determines unfavorable pregnancy outcome.

Vitamins

Maintenance of health during the course of pregnancy requires an adequate supply of vitamins and minerals, some of which have particular significance. In some instances, this is accomplished by increasing dietary intake; in others, vitamin-mineral supplementation is initiated. One study of periconceptional multivitamin supplementation showed that it reduced the risk of heart defects in infants by 43%; this protective effect was not conferred when multivitamin supplementation was begun in the second month of pregnancy or later (Bolto et al., 1996).

FOLIC ACID. Folic acid needs increase during pregnancy in response to the demands of maternal erythropoiesis and fetal and placental growth. The 1998 RDA is 600 mcg which includes a 200 mcg increase over the RDA for nonpregnant females. The Institute of Medicine goes on to recommend that 400 mcg per day come from fortified foods or supplements in addition to the folate in food and drink (Institute of Medicine, 1998). A Tolerable Upper Intake Level (UL) was also set at 800–1000 mcg per day from fortified foods or supplements.

Folic acid deficiency is marked by a reduced rate of DNA synthesis and mitotic activity in individual cells. Clinical detection of megaloblastic anemia may not occur until the third trimester; however, preliminary morphologic and biochemical signs of deficiency may precede this state. (See Chapter 35.)

The consequences of folic acid deficiency in the absence of anemia are currently the focus of much scientific interest. Maternal folic acid deficiency in experimental animals is associated with an increased incidence of pregnancy-related problems, including congenital malformations in the offspring. Malformations have been noted in the offspring of women using folate antagonist drugs, such as methotrexate and valproic acid. Limited evidence in humans also suggests that deficiency of this vitamin may be associated with spontaneous abortion and obstetric complications, such as preterm labor and LBW. In one study, women with a folate intake of 240 mg/day or less were found to have double the risk of bearing an LBW infant or a premature infant (Scholl et al., 1996).

Perhaps the greatest significance of folic acid and its potential influence on pregnancy outcome is its role in preventing **neural tube defects,** such as spina bifida and anencephaly. Neural tube defects are among the most common birth defects, with approximately 2500 new cases occurring in the United States each year. Moreover, neural tube defects have a fairly high recurrence rate, approximately 2% to 10%.

Two randomized trials in Europe have strengthened the association between periconceptional supplementation with folic acid and the prevention of neural tube defects. In the Medical Research Council (MRC) Vitamin Study, 1817 women who had had an infant with a neural tube defect were randomized at 33 study sites to receive either a folic acid supplement, a multivitamin supplement, folic acid plus the multivitamins, or a placebo. The group that received the folic acid supplement showed a 72% reduction in the risk of recurrence of neural tube defects. So striking were the results that the trial was halted early (MRC, 1991). The second study of 5520 European pregnant women showed that periconceptual supplementation with a multivitamin containing 800 mcg of folic acid reduced the incidence of neural tube defects in the infants born (Czeizel et al., 1994). In both of these studies, folic acid supplementation was associated not only with a significant reduction in birth defects, but also with an increase in recognized spontaneous abortions. It may be that folic acid acts through an unusual mechanism—**terathanasia**—the selective promotion of spontaneous abortion of defective fetuses (Hook and Czeizel, 1997).

Studies have shown that red cell folate levels exceeding 906 mmol/L (400 ng/mL) are best for preventing neural tube defects. In a study of 189 healthy women attempting to become pregnant, only 1 in 4 women had red cell folate levels greater than this level. Women who consumed only naturally occurring sources of folate had the lowest levels of folate intake and the lowest frequency of red cell folate levels considered to be protective. Only those women who consumed folic acid supplements achieved red cell folate levels that were considered to be optimal for protection against neural tube defects (Brown et al., 1997).

Based on these remarkable results, the CDC have recommended that all women of childbearing years increase their intake of folic acid (CDC, 1992). It is crucial to note that, because the neural tube closes by 28 days of gestation (before most women realize they are pregnant), supplementation with folic acid should ideally occur prior to conception—hence, the CDC's recommendation to increase intake throughout the childbearing years. One way to accomplish this is by fortifying food with folic acid. The Food and Drug Administration (FDA) has ruled that, effective January of 1998, products made with enriched flour or grain products, such as bread, rice, and pasta should contain additional folic acid, just as they now contain additional iron, niacin, and other vitamins. Women of childbearing age should be encouraged to include generous amounts of folic acid sources in their diets—that is, foods such as dark green, leafy vegetables; legumes; orange juice; soy; wheat germ; almonds; and peanuts (see Appendix 41). In addition, women planning a pregnancy should begin periconceptional supplementation with folic acid at levels of 400 to 800 mcg per day (CDC, 1992).

Certain groups of women who smoke, consume moderate or heavy amounts of alcohol, or use recreational drugs are at risk for marginal folate status. Additionally, users of oral contraceptives, antiepileptic medications, and some other prescription drugs, as well as those with malabsorption syndromes, may have low serum or red blood cell folate levels.

It is alarming to learn that, in a 1997 Gallup survey sponsored by the March of Dimes, only 6% of the respondents—women aged 18 to 45 years—knew that folic acid should be taken before pregnancy (Johnston and Staples, 1997).

VITAMIN B_6. The 1998 RDA for vitamin B_6 during pregnancy is 1.9 mg per day. The additional 0.6 mg above the recommendation for nonpregnant adult women provides for increased needs associated with synthesis of nonessential amino acids in growth and vitamin B_6–dependent niacin synthesis from tryptophan. In 1998 a UL for vitamin B_6 was also set at 80–100 mg/day (Institute of Medicine, 1998).

The apparent alterations in vitamin B_6 status are regarded as indicative of some poorly understood physiologic adjustment to pregnancy. However, in some studies of infants born to mothers with varying vitamin B_6 status, unsatisfactory Apgar scores were associated with lower levels of the vitamin in both maternal and cord serum and breast milk (Roepke and Kirksey, 1981; Schuster et al., 1981).

Vitamin B_6 has also been used to manage severe nausea and vomiting in pregnant women. Although this vitamin catalyzes a number of reactions involving neurotransmitter production, it is not known whether this function is involved in the relief that sometimes follows its administration. The amount of vitamin B_6 that is necessary to achieve this antiemetic effect is massive (25 mg t.i.d.), so if used for this purpose, its administration should be closely monitored (Sahakian et al., 1991).

ASCORBIC ACID. An extra 10 mg/day of vitamin C is recommended for pregnant women. The total recommendation of 70 mg/day is easily met by the typical American diet.

Although ascorbic acid deficiency has not been associated with adverse pregnancy outcome in large population studies, a few studies have suggested an association between low plasma levels of vitamin C and preeclampsia, as well as premature rupture of the membranes (Casanueva et al., 1993).

VITAMIN A. The RDA of 4000 IU (or 800 retinol equivalents [RE]) for vitamin A is not increased for pregnancy in view of maternal stores that easily meet the fetal accretion rate. Vitamin A deficiency is teratogenic in lower animals, but confirmatory evidence of its teratogenicity in humans is lacking. However, excessive consumption of vitamin A does appear to be teratogenic. At least seven case reports of adverse pregnancy outcome have been associated with a daily ingestion of 25,000 IU (7500 RE) or more (Rosa et al., 1986). In addition, epidemiologic evidence indicates that the drug isotretinoin, a vitamin A analogue used for treatment of cystic acne, causes major malformations involving craniofacial, central nervous system, cardiac, and thymic changes (Lammer et al., 1985).

More disturbing is the finding that pregnant women who take vitamin A supplements at levels as low as 2.5 times the RDA—10,000 IU per day, an amount easily available in a general multiple vitamin supplement—increase their risk of delivering a baby with a cranial neural crest defect five times over that of women who take 5000 IU or less per day (Rothman et al., 1995). These findings do not apply to beta-carotene, a precursor of vitamin A. Vitamin A poses the most danger when taken in these amounts 2 weeks prior to conception and during the first 2 months of gestation. Because animal liver contains 9000 IU of vitamin A per 3-oz portion, women contemplating a pregnancy, or in the early stages should eat only small amounts of liver infrequently. See Appendix 41 or Table 4–4 for vitamin A content of foods.

The Teratology Society (1987) advocates informing women in their reproductive years that the excessive use of vitamin A shortly before and during pregnancy could be harmful to their babies. This group also suggests that manufacturers of vitamin A–containing supplements lower the maximum amount of vitamin A per unit dosage to 5000 to 8000 IU (about 1500 to 2400 RE) and identify the source of the vitamin. They further support the practice of labeling products containing vitamin A to indicate that consumption of excessive amounts may be hazardous to the embryo or fetus when taken during pregnancy. Women of childbearing age should consult with their physicians before consuming these products.

VITAMIN D. The AI for vitamin D is 5 mcg (200 IU)/day, the same as that for nonpregnant women. The Dietary Reference Intakes (DRIs) also include a UL of 50 mcg/day during pregnancy (Institute of Medicine, 1997).

Vitamin D has long been appreciated for its positive effects on calcium balance during pregnancy. This vitamin and its metabolites cross the placenta and appear in fetal blood in the same concentration as found in maternal circulation.

Maternal deficiency of vitamin D and the subsequent limitation in placental transport to the fetus have been associated with neonatal hypocalcemia or enamel hypoplasia, or both. Vitamin D levels are often low in such infants. However, excessive amounts of vitamin D may be harmful during gestation. Severe infantile hypercalcemia has been reported in newborn animals and in human infants.

VITAMIN E. Vitamin E needs are believed to increase somewhat during pregnancy, but vitamin E deficiency in humans is rare and has not been linked with either damage to offspring or reduced fertility. However, the 1989 RDA of 10 mg of alpha-tocopherol equivalents (alpha-TE) includes a daily increase of 2 mg of alpha-TE to compensate for the amount deposited in the fetus.

Vitamin E deficiency has long been associated with spontaneous abortion in experimental animals. However, studies have failed to support the use of this vitamin as an abortion-preventing agent in humans.

VITAMIN K. No RDA for vitamin K during pregnancy has been established because information is lacking. Therefore, the recommendation of 65 mg for adult women aged 25 to 50 applies to pregnant women as well. Usual diets provide adequate amounts of vitamin K.

Minerals

CALCIUM. The pregnant woman routinely exhibits extensive adjustments in calcium metabolism, largely as a result of the influence of hormonal factors. Human chorionic somatomammotropin from the placenta progressively increases the rate of bone turnover. Estrogen, also largely derived from the placenta, inhibits bone resorption, provoking a compensatory release of parathyroid hormone, which maintains the serum calcium level while enhancing intestinal absorption. The net effect of these changes, which predate fetal skeletal mineralization, is the promotion of progressive calcium retention to meet progressively increasing fetal skeletal demands for mineralization. Fetal hypercalcemia and subsequent endocrine adjustments ultimately stimulate the mineralization process.

Approximately 30 g of calcium is accumulated during pregnancy, almost all of it in the fetal skeleton (25 g). The remainder is stored in the maternal skeleton, presumably held in reserve for the calcium demands of lactation. Most accretion occurs during the latter part of pregnancy, with an estimated average of 300 mg per day being deposited during the last trimester.

The new AI for calcium during pregnancy is 1300 mg/day for women younger than 19 years of age and 1000 mg/day for adult women. This new recommendation reflects no increase over the AI for nonpregnant females because of the effect of maternal hormones on increasing the absorption and utilization of calcium. Intakes lower than this may cause calcium to leach from the calcium reservoir in the maternal skeleton, of which the total requirement of pregnancy (30 g) amounts to about 2.5%. Multiparous women with poor calcium intake can exhibit evidence of clinical osteomalacia, and neonatal bone density may relate to the adequacy of maternal calcium consumption during pregnancy. Typical diets of other cultures are often lower in protein, which would reduce urinary calcium losses and, therefore, calcium requirements (see Chapter 5). Tolerable Upper Intake Levels (UL) were also determined. The UL for calcium during pregnancy is 2500 mg per day.

PHOSPHORUS. The RDA for phosphorus is the same for pregnant women as for nonpregnant women: 1250 mg/day for women younger than 19 years of age and 700 mg/day for those 19 and older. Phosphorus is found in such a wide variety of foods that deficiency is rare. The UL during pregnancy is 3500 mg/day.

IRON. A marked increase in the maternal blood supply during pregnancy greatly increases the demand for iron. With the availability of this mineral, either from the diet or supplements, total erythrocyte volume increases by 20% to 30%. Active bone marrow may utilize an extra 500 mg of elemental iron during pregnancy, and the term fetus and placenta accumulate 250 to 300 mg of elemental iron. Overall, the pregnant woman must have between 700 and 800 mg of extra iron, most of which is needed during the last half of pregnancy when the heaviest maternal and fetal demands occur. Averaged over the entire pregnancy, this amounts to a daily increment of 15 mg of iron. Adding this amount to the recommended intake of 15 mg/day in the nonpregnant state brings the 1989 RDA for iron during pregnancy to a total of 30 mg/day.

Only rarely do women enter pregnancy with iron stores sufficient to cover all needs without compromising maternal well-being. Iron supplementation, usually in the form of ferrous salts, is thus often acknowledged as a necessary means of preventing iron deficiency anemia.

Maternal anemia, defined by a hematocrit value of less than 32% and a hemoglobin level of less than 11 g/dL, occurs in some pregnant women who do not use iron supplements. An anemic woman is clearly less able to tolerate hemorrhage with delivery and is more prone to develop puerperal infection; however, the fetal effects of maternal anemia are poorly understood. Some data suggest that fetal effects are relatively mild, but several reports suggest that pregnancy outcome may be compromised. It might be hypothesized that poor iron consumption leads to poor hemoglobin production, followed by compromised delivery of oxygen to the uterus, placenta, and developing fetus. If maternal cardiac output increases to accommodate the insufficiency in hemoglobin content, the added workload undertaken by the heart could unduly stress maternal systems.

The Institute of Medicine recommends that all pregnant women eating a well-balanced diet should take 30 mg of ferrous iron supplement daily during the second and third trimesters. Further, for optimal absorption, the iron supplement should ideally be taken between meals and not with milk, tea, or coffee. If iron deficiency anemia is detected by routine testing, therapy should consist of 60 to 120 mg of ferrous iron in divided doses throughout the day. When hemoglobin returns to a level appropriate for the women's stage of pregnancy, the 30 mg/day regimen may be resumed (IOM, 1990).

Elevated maternal hemoglobin levels (greater than 13.2 g/dL) have been associated with increased fetal risk, as well as increased maternal hypertension, possibly reflecting a failure in plasma volume expansion or the harmful effect of high hemoglobin levels on uteroplacental circulation (Murphy et al., 1986).

ZINC. The 1989 RDA for zinc is 15 mg/day during pregnancy; this represents an additional 3 mg above the RDA for the nongravid woman. The average zinc intake of pregnant women is 11.1 mg/day (Murtaugh and Weingart, 1995). Because zinc stored in maternal bones is somewhat unavailable, a zinc-deficient diet does not effectively lead to zinc's mobilization. As a result, a dietary deficiency is quickly reflected in the maternal mineral balance.

Animal studies of zinc levels in gestation have shown that zinc deficiency is highly teratogenic in rats and leads to the development of a variety of congenital malformations. Nonhuman primates are also affected, and abnormal brain development and behavior have been described in offspring of zinc-deficient monkeys. Zinc supplementation in women with low prepregnant weights and low plasma zinc levels resulted in an increase in infant birthweight (Goldenberg et al., 1995).

Maternal zinc status may be inversely related to the level of prenatal iron supplementation, as excess iron inhibits zinc absorption (IOM, 1990).

COPPER. The copper content of many diets of pregnant women is only marginal; however, it is currently unknown whether moderate dietary copper deficiency is of consequence to the developing human fetus. Inasmuch as copper deficiency has been found to be teratogenic in animals, copper deficiency may also compromise pregnancy outcome in humans. Excess iron supplementation inhibits copper absorption.

SODIUM. Sodium metabolism is altered during pregnancy under the stimulus of a modified hormonal milieu. Glomerular filtration of the increased maternal blood volume typically leads to the filtration of an additional sodium load of 5000 to 10,000 mEq/day. Compensatory mechanisms maintain fluid and electrolyte balance.

Restriction of dietary sodium has been common in the past among pregnant women who have edema; however, moderate edema appears to be a normal consequence of pregnancy and is no longer treated with diuretics or low-sodium diets. In fact, the increased fluid retention that is normal during pregnancy actually increases the body's demand for sodium. Rigorous sodium restriction in pregnant animals stresses the renin-angiotensin-aldosterone system to the point of breakdown; such animals tend to develop water intoxication along with renal and adrenal tissue degeneration. Neonatal hyponatremia (low blood sodium) has been observed in offspring of women who unduly restricted sodium intake before delivery.

Although moderation in the use of salt and other sodium-rich foods is appropriate for everyone, *aggressive restriction is usually unwarranted in pregnancy, and consumption of sodium should not be less than 2 to 3 g/day.*

MAGNESIUM. The new RDA of 360–400 mg of magnesium in pregnancy includes an increase of 40–90 mg to meet the needs of fetal and maternal tissue growth. The term fetus accumulates 1 g of magnesium during gestation. The Institute of Medicine has noted that magnesium supplementation during pregnancy has been linked to reduced incidence of preeclampsia and intrauterine growth retardation. However, the IOM has also set a Tolerable Upper Intake Level (UL) for magnesium from supplements or pharmacological agents (outside of food and drink) during pregnancy at 350 mg/day. (Institute of Medicine, 1997.) (See the section on edema and leg cramps, p. 183, for a further discussion of the role of magnesium.)

FLUORIDE. The role of fluoride in prenatal development is somewhat controversial. Development of the primary dentition begins at 10 to 12 weeks of pregnancy; from the sixth to the ninth month, the first four per[illegible]anent molars and eight of the permanent inci[illegible] begin to form. Thus, 32 teeth are formin[illegible]leveloping during gestation. Questions invol[illegible]xtent to which fluoride is transported acros[illegible]icenta and its value in utero in the develop[illegible] caries-resistant permanent teeth (see Cha[illegible] The Adequate Intake (AI) for fluoride in p[illegible] is 3 mg/day and the UL is 10 mg/day (Inst[illegible]Medicine, 1997).

Io[illegible] additional increment of 25 mg/day of iodi[illegible]he RDA of 175 mg/day has been propose[illegible]quate to cover the extra demands of the fetu[illegible]ne.

M[illegible] iodine deficiency has long been recogniz[illegible]ause of cretinism in offspring. Data also sug[illegible]t suboptimal iodine nutrition of the mo[illegible] compromise development of the fetus, eve[illegible]retinism does not occur (Connolly et al., 19[illegible]ings indicate that iodine deficiency may lea[illegible]pectrum of subclinical deficits that place th[illegible] a developmental disadvantage.

[illegible] studies have established that iodine su[illegible]tation before conception can prevent ende[illegible]inism, but recent findings indicate that, in[illegible]s where preconception iodine intake cann[illegible]ured, supplementation before the end of th[illegible] trimester can also protect the fetal brain fr[illegible]effects of iodine deficiency (Xue-Yi et al., 1[illegible] Chapter 5).

Guide for Eating During Pregnancy

Recommended Food Intake

The increased requirements of pregnancy can be met by following the Daily Food Guide presented in Table 7–5.

Three 1-cup servings of milk per day provide more than the additional 10 to 16 g of high-quality protein needed, increase the calcium intake to 900 mg, and provide an additional 270 kcal (if skim milk) or 480 kcal (if whole milk). A number of choices are available: whole milk, low-fat milk, skim milk, nonfat powdered milk, buttermilk, acidophilus milk, lactaid-treated milk, evaporated milk, enriched soy milk, and yogurt. If preferred, the required amount can be used in soups, custards, puddings, ice cream, or flavored beverages. Nonfat milk powder can be added during the preparation of meat loaf, soups, scrambled eggs, mashed and scalloped potatoes, sandwich spreads, cooked cereals, homemade breads, cookies, or pastries. Approximately 1/3 cup of dried skim milk is equivalent to 1 cup of fluid milk. Milk can be made richer in calcium, protein, and calories by adding 2 tablespoons of dried nonfat milk to a glass of fluid milk. Three cups of milk either soy or cow's fortified with vitamin D provide 7.5 μg of cholecalciferol (300 IU). If fluid milk is used in limited amounts, a vitamin D supplement may be desirable, especially if exposure to sunlight is limited.

Many women, primarily non-Caucasian women, are unable to digest the lactose in milk (see Chapter 31) unless it is taken in small amounts at a time. Commercial enzyme preparations, such as Lactaid, can be added to fluid milk and are readily available. Cheese or yogurt, which contain only small

TABLE 7–5 DAILY FOOD GUIDE FOR WOMEN

	MINIMUM NUMBER OF SERVINGS		
FOOD GROUP	Nonpregnant 11–24 yr old	Nonpregnant 25–50 yr old	Pregnant/ Lactating 11–50 yr old
Protein foods	5*	5*	7†
Milk products	3	2	3
Breads, grains	7	6	7
Whole-grain	4	4	4
Enriched	3	2	3
Fruits, vegetables	5	5	5
Vitamin C–rich	1	1	1
Beta-carotene–rich	1	1	1
Folate-rich	1	1	1
Other	2	2	2
Unsaturated fats	3	3	3

(Adapted from Nutrition During Pregnancy and the Postpartum Period: a Manual for Health Care Professionals. California Department of Health Services, Maternal Child Health Branch, 1990.)

*Equivalent in protein to 5 oz of animal protein; at least three servings per week should be from the vegetable proteins.

†Equivalent in protein to 7 oz of animal protein; at least one of these servings should be a vegetable protein.

amounts of lactose, or soy milk which is lactose-free can be substituted. If necessary, preparations, such as calcium lactate or calcium carbonate, may be prescribed (see Chapter 31).

Daily consumption of whole-grain breads and cereals, leafy green and yellow vegetables, and fresh and dried fruits should be encouraged to provide additional minerals, vitamins, and fiber. Careful attention to the selection of foods that are good sources of iron and folic acid is important (see Appendix Table 41). Table 7–6 offers a sample menu that meets the needs of the normal pregnant woman.

Drinking six to eight glasses of fluid daily is encouraged. Intestinal stasis often occurs as a result of the necessary restrictions of activities and the pressure of the enlarging uterus. However, for most individuals, the bulky content of the protective diet plus the suggested fluid intake tend to counteract any difficulty with constipation. Sometimes, though, a fiber supplement is necessary.

Pregnant women are usually highly motivated and very receptive to well-presented nutritional advice. A full discussion of individual needs and involvement of the mother (and, perhaps, the father) in planning the dietary changes are usually effective strategies (Fig. 7–5).

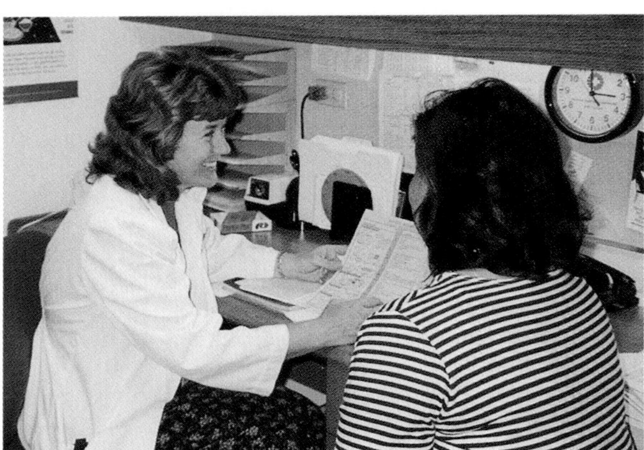

FIGURE 7–5 A prospective mother learns about nutrition for her pregnancy.

TABLE 7–6 SUGGESTED MENU FOR A PREGNANT WOMAN*

Breakfast
Orange juice, ½ cup
Oatmeal, ½ cup
Whole grain or enriched toast, 1 slice
Peanut butter, 2 tsp
Decaffeinated coffee or tea

Midmorning Snack
Apple
High-bran cereal, ¼ cup
Nonfat or reduced-fat milk, ½ cup

Lunch
Turkey (2 oz) sandwich on rye or whole grain bread with lettuce and tomato and 1 tsp mayonnaise
Green salad
Salad dressing, 2 tsp
Fresh peach
Nonfat or low-fat milk, 1 cup

Midafternoon Snack
Nonfat or low-fat milk, 1 cup
Graham crackers, 4 squares

Dinner
Baked chicken breast, 3 oz
Baked potato with 2 T sour cream
Peas and carrots, ½ cup
Green salad
Salad dressing, 2 tsp

Evening Snack
Nonfat yogurt, ½ cup
Fresh strawberries

*Quantities of food should be adjusted to meet individual energy needs to promote appropriate weight gain. The pregnant adolescent, very active woman, or underweight woman will require greater quantities.

Alcohol

Abundant evidence from both animal studies and human experience has linked heavy alcohol consumption with teratogenicity. A pattern of abnormalities identified in affected offspring has been labeled the **fetal alcohol syndrome** (Streissguth et al., 1980). Features of this syndrome include prenatal and postnatal growth failure; developmental delay; microcephaly; eye changes, including involvement of the epicanthal fold; facial abnormalities; and skeletal joint abnormalities (Fig. 7–6). Infants born to moderately heavy drinkers may display limited features of the syndrome (*fetal alcohol effects*). Use of alcohol during pregnancy has been associated with an increased rate of spontaneous abortion, abruptio placentae, and LBW delivery (Council on Scientific Affairs, 1983). Some evidence also suggests a relationship between paternal alcohol use and the size of the offspring (Little and Sing, 1986).

The impact of binge drinking has never been satisfactorily evaluated. Owing to the different tolerance levels of individuals for alcohol, the question of how much moderate drinking is safe during pregnancy has not been answered. A 1995 survey of women who were pregnant or of childbearing age indicated an increasing pattern of alcohol consumption in the United States (Zuger, 1997). Because data are insufficient at this time to recommend any safe level of alcohol consumption during pregnancy, health care providers should heighten their efforts to promote abstinence from alcohol among women who are pregnant or planning a pregnancy.

The mechanisms by which alcohol affects the fetus are not completely understood. As alcohol crosses the placenta, it may accumulate to toxic levels that are particularly damaging during blastogenesis and cell differentiation (Fig. 7–7). Fetal damage may also be caused by dietary deficiencies or altered

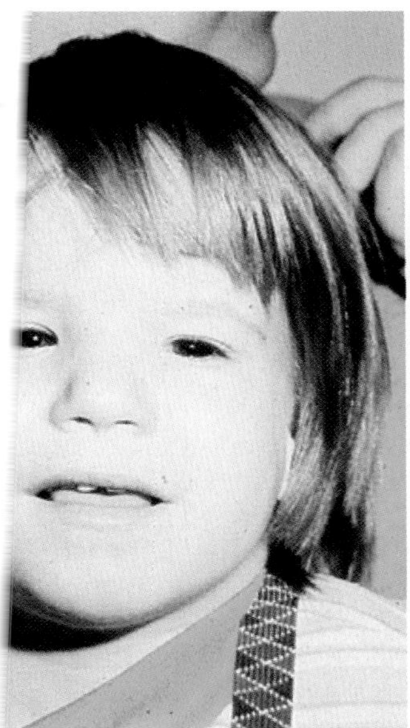

FIGURE ... with fetal alcohol syndrome at 1 year of age. (Reprinted ... nission from Streissguth, A.P., Landesman-Dwyer, S., ..., & Smith, D.W. (1980). Teratogenic effects of alcohol in ... laboratory animals. Science, 209:353–361.)

metabo... ey nutrients among drinkers, most notably ... , magnesium, and zinc.

There ... nce that the course and outcome of pregna... be significantly improved if problem drinker ... their habits, even after conception has occ... osett et al., 1983). However, those who re... eliminate alcohol consumption are usually ... oderate drinkers, not the heavy drinke... sguth et al., 1983).

Non-Nutritive Substances in Foods

CAFFEINE. The effect of caffeine on pregnancy has been extensively researched. Recent conclusions indicate that caffeine alone does not seem to pose a risk to the fetus or to the pregnant woman. Researchers from Howard University conducted a critical review of the literature on four pregnancy outcome variables—birthweight, preterm labor and delivery, spontaneous abortion, and congenital malformation—and found that "caffeine may interact with genetic and pharmacokinetic factors or socioeconomic influences and life-style choices, such as use of alcohol, tobacco, and other drugs, to increase the probability of adverse outcome . . ." (Hinds et al., 1996). Although it appears to be sensible to limit coffee and caffeine intake during pregnancy, there are insufficient data for making a specific recommendation (Nehlig and Debry, 1994).

In 1989, caffeine was linked to infertility in a group of healthy women studied by the National Institute of Environmental Health Sciences. Women who consumed more caffeine per day than the amount in 1 cup of coffee (or 3 cans of caffeinated soda pop) were 50% less likely to conceive during a given menstrual cycle than women who consumed less caffeine (Christianson et al., 1989). A more recent study provided some evidence of the association between coffee consumption and delayed conception, but raised questions about the effect of caffeine intake in relation to other job- and life-related stress variables (Bolumar et al., 1997).

ARTIFICIAL SWEETENERS. There are three types of artificial sweeteners sold in the U.S.; their chemical names are saccharin, acesulfame-K, and aspartame.

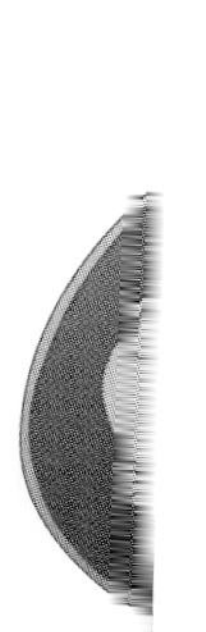

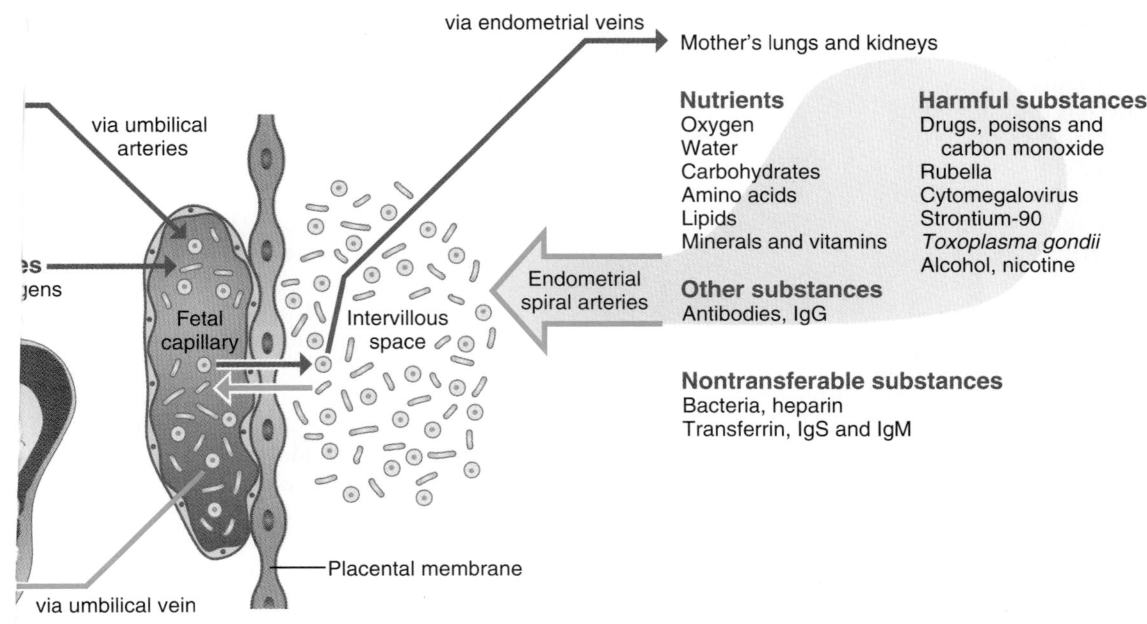

URE 7–7 Diagram illustrating transfer of substances across the placental membrane. *Ig,* immunoglobulin.

Saccharin has not been identified as a **teratogen,** but because it has been shown to be weakly carcinogenic in rats, moderate consumption seems appropriate. Acesulfame-K is currently considered to be safe for consumption; however, there have been inadequate long-term studies in humans during pregnancy. Both saccharin and acesulfame-K cross the placenta and appear in breastmilk, but have no known effect.

Questions about the safety of aspartame use during pregnancy relate to the release of phenylalanine, an amino acid product of its metabolism. In most people, phenylalanine is rapidly broken down into a relatively harmless substance; however, persons with phenylketonuria (PKU) lack the enzyme necessary for its conversion, and can suffer brain damage as a consequence of the high levels of phenylalanine that accumulate in the blood (see Chapter 44). High circulating levels of this amino acid are known to damage the fetal brain; however, the amount of phenylalanine accumulating in the blood of a pregnant woman who does not suffer from PKU is extremely small. The amount of aspartame necessary to raise serum phenylalanine levels to potentially dangerous ranges would require the consumption of one 12-oz can of diet soda every 8 minutes, 24 hours per day. In view of these practical considerations and the fact that there are no conclusive data suggesting increased risk, it seems unreasonable to counsel avoidance of this artificial sweetener during pregnancy (Sturtevant, 1985). However, artificially sweetened soft drinks may serve as substitutes for other beverages, such as milk or juices, that have greater nutritional value.

CONTAMINANTS. A number of contaminants are found in food, some of which may adversely affect the course and outcome of pregnancy if consumed in sufficient amounts. Most heavy metals are embryotoxic, but only mercury, lead, cadmium, and possibly, nickel and selenium have been implicated in this regard. Lead toxicity has been associated with abortion and menstrual disorders; researchers have reported a correlation between atmospheric lead levels and congenital malformations. Pregnant women taking calcium supplements should be advised against using dolomite, which has been found to contain lead.

Beliefs, Avoidances, Cravings, and Aversions

Most women change their diets during their pregnancies. Some changes are based on medical advice, others on folk medicine beliefs or changes in preferences and appetite that may be idiosyncratic or culturally patterned. As the latter affect a woman's willingness to follow prescribed dietary regimens, the health care provider should be aware of their existence.

One important group of *beliefs* espouses the use of dietary means to ensure an easier delivery. Of these, perhaps the most potentially harmful ones are those that involve the elimination of animal proteins or the avoidance of "excessive" weight gain. According to this system of beliefs, low weight gain is deemed desirable because a smaller fetus is believed to be easier to deliver, it is assumed that the baby can "catch up" in terms of growth after birth.

Food avoidances reflect a mother's conscious choice not to consume certain foods during her pregnancy, usually for a reason she can articulate and that seems reasonable to her. The four most commonly avoided foods are sources of animal protein: milk, lean meats, pork, and liver.

Cravings and aversions are powerful urges toward or away from foods, including foods about which women experience no unusual attitudes when not pregnant. The most commonly craved foods are sweets and dairy products. The most common aversions reported are to alcohol, coffee, other caffeinated drinks, and meats. However, cravings and aversions are not limited to any particular foods or food groups.

The significance of these behaviors is difficult to evaluate, as much of the information is anecdotal. The nutritional importance of such practices cannot be assessed without reference to the rest of the individual's diet. Cravings and aversions are not necessarily deleterious.

PICA. **Pica** refers to a compulsion for persistent ingestion of unsuitable substances that have little or no nutritional value. Pica of pregnancy most often involves consumption of dirt or clay **(geophagia)** or starch **(amylophagia),** such as laundry starch. However, nonfood substances subject to compulsive consumption include a bizarre variety of nonfoods, such as ice, paper, burnt matches, stones or gravel, charcoal, soot, cigarette ashes, antacid tablets, milk of magnesia, baking soda, and coffee grounds. The incidence of pica is not limited to any one geographic area, race, sex, culture, or social status, nor is it limited to pregnancy. A familiar example of pica is the consumption of lead paint chips by young children who are hungry and who find the sweet-tasting lead paint chips appealing

Malnutrition is among the medical consequences of pica, as nonfood substances displace essential nutrients in the diet. Starch in excessive amounts can contribute to obesity. Some substances contain toxic compounds, such as heavy metals; others can interfere with the absorption of minerals such as iron. Starch and clay in gross amounts can lead to intestinal obstruction.

The etiology of pica is poorly understood. One theory suggests that the ingestion of nonfood substances relieves nausea and vomiting. It has also been hypothesized that a deficiency of an essential nutrient, such as calcium or iron, results in the eating of nonfood substances that contain these nutrients (Rainville, 1998). Much of this behavior appears to be based on superstitions, customs and traditions that are often passed from mother to daughter.

Table 7–7 presents a summary of nutritional care for the pregnant woman.

TABLE 7–7 SUMMARY OF NUTRITIONAL CARE FOR THE PREGNANT WOMAN

1. Energy intake to meet nutritional needs and allow for about a 0.4 kg (14 oz) weight gain per week during the last 30 weeks of pregnancy
2. Protein intake to meet nutritional needs (about an additional 10–16 g/day)
3. Sodium intake should not be excessive, but should be no less than 2 g/day.
4. Mineral and vitamin intakes to meet the RDA. For folic acid, this will require supplementation and for iron it will likely require supplementation.
5. Alcohol should be omitted.
6. Caffeine can be consumed in moderation: less than 200 mg/day—equivalent of 2 cups of coffee.

Diet-Related Complications of Pregnancy

Nausea and Vomiting

Morning sickness or nausea is common during the early months of pregnancy, but the condition usually disappears as spontaneously as it appears. However, when early pregnancy is characterized by excessive vomiting, an acute protein and energy deficit, as well as a loss of minerals, vitamins, and electrolytes may result.

For the more common form of morning sickness, some dietary measures may help. Small, frequent, dry meals of easily digested carbohydrate-containing foods are usually best tolerated. Liquids are best taken between meals. Fats are often a problem, as they are relatively hard to digest. Unfortunately, there is no cure-all. One author suggests that the woman suffering with nausea should eat whatever makes her feel good and avoid odors that trigger nausea (Erick, 1994).

The pregnant woman should be advised of the importance of eating and be encouraged to eat as much as possible when she is not nauseated. Although anecdotal data indicate that vitamin B_6 has sometimes successfully relieved the nausea of pregnancy, its use is not routinely recommended.

Prolonged, persistent vomiting **(hyperemesis gravidarum)** develops in about 2% of pregnant women (Erick, 1995). Hospitalization is usually indicated, with intravenous fluid and electrolyte replacement required to prevent complications of dehydration. Parenteral nutritional support may be required in the rare persistent case. Tube feeding may be successful, and if so, should be used because of the relatively fewer complications associated with it compared to parenteral nutrition support. See Chapter 22.

Heartburn

Heartburn is a common complaint during the latter part of pregnancy. In most cases, this is an effect of pressure of the enlarged uterus on the stomach which, in combination with the relaxation of the esophageal sphincter, results in occasional regurgitation of stomach contents into the esophagus. This can usually be relieved by limiting the amount of food consumed at one time, and drinking fluids between meals rather than with meals. Attention to wearing loose clothing around the waist, eating slowly, and sitting upright after meals for at least 3 hours before lying down may also help.

Constipation and Hemorrhoids

Pregnant women may develop constipation, most frequently during the latter stages of pregnancy. Causes of this problem include reduced gut motility, physical inactivity, and pressure exerted on the bowel by the enlarged uterus. The weight of the fetus and downward pressure on the veins also may lead to the development of hemorrhoids during this period. Increased consumption of fluids, fiber-rich foods, and dried fruits (especially prunes and figs) usually controls these problems, but some women may also require a bulking type of stool softener (see Chapter 31).

Edema and Leg Cramps

Mild, physiologic edema is usually present in the extremities in the third trimester and should not be confused with the pathologic, generalized edema associated with pregnancy-induced hypertension. The swelling of the lower extremities may be caused by the pressure of the enlarging uterus on the veins returning fluid from the legs. Extravascular fluid is often mobilized in the evening when the woman is lying down, resulting in a tendency to urinate during the night. This normal edema requires no sodium restriction or other dietary change.

The common occurrence of leg cramps during pregnancy, manifested nocturnally by sudden contractions of the gastrocnemius muscle, is thought to be related to a decline in serum calcium levels related to a calcium-phosphorus imbalance. Prevention or relief of these leg cramps has been reported with reduction of milk (a high-phosphorus, high-calcium beverage) intake and supplementation with nonphosphate calcium salts. Although several studies confirmed the benefit of these measures in terms of the total serum calcium level in affected women, other controlled and double-blind studies have failed to indicate a correlation between leg cramps and either the intake of dairy products or calcium supplementation.

Magnesium is another mineral with the potential for relieving leg cramps. Pregnancy or lactation can lead to a secondary magnesium deficiency as evidenced by low serum magnesium levels (Hammar and Berg, 1988; Dahle et al., 1995). Because signs of magnesium deficiency include muscle tremor, ataxia, tetany, and cramps, it makes sense that additional magnesium may relieve the leg cramps associated with pregnancy or lactation. In fact, in a placebo-controlled study, women with pregnancy-related leg cramps were found to have low serum magnesium levels. With the administration of 122 mg of magnesium (as the lactate and citrate) in the morning and 244 mg in the evening, the magnesium-treated group reported a significantly greater reduction of distress than did the control group. Interestingly, however, the low serum magnesium level initially detected in the magnesium-treated group did not return to normal levels, even though leg cramps improved. Perhaps this is attributable to the fact that only 0.5% of the body magnesium is extracellular, so treatment benefits might better correlate with changes in the level of serum ionized magnesium or intracellular magnesium (Dahle et al., 1995).

Diabetes Mellitus

Individualized, expert care is needed for the nutritional management of the pregnant woman with diabetes. On the basis of nutritional history and assessment early in pregnancy, and preferably prior to conception, an individually adapted meal plan should be developed by a skilled nutritionist as part of the health care team (see Chapter 34).

The incidence of preeclampsia is high in the pregnant woman with diabetes, and fetal morbidity and mortality are significantly greater than in normal pregnancy. Preconception and early prenatal care provided by a team of professionals, including a clinical nutritionist, is important in preventing unfavorable outcomes. With good specialized care, the risk of complications can be reduced to the same level as seen in pregnancies in nondiabetic women (Cousins, 1991).

Infants born to women with diabetes are usually larger than those of women who do not have diabetes. This is most likely caused by in utero exposure of the infant to supernormal levels of its own insulin, which is a growth promoting hormone. High fetal insulin levels reflect hyperglycemia in the mother, allowing high levels of glucose to cross the placenta. Infants of mothers with diabetes also tend to become hypoglycemic shortly after birth because of the insulin they have produced and the sudden loss of glucose supply from the mother.

Successful pregnancy requires adequate dietary intake to meet the growth needs of the fetus, prevent ketosis, and prevent depletion of the mother's nutritional stores. Maintenance of optimal blood glucose levels, monitored by frequent glucose measurement, and appropriate insulin adjustments are crucial. Insulin requirements decrease in the first half of pregnancy because of fetal use of glucose, and the mother may need only two thirds of her usual amount. In the second half of pregnancy, hormone changes induce an increase in insulin requirements of 70% to 100% over prepregnancy requirements. This increase occurs rather abruptly during the fifth month and may last through the ninth month. It is at this point that the demands of pregnancy may impose a need for insulin in a pregnant woman with diabetes whose condition was adequately controlled by diet alone in the nonpregnant state. Frequent changes in diet and in insulin dosage may be necessary.

Diabetes may occur only in response to the stress of pregnancy and may resolve itself after delivery, a condition called **gestational diabetes.** This form of diabetes, usually arising after 20 weeks' gestation, may affect as many as 5% to 10% of all pregnant women. Although symptoms are similar to those of diabetes mellitus, including glycosuria and elevated blood glucose levels, the hyperglycemia does not usually reach the markedly high levels of classic diabetes mellitus. Infants born to women who present with gestational diabetes are at increased risk for perinatal mortality, as well as for prematurity with its attendant complications. If the mother's blood glucose is not well controlled, the infant is at risk for macrosomia. In addition, women who have experienced gestational diabetes are at risk for type 2 diabetes mellitus later in life.

Currently, most obstetrical health care providers perform a routine 50-g oral glucose challenge in patients at 24 to 28 weeks' gestation to screen for gestational diabetes. If the results are questionable, an oral glucose tolerance test is scheduled to confirm the diagnosis. Gestational diabetes is treated largely through dietary changes (some calorie restriction may be necessary), and moderate exercise to achieve weight control. Insulin is rarely administered, but blood glucose levels are monitored daily. Through these venues, gestational diabetes can be controlled, resulting in a favorable pregnancy outcome.

Pregnancy-Induced Hypertension (Preeclampsia and Eclampsia)

Pregnancy-induced hypertension (PIH) is a syndrome characterized by hypertension, proteinuria, and edema. Hypoalbuminemia, hypovolemia, and subsequent hemoconcentration are also present. The condition usually develops in the third trimester, affecting about 7% to 8% of the obstetric population, particularly those who are young, pregnant for the first time, or of low socioeconomic status. The terms **preeclampsia** and **eclampsia** refer to the nature and degree of the symptoms involved. Eclampsia is an extension of preeclampsia, with grand mal seizures occurring near the time of labor; it can also occur postpartum.

PIH is usually defined by a systolic blood pressure of 140 mm Hg or a diastolic pressure of 90 mm Hg, or both. However, because young women—the typical group to experience eclampsia—often have very low prepregnant blood pressures (ranging from 90/60 to 120/80 mm Hg), it is advisable to look at the blood pressure *change* during pregnancy. A rise of 20 to 30 mm Hg in systolic pressure or 10 to 15 mm Hg in diastolic pressure, or both, documented on two or more occasions 6 hours apart, is diagnostic.

The extent of proteinuria varies with the degree of PIH. Often, it is fluctuating or transient, and may be minimal, even in severe cases. The presence of 500 mg of protein in a 24-hour urine sample or a 2+ protein test result on random urine collection confirms the condition of PIH. Eclampsia is defined by a level of 5 g of protein in a 24-hour urine specimen or a 3+ to 4+ protein test result on random urine collection.

When edema is generalized, it indicates that the kidneys are reabsorbing large amounts of sodium and there is no control of the extracellular fluid volume. With increased sensitivity to renin, some hypertension can be expected to develop. The edema of PIH may also be associated with dizziness, headache, visual disturbances, facial edema, anorexia, nausea, and vomiting. In the severe state of eclampsia, convulsions occur near the time of labor.

The etiology of PIH is still unknown, but its development is associated with poverty, lack of prenatal care, and poor nutritional status. Most researchers agree that it is associated with decreased uterine blood flow, leading to reduced fetal nourishment. Of the proposed nutritional causes, protein deficiency has been the most popular. The link between protein intake and PIH is not clear, however, and evidence of the benefit of a high-protein diet in preventing the disorder is inconclusive.

An association between calcium deficiency and PIH was proposed in the late 1980s. A recent trial study of calcium supplementation in healthy, nulliparous women revealed that calcium supplementation alone during pregnancy did not prevent preeclampsia or PIH (Levine et al., 1997). However, another earlier trial of calcium supplementation did show a lowering of systolic and diastolic blood pressure (Bucher et al., 1996).

Magnesium supplementation is also recommended to prevent and treat preeclampsia and eclampsia (Roberts, 1995). Magnesium sulfate has even been shown to be superior to phenytoin for managing convulsions in eclamptic women (Lucas, 1995).

Previous attempts to treat PIH have focused on sodium restriction and diuretics. Sodium restriction has failed to alter blood pressure, weight gain, or proteinuria significantly in gravid women, and seems to have no place in the treatment or prevention of PIH. The same can be said for diuretics; use of these drugs does not lower the incidence of PIH or aid in its management. In fact, it may be dangerous to recommend diuretics for women with PIH because they are known to have a subnormal intravascular volume secondary to peripheral vasoconstriction. Diuretics would restrict intravascular volume even further through forced kidney diuresis of sodium and water. As with diuretics and sodium restriction, restricted energy intake has not been found to prevent preeclampsia in pregnant women with large weight gains.

LACTATION

Research conducted over the last 30 years has unequivocally demonstrated that exclusive breast-feeding is the preferred method of infant feeding for the first 4 to 6 months of life. Both the American Dietetic Association and the American Academy of Pediatrics have issued position statements in support of breast-feeding. Some of the distinct advantages of breast-feeding are listed in Table 7–8.

The fact that human milk is superior to formula for infants has influenced a number of health promotion strategies. In the United States, the Surgeon General recommended that, by the year 2000, 75% of all women should be breast-feeding when they leave the hospital, and 50% should still be breast-feeding when the baby is 6 months of age (Britt, 1990). In the early 1980s, as many as 62% of women giving birth in the United States left the hospital breast-feeding. However, in the 1990s, this rate declined dramatically; only slightly more than 50% of all women left the hospital breast-feeding their babies. To reach the Surgeon General's goal, efforts to promote the practice and duration of breast-feeding need to be strengthened in hospitals, health maintenance organizations, private doctor's offices, and public health clinics.

On an international level, in 1990, the World Health Organization (WHO) and UNICEF jointly adopted the Baby Friendly Hospital Initiative (BFHI), a global effort to increase the incidence and duration of breast-feeding. To become "baby friendly," a hospital must agree to implement the "Ten Steps to Successful Breast-feeding." The 10 steps include guidelines for mother-baby management in the hospital, such as provisions for training hospital staff in breast-feeding education and prohibiting supplementary bottles of formula to breast-feeding babies unless *medically* indicated (Ebrahim, 1993) (see the accompanying box, "*Clinical Insight:* The Baby Friendly Hospital Initiative").

Physiology of Lactation

The mammary glands prepare for **lactation** through a series of developmental steps that occur during adolescence and pregnancy. Hormonal

TABLE 7–8 ADVANTAGES OF BREAST-FEEDING

1. Breast milk is nutritionally superior to any alternative.
2. Breast milk is bacteriologically safe and always fresh.
3. Breast milk contains a variety of anti-infectious factors and immune cells.
4. Breast milk is the least allergenic of any infant food.
5. Breast-fed babies are least likely to be overfed.
6. Breast-feeding promotes good jaw and tooth development.
7. Breast-feeding generally costs less than the commercial infant formulas currently available.
8. Breast-feeding automatically promotes close mother–child contact.
9. Breast-feeding is generally more convenient once the process is established.

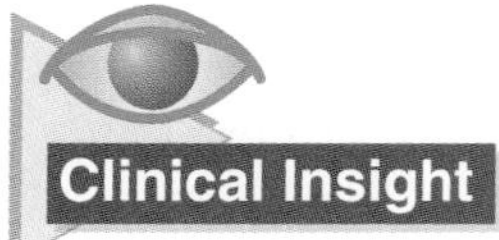

The Baby Friendly Hospital Initiative

Ten Steps to Successful Breast-Feeding

1. Have a written breast-feeding policy that is routinely communicated to all health care staff.
2. Train all health care staff in the skills necessary to implement this policy.
3. Inform all pregnant women about the benefits and management of breast-feeding.
4. Help the mother initiate breast-feeding within a half hour of birth.
5. Show mothers how to breast-feed and how to maintain lactation, even if they are separated from their infants.
6. Give newborn infants no food or drink other than breast milk unless medically indicated.
7. Practice rooming-in; allow mothers and infants to remain together 24 hours a day.
8. Encourage breast-feeding on demand.
9. Give no artificial teats or pacifiers (also called dummies or soothers) to breast-feeding infants.
10. Foster the establishment of breast-feeding support groups and refer mothers to them on discharge from the hospital or clinic.

(From Ebrahim GJ. The Baby Friendly Hospital Initiative. J Trop Pediatr 39:2, 1993.)

changes markedly increase breast, areola, and nipple size. The principal feature of mammary growth in pregnancy is a great increase in ducts and alveoli under the influence of many hormones. Late in pregnancy, the lobules of the alveolar system are maximally developed and small amounts of colostrum may be released for several months before delivery. Anatomic features of the human mammary gland are illustrated in Figure 7–8. Delivery of the infant is followed by a dramatic change in the hormonal pattern of the mother. A sudden drop in circulating levels of estrogen and progesterone accompanies a rapid rise in the secretion of *prolactin*. These changes and others set the stage for the formal onset of lactation.

The typical stimulus for milk production and secretion is the suck of the infant at the mother's breast. Nerves beneath the skin of the areola send a message via the spinal cord to the hypothalamus, which in turn, transmits a message to the pituitary gland, where both the anterior and posterior areas are stimulated to release their respective hormones. **Prolactin** from the anterior pituitary stimulates milk production by alveolar cells in the mammary tissue, as shown in Figure 7–9. **Oxytocin** from the posterior pituitary stimulates the myoepithelial cells of the mammary gland to contract, causing movement of milk through the duct system and lactiferous sinuses for ultimate depostition in the mouth of the infant. This latter process, referred to as **let-down,** is accompanied in the woman by a distinct sensation described as a "tingling feeling." Because oxytocin also stimulates the muscle cells of the uterus to contract, lactation immediately following delivery is considered useful in promoting rapid shutdown of bleeding from this tissue.

The process of let-down appears to be sensitive to small changes in circulating oxytocin levels; minor emotional disturbances or environmental stresses may influence the ease with which breast milk is provided to the infant. Stress from labor and delivery can delay lactogenesis (Chen, 1998). The attitude of the mother toward the process of breast-feeding is a powerful factor in determining her success at lactation. The support of the father, physician, nurse, extended family, and friends is also an important determinant of the degree of satisfaction and success derived from the breast-feeding experience.

FIGURE 7–8 Structural features of the human mammary gland showing the terminal glandular (alveolar) tissue of each lobule leading into the duct system, which enlarges eventually into the lactiferous duct and lactiferous sinus. The lactiferous sinuses rest beneath the areola and converge at the nipple pore.

Nutritional Requirements of Lactation

The process of lactation is nutritionally demanding, especially for the woman who nurses her infant exclusively for a number of months. Increased intake of most nutrients is advised, as Table 7–4 indicates.

Milk volume is not likely to be affected by the mother's daily intake. Rather, the primary influ-

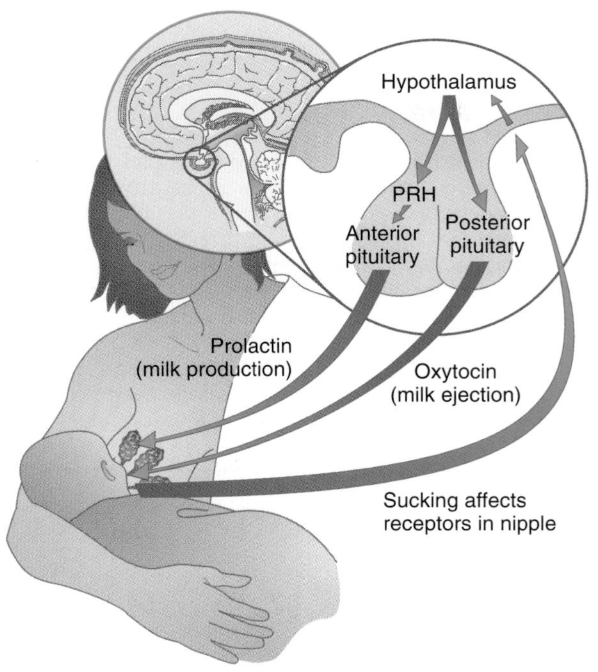

FIGURE 7–9 Physiology of milk production and the let-down reflex. *PRH,* prolactin-releasing hormone.

ence on milk volume is the frequency of infant feeding.

Milk composition, on the other hand, may vary according to the mother's diet. For example, the fatty acid composition of a mother's milk reflects her dietary intake. Additionally, milk levels of selenium, iodine, and some of the water-soluble B vitamins may be low if maternal intake is very low. The other nutrients seem to be present at remarkably constant levels, regardless of maternal diet. One study, however, suggests that important proteins provided by human milk may be secreted in reduced amounts if the mother is malnourished (Chang, 1990).

Energy

Milk is produced with about 80% efficiency; production of 100 mL of milk (about 67 kcal) requires an 85-kcal expenditure. Average milk production in the first 6 months is 750 mL/day, with a range of 550 to more than 1200 mL/day (IOM, 1991). Recall that milk volume is a function of the frequency of infant feeding. Therefore, infants who feed often are likely to stimulate the production of larger volumes of milk.

During the second 6 months of lactation, production generally drops to an average of 600 mL/day. During this time, most infants are also consuming solid foods, so the frequency of breast-feeding usually declines.

The RDA for energy needs during lactation provides for an extra 500 kcal/day above the level for nonpregnant women. The woman who was obese prior to pregnancy or who had excessive weight gain during her pregnancy may not require the full 500 kcal/day. Maternal fat stores accumulated during pregnancy provide about 100 to 150 kcal/day during the early months of lactation. When the reserve fat pad has been depleted, dietary energy support for lactation must be increased if the mother intends to provide all or most of her infant's nutrition through breast milk alone.

The major effect on lactation of maternal undernutrition is the production of less milk each day. This happens with the nursing mother who takes on a rigorous weight-reduction diet while attempting to breast-feed her infant. Once lactation is well established, the mother can reduce her energy intake modestly to increase the rate of fat utilization without an adverse impact on milk production.

One study showed that healthy breast-feeding women could lose as much as 1 lb/week while supplying enough milk to maintain their infant's growth (Dusdieker et al., 1994). Breast-feeding women should be reminded of the energy drain of lactation, and the fact that women who are breast-feeding exclusively lose body fat with no reduction in caloric intake (Dewey et al., 1993). Women who are already lean may be at risk for reduced milk production if they restrict their energy intake. It is generally advisable for lactating women not to restrict their energy intake to less than 1800 kcal/day (Dewey and McCrory, 1994).

Suboptimal quantity of milk production may also result from inadequate fluid intake by the mother. Breast-feeding mothers should be encouraged to consume 2 to 3 quarts of fluid daily, perhaps more in very hot weather. They should also be advised that oral contraceptives may suppress lactation, especially in the first 6 to 10 weeks.

Protein

The RDA provides for an additional 15 g of protein during the first 6 months of lactation and 12 g during the second 6 months, when less milk is produced. The average protein requirement for lactation is estimated from milk composition data and the mean volume of 750 mL produced daily, assuming an efficiency of 70% in conversion of dietary protein to milk protein.

Lipids

The fat in breast milk directly reflects both the amount and saturation pattern of fat in the maternal diet. Severe restriction of energy intake results in mobilization of body fat, with the result that the milk produced has a fatty acid composition resembling that of the mother's depot fat.

Human milk contains 10 to 20 mg/dL of cholesterol, resulting in an approximate daily consumption of 100 mg/day by the infant. The amount of cholesterol in milk does not seem to be influenced

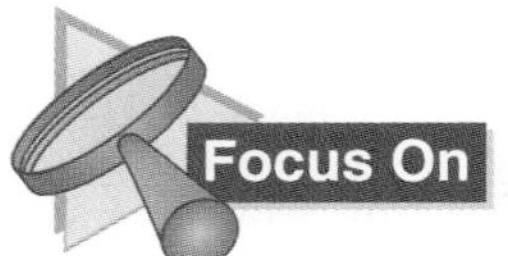

Omega-3 Fats and Infant Brain Development and Lactation

Docosahexaenoic acid (DHA) is a long-chain polyunsaturated fatty acid of the omega-3 type and is commonly written as 22:6n-3. It is found in large amounts in the brain (Hachey, 1994). Because DHA is important for the growth and development of the fetal central nervous system, it has been suggested that the prenatal diet should include adequate amounts of preformed DHA (Crawford, 1993; Monique et al., 1996).

It is presumed that if adequate amounts of dietary n-3 fatty acids, most commonly derived from fish, are provided in the prenatal diet, adequate amounts of DHA will be stored in the fetal adipose tissue. This will allow fetal and early infant brain development, which requires DHA, to proceed optimally, because there will be adequate DHA in these adipose stores, especially in the infant who is not breast-fed (Nettleton, 1993). Two to three fish meals per week during pregnancy seem to provide adequate amounts of DHA (Olsen et al., 1993). Vegetable sources of omega-3 fats include flax seeds and nuts. The breast-fed infant conceivably could receive additional DHA if the mother is consuming omega-3 fatty acids in her diet. The Food and Drug Administration (FDA) is presently considering requiring the addition of omega-3 fatty acids to infant formula. (See Chapter 8.)

by the mother's diet; however, the cholesterol content of the milk is reduced as lactation progresses.

Certain lipids that affect brain development are more important than initially believed. See the accompanying box, "*Focus On:* Omega-3 Fats."

Vitamins and Minerals

Some mineral and vitamin concentrations in breast milk are sensitive to maternal intake. For example, zinc supplementation in mothers results in increased zinc concentrations in their milk. In the process of normal lactation, the zinc content of breast milk drops dramatically during the first few months from 2 to 3 mg zinc per day to 1 mg/day by the third postpartum month. The requirements for zinc during lactation are greater than those during pregnancy (Krebs, 1998).

The selenium content of milk appears to be strongly related to maternal selenium status. The vitamin D content of milk is related to the maternal vitamin D intake and the amount of sun exposure. The calcium content is not related to maternal intake (Kalkwarf, 1997). There also is no convincing evidence that maternal changes in bone mineral density are influenced by the level of calcium intake across a broad range of intakes (up to 1600 mg/day). Typically, during 3 to 6 months of lactation, there is a 1% to 2% decrease in whole body bone mineral density evidenced by a 3% to 5% reduction in lumbar spine density. However, these losses are reversed as lactation continues and after weaning (Kalkwarf et al., 1997; Prentice, 1997). This is the reason that the AI for calcium during pregnancy and lactation is the same as for nonpregnant, nonlactating women—1300 mg/day for 9- to 18-year olds, and 1000 mg/day for 19- to 50-year-old women. The UL is also the same at 2500 mg/day (Institute of Medicine, 1997). The Dietary Reference Intakes for lactating women are presented in Table 7–4.

Breast-Feeding an Infant

Preparation

The advantages of breast-feeding should be presented throughout the childbearing years. The process of lactation and the benefits of breast-feeding should be a part of high school family and health curricula. Women should be encouraged to express and discuss their opinions and feelings so that any misinformation can be corrected. During the last months of pregnancy, counseling on the process of lactation should be made available to women who have decided to breast-feed. Fathers should be encouraged to participate in counseling sessions, as the emotional support they provide contributes to the success of lactation. Many mothers have never seen a woman nursing an infant; therefore, they may find it especially helpful to confer with a woman who is successfully nursing a baby and who can answer questions and provide positive reinforcement.

The Technique

The baby should be put to the breast as soon after birth as the mother feels ready. It is not essential that suckling occur immediately after delivery, but for mothers who want this experience, their wishes should be accommodated if possible. Milk may be expected to flow within 48 to 96 hours after delivery. Before this time, the thin yellow fluid called **colostrum** should appear. Higher in protein and lower in fat and carbohydrate than mature milk, colostrum provides approximately 15 kcal/oz and is a rich source of antibodies. As it is replaced by transitional and mature milk, the breasts become enlarged and firm as they fill with milk.

For breast-feeding to be successful, it is important that both mother and infant get into a comfortable position, either sitting or lying down. The mother should hold the baby close, cradling the baby in her arm to support the head if she is sitting up. If the baby's cheek is touched, the baby will turn toward that side (the *rooting reflex*). The mother should hold her breast so that the areola and nipple are in the baby's mouth as much as possible. If the breast is very full, it helps to press it gently away from the baby's nose so that the infant can breathe more easily. Alternatively, it may be helpful for the mother to express a little milk before letting the baby nurse. The baby should be allowed to nurse for at least 10 minutes on each side initially, then longer if both mother and infant wish. Length of time at the breast should not be unduly limited as this may prevent establishment of successful lactation.

Lactating women experience a tingling sensation in the breast which is being suckled, signaling the let-down reflex. This is often accompanied by milk dripping from the other breast and, occasionally, by uterine cramps. It may take some time for the let-down reflex to become fully functional and conditioned. Some women never feel the let-down, but swallowing by the baby is a definite sign that it has occurred. Rest or a hot shower before nursing may facilitate the let-down reflex. If the woman has too much milk, the baby may need to nurse on only one side at a feeding for awhile. This reduces overall stimulation and, eventually, the milk supply. This is also an ideal opportunity for the mother to express milk from the other breast so it can be stored for a future feeding when the mother needs to be away.

To remove the baby from the breast, a finger is placed in the corner of the baby's mouth until the suction is broken. The breast can then be removed from the infant's mouth comfortably. Most babies need to be burped before they are fed from the second breast; the need for burping, however, is highly individual.

Because breast milk is more easily digested than other infant feeding solutions, breast-fed infants may wish to feed more often than formula-fed babies. If the baby wants to nurse, there is no reason not to let him or her do so; breast-fed babies consume what they need when they need it. Breast-feeding whenever the baby is hungry is easy to do because the milk is always ready. Some babies may be hungry as frequently as every hour or two on some days, whereas others may not become hungry until 4 hours after the previous feeding. The more often the baby nurses, the more milk the breasts produce; thus, whenever a woman's supply is low (e.g., during or after an illness, provided there is no risk of the baby contracting the disease through breast-feeding), she should nurse more often.

Parents should realize that crying does not always mean that the baby is hungry. He or she may be physically uncomfortable or just want to be held, burped, or changed. Parents usually learn to distinguish the different needs of their infants.

Feeding time is perfectly suited for establishing and maintaining close mother–child interactions (Fig. 7–10). The mother, however, need not be tied to her infant all of the time. On occasions when she wants or needs to be away at the usual time of feeding, a bottle of breast milk that has been expressed earlier, or a commercial baby formula, can be given. It is best to avoid supplemental bottles until the woman is satisfied that her milk supply is well established and regulated, usually around 6 weeks postpartum.

Infants who are introduced to artificial nipples in the first few weeks of life may experience "nipple confusion." Because the muscle action required by the infant to empty a bottle is quite different from that needed to nurse at the breast, the very young infant may be easily confused if both feeding methods are offered. As it is more work to suck at the breast, infants in such situations may refuse the breast, leading to lactation failure. Because babies are easily portable during the early weeks of life, the mother may choose to take the infant along on shopping trips and other outings, thus minimizing mother–baby separation. There is no need to offer breast-fed babies additional water from a bottle; human milk usually provides all the fluid the baby needs.

Duration of Breast-Feeding

The length of time a woman breast-feeds her infant depends on her own feelings and situation. If she is working, she can continue to breast-feed by expressing milk and instructing a caregiver to give it in a bottle. Milk will continue to be produced as long as there is demand for it and it is taken from

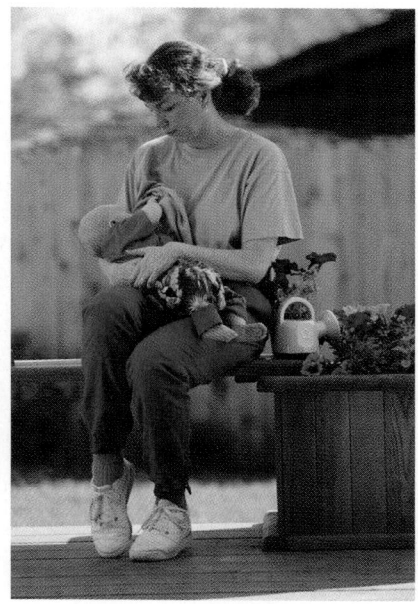

FIGURE 7–10 A mother and her baby enjoy close physical contact while nursing. (© by Kathryn Abbe, New York.)

the breast, although a breast may not be emptied at any given feeding.

Some mothers prefer to breast-feed until the baby is weaned to a cup (thus avoiding bottles altogether); this can be accomplished when the baby is about 9 to 10 months of age. Some mothers choose to breast-feed much longer—some for several years—letting the baby decide when to be weaned. There is a wide variability in ease of weaning, depending on the baby's overall interest in nursing, the relationship between mother and child, and the use of bottles. Babies who have had frequent supplemental bottles from birth are likely to wean themselves at an early age.

When a mother decides to wean her baby, it should be done gradually over a period of several weeks. At first, one feeding can be omitted for several days; two feedings may then be skipped, and so on until the baby is down to one feeding a day (usually the night or early morning feeding). Eventually, this last feeding can be discontinued. Weaning in this gradual manner is easier on the mother, as it avoids engorgement of her breasts, and it eases the baby's transition to the new routine.

Exercise and Breast-Feeding

The breast-feeding mother should be encouraged to get back to exercise a few weeks postpartum, after lactation is well established. Aerobic exercise at 60% to 70% of maximal heart rate has no adverse effect on lactation; infants gain weight at the same rate, and the mother's cardiovascular fitness improves (Dewey et al., 1994). However, strenuous exercise resulting in lactic acid production is not recommended. In some women, lactic acid levels rise in their breast milk and remain high for 90 minutes after strenuous exercise, giving the milk a sour taste that babies may not like (Wallace, 1992). Women who want to do anaerobic exercise should nurse beforehand, and not again until at least 1½ hours afterward.

Common Problems

The inexperienced nursing mother may encounter some problems in adjusting to the breast-feeding experience. Success or failure at breast-feeding depends mainly on the availability of help in the early weeks and the support of a clinician or friend who can provide useful tips. Table 7–9 summarizes some of the initial difficulties, along with comments about counseling strategies.

ENGORGED BREASTS. If nursing has been on demand since birth, painful engorgement of the breasts is not likely to occur. If the breasts become engorged, the discomfort can be relieved by applying wet cloths, as hot as can be endured, to the whole breast and, at the same time, expressing milk from the nipple. As the wet cloth cools, it should be replaced with another hot one.

To express milk by hand, the thumb and forefinger are placed on opposite sides of the breast just outside the areola, pressed into the rib cage, and then squeezed together and downward; the nipple should not be pulled outward. The procedure is repeated, moving the thumb and forefinger around the nipple until as much milk as desired has been expressed. Breast massage before the milk is expressed sometimes helps; this is done by putting the thumbs together on top of the breast and the remaining fingers under the breast. Gentle massage is then exerted from around the breast toward the nipple. If the milk is to be used later, it should be expressed into a sterile bottle and refrigerated. Milk expression is not easy for some women at first, but persistence usually brings success if the mother takes the time.

SORE NIPPLES. The nipples may become sore at the beginning of breast-feeding. Sore nipples, usually caused by incorrect positioning of the baby at the breast, are easily treated. The mother should make sure that the baby's mouth is open wide prior to latch-on. A large portion of the areola should extend into the baby's mouth, and the baby's lower lip should be rolled slightly outward. Failure to do this can result in the baby chewing on the nipple, which not only causes the mother intense discomfort, but can also lead to inefficient milk extraction. A substance secreted by the breasts serves to lubricate the nipple. It is not necessary to "toughen up the nipple," as was formerly advised. In fact, rubbing a towel against a nipple may remove some of this important lubricant and make nipples more prone to soreness.

TABLE 7–9 MANAGEMENT OF BREAST-FEEDING PROBLEMS

PROBLEM	APPROACHES TO MANAGEMENT
Retracted nipple(s)	Before feeding the infant, roll the nipple gently between the fingers until erect.
Baby's mouth not open wide enough	Before feeding, depress the infant's lower jaw with one finger as the nipple is guided into the mouth.
Baby sucks poorly	Stimulate sucking motions by pressing upward under the baby's chin. Expression of colostrum often occurs, and the taste may stimulate sucking.
Baby demonstrates rooting but does not grasp the nipple; eventually cries in frustration	Interrupt the feeding, comfort the infant; the mother should take time to relax before trying again.
Baby falls asleep while nursing	If the infant falls asleep early in the feeding, the mother should awaken the infant by holding him or her upright, rubbing his or her back, talking to him or her, or providing similar quiet stimuli; another effort at feeding can then be made. If the baby falls asleep again, the feeding should be postponed.

If soreness occurs, it is always temporary, and only lasts until the nipples become accustomed to the baby's sucking. One of the best ways to relieve the soreness is to expose the nipples to the air. This is done by removing the bra and wearing a loose cotton blouse or shirt. It is also helpful to expose the bare nipples briefly to the heat of a sunlamp, the sun, or a hand-held electric hair dryer on a low setting. Although a variety of creams are touted to aid sore nipples, the mother must be cautious; many of them contain lanolin, and the mother should not use these if she is allergic to wool. Additionally, many infants find the taste of the cream unacceptable and may refuse to nurse. Persistence in breast-feeding is important, as the soreness will resolve, particularly if a proper nursing position is used. Until soreness subsides, nursing should be initiated on the side that feels the best. Limiting sucking leads to engorgement and increases soreness. Nursing should not be limited during the first few days and weeks of life to prevent sore nipples, as this can lead to lactation failure from lack of appropriate breast stimulation.

If a woman experiences intensely sore nipples, particularly a shooting pain in the breast after several weeks or months of successful breast-feeding, it may be a sign of a thrush infection. In such cases, she needs to seek care from her health care provider. She may continue breast-feeding, but it is important to note that, if thrush is diagnosed, both mother and baby need to be treated, even if the baby shows no classic signs of infection.

Inverted (Retracted) and Flat Nipples. Most nipples protrude a bit from the surrounding areola. Sometimes, however, they look flat, or even go inward, either partially or completely. These are called inverted or "turned in" nipples. Careful examination will determine whether or not the nipples are truly inverted.

Inverted nipples can cause serious difficulties, but they are rare. Most apparently inverted nipples are merely flat, and with patience and care during pregnancy and the first phase of breast-feeding, they will become normal. If the nipple is pulled out (protracted), but slips away as if it is fastened to the tissues beneath the skin, it is potentially functional. If it is truly inverted, it cannot be protracted at all. Usually, it is possible to pull the nipple out a short way, and such a nipple stretches when the baby sucks from it. Some flat-looking nipples protract very well.

A truly inverted (nonprotractible) nipple can be quite difficult to manage, but must be treated if breast-feeding is to be attempted. The first step is to obtain plastic breast shields or something similar to wear inside the bra. The woman should wear these shields daily over her nipples from the seventh month of pregnancy until term. She must also do the "pulling exercise"—repeatedly pulling the nipple away from the areola.

The use of nipple shields has been associated with numerous cases of lactation failure. The shape and texture of the shields can make efficient milk extraction nearly impossible. If a nipple shield is used, it should be only a soft, silicone one, not the hard plastic variety. Women with flat but protractable nipples may also use nipple shields, but generally find them unnecessary as the nipple usually becomes erect when nursing is initiated.

Plugged Ducts. Occasionally, a milk duct becomes plugged, creating a tender spot on the breast that may even appear to be lumpy and hot to the touch. This can result from inadequate emptying of the milk ducts or wearing a bra that is too tight. Should a plugged duct develop, the following approaches may be helpful:

1. Offer the sore breast to the baby first, so that it will be emptied more completely.
2. Nurse longer and more often; if the breast gets too full, the plugged duct becomes worse and an infection may develop.
3. Change positions at every feeding so that the pressure of the nursing will be applied to different places on the breast.
4. Apply warm compresses to the breasts between feedings.

Infection. If breast tenderness is accompanied by fever and a general flu-like feeling, a breast infection is probably present. Treatment involves bed rest, continued nursing (offering the sore breast first), application of heat with a hot water bottle or heating pad, supporting the breasts with a firm bra, and consulting a health practitioner. Antibiotics are frequently prescribed.

There is no danger of the baby becoming ill from nursing on an infected breast. The infection resides in the breast tissue and not in the milk. The baby can and should continue to nurse on the affected breast (breast infections are usually unilateral).

Breast infections are sometimes complicated by localized pus accumulation; this is referred to as a breast abscess and may require surgical opening and drainage, in addition to antibiotics. Women are advised not to nurse on the affected side until the abscess heals. During the interval when the woman is not nursing, the milk should be expressed frequently by hand from the affected breast.

Leaking. Some mothers are bothered by leaking breasts, either during or between feedings. Although this may help relieve fullness in the early weeks of lactation, it soon becomes a nuisance. It can be stopped by pressing firmly with the palm of the hand against the leaking nipple. A less obvious way to stop both breasts from leaking is for the woman to cross her arms against her breasts and press firmly. Cotton pads with an outside plastic coat may be inserted inside the bra to catch any milk that may be released. If this is done, the pads should be changed frequently.

Failure to Thrive in the Breast-Feeding Infant. Insufficient milk supply is rarely a problem for the well-fed mother. Because sucking stimulates the flow of milk, feeding on demand for adequate duration should supply ample amounts of milk to the infant. If the baby continues steadily to gain weight and length, has at least six to eight wet diapers daily, and has frequent stools, the milk supply is probably adequate.

Occasionally, an infant fails to thrive while seeming to nurse properly. A variety of circumstances can be explored as likely bases for the unsatisfactory breast-feeding experience. The diagram in Figure 7–11 illustrates potential problems in the mother or the infant that should be investigated during the course of evaluation. If the cause of the problem cannot be identified, or the defined problem cannot be corrected, it may be necessary to encourage the mother to use commercial infant formula for at least partial nutritional support of the infant.

Relactation and Induced Lactation

Occasionally, a mother starts breast-feeding late or discontinues nursing, but decides at a much later date to begin again. She can attempt relactation through providing the infant substantial opportunities to suck at the breast. With much sucking stimulus over several days, many patient and persistent women can initiate the lactation process late, or once again. Their volume of milk production may be less than the infant demands, in which case a supplemental feeding following nursing may be necessary. Alternatively, some women find that a nursing trainer complements their own milk production. While the baby sucks at the breast, he or she also obtains milk via suction through a small tube leading to a bag of fresh formula clipped to the mother's bra. While sucking, the baby simultaneously builds up the mother's milk supply and receives adequate nutrition through the feeding device.

After adopting an infant, a few adoptive mothers decide to attempt lactation. Some of these women have never done so before, and others have breastfed a previous baby of their own. With much sucking stimulus, lactation can often be induced, but only with great perseverance and, in most cases, only if a woman has once carried a pregnancy well

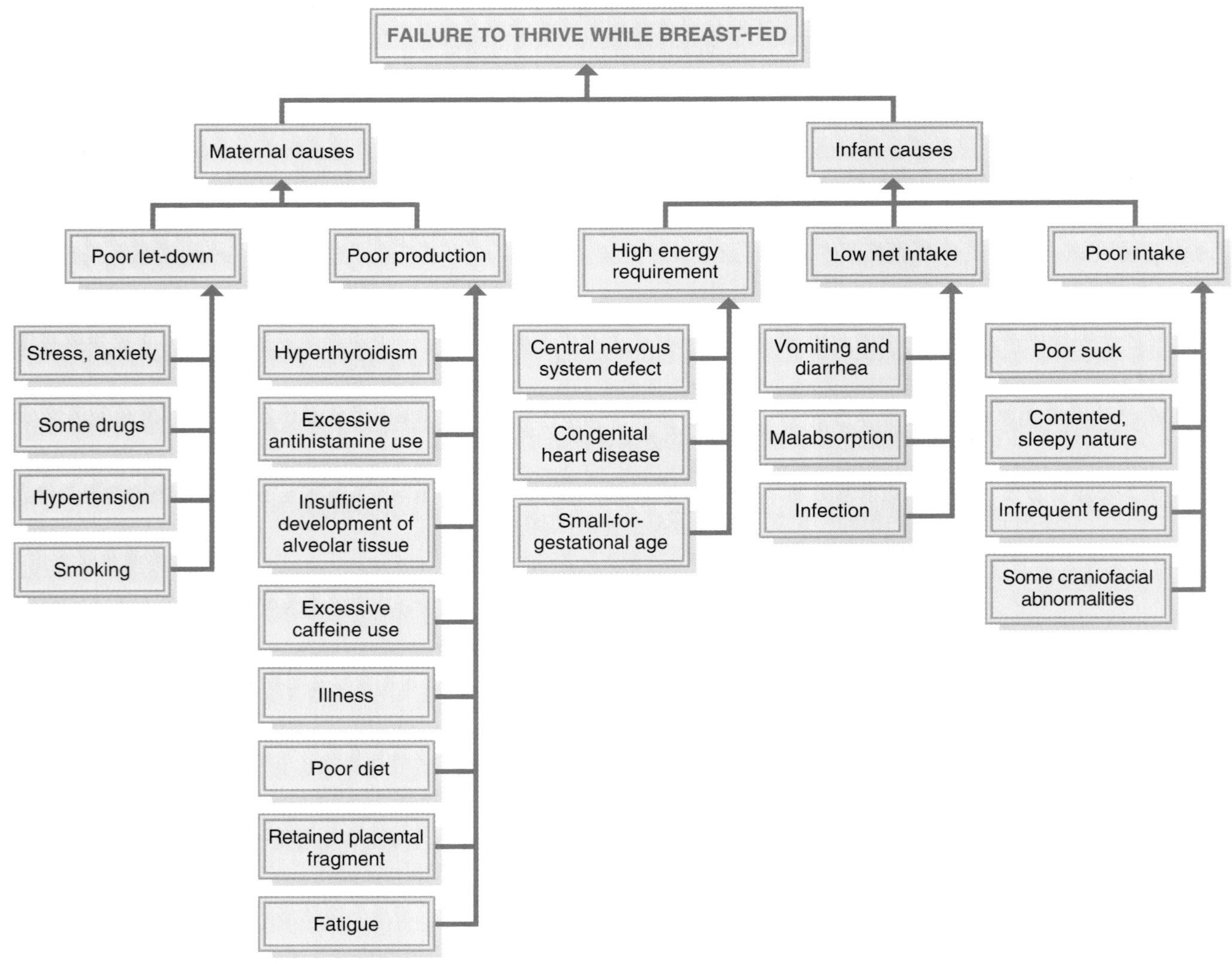

FIGURE 7–11 Diagnostic flow chart for failure to thrive.

into the second trimester. Because the mammary glands complete their development for lactation during the first 6 months of pregnancy, a woman who has never been pregnant or never carried a pregnancy beyond the first trimester is a poor candidate for successful induction of lactation.

Breast Pumping and Milk Storage

Mothers may wish to remove milk from their breasts for a number of reasons: to save it for a later feeding, to take it to their hospitalized neonate, to donate it to a milk bank, or other reasons. Under such circumstances, some women find it satisfactory to express milk by hand, whereas others find that a manual or electric breast pump provides a better stimulus for milk flow and a more efficient mode of milk collection. Instructions for use accompany each of these pumps, but individual counseling by a skilled clinician or experienced nursing mother can greatly simplify the process of learning to pump.

Milk storage times vary. For example, milk left in a refrigerator should be used within 24 hours; if frozen, it may keep for 3 weeks. A variety of milk storage bags are available, but they should all be labeled with the date that the milk was collected. When thawing frozen milk, the contents should be left in the bag and held under a stream of cool water. Breast milk should never be thawed in the microwave.

NUTRITION, FERTILITY, AND CONCEPTION

Although most American women have access to sufficient food sources of energy, protein, and micronutrients, individual circumstances sometimes prevent a woman from achieving nutritional well-being. The problem may be one of limited resources, but it is just as likely that self-selected behaviors will lead to nutritional imbalances over time. Should poor dietary practices occur during childhood or adolescence, growth and development can be temporarily or permanently limited. Stunted linear growth or incomplete development of the pelvic girdle may interfere later with normal fetal development owing to restricted maternal space. Chronic dieting may lead to amenorrhea, with the obvious consequence of reduced fertility. Deficiencies of specific nutrients may lead to eventual depletion of nutrient stores, adversely affecting the function of many physiologic and biochemical processes. Resistance to disease may decrease, and energy to perform daily activities may wane. Overeating associated with lack of exercise may lead to excessive deposition of body fat and dysmenorrhea. Massive obesity poses a serious risk to the well-being of both mother and child during and after pregnancy.

The Dietary Guidelines for Americans provide an appropriate base for counseling women of reproductive age (see Chapter 15). Although the food industry is making an effort to assist consumers with dietary change, only minimal signs of dietary improvement have been observed recently. Clearly, there is need for continued focus on individualized nutrition counseling for women of reproductive age. Whether defined problems are attributable to lack of resources, lack of nutrition knowledge, self-imposed dietary manipulations, genetic idiosyncrasies, or a combination of these factors, solutions to defined problems can often be found. Although the value of nutritional counseling may not be measurable immediately, the ultimate result may be improved preparation for reproduction and the accompanying responsibilities of parenting.

CASE STUDY 1

Melissa E. is a 15-year-old primagravida who is in her 12th week of pregnancy. She is 5'5" tall and weighs 120 lb. Her pregravid weight was 118 lb. Her diet history reveals that she does not have a regular eating pattern, and her food choices usually consist of convenience foods and carbonated beverages. She is single and still living with her parents. The physician has prescribed a prenatal vitamin and mineral supplement, as well as nutrition counseling. Her hemoglobin and hematocrit values are within normal limits.

1. What are your weight gain goals for this pregnant adolescent?
2. What nutritional advice would you give her for a healthy pregnancy?
3. How would you design an eating plan for Melissa that she can follow?

CASE STUDY 2

Claire L., a 23-year-old primipara who is 10 days postpartum, has come to the WIC clinic for certification as a breast-feeding mother. She is breast-feeding her baby every 3 hours, but is concerned that he may not be getting enough milk. While with the nutritionist in the clinic, she begins to cry, citing sore nipples, profound fatigue, and worry. A 24-hour recall from the day before shows that C. L. skipped breakfast and ate some microwaved meals for lunch and dinner.

The nutritionist asks permission to watch Claire nurse her baby. Because she is not supporting the baby's back and buttocks firmly, the baby tugs at the nipple, causing the soreness.

The nutritionist then weighs the baby and finds that he has already regained his birth weight. This reassures Claire that her baby is, indeed, getting enough milk.

1. What would you recommend to improve the baby's position during nursing? How will this improve the nursing experience?
2. What advice would you give Claire about her fatigue?
3. How would you design an eating plan for Claire that she can follow?

CITED REFERENCES

Abrams BF, Laros RK. Prepregnancy weight, weight gain and birth weight. Am J Obstet Gynecol 154:503, 1986.

American College of Obstetrics and Gynecology (ACOG). Exercise during pregnancy and the postpartum period. ACOG Tech Bull (No. 189), February, 1994.

Barker DJP. Fetal origins of coronary heart disease. Br Med J 311:171, 1995.

Bolto LD, et al. Periconceptual multivitamin use and the occurrence of conotruncal heart defects: Results from a population-based case control study. Pediatrics 98:911, 1996.

Bolumar F, et al. Caffeine intake and delayed conception: A European multicenter study on infertility and subfecundity. Am J Epidemiol 145:324, 1997.

Britt EC. Healthy People 2000. J Nutr Educ 22:239, 1990.

Brown JE, et al. Predictors of red cell folate level in women attempting pregnancy. JAMA 277:548, 1997.

Brown JE, Toma RB. Taste changes during pregnancy. Am J Clin Nutr 43:414, 1986.

Bucher HC, et al. Effect of calcium supplementation on pregnancy-induced hypertension and preeclampsia. JAMA 275:1113, 1996.

Casanueva E, et al. Incidence of premature rupture of membranes of pregnant women with low leukocyte levels of vitamin C. Eur J Clin Nutr 45:401, 1991.

Casanueva E, et al. Premature rupture of amniotic membranes as functional assessment of vitamin C status during pregnancy. Ann NY Acad Sci 678:369, 1993.

Caulfield LE, et al. Determinants of gestational weight gain outside the recommended ranges among black and white women. Obstet Gynecol 87:760, 1996.

Centers for Disease Control. Recommendations for use of folic acid to reduce the number of cases of spina bifida and other neural tube defects. MMWR 41:1, 1992.

Chang S-J. Antimicrobial proteins of maternal and cord sera and human milk in relation to maternal nutritional status. Am J Clin Nutr 51:183, 1990.

Chen DC, et al. Stress during labor and delivery and early lactation performance. Am J Clin Nutr 68:335, 1998.

Christianson RE, et al. Caffeinated beverages and decreased fertility. Lancet 1:378, 1989.

Clapp JF. Exercise in pregnancy—Good, bad or indifferent? In: Lee RV, Barron WB, Cotton DB, Coustan D (eds.). Current Obstetric Medicine, vol 3. Chicago: CV Mosby, 1993, p. 4.

Clapp JF, Little KD. Effect of recreational exercise on pregnancy weight gain and subcutaneous fat deposition. Med Sci Sports Exerc 27:170, 1995.

Cnattingius S, et al. Prepregnancy weight and the risk of adverse pregnancy outcomes. N Engl J Med 337:147, 1998.

Connolly KJ, et al. Fetal iodine deficiency and motor performance during childhood. Lancet 2:1149, 1979.

Council on Scientific Affairs, American Medical Association. Fetal effects of maternal alcohol use. JAMA 249:2517, 1983.

Cousins L. The California Diabetes and Pregnancy Program: A statewide collaborative program for the preconception and prenatal care of diabetic women. Clin Obstet Gynecol 5:443, 1991.

Crawford MA. The role of essential fatty acids in neural devlopment: Implications for perinatal nutrition. Am J Clin Nutr 57:703, 1993.

Czeizel AE, et al. Pregnancy outcomes in a randomized controlled trial of periconceptional multivitamin supplementation. Arch Gynecol Obstet 255:131, 1994.

Dahle LO, et al. The effect of oral magnesium substitution on pregnancy-induced leg cramps. Am J Obstet Gynecol 173:175, 1995.

Dewey KG, et al. Maternal weight-loss patterns during prolonged lactation. Am J Clin Nutr 58:162, 1993.

Dewey KG, et al. A randomized study of the effects of aerobic exercise by lactating women on breast-milk volume and composition. N Engl J Med 330:449, 1994.

Dewey KG, McCory MA. Effects of dieting and physical activity on pregnancy and lactation. Am J Clin Nutr 59(suppl):446S, 1994.

Dusdieker LB, et al. Is milk production impaired by dieting during lactation? Am J Clin Nutr 59:833, 1994.

Ebrahim GJ. The baby friendly hospital initiative (Editorial). J Trop Pediatr 39:2, 1993.

Edwards LE, et al. Pregnancy complications and birth outcomes in obese and normal-weight women: Effects of gestational weight change. Obstet Gynecol 87:389, 1996.

Edwards LE, et al. Pregnancy in the underweight woman: Course, outcome and growth patterns of the infant. Am J Obstet Gynecol 135:297, 1979.

Erick M. Battling morning (noon and night) sickness: New approaches for an age-old problem. J Am Diet Assoc 94:147, 1994.

Erick M. Hyperolfaction and hyperemesis gravidarum: What is the relationship? Nutr Rev 53:289, 1995.

Eskenazi B, et al. A multivariate analysis of risk factors for preeclampsia. JAMA 266:237, 1991.

Food and Nutrition Board, National Research Council, National Academy of Sciences. Recommended Dietary Allowances, 10th ed. Washington, DC: National Academy Press, 1989.

Goldenberg RL, et al. The effect of zinc supplementation on pregnancy outcome. JAMA 274:463, 1995.

Hachey DL. Benefits and risks of modifying maternal fat intake in pregnancy and lactation. Am J Clin Nutr 59:454, 1994.

Hammar M, Berg G. Serum calcium and magnesium status in women with leg cramps during pregnancy. In: Berger H (ed.). Vitamins and Minerals in Pregnancy and Lactation, Nestle Nutrition Workshop Series, vol. 16. New York: Raven, 1988, p. 147.

Hickey LE. Energy Expenditure and Body Composition During Pregnancy: A Longitudinal Study. Unpublished doctoral dissertation. University of California, Berkeley, CA, 1994.

Hinds TS, et al. The effect of caffeine on pregnancy outcome variable. Nutr Rev 54:203, 1996.

Hook EB, Czeizel AE. Can terathanasia explain the protective effect of folic acid supplementation on birth defects? Lancet 350:513, 1997.

Hytton FE, Leitch I. The Physiology of Human Pregnancy, 2nd ed. Oxford: Blackwell Scientific Publications, 1971.

Institute of Medicine. Preventing Low Birthweight. Washington, DC: National Academy Press, 1985.

Institute of Medicine, Food and Nutrition Board. Dietary Reference Intakes for Calcium, Phosphorus, Magnesium, Vitamin D and Fluoride. Washington, D.C.: National Academy Press, 1997.

Institute of Medicine, Food and Nutrition Board. Nutrition During Pregnancy, Parts I and II. Washington, DC: National Academy Press, 1990.

Institute of Medicine, Food and Nutrition Board. Dietary Reference Intakes for Thiamin, Riboflavin, Niacin, Vitamin B_6, Folate, Vitamin B_{12}, Pantothenic Acid, Biotin and Choline. Washington, D.C.: National Academy Press, 1998.

Johnston RB, Staples DA. Knolwedge and use of folic acid by women of childbearing age—United States, 1997. MMWR 46:721, 1997.

Kalkwarf HJ, et al. The effect of calcium supplementation on bone density during lactation and after weaning. N Engl J Med 337:523, 1997.

King JC, et al. Energy metabolism during pregnancy: Influence of maternal energy status. Am J Clin Nutr 59(suppl):439S, 1994.

Konzelmann K. Consider the facts for pregnant adolescents. Perinat Nutr Rep 3(2):1, 1996.

Kramer MS. Intrauterine growth and gestational duration determinants. Pediatrics 80:502, 1987.

Krebs NF. Zinc supplementation during lactation. Am J Clin Nutr 68 (suppl2):509S, 1998.

Kuczmarski RJ, et al. Increasing prevalence of overweight among U.S. adults: The National Health and Nutrition Examination Surveys 1960 to 1991. JAMA 272:205, 1994.

Lammer EJ, et al. Retinoic acid embryopathy. N Engl J Med 313:837, 1985.

Lechtig A, et al. Effect of food supplementation during pregnancy on birth weight. Pediatrics 56:508, 1975a.

Lechtig A, et al. Effect of moderate maternal malnutrition on the placenta. Am J Obstet Gynecol 123:191, 1975b.

Lederman SA. Preliminary data presented at the Maternal Weight Gain Meeting, McLean, Virginia. National Center for Education in MCH, U.S. Department of Health and Human Services, 1996.

Levine R, et al. Trial of calcium to prevent preeclampsia. N Engl J Med 337:69, 1997.

Little RE, Sing CF. Association of father's drinking and infant's birth weight. N Engl J Med 314:1644, 1986.

Lucas M, et al. A comparison of magnesium sulfate with phenytoin for the prevention of eclampsia. N Engl J Med. 333:201, 1995.

Luke B. The changing pattern of multiple births in the United States: Maternal and infant characteristics, 1973 and 1990. Obstet Gynecol 84:101, 1994.

Luke B, et al. Prenatal weight gain and the birthweight of triplets. Acta Genet Med Gemellol 44:93, 1995.

Luke B, et al. A consideration of height as a function of prepregnancy nutritional background and its potential influence on birth weight. J Am Diet Assoc 84:176, 1984.

Luke B, Leurgans S. Maternal weight gains in ideal twin outcomes. J Am Diet Assoc 96:178, 1996.

Monique A, et al. Fat intake of women during normal pregnancy—Relationships with maternal and neonatal essential fatty acid status. J Am Coll Nutr 15:49, 1996.

MRC Vitamin Study Research Group. Prevention of neural tube defects: Results of the Medical Research Council vitamin study. Lancet 338:131, 1991.

Murphy JF, et al. Relation of haemoglobin levels in first and second trimesters to outcome of pregnancy. Lancet 1:992, 1986.

Murtaugh MA, Weingart J. Individual nutrient effects on length of gestation and pregnancy outcome. Semin Perinatol 19:197, 1995.

Naeye RL. Teenaged and pre-teenaged pregnancies: Consequences of the fetal-maternal competition for nutrients. Pediatrics 67:146, 1981.

Naeye RL. Weight gain and the outcome of pregnancy. Am J Obstet Gynecol 135:3, 1979.

Nehlig A, Debry G. Potential teratogenic and neurodevelopmental consequences of coffee and caffeine exposure: A review of human and animal data. Neurotox Teratol 16:531, 1994.

Nettleton JA. Are n-3 fatty acids essential nutrients for fetal and infant development? J Am Diet Assoc 93:58, 1993.

Olsen SF, et al. Frequency of seafood intake in pregnancy as a determinant of birthweight: Evidence for a dose-dependant relationship. J Epidemiol Comm Hlth 47:436, 1993.

Owen AL, Owen GM. Twenty years of WIC: A review of some effects of the program. J Am Diet Assoc 97:777, 1997.

Prentice A. Calcium supplementation during breastfeeding. N Engl J Med 337:558, 1997.

Rainville A. Pica practices of pregnant women are associated with lower maternal hemoglobin level at delivery. J Am Diet Assoc 98:293, 1998.

Revelli A, et al. Exercise and pregnancy: A review of maternal and fetal effects. Obstet Gynecol Surv 47(6):355, 1992.

Roberts J. Magnesium for preeclampsia and eclampsia. N Engl J Med 333:250, 1995.

Roepke JLB, Kirksey A. Effects of vitamin B_6 supplementation during pregnancy on the vitamin B_6 nutriture of previous long-term oral contraceptive users and nonusers. Fed Proc 40:863, 1981.

Rosa FW, et al. Vitamin A congeners. Teratology 33:355, 1986.

Rosett HL, et al. Treatment experience with pregnant problem drinkers. JAMA 249:2029, 1983.

Rothman KJ, et al. Teratogenicity of high vitamin A intake. N Engl J Med 333:1369, 1995.

Sahakian V, et al. Vitamin B_6 is effective therapy for nausea and vomiting of pregnancy: A randomized, double-blind, placebo controlled study. Obstet Gynecol 78:33, 1991.

Scholl TO, et al. Dietary and serum folate: Their influence on the outcome of pregnancy. Am J Clin Nutr 63:520, 1996.

Schuster K, et al. Vitamin B_6 status of low income adolescent and adult pregnant women and the condition of their infants at birth. Am J Clin Nutr 34:1731, 1981.

Shaw GM, et al. Risk of neural tube defect–affected pregnancies among obese women. JAMA 275:1093, 1996.

Smith GFD. Effects of the state of nutrition of the mother during pregnancy and labour on the condition of the child at birth and for the first few days of life. Lancet 2:54, 1916.

Stone JL, et al. Risk factors for severe preeclampsia. Obstet Gynecol 93:357, 1994.

Story M (ed.). Nutrition Management of the Pregnant Adolescent. Washington, DC: U.S. Department of Agriculture and Health and Human Services; March of Dimes Birth Defects Foundation, National Clearing House, 1990.

Streissguth AP, et al. Comparison of drinking and smoking patterns during pregnancy over a six-year interval. Am J Obstet Gynecol 145:716, 1983.

Streissguth AP, et al. Teratogenic effects of alcohol in humans and laboratory animals. Science 209:353, 1980.

Sturtevant FM. Use of aspartame in pregnancy. Int J Fertil 30:85, 1985.

Susser M, Smith Z. Timing in prenatal nutrition: A reprise of the Dutch Famine Study. Nutr Rev 52:84, 1994.

Teratology Society. Teratology Society position paper: Recommendations for vitamin A use during pregnancy. Teratology 35:269, 1987.

Wallace JP, et al. Infant acceptance of postexercise breast milk. Pediatrics 89:1245, 1992.

Werler MM, et al. Prepregnant weight in relation to risk of neural tube defects. JAMA 275:1089, 1996.

Worthington-Roberts BS, Williams SR. Nutrition in Pregnancy and Lactation, 5th ed. St Louis: CV Mosby, 1993.

Xue-Yi C, et al. Timing of vulnerability of the brain to iodine deficiency in endemic cretinism. N Engl J Med 331:1739, 1994.

Zlatnick FJ, Burmeister LF. Dietary protein in pregnancy: Effect on anthropometric indices of the newborn infant. Am J Obstet Gynecol 146:199, 1983.

Zuger A. Alcohol consumption among pregnant and childbearing-aged women: United States, 1991 and 1995. MMWR 46:346, April 25, 1997.

ADDITIONAL REFERENCES

Pregnancy

Allen LH (ed.). Recent developments in maternal nutrition and their implication for practitioners. Am J Clin Nutr 59 (suppl 2), 1994.

American College of Obstetrics and Gynecology (ACOG). Nutrition during pregnancy. ACOG Technical Bulletin No. 179. Int J Gynecol Obstet 43:67, 1993.

American Dietetic Association. Position of The American Dietetic Association: Nutrition care for pregnant adolescents. J Am Diet Assoc 94:450, 1994.

Barclay B. Experience with enteral nutrition in the treatment of hyperemesis gravidarum. Nutr Clin Pract 4:153, 1990.

Barrett J, et al. Absorption of non-heme iron from food during normal pregnancy. Br Med J 309:79, 1994.

Bunin G, et al. Relation between maternal diet and subsequent primitive neuroectodermal brain tumors in young children. N Engl J Med 329:536, 1993.

Dewey KG, McCrory MA. Effects of dieting and physical activity on pregnancy and lactation. Am J Clin Nutr 59(suppl):446S, 1994.

Duque AG. The role of lipids in fetal brain development. Perinatol Nutr Rep. Spring: p. 4, 1997.

Durnin JVGA. Energy requirements of pregnancy: An integration of the longitudinal data from the 5-country study, Nestle Foundation Annual Report. Lausanne, Switzerland: Nestle Foundation, 1986.

Erick M. No More Morning Sickness. Penguin Books, USA, Inc., 1993.

Eskes TKAB. Open or closed? A world of difference: A history of homocysteine research. Nutr Rev 56:236, 1998.

Fraser A, et al. Association of young maternal age with adverse reproductive outcomes. J Am Diet Assoc 332:1113, 1995.

Frequent alcohol consumption among women of childbearing age. Behavioral Risk Factor Surveillance System. MMWR 48:328, 1994.

Glenn FB, et al. Fluoride tablet supplementation during pregnancy for caries immunity: A study of the offspring produced. Am J Obstet Gynecol 143:560, 1982.

Harsham J, et al. Growth patterns of infants exposed to cocaine and other drugs in utero. J Am Diet Assoc 94:999, 1994.

Hatch, et al. Maternal exercise during pregnancy, physical fitness, and fetal growth. Am J Epidemiol 137:1105, 1993.

Kritz-Silverstein D, et al. Relation of pregnancy history to insulin levels in older, nondiabetic women. Am J Epidemiol 140:375, 1994.

Laurence KM, et al. Double-blind randomized controlled trial of folate treatment before conception to prevent recurrence of neural tube defects. Br Med J 282:1509, 1981.

Lenders C, et al. Gestational age and infant size at birth are associated with dietary sugar intake among pregnant adolescents. J Nutr 127:1113, 1997.

Mills J, et al. Moderate caffeine use and the risk of spontaneous abortion and intrauterine growth retardation. JAMA 269:593, 1993.

Oakley GP, Erickson JO. Vitamin A and birth defects (Editorial). N Engl J Med 333:1414, 1995.

Of caffeine and miscarriages. Tufts Univ Diet Nutr Lett 11(12):1, 1994.

Pettit D, et al. Comparison of World Health Organization and National Diabetes Group procedure to detect abnormalities of glucose tolerance during pregnancy. Diabetes Care 17:1264, 1994.

Smithells RW, et al. Further experience of vitamin supplementation for prevention of neural tube defect recurrences. Lancet 1:1027, 1983.

Strode MA, et al. Effects of short-term caloric restriction on lactational performance of well-nourished women. Acta Paediatr Scand 75:222, 1986.

Wolfe H. High prepregnancy body-mass index—A maternal-fetal risk factor (Editorial). N Engl J Med 338:191, 1998.

Wolfe L, Mottola M. Aerobic exercise in pregnancy: An update. Can J Appl Physiol 18:119, 1993.

Lactation

American Dietetic Association. Position of The American Dietetic Association: Promotion and support of breast feeding. J Am Diet Assoc 97:662, 1997.

Bagwell J, et al. Knowledge and attitudes toward breast-feeding: Differences among dietitians, nurses and physicians working with WIC clients. J Am Diet Assoc 93:801, 1993.

Benke PJ. The isotretinoin teratogen syndrome. JAMA 251:3267, 1984.

Fly AD et al. Major mineral concentrations in human milk do not change after maximal exercise testing. Am J Clin Nutr 68:345, 1998.

Freed G, et al. National assessment of physicians' breast-feeding knowledge, attitudes, training and experience. JAMA 273:472, 1995.

Grummer-Strawn L. Does prolonged breast-feeding impair child growth? Pediatrics 91:766, 1993.

Hilson J, et al. Maternal obesity and breast-feeding success in a rural population of white women. Am J Clin Nutr 66:1371, 1997.

Huggins K, Ziedrich L. The Nursing Mother's Guide to Weaning. Boston, MA: The Harvard Common Press, 1994.

Institute of Medicine, Food and Nutrition Board. Nutrition During Lactation. Washington, DC: National Academy Press, 1991.

Krebs N, et al. Bone mineral density changes during lactation: Maternal, dietary, and biochemical correlates. Am J Clin Nutr 65:1738, 1997.

Mackey A, et al. Self-selected diets of lactating women often fail to meet dietary recommendations. J Am Diet Assoc 98:297, 1998.

Mannan S, Picciano MF. Influence of maternal selenium status on human milk selenium concentration and glutathione peroxidase activity. Am J Clin Nutr 46:95, 1987.

Sharma M, Petosa R. Impact of expectant fathers in breast-feeding decisions. J Am Diet Assoc 97:1311, 1997.

Stacy L, Mizumoto D. Breast-Feeding: Nature's Best for You and Your Baby. Chicago, IL: The American Dietetic Association, 1993.

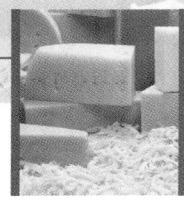

CHAPTER 8

Nutrition in Infancy*

CRISTINE M. TRAHMS, MS, RD, FADA

CHAPTER OUTLINE

- Physiologic Development
- Nutrient Needs of Infants
- Milk for Infants
- Foods for Infants
- Feeding the Infant

Key Terms

ARACHIDONIC ACID—a very-long-chain fatty acid (C20: 4n–6), known to be a derivative of linoleic, that is found in breast milk
CASEIN—the principle protein in cow's milk
CASEIN HYDROLYSATE—casein that has been split into smaller components by acid, alkali, or enzyme
CATCH-UP—the growth phenomenon in the first year of life that occurs when the rate of growth shifts upward to the genetic potential
COLIC—severe abdominal pain in infants
DOCOSAHEXAENOIC ACID—a very-long-chain fatty acid (C22: 6n–3), known to be a derivative of linolenic acids, that is found in breast milk
ELECTROLYTICALLY REDUCED IRON—iron that has been fractionated into small particles for improved absorption; used in the fortification of foods
HEMORRHAGIC DISEASE OF THE NEWBORN—a self-limited hemorrhagic disorder, occurring during the first few days of life, that is caused by a deficiency of vitamin K; occurs more frequently in breast-fed than in formula-fed infants
LACTALBUMIN—an easy-to-digest protein found in milk
LAG DOWN—the growth phenomenon in the first year of life that occurs when the rate of growth shifts downward to the genetic potential
PALMAR GRASP—an immature way of holding an object involving use of the palm
PINCER GRASP—a more refined and mature way of holding an object involving the use of the fingers
RENAL SOLUTE LOAD—the amount of nitrogenous waste and minerals that must be excreted by the kidney
WHEY PROTEINS—the proteins remaining in the watery fraction of milk after the curd and cream have been removed

The first 2 years of life, characterized by rapid physical and social growth and development, is a period in which many changes that affect feeding and nutrient intake occur. The adequacy of infants' nutrient intakes affects their interaction with their environment. Healthy, well-nourished infants have the energy to respond to and learn from the stimuli in their environment and to interact with their parents and caregivers in a manner that encourages bonding and attachment.

PHYSIOLOGIC DEVELOPMENT

An infant's birth weight is determined by the length of gestation, the mother's prepregnancy weight, and the mother's weight gain during gestation. After birth, genetic influences begin seeking their predetermined growth channel (Fig. 8–1). Most infants who are genetically determined to be larger reach their growth channel at between 3 and 6 months of age. However, many infants born at or below the 10th percentile for height may not reach their appropriate growth channel until 1 year of age. Larger infants at birth who are genetically determined to be smaller grow at their fetal rate for several months. Often, they do not reach their growth channel until 13 months of age.

Infants lose weight during the first few days of life, but birth weight is usually regained by the 7th to 10th day of life. Growth thereafter proceeds at a rapid but decelerating rate. Infants usually double their birth weight by 4 to 6 months of age, tripling it by the age of 1 year. The number of pounds gained during the second year approximates the

*This chapter is a revision of a chapter, written by Peggy L. Pipes, MA, MPH, RD, that appeared in the previous edition.

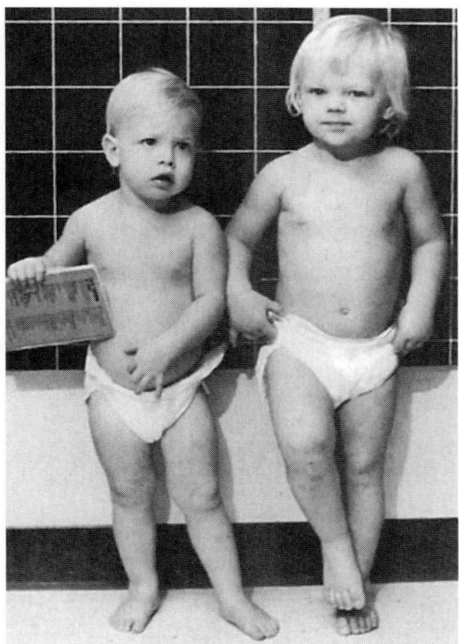

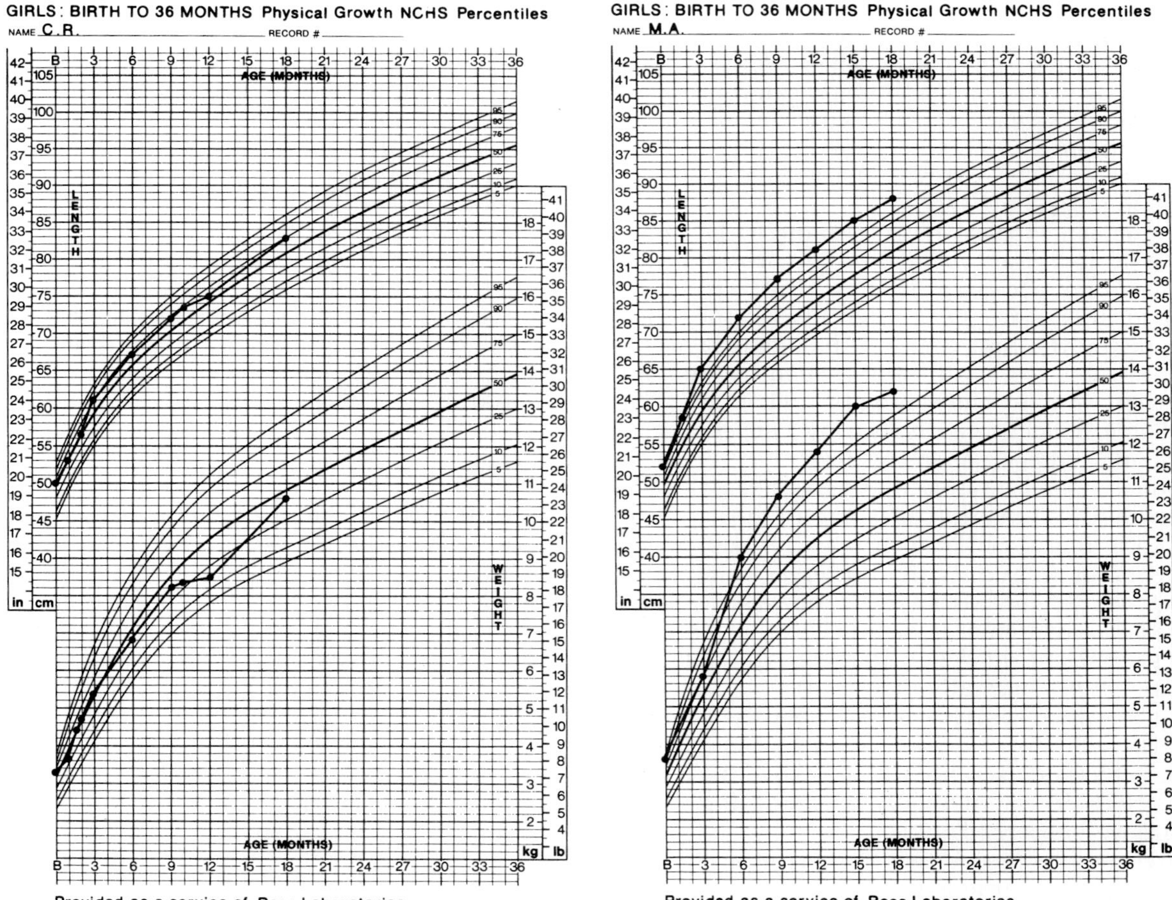

FIGURE 8–1 These two little girls, born just 1 month apart with only a 1-lb difference in birth weight, show a marked difference in rates of growth and appearance. Note the early catch-up growth shown in the growth chart for M.A. to above the 95th percentile for height and weight prior to 3 months of age. Also note the effect of illness on both weight gain and linear growth in C.R. at the age of 12 months, as well as the subsequent catch-up growth. The photograph shows the two girls at approximately 20 months of age. (Growth charts adapted from National Center for Health Statistics: NCHS Growth Charts, 1976. Monthly Vital Statistics Report, Vol. 25, No. 3, Suppl. (NRA) 76–1120. Health Resources Administration, Rockville, MD, June 1976. Data from The Fels Research Institute, Yellow Springs, OH. Courtesy of Ross Laboratories, Columbus, OH.)

birth weight. Infants increase their length by 50% during the first year of life and double it by 4 years of age. Total body fat increases rapidly during the first 9 months, after which the rate of fat gain tapers off throughout the rest of childhood. Total body water decreases throughout infancy from 70% at birth to 60% at 1 year. The decrease is almost all in extracellular water, which declines from 42% at birth to 32% at 1 year of age (See Fig. 6–1 on page 154).

The neonate has a functional but physiologically immature kidney that increases in size and concentrating capacity in the early weeks of life. This organ doubles its weight by 6 months and triples its weight at 1 year. The last renal tubule is estimated to form between the eighth fetal month and the end of the first postnatal month. The glomerular tuft is covered by a much thicker layer of cells throughout neonatal life than at any later time, which may explain why the glomerular filtration rate is lower during the first 9 months than it is in later childhood and adulthood. In the neonatal period, the ability to form acid urine and concentrated solutes is often limited. The concentrating capacity at birth may be limited to as little as 700 mOsm/L in some infants. Others have the concentrating capacity of adults (1200 to 1400 mOsm/L). By 6 weeks, most infants can concentrate urine at adult levels. Renal function in the normal newborn infant is rarely a concern; however, difficulties may arise in infants with diarrhea or when formula is prepared improperly.

The stomach capacity of infants increases from a range of 10 to 20 mL at birth to 200 mL by 1 year, enabling infants to consume more food at a given time, and at less frequent intervals, as they grow older. During the first weeks of life, gastric acidity decreases and, for the first few months, remains lower than that of older infants and adults. The rate of emptying is relatively slow, depending on the size and composition of the meal.

Although gastric secretion of pepsin remains low during the first 3 months, it is not a limiting factor for protein digestion. Trypsin activity in duodenal fluids is lower in infants than in older children, as is the activity of enterokinase (the enzyme responsible for the activation of trypsin). The enzymatic activity is sufficient, however, to digest the milk protein that infants normally ingest.

Fat absorption varies in the neonate. Human milk fat is well absorbed, but butter fat is poorly absorbed, with fecal excretions of 20% to 48%. The fat combinations in commercially prepared infant formula are well absorbed.

Human milk contains two lipases. One of these, found in the lipid fraction of milk, is essential for the milk lipid formation in the mammary gland, but is of no known nutritional importance to the baby. The other—*bile-stimulated lipase*—hydrolyzes triglycerides into three fatty acids and glycerol. The infant's lingual and gastric lipases hydrolyze short- and medium-chain fatty acids in the stomach. Gastric lipase hydrolyzes long-chain fatty acids.

Most long-chain triglycerides pass unhydrolyzed into the small intestine, where they are broken down by pancreatic lipase. Bile salt–stimulated lipase in human milk also stimulates the hydrolysis of triglycerides in the small intestine. Bile salts, which are effective emulsifiers when combined with monoglycerides, fatty acids, and lecithin, aid in the intestinal digestion of fat.

The activities of the enzymes responsible for the digestion of disaccharides maltase, isomaltase, and sucrase reach adult levels by 28 to 32 weeks of gestation. Lactase activity (responsible for digesting the disaccharide in milk) increases near term and reaches adult levels by birth, whereas pancreatic amylase, which digests starch, continues to remain low during the first 6 months after birth. If starch is fed before this time, increased activity of salivary amylase and digestion in the colon usually compensate. (See Fig. 1–6.)

NUTRIENT NEEDS OF INFANTS

Nutrient needs of infants reflect rates of growth, energy expended in activity, basal metabolic needs, and the interaction of the nutrients consumed. Balance studies have defined minimal acceptable levels of intakes for a few nutrients, but for most nutrients, the suggested intakes have been extrapolated from the intakes of normal, thriving infants. The Dietary Reference Intakes (DRIs) for infants are shown in Table 8–1. The Food and Nutrition Board of the National Academy of Sciences (NAS) has reevaluated the calcium, phosphorus, and magnesium needs of infants and has established Adequate Intakes (AIs), which are based on mean nutrient intakes needed for optimal health and are less than the previous Recommended Dietary Allowances (RDAs). This is true for several vitamins also.

Energy

Normal infants who are breast-fed to satiety, and infants who are fed a standard 20-kcal/oz formula and whose mothers are sensitive to their cues of hunger and satiety, generally adjust their intake to meet their energy needs. The best method for determining the adequacy of infants' energy intakes is to carefully monitor their gain in length by plotting it on the growth charts shown in Appendix Tables 6, 7, 10, and 11. It is important to recognize that, during the first year, a **catch-up** or **lag down** period in growth may be noted.

Growth in length should proceed at approximately the same rate. If an infant begins to reduce his or her rate of weight gain, does not gain weight, or loses weight, the energy and nutrient intake should be monitored carefully. If the rate of growth in length is reduced or ceases, the probability of malnutrition or undetected disease, or both, should be investigated thoroughly. If weight gain proceeds at a much more rapid rate than growth in length, the energy concentration of the formula, the quantity of formula consumed, and the amount and type

TABLE 8–1 DIETARY REFERENCE INTAKES: RECOMMENDED DIETARY ALLOWANCES (RDA) AND ADEQUATE INTAKES (AI) FOR INFANTS AND CHILDREN, BIRTH TO AGE 3 YEARS

	AGE (YR)		
NUTRIENT	**0.0–0.5**	**0.5–1.0**	**1–3**
Energy needs (kcal)	weight (kg) × 108	weight (kg) × 98	weight (kg) × 102
Protein (g)	weight (kg) × 2.2	weight (kg) × 1.6	weight (kg) × 1.2
Vitamin A (μg RE)*	375	375	400
Vitamin D (μg)†			
RDA	5	5	5
AI			
Vitamin E (mg)‡	3	4	6
Vitamin K (μg)	5	10	15
Vitamin C (mg)	30	35	40
Thiamine (mg)			
RDA			0.5
AI	0.2	0.3	
Riboflavin (mg)			
RDA			0.5
AI	0.3	0.4	
Niacin (mg NE)§			
RDA			6
AI	2	4	
Vitamin B_6 (mg)			
RDA	0.1	0.3	0.5
AI			
Folic acid (μg)**			
RDA			150
AI	65	80	
Vitamin B_{12} (μg)			
RDA			0.9
AI	0.4	0.5	
Pantothenic acid (mg)			
AI	1.7	1.8	2
Biotin (μg)			
AI	5	6	8
Choline (mg)			
AI	125	150	200
Calcium (mg)‖			
AI	210	270	500
Phosphorus (mg)			
RDA			460
AI	100	275	
Magnesium (mg)			
RDA			80
AI	30	75	
Iron (mg)			
RDA	6	10	10
Zinc (mg)			
RDA	5	5	10
Iodine (μg)			
RDA	40	50	70
Selenium (μg)			
RDA	10	15	20
Fluoride (mg)			
AI	.01	.5	.7

(Reprinted with permission from Recommended Dietary Allowances, 10th edition, © 1989 by the National Academy of Sciences. Published by National Academy Press, Washington, DC. Data from Institute of Medicine, Food and Nutrition Board: Dietary Reference Intakes for Thiamin, Riboflavin, Niacin, Vitamin B-6, Folate, Vitamin B-12, Pantothenic Acid, Biotin and Choline, Washington, DC, National Academy Press, 1998; Institute of Medicine, Food and Nutrition Board: Dietary Reference Intakes for Calcium, Phosphorus, Magnesium, Vitamin D and Fluoride, Washington, DC, National Academy Press, 1997.)

**RE* = retinol equivalent; 1 RE = 1 μg retinol, or 6 μg β-carotene.

†As cholecalciferol; 10 mg cholecalciferol = 400 IU of vitamin D.

‡α-Tocopherol equivalents (TE); 1 mg d,a-tocopherol = 1 α-TE.

§NE = niacin equivalent.

**Dietary folate equivalent (DFE), 1 DFE = 1 μg food folate = .6 μg folic acid (from fortified food or supplement) consumed with food.

‖National Academy of Sciences, Food and Nutrition Board, 1997.

RDAs are set to meet the needs of almost all (97 to 98%) individuals in a group.

AIs are the mean intakes for healthy breast-fed infants. The AI for other life-stage groups is believed to cover needs of all individuals in the group, but lack of data prevent being able to specify the percentage of persons covered by this intake.

of semi-solids and table food offered should be evaluated. The activity level of the infant should also be assessed.

Formula-fed infants consume more calories of energy per unit of body size than do breast-fed infants during the first year. Gains in weight are greater in formula-fed infants, as are increases in body mass per gram of protein intake. However, no functional advantage has been ascribed to the more rapid growth (Heinig et al., 1993).

Presently, the RDAs for energy for infants are being reevaluated. Based on newer methodology and data, it appears that the current RDAs overestimate infants' energy needs by about 15%, and there is little dispute that they need to be modified (Cryan and Johnson, 1997; see Chapter 2).

Protein

Protein is needed for tissue replacement, as well as for growth. Protein requirements during the rapid growth of infancy are higher, on a per kilogram of weight basis, than those for the adult or older child. Recommendations are based on the composition of human milk, assuming the efficiency of utilization of mother's milk to be 100%. Table 8–1 lists the RDAs for protein in terms of grams per kilogram of body weight for children from birth to 3 years of age. On the basis of grams per kilocalorie of energy, advisable intakes are 1.9 g/100 kcal for infants 0 to 4 months of age; 1.7 g/100 kcal for infants 4 to 12 months of age; and 1.4 g/kg/day for infants 12 to 36 months of age (Fomon, 1993). These figures are calculated to be about 15% lower for infants receiving breast milk because of the higher biologic value of human milk protein.

Essential amino acid needs are the same for infants as for adults except that *histidine* appears to be an essential amino acid for infants, but not for adults. Tyrosine, cystine, and taurine may also be essential for the premature infant.

Human milk or formula provides the major portion of protein during the first year of life. The amount of protein in human milk is adequate for the first 6 months of the infant's life, even though the protein in human milk is considerably less than in infant formula. In the last 6 months of the first year, diets of breast-fed infants should be supplemented with additional sources of high-quality protein, such as yogurt, strained meats, or cereal mixed with milk.

Inadequate intakes of protein may be the result of excessive dilution of formula, continuation of a regimen designed to treat diarrhea after an enteric illness, extreme vegetarian food patterns, multiple food allergies, or the deprivation associated with extreme poverty.

Lipid

It is recommended that infants consume a minimum of 3.8 g/100 kcal and a maximum of 6 g/100 kcal of fat (constituting 30% to 54% of calories of energy). This quantity is present in human milk and all formulas prepared for infants. Significantly lower intakes, as with skim milk feedings, may result in an inadequate energy intake. Infants may try to correct the deficit by increasing the volume of milk, but they usually cannot make up the entire amount. Increasing the intake of skim milk furnishes energy, but the accompanying excesses of protein, calcium, and phosphorus contribute to a high renal solute load and subsequent dehydration.

Linoleic acid, which is essential for growth and dermal integrity, should provide 3% of the total kilocalories or .5–1.0 g/kg daily (Heird, 1996). Smaller amounts of *α-linolenic acid,* a precursor of the n-3 fatty acids docosahexaenoic acid (DHA) and eicosapentaenoic acid (EPA), should be included. Five percent of the kilocalories of energy in human milk and 10% in most infant formulas are derived from linoleic acid. Table 8–2 indicates the linoleic acid content of infant formulas.

Carbohydrate

Carbohydrates should supply 30% to 60% of the energy intake during infancy. Thirty-seven percent of the energy in human milk and 40% to 50% of the energy in commercial formulas is derived from lactose or other carbohydrates. The rare infant who cannot tolerate lactose requires a special diet, as discussed in Chapters 31 and 44.

Botulism in infancy is caused by ingestion of *Clostridium botulinum* spores, which germinate and produce toxin in the lumen of the bowel. Honey and corn syrup, sometimes used in home-prepared foods, have been identified as the only food sources of these spores in infants' diets. The spores are extremely resistant to heat treatment and are not destroyed by present methods of processing. Thus, honey and corn syrup should not be fed to infants younger than 1 year of age as they do not yet have the immunity required to resist botulism spore development.

TABLE 8–2 LINOLEIC ACID CONTENT OF SELECTED INFANT FORMULAS

FORMULA	LINOLEIC ACID IN MG PER 100 KCAL OF ENERGY
Similac (Ross)	1000
Enfamil (Mead Johnson)	860
Good Start (Carnation)	850
Prosobee (Mead Johnson)	860
Isomil (Ross)	1000
LactoFree (Mead Johnson)	860
Alsoy (Carnation)	920
Alimentum (Ross)	1600
Follow-Up (Carnation)	680
Follow-Up Soy (Carnation)	720
Next Step (Mead Johnson)	810
Next Step Soy (Mead Johnson)	720

Water

The water requirement for infants is determined by the amount lost from the skin and lungs and in the feces and urine, plus a small amount needed for growth. The National Research Council recommends an intake of 1.5 mL/kcal/day. Water requirements per kilogram of body weight are shown in Table 8–3.

Because the renal concentrating capacity of young infants may be less than that of older children and adults, they may be vulnerable to water imbalance. Under ordinary conditions, human milk and formula that is properly prepared will supply adequate amounts of water. When a formula is boiled, however, the water evaporates and solutes become concentrated; boiled milk or formulas are, therefore, inappropriate for infants. In very hot, humid environments, infants may require additional water. When other than renal losses of water are high, as in cases of vomiting and diarrhea, infants should be monitored carefully to detect any fluid electrolyte imbalance.

Water intoxication results in hyponatremia, restlessness, nausea, vomiting, diarrhea, and polyuria or oliguria. Seizures can also result. This condition may occur if water is fed as a replacement for milk; if the formula is excessively diluted; or if bottled water, instead of an electrolyte solution, is given as treatment for diarrhea ("Tapping the Market for Bottled Baby Water," 1995).

Minerals

Calcium

For calcium, the old RDA of 400 to 800 mg/day was set to meet the needs of infants fed cow's milk–based formula, in whom approximately 25% to 30% of the intake is retained. This amount is not applicable to breast-fed infants, who retain approximately two thirds of their intake of calcium. The new AI of 210 to 500 mg/day is the mean intake of healthy breast-fed infants. The calcium:phosphorus ratio in an infant's diet is no longer thought to be important.

TABLE 8–3 WATER REQUIREMENTS OF INFANTS AND CHILDREN

AGE	WATER REQUIREMENT (ml/kg/day)
10 days	125–150
3 months	140–160
6 months	130–155
1 year	120–135
2 years	115–125
6 years	90–100
10 years	70–85
14 years	50–60

(From Barness LA. Nutrition and nutritional disorders. In: Behrman RE, Kliegman RM. Nelson Textbook of Pediatrics, 14th ed. Philadelphia: WB Saunders, 1992.)

Iron

Normal infants have adequate stores of iron for growth up to a doubling of their birth weight. This weight doubling occurs at approximately 4 months of age in full-term infants, and much earlier in prematurely born infants. Recommended intakes of iron increase from 6 mg/day in the first 6 months to 10 mg/day until 3 years of age. Infants who are fed only breast milk are at risk of a negative iron balance, beginning at 4 to 6 months of age, and may deplete their reserves by 6 to 9 months (Kim et al., 1996). Iron in human milk is highly bioavailable; however, both breast-fed and formula-fed infants should receive an additional source of iron by 4 to 6 months of age. Iron-fortified cereals and infant formula are common food sources.

Iron deficiency and iron deficiency anemia are common health concerns for the older infant. Recent data suggest that, for children 1 to 2 years of age who are living in the United States, the prevalence of iron deficiency is 9%, and of iron deficiency anemia is 3% (Looker et al., 1997).

The iron status of infants fed whole milk during the first year is less satisfactory than that of breast-fed infants or those fed formula with iron. Not only is milk a poor source of iron, it also contains factors that inhibit absorption (Fuchs et al., 1993).

Zinc

Normal newborn infants have no reserves of zinc and are, therefore, immediately dependent on a dietary source. Zinc is better absorbed from human milk than from infant formula, as evidenced by higher concentrations of zinc in breast-fed than in formula-fed babies. Human milk and infant formulas provide adequate zinc (0.3 to 0.5 mg/kg body weight) for the first year of life; other foods should provide most of the zinc required during the second year. See Table 8–1 for the RDAs established for zinc.

Fluoride

The importance of fluoride in preventing dental caries has been well documented. However, fluoride can also cause dental fluorosis (ranging from fine white lines to entirely chalky teeth) at intake levels of 4 to 1000 mg/day (see Chapter 29).

Breast milk has a very low fluoride content. Powdered formulas have higher concentrations than do concentrated formulas. Commercially prepared infant cereals, wet pack cereals, and fruit juice produced with fluoridated water are significant sources of fluoride in infancy.

Some evidence suggests that supplementation with fluoride, as previously recommended, may increase the risk of fluorosis in some children. Currently no fluoride supplementation is recommended for infants younger than 6 months of age. After tooth eruption, it is recommended that fluoridated water be offered several times per day to breast-fed infants, to those who receive cow's milk, and to those fed formulas made with water that contains less than 0.3 mg of fluoride/L (Committee on Nutrition, 1998).

Vitamins

Milk derived from an adequately fed, lactating mother supplies all the vitamins that the term infant needs except for vitamin D, since human milk contains only 40 to 50 IU/L of vitamin D. Breast-fed infants should receive a vitamin D supplement or be exposed regularly to sunlight. Exposure for 30 minutes per week, with the infant wearing only a diaper, or 2 hours per week, if fully clothed without a hat, is sufficient to meet vitamin D needs (Specker et al., 1985). Cases of rickets have often been diagnosed in breast-fed infants with dark skin and little exposure to sunlight (Gessner et al., 1997; Ahmed et al., 1995). Commercially prepared infant formulas are fortified with all necessary vitamins. Both evaporated and homogenized cow's milk are fortified with vitamin D, but contain very little vitamin C. Fresh goat's milk is deficient in vitamin D, vitamin C, and folate.

Vitamin deficiencies have been reported in infants fed formula products in which nutrients were destroyed or omitted during processing, and in infants who were fed by a lactating mother whose diet was inadequate and who was not receiving appropriate vitamin supplements. In the early 1950s, infants fed a formula in which vitamin B_6 was destroyed during processing were found to be pyridoxine-deficient (Coursin, 1954). A similar incident was reported again in the early 1980s, when a manufacturer neglected to add vitamin B_6 during manufacturing of the formula. Fortunately, very few such instances occur; however, when symptoms of vitamin deficiency are noted in formula-fed infants, such errors in processing must be considered.

Most infants can tolerate cow's milk or soy formulas. However, a small number of infants with multiple food intolerances can tolerate only goat's milk for long periods in infancy. When their diets are not supplemented with folate, these infants fail to thrive.

Milk from lactating mothers who follow a strict vegan diet may be vitamin B_{12}–deficient, especially if the mother has followed the regimen for a long time before and during the pregnancy. Vitamin B_{12} deficiency has also been diagnosed in an infant breast-fed by a mother with pernicious anemia (Higgenbottom et al., 1978; Johnson and Roloff, 1982).

The vitamin K nutriture of the neonate requires special attention. Deficiency may result in bleeding or **hemorrhagic disease of the newborn.** This condition is more common in breast-fed infants than in other infants because breast milk contains only 15 μg/L of vitamin K, whereas cow's milk and cow's milk–based formulas contain approximately four times that amount. Breast-fed infants consume less milk during the first few days of life than do formula-fed infants, which also accounts for their low vitamin K intake. It is recommended that all formulas contain a minimum of 4 μg of vitamin K per 100 kcal of formula. The suggested intake of 5 to 15 μg/day can be supplied by mature breast milk (15 μg/L), although perhaps not during the first few days to 1 week of life. Vitamin K supplementation may be necessary during that time. Many states require that infants receive an injection of vitamin K as a prophylactic measure while they are in the nursery. Previous reports that vitamin K injections may increase the risk of leukemia or cause cancer have not been supported by recent studies (Greer, 1995) (see Chapter 4).

Vitamin and mineral supplements should be prescribed only after careful evaluation of the infant's intake and exposure to sunlight. Infants who are fed commercially prepared formula rarely need supplements. Breast-fed infants need additional vitamin D supplementation by 2 months of age. Infants who are fed homogenized milk or an evaporated milk formula need a food source or supplement of vitamin C, and those who are fed fresh goat's milk need food sources or supplements of vitamin C, folate, and vitamin D. (Evaporated goat's milk is fortified with vitamin D.) Chapter 9 discusses the feeding of premature or high-risk infants and their special needs.

MILK FOR INFANTS

Human milk is unquestionably the food of choice for the infant. Its composition is designed to provide the necessary energy and nutrients in appropriate amounts. It contains factors that provide protection against certain bacteriologic infections, diarrhea, and otitis media (Scariati et al., 1997; American Academy of Pediatrics, 1997). Allergic reactions to human milk are relatively rare. Moreover, the closeness of the mother and infant during breast-feeding facilitates attachment and bonding (see Figure 7–10).

In fact, the Healthy Children 2000 Objectives propose to support breast-feeding among mothers of newborn infants (see "*Focus On:* Healthy Children 2000 Objectives: Nourishment of Infants").

Both the American Dietetic Association (ADA) and the American Academy of Pediatrics support exclusive breast-feeding for the first 4 to 6 months of life, and breast-feeding supplemented by weaning foods for at least 12 months (ADA Position Paper, 1997; American Academy of Pediatrics, 1997). This timing is important to note because the early addition of other foods promotes a decrease in breast milk intake and early weaning (Hill et al., 1997).

Unmodified cow's milk is inappropriate for infants. The tough, hard curd is difficult for young infants to digest, and a lesser amount of fat is ab-

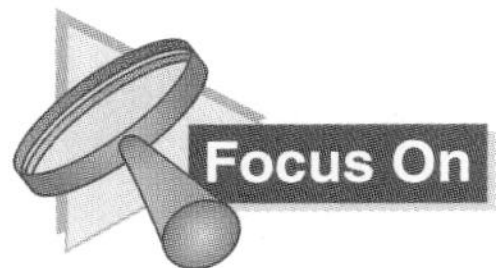

Healthy Children 2000 Objectives: Nourishment of Infants

2.4 Reduce growth retardation among low-income children aged 5 years and younger to less than 10 percent.

2.10 Reduce iron deficiency to less than 3 percent among children aged 1 to 4 years.

2.11 Increase to at least 75 percent the proportion of mothers who breast-feed their babies in the early postpartum period and to at least 50 percent the proportion who continue breast-feeding until their babies are 5 to 6 months old.

2.12 Increase to at least 75 percent the proportion of parents and caregivers who use feeding practices that prevent baby bottle tooth decay.

sorbed from cow's milk than from human milk. The much higher protein and ash content of cow's milk results in a higher **renal solute load,** which is the amount of nitrogenous waste and minerals that must be excreted by the kidney. Ingestion of goat's milk contributes to an even higher renal solute load.

Commercial formulas made from heat-treated nonfat milk are designed to provide necessary nutrients in a well-absorbed form. The manufacture of infant formulas is regulated by the Food and Drug Administration (FDA) through the Infant Formula Act (Nutrient Requirements for Infant Formulas, 1985). By law, infant formulas are required to provide a nutrient level that is consistent with these guidelines, as presented in Table 8–4.

Composition of Human and Cow's Milk

The composition of human milk is different from that of cow's milk; for this reason, cow's milk is not recommended for the human infant until at least 1 year of age. Both provide 20 kcal/oz; however, the nutrient sources of the energy are different. For example, protein provides 6% to 7% of the energy in human milk and 20% of the energy in cow's milk. Human milk is 60% whey and 40% casein; by contrast, cow's milk is 20% whey and 80% casein. **Casein** forms a tough, hard-to-digest curd in the infant's stomach, whereas **lactalbumin** forms soft, flocculent, easy-to-digest curds. The amino acids taurine and cystine are present in higher concentrations in human milk than in cow's milk. These amino acids may be essential for premature infants. Lactose provides 42% of the energy in human milk and only 30% of the energy in cow's milk.

Lipids provide 50% of the energy in both human and cow's milk. Monounsaturated oleic acid is the predominant fatty acid in both milks. Linoleic acid, the essential fatty acid, provides 4% of the energy in human milk and only 1% of that in cow's milk. The cholesterol content of human milk is 7 to 47 mg/dL, compared to 10 to 35 mg/dL in cow's milk. An additional lipase in the nonfat fraction of human milk is stimulated by bile salts and contributes significantly to the hydrolysis of milk triglycerides.

All of the water-soluble vitamins in human milk reflect maternal intake. Cow's milk contains adequate quantities of the B complex vitamins, but very little vitamin C. Both milks provide sufficient vitamin A. Human milk, which provides 2 IU/L, is a richer source of vitamin E than cow's milk. Human milk contains five metabolites of vitamin D, providing 40 to 50 IU/L of vitamin D activity; however,

TABLE 8–4 NUTRIENT LEVELS IN INFANT FORMULAS AS SPECIFIED BY THE INFANT FORMULA ACT

SPECIFIED NUTRIENT COMPONENT	MINIMUM LEVEL REQUIRED PER 100 KCAL OF ENERGY
Protein (g)	1.8
Fat (g)	3.3
Percent of calories	30
Linoleic acid (mg)	300
Percent of calories	2.7
Vitamin A (IU)	250
Vitamin E (IU)	0.7
Vitamin D (IU)	40
Vitamin K (μg)	4
Thiamin (μg)	40
Riboflavin (μg)	60
Niacin (μg)	250
Ascorbic acid (mg)	8
Pyridoxine (μg)	35
Vitamin B_{12} (μg)	0.15
Folic acid (μg)	4
Biotin (μg) (non–milk-based formulas only)	1.5
Pantothenic acid (μg)	300
Choline (mg) (non–milk-based formulas only)	7
Inositol (mg) (non–milk-based formulas only)	4
Calcium (mg)	60
Phosphorus (mg)	30
Iron (mg)	0.15
Zinc (mg)	0.5
Magnesium (mg)	6
Manganese (μg)	5
Sodium (mg)	20
Potassium (mg)	80
Iodine (μg)	5
Chloride (mg)	55
Copper (μg)	60

(From Nutrient Requirements for Infant Formulas, Final Rule. (21 CFR 107). Federal Register 50:45106, 1985.)

the need for additional vitamin D becomes progressively important with increasing age. Cow's milk is usually fortified with 400 IU/L of vitamin D.

The quantity of iron in human and cow's milk is small (0.3 mg/L). Forty-nine percent of the iron in human milk, but less than 1% of the iron in cow's milk, is absorbed. The bioavailability of zinc in human milk is higher than in cow's milk. Cow's milk contains three times as much calcium and six times as much phosphorus, and the fluoride concentration is twice that of human milk.

The sodium and potassium concentrations in human milk are about one third those in cow's milk, thus reducing the renal solute load. The osmolality of human milk averages 286 mOsm/kg, whereas that of cow's milk is 400 mOsm/kg.

Anti-infective Factors

Human milk and colostrum contain antibodies and anti-infective factors that are not present in cow's milk. Secretory immunoglobulin A (IgA) is the predominant immunoglobulin in human milk, and it plays a role in protecting the infant's immature gut from infection. However, research indicates that breast-feeding must be maintained until the infant is at least 3 months of age in order for this protection to be conferred.

The iron-binding protein lactoferrin in human milk deprives bacteria of iron and thus slows their growth. Lysozymes, which are bacteriolytic enzymes found in human milk, destroy the cell membranes of bacteria after they have been inactivated by the peroxides and ascorbic acid that are also present in human milk. Breast milk enhances the growth of the bacterium *Lactobacillus bifidus,* which produces an acidic gastrointestinal environment that interferes with the growth of certain pathogenic organisms. Because of these anti-infective factors, the incidence of infections is lower in breast-fed infants than in bottle-fed babies.

Formulas

Infants whose mothers are unwilling or unable to breast-feed are usually fed a formula based on cow's milk or a soy product. Those who have special requirements receive specially designed products.

Nonfat milk formulas available for normal infants are formulated to approximate, as closely as possible, the composition of human milk. For example, Enfamil has been modified to provide a whey: casein protein ratio similar to that of human milk. Similac and Gerber formulas are subjected to heat treatment, which serves to reduce the curd tension. Good Start formula contains reduced-mineral whey. It is higher in protein and lower in fat than other commercially available formulas. Vegetable oils are added to ensure fat absorption similar to that from human milk, and vitamins and minerals are added to meet the recommended intake for infants.

Formulas are also available for the older infant (e.g., Follow-Up and Follow-Up soy formulas). Formulas are also available for toddlers (e.g., Next Step and Next Step soy formulas). However, most pediatricians believe there is no need for "older infant" formulas unless toddlers are receiving inadequate amounts of solid feedings (Committee on Nutrition, 1989c).

The declining prevalence of anemia in infants is credited to the use of iron-fortified formula; for this reason, the American Academy of Pediatrics recommends iron-fortified formulas for all infants. The widespread theory that iron-fortified formula causes constipation, loose stools, colic, and spitting up in some infants has not been confirmed by clinical studies (Committee on Nutrition, 1989b; Committee on Nutrition, 1998). Formulas are available with and without additional iron. Table 8–5 shows the composition of various formulas, human milk, and cow's milk.

Recently, soy-based formulas have come under scrutiny. Infants ingesting soy formulas grow as well as, and absorb minerals at a rate equivalent to, infants fed cow's milk–based formulas. The concern about soy formulas stems from infants' exposure to phytoestrogens (see Chapter 12) or isoflavones, which is several thousand times higher than the exposure from breast milk or cow's milk–based formulas (Setchell et al., 1997), and whether or not this exposure poses a developmental hazard. The amount of soy protein isolate used in the manufacture of soy-based infant formulas determines the isoflavone content. From one study it is estimated that a typical 4-month-old infant ingesting soy formula would be exposed to 28 to 47 mg of isoflavones/day. Plasma concentrations in the study infants receiving soy-based formula were significantly greater than in infants fed breast milk or cow's milk–based formulas (Irvine et al., 1998). The biological impact of these elevated isoflavone levels on long-term infant development is not yet understood.

In an ongoing effort to manufacture infant formulas that closely approximate breast milk, the long-chain polyunsaturated fatty acid intake of formula-fed infants has been evaluated (Auestad et al., 1997; Jensen et al., 1997; Koletzko et al., 1996). **Arachidonic acid** and **docosahexaenoic acid** (DHA) are found in breast milk but not in cow's milk. Current research indicates that these very-long-chain fatty acids may be associated with accelerated cognition and vision. However, there is no current documentation that formula-fed infants are compromised, in terms of growth or development, when fed formulas without arachidonic acid or DHA supplementation.

A variety of products are available for infants who do not tolerate the milk in cow's milk–based formulas. Soy products designed to meet all nutrient needs are recommended for (1) children of vegetarian families; (2) children with galactosemia or primary lactase deficiency, as well as those recovering from secondary lactose intolerance; and (3) in-

TABLE 8–5 COMPOSITION OF SELECTED INFANT FORMULAS PER LITER

MILK/FORMULA	ENERGY (KCAL)	PROTEIN (G)	FAT (G)	CARBOHYDRATE (G)	CALCIUM (MG)	PHOSPHORUS (MG)	SODIUM		POTASSIUM		IRON (MG)	PROTEIN SOURCE	FAT SOURCE	CARBOHYDRATE SOURCE	COMMENT(S)
							MG	MEQ	MG	MEQ					
Human Milk	750	11	45	70	340	140	161	7	570	15	0.2	Lactalbumin, casein	Human fat	Lactose	Protein readily digested; adequate in all nutrients except vitamin D and fluoride
Milk-Based Infant Formulas															
Similac (Ross)	676	13.9	36.5	72.3	527	284	162	7.1	710	18.2	12.2/1.5*	Nonfat milk, whey	High oleic safflower, soy, coconut oils	Lactose	Vitamins and minerals added
Enfamil (Mead Johnson)	676	14.2	35.8	73.7	527	358	183	8	730	18.7	12.2/4.7*	Reduced-mineral whey, nonfat milk	Palm olein, soy, coconut, high oleic safflower oils	Lactose	Vitamins and minerals added
LactoFree (Mead Johnson)	676	14.9	37.2	70.3	554	372	203	8.8	744	19.1	12.2	Milk protein isolate	Palm olein, soy, coconut, high oleic sunflower oils	Corn syrup solids	Vitamins and minerals added
Good Start (Carnation)	676	16.2	34.5	74.4	433	243	162	7	662	17	10.1	Enzymatically hydrolyzed reduced-mineral whey	Palm olein, soy, coconut, high oleic safflower oils	Lactose, maltodextrin	Whey-predominant formula for normal infants; vitamins and minerals added
Cow's Milk															
Skim	357	35	2	50	1256	1028	524	23	1689	43	Trace	Casein	None	Lactose	Inappropriate for infants
2%	503	34	20	49	1236	965	508	22	1568	40	Trace	Casein	Butterfat	Lactose	Inappropriate for infants
Whole	624	33	34	47	1211	948	499	22	1539	39	Trace	Casein	Butterfat	Lactose	Inappropriate for infants younger than 12 months of age
Soy-Based Infant Formulas															
Prosobee (Mead Johnson)	676	20	35.8	67.6	710	561	243	10.6	811	20.8	12.2	Soy protein isolate with L-methionine	Palm olein, soy, coconut, high oleic sunflower oils	Corn syrup solids	Vitamins and minerals added
Isomil (Ross)	676	18	36.9	68	710	507	297	12.9	720	18.7	12.2	Soy protein isolate with L-methionine	Soy, coconut oils	Corn syrup, sucrose	Vitamins and minerals added
Alsoy (Carnation)	676	18.6	33.4	75	710	412	233	10	784	17.1	12.2	Soy protein isolate with L-methionine	Palm olein, soy, coconut, high oleic safflower oils	Corn maltodextrin, sucrose	Vitamins and minerals added

(continued)

TABLE 8–5 COMPOSITION OF SELECTED INFANT FORMULAS PER LITER (continued)

MILK/FORMULA	ENERGY (KCAL)	PROTEIN (G)	FAT (G)	CARBOHYDRATE (G)	CALCIUM (MG)	PHOSPHORUS (MG)	SODIUM MG	SODIUM MEQ	POTASSIUM MG	POTASSIUM MEQ	IRON (MG)	PROTEIN SOURCE	FAT SOURCE	CARBOHYDRATE SOURCE	COMMENT(S)
Casein Hydrolysate Formulas															
Nutramigen (Mead Johnson)	676	18.9	33.8	74.4	635	426	318	13.8	744	19.1	13	Casein hydrolysate with added amino acids	Palm olein, soy, coconut, high oleic sunflower oils	Corn syrup solids, modified cornstarch	Vitamins and minerals added
Pregestimal (Mead Johnson)	676	18.9	37.9	69.4	635	426	264	11.5	737	18.9	12.7	Casein hydrolysate with added amino acids	MCT (55%), corn, soy, high oleic safflower oils	Corn syrup solids, dextrose, modified cornstarch	Vitamins and minerals added
Alimentum (Ross)	676	18.6	37.5	68.9	710	507	297	12.9	798	20.5	12.2	Casein hydrolysate with added amino acids	MCT (50%), safflower, soy oils	Sucrose, modified tapioca starch	Vitamins and minerals added
Formulas for Feeding Beyond 4 to 6 months of Age															
Follow-Up (Carnation)	676	16.2	34.5	74.3	432	243	162	17.1	662	16.9	10.1	Nonfat milk	Palm olein, soy, coconut, high oleic safflower oils	Corn syrup solids, lactose	Vitamins and minerals added
Follow-Up Soy (Carnation)	676	20.9	29.7	81.1	912	608	284	12.3	797	20.4	12.2	Soy protein isolate with L-methionine	Palm olein, soy, coconut, high oleic safflower oils	Corn syrup solids, maltodextrin, sucrose	Vitamins and minerals added
Formulas for Feeding Beyond 1 Year of Age															
Next Step (Mead Johnson)	676	17.6	33.8	75	811	568	277	12	879	22.5	12.2	Nonfat milk	Palm olein, soy, coconut, high oleic sunflower oils	Lactose, corn syrup solids	Vitamins and minerals added
Next Step Soy (Mead Johnson)	676	22.3	29.7	79.7	777	608	304	13.2	1014	26.1	12.2	Soy protein isolate with L-methionine	Palm olein, soy, coconut, high oleic sunflower oils	Corn syrup solids, sucrose	Vitamins and minerals added

MCT, medium-chain triglycerides.
*Level depends on whether or not iron is added.

fants who are potentially allergic to cow's milk but who have not shown clinical manifestations of allergy. These products are not recommended for children known to have food allergies, as many infants who are allergic to cow's milk also develop allergy to soy milk (Committee on Nutrition, 1989a).

Infants who are intolerant of soy products may be fed formulas made from a **casein hydrolysate** (Nutramigen, Pregestimil, or Alimentum). Other formulas are available for children with specific problems, such as malabsorption or metabolic disorders (e.g., phenylketonuria).

Infants who receive adequate breast milk and/or infant formula require minimal supplemental nutrients (see "*Focus On:* Recommendations for Vitamin and Mineral Supplementation in Full-Term Infants").

Whole Cow's Milk

Although it is generally recommended that infants receive human milk or iron-fortified formula for the first year of life, many parents make the transition from formula to fresh cow's milk when the infant is between 5 and 9 months of age. The Committee on Nutrition of the American Academy of Pediatrics, however, has concluded that infants should not be fed whole cow's milk during the first year of life (Committee on Nutrition, 1998). Infants who are fed whole cow's milk have been found to have lowered intakes of iron, linoleic acid, and vitamin E, and excessive intakes of sodium, potassium, and protein. Cow's milk may cause a small gastrointestinal blood loss.

Low-fat (2%) and nonfat milk are also inappropriate for infants during the first 2 years of life. In addition, substitute or imitation milks are inappropriate, and should not be fed to infants.

Formula Preparation

Commercial formulas are available in ready-to-feed forms requiring no preparation, as concentrates prepared by mixing the formula with equal parts of water, and in powder form, designed to be mixed with 2 oz of water per level tablespoon or scoop of the powder.

In most households that maintain a reasonable level of sanitation, formulas are seldom sterilized. However, care should be taken to maintain a very clean environment when formulas are made. All equipment, including bottles, nipples, mixers, and the top of the can of milk, should be thoroughly washed. The infant should be fed immediately after the formula is prepared, and any milk not consumed at that feeding should be discarded. Any opened cans of formula should be covered and refrigerated.

FOODS FOR INFANTS

A variety of commercially prepared foods, as well as organically grown products, are available for infants. These vary widely in nutrient value.

Ready-to-serve dry infant cereals are fortified with **electrolytically reduced iron.** Three level tablespoons of cereal provide about 5 mg of iron, or from one half to one third the amount the infant requires. Cereal is, therefore, usually the first food added to the infant's diet. Cereal and fruit mixtures in jars are fortified with ferrous sulfate to provide 7 to 9 mg of iron per 4.5-oz jar.

Strained and junior vegetables and fruits provide carbohydrate and variable amounts of vitamins A and C. Vitamin C is added to a number of fruits and all fruit juices. Tapioca is added to a number of the fruits. Milk is added to creamed vegetables, and wheat is incorporated into the mixed vegetables.

Strained and junior meats are prepared with only water, except for lamb, to which lemon juice is added. Strained meats, which have the highest energy density of any of the commercial baby foods, are an excellent source of high-quality protein and heme iron.

A number of dessert items are also available, including puddings and fruit desserts. The nutrient composition of these products varies, but all contain

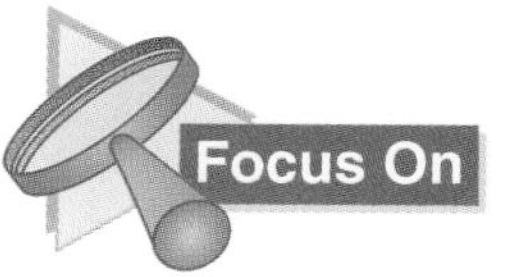

Recommendations for Vitamin and Mineral Supplementation in Full-Term Infants

Iron	*Breast-fed infants:* about 1 mg/kg/day by 4–6 months of age, preferably from supplemental foods *For breast-fed infants younger than 12 months:* only iron-fortified formulas for weaning or supplementing breast milk *Formula-fed infants:* only iron-fortified formula during the first year of life
Vitamin D	An intake of 400 IU/day is recommended; most formulas contain 62 IU/100 calories to meet this recommendation. Adequate sun exposure for white infants is 30 min/week if clothed in diaper only, or 2 hours/week if fully clothed (no hat).
Vitamin K	Supplementation soon after birth to prevent hemorrhagic disease of the newborn.
Fluoride	Intake of 0.25 mg/day after 6 months of age if water contains <0.3 ppm.

(Adapted with permission from Committee on Nutrition, American Academy of Pediatrics: Handbook of Pediatric Nutrition, 4th ed. Elk Grove Village, IL, 1998.)

TABLE 8–6 DIRECTIONS FOR HOME PREPARATION OF INFANT FOODS

1. Select fresh, high-quality fruits, vegetables, or meats.
2. Be sure that all utensils, including cutting boards, grinder, knives, and the like, are thoroughly cleaned.
3. Wash hands before preparing the food.
4. Clean, wash, and trim the food in as little water as possible.
5. Cook the foods until tender in as little water as possible. Avoid overcooking, which may destroy heat-sensitive nutrients.
6. Do not add salt. Add sugar sparingly. Do not add honey or corn syrup to food intended for infants younger than 1 year of age.*
7. Add enough water for the food to be easily puréed.
8. Strain or purée the food using an electric blender, a food mill, a baby food grinder, or a kitchen strainer.
9. Pour purée into an ice cube tray and freeze.
10. When the food is frozen hard, remove the cubes and store in freezer bags.
11. When ready to serve, defrost and heat in a serving container the amount of food that will be consumed at a single feeding.

*Botulism spores have been reported in honey and corn syrup, and young infants do not have the immune capacity to resist this infection.

sugar and modified corn or tapioca starch. Most infants do not require this excess energy.

Mothers who wish to make their own baby food can easily do so, following the directions in Table 8–6. Home-prepared foods are generally more concentrated in nutrients than commercially prepared ones because less water is used. Salt should not be added to foods prepared for infants, and sugar should be added sparingly.

FEEDING THE INFANT

Early Feeding Patterns

Because milk from a mother who consumes an adequate diet is uniquely designed to meet the needs of the human infant, breast-feeding for the first 6 months of life is strongly recommended. Most chronic medical conditions do not contraindicate breast-feeding.

A mother should be encouraged to nurse her infant immediately after birth. Those who care for and counsel parents during the first postpartum days should acquaint themselves with ways in which they can be supportive. Ideally, counseling and preparation start in the last few months or weeks of pregnancy, as is discussed in Chapter 7.

During the first few days of life, the breast-feeding baby receives colostrum, a yellow transparent fluid that meets the infant's needs during the first week. It contains less fat and carbohydrate, but more protein and greater concentrations of sodium, potassium, and chloride, than mature milk.

Infants who are bottle-fed will most likely receive ready-to-feed formula in the hospital. At home, products such as concentrated formulas that have been refrigerated should be mixed with warm water or heated to body temperature in a water bath. Refrigerated, read-to-feed formula also needs to be warmed. Microwave heating is not recommended because of the risk of burns from formula that is too hot.

Regardless of whether infants are breast- or bottle-fed, they should be held and cuddled during feeding. Once a feeding rhythm is established, infants will become fussy or cry to indicate hunger; often, they smile and fall asleep when they are satisfied (Table 8–7). Infants, not adults, should establish their feeding schedules. Initially, most infants feed at intervals of 2 to 3 hours; by 4 weeks of age, most extend the intervals between feedings to 4 hours. By 2 to 4 months of age, sufficient maturation has usually occurred to omit the night feeding.

Baby Bottle Tooth Decay

A pattern of tooth decay that involves the upper anterior and, sometimes, lower posterior teeth is common among infants and children who are given sugar-sweetened beverages or fruit juice in a bottle at bedtime (see Chapter 29 and Fig. 29–5). Infants should be fed, burped, and put to bed without milk, juice, or food.

Development of Feeding Skills

At birth, infants coordinate sucking, breathing, and swallowing, and are prepared to suck or suckle liquids, but not foods with texture. During the first year, normal infants develop head control, the ability to move into and sustain a sitting posture, and the ability to grasp, first with a **palmar grasp,** and then with a refined **pincer grasp** (Fig. 8–2). They develop a mature suck and rotary chewing, and

TABLE 8–7 SATIETY BEHAVIORS IN INFANTS

AGE (WEEKS)	BEHAVIOR
4–12	Draws head away from the nipple Falls asleep When nipple is reinserted, the infant closes lips tightly. Bites nipple, purses lips, or smiles and lets go
16–24	Releases nipple and withdraws head Fusses or cries Obstructs mouth with hands Pays increased attention to surroundings Bites nipple
28–36	Changes posture Keeps mouth tightly closed Shakes head as if to say "no" Plays with utensils Hands become more active Throws utensils
40–52	Behaviors listed for previous age range Sputters with tongue and lips Hands bottle or cup to mother

(Adapted from Gesell A, Ilg FL. Feeding Behavior of Infants. Philadelphia: JB Lippincott, 1937. Reprinted with permission from Pipes PL. Health care professionals. In: Garwood G, Fewell R (eds.). Educating Handicapped Infants. Rockville, MD: Aspen Systems, 1982.)

progress from being fed to feeding themselves using their fingers. In the second year, they learn to feed themselves independently with a spoon. They learn to walk and seek food for themselves.

Addition of Semi-Solid Foods

Developmental readiness and nutrient needs have been the criteria that determine appropriate times for the addition of various foods. Table 8–8 lists developmental landmarks and their indications for progression in semi-solid and table food introduction. During the first 4 months of life, the infant attains head and neck control, and oral motor patterns change from a suck to a suckling to the beginnings of a mature sucking pattern. Puréed foods fed during this phase are consumed in the same manner as liquids, with each suckle followed by a tongue-thrust swallow.

Between 4 and 6 months of age, when the mature suck is refined and munching movements (up and down chopping motions) begin, the introduction of strained foods is appropriate. Infant cereal is usually introduced first. Thereafter, a variety of commercially or home-prepared foods may be offered. The sequence in which these foods are introduced is not important; however, it is important that only one food (e.g., peaches rather than peach cobbler with many ingredients) be introduced at a time. This helps parents to identify any allergies or intolerances to particular foods. Introducing vegetables before fruits may increase vegetable acceptance.

Infants gradually increase their acceptance of new foods by slowly increasing the quantity they accept. Breast-fed infants appear to accept greater quantities than do formula-fed infants (Sullivan and Birch, 1994).

As oral–motor maturation proceeds, infants' rotary chewing develops, indicating a readiness for more textured foods, such as well-cooked mashed vegetables, casseroles, and pasta from the family menu. Learning to grasp—first with a palmar grasp, then an inferior pincer grasp, and finally, a refined pincer grasp—indicates a readiness for finger foods, such as oven-dried toast, arrowroot biscuits, or cheese sticks (see Fig. 8–2). Table 8–9 presents recommendations for adding foods to the infant's diet. Hot dogs, grapes, and bread that has been spread with peanut butter can cause choking, and so should not be offered at this age unless cut into small pieces.

During the last quarter of the first year, babies can approximate their lips to the rim of the cup and can drink if the cup is held for them. During the second year, they gain the ability to rotate their wrists and elevate their elbows, thus allowing them to hold the cup themselves. They feed very messily at first, but by 2 years of age, most normal children are skillful self-feeders (Fig. 8–3).

TABLE 8–8 DEVELOPMENTAL STAGES OF READINESS TO PROGRESS IN FEEDING BEHAVIORS DURING FIRST 2 YEARS OF LIFE

DEVELOPMENTAL LANDMARKS	CHANGE INDICATED	EXAMPLE OF APPROPRIATE FOODS
Tongue laterally transfers food in the mouth Voluntary and independent movements of the tongue and lips Sitting posture that can be sustained Beginning of chewing movements (up and down movements of the jaw)	Introduction of soft, mashed table food	Tuna fish; mashed potatoes; well-cooked, mashed vegetables; ground meats in gravy and sauces; soft, diced fruit, such as bananas, peaches, and pears; flavored yogurt
Reaches for and grasps objects with scissors (palmar) grasp Brings hand to mouth	Finger feeding (large pieces of food)	Oven-dried toast, teething biscuits, cheese sticks (Food should be soluble in the mouth to prevent choking.)
Voluntary release (refined digital [pincer] grasp)	Finger feeding (small pieces of food)	Bits of cottage cheese, dry cereal, peas and other bite-size vegetables, small pieces of meat
Rotary chewing pattern	Introduction of food of varied texture from family menu	Well-cooked, chopped meats and casseroles, cooked vegetables and canned fruit (not mashed), toast, potatoes, macaroni, spaghetti, peeled ripe fruit
Approximates lips to rim of the cup	Introduction of cup for sipping liquids	
Understands relationship of container and its contents	Beginning of self-feeding (though messiness should be expected)	Food that, when scooped, adheres to the spoon, such as applesauce, cooked cereal, mashed potatoes, cottage cheese, yogurt
Increased movements of the jaw Development of ulnar deviation of the wrist	More skilled at cup and spoon feeding	Chopped, fibrous meats, such as roast and steak Raw vegetables and fruit (introduced gradually)
Walks alone	May seek food and obtain food independently	Foods of high nutrient value should be available.
Names food, expresses preferences; prefers unmixed foods Goes on food jags Appetite appears to decrease.		Balanced food intake should be offered, and the child should be permitted to develop food preferences. Parents should not be concerned that these preferences will last forever.

(Adapted from Trahms CM, Pipes P. Nutrition in Infancy and Childhood, 6th ed. New York: McGraw-Hill, 1997.)

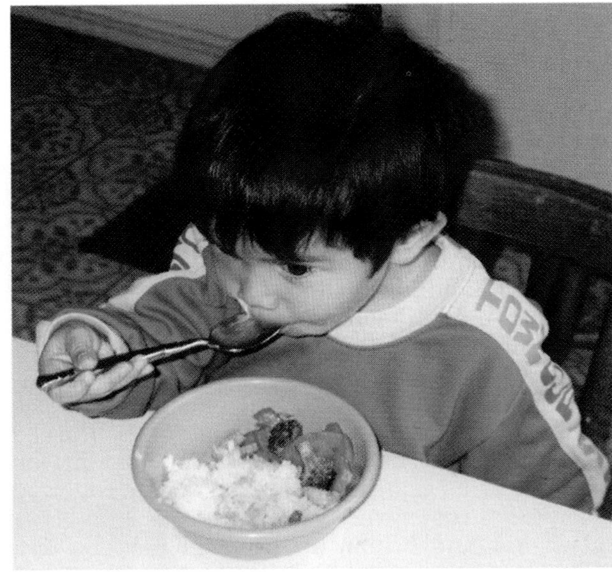

B

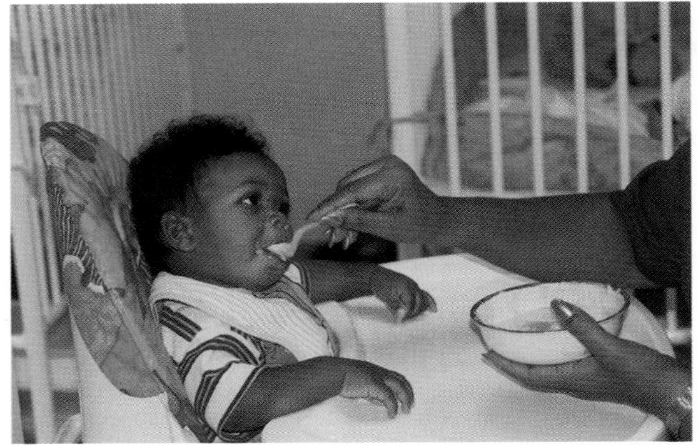

A

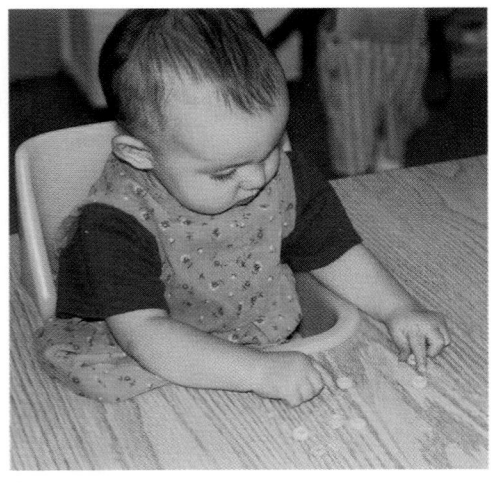

C

FIGURE 8–2 Development of feeding skills in infants and toddlers. *A.* At 7 months, this child shows beginning involvement with feeding by anticipating the spoon. *B.* At 9 months, this little boy is beginning to use his spoon independently, although he is not yet able to rotate his wrist to keep food on it. *C.* This 9-month-old little girl demonstrates a refined pincer grasp that is used to pick up food.

TABLE 8–9 SUGGESTED AGES FOR THE INTRODUCTION OF JUICE, SEMI-SOLID FOODS, AND TABLE FOODS

	AGE (MONTHS)		
FOOD	**4–6**	**6–8**	**9–12**
Iron-fortified cereals for infants	Add		
Vegetables		Add strained	Gradually eliminate strained foods and introduce table foods.
Fruits		Add strained	Gradually eliminate strained foods; introduce chopped, well-cooked or canned foods.
Meats		Add strained or finely chopped table meats.	Decrease the use of strained meats; increase the varieties of table meats offered.
Finger foods, such as arrowroot biscuits, oven-dried toast		Add those foods that can be secured with a palmar grasp.	Increase the use of small finger foods as the pincer grasp develops.
Well-cooked mashed or chopped table foods, prepared without added salt or sugar			Add
Juice or formula by cup			Add

(From Trahms CM, Pipes P. Nutrition in Infancy and Childhood, 6th ed. New York: McGraw-Hill, 1997.)

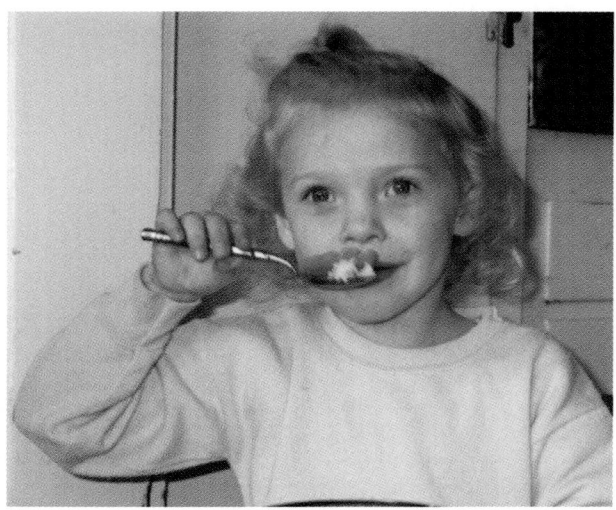

FIGURE 8–3 This 2-year-old is skilled at self-feeding, having the ability to both rotate the wrist and elevate the elbow to keep food on the spoon.

Feeding the Older Infant

As maturation proceeds and the rate of growth slows down, infants' interest in and approach to food change. Between 9 and 18 months of age, most reduce their milk intake. They become finicky about what and how much they will eat, and they may go on food jags. These are rarely dangerous, however, and should not be major concerns (see "*Clinical Insight:* Self-Selected Diets of Infants and Young Children").

In the weaning stage, infants have to learn many manipulative skills, including the chewing and swallowing of solid food and the use of utensils. They learn to eat a variety of textures and flavors of food, to finger feed, and then to feed themselves with a utensil. Very young children should be encouraged to feed themselves.

At the beginning of a meal, children are hungry and should be allowed to feed themselves; when they become tired, they can be helped quietly. Emphasis on table manners and the fine points of eating should be left until later, when they have the necessary maturity and developmental readiness for such considerations.

The food should be in a form that is easy to handle and eat. Meat should be cut into bite-sized pieces. Potatoes and vegetables should be mashed so that a spoon can be used easily. Raw fruits and vegetables should be in sizes that can be picked up easily. In addition, the utensils should be small and manageable. The cup should be easy to hold, and dishes should be designed so that they do not tip over easily.

Size of Servings

The size of servings offered a child is very important. At 1 year, babies will eat one third to one half the amount an adult normally consumes. This proportion increases to one half an adult portion or a little more by the time the child reaches 3 years of age, and increases further—to about two thirds—by 6 years of age. Little children should not be served a large plateful of food; the size of the plate and the amount should be kept in proportion to their age. A tablespoon (not heaping!) of each food offered for each year of age is a good guide to follow. Serving less than is thought or hoped will be

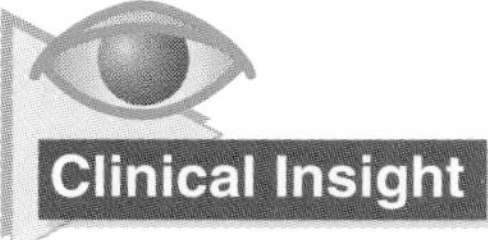

Self-Selected Diets of Infants and Young Children

Young children, if left to their own devices with a wide variety of wholesome foods at their disposal, instinctively choose an adequate diet. This was documented by research conducted in the late 1920s by Davis, who was attempting to demonstrate that the prevailing practice of withholding solid foods until 1 year of age was not in the best interest of the child (Davis, 1928). At the onset of the study, Davis studied three children, aged 7 to 9 months, for 6 months to 1 year. Later, she studied 12 additional children for 6 months to 4½ years, during which time their diets were entirely self-selected. They were offered a variety of fresh, unprocessed, and unseasoned foods, and were allowed to eat as little or as much as they pleased of any or all items (Davis, 1939). A modern evaluation of their intakes indicates that the foods consumed equaled or exceeded the RDA for all nutrients except iron.

It appears to be difficult for a child with a normal appetite to fail to obtain an adequate diet with choices limited to the following: beef, lamb, chicken, liver, kidney, brains, sweetbreads, haddock; whole wheat, oatmeal, barley, cornmeal, Ry-Krisp; bone marrow, bone jelly, eggs, raw milk; apples, oranges, bananas, peaches, pineapples; lettuce, cabbage, spinach, cauliflower, peas, beets, carrots, turnips, potatoes, tomatoes; and sea salt.

Items not included were any of the desserts or snacks common to the period, and certainly none of the highly refined, energy-rich, and nutrient-dilute foods available today.

A preference for sweetness that is present at birth and persists throughout childhood suggests that infants who are confronted with dietary selections that include desserts and sweetened snack foods would be unable to make the choices appropriate for a nutritious diet (Story and Brown, 1987).

However, it must also be noted that a similar study of children, aged ½ to 4 years, who were presented with wholesome foods common today also demonstrated the ability to select foods to meet their energy requirements. Unfortunately, the nutrient adequacy of their selected diets was not determined (Birch, 1991).

eaten helps children to eat successfully and happily. They will ask for more food if their appetite is not satisfied.

Type of Food

In general, children prefer simple, uncomplicated foods (Lowenberg, 1997). Food from the family meal may be adapted for the child and served in child-sized portions. Children younger than 6 years of age usually prefer mild-flavored foods. Because the young child's stomach is small, a snack may be required between meals. Fruit, cheese, crackers, fruit juices, and milk contribute nutrients as well as energy. Children aged 2 to 6 years often prefer raw instead of cooked vegetables and fruits.

It is especially desirable that babies be offered foods that vary in both texture and flavor. The infant who is accustomed to many kinds of foods is less likely to grow up with definite food dislikes. To add variety to the infant's diet, different vegetables and fruits may be added to cereal feedings. It is important to offer a variety of dishes and not to allow the youngster to continue on a diet consisting of one or two favorite foods. Older infants generally reject unfamiliar foods the first time they are offered. If the parent continues to offer small portions of these foods without comment, the infant will become familiar with the item and will often accept it. It is important that the child's intake of fruit juice does not replace the intake of more energy-dense foods. If excessive amounts are consumed, children may "fail to thrive," as discussed in Chapter 10.

Forced Feeding

Children should not be forced to eat; instead, the cause for the unwillingness to eat should be determined. A normal, healthy child will eat without coaxing. A child may refuse food because he or she is too inactive to be hungry, or too active and overtired. Fatigue can be avoided by planning a short rest period for the child before meals, or by providing a picture book for the child's quiet enjoyment. A child who is fed snacks or given a bottle too close to mealtime will not be hungry, and so may refuse the meal that is offered. Omitting all eating or drinking for 1 to 1½ hours before a meal helps solve the problem.

An overanxious parent can affect the appetite of the infant or the child. Emotions can retard the flow of gastric juice and inhibit digestion. Refusal to eat may also be the result of too much attention. Children enjoy the attention of their parents and soon learn that refusal to eat is one way to obtain it.

If a child refuses to eat, the family meal should be completed without comment and the plate should be removed. This procedure is usually harder on the parent than on the child. At the next mealtime, the child will be hungry enough to enjoy the food presented.

CASE STUDY

Lela M, a 12-week-old female infant born by cesarean section at 42 weeks' gestation to an 18-year-old gravida 1 para 1 single mother who participated in the WIC program prenatally and postnatally, is found to plot weight for length at the 95th percentile. Her mother gained 70 lb prenatally. As can be noted, the baby's length and weight remain in the same channel as when she was born.

The decision was made prenatally to feed the infant formula, rather than to breast-feed, because it was thought to be more convenient for the mother. The mother's choice of formula is powdered Similac with Iron. The formula is prepared with 1 measure of powder mixed in 2 oz of water. At 12 weeks of age, Lela consumes about six 8-oz bottles per day. Her mother reports no schedule, but feeds Lela on demand. Most often, the baby sleeps during the night, but if she is fussy, her mother gives her small amounts of commercially prepared infant cereal, vegetables, and fruit. According to the mother, "She really likes applesauce."

1. To get an accurate assessment of this infant's intake, what additional information is needed?
2. Is Lela growing appropriately? Explain your answer.
3. What is Lela's estimated energy intake? Is this appropriate?
4. Would you guess that this infant is ready for semisolid foods? What would you look for in a feeding evaluation?

Where the Child Should Eat

Children should eat their meals at the family table. They then have an opportunity to learn table manners while enjoying meals with a family group. Sharing the family fare strengthens ties and makes mealtime a pleasant period. However, if the adult meal is delayed or if adult guests are present, the children should receive their meal at the usual time. When children eat with the family, everyone must be careful not to make unfavorable comments about any food. Children are great imitators of the people they admire; thus, if the father or older siblings turn up their noses at squash, for example, they are likely to do the same.

CITED REFERENCES

Ahmed I, et al. Vitamin D deficiency rickets in breast-fed infants presenting with hypocalaemia. Acta Paediatr 82:941, 1995.

American Academy of Pediatrics Work Group on Breastfeeding: Breastfeeding and the use of human milk. Pediatrics 100:1035, 1997.

American Dietetic Association Position Paper. Promotion of breastfeeding. J Am Diet Assoc 97:662, 1997.

Auestad N, et al. Visual acuity, erythrocyte fatty acid composition and growth in term infants fed formula with long chain polyunsaturated fatty acids for one year. Pediatr Res 41:1, 1997.

Birch L, et al. The variability of young children's energy intake. N Engl J Med 324:232, 1991.

Committee on Nutrition, American Academy of Pediatrics. (AAP) Handbook of Pediatric Nutrition, 4th ed. Elk Grove Village, IL. AAP, 1998.

Committee on Nutrition, American Academy of Pediatrics. Follow-up on weaning formulas. Pediatrics 83:1067, 1989c.

Committee on Nutrition, American Academy of Pediatrics. Hypoallergenic infant formulas. Pediatrics 83:1383, 1989a.

Committee on Nutrition, American Academy of Pediatrics. Iron-fortified infant formulas. Pediatrics 84:1114, 1989b.

Coursin DB. Convulsive seizures in infants with pyridoxine deficient diet. JAMA 154:406, 1954.

Cryan J, Johnson RK. Should the current recommendations for energy intake in infants and young children be lowered? Nutr Today 32:69, 1997.

Davis CM. Results of the self-selection of diets by young children. Can Med Assoc J 41:257, 1939.

Davis CM. Self-selection of diet by newly weaned infants: An experimental study. Am J Dis Child 36:651, 1928.

Fomon SJ. Nutrition of Normal Infants. St Louis: CV Mosby, 1993.

Fuchs GJ, et al. Iron status and intake of older infants fed formula vs cow milk with cereal. Am J Clin Nutr 58:343, 1993.

Gessner BB, et al. Nutritional rickets among breastfed black and Alaska Native children. Alaska Med 39:119, 1997.

Greer FR. Vitamin K deficiency and hemorrhage in infancy. Clin Perinatol 22:759, 1995.

Heinig MJ, et al. Energy and protein intakes of breast-fed and formula-fed infants during the first year of life and their association with growth velocity: The DARLING STUDY. Am J Clin Nutr 58:152, 1993.

Heird, WC. Nutritional Requirements during infancy. In: Ziegler EE and Filer LJ (ed). Present Knowledge in Nutrition, 7th ed. Washington, DC, ILSI Press, 1996.

Higgenbottom L. A syndrome of megaloblastic anemia and neurological abnormalities of a vitamin B_{12} deficient breast fed infant of a strict vegetarian. N Engl J Med 299:317, 1978.

Hill PD, et al. Does early supplementation affect long-term breastfeeding? Clin Pediatr 56:345, 1997.

Irvine CH, et al. Phyto-estrogens in soy-based infant foods: Concentrations, daily intake, and possible biological effects. Proc Soc Exp Biol Med 217:247, 1998.

Jensen CL, et al. Effect of dietary linoleic/alpha-linolenic acid ratio on growth and visual function in term infants. J Pediatr 131:200, 1997.

Johnson PR, Roloff JS. Vitamin B_{12} deficiency in an infant strictly breast-fed by a mother with latent pernicious anemia. J Pediatr 100:917, 1982.

Kim SK, et al. Red blood cell indices and iron status according to feeding practices in infants and young children. Acta Paediatr 85:139, 1996.

Koletzko B, et al. Arachidonic acid supply and metabolism in human infants born at full term. Lipids 31:79, 1996.

Looker AC, et al. Prevalence of iron deficiency in the United States. JAMA 277:973, 1997.

Lowenberg M. The development of food patterns in young children. In: Trahms CM, Pipes P. Nutrition in Infancy and Childhood, 6th ed. McGraw-Hill, 1997.

Nutrient Requirements for Infant Formulas, Final Rule (21 CFR 107). Federal Register 50:45106, 1985.

Scariati PD, et al. Longitudinal analysis of infant morbidity and the extent of breastfeeding in the United States. Pediatrics 99:E51, 1997.

Setchell KD, et al. Exposure of infants to phtyoestrogens from soy based formula. Lancet 350:23, 1997.

Specker B, et al. Sunshine exposure and serum-25-hydroxyvitamin D concentrations in exclusively breast-fed infants. J Pediatr 107:372, 1985.

Story M, Brown JE. Do young children instinctively know what to eat? N Engl J Med 316:103, 1987.

Sullivan SA, Birch LL. Infant dietary experience and acceptance of solid foods. Pediatrics 93:271, 1994.

Tapping the market for bottled baby water. Tufts Univ Diet Nutr Lett 13(1):6, 1995.

U.S. Department of Health and Human Services, Public Health Service and United States Maternal and Child Health Bureau. Healthy Children 2000: National Health Promotion and Disease Prevention Objectives Related to Mothers, Infants, Children, Adolescents, and Youth. Washington DC: U.S. Government Printing Office (DHHS Publication HRSA-M-CH-91-2), 1991.

ADDITIONAL REFERENCES

Bachrach S, et al. An outbreak of vitamin D deficiency rickets in a susceptible population. Pediatrics 64:871, 1979.

Calvo EB, et al. Iron status in exclusively breast fed infants. Pediatrics 90:375, 1992.

Churella H, et al. Growth and protein status of term infants fed soy protein formulas differing in protein content. J Am Coll Nutr 13:262, 1994.

Committee on Nutrition, American Academy of Pediatrics. Soy-protein formulas: Recommendations for use in infant feeding. Pediatrics 72:359, 1983.

Committee on Nutrition, American Academy of Pediatrics. Imitation and substitute milks. Pediatrics 73:876, 1984.

Committee on Nutrition, American Academy of Pediatrics. The use of whole cow's milk in infancy. Pediatrics 91:515, 1992.

Dewey KG, et al. Breast-fed infants are leaner than formula-fed infants at 1 y of age: The DARLING study. Am J Clin Nutr 57:140, 1993.

Food and Nutrition Board, National Research Council, National Academy of Sciences: Recommended Dietary Allowances, 10th ed. Washington, DC: National Academy Press, 1989.

Garza C, Frongillo EA. Infant feeding recommendations (Editorial). Am J Clin Nutr 67:815, 1998.

Harris CS, et al. Childhood asphyxiation by food: A national analysis and overlook. JAMA 251:231, 1984.

Holman SR. Infant feeding in Roman antiquity. Nutr Today, 33:113, 1998.

Howie PW, et al. Protective effect of breast feeding against infection. Br Med J 300:11, 1990.

Johnson CE, et al. Selenium status of term infants fed human milk or selenium-supplemented soy formula. J Pediatr 122:739, 1993.

Kauter DA, et al. *Clostridium botulinum* spores in infant foods: A survey. J Food Protect 45:1028, 1982.

Klebanoff MA, et al. The risk of childhood cancer after neonatal exposure to vitamin K. N Engl J Med 329:905, 1993.

Lack of adverse reactions to iron-fortified formula. Nutr Rev 47:41, 1989.

Mehta KC, et al. Trial on timing of introduction to solids and food type on infant growth. Pediatrics 102:569, 1998.

Michaelsen FK, et al. The Copenhagen cohort study on infant nutrition and growth: Breast-milk intake, human milk macronutrient content, and influencing factors. Am J Clin Nutr 59:600, 1994.

Neuringer MD, Connor WE. N-3 fatty acids in the brain and retina: Evidence for their essentiality. Nutr Rev. 44:285, 1986.

Smith D, et al. Shifting linear growth during infancy: Illustration of genetic factors in growth from fetal life through infancy. J Pediatr 89:225, 1976.

Smith MM, Lifshitz F. Excess fruit juice consumption as a contributing factor in nonorganic failure to thrive. Pediatrics 93:438, 1994.

Trahms C, Pipes P. Nutrition in Infancy and Childhood, 6th ed. New York: McGraw-Hill, 1997.

Work Group on Cow's Milk Protein and Diabetes Mellitus, American Academy of Pediatrics. Infant feeding practices and their possible relationship to the etiology of diabetes mellitus. Pediatrics 94:752, 1994.

Ziegler EE. Milk and formulas for older infants. J Pediatr 117 (suppl):S76, 1990.

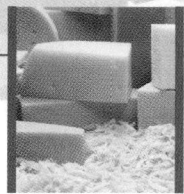

CHAPTER 9

Nutrition for the Low–Birth-Weight Infant

DIANE M. ANDERSON, PhD, RD, CSP, FADA

Chapter Outline

- Characteristics of Low–Birth-Weight Infants
- Parenteral Nutrition
- Transition from Parenteral to Enteral Nutrition
- Enteral Nutrition
- Growth and Nutritional Assessment
- Discharge Care
- Neurodevelopmental Outcome

Key Terms

ANTENATAL—the period of time before birth

APPROPRIATE FOR GESTATIONAL AGE—describing the infant whose birth weight is between the 10th and 90th percentiles for gestational age on an intrauterine growth grid

EXTREMELY LOW BIRTH WEIGHT (ELBW)—referring to an infant who weighs less than 1000 g (2¼ lb) at birth

GASTRIC GAVAGE—a feeding method that involves inserting a soft feeding tube through the mouth or nose into the stomach

GESTATIONAL AGE—the age of the infant at birth, as determined by the length of the pregnancy (the number of weeks since the last menstrual period); it can also be determined by clinical assessment

GLUCOSE LOAD—the amount of glucose received intravenously

HEMOLYTIC ANEMIA—anemia secondary to oxidative destruction of mature red blood cells; sometimes caused by vitamin E deficiency

HUMAN MILK FORTIFIER—a supplement of protein, carbohydrate, fat, minerals, and vitamins added to human milk to meet the increased nutrient needs of the premature infant

INFANCY—birth to 1 year of age

INFANT MORTALITY RATE—number of infant deaths in the first year of life per 1000 live births

LARGE FOR GESTATIONAL AGE—referring to an infant whose birth weight is above the 90th percentile of the standard weight for gestational age (the intrauterine growth chart)

LOW BIRTH WEIGHT (LBW)—referring to an infant who weighs less than 2500 g (5½ lb) at birth

NECROTIZING ENTEROCOLITIS—inflammation or death of the gastrointestinal tract

NEONATAL PERIOD—first 28 days of life

NEUTRAL THERMAL ENVIRONMENT—the environmental temperature at which the infant expends the least amount of energy to maintain body temperature

OSTEOPENIA OF PREMATURITY—reduced bone mass in the premature infant resulting from a decreased rate of bone synthesis; often attributable to inadequate calcium and phosphorus intake

PERIVENTRICULAR LEUKOMALACIA—necrosis of the cerebral white matter that occurs when blood flow is decreased to the brain; can result in neurologic abnormalities, including intellectual deficits

RESPIRATORY DISTRESS SYNDROME—lung disease, secondary to a surfactant deficiency, which presents shortly after birth and is common in preterm infants

POSTNATAL PERIOD—from 28 days of age to the first birthday

PERINATAL PERIOD—from 28 weeks of gestation to 4 weeks after birth

PREMATURE (PRETERM)—referring to an infant born before 37 weeks' gestation

SMALL FOR GESTATIONAL AGE (SGA)—referring to an infant who weighs less than the 10th percentile of the standard weight for gestational age

SURFACTANT—a mixture of lipoproteins, secreted by alveolar cells into the alveoli and respiratory air passages, that contributes to the elastic properties of pulmonary tissue

TERM INFANT—an infant born between the 37th and 42nd week of gestation

VERY LOW BIRTH WEIGHT (VLBW)—referring to an infant who weighs less than 1500 g (3⅓ lb) at birth

The management of low-birth-weight (LBW) infants requiring intensive care continues to improve dramatically. With new technologies, improved understanding of perinatal pathophysiology, current nutrition management principles, and regionalization of perinatal care, the infant mortality rates continue to decrease in the United States (American Academy of Pediatrics and American College of Obstetrics and Gynecology, 1997). In particular, the development and use of surfactant have increased the survival of preterm infants, as has the use of antepartum corticosteroids (Modanlou et al., 1996). Studies indicate that most LBW infants have the potential for long and productive lives (Bregman and Kimberlin, 1993).

There are many methods by which nutrition can be provided to LBW infants, each having certain benefits and limitations. The infant's size, age, and clinical condition dictate the nutritional requirements and how they can be provided. Because of the complexities involved in the neonatal intensive care setting, a team that includes a registered dietitian trained in neonatal nutrition should make the decisions necessary to facilitate optimal nutrition. Within a regionalized perinatal care system, the neonatal nutritionist may also consult with health care providers in community hospitals and public health settings (visit www.pediatrics.org).

CHARACTERISTICS OF LOW–BIRTH-WEIGHT INFANTS

Gestational Age and Size

At birth, an infant who weighs less than 2500 g (5½ lb) is classified as being of **low birth weight;** the infant weighing less than 1500 g (3⅓ lb) is referred to as a **very low birth weight (VLBW)** infant; and the infant weighing less than 1000 g (2¼ lb) is defined as an **extremely low birth weight (ELBW)** infant. LBW may be attributable to a shortened period of gestation, which is prematurity, or a retarded intrauterine growth rate, which makes the infant small for gestational age.

The **term infant** is born between the 37th and 42nd week of gestation. A **premature** infant is one who is born before 37 weeks of gestation, whereas a *post-term* infant is born after 42 weeks of gestation.

Antenatally, an estimate of the infant's **gestational age** is based on the date of the mother's last menstrual period, clinical parameters of uterine fundal height, the presence of quickening, fetal heart tones, or ultrasound evaluations. After birth, gestational age is determined by clinical assessment. Clinical parameters fall into two groups: (1) a series of neurologic signs, dependent mainly on postures and tone, and (2) a series of external characteristics that reflect the physical maturity of the infant. The New Ballard Score (Ballard et al., 1991) examination is one clinical assessment tool that is frequently used. Accurate assessment of gestational age is important in establishing nutritional goals for individual infants and in differentiating the premature infant from the term SGA infant.

A **small for gestational age (SGA)** infant is defined as one who weighs less than the 10th percentile of the standard weight for that gestational age. An SGA infant whose intrauterine weight gain is poor, but whose linear and head growth are between the 10th and 90th percentiles on the intrauterine growth grid, is said to have experienced *asymmetrical intrauterine growth retardation* (IUGR). An SGA infant whose length and occipital frontal circumference are also below the 10th percentile of the standards is said to have *symmetrical* IUGR. Symmetrical IUGR, usually reflecting early and prolonged intrauterine deficit, is apparently more detrimental to later growth and development. The **appropriate for gestational age (AGA)** infant has a birth weight between the 10th and 90th percentiles on the intrauterine growth chart. The infant whose birth weight is above the 90th percentile on the intrauterine growth chart is **large for gestational age (LGA).** Fig. 9–1 shows the classification of neonates based on maturity and intrauterine growth.

Infant Mortality and Statistics

Although the **infant mortality rate** in the United States continues to decrease, it is still higher than in many Western countries (see "*New Directions*: De-

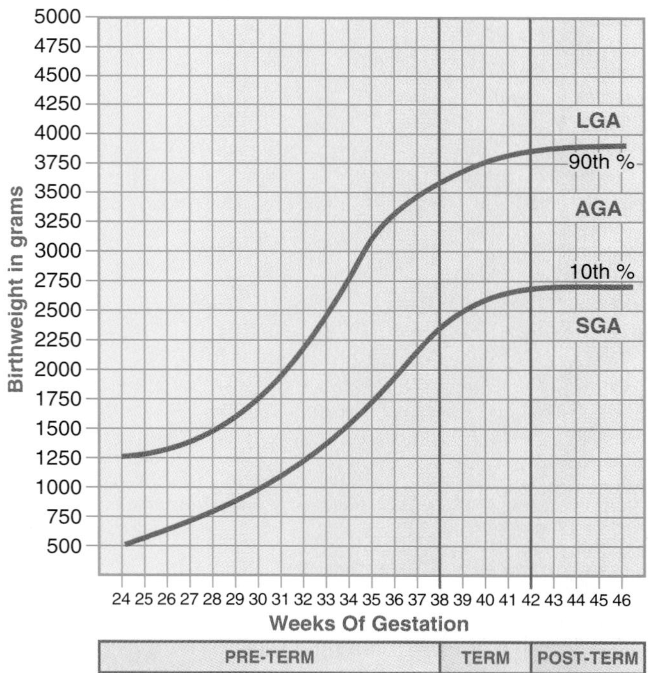

FIGURE 9–1 Classification of neonates based on maturity and intrauterine growth. *SGA*, small for gestational age; *AGA*, appropriate for gestational age; *LGA*, large for gestational age. (From Battaglia FC, Lubchenco LO. A practical classification of newborn infants by weight and gestational age. J Pediatr 71:159, 1967.)

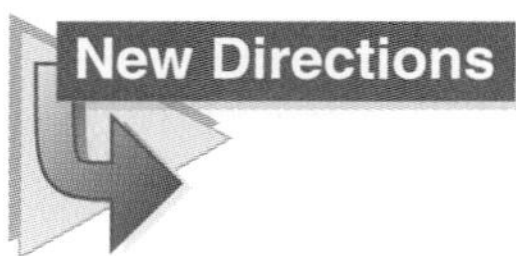

Demographics of Infant Mortality

The *infant mortality rate*, defined as the number of infant deaths in the first year of life per 1000 live births, has declined in the United States to a low of 7.2 in 1996. This rate is the lowest recorded rate for the United States and represents a greater than 60% decrease since 1970 (Guyer et al., 1997). In 1996, the U.S. infant mortality rate was 6.0 for the white population and 14.2 for the black population, for a total infant mortality rate of 7.2. This racial difference may be explained by the increased number of LBW and VLBW infants born to black mothers.

In 1995, 19 developed countries with populations greater than 2.5 million had infant mortality rates lower than that of the United States, as shown in the accompanying table. The range from the lowest to the highest represented a difference of 4.2 deaths per 1000 live births. In this ranking of the world's nations, Sweden had the lowest infant mortality rate, at 3.7.

All of the 19 countries with infant mortality rates lower than that of the United States have populations 47% or less of the U.S. population. Some of these countries even have populations smaller than the major U.S. cities of New York and Los Angeles. This can make a difference in accessibility to prenatal care.

Birth rate, or the number of births per 1000 population, in the 21 countries was lowest in Spain (9.0). The United States has one of the highest birth rates (14.8/1000 population) of the countries listed, second only to New Zealand and Singapore, with birth rates of 16.3/1000 and 16.0/1000 population, respectively.

During the 1990s, the teen pregnancy rate in the United States decreased to an average of 56.8 pregnancies per 1000 teens (Ventura et al., 1997). This rate is still higher than the low of 50 to 53 per 1000 teens reported in 1985 (Ventura et al., 1997). The rate of low birth weight (LBW) has been found to be inversely correlated with the age of the mother, with an incidence of 16.2% for mothers younger than 15 years of age and 12.0% for mothers aged 20 to 24 years (Ventura et al., 1997).

BIRTH RATE AND INFANT MORTALITY (IM) RATE OF COUNTRIES WITH A POPULATION ≥ 2.5 MILLION AND AN IM RATE ≤ THE UNITED STATES

COUNTRY	BIRTH RATE* (1995 OR 1996)	INFANT MORTALITY RATE (1995)†	COUNTRY'S POPULATION AS A % OF U.S. POPULATION
Sweden	10.8	3.7	3
Finland	11.7	3.9	2
Singapore	16.0	4.0	1
Japan	9.6	4.3	47
Hong Kong	10.2	4.6	2
Switzerland	11.7	4.8§	3
France	12.6	4.9	22
Denmark	12.9	5.3	2
Germany	9.4‡	5.3	31
Netherlands	11.9	5.4§	6
Austria	10.8	5.5	3
Spain	9.0	5.6	15
Australia	14.2‡	5.7	7
Canada	12.5	6.1	11
Belgium	11.4‡	6.1	4
United Kingdom	12.5‡	6.2	22
Italy	9.1‡	6.2	21
Ireland	13.5‡	6.4	1
New Zealand	16.3‡	6.7	1
Greece	9.7	7.9	4
United States	14.8	7.9	100

(Data from Guyer B, Martin JA, MacDorman MF, et al. Annual Summary of Vital Statistics—1996. Pediatrics 100:905, 1997; and The World Almanac and Book of Facts—1998. Mahwah, NJ: Funk and Wagnalls, 1997.)

*Birth rate per 1000 population.

†Infant mortality rate per 1000 live births.

‡Rate is for 1995.

§Rate is for 1996; the rate for 1995 was not reported.

mographics of Infant Mortality"). This discrepancy may be attributable to the inconsistent collection of mortality data among nations, which may falsely lower mortality rates in other countries. However, the high incidence of LBW infants born in the United States contributes to this high infant mortality rate. Greater than 63% of the infant mortality rate is linked to LBW infants (Guyer et al., 1997). There is an inverse relationship between birth weight and infant mortality rate (Ventura et al., 1997). LBW infants with a birth weight of 1500 g to 2499 g have a risk of infant mortality that is fivefold greater than that in infants with a birth weight of 2500 g or greater. As the birth weight drops to less than 1500 g, the infant mortality rate increases 65 times. Even though the United States has a high incidence of LBW and VLBW infants, this country still has one of the best birth weight–specific survival rates (American Academy of Pediatrics and American College of Obstetrics and Gynecology, 1997). The high incidence of teenaged pregnancy also contributes to the high infant mortality rate, for there is a 10% increase in incidence of LBW associated with teen pregnancy (Ventura et al., 1997).

The incidence of multiple births has increased, which is also associated with a higher infant mortality rate. Multiple births are nine times more likely to result in LBW than a singleton birth (Ventura et al., 1997). In 1995, as compared to 1980, the number of twin births rose 42% and the number of triplets or greater gestations soared 272% (Ventura et al., 1997). This growth in the number of multiple births is related to women delaying childbirth, because multiple gestations are associated with mothers of older ages. In addition, fertility-enhancing therapies are frequently used.

Problems of Immaturity

The premature or LBW infant has not had the chance to develop fully in utero and is physiologically different from the term infant (Fig. 9–2). Because of this, LBW infants have a variety of clinical problems in the early **neonatal period,** depending on their intrauterine environment, degree of prematurity, birth-related trauma, and function of immature or stressed organ systems. Certain problems, presented in Table 9–1, occur with such frequency that they are considered to be typical of prematurity. Premature infants are at high nutritional risk because of poor nutrient stores; physiological immaturity; illness, which may interfere with nutritional management and needs; and the nutrient demands required for growth.

Decreased Metabolic Reserves

Most fetal nutrient stores are deposited during the last 3 months of pregnancy; therefore, the premature infant begins life in a compromised nutritional state. Because metabolic (energy) stores are limited, nutritional support in the form of parenteral and/or enteral nutrition should be initiated as soon as possible. In the preterm infant weighing 1000 g, fat constitutes only 1% of total body weight; by contrast, the term infant (3500 g) has a fat percentage of about 16%. The 1000-g AGA premature infant, for example, has a glycogen and fat reserve equivalent to about 110 kcal/kg of body weight. With basal metabolic needs of approximately 50 kcal/kg/day, it is obvious that this infant will rapidly run out of fat and carbohydrate fuel unless adequate nutritional support is established. Therefore, the depletion time will be even shorter for preterm infants weighing less than 1000 g at birth. Nutrient reserves are depleted most quickly by tiny infants who have IUGR as a result of their increased basal metabolic rate.

It is often difficult, however, to provide adequate nutritional intake during the first several days of

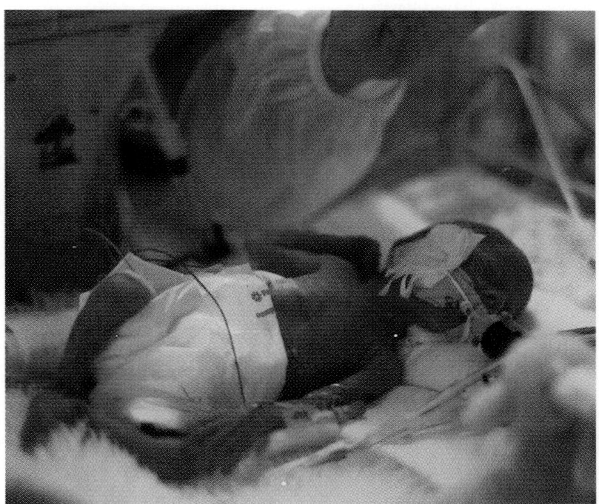

FIGURE 9–2 A.R., born at 27 weeks' gestation, had a birth weight of 870 g (1 lb 14 oz).

TABLE 9–1 PROBLEMS COMMON TO PREMATURE INFANTS

SYSTEM	PROBLEM
Respiratory	Respiratory distress syndrome, chronic lung disease (bronchopulmonary dysplasia)
Cardiovascular	Patent ductus arteriosus
Renal	Fluid and electrolyte imbalance
Neurologic	Intraventricular hemorrhage, periventricular leukomalacia
Metabolic	Hypoglycemia, hyperlgycemia, hypocalcemia, metabolic acidosis
Gastrointestinal	Hyperbilirubinemia, feeding intolerance, necrotizing enterocolitis
Hematologic	Anemia
Immunologic	Sepsis, pneumonia, meningitis
Other	Apnea, bradycardia, cyanosis, osteopenia

(Adapted from Zerzan J, O'Leary MJ. Nutrition for preterm and low-birth-weight infants. In: Trahms CM, Pipes PL (eds.). Nutrition in Infancy and Childhood, 6th ed. New York: WCB/McGraw-Hill, 1997.)

TABLE 9–2 EXPECTED SURVIVAL TIME OF INFANTS IN STARVATION (H_2O ONLY) AND SEMISTARVATION ($D_{10}W$)

	ESTIMATED SURVIVAL TIME (DAYS)*	
BIRTH WEIGHT (g)	H_2O	$D_{10}W$
1000	4	11
2000	12	30
3500	32	80

*Data from Heird WC, Driscoll JM, Schullinger JN, et al. Intravenous alimentation in pediatric patients. J Pediatr 80:351, 1972.

life because of immaturity of the organ systems and severe medical problems. When adequate dietary intake cannot be achieved, and fat and glycogen reserves have been exhausted, the infant begins to catabolize vital body protein tissue for energy. Theoretical estimates of survival time of starved and semi-starved infants are shown in Table 9–2. These estimates assume depletion of all glycogen and fat and about one third of body protein tissue, at a rate of 50 kcal/kg/day. The effects of fluids, such as intravenous water (no exogenous calories) and 10% dextrose solution ($D_{10}W$), are shown. Even with protein tissue catabolism, the projected survival times are alarmingly short.

The small premature infant is particularly vulnerable to undernutrition. Malnutrition in premature infants may increase the risk of infection, prolong chronic illness, and adversely affect brain growth and function. In fact, Lucas et al. (1994) reported that the type of milk used for the neonatal diet may be directly linked to neurodevelopment at 18 months of age.

PARENTERAL NUTRITION

Many critically ill preterm infants have difficulty working up to full enteral feedings in the first several days or even weeks of life. The infant's small stomach capacity, immature gastrointestinal tract, and illness make the progression of enteral feedings difficult (Fig. 9–3). Parenteral nutrition (PN) becomes essential for nutrition support, either as a supplement to enteral feedings or as the total source of nutrition. Chapter 22 offers a complete discussion of PN; only those aspects relating to feeding of the preterm infant are presented here.

Fluid

Because fluid needs are extremely variable for preterm infants, fluid balance must be monitored. Inadequate intake can lead to dehydration, electrolyte imbalances, and hypotension. Excessive intake, on the other hand, can lead to edema, congestive heart failure, and possible opening of the ductus arteriosus. Additional neonatal clinical complications reported with high fluid intakes include necrotizing enterocolitis, bronchopulmonary dysplasia (BPD) (see Chapter 37), and intraventricular hemorrhage. The premature infant has a greater percentage of body water (especially extracellular water) than the term infant. (See Fig. 6–1.) Extracellular water should decrease in all infants during the first few days of life. This reduction is accompanied by a normal loss of 10% to 15% of body weight and improved renal function. ELBW infants often lose up to 20% of their birth weight without complications (Bell and Oh, 1994). Failure of this transition in fluid dynamics and lack of diuresis may complicate the course of preterm infants with respiratory disease.

Water requirements are estimated by the sum of the predicted losses from the lungs and skin, urine, and stool and the water needed for growth. A major route of water loss in preterm infants is evaporation through the skin and respiratory tract. This insensible water loss is highest in the smallest and least mature infants owing to their larger body surface area relative to body weight, increased permeability of the skin epidermis to water, and greater skin blood flow relative to metabolic rate. Insensible water loss is increased by radiant warmers and phototherapy lights and decreased by heat shields, thermal blankets, and humidified incubators. Insensible water loss can vary from 50 to 100 mL/kg/day on the first day of life, and increase up to 120 to 200 mL/kg/day, depending on the infant's size, gestational age, day of life, and environment (Yu, 1992). Decreasing insensible water loss with the use of humidified incubators can reduce fluid requirements to no more than 180 mL/kg/day (Costarino and Baumgart, 1993).

Excretion of urine, the other major route of water loss, varies from 40 to 85 mL/kg/day (Bell and Oh, 1994). This loss depends on the fluid volume and solute load presented to the kidneys. The infant's ability to concentrate urine increases with maturity. Stool water loss is generally 5 to 10 mL/kg/day, and 10 mL/kg/day is suggested as optimal for growth (Bell and Oh, 1994).

Because of the many variables affecting neonatal fluid losses, fluid needs must be determined on an individual basis. Usually, fluid is administered at a rate of 80 to 105 mL/kg/day the first day of life in order to meet insensible losses and urine output. Fluid needs are then evaluated by assessing fluid intake and comparing it to the clinical parameters of urine volume output, specific gravity or osmolality, and serum electrolytes, creatinine, and urea nitrogen levels. Assessment of weight, blood pressure, peripheral perfusion, skin turgor, and mucous membrane moisture is performed daily. Daily fluid administration is generally increased by 10 to 20 mL/kg/day. By the end of the second week of life, preterm infants may receive fluids at a rate of 140 to 160 mL/kg/day (Lorenz et al., 1995; Costarino and Baumgart, 1993). Fluid restriction may be necessary in preterm infants with patent ductus arte-

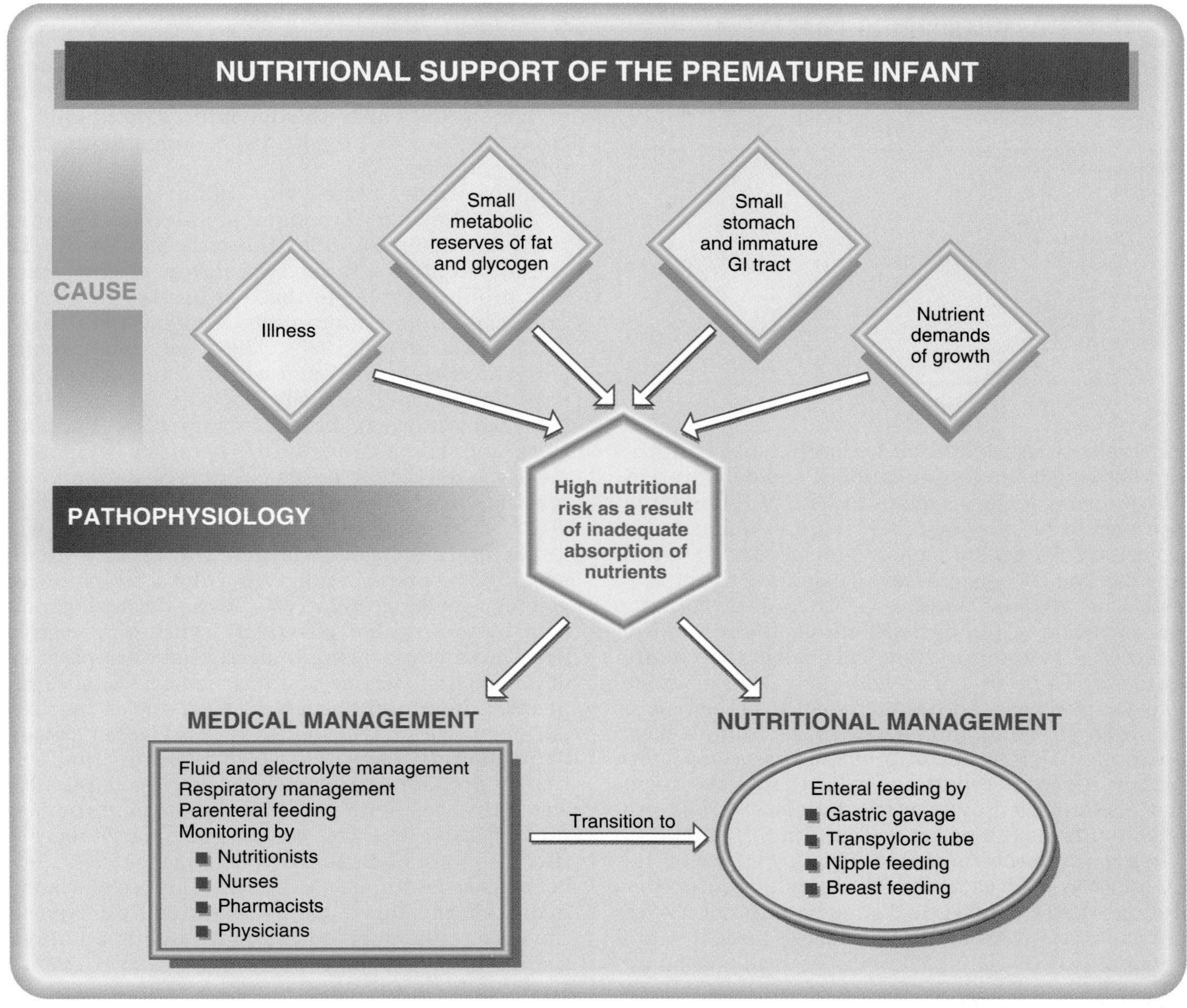

FIGURE 9–3 Pathophysiology algorithm—nutritional support of premature infants. (Algorithm content developed by John Anderson, Ph.D., and Stanford C. Garner, Ph.D., 2000.)

riosus (PDA), congestive heart failure, renal failure, or cerebral edema. An increase in fluids is indicated when the preterm infant is placed under phototherapy lights or a radiant warmer, or when environmental or body temperature is elevated.

Energy

The energy needs of preterm infants fed parenterally are less than those of enterally fed infants because absorption loss does not occur when nutritional intake bypasses the intestinal tract. Enterally fed preterm infants usually require 105 to 130 kcal/kg/day to grow, whereas parenterally fed premature neonates can grow well on 80 to 90 kcal/kg/day (Hansen, 1993). Minimal maintenance energy needs and adequate protein should be provided as early as possible to prevent tissue catabolism. Rivera et al. (1993) have demonstrated that providing VLBW infants 1.5 g of protein and 35 to 54 kcal/kg/day promotes nitrogen balance during the first 3 days of life. Energy and protein intake should be increased as the infant's condition stabilizes and growth becomes the goal (Table 9–3).

Glucose

Glucose or dextrose is the principal energy source (3.4 kcal/g). However, glucose tolerance is limited in premature infants, especially in VLBW infants. The reasons for this intolerance are inadequate insulin production, insulin resistance, and continued hepatic glucose release while intravenous glucose is infusing. Hyperglycemia is less likely when glucose is administered with amino acids than when it is infused alone. Amino acids exert a stimulatory effect on in-

TABLE 9–3 COMPARISON OF PARENTERAL AND ENTERAL ENERGY NEEDS OF PREMATURE INFANTS

	PARENTERAL	ENTERAL
Maintenance		
Gradually increase intake to meet energy needs by the end of the first week.	40–60 kcal/kg/day	50 kcal/kg/day
Growth		
Meet energy needs as soon as the infant is stable.	80–90 kcal/kg/day	105–130 kcal/kg/day

sulin release. Avoidance of hyperglycemia is important because it can lead to diuresis and dehydration.

To prevent hyperglycemia in VLBW infants, glucose should be administered in small amounts. To accurately determine the amount of glucose an infant receives, it is necessary to calculate the glucose load. The **glucose load** is a function of both the concentration of the dextrose infusion and the rate at which it is administered. This calculation is presented in Table 9–4. The administration of exogenous insulin may be necessary with persistent or very high glycemia, but swings in the infant's blood glucose level are common problems associated with its use. A recent report suggests that protein synthesis is inhibited by insulin administration in premature infants (Poindexter et al., 1998).

In general, preterm infants should receive an initial glucose load of less than 6 mg/kg/min, with a gradual increase to 11 to 14 mg/kg/min. ELBW infants tolerate a lower initial glucose load of 4 to 6 mg/kg/min (Yu, 1992). The glucose load can be advanced by 1 to 2 mg/kg/min (Sapsford, 1994). Hypoglycemia is not as common a problem as hyperglycemia, but it may occur if the glucose infusion is abruptly decreased or interrupted.

Amino Acids

Protein guidelines range from 2.5 to 3.5 g/kg/day. However, an intrauterine growth rate of protein accretion can be achieved at 3.0 g/kg/day (Hanning and Zlotkin, 1997). ELBW infants may need as much as 3 to 4 g/kg/day (Hanning and Zlotkin, 1997). Protein in excess of these parenteral requirements should not be administered, as additional protein offers no apparent advantage and increases the risk of metabolic problems. In practice, preterm infants are usually given a small amount of amino acids (1.0 to 1.5 g/kg/day) within the first few days of life, after which the amount is gradually increased by 0.5 to 1.0 g/kg/day to a maximum of 3.5 to 3.8 g/kg/day.

In the United States, two pediatric solutions are in use. They are Trophamine (McGaw Laboratories), and Aminosyn PF (Abbott Laboratories). The use of pediatric solutions results in plasma amino acid profiles similar to those of healthy infants fed breast milk, and appropriate acid–base status has been noted (Heird, 1995). These solutions promote adequate weight gain and nitrogen retention. Standard amino acid solutions, such as Aminosyn (Abbott Laboratories), FreAmine (McGaw Laboratories), and Travasol (Clintec), were not designed to meet the particular needs of immature infants and may provoke imbalances in plasma amino acid levels. For example, cysteine, tyrosine, and taurine levels in these solutions are low relative to the needs of the preterm infant, but the methionine and glycine levels are relatively high. Because premature infants do not effectively synthesize cysteine from methionine owing to decreased concentrations of the hepatic enzyme cystathionase, a cysteine supplement has been suggested. Cysteine is insoluble and unstable in solution, so it is added as cysteine hydrochloride when the parenteral nutrition solution is prepared. In one study, nitrogen retention was increased with cysteine supplementation, although this has not consistently been reported (Rivera et al., 1993; Heird and Gomez, 1996). Metabolic acidosis can also occur with the use of cysteine hydrochloride, but it can be corrected by decreasing the dose of the supplement or by adding additional acetate to the solution (Uauy et al., 1993).

In addition to plasma amino acid imbalances, other metabolic problems associated with amino acid infusions in preterm infants include metabolic acidosis, hyperammonemia, and azotemia. These problems can be minimized by using the crystalline amino acid products that are available today, and by keeping the protein load within the recommended guidelines, as shown in Table 9–5.

Lipid

Intravenous fat emulsions are used for two reasons: (1) to meet essential fatty acid (EFA) requirements and (2) to provide a concentrated source of energy.

TABLE 9–4 GUIDELINES FOR GLUCOSE LOAD IN PREMATURE INFANTS

BIRTH WEIGHT (g)	INITIAL LOAD (mg/kg/min*)	DAILY INCREMENTS (mg/kg/min)	MAXIMUM LOAD (mg/kg/min)
<1000	4–6	1–2	11–12
1001–2000	≤6	1–2	11–12

*Use the following formula to calculate glucose load: (% glucose × mL/kg/day) × (1000 mg/g glucose) ÷ (1440 minutes/day) = glucose load
Example: (0.10 × 150 mL/kg/day) × (1000 mg/g glucose) ÷ (1440 minutes/day) = 10.4 mg/kg/min

TABLE 9–5 GUIDELINES FOR ADMINISTRATION OF PARENTERAL AMINO ACIDS IN PREMATURE INFANTS

INITIAL RATE (g/kg/day*)	INCREMENTS (g/kg/day)	MAXIMUM RATE (g/kg/day)
1.5	0.5–1.0	3.5–3.8†

(From Hansen JW. Appendix Table A.1. Consensus recommendations. In: Tsang RC, Lucas A, Uauy R, Zlotkin S (eds.). Nutritional Needs of the Preterm Infant. Baltimore: Williams & Wilkins, 1993, p. 287.)

*Use the following formula to calculate protein load: % protein × mL/kg/day = g protein/kg

Example: 0.02 × 150 mL/kg = 3 g/kg/day

†3.8 g/kg/day is recommended for infants weighing < 1000 g.

EFA needs can be met by providing 0.5 to 1.0 g/kg/day of lipids. Biochemical evidence of EFA deficiency has been noted during the first week of life in VLBW infants fed parenterally without fat. The clinical consequences of EFA deficiency may include coagulation abnormalities, abnormal pulmonary surfactant, and adverse effects on lung metabolism.

Lipid should be introduced slowly in preterm infants, with periodic monitoring of plasma triglyceride levels, which should remain less than 150 mg/dL. Elevated plasma triglyceride levels may occur in the infant with decreased ability to hydrolyze triglycerides. This problem is most commonly seen with decreasing gestational age, in SGA infants, and with infection, surgical stress, and malnutrition. Under these conditions, close monitoring of serum triglyceride levels is indicated, and less than 3 g/kg/day of fat may need to be provided. Further, hyperbilirubinemia can increase the risk of lipid toxicity. Kernicterus can occur in infants with hyperbilirubinemia if free fatty acids displace bilirubin from albumin-binding sites, raising the level of free bilirubin in the blood. In preterm infants with hyperbilirubinemia, initial lipid loads should not exceed EFA needs so as to avoid possible complications. Once the infant is medically stable and additional energy is needed for growth, lipid loads can slowly be increased.

Lipid should be administered over 24 hours at a maximum rate of 0.8 to 0.12 g/kg/hr to prevent a rise in triglycerides and free fatty acids (Heird and Gomez, 1996). A daily increment of 0.5 g/kg/day is provided until a rate of 3 g/kg/day is achieved (Innis, 1993) (see Table 9–6). Total lipid load is usually less than 30% to 40% of nonprotein calories, but it should not exceed 60% of nonprotein calories. The lipid emulsions presently in use are described in Chapter 22. In preterm infants, 20% solutions providing 2 kcal/cc are recommended because plasma triglyceride, cholesterol, and phospholipid levels are generally lower with these than with the 10% emulsions. The lower plasma fat levels may be attributable to a decreased phospholipid load per gram of fat in the 20% emulsion. Lipid emulsions that contain medium-chain triglycerides (MCTs) are available in Europe, but their use in neonates requires additional investigation (Koletzko, 1997).

TABLE 9–6 GUIDELINES FOR ADMINISTRATION OF PARENTERAL LIPIDS IN PREMATURE INFANTS

INITIAL RATE (g/kg/day*)	INCREMENTS (g/kg/day)	MAXIMUM RATE (g/kg/day)
0.5	0.5	3.0

*Use this formula to calculate lipid load: 20% lipid = 20 g/100 mL
% lipid × mL/kg/day = g lipid/kg

Example: 0.02 × 15 mL/kg = 3 g lipid/kg/day

It has been suggested that continuous administration of heparin to infants receiving parenteral lipid may improve lipid clearance by stimulating the release of the enzymes lipoprotein lipase and hepatic lipase into the circulation, thus promoting the intravascular lipolysis of fat. Heparin is commonly administered at 1 U/mL. Higher heparin concentrations may lead to increased serum free fatty acids. Heparin also prevents thrombosis formation and, with the administration of lipids, prolongs the life of peripheral veins.

Also under consideration is the supplemental use of *carnitine* in preterm infants receiving PN. Carnitine facilitates the mechanism by which fatty acids are transported across the mitochondrial membrane, allowing their oxidation to provide energy. Enhanced lipid utilization has been documented with carnitine supplementation in LBW infants receiving PN for longer than 1 month (Christensen et al., 1989). Other short-term investigations have failed to show an improvement in fatty acid oxidation. One study reported increased protein oxidation and decreased weight gain (Sulkers et al., 1990). Carnitine supplementation may be helpful for preterm infants who are receiving only PN at 1 month of age.

Electrolytes

After the first few days of life, sodium, potassium, and chloride are added to parenteral solutions to compensate for the loss of extracellular fluid. Potassium should be withheld until renal flow is demonstrated so as to prevent hyperkalemia and cardiac arrhythmia. In general, the preterm infant has the same electrolyte requirements as the term infant, but actual requirements vary, depending on factors such as renal function, state of hydration, and the use of diuretics (Table 9–7). Very immature infants

TABLE 9–7 GUIDELINES FOR ADMINISTRATION OF PARENTERAL ELECTROLYTES IN PREMATURE INFANTS

ELECTROLYTE	mEq/kg/day
Sodium	2–3
Chloride	2–3
Potassium	2–3

may have a limited ability to conserve sodium and so may require increased amounts of sodium to maintain a normal serum sodium concentration. Serum electrolyte levels should be monitored periodically. Urine electrolytes should be quantified when serum levels are abnormal in order to detect inappropriate electrolyte excretion.

Minerals

Calcium and phosphorus are important components of the PN solution. Premature infants who receive PN with low calcium and phosphorus concentrations are at risk for developing osteopenia of prematurity. This poor bone mineralization is most likely to occur in VLBW infants who are maintained on PN for prolonged periods. Calcium and phosphorus status should be monitored using serum calcium, phosphorus, and alkaline phosphatase levels, as well as radiographic bone studies.

Preterm infants have higher calcium and phosphorus needs than term infants. It is difficult to add enough calcium and phosphorus to parenteral solutions to meet these higher requirements, however, without causing precipitation of the minerals. Calcium and phosphorus should be provided simultaneously in PN solutions. Alternate-day infusions are not recommended because abnormal serum mineral levels and decreased mineral retention occurs.

Current recommendations for parenteral administration of increased amounts of calcium, phosphorus, and magnesium are presented in Table 9–8. The intakes are expressed per liter of solution, at a rate of 120 to 150 mL/kg/day, with 2.5 g of protein. Lower fluid volumes or lower protein concentrations may cause the minerals to precipitate out of solution.

Trace Elements

Zinc should be given to all preterm infants receiving PN. If enteral feedings cannot be started by 2 weeks of age, then additional trace elements should be added. However, the amounts of copper and manganese should be reduced for infants with obstructive jaundice, and the amounts of selenium, chromium, and molybdenum should be reduced in infants with renal dysfunction. Parenteral iron is not routinely provided, as treated infants often receive blood transfusions in the early period of life, and enteral feedings, which provide a source of iron, can often be initiated. The dosage for parenteral iron is approximately 10% of the enteral dosage. Guidelines range from 0.1 to 0.2 mg/kg/day (Greene et al., 1988). Recommended guidelines have not yet been established for parenteral administration of fluoride to preterm infants (Table 9–9).

TABLE 9–8 GUIDELINES FOR ADMINISTRATION OF PARENTERAL MINERALS IN PREMATURE INFANTS

MINERALS	mg/L*
Calcium	500–600
Phosphorus	400–450
Magnesium	50–70

(Adapted from Greene HL, et al. Guidelines for the use of vitamins, trace elements, calcium, magnesium and phosphorus in infants and children receiving total parenteral nutrition: Report of the Subcommittee on Pediatric Parenteral Nutrient Requirements from the Committee on Clinical Practice Issues of the American Society for Clinical Nutrition. Am J Clin Nutr 48(5):1324, 1988.)

*Guidelines are given per liter to prevent administration of excessively high concentrations of calcium and phosphorus with intakes expressed per kilogram of body weight or with fluid restriction.

These recommendations assume an average fluid intake of 120 to 150 mL/kg/day with 2.5 g of amino acids per 100 mL. These dosages should be administered only by central venous infusion.

TABLE 9–9 GUIDELINES FOR ADMINISTRATION OF PARENTERAL TRACE ELEMENTS IN PREMATURE INFANTS

TRACE ELEMENTS	μg/kg/day
Zinc	400.0
Copper	20.0*
Manganese	1.0*
Selenium	2.0†
Chromium	0.2†
Molybdenum	0.25†
Iodine	1.0

(Adapted from Greene HL, Hambidge KM, Schanler R, et al. Guidelines for the use of vitamins, trace elements, calcium, magnesium and phosphorus in infants and children receiving total parenteral nutrition: Report of the Subcommittee on Pediatric Parenteral Nutrient Requirements from the Committee on Clinical Practice Issues of the American Society for Clinical Nutrition. Am J Clin Nutr 48(5):1324, 1988.)

*Reduce or omit in infants with obstructive jaundice.

†Reduce or omit in infants with renal dysfunction.

Vitamins

Shortly after birth, all newborn infants receive a single dose of vitamin K intramuscularly at 0.3 to 1.0 mg/day. This injection is to prevent hemorrhagic disease of the newborn secondary to vitamin K deficiency. Stores of vitamin K are low in newborn infants, and little intestinal bacterial production of vitamin K occurs until bacterial colonization takes place. Because initial dietary intake of vitamin K may be limited, neonates would be at nutritional risk if they did not receive this intramuscular supplement.

The only intravenous multivitamin preparation currently approved and designed for use in infants and children is MVI-Pediatric (Armour Pharmaceutical Co.). The American Academy of Pediatrics (1998) recommends using the American Society of Clinical Nutrition's guideline of 40% of the 5 mL MVI-Pediatric vial per kg of weight. The maximum dose of 5 mL would be achieved at a weight of 2.5 kg (Greene et al., 1988).

Large supplemental doses of vitamin A have been suggested for the prevention of BPD because of the vitamin's role in facilitating tissue repair and because there have been reports of preterm infants having low vitamin A stores. Shenai et al. (1987) reported a significant decrease in the incidence of BPD with intramuscular injections of vitamin A to preterm infants, but Pearson et al. (1992) found no significant reduction in BPD incidence with vitamin A supplementation. Robbins and Fletcher (1993) have suggested that supplemental intramuscular vitamin A may be helpful only in preterm infants with poor vitamin A status. Interesting, BPD has been reported in infants determined to have sufficient stores of vitamin A (Walsh and Hazinski, 1996). Presently, vitamin A supplementation is not recommended.

The sugar *inositol* is present in human milk and infant formula, but only in low concentrations in PN solutions. It functions as a component of membrane phospholipids and may be involved in signal transduction (Krug-Wispe, 1994). Hallman et al. (1992) reported that the addition of inositol to PN solutions was associated with increased survival and a decreased incidence of both BPD and retinopathy of prematurity in preterm infants with respiratory distress syndrome. However, inositol is not yet approved for clinical use because its effectiveness has not been definitively established.

TRANSITION FROM PARENTERAL TO ENTERAL NUTRITION

It is desirable to begin enteral feedings in preterm infants as early as possible because feedings stimulate gastrointestinal enzymatic development and activity, promote bile flow, and increase villous growth in the small intestine. These early enteral feedings can also decrease the incidence of cholestatic jaundice and the duration of physiologic jaundice, and can improve subsequent feeding tolerance in preterm infants. At times, small, initial feedings are used only to prime the gut, and are not intended to optimize enteral nutrient intake until the infant demonstrates feeding tolerance or is clinically stable.

When making the transition from parenteral to enteral feeding, it is important to maintain parenteral feeding until enteral feeding is well established so as to maintain adequate net intake of fluid and nutrients (Table 9–10). In VLBW infants, it may take 7 to 14 days to achieve full enteral feeding; it may take longer for infants with feeding intolerance or illness. The smallest, sickest infants are usually limited to increments of only 10 mL/kg/day. Larger, more stable, preterm infants may tolerate increments of 20 mL/kg/day. See Chapter 22 for a further discussion of transitional feeding.

ENTERAL NUTRITION

Enteral alimentation is preferred for preterm infants because this approach is more physiologic than parenteral alimentation and provides a superior nutritional intake. Initiating a tiny amount of an appropriate milk feeding whenever possible is beneficial. However, determining when and how to advance enteral feedings is often difficult, and involves consideration of the degree of prematurity, history of perinatal insults, current medical condition, function of the gastrointestinal tract, respiratory status, and several other individual concerns. Table 9–11 summarizes factors to consider before initiating or advancing enteral feedings.

TABLE 9–10 GUIDELINES FOR ADMINISTRATION OF PARENTERAL VITAMINS IN PREMATURE INFANTS

	PRETERM	<1000 g*	1001–3000 g*	>3000 g*
% of one 5-mL vial of MVI-Pediatric†	40%/kg	30%/day	65%/day	100%/day

(Data from Greene HL, Hambidge KM, Schanler R, et al. Guidelines for the use of vitamins, trace elements, calcium, magnesium and phosphorus in infants and children receiving total parenteral nutrition: Report of the Subcommittee on Pediatric Parenteral Nutrient Requirements from the Committee on Clinical Practice Issues of the American Society for Clinical Nutrition. Am J Clin Nutr 48(5):1324, 1988.)

*Data from MVI-Pediatric Insert, Amour Pharmaceutical, 1996.

†MVI-Pediatric (5 mL) contains the following vitamins: 80 mg of ascorbic acid, 0.7 mg of vitamin A, 10 μg of vitamin D, 1.2 mg of thiamine, 1.4 mg of riboflavin, 1 mg of vitamin B_6, 17 mg of niacin, 5 mg of pantothenic acid, 7 mg of vitamin E, 20 μg of biotin, 140 μg of folic acid, 1 μg of vitamin B_{12}, and 200 μg of vitamin K.

Nutritional Requirements

Preterm infants should be fed enough to promote growth similar to that of a fetus at the same gestational age, but not so much as to cause nutrient toxicity. Although the exact nutrient requirements are unknown for preterm infants, several useful guidelines exist. In general, the requirements of premature infants are higher than those of term infants because the preterm infant has smaller nutrient stores, decreased digestion and absorption capabili-

TABLE 9–11 FACTORS TO CONSIDER BEFORE INITIATING OR ADVANCING ENTERAL FEEDINGS

CATEGORY	FACTORS
Perinatal	Birth asphyxia
Respiratory	Stability of ventilation, blood gases, apnea, bradycardia, cyanosis
Medical	Vital signs (heart rate, respiratory rate, blood pressure, temperature)
Gastrointestinal	Anomalies (gastroschisis, omphalocele), patency, GI tract function (bowel sounds present, passage of stool), risk of necrotizing enterocolitis
Equipment or procedures	Umbilical artery catheter, and intubation or extubation, other

(Adapted from Zerzan J, O'Leary MJ. Nutrition for preterm and low-birth-weight infants. In: Trahms CM, Pipes PL (eds.). Nutrition in Infancy and Childhood, 6th ed. New York: WCB/McGraw-Hill, 1997.)

ties, and a rapid growth rate. Stress, illness, and certain therapies for illness may further influence nutrient requirements. It is also important to keep in mind that in general enteral nutrient requirements are different from parenteral requirements.

Energy

The energy requirement of premature infants varies with individual biologic and environmental factors. It has been estimated that an intake of 50 kcal/kg/day is required to meet maintenance energy needs, compared with 105 to 130 kcal/kg/day for growth, as shown in Table 9–12. However, energy needs may be increased by stress, illness, and rapid growth. Likewise, energy needs may be decreased if the infant is placed in a neutral thermal environment. It is important to consider the infant's rate of growth in relation to average energy intakes. Some premature infants may need at least 130 to 150 kcal/kg/day to sustain an appropriate rate of growth. SGA infants, or those with BPD, often require such increased amounts. To achieve these high caloric intakes in infants with limited capacities to tolerate large fluid volumes, it may be necessary to concentrate the feedings to a level of more than 24 kcal/oz.

Protein

The amount and quality of protein must be considered when establishing protein requirements for the preterm infant. Amino acids must be provided at a level that meets demands without inducing amino acid or protein toxicity.

AMOUNT. A reference fetus model has been used to determine the amount of protein that would need to be ingested to match the quantity of protein deposited into newly formed fetal tissue (Ziegler et al., 1976). To achieve these fetal accretion rates, additional protein must be supplied to compensate for intestinal losses and obligatory losses in the urine and skin.

TABLE 9–12 ESTIMATES OF ENERGY REQUIREMENTS FOR ENTERALLY FED PREMATURE INFANTS

	AVERAGE ESTIMATE (kcal/kg/day)
Energy expended	40–60
Resting metabolic rate	40–50
Activity	0–5*
Thermoregulation	0–5*
Synthesis	15†
Energy stored	20–30†
Energy excreted	15
Energy intake	90–120

(Adapted from American Academy of Pediatrics, Committee on Nutrition: Nutritional needs of preterm infants. In: Kleinman RE (ed.). Pediatric Nutrition Handbook, 4th ed. Elk Grove, IL: American Academy of Pediatrics, 1998, p. 55.)

*Energy for maintenance.

†Energy for growth.

Based on this method for determining protein needs, the advisable protein intake is 3.5 to 4 g/kg/day. This amount of protein is apparently well tolerated by stable infants who are growing rapidly. There is concern, however, that this amount of protein may cause additional stress to sick infants who are not growing.

TYPE. The quality or type of protein is an important consideration, as premature infants have different amino acid needs than do term infants owing to immature hepatic enzyme pathways. The amino acid composition of *whey protein,* which differs from that of casein (see key terms, Chapter 8), is more appropriate for premature infants. Higher levels of the essential amino acid cysteine are present in the preterm infant, whereas levels of the amino acids phenylalanine and tyrosine, which the preterm infant has difficulty oxidizing, are comparatively lower. Further, metabolic acidosis decreases with consumption of whey-predominant formulas. Because of the advantages of whey protein for premature infants, mother's milk or formulas containing whey-predominant proteins should be chosen whenever possible.

Taurine is a sulfonic amino acid that may be important for preterm infants. Human milk is a rich source of taurine, and taurine is added to most infant formulas. Term and preterm infants develop low plasma and urine concentrations of taurine without a dietary supply, but the clinical significance of this requires further study.

Energy must be provided at sufficient levels to allow protein to be utilized for growth and not merely energy expenditure. A range of 10.2% to 12.4% of calories from protein has been suggested. Kashyap and co-workers (1988) reported that 3 g of protein per 100 kcal is the upper limit at which protein is effectively deposited. Inadequate protein intake is growth-limiting, whereas excessive intake causes elevated plasma amino acid levels, azotemia, and acidosis.

Lipid

AMOUNT. The growing preterm infant needs an adequate intake of well-absorbed dietary fat to help meet the high energy needs of growth, provide essential fatty acids, and facilitate absorption of other important nutrients, such as the fat-soluble vitamins and calcium. However, neonates in general, and premature and SGA infants in particular, digest and absorb lipid inefficiently.

The percentage of total calories as fat relative to carbohydrate and protein is another important consideration. Fat should constitute 40% to 50% of total calories. Furthermore, a diet that is high in fat and low in protein may yield more fat deposition than is desirable for the growing preterm infant. *Linoleic acid* should comprise 3% to 5% of the total calories, and 1% of the total calories should be *linolenic acid*, to meet essential fatty acid needs. Additional longer-chain fatty acids—arachidonic acid and docosahexaenoic acid—are present in human milk, and their potential role and efficacy in infant formulas are currently being investigated (Heird, 1997). Both of these fatty acids may play a role in visual and neurologic development and physical growth.

TYPE. Preterm infants have a low level of pancreatic lipase and bile salts; this decreases their ability to digest and absorb fat. *Lipases* are needed for triglyceride breakdown, and bile salts solubilize fat for ease of digestion and absorption. Because MCTs do not require pancreatic lipase and bile acids for digestion and absorption, they have been added to the fat mixture in premature infant formulas.

Human milk and vegetable oils contain the EFA linoleic acid, but MCT oil does not. Premature infant formulas must contain vegetable oil, along with MCT oil, to provide the essential long-chain fatty acids.

The composition of dietary fat also plays a role in the digestion and absorption of lipid. Infants absorb vegetable oils more efficiently than saturated animal fats. One exception is the saturated fat in human milk. Infants show better digestion and absorption of human milk fat than the saturated fat in cow's milk, or even the vegetable oil in standard infant formulas. This is because human milk contains two lipases that facilitate fat digestion and has a special fatty acid composition that aids absorption.

Carbohydrate

Carbohydrate is an important source of energy, and the enzymes for endogenous production of glucose from carbohydrate and protein are present in preterm infants.

AMOUNT. Approximately 40% of the total calories in human milk and standard infant formulas is derived from carbohydrate. Too little carbohydrate may lead to hypoglycemia, whereas too much may provoke osmotic diuresis or loose stools. The recommended range for carbohydrate intake is 40% to 50% of total calories.

TYPE. *Lactose,* a disaccharide composed of glucose and galactose, is the predominant carbohydrate in almost all mammalian milks, and may be important to the neonate in glucose homeostasis. This control may be related to the fact that galactose can either be utilized for glucose production or glycogen storage (Kliegmen and Sparks, 1985). Galactose generally is used for glycogen formation first, and then it becomes available for glucose production as blood glucose levels decrease (Thureen and Hay, 1993). Because infants born before 28 to 34 weeks of gestation have low lactase activity, there is concern that the premature infant's ability to digest lactose may be marginal. In practice, malabsorption is not a clinical problem, but whether the lactose is hydrolyzed in the intestine or fermented in the colon is a controversial issue (Kien, 1993). *Sucrose* is another disaccharide that is commonly found in commercial infant formula products. Because sucrase activity early in the third trimester is at 70% of newborn levels, sucrose is well tolerated by most premature infants. Both sucrase and lactase are sensitive to changes in the intestinal milieu. Infants who have diarrhea, are undergoing antibiotic therapy, or are undernourished may develop temporary intolerances to lactose and sucrose.

Glucose polymers are common carbohydrates in the preterm infant's diet. These polymers, consisting mainly of chains of five to nine glucose units linked together, are used to achieve the iso-osmolality of certain specialized formulas. *Glucosidase enzymes* for digesting glucose polymers are active in small preterm infants.

Minerals and Vitamins

Premature infants require the same vitamins and minerals as term infants, but poor body stores, physiologic immaturity, illness, and rapid growth increase their needs (Table 9–13). Formulas and **human milk fortifiers,** developed especially for preterm infants, contain increased vitamin and mineral concentrations to meet the needs of the infant, obviating the need for additional supplementation in most cases. The major exception is the infant receiving human milk that is fortified, as the fortifiers do not contain iron. An iron supplement of 2 to 4 mg/kg/day should be sufficient to meet this infant's needs (American Academy of Pediatrics, 1998).

CALCIUM AND PHOSPHORUS. Calcium and phosphorus are just two of many nutrients that growing premature infants require for optimal bone mineralization. Intake guidelines have been established at levels that promote the bone mineralization rate that would occur with the fetus. An intake of 175 mg/100 kcal/day of calcium and 91.5 mg/100 kcal/day of

TABLE 9–13 RECOMMENDATIONS FOR ENTERAL ADMINISTRATION OF VITAMINS IN THE PREMATURE INFANT

VITAMIN	AMOUNT (kg/day)
Vitamin A	700–1500 IU
Vitamin D	150–400 IU
Vitamin E	6–12 IU
Vitamin K	8–10 μg
Ascorbic acid	18–24 mg
Thiamin	180–240 μg
Riboflavin	250–360 μg
Pyridoxine	150–210 μg
Niacin	3.6–4.8 mg
Pantothenate	1.2–1.7 μg
Biotin	3.6–6.0 μg
Folate	25–50 μg
Vitamin B_{12}	0.3 μg

(Adapted from Hansen JW. Appendix Table A.1. Consensus recommendations. In: Tsang RC, Lucas A, Uauy R, Zlotkin S (eds.). Nutritional Needs of the Preterm Infant. Baltimore: Williams & Wilkins, 1993, p. 287.)

phosphorus is recommended. Two thirds of the calcium and phosphorus body content of the term neonate is accumulated through active transport mechanisms during the last trimester of pregnancy. The infant who is born prematurely is deprived of this important intrauterine mineral deposition. With poor mineral stores and low dietary intake, preterm infants can develop **osteopenia of prematurity.** This disease is characterized by demineralization of growing bones and is documented by radiologic evidence of "washed-out" bones. Very immature babies are particularly susceptible to osteopenia and may develop bone fractures or florid rickets if dietary deficiency is prolonged. Osteopenia of prematurity is most likely to occur in preterm infants who (1) are fed infant formula that is not specifically formulated for preterm infants, (2) are fed human milk that is not supplemented with calcium and phosphorus, or (3) are receiving long-term PN without enteral feedings.

VITAMIN D. Human milk with human milk fortifier or infant formula for preterm infants provides adequate vitamin D when full calorie intakes are achieved. It was once common practice to provide 400 to 1000 IU/day as a supplement to prevent osteopenia of prematurity, but this was later shown not to be effective. In fact, the present recommendations for intake range from 150 to 400 IU/day for the preterm infant.

VITAMIN E. Preterm infants require more vitamin E than term infants because of their limited tissue stores, decreased absorption of fat-soluble vitamins, and rapid growth. Vitamin E deficiency is exacerbated by a high intake of iron or polyunsaturated fatty acids (PUFAs), either of which increases the vitamin E requirement. An important function of vitamin E is its protection of biologic membranes against oxidative breakdown of lipids. Requirements for vitamin E increase when the diet is high in PUFAs. The PUFAs are incorporated into the red blood cell membranes and are more susceptible to oxidative damage than when saturated fatty acids comprise the membranes. Because iron is a biologic oxidant, a diet high in either iron or PUFAs increases the risk of vitamin E deficiency.

A premature infant with vitamin E deficiency may experience **hemolytic anemia** (oxidative destruction of red blood cells). This anemia is uncommon today, however, owing to changes that have been made in infant formula composition. The fat blends in human milk and premature infant formulas now contain appropriate vitamin E:PUFA ratios for preventing hemolytic anemia. Preterm infants do not generally receive additional iron, except during recombinant erythropoietin therapy. In such cases, supplementation with vitamin E at 15 IU per day is indicated (Shannon et al., 1995).

Because the dietary requirement for vitamin E depends on the PUFA content of the diet, the recommended intake of vitamin E is commonly expressed as a ratio of vitamin E to PUFA. The recommendation for vitamin E is 0.7 IU (0.5 mg of d-alpha-tocopherol) per 100 kcal, and at least 1.0 IU of vitamin E per gram of linoleic acid.

Pharmacologic dosing of vitamin E (50 to 100 mg/kg/day) has not proven to be helpful in preventing BPD or retinopathy of prematurity by reducing the toxic effects of oxygen. Furthermore, high doses of vitamin E have been associated with intraventricular hemorrhage, sepsis, necrotizing enterocolitis, liver and renal failure, and death.

IRON. Preterm infants are at risk for iron deficiency anemia because of the reduced iron stores associated with early birth. At birth, most of the available iron is in the circulating hemoglobin. Thus, frequent blood sampling further depletes the amount of iron available for erythropoiesis. Transfusions of red blood cells are often needed to treat the early physiologic anemia of prematurity. The use of recombinant erythropoietin therapy is being investigated as another potential means of treating this anemia. Iron supplementation is indicated to facilitate red blood cell production, and a dosage of 6 mg/kg/day of enteral iron has been used (Shannon et al., 1995).

In general, the recommendation for iron intake is 2 to 4 mg/kg/day. Infants fed human milk should be given ferrous sulfate drops. Formulas fortified with iron usually contain sufficient iron for preterm infants. The optimal time to introduce iron into the preterm infant's diet is unclear; suggestions range from 2 weeks to 2 months of age (American Academy of Pediatrics, 1998).

FOLIC ACID. Premature infants seem to have higher folic acid needs than infants born at term. Although serum folate levels are high at birth, they decrease dramatically, probably as a result of high utilization of folic acid by the premature infant for DNA and the tissue synthesis needed for rapid growth.

A mild form of folic acid deficiency, manifested by low serum folate concentrations and hypersegmentation of neutrophils, is not unusual in premature infants. Megaloblastic anemia is much less commonly observed. A daily folic acid intake of 25 to 50 mg effectively maintains normal serum folate concentrations. Fortified human milk and formulas for premature infants meet these guidelines when full enteral feedings are established.

SODIUM. Preterm infants, especially those with VLBW, are susceptible to hyponatremia during the neonatal period. These infants may have excessive urinary sodium losses because of renal immaturity and an inability to conserve adequate sodium. Furthermore, their sodium needs are high because of their rapid growth rate.

Daily sodium intakes of 4 to 8 mEq/kg or more may be required by some infants to avoid hyponatremia. Routine sodium supplementation of fortified human milk and infant formulas is not necessary. However, it is important to consider the possibility of hyponatremia and to monitor infants by assessing serum or urinary sodium concentrations. Milks can be supplemented with sodium if repletion is necessary (Kloiber et al., 1996).

Methods of Feeding

Decisions about breast-, bottle-, or tube-feeding depend on the gestational age and the clinical condition of the preterm infant. The goal is to feed the infant via the most physiologic method possible by supplying nutrition for growth without inducing clinical complications.

Gastric Gavage

Gastric gavage by the *oral route* is often chosen for infants who are unable to suck because of immaturity or insults to the central nervous system. Infants of less than 32 to 34 weeks gestational age, regardless of birth weight, may be expected to have poorly coordinated sucking and swallowing activity related to their developmental immaturity; consequently, they have difficulty with nipple feeding. Using the oral **gastric gavage** method, a soft feeding tube is inserted through the mouth and into the infant's stomach. The major risks of this technique include aspiration and gastric distention. Because of weak or absent cough reflexes and poorly developed respiratory muscles, the tiny infant may not be able to dislodge milk from the upper airway, which can cause reflex bradycardia or airway obstruction. However, electronic monitoring of vital functions and proper positioning of the infant during feeding minimize the risk of aspiration from regurgitation of stomach contents. Gastric distention and vagal nerve stimulation, with resultant bradycardia, are potential problems when oral gastric gavage feedings are delivered on an intermittent bolus schedule. Occasionally, elimination of the distention and vagal bradycardia requires the use of an indwelling tube for continuous gastric gavage feedings, rather than intermittent administration of boluses. Continuous drip feedings are sometimes preferred for tiny, immature infants whose small gastric capacity and slow intestinal motility may impede the tolerance of large-volume bolus feeds. *Nasal gastric gavage* is sometimes better tolerated than oral tube feeding. However, because neonates are obligatory nose breathers, this technique may compromise the nasal airway in preterm infants, causing an associated deterioration in respiratory function. This method is helpful, however, for the infant learning to nipple feed. Use of a nasal gastric tube allows the infant to form a tight seal on the bottle nipple, which can be difficult if an oral feeding tube is in place during feedings.

Transpyloric Feeding

Transpyloric tube feeding is indicated for infants who are at risk for formula aspiration into the lungs or who have slow gastric emptying. The goal of this method is to circumvent the often slow gastric emptying of the immature infant by passing the feeding tube through the stomach and pylorus and locating its tip within the duodenum or jejunum. The infant with severe gastrointestinal reflux does well with this method, which prevents aspiration of feedings into the lungs. This method is also used for infants whose respiratory function is compromised and who are at risk for formula aspiration. The possible disadvantages of transpyloric feedings include decreased fat absorption, diarrhea, dumping syndrome, alterations of the intestinal microflora, intestinal perforation, and bilious fluid in the stomach. The placement of transpyloric tubes also requires considerable expertise, as well as radiographic confirmation of the location of the catheter tip. Although associated with many possible complications, transpyloric feedings are used when gastric feeds are not successful (Pereira, 1995).

Nipple-Feeding

Nipple-feeding may be attempted in infants whose gestational age is greater than 32 weeks. Prior to this time, the infant is unable to coordinate sucking, swallowing, and breathing. The ability to nipple-feed is usually indicated by evidence of an established sucking reflex and sucking motion. Because sucking requires effort by the infant, any stress from other causes, such as hypothermia or hypoxemia, diminishes sucking ability. Therefore, nipple-feeding should be initiated only when the infant is under minimal stress and is sufficiently mature and strong to sustain the sucking effort. Initial bottle-feedings may be limited to one to three times per day to prevent undue fatigue or the expending of too much energy, either of which can result in a decreased rate of weight gain.

Breast-Feeding

When the mother of a premature infant chooses to breast-feed, it is desirable that the infant begin nursing at the breast as soon as the infant is ready to begin nippling. Before this time, the mother must express her milk so that it can be tube-fed to her infant. These mothers need emotional and educational support to facilitate lactation. Better coordination of sucking, swallowing, and breathing and less disruption in ventilation have been seen in premature infants who were breast-fed compared with those who were bottle-fed (Meier and Anderson, 1987). So-called kangaroo baby care—allowing the mother to hold her infant with skin-to-skin contact—facilitates her lactation (Hurst et al., 1997). In addition, this contact promotes continuation of breast-feeding and enhances the mother's confidence in caring for her high-risk infant. The latter benefit may also apply to fathers who engage in kangaroo care with their infants.

Cup-feeding, instead of bottle supplements, has recently been suggested for the preterm infant, based on the rationale that it may prevent confusion on the part of the infant between nursing at the breast and the bottle (Lang et al., 1994). Additional research is needed in this area, however, to document the benefits and complications of this practice. Milk aspiration and the refusal to breast-feed are two possible problems (Thorley, 1997).

Volume of Feeding

The appropriate amount of milk preterm infants should be fed is unknown. Most nurseries initiate feedings with small volumes and advance the amount fed as tolerated. In general, volume size decreases with lower birth weights. Although gastric capacity increases with postnatal age, individual infants vary in their ability to tolerate enteral volumes and should be monitored by periodic measurement of gastric residuals.

Tolerance of Feedings

All preterm babies receiving enteral nutrition should be monitored for signs of feeding intolerance. Vomiting of feedings usually signals the infant's inability to retain that amount of milk. When not associated with other signs of a systemic illness, vomiting may indicate a too rapid increase in feeding volumes or an excessive volume for the infant's size and maturity. Reducing the volume may be all that is required. If this does not eliminate vomiting, or if signs of a systemic illness coexist, feedings may need to be interrupted until the infant's condition has stabilized. Bile-stained emesis may indicate intestinal blockage and the need for further evaluation.

Abdominal distention may be caused by excessive feeding, organic obstruction, excessive swallowing of air, resuscitation, or sepsis (i.e., systemic infection). Observing the infant for abdominal distention should be a routine practice for the nurse caring for such infants. Intermittent measurement of abdominal circumference will aid in the early detection of distention. This symptom often indicates the need to interrupt feeding until the cause of the distention is determined and the abdomen is once again soft and nondistended.

Gastric residuals, measured by aspiration of the stomach contents, should be determined routinely before each bolus gavage feeding, and intermittently in all continuous-drip feedings. Whether or not a residual amount is significant depends partly on its volume in relation to the total volume of the feeding. For emample, a residual whose volume is more than 50% of a bolus feeding, or is equal to the continuous infusion rate, might be a sign of feeding intolerance. When interpreting the significance of a gastric residual measurement, however, it is important to consider other concurrent signs of feeding intolerance and the previous pattern of residual volumes established for that infant. Bloody or bilious gastric residuals are more alarming than those that appear to be undigested milk.

The *frequency and consistency of bowel movements* require constant attention when feeding preterm infants. Simple inspection can detect the presence of gross blood. However, occult blood is not always visible, and so should be investigated by a specific assay to detect small amounts of blood in the stool.

No one method of feeding is without hazard for preterm infants, and unless close attention is paid to symptoms that indicate poor feeding tolerance, serious complications may ensue. Certain diseases can be recognized clinically by determining signs of feeding intolerance. For example, **necrotizing enterocolitis** is a serious and potentially fatal disease associated with specific signs, such as abdominal distention and tenderness, abnormal gastric residuals, and grossly bloody stools.

Composition of Feedings

Human Milk

Human milk is the ideal food for healthy term infants and for premature infants. Although human milk requires nutrient supplementation to meet the increased needs of the premature infant, the benefits of human milk are numerous for the infant. Intriguingly, during the first month of lactation, the composition of milk from mothers delivering prematurely differs from that of mothers who deliver at term. When premature infants are fed their own mother's milk, they grow more rapidly than infants fed banked breast milk (mature breast milk) (Gross, 1983).

In addition to its nutrient concentration, human milk offers nutritional benefits related to its unique composition of amino acids and long-chain fatty acids. The zinc and iron in human milk are more readily absorbed, and fat is more easily digested because of the presence of lipases. Moreover, human milk contains factors that are not present in formulas. These components include (1) live cells, macrophages, and T and B lymphocytes; (2) antimicrobial factors, SIgA, lactoferrin, and others; (3) hormones; (4) enzymes; and (5) growth factors. The significance of many of these factors is currently being investigated. It has also been suggested that human milk fed to preterm infants reduces the incidence of necrotizing enterocolitis and improves neurodevelopment (Lucas et al., 1994).

There is, however, one well-documented problem associated with feeding human milk to preterm infants. Whether preterm, term, or mature, human milk does not meet the calcium and phosphorus needs for normal bone mineralization in infants born prematurely. For this reason, calcium and phosphorus supplements are recommended for rapidly growing preterm infants who are fed predominantly human milk. Currently, two human milk fortifiers are available: Similac Natural Care (Ross Laboratories), which is available in liquid form, and Enfamil Human Milk Fortifier (Mead Johnson Nutritionals), which is available in powdered form. These contain calcium and phosphorus, along with protein, carbohydrate, fat, vitamins, and minerals, and are designed to be added to expressed breast milk fed to premature infants.

Providing human milk to the premature infant can be a very positive experience for the mother, one that promotes maternal involvement and interaction. Because many preterm infants are neither strong enough nor mature enough to nurse at their mother's breast in the early neonatal period, these mothers usually express their milk for several days (and sometimes, several weeks) before nursing can be established. The proper technique of expression, storage, and transport of milk should be reviewed with the mother (see Chapter 7). Many summaries of the special considerations for nursing a preterm infant have been published (Hopkinson et al., 1997; Lawrence, 1994).

Premature Infant Formulas

Formula preparations have been developed to meet the unique nutrient and physiological needs of growing preterm infants. The quantity and quality of nutrients in these products promote growth at intrauterine rates. These formulas, which have caloric densities of 20 and 24 kcal/oz, are available only in the ready-to-feed form, which prohibits further concentration. These premature formulas differ in many respects from standard cow's-milk–based formulas (Table 9–14). The types of carbohydrate, protein, and fat differ in order to facilitate digestion and absorption of nutrients. These formulas also have increased concentrations of protein, minerals, and vitamins to meet the higher nutritional requirements of preterm infants.

Transitional Infant Formulas

Formulas containing 22 kcal/oz have been designed for the premature infant as transition formulas. The nutrient content of these preparations lies between that of the nutrient-dense premature infant formulas and the standard infant formula, as shown in Table 9–14. These formulas can be initiated when the infant reaches a weight of 1800 g or more, and their use can be continued until the infant reaches a weight of 2500 to 3600 g. Transitional formulas are available in powder form for home use, and in ready-to-feed form for use in hospitals. One study has suggested that weight and length gain is improved in infants who receive these formulas until 9 months of age (Lucas et al., 1992).

Selection of Enteral Feeding

During the initial period of feeding, premature infants may often require additional time to adjust to enteral nutrition, and may experience concurrent stress, weight loss, and diuresis. The primary goal of enteral feeding during this initial period is to facilitate tolerance to the milk provided. When aggressive nutritional support is expected from the onset of enteral feeding, the effort often fails. These infants appear to be unable to assimilate a large volume and concentration of nutrients until a period of adjustment has ensued. Thus, enteral feedings often require supplementation with parenteral fluids until an adequate oral volume is tolerated.

After the initial period of adjustment, the goal of enteral feeding changes to the provision of complete nutrition so as to promote growth and rapid organ development. All essential nutrients should be provided in quantities that support sustained growth in all parameters. For this effect, the following feeding choices are appropriate: (1) human milk supplemented with human milk fortifier and iron, (2) iron-fortified premature infant formula for infants who weigh less than 2 kg, or (3) iron-fortified standard infant formula for infants who weigh more than 2 kg.

TABLE 9–14 COMPARISON OF THE NUTRITIONAL CONTENT OF HUMAN MILK, STANDARD FORMULAS, AND PREMATURE INFANT FORMULAS

	HUMAN MILK	STANDARD FORMULA*	TRANSITIONAL FORMULA†	PREMATURE FORMULA‡
Caloric density (kcal/oz)	20	20	22	20, 24
Protein whey/casein	70:30	60:40 48:52 100:0	60:40 50:50	60:40
Protein (g/L)	10–14	14–16	19–21	18–24
Carbohydrate	Lactose	Lactose	Lactose, glucose polymers	Lactose, glucose polymers
Carbohydrate (g/L)	66–72	73–74	77–79	72–90
Fat	Human fat	Vegetable	Vegetable, MCT oil	Vegetable, MCT oil
Fat (g/L)	39	35–37	39–41	35–44
Calcium (mg/L)	250–279	432–527	780–890	1115–1452
Phosphorus (mg/L)	130–143	243–378	460–490	561–806
Vitamin D (IU/L)	20	405	590–600	1014–2177
Vitamin E (IU/L)	3.4–11.0	13.5–20.3	27.0–30.0	27.0–50.8
Folic acid (μg/L)	33–50	61–108	187–192	237–298
Sodium (mEq/L)	7.7–10.9	7.1–7.9	10.8–11.3	11.5–15.1

MCT, medium-chain triglyceride.
*Based on the composition of Enfamil, Good Start, and Similac formulas.
†Based on the composition of Enfamil 22 and Similac NeoSure formulas.
‡Based on the composition of Enfamil Premature Formula and Similac Special Care formulas.

Premature infants can be discharged home on a transitional formula unless osteopenia is present. In the latter case, calcium and phosphorus–enriched premature infant formula should be provided until the osteopenia resolves. The breast-fed infant who has osteopenia should also receive supplementation from bottles of fortified human milk or premature infant formula. Breast-fed babies without osteopenia should receive a multivitamin/mineral supplement that contains vitamin D and iron.

Formula Manipulations

Occasionally, it may be desirable to increase the energy content of the formulas fed to small infants. This may be appropriate when the infant is not growing at a desirable rate and is already ingesting a maximum volume of fluid.

Concentration of Formulas

One approach to providing hypercaloric formula is to prepare formula with less water, thus concentrating all nutrients, including energy. Concentrated infant formulas with energy contents of 24 or 27 kcal/oz are available to hospitals as ready-to-feed nursettes. When these concentrated formulas are used, however, it is important to consider the infant's fluid intake and fluid losses in relation to the renal solute load of the concentrated feeding in order to ensure that positive water balance is maintained. This method of increasing formula density is often preferred because nutrient balance remains the same, and the infant who has an increased energy requirement also has an increased need for additional nutrients.

Caloric Supplements

Another approach to increasing the energy content of a formula involves the use of caloric supplements, such as MCT oil (Mead Johnson Nutritionals), and glucose polymers, such as Polycose (Ross Laboratories). These supplements increase the caloric density without markedly altering solute load or osmolality. However, they do alter the relative distribution of total calories derived from protein, carbohydrate, and fat. Because even small amounts of MCT oil or Polycose adversely dilute the percentage of calories derived from protein, adding these supplements to human milk or standard (20 kcal/oz) formulas is not advised. Caloric supplements are used when the formula meets the infant's nutrient requirements except for energy, or when the renal solute load is a concern (Sapsford, 1994). Because premature infant formulas are available only as ready-to-feed preparations, altering the concentration by preparing them with less water is not possible. Instead, these premature formulas should be advanced in volume as tolerated, and then caloric supplements added. The transitional formulas are available in both ready-to-feed and powder form, and can be concentrated to 27 and 30 kcal/oz. However, this formula would still be inadequate for infants with an increased calcium requirement (e.g., infants with osteopenia).

When a high-energy formula is appropriate, MCT oil and Polycose can be added to a base that has a concentration of 24 kcal/oz or greater (either full-strength premature formula or a concentrated standard formula), to a maximum of 50% of total calories derived from fat, and a minimum of 9% of total calories supplied as protein. For the infant who can tolerate long-chain fatty acids, an emulsified fatty acid product (Microlipid, Sherwood Medical) may be appropriate, as this product stays in solution better than the MCT oil, which clings to the sides of the container.

GROWTH AND NUTRITIONAL ASSESSMENT

Growth Rates and Growth Charts

All neonates typically lose some weight after birth. This is particularly true for preterm infants, who are born with more extracellular water than term infants and thus tend to lose more weight. However, postnatal weight loss should not be excessive. Preterm infants who lose more than about 15% to 20% of their birth weight may become dehydrated as a result of inadequate fluid intake, or they may experience tissue wasting from poor energy intake. Birth weight should be regained by the second or third week of life. The smallest and sickest infants will take the longest time to regain their birth weights.

During the first 40 days of life, the Hall growth chart is commonly used to assess weight progress. This chart, shown in Figure 9–4, longitudinally de-

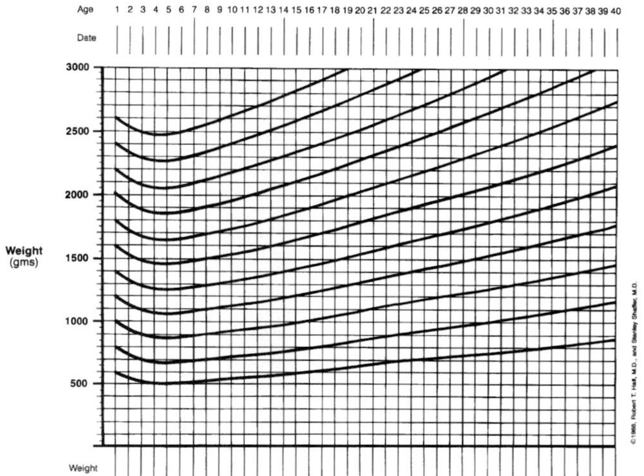

FIGURE 9–4 Weight chart for premature infants based on actual growth data. (From Shaffer SG, et al. Postnatal weight changes in low-birth-weight infants. Pediatrics 79:702, 1987.)

picts daily weight changes and actual growth curves for more than 300 infants with various neonatal medical problems requiring care in a neonatal intensive care unit (Shaffer et al., 1987).

Intrauterine growth curves have also been developed using birth weight data of infants born at successive weeks of gestation. These curves do not depict the initial period of postnatal weight loss, however, and probably represent unrealistic goals for preterm infants in the neonatal period. Once the infant's condition stabilizes and full nutrient intake is possible, the infant may be able to grow at a rate that parallels these curves. An intrauterine weight gain of 15 g/kg/day can be achieved prior to 38 weeks' gestation (Wright et al., 1993).

Although weight is an important anthropometric parameter, measurements of length and head circumference can also be helpful. Growth curves, such as those shown in Figure 9–5, can be used to evaluate the adequacy of growth in all three parameters. This chart has the benefit of a built-in correction factor for prematurity, and the infant's growth can be followed on one chart through the first year of corrected age. This chart represents cross-sectional data constructed from the anthropometric measurements taken at birth of infants with different gestational ages and of infants followed in a health maintenance program (Babson and Benda, 1976).

The National Center for Health Statistics curves for full-term infants from birth to 3 years of age can also be used for preterm infants after 40 weeks of gestation, as long as age is corrected (or adjusted) for prematurity (Bernstein et al., 1998). For example, the infant born at 28 weeks' gestation is 12 weeks premature (40 weeks – 28 weeks birth gestation). At 4 months postnatal age, the growth parameters of a premature infant born at 28 weeks' gestation can be compared with those of a 1-month-old infant born at term (see Table 9–15 for calculations). When using growth grids, age should be adjusted for prematurity until at least 2½ to 3 years' corrected age (Bernstein et al., 1998). In Figure 9–6, A.R.'s pattern of growth is shown up to 14 years of age.

TABLE 9–15 STEPS FOR CORRECTING OR ADJUSTING AGE FOR PREMATURITY

1. Calculate the number of weeks the infant was premature: 40 weeks (term) – birth gestation.
2. Number of weeks early = the correction factor.
3. Chronological age – correction factor = adjusted age for prematurity.

Example:

1. 40 weeks – 28 weeks gestation = 12 weeks early.
2. 12 weeks or 3 months is the correction factor.
3. 4 months (chronological age) – 3 months corrected factor = 1 month adjusted age.

Casey and associates (1991) have reported longitudinal growth data on premature infants from birth to 3 years of age. After 4 months of age, preterm infants were found to grow at rates similar to those of full-term infants (see "*Focus On:* Long-Term Outcome for Premature Infants").

Laboratory Indices

Laboratory assessment usually involves measuring the following parameters: (1) fluid and electrolyte balance, (2) parenteral nutrition tolerance, (3) bone

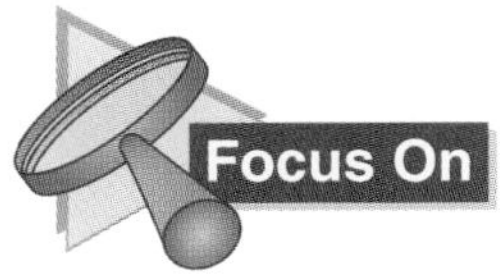

Long-Term Outcome for Premature Infants

As the survival of premature infants continues to improve, their physical growth, mental development, health, and quality of life are being investigated. Previously, it was believed that if premature infants were to achieve catch-up growth, it would only occur during the first few years of life. However, catch-up growth for weight, length, and head circumference can continue through the first 18 years of life (Hirata and Bosque, 1998). In fact, even extremely-low-birth-weight (ELBW) infants can reach their predicted genetic height.

Only recently have tools been developed and validated to assess how children report their health status and quality of life. Saigal and group (1996) compared two groups of adolescents ranging in age from 12 to 16 years. The first group included 150 children who were born premature with ELBW. The second group consisted of 124 children who were born at term and were not low-birth-weight (LBW) infants. All children were interviewed in the same fashion except for nine ELBW children who were severely neurologically impaired. The parents of these nine children completed the interviews on their behalf. Neuorsensory impairments were present in 27% of the premature children and 1.6% of the term children. The impairments included cerebral palsy, hydrocephalus, cognitive impairments, autism, blindness, and deafness. Thirty-four percent of the preterm children, compared to 58% of the term children, rated their health as perfect. Quality of life was rated lower by the premature children. However, when the parents' scores for the nine neurologically impaired teens were deleted, there was no difference between the two groups in terms of their assessment of quality of life. Although premature children may suffer more frequently from neurosensory impairment, their perception is optimistic for their quality of life.

Not only has survival of premature infants increased, but these children are enjoying life. The medical and nutritional care in the nursery continues to be advanced, which improves the infant's outcome in the nursery and sets the stage for later development.

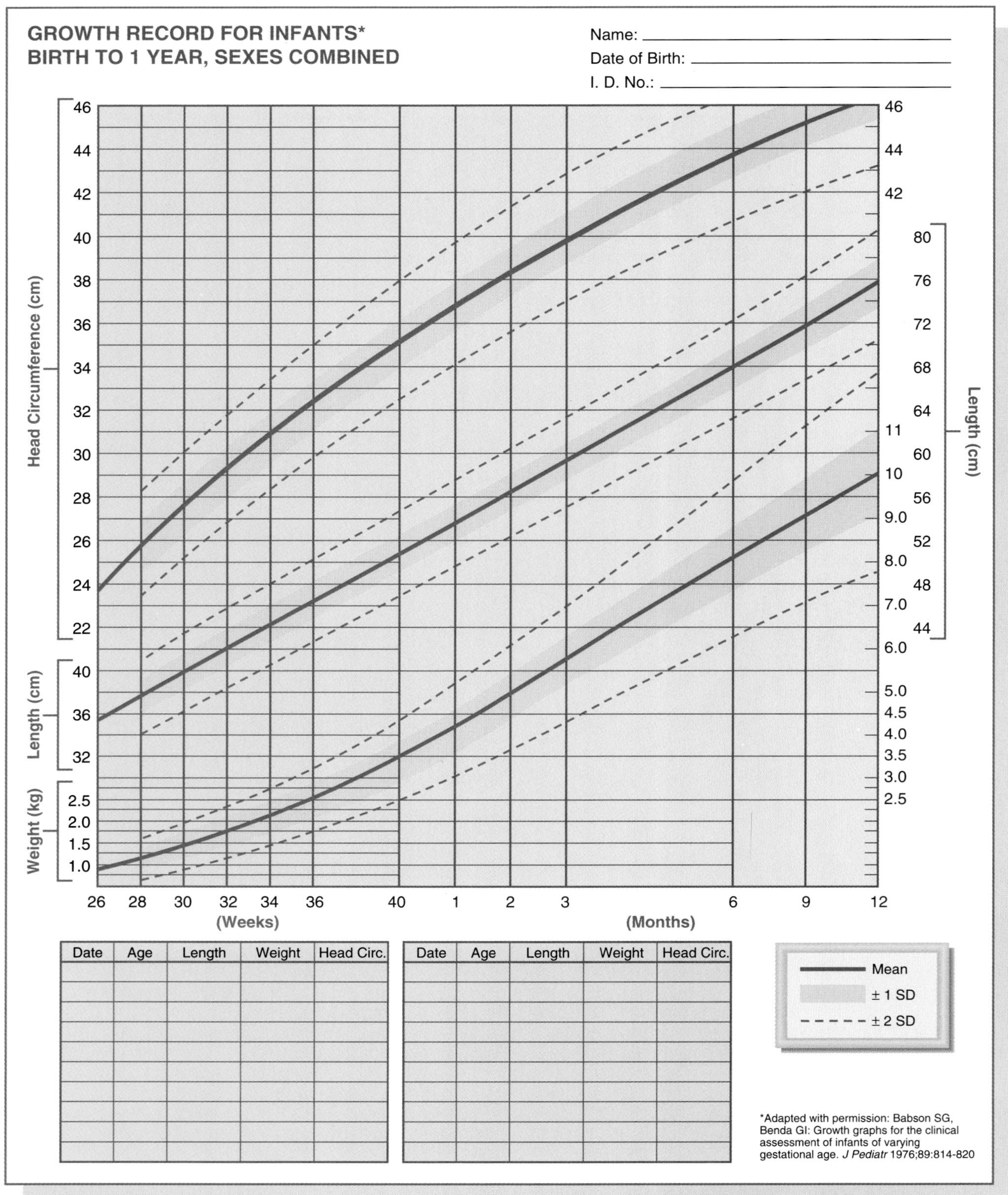

FIGURE 9–5 An example of a growth record of weight, length, and head circumference for infants from 26 weeks' gestation to 1 year of age. This chart has a built-in correction factor for prematurity. (From Babson SG, Benda GI. Growth graphs for the clinical assessment of infants of varying gestational age. J Pediatr 89:814, 1976.)

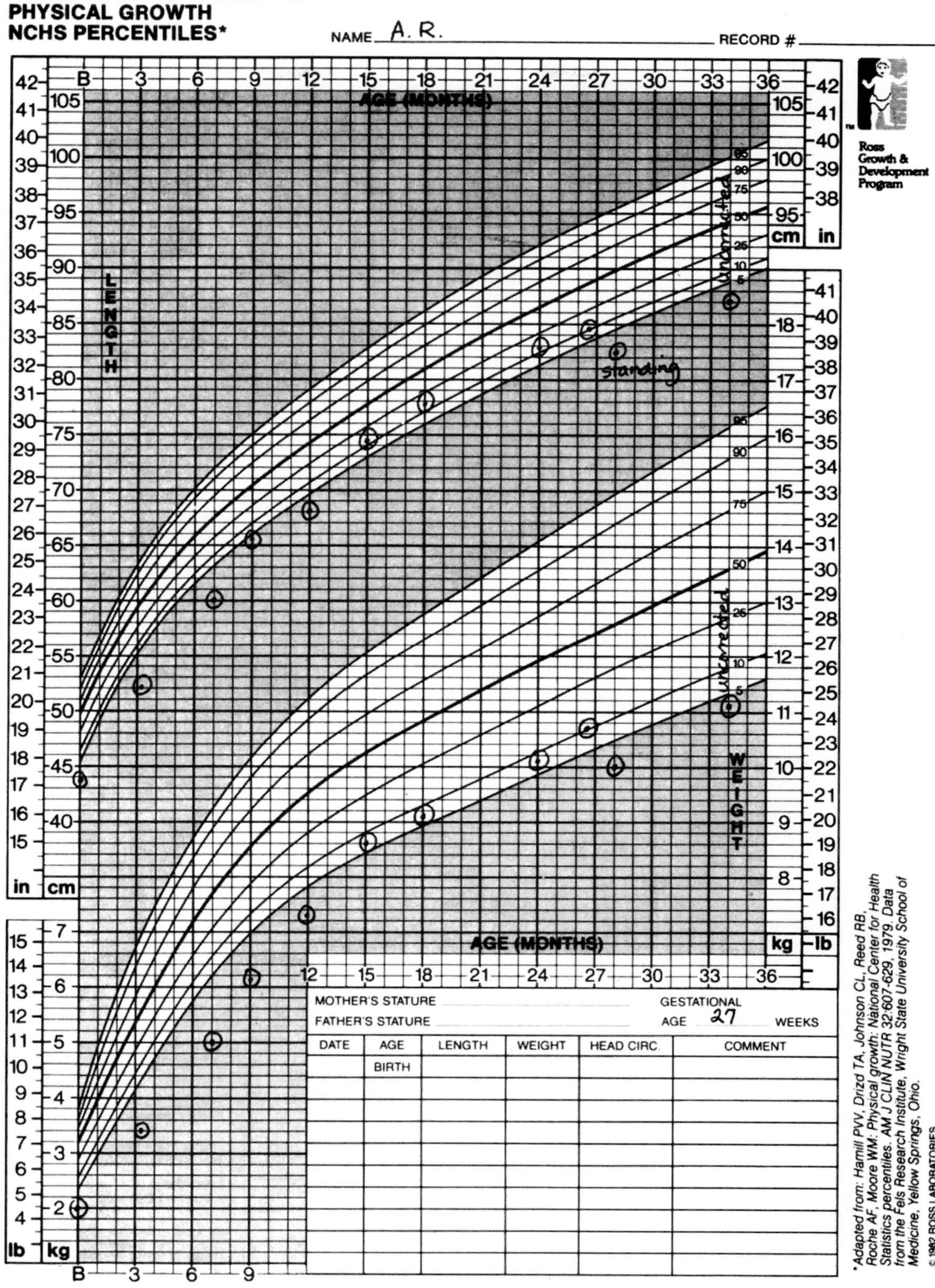

A

FIGURE 9–6 *A*, These graphs show how “A.R.”, a 27-week-old premature infant, grew after leaving the neonatal unit 1 day before her due date at a weight of 4½ lb. Heights and weights up to the age of 28 months were plotted on the grid at “corrected age” points, and thereafter at “uncorrected age” points. She exhibited catch-up growth during the first 15 months.

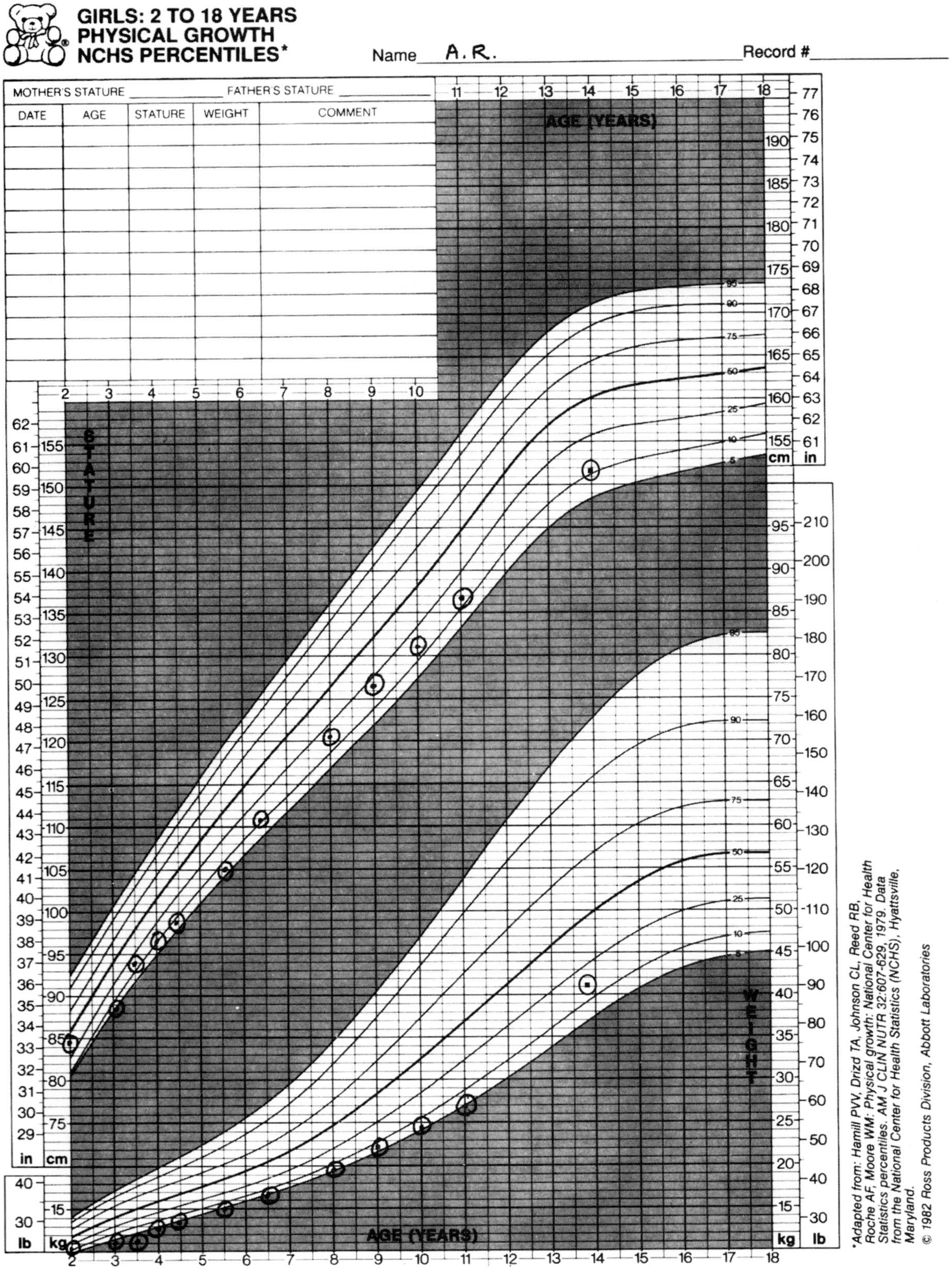

GIRLS: 2 TO 18 YEARS
PHYSICAL GROWTH
NCHS PERCENTILES*
Name A. R.
Record #
MOTHER'S STATURE
FATHER'S STATURE
DATE
AGE
STATURE
WEIGHT
COMMENT
AGE (YEARS)
STATURE
WEIGHT
in
cm
lb
kg
*Adapted from: Hamill PVV, Drizd TA, Johnson CL, Reed RB, Roche AF, Moore WM: Physical growth: National Center for Health Statistics percentiles. AM J CLIN NUTR 32:607-629, 1979. Data from the National Center for Health Statistics (NCHS), Hyattsville, Maryland.
© 1982 Ross Products Division, Abbott Laboratories

B

FIGURE 9–6 *B*, A.R.'s growth pattern is shown from the age of 2 to 14 years. During the first 10 years, she appears to be growing at the 5th percentile for weight and the 10th percentile for height. She is following her channel of growth, but not exhibiting catch-up growth. Between the ages of 10 and 14 years, she changed growth channels for both height and weight, reaching the 25th percentile for height and the 10th percentile for weight.

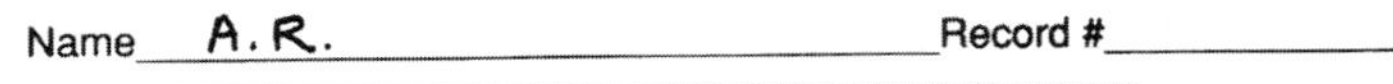

mineralization status, and (4) hematologic status. In addition, serum protein, prealbumin, and retinol-binding protein levels may reflect recent changes in nutritional intake. However, it must be remembered that these levels are also influenced by the infant's gestational age, the presence or absence of illness, the infant's level of stress, and vitamin A and zinc status.

DISCHARGE CARE

Successful feeding is the pivotal factor involved in the decision to discharge the preterm infant from the nursery to home. Preterm infants must be able to (1) tolerate and, in most cases, nipple all of their feeds, (2) grow adequately on a modified-demand feeding schedule (usually every 3 to 4 hours during the day or every 2 to 3 hours for the breast-fed infant), and (3) maintain their body temperature outside of an incubator. In addition, it is important that any ongoing chronic illness, including nutritional problems, be manageable at home. Most important, the parents must be ready to care for their infant. Twenty-four-hour nursery visitation can facilitate the parents' role in managing their infant's care at home and developing their caregiving skills. Often, parents are permitted to "room in" with their infant prior to discharge, which helps build their confidence in caring for their high-risk infant (see Fig. 9–7).

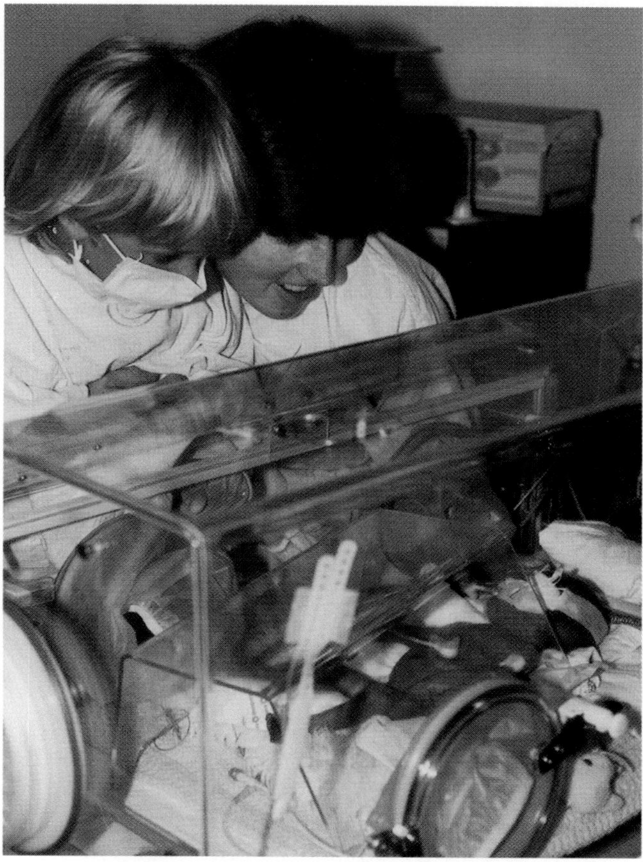

FIGURE 9–7 Photograph of a family in the nursery with their premature infant before discharge.

Many preterm infants are discharged from the hospital weighing less than 5½ lb. Although these infants must meet discharge criteria before they can go home, the stress of a new environment may lead to setbacks. Small preterm infants should be followed very closely during the first month after discharge, and parents should be given as much information and support as possible. Within the first week of discharge, a home visit by a nurse and/or nutritionist and an office visit to the pediatrician are highly desirable in terms of education and early intervention.

Factors that affect the feeding skills and behavior of preterm infants are particularly important in discharge care. Physical factors, such as variable heart rate, rapid respiratory rate, and tremulousness, are examples of physiological events that interfere with feeding. Infants weighing less than 5½ lb have poor muscle tone. Although muscle tone gradually improves as an infant becomes larger and more mature, it can decline quickly in infants who are tired or weak. Feeding is often difficult for infants who have limited muscle flexion and strength and poor head and neck control, which is important in maintaining good feeding posture. Positioning these infants in a manner that supports normal body flexion and ensures proper alignment of the head and neck during the course of the feeding may be helpful. The premature infant may also require support of the chin and cheeks during bottle-feedings.

Small infants tend to sleep more than larger, term infants. It is much easier for preterm infants to feed effectively if they are fully awake before feeding. To awaken a preterm infant, one should provide one type of gentle stimulation for a few minutes, then change to a different activity, and so on, until the infant is fully awake. Lightly swaddling the infant and placing him or her in a semiupright position may also facilitate awakening.

In addition, the feeding environment should be as quiet as possible. Preterm infants are easily distracted and have difficulty focusing on feeding when noises or movements interrupt their attention. They also tire quickly and are easily overstimulated. When this happens, they may show only subtle signs of distress. It is important to teach parents of premature infants to recognize these subtle cues that indicate the need for rest or comfort, and to respond to them appropriately.

After discharge, most preterm infants need at least 165 to 180 mL/kg/day (or 2½ to 2⅔ oz/lb/day) of breast milk or standard infant formula containing 20 kcal/oz. This amount of milk provides 110 to 120 kcal/kg/day (or 50 to 55 kcal/lb/day). Alternatively, transitional formula having a concentration of 22 kcal/oz can be provided at a rate of 155 to 170 mL/kg/day (or 2½ oz/lb/day). The best way to de-

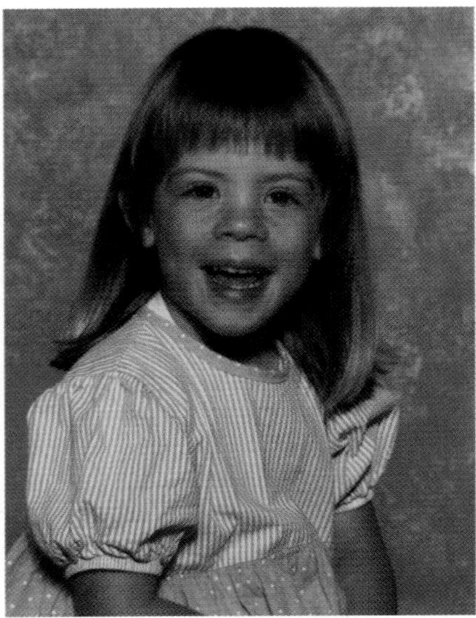

A

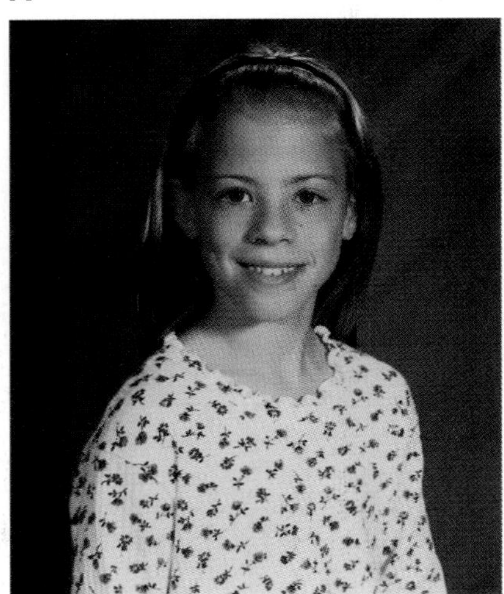

B

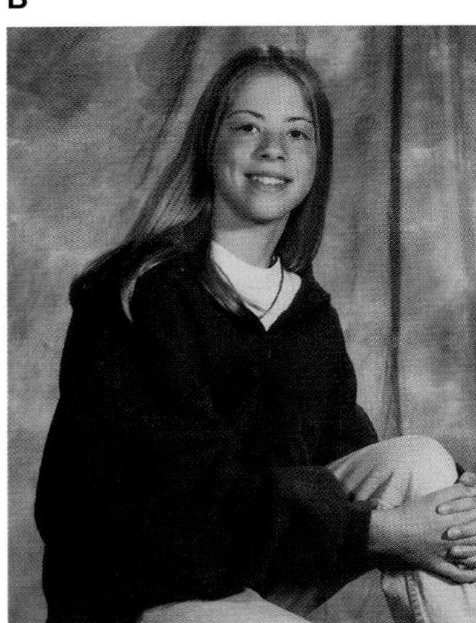

C

FIGURE 9–8 *A,* This photograph shows the premature baby "A.R." (as in Figure 9–2) at a healthy 3½ years of age. *B,* A.R. at 10 years of age. *C,* A.R. at almost 14 years of age.

termine whether these amounts are adequate for individual infants is to compare intake with growth progress over time. In some cases, a formula that provides 24 kcal/oz may be necessary. Powdered transitional formula can be readily altered to provide a concentration of 24 kcal/oz. Ready-to-feed premature formulas providing 24 kcal/oz should be used for the premature infant who has osteopenia.

It is important to evaluate needs based on the three growth parameters: weight, length, and head circumference. Patterns of growth should be assessed to determine whether (1) individual curves at least parallel reference curves, (2) growth curves are shifting inappropriately across growth percentiles, (3) weight is appropriate for length, and (4) growth is proportionate in all three parameters.

CASE STUDY

Sara S., a 26-week gestation infant was admitted to the neonatal intensive care unit. Birth weight was 850 g, which classified the infant as appropriate for gestational age. The infant presented with respiratory distress syndrome and required intubation for mechanical ventilation. During the first few hours of life, surfactant was given, and ventilator settings were lowered. The infant was placed in a humidified incubator. Intravenous $D_{10}W$ was started at 100 mL/kg/day. On day 2 of life, the infant had gained 20 g, and serum sodium and urine volume output were low. A patent ductus arteriosus was diagnosed. Indomethacin was administered to close the ductus arteriosus. On day 4 of life, body weight had decreased 50 g, or 6% of birth weight, and serum electrolytes were normal. Parenteral fluids were optimized by increasing the protein concentration, and the volume of intravenous fat was advanced. By day 6 of life, the infant was clinically stable. Feedings of milk from the infant's own mother were begun at 0.7 mL every 2 hours, delivered by bolus oral gastric tube. This volume provided 10 mL/kg of birth weight. Feedings were well tolerated. Human milk was advanced by 10 mL/kg/day, and parenteral fluids were decreased concurrently. The infant was successfully extubated to room air after full enteral feedings were established.

1. On day 2 of life, this infant's intravenous fluid volume should be
   a. increased, for the infant requires more calories.
   b. decreased, as the infant is overhydrated.
   c. changed to enteral feedings because the infant is clinically stable.
2. Intravenous fat should be provided to this premature infant
   a. using a 10% emulsion.
   b. using a 20% emulsion.
   c. using a 24-hour infusion rate.
   d. b and c.
3. Milk from this premature infant's mother may be inadequate in which nutrients? What would be your recommendations?
4. By day 6, is Sara's intake of protein adequate? If not, what would you recommend?

NEURODEVELOPMENTAL OUTCOME

It is possible to meet the metabolic and nutritional needs of premature infants sufficiently to sustain life and promote growth and development. In fact, more tiny immature infants are surviving than ever before, given adequate nutritional support and the recent advances in neonatal intensive care technology. However, the incidence of neurosensory and developmental handicaps has remained constant, despite the increase in the total number of surviving children (Hack, 1997).

The increased survival rate of VLBW infants has given rise to increased concern about the short- and long-term neurodevelopmental outcome of these babies. Many questions have been posed about the quality of life awaiting infants who receive neonatal intensive care. As a rule, VLBW infants should be referred to a follow-up clinic to evaluate development and growth and to facilitate early interventions. Surviving ELBW infants, particularly those with birth weights of less than 750 g, have an increased risk of developing central nervous system handicapping conditions of varying severity and functional impairment (Hack et al., 1994). Despite this risk, however, many of these premature babies reach childhood without evidence of any disability (Fig. 9–8) (see the accompanying Case Study).

CITED REFERENCES

American Academy of Pediatrics and American College of Obstetricians and Gynecologists: Introduction. In: Guidelines for Perinatal Care, 4th ed. Evanston, IL: American Academy of Pediatrics, 1997, p. xvii.

American Academy of Pediatrics, Committee on Nutrition: Nutritional needs of preterm infants. In: Kleinman RE (ed.). Pediatric Nutrition Handbook, 4th ed. Elk Grove, IL: American Academy of Pediatrics, 1998, p. 55

Babson SG, Benda GI. Growth graphs for the clinical assessment of infants of varying gestational age. J Pediatr 89(5):814, 1976.

Ballard JL, et al. New Ballard score, expanded to include extremely premature infants. J Pediatr 119:417, 1991.

Bell EF, Oh W. Fluid and electrolyte management. In: Avery GB, Fletcher MA, MacDonald (eds.). Neonatology: Pathophysiology and Management of the Newborn, 4th ed. Philadelphia: JB Lippincott, 1994, p. 312.

Bernstein S, et al. Approaching the management of the neonatal intensive care unit graduate through history and physical assessment. Pediatr Clin North Am 45(1):79, 1998.

Bregman J, Kimberlin LVS. Developmental outcome in extremely premature infants. Impact of surfactant. Pediatr Clin North Am 40(5):937, 1993.

Casey PH, et al. Growth status and growth rates of a varied sample of low birth weight, preterm infants: A longitudinal cohort from birth to three years of age. J Pediatr 119:599, 1991.

Christensen ML, et al. Plasma carnitine concentration and lipid metabolism in infants receiving parenteral nutrition. J Pediatr 115:794, 1989.

Costarino AT, Baumgart S. Water as nutrition. In: Tsang RC, Lucas A, Uauy R, Zlotkin S (eds.). Nutritional Needs of the Preterm Infant. Baltimore: Williams & Wilkins, 1993, p. 1.

Greene HL, et al. Guidelines for the use of vitamins, trace elements, calcium, magnesium, and phosphorus in infants and children receiving total parenteral nutrition: Report of the Subcommittee on Pediatric Parenteral Nutrient Requirements from the Committee on Clinical Practice Issues of the American Society for Clinical Nutrition. Am J Clin Nutr 48(5):1324, 1988.

Gross, SJ. Growth and biochemical response of preterm infants fed human milk or modified infant formula. N Engl J Med 308:237, 1983.

Guyer B, et al. Annual summary of vital statistics—1996. Pediatrics 100:905, 1997.

Hack M. The outcome of neonatal intensive care. In: Klaus MH, Fanaroff AA (eds.). Care of the High Risk Noenate. Philadelphia: WB Saunders, 1993.

Hack M. Follow-up for high-risk noenates. In: Fanaroff AA, Martin RJ (eds.). Neonatal-Perinatal Medicine Diseases of the Fetus and Infant, vol. 2. 6th ed. St. Louis: CV Mosby, 1997, p. 952.

Hack M, et al. School-age outcomes in children with birth weights under 750 g. N Engl J Med 331:753, 1994.

Hallman M, et al. Inositol supplementation in premature infants with respiratory distress syndrome. N Engl J Med 326:1233, 1992.

Hanning RM, Zlotkin SA. Parenteral proteins. In: Baker RD, Baker SS, Davis A. Pediatric Parenteral Nutrition. New York: Chapman & Hall, 1997, p. 128.

Hansen JW. Appendix Table A.1. Consensus recommendations. In: Tsang RC, Lucas A, Uauy R, Zlotkin S (eds.). Nutritional Needs of the Preterm Infant. Baltimore: Williams & Wilkins, 1993, p. 287.

Heird WC. Amino acid and energy needs of pediatric patients receiving parenteral nutrition. Pediatr Clin North Am 42(4):765, 1995.

Heird WC. Statistically significant versus biologically significant effect of long-chain polyunsaturated fatty acids on growth. In: Dobbing J, London UK (eds.). Developing Brain and Behavior. London: Academic Press, Ltd., 1997, p. 169.

Heird WC, Gomez MR. Parenteral nutrition in low-birth-weight infants. Ann Rev Nutr 16:471, 1996.

Hirata T, Bosque E. When they grow up: The growth of extremely low birth weight (<1000 gm) infants at adolescence. J Pediatr 132:1033, 1998.

Hopkinson J, et al. Management of breast-feeding. In: Tsang RC, Zlotkin SH, Nicholas BL, Hansen JW (eds.). Nutrition During Infancy: Principles and Practice, 2nd ed. Cincinnati: Digital Educational Publishing, Inc., 1997, p. 381.

Hurst NM, et al. Skin-to-skin holding in the neonatal intensive care unit influences maternal milk volume. J Perinatol 17:213, 1997.

Innis SM. Fat. In: Tsang RC, Lucas A, Uauy R, Zlotkin S (eds.). Nutritional Needs of the Preterm Infant. Baltimore: Williams & Wilkins, 1993, p. 65.

Kashyap S, et al. Growth, nutrient retention, and metabolic response in low birth weight infants fed varying intakes of protein and energy. J Pediatr 113:713, 1988.

Kien CL. Carbohydrate. In: Tsang RC, Lucas A, Uauy R, Zlotkin S (eds.). Nutritional Needs of the Preterm Infant. Baltimore: Williams & Wilkins, 1993, p. 47.

Kliegman RM, Sparks JW. Perinatal galactose metabolism. J Pediatr 107:831, 1985.

Kloiber LL, et al. Late hyponatremia in very-low-birth weight infants: Incidence and associated risk factors. J Am Diet Assoc 96:880, 1996.

Koletzko B. Importance of dietary lipids. In: Tsang RC, Zoltkin SH, Nichols BL, Hansen JW (eds.). Nutrition During Infancy: Principles and Practice, 2nd ed. Cincinnati: Digital Educational Publishing, Inc., 1997, p. 123.

Koo WWK, et al. Effect of three levels of vitamin D intake in preterm infants receiving high mineral-containing milk. J Pediatr Gastroenterol Nutr 21:182, 1995.

Krug-Wispe SK. Vitamins, minerals, and trace elements. In: Groh-Wargo S, Thompson M, Cox JH (eds.). Nutritional Care for High-Risk Newborns, rev. ed. Chicago: Precept Press, Inc., 1994, p. 94.

Lang S, et al. Cup feeding: An alternative of infant feeding. Arch Dis Child 71:365, 1994.

Lawrence RA. Breastfeeding: A Guide for the Medical Profession, 4th ed. St. Louis: CV Mosby, 1994.

Lorenz JM, et al. Phases of fluid and electrolyte homeostasis in the extremely low birth weight infant. Pediatrics 96:484, 1995.

Lucas A, et al. Randomized trial of nutrition for preterm infants after discharge. Arch Dis Child 67:324, 1992.

Lucas A, et al. A randomized multicenter study of human milk versus formula and later development in preterm infants. Arch Dis Child 70(2):F141–F146, 1994.

Meier P, Anderson GC. Responses of small preterm infants to bottle- and breast-feeding. Matern Child Nurs 12:97, 1987.

Modanlou HD, et al. Combined effects of antenatal corticosteroids and surfactant supplementation on the outcome of very low birth weight infants. J Perinatol 16:422, 1996.

Pearson E, et al. Trial of vitamin A supplementation in very low birth weight infants at risk for bronchopulmonary dysplasia. J Pediatr 121:420, 1992.

Pereira GR. Nutritional care of the extremely premature infant. Clin Perinatol 22(1):61, 1995.

Poindexter BB, et al. Exogenous insulin reduces proteolysis and protein synthesis in extemely low birth weight infants. J Pediatr 132:948, 1998.

Rivera A, et al. Effect of intravenous amino acids on protein metabolism of preterm infants during the first three days of life. Pediatr Res 33:106, 1993.

Robbins ST, Fletcher AB. Early vs delayed vitamin A supplementation in very-low-birth-weight infants. J Parenter Enteral Nutr 17:220, 1993.

Saigal S, et al. Self-perceived health status and health-related quality of life of extremely low birth-weight infants at adolescence. JAMA 276:453, 1996.

Sapsford AL. Energy, carbohydrate, protein and fat. In: Groh-Wargo S,

Thompson M, Cox JH (eds.). Nutritional Care for High-Risk Newborns, rev. ed. Chicago: Precept Press, Inc., 1994, p. 71.
Shaffer SG, et al. Postnatal weight changes in low birth weight infants. Pediatrics 79:702, 1987.
Shannon KM, et al. Recombinant human erythropoietin stimulates erythroiesis and reduces erythrocyte transfusions in very low birth weight preterm infants. Pediatrics 95:1, 1995.
Shenai JP, et al. Clinical trial of vitamin A supplementation in infants susceptible to bronchopulmonary dysplasia. J Pediatr 111:269, 1987.
Sulkers EJ, et al. Effects of high carnitine supplementation on substrate utilization in low-birth-weight infants receiving total parenteral nutrition. Am J Clin Nutr 52:889, 1990.
Thorley V. Cup feeding: Problems created by incorrect use. J Hum Lact 13(1):54, 1997.
Thureen PJ, Hay WW. Conditions requiring special nutritional management. In: Tsang RC, Lucas A, Uauy R, Zlotkin S (eds.). Nutritional Needs of the Preterm Infant. Baltimore: Williams & Wilkins, 1993, p. 243.
Uauy R, et al. Conditional nutrients. In: Tsang RC, Lucas A, Uauy R, Zlotkin S (eds.). Nutritional Needs of the Preterm Infant. Baltimore: Williams & Wilkins, 1993, p. 267.
Ventura SJ, et al. Report of final natality statistics, 1995. Monthly Vital Statistics Report. 45(11)(suppl):1, 1997.
Walsh WF, Hazinski TA. Bronchopulmonary dysplasia. In: Spitzer AR (ed.). Intensive Care of the Fetus and Neonate. St. Louis: CV Mosby, 1996, p. 641.
Wright K, et al. New postnatal growth grids for very low birth weight infants. Pediatrics 91:922, 1993.
Yu VYH. Intravenous feeding in the preterm neonate. In: Yu VYH, MacMahon RA (eds.). Intravenous Feeding of the Neonate. London: Edward Arnold, A Division of Hodder & Stoughton, 1992, p. 240.
Ziegler EE, et al. Body composition of the reference fetus. Growth 40:329, 1976.

ADDITIONAL REFERENCES

American Academy of Pediatrics. Work Group on Breastfeeding: Breastfeeding and the use of human milk. Pediatrics 100:1035, 1997.
American Dietetic Association. Position of the American Dietetic Association: Promotion of breast-feeding. J Am Diet Assoc 97:662, 1997.
Amorde-Spalding K, D'Harlingue AE, Phillips BL, et al. Tocopherol levels in infants ≤ 1000 grams receiving MVI Pediatric. Pediatrics 90:992, 1992.
Anderson DM, Pittard WB. Update on neonatal nutrition therapy. Top in Clin Nutr 13(1):8, 1997.
ASPEN Board of Directors: Guidelines for the use of parenteral and enteral nutrition in adult and pediatric patients. Section VII. Nutrition support for low-birth-weight infant. J Parenter Enteral Nutr 17(suppl):33SA, 1993.
Balistreri WF, Farrell MK, Bove KE. Lessons from the E-Ferol tragedy. Pediatrics 78:503, 1986.
Berry MA, Conrod H, Usher RH. Growth of very premature infants fed intravenous hyperalimentation and calcium-supplemented formula. J Pediatr 100:647, 1997.
Berseth CL. Minimal enteral feedings. Clin Perinatol 22(1):195, 1995.
Berseth CL. Gastrointestinal motility in the neonate. Clin Perinatol 23(2):179, 1996.
Borum PR. Medium-chain triglycerides in formula for preterm neonates: Implications for hepatic and extrahepatic metabolism. J Pediatr 120:S139, 1992.
Chamberlin JL. Assessment and treatment of feeding problems/dysfunction. In: Groh-Wargo S, Thompson M, Cox JH (eds.). Nutritional Care for High-Risk Newborns, rev. ed. Chicago: Precept Press, Inc., 1994, p. 220.
Chan GM. Growth and bone mineral status of discharged very low birth weight infants fed different formulas or human milk. J Pediatr 123:439, 1993.
Gross SJ. Vitamin E. In: Tsang RC, Lucas A, Uauy R, Zlotkin S (eds.). Nutritional Needs of the Preterm Infant. Baltimore: Williams & Wilkins, 1993, p. 101.
Hack M, et al. Effect of very low birth weight and subnormal head size on cognitive abilities at school age. N Engl J Med 325:231, 1991.
Hall RT, et al. Feeding iron-fortified premature formula during initial hospitalization to infants less than 1800 grams birth weight. Pediatrics 92:409, 1993.
Haumont D, et al. Plasma lipid and plasma lipoprotein concentrations in low birth weight infants given parenteral nutrition with twenty or ten percent lipid emulsion. J Pediatr 115:787, 1989.
Heird WC, et al. Intravenous alimentation in pediatric patients. J Pediatr 80:351, 1972.
Lucas A. Enteral feeding. In: Tsang RC, Lucas A, Uauy R, Zlotkin S (eds.). Nutritional Needs of the Preterm Infant. Baltimore: Williams & Wilkins, 1993, p. 209.
Lucas A, Cole TJ. Breast milk and neonatal necrotizing enterocolitis. Lancet 336:1519, 1990.
Meetze WH, et al. Gastrointestinal priming prior to full enteral nutrition in very low birth weight infants. J Pediatr Gastroenterol Nutr 15:163, 1992.
Moro GE, et al. Fortification of human milk: Evaluation of a novel fortification scheme and of a new fortifier. J Pediatr Gastroenterol Nutr 20:162, 1995.
Moyer-Mileur L, et al. Evaluation of liquid or powdered fortification of human milk on growth and bone mineralization status of preterm infants. J Pediatr Gastroenterol Nutr 15:370, 1992.
Schanler RJ. Suitability of human milk for the low-birthweight infant. Clin Perinatol 22(1):207, 1995.
Tyson JE, Broyles RS. Progress in assessing the long-term outcome of extremely low-birthweight infants. JAMA 276:492, 1996.
Valentine CJ, et al. Hindmilk improves weight gain in low-birth-weight infants fed human milk. J Pediatr Gastroenterol Nutr 18:474, 1994.
van Goudoever JB, Colen T, Wattimena JLD, et al. Immediate commencement of amino acid supplementation in preterm infants. J Pediatr 127:458, 1995.
Ziegler EE. Protein in premature feeding. Nutrition (1):69, 1994.

CHAPTER 10

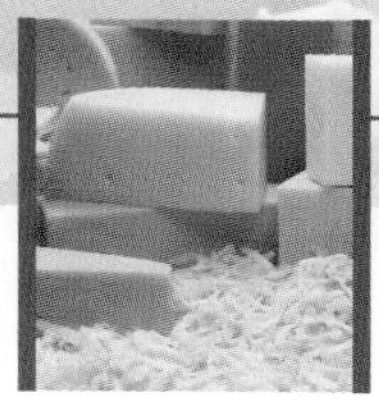

Nutrition in Childhood

BETTY LUCAS, MPH, RD, CD

Chapter Outline

- Growth and Development
- Nutrient Needs
- Providing an Adequate Diet
- Preventing Chronic Disease
- Nutritional Concerns
- Nutrition Education

Key Terms

ADIPOSITY REBOUND—a phenomenon of normal growth, occurring at around 6 years of age, when a child's body fat increases

APPETITE—a natural desire to eat, especially when food is present

CATCH-UP GROWTH—a higher-than-normal growth rate to recover a previous growth curve following a period of growth suppression as a result of extended illness or deprivation

FAILURE TO THRIVE—weight loss or lack of weight gain in a child due to acute or chronic illness, a restricted diet, poor appetite, lack of food, lack of social interaction, or a harsh or disruptive environment

FOOD INSECURITY—limited or uncertain availability of nutritionally adequate and safe foods, or a limited ability to acquire acceptable foods in socially acceptable ways

FOOD JAG—a period during which foods that were previously liked are refused or a particular food is requested at every meal; commonly seen in children aged 2 to 6 years

GROWTH CHANNEL—a curve of weight and height gain throughout the period of growth; stated as a percentile based on a standard growth chart

The period from 1 year of age to puberty is often referred to as the "latent" or "quiescent" period of growth, in contrast to the dramatic changes that occur in infancy and adolescence. Although physical growth may be less remarkable and proceed at a steadier pace than during the first year, these preschool and middle school years are a time of significant growth in the social, cognitive, and emotional areas.

GROWTH AND DEVELOPMENT

Physical Growth

The rate of growth slows considerably after the first year of life. In contrast to the tripling of birth weight that occurs in the first 12 months, another year passes before birth weight is quadrupled. Likewise, birth length increases by 50% in the first year, but is not doubled until approximately the age of 4 years. The actual increments of change are small compared with those of infancy and adolescence. Weight typically increases an average of 2 to 3 kg (4½ to 6½ lb) per year until the child is 9 or 10 years old. At this time, the rate increases, signaling the approach of puberty. Height increments average 6 to 8 cm (2½ to 3½ in) per year from 2 years of age until the pubertal acceleration.

In general, growth is steady and slow during the preschool and school-age years, but it can be erratic in individual children. Some small children may appear to be in a "holding pattern" for several months, after which they exhibit a spurt in height and weight. Interestingly, these patterns usually parallel similar changes in appetite and food intake. For parents who are not knowledgeable about these trends (and even for some who are), periods of slow growth and poor appetite can cause anxiety, which may lead to mealtime struggles.

The body proportions of young children change significantly after the first year. There is little head growth, trunk growth slows substantially, and the limbs lengthen considerably, all of which impart a more mature body proportion. With increased physical activity and walking, the legs straighten while the abdominal and back muscles tighten to support the now erect child. These changes are gradual and subtle, occurring over a period of years.

Body composition in preschool and school-aged children remains relatively constant. Fat gradually decreases during the early childhood years, reaching a minimum at approximately 6 years of age. After that, it increases (termed the **adiposity rebound**) in preparation for the pubertal growth spurt (Deitz, 1994). Sex differences are apparent early, with boys having more lean body mass per centimeter of height. Girls have a higher percentage of weight as fat, even in the early years, but these sex differences in lean body mass and fat do not become significant until adolescence.

Catch-Up Growth

A child who is recovering from an illness or undernutrition and whose growth has slowed or ceased will experience a greater-than-expected rate of recovery. This is referred to as **catch-up growth**, a period during which the body strives to catch up to the child's normal growth curve. The degree of growth suppression is influenced by the timing, severity, and duration of the precipitating cause; that is, a severe illness or prolonged nutritional deprivation during a period of rapid growth will have the most dramatic effect.

Early studies supported the thesis that malnourished infants who did not experience immediate catch-up growth would have permanent growth retardation. However, studies of malnourished children from developing countries who subsequently received adequate nourishment, as well as reports of children who were malnourished because of chronic diseases, such as celiac disease or cystic fibrosis, have demonstrated complete catch-up growth after the first year or two of life.

Rates of catch-up in weight gain can be 20 times faster than normal in children who are both stunted (low length/height for age) and wasted (low weight for height); that is, their weight deficit is greater than their length deficit. Once catch-up growth has reached an appropriate weight for length, the rate of weight gain is approximately three times the usual rate expected for age. The catch-up in linear growth reaches its peak about 1 to 3 months after treatment starts, whereas weight gain begins immediately (Ashworth and Millward, 1986).

Nutrient requirements, especially for energy and protein, vary depending on the rate and stage of catch-up. For instance, more protein and energy are needed during the very rapid weight gain period and in cases in which lean tissue is the major component of the weight gain. Guidelines for determining nutrient requirements are discussed in the accompanying box ("*Clinical Insight:* Obtaining Optimal Catch-Up Growth").

Assessing Growth

Because children are constantly growing and changing, periodic assessment of their progress allows any problems to be detected and treated early. Many children are seen by health care professionals only when they are ill, at which time growth and development may not be the focus of care.

A complete assessment of nutritional status includes the collection of anthropometric data. This includes length or height, weight, weight for height, and/or body mass index (BMI), all of which are plotted as percentiles on the National Center for Health Statistics (NCHS) growth charts (see Appendices 6 through 13). Other measurements, which are less commonly used but which provide estimates of body composition, include upper arm circumference, and triceps or subscapular fat folds. Care should be taken to use standardized equipment and techniques for obtaining and plotting growth measurements (Lohman et al., 1991). For instance, the charts designed for birth to 36 months of age are based on length measurements and nude weights, whereas the charts used for 2- to 18-year-olds are based on norms for standing height and weight with light clothing and without shoes (see Chapter 16).

Growth measurements must be recorded at regular intervals to indicate growth patterns. Height and weight measurements, if taken only once, do not lend themselves to an interpretation of growth status. Children generally maintain their heights and weights in the same **growth channels** during the preschool and early childhood years, although these channels are not well established until after 2 years of age. Individual children sometimes grow at faster or slower rates; nonetheless, they should follow along their same channels.

The height and weight of a child should be in proportion. This can be assessed by plotting the weight for height on the NCHS growth charts, or by determining BMI (see Appendix 20) and comparing this to norms for age (Rosner et al., 1998). A gross assessment can also be made by noting the difference between the height and weight channels; a difference of more than two channels suggests that the child is overweight or underweight and warrents further investigation. Midarm circumference and fat skinfold measurements yield more specific information regarding the composition of the child's weight.

Regular monitoring of growth enables trends to be identified early and intervention or education to be initiated so that long-term growth is not compromised. Weight that increases at a rapid rate and crosses growth channels suggests the development of obesity. Lack of weight gain or loss of weight over a period of months may be a result of undernutrition, an acute illness, an undiagnosed chronic disease, or significant emotional or family problems. Figure 10–1 demonstrates these changes in growth parameters.

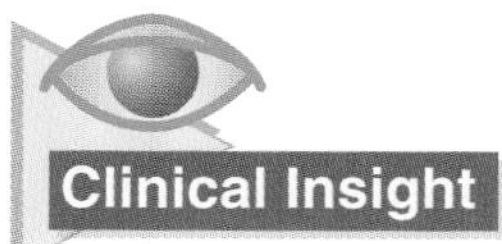

Obtaining Optimal Catch-Up Growth

Clinical management of a child who is growth retarded as a result of malnourishment, chronic disorder, or malabsorptive disease begins initially with a thorough assessment. This assessment includes determining the nature, severity, and duration of the nutritional insult, as well as the usual components of nutritional assessment (anthropometric, dietary, biochemical, clinical, and social/environmental assessments). Growth data (height, weight, BMI, and weight for height) are important criteria to follow over time, and arm circumference and triceps fatfold can provide estimates of body composition.

The nutritional goals depend on whether the child is stunted and chronically malnourished or primarily wasted (i.e., the weight deficit exceeds the length deficit). In the former case, the child may not be expected to gain more than 2 to 3 g/kg/day, whereas in the latter case, the child may gain as much as 20 g/kg/day (Ashworth and Millward, 1986). Once a child who is wasted "catches up" in weight, dietary management changes to facilitate a slower catch-up rate in both weight and linear growth.

The following table illustrates the varying requirements for energy and protein at different rates of weight gain. Generally, the protein need increases proportionately more than the energy need when the gain is greater.

Milk or a milk-based formula often provides the basis of the diet for young children during catch-up, along with developmentally appropriate foods. Frequent, small feedings are usually better tolerated than infrequent, large ones. Because total volume and the child's stomach capacity can be limiting factors, energy and nutrients can be concentrated or adjusted through the use of commercial liquid or powder supplements, formula concentration, increased use of fats and oils, or the addition of glucose polymers and medium-chain-triglyceride oil.

Growth and nutritional status should be monitored frequently, and dietary management can be modified as needed. In all cases, medical, social, and environmental concerns related to the growth retardation must be addressed and resolved.

DIETARY REQUIREMENTS FOR ENERGY AND PROTEIN AT DIFFERENT RATES OF WEIGHT GAIN*

RATE OF WEIGHT GAIN (g/kg/day)	ENERGY* (kcal/kg/day)	PROTEIN† (g/kg/day)	PROTEIN† (g of protein/100 kcal)	NO. OF WEEKS NEEDED TO RENOURISH WASTED CHILD‡
—	85	0.62	0.73	NA
1	90	0.83	0.92	50
2	94	1.04	1.11	25
5	108	1.67	1.55	10
10	130	2.72	2.09	5
20	174	4.82	2.77	2.5

(From Ashworth A, Millward DJ. Catch-up growth in children. Nutr Rev 44:157, 1986.)

NA, not applicable.

*This assumes that the intake for zero energy balance is 85.5 kcal/kg/day, and the cost of weight gain is 4.4 kcal/kg, which indicates that the composition of the tissue deposited is 73.5% lean and 26.5% fat.

†This assumes that the intake for zero N balance is 100 mg of N/kg/day, the protein content of weight gain is 14.7%, and the efficiency of dietary protein utilization for tissue deposition is 70%.

‡This assumes that the child has an initial weight deficit of 3 kg and an average body weight, during rehabilitation, of 8.5 kg.

NUTRIENT NEEDS

Because children are growing and developing bones, teeth, muscles, and blood, they need more nutritious food in proportion to their weight than do adults. They can become at risk for malnutrition when they have poor appetite of long duration, accept a limited number of foods, or dilute their diets significantly with nutrient-poor foods.

The Dietary Reference Intakes (DRIs), which replace the periodic revisions of the Recommended Dietary Allowances (RDAs), are based on current knowledge of nutrient intakes needed for optimal health (Food and Nutrition Board, 1989; Institute of Medicine, 1997 and 1998). The DRIs include Estimated Average Requirements (EARs), RDAs, Adequate Intakes (AIs), and Tolerable Upper Intake Levels (ULs). Most data for preschool and school-aged children are values interpolated from data on infants and adults. (See Table 8–1 and Table 15–1.) Because they provide a margin of safety (except for energy) above the physiologic requirement for most children in the United States, they cannot be applied appropriately to individual children. Thus, when intake falls below the recommended level, one cannot necessarily assume the child is inadequately nourished.

Energy

The energy needs of a child are determined on the basis of basal metabolism, rate of growth, and activity. Dietary energy must be sufficient to ensure growth and spare protein from being used for energy, without being so excessive that obesity results. A suggested proportion of energy is 50% to

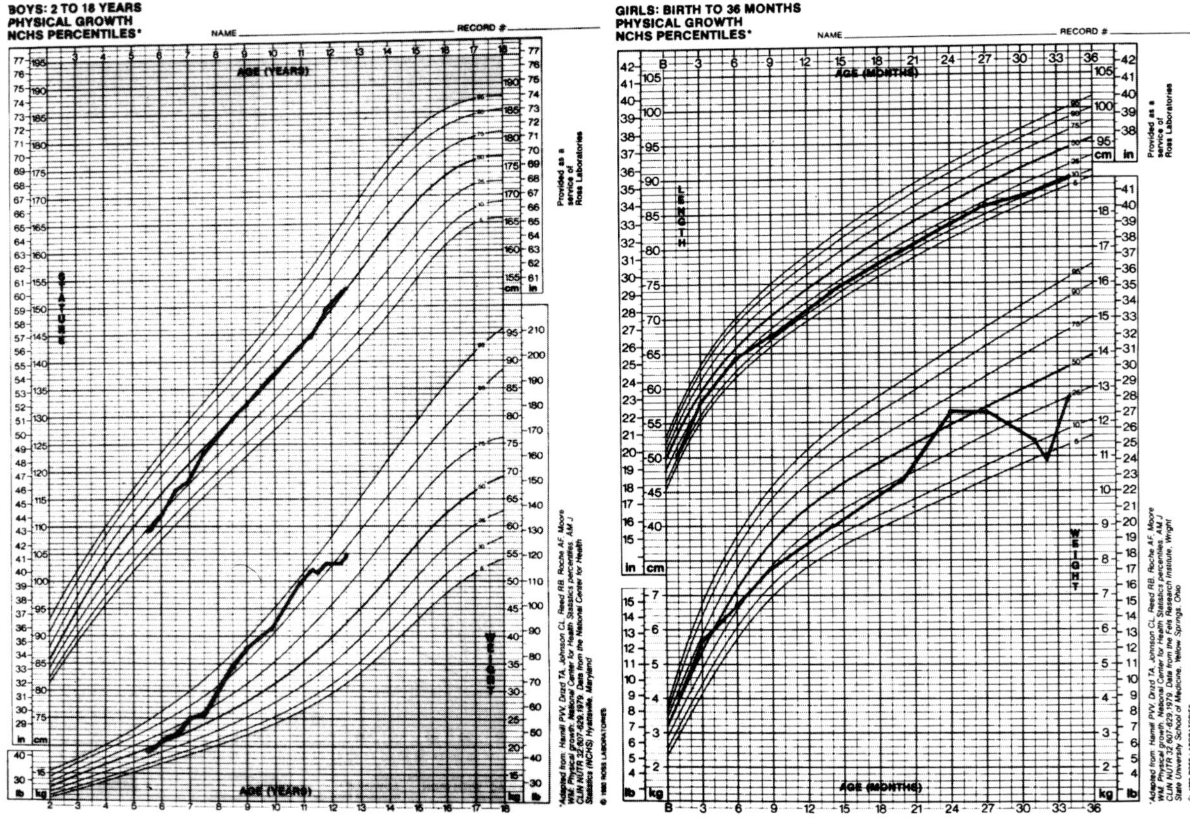

FIGURE 10–1 *A*, Excessive weight gain was noted in an 8-year-old boy after leg surgery that kept him immobilized in a body cast for 2 months. This was followed by a long period of stress due to family problems. After the age of 11 years, he became involved in a weight management clinic. *B*, Significant weight loss occurred in a 2-year-old girl during a prolonged period of diarrhea and feeding problems. After a diagnosis of celiac disease was established and a gluten-free diet was initiated, rebound weight gain was seen.

60% as carbohydrate, 25% to 35% as fat, and 10% to 15% as protein.

Newer techniques for assessing energy expenditure suggest that the RDAs for energy (Table 10–1) may be set too high. Using a doubly labeled water determination, the RDAs for infants may be overestimated by about 15%, and for children, by up to 25% (Cryan and Johnson, 1997). (See Chapter 2.)

Energy intakes of healthy, growing children of the same age and sex vary depending mainly on their activity level. A 7-year-old boy and a 10½-year-old girl approaching the age of puberty have significantly different factors determining their energy needs, even though they are in the same RDA age category. It is useful to determine energy requirements on an individual basis using kilocalories per kilogram of weight or per centimeter of height (Beal, 1970). Until modified, the RDA should be used as a guide for determining appropriate energy intakes for child nutrition programs.

TABLE 10–1 RECOMMENDED DIETARY ALLOWANCES FOR ENERGY AND PROTEIN FOR CHILDREN

	KCAL			G OF PROTEIN	
AGE (yrs)	Daily	Per kg	Per cm	Daily	Per kg
1–3	1300	102	14.4	16	1.2
4–6	1800	90	16.0	24	1.1
7–10	2000	70	15.2	28	1.0

(Reprinted with permission from Recommended Dietary Allowances, 10th ed. © 1989 by the National Academy of Sciences. Published by National Academy Press, Washington, DC.)

Protein

The need for protein per kilogram of body weight decreases from approximately 1.2 g in early childhood to 1 g in late childhood (see Table 10–1). Reported intakes from national surveys have shown that protein intakes are considerably higher, in the range of 10% to 16% of kcal (USDA, 1997).

Protein deficiency is uncommon in American children, partly because of our cultural emphasis on protein foods. Children who are most likely to be at risk for inadequate protein intake are those on strict vegan diets, those who have multiple food allergies, or those who have limited food selections because of fad diets, behavioral problems, or limited access to food.

Minerals and Vitamins

Minerals and vitamins are necessary for normal growth and development. Insufficient intake can cause impaired growth and result in deficiency diseases, as described in Chapters 4 and 5. The RDAs for different age groups are listed in Table 8–1 and Table 15–1.

Children between 1 and 3 years of age are at high risk for iron deficiency anemia. The rapid growth period of infancy is marked by an increase in both hemoglobin and total iron mass. In addition, the child's diet may not be rich in iron-containing foods. Recommended intakes must consider the relative absorbability, as well as the quantity, of iron in foods, especially those of plant origin. (See Chapters 5 and 35 for further discussions of iron.)

For this age group, calcium is needed for adequate mineralization and maintenance of growing bone. The new AI recommendations from the Food and Nutrition Board call for increased levels of calcium for older school-aged children (1300 mg of calcium per day for children 9 to 18 years of age), reflecting the need to support optimal bone mineralization (Institute of Medicine, 1997). The AI recommendations for 1- to 3-year-olds is 500 mg/day; an AI of 800 mg/day has been recommended for children 4 to 8 years of age. Actual need depends on individual absorption rates and dietary factors, such as quantities of protein, vitamin D, and phosphorus. Calcium retention in children between 2 and 8 years of age totals approximately 100 mg/day. Because calcium intake has very little influence on the degree of urinary calcium excretion during periods of rapid growth, children need two to four times as much calcium per kilogram as do adults (Matkovic, 1991). Because milk and other dairy products are the primary sources of calcium, children who consume none or limited amounts of these foods are at risk for calcium deficiency (Fig. 10–2).

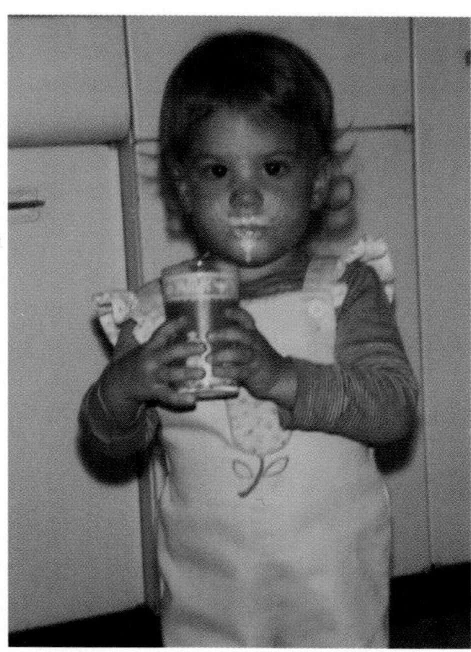

FIGURE 10–2 Milk and other dairy products supply the preschool child with the calcium and vitamin D needed for growing bones.

Vitamin D is needed for calcium absorption and for deposition of calcium in the bones. Because this nutrient is also available from the action of sunlight on subcutaneous tissues, the amount required from dietary sources depends on nondietary factors, such as geographical location and time spent outside. Children living in tropical areas may need no dietary vitamin D, or only 2.5 μg (100 IU) or less for optimal utilization of calcium (see "*Focus On:* Sunshine, Vitamin D, and Fortification" in Chapter 4). In the temperate zones, however, some dietary source is needed, and the RDA has been established at 10 μg (400 IU) for children. Vitamin D–fortified milk is the main source of this nutrient. Dairy products, such as cheese and yogurt, are not usually made from fortified milk, however.

Zinc is essential for growth; a deficiency results in growth failure, poor appetite, decreased taste acuity, and poor wound healing. An allowance of 10 mg/day of zinc is recommended, but because the best sources of zinc are meats and seafood, some children may regularly have a lower intake. Marginal zinc deficiency has been reported in preschool and school-aged children from both middle- and low-income families (Buzina et al., 1980; Hambidge et al., 1976). Diagnosis may be difficult because of variations in laboratory methods and values. Laboratory parameters, including plasma, serum, erythrocyte, hair, and urine levels, are of limited value in diagnosing zinc deficiency. Therefore, in many cases, a carefully controlled, short-term trial of zinc supplementation may be the only conclusive way to diagnose a problem (Krebs and Hambidge, 1996) (see Chapter 5).

Vitamin–Mineral Supplements

More than 50% of preschool children use supplements, most commonly a multivitamin–mineral with iron. The use of supplements usually decreases in older children. The highest rates of supplement use are found in families with more education, insurance coverage, and higher incomes, which may not be the families that are at greatest risk for inadequate diets (Yu et al., 1997). Supplements do not necessarily fulfill specific nutrient needs, however. For instance, significant levels of calcium, which is often consumed at levels below those recommended, is not commonly included in children's vitamin/mineral supplements.

The American Academy of Pediatrics does not support routine vitamin/mineral supplementation for normal children, except for fluoride supplements in unfluoridated areas. However, children at nutritional risk who may benefit from supplementation include (1) those from deprived families; (2) those with anorexia, poor appetites, and poor eating habits; (3) those with chronic diseases, such as cystic fibrosis or liver disease; (4) those enrolled in dietary programs for weight management; and (5) those consuming vegetarian diets without adequate intake of dairy products (Am. Academy of Pediatrics, 1998b).

Children who routinely take a multiple vitamin or vitamin–mineral will not incur risk if the supplement contains nutrients in amounts that do not exceed the RDA. However, megadoses should be avoided, particularly of the fat-soluble vitamins, large amounts of which can result in toxicity (see Chapter 4).

PROVIDING AN ADEQUATE DIET

Food and eating mean more than the provision of nutrients for body growth and maintenance. The development of feeding skills, food habits, and nutrition knowledge parallels the cognitive development that takes place in a series of stages, each laying the groundwork for the next. Table 10–2 outlines the development of feeding skills in terms of Piaget's theory of child psychology and development.

Patterns of Intake

The nutrients whose levels are most likely to be low or deficient in children's diets are calcium, iron, zinc, vitamin B_6, and vitamin A (Alaimo K et al., 1994; Nicklas, 1993b; Kennedy and Goldberg, 1995; USDA, 1997). Clinical signs of malnutrition in American children, however, are rare.

Studies of children have shown changing trends in their food patterns. These include an increased use of low-fat and nonfat milk, decreased intake of whole milk and eggs, increased snacking, and an increased tendency to consume food away from home (USDA, 1997; Nicklas, 1993b).

A recent analysis of national food intake data from studies of children and adolescents indicates that, in most cases, dietary intake does not meet the national recommendations for food groups as presented in the U.S. Dietary Guidelines and Food Guide Pyramid. Except for the dairy group, mean

TABLE 10–2 PIAGET'S THEORY OF COGNITIVE DEVELOPMENT IN RELATION TO FEEDING AND NUTRITION

DEVELOPMENTAL PERIOD	COGNITIVE CHARACTERISTICS	RELATIONSHIPS TO FEEDING AND NUTRITION
Sensorimotor (Birth–2 years)	Progression from neonate with automatic reflexes to intentional interaction with the environment and the beginning use of symbols	Progression is made from sucking and rooting reflexes to the acquisition of self-feeding skills.
		Food is used primarily to satisfy hunger, as a medium to explore the environment, and as an opportunity to practice fine motor skills.
Preoperational (2–7 years)	Thought processes become internalized; they are unsystematic and intuitive.	Eating becomes less the center of attention and secondary to social, language, and cognitive growth.
	Use of symbols increases.	Food is described by color, shape, and quantity, but there is only a limited ability to classify food into "groups."
	Reasoning is based on appearances and happenstance.	
	The child's approach to classification is functional and unsystematic.	Foods tend to be classed as "like" and "don't like."
	The child's world is viewed egocentrically.	Foods can be identified as "good for you," but reasons are unknown or mistaken.
Concrete operations (7–11 years)	The child can focus on several aspects of a situation simultaneously.	There is a beginning realization that nutritious food has a positive effect on growth and health, but limited understanding of how or why this occurs.
	Cause-and-effect reasoning becomes more rational and systematic.	
	The ability to classify, reclassify, and generalize emerges.	
	A decrease in egocentrism permits the child to take another's view.	Mealtimes take on a social significance.
		The expanding environment increases both the opportunities for and the influences on food selection (e.g., peer influence rises).
Formal operations (11 years and beyond)	Both hypothetical and abstract thought expand.	The concept of nutrients from food functioning at physiologic and biochemical levels can be understood.
	The child's understanding of scientific and theoretical processes deepens.	Conflicts in making food choices may be realized (i.e., knowledge of the nutritious value of foods may conflict with preferences and nonnutritive influences).

numbers of servings reported were less than the minimum recommendations for children aged 2 to 11 years. Only about 30% of this group met the recommendations for fruit, grain, and meat; 36% met vegetable recommendations. Total fat intake averaged 35% of energy intake (Munoz et al., 1997).

Population studies of nutritional status have reported an increased frequency of low nutrient intake in children from low-income families (USDA, 1987; Cook and Martin, 1997). In addition, studies have demonstrated an increased rate of poor dietary intake in certain populations, such as inner-city, low-income children and homeless children (Emmons, 1986; Taylor and Koblinsky, 1993).

Just as physical growth is not smooth and consistent, neither is food intake. **Appetite,** although subjective, usually follows the rate of growth and nutrient needs. A "good" appetite in infancy often becomes a "fair to poor" appetite in the young preschool-aged child, frequently causing parental anxiety.

By a child's first birthday, milk consumption has declined and will continue to do so in the next year. Vegetable intake decreases, and intakes of cereals, grain products, and sweets increase. Ground beef and hot dogs are preferred to meats that are harder to chew.

Changes in food consumption are reflected in nutrient intakes. Compared with nutrient intake in infancy, that in the early preschool years shows a decrease in calcium, phosphorus, riboflavin, iron, and vitamin A. Most other key nutrients remain relatively stable. During the early school years, a pattern of consistent and steady increases in all nutrients is seen until adolescence. For any age and sex group, a wide variability of nutrient intake is seen in healthy children.

Factors Influencing Food Intake

Numerous influences, some obvious and some subtle, determine the food intake and habits of children. It is well known that habits, likes, and dislikes are established in the early years and are carried through to adulthood, when change is often met with resistance and difficulty. The major influences on food intake in the developing years include family environment, societal trends, the media, peer pressure, and illness or disease.

Family Environment

For toddlers and preschool children, the family is the primary influence in the development of food habits. Parents and older siblings are significant models for young children as they learn, and imitate the individuals in their immediate environment. Food attitudes of parents have been shown to be strong predictors of food likes and dislikes, as well as of diet complexity, in children of primary school age. It is still not clear how much of the similarity between children's and their parents' food preferences is attributable to genetic influences and how much to environmental factors. One report suggests that food preferences are dictated, at least in part, by genetics. Monozygotic twins, aged 9 to 10 years, had more similarity in their food preferences than did dizygotic twins of the same sex (Falcigia and Norton, 1994).

Contrary to common belief, young children do not have the innate ability to choose a balanced, nutritious diet (see Chapter 8, "*Focus On:* Self-Selected Diets of Infants and Young Children"). Thus, parents and other adults are responsible for offering a variety of nutritious and developmentally appropriate foods. A positive feeding relationship includes a division of responsibility between parent and children. The parent provides safe, nutritious food as regular meals and snacks, and the children decide how much, if any, they eat.

The atmosphere around food and mealtime is also an important factor that influences attitudes toward food and eating. High expectations for a child's mealtime manners, with the threat of reprimand, can make dinner a dreaded time. Arguments and other emotional stress can also have a negative effect. Meals that are rushed create a hectic atmosphere and reinforce the tendency to eat too fast. A positive environment is one in which sufficient time is set aside to eat, occasional spills are tolerated, and conversation that includes all family members is encouraged (see Fig. 10–3).

Societal Trends

In recent decades, the nuclear family has changed from the traditional two-parent, one-income family. Almost three fourths of women with school-aged children are employed outside the home. Children, therefore, eat one or more meals at child care homes, day care centers, or schools. Because of time constraints, food purchasing and meal preparation routines may be modified to include proportionately more convenience or fast foods. The employment of mothers per se, however, does not appear to affect children's dietary intakes negatively (Johnson et al., 1993).

Recent increases in poverty rates now mean that one fifth of American children live in families with incomes below the poverty line, but these children constitute 40% of all the poor. In addition, the increasing numbers of single-parent households are predominantly headed by women, which usually means a lower income and less money for all expenses, including food, compared to households headed by men. The 1996 census reported a poverty rate of 59% for children younger than 6 years old who were living in families headed by a single female (Community Nutrition Institute, 1997). This "feminization of poverty" makes these families increasingly vulnerable to multiple stresses, including marginal health and nutritional status, owing in part to lack of jobs, child care, adequate housing, and health insurance (Luder and Bonforte, 1992).

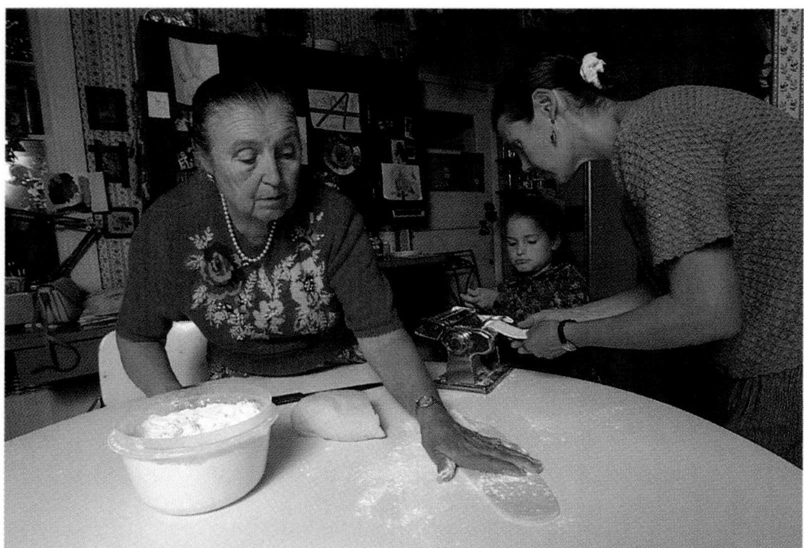

FIGURE 10–3 Three generations of Italian-Americans make a pasta dinner. The custom of eating authentically prepared foods gives mealtime a place of prominence in this home, not to be exchanged for "eating fast foods on the run." (From Leahy J, Kisilay P. Foundations of Nursing Practice: A Nursing Process Approach. Philadelphia: WB Saunders, 1998.)

Moreover, recent studies suggest that episodic hunger in American children is associated with poor psychosocial function (see "*Focus On:* Childhood Hunger: Effect on Behavioral and Emotional Function").

Media Messages

By the time the average American child has graduated from high school, he or she will have watched 15,000 hours of television and spent 11,000 hours in the classroom. School-aged children watch an average of more than 23 hours per week, whereas preschool children average 27 hours per week. One half of all commercials in children's programs advertise food, with a food commercial appearing approximately every 5 minutes (Kotz and Story, 1994). Most of the advertisements targeted toward children are for foods low in fiber and high in sugar, fat, or sodium.

Preschool children are generally unable to distinguish commercial messages from the regular program; in fact, they often pay more attention to the former. Many schools include a short television segment as part of the school day; however, the content is accompanied by advertisements aimed at chil-

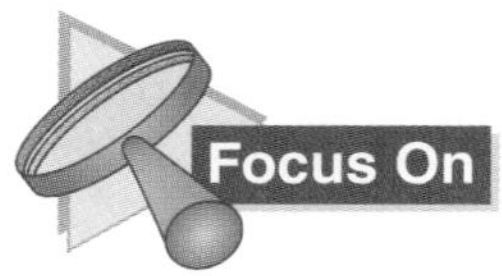

Childhood Hunger: Effect on Behavioral and Emotional Function

It is well accepted that malnourished children are less responsive, less inquisitive, and show decreased exploratory behavior. Specific nutrient deficiencies, such as iron-deficiency anemia, can also result in persistent decreased attention and problem-solving ability. Less clear is the impact of periodic hunger or **food insecurity** on a child's behavior or functioning. With recent federal welfare reform legislation, an increasing number of low-income children and their families are at risk for limited food resources.

The Community Childhood Hunger Identification Project (CCHIP) conducts surveys using standardized questions and large, rigorously selected samples to categorize families as "hungry," "at-risk for hunger," or "not hungry" (Kleinman et al., 1998). Results estimate that 8% of the children younger than 12 years of age living in the U.S. experience prolonged periodic food insufficiency each year. In one study, a group of 328 parents from a larger CCHIP study were asked to complete a Pediatric Symptom Checklist related to their child's emotional and behavioral symptoms. "Hungry" children were three times more likely than "at-risk for hunger" children, and seven times more likely than "not hungry" children, to have scores indicative of clinical dysfunction, such as aggression, irritability, oppositional behavior, and anxiety (Kleinman et al., 1998). In a similar CCHIP study, 204 school-aged children, their parents, and teachers provided information on psychosocial function using the parent Child Behavior Checklist (CBCL), the Connors Teacher Rating Scale, and a global assessment scale (Murphy JM, et al., 1998). Results showed that "hungry" and "at-risk for hunger" children were twice as likely as "not hungry" children to be considered functionally impaired, with a significant association between hunger and CBCL scores. Teachers reported an increased incidence of hyperactivity, absenteeism, and tardiness in the "hungry" and "at-risk for hunger" children. Although these studies have limitations because of other factors (i.e., stress, family dysfunction, or substance abuse) that may affect a child's function, there is a correlation between children's food insufficiency and their behavioral and academic function. If future studies support this relationship, implications would be clear for social policies that assure children their basic needs for optimal growth and development.

dren. As children get older, they gain knowledge about the purpose of commercial advertising and become more critical of its validity. However, they are still susceptible to the commercial message.

Television can also be detrimental to growth and development in that it encourages inactivity and passive use of leisure time. Indeed, television viewing, along with multiple media cues to eat, has been suggested as a factor contributing to excessive weight gain in children aged 6 to 17 years (Dietz and Gortmaker, 1985). However, a longitudinal and cross-sectional study of a large number of middle school girls found no significant association between television viewing and physical inactivity and obesity (Robinson, 1993).

Peer Influence

As children grow, their world expands and their social contacts increase in importance. Peer influence increases with age and extends to food attitudes and choices. This may be manifested by a sudden refusal of a food or a request for a current "popular" food. Decisions as to whether to participate in school lunch programs may be made more on the basis of what friends choose to do than on the menu offered. Such behaviors usually represent a phase that will change. Positive behaviors, such as a willingness to try new foods, can be reinforced. Parents need to set limits for undesirable influences, but also need to be realistic; struggles over food are self-defeating.

Illness or Disease

Children who are ill usually have a decreased appetite and limited food intake. Acute viral or bacterial illnesses are often of short duration, but may require an increase in fluids, protein, or other nutrients. Chronic conditions, such as asthma, congenital heart disease, and cystic fibrosis, may make it difficult to obtain nutrients for optimal growth. Children with these types of conditions are more likely to have behavior problems or family struggles around food. Children requiring special diets (e.g., those who have diabetes or phenylketonuria) not only have to adjust to the limits of foods allowed, but also have to deal with issues of independence and peer acceptance as they grow older. Some rebellion against the prescribed diet is typical, especially as the child approaches puberty.

Feeding the Preschool Child

The period from 1 to 6 years of age is marked by vast development and the acquisition of skills. The child learns to talk, run, and become a social being. The 1-year-old child primarily uses fingers to eat and may need assistance with a cup. By 2 years of age, he or she can hold a cup in one hand and use a spoon well (see Fig. 8–3), but the child may still prefer to use his or her hands at times. The 6-year-old child has refined skills and is beginning to use a knife for cutting as well as for spreading.

Because growth is slower during these years, appetite also decreases, often causing parental concern. Children have a decreased interest in food and an increased interest in the world around them. They develop **food jags** during this time, refusing previously accepted food, or asking for one particular food at each meal. This behavior may be attributable to boredom with the usual foods, or it may be a means of asserting newly discovered independence.

This is often a difficult time for parents, who may have concerns about the adequacy of their child's diet and who may be frustrated with their child's seemingly irrational food behavior. Struggles over control of the eating situation are fruitless; no child can be forced to eat. Parents need to understand that this period is developmental and temporary. They will still retain control over what foods are offered, and they will still have the opportunity to set limits on inappropriate behaviors. Neither rigid control nor a laissez-faire approach is likely to succeed. Parents and other caregivers should continue to offer a variety of foods, including the child's favorite ones, and substitutions for those foods that are refused should be made within the same food group. As Birch and colleagues (1991) have documented, preschool children tend to vary considerably in their meal intakes during the day, but their total daily energy intake remains fairly constant.

Preschool children, because of their smaller capacity and variable appetites, do best with small servings of food offered several times a day. Sizes of portions will appear small by adult standards. A general rule of thumb is to offer 1 tablespoon of each food for every year of age, and to serve more food according to appetite. Table 10–3 is a guide for food and portion sizes designed to provide an adequate diet for preschoolers. Most children eat four to six times a day, making snacks as important as meals in terms of their contribution to the total daily nutrient intake. Their snacks should be chosen carefully so that they are dense in nutrients; they should be not limited to cookies, soda pop, and chips. Likewise, foods least likely to promote dental caries should be selected. Wholesome snacks enjoyed by many young children include fresh fruit, cheese, raw vegetable sticks, milk, fruit juices, whole-grain crackers, and peanut butter sandwiches.

Senses other than taste play an important part in food acceptance by young children. Extreme temperatures are generally avoided, and many children actually prefer their food lukewarm. Some foods are rejected because of odor rather than taste. A sense of order in the food presentation is often required. Many children will not accept foods that touch each other on the plate, and casseroles and mixed dishes are not popular, except for spaghetti, macaroni and cheese, and pizza. It is not unusual for broken crackers to go uneaten or a sandwich to be refused

TABLE 10–3 FEEDING GUIDE FOR PRESCHOOL CHILDREN*

	2- TO 3-YEAR-OLDS		4- TO 6-YEAR-OLDS		
FOOD	**Portion Size**	**No. of Servings**	**Portion Size**	**No. of Servings**	**COMMENTS**
Milk and dairy products	½ cup (4 oz.)	4–5	½–¾ cup	3–4 (4–6 oz)	The following may be substituted for ½ cup of liquid milk: ½–¾ oz cheese, ½ cup yogurt, 2½ T nonfat dry milk powder.
Meat, fish, poultry, or equivalent	1–2 oz	2	1–2 oz	2	The following may be substituted for 1 oz of meat, fish, or poultry: 1 egg, 2 T peanut butter, 4–5 T cooked legumes.
Fruits and vegetables		4–5		4–5	Include one green leafy or yellow vegetable for vitamin A, such as spinach, carrots, broccoli, or winter squash.
Vegetables					
Cooked	2–3 T		3–4 T		
Raw†	Few pieces		Few pieces		
Fruit					Include one vitamin C–rich fruit, vegetable, or juice, such as citrus juices, orange, grapefruit sections, strawberries, melon in season, tomato, or broccoli.
Raw	½–1 small		½–1 small		
Canned	2–4 T		4–6 T		
Juice	3–4 oz		4 oz		
Bread and grain products		3		3	The following may be substituted for 1 slice of bread: ½ cup spaghetti, macaroni, noodles, or rice; 5 saltines, 1 tortilla, or ½ bagel.
Whole-grain or enriched bread	½–1 slice		1 slice		
Cooked cereal	¼–½ cup		½ cup		
Dry cereal	½–1 cup		1 cup		

(Adapted from Lowenberg ME. Development of food patterns in young children. In: Trahms CM, Pipes P. Nutrition in Infancy and Childhood, 6th ed. St Louis: WCB/McGraw-Hill, 1997.)

*This is a guide to a basic diet. Fats, oils, sauces, desserts, and snack foods provide additional kilocalories to meet the needs of a growing child. Foods can be selected from this pattern for both meals and snacks.

†Do not give to children until they can chew well.

because it is "cut the wrong way." Many young children are keenly sensitive to food palatability and can readily detect off-flavors or reject overcooked vegetables.

The physical setting of children's meals is as important as the emotional atmosphere. Children should not be made to eat with feet dangling and arms reaching up to a table at chest height. Rather, sturdy, child-sized tables and chairs are ideal; if children eat at a standard table with the family, a high chair, "booster chair," or other similar modification should be used to make them comfortable. Bowls, plates, and cups should be nonbreakable and heavy enough to resist spilling. For very young children, a shallow bowl is often better than a plate, to facilitate scooping. Thick, short-handled spoons and forks allow for an easier, less tiring grasp.

Young children usually do not eat well if they are tired, and this needs to be considered when meal and play times are scheduled. A quiet activity or rest immediately before eating is conducive to a relaxed, enjoyable meal. To stimulate a good appetite, however, children need active, large motor activity and time spent outside in the fresh air.

Children should not be given any food or drink within 1½ hours of a meal. It does not take much to satisfy a young child's appetite, and even small snacks may result in poor eating at mealtime.

Clinical experience suggests that fruit juices, especially apple juice and juice drinks, are an increasingly common beverage for young children, both at home and in group settings. These juices frequently replace water and milk in a child's diet. In addition to nutritional concerns, this practice may have other effects. One study of healthy children and those with chronic, nonspecific diarrhea revealed that ingestion of fruit juices often resulted in carbohydrate malabsorption (Hyams et al., 1988). Pear and apple juice, in particular, have been implicated (Smith et al., 1995). This information suggests that these juices should be avoided when treating acute diarrhea with clear liquids. For children with chronic diarrhea, a trial of restricting fruit juices may be warranted before more costly diagnostic tests are done.

Excessive fruit juice consumption (12 to 30 oz/day) has been identified as a contributing factor in some cases of failure to thrive in toddlers. A reduction in juice intake, along with nutritional education designed to increase total energy intake, resulted in improved growth (Smith and Lifshitz, 1994). A recent report of children aged 2 and 5 years linked excess fruit juice intake (>12 oz/day) to short stature and obesity (Dennison et al., 1997). However, study design and methodology prevented cause-and-effect conclusions to be drawn. It is quite possible that excess juice intake in young preschool children replaces intake of higher-energy foods and can take the edge off a child's appetite, resulting in decreased intake and poor growth. It is also possible that a large volume of juice, in addition to other dietary and activity factors, may contribute to or sustain an overweight condition in a child. Practical guidelines for parents suggest a juice intake of 4 oz or less per day for infants, and a limit of 12 oz daily for older children.

Group Feeding

A generation ago, the food experiences of most preschool children centered on home and family. Today, because of changing family life-styles, many children spend part or most of their days in day care centers, preschools, or Head Start programs. At such places, they may consume only a snack, or as many as two meals and two snacks per day, depending on the time involved. For many children, therefore, more than half of their nutrients may be provided in these settings.

Food service in group feeding settings, such as day care centers, Head Start programs, and preschool programs in elementary schools, is regulated by federal or state guidelines. Many facilities and some day care homes may participate in USDA-sponsored child nutrition programs. The quality of meals and snacks can vary greatly; parents should investigate this aspect of care when selecting a placement for their child. In addition to providing the child with optimal nutrients, a program should offer food that is appealing, safely prepared, and appropriate, considering cultural and developmental patterns.

Because of peer pressure, children usually eat well in group settings (Fig. 10–4). These settings are also ideal environments for nutrition education programs, both at mealtimes and as the focus for various learning activities. Experiencing new foods, participating in simple food preparation, and planting a garden are activities that develop and enhance positive food habits and attitudes.

Feeding the School-Aged Child

Growth during the school-age years (ages 6 to 12) is slow but steady, paralleled by a constant increase in food intake. In addition to being in school a greater part of the day, the child is also likely to begin participating in clubs and group activities, sports, and recreational programs. The influence of peers and significant adults, such as teachers, coaches, or sports idols, is increased. Friendships and other social contacts become more important. Except for severe cases, most behavioral problems connected with food have been resolved by this age, and the child enjoys eating to alleviate hunger and obtain social satisfaction.

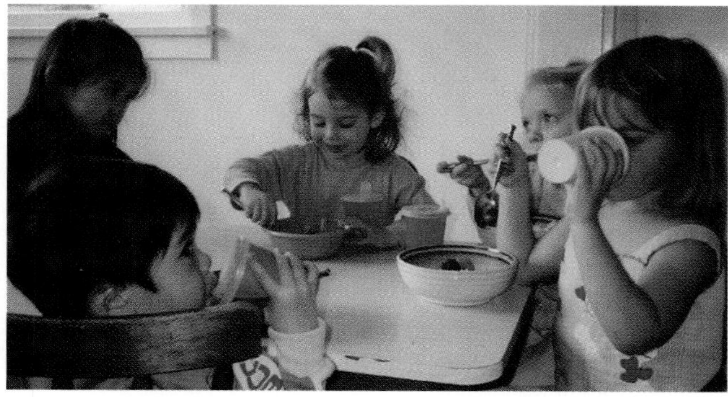

FIGURE 10–4 Children who eat with each other in an appropriate environment often eat better and try a wider variety of foods than they do when alone.

The school-aged child may participate in the school lunch program or may carry a lunch from home. The National School Lunch Program, administered by the U.S. Department of Agriculture (USDA), provides approximately one third of the RDA for students. Children from low-income families are eligible for free or reduced-price meals. In addition, the School Breakfast Program has been expanded to include about 70% of the schools participating in the lunch program.

Efforts have been made to decrease plate waste by altering menus to accommodate student preferences, allowing students to decline one or two menu items, and offering salad bars. However, there is still concern over excessive amounts of fat, salt, and sugar in school meals (Nicklas, 1995; Burghardt et al., 1995). This concern has resulted in a move to incorporate the U.S. Dietary Guidelines into child nutrition programs by reducing the fat content of recipes and offering a greater variety of fresh fruits and vegetables, whole grain products, and fewer baked desserts (USDA, 1995) (see Chapter 14). Children requiring special diets (e.g., low-fat, allergy, or low-sodium, diets) will need to have the menus modified to meet their needs. Children receiving special education services who participate in school meals are eligible for modified meals, as indicated by their diagnosis or feeding abilities (Horsley et al., 1996).

Consumption of school meals is also affected by the daily school schedule, and the amount of time allotted for children to eat. A recent study of elementary school students found that plate waste was significantly decreased when recess was scheduled before, rather than after, the lunch period (Getlinger et al., 1996).

Studies of lunches packed at home indicate that they usually provide fewer nutrients but less fat than the school lunch meal. Favorite foods tend to be packed, and less variety is seen. Food choices are limited to those that travel well and require no heating or refrigeration. A typical well-balanced lunch brought from home would include a sandwich with whole-grain bread and a protein-rich filling (lean meat, egg, cheese, peanut butter), fresh fruit and/or vegetable, low-fat milk, and an optional cookie, graham cracker, or other simple dessert. Food safety measures (e.g., keeping perishable foods well chilled) must be observed when packing lunches for school.

Because of changes in family life-styles, many school-aged children are responsible for preparing their own breakfasts. It is not uncommon for children to skip this meal altogether, even in the primary grades. Children who skip breakfast tend to consume less energy and fewer nutrients than those

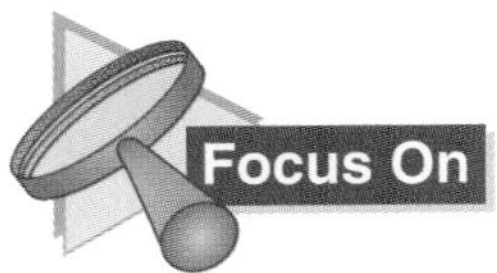

Breakfast: Does It Impact Learning?

The educational benefits of school feeding programs, particularly the role of breakfast in school performance, have been debated and discussed for decades. Experimental studies of healthy children, aged 9 to 11 years, have shown that those who fasted overnight (i.e., skipped breakfast) and were then given a variety of tests had increased errors, slower stimulus discrimination, and slower memory recall (Pollitt et al., 1998a). Similar studies in other countries with children who were at nutritional risk (i.e., wasted and stunted) have demonstrated even poorer performance on the learning tasks without breakfast (Pollitt et al., 1998a). These studies suggest that brain function is sensitive to short-term variations in nutrient availability. A short fast may impose greater stress on young children than adults, resulting in metabolic alterations as various homeostatic mechanisms work to maintain circulating glucose concentrations (Pollitt et al., 1998a). A recent report on breakfast and cognitive function in elementary school children suggests that timing of the meal may be a factor (Vaisman et al., 1996). Those receiving breakfast 30 minutes before testing scored higher than baseline testing compared to those who had breakfast 2 hours before testing. Although this may be related to glucose concentration, further controlled studies relating to meal timing are needed.

A field study in a predominantly low-income school district compared academic achievement before and after introducing the School Breakfast Program. The children who received the school breakfast had significantly improved basic skills test scores and less tardiness than those who did not receive the breakfast (Meyers et al., 1989). Similar school-based studies in Jamaica and Peru have also shown the introduction of breakfast programs to result in better school performance and attendance (Pollitt, 1995).

This knowledge underscores the potential benefits of school feeding programs that include breakfast, not only for low-income and at-risk children, but for all school children. A recent summary outlines the breakfast and cognition issue, including challenges of research design, appropriate cognitive and biochemical measures, and relevance to nutrition public policy (Pollitt and Mathews, 1998).

who eat breakfast (Nicklas et al., 1993a). A review of the effects of breakfast on cognition and school performance suggests that children who go to school without breakfast are more likely to experience deficits in their performance than those who eat breakfast (Pollitt, 1995) (see "*Focus On:* Breakfast: Does It Impact Learning?").

Snacks are commonly consumed by school-aged children, primarily after school and in the evening. As children grow older and acquire money to spend, they tend to consume more snacks from vending machines, fast-food restaurants, and neighborhood groceries. Families can continue to offer wholesome snacks at home and support nutrition education efforts in the school. In most cases, good eating habits established in the first few years carry a child through this period of decision making and responsibility.

PREVENTING CHRONIC DISEASE

To help decrease the prevalence of chronic conditions, such as heart disease, cancer, diabetes, and obesity in Americans, governmental and nonprofit agencies have promoted healthy eating habits. Their recommendations include the Dietary Guidelines for Americans, the USDA Food Guide Pyramid, the National Cholesterol Education Program (NCEP), and the National Cancer Institute Dietary Guidelines (see Chapter 15).

The NCEP recommendations for children older than 2 years of age are the same as those for adults: (1) no more than 30% of calories from fat (10% or less from saturated fat, up to 10% from unsaturated fat, and 10% to 15% from monosaturated fat), and (2) no more than 300 mg of cholesterol per day. Cholesterol screening is also recommended for children with family risk factors: parents or grandparents who have had a cardiac event before the age of 55 years or at least one parent with a cholesterol level of 250 mg/dL or more (NHLBI, 1991) (see Chapter 26).

Although controversy remains regarding the rationale and long-term consequences of reducing cholesterol levels in children, evidence supports selective cholesterol screening (Gidding, 1993). The American Academy of Pediatrics (1998a) does not advise following a diet that restricts intake to less than 30% of calories from fat. Although severe calorie and fat reduction will result in failure to thrive, one study of preschool children showed that stature and growth were no different between those with the lowest (27.1%) and those with the highest (38.4%) total dietary fat (Shea et al., 1993). Dietary trends have demonstrated decreases in total fat, saturated fat, and percentage of calories from fat (36% in 1987 to 1988 and 32% to 33% in 1994 to 1996) in children's diets, but these levels have not yet met the NCEP guidelines (Nicklas, 1993b; USDA, 1997).

Reports have shown that, from the age of 4 years to adolescence, children can consume diets that comply with the NCEP guidelines without compromising energy or nutrient intake (Dixon et al., 1997). On the other hand, studies using low-fat diets with children have shown little effect on blood cholesterol levels, blood pressure measurements, or body weight (Leupker et al., 1996; Dietary Intervention Study in Children, 1995). Some critics warn of the risks from broad implementation of low-fat diets for children (Olson, 1995). Canadian pediatricians suggest a gradual decrease in fat to reach the goal of no more than 30% of energy from fat by the time linear growth is reached in adolescence (Joint Working Group, 1995).

As there are no apparent risks to growth or nutrient intake for children who consume a diet meeting the NCEP guidelines, a gradual transition to a lower-fat diet after the age of 2 years is appropriate. Health practitioners should screen for dietary fat intake in children with poor growth, and inquire about excessive use of low-fat and nonfat foods, especially in young children.

Osteoporosis is a disease of the elderly, but its prevention begins in childhood by maximizing calcium retention and bone density in the growing years. Balance studies of adolescent girls suggest that, to reach maximum calcium balance, young teenaged girls may need to consume more than the recommended amounts (Matkovic and Heany, 1992). Even in prepubertal children, calcium supplementation, when coupled with an average calcium dietary intake, was found to increase bone mineral density significantly (Johnston et al., 1992). This evidence supports the recent increase to 1300 mg/day in the AI for calcium for children and adolescents 9 to 18 years of age (Institute of Medicine, 1997). Because recent food consumption surveys show an increased intake of soft drinks and noncitrus juices among children, as well as a decrease in total milk consumption, education is needed to encourage young people to achieve an appropriate intake of calcium food sources (USDA, 1997).

Education about dietary fiber and disease prevention has mainly been focused on the adult population, and only limited information is available on dietary fiber intake of children. Recent national survey data indicate that 3- to 5-year-olds consume a mean of 10.7 g of dietary fiber per day, up slightly from the late 1980s; school-aged children consume approximately 13 g per day (USDA, 1997). To promote dietary fiber intake for health and normal laxation in children, a recent recommendation suggests that children older than 2 years of age should consume, at a minimum, an amount of dietary fiber that is equivalent to their age plus 5 g per day; indeed, they can safely consume an amount equal to their age plus 10 g per day (Williams, 1995). This recommendation has been endorsed by several national child health organizations. Educational efforts are needed, however, to increase fiber intake in older school-aged children.

A decreased level of physical activity in children has been noted for several decades, and this is thought to be a substantial contributor to pediatric obesity. Participation in school physical education programs generally decreases with increasing grades, with high school girls having the lowest participation rates (Kohl and Hobbs, 1998). Regular physical activity not only helps control excess weight gain, but also improves strength and endurance, enhances self-esteem, and reduces anxiety and stress. Activity, combined with an optimal calcium intake, is associated with increased bone mineral density in children and adolescents (Gunnes and Lehmann, 1996). The Council on Physical Education for Children has recommended that elementary school children be active for at least a cumulative 60 minutes a day, including moderate to vigorous activity (Corbin and Pangrazi, 1998). The Centers for Disease Control (CDC) and Prevention have recently developed guidelines for school and community programs to promote lifelong physical activity among young people (CDC, 1997) (www.cdc.gov/needphp/dnpa).

In an effort to promote dietary habits that can reduce the incidence of chronic diseases later in life, the Dietary Guidelines for Americans and the Food Guide Pyramid have been applied to children as well as their parents. Some experts and professional groups, however, support the development of separate dietary guidelines for children so as to ensure that their primary nutritional needs for growth and development are met, and secondarily, to prevent disease (The American Dietetic Association, 1995; National Dairy Council, 1996).

Overall, a child's diet should provide adequate energy to support optimal growth and development without excess fatness. Emphasis should be placed on intake of fruits and vegetables, whole-grain products, low-fat dairy products, legumes, and lean meat, fish, and poultry. Fermentable carbohydrate intake should be controlled for good dental health. Adherence to these general dietary guidelines is beneficial for children in that total fat is reduced and intake of dietary fiber and beta-carotene and other phytochemicals is increased (see Chapter 12), resulting in a more nutrient-dense diet.

NUTRITIONAL CONCERNS

Obesity

The increasing prevalence of obesity in children is a significant public health problem. The NHANES III survey (1988–1991), using BMIs as criteria, documented an overweight prevalence in children and adolescents of 11%, based on the 95th percentile cutoff, with an additional 14% having BMIs between the 85th and 95th percentiles (Troiano and Flegal, 1998). A similar increasing prevalence of obesity among low-income preschool children has recently been reported from the national Pediatric Nutrition Surveillance System. Using weight-for-height criteria, 10.2% of children younger than 5 years of age were overweight based on the 95th percentile cutoff, and 21.6% were overweight based on an 85th percentile cutoff (Mei et al., 1998). These prevalences have continued to increase since the mid-1960s and especially since the late 1970s. Although there is increased appreciation of the role of inheritability in obesity development, based on studies of molecular genetics and animal obesity phenotypes, these recent increases in overweight prevalence cannot be explained by genetics alone (Rosenbaum and Leibel, 1998).

Obesity in childhood is usually not a benign condition, despite the popular belief that overweight children will "outgrow" their condition. The longer a child has been overweight, the more likely that that state will continue into adolescence and adulthood. Consequences of obesity in childhood include psychosocial difficulties (discrimination, negative self-image, decreased socialization), increased height with possible inappropriate societal expectations, and increased frequency of hyperlipidemia, hypertension, and abnormal glucose tolerance.

Children whose normal growth adiposity rebound occurs before 5½ years of age are more likely to be fatter at adulthood than those whose adiposity rebound occurs after 7 years of age (Rolland-Cachera et al., 1987). The timing of the adiposity rebound and excess fatness in adolescence are two critical factors in the development of obesity in childhood, with the later period being the most predictive of adult obesity and related morbidity (Dietz, 1994).

Energy intakes have remained stable over the past 20 years, suggesting that diet is not a major contributor to the increased prevalence of obesity (Kennedy and Goldberg, 1995). Inactivity, however, plays a major role in obesity development, whether it results from television and computer use, limited opportunities for physical activity, or safety concerns that prevent children from enjoying free play outdoors. Two studies have suggested metabolic changes in children who watch television. Klesges and co-workers (1993) demonstrated a metabolic rate lower than resting rate in 8- to 12-year-old children who were watching television. The decrease in metabolic rate appeared to be more pronounced in obese children. Another study documented excessive television viewing in children whose cholesterol levels were greater than 200 mg/dL; those watching more than 4 hours per day had the highest relative risk for high cholesterol levels (Wong, 1992).

Determining obesity in growing children is difficult. Some excess fatness may occur at either end of the childhood spectrum; that is, the 1-year-old toddler and the prepubertal child may be heavier and fatter for developmental and physiologic reasons, but this is not often permanent. Height and weight alone do not allow for the highly muscled child. BMI, which is a useful clinical tool for assessing weight in comparison to height, has its limitations in determining obesity owing to variability related to sex, race, and maturation stage (Daniels et al., 1997). Children at risk for obesity should be monitored frequently so that early intervention can be provided.

Management of obesity in children should include consideration of nutrient needs for growth. Success is most likely to result from a program that includes family involvement, dietary modifications, nutrition information, activity planning, and behavioral components (Mahan, 1987) (see Case Study, p. 254). A follow-up study of 158 obese children who participated in regular, long-term group meetings revealed that, 10 years after treatment, 30% were not obese, and 34% had decreased their percentage of overweight by 20% or more (Epstein et al., 1994). The best outcomes were seen in children who participated in programs that were family-based and included a physical activity component. These long-term outcomes were better than those seen in similar programs for adults. Depending on the child, goals for weight change may include a decrease in the rate of weight gain, maintenance of weight, or, in severe cases, a slow weight loss (see Chapter 23).

Prevention of childhood obesity needs to be addressed as an important public health policy in the United States. In addition to studies of etiologic factors, prevention will require family/child anticipatory education, school and community support for physical activity opportunities in which personal safety is assured, and federal guidance for clinical assessment and ongoing research. Care is needed to avoid overdiagnosis and overtreatment of these children. The hazards of treating children who are overweight or obese include the following: alternate undereating and overeating, feelings of failure in meeting external expectations, ignoring of internal cues for appetite and satiation, feelings of deprivation and isolation, an increased risk for disordered eating, and increasingly poor or sustained poor self-image. Satter (1996) has suggested a new paradigm for pediatric obesity that emphasizes "trust" over "control." This approach can be applied both clinically and in broad prevention programs.

Underweight/Failure to Thrive

Weight loss, lack of weight gain, or **failure to thrive** can be caused by an acute or chronic illness, a restricted diet, poor appetite, poor appetite secondary to constipation or medication, deprivation, or simple lack of food. Careful assessment is critical and must include the social and emotional environment of the child, as well as physical findings. If the child is also short in stature, the possibility of a zinc deficiency should be investigated.

Reports have documented growth failure in children that is the result of contemporary life-style factors. Poor weight gain, short stature, and delayed puberty were noted in boys and girls 9 to 17 years of age who deliberately restricted their energy intake for fear of becoming obese (Pugliese et al., 1983). Surveys of preadolescent children indicate that many have the same body image concerns (wanting to be thinner), dieting patterns, and eating patterns (frequent consumption of diet soft drinks) as adolescents (Gustafson-Larson and Terry, 1992). In other reports, failure to thrive in preschool children was associated with food restriction stemming from parents' overconcern regarding obesity, atherosclerosis, or other potential health problems, and with excess fruit juice intake (Pugliese et al., 1987; Smith and Lifshitz, 1994).

Lack of fiber in the diet or poor bowel habits that lead to chronic constipation can result in poor appetite, diminished intake and failure to thrive. In such cases, relieving the constipation by adding fruits (especially dried ones) and vegetables, high-fiber breakfast cereals, and/or bran muffins and legumes to the diet will help to relieve constipation and improve the appetite and, eventually, promote weight gain. Because fiber intake is often low in children, especially those who are "picky" eaters, this should always be addressed in the evaluation.

The provision of adequate energy and nutrients, as well as nutrition education, should be among the goals of the management plan. Attempts should be made to increase appetite and modify the environment to ensure optimal intake.

Iron Deficiency

Iron deficiency is one of the most common nutrient disorders of childhood, affecting approximately 9% of 1- to 3-year-olds. Certain low-income populations and other groups, such as Native Alaskans, have exhibited an increased incidence of iron deficiency, even in older children. Possible factors associated with iron deficiency, with or without anemia, include parents' educational level and lack of medical care, as well as dietary intake.

In addition to children's growth and their increased physiologic need for iron, dietary factors also play a role. A 1-year-old child may continue to consume a large quantity of milk, to the exclusion of other foods, resulting in "milk anemia." Many young preschool children do not like meat, so most of their iron intake is in the nonheme form, which is absorbed less efficiently. Iron deficiency is less of a problem in older preschool and school-aged children.

Infants with iron deficiency, both with and without anemia, tend to score lower on standardized tests of mental development and have demonstrated decreased attention to relevant information needed for problem-solving (Pollitt et al., 1986). As reported in one study, the impact of iron deficiency occurring in infancy can still be observed at the age of 5 years, as evidenced by poor performance on developmental tests (Lozoff et al., 1991). These data have clinical significance in terms of assessing the nutrient quality of individual diets, as well as in terms of policy-making decisions intended to address the nutritional needs of low-income, high-risk children.

Attention to good dietary sources of iron can help prevent iron deficiency anemia. To enhance absorbability of nonheme iron sources, education should be aimed at increasing the amount of ascorbic acid and meat, fish, and poultry in the diet. See Chapter 35 for a further discussion of anemia.

Dental Caries

Nutrition and eating habits are important factors affecting dental health. Optimal nutrient intake is needed to produce strong teeth and healthy gums. The composition of the diet and an individual's eating habits (i.e., dietary carbohydrate intake, retentiveness of foods, and frequency of eating) are significant factors in the development of dental caries. Infants and young children who drink sweetened liquids from a bottle, at bedtime or frequently throughout the day, are susceptible to baby bottle tooth decay (BBTD) (discussed in Chapter 29).

Because children tend to consume snacks regularly, those that are least cariogenic should be emphasized. When eaten with high-sugar foods, protein foods, such as cheese, nuts, and meats, do not cause a decrease in plaque pH and may help protect against caries.

Desserts and sweet foods should be consumed infrequently and incorporated into meals to reduce their cariogenicity. Parents provide strong role models for their children in terms of practicing positive food habits and good dental hygiene. A toothbrush should be introduced in the toddler period, and daily oral hygiene should be performed. As fluoride is highly effective in caries prevention, it should be supplied to children via a fluoridated water supply or a fluoride supplement (see Chapter 29).

Allergies

Food allergies usually manifest themselves in infancy and childhood and occur more frequently when there is a family history of allergies. Allergic responses most often include respiratory or gastrointestinal symptoms and skin reactions, but in some cases they may be more vague, such as fatigue, lethargy, and behavior changes. Controversy exists over the true definition of food allergy, and tests for allergies to food are not specific and unequivocal. See Chapter 41 for further discussion of this topic.

Attention-Deficit Hyperactivity Disorder

Attention-deficit hyperactivity disorder (ADHD), commonly called hyperactivity, is a clinical diagnosis based on specific criteria (i.e., excessive motor activity, impulsiveness, short attention span, low tolerance to frustration, and onset before 7 years of age). Because some dietary factors have been suggested as causes of this disorder, various dietary treatments have been promoted, such as the Feingold diet, omission of sugar, allergy elimination diets, and megavitamin therapy.

In the early 1970s, Feingold proposed that many children were hyperactive because they were sensitive to salicylates and artificial colorings and flavorings in their food. His popular treatment was to remove those substances from the child's diet; later, the preservatives BHA and BHT were eliminated. Although early anecdotal reports were positive, studies using controlled double-blind dietary challenges and objective behavior rating scales have not supported the Feingold hypothesis (Lipton and Mayo, 1983). Of the hyperactive children who seemed to respond most favorably to the diet (about 5% to 10%), most were preschoolers. One study of preschool hyperactive boys, involving total diet replacement (Feingold diet plus elimination of specific foods believed to bother the children) with crossover between experimental and control diets, revealed a more positive impact of the diet (Kaplan et al., 1989). In this study, almost 50% of the boys showed some improvement in behavior, based on accepted rating scales.

These conflicting study results may be explained in part by a placebo effect or by altered interactions between the family and the child with ADHD. For the family who wishes to try the diet, however, there is little nutritional risk. Periodic nutritional counseling should be provided, and the families should be urged to consider other helpful treatments for their child's disorder, such as behavioral management, special education, and medication.

Although sugar has popularly been implicated as a cause of hyperactive behavior in children, controlled challenge studies have not demonstrated any negative behavioral effects (Wolraich et al., 1995). In one study, the children who consumed sugar were actually quieter and less active than those receiving the placebo (Behar et al., 1984). Although there is little evidence to support a sugar-induced behavioral effect, the benefits of decreasing sugar consumption (e.g., improved dental health and a more nutrient-dense diet) should be emphasized.

Another theory proposes that altered fatty acid metabolism is a factor in ADHD. One study found significantly lower concentrations of key fatty acids, including *docosahexaenoic acid (DHA)* and *arachidonic acid,* in boys with ADHD compared to those in controls (Stevens et al., 1995). Some of the subjects also showed general symptoms of essential fatty acid deficiency, but dietary intake of fatty acids was not low. Nearly half of the subjects with ADHD were also receiving stimulant medication. No cause-and-effect relationship between fatty acid metabolism and ADHD has been documented, and limited supplementation studies have not demonstrated significant benefit.

Children who have allergies may exhibit some of the behaviors (e.g., irritability, poor attention) that are seen in children with ADHD, but it remains questionable whether elimination diets can alleviate these symptoms or alter negative behaviors. Likewise, the value of megavitamin therapy for ADHD has not been supported in controlled studies (Haslam et al., 1984).

NUTRITION EDUCATION

As children grow, they acquire knowledge and assimilate concepts by leaps and bounds. These early years are ideal for providing nutrition information and promoting positive attitudes about all foods. This learning can be informal and natural and can take place in the home, with parents as behavioral models and with provision of a diet representing a wide variety of foods. Food can be used in daily experiences for the toddler and preschooler, and can be used to promote the development of language, cognition, and self-help behaviors (i.e., labeling; describing size, shape, and color; sorting; assisting in preparation; and tasting).

More formal nutrition education is provided at preschools, in Head Start programs, in schools, and at websites such as that of the National Center for Education in Maternal and Child Health (www.ncemch.org). Attempts to teach children nutrition concepts and information should take into account their developmental level. The play approach, based on Piaget's theory of learning, is a method for teaching nutrition and fitness to school-aged children (Rickard et al., 1995).

The concept of nutrients is abstract, and so is lost on preschoolers and most primary school children. Some nutrition curricula are too sophisticated for the children's conceptual abilities, and modifications may be necessary to make the educational experiences meaningful. Activities and information that focus on children's real-world relationships with food are most likely to yield positive results.

CASE STUDY

Brian J. is a 7-year, 4-month-old boy who gained 15 lb during the last school year. Evaluation revealed that Brian moved to a new home and school a year ago following his parents' divorce. After-school care was provided by an elderly neighbor who loved to bake for Brian. Because he had no friends in the neighborhood, his main leisure activities were watching television and playing video games. His mother reports relying more on take-out and fast-food meals because of the time constraints of her full-time job (as well as weight gain for herself), but she has recently started an aerobics class with a friend and is interested in developing healthier eating habits.

Following joint sessions with Brian and his mother, the following priorities were identified by the family: (1) explore after-school care at the local community center, which includes sports and crafts; (2) alter shopping and food preparation to emphasize the Food Guide Pyramid and low-fat choices; (3) begin weekend swimming or bicycling for the family; and (4) limit TV and video games to no more than 2 hours daily.

Three months later, most changes had been made except for the weekend family activity and less television on the weekends. However, Brian was now playing soccer, had lost 4 lb, and had grown taller.

1. What recommendations should be made to prevent relapse for Brian?
2. What other activities can Brian try as a means of avoiding or reducing the tendency to overeat?
3. How can his mother alter some favorite recipes to lower the fat content (e.g., his favorite meal is fried chicken with gravy, mashed potatoes, and ice cream)?

Meals, snacks, and food preparation activities at preschools, Head Start programs, and school cafeterias provide children an opportunity to practice and reinforce their nutrition knowledge, as well as to demonstrate their cognitive learning. Parental involvement in nutrition education projects can also produce positive outcomes, with subsequent carryover into the home.

CITED REFERENCES

Alaimo K, et al. Dietary intake of vitamins, minerals, and fiber of persons ages 2 months and over in the United States: Third national health and nutrition examination survey, phase I, 1988–1991, Advance Data from Vital Statistics; No. 258 (PHS) 95-1250. Hyattsville, MD: National Center for Health Statistics, 1994.

American Academy of Pediatrics. Committee on Nutrition: Cholesterol in childhood. Pediatrics 101:141, 1998a.

American Academy of Pediatrics. Pediatric Nutrition Handbook. 4th ed. Elk Grove Village, IL: American Academy of Pediatrics, 1998b.

American Dietetic Association. Timely statement of The American Dietetic Association: Dietary guidance for healthy children. J Am Diet Assoc 95:370, 1995.

Ashworth A, Millward DJ. Catch-up growth in children. Nutr Rev 44:157, 1986.

Beal VA. Nutritional intake. In: McCammon RW (ed.). Human Growth and Development. Springfield, IL: Charles C Thomas, 1970.

Behar D, et al. Sugar challenge testing with children considered behaviorally "sugar reactive." Nutr Behav 1:277, 1984.

Birch LL, et al. The variability of young children's energy intake. N Engl J Med 324:232, 1991.

Burghardt JA, et al. Meals offered in the National School Lunch Program and the School Breakfast Program. Am J Clin Nutr 61(suppl): 187S, 1995.

Buzina R, et al. Zinc nutrition and taste acuity in school children with impaired growth. Am J Clin Nutr 33:2262, 1980.

Centers for Disease Control, National Center for Chronic Disease Prevention and Health Promotion. Guidelines for School and Community Programs to Promote Lifelong Physical Activity Among Young People, 1997. [On-line]. Available: <http://www.cdc.gov/nccdphp/dash/activity.htm

Community Nutrition Institute. Rich a little richer, poor a little poorer in 1996 as the U.S. income gap expands. Week 26(38):1, Oct. 3, 1997.

Cook JT, Martin LS. Differences in nutrient adequacy among poor and non-poor children. Medford, MA, May 1995. Tufts University School of Nutrition, Center on Hunger, Poverty and Nutrition Policy, 1997.

Corbin CB, Pangrazi RP. Physical Activity for Children: A Statement of Guidelines. Ruston, VA: National Association for Sport and Physical Education, Council on Physical Education for Children, 1998.

Cryan J, Johnson RK. Should the current recommendations for energy intake in infants and young children be lowered? Nutr Today 32:69, 1997.

Daniels SR, et al. The utility of body mass index as a measure of body fatness in children and adolescents: Differences by race and gender. Pediatrics 99:804, 1997.

Dennison BA, et al. Fruit juice consumption by preschool-aged children is associated with short stature and obesity. Pediatrics 99:15, 1997.

Dietary Intervention Study in Children (DISC) by the Writing Group. Efficacy and safety of lowering dietary intake of fat and cholesterol in children with elevated low-density lipoprotein cholesterol. JAMA 273:1429, 1995.

Dietz WH. Critical periods in childhood for the development of obesity. Am J Clin Nutr 59:955, 1994.

Dietz WH, Gortmaker SL. Do we fatten our children at the TV set? Television viewing and obesity in children and adolescents. Pediatrics 75:807, 1985.

Dixon LB, et al. The effect of changes in dietary fat on the food group and nutrient intake of 4- to 10-year-old children. Pediatrics 100:863, 1997.

Emmons L. Food procurement and the nutritional adequacy of diets of low-income families. J Am Diet Assoc 86:1684, 1986.

Epstein LH, et al. Ten-year outcomes of behavioral family-based treatment for childhood obesity. Health Psychol 13:373, 1994.

Falcigia GA, Norton PA. Evidence for a genetic influence on preference for some foods. J Am Diet Assoc 94:154, 1994.

Food and Nutrition Board, National Research Council, NAS. Recommended Dietary Allowances, 10th ed. Washington, DC: National Academy Press, 1989.

Getlinger MJ, et al. Food waste is reduced when elementary-school children have recess before lunch. J Am Diet Assoc 96:906, 1996.

Gidding SS. The rationale for lowering serum cholesterol levels in American children. Am J Dis Child 147:386, 1993.

Gunnes M, Lehmann EH. Physical activity and dietary constituents as predictors of forearm cortical and trabecular bone gain in healthy children and adolescents: A prospective study. Acta Paediatr 85:19, 1996.

Gustafson-Larson AM, Terry RD. Weight-related behaviors and concerns of fourth-grade children. J Am Diet Assoc 92:818, 1992.

Hambidge KM, et al. Zinc nutrition of preschool children in the Denver Head Start Program. Am J Clin Nutr 29:734, 1976.

Haslam RHA, et al. Effects of megavitamin therapy on children with attention deficit disorders. Pediatrics 74:103, 1984.

Horsley JW, et al. Nutrition Management of School Age Children with Special Needs: A Resource Manual for School Personnel, Families and Health Professionals, 2nd ed. Richmond, VA: Virginia Department of Health and Virginia Department of Education, 1996.

Hyams JS, et al. Carbohydrate malabsorption following fruit juice ingestion in young children. Pediatrics 84:64, 1988.

Institute of Medicine, Food and Nutrition Board. Dietary Reference Intakes for Thiamin, Riboflavin, Niacin, Vitamin B_6, Folate, Vitamin B_{12}, Pantothenic Acid, Biotin, and Choline. Washington, DC: National Academy Press, 1998.

Institute of Medicine, Food and Nutrition Board. Dietary Reference Intakes for Calcium, Phosphorus, Magnesium, Vitamin D, and Fluoride. Washington, DC: National Academy Press, 1997.

Johnson RK, et al. Effects of maternal employment on family food consumption patterns and children's diets. J Nutr Educ 25:130, 1993.

Johnston CC, et al. Calcium supplementation and increases in bone mineral density in children. N Engl J Med 327:82, 1992.

Joint Working Group of the Canadian Paediatric Society and Health Canada. Nutrition recommendations update: Dietary fats and children. Nutr Rev 53:367, 1995.

Kaplan BJ, et al. Dietary replacement in preschool-aged hyperactive boys. Pediatrics 83:7, 1989.

Kennedy E, Goldberg J. What are American children eating? Implications for public policy. Nutr Rev 53:111, 1995.

Kleinman RE, et al. Hunger in children in the United States: Potential behavioral and emotional correlates. Pediatrics 101:e3,1998.

Klesges RC, et al. Effects of television on metabolic rate: Potential implications for childhood obesity. Pediatrics 91:281, 1993.

Kohl HW, Hobbs KE. Development of physical activity behaviors among children and adolescents. Pediatrics 101:549, 1998.

Kotz K, Story M. Food advertisements during children's Saturday morning television programming: Are they consistent with dietary recommendations? J Am Diet Assoc 94:1296, 1994.

Krebs NF, Hambidge KM. Trace elements in human nutrition. In: Walker WA, Watkins JB. Nutrition in Pediatrics, 2nd ed. Hamilton, Ontario: B.C. Decker Inc., 1996.

Lipton MA, Mayo JP. Diet and hyperkinesis—An update. J Am Diet Assoc 83:132, 1983.

Lohman TG, Roche AF, Martorell R (eds.). Anthropometric Standardization Reference Manual. Champaign, IL: Human Kinetics Books, 1991.

Lozoff B, et al. Long-term development outcome of infants with iron deficiency. N Engl J Med 325:687, 1991.

Luder E, Bonforte RJ. Children—An endangered species. Top Clin Nutr 8(1):1, 1992.

Luepker RV, et al. Outcomes of a field trial to improve children's dietary patterns and physical activity. The Child and Adolescent Trial for Cardiovascular Health (CATCH). JAMA 275:768, 1996.

Mahan LK. Family-focused behavioral approach to weight control in children. Pediatr Clin North Am 34:983, 1987.

Matkovic V. Calcium metabolism and calcium requirements during skeletal modeling and consolidation of bone mass. Am J Clin Nutr 54:S245, 1991.

Matkovic V, Heany RP. Calcium balance during human growth: Evidence for threshold behavior. Am J Clin Nutr 55:992, 1992.

Mei Z, et al. Increasing prevalence of overweight among U.S. low-income preschool children: The Centers for Disease Control and Prevention Pediatric Nutrition Surveillance, 1983–1995. Pediatrics 101:e12, 1998.

Meyers AF, et al. School breakfast program and school performance. Am J Dis Child 143:1234, 1989.

Munoz KA, et al. Food intakes of U.S. children and adolescents compared with recommendations. Pediatrics 100:323, 1997.

Murphy JM, et al. Relationship between hunger and psychosocial functioning in low-income American children. J Am Acad Child Adolesc Psychiatry 37:163, 1998.

National Dairy Council. They're Not Little Adults. A Backgrounder for Health Professionals: Children's Nutrition and Dietary Guidelines. Rosemont, IL: National Dairy Council, 1996.

National Heart, Lung, and Blood Institute, National Cholesterol Education Program: Report of the Expert Panel on Blood Cholesterol Levels in Children and Adolescents. Bethesda, MD: National Heart, Lung, and Blood Institute, 1991.

Nicklas TA. Dietary studies of children: The Bogalusa Heart Study Experience. J Am Diet Assoc 95:1127, 1995.

Nicklas TA, et al. Breakfast consumption affects adequacy of total daily intake in children. J Am Diet Assoc 93:886, 1993a.

Nicklas TA, et al. Secular trends in dietary intakes and cardiovascular

risk factors of 10-year-old children, 1973–1988. Am J Clin Nutr 57:930, 1993b.
Olson, RE. The folly of restricting fat in the diet of children. Nutr Today 30(6):234, 1995.
Pollitt E. Does breakfast make a difference in school? J Am Diet Assoc 95:1134, 1995.
Pollitt E, et al. Fasting and cognition in well- and undernourished school children: A review of three experimental studies. Am J Clin Nutr 67(suppl):779S, 1998a.
Pollitt E, Mathews R. Breakfast and cognition: An integrative summary. Am J Clin Nutr 67(suppl):804S, 1998b.
Pollitt E, et al. Iron deficiency and behavioral development in infants and preschool children. Am J Clin Nutr 43:555, 1986.
Pugliese MT, et al. Fear of obesity: A cause of short stature and delayed puberty. N Engl J Med 309:513, 1983.
Pugliese MT, et al. Parental health beliefs as a cause of nonorganic failure to thrive. Pediatrics 80:175, 1987.
Rickard KA, et al. The play approach to learning in the context of families and schools: An alternative paradigm for nutrition and fitness education in the 21st century. J Am Diet Assoc 95:1121, 1995.
Robinson TN, et al. Does television viewing increase obesity and reduce physical activity? Cross-sectional and longitudinal analyses among adolescent girls. Pediatrics 91:273, 1993.
Rolland-Cachera M-F, et al. Tracking the development of adiposity from one month of age to adulthood. Ann Hum Biol 14:219, 1987.
Rosenbaum MD, Leibel RL. The physiology of body weight regulation: Relevance to the etiology of obesity in children. Pediatrics 101:525, 1998.
Rosner B, et al. Percentiles for body mass index in U.S. children 5 to 17 years of age. J Pediatr 132:211, 1998.
Satter EM. Internal regulation and the evolution of normal growth as the basis for prevention of obesity in children. J Am Diet Assoc 96:860, 1996.
Shea S, et al. Is there a relationship between dietary fat and stature or growth in children three to five years of age? Pediatrics 92:579, 1993.
Smith MM, et al. Carbohydrate absorption from fruit juice in young children. Pediatrics 95:340, 1995.
Smith MM, Lifshitz F. Excess fruit juice consumption as a contributing factor in nonorganic failure to thrive. Pediatrics 93:438, 1994.
Stevens LJ, et al. Essential fatty acid metabolism in boys with attention-deficit hyperactivity disorder. Am J Clin Nutr 62:761, 1995.
Taylor MT, Koblinsky SA. Dietary intake and growth status of young homeless children. J Am Diet Assoc 93:464, 1993.
Troiano RP, Flegal KM. Overweight children and adolescents: Description, epidemiology, and demographics. Pediatrics 101:497, 1998.
USDA: Agricultural Research Service Food Surveys Research Group. 1997 Data Tables: Results from USDA's 1994–96 Continuing Survey of Food Intakes by Individuals and 1994–96 Diet and Health Knowledge Survey. [On-line]. Available (under "Releases"): <http://www.barc.usda.gov/bhnrc/foodsurvey/home.htm>
USDA: Child Nutrition Programs: School Meal Initiatives for Healthy Children. Federal Register, 7 CFR, Part 220, Food and Consumer Service, USDA, June 13, 1995.
USDA. Nationwide Food Consumption Survey. Continuing Survey of Food Intakes by Individuals: Women 19-50 years and children 1-5 years, 1 day, 1986, Report No. 86-1. Hyattsville, MD: Nutrition Monitoring Division, Human Nutrition Information Service, USDA, 1987.
Vaisman N, et al. Effect of breakfast timing on the cognitive functions of elementary school students. Arch Pediatr Adolesc Med 150:1089, 1996.
Williams CL, et al. A new recommendation for dietary fiber in childhood. Pediatrics 96(suppl):985, 1995.
Wolraich ML, et al. The effect of sugar on behavior or cognition in children: A meta-analysis. JAMA 274:1617, 1995.
Wong ND, et al. Television viewing and pediatric hypercholesterolemia. Pediatrics 90:75, 1992.
Yu SM, et al. Vitamin-mineral supplement use among preschool children in the United States. Pediatrics 100:e4, 1997.

ADDITIONAL REFERENCES

Albertson AM, et al. Nutrient intakes of 2- to 10-year-old American children: 10-year trends. J Am Diet Assoc 92:1492, 1992.
American Dietetic Association. Position of The American Dietetic Association: Child and adolescent food and nutrition services. J Am Diet Assoc 96:913, 1996.
American Dietetic Association. Position of ADA, SNE, ASFSA: School-based nutrition programs and services. J Am Diet Assoc 95:367, 1995.
American Dietetic Association. Position of the American Dietetic Association: Vitamin and mineral supplementation. J Am Diet Assoc 96:73, 1996.
Barr DGD, et al. Catch-up growth in malnutrition, studied in celiac disease after institution of gluten-free diet. Pediatr Res 6:521, 1972.
Birch L. Children's preferences for high fat foods. Nutr Rev 50:249, 1992.
Conners CK, Blouin AG. Nutritional effects on behavior of children. J Psychiatr Res 17:169, 1982/1983.
Contento I, et al. The effectiveness of nutrition education and implications for nutrition education and policy, programs, and research: A review of research. J Nutr Educ 27:298, 1995.
Dennison B, et al. Challenges to implementing the current pediatric screening guidelines into practice. Pediatrics 94:296, 1994.
Dietz, WH. Health consequences of obesity in youth: Childhood predictors of adult disease. Pediatrics 101:518, 1998.
Edelstein S. The Healthy Young Child. Minneapolis, MN: West Publishing Co., 1995.
Fomon SJ, et al. Body composition of reference children from birth to age 10 years. Am J Clin Nutr 35:1169, 1982.
Ho CS, et al. Evaluation of the nutrient content of school, sack and vending lunch of junior high students. Sch Food Serv Res Rev 15:85, 1991.
Johnson S, Birch L. Parents' and children's adiposity and eating style. Pediatrics 94:653, 1994.
Leung A, Robson W. The toddler who does not eat. Am Fam Phys 49:1789, 1994.
Miller J, Korenman S. Poverty and children's nutritional status. Am J Epidemiol 140:233, 1994.
Pilant VB. Current issues in child nutrition programs. Top Clin Nutr 9(4):1, 1994.
Queen PM, Lang CE (eds.). Handbook of Pediatric Nutrition. Gaithersburg, MD: Aspen Publishers Inc., 1993.
Satter EM. Childhood eating disorders. J Am Diet Assoc 86:357, 1986.
Satter EM. How to Get Your Kid to Eat . . . But Not Too Much. Palo Alto, CA: Bull Publishing Company, 1987.
Satter EM. The feeding relationship. J Am Diet Assoc 86:352, 1986.
Schlicker SA, et al. The weight and fitness status of United States children. Nutr Rev 52:11, 1994.
Shea S, et al. The rate of increase in blood pressure in children 5 years of age is related to changes in aerobic fitness and body mass index. Pediatrics 94:465, 1994.
Simeon DT, Grantham-McGregor S. Effects of missing breakfast on the cognitive functions of school children of differing nutritional status. Am J Clin Nutr 49:646, 1989.
Similarity of children's and their parents' food preferences. Nutr Rev 45:134, 1987.
Stoch MB, Smythe PM. 15-year developmental study of effects of severe undernutrition on subsequent physical growth and intellectual functioning. Arch Dis Child 51:327, 1976.
Trahms CT, Pipes PL. Nutrition in Infancy and Childhood, 6th ed. St. Louis: WCB/McGraw-Hill, 1997.

CHAPTER 11

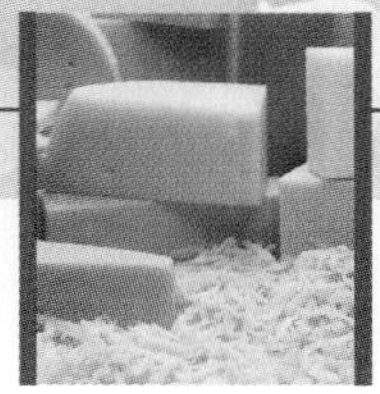

Nutrition in Adolescence

BONNIE A. SPEAR, PHD, RD

CHAPTER OUTLINE

- Growth and Development
- Nutritional Requirements
- Food Habits
- Situations with Special Needs
- Strategies for Improving Nutritional Well-Being

Key Terms

ADOLESCENCE—the period of life beginning with the appearance of secondary sex characteristics and ending with the cessation of somatic growth

BODY IMAGE—a mental self-concept related to rate of growth and change in body proportions

EATING DISORDER—abnormal behaviors related to food and eating that may include starving, bingeing, vomiting, laxative abuse, or excessive exercise accompanied by unrealistic ideas about food, distorted body image, and psychological and developmental abnormalities

GROWTH SPURT—the 18- to 24-month period of adolescence when growth rate is the fastest

GYNECOLOGIC AGE—the number of years between the onset of menses and the date of conception in the pregnant adolescent

MENARCHE—onset of menses in the female

PEAK HEIGHT GAIN VELOCITY—the fastest rate of growth during the growth spurt

PUBERTY—the period during which the secondary sex characteristics begin to develop and the capability of sexual reproduction is attained

SEXUAL MATURITY RATING—a method of assessing the stage of sexual development, usually stated as sexual maturation or Tanner stages

TASKS OF ADOLESCENCE—the accomplishments expected in adolescence in order to achieve maturity in emotional and intellectual development

Adolescence is one of the most challenging periods in human development. The relatively uniform growth of childhood is suddenly altered by an increase in the velocity of growth. These sudden changes create special nutritional needs. The adolescence is considered especially vulnerable nutritionally for several reasons. First, there is an increased demand for nutrients related to the dramatic increase in physical growth and development. Second, the change of life-style and food habits of adolescents affect both nutrient intake and needs. Third, there are special nutrient needs associated with participation in sports, pregnancy, development of an eating disorder, excessive dieting, use of alcohol and drugs, or other situations common to adolescents (Spear, 1996).

GROWTH AND DEVELOPMENT

Physiological Changes

Puberty, the process of physically developing from a child to an adult, is initiated by physiological factors and includes maturation of the total body. Adolescence is the only time following birth when the rate of growth actually increases. Figure 11–1 shows the rate of linear growth during the teenage years compared with that during the childhood years. The adolescent gains about 20% of adult height and 50% of weight during this period.

This growth continues throughout the approximately 5 to 7 years of pubertal development. A great percentage of this height will be gained during the 18- to 24-month period of the **growth spurt. Peak height gain velocity** occurs at different ages for different individuals, as does the initiation of puberty. For example, Figure 11–2 shows a group of adolescent males, all of whom are 13 years of age; all are at different levels of maturation and, therefore, have different nutritional needs.

In general, girls began the pubertal process approximately 2 years earlier than boys. Factors known about the timing and milestones of pubertal development are summarized in Figure 11–3 and Appendices 14 and 15. Although growth slows following the achievement of sexual maturity, linear

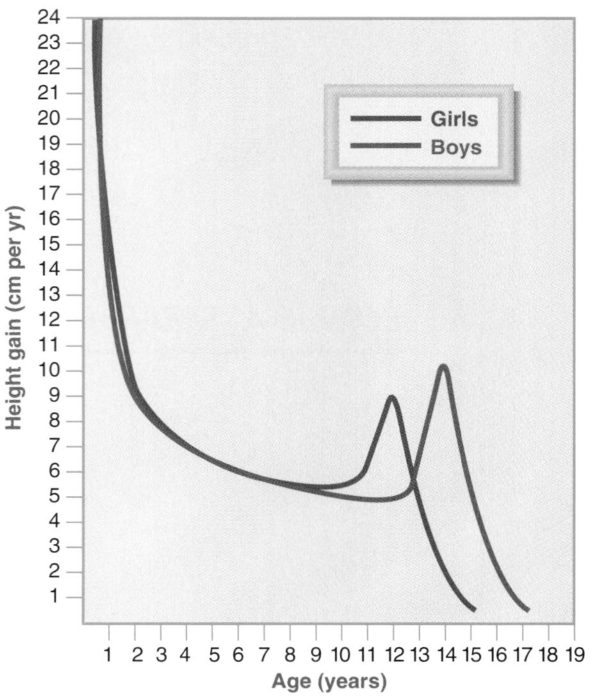

FIGURE 11–1 Typical individual velocity curves for supine length or height in boys and girls. The curves represent the velocity of growth of the typical boy and girl at any given age.

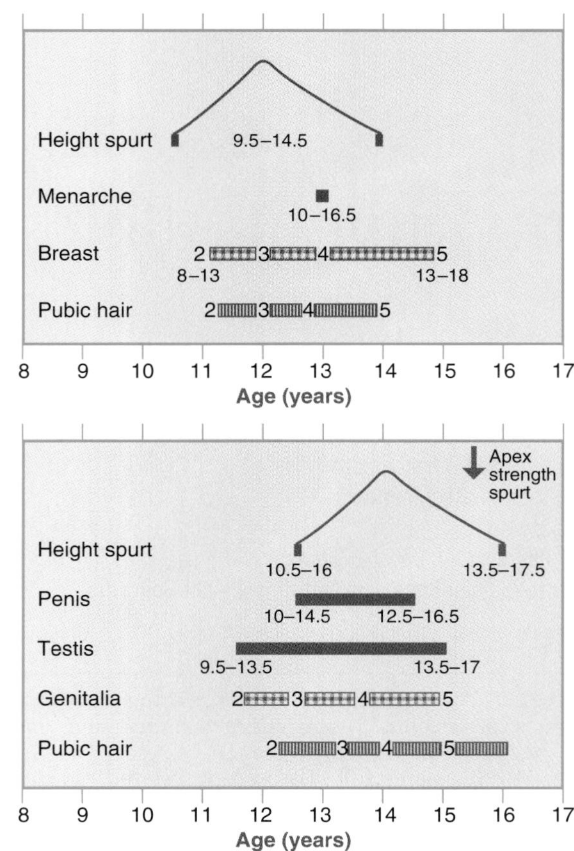

FIGURE 11–3 Diagram of the sequence of events at puberty in girls (*upper chart*) and boys (*lower chart*). The breast, genitalia, and pubic hair development are numbered 2–5 based on Tanner developmental stages. (From Marshall WA, Tanner JM. Variations in the pattern of pubertal changes in boys. Arch Dis Child 45:13, 1970.)

growth and weight acquisition continue into the late teens for females and early twenties for males. Most females gain no more than 2 to 3 inches following **menarche,** although girls who have early menarche tend to grow more after the onset of menstruation than do those having later menarche.

In the process of total body maturation, the composition of the body changes. In the prepubertal period, the proportion of fat and muscle in males and females tends to be similar, with body fat averaging about 15% and 19%, respectively. Girls gain more fat than boys during puberty, and in adulthood, they have about 22% to 26% body fat, compared with around 15% to 18% in men. During puberty, men gain twice as much lean tissue as do women.

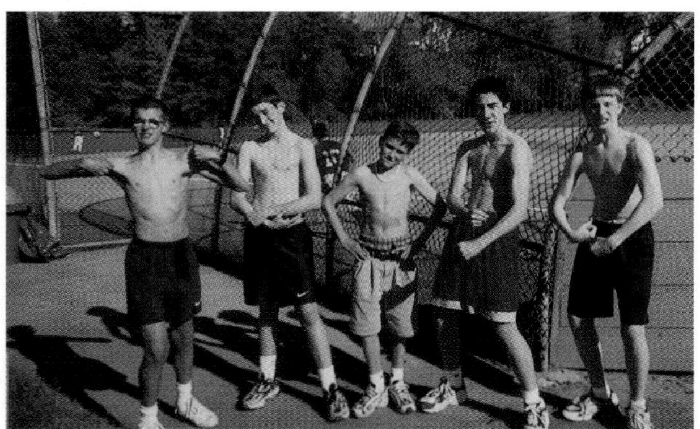

FIGURE 11–2 These boys are all 13 years old, but their energy needs vary according to their individual growth rates.

Assessment of Growth

Weight and height can be plotted on growth grids to determine whether individuals are maintaining their growth pattern or growth channel. The relationship between weight and height can be evaluated by using the detailed tables of the National Center for Health Statistics (Appendix Tables 8 and 12). Appropriate weights for height, according to age and sex, lie between the 25th and 75th percentiles, a range that allows for individual differences in body build (Mahan and Rees, 1984).

Use of body mass index (BMI), which is highly correlated with body fatness, can also indicate weight status. An adolescent's BMI is calculated by dividing body weight (expressed in kilograms), by the square of the adolescent's height (in meters); that is, BMI = kg/m^2. The BMI table (Table 11–1) can be used to determine the adolescent's weight status. Adolescents with BMIs below the 5th percentile should be assessed for organic diseases or eating disorders. Adolescents with BMIs between the 85th percentile and the 95th percentile are at risk for overweight and a nutritional assessment

TABLE 11–1 RECOMMENDED MAXIMUM VALUES FOR BODY MASS INDEX (BMI, IN kg/m²) FOR ADOLESCENTS WHO ARE OVERWEIGHT OR AT RISK OF OVERWEIGHT DURING ADOLESCENCE

	AT RISK OF OVERWEIGHT (≥85th and ≤95th percentile)		OVERWEIGHT (≥95th percentile)	
AGE (yrs)	Males	Females	Males	Females
10	20	20	23	23
11	20	21	24	25
12	21	22	25	26
13	22	23	26	27
14	23	24	27	28
15	24	24	28	29
16	24	25	29	29
17	25	25	29	30
18	26	26	30	30
19	26	26	30	30
20–24	27	26	30	30

(From Himes JH, Dietz WH. Guidelines for overweight in adolescent preventive services: Recommendations from an expert committee. Am J Clin Nutr 59:307, 1994.)

should be performed to determine health risk. Adolescents with BMIs at the 95th percentile or greater for age and gender are overweight and should have an in-depth medical assessment (WHO, 1995) (see page 265 and Chapter 23).

A skinfold evaluation yields a further degree of precision. For example, a low skinfold measurement in an individual who is above the 75th percentile in weight for height indicates a state of being overweight, but *not* overfat. An assessment of muscle and arm circumference can confirm the muscular composition. However, a skinfold in the 90th percentile or greater suggests obesity. Measurement of skinfolds is further discussed in Chapter 16.

Sexual Maturity Rating

Because adolescents of the same age often differ markedly in size (see Fig. 11–2), it is impossible to use age alone in evaluating pubertal growth. An assessment of the degree of maturation of secondary sexual characteristics is useful, not only in evaluating physical growth, but also in detecting certain diseases and disorders associated with adolescence. **Sexual maturity ratings** (SMRs), often called Tanner stages, are widely used to evaluate growth and developmental age during adolescence. These ratings are based on the development of secondary sex characteristics and are assigned on a scale of 1 (prepubertal) to 5 (adult). For boys, this scale is based on the progression of genital and pubic hair development (Appendix 14); for girls, the rating is based on the stage of breast and pubic hair development. These stages of growth correlate highly with other pubertal events. Table 11–2 shows the changes in the secondary sex characteristics. Because nutrition professionals are often unable to evaluate breast and genital development, Table 11–2 also gives other characteristics that correspond with each SMR level. Knowledge of the relationship between these milestones and physical growth enables the clinician to assess the progress of growth in an adolescent at a particular time, give some indication of the extent of future growth, and provide clinical counseling that is geared to individual needs for growth and development.

Excessive or less-than-normal growth can be detected by plotting height changes on the grids in Appendices 8 and 12. The major cause of short stature during adolescence is genetically late initiation of puberty, although other conditions, such as chronic disease or skeletal and chromosomal abnormalities, also can account for certain children being shorter than normal. Hormonal imbalances leading to abnormal growth are rare.

Psychological Changes

Adolescence is a period of maturation for both mind and body. Along with the physical growth of puberty, emotional and intellectual development are rapid. Adolescents' capacity for abstract thinking, as opposed to the concrete thought patterns of childhood, enables them to accomplish the **tasks of adolescence** (Table 11–3). Many of these tasks have implications for their nutritional well-being.

Cognitive and emotional development can be divided into early, middle, and late adolescence. Determining the adolescent's stage can be very helpful in providing nutritional counseling as well as in designing educational programs.

In *early adolescence,* the adolescent:

- is preoccupied with body and body image
- trusts and respects adults
- is anxious about peer relationships
- is ambivalent about autonomy

The nutritional implications are that adolescents in this stage are willing to do or try anything that will make them look better or improve their body image. However, adolescents at this stage want immediate results, so nutrition counseling should be geared to

TABLE 11–2 RATINGS OF SEXUAL MATURATION†

	PUBIC HAIR	GENITALIA	CORRESPONDING CHANGES
Boys			
Stage 1	None	Pre-pubertal	
Stage 2	Small amount at outer edges of pubis; slight darkening	Beginning penile enlargement Testes enlarged to 5-mL volume Scrotum reddened and changed in texture	Increased activity of sweat glands
Stage 3	Covers pubis	Penis lengthening Testes enlarged to 8–10 mL Scrotum further enlarged	Voice begins to change Faint mustache/facial hair appears Axillary hair present Beginning of peak height velocity (PHV) (growth spurt of 6–8 inches)
Stage 4	Adult type, does not extend to the thighs	Penis is wider and longer. Testes enlarged to 12 mL Scrotal skin darker	End of PHV Voice deepens Acne may be severe Facial hair increases Hair on legs becomes darker
Stage 5	Adult type, now spreads to the thighs	Adult penis Testes enlarged to 15 mL	Muscle mass increases significantly
Girls			
Stage 1	None	No change from childhood	
Stage 2	Small amount, downy, on medial labia	Breast bud	Increased activity of sweat glands Beginning of peak height velocity (PHV) (growth spurt of 3–5 inches)
Stage 3	Increased, darker, and curly	Larger, but no separation of the nipple and the areola	End of PHV Beginning of acne Axillary hair present
Stage 4	More abundant, coarse texture	Increased size Areola and nipple form secondary mound	Acne may be severe Menarche begins
Stage 5	Adult, spreads to medial thighs	Adult distribution of breast tissue, continuous outline	Increase in fat and muscle mass

(Adapted from Tanner JM. Growth at Adolescence, 2nd ed. Oxford: Blackwell Scientific Publications, 1962.)
†See Appendix Table 14.

short-term goals and to addressing nutritional concerns that impact the teen's appearance or performance, in (e.g., dance, sports), or both.

A teen in *middle adolescence:*

- is greatly influenced by his or her peer group
- is mistrustful of adults
- sees independence as being very important
- experiences significant cognitive development

During this stage, the teen will listen to peers more than to parents or other adults. Teens are becoming more in charge of the foods they eat. The drive toward independence often results in temporary rejection of the family dietary patterns. Nutritional counseling should include making wise decisions when eating away from home.

The teen in *late adolescence:*

- has established a body image
- is oriented toward the future and is making plans
- is increasingly independent
- is more consistent in his or her values and beliefs
- is developing intimacy and permanent relationships

TABLE 11–3 DEVELOPMENTAL TASKS IN ADOLESCENCE

Developmental Task
1. Forming more mature relationships with peers of both sexes
2. Establishing a male or female social role
3. Accepting one's physique and using one's body effectively
4. Becoming emancipated from parents and other adults
5. Preparing for marriage and family life
6. Choosing a vocation and preparing for that career
7. Developing standards and value systems as a guide to behavior
8. Developing social intelligence and a commitment to responsible citizenship
9. Developing conceptual and problem-solving, decision-making skills

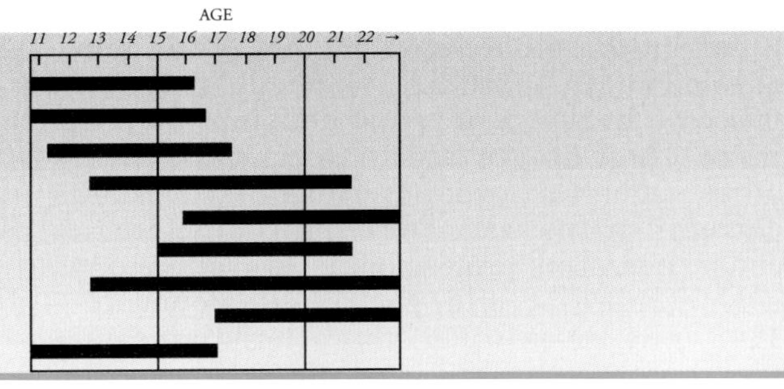

(Adapted from Mahan LK, Rees JM. Nutrition in Adolescence. St Louis: CV Mosby, 1984; and Thornburg H. Contemporary Adolescence: Readings, 2nd ed. Monterey, CA. Brooks/Cole, 1975, p 7.)

By late adolescence, teens are thinking about the future and are interested in improving their overall health. Nutritional counseling during this stage can address long-term goals. Adolescents in this stage still want to make their own decisions, but are open to information provided by health care providers. Nutritional counselors should not only present current recommendations, but should also explain the rationale behind them.

As adolescents strive for independence, they often take risks. Many of these risks are important to becoming independent (e.g., trying out for a sports team, applying to college, dating), but many risk behaviors can be dangerous. Resnick et al. (1993) found that serious behaviors, termed *acting out behaviors,* can be grouped together and include the following: drug use, school absenteeism, and unintended injury risk, such as drinking and driving, not wearing seatbelts, and not using a bicycle helmet. The second group of serious behaviors, termed *quietly disturbed behaviors,* are of concern to nutritionists because these behaviors include the following: poor body image; disordered eating, including bingeing, bulimia, and chronic dieting; fear of loss of control over eating; emotional stress; and suicidal ideation.

Body Image

Developing a **body image,** an image of the physical self that includes an adult body, is an intellectual and emotional task that is intertwined with nutritional issues. Adolescents often feel uncomfortable with their rapidly changing bodies, yet at the same time, they want to be like their most perfect peers and cultural idols (see "*Clinical Insight:* Body Image and Dieting Practices of Adolescents"). Their sense of worth may be derived from feelings about their own physical attributes, a trait that causes them to be vulnerable to severe distortions if an eating disorder develops.

The desire to change their rate of growth or body proportions can lead adolescents to dietary manipulations that may have negative consequences and be subject to exploitation by commercial interests. Rapid weight gain accompanying the development of secondary sexual characteristics causes many young women to restrict the amount of food they eat unnecessarily. Young men are tempted to use nutritional supplements, hoping to achieve the muscular appearance of adults. The importance to teens of fitting in, having body images they think will help them fit in, cannot be overlooked in nutritional counseling.

Clinical Insight

Body Image and Dieting Practices of Adolescents

Regardless of how they look to others, adolescents are seldom satisfied with their appearance. As might be expected, girls often view their weight and body shape with disfavor, but boys also visualize enviable masculine physiques that often do not coincide with their own. This disparity between the perceived and the desired often leads to inappropriate eating behavior. The Youth Risk Behavior Survey of 1995 obtained information from 10,904 students about their body image and their behavior to change it. The survey included a self-administered, 75-item questionnaire given to a random sample of high school students from public and private schools in grades 9 through 12 that were representative of the U.S. high school population. As previous studies (Moore, 1988, 1990) had shown, the survey revealed large differences in how females and males viewed themselves.

Female adolescents (34%) were twice as likely as their male counterparts (15%) to view themselves as "too fat." The boys were twice as likely to view themselves as "too thin" (16% versus 7%). Both male and female black students were less likely to view themselves as "too fat." It seems that greater body weight does not carry the same stigma among blacks that it does among whites (Desmond, 1989). Overall, white and Hispanic students (29% and 32%, respectively) were significantly more likely than black students (21%) to identify themselves as being overweight (Kann et al., 1996).

Among the female students, 60% were attempting to lose weight at the time of the survey, whereas only 24% of the male students were attempting weight loss. Even more disturbing is the fact that 25% of those girls who considered themselves to be the "right weight" were still trying to lose weight. They appear never to be satisfied. Of the boys, 24% were trying to lose weight, but an even greater proportion (26%) were trying to gain weight. Overall, white and Hispanic students (43% and 45%, respectively) were significantly more likely than black students (33%) to be attempting weight loss (Kann et al., 1996).

The most popular method for losing weight was exercising, followed closely by skipping meals, particularly among the female students. White students were more likely to report exercise as a method of weight control than black students. Eight percent of the female students and 2% of the male students reported using vomiting or laxatives to control their weight during the 7 days preceding the survey, but the numbers jumped to 14% and 4%, respectively, when they are asked, "Have you ever used vomiting to manage you weight?" Additionally, 9% of the female students and 2% of the male students had taken diet pills to lose weight.

As these studies show, the adolescent with a normal-appearing physique may have a very different body image. This leads to dissatisfaction and inappropriate behaviors in an effort to change one's shape. Clinicians need to be aware of this disparity in some teens and may need to probe further to determine the extent of inappropriate eating and exercise behaviors. Adolescents may be dieting even when they are not overweight, and they need help to accept more realistic body weights (Emmons, 1994).

NUTRITIONAL REQUIREMENTS

Recommendations for fulfilling the nutritional needs of adolescents arise from a small research base. Often, the amounts recommended are extrapolated from studies in adults or children. Part of the difficulty lies in the fact that studies of requirements must consider not only age, but also stage of physical maturity or SMR. The Dietary Reference Intakes (DRIs) which include the Recommended Dietary Allowances (RDAs), Adequate Intakes (AIs), and Tolerable Upper Intake Levels (ULs) for adolescents are stated for three age groups, as shown in Table 15–1.

Energy

The RDAs for energy for teenagers of various chronological ages and for each sex are shown in Table 11–4. As with other nutrients, the RDAs for energy do not include a safety factor for increased energy needs (e.g., during periods of illness, trauma, stress) and thus are considered to be only average needs. Actual needs for adolescents will vary with level of physical activity and stage of maturation.

In order to compensate for differences in growth by age, calories per unit of height is the preferred index for determining caloric needs. The use of kcal/cm can be used as a rough predictor of energy needs. Table 11–4 shows the RDAs for age, as well as the recommended kcal/cm. The recommended range of energy intake for adolescence shown in Table 11–4 reflects the different needs of teenagers. Growth rate, as well as level of exercise, must be considered in determining the needs of the individual.

Protein

During adolescence, protein needs, like those for energy, correlate more closely with the growth pattern than with chronological age. Using the RDA for protein in relation to height is probably the most useful method of estimating need (see Table 11–4). Average intakes of protein are well above the RDA (range of 45 to 72 g/day) for all age groups. In fact, when comparing protein intakes of adolescents from the United States with teens from other countries, studies show that U.S. adolescents have a much higher intake of protein. There is little evidence to show that insufficient protein intake is common in the adolescent population. However, if energy intake is inadequate for any reason (e.g., economic problems, chronic illness, or attempts to lose weight), dietary protein may be used to meet energy needs and will, therefore, be unavailable for synthesis of new tissue or for tissue repair. This may result in a state of insufficient protein, which will lead to a reduction in growth rate and a decrease in lean body mass. Current dieting patterns in some adolescent females can result in restricted calorie intakes that are potentially harmful, especially when protein sources are used to meet energy needs.

Excessive intakes of protein can also have an impact on nutritional status. For example, a high protein intake can interfere with calcium metabolism (see Chapters 4 and 28) and increase fluid needs. These increased fluid needs may put adolescent athletes at high risk for dehydration.

TABLE 11–4 RECOMMENDED ENERGY AND PROTEIN ALLOWANCES

AGE (yrs)	Kcal/day	Kcal/kg	Kcal/cm	PROTEIN g/day	PROTEIN g/cm
Females					
11–14	2200	47	14.0	46	0.29
15–18	2200	40	13.5	44	0.26
19–24	2200	38	13.4	46	0.28
Males					
11–14	2500	55	16.0	45	0.28
15–18	3000	45	17.0	59	0.33
19–24	2900	40	16.4	58	0.33

(Reprinted with permission from Recommended Dietary Allowances, 10th ed. © 1989 by the National Academy of Sciences. Published by National Academy Press, Washington, DC.)

Micronutrients

Micronutrients (vitamins and minerals) play an important role in the growth and health of adolescents. Inadequate fruit and vegetable consumption has been linked to certain types of cancer and other diseases. Because of the many health benefits associated with fruits and vegetables, national recommendations support increased consumption of these foods. The national recommendations are to eat five servings of fruits and vegetables per day. Unfortunately, surveys show that, for adolescents, there are significant gaps between actual intake and these recommendations. The 1995 Youth Risk Behavior Survey revealed that, on the day of evaluation, 41% of the adolescents ate no fruit and vegetables, and only 9% ate five servings (Kann, 1996). This inadequate intake has a tremendous impact on the vitamins and minerals adolescents need for growth.

MINERALS

Adolescents incorporate twice the amount of calcium, iron, zinc, and magnesium into their bodies during the years of their growth spurt than at other times.

CALCIUM. Because of accelerated muscular, skeletal, and endocrine development, calcium needs are greater during puberty and adolescence than in childhood or during the adult years. At the peak of the growth spurt, the daily deposition of calcium can be twice that of the average during the rest of the adolescent period. In fact, 45% of the skeletal mass is added during adolescence.

The DRI for calcium is 1300 mg for all adolescents (Yates, 1998). Calcium requirements are expressed as Adequate Intakes (AIs). The AI is believed to cover needs of all individuals in a group, but lack of data or uncertainty in the data preclude specifying, with confidence, the percentage of persons covered by this intake (Institute of Medicine, 1997). This is especially true for adolescents. The National Institutes of Health Consensus Development Conference Statement on Optimal Calcium Intake (NIH, 1994) recommended 1200 to 1500 mg of calcium per day for adolescents 11 to 24 years of age. In their statement, the committee acknowledged that there appears to be a certain threshold level of dietary calcium that is necessary to allow growing adolescents to achieve their genetically predetermined peak bone mass. Dietary survey data indicate that adolescents, particularly females, are at greatest risk for inadequate calcium intake (Alaimo, 1994). Calcium intake tends to decline among females 10 to 17 years of age. Consumption surveys show an average intake for females to be 780 to 820 mg per day. In male adolescents, the average intake is 800 to 920 mg per day. NHANES has also shown a decline in dietary intakes of adolescents from NHANES II (1976–80) to NHANES III (1988–91) (Albertson, 1997), as shown in the following chart:

Calcium Intakes

Age (yrs)	NHANES II (1976–1980)	NHANES III (1988–1991)
6–11	1209	867
12–15	854	796
16–19	725	822

Additionally, there is evidence to suggest that high soft drink consumption in the adolescent population contributes to low calcium intake in this age group because of the likelihood that soda is being substituted for milk. It is estimated that 14% of the total caloric intake in male adolescents and 15% of total caloric intake in female adolescents can be attributed to soft drink consumption. Male adolescents average $2\frac{1}{2}$ 12-oz servings of soft drinks per day, but only $1\frac{1}{2}$ cups of milk per day; by comparison, female adolescents average $1\frac{3}{4}$ 12-oz servings of soft drinks per day, but less than 1 cup of milk per day. Pronounced bone loss in animals has been observed with excess phosphorus or insufficient calcium intakes. Teenagers may have low Ca:P ratios secondary to excess consumption of high-phosphorus soft drinks, but additional research is needed to determine the combined effect of decreased milk intake and increased intake of soft drinks and processed foods that are high in phosphorus.

Iron. Both male and female adolescents have high requirements for iron. In the male adolescent population, the build-up of muscle mass is accompanied by greater blood volume; in female adolescents, iron is lost monthly with the onset of menses. During adolescence, anemia secondary to iron deficiency may impair the immune response and decrease resistance to infection. Iron deficiency anemia can also affect learning, as evidenced by studies showing that children and adolescents with anemia have problems with short-term memory. (See Chapter 35.)

Zinc. *Zinc* is known to be essential for growth and sexual maturation. Although plasma zinc levels decline during pubertal development, retention of zinc increases significantly during the growth spurt. This increased utilization may lead to more efficient use of dietary sources. However, limited intake of zinc-containing foods may affect physical growth, as well as the development of secondary sex characteristics. Although there is limited research in this area, there is some evidence that adolescents with low serum zinc levels may have increased problems with acne (see the section on acne, page 267).

Other Minerals. Although the role of other minerals in the nutriture of adolescents has not been studied extensively, the importance of *magnesium, iodine, phosphorus, copper, chromium, cobalt,* and *fluoride* is well recognized. The possibility of interactions among these nutrients cannot be overlooked. Recommendations for estimated safe and adequate dietary intakes, listed in Table 15–2, are made on the basis of the best data presently available.

VITAMINS

The need for vitamins is increased during adolescence. Because of increased energy demands during this period, increased quantities of thiamine, riboflavin, and niacin are required for the release of energy from carbohydrates. With tissue synthesis, there is an increased demand for vitamin B_6, folic acid, and vitamin B_{12}. There is also an increased requirement for vitamin D (for rapid skeletal growth), and vitamins A, C, and E are needed for new cell growth. Although there are few reports of low serum vitamin C levels in teens, those who habitually avoid fruits and vegetables and those who smoke cigarettes may be at increased risk for deficiency. As with other nutrients, vitamin needs are primarily determined by an individual's degree of maturity, rather than chronological age, owing to the demands of growth. In most cases, sufficient vitamin intake can be achieved by a well-chosen diet, without the need for vitamin supplements. Adolescents who diet, have an eating disorder or chronic disease, or chronically make poor food choices are the exceptions to this rule.

Potential Nutritional Inadequacies

Surveys of nutrient intakes have shown that adolescents are likely to obtain less vitamin A, vitamin B_6, folate, riboflavin, iron, calcium, and zinc than recommended. Young women are also likely to obtain less magnesium, copper, and manganese than recommended (Alaimo et al., 1994).

Studies also show that teens' intakes are higher than optimal in fat, saturated fat, protein, and sodium. The School Nutrition Dietary Assessment Study revealed that dietary fat represented 33% to 35% of energy intake, and that the intake of saturated fat was 12% to 13%, higher than the recommended level of 10% (Devaney et al., 1995). Although the intake of fat, as a percentage of calories, has decreased from 37% to around 33% or 34%, the levels still remain higher than the recommended 30%. Even though the fat intakes of adolescents appear to be decreasing, the incidence of obesity in this population continues to increase.

TABLE 11–5 SITUATIONS AND FEELINGS ASSOCIATED WITH EATING "JUNK" FOODS AND "HEALTHY" FOODS

"JUNK" FOODS	"HEALTHY" FOODS
Being with friends	Being with parents
Being away from home/parents	Staying home
Enjoyment/pleasure	Being concerned with weight and appearance
Being at the mall/store	
Snacks	Meals
Not being in control, overeating, guilt, disgust	Self-control

(Adapted and used by permission from Chapman G, Maclean H. "Junk food" and "healthy food": Meanings of food in adolescent women's culture. J Nutr Educ 25:108, 1993.)

FOOD HABITS

Adolescents are not only maturing physically, but also cognitively and psychosocially. They search for identity, strive for independence and acceptance, and are concerned about appearance. Irregular meals, snacking, eating away from home, and following alternative dietary patterns characterize the food habits of adolescents. These habits are further influenced by family, peers, and the media.

Irregular Meals and Snacking

Meal patterns of adolescents are often chaotic. Teenagers miss an increasing number of meals at home as they get older. Breakfast and lunch are often the meals most frequently missed, but social and school activities may cause a teen to miss an evening meal as well. Female adolescents tend to miss more meals than their male counterparts.

Although concern has been expressed about the habit of snacking, teenagers may obtain substantial nourishment from foods eaten outside traditional meals. Thus, the choice of foods is more important than the time or place of eating.

As a result of health and science education at school, most adolescents know what they should and should not eat (Story and Resnick, 1986). However, overcoming barriers to act on that knowledge is the concern. Teens identify the biggest barrier as time. Teens perceive themselves as too busy to worry about food, nutrition, meal planning, or eating right. Additionally, adolescents tend to form different associations with healthy foods and junk foods. As shown in Table 11–5, adolescents form mainly negative associations with healthy foods, but positive associations with junk foods (Chapman and Maclean, 1993). In order for adolescents to change their eating habits to better behaviors, counseling must center on fitting proper nutrition into allowable time, making selection of healthy foods easier, and making healthy foods appealing to teens and their peers.

During the time of peak growth velocity, adolescents usually need to eat large amounts of food often. They are able to use foods with a high concentration of energy; however, they need to be increasingly careful of the amounts and frequency of eating when growth has slowed. Habits of overeating adopted during adolescence may ultimately contribute to a number of debilitating diseases.

Fast Foods and the Media

The use of fast foods for meals or snacks is especially popular with busy adolescents. So-called fast foods include foods from vending machines, self-service restaurants, convenience groceries, and franchised food restaurants. Fast foods tend to be low in iron, calcium, riboflavin, and vitamin A, and there are few sources of folic acid. The vitamin C content of fast foods is also low unless fruit or fruit juice is consumed. Although most places offer a selection of healthy foods, most of the food items provide more than 50% of their calories from fat. Adolescents should be counseled on how to make wise and healthy choices when eating in one of these establishments.

Television and magazines probably have a greater influence on adolescents' eating habits than any other form of mass media. It is estimated that, by the time the average child reaches the teen years, he or she has viewed 100,000 food commercials, most of them for products with high concentrations of fat and simple carbohydrates. More than 65% of food advertisements promote beverages (primarily alcohol) and sweets (Brown, 1998).

SITUATIONS WITH SPECIAL NEEDS

Pregnancy

Recommended weight gains during pregnancy may be slightly higher for the teenager than for the adult. The current recommendation is that pregnant adolescents should gain weight within the upper range of that currently recommended for adults (i.e., 30 to 35 lb) (Institute of Medicine, 1990). For adolescents with a below-normal prepregnancy weight, a 35- to 40-lb weight gain may be desirable (Institute of Medicine, 1990; Story and Alton, 1992) (see Chapter 7).

Pregnant adolescents who are of young **gynecologic age** (defined as the number of years between the onset of menses and the date of conception) or who are undernourished at the time of conception have the greatest nutritional needs. A young woman who conceives soon after her first menstrual period is at greatest physiologic risk. It was once thought that adolescents with advanced physiologic maturity had no more physical complications during pregnancy than adult women, but the Camden study (Scholl, 1998) has shown that both these adolescents and their infants are at increased risk. This longitudinal study sought to explain why, with increasing maternal weight gains in adolescent mothers, the infant birth weights remained low. This increased risk of fetal growth restriction may be attributed to disruption in the fetal-placental blood flow and in the transmission of nutrients to the fetus as a result of the physiology associated with maternal growth. Perhaps the increased concentrations of insulin, human growth hormone, and insulin-like growth factors that are characteristic of adolescent growth (even into late adolescence), when superimposed on the normal milieu of pregnancy, enhance accrual of fat stores and maternal weight gain but diminish circulating nutrients, ultimately impairing fetal growth.

Aside from the consequences to the outcome of pregnancy, adolescents who begin their childbearing early (while still growing themselves), may be at particular risk for overweight and obesity. The Camden Study (Hediger et al., 1998) has documented that the excessive accrual of subcutaneous fat stores at central body sites often, in later life, leads to the development of cardiovascular disease, non–insulin-dependent diabetes mellitus, and hypertension.

A clinically practical method of ensuring nutritional adequacy is to encourage the pregnant adolescent to gain the recommended amount of weight by consuming nutrient-rich foods. Most important, contact with health professionals during prenatal care provides the opportunity to teach adolescents about feeding themselves and their families (American Dietetic Association, 1994). Because of the economic instability of the pregnant adolescent, it is impossible to assume that she will have an adequate food supply. Health professionals can help provide access to and information about resources, such as food stamps, food banks, and the Women, Infants, and Children (WIC) program. Table 7–4 lists recommended amounts of nutrients during pregnancy.

Eating Disorders

Eating disorders and unhealthy eating behaviors, such as restrictive dieting, overeating, and the use of harmful weight-control behaviors (e.g., vomiting, overuse of laxatives) represent major health concerns affecting adolescents, predominantly female adolescents (although there has been an increase in eating disorders among males recently). Eating disorders typically begin between the ages of 14 and 20 years (Striegel-Moore, 1997). It is estimated that, for adolescents, eating disorders constitute the third most common chronic disease after obesity and asthma (Golden, 1997).

Just as adolescents are at increased risk for developing eating disorders, they are also more vulnerable to the complications of these disorders. The impact of malnutrition on linear growth, brain development, and bone acquisition can be long-standing and irreversible. Yet, with early and aggressive treatment, there is potential for a better outcome than in adults who have more long-standing disease (Golden, 1997).

Early identification of adolescents with disordered eating habits has been linked to improved long-term outcome, but this is difficult to accomplish. Often, parents will bring an affected teen in for another reason—gastrointestinal complaints, amenorrhea, or unexplained weight loss. A screen for disordered eating can easily be done, and this should include questions about fear of becoming fat, amount of dieting, use of laxatives, fasting or frequent meal skipping to lose weight, and excessive exercise.

Because adolescence is the greatest period of risk for development of an eating disorder, efforts must be made to reduce the incidence of malnutrition, or at least provide early intervention to prevent its serious complications (Striegel-Moore, 1997). This subject is discussed in greater detail in Chapter 24 (also see Eating Disorders Awareness and Prevention at http://members.aol.com/edapinc).

Obesity

Obesity in teenagers seems to be on the rise. Among 12- to 19-year-olds in the United States, the prevalence of overweight is up to 21%, an increase of 6% in the past decade. Although the underlying causes of obesity are not fully understood, obesity appears to be a complex, multifactorial, chronic disease. Contributing factors include genetics, metabolic physiology, and environmental and psychosocial factors. The eating habits and physical inactivity patterns of adolescents both have contributed to the rise in adolescent obesity (Christoffel and Ariza, 1998; Troiano and Flegal, 1998). However, teenagers are merely tracking recent trends in the adult population, which include a similar increase in overweight during the past decade (Troiano et al., 1995).

This is a disturbing trend that warrants the attention of health professionals, as overweight in adolescence appears to be associated with a range of adverse physical health effects that are independent of adult weight. This fact was demonstrated in a 55-year follow-up of the Harvard Growth Study. An increased risk of morbidity from coronary heart disease and atherosclerosis was found in both men and women who were overweight as teens. In men who were overweight during adolescence, the risk of colorectal cancer and gout was increased, whereas in women who were overweight in their youth, the risk of arthritis was increased over that of their leaner counterparts (Must et al., 1992).

The social and economic consequences of overweight in adolescence are, perhaps, even greater than the long-term physical health effects. In fact, the former appear to be greater than those experienced by teens with chronic diseases, such as asthma, musculoskeletal abnormalities, diabetes, and epilepsy, and the consequences are more severe in women than in men (Gortmaker et al., 1993; Stunkard, 1993). Remaining unmarried, earning a low income, and obtaining fewer years of education have been found to be related to the incidence of obesity and to the persistence of discrimination against the obese that continues in our society (see Chapter 23).

The obese teenager may gain weight as a result of a combination of psychological, physiologic, and cultural factors, as discussed in Chapter 23. It appears that the longer teenagers have been obese for any reason, the greater the chance that their bodies will be subject to processes that tend to maintain the obese state. By adolescence, they often have adopted the restricted life-style characteristic of the obese. Commonly, they do not want to be seen in settings requiring vigorous exercise, and they are often subjected to real or imagined social rejection.

Accurate identification of the overweight adolescent is important because early, family-centered, behavior-based treatment can be successful (Williams, 1998). The adolescent can be evaluated based on BMI (weight/height^2 or kg/m^2) as shown in Table 11–1 and Appendix Table 20. Adolescents with BMIs at or above the 95th percentile for age and sex, or those with BMIs above 30 (whichever is smaller), should be considered overweight for screening purposes (see Table 11–1). These adolescents should be referred for further in-depth medical assessment and treatment. Those adolescents with BMIs at or above the 85th percentile for age and sex, but less than the 95th percentile or equal to 30 (whichever is smaller), are considered to be at risk of overweight. These teens should be referred for second-level screening, which includes data on family history, blood pressure, total cholesterol level, any major change in BMI, and concern about weight (Himes and Dietz, 1994). Figure 11–4 outlines the established screening guidelines for overweight adolescents.

Teenagers are vulnerable to unrealistic attitudes about the amount of time and effort necessary for effective weight management. Diet fads, drugs, and equipment appear to them to provide the quick remedy they seek. Meanwhile, realistic educational and comprehensive therapeutic programs are scarce. Thus, the obese teenager is very likely to be obese throughout life.

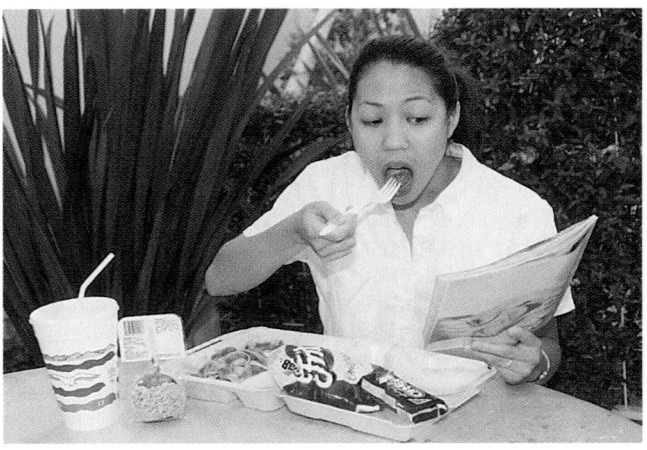

FIGURE 11–4 The choice of foods is more important than the time or place of eating for teenagers who obtain nourishment outside traditional meals. (From Bowden VR, Dickey SB, Greenberg CS. Children and Their Families: The Continuum of Care. Philadelphia: WB Saunders, 1998, p. 2032).

Education about weight control can be designed effectively for a wide range of audiences in a variety of settings, including youth programs and organizations. To be successful, therapeutic programs must include an individualized nutrition plan, a physical activity plan, and psychologically supportive components involving families as well as the individual adolescent (Williams, 1998). Family therapy is an important factor in preventing progression from obesity in childhood to severe obesity in adolescence (Flodmark et al., 1993).

Hyperlipidemias

Pediatric epidemiology programs have established that the major adult cardiovascular diseases—coronary artery disease and essential hypertension—begin in childhood. Cardiovascular risk factors change during periods of growth and development, and there are distinct ethnic (black-white) and male-female differences that relate to adult heart disease (Spotlight on Research, 1994). These risk factors have been shown to "track" over a 15-year period and are predictive of adult levels (Berenson, 1998). Cardiovascular risk factors also tend to cluster; for example, obesity correlates with high blood pressure and with adverse serum lipoprotein changes. Adolescents with high blood cholesterol levels are also likely to have elevated cholesterol levels as adults. Attention should be paid to screening children and adolescents in families with a history of premature cardiovascular disease or parental hypercholesterolemia (NCEP, 1991). Among the individuals who should be screened are: (1) children and adolescents whose parents or grandparents, at age 55 years or less, were found to have coronary atherosclerosis through diagnostic coronary arteriography, or who suffered a documented cardiovascular or cerebrovascular event or sudden cardiac death; (2) children and adolescents with a parent who has an elevated blood cholesterol level; and (3) adolescents who are at high risk because they smoke or because they are obese.

The nutritional recommendations of the National Cholesterol Education Program (NCEP), discussed in detail in Chapter 26, are appropriate for all children older than 2 years of age. Helping adolescents understand the importance of current life-style factors on later disease processes is a challenge, but not impossible. The challenge is in making the information practical in the adolescent's hectic life-style, much of which revolves around consuming food that is high in fat, low in fiber and nutrients, and of limited variety. Promoting healthy life-style behaviors should include a discussion not only of food choices, but also of the risks of smoking and alcohol use and the benefits of increased physical activity.

The Child and Adolescent Trial of Cardiovascular Health (CATCH), initiated in 1987, is a study of 12,000 elementary school children and adolescents and is designed to evaluate school-based interventions in reducing subsequent cardiovascular risk (Nicklas et al., 1998). The results of this program have demonstrated that a school-based program involving school food service, physical education, classroom curricula, and the family can help children and adolescents make healthful changes in behavior. If these changes can be continued for several years, there is considerable potential for producing cardiovascular health benefits.

Sports Nutrition

Young athletes are particularly vulnerable to nutritional misinformation and unsafe practices that promise enhanced performance. Pressures to achieve optimal performance encourage athletes to experiment with supplements and ergogenic aids in order to achieve the "competitive edge." (See Chapter 25.) Inappropriate use of supplements, unsafe weight loss practices, and inadequate nutrient intakes can adversely affect the adolescent's health and limit growth.

Adequate fluid intake and prevention of dehydration are critical for young athletes. This is especially true for the younger adolescent. In fact, heat illness ranks second to head injury as a cause of reported noncardiac causes of death in secondary school athletes. Compared to adults, children and young adolescents are at higher risk for becoming dehydrated and developing hyperthermia because of the following factors (Steen, 1996):

- They sweat less (absolute and per sweat gland), which potentially decreases their capacity to dissipate heat through the evaporation of the sweat.
- They experience greater heat production during exercise but have less ability to transfer heat from the muscles to the skin.
- They have a greater body surface area, which can result in excessive heat gain in extreme heat and excessive heat loss in the cold.
- They have a lower cardiac output, which reduces their capacity for heat transport from the core to the skin during strenuous exercise.
- They acclimatize to exercising in heat more gradually than adults. A young adolescent may require five to six sessions to achieve the same degree of acclimatization acquired by an adult in 2 to 3 sessions in the same environment.

It should be remembered that not only the actual temperature, but also the degree of humidity, affects an individual's ability to dissipate heat. The higher the humidity, the less sweat that will be evaporated from the skin; this decreases the body's ability to cool itself and increases the risk of heat-related illness.

Adolescents with certain diseases or medical conditions are at increased risk for developing heat-related illness. Excessive fluid loss may occur in children or adolescents with bulimia, congenital heart disease, diabetes mellitus, gastroenteritis, fever, or obesity. Additionally, insufficient fluid intake may occur in persons with anorexia nervosa, cystic fibrosis, mental retardation, or kidney disease. Children who are obese experience heat-related illness more frequently than children of normal weight because: (1) only a small amount of heat is needed to increase the temperature of a large amount of fat mass; (2) fat mass has a lower water content than lean body mass (so a greater amount of fluid is lost in persons with high fat mass; and (3) obese children expend greater effort than lean children, given the same intensity of exercise, which increases their overall body temperature more quickly.

Teens with these conditions should be considered to be at high risk, and should be watched more closely when they are physically active, but they should not be kept from participating in activities. If kept properly hydrated, these children's medical conditions can often be improved with a consistent physical activity program.

As with adults, adolescent athletes need a diet high in carbohydrates for energy, with adequate amounts of protein (see Chapter 25). Recommended levels include 55% to 60% carbohydrate, 15% to 20% protein, and 25% to 30% fat. Supplements promising increased muscle mass, increased strength, and improved ability should be used with caution, and in most cases, should be avoided. Many of these supplements increase the risk for dehydration and have little impact on the development of muscle mass.

Acne

Dermatologic complaints account for as many as 50% of adolescent contacts with health professionals. Acne is a normal characteristic of development that occurs with varying degrees of severity. It is initiated by the influence of testosterone on the sebaceous gland and is mediated by other factors, such as stress, stage of menstrual cycle, and composition of the affected tissues in the individual. Dietary factors have traditionally been blamed, but carefully controlled studies have shown no correlation between the ingestion of foods and the appearance or degree of acne. Teenagers should be supported in their efforts to deal with this problem by discussing the physiologic basis for its development and control.

Effective medications include oral antibiotics and topical applications of benzoyl peroxide, and tretinoin (Retin-A), an oral synthetic retinoid 13-*cis*-retinoic acid (Accutane), and a vitamin A derivative. Although very effective in treating acne, tretinoin can cause an increase in serum triglyceride and total cholesterol levels that is reversed after medication is discontinued. Adolescents taking Accutane should have their lipid levels checked before and during treatment, and appropriate diet therapy should be started if necessary. Women should also avoid unprotected sexual activity, because tretinoin is a teratogen and mutagen.

Vitamin A is the most effective vitamin for treating acne because it reduces the production of sebum (the white fatty substance found in the body's pores). Vitamin A is the base for many topical acne products, including Accutane. It is important to remember, however, that large amounts of vitamin A may be toxic. Vitamin E helps to regulate the level of vitamin A. Laboratory studies have shown that animals deficient in vitamin E have difficulty processing vitamin A. Adolescents should be encouraged to consume diets with adequate amounts of vitamins A and E (Hurwitz, 1995).

The role of zinc in the development and treatment of acne is confusing. If a role does exist, it may be related to the free fatty acid production of the pilosebaceous follicle. One study found low levels of serum zinc in those suffering most from acne, suggesting that zinc deficiency exacerbates the condition (Michaelson et al., 1977).

Substance Use

Use of tobacco, alcohol, marijuana, and other drugs is a major public health problem. The effect of these chemicals on nutritional status depends on the amount and length of use, as well as on the individual's general state of health. Studies have indicated that although adolescent alcohol and drug abusers generally consume adequate quantities of principal nutrients and do not develop nutrient deficiencies, they obtain these nutrients from a narrower range of foods than nonabusers.

Juvenile Incarceration

Teens involved with the juvenile justice system are at increased risk for nutritional problems. These teens often engage in risk-taking behaviors that interfere with adequate nutritional intake, and thus are often affected by social conditions that make appropriate food unavailable. Of concern to nutritional health professionals working within the juvenile justice system is the level of nutritional care once a teen is adjudicated. It has been noticed that many teens (especially male adolescents during their peak height velocity) lose a significant amount of weight when they are incarcerated. When these teens are interviewed, they state that they are always hungry. National guidelines established for correctional facilities provide for approximately 2200 calories per day. Although this caloric intake is sufficient for younger adolescents, it is inadequate for growing teens. There are many reasons why nutritional problems exist in juvenile facilities, among them limited resources for food, lack of understanding of the nutritional needs of adolescents on the part of food service employees and administrative staff, lack of consultation from trained nutritional professionals, and teens' dislike of foods served in the facility.

STRATEGIES FOR IMPROVING NUTRITIONAL WELL-BEING

Assessment of Nutritional Status

Assessment of nutritional status in adolescents follows normal procedures, but with some exceptions (See Chapters 16 and 17.) It is important to use an age-specific data base for each aspect of nutritional assessment. Standards based on stage of maturity are even more exact, and should be used if available.

Nutritional assessment also should include an evaluation of the nutritional environment, including parental, peer, school, cultural, and personal lifestyle factors. The attitude of the adolescent toward food and nutrition is also a primary component of a comprehensive evaluation. A prime component of nutritional counseling for adolescents is helping them overcome their perceived barriers to eating well (see earlier section on Food Habits).

TABLE 11–6 RECOMMENDED DAILY EATING GUIDE FOR ADOLESCENTS

- 3–4 cups of nonfat or low-fat milk or yogurt—to provide calcium, vitamin D, riboflavin, and, in some vegetarian teens, adequate protein intake
- 5 or more servings of fresh, frozen, dried, raw, or cooked fruits and/or vegetables, mostly yellow, orange, dark green, or red
- 2 servings (2–3 oz each) of lean protein foods, such as chicken, turkey, fish, lean beef, or lean pork
- 6–11 servings of grains, breads, and cereals (preferably whole-grain), rolls, pasta, rice, potatoes, and other starches to meet energy needs
- Small amounts, perhaps once per day, of high-fat, high-sugar items, such as desserts, soda, candy, cookies, and pastries, which have little nutritional value

CASE STUDY 1

Male Adolescent

Joe Y. is a 17-year-old adolescent who lives at home with his parents and younger sister. He has no prior medical problems, but recently complained about lack of energy during sports and athletic activities at school. He has been scheduled to meet with you, a nutrition counselor, because his pediatrician recommended it. Upon arrival, he shares his food diary with you, which indicates that he skips lunch on the days that he will be wrestling after school. Otherwise, he eats the same meals each day—sugar-sweetened cereals with whole milk and black coffee for breakfast; a luncheon meat sandwich with two candy bars on days when he eats lunch; and a typical family meal for dinner.

1. What suggestions will you make about his breakfast and lunch meals?
2. How much calcium does he need at the age of 17 years? If he drinks only one glass of milk each day, what percentage of his daily requirement is he missing?
3. What other nutrients might be low in Joe's diet? How can he change his diet to include the proper types of foods that he needs at his age?

Prerequisites for Change

Especially because of their growing independence, any attempt to help adolescents improve their nutritional status will require careful planning. For a plan to succeed, the adolescent must be willing to change. An assessment of the teen's desire to change is essential. Encouraging the desire to change usually requires most of the nutrition counselor's attention. A recommended eating plan for meeting adolescents' nutritional needs is presented in Table 11–6.

Knowledge, attitude, and behavior must be addressed when guiding adolescents toward acquiring healthful food habits. Information can be provided in a variety of settings, ranging from the classroom to a hospital bedside.The clinician must understand the change process and how to communicate that process in a meaningful way (see Chapter 21). Parents must be included in the process and encouraged to be supportive but not intrusive.

CASE STUDY 2

Female Adolescent

Carly R. is a 14-year-old girl who has been referred to you by her mother and her family physician. Mom is concerned that Carly is not eating right, and her doctor wants you to give her some nutritional advice, especially because she has expressed a desire to be a vegetarian. She has heard that red meat contains a lot of fat and she "does not want to get fat." A physical examination by her physician shows that she is between Tanner stage 1 and 2 for development, she weighs 89 lb, and she is 5 feet tall. She is extremely active, spending every afternoon after school playing some kind of sport—basketball, swimming, track, or soccer.

1. List at least four questions you would include in your assessment session with this young person. Why would you include these questions?
2. What are the particular nutritional requirements for a teenaged girl in Tanner stage 1?
3. How would you address this girl's concern about meat and her desire to be a vegetarian?
4. How would you counsel this young person regarding her desire not to get fat?
5. What advice would you give this teen's parents regarding their food-related interactions with her?

CITED REFERENCES

Alaimo K, et al. Dietary intake of vitamins, minerals and fiber of persons ages 2 months and over in the United States: Third National Health and Nutrition Examination Survey, Phase 1, 1988–91. Advance data from vital and health statistics, No. 258. Hyattsville, MD: National Center for Health Statistics, 1994.

Albertson AM, et al. Estimated dietary calcium intake and food sources for adolescent females: 1980–92. J Adol Health Care 20:20, 1997.

American Dietetic Association. Position on nutrition care for pregnant adolescents. J Am Diet Assoc 94:449, 1994.

Berenson GS, et al. Precursors of cardiovascular risk in young adults from a biracial (black-white) population: The Bogalusa Heart Study. In: Jacobson MS, Rees JM, Golden NH, Irwin CE (eds.). Adolescent Nutritional Disorders: Prevention and Treatment. New York: The New York Academy of Science, 1998.

Brown JD, Witherspoon EM. The mass media and American adolescents' health. Proceedings of the Health Futures of Youth! Pathways to Adolescent Health Conference. Annapolis, MD, September 14, 1998.

Chapman G, Maclean H. "Junk food" and "healthy food": Meanings of food in adolescent women's culture. J Nutr Educ. 25:108, 1993.

Christoffel KK, Ariza A. The epidemiology of overweight in children: Relevance for clinical care. Pediatrics 101:103, 1998.

Desmond SM, et al. Black and white adolescents' perceptions of their weight. J School Health 59:353, 1989.

Devaney BL, et al. Dietary intakes of students. Am J Clin Nutr 61(suppl): 205, 1995.

Driskell JA, Clark AJ, Moak SW. Longitudinal assessment of vitamin B_6 status in Southern adolescent girls. J Am Diet Assoc 87:307, 1987.

Emmons L. Predisposing factors differentiating adolescent dieters and nondieters. J Am Diet Assoc 94:725, 1994.

Flodmark C-E, et al. Prevention of progression to severe obesity in a group of obese schoolchildren treated with family therapy. Pediatrics 91:880, 1993.

Golden N. The adolescent: Vulnerable to develop an eating disorder and at high risk for long-term sequelae. In: Jacobson MS, Rees JM, Golden N, Irwin C (eds.). Adolescent Nutritional Disorders: Prevention and Treatment. New York: Annals of the New York Academy of Sciences, 1997, pp. 94.

Gortmaker SL, et al. Social and economic consequences of overweight in adolescence and young adulthood. N Engl J Med 329:1008, 1993.

Hediger ML, et al. Implications of the Camden Study of Adolescent Pregnancy: Interactions among maternal growth, nutrition status, and body composition. In: Jacobson MS, Rees JM, Golden NH, Irwin CE (eds.). Adolescent Nutritional Disorders: Prevention and Treatment. New York: The New York Academy of Science, 1998.

Himes JH, Dietz WH. Guidelines for overweight in adolescent preventive services: Recommendations from an expert committee. Am J Clin Nutr 59:307, 1994.

Hurwitz S. Acne treatment for the '90s. Contemporary Pediatrics 12(8):19, 1995.

Institute of Medicine, Committee on Nutrition Status During Pregnancy and Lactation: Nutrition During Pregnancy, Pt. 1. Weight gain. Washington, DC: National Academy Press, 1990.

Institute of Medicine, Food and Nutrition Board. Dietary Reference Intakes for Calcium, Phosphorus, Magnesium, Vitamin D, and Fluoride. Washington, DC: National Academy Press, 1997.

Kann L, et al. Youth risk behavior surveillance: United States, 1995. J School Health 66:365, 1996.

Mahan LK, Rees JR. Nutrition in Adolescence. St. Louis: Times/Mirror Mosby, 1984.

Marshall WA, Tanner JM. Variations in the pattern of pubertal changes in boys. Arch Dis Child 45:13, 1970.

Michaelson G, et al. Effects of oral zinc and vitamin A in acne. Arch Dermatol 113:31, 1977.

Moore DC. Body image and eating behavior in adolescent boys. Am J Dis Child 144:475, 1990.

Moore DC. Body image and eating behavior in adolescent girls. Am J Dis Child 142:144, 1988.

Must A, et al. Long-term morbidity and mortality of overweight adolescents. N Engl J Med 327:1350, 1992.

National Cholesterol Education Program (NCEP): Report of the Expert Panel on Blood Cholesterol Levels in Children and Adolescents. NIH Publication No. 91-2732. National Heart, Lung and Blood Institute, Public Health Service, September, 1991.

Nicklas TA, et al. School-based programs for health-risk reduction. In: Jacobson MS, Rees JM, Golden NH, Irwin CE (eds.). Adolescent Nutritional Disorders: Prevention and Treatment. New York: The New York Academy of Science, 1998.

Recommended Dietary Allowances, 10th ed. Washington, DC: National Academy of Sciences/National Academy Press, 1989.

Resnick, MD, et al. Health and risk behaviors of urban adolescent males involved in pregnancy. Families in Society: The Journal of Contemporary Human Services 74:366,1993.

Scholl TO, et al. Maternal growth and fetal growth: Pregnancy course and outcome in the Camden Study. In: Jacobson MS, Rees JM, Golden NH, Irwin CE (eds.). Adolescent Nutritional Disorders: Prevention and Treatment. New York: The New York Academy of Science, 1998.

Serdula MK, et al. Weight control practices of U.S. adolescents and adults. Ann Intern Med 119 (no. 7, pt. 2):667, 1993.

Spear BA. Adolescent growth and development. In: Rickert VI (ed.). Adolescent Nutrition: Assessment and Management. New York: Chapman and Hall, 1996, pp. 3–24.

Spotlight on Research: Heart Memo, Special Edition, 1994. Bethesda, MD: Office of Prevention, Education and Control, National Heart, Lung and Blood Institute, Public Health Service, National Institutes of Health, 1994.

Steen SN. Timely statement of the American Dietetic Association: Nutrition guidance for adolescent athletes in organized sports. J Am Diet Assoc 96:610, 1996.

Story M, Alton I. Nutrition management of the pregnant adolescent. Nutr MD 18:1, 1992.

Story M, Resnick MD. Adolescents' views on food and nutrition. J Nutr Educ 18:188, 1986.

Striegel-Moore R. Risk factors for eating disorders. In: Jacobson MS, Rees JM, Golden N, Irwin C (eds.). Adolescent Nutritional Disorders: Prevention and Treatment. New York: Annals of the New York Academy of Sciences, 1997, pp. 98–109.

Stunkard AJ, Sorensen TIA. Obesity and socioeconomic status—A complex relation. N Engl J Med 329:1036, 1993.

Thornburg H. Contemporary Adolescence: Readings, 2nd ed. Monterey, CA: Brooks/Cole, 1975, p. 7.

Troiano RP, Flegal KM. Overweight children and adolescents: Description, epidemiology and demographics. Pediatr 101(suppl):497, 1998.

Troiano RP, et al. Overweight prevalence and trends for children and adolescents. The National Health and Nutrition Examination Surveys, 1963–1991. Arch Pediatr Adolesc Med 149:1085, 1995.

Williams CL, et al. Management of childhood obesity in pediatric practice. In: Jacobson MS, Rees JM, Golden NH, Irwin CE. Adolescent Nutritional Disorders: Prevention and Treatment. New York: The New York Academy of Science, 1998.

World Health Organization (WHO). Physical status: The use and interpretation of anthropometry. Report of a WHO Expert Committee. WHO Tech Rep Ser 854:1–452, 1995.

Yates AM, et al. Dietary Reference Intakes: The new basis for recommendations for calcium and related nutrients, B vitamins and choline. J Am Diet Assoc 98:699,1998.

ADDITIONAL REFERENCES

Frisancho AR, et al. Developmental and nutritional determinants of pregnancy outcome among teenagers. Am J Phys Anthropol 66:247, 1985.

Frisch RE. Fatness of girls from menarche to age 18 years, with a nomogram. Hum Biol 48:353, 1976.

Gong E, Heald FT. Diet, nutrition and adolescence. In: Shils ME, Olson JA, Shike M (eds.). Modern Nutrition in Health and Disease, 8th ed. Philadelphia: Lea & Febiger, 1994.

Gong EJ, Spear BA. Adolescent growth and development: Implications for nutritional needs. J Nutr Educ 20:273, 1988.

Hammer LD, et al. Standardized percentile curves of body-mass index for children and adolescents. Am J Dis Child 145:259, 1991.

Johnson RK, et al. Characterizing nutrient intakes of adolescents by sociodemographic factors. J Adol Health 15:149, 1994.

Merzenich H, et al. Dietary fat and sports activity as determinants for age at menarche. Am J Epidemiol 138:217, 1993.

Meserole LP, et al. Prenatal weight gain and postpartum weight loss pattern in adolescents. J Adol Health Care 5:21, 1984.

Must A, et al. Reference data for obesity: 85th and 95th percentiles of body mass index (wt/ht_2) and triceps skinfold thickness. Am J Clin Nutr 53:839, 1991.

Must A, et al. Reference data for obesity: 85th and 95th percentiles of body mass index (wt/ht_2)—A correction. Am J Clin Nutr 54:773, 1991 (rapid communication).

National Institute of Health, Consensus Development Conference Statement, optimal calcium intake. Bethesda, MD. June 6–8, 1994.

Results from the National Adolescent Student Health Survey. JAMA 261:2025, 1989.

Schlicker SA, et al. The weight and fitness status of United States children. Nutr Rev 52:11, 1994.

Tanner JM. Foetus into Man: Physical Growth from Conception to Maturity. Cambridge, MA: Harvard University Press, 1978.

Thompson P, et al. Zinc status and sexual development in adolescent girls. J Am Diet Assoc 86:892, 1986.

Wright LS. Physiological development in adolescence. In: Mahan LK, Rees JM. Nutrition in Adolescence. St. Louis: Times/Mirror Mosby, 1984.

CHAPTER 12

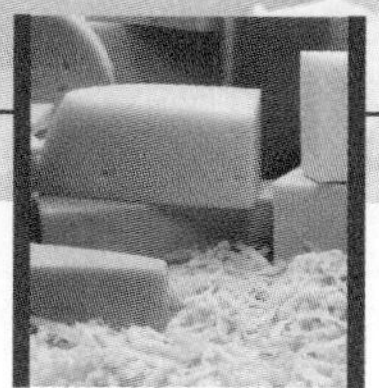

Nutrition in the Adult Years

KIMBERLY MATHAI, RD, MS

Chapter Outline

- Physiological and Psychosocial Changes
- Defensive Nutrition Paradigm
- Plant-Based Foods: Phytochemicals
- Intestinal Integrity
- Detoxification
- Guidelines for the Defensive Nutrition Paradigm

Key Terms

ALLYL SULFIDES—organosulfur phytochemicals found in allium vegetables; may act as cancer-blocking or cancer-suppressing agents

BUTYRATE (BUTYRIC ACID)—a short-chain fatty acid that is the preferred fuel of intestinal cells; produced by bacterial fermentation of dietary fiber

CAROTENOIDS—a subclass of terpene phytochemicals found in some vegetables, including tomatoes, parsley, oranges, pink grapefruit, and spinach

CYTOCHROME P-450 (MIXED-FUNCTION OXIDASE SYSTEM)—a family of enzymes involved in phase I of the liver detoxification system

DEFENSIVE NUTRITION PARADIGM—a nutrition plan that includes plant-based foods and balancing the intake of healthy fats in order to prevent disease and promote wellness

DETOXIFICATION—a process that decreases the negative impact of xenobiotics or toxins on the body

DITHIOLTHIONES, INDOLES, ISOTHIOCYANATES—organosulfur phytochemicals; a subclass of thiols found in cruciferous vegetables

DYSBIOSIS—an imbalance in gut microflora that may produce harmful effects

FLAVONOIDS—a subclass of phenol phytochemicals that are pigments and that act as free radical scavengers in plants

GENISTEIN—an isoflavone found in soy products

GENOME—the complete set of hereditary factors contained in a haploid set of chromosomes

GLYCEMIC INDEX—a ranking of the effect on blood glucose of the consumption of a single food relative to a reference carbohydrate (e.g., white bread or glucose)

GUT-ASSOCIATED LYMPHOID TISSUE (GALT)—lymphoid tissue surrounding the digestive tract

ISOFLAVONES—a subclass of phenol phytochemicals, found in beans and other legumes (especially soybeans), that may have cancer-preventing properties, especially against hormone-driven cancers

LACTOBACILLUS—a beneficial intestinal organism that produces organic acids which retard the growth of pathogenic bacteria

LIGNANS—phytoestrogens, found in flaxseeds, wheat bran, and other whole grains, that affect sex hormone metabolism and may reduce the risk of hormone-linked cancer

LIMONOIDS—a subclass of terpenes found in citrus fruits; identified as chemopreventive agents that induce enzymes in the liver's phase I and II enzyme detoxification system

LYCOPENE—one of the carotenoid phytochemicals found in tomatoes that acts as a free radical scavenger

PHASE I AND PHASE II DETOXIFICATION—the sequential two-stage enzyme detoxification process of the liver, whereby toxic molecules are biotransformed from lipid-soluble substances into water-soluble molecules that can then be excreted from the body

PHENOLS—a class of phytochemicals that function in plants as blue, blue-red, and violet pigments and that provide protection against oxidative damage

PHYTOCHEMICALS—biologically active, naturally occurring substances in plants that act as natural defense systems in plants and that show potential for reducing risk for cancer and cardiovascular disease

PHYTOESTROGENS—phytochemicals that are non-steroidal estrogens of dietary origins; structurally similar to estrogens, they act in the body as weak estrogens and antiestrogens

PLANT-BASED DIET—an eating plan in which plant foods provide a significant portion of the nutrients and calories, as presented in the food guide pyramid

PREBIOTICS—nondigestible food products that stimulate the growth of symbiotic bacterial species already present in the colon; they help to improve the health of the host

PREMENSTRUAL SYNDROME—symptoms occurring around the time of menses that may include anxiety, mood swings, depression, fatigue, breast tenderness, weight gain, cramps, and backache

PROBIOTICS—microbial foods or supplements that can be used to change or reestablish the intestinal flora and improve the health of the host

SYNDROME X—a cluster of metabolic disorders, including non–insulin-dependent diabetes mellitus, hypertension, and dyslipidemia, that is characterized by insulin resistance

TERPENES—the largest class of phytochemicals; found in a wide variety of plants

THIOL—a sulfur-containing phytonutrient found in cruciferous vegetables

Nutrition in the adult years emphasizes the importance of diet in maintaining wellness and preventing disease. The role of nutrition has expanded significantly, and it is now viewed as a tool that can be used not just to prevent deficiency diseases but as a defense against chronic disease. A U.S. Department of Health and Human Services (DHHS) report, "Healthy People 2000: National Health Promotion and Disease Prevention Objectives," states that 50% of the mortality from chronic disease may be modified by life-style factors, such as nutrition (U.S. DHHS, 1990). The report of the American Institute for Cancer Research, "Food Nutrition and the Prevention of Cancer: A Global Perspective" reviews more than 4500 research studies and estimates that cancer rates would drop by as much as 20% if people would eat five or more servings of fruits and vegetables per day (American Institute for Cancer Research, 1997). This link between diet and disease is important in adulthood, even though the symptoms of disease may not appear until the sixth or seventh decades of life.

PHYSIOLOGICAL AND PSYCHOSOCIAL CHANGES

Physiological Changes

There are significant physiologic and psychosocial changes that occur in the adulthood years from ages 25 to 55. The outstanding physiologic change in many adults during this time is weight gain, involving body composition shifts with a lessening of lean body mass and an accumulation of larger fat stores. More than 50% of Americans are somewhat overweight; 33% are obese (Rippe, 1998). (See Chapter 23.) Two factors that significantly impact weight gain are excessive caloric intake, which may lead to increased fat stores, and a lack of physical activity, which results in a decline in lean body mass. The physiologic changes that result from weight gain have important health consequences. With an increase in body weight, adult health can shift from wellness and progress to chronic disease. Comorbid conditions associated with obesity include Type 2

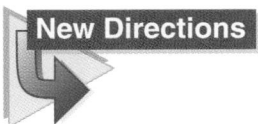

Role for Nutrition in Genetics and Immunity

Scientists at the frontiers of nutrition research are examining the links between disease and genetics and advancing our understanding of how disease resulting from loss of cellular control can be managed or prevented. As research continues to study how the human genome works (e.g., Who is likely to develop colon cancer or breast cancer? Who is at risk for type 2 diabetes because of a PC-1 gene?), health care professionals may soon be able to develop individualized nutrition interventions, pharmacotherapy, or life-style modifications based on an individual's genetic uniqueness and biochemical individuality.

Many genetic characteristics exhibit pleomorphism, which means that they can be expressed in different ways depending upon internal and external triggers. This gene plasticity explains that while specific diseases such as heart disease, arthritis, and cancer may have a genetic component, persons may also have protection from these diseases because of other genetic characteristics. Modifications of gene expression may be related to endo- and exotoxins, such as infectious organisms, stress, radiation, trauma, and other factors including nutrition and activity and exercise patterns (Bland, 1999). An individual's phenotype (and thus health) results from an interaction between the genome and these triggers. These triggers act by causing cells to release intercellular communication agents such as hormones, prostaglandins, neurotransmitters, and endorphins. Because these agents are produced by many types of cells and the result of altered gene expression is altered protein synthesis, the function of many organ systems can be modified. Imbalances of these agents in response to a trigger result in signs and symptoms of illness. New research is giving us a deeper understanding of the role of life-style, nutrition, and environment in determining which intercellular communication agents are expressed at any one time from a person's genes.

Nutrients affect cell recognition, receptor site function, and genetic expression. For example, zinc influences the enzyme which is involved in the production of messenger RNA, and a deficiency in this mineral can alter gene expression and protein synthesis (Bland, 1998). Other dietary components that interact with receptors and activate their gene regulatory networks are specific fatty acids such as DHA, vitamin A, and 1,25-dihydroxy Vit D3 (DeLuca, 1998; Gustafsson, 1998). The recognition of the impact of nutrition in support or suppression of genetic factors has profound consequences. Appropriate nutrition interventions can alter the consequences of genetic expression which promote chronic disease. And ultimately these nutrition interventions may slow down biological aging.

diabetes, impaired glucose tolerance, hyperinsulinemia, dyslipidemia, cardiovascular disease, hypertension, sleep apnea, gallbladder disease, osteoarthritis of weight-bearing joints, reduced fertility, and some cancers (Rippe, 1998). (See *"New Direction:* Role for Nutrition in Genetics and Immunity."

For women, the adult years include monthly hormonal shifts that trigger the female reproductive cycle. These hormones, including estrogen and progesterone, signal physiologic changes in the ovaries and uterus that prepare these organs for possible fertilization. (See *"Clinical Insight:* Premenstrual Syndrome.")

Perimenopause and menopause typically begin when a woman enters her late 40s. During menopause, estrogen production declines, and bone mass decreases. Osteoporosis, a bone-thinning disease, may occur in the menopausal and postmenopausal years. (See Chapter 28.) By the year 2010, an estimated 21 million women will reach age 50 and become menopausal; the average American woman lives at least one third of her life in the postmenopausal stage (Menopause, 1994).

Psychosocial Changes

Various social models exist for American adults—single adulthood, partnered adulthood without children, single-parent adulthood, adulthood in a two-parent working family, and adulthood in a two-parent family with one parent at home as caretaker. These varied social models influence food shopping, food preparation, and the frequency of sit-down meals in a home environment. Responsibilities of working or single parents, and stresses related to long working or commuting hours, affect eating habits. Too little time for food planning may lead to meal patterns that rely heavily on processed foods, take-out foods, or restaurant-prepared meals, with only sporadic meals prepared and eaten at home. These psychosocial factors contribute to food choices that may lead to steady weight gain in adults.

Food Patterns

Information about the prevalent food patterns of adults in the United States can be culled from government surveys, such as the United States Department of Agriculture's (USDA's) Continuing Survey of Food Intake by Individuals. This survey, also known as "What We Eat in America," measures the kind and amount of foods eaten by Americans. The 1994–1996 survey noted the following (Williams, 1997):

- About 25% of the calories consumed by both men and women 20 years of age and older are from foods obtained and eaten away from home.
- Snacks (including alcoholic beverages and other beverage categories) account for 17% of the total calories that Americans consume.

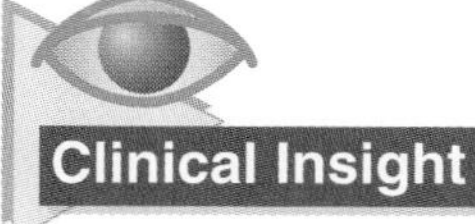

Premenstrual Syndrome

Many women experience menses-related mood fluctuations and general discomfort. For about 10% to 20% of these women, the symptoms are sufficiently severe to create personal hardship. The most common symptoms include anxiety, depression, mood swings, fatigue, weight gain, swelling, breast pain, cramps, and backache. This complex of physical and psychological symptoms, labeled **premenstrual syndrome** (PMS), generally begins 7 to 10 days prior to the onset of menses, increasing in severity as the menses approaches. Because peak severity usually occurs during menses, the term *perimenstrual symptoms* has been proposed to describe more accurately what most women experience.

No one consistent imbalance or deficiency has been identified to explain the etiology of PMS, although there are some promising theories related to hormone imbalance (estrogen and progesterone), neurotransmitter synthesis defects, disorders of essential fatty acid metabolism, and nutrient deficiencies.

Results of clinical trials examining the efficacy of various therapies are mixed. A number of studies have examined the effect of vitamin B_6 on symptoms of PMS; in one study, depression, irritability, and fatigue were improved with administration of 50 mg per day of vitamin B_6, but there was no improvement in other symptoms (Doll et al., 1989). Research into the role of essential fatty acids in the treatment of PMS has produced some positive outcomes in relieving symptoms, especially cyclical mastalgia (breast pain). In a series of double-blind trials, supplementation with 1 to 2 g of evening primrose oil (a source of the essential fatty acid gamma-linolenic acid) significantly reduced PMS symptoms, with the greatest impact being reported for mastalgia (Horrobin and Manku, 1989). In a study that examined the relationship between PMS symptoms and calcium regulation, women who took 1200 mg of calcium daily, in the form of calcium carbonate, throughout the course of three menstrual cycles reported significantly lower incidence of PMS symptoms compared to the placebo group (Thys-Jacobs et al., 1998).

Nutrition and stress reduction may also positively impact premenstrual symptoms. Women who experience PMS symptoms report higher intakes of refined carbohydrates, refined sugar, sodium, and dairy products than women without PMS (Abraham, 1987). A healthy diet that includes fruits and vegetables (especially dark green ones), whole grains, legumes, and quality fats and proteins, when combined with regular exercise and stress reduction or relaxation techniques, can help women cope with premenstrual syndrome.

- The average daily sodium intake from foods alone is more than 4000 mg for men and almost 3000 mg for women.
- Fifty percent of all Americans drink carbonated soft drinks on any given day.
- Twenty-five percent of all Americans eat fried potatoes on any given day.

The intake of fruits and vegetables among Americans is low; researchers in one study found that only 1 in 11 Americans has five or more servings of fruits and vegetables in a day. One in nine of those surveyed ate no fruit or vegetable on the interview day (Patterson et al., 1990). The average American has been shown to eat only about 1.5 servings of vegetables and 1 serving of fruit per day (Craig, 1997).

DEFENSIVE NUTRITION PARADIGM

A nutrition plan for adults that focuses on the promotion of health-building and health-sustaining dietary patterns to support continued full functioning during aging is a **defensive nutrition paradigm.** The goal of the defensive nutrition paradigm is to prevent disease and promote wellness by optimizing the intake of plant-based foods, such as fruits, vegetables, grains, and legumes. Balancing healthy fats, including the omega-6 and omega-3 essential fatty acids, while minimizing the intake of saturated fats is important in this plan. Consumption of meat, particularly red meat (beef, pork, and lamb), should be limited, if used at all. Red meat is a significant source of saturated animal fat and has been linked with increased risk of cancer, including colon and rectal cancer and, possibly, breast, pancreatic, and prostate cancer (American Institute for Cancer Research, 1997). Consumption of moderate portions of fish, poultry, and other forms of meat, such as wild game, is preferred in a **plant-based diet.** A food program that emphasizes plant-based foods, combined with a regular exercise program and maintenance of a healthy weight, may have a significant and positive impact on health by reducing the risk of cancer, cardiovascular disease, diabetes, and other chronic diseases.

Plant-based foods provide nutritional support for organ systems that help defend the body against chronic disease. These systems include (1) the gastrointestinal (GI) system, which absorbs nutrients for the body, protects the body from toxins, and acts as part of the body's immune system, and (2) the liver, with a two-phase enzyme detoxification system that acts as a disposal system for procarcinogens and other toxins.

PLANT-BASED FOODS: PHYTOCHEMICALS

Plant foods contain not only major components (e.g., protein, fat, carbohydrate, fiber, and micronutrients, such as vitamins and minerals) but also large numbers of nonnutrient compounds—**phytochemicals.** Phytochemicals (from the Greek word *phyto,* meaning plant), are biologically active, naturally occurring chemical components in plant foods. In plants, phytochemicals act as natural defense systems for their host plants, protecting the plants from infections and microbial invasions and giving color, aroma, and flavor. More than 2000 plant pigments are phytochemicals, such as flavonoids, carotenoids, and anthocyanins. Dietary sources of phytochemicals include fruits, vegetables, legumes, whole grains, nuts, seeds, fungi, herbs, and spices (Craig, 1997; King, 1999).

Phytochemicals are the subject of intense scientific research focusing on the prevention or treatment of chronic disease, especially cancer and heart disease (www.ncbi.nlm.nih.gov). As protection against cancer, plant-based chemicals act to detoxify drug toxins, carcinogens, and mutagens. These detoxification actions have overlapping and complementary mechanisms that include neutralizing free radicals, inhibiting enzymes that activate carcinogens, and inducing enzymes that detoxify carcinogens (Lampe, 1997; Steinmetz and Potter, 1996). Phytochemicals appear to reduce the risk of coronary heart disease by protecting low-density lipoprotein (LDL) cholesterol from oxidation, reducing the synthesis or absorption of cholesterol, and affecting blood pressure and clotting (A garden of phytochemicals, 1995).

Phytochemicals may act as blocking or suppressing agents to reduce the risk of cancer. Blocking agents prevent the active carcinogen or tumor promoter from reaching the target tissue by several mechanisms, or a combination of mechanisms: (1) by inducing activities of enzyme systems that detoxify carcinogens, (2) by trapping and sequestering reactive carcinogens, or (3) by blocking cellular events required for tumor promotion. Suppressing agents, whose actions are less well defined, may arrest carcinogenesis by acting on the cellular level, preventing malignant expression of cells that have been exposed to cancer-causing agents (Wattenberg, 1992).

A review of 156 dietary studies revealed that, in 82% of these studies, fruit and vegetable consumption reduced the risk of cancer by more than 50%. These researchers concluded that "For most cancer sites, persons with low fruit and vegetable intake (at least the lower one-fourth of the population) experience about twice the risk of cancer compared with those with high intake, even after controlling for potentially confounding factors" (Block, 1992).

Phytochemicals are grouped into classes on the basis of their similar protective functions, as well as their individual physical and chemical characteristics. Some of the major classes of phytochemicals are the terpenes, phenols, and thiols (Table 12–1).

Terpenes

Terpenes, one of the largest classes of phytonutrients, are found in a wide variety of plant foods and act as powerful antioxidants. **Carotenoids** are one

TABLE 12–1 PHYTOCHEMICALS AND THEIR SOURCES

PHYTOCHEMICAL	SOURCE
Butyrate	Fruits, vegetables, legumes
Carotenoids	Dark yellow and orange and deep green vegetables and fruit
Diallyl sulfide	Onions, garlic, scallions, leeks, chives
Flavonoids and phenols	Parsley, carrots, citrus fruits, broccoli, cabbage, cucumbers, squash, yams, tomatoes, eggplant, peppers, soy products, berries, potatoes, broad beans, pea pods, colored onions, radishes, horseradish, tea, onions, apples
Indoles	Cabbage, Brussels sprouts, cauliflower, spinach, broccoli
Isoflavones	Soybeans and soybean products
Isothiocyanates	Cabbage, cauliflower, broccoli, Brussels sprouts, mustard, horseradish, radishes
Flavonoids	Fruits, vegetables, wine, green tea, onions, apples, kale, beans
Lignans	Flaxseed, whole grain products
Limonone	Citrus oil
Lycopenes	Tomatoes, red grapefruit, guava, dried apricots
Organosulfuric compounds	Garlic, onions, chives, citrus fruits, broccoli, cabbage, cauliflower, Brussels sprouts
Terpenes and monoterpenes	Citrus, citrus fruits, parsley, carrots, celery, broccoli, cabbage, cauliflower, cucumbers, squash, yams, tomatoes, eggplant, peppers, mint, basil, caraway seeds

subclass of terpenes that has been studied extensively. There are more than 600 naturally occurring carotenoids, which are yellow, orange, and red plant pigments. Vegetables that contain carotenoids include tomatoes, parsley, oranges, pink grapefruit, and spinach.

Lycopene, a carotenoid found in tomatoes, has been called one of the most effective biological singlet–oxygen quenchers, two times as powerful as betacarotene in the destruction of free radicals (DiMascio et al., 1989). Researchers examined the effect of tomato-based foods on cancer and reported that men who ate 10 or more servings of these lycopene-rich foods per week had a 45% reduced risk of prostate cancer development (Giovanucci et al., 1995).

Limonoids are another subclass of terpenes (monoterpenes) found in citrus fruits like grapefruit and orange juice. The liminoids have been identified as chemopreventive agents that induce enzymes in the liver's phase I and II enzyme detoxification system. This system detoxifies carcinogens by making them more water-soluble for excretion from the body (Craig, 1997).

Phenols

Phenols are phytochemicals that protect plants from oxidative damage; they include the subclass **flavonoids.** More than 800 flavonoids, which are the blue, blue-red, and violet plant pigments, have been identified. Flavonoids scavenge free radical compounds, such as superoxide anion and singlet oxygen, and sequester metal ions. One of the major flavonoids, *quercetin,* inhibits oxidation and cytotoxicity of LDL; it occurs in foods such as red and yellow onions, kale, broccoli, red grapes, apples, and cereals. By scavenging activated mutagens and carcinogens, flavonoids may also decrease the risk of cancer (Peterson and Dwyer, 1998).

Phenolic flavonoids, found in foods like grape juice and red wine, have been shown to reduce the risk of heart disease by acting as antioxidants to protect LDL cholesterol from oxidation and by inhibiting platelet aggregation (Craig, 1997). Elderly men participating in a clinical trial that involved consumption of increased levels of flavonoids from tea, onions, and apples had a decreased incidence of coronary heart disease (Hertog et al., 1993).

Phytochemicals in wine may partly explain why, in regions of France where saturated fat intake is high, there are low rates of cardiovascular disease, a phenomenon termed the "French Paradox." Researchers studying this population have found that the phenolic compounds in red wine may have a heart-protective effect (Frankel et al., 1993).

Isoflavones are a phenol subclass found in beans and other legumes, especially soybeans and soy foods. Some isoflavones are **phytoestrogens** (also known as phytosterols), which are weak, nonsteroidal versions of estrogens (structurally similar to steroidal estrogens). They function both as weak estrogens (agonists) and as antiestrogens (antagonists) (Lampe, 1997). Phytoestrogens have a wide range of health effects, including reduction of the risk of heart disease. Elevated serum cholesterol, one risk factor associated with heart disease, can be significantly lowered with an intake of soy protein. A meta-analysis of 38 research studies on the effect of soy on blood lipids revealed that, in persons with hypercholesterolemia, intake of 25 to 50 g of soy protein daily decreases LDL cholesterol levels by approximately 10% (Anderson et al., 1995) (see Table 12–2). Other heart-protective effects of soy include improved arterial elasticity and protection of LDL from oxidation (Messina, 1998).

Phytoestrogens found in soy foods act as antioxidants, carcinogen blockers, or tumor suppressors,

TABLE 12–2 ISOFLAVONE CONTENT OF SOY FOODS

SOY FOOD	ISOFLAVONES (mg)
Mature soybeans, dried, ½ cup	176
Soybeans, roasted, ½ cup	167
Tempeh, uncooked, ½ cup	61
Soy flour, ¼ cup	44
Tofu, fresh, ½ cup	38
Textured soy protein, dry, ¼ cup	28
Soy milk, 1 cup	20

*Average isoflavone content; amounts vary depending upon variety of soybean used and manufacturing process.

and may exert a protective effect against hormone-related cancers (e.g., breast cancer) by reducing estrogen binding at receptor sites (Messina et al., 1994). Phytoestrogens may be useful in preventing or surviving prostate cancer, as these compounds may act as estrogen-like agonists, preventing testosterone from accelerating tumor growth. In animal studies, soy isoflavones prolong the time of appearance of prostate cancer tumors (Messina, 1998). Epidemiologic studies have shown that, in populations in which phytoestrogen intake is high, there is a decreased incidence of hormone-related breast and prostate cancers (Adlercreutz, 1995). (See "*Focus On:* Soy.")

Thiols

Thiol is a sulfur-containing phytonutrient found in cruciferous vegetables, such as broccoli, cauliflower, brussels sprouts, kale, and cabbage. Cruciferous vegetables contain subclasses of thiols identified as **indoles, dithiolthiones,** and **isothiocyanates.** These organosulfuric compounds upregulate enzymes involved in the detoxification of carcinogens and other foreign compounds (American Dietetic Association, 1995).

In both cohort and case control studies, researchers have found an inverse relationship between the consumption of broccoli, cabbage, and cauliflower and the risk of cancer. The association between increased vegetable consumption and cancer risk is most consistent for cancers of the lung, stomach, colon, and rectum (Verhoeven et al., 1996).

Organosulfur compounds are also found in the allium or onion family, which includes garlic, shallots, and leeks. The phytochemicals in garlic, the **allyl sulfides,** and other organosulfur compounds appear to prevent carcinogen activation. Allyl sulfides have several actions, including (1) increasing the production of glutathione S transferase, a phase II enzyme of the liver's detoxification system, (2) inhibiting mutagenesis, and (3) increasing the activity of macrophages and T lymphocytes (Wattenberg, 1985; Warshafsky et al., 1993).

Lignans

Lignans, phytochemicals found in flaxseeds, wheat bran, rye meal, buckwheat, oatmeal, and barley, are the focus of research for their anticancer and phytoestrogen properties. The richest source of lignans is flaxseeds, which contain 75 to 800 times more lignans than any other plant food (Serraino and Thompson, 1992). These plant lignans are converted to mammalian lignans by gut bacteria and have biological properties that include antimitotic and antioxidant activity.

Lignans are phytoestrogens that may have a protective effect against hormone-sensitive cancers by virtue of their interference with sex hormone metabolism. Animal studies have revealed that sex hormone–binding globulin, which enhances clearance of circulating estrogen and may reduce risk for hormone-driven cancers, is upregulated by lignans (Adlercreutz et al., 1980).

In summary, phytochemicals in plant-based foods function as powerful antioxidants and metabolism regulators that may offer protection against the development of chronic disease that can begin in adulthood. These plant-based foods are the core of a defensive nutritional plan that focuses on disease prevention and promotion of optimal wellness throughout the adult years.

INTESTINAL INTEGRITY

Plant-based foods also function in the defensive nutrition paradigm to support intestinal integrity. Intestinal integrity relates to the unique function of

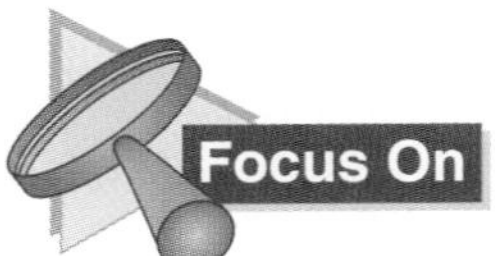

Soy

Soy foods are the richest source of isoflavones (soy phytochemicals), and genistein, daidzein, and glycitein are the major isoflavones in soy. These isoflavones are a class of phytoestrogens with documented health benefits, including reduction of hypercholesterolemia, support for prostate health, and possibly, increased bone density and reduction of the risk of hormone-dependent cancers (Messina and Erdman, 1998).

The ancient Chinese considered soy, which is native to eastern Asia, to be one of the five sacred grains vital for life. The United States is now the world's largest producer of soybeans. Soybeans are 13% to 25% oil, 30% to 50% protein, and 14% to 24% carbohydrate, including 2% to 5% fiber. Soy protein is nutritionally equivalent to proteins derived from animal sources, including egg, milk, and meat (Young et al., 1984).

Asian populations are known to have decreased incidence of breast, prostate, and other cancers, which epidemiologists hypothesize may be attributable to the average daily intake of one serving of soy (equal to approximately 40 mg of isoflavones). Japanese women have a high intake of soy foods, which may account for their lower rate of menopausal symptoms (Adlercreutz et al., 1991). Studies investigating the health benefits of soy foods have involved the intake of 45 to 90 mg of isoflavones per day (equivalent to 2 to 3 servings of soy foods).

Although the exact amount of soy foods needed to reduce the risk of diseases, such as cancer and cardiovascular disease, or to reduce menopausal symptoms remains speculative, adding one or more servings of soy foods per day could promote overall better health (see Table 12–2).

the gut to act both as a conduit for nutrients into systemic circulation, and as a barrier against toxins from a variety of sources, including exotoxins, like drugs and chemicals, and endotoxins, such as bacterial waste, food antigens (foreign proteins), and the breakdown products of metabolism. When intestinal integrity is compromised, the permeability of the gut may be altered and the ability of the gut to act as a barrier against antigens or other pathogens is eroded. Two factors that influence intestinal integrity are the bacterial populations in the gut and the health of the gut mucosa, both of which are influenced by nutrition (O'Dwyer, 1988).

Intestinal Ecology: Bacteria

Intestinal microflora, estimated at 100 trillion bacteria, is comprised of hundreds of different species of microbiota that have a significant impact on human health (Gibson and Roberfroid, 1995). The large intestine hosts the largest population of microorganisms, with more than 500 species; 35% to 50% of the contents of the human colon is composed of bacteria. Bacteria that are both pathogenic (e.g., hemolytic *Escherichia coli, Clostridium perfringens, Campylobacter,* and *Listeria*) and beneficial (e.g., bifidobacteria, *Lactobacillus,* and *E. coli* [nonpathogenic strain]) exist in the gut. In an optimally functioning gut, there is a balance between these two populations.

Healthy GI microflora function to (1) form a barrier against invading organisms by enhancing the host's defense mechanisms against pathogens, (2) improve gut immunity by adhering to the intestinal mucosa and stimulating local immune responses, and (3) help digest foods and produce certain vitamins (Salminen et al., 1995). Table 12–3 outlines some properties, functions, and effects on the host of intestinal microflora.

An imbalance in gut microflora that produces harmful effects is termed **dysbiosis,** a term popularized in the late 19th century in Europe (Galland and Barrie, 1993). The link between dysbiosis and the development of certain diseases is just begin-

TABLE 12–3 THE IMPORTANCE OF INTESTINAL MICROFLORA AND THEIR FUNCTIONS*

SOME FUNCTIONS OF THE INTESTINAL MICROFLORA	EFFECTS ON THE HOST	SOME PRIMARY BACTERIA INVOLVED AND THEIR PROPERTIES†
Healthful Properties		
1. Produce vitamins, short-chain fatty acids, and protein, which are partly absorbed and utilized by the host	Maintain good health	
2. Supplement the digestive and absorptive process	Maintain good health	**Predominantly Healthful Properties**
3. Protect the host from overgrowth and infection by exogenous organisms, such as pathogenic bacteria and yeasts	Maintain good health	Bifidobacteria (1,2,3,4) *Lactobacillus* (3) *Eubacterium* (3)
4. Stimulate the immune system	Maintain good health	**Combination of Healthful and Virulent Properties** Bacteroidaceae (1,2,3,4,5,7,8) Peptococcaecea (3,8) *Escherichia coli* (4,5,6,7,8) *Streptococcus* (3,8)
Virulent Properties		
5. Produce certain putrefactive substances (ammonia, hydrogen sulfide, amines, phenols, indoles, etc.) and secondary bile acids	These substances may cause diarrhea, constipation, and growth inhibition. They may also injure the intestine directly and be partially absorbed, potentially contributing throughout the host's life to aging and geriatric diseases, such as arteriosclerosis, hypertension, liver disorders, autoimmune diseases, and immunosuppression	
6. Produce other toxins		
7. Produce carcinogens	May produce cancer	**Predominantly Virulent Properties**
8. Stimulate pathogenicity	May contribute to the establishment of a pathologic condition (i.e., spontaneous infections, such as diarrhea, gastroenteritis, superinfection [cerebromeningitis, endocarditis, septicemia, urinary tract infection, brain abscess, liver abscess, pulmonary abscess])	*Veillonella* (8) *Clostridium perfringens* (7,8) *Staphylococcus* (7,8) *Proteus* (7,8)

(Adapted from Percival M. Intestinal health. Clin Nutr Insights 5:1, 1997. Published by the Foundation for the Advancement of Nutritional Education, Metagenics Northwest, 1010 Tyinn St., Suite 26, Eugene, OR 97402.)

*It is important to maintain balance in the intestinal flora. If an imbalance occurs in favor of bacteria with virulent properties, illness can result.

†The numbers that follow the name of the bacteria identify their functions as defined in the first column.

ning to be explored. For example, the role of GI bacteria in the development of cancer was studied by the U.S. Environmental Protection Agency. Researchers found that potentially carcinogenic agents (food dyes, aflatoxins, pesticides, nitrites) and cancer-causing agents in nonfoods (smokeless tobaccos, prescription medications) were bioactivated by enzyme systems in gut bacteria. These bioactivations, which can lead to cancer, are promoted at a higher rate in GI systems with imbalanced floral populations (Chadwick et al., 1992).

Nutritional Support for Beneficial Microflora

Healthy microflora can be supported by two interventions: prebiotics and probiotics. **Prebiotics** are nondigestible food products that stimulate the growth of symbiotic bacterial species, already in the colon, that improve the health of the host. **Probiotics** are defined as microbial foods or supplements that can be used to change or improve intestinal bacterial balance to improve the health of the host (Gibson and Roberfroid, 1995).

Prebiotics include foods that contain substrates that nourish beneficial gut microbiota. These substrates include dietary fiber and fructo-oligosaccharides (FOS). FOSs are short-chain simple sugars (neosugars) that are 3 to 10 sugar units in length, of which at least 2 units are fructose. They are divided into three categories based on the number of fructose units they contain. The sugars of FOSs are linked together by indigestible bonds that cannot be hydrolyzed by enzymes in the small intestine, so carbohydrates from FOSs pass undigested into the large intestine. Food sources of these FOSs include honey, beer, onion, burdock root, asparagus, rye, Jerusalem artichoke, banana, maple sugar, oats, and Chinese chives (Levin, 1994).

FOSs have been shown to selectively stimulate the growth of beneficial bacteria, including bifidobacteria and ***Lactobacillus,*** which results in the reduction of pathogenic bacteria, such as *Salmonella* and *clostridia* in the GI tract. One study revealed that increasing these neosugars causes an increase in bifidobacteria and a decrease in the activity of β-glucuronidase, an enzyme which converts procarcinogens to carcinogens in the bowel (Buddington et al., 1996). Components of dietary fiber, including pectin, hemicellulose, and inulin, a storage carbohydrate that occurs in chicory, onions, asparagus, and Jerusalem artichokes, also function as prebiotics and stimulate the production of short chain fatty acids (SCFAs). (See below.)

A second avenue to support intestinal integrity is direct repopulation of the intestinal milieu with probiotics, that is, organisms and substances that contribute to intestinal microbial balance. The most common forms of probiotics include *Lactobacillus* and bifidobacteria, which support intestinal health by inhibiting the overgrowth of toxic bacteria. By competing for attachment sites and nutrients, these beneficial bacteria inhibit the proliferation of nonbeneficial organisms.

Lactobacillus and bifidobacteria also produce organic acids that reduce intestinal pH and retard the growth of pathogenic acid-sensitive bacteria. At optimal pH, the organic acids produced by beneficial bacteria solubilize in the cell membrane of pathogenic bacteria, block transport of their necessary growth substances, acidify the cell interiors, and exert other inhibitory influences on their growth (Schauss, 1990).

Fermented dairy products, including live culture yogurts, kefir, and commercial probiotic preparations, contain *Lactobacillus,* bifidobacteria, and other forms of benefical bacteria. Other forms of fermented foods, such as sauerkraut, miso, and tempeh, may also be cultured with *Lactobacillus* strains. However, the potency and number of viable organisms in commercial probiotic products varies widely. An analysis of the concentration and viability of the *L. acidophilus* bacteria in 11 commercial *L. acidophilus* supplement products showed that only two of the products actually contained *L. acidophilus* (Hughes et al., 1990).

Intestinal Mucosa: Nutritional Support

Gut integrity is linked not only to a balance of intestinal bacteria but also to the healthy nourishment of enterocytes and colonocytes, the intestinal mucosal cells. One of the major functions of the intestinal mucosa is its barrier activity, which prevents antigenic or pathogenic molecules or microorganisms from entering the systemic circulation. The GI mucosa is composed of epithelial cells that are close-fitting, thin, and semipermeable, with tight junctures between the cells. When the mucosa is disrupted, altered intestinal permeability may result, and bacteria from the gut, undigested food, or toxins may translocate across this barrier.

The exact etiology of altered intestinal permeability is unclear, but dietary intake and bacterial imbalance in the gut have been suggested as factors. Conditions relating to dietary intake that have been linked to excessive gut permeability include (1) delayed transit of food through the intestine and (2) delayed peristalsis (Levin, 1994). Both of these conditions are linked to a lack of dietary fiber, which not only improves bowel transit time and intestinal muscle activity but also protects gut integrity by nourishing intestinal cells. (See Chapters 1, 3, and 31 for further discussion of fiber.)

Butyrate, acetate, and propionate, all of which are SCFAs, are the preferred "fuels" of the intestinal cells. Sources of these fuels include dietary fiber, particularly soluble fiber. In the colon, beneficial gut bacteria, primarily the bifidobacteria, metabolize SCFAs from indigestible carbohydrates in dietary fiber (Evans and Shronts, 1992). **Butyric acid** or **butyrate** is the preferred food of the cells of the large intestine and is produced only by fermentation action of gut bacteria on dietary fiber. The

SCFAs proprionate and acetate are used primarily by the liver for energy production, but the by-products of that metabolism, including glutamine, glutamate, and acetoacetate, are preferred over glucose as fuels for enterocytes, the cells of the small intestine (Windmueller and Spaeth, 1990).

The use of broad-spectrum antibiotics negatively impacts intestinal integrity. Antibiotics are antimicrobial agents that prevent serious bacterial infections from becoming life-threatening, but they kill both beneficial and pathogenic bacterial populations. Antibiotics cause changes in intestinal microflora and may alter the balance between beneficial and pathogenic microflora. Thus, when the gut is in recovery from antibiotics, both forms of bacteria compete for food and attachment sites. Bacteria have been shown to have very short times for doubling (*E. coli* about 20 minutes). This rapid adaptation to dietary change may lead to a proliferation of pathogenic organisms in the colon (Adlercreutz, 1998). Probiotics may be used to reestablish healthy microflora populations when these populations have been devastated by the use of antibiotics.

DETOXIFICATION

Optimal health is a function of the body's ability not only to assimilate nutrients but to limit the accumulation of potentially harmful toxins, both endogenous and exogenous. The body has a measure of protection from xenobiotics (compounds foreign to the body) by its natural barriers, which include the GI system, the lungs, and the skin. However, foreign compounds that cross these barriers are shuttled to the body's **detoxification** systems, which decrease the negative impact of xenobiotics or toxins on the biochemistry and cellular integrity of the body. Two major detoxification pathways in the body are (1) the immune tissue located in the gut and (2) the enzyme systems in the liver. Food and nutrients have significant effects on both of these pathways.

Gut-Associated Lymphoid Tissue (GALT)

The GI tract plays a major role in keeping endogenous and exogenous toxins from entering the systemic circulation by the barrier function of the gut mucosa. If toxins breach this barrier, further migration of these compounds is arrested by the action of **gut-associated lymphoid tissue (GALT).**

The gut is the largest lymphoid organ in the body, as more than 50% to 60% of the body's lymphoid tissue surrounds the digestive tract. GALT generates almost 70% of the body's antibodies and contains the greatest number of lymphocytes in the body (Mayer et al., 1996).

This major immune system in the gut is composed of secretory immunoglobulin A (sIgA), which often operates separately from the systemic immune system (Walker, 1994). GALT immunoglobulins attach to bacteria, viruses, and other foreign particles to prevent absorption of these compounds into the body. Additionally, bacterial enzymes and toxins (e.g., *E. coli* [pathogenic]) are directly inactivated by sIgA (Lukaczer, 1996b).

Increased production of sIgA levels is promoted by certain strains of beneficial bacteria, such as bifidobacteria (Yasui et al., 1992). *Saccharomyces boulardii* is a beneficial yeast that also appears to stimulate the intestinal production of natural sIgA (Buts et al., 1990).

Phases I and II of the Detoxification System of the Liver

The digestive tract is the first line of defense for excluding foreign materials from the systemic circulation. Antigens or toxins not processed by the intestinal lumen or gut bacteria are delivered via the hepatic portal vein to the liver for detoxification. The liver's actions on these toxins, termed *biotransformations,* involve two sequential phases (**phase I and phase II detoxification**) whereby toxic molecules are transformed from lipid-soluble substances into water-soluble molecules that can be excreted from the body.

In phase I, the **cytochrome P-450,** or **mixed-function oxidase system** (MFOS), a family of enzymes, is activated. In this phase, endogenous compounds (e.g., hormones and prostaglandins produced in the body) and xenobiotics are transformed by biochemical reactions, primarily by glutathione conjugation, to more water-soluble compounds (Bland, 1997).

In phase II, the metabolites produced in phase I are conjugated in a series of reactions controlled by a different series of enzymes, termed conjugases. These enzymes attach a substance to the phase I biotransfomed compounds to make them less toxic and more easily eliminated. Conjugators involved in phase II reactions include glucuronic acid, glutathione, and glycine. Enzymes that catalyze phase II reactions include glutathione S transferase and nicotinamide-adenine-dinucleotide phosphate (NADPH) quinone reductase (Wattenberg, 1992). The conjugated water-soluble metabolites produced by phase II are excreted in the urine or feces.

Achieving a balance between these two phases of detoxification is critical, as phase I metabolites that are not biotransformed by phase II agents can be more toxic than the parent molecule. For example, a component of cigarette smoke that is relatively harmless is transformed during phase I into a metabolically activated carcinogen, but in phase II, the metabolite is biotransformed and detoxified (Percival, 1997).

Phase I and phase II balance is also important in minimizing the free radical damage produced by cytochrome P-450 activity. The more efficiently these metabolites are processed by the two-phase system, the less likely cell or tissue damage by free radicals will occur (Lukaczer, 1996a) (Fig. 12–1).

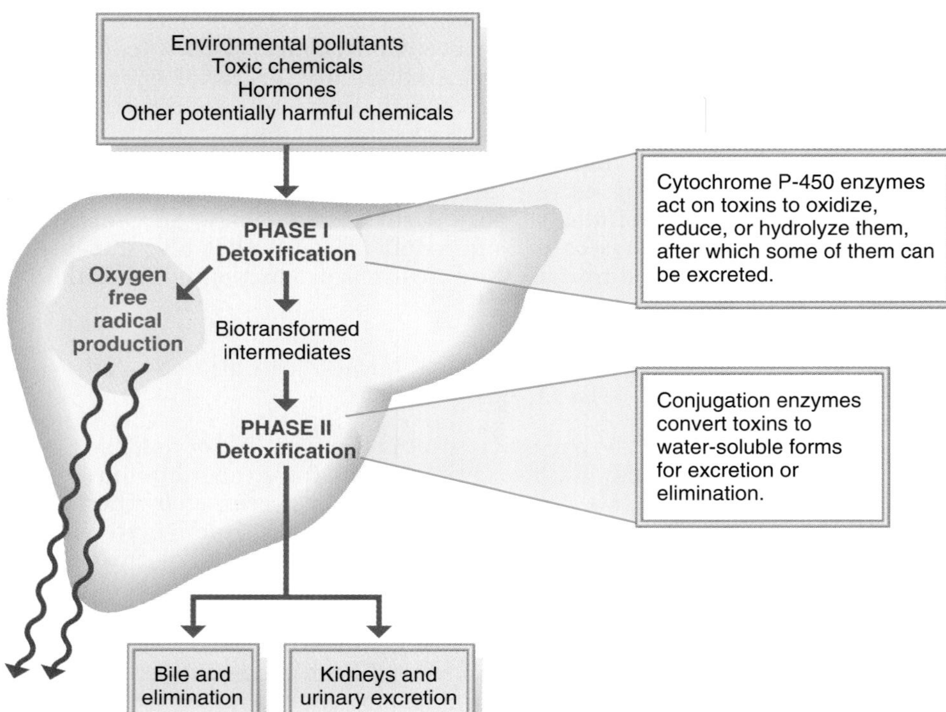

FIGURE 12–1 Detoxification in the liver. (Adapted from Percival M. Phytonutrients and detoxification. Clin Insights 5:3, 1997. Published by the Foundation for the Advancement of Nutritional Education, Metagenics Northwest, Eugene, OR.)

Nutritional Support for Liver Detoxification

An individual's nutritional status and the presence of nutrients drive both phase I and phase II detoxification; nutrient deficiencies will affect the optimal function of these systems. Foods, especially those high in specific phytochemicals, provide key nutrients that support these detoxification pathways.

Indoles, phytochemicals found in broccoli, cauliflower, and other cruciferous vegetables, markedly enhance phase I pathways (Anderson and Dappas, 1991). The dithiolthiones and isothiocyanates, other phytochemicals in the cruciferous family, and the liminoids, phytochemicals in citrus, increase phase II enzymes, including glutathione S transferase, which blocks carcinogens from damaging cellular DNA (Craig, 1997).

The organosulfuric compounds found in vegetables of the allium family—garlic, onions, shallots, and leeks—have also been shown to induce phase II enzymes (Wattenberg, 1985). Additionally, curcumin, an ingredient in the spice tumeric, is known to markedly increase the activity of phase II enzymes, and animal studies have shown that it decreases tumor incidence significantly (Azuine and Bhide, 1992).

Phytochemicals in certain foods can also function as agents to retard the detoxification process. Grapefruit juice contains the flavonoid, naringenin, which is one compound that acts as a blocking agent in the cytochrome P-450 system. This downregulation of the P-450 system allows certain drugs to have a slower clearance rate, increasing their therapeutic activity (Yee et al., 1995). For example, cholesterol-lowering "statin" drugs have a 12 times higher concentration in the blood when taken with grapefruit juice. Calcium channel blockers, tranquilizers (the benzodiazepines), and some antihistamines are also affected by grapefruit juice (Fuhr, 1998) (see Chapter 18).

GUIDELINES FOR THE DEFENSIVE NUTRITION PARADIGM

Nutritional needs change during the adult years. A nutrition model that features foods that maximize outcomes for disease prevention should be flexible so as to address changes in both the physiology and psychology of the maturing adult. Basic energy requirements may be determined using equations for estimating total energy expenditure that factor basal energy expenditure, sleep, and activity factors (see Chapter 2).

Guidelines for maintaining a nutrient-dense, phytochemical-rich food plan can be based on the recommendations of the Food Guide Pyramid. Defensive nutrition guidelines include daily consumption of five to nine servings of fruits and vegetables (particularly dark yellow, green, and red vegetables, roots, and hard-shelled squashes); six to eleven servings of bread, cereal, grains, rice, and pasta (mostly unrefined whole grain); three glasses of nonfat or low-fat milk, yogurt, or cheese or other calcium-rich foods (such as dark leafy greens, corn tortillas, calcium-fortified soy beverage); and two to three servings of dry beans, soyfoods (such as tofu, tempeh, or soy protein powder), nuts, fish, poultry, eggs, or extra-lean meat per day (see Chapter 15).

Early Adulthood

In early adulthood, nutrition plays a pivotal role in establishment of eating patterns. Meal patterns that support optimal nutrition intake and health include:

- Consumption of five to nine servings of fruits and vegetables each day
- A balanced intake of foods with essential fatty acids (omega-6 and omega-3 fatty acids)
- Avoidance of foods high in saturated fats and trans-fatty acids
- Inclusion of high-fiber foods, especially foods high in lignans and FOS
- Limited intake of refined carbohydrates
- Increased water consumption—at least eight 8-oz glasses of water per day
- Targeted daily vitamin/mineral supplementation to compensate for inadequacies in the diet

Optimally, the diet of young adults should include a wealth of plant-based foods that are rich in phytochemicals and other nutrients that support intestinal integrity and detoxification pathways.

Fruits and Vegetables

Studies have shown that Americans eat too few fruits and vegetables. The challenge for nutrition professionals is to assist young adults to develop eating patterns that include regular intake of fruits and vegetables. Young adults may have food intake patterns that rely on restaurant or take-out convenience foods, which are typically high in fat, sugar, and sodium. Indeed, one survey found that, of more than 18,000 persons who frequented restaurants three or more times per week, more than 20% were in their 20s (Leach, 1998).

Increased consumption of fruits and vegetables, with a minimum of five servings of fruits or vegetables daily, is a useful target for meal plans. Strategies for increasing fruit and vegetable intake may include: (1) trying one new fruit or vegetable each week, (2) doubling the normal serving size for vegetables, (3) eating fruit on cereal or muesli, (4) consuming all–vegetable-based meals (e.g., vegetable chili or stew) on a regular basis, (5) eating fruit as a snack, and (6) adding vegetables to favorite entrees (e.g., tacos, pizza, lasagna) (Steinmetz and Potter, 1996).

When fruits and vegetables form the core of meal plans, they can play an important role in preventing chronic disease, especially cancer. Cancer is one of the leading causes of death among Americans; men have a one in two risk of developing cancer, and women have a one in three risk. Combining fruit and vegetable intake with physical activity, maintenance of a healthy weight, and abstinence from smoking may reduce cancer risk by 60% to 70% (American Institute for Cancer Research, 1997).

Omega-3 Fatty Acids

A balanced intake of the essential fatty acids—omega-6 (n-6) and omega-3 (n-3) fatty acids—is an important component of a nutrition plan for optimal wellness. Omega-3 fatty acids, including alpha-linolenic acid (ALA), eicosapentaenoic acid (EPA), and docosahexaenoic acid (DHA), constitute less than 1% of the total fatty acids in the U.S. food supply, whereas foods high in omega-6 fatty acids (linoleic acid and gamma-linolenic acid) constitute a significant majority (Raper et al., 1992). Because humans cannot interconvert n-6 and n-3 essential fatty acids (their metabolism uses the same desaturation enzymes), there is competition between the two essential fatty acid families, and n-6:n-3 imbalances may occur. Current n-6:n-3 dietary ratios range from 10:1 to 25:1 (Simopoulos, 1991).

Although the Food and Nutrition Board of the National Research Council has not specified an optimal n-6:n-3 fatty acid ratio, the Canadian Health Board recommends a ratio of 4:1 to 10:1 (Health and Welfare Canada, 1990). The intake of n-3 fatty acids needs to be increased for optimal health. Flaxseed is the richest source of ALA, an omega-3 fatty acid, which can be converted in the body to other omega-3 fatty acids, EPA, and DHA. Other sources include canola and soybean oils, walnuts, butternuts, and red and black currant seeds. Fatty marine fish, such as salmon, mackerel, and herring, are rich in the preformed n-3 fatty acids EPA and DHA (Nettleton, 1991). These long-chain omega-3 fatty acids downregulate inflammatory prostaglandins, and may have a beneficial effect against autoimmune diseases like arthritis, lupus, and other inflammatory conditions (Carter, 1993).

Results of epidemiologic studies suggest that ALA has a specific preventive effect against cardiovascular heart disease (CHD). In the Multiple Risk Factor Intervention Trial (MRFIT), intake of ALA as a percentage of total calories was inversely associated with mortality from CHD in men who had high risk of developing CHD owing to their smoking, blood pressure, and blood cholesterol status (Dolecek, 1992).

Current recommendations for essential fatty acids suggest a minimum of 3% of calories from n-6 fats with 60 calories of pure linoleic acid, and a minimum of 0.5% of calories from n-3 fats with 10 calories of pure ALA (1.1 g) (Bjerve et al., 1987). In a 2000-kcal diet, 1.1 g of n-3 fatty acids would be provided by either 1/2 tsp. of flax oil, 2 tsp. of flaxseed meal, 3 T. of walnuts, or 1 T. canola or soybean oil (Davis et al., 1995).

Vitamin/Mineral Supplementation

Studies have shown that few Americans are able to meet recommended nutritional guidelines promoted by programs such as "Five A Day," which encourage the daily intake of five or more servings of fruits and vegetables. A telephone survey of 24,000 adults in 16 states found that only 20% of the respondents had eaten the recommended five or more daily servings of fruits and vegetables (Serdula et al., 1995).

A study of the nutrient intake levels of the offspring of subjects involved in the Framingham Heart Study revealed that only 50% of the study's 2520 subjects met the RDA for vitamins A, E, and B_6; only 25% of the women in the study had daily intakes of 800 mg of calcium or more; and 75% of the population fell short of the suggested intake level of betacarotene. These researchers concluded that "... large proportions of adults fall short of the guidelines for some key nutrients" (Millen et al., 1997).

Many adults recognize the inadequacy of their daily diets in providing necessary vitamins and minerals and compensate by taking vitamin and mineral supplements. A national survey conducted by the National Center for Health Statisics in collaboration with the Food and Drug Administration (FDA) revealed that 32% of the men and 45% of the women surveyed reported having taken nutritional supplements in the 2 weeks prior to the interview (Moss et al., 1989). Health care professionals, including dietitians and cardiologists, may take dietary supplements, including vitamin, mineral, and herbal supplements. In two surveys of registered dietitians, 50% to 80% took nutritional supplements (Worthington-Roberts and Breskin, 1984; Mathai, 1995). In a sample of 181 cardiologists, 44% took one or more vitamins with antioxidant activity (Mehta, 1997).

Dietary supplementation is an established practice among many Americans, and dietetic professionals should be prepared (1) to assess and recommend appropriate nutrients in supplemental forms when necessary, and (2) to educate supplement users that supplements may meet certain nutrient needs, but should be used in addition to a healthy diet, not in place of it. An excellent guide to reliable nutrition information is www.navigator.tufts.edu.

Mid-Adulthood

During the mid-adulthood years, many Americans experience an increase in weight above the ideal. (See Chapter 23.) An estimated 33% of Americans are obese, and obesity-related medical conditions are the second leading cause of death in the United States. Overweight adults are at increased risk for many acute and chronic diseases, including hypertension, dyslipidemia, coronary heart disease, gallbladder disease, and some types of cancer. Over 300,000 Americans die each year from obesity-related diseases, and health care costs related to obesity are estimated at $70 billion annually (American Dietetic Association, 1997).

One cause of weight gain in middle-aged Americans is an increase in daily caloric intake. The Third National Health and Nutritional Examination Survey (NHANES III 1988–1994) revealed that Americans have increased their daily energy intake by an additional 100 to 300 kcal over what it was in the NHANES II study (Daily Dietary Fat ..., 1993). Another factor in weight gain is sedentary living; too few Americans have regular exercise programs. The Centers for Disease Control found that, of 87,000 adults aged 18 years and older, 58.1% reported no or irregular physical activity (1993 Prevalence ..., 1993).

A nutrition program built on the healthy nutritional fundamentals introduced in the young adult years, combined with a regular exercise program, can help middle-aged adults to realize and maintain healthy body weights.

Hyperinsulinemia and Syndrome X

Mid-adulthood can also bring the onset of **syndrome X,** a clinical condition which is increasingly prevalent in the United States. Syndrome X refers to a cluster of metabolic disorders, including type 2 diabetes mellitus (NIDDM), hypertension, and dyslipidemia, and often includes obesity, although it can also present in persons who are not obese (Reaven, 1995). A major factor in syndrome X is a defect in glucose metabolism, termed *insulin resistance,* which is cellular resistance to insulin that results in secretion of excessive insulin by the body in an attempt to regulate blood sugar (hyperinsulinemia) (Fig. 12–2).

Hyperinsulinemia and impaired glucose tolerance are characteristic of type 2 diabetes mellitus, but are not restricted to persons who have demonstrated type 2 diabetes. (See Chapter 34 for a further discussion of diabetes mellitus.) Resistance to insulin-mediated glucose uptake may be more common than currently understood, and may be present in a substantial proportion of an apparently healthy population (Reaven, 1995).

Diet plays an important role in improving insulin resistance and moderating hyperinsulinemia. Factors that have a positive impact on insulin include exercising, reducing caloric intake, and reducing body weight (Coulston, 1997).

A defensive nutrition plan for middle-aged adults emphasizes foods that supply glucose to the cells at a steady rate and moderate insulin demands. One useful tool for measuring the rate at which foods provide glucose to the blood and thus stimulate insulin release is the **glycemic index (GI).** The glycemic index measures the effect on blood glucose of equivalent amounts of carbohydrate contained in different foods (Wolever, 1990). Some carbohydrate-containing foods cause blood glucose levels to rise quite rapidly; other foods allow the body to maintain a "steady state" relative to the release of insulin to control blood sugar levels.

The glycemic index ranks the effect of a single food on blood glucose levels relative to a reference carbohydrate, such as white bread (see Appendix Table 54). Factors that influence the glycemic index

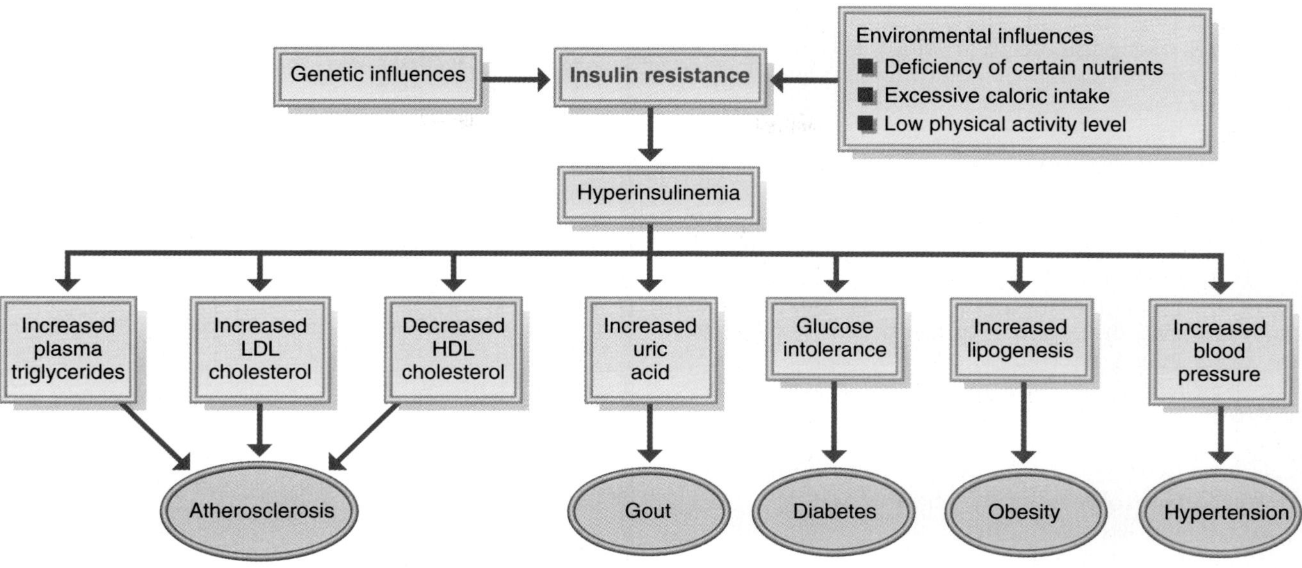

FIGURE 12–2 Pathophysiology of insulin resistance.

of a food include (1) the type of fiber in the food (e.g., foods with soluble [gel-forming] fiber, such as beans, have a low glycemic index); (2) the form in which the food is eaten (e.g., rice cakes have a higher glycemic index than cooked rice); (3) the presence of fat; (4) the form of sugar in the food (e.g., fructose causes less of an increase in blood glucose level than sucrose or glucose); (5) the effect of protein and fat eaten with the carbohydrate food; and (6) the starch structure of the carbohydrate in the food (e.g., foods with greater amylose content have lower glycemic indexes) (Wolever, 1990; Foster-Powell and Brand Miller, 1995).

In general, high-fiber foods with low glycemic indices (e.g., beans, vegetables, whole fruit, and whole grains, such as oatmeal, basmati rice, and barley) are the preferred forms of carbohydrates in a defensive nutrition plan. Meal combination is also an important factor in managing blood glucose levels. Combining protein, fat, and carbohydrate at meals and snacks (i.e., small serving of nuts and a piece of fruit) can lead to better control of blood glucose levels and less insulin release than meals or snacks that consist mainly of carbohydrate (i.e., a bagel with jelly). (See *"Focus On:* Chromium.")

Women's Health: Special Concerns in Mid-Adulthood

Women have special health and nutrition concerns in their later adult years due to perimenopause and menopause. In menopause, which the average woman experiences at about age 50, estrogen production declines (endogenous estrogen circulation declines about 60%), signaling the end of the repro-

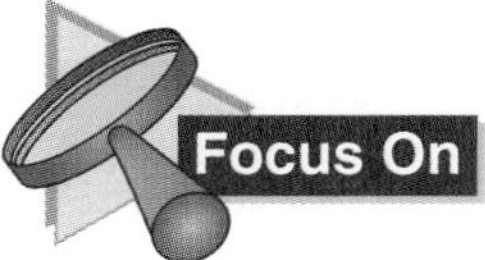

CHROMIUM

Chromium is a part of glucose tolerance factor (GTF), which prevents glucose intolerance (Linder, 1991). As an essential cofactor for insulin, chromium acts, either directly or indirectly, to enhance the effectiveness of insulin in binding to cells. The effect of chromium on insulin was discovered in 1957 by Klaus Schwartz and Walter Mertz, who found that animals fed commercial diets developed an inability to metabolize sugar; they developed a glucose intolerance. Adding brewers' yeast, which contains chromium, to the animals' diets normalized their blood sugar level (Mertz, 1969).

A double-blind, placebo-controlled study examined the effect of supplemental chromium at dosages of 200 μg and 1000 μg on persons with type 2 diabetes. Patients who received supplemental chromium showed significant beneficial effects in terms of HgbA1c and blood glucose, insulin, and cholesterol variables. The beneficial effects of chromium in individuals with diabetes were observed at levels higher than the upper limit established for estimated safe and adequate daily dietary intake (50 to 200 μg per day) (Anderson and Cheng, 1997).

For individuals with hyperinsulinemia, type 2 diabetes, or milder forms of insulin resistance, chromium supplementation at 200 μg per day, or a daily intake of chromium-rich foods, should be considered (see Chapters 5 and 34).

ductive period (Dwyer et al., 1994). However, women are not completely without estrogen, even after the ovaries cease production, as the adrenal glands continue to produce weaker forms of estrogens.

With diminished production of estrogen, women may experience symptoms associated with menopause, including vasomotor symptoms, such as hot flashes. Bone health is also affected as a result of the decline in circulating estrogen, as the body's ability to keep up with the natural process of bone turnover slows in response to the decrease of estrogen. Bone mass decreases, and osteoporosis may occur (see Chapter 28). Lowered levels of circulating estrogen also affect blood lipids, resulting in an increase in total cholesterol and LDL cholesterol levels and a decrease in high-density lipoprotein (HDL) cholesterol levels (see Chapter 26).

Plant-based estrogens, or phytoestrogens, as adjunctive therapy for alleviating the symptoms of menopause, are the subject of increasing research. Phytoestrogens are nonsteroidal estrogens of dietary origin. They have 1/100,000 to 1/1000 the strength of steroidal estrogens, and they exert biological effects as they fit estrogen receptor sites. Phytoestrogens include (1) isoflavones, found primarily in soy; (2) lignans, which are in highest concentrations in flax; and (3) coumestans, found in alfalfa and bean sprouts.

Phytoestrogens in soy may reduce the incidence of hot flashes, one symptom of menopause. In a double-blind study, women who ate 60 g of soy protein daily for 12 weeks had 45% fewer hot flashes than the placebo-treated group (Albertazzi et al., 1998). Soy isoflavones may also protect women against osteoporosis by the action of **genistein,** which has an effect similar to estrogen. It stimulates osteoblasts, the bone-forming cells. In animal studies, isoflavones reduced bone loss to a degree comparable to estrogen (Arjmandi et al., 1996). In a group of postmenopausal women treated daily with 40 g of soy protein isolate, a significant increase in lumbar spine bone mineral content (2%) was noted in the treatment group after 26 weeks (Potter et al., 1998). Furthermore, plant-based estrogens appear to bind to estrogen receptor sites, competing with more potent estrogens to inhibit hormone-promoted cancers (Dwyer, 1994).

To summarize, in the adult years, people create and build careers, nurture families, contribute to the community, realize goals, and plan their postwork lives. Nutrition in the adult years focuses on maintaining health by using foods, particularly plant-based foods and their constituents (phytonutrients), to optimize the functions of the digestive and liver detoxification systems, as well as other organ systems of the body, including the immune system. With a nutrition program based on the principles of a defensive nutrition paradigm, persons in all stages of adulthood can maintain and promote health and productivity while preventing disease.

CASE STUDY

JoAnn H. is a 48-year-old woman who works full-time and is the single parent of two teenagers. She is 5 feet 9 inches tall and currently weighs 175 lb. In the past 2 years, she has gained 10 lb. Her recent blood glucose test results were borderline high, and there is a history of both diabetes and cancer in her family. She has recently completed a course of antibiotics for an ear infection and has been experiencing symptoms of mood swings and night sweats, which she thinks may be related to perimenopause.

JoAnn has called to make an appointment for dietary counseling and has expressed interest in getting more information about how diet can help her to maintain her health, to manage her risk of diabetes and cancer, and to prevent any further weight gain. Her typical meals are as follows: a bagel, coffee, and orange juice for breakfast; a sandwich with ham and cheese, lettuce, tomato, and mayonnaise and fat-free cookies for lunch; and pasta with chicken and carrots, a green salad with blue cheese dressing, and a small slice of cake or a dish of ice cream for dinner. Beverages include diet colas, and snacks are rice cakes or popcorn. She has no regular exercise program.

1. Assess what kinds of foods are lacking in JoAnn's diet that could help (1) manage her blood glucose levels, (2) relieve her perimenopausal symptoms, and (3) help reduce her risk of cancer.
2. Outline your presentation to JoAnn to explain how adding or increasing certain foods in her diet may help to address her concerns. What background information would you give her so that she will appreciate the rationale for your recommendations?
3. Along with JoAnn, design a 3-day meal plan that reflects these concepts. Plan the menus for all breakfasts eaten at home, lunches prepared at home and taken to work, and two dinners, one prepared at home and one eaten at a restaurant.
4. Would you recommend any dietary supplements for JoAnn? What information or assessment tools would you use to determine the necessity of such supplementation?
5. Describe how you would help JoAnn formulate goals for an exercise program.

CITED REFERENCES

Abraham GE. Role of nutrition in managing the premenstrual tension syndromes. J Reprod Med 32:405, 1987.

Adlercreutz H. Evolution, nutrition, intestinal microflora and prevention of cancer: A hypothesis. Soc Exper Biol Med 217:241, 1998.

Adlercreutz H. Phytoestrogens: Epidemiology and a possible role in cancer protection. Environ Health Perspect 103 (Suppl 7):103, 1995.

Adlercreutz H, et al. Urinary excretion of lignans and isoflavonoid phytoestrogens in Japanese men and women consuming a traditional Japanese diet. Am J Clin Nutr 54:1093, 1991.

Adlercreutz H, et al. Biliary excretion and intestinal metabolism of progesterone and estrogens in man. J Steroid Biochem 25:791, 1980.

A garden of phytochemicals. Berkeley Wellness Lett 12:6, 1995.

Albertazzi P, et al. The effect of dietary soy supplementation on hot flashes. Obstet Gynecol 91:6, 1998.

American Dietetic Association. Phytochemicals and functional foods. J Am Diet Assoc 95:493, 1995.

American Dietetic Association. Weight management. J Am Diet Assoc 97:71, 1997.

American Institute for Cancer Research. Food, nutrition and the prevention of cancer: A global perspective. Washington, DC: American Institute for Cancer Research, 1997.

Anderson J, et al. Meta-analysis of the effects of soy protein on serum lipids. N Engl J Med 333:276, 1995.

Anderson KE, Dappas A. Dietary regulation of cytochrome P-450. Annu Rev Nutr 11:141, 1991.

Anderson RA, Cheng N. Elevated intakes of supplemental chromium improve glucose and insulin variables in individuals with type 2 diabetes. Diabetes 46:1786, 1997.

Arjmandi BH, et al. Dietary soybean protein prevents bone loss in an ovarectomized rat model of osteoporosis. J Nutr 126:161, 1996.

Azuine M, Bhide S. Chemopreventive effect of turmeric against stomach and skin tumors induced by chemical carcinogens in Swiss mice. Nutr Cancer 17:77, 1992.

Bjerve KS, et al. Alpha-linoleic acid deficiency in patients on long-term gastric tube feeding: Estimation of linolenic acid and long-chain unsaturated n-3 fatty acid requirement in man. Am J Clin Nutr 45:66, 1987.

Bland J. Improving intercellular communication in managing chronic illness. 1999 Seminar Series. HealthComm International, Inc., Gig Harbor, WA, 1999.

Bland J. Improving genetic expression in the prevention of the disease of aging. Institute for Functional Medicine Inc. Health Comm International Inc. Gig Harbor, WA, 1998.

Bland J. Nutritional Improvement of Health Outcomes: The Inflammatory Disorders. HealthComm Seminar Series. Gig Harbor, WA: HealthComm International, 1997.

Block G, et al. Fruit, vegetables and cancer prevention: A review of the epidemiological evidence. Nutr Cancer 18:1, 1992.

Buddington RK, et al. Dietary supplement of neosugar alters the fecal flora and decreases activities of some reductive enzymes in human subjects. Am J Clin Nutr 63:709, 1996.

Buts J, et al. Stimulation of secretory IgA and secretory component of immunoglobulins in small intestine of rats treated with *Saccharomyces boulardii.* Dig Dis Sci 35:251, 1990.

Carter JF. Potential of flaxseed in baked foods and other products in human nutrition. Cereal Foods World 38:753, 1993.

Chadwick RW, et al. Role of GI mucosa and microflora in the bioactivation of dietary and environmental mutagens or carcinogens. Drug Metab Rev 24:425, 1992.

Coulston A. Insulin resistance: Its role in health and disease and implications for nutrition management. Top Nutr (Hershey Foods Corporation) 6:1, 1997.

Craig W. Phytochemicals: Guardians of our health. J Am Diet Assoc 97(Suppl 2):S199, 1997.

Daily Dietary Fat and Total Food Energy Intakes—NHANES Phase 1, 1988–91. MMWR 7:116, 1993.

Davis B, et al. Becoming Vegetarian. Summertown, TN: Book Publishing Co., 1995, p. 118.

DeLuca HF, Zierold C. Mechanisms and functions of vitamin D. Seventeenth Marabou Symposium. Diet and Genetic Interactions. Nutr Rev 56(2, pt II):S4, 1998.

DiMascio P, et al. Lycopene as the most efficient biological carotenoid singlet-oxygen quencher. Arch Biochem Biophys 272:532, 1989.

Dolecek TA. Epidemiological evidence of relationships between dietary polyunsaturated fatty acids and mortality in the multiple risk factor intervention trial. Proc Soc Exp Biol Med 200:177, 1992.

Doll H, et al. Pyridoxine (vitamin B_6) and the premenstrual syndrome: A randomized crossover trial. J R Coll Gen Pract 39:364, 1989.

Dwyer JT, et al: Tofu and soy drinks contain phytoestrogens. J Am Diet Assoc 94:739, 1994.

Evans MA, Shronts EP. Intestinal fuels: Glutamine, short-chain fatty acids, and dietary fiber. J Am Diet Assoc 92:1239, 1249, 1992.

Foster-Powell K, Brand Miller J. International tables of glycemic index. Am J Clin Nutr 62:871S, 1995.

Frankel EN, et al. Inhibition of oxidation of human low-density lipoprotein by phenolic substances in red wine. Lancet 341:453, 1993.

Fuhr U. Drug interactions with grapefruit juice. Extent, probable mechanism and clinical relevance. Drug Safety 18:251, 1998.

Galland L, Barrie S. Intestinal dysbiosis and the causes of disease. J Adv Med 6:67, 1993.

Gibson GR, Roberfroid MB. Dietary modulation of the human colonic microbiota: Introducing the concept of prebiotics. J Nutr 125:1401, 1995.

Giovanucci E, et al. Intake of carotenoids and retinol in relation to risk of prostate cancer. J Natl Cancer Inst 87:1767, 1995.

Gustafsson J-A. Fatty acids in control of gene expression. Seventeenth Marabou Symposium. Diet and Genetic Interactions. Nutr Rev 56(2, pt II):S20, 1998.

Health and Welfare Canada. Nutrition Recommendations. The Report of the Scientific Review Committee. Department of Supply and Services. Cat. No. H49-42/1990E. Ottawa, Ontario, Canada. 1990.

Hertog MG, et al. Dietary antioxidant flavonoids and risk of coronary heart disease: The Zutfan elderly study. Lancet 342:1007, 1993.

Horrobin DF, Manku MS. PMS and PMS breast pain (cyclical mastalgia): Disorders of EFA metabolism. Prostaglandins, Leukotrienes and Essential Fatty Acid Rev 37:255, 1989.

Hughes VL, Hiller SL. Microbiologic characteristics of Lactobacillus products used for colonization of the vagina. Obstet Gynecol 75:244, 1990.

King A, Young G. Characteristics and occurrence of phenolic phytochemicals. J Am Diet Assoc. 99:213, 1999.

Krauss R. Genetic influences on lipoprotein response to dietary fat and cholesterol: Proceedings of a symposuim held in Anaheim, CA, April 26, 1994. Am J Clin Nutr 62:457S, 1995.

Lampe J. Functional Foods and Health Claims: Separating the Wheat from the Chaff. Presentation at the Annual Meeting, Washington State Dietetic Association, February 20, 1997.

Leach P. New survey targets eating trends. The Wall Street Journal, April 17, 1998.

Levin B. Intestinal permeability and nutritional support of intestinal integrity. Q Rev Nat Med Summer:141, 1994.

Linder M. Nutritional Biochemistry and Metabolism with Clinical Applications, 2nd ed. Norwalk, CT: Appleton and Lange, 1991, pp. 248–249.

Lukaczer D. Assessing hepatic detoxification. Q Rev Nat Med Spring:67, 1996a.

Lukaczer D. Secretory IgA and gastrointestinal barrier competence. Q Rev Nat Med Fall:227, 1996b.

Mathai, K. Dietary supplementation and meal planning patterns among Washington State dietitians. Unpublished master's thesis, Bastyr University, 1995.

Mayer L, et al. Antigen trafficking in the intestine. Ann NY Acad Sci 778: 28, 1996.

Mehta J. Intake of antioxidants among American cardiologists. Am J Cardiol 79:1558, 1997.

Menopause. Harvard Women's Health Lett 6(2):2, 1994.

Mertz W. Chromium occurrence and function in biological systems. Physiol Rev 49:163, 1969.

Messina M. For your information. J Am Diet Assoc 98:974, 1998.

Messina M, Erdman JW (eds.). The role of soy in preventing and treating chronic disease. Am J Clin Nutr 68(Suppl 6):1329S, 1998.

Messina MJ, et al. Soy intake and cancer risk: A review of the in vitro and in vivo data. Nutr Cancer 21:113, 1994.

Millen BE, et al. Population nutrient intake approaches dietary recommendations: 1991–1995 Framingham Nutrition Studies. J Am Diet Assoc 97:742, 1997.

Moss AJ, et al. Use of vitamin and mineral supplements in the United States: Current users, types of products and nutrients. Adv Data Vital Health Stat 74, DHHS Publication No. PHS 89-1250, 1989.

Nettleton JA. n-3 fatty acids: Comparison of plant and seafood sources in human nutrition. J Am Diet Assoc 91:331, 1991.

1993 Prevalence of sedentary lifestyle—Behavioral risk factor surveillance system, United States, 1991. MMWR 29:576, 1993.

O'Dwyer ST, et al. A single dose of endotoxin increases intestinal permeability in healthy humans. Arch Surg 123:1459, 1988.

Patterson B, et al. Fruit and vegetables in the American diet. Data from the NHANES II survey. Am J Public Health 80:1443, 1990.

Percival M. Phytonutrients and detoxification. Clin Nutr Insights 5:1, 1997.

Peterson J, Dwyer J. Taxonomic classification helps identify flavonoid-containing foods on a semiquantitative food frequency questionnaire. J Am Diet Assoc 98:677, 685, 1998.

Potter SM, et al. Soy protein and isoflavones: Their effects on blood lipids and bone density in postmenopausal women. Am J Clin Nutr 68(suppl 6):1375S, 1998.

Raper NR, et al. Omega-3 fatty acid content in the U.S. food supply. J Am Coll Nutr 11:304, 1992.

Reaven G. Pathophysiology of insulin resistance in human disease. Physiol Rev 75:473, 1995.

Rippe J. The obesity epidemic: Challenges and opportunities. J Am Diet Assoc 98(Suppl 2):S5, 1998.

Salminen S, et al. Gut flora in normal and disordered states. Chemotherapy 41(Suppl 1):5, 1995.

Schauss AG. *Lactobacillus acidophilus*: Method of action, clinical application and toxicity data. J Adv Med 3:163, 1990.

Serdula M, et al. Fruit and vegetable intake among adults in 16 states: Results of a brief telephone survey. Am J Public Health 85:236, 1995.

Serraino M, Thompson LU. Flaxseed supplementation and early markers of colon carcinogenesis. Cancer Lett 63:159, 1992.

Simopoulos AP. Omega-3 fatty acids in health and disease and in growth and development. Am J Clin Nutr 54:438, 1991.

Steinmetz K, Potter J. Vegetables, fruit and cancer prevention: A review. J Am Diet Assoc 96:1027, 1996.

Thys-Jacobs S, et al. Calcium carbonate and the premenstrual syndrome: Effects on premenstrual and menstrual symptoms. Premenstrual Syndrome Study Group. Am J Obstet Gynecol 179:444, 1998.

U.S. Department of Health and Human Services (DHHS). Healthy People 2000: National Health Promotion and Disease Prevention Objectives. Washington, DC: DHHS (PHS), Publication No. 91-50213, 1990.

Verhoeven DT, et al. Epidemiological studies on brasssica vegetables and cancer risk. Cancer Epidemiol Biomarkers Prev 5:733, 1996.

Walker W. Uptake of antigens: Role in gastrointestinal disease. Acta Paediatr Jpn 36:597, 1994.

Warshafsky S, et al. Effect of garlic on total serum cholesterol: A meta-analysis. Ann Intern Med 119:599, 1993.

Wattenberg L. Chemoprevention of cancer. Cancer Res 45:1, 1985.

Wattenberg L. Inhibition of carcinogenesis by minor dietary constituents. Cancer Res 52(Suppl):2085S, 1992.

Williams W. What we eat in America survey. Nutr Today 32:37, 1997.
Windmueller H, Spaeth A. Uptake and metabolism of plasma glutamine by the small intestine. Nutr Rev 48:310, 1990.
Wolever T. The glycemic index. In: Bourne GH (ed.). Aspects of Some Vitamin, Minerals and Enzymes in Health and Disease. World Rev Nutr Diet. Basel: S Karger, 62:120, 1990.
Worthington-Roberts B, Breskin M. Supplement patterns of Washington State dietitians. J Am Diet Assoc 84:795, 1984.
Yasui I, et al. Detection of Bifidobacterium that induce large quantities of IgA. Microbial Ecol Health Dis 5:155, 1992.
Yee GC, et al. Effect of grapefruit juice on blood cyclosporin concentration. Lancet 345:955, 1995.
Young VR, et al. Evaluation of the protein quality of an isolated soy protein in young men: Relative nitrogen requirements and effect of methionine supplementation. Am J Clin Nutr 39:16, 1984.

ADDITIONAL REFERENCES

Albanese C, et al. Effect of secretory IgA on transepithelial passage of bacteria across the intact ileum in vitro. J Am Coll Surg 179:679, 1994.
Caragay AB. Cancer-preventive foods and ingredients. Food Res 46:65, 1992.
Fortes C, et al. The effect of zinc and vitamin A supplementation on immune responses in an older population. J Am Geriatr Soc 46:19, 1998.
Hahn NI. Are phytoestrogens nature's cure for what ails us? A look at the research. J Am Diet Assoc 98:9, 1998.
Heuser MD, Adler W. Immunological aspects of aging and malnutrition. Clin Geriatr Med 13:697, 1997.
Kim S. Dietetics professionals and women's health research at the National Institutes of Health. J Am Diet Assoc 98:133, 1998.
Kubena K, McMurray D. Nutrition and the immune system: A review of nutrient-nutrient interactions. J Am Diet Assoc 96:1156, 1996.
Opara J, Levine J. The deadly quartet—The insulin resistance syndrome. South Med J 90:1162, 1997.
Percival M. Intestinal health. Clin Nutr Insights 5:1, 1997.
Poehlam E, et al. Changes in energy balance and body composition at menopause: A controlled longitudinal study. Ann Intern Med 123:673, 1995.
Pszcola D. Fruit and vegetable ingredients: Advancing the 5-a-day message. Food Technol 51:127, 1997.
Rao N. Bioactive chemicals in Indian foods. Nat Foundation India Bull 16:1, 1995.
Seventeenth Marabou Symposium. Diet and Genetic Interactions. Nutr Rev, 56(2, pt II), 1998.
Sloan A. Food industry forecast: Consumer trends to 2020 and beyond. Food Technol 52:37, 1998.

CHAPTER 13

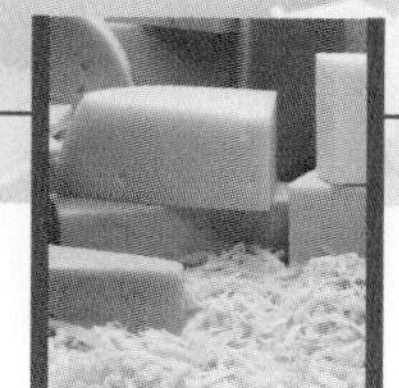

Nutrition in Aging

NANCY G. HARRIS MS, RD, LDN

Chapter Outline

- Life Span
- The Aging Process
- Nutritional Requirements of the Elderly
- Nutritional Care of the Elderly
- Nutritional Care in Assisted Living and Skilled Care Facilities
- The Nutrition Screening Initiative

Key Terms

AGED—persons 75 to 84 years of age
CELLULAR THEORY—a theory that relates aging to the creation of cross-linkages between macromolecules
CENTENARIANS—those (human longevity outliers) living to 100 years of age or beyond the age of current life span records
DYSGEUSIA—loss of sense of taste
ELDERLY NUTRITION PROGRAM (ENP)—a program, covered by Title III, parts C-1 and C-2, and Title VI of the Older Americans Act, which provides funds for nutritional services to older individuals in the community
ERROR THEORY—a theory that relates aging to environmental damage to the DNA template, leading to errors in the genetic program
FREE-RADICAL THEORY—a theory that relates aging to cellular damage caused by free radicals
HYPOCHLORHYDRIA—deficiency of hydrochloric acid in the gastric juice
HYPOSMIA—diminished sense of smell
LIFE EXPECTANCY—the average length of life projected for a population of a given age
LIFE SPAN—the maximum number of years of life that humans have lived
NUTRITION SCREENING INITIATIVE—a screening program established to promote timely nutritional screening and intervention in the United States
OBRA (OMNIBUS BUDGET RECONCILIATION ACT OF 1987)—refers to the federal regulations that govern skilled nursing care facilities
OLDEST-OLD—persons 85 years of age and older
PROGRAM THEORY—a theory of aging that proposes that cells are capable of reproducing themselves for a programmed, finite number of times, after which they die
SARCOPENIA—age-related loss of skeletal muscle
XEROSTOMIA—dry mouth from decreased salivation
YOUNG-OLD—persons 65 to 74 years of age

Over the past century, the United States has witnessed a challenging shift in the age distribution of its population. Improvements in health care technology have resulted in decreased infant mortality and reduced morbidity from disease. The number of persons older than 65 years of age has increased from 4% of the population in 1900 to 13% of the population in 1990, and this figure is expected to reach 20% by the year 2030 (Rubenstein, 1990). The most rapidly growing age bracket is the over-85 segment, which currently includes 3.5 million Americans. It is estimated that this figure will approach 20 million by the year 2050 (Dychtwald, 1989; Day, 1993) (Fig. 13–1). These population trends will have a significant impact on the future of health care and other services (Schlenker, 1998).

Traditionally, in the United States, the "elderly" population has been defined as that segment of the population that is 65 years of age or older. This definition, however, fails to recognize the physical and socioeconomic changes experienced by older people as they age. Additionally, the rapidly increasing number of people included in this elderly group has led to the need for more definitive age groupings. Thus, the specific age groups of 65 to 74 years, 75 to 84 years, and 85 and older are often referred to, respectively, as the **young-old,** the **aged,** and the **oldest-old** (Schlenker, 1998). Researchers continue to investigate variations in physical health, mental alertness, and vitality among the elderly.

This chapter is a revision of a chapter, contributed by Jill M. Shuman, MS, RD, that appeared in the previous edition.

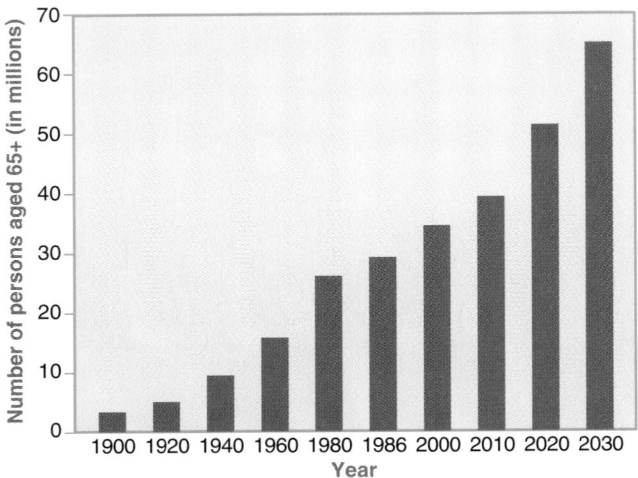

FIGURE 13–1 Number of persons aged 65 and older from 1900 to 2030. Increments in years on horizontal scale are uneven. (Data from US Bureau of the Census.)

More than ever before, increased emphasis is being placed on identifying the factors that promote wellness, including health, nutritional status, and fitness (see "*New Directions:* Physical Fitness and the Elderly"). Positive nutritional habits throughout life can clearly influence the quality of life a person may expect in later years.

LIFE SPAN

Discussions about length of life are frequently mired in confusion because the terms life span and life expectancy are often used interchangeably. **Life span** defines the maximum number of years of life that humans have lived. Although gerontologists continue to debate the limits of the human life span, there is evidence that the upper natural range is somewhere between 120 and 140 years (Dychtwald, 1989). The maximum human life span will continue to increase as more **centenarians,** or "human longevity outliers," survive to challenge today's record (Smith, 1997). Gains in life span have not been equal in both gender groups, but the differences are narrowing (Schlenker, 1998).

Life expectancy, by contrast, is the average length of life projected for a population of a given age. In terms of life expectancy determined at birth, it is the number of years an infant born at a particular time may expect to live, assuming that prevailing conditions will remain the same. Life expectancy, or the length of time a person can be expected to live based on certain variables, is subject to environmental influences, and it has continued to increase. In 1996, the estimated life expectancy at birth was 76.1 years (NCHS, 1996).

Increased life expectancy can be attributed largely to improvements in infant and childhood morbidity and mortality. Twice as many infants now survive until their first birthday as compared to those born at the turn of the century. Improved standards of living, availability of health services, and improvements in medical technology have reduced the threat of many childhood diseases.

Nutritional status can positively affect life expectancy; improved nutritional intake and disease control have clearly increased the number of people in the general population who reach an age that approaches the maximum recorded life span. Most recently, the period of middle to late-middle age has been marked by increased longevity. Beginning in 1930 for women, but only in the last 10 years for men, the life expectancy of individuals who reach middle age or older has increased in technologically advanced countries. The reduced or delayed mortality in this group is a result of the postponing of the degenerative diseases that typically affect this age group.

Factors involved in increased life expectancy include improved medical care, higher standards of living, and, to a large degree, improved nutrition.

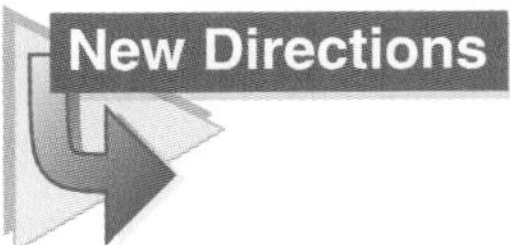

Physical Fitness and the Elderly

Many of the diseases associated with age and aging can be positively affected by an active life-style. Cardiopulmonary, musculoskeletal, and endocrine changes associated with age and disease show a decline in progression with regular physical activity. Physical activity in older people, however, is often restricted by weakness and muscle loss. Energy expenditures have been found to differ, too. In one study, elderly women were found to walk less efficiently than their middle-aged counterparts, and so needed more total calories for the same activity (Voorrips et al., 1993).

Many factors, including chronic illness, sedentary life-style, nutritional inadequacy or deficiencies, and aging itself, may contribute to muscle weakness and the loss of skeletal muscle mass in people of advanced age. Exercise training in elderly subjects has proved to be beneficial in improving gait velocity, range of motion, and endurance. Studies continue to show that exercise training can improve the functional capacity of older adults.

Perhaps the most exciting finding of these studies is the fact that not only does the aging musculoskeletal system appear to retain its responsiveness to progressive resistance training, it also significantly improves in functional mobility and overall activity. In addition, metabolic function improves due to the increased muscle tissue (Evans and Cyr-Campbell, 1997; Hakim 1998; Ades et al., 1996).

The increased awareness of the relationship of nutrition and other life-style practices to the occurrence of diseases with aging may lead to further increases in life expectancy. The three leading causes of death in the United States in 1996—heart disease, cancer, and cerebrovascular disease—all have nutrition-related risk factors (NCHS, 1996). Those reaching 65 years of age can expect to live another 17 years (Kannel, 1988).

Since 1968, life expectancy has increased by 3 to 4 years as the result of a 30% decrease in mortality from coronary artery disease and a 50% decrease in stroke mortality (Leaf, 1988). Although this increase is partly attributable to improved medical treatment and care, it is mainly related to changes in life-style, including avoidance of nutritional practices thought to promote atherosclerosis and hypertension. Considerable epidemiologic evidence has implicated nutritional status as a factor in certain types of cancer, osteoporosis, exogenous obesity, hypertension, cardiovascular disease, and type 2 diabetes mellitus.

Theories of Aging

Aging is a process that involves the whole body. Each organ independently loses its function, and the body becomes senescent. Individuals are known to age at different rates, but the processes that control the rate at which people age, and how this senescence affects the development of chronic diseases, are poorly understood (Mitchell, 1997). Although the degenerative changes that accompany aging are not well understood, a number of theories have been proposed to account for the deterioration, at least in part. The changes associated with aging are partly influenced by genetics, race, and gender. The role of environmental, psychosocial, and life-style factors on the pathology of disease is uncertain.

Support for the **program theory** of aging has been derived from laboratory cultures of embryonic cells, which have been found to reproduce themselves a finite number of times and then die. If cell reproduction is temporarily halted and then resumed, reproduction continues only until the established number has been reached.

The **error theory** of aging suggests that environmental damage to the DNA template results in errors in the genetic program. Subsequent production of abnormal proteins gives rise to mutations and teratogens.

The **cellular theory** of aging is based on the premise that environmental factors cause degenerative changes in cellular components, with cross-linkages subsequently forming between macromolecules. Altering the form and function of collagen affects sensitive processes, such as the passage of substances across cell membranes. Similar cross-linkages in DNA could introduce errors into the genetic program. Consonant with this "wear-and-tear" theory is the fact that maximum life span in different species correlates with the metabolic level and the length of time necessary to reach reproductive maturity. Insects and shrews, for example, have extremely rapid metabolic rates and short life spans.

One prominent theory of aging—the **free-radical theory**—involves the continuous formation of free radicals as a result of exposure to oxygen, background radiation, and other environmental factors. These highly reactive substances are thought to damage cellular components. A variety of antioxidants, including tocopherols, superoxide dismutase, and glutathione peroxidase, are able to repair damage caused by free radicals. Disappointingly, however, antioxidant therapy has failed to extend the life span of mammals significantly.

The only nutritional model that has actually been successful in prolonging life in mammalian species, involves severe dietary restriction of energy (Sohal and Weindrich, 1996; Masoro, 1990). The original studies in this area demonstrated that dietary restriction in rats increased longevity, but led to diminished sexual maturation and fertility (McCay et al., 1941). Subsequent studies involving less severe dietary restriction (a 50% to 60% lower energy intake than animals allowed to eat ad lib) have revealed increased longevity in rats, mice, and hamsters without the previously observed developmental abnormalities (Merry and Holehan, 1988). Moreover, susceptibility to the degenerative diseases of aging was found to be decreased, and many age-associated physiologic changes were delayed. Although the animals in these studies were leaner than the control animals, the results do not point to reduction of body fat as the mechanism by which food restriction extends length of life.

There is growing evidence that food restriction may influence the aging process by protecting against free-radical damage (Koizumi et al., 1987; Emerit and Chance, 1992). Other research indicates that the effects of food restriction on the aging process may be attributable to modulation of the age-related changes in gene expression (Richardson et al., 1987).

The results of these experiments cannot necessarily be applied to humans. These animal studies involve change in a single variable—energy intake—whereas human longevity is influenced by a variety of interacting factors. Even if people were willing to accept drastic restrictions in energy intake and the concomitant reduced quality of life, there is no evidence that lifelong food restriction would be safe (Masoro, 1990). Furthermore, there is nothing to suggest that such restriction would prolong life beyond the maximum current life span of approximately 115 years.

THE AGING PROCESS

Aging is a normal process that begins at conception and ends at death. During periods of growth, anabolic processes exceed catabolic changes. Once the body reaches physiologic maturity, the rate of catabolic or degenerative change becomes greater than the rate of anabolic cell regeneration. The resultant loss of cells leads to varying degrees of decreased efficiency and impaired organ function.

Aging is marked by a progressive loss of lean body mass, as well as changes in most body systems. Which, if any, of these changes are the inevitable outcome of genetically programmed events or of prolonged environmental influences is a matter of debate. Although precise data on the effect of nutrition on the health of the elderly are lacking, in general, the aged appear to be subject to the same influences that govern nutritional status in the younger population.

Sensory Losses

The senses of taste, smell, sight, hearing, and touch diminish at individualized rates. Reduced senses of taste (**dysgeusia**) and smell (**hyposmia**) are common in the elderly and may result from a variety of factors, including normal aging; certain diseases, such as Alzheimer's disease; medications; surgical interventions; radiation therapy; and environmental exposure (Table 13–1). Taste and smell dysfunction tends to begin at around 60 years of age, and becomes more severe in persons older than 70 years of age (Schiffman, 1994). A reduced ability to detect odors and identify foods eaten is important. Loss of taste and smell senses may not only reduce the pleasure and comfort associated with food, but may also pose a risk factor for food poisoning or for overexposure to environmentally hazardous chemicals that would otherwise be detectable by taste and smell (Schiffman, 1997). Because taste and smell stimulation induces metabolic changes, such as salivary, gastric acid, and pancreatic secretions, as well as increases in plasma levels of insulin, decreased sensory stimulation may impair these metabolic processes (Schiffman and Warwick, 1992).

Hearing loss, impaired vision, and loss of functional status are also common in elderly persons and may lead to diminished food intake as a result of decreased appetite, food recognition, and self-feeding ability.

TABLE 13–1 MEDICAL CONDITIONS THAT AFFECT THE SENSE OF TASTE

Nervous System Disorders	**Localized Disease Processes**
Bell's palsy	Facial hypoplasia
Damage to chorda tympani	Glossitis and other oral disorders
Familial dysautonomia	Leprosy
Head trauma	Oral Crohn's disease
Multiple sclerosis	Radiation therapy
Raeder's paratrigeminal syndrome	Sjögren's syndrome
Diseases or Disorders Affecting Nutritional Status	**Other**
Cancer	Hypertension
Chronic renal failure	Influenza-like infections
Liver disease, including cirrhosis	Laryngectomy
Niacin (vitamin B_3) deficiency	
Thermal burn	
Zinc deficiency	
Endocrine System Disorders	
Adrenocortical insufficiency	
Congenital adrenal hyperplasia	
Pseudohypoparathyroidism	
Panhypopituitarism	
Cushing's syndrome	
Cretinism	
Hyothyroidism	
Diabetes mellitus	
Gonadal dysgenesis (Turner's syndrome)	

(Reprinted with permission from Schiffman SS. Changes in taste and smell: Drug interactions and food preferences. Nutr Rev 52:S11, 1994.)

Oral Health Status

Xerostomia, the subjective feeling of dry mouth caused by hyposalivation, is a common problem among the elderly (Bivona, 1998). Indeed, xerostomia affects more than 70% of the elderly, and can significantly affect nutrient intake (Davis and Sherer, 1994). Geriatric persons with xerostomia have been shown to have difficulty chewing and swallowing, and as a result, they tend to avoid certain foods, particularly crunchy, dry, and sticky foods (Loesche et al., 1995).

Untreated dental caries and periodontitis are major causes of tooth loss in the elderly, leading to edentulousness and the wearing of dentures. Generally, people who wear dentures chew 75% to 85% less efficiently than those with natural teeth (Martin, 1991), which may lead to decreased consumption of meats and fresh fruits and vegetables. In turn, this can result in an inadequate intake of energy, iron, and vitamins, particularly vitamin C, folate, and beta-carotene.

Gastrointestinal Function

A number of changes affecting nutrient intake, digestion, and absorption occur in the gastrointestinal system during the aging process (Lovat, 1996). Human adult-onset lactase decline, which interferes with digestion and absorption of the lactose in dairy products, is frequently a characteristic of the aging intestine. This can be a risk factor for developing osteoporosis (Lee and Krasinski, 1998).

One of the most remarkable changes that occurs with aging is the frequent development of atrophic gastritis and the inability to secrete gastric acid (Saltzman and Russell, 1998). Gastric **hypochlorhydria** affects approximately one third of older Americans and can cause malabsorption due to small bowel bacterial overgrowth and diminished absorption of nutrients, such as vitamin B_{12}, which can result in pernicious anemia (Russell, 1997).

Aging alters the metabolism of calcium and vitamin D in several ways that can contribute to accelerated bone loss and the development of senile osteoporosis (Bouillon et al., 1997). Calcitriol synthesis and activity in calcium absorption by the small intestine are decreased with aging. Calcium availability is affected by poor dietary intake of calcium and vitamin D, but also by reduced production of provitamin D by the skin through solar exposure (Wemeau, 1995).

Constipation, one of the most common digestive complaints, increases in frequency in the elderly (Duffy et al., 1995). Constipation is often attributable to prolonged rectosigmoid transit, which can be caused by deficient fluid intake, inadequate dietary fiber intake, and a sedentary life-style. In the elderly, it may also be related to inadequate energy intake, rather than to inadequate fiber consumption alone, as well as to psychological distress factors (Evans et al., 1998). Low energy intake, fewer meals per day, low fluid intake, and depression were found to be the most relevant factors. Constipation can often be reduced by increasing intake of dietary fiber, fluid, and kilocalories, as well as by increasing physical activity. However, care should be taken to monitor calcium status when a very-high-fiber diet is prescribed. If an elderly person reports constipation, it is important to complete a careful physical, psychological, and bowel history rather than immediately conclude that a laxative is indicated (Harari, 1998). Laxatives are used by 8.8% of elderly persons living in the community and by 74.6% of those residing in nursing homes (Pahor et al., 1994). Laxative use increases with increasing age and is independently associated with hypoalbuminemia. Use of laxatives and increased fiber intake have been shown to produce an overall increase in the frequency of bowel elimination amounting to 1.4 bowel movements per week (95% confidence interval) (Tramonte, 1997). Biofeedback has been suggested as an effective long-term treatment alternative for idiopathic constipation that is unresponsive to traditional therapies (Chiotakakou-Faliakou et al., 1998).

Metabolic Function

The decrease in glucose tolerance associated with the aging process leads to an increase in plasma glucose levels of 1.5 mg/dL per decade. Whether this impaired glucose tolerance results from deficient insulin production or from deficient action is still a matter of debate. Retrospective studies indicate that good glucose control reduces the incidence and severity of complications from diabetes. Treatment of glucose intolerance in the elderly usually involves dietary modifications, exercise, and oral pharmacologic agents (Samos and Roos, 1998).

Resting metabolic rate decreases approximately 15% to 20% over the life span, primarily due to changes in body composition and reductions in physical activity. Basal metabolic rate can be predicted in healthy, older women within an average of 116 kcal per day (Taaffe et al., 1995). Where height measurement is hard to determine, knee height is especially helpful in assessing height in the elderly, as it does not decrease with age as does stature (Harari et al., 1996) (see Chapter 16).

Cardiovascular Function

Cardiovascular disease continues to be one of the leading causes of death in the United States. The risk factors that influence the occurrence of cardiovascular disease in the elderly are similar to those for persons who are middle-aged. Moreover, targeting the elderly for treatment has been shown to be cost-effective (Kannel, 1997).

During the aging process, blood vessels become less elastic and total peripheral resistance increases, leading to an increased risk and prevalence of hypertension. Blood pressure continues to increase in women older than 80 years of age, but declines substantially in older men. Serum cholesterol levels in men tend to peak at 60 years of age, but total cholesterol levels as well as the low-density lipoprotein (LDL) fraction, continue to rise in women until the age of 70 years (Kannel, 1988). Waist-to-hip ratio, alcohol intake, smoking, and fasting plasma glucose and plasma insulin levels are significant predictors of serum triglyceride levels in postmenopausal women (Laws et al., 1993).

Although low cholesterol levels may be predictive of future cognitive dysfunction, and despite the fact that there appears to be no clear rationale for lowering cholesterol levels by severe dietary restrictions in the elderly (Morley and Solomon, 1994), it cannot be assumed that dietary treatment of hypercholesterolemia is without merit. Correction of hypertension and hyperlipidemia have been shown to reduce cardiovascular morbidity and mortality in the elderly. The beneficial effects of other strategies, such as lowering homocysteine and fibrinogen levels, have not been well established in this age group (Kannel, 1997).

Renal Function

Renal function and glomerular filtration rate can diminish as much as 60% between the ages of 30 and 80 years, primarily owing to certain chronic conditions, a reduction in the number of nephrons, and reduced blood flow. This makes the elderly person less able to respond to changes in fluid status and to challenges to the acid-base balance. Excessive amounts of protein waste products and electrolytes may become increasingly difficult to metabolize. Geriatric nephropathy may be the result of chronic protein overnutrition (Rudman, 1988). According to consumer studies, the average American consumption of protein is 1.5% greater than the RDA.

Musculoskeletal Function

Aging is associated with remarkable body composition changes, including a reduction in lean body mass and an increase in body fat (Hurley et al.,

1997). **Sarcopenia,** an age-related loss in skeletal muscle, is the result of a decline in muscle strength. Sarcopenia contributes to changes in gait and balance, loss of physical function, and risk for chronic diseases (Dutta, 1997). Lean body mass declines approximately 2% to 3% per decade. The average body fat percentage in males increases from about 15% when young to 25% at the age of 60 years. In women, it increases from 18% to 23% when young to 32% at the age of 60 years. This change in body fat is attributable to less intense physical activity and to an alteration in testosterone and growth hormone production that affects anabolism and lean tissue growth.

Body protein level in the healthy elderly is 30% to 40% less than that in young adults. Loss in muscle mass accounts for the age-associated decreases in basal metabolic rate, muscle strength, and activity levels. Increased body fatness, especially as manifested by abdominal obesity, is associated with increased risk for several chronic diseases (Evans and Cyr-Campbell, 1997).

Older women have a higher body mass index and lower waist-to-hip ratio than men of the same age. Table 13–2 presents appropriate weights in relation to height for adults aged 65 years and older. These recommendations illustrate the wide ranges of weight associated with health and longevity in the elderly.

Older women tend to reduce their energy intakes less so than men, which has negative implications for them in relation to weight management, type 2 diabetes mellitus, and other chronic diseases. Sufficient dietary protein intake can reduce whole-body protein turnover in the elderly.

Physical activity has been shown to help maintain the integrity of both muscle and bone (Evans and Cyr-Campbell, 1997). Walking is especially beneficial (Hakim et al., 1998). Strength and resistance training positively influence protein synthesis and breakdown. Moreover, resistance training has been shown to restore muscle tissue and enhance functional status in elderly individuals (Ades et al., 1996). Figures 13–2 and 13–3 provide examples of safe aerobic activity for the older population.

Neurologic Function

The confusional states that arise in some elderly persons have numerous causes. Of great interest in this area is the experimental use of substances—specifically, tyrosine, tryptophan, and choline—that

TABLE 13–2 HEIGHT/WEIGHT TABLES FOR INDIVIDUALS AGED 65 TO 94 YEARS

HEIGHT (in)*	RECOMMENDED WEIGHTS (lbs) ACCORDING TO AGE (yrs)					
	65–69	70–74	75–79	80–84	85–89	90–94
Men Aged 65 Years and Older						
61	128–156	125–153	123–151			
62	130–158	127–155	125–153	122–148		
63	131–161	129–157	127–155	122–150	120–146	
64	134–164	131–161	129–157	124–152	122–148	
65	136–166	134–164	130–160	127–155	125–153	117–143
66	139–169	137–167	133–163	130–158	128–156	120–146
67	140–172	140–170	136–166	132–162	130–160	122–150
68	143–175	142–174	139–169	135–165	133–163	126–154
69	147–179	146–178	142–174	139–169	137–167	130–158
70	150–184	148–182	146–178	143–175	140–172	134–164
71	155–189	152–186	149–183	148–180	144–176	139–169
72	159–195	156–190	154–188	153–187	148–182	
73	164–200	160–196	158–192			
Women Aged 65 Years and Older						
58	120–146	112–138	111–135			
59	121–147	114–140	112–136	100–122	99–121	
60	122–148	116–142	113–139	106–130	102–124	
61	123–151	118–144	115–141	109–133	104–128	
62	125–153	121–147	118–144	112–136	108–132	107–131
63	127–155	123–151	121–147	115–141	112–136	107–131
64	130–158	126–154	123–151	119–145	115–141	108–132
65	132–162	130–158	126–154	122–150	120–146	112–136
66	136–166	132–162	128–157	126–154	124–152	116–142
67	140–170	136–166	131–161	130–158	128–156	
68	143–175	140–170				
69	148–180	144–176				

(Adapted from Master AM, Laser RP, Beckman G. Weight and height tables for the elderly. JAMA 172:658–662. Copyright 1960, American Medical Association. *Source:* Chumlea W. Nutritional assessment of the elderly through anthropometry. Columbus, OH: Ross Laboratories, 1984, p. 10.)

*The formula for calculating stature from knee height in men is 64.19 – (0.04 [3 age]) + (2.02 [knee height]). In women, it is 84.88 – (0.24 [age]) + (1.83 [knee height]).

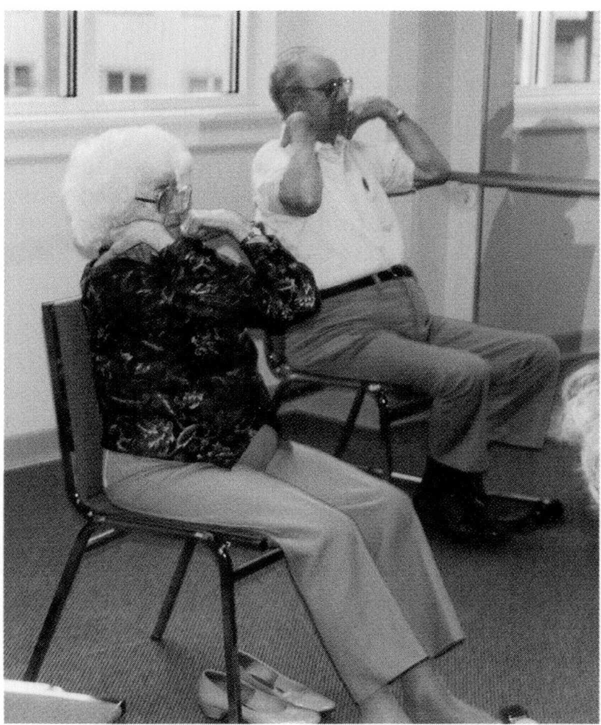

FIGURE 13–2 Armchair aerobics programs provide an opportunity for both safe exercise and socialization. (Courtesy of Cypress Glen Retirement Community, Greenville, North Carolina.)

serve as precursors of brain neurotransmitters involved in abnormalities such as Parkinson's disease and Alzheimer's disease. The specific roles of these nutrients in the etiology and treatment of Parkinson's and Alzheimer's disease remain to be determined.

There are some suggestions that a high-carbohydrate diet, when accompanied by insufficient protein intake, may lead to poor attention and decreased alertness in older people, possibly as a result of decreased synthesis of serotonin. Carnitine, derived from the amino acids lysine and methionine, may be effective in slowing the mental deterioration in Alzheimer's disease (Berry, 1994).

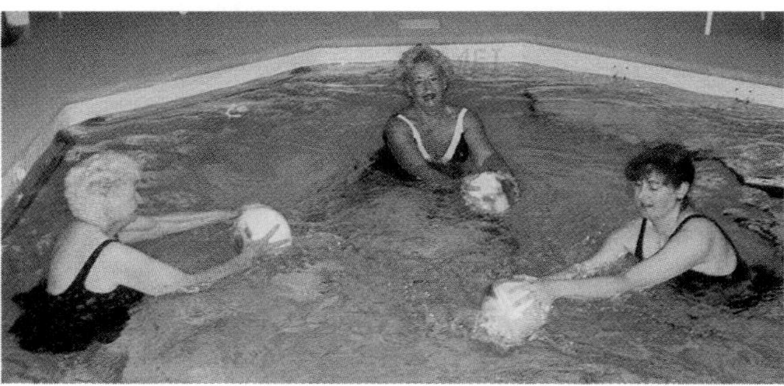

FIGURE 13–3 Aqua aerobics can improve cardiovascular, skeletal, and muscular function. (Courtesy of Cypress Glen Retirement Community, Greenville, North Carolina.)

The role of antioxidants has been studied extensively in connection with the many processes related to aging and cognitive function. Beta-carotene and carotenoids seem to play a protective role, whereas vitamins C and E are not as strongly related (Warsama Jama et al., 1996; Ortega et al., 1997).

Immunocompetence

Immune function declines with age. Both humoral and cell-mediated immunities are affected. These changes result in a diminished ability to fight infections, leading to an increased prevalence of infections in the elderly. Reduced immunosurveillance may also help to explain the increased prevalence of malignant disease in this population (Good and Lorenz, 1988).

Some preliminary studies have been conducted on the effects of supplementation with various nutrients on the immune function of the elderly. For example, vitamin E supplementation, instituted for a few months in a group of elderly, was found to enhance the immune function of the subjects (Meydani, 1990). Zinc status in the elderly may also be an important factor in immune function (Roebothan and Chandra, 1994). In another study, natural killer (NK) activity in cells was enhanced by a high intake of polyunsaturated fatty acids (Rasmussen et al., 1994). Further studies are underway, including some that demonstrate that multivitamin supplementation enhances delayed-hypersensitivity skin test responses in healthy older persons (Bogden et al., 1994).

Psychosocial Factors

Depression can affect appetite, digestion, energy level, weight, and well-being. In the elderly, depression may be associated with an inability to perform daily tasks, loss of relatives and friends, a feeling of nonproductivity, social isolation, financial concerns, or a decline in cognitive function.

Loneliness and changes in daily routines, especially those related to food purchasing, preparation, and consumption, are common in widowhood. Widowed persons who enjoy mealtimes, have high-quality diets and good appetites, and who receive social support generally experience more rapid grief resolution with fewer health consequences than do those without these characteristics (Rosenbloom and Whittington, 1993).

Loss of independence and mobility can become stressful issues for the elderly. These circumstances may also make purchasing food and preparing meals very difficult. An inability to drive safely to the local grocery store or to transport groceries home can result in an inadequate or limited availability of food.

Elderly persons may also become homebound out of fear of being victimized. This is particularly a problem in poor, crime-ridden areas. Failing health may further increase the problems of fearfulness, isolation, and immobility.

Financial status is often compromised in retired elderly persons. This may necessitate reductions in budget allocations for food and/or services. Moreover, elderly persons who may be eligible for food stamps are not always comfortable taking advantage of the service.

NUTRITIONAL REQUIREMENTS OF THE ELDERLY

Energy

Although obesity in humans is associated with a shortened life expectancy, the extent of its effect is somewhat controversial. Some data have indicated that being underweight is associated with as high a mortality rate as moderate obesity, particularly in those older than 60 years of age. The increase in body fat and corresponding obesity that occurs with aging is actually accompanied by a decline in dietary intake. Older persons can develop both physiologic and pathologic anorexia of aging, which increases the risk of protein-energy malnutrition. Despite its prevalence, protein-energy malnutrition in the elderly is often missed as a diagnosis and is seldom treated. Recently, screening tools have been made available to better detect such problems in the elderly population (Morley, 1997).

Energy requirements generally decrease with age due to a decline in basal metabolic rate and a reduction in physical activity. The 1989 Recommended Dietary Allowances (RDAs) call for a reduction in average daily energy allowances for those 51 years of age or older amounting to 600 kcal/day for men and 300 kcal for women (Food and Nutrition Board, 1989). Meeting the nutritional needs of the elderly is challenging because, although their energy requirements decrease, their requirements for protein, vitamins, and minerals either do not diminish or actually increase. Average caloric intake for persons 51 years and older is 2300 kcal per day for men and 1900 kcal per day for women. Health problems arise when intakes total less than 1500 kcal per day.

Surveys, such as the USDA Food Consumption Survey and the National Health and Nutrition Examination Survey (HANES) I and II, report that the elderly are at nutritional risk. Indeed, the elderly often consume less than two thirds of the RDA for several nutrients. Inadequate intake of the following nutrients was recently identified as posing the greatest risk in the elderly: protein, riboflavin, folate, vitamin B_{12}, vitamin B_6, vitamin C, zinc, and carotenoids, such as lutein and zeaxanthin (Blumberg, 1997).

Protein

As people age and experience a decrease in skeletal tissue mass, the store of protein provided by skeletal muscle may be inadequate to meet the needs for protein synthesis, making dietary protein intake more important to meet essential needs. In 1989, the Food and Nutrition Board concluded that the protein RDA of 0.8 g per kilogram of body weight was appropriate for adults of all ages (Food and Nutrition Board, 1989). However, subsequent studies have demonstrated that this is not adequate to maintain nitrogen equilibrium in elderly adults. It is now thought that an intake of 1.0 g per kilogram is needed to maintain a positive nitrogen balance in the elderly (Campbell, 1996). A protein intake of 1.0 to 1.25 g per kilogram is generally safe for older adults.

The serum albumin level is the most reliable indicator of protein nutriture. Other serum protein values, such as transferrin, urea nitrogen, and total protein, are less reliable. Low serum albumin levels often correlate with the onset of pressure ulcers (Gilmore et al., 1995).

Protein needs increase in relation to the acuity and chronicity of disease. Stressful physical and psychological stimuli can induce a negative nitrogen balance. Infection, altered gastrointestinal function, and metabolic changes caused by chronic disease can reduce the efficiency of dietary nitrogen utilization and increase nitrogen excretion.

Carbohydrate

An impaired glucose tolerance in the elderly can lead to hypoglycemia, hyperglycemia, and type 2 diabetes mellitus. Insulin sensitivity can be enhanced by balanced energy intake, weight management, and regular physical activity (see Chapter 34).

Diminished lactase secretion can result in lactose intolerance and gastrointestinal complaints. Dietary modifications, including controlled intake of lactose-containing products, substitution of less problematic dairy products, and utilization of lactase-treated products, can help alleviate discomfort with cramping, flatulence, and diarrhea. Care should be taken to include calcium-rich dairy products in the diet (see Chapter 31).

There is no established Recommended Dietary Allowance (RDA) for carbohydrates. Current dietary guidelines recommend that 50% to 60% of total daily calories should come from carbohydrates. Emphasis should be placed on increasing the intake of complex carbohydrates, including dietary fibers, and controlling the intake of simple sugars.

Lipids

There is no established RDA for lipids. Current dietary guidelines recommend that no more than 30% of the total daily caloric intake come from lipids. Emphasis should be placed on reducing the intake of saturated fat and choosing monounsaturated or polyunsaturated fat sources. Coronary heart disease is the number one cause of death in the United States. Although there is no direct available evidence that dietary changes can reduce the risk of cardiovascular events in the elderly, there is no reason to believe that the same environmental factors leading to decreased risk in the younger population will not continue to be effective in later years. The recommended reduction of dietary fat to no more than 30% of total kilocalories also supports principles of weight control and cancer prevention. Conversely, over-restriction of dietary fat to less than 20% of the caloric intake may affect the overall quality of the diet.

Minerals

Aging produces physiologic changes that affect the need for several essential nutrients. Nutritional surveys of the elderly have shown a relatively low prevalence of severe nutrient deficiencies, but they have shown evidence of subclinical nutrient deficiencies that can affect function. Poor mineral status in the elderly is attributable, in part, to low dietary intake. In addition, there is inadequate information available about mineral nutriture and metabolism in the very old. New dietary guidelines for the elderly should emphasize the value of high quality, nutrient-dense foods.

Bone loss resulting in osteoporosis, the presence of hypochlorhydria, and the attendant failure to absorb calcium efficiently suggest the need for increased calcium intakes. The 1998 Adequate Intake (AI) for calcium intake reflects an increase in recommendations to 1200 mg per day for men and women aged 51 and older. Phosphorus recommendations have been decreased to 700 mg per day for the same groups.

Iron stores tend to increase with increasing age. Thus, iron-deficiency anemia in the older population is most likely to be related to gastrointestinal blood loss from malignant disease, peptic ulcer disease, or use of nonsteroidal anti-inflammatory drugs (NSAIDs).

Intakes of zinc in the elderly decline in relation to the decrease in energy intake and are much lower than the recommended level of 15 mg/day for men and 12 mg/day for women. Definite indicators of zinc status are not available; this impedes assessment in the elderly. Older people who avoid flesh foods may be at increased risk of poor zinc status owing to the reduced bioavailabilty of zinc from other food sources. Zinc deficiency is associated with impaired immune function, anorexia, dysgeusia, delayed wound healing, and pressure ulcer development.

There is no RDA established for sodium. Sodium intake is often associated with hypertension, but it is difficult to identify those hypertensive individuals who are sensitive to sodium. Therefore, it is prudent to limit dietary sodium intake to approximately 2 to 4 g per day. However, hyponatremia is a common finding among hospitalized and institutionalized elderly, so the possibility of deficient sodium intake should be considered in this population.

Although selenium levels tend to decline with age, the RDA for selenium is the same as that for younger adults (see Table 13–3).

TABLE 13–3 DIETARY REFERENCE INTAKES: RECOMMENDED DIETARY ALLOWANCES AND ADEQUATE INTAKES

	MEN	WOMEN
Energy (kcal)	2300	1900
Protein (g)	63	50
Vitamin A (mcg RE)	1000	800
Vitamin D (mcg)*		
51–70 years of age	10	10
>70 years of age	15	15
Vitamin E (mg α-TE)	10	8
Vitamin K (mg)	80	65
Thiamin (mg)	1.2	1.1
Riboflavin (mg)	1.3	1.1
Niacin (mg NE)	16	14
Vitamin B_6 (mg)	1.7	1.5
Folate $(\mu g)_{12}$	400	400
Vitamin B12 (μg)	2.4	2.4
Calcium (mg)*	1200	1200
Phosphorus (mg)	700	700
Magnesium (mg)	420	320
Iron (mg)	10	10
Zinc (mg)	15	12
Iodine (mcg)	150	150
Selenium (mcg)	70	55

(Reprinted with permission from Food and Nutrition Board National Research Council. Recommended Dietary Allowances, 10th edition, © 1989 by the National Academy of Sciences. Published by National Academy Press; and Dietary Reference Intakes: Recommended Levels for Individual Intake, Food and Nutrition Board, Institute of Medicine, National Academy of Sciences, © 1998.)

RE, retinol equivalents; *α-TE*, alpha-tocopherol equivalents; *NE*, niacin equivalents.
*Adequate intakes

Vitamins

Much remains to be learned about vitamin requirements and the efficiency of vitamin absorption, utilization, and excretion in the elderly. However, it is rare to identify vitamin A deficiency in older adults. Indeed, chronic hypervitaminosis A may be a problem in elderly people who take large doses of supplementary vitamin A. Over supplementation with vitamin A has been associated with increased levels of circulating retinyl esters, which may indicate vitamin toxicity or liver damage.

The requirement for vitamin D is dependent on the concentration of calcium and phosphorus in the diet; the person's age, sex, degree of exposure to sunlight; and the amount of skin pigmentation. Elderly people are at risk for vitamin D deficiency because of inadequate diets (Fig. 13–4). Whether age influences vitamin D absorption from the gastrointestinal tract is not clear. The lower levels of vitamin D in institutionalized and homebound elderly may result from decreased exposure to sunlight, resulting in less efficient synthesis of vitamin D in the skin, or from a decrease in renal mass (Ryan et al., 1995). A decline in skin thickness is partially related to the lower levels of 25-hydroxyvitamin D levels that occur with aging (Need et al., 1993). Seasonal variations in serum vitamin D levels are greater in lean than in fat subjects. The 1998 AI for

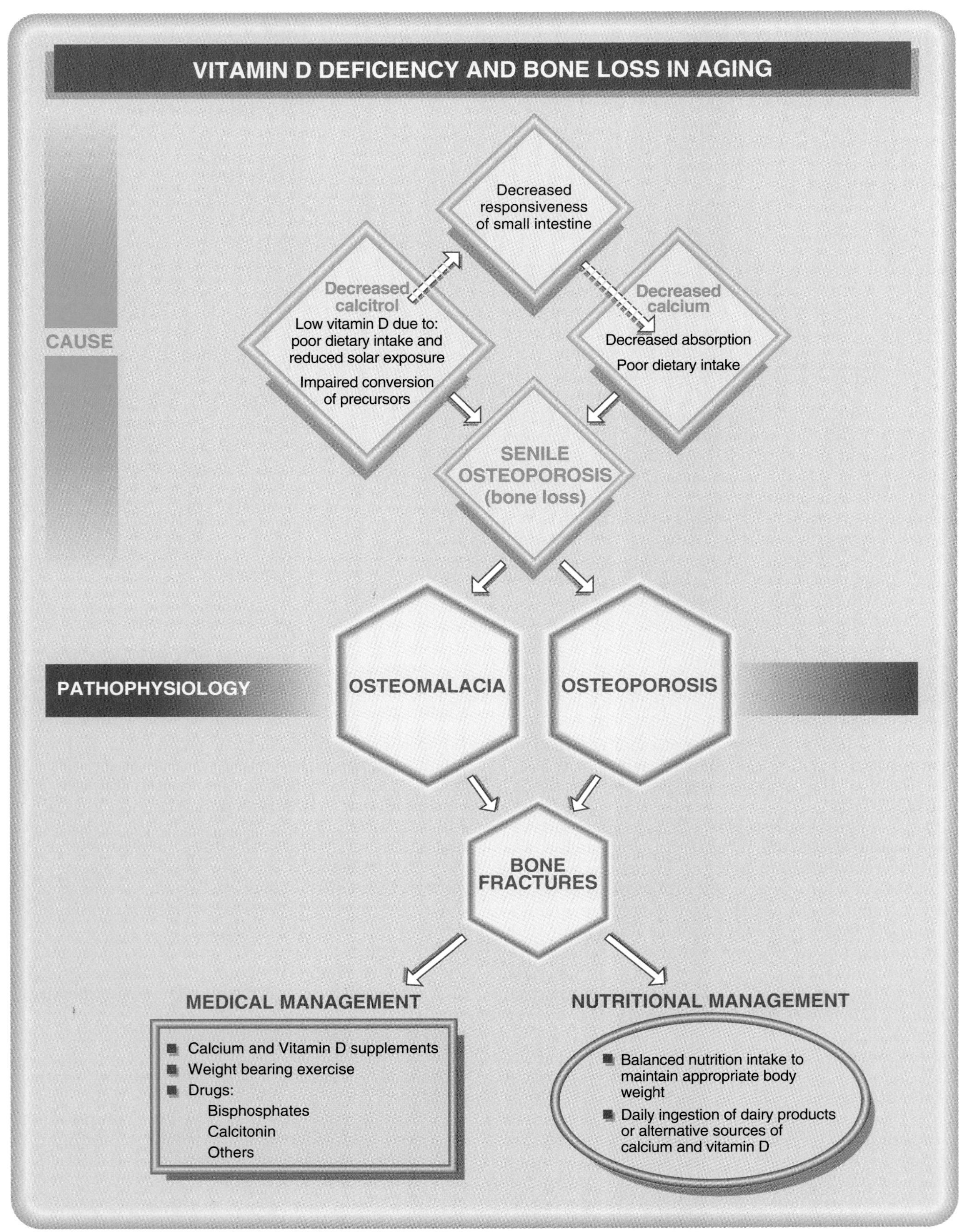

FIGURE 13–4 Pathology algorithm—vitamin D deficiency and bone loss in aging. (Algorithm content developed by John Anderson, Ph.D., and Stanford C. Garner, Ph.D., 2000.)

vitamin D is 10 and 15 mcg per day for those aged 51–70 years and older than 70 years, respectively.

Exposure of the skin to sunlight appears to be an important factor in maintaining appropriate vitamin D status in the elderly. Vitamin D supplementation should be considered for housebound or institutionalized elderly people. There is evidence to suggest that there is impaired conversion of vitamin D precursors in the liver and kidney, which can affect vitamin D status. Lack of adequate vitamin D and calcium are associated with osteoporosis and osteomalacia. Vitamin D malnutrition is prevalent among elderly patients in long-term care facilities. A negative correlation has been found between vitamin D intake and fractures, for which nursing home residents should be monitored carefully (Komar et al., 1993). Vitamin D may help in healing skin lesions, especially psoriasis, hyperproliferative disorders of cancer, and actinic keratoses (Holick, 1994). Prudent dietary supplementation with calcium and vitamin D improves bone density and may prevent fractures in a healthy elderly population (Dawson-Hughes et al., 1997).

Elderly subjects often have lower blood, plasma, and serum levels of vitamin C than younger adults. However, there does not appear to be any age-related alterations in the absorption or utilization of vitamin C. Stress, smoking, and some medications can increase vitamin C requirements, so an assessment of dietary intake is especially important in individuals who may be at risk. Encouraging the consumption of vitamin C–rich foods may be the most effective way of improving vitamin C status in the elderly. The current RDA is 60 mg for both men and women older than 51 years of age who do not smoke, and 100 mg per day in individuals who do smoke.

The antioxidant vitamins, such as vitamin E, carotenoids, and vitamin C, have been promoted as agents that enhance the health of the elderly. The role of high antioxidant serum levels in reducing the risk for age-related macular degeneration, the leading cause of irreversible blindness in the United States, has been studied. Preliminary studies have yielded promising results (Eye Disease Case-Control Study Group, 1993; Seddon and Hennekens, 1994; West et al., 1994). Vitamin C may be protective against cataract at an intake level of between 150 and 250 mg per day, which is possible to achieve from dietary sources alone (Jacques et al., 1997). In one study, elderly persons with the highest dietary intake of carotenoids had a 43% lower risk for macular degeneration than did those in the lowest quintile (Seddon et al., 1994). Vitamin E has also been found to be a potent nutrient for reducing the decline in cellular immunity that occurs in the elderly (Moriguchi, 1998).

Many studies have demonstrated an inadequate intake of vitamin B_6 among the elderly. Requirements for the vitamin are increased in many elderly persons owing to atrophic gastritis, which interferes with absorption. Alcoholism and liver dysfunction are additional risk factors for a deficiency of vitamin B_6. The 1998 RDA has established 1.7 mg per day for men and 1.5 mg per day for women 51 years and older as the recommended intake level.

There is no specific age-related impact on folate requirements in the elderly. However, alcoholism is a risk factor for folate deficiency. Severe deficiencies of folic acid in the elderly may result in anemias and elevated serum homocysteine levels, a risk factor for cardiac disease. The 1998 RDA is 400 mcg per day for both men and women 51 years and older. Diets are often lacking in folate, so consumption of folate-fortified foods (e.g., cereals, flour products) or folate-rich foods (e.g., liver, dried beans, broccoli, avocados, asparagus, spinach) should be encouraged.

The usual causes of vitamin B_{12} deficiency are atrophic gastritis and bacterial overgrowth, which decrease absorption and can lead to pernicious anemia. Persons with these conditions may require a higher dietary vitamin B_{12} intake through oral or injectable vitamin supplementation (see Chapter 35). While a low serum B_{12} may be associated with cognitive impairment, recent studies have not confirmed causation; B_{12} screening in the elderly is suggested (Bernard et al., 1998).

Recent research has shown that increased serum levels of vitamins B_6, B_{12}, and folate confer protection against elevated serum homocysteine, an independent risk factor for cardiovascular disease, depression, and certain neurologic deficits (Stampfer, 1992; Selhub et al., 1993). For many elderly persons, nutritional status relating to these nutrients is less than optimal and warrants special attention (Joosten et al., 1993).

Although overt malnutrition is relatively uncommon in the healthy elderly population, a maintenance-level multivitamin and mineral supplement may enhance immunity (Chandra, 1997) and may cure latent nutritional deficiency states that may be the basis for common complaints by some individuals. On the other hand, some studies indicate that 39% to 69% of elderly Americans, especially women, take higher levels of vitamin or mineral supplements (Hartz et al., 1988; Chandra et al., 1991) than the general adult population, and many are taking potentially toxic doses. Questions about nutrient supplementation should always be included in a nutritional assessment.

Water

Water accounts for approximately 50% of an older person's weight. This represents a decline of 10% from young adulthood, and is associated with a corresponding decline in lean body mass. Daily fluid replacement is essential, particularly in those who exercise regularly, consume large amounts of protein, use laxatives or diuretics, or live in areas with high temperatures. Hydration status in incontinent persons should be monitored carefully. Dehydration is the most common cause of fluid and electrolyte disturbances in the elderly (Chernoff, 1994). Reduced thirst sensation, reduced fluid intake, limited access to water, and diminished water conservation by the kidneys are important contributing factors to potential dehydration. Deficient fluid intake in the presence of diarrhea or fever can lead to clinical dehydration requiring hospitalization.

Fluid status is a critical component of the initial and ongoing assessment of an elderly person. Fluid needs are affected by variations in activity, insensible water losses, and urinary solute load. Generally, a daily fluid intake of 30 to 35 mL per kilogram of actual body weight and a minimum of 1500 mL per day or 1.0 to 1.5 mL per kilocalorie is adequate.

Overall Nutritional Status

Subgroups within the aging population are at risk of malnutrition for a variety of reasons (Table 13–4). These include lack of nutrition education, financial constraints, declining physical and psychological functional abilities, social isolation, and treatments for multiple, concomitant disorders or diseases. Secondary causes of malnutrition include anorexia, malabsorption secondary to gastrointestinal dysfunction, increased nutrient demand as a result of injury or disease, drug-nutrient interactions resulting from polypharmy, and substance abuse, such as alcoholism. When alcohol is substituted for nutritious foods, it may interfere with absorption of some nutrients, notably folic acid.

A cross-sectional survey of 200 elderly residents in long-term care facilities revealed a high level of undernutrition (Keller, 1993). Severe undernutrition was present in 18% of the residents; 10% were severely overnourished. Mild to moderate undernutrition was found in another 27.5%. Overnutrition was associated with the presence of disease, multiple medications, feeding impairments, high protein intake, and mental state. Undernutrition was associated with dysphagia, slow eating, low protein intake, poor appetite, feeding tube use, and age.

Most older Americans live at home and are independent (14 million). However, 6 million are impaired but still living alone, 3 to 4 million are confined to home or assisted living centers, and 1.4 million live in nursing homes or skilled care facilities. Institutionalized older adults are at higher risk for malnutrition than those living at home (Kerstetter et al., 1992), probably because they are sicker. Cancer-related cachexia accounts for about 50% of the cases of malnutrition in the institutionalized adult. Pressure ulcers, particularly in nonambulatory people, increase nutrient needs and can pose a serious threat.

TABLE 13–4 POSSIBLE CAUSES OF UNDERNUTRITION IN THE ELDERLY

Depression or feelings of worthlessness
Polypharmacy that affects appetite, food intake, or the absorption, utilization, or excretion of nutrients
Loss of income, poverty
Social isolation, loss of loved ones, loneliness
Diseases that reduce appetite, decrease absorption or utilization of nutrients, or increase requirements for nutrients
Lack of education about proper nutrition
Dental problems or gum disease
Mental problems or dementia
Decreased functional ability
Substance abuse

NUTRITIONAL CARE OF THE ELDERLY

Dietary Planning

The general principles for planning a nutritious diet for the elderly are similar to those for younger adults. However, modifications may be necessary because of certain characteristics inherent to the process of aging. The most important guideline is to provide meals and snacks that are nutrient-dense, visually appealing, tasteful, and of the appropriate consistency. Four or five smaller meals are often more acceptable than three substantial ones.

The importance of a balanced intake of foods from all food groups should be emphasized. When significant nutrient sources, such as milk, are voluntarily eliminated from the diet, alternatives that supply the missing nutrients should be substituted. Supplementation may be indicated if entire food groups are eliminated. Improvements in serum albumin, total lymphocyte count, serum cholesterol, and hemoglobin levels, as well as in weight status, have been noted when oral liquid supplements are given to elderly nursing home patients (Johnson et al., 1993).

Special attention must be paid to the variety of situations that can prevent elderly persons from meeting their nutritional needs. If mastication or deglutition are problems, modification of food and beverage consistency may be indicated. Tolerable consistencies of solid foods and liquids are critical. The danger in dysphagia is that the person may choke on foods or beverages that are swallowed too rapidly. Aspiration pneumonia is the greatest risk in such cases (see "*Clinical Insight:* Dietary Strategies for Management of Dysphagia"). If food purchasing or meal preparation is a problem, supportive services should be identified. If the elderly person experiences difficulty utilizing eating utensils, modified utensils can be made or purchased.

Community Nutrition Programs

Community-based nutrition programs for the elderly are administered by governmental, private, nonprofit, and volunteer agencies throughout the United States. Nutrition services, funded under Title III, Parts C-1 and C-2, and Title VI of the

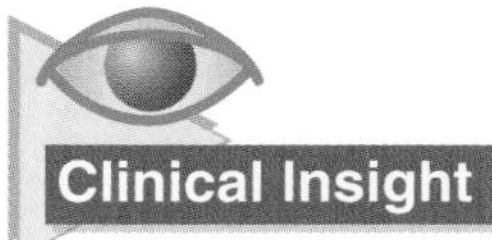

Dietary Strategies for Management of Dysphagia

For many elderly persons, swallowing difficulty occurs as a result of poor dentition, stroke, Alzheimer's disease or other dementias, traumatic brain injury, parkinsonism, amyotrophic lateral sclerosis, multiple sclerosis, debilitation after cardiac surgery, recurrent pneumonias, esophageal reflex or cancer, brain surgery, or prolonged intubation. A wet gurgly voice, coughing or choking when eating or drinking, drooling, pocketing of food, difficulty initiating the swallowing process, poor lip closure, poor head control, slurred speech, and excessively long eating time are indicators of swallowing difficulty. If any of these conditions persist, consultation by a speech therapist is warranted, and modifications in food and liquid consistencies may be indicated.

Thin liquids (other than pure water taken alone in small sips) may need to be avoided. In an institutional setting, the food service or nursing staff can thicken liquids with noncommercial products, such as oatmeal, cream of rice, cream of wheat, grits, instant mashed potatoes, bread crumbs, skim milk powder, gelatin, cornstarch, yogurt, applesauce, or instant pudding. Commercial thickeners are also available, and these are usually made from modified food starch or vegetable gum bases. Several products are available, such as Thick-It Original and Thick-It 2. Different products and consistencies for thickening food and liquids should be tried until the best tolerated texture for the individual's swallowing function is found. Most speech therapists recommend either fluid nectar (apricot juice consistency), soft (honey) consistency, or firm (pudding) consistency depending on the client's abilities and functional recovery. One common concern is dehydration, which can occur if liquids are not consumed in adequate amounts. In some clients, the ability to tolerate food or liquids declines to the point that tube feeding is required to replace all oral feedings.

In the outpatient or home setting, the nurse and dietitian play essential roles in communicating any changes in swallowing status to the physician so that texture and thickness modifications can be implemented. A thorough initial nutritional assessment and frequent reassessments are necessary to maintain a desirable quality of life.

Older Americans Act and collectively called the **Elderly Nutrition Program (ENP),** are valuable services that assist older individuals to remain independent and living at home in the community. This program authorizes funds for congregate and home-delivered nutrition programs for the elderly. Through this program, one meal that provides one third of the RDA for persons older than 50 years of age is served weekdays to senior citizens in congregate meal settings or in the home for those unable to come to the sites.

To be eligible to receive services at the congregate meal sites, participants must be 60 years of age or older or be the spouse or primary caretaker of an eligible participant. Other services, including outreach, transportation, nutrition education, and recreational activities, are provided. A donation or contribution for the meals is often requested, but not required. Food stamps are accepted as donations. Many of the advantages of this program are related to the social interaction encountered at the meal sites. Surveys comparing the intake of food program participants to that of nonparticipants have revealed that intakes of energy and protein were increased in the former, as were intakes of vitamins and minerals, notably calcium.

Other community resources include home health care agencies, hospice organizations, commodity food sources, food banks, food co-ops, and home-delivered grocery services. Chore services may be secured for shopping and meal preparation for senior citizens who are unable to shop or prepare their own meals. Internet websites relevant for the elderly include the Administration on Aging at http://www.nih.gov/nia/ and http://www.fiu.edu/~nuteldr/AoAdoc.htm.

Nutritional Needs During Prolonged Illness

Energy and nutrient requirements vary greatly with physiologic and pathologic conditions. Negative nitrogen balance occurs in catabolic states associated with injury, surgery (see Chapter 33), or acute and chronic diseases of the elderly, such as emphysema and bronchitis, cancer, organic brain syndromes, cirrhosis, and maldigestion or malabsorption syndromes. In these conditions, negative nitrogen balance can be reduced if aggressive nutritional support is provided. Careful consideration must be given to meeting the increased nutritional requirements resulting from the disease, as well as from the compromised organ and cell function associated with aging.

Enteral or parenteral nutrition may be necessary when a person is unable to consume adequate calories and nutrients through normal feeding methods. Malnutrition is associated with higher morbidity and mortality, as well as a poor quality of life. Because it is more difficult to correct nutritional status once it has deteriorated, early detection of malnutrition is very important. When malnutrition is detected with proper screening techniques, nutritional intervention can be started early and further deterioration can be prevented.

NUTRITIONAL CARE IN ASSISTED LIVING AND SKILLED CARE FACILITIES

As the size of the geriatric population increases and the needs of this population change, new housing and health care alternatives arise that combine independence with personal care in a supportive, dignified, community setting. Assisted living is a combination of safe housing, personalized supportive services, and health care designed to meet the needs of those who need assistance with activities of daily living. Assisted living residences offer cost-effective, quality care that fosters independence for each resident. Residents are treated with dignity and respect and individuality is promoted. Assisted living residents maintain active social lives with planned activities, exercise classes, religious and social functions, and field trips directed by the facilities (Figure 13–5).

Other elders who require skilled care may reside in nursing homes or skilled care units in retirement centers. Newly admitted nursing home residents are often transferred from an acute-care hospital after treatment. They are often weak, in poor health, and nutritionally depleted upon arrival at the institution. However, data do not support the premise that institutionalization itself leads to malnutrition. In a study conducted in 15 long-term care facilities in the Boston area, subjects free from clinically apparent terminal or wasting illness were studied. Nutritional intakes were comparable to those found in a simultaneously studied free-living population (Sayhoun et al., 1988). Most biochemical markers of nutritional status were equal to those of free-living populations. However, some were lower, most commonly, markers of vitamin B_{12}, folate, and vitamin B_6 status (Drinka and Goodwin, 1991). Drinka and colleagues have recommended that all nursing home residents be provided a daily multivitamin supplement with 400 mcg of folic acid (Drinka et al., 1993). This is an inexpensive provision that may have many benefits that are not yet fully understood.

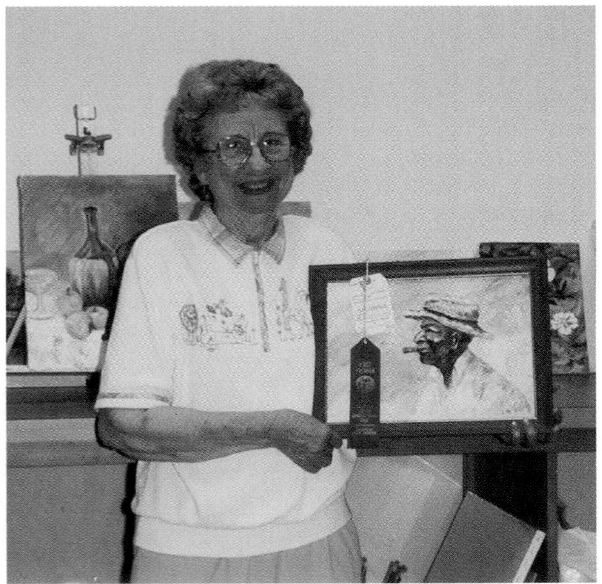

FIGURE 13–5 Seniors benefit from sensory stimulation afforded by programs, such as art therapy. (Courtesy of Cypress Glen Retirement Community, Greenville, North Carolina.)

Caregivers in long-term care facilities should consider a few issues when planning care and services under the **Omnibus Budget Reconciliation Act (OBRA) of 1987**, which is intended to standardize the quality of care provided in nursing homes nationwide. Surveyors from state regulatory agencies use specific criteria to audit the care given in nursing homes, and they have the authority to close down a facility immediately if many violations are noted (Table 13–5). For consultant dietitians, it may be difficult to provide all the necessary services if on-site time is limited. Facilities are now often encouraged to hire full-time registered dietitians to provide more thorough nutritional assessments and follow-up care. Table 13–6 provides an overview of multidisciplinary care roles.

The nutritional care of institutionalized elderly persons must be directed toward identifying and responding to changing physiologic and psychological needs on a long-term basis. It is important to comply with resident assessment and intervention protocols. Periodic reassessment of nutritional status is critical in avoiding unnecessary dietary restrictions or missing important, unmet nutritional needs.

Body weight history is an indicator of nutritional status. Weights should be monitored on a frequent basis so that variances can be identified and investigated. Because of gradual loss of stature (1.2 cm for each 20 years of maturity), the elderly weigh more per unit of height than younger adults. Therefore, it is important to utilize standards specific for this population (see Table 13–2).

Depression was identified as the single most common cause of weight loss in one nursing home study. Other factors included medications, reduction in or tapering of the use of psychotropic drugs, swallowing disorders, paranoia, dementia, gallstones, and obsessive-compulsive disorders (Morley and Kraenzle, 1994). Observing and recording food, beverage, and supplement consumption of residents are important aspects of providing quality nutritional care. Improving the dietary intake of the elderly resident requires special care and attention on the part of all dietary, health care, and allied health staff.

Two common problems of residents in nursing homes are urinary tract infections, especially in women, and pressure ulcers. Special attention must be directed to the prevention and immediate correction of these conditions (see the accompanying boxes, "*Clinical Insight:* Elderly Women and Urinary Tract Infections" and "*Clinical Insight:* Pressure Ulcers and The Role of Nutrition"). Aggressive

TABLE 13–5 OBRA '87*: ISSUES TO CONSIDER FOR CAREFUL PLANNING IN NURSING HOMES

Key issues that differentiate nursing homes from other types of facilities include the following:

1. Nursing homes have residents rather than patients; often, they live there for years.
2. Chemical or physical restraints must not be used for discipline or convenience, but may be used to prevent injury to the resident or to others. The doctor must include relevant documentation for the rationale for restraint use. Care plans must also include appropriate measures to be used with restraints (e.g., keeping water close at hand if siderails are used, etc.) Constipation or other consequences must be evaluated and treated.
3. A comprehensive assessment performed by staff from all key disciplines must be completed within 4 days of admission. The minimum data set (MDS) is then reviewed by state surveyors and payors to determine if resource utilization has been appropriate.
4. Care plans must be completed within days after admission and reviewed every 14 days, or as status changes. For example, development of a pressure ulcer warrants a status change in the care plan.
5. Quality of care is intended to attain and maintain the highest possible level of physical, mental, and psychosocial well-being for the resident. Surveyors look for the presence of pressure ulcers (especially those that are nosocomial, or developed on-site); avoidance of catheters when possible; decreased range of motion without appropriate treatments; automatic use of feeding tubes; decreased weight or protein levels; and dehydration. Any of these factors may indicate that the resident is not receiving the optimal level of care and service.
6. Psychotropic drug use is monitored carefully. Psychotic or agitated behavior that endangers the resident or others must be documented as just cause for such drug use. Gradual reduction in the quantities of drugs used, drug holidays, and other behavioral programs are suggested.
7. Rehabilitation services must be available to every resident. Physical therapists and occupational therapists generally screen new residents upon admission.
8. Routine dental care and emergency care must be available.
9. Pharmacy reviews must be conducted, with notations to the attending physician as appropriate.
10. A resident can refuse care and treatment, but such refusal must be documented. Aggressive efforts to counsel or offer alternatives should be charted, and refusal of care must be documented in the chart.

*OBRA '87 refers to the Omnibus Budget Reconciliation Act of 1987, the federal regulations that govern skilled nursing care facilities. Final implementation occurred in 1990.

refeeding with oral supplements has been demonstrated to reduce mortality in malnourished older persons, especially those who have pressure ulcers or hip fractures (Morley and Solomon, 1994). In addition, serving attractive and palatable food in an atmosphere that encourages independence in eating or provides assistance when necessary helps to promote the nutritional well-being of the residents.

TABLE 13–6 MULTIDISCIPLINARY GERIATRIC ASSESSMENT

PROVIDER	ACTIVITY
Medical Staff	Physical and geropsychiatric assessments
	Geriodontics
	Sensorimotor assessment
	Pharmacologic assessment
Nurse	Functional ability assessment
	Identification and monitoring of risk indicators
	Compliance surveillance
Registered Dietitian	Nutritional screening
	Nutritional assessment
	Nutrition interventions
	Nutrition surveillance
Social Worker	Activities of daily living (ADL) assessment
	Identification of and referral to resources
	Socioeconomic assessment
	Coordination of activities and support services
Physical Therapist	Agility and gait assessments
	Balance assessment
	Strength assessment
	Endurance assessment
Occupational Therapist	Kitchen safety/ability assessment
	Driving safety assessment
	ADL adaptations
Psychologist	Cognitive assessment
	Visual-spatial assessment
Speech Therapist	Dysphagia assessment
	Speech assessment

THE NUTRITION SCREENING INITIATIVE

The **Nutrition Screening Initiative (NSI)** was established in early 1990 as a 5-year, multifaceted campaign to promote nutritional screening and improve nutritional care in the United States (Nutrition Screening Initiative, 1991). This was established in direct response to the 1988 U.S. Surgeon General's Workshop on Health Promotion and Aging and the U.S. Department of Health and Human Services' Report, *Healthy People 2000,* which called for increased nutritional screening. The initiative has continued as a joint project of the American Dietetic Association, the American Academy of Family Physicians, and the National Council on the Aging, Inc. Serving as advisers and providing technical support is an advisory committee comprising more than 30 major national organizations concerned with medicine, health, nutrition, and aging.

The initiative's premise is that better nutrition can improve quality of life, facilitate "aging in place," promote health, and improve outcomes after illness or injury. Good nutritional status can shorten hospital stays and delay entry into nursing homes. Through research, professional education, consumer outreach, and policy strategies, the initiative is working to accelerate the rate at which nutrition screening and care are incorporated into the country's health and social service programs. The NSI indicates that 24% of the elderly are at high nutritional risk, and 38% are at moderate risk. Patients with good nutritional status generally have

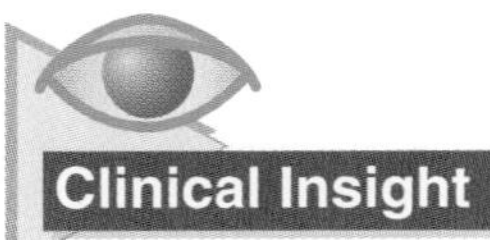

Elderly Women and Urinary Tract Infections

Elderly women, especially those who are hospitalized or institutionalized, are prone to develop recurrent urinary tract infections. The use of cranberry juice as a bacteriostatic beverage has long been advocated as a folk remedy for such infections. Recent studies however, suggest that there may actually be some benefit derived from its use, probably from its role in acidifying urine. According to these studies, either the hippuric acid may be beneficial, or another substance in cranberry juice may prevent the adhesion of bacteria to the epithelial cells of the urinary tract (Avorn et al., 1994). Although it has not been concluded that cranberry juice should be used as a preventive agent for urinary tract infections, the frequent need to increase fluid intake in the elderly may warrant its inclusion as a regular choice (see Chapter 38).

better hospital outcomes, shorter stays, and less mortality than do those with less optimal nutriture (Saffel-Shrier and Athas, 1993).

By obtaining consensus among nutrition experts on risk factors and indicators of poor nutritional status in older Americans, the initiative developed and distributed three screening tools: "Determine Your Nutritional Health Checklist" and Levels I and II nutrition screens. The "Determine Your Nutritional Health Checklist" is a public awareness tool listing the warning signs of poor nutritional status in older Americans. These include disease, poor eating habits, tooth loss or tooth pain, economic hardship, reduced social contact, multiple medicines, involuntary weight loss or gain, needs assistance in self-care, and an age older than 80 years. Using the checklist, individuals can identify and score various factors associated with nutritional risk. Checklists have been put into circulation nationwide, either by direct distribution to individuals or through distribution by health and social service providers in all elderly care settings, including meal programs, senior and adult day care centers, physicians' offices, hospitals, and nursing homes and other extended care facilities. The checklists are the first step in identifying individuals who are at moderate or high risk for poor nutritional status and who will benefit from nutritional intervention.

In 1992, the NSI convened an Interventions Roundtable in Washington, DC to identify nutritional interventions that would address the findings derived from the checklists and screens. The initiative specified six interdisciplinary interventions that were published in the *Nutrition Interventions Manual for Professionals Caring for Older Americans* (Blackburn et al, 1992). The interventions manual contains the Checklist and the Level I and Level II Screens, in addition to guidelines for administering these tools in a variety of settings. The manual also summarizes practical steps to be taken to improve nutritional health and treat nutritional problems in six key intervention areas: social services, oral health, mental health, medications use, nutrition education, and nutrition support.

The Six Intervention Areas

The six areas of intervention identified by the manual and their respective roles in supporting nutrition are as follows:

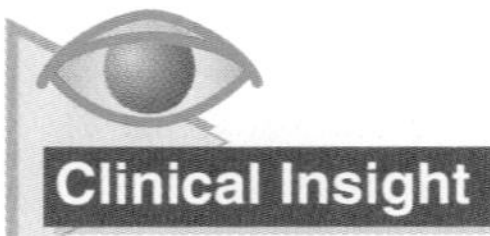

Pressure Ulcers and the Role of Nutrition

Pressure ulcers occur over a bony prominence as a result of continued pressure on the tissue covering the bone. Persons who are confined to a chair or bed and who infrequently change positions are at increased risk of developing pressure ulcers. Cancer, diabetes, and renal and cardiovascular disease may decrease the blood supply to vulnerable areas, such as the coccyx, elbows, heels, and back of the head. In institutions, the nursing staff has strict protocols for repositioning residents every 2 hours. At home, an individual may be at increased risk if he or she is unaware of the importance of changing positions.

Nutritionally compromised elderly individuals are also at risk. Studies have noted that low serum albumin levels often correlate directly with pressure ulcer development. Persons who are malnourished should be offered small, frequent meals with fortified foods, snacks, or supplements as needed. The nutrient composition of tube feedings should be reviewed regularly for adequacy of protein and kilocalorie content. Protein and kilocalorie needs are increased in the individual with pressure ulcers. Intake of vitamin C, vitamin A, and zinc should also be monitored. Requirements for protein and calories are increased even further with multiple draining sores.

In many respects, the nutritional care of pressure ulcers must be as carefully planned as that for a burn. Pressure ulcer tissue is as delicate as eye tissue; nothing other than normal saline should be poured onto the wound. The dietitian plays an essential role, along with other team members, in preventing and managing pressure ulcers. Weekly assessments of residents with pressure ulcers, conducted by nursing and nutrition staff, can facilitate timely responses to changes in status.

1. Social service interventions are fundamental in assisting older people to obtain, prepare, and eat an appropriate diet. Food stamps, meal programs, transportation, and home services are examples of social service interventions.
2. Oral health profoundly affects a person's food intake, diet quality, and socialization. An oral health checklist is included in the interventions manual.
3. Mental health plays a central role in a person's motivation and ability to meet nutritional needs. Interventions address dementia, depression, alcoholism, and other common mental health problems affecting older people.
4. The use of medications may alter nutrient needs and the body's response to nutrients. Drug-nutrient and drug-drug interactions are outlined, and a medication use checklist and drug-nutrient screening tool are also included.
5. Nutrition education and counseling for the older person can play vital roles in changing eating habits. Older persons have sets of health, personal, and life-cycle factors that warrant a unique, specialized approach to nutrition education. A built-in monitoring system is needed to assist the rural elderly with special diet prescriptions, for example.
6. Nutritional support interventions should be considered for those persons who cannot or will not eat a regular balanced diet. Such support may include increasing or decreasing nutrients in the diet; changing the timing, size, or composition of meals; modifying food texture; or in extreme circumstances, changing the route of administration.

In 1993, a follow-up national conference highlighted the most effective programs that addressed the six previously identified interventions. Networks were established among physicians, dietitians, dentists, social workers, and psychologists to provide more accessible and cost-effective care (Gallagher-Alfred, 1993).

Health professionals view the lack of third-party reimbursement as a primary obstacle to routine screening and treatment. Because there is broad consensus that nutritional screening and treatment should be included as part of a reimbursable basic benefits package, the initiative team is working on several approaches to expand reimbursement for nutrition screening and services. The NSI is promoting the importance of nutrition screening and building alliances to ensure that nutritional status is considered a fundamental component of health care (Wellman, 1994).

CASE STUDY

Marion K. is an 85-year-old black female who has recently moved from her home into a long-term, skilled care facility. She has controlled type I diabetes mellitus and hypertension, but has recently been diagnosed as having mild renal failure. Her diet prescription controls all of these factors well. She knows her dietary restrictions (60 g of protein, no added salt, no concentrated sweets) and can quote the proper portions and types of foods that she is allowed to eat. Her newly identified problem is a difficulty swallowing fluids.

1. What recommendations do you have for changing her diet, knowing that it controls her diseases so well?
2. Because fluids are now difficult for her to swallow, what changes will you make to accommodate her in the facility dining room?
3. Marion needs a snack in the afternoon and at bedtime to keep her blood glucose level within an acceptable range. What are some suggestions for snack foods?

CITED REFERENCES

Ades PA, et al. Weight training improves walking endurance in healthy elderly persons. Ann Intern Med 124:568, 1996.

Avorn J, et al. Reduction of bacteriuria and pyuria after ingestion of cranberry juice. JAMA 271:751, 1994.

Bernard MA, et al. The effect of vitamin B_{12} deficiency on older veterans and its relationship to health. J Am Geriatr Soc 46:1199, 1998.

Berry E. Chronic disease: How can nutrition moderate the effects? Nutr Rev 52:S28, 1994.

Bivona PL. Xerostomia. A common problem among the elderly. NYS Dent J 64:46, 1998.

Blackburn GL, Dwyer JT, Wellman NS (eds.). Nutrition Interventions Manual for Professionals Caring for Older Americans. Washington, DC: Nutrition Screening Initiative, 1992.

Blumberg J. Nutritional needs of seniors. J Am Coll Nutr 16:577, 1997.

Bogden J, et al. Daily micronutrient supplements enhance delayed hypersensitivity skin test responses in older people. Am J Clin Nutr 60:437, 1994.

Bouillon R, et al. Aging and calcium metabolism. Clin Endocrinol Metab 11:341, 1997.

Campbell W. Dietary protein requirements of older people: Is the RDA adequate? Nutr Today 31:192, 1996.

Chandra RK. Graying of the immune system. J Am Med Assoc 277:1398, 1997.

Chandra RK, et al. Nutrition of the elderly. Can Med Assoc J 145:1475, 1991.

Chernoff R. Thirst and fluid requirements. Nutr Rev 52(8, part II):S3, 1994.

Chiotakakou-Faliakou E, et al. Biofeedback provides long-term benefit for patients with intractable, slow and normal transit constipation. Gut 42:517, 1998.

Davis J, Sherer K. Applied nutrition and diet therapy for nurses. Philadelphia: WB Saunders Co., 1994.

Dawson-Hughes B, et al. Effect of calcium and vitamin D supplementation on bone density in men and women 65 years of age or older. N Engl J Med 337:670, 1997.

Day JC. Bureau of the Census. Current Population Reports. Population Projections of the United States By Age, Sex, Race and Hispanic origin: 1993 to 2050 (middle series). Washington, DC: US Government Printing Office, 1993, p. 25.

Drinka P, Goodwin S. Prevalence and consequences of vitamin deficiency in the nursing home: A critical review. J Am Geriatr Soc 39:1008, 1991.

Drinka PJ, et al. Low serum folic acid levels in a nursing home population: A clinical experience. J Am Coll Nutr 12:186, 1993.

Duffy V et al. Olfactory dysfunction and related nutritional risk in free-living, elderly women. J Am Diet Assoc 95:89, 1995.

Dutta C. Significance of sarcopenia in the elderly. J Nutr 127(suppl):992S, 1997.

Dychtwald K. Age Wave. Los Angeles: Jeremy P. Tarcher, Inc., 1989.

Emerit I, Chance B. Free Radicals and Aging. Basel, Switzerland: Birkhauser Verlag, 1992.

Evans J, et al. Relation of colonic transit to functional bowel disease in older people: A population-based study. J Am Geriatr Soc 46:83, 1998.

Evans WJ, Cyr-Campbell D. Nutrition, exercise, and healthy aging. J Am Diet Assoc 97:632, 1997.

Eye Disease Case-Control Study Group: Antioxidant status and neovascular age-related macular degeneration. Arch Ophthalmol 111:104, 1993.

Food and Nutrition Board, National Research Council: Recommended Dietary Allowances, 10th ed. Washington, DC: National Academy of Sciences, 1989.

Gallagher-Alfred CR. Implementing nutrition screening and interventions strategies. Washington, DC: Nutrition Screening Initiative, 1993.
Gilmore S, et al. Clinical indicators associated with unintentional weight loss and pressure ulcers in elderly residents of nursing facilities. J Am Diet Assoc 95:984, 1995.
Good RA, Lorenz E. Nutrition, immunity, aging, and cancer. Nutr Rev 46:62, 1988.
Hakim A, et al. Effects of walking on mortality among nonsmoking retired men. N Engl J Med 338:94, 1998.
Harari D, et al. Bowel habit in relation to age and gender. Findings from the National Health Interview Survey and clinical implications. Arch Intern Med 156:315, 1996.
Hartz SC, et al. Nutrient supplement use by healthy elderly. J Am Coll Nutr 7:119, 1988.
Holick M. McCollum Award Lecture, 1994. Vitamin D: New Horizons for the 21st century. Am J Clin Nutr 60:619, 1994.
Hurley R, et al. Comparative evaluation of body composition in medically stable elderly. J Am Diet Assoc 97:1105, 1997.
Jacques P, et al. Long-term vitamin C supplement use and prevalence of early age-related lens opacities. Am J Clin Nutr 66:911, 1997.
Johnson L, et al. Oral nutritional supplement use in elderly nursing home patients. J Am Geriatr Soc 41:947, 1993.
Joosten E, et al. Metabolic evidence that deficiencies of vitamin B-12 (cobalamin), folate, and vitamin B-6 occur commonly in elderly people. Am J Clin Nutr 58:468, 1993.
Kannel WB. Cardiovascular risk factors in the elderly. Coronary Artery Dis 8:565, 1997.
Kannel WB. Nutrition and the occurrence and prevention of cardiovascular disease in the elderly. Nutr Rev 46:68, 1988.
Keller H. Malnutrition in institutionalized elderly: How and why? J Am Geriatr Soc 41:1212, 1993.
Kerstetter J, et al. Malnutrition in the institutionalized older adult. J Am Diet Assoc 92:1109, 1992.
Koizumi A, et al. Influences of dietary restriction and age on liver enzyme activities and lipid peroxidation in mice. J Nutr 117:361, 1987.
Komar L, et al. Calcium homeostasis of an elderly population upon admission to a nursing home. J Am Geriatr Soc 41:1057, 1993.
Laws A, et al. Metabolic and behavioral covariates of high-density lipoprotein cholesterol and triglyceride concentrations in postmenopausal women. J Am Geriatr Soc 41:1289, 1993.
Leaf A. The aging process: Lessons from observations in man. Nutr Rev 46:40, 1988.
Lee MF, Krasinski SD. Human adult-onset lactase decline: An update. Nutr Rev 56(1, part 1):1, 1998.
Loesche W, et al. Xerostomia, xerogenic medications and food avoidances in selected geriatric groups. J Am Geriatr Soc 43:401, 1995.
Lovat LB. Age related changes in gut physiology and nutritional status. Gut 38:306, 1996.
Martin W. Oral health in the elderly. In: Chernoff R (ed.). Geriatric Nutrition: The Health Professional's Handbook. Gaithersburg, MD: Aspen, 1991.
Masoro E. Nutrition and longevity. In: Morley J, Glick Z, Rubenstein Z (eds.). Geriatric Nutrition: A Comprehensive Review. New York: Raven Press, 1990.
McCay CM, et al. Nutrition requirements during the latter half of life. J Nutr 21:4, 1941.
Merry BJ, Holehan AM. Effects of diet on aging. In: Timiras PS (ed.). Physiological Basis of Geriatrics. New York: Macmillan, 1988.
Meydani SN, et al. Vitamin E supplementation enhances cell-mediated immunity in healthy elderly. Am J Clin Nutr 52:557, 1990.
Mitchell MK. Nutrition Across the Life Span. Philadelphia: WB Saunders, 1997.
Moriguchi S. The role of vitamin E in T-cell differentiation and the decrease of cellular immunity with aging. Biofactors 7:77, 1998.
Morley J. Anorexia of aging: Physiologic and pathologic. Am J Clin Nutr 66: 760, 1997.
Morley J, Kraenzle D. Causes of weight loss in a community nursing home. J Am Geriatr Soc 42:583, 1994.
Morley J, Solomon D. Major issues in geriatrics over the last five years. J Am Geriatr Soc 42:218, 1994.
NCHS (National Center for Health Statistics): Births and Deaths: United States. Monthly Vital Statistics Report 1996, Vol. 46, No. 1(S2).
Need A, et al. Effects of skin thickness, age, body fat and sunlight on serum 25-hydroxyvitamin D. Am J Clin Nutr 58:882, 1993.
Nutrition Screening Initiative: Nutrition Screening Manual for Professionals Caring for Older Americans. Washington, DC: Nutrition Screening Initiative, 1991.
Ortega R, et al. Dietary intake and cognitive function in a group of elderly people. Am J Clin Nutr 66:883, 1997.
Pahor M, et al. Use of laxative medication in older persons and associations with low serum albumin. J Am Geriatr Soc 42:50, 1994.
Rasmussen L, et al. Effect of diet and plasma fatty acid composition on immune status in elderly men. Am J Clin Nutr 59:572, 1994.
Richardson A, et al. Effect of age and dietary restriction on the expression of alpha-2m-globulin. J Biol Chem 262:12821, 1987.
Roebothan BV, Chandra RK. Relationship between nutritional status and immune function of elderly people. Age Aging 23(1):49, 1994.
Rosenbloom C, Whittington F. The effects of bereavement on eating behaviors and nutrient intakes in elderly widowed persons. J Gerontol 48:S223, 1993.
Rubenstein LZ. An overview of aging—demographics, epidemiology, and health services. In: Morley J, Glick Z, Rubenstein Z (eds.). Geriatric Nutrition: A Comprehensive Review. New York: Raven Press, 1990, p 1.
Rudman D. Kidney senescence: A model for aging. Nutr Rev 46:209, 1988.
Russell RM. Gastric hypochlorhydria and achlorhydria in older adults. JAMA 278:1659, 1997.
Russell R. New views on the RDAs for older adults. J Am Diet Assoc 97:515, 1997.
Ryan C, Eleazer P, Egbert J. Vitamin D in the elderly. Nutr Today 30:228, 1995.
Saffel-Shrier S, Athas B. Effective provision of comprehensive nutrition case management for the elderly. J Am Diet Assoc 93:439, 1993.
Saltzman JR, Russell RM. The aging gut. Nutritional issues. Gastroenterol Clin North Am 27:309, 1998.
Samos LF, Roos BA. Diabetes mellitus in older persons. Med Clin North Am 82:791, 1998.
Sayhoun NR, et al. Dietary intakes and biochemical indicators of nutritional status in an elderly, institutionalized population. Am J Clin Nutr 47:524, 1988.
Schiffman SS. Changes in taste and smell: Drug interactions and food preferences. Nutr Rev 52:S11, 1994.
Schiffman SS. Taste and smell losses in normal aging and disease. JAMA 278:1357, 1997.
Schiffman SS, Warwick ZS. Effect of flavor enhancement of foods for the elderly on nutritional status: Food intake, biochemical indices, and anthropometric measures. Physiol Behav 53:395, 1992.
Schlenker ED. Who are the aging? In: Malinee, V (ed.). Nutrition in Aging, 3rd ed. Boston: McGraw-Hill, 1998, pp. 2–5.
Seddon JM, et al. Dietary carotenoids, vitamins A, C, and E, and advanced age-related macular degeneration. JAMA 272:1413, 1994.
Seddon JM, Hennekens CH. Vitamins, minerals and macular degeneration. Arch Ophthalmol 112:176, 1994.
Selhub J, et al. Vitamin status and intake as primary determinants of homocysteinemia in an elderly population. J Am Med Assoc 270:2693, 1993.
Smith DW. Centenarians: Human longevity outliers. Gerontologist 37:200, 1997.
Sohal RS, Weindrich R. Oxidative stress, caloric restriction and aging. Science 273:59, 1996.
Stampfer M, et al. A prospective study of plasma homocystein and risk of myocardial infarction in U.S. physicians. JAMA 268:877, 1992.
Taaffe DR, et al. Accuracy of equations to predict basal metabolic rate in older women. J Am Diet Assoc 95:1387, 1995.
Tramonte SM, et al. The treatment of chronic constipation in adults. A systematic review. J Gen Intern Med 12:15, 1997.
Warsama Jama J, et al. Dietary antioxidants and cognitive function in a population-based sample of older persons. Am J Epidemiol 144:275, 1996.
Wemeau JL. Calciotropic hormones and ageing. Horm Res 43:76, 1995.
Wellman N. The Nutrition Screening Initiative. Nutr Rev 52:544, 1994.
West S, et al. Are antioxidants or supplements protective for age-related macular degeneration? Arch Ophthalmol 112:222, 1994.

ADDITIONAL REFERENCES

American Dietetic Association. Position of The American Dietetic Association: Liberalized diets for older adults in long-term care. J Am Diet Assoc 98:201, 1998.
American Dietetic Association. Position of The American Dietetic Association: Nutrition, aging and the continuum of care. J Am Diet Assoc 96:1048, 1996.
Bernard M, et al. Common health problems among minority elders. J Am Diet Assoc 97:771, 1997.
Blaum C, et al. Validity of the minimum data set for assessing nutritional status in nursing home residents. Am J Clin Nutr 66:787m, 1997.
Chidester J, Spangler A. Fluid intake in the institutionalized elderly. J Am Diet Assoc 97:23, 1997.
Chumlea W, et al. Stature prediction equations for elderly non-Hispanic white, non-Hispanic black, and Mexican-American persons developed from NHANES III data. J Am Diet Assoc 98:137, 1998.
Fabiny A, Kiel D. Assessing and treating weight loss in nursing home residents. Clin Geriatr Med 13:737, 1997.
Fortes C, et al. The effect of zinc and vitamin A supplementation on immune response in an older person. J Am Geriatr Soc 46:19, 1998.
Heuser M, Adler W. Immunological aspects of aging and malnutrition. Clin Geriatr Med 13:697, 1997.
Hurley R, et al. Comparative evaluation of body composition in medically stable elderly. J Am Diet Assoc 97:1105, 1997.
Katz I, DiFilippo S. Neuropsychiatric aspects of failure to thrive in late life. Clin Geriatr Med 13:623, 1997.

Klein G, et al. Nutrition and health for older persons in rural America: A managed care model. J Am Diet Assoc 97:885, 1997.

LaRue A, et al. Nutritional status and cognitive functioning in a normally aging sample: A 6-yr reassessment. Am J Clin Nutr 65:20, 1997.

Losonczy K, et al. Vitamin E and vitamin C supplement use and risk of all-cause mortality in older persons. The Established Populations for Epidemiologic Studies of the Elderly. Am J Clin Nutr 64:190, 1996.

Markson E. Functional, social, and psychological disability as causes of loss of weight and independence in older community-living people. Clin Geriatr Med 13:639, 1997.

Meydani S, et al. Vitamin E supplementation and in vivo immune response in healthy elderly subjects: A randomized controlled trial. JAMA 277:1380, 1997.

Mouton C. Special health considerations in African-American elders. Am Fam Physician 55:1243, 1997.

Obisesan T, et al. Moderate wine consumption is associated with decreased odds of developing age-related macular degeneration in NHANES-1. J Am Geriatr Soc 46:1, 1998.

Perrig W, et al. The relation between antioxidants and memory performance in the old and very old. J Am Geriatr Soc 45:718, 1997.

Ponza M, et al. Serving elders at risk: The Older Americans Act Nutrition Programs, National Evaluation of the Elderly Nutrition Program, 1993–1995. Washington, DC: Mathematica Policy Research, Inc., 1996.

Reuben D, et al. Correlates of hypoalbuminemia in community-dwelling older persons. Am J Clin Nutr 66:38, 1997.

Ritchie C, et al. Nutritional status of urban homebound older adults. Am J Clin Nutr 66:815, 1997.

Roubenoff R, Harris T. Failure to thrive, sarcopenia, and functional decline in the elderly. Clin Geriatr Med 13:613, 1997.

Sayhoun N, et al. Nutrition Screening Initiative checklist may be a better awareness/educational tool than a screening one. J Am Diet Assoc 97:760, 1997.

Stabler S, et al. Vitamin B_{12} deficiency in the elderly: Current dilemmas. Am J Clin Nutr 66:741, 1997.

Stevens J, et al. The effect of age on the association between body-mass index and mortality. N Engl J Med 338:1, 1998.

Suleiman S, et al. Effect of calcium intake and physical activity level on bone mass and turnover in healthy, white postmenopausal women. Am J Clin Nutr 66:937, 1997.

Sullivan D, Lipschitz D. Evaluating and treating nutritional problems in older patients. Clin Geriatr Med 13:753, 1997.

Thun M, et al. Alcohol consumption and mortality among middle-aged and elderly U.S. adults. N Engl J Med 337:1705, 1997.

Tripp F. The use of dietary supplements in the elderly: Current issues and recommendations. J Am Diet Assoc 97:S181, 1997.

Verdery R. Clinical evaluation of failure to thrive in older people. Clin Geriatr Med 13:769, 1997.

Wallace J, Schwartz R. Involuntary weight loss in elderly outpatients: Recognition, etiologies and treatment. Clin Geriatr Med 13:717, 1997.

Wang S, et al. Longitudinal weight changes, length of survival, and energy requirements of long-term care residents with dementia. J Am Geriatr Soc 45:1189, 1997.

Wellman N, et al. Elder insecurities: Poverty, hunger and malnutrition. J Am Diet Assoc 97:S120, 1997.

Wilkinson T, et al. The response to treatment of subclinical thiamine deficiency in the elderly. Am J Clin Nutr 66:925, 1997.

PART 3

Nutrition Care

Part 3 includes background chapters related to the nutritional care process, starting with the population in general (i.e., community nutrition) and methods for dietary planning. The nutrition assessment of the individual is covered in chapters on dietary and clinical evaluation and biochemical assessment, use of herbals/botanicals and phytochemicals. Nutritional care is discussed in the chapters on the nutritional care process, methods of nutritional support, and drug–nutrient interaction. The inclusion of the chapter on complementary therapy and the use of herbs and phytonutrients is important because of the rapidly growing interest and knowledge in this field related to health.

The reader is encouraged to refer to these chapters for appropriate suggestions as work is completed for either population groups or individuals. Although it is essential to assess a person individually, one must also be aware that certain parameters are meaningful for groups of people with specific diagnoses. Knowledge of common problems or symptoms related to diseases provides the practitioner with the basic skills needed to prepare an effective nutritional care plan and to evaluate or alter it throughout the intervention.

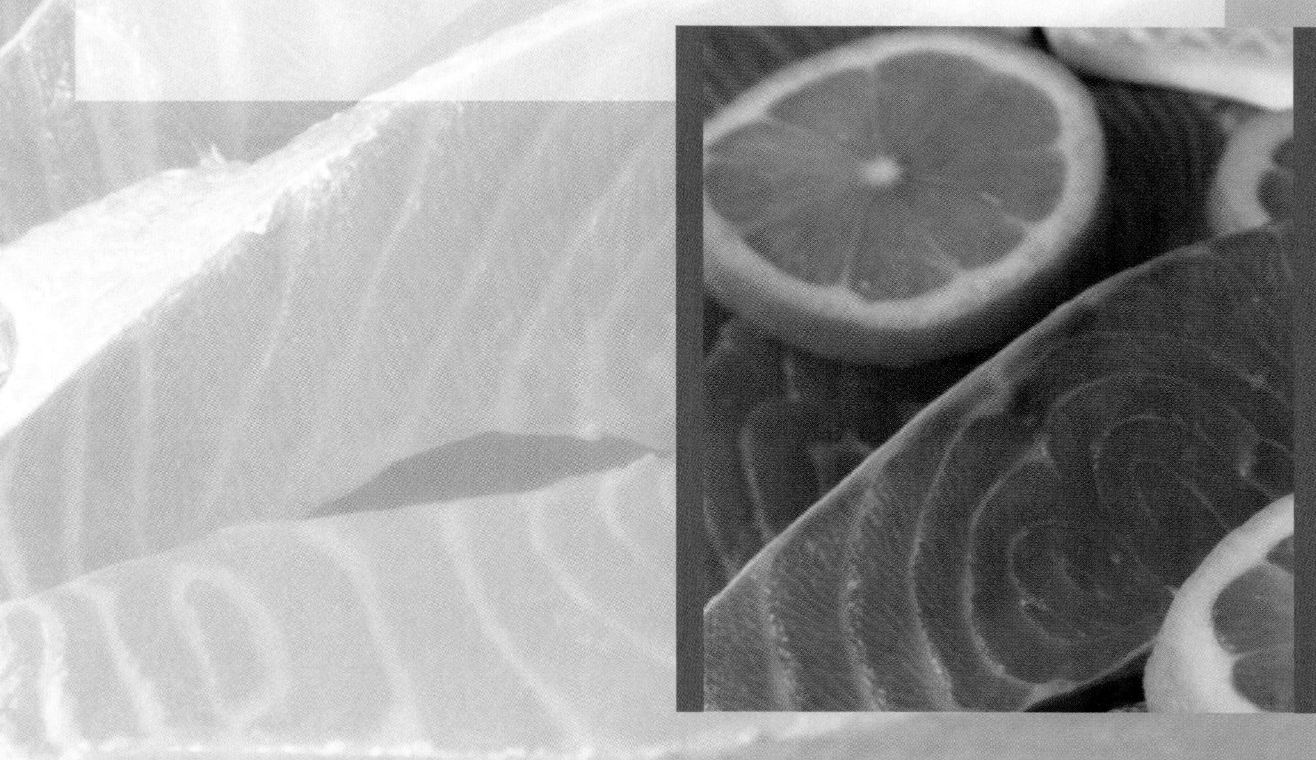

CHAPTER 14

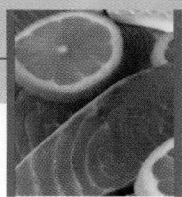

Nutrition in the Community

CYNTHIA TAFT BAYERL, MS, RD

Chapter Outline

Key Terms

ACCEPTABLE DAILY INTAKE (ADI)—the amount of a chemical or nutrient that, if ingested daily over a lifetime, appears to be without appreciable risk

ADULT CARE FOOD PROGRAM—a federal program established in 1965 by the Older Americans Act, Title VII section under the Elderly Nutrition Program for congregate dining and home-delivered meals for senior citizens; later folded into the Title III program in 1978

CHILD NUTRITION PROGRAMS—federally funded programs aimed at improving the nutritional status of children in the United States, including school lunch and breakfast programs, Head Start, summer feeding programs, and the WIC program

COMMODITY FOOD PROGRAM—Donated Food (Commodities) Program administered by the State Department of Agriculture and Consumer Services and which makes donated foods from the U.S. Department of Agriculture available to eligible schools, institutions, summer camps, summer feeding programs, and soup kitchens

COMMUNITY ASSESSMENT—one of the three public health core functions that involves all the activities related to the concept of community diagnosis (i.e., surveillance, identifying needs, analyzing the causes of problems, collecting and interpreting data, case-finding, monitoring and forecasting trends, research, and evaluation of outcomes)

CONTINUING SURVEY OF FOOD INTAKE OF INDIVIDUALS (CSFII)—part of the National Nutrition Monitoring System food consumption survey conducted by the U.S. Department of Agriculture; the first nationwide dietary intake survey designed to be conducted bi-annually

DELANEY CLAUSE—a clause of the Food Additive Amendment of 1959 that prohibits the use in food of any substance shown to cause cancer in animals or humans; repealed for pesticides in 1996 with passage of The Food Quality Protection Act

FOOD ADDITIVE—any natural or synthetic material other than the basic raw ingredients, used in the production of a food item to enhance the final product

FOOD BORNE ILLNESS—called food poisoning, usually with gastrointestinal symptoms, caused by organisms or their toxins carried in ingested food

FOOD IRRADIATION—the exposure of food to sufficient radient energy to destroy insects and microorganisms; used in food protection or preservation; also called cold pasteurization

FOOD SECURITY—access by individuals at all times to a readily available supply of nutritionally adequate and safe foods and an ensured ability to acquire acceptable foods in socially acceptable ways (American Dietetic Association, 1998)

FOOD STAMP PROGRAM—a federal entitlement program established in 1964 to provide more food-buying power to low-income persons or families through monthly allotments of stamps made available at a cost, which translates into reduced-price groceries; administered by the U.S. Department of Agriculture

FUNCTIONAL FOODS—substances or parts of a food that may be considered to provide medical or health benefits beyond basic nutrition; formerly known as nutraceuticals

GENERALLY RECOGNIZED AS SAFE (GRAS)—descriptive of 675 commonly used food ingredients that were already considered safe and in use when the 1959 Food Additives Amendment was enacted

HEAD START—a comprehensive child development program targeted primarily to low-income preschool children and their families

NATIONAL HEALTH AND NUTRITION EXAMINATION SURVEY (NHANES)—a series of surveys that include information from medical history, physical measurements, biochemical evaluation, physical examination, and dietary intake of a representative sample of the U.S. population groups within the United States; a responsibility of the U.S. Department of Health and Human Services

NATIONAL SCHOOL LUNCH PROGRAM—a child nutrition program started in 1946 that makes available cash reimbursement so that schools can provide a free or reduced-price lunch that meets specified nutritional requirements; may also provide commodity foods

NATIONWIDE FOOD CONSUMPTION SURVEY (NFCS)—a survey conducted approximately every 10 years by the USDA to monitor the nutrient intake of a cross-section of the U.S. public

NUTRITION EPIDEMIOLOGY—the study of nutrition and diet as they relate to the etiology, pathogenesis, and prevention of disease (e.g., diet and heart disease, diet and cancer)

NUTRITION SCREENING INITIATIVE (NSI)—screening among the noninstitutionalized elderly to evaluate nutritional risks as targets for early preventive efforts; sponsored by the American Dietetic Association, the American Academy of Family Physicians, and the National Council on the Aging

NUTRITION SURVEILLANCE—the ongoing monitoring of the nutritional status of population groups, including dietary intake data, anthropometric, biochemical, clinical, and environmental data

POLICY DEVELOPMENT—the last of the three public health core functions, which is the process by which society makes decisions about problems, chooses goals and prepares the means to reach them, handles conflicting views about what should be done, and allocates resources

PRIMARY PREVENTION—a disease prevention strategy that targets generally healthy individuals to decrease the probability that they will develop a disease or disability

PUBLIC HEALTH ASSURANCE—one of the three core public health functions, which addresses the implementation of legislative mandates, maintenance of statutory responsibilities, support of crucial services, regulation of services and products provided in both the public and private sector, and maintenance of accountability

SECONDARY PREVENTION—a disease prevention strategy that focuses on detection, diagnosis, and intervention early in the disease process to minimize detrimental and disabling effects

TERTIARY PREVENTION—rehabilitation of an individual to optimum function by fixing or ameliorating the health defect or disability; may involve medical treatment

TOTAL DIET STUDY (MARKET BASKET SAMPLE)—analysis of 234 food items purchased throughout the United States and representing the diets of consumers for comparison with acceptable daily intakes

WIC—the Special Supplemental Nutrition Program for Women, Infants, and Children, established in 1972 to provide supplemental food and nutrition education and to improve the nutritional status of medically high-risk pregnant and lactating women and children up to 5 years of age from low-income families; funding is through the U.S. Department of Agriculture

---

Nutrition services or medical nutrition therapy in community and public health agencies offer exciting opportunities for nutritionists interested in a range of activities, from direct care services including counseling of individuals to broader based administrative roles such as managing a health promotion program or developing and implementing public policy. Public health nutrition services provided in community-based settings are built on legislation and regulations that serve as the foundation of their existence.

WHAT IS COMMUNITY OR PUBLIC HEALTH NUTRITION?

The nutritional status of the public or "community" is commonly referred to as public health nutrition. *Public health* is defined as "the science and art of preventing disease, prolonging life, and promoting health and efficiency through organized community effort, so organizing these benefits as to enable every citizen to realize his birthright of health and longevity" (Winslow, 1920).

Public health is "public" because it involves "organized community effort." An example of this is the public health campaign to decrease mortality and morbidity due to cigarette smoking. This campaign has had many successes such as limiting smoking in public places as a result of organized community efforts to adopt laws and regulations restricting smoking.

The mission of public health is to ensure that organized approaches are mobilized when they are needed. Public health has been envisioned as the scientific diagnosis and treatment of the community, which is defined as a geopolitical entity. In this vision the community rather than the individual is seen as the client.

Health and well-being in the community encompass factors beyond those commonly thought of in a traditional sense of physical or mental health. They include adequate food, housing, income, employment, education, and safety for all persons living in that community. This public health approach, also referred to as a population-based or **epidemiologic** approach, is different from the clinical or individual patient care approach traditionally seen in hospitals and other clinical settings. This approach is also considered to be **primary prevention** (health promotion) as opposed to **secondary prevention** (risk reduction) or **tertiary prevention** (treatment and rehabilitation) (Kaufman, 1990).

To adequately address the health needs of the community involves participation by many community-based providers. Collaboration by community-based agencies and individuals, including the public health agency, nonprofit and for-profit agencies, is needed, because one agency alone cannot necessarily deliver all the services.

NATIONAL FOOD AND NUTRITION DATA SOURCES

Nutrition programs rely on data from nutrition and health surveys to identify the needs of those to be served. Although an increasing number of states have begun to conduct their own assessments, national statistics are still needed. Data from national surveys are used to monitor the dietary status of the population, assess the nutritional adequacy of the food supply, measure the economics of food consumption, evaluate the effects of food assistance and regulatory programs, and provide the public guidelines for food selection. The data are also used to direct program development and to determine national, state, and local funding.

Until the late 1960s, the only information about food and nutrient consumption at a national level was provided by the surveys conducted by the U.S. Department of Agriculture (USDA). Since then, the proliferation of increasingly sophisticated nutrition-oriented surveys testifies to the elevated interest about food, nutrition, and health in the past 30 years.

National Health and Nutrition Examination Surveys

The first **National Health and Nutrition Examination Survey (NHANES)** was conducted from 1971 to 1974 by the U.S. Department of Health, Education, and Welfare (National Center for Health Statistics, 1977) (Table 14–1). This agency, renamed the Department of Health and Human Services (DHHS) in 1980, has continued the NHANES surveys approximately every 5 years, with NHANES II (1976–1980) and Hispanic HANES (1982–1984) (Carroll et al., 1983; Woteki et al., 1988). NHANES III (1988–1994) studied 30,000 persons, with a large proportion of persons age 65 years and older. Surveys are listed in Table 14–1.

Unique to NHANES III is the absence of an upper age limit, making it particularly useful for the study of aging related to nutritional issues. Monitoring nutrition and setting policy from survey findings are ongoing operations. Figure 14–1 indicates how these facets are correlated.

In addition to nutrient intake data, the NHANES surveys provide information on the health status of the nation. Survey data on individuals include (1) medical history, (2) physical measurements, (3) biochemical evaluation, (4) physical signs and symptoms, and (5) diet information from food frequency questionnaires and 24-hour recalls.

NHANES reports provide a health profile of the community with respect to 30 topics including blood pressures and the prevalence of hypertension; cholesterol levels and cardiovascular risk factors; measurements of height and weight and prevalence of overweight and obesity; and levels of energy and nutrient intakes and iron status and other hematologic data.

Nationwide Food Consumption Survey

The **Nationwide Food Consumption Survey (NFCS)** has been conducted by the USDA approximately every 10 years since 1935. It monitors the nutrient intake of a cross section of the American public by collecting information on food consumption of households and selected individuals. As such, it is a resource of data on national food habits and trends.

In most recent NFCS (1987–1988), 37% (4495 households) completed the household food use questionnaire. In this part of the survey respondents were asked to provide information on food use by the household for a 1-week period and on the cost of

TABLE 14–1 FOOD, NUTRITION, AND HEALTH SURVEYS

NAME OF SURVEY	TIMING	AGENCY*	PURPOSE/COMMENTS
Ten State Nutrition Survey	1968–1970	DHEW	To evaluate dietary intake, nutritional, and economic status
Preschool Nutrition	1968–1970	DHEW	To evaluate dietary intake, nutritional, and economic status in children 1–6 y in 36 states
National Health and Nutrition Examination Survey (NHANES)	1971–1974	DHEW	First nationwide health survey to include nutrition; ages 1–74 y included
NHANES II	1976–1980	DHEW	Ages 6 mo to 74 y included
Hispanic HANES (HHANES)	1982–1984	DHHS	To remedy underreporting of Hispanics
NHANES III	1988–1994	DHHS	Ages 2 mo and older; to monitor health and nutrition over time, especially in the elderly
Continuing Survey of Food Intakes by Individuals	1985–1986	USDA	Women 19–50 y and their children; men 19–50 y
CSFII	1989+	USDA	US 1 low-income sample included
National Food Consumption Survey	1987–1988; every 10 y	USDA	US 1 low-income sample included
Total Diet Study	Ongoing	DHHS/FDA	Specific age-sex groups; market basket sample
Food Disappearance Data	Annual	USDA	To monitor total available food used; waste not accounted for
Cholesterol Awareness Study	1986	DHHS/NIH	To assess cholesterol knowledge of consumers
Pregnancy and Infant Feeding Survey	1988–1989	DHHS/FDA	To assess feeding practices of pregnant women and infants
Coordinated State Surveillance System	Ongoing	DHHS/CDC	Pregnant women, children included

*Agencies: CDC, Centers for Disease Control and Prevention; DHEW, Department of Health, Education and Welfare until 1980, then renamed DHHS; DHHS, Department of Health and Human Services; FDA, Food and Drug Administration; HNIS, Human Nutrition Information Service; NIH, National Institutes of Health; USDA, United States Department of Agriculture.

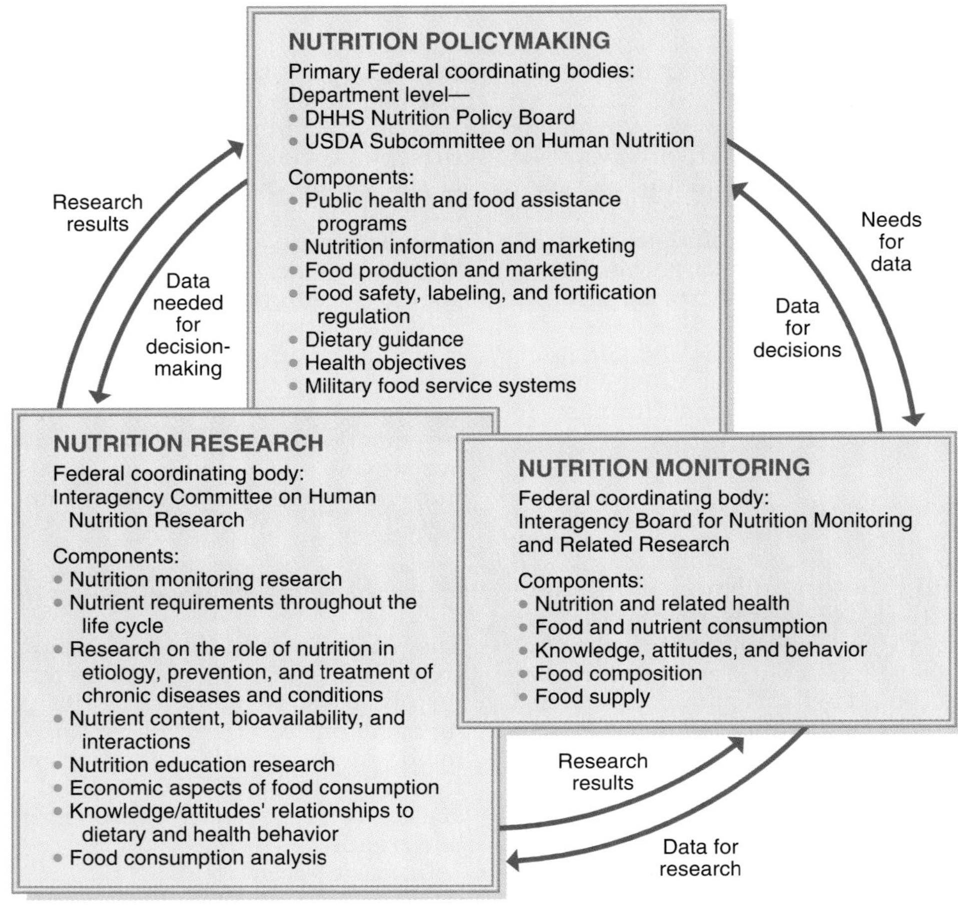

NUTRITION POLICYMAKING
Primary Federal coordinating bodies:
Department level—
• DHHS Nutrition Policy Board
• USDA Subcommittee on Human Nutrition
Components:
• Public health and food assistance programs
• Nutrition information and marketing
• Food production and marketing
• Food safety, labeling, and fortification regulation
• Dietary guidance
• Health objectives
• Military food service systems
Research results
Data needed for decision-making
Needs for data
Data for decisions
NUTRITION RESEARCH
Federal coordinating body:
Interagency Committee on Human Nutrition Research
Components:
• Nutrition monitoring research
• Nutrient requirements throughout the life cycle
• Research on the role of nutrition in etiology, prevention, and treatment of chronic diseases and conditions
• Nutrient content, bioavailability, and interactions
• Nutrition education research
• Economic aspects of food consumption
• Knowledge/attitudes' relationships to dietary and health behavior
• Food consumption analysis
NUTRITION MONITORING
Federal coordinating body:
Interagency Board for Nutrition Monitoring and Related Research
Components:
• Nutrition and related health
• Food and nutrient consumption
• Knowledge, attitudes, and behavior
• Food composition
• Food supply
Research results
Data for research

FIGURE 14–1 Relationships among nutrition policy-making, research, and monitoring. (From Wotecki C. Nutrition monitoring research, Research Agenda Conference Proceedings. Chicago: American Dietetic Association, 1992, p. 42.)

that food. Thirty-one percent of individual household members (10,172 individuals) provided day 1 intake information. Household members were asked to provide 3 days of information on their food intake through a 24-hour food recall and 24 hours of a food diary.

Continuing Survey of Food Intake of Individuals: Diet and Health Knowledge Survey

In 1985 to 1986 the **Continuing Survey of Food Intake of Individuals (CSFII)** was created and later became part of the National Nutrition Monitoring System of the USDA, established in 1990. It is the first nationwide dietary intake survey designed to be conducted annually.

The Diet and Health Knowledge Survey (DHKS), which is a telephone follow-up to CFSII, was initiated in 1989. The survey is designed so that individuals' attitudes and knowledge about healthy eating can be linked with their food choices and nutrient intake. Together, these two surveys are known as the *What We Eat In America* survey. This survey reports the kinds and amounts of foods eaten, and they also measure attitudes and knowledge about diet and health among Americans.

The CFSII collected data on women age 19 to 50 years and their children age 1 to 5 years in 1985, a similar sample of low-income women and their children aged 1 to 5 years in 1986, and men aged 19 to 50 years in 1986 (Joint Nutrition Monitoring Evaluation Committee, 1986; Nutrition Monitoring Division, 1986, 1987, 1989; USDA, 1985).

The latest report from the CFSII was released in 1998, regarding intakes from 1994 through 1996. Data are available on CD-Rom or magnetic data tape through USDA's Agricultural Research Service, Food Surveys Research Group at http://www.barc.usda.gov/bhnrc/foodsurvey/home.htm.

Results from this survey show that adult women fail to meet the recommended dietary allowances (RDAs) for calcium, vitamin E, vitamin B_6, magnesium, and zinc; adult men fail to meet RDA levels for vitamin E, magnesium, and zinc. Fat accounts for 33% of calories in the American diet, a continued decrease from 34% in 1989 to 1991 and 40% in 1977 to 1978. One third of adults are overweight, and vegetable consumption is decreasing slightly, while the consumption of grain-based products is on the rise. About 57% of Americans eat away from home on any given day. Consumption of fluid milk among young children has decreased by 16% since the late 1970s (USDA, 1998).

Household data for these studies are determined by calculating the nutrient content of foods reported to be used in the home during the survey week, and comparing the results with the RDAs for persons of the same age and sex as those in the households.

The data derived from the CSFII and DHKS are used by federal and state decision makers and researchers in monitoring the nutritional adequacy of American diets, measuring the impact of food fortification on nutrient intakes, and developing dietary guidance and related programs.

Supplemental Children's Survey

The Food Quality Protection Act of 1996 requires the Secretary of Agriculture to provide the Environmental Protection Agency (EPA) with information on food consumption patterns of a statistically valid sample of infants and children. The USDA is conducting the *Supplemental Children's Survey (SCS)* to meet this mandate.

The SCS will provide intakes on approximately 5000 children through 9 years of age. The sample design and the data collection procedures are the same as those used for the 1994 to 1996 CFSII so the two data sets can be merged. Data collection took place from December 1997 through November 1998 and will be reported in the near future.

National Nutrition Monitoring and Related Research Act

The 101st Congress passed Public Law 101-445, the *National Nutrition Monitoring and Related Research (NNMRR)* Act, in October, 1990. This law is intended to provide consistency and unification of survey methods for monitoring the eating habits and nutrition of Americans, especially for setting public policy (Sims, 1993). Key provisions of the act include planning and coordinating the 22 federal agencies that review and implement nutritional surveys or services. A National Nutrition Monitoring Advisory Council was established to complete this function (Kuczmarski et al., 1994).

In the Third Report on Nutrition Monitoring in the United States: Executive Summary (Interagency Board for Nutrition Monitoring and Related Research, 1995), the prevalence of overweight continues to be a concern; the intake of total fat and saturated fatty acids remains above recommended levels for a majority of the population; anemia continues to be a concern among children aged 1 to 2, girls 12 to 19, and women 20 to 59 years of age; and 9% to 13% of people living in low-income households experience some degree of food insufficiency. See Chapter 15.

Nutrition Screening Initiative

The **Nutrition Screening Initiative (NSI)** was designed by the American Dietetic Association (ADA) in cooperation with the American Academy of Family Physicians and the National Council on the Aging, to provide a tool to assess senior citizens who are living independently. The level 1 screen is designed to identify warning signs of nutritional risk. The level 1 screen evaluates risk factors such as body weight, eating habits, living environment, and functional status. Level 2 screening, a more comprehensive nutritional assessment, includes more diagnostic information.

The screening tool has been used with more than 300,000 individuals nationwide. When nutritional deficits are identified and corrected early, it is possible to reduce the negative consequences of hospitalizations and poor health outcomes. More information is available from the NSI at (202) 625-1662 and Chapter 13 describes the NSI in greater detail.

National Nutrient Data Bank

The *National Nutrient Data Bank* is the United States' primary resource of information on the nutrient content of foods. The data comes from private industry as well as academic and government laboratories. Until recently, most of this information was published in the form of Agriculture Handbook 8 (AH-8). However, AH-8 is no longer available in printed form.

The information found in AH-8 is now provided in the USDA Nutrient Database for Standard Reference (SR) on the Internet. The most recent release of SR, number 11, was released in September, 1996. It contains nutrient analysis of 5900 foods. The web site address is http://www.nal.usda.gov/fnic/foodcomp.html.

NATIONAL NUTRITION GUIDELINES AND GOALS

Initially, most of the nutrition education materials available to the public were produced by the USDA. The first dietary guidance pamphlet, *Food for Young Children,* was issued in 1916. The initial version of what eventually evolved into the Daily Food Guide based on food groups was published in 1917. It began with five food groups and evolved through seven groups to become the familiar "Basic Four" groups in *Food for Fitness, A Daily Food Guide,* and finally, in 1992, the *Food Guide Pyramid* (see Chapter 15) (Human Nutrition Information Service, 1992). Canadian dietary guidelines have also been published (see the accompanying box, "*Focus On:* Canadian Dietary Studies").

The RDAs were formulated in 1943 by the Food and Nutrition Board of the National Research Council, National Academy of Sciences (Food and Nutrition Board, 1989). The first guidelines were

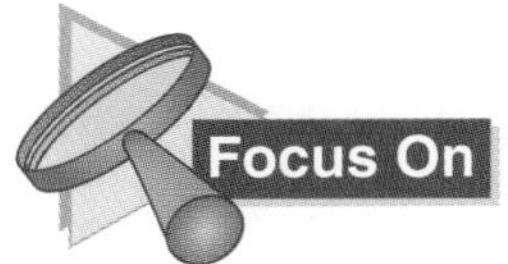

Canadian Dietary Studies

Dietary intake studies have been compiled, and their results released, on the food consumption patterns of the three Canadian provinces of Ontario, Nova Scotia, and Quebec. Thousands of Canadian citizens participated in a survey that reviewed dietary intakes. Over 90% of adolescents in this study reported intakes of fat greater than 30% of total calories; 50% consume more than half of their calories as fat. In the adults, 10% of men and 16% of women consumed less than 30% of their daily intake as fat. Complex carbohydrate intakes did not meet the desired level of 55% of calories consumed; less than 25% of all age groups met this dietary goal. Obesity was identified in 24% of adult women and 17% of men.

One fifth of the women and one fourth of the men consumed more than 25g of fiber daily. In Nova Scotia, 20% of the 2212 respondents over age 18 had at least one risk factor for heart disease that was modifiable, such as cholesterol or saturated fat intake. Protein intakes exceeded suggested levels except for women over age 65. Of all respondents, 67% reported use of some type of alcoholic beverage weekly, with a slightly higher rate for men; use overall declined with age.

In Quebec, grain products accounted for 35% of total carbohydrate intake and provided a major source of dietary fiber. Cholesterol intakes averaged 350 mg for men and 263 mg for women. Calcium and vitamin D intakes were low, particularly for those over age 50. Iron was low for women, and vitamin C supplements were commonly used by 20% of the population (Canadian National Institute of Nutrition, Rapport 8(4): 1993).

These Canadian studies are of interest as the NHANES III data are gradually being published in the United States. Comparisons between the two countries are of interest to nutrition counselors.

based on achievement of optimal health through avoidance of nutrient deficiencies and on attainment of nutrient intakes as specified in the RDA. However, the distinct trend of more recent goals has been toward preventing nutrition-related disease (Ostenso, 1988). New dietary reference intakes (DRIs) and related guidelines for some specific nutrients have been published (Pennington and Hubbard, 1997); see Chapter 15 for more detail.

The Senate Select Committee on Nutrition and Human Needs presented the first *Dietary Goals for the United States* in 1977 (Senate Select Committee, 1977, 1978). In 1980 these were modified and issued jointly as *Dietary Guidelines for Americans* by the DHHS and the USDA, and revised again in 1985 and 1990 (Nutrition and Your Health, 1980, 1990). Their emphasis on nutrient intakes and excesses reflects the increasing national concern over obesity, cancer, hypertension, and coronary artery disease. (Dietary Guidelines are discussed in detail in Chapter 15.)

Early dietary guidelines, based on a philosophy of preventive nutrition, were formulated by the American Heart Association. Originally, these were directed toward persons at risk for hypertension and coronary artery disease; more recently, their recommendations have been extended to the general public. The *National Cholesterol Education Program* of the National Heart, Lung, and Blood Institute in 1987 provided specific guidelines for identifying and treating hyperlipoproteinemia (National Cholesterol Education Program, 1988); see Chapter 26.

Following publication of *Diet, Nutrition and Cancer* (Committee on Diet, Nutrition and Cancer, 1982), the National Cancer Institute in 1988 issued the *Dietary Guidelines for Cancer Prevention*. In 1991, the National Cancer Institute collaborated with the National Institutes of Health (NIH) to produce the *5-A-Day Program for Better Health* (U.S. Department of Health and Human Services, 1991). See Chapter 39 for further discussion of cancer.

Diets that are high in fat and low in fiber and fruit/vegetable intake have been associated with increased incidence and mortality from cancer. The 5-A-Day Program promotes the consumption on a daily basis of fruits and vegetables, especially those rich in vitamin A, ascorbic acid, and fiber. Cruciferous vegetables from the cabbage family are recommended several times a week. See Chapter 12 for further discussion of phytonutrients and their role in cancer prevention. Table 14–2 lists some of the dietary reports that have influenced the development of guidelines or affected the manner in which health priorities are determined.

The Surgeon General's Report on Nutrition and Health (The Surgeon, 1988) included comprehensive documentation of the scientific basis for the recommendations. The detailed report examined current knowledge of specific dietary practices and specific disease conditions and states the implications for the individual as well as for future public health policy decisions (Table 14–3).

Healthy People

Healthy People is the prevention agenda for the nation. Publication of *Healthy People* (1979), the Surgeon General's first report on health promotion and disease prevention, eventually led to the formulation of health objectives addressing specific issues in the priority areas identified. Strategies for achieving the 1990 objectives were outlined in the

TABLE 14–2 HISTORY OF DIETARY RECOMMENDATIONS FOR THE U.S. PUBLIC

PUBLICATION	YEAR	ORGANIZATION OR AGENCY*	RECOMMENDATION
Food for Young Children	1916	USDA	First U.S. government dietary guidance pamphlet
Food Guide	1917	USDA	5 food groups: flesh, starches, fats, watery fruits and vegetables, sweets
Food Guide	1933	USDA	12 food groups
RDA	1941	FNB/NAS	Recommended intakes for known nutrients
Food Guide	1946	USDA	"Basic 7" food groups
Food for Fitness (Daily food guide)	1958	USDA	"Basic 4" food groups based on RDA[†]
Dietary Goals for the U.S., 1st ed	1977	Senate Select Committee on Nutrition and Human Needs	First government publication to address macronutrient intake and excess
Dietary Goals for the U.S., 2nd ed	1978	Senate Select Committee on Nutrition and Human Needs	Refined recommendations of 1st edition
Nutrition and Your Health: Dietary Guidelines for Americans	1980	USDA/DHHS	Generic recommendations similar in content to the Dietary Goals without specified amounts
Toward Healthful Diets	1980	FNB/NAS	Similar to Guidelines and goals except for fat recommendations
Various guidelines on nutrition	1980	AMA, AHA, NCI, American Society for Clinical Nutrition, NAS	Several organizations published similar recommendations
Diet, Nutrition, and Cancer	1982	Committee on Diet, Nutrition and Cancer, NRC, NAS	Dietary guidelines to reduce risk of cancer
Nutrition and Your Health: Dietary Guidelines for Americans, 2nd ed	1985	USDA/DHHS	
National Cholesterol Education Program	1987	DHHS/NHLBI	Guidelines for cholesterol education
NCI Dietary Guidelines: Rationale	1988	DHHS/NCI	Recommendations to reduce risk of cancer
Nutrition and Your Health: Dietary Guidelines for Americans, 3rd ed	1990	USDA/DHHS	
Food Guide Pyramid	1992	USDA/HNIS	New eating guide based on RDA that also considers salt, fat, and sugar
National Cholesterol Education Program–Updated Guidelines	1994	DHHS/NHLBI	Updated guidelines to further target the asterisked population
Dietary Guidelines for Americans, 4th ed	1995	USDA/DHHS	New guidelines due in 2000

*AHA, American Heart Association; AMA, American Medical Association; DHHS, Department of Health and Human Services; FNB, Food and Nutrition Board; HNIS, Human Nutrition and Information Services; NAS, National Academy of Sciences; NCI, National Cancer Institute; NHLBI, National Heart, Lung and Blood Institute; NRC, National Research Council; USDA, U.S. Department of Agriculture.

[†]RDA, Recommended Dietary Allowances; revised approximately every 5 years since 1943.

U.S. Public Health Service publication *Promoting Health/Preventing Disease: Objectives for the Nation* (Promoting Health/Preventing Disease, 1980). Initiatives for *Healthy People 2000* were written in 1990 with 319 objectives, 19 of which were nutritional goals.

Following is an example of one specific nutritional directive: Reduce prevalence of overweight to no more than 20% of persons over 20 years of age and 15% among adolescents (*Healthy People 2000,* 1990). A status review from this report suggested that obesity is still a concern. Although people are eating less fat, they are not actually achieving ideal body weight. A greater percentage are overweight (McGinnis and Lee, 1995).

The goals for this initiative have been updated and are currently referred to as *Healthy People 2010* (Table 14–4). Current updates may be found at website http://web.health.gov/healthypeople or by calling the Office of Disease Prevention and Health Promotion at (202) 205-8583.

FOOD ASSISTANCE AND NUTRITION PROGRAMS

Providing guidelines or food selection information does not guarantee optimal nutrition without access to adequate food or money to buy it. An increasing variety of food and nutrition programs have become available to assist the consumer in obtaining a safe and wholesome food supply available continuously in adequate amounts. Over the years these programs have come primarily from the USDA. Programs currently under the direction of that organization are listed in Table 14–5.

It is evident from NHANES studies that foods from the tip of the Food Pyramid (i.e., fats, sweets, alcohol) often displace nutrient-dense foods in the American diet; 33% of energy intake is often from this "other category" (Kant and Schtzkin, 1994). The public may have difficulty choosing a diet that meets both the dietary guidelines and the RDAs

TABLE 14–3 RECOMMENDATIONS OF THE SURGEON GENERAL'S REPORT ON NUTRITION AND HEALTH

ISSUES FOR MOST PEOPLE

- *Fats and cholesterol:* Reduce consumption of fat (especially saturated fat) and cholesterol. Choose foods relatively low in these substances, such as vegetables, fruits, whole grain foods, fish, poultry, lean meats, and low-fat dairy products. Use food preparation methods that add little or no fat.
- *Energy and weight control:* Achieve and maintain a desirable body weight. To do so, choose a dietary pattern in which energy (caloric) intake is consistent with energy expenditure. To reduce energy intake, limit consumption of foods relatively high in calories, fats, and sugars, and minimize alcohol consumption. Increase energy expenditure through regular and sustained physical activity.
- *Complex carbohydrates and fiber:* Increase consumption of whole-grain foods and cereal products, vegetables (including dried beans and peas), and fruits.
- *Sodium:* Reduce intake of sodium by choosing foods relatively low in sodium and limiting the amount of salt added in food preparation and at the table.
- *Alcohol:* To reduce the risk for chronic disease, take alcohol only in moderation (no more than two drinks a day), if at all. Avoid drinking any alcohol before or while driving, operating machinery, taking medications, or engaging in any other activity requiring judgment. Avoid drinking alcohol while pregnant to lessen the risk of birth defects.

OTHER ISSUES FOR SOME PEOPLE

- *Fluoride:* Community water systems should contain fluoride at optimal levels for prevention of tooth decay. If such water is not available, use other appropriate sources of fluoride.
- *Sugars:* Those who are particularly vulnerable to dental caries (cavities), especially children, should limit their consumption and frequency of use of foods high in sugars.
- *Calcium:* Adolescent girls and adult women should increase consumption of foods high in calcium, including low-fat dairy products.
- *Iron:* Children, adolescents, and women of childbearing age should be sure to consume foods that are good sources of iron, such as lean meats, fish, certain beans, and iron-enriched cereals and whole-grain products. This issue is of special concern for low-income families.

(From The Surgeon General's Report on Nutrition and Health—Summary and Recommendations. USDHHS (PHS) Publ 88-50211. Washington, DC: U.S. Government Printing Office, 1988.)

without individualized education (Dollahite et al., 1995), such as that provided by the USDA's Cooperative Extension and other agencies.

Foods eaten between meals make a significant contribution to total food intake and should be part of the nutrition message that is targeted for all age groups. Over $12 billion may be spent annually on snack foods alone (Cross et al., 1994). Changes in eating patterns and food purchasing behaviors often lag behind shifts in consumer life-styles and attitudes: 9 of top 10 entrees eaten at home in 1996 were the same items as those selected in 1987, just in a different order (Sloan, 1998). Home-meal replacements, pre-prepared fresh products, and home-delivered meals are now important, based on longer working hours. Lunch breaks are becoming shorter or filled with errands. More meals are eaten on the job or in the car; more vending sales and hand-held foods are needed that are healthy choices. Clearly, consumers need guidance in making effective food choices.

TABLE 14–4 HEALTHY PEOPLE 2010 DRAFT NUTRITION OBJECTIVES

Goal: To promote health and reduce chronic disease risk, disease progression, debilitation, and premature death associated with dietary factors and nutritional status among all people in the United States

Objectives: Twenty measurable nutrition objectives cover a wide range of issues:

1. Healthy weight
2. Obesity in adults
3. Overweight and obesity in children and adolescents
4. Growth retardation
5. Fat intake
6. Saturated fat intake
7. Vegetable and fruit intake
8. Grain product intake
9. Calcium intake
10. Sodium intake
11. Iron deficiency
12. Anemia among low-income pregnant women
13. School meals and snacks
14. Nutrition education—elementary schools
15. Nutrition education—middle/junior high schools
16. Nutrition education—senior high schools
17. Worksite nutrition education and weight management programs
18. Nutrition assessment and planning
19. Nutrition counseling
20. Food security

(From The American Dietetic Association ADA Courier. Chicago: ADA, January 1999.)

Recognizing that there are also problems of undernutrition, the American Dietetic Association addressed domestic food and nutrition security through a position paper and through varying efforts at all levels (American Dietetic Association, 1998a). This paper describes the impact of hunger and undernutrition on vulnerable groups such as infants, children, pregnant women, and the elderly. Dietary patterns characterized by omission of food groups are associated with risk of mortality from all causes in both men and women (Kant et al., 1993). The goal is **food security** for all Americans (Kendall et al., 1996). More information is available through www.iglou.com/why.

A wide variety of health-related programs conducted by the USDA and the DHHS significantly affect the nutritional status of the population, from the newborn infant to the elderly. Among some of the landmark programs are the National School Lunch Program, the WIC program, the Food Stamp

TABLE 14–5 FOOD PROGRAMS ADMINISTERED BY THE USDA

PROGRAM AND YEAR STARTED	ELIGIBLE INDIVIDUALS OR GROUPS	OBJECTIVES OF PROGRAM	COMPONENTS OF PROGRAM
Food Distribution Program (Donatable Foods), 1930s	Supplemental food program for mothers and infants; elderly feeding program; schools and institutions	To distribute surplus food to individuals and institutions to help agricultural support program	Distribution of surplus food; previously, to needy families but at present, only to eligible schools, institutions, and persons in U.S. Trust territories
National School Lunch Program (NSLP), 1946	All children enrolled at participating schools, residential child care institutions, including homes for developmentally disabled up to 21 y old, juvenile detention centers, and orphanages	To provide a nutritious lunch (one that has as its objective to provide one third of the RDA for a child) at a reasonable cost to school children; to provide reduced-price or free lunches to needy eligible children	Donated food to participating schools; federal monetary support
Food Stamp Program, 1964	Needy families and individuals in participating counties (almost all counties); entitlement program based on income for all Americans	To supplement an individual's or a family's food-buying power	Limited monthly allotment of food vouchers at a reduced price, depending on income; coupons are used to pay for food
Child Care Food Program (CCFP), 1968	Preschool children in nonprofit facilities such as day care centers, Head Start centers, and family day care homes	To provide meal service for children in full-time day care centers and Head Start programs and after school care programs	Federal monetary support; cash in lieu of commodities available
Special Milk Program,* 1968	Schools, child care centers, summer camps, and institutions	To reduce the cost of milk to children or provide it free to children who are also eligible for free meals	Federal reimbursement to schools or centers for all or part of the cost of the milk served
Summer Food Service Program for Children, 1968	Public agency sponsored programs for preschool and school-age children in schools, recreation centers and summer camps, and during vacations in areas with a continuous school calendar	To provide free lunches to children in summer programs	Federal monetary support
School Breakfast Program, 1973	All children enrolled in participating schools	To provide children a nutritious breakfast at a low cost	Donated food to participating schools; federal monetary support
Supplemental Nutrition Program for Women, Infants, and Children (WIC), 1974 (renamed "Nutrition" versus "Food" in 1993/4)	Pregnant and lactating women and infants and children up to 5 y old who are judged to be at nutritional risk because of inadequate nutrition and income	To improve the nutritional status of pregnant and lactating women and children up to 5 y old in low-income areas	Cash grants to state health departments and comparable agencies who make available supplemental foods through participating health clinics; health clinics provide specified nutritious food supplements or vouchers for these foods; regular health examination of the mother and the children and nutrition education required

RDA, Recommended Dietary Allowances.
*If a school is on the School Lunch Program, it cannot receive the Special Milk Program and vice versa.

Program, Cooperative Extension, Senior Adult Meals, and child care food programs.

National School Lunch Program

School food programs for children began to a limited degree in the early 1900s at the time when free, compulsory, and universal education was established. The first widely scattered efforts were conducted by philanthropic organizations, local school districts, and private individuals; some of these organizations began as early as 1853. States and municipalities gradually expanded the number of feeding programs with increasing federal involvement, primarily in the form of donations from the accumulation of surplus foods.

Legislation establishing the **National School Lunch Program** under the direction of the USDA was passed in 1946. Under the program, federal cash reimbursement and donated foods from the **Commodity Food Program** are provided to schools that serve a lunch meeting specified nutritional requirements. Modifications in 1971 established the provision that children from families with incomes at the poverty level are eligible for a free lunch and children in families with incomes between 130% and 185% of the poverty level are eligible for a reduced-price lunch (see http://schoolmeals.nal.usda.gov).

In addition, a small reimbursement is provided to the school for all lunches, but children from families with incomes above 185% of the poverty level pay the established price. In fiscal year 1997 more than 26 million children each day participated in meals supported by the National School Lunch Program (USDA, 1998).

In 1994, the Food and Nutrition Service (formerly Food and Consumer Service) launched the *School Meals Initiative for Healthy Children.* The purpose of this initiative is twofold: (1) education for children on the importance of making healthy food choices and (2) support for school food service professionals to offer healthy school meals that meet the Dietary Guidelines for Americans. Starting at the beginning of the 1996–1997 school year the initiative was implemented in schools throughout the United States (USDA, 1998).

Special Milk Program

The *Special Milk Program,* established in 1955 by the USDA, provides reimbursement for milk served to children. It is available to schools and child care institutions that are not eligible for other federal child nutrition service programs. Children whose families are eligible for free school lunch or breakfast are eligible for free milk through this program.

In fiscal year 1997, 140 million half pints of milk were served through the Special Milk Program. Because of the expansions made in the National School Lunch Programs there has been a substantial decrease in the Special Milk Program since the 1960s.

School Breakfast Program

The *School Breakfast Program* began as a pilot project in 1966 and was made permanent in 1975. Eligibility criteria are the same as for the School Lunch Program. Children who participated in the School Breakfast Program have higher standardized achievement test scores than eligible nonparticipants. See Chapter 10 for the further discussion of children and breakfast.

In fiscal year 1997 an average of 6.9 million children participated in the School Breakfast Program daily and, of those, 5.5 million received the meals at a free or reduced price (USDA, 1998).

Summer Food Service Program

The *Summer Food Service Program* was established in 1975 after a pilot program in 1968. The program provides free, nutritious meals to low-income children during school vacations. It is offered in areas or at activity programs such as day camps where at least half of the children are from households with incomes below 185% of the poverty level.

The program provides one to two meals per day except in special conditions when three meals are provided daily. All meals are served free to eligible participants. The sites are reimbursed by the USDA for the meals served. During the summer of 1997, 2.3 million children participated in this program (USDA, 1998).

WIC Program

The **WIC** program (formally the Special Supplemental Nutrition Program for Women, Infants, and Children) is funded as part of the Child Nutrition Program legislation. The WIC program, administered by the USDA, was established in 1974 to provide nutrition education and to improve the nutritional status of pregnant and lactating women and children up to 5 years of age from low-income families.

The program involves cash grants to state health departments and comparable agencies that make available supplemental foods and nutrition education through participating health clinics. It is intended to assist low-income persons at high risk medically. A 1990 study showed that participants had lower medical costs for themselves and their babies, longer gestation periods, and higher birth weights; lower infant mortality have also resulted (www.usda.gov/fes/ogapi/wicunf~l.htm).

Head Start Program

The **Head Start** program is a comprehensive child-health development program targeted for children between the ages of 3 and 5 from families that meet the federal poverty guidelines. The Head Start Act of 1965 established this program, which provides all enrolled children with a broad array of services including education, health (medical, nutrition, dental, and mental health), social services, parent involvement activities, and special services to children with disabilities. In addition to services to families the Head Start Program has an early childhood clearinghouse (www.acf.dhhs.gov/programs/hsb/faq.htm).

Food Stamp Program

The **Food Stamp Program** was established in 1964 to supplement the food-buying power of needy individuals and families in a way that gave them freedom of choice. Monthly allotments of stamps to be used for food purchase are available at a cost that translates into reduced-price groceries. Bonus stamps are provided free to purchasers of food stamps under specified circumstances.

Senior Adult Meals

A federal program was established in 1965 for congregate dining and home-delivered meals for senior citizens. The *Title III Elderly Nutrition Program of the Older Americans Act* authorizes supportive and nutrition services. Meals are to provide one third of the daily RDAs for older adults. For most of the participants, nutrient intake improves significantly. The last reauthorization added the consultation of nutrition professionals to the program's regulations.

Cooperative Extension, Expanded Food and Nutrition Education Program (EFNEP), and Nutrition Education Training (NET) Programs

Other important programs that provide food or nutrition services include the *Cooperative Extension* program, which provides hands-on training in homes and community settings for the residents of each community, often through a state university. This program is funded under the USDA through land-grant colleges and universities (see www.ceeusda.gov).

One component of Cooperative Extension is the *Expanded Food and Nutrition Education Program* (EFNEP), which provides education tailored for low-income families. EFNEP has been in place since 1969.

The *Nutrition Education and Training Act* (NET) is another program that provides specialized funding for the school systems to help teachers adapt nutrition into their curricula.

FOOD SAFETY: LAWS, REGULATIONS, AND ISSUES

One of the major responsibilities of the public health system is to ensure the safety of the food supply. A multitiered approach to enhance safety and to monitor systems to prevent epidemics of **food borne illness** involves both public agencies (e.g., community/local and state public health agencies, federal regulatory agencies) and private agencies (e.g., food producers and manufacturers) for the most effective approach.

A health promotion/disease prevention approach supported by the public and private sectors would greatly enhance efforts to help educate consumers as well as food manufacturers on the latest technologies and regulations in food safety. The epidemiology of food borne illness is changing.

In the past food borne illness was described in the literature after a large local event such as a cookout or a wedding reception. The food borne outbreak occurred when foods were handled improperly or remained unrefrigerated for too long, leading to bacterial contamination of a single food item (e.g., potato salad or undercooked meat). The contaminated food was ingested by a limited number of persons attending the event.

Recent studies have described new pathogens that have emerged, some of which have spread worldwide. Examples of pathogens that have reservoirs in healthy animals and foods that can be spread to other foods are *Salmonella, Staphylococcus Aureus, Escherichia coli* (157:H7), *Camphylobacter,* and *Yersinia enterocolitica.* These pathogens have caused millions of cases of sporadic illness and chronic complications over many states and nations.

Improved surveillance systems that combine rapid systems to identify the offending organism include: sub-typing methods, cluster identification and collaborative investigation that can identify and halt large outbreaks. Research into ways that pathogens can persist in animal reservoirs is important to long-term prevention of outbreaks. In the past the focus was on prevention of contamination of human food with sewage or animal manure. In the future prevention of food borne disease will depend on controlling the contamination of feed and water consumed by the animals and passed on to humans (Tauxe, 1997). In addition, sanitation problems such as cross-contamination of work surfaces, poor hygiene and handwashing, lack of hair restraints, and other practices by food handlers can spread food borne illnesses rapidly. More current information on food safety is available at web site http:/ificinfo.health.org and from the USDA, including information from the consumer FIGHT BAC™ program, and from the FDA.

Surveillance Systems

The public health surveillance and response systems involve local, state, and national agencies. At the local level the county or city health department is usually the first agency to be used to provide the most basic surveillance, investigation, and prevention activities. At the state level, epidemiologists from the public health laboratories, sanitarians, and educators conduct statewide surveillance and prevention activities in conjunction with local authorities.

Local, state, and federal agencies work closely together to investigate food borne illness for two major reasons. The local health agency would be the first to identify and control the ongoing source of contamination by emergency action (e.g., restaurant closing, product recall), and then would examine ways to prevent similar outbreaks in the future.

Regulatory Agencies

At the national level, several agencies under DHHS manage different aspects of food safety. These include the Centers for Disease Control and Prevention (CDC), the Food and Drug Administration (FDA), and the Food Safety Inspection Service (FSIS) of the USDA. Laws and rules regulating food safety and quality are found in Table 14–6.

The CDC is the primary agency responsible for risk assessment for public health hazards. The CDC conducts the primary national surveillance and supports state health departments in managing their response to state epidemic outbreaks.

The FDA and the USDA are the primary agencies

TABLE 14–6 HISTORY OF LAWS AND RULES REGULATING FOOD SAFETY AND QUALITY IN THE UNITED STATES

NAME OF ACT AND DATE PASSED	CONTENT OF LEGISLATION
Wiley Act or "pure food and drug law." Passed 1906. The act itself was repealed 1938, but not all of amendments	"An act for preventing the manufacture, sale or transportation of adulterated or misbranded or poisonous or deleterious foods, drugs, medicines and liquors, and for other purposes."
Meat Inspection Act, passed 1907	Requires that "all meat and meat food products in interstate commerce be prepared under the supervision of the USDA."
Weight and Measure Amendment to Wiley Act, passed 1913	Clarifies rules about stating the quantity of the contents of packaged foods.
Kenyon Amendment to Wiley Act, passed 1919	Extends the weight and measure amendment to cover packaged meats.
McNary–Napes Amendment to Wiley Act, passed 1930	Authorizes the USDA to establish minimum standards for the quality, condition, and amounts of foods in containers, to be required of all canned foods except meat and milk.
Seafood Inspection Amendment to the Wiley Act, passed 1935	Authorizes the USDA "to provide government inspection of the packaging of any seafood which might enter into interstate commerce" for those packers desiring such inspection service.
Food, Drug and Cosmetic Act, passed 1938	Authorizes the Food and Drug Administration (FDA) to carry out the intent of Congress to ensure that foods are safe, pure, and wholesome, are made or processed under sanitary conditions, and are honestly labeled and packaged; to carry on research and public education; to set regulations governing the definitions and standards of identity of foods, containers, and labeling; and to promote honesty and fair dealing in the interest of the consumer. Standards of identity can be obtained from the FDA free of charge. Minimum standards of quality were set for tenderness, color, and freedom from defects. Standards for enrichment were set. Products labeled "enriched" or "fortified" must contain the exact specified amount of added nutrients.
Miller Pesticide Amendment, passed 1954	Establishes acceptable or relatively harmless levels for pesticide and chemical residues on raw agricultural commodities. The applicant must demonstrate the "usefulness" of a pesticide to the USDA's satisfaction and its "safety" to the FDA before its use.
Poultry Products Inspection Act, passed 1956	Makes continuous inspection compulsory for fresh, frozen, ready-to-eat, and canned poultry products. Labeling regulations were established for poultry products and enforcement powers were given to the USDA.
Food Additives Amendment to the Food, Drug and Cosmetic Act, passed 1958	Requires that the safety of chemicals used in processing be proved by industry to be safe before being sold for use in foods. Previously the government was responsible for proving a chemical unsafe *after* it was on the market, often requiring court action for removal. Chemicals in use prior to 1959 were considered Generally Recognized as Safe (GRAS) and use was allowed to continue. The Delaney Clause prohibits use of any food additive found to produce cancer when ingested in any amount by test animals of any species. Extended in 1968 to cover residues of animal drugs in meat, eggs, milk. Recently, pesticides were separated by the passage of The Food Quality Protection Act in 1996.
Color Additive Amendment to the Food, Drug and Cosmetic Act, passed 1960	Requires manufacturers to prove that their color additives are safe, and authorizes the FDA to establish and enforce tolerances for the use of color additives in foods, drugs, and cosmetics.
Fair Packaging and Labeling Act, passed 1967	Requires prominent labels on packaged foods and the following information: (1) statement of the food's identity must appear on the principal display panel in bold type; (2) name and address of manufacturer, packer, and distributor must be conspicuously stated; (3) statement of the net contents must appear in concise standard measure. (No qualifying terms such as "giant quart" may appear.); (4) statement listing ingredients, when required, must appear in type of legible size on a single panel of the label. The common names of ingredients must appear in decreasing order of predominance. These regulations include proposals for special diet foods, with particular reference to vitamin and mineral supplementation and low-calorie foods.
Nutrition Education and Labeling Act, passed 1990	Requires mandatory nutrition labeling on all FDA-regulated foods and voluntary labeling of fruits, vegetables, and raw fish. It also requires the Secretary to carry out activities to educate the consumers about the availability of nutrition information on the label and the importance of this information in maintaining healthy dietary practices.
Food Quality Protection Act, passed 1996	Requires new systems for maintaining food safety and outbreaks of food borne illnesses.

responsible for regulating food safety. Each agency has specific responsibilities regarding the nation's food and water; in some cases these responsibilities overlap.

In some respects the FDA may be the most well known of the agencies to the general public. The FDA policies and work touch the lives of virtually every American every day because this is the agency primarily responsible for seeing that the food we eat is safe and wholesome (Figures 14–2 and 14–3).

The FDA also oversees the safety of the cosmetics we use and ensures that the medicines and medical devices we use are safe and effective. The FDA also is responsible for the safety of the radiation-emitting products we use daily such as microwave

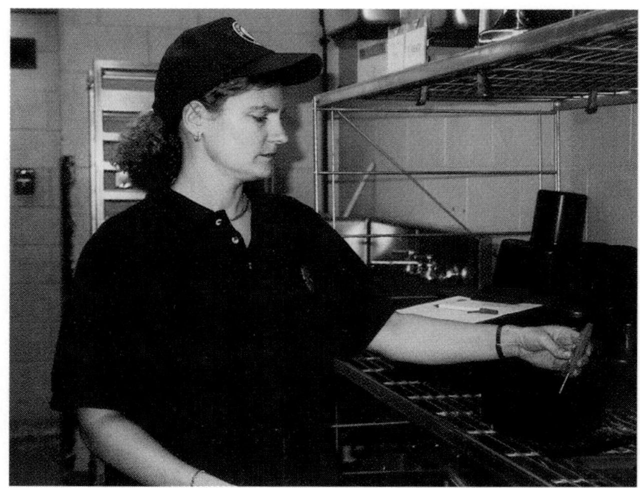

FIGURE 14–2 Food and Drug Administration staff inspecting food.

ovens. The FDA also regulates low-acid canned foods, imported foods, pasteurized milk, many seafoods, rabbits that are raised for meat, and food and water provided on aircraft and trains. In addition the FDA monitors foods and drugs for pets and farm animals.

The USDA regulates meat and poultry, including primary slaughter and further processing, and pasteurized eggs; investigates animal and plant disease; and maintains the County Extension outreach programs.

Of course, there are examples where more than one agency overlaps in assignments. A prime example the activities of two agencies overlapping is monitoring eggs in the shell. The USDA regulates the grading of shell eggs for quality, but the FDA has responsibility for the microbiologic safety of shell eggs.

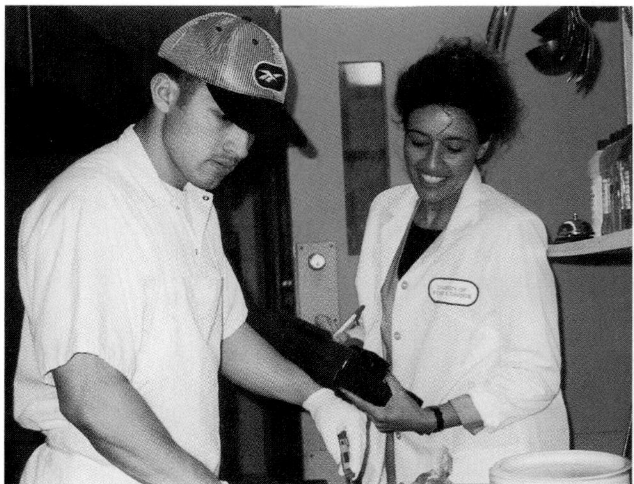

FIGURE 14–3 Food and Drug Administration inspectors.

With the increasing emergence of new foods, as well as the increasing number of foods imported from other countries, there are newer approaches to food safety for the future FDA.

Approaches to the Prevention of Food Borne Illnesses

Preventing food borne illness is a unique opportunity for public health and community agencies to collaborate with industry to make foods safe and to keep them safe throughout the chain of production and consumption. The USDA/FDA Foodborne Illness Education Information Center is a major national resource center that provides information about food borne illness prevention to educators, trainers, and organizations developing education and training materials for food workers and consumers. The center is part of an interagency agreement between the FSIS of the USDA and the FDA of the DHHS.

The USDA and FDA established the center as part of a national campaign to reduce the risk of food borne illness and to increase knowledge of food-related risks from production through consumption. The Center's primary function is the development and maintenance of two databases that compile many sources of educational materials including software, audiovisuals, and printed information for a wide range of audiences including school children, managers, retail workers, educators and more (see foodborne@nal.usda.gov). The center also manages databases that list resources and training on the most up-to-date programs on food safety including the *Hazard Analysis Critical Control Points (HACCP)*.

The HACCP is a major program offered by the Foodborne Illness Education Information Center that focuses on strategies to identify and control key points in the food production chain from the farmers working in the field, to foods prepared for service at the dinner table. The HACCP system replaces an older strategy of inspection of the final food product.

HACCP builds in strategies aimed at prevention of food borne illness rather than control of it. Persons working with food are trained to implement the strategies at critical points in the operation. To decrease the bacterial overgrowth on imported fresh fruits, an HACCP strategy would be (1) to refrigerate or chill the fruit and (2) to use bottled or distilled water for the ice cubes used in chilling the fruit, rather than using potentially polluted river water.

Another example of a HACCP strategy that has received much press coverage is reducing the risk of *E. coli* contamination in ground beef by heating it to a higher temperature than previously thought necessary. Use of a combination of several HACCP strategies in managing the safety of ground beef would include improved sanitation of the plant equipment; handwashing with soap and water; inspections of the slaughterhouse; keeping the cows healthy; irradiating the meat after slaughter; and thoroughly cooking the beef.

To prepare for food safety in the future, the nation must further improve and enhance the successes of the present food safety systems. To do this, enhancement of the present surveillance systems, continuation of applied research to better understand the changing environment, and building systems for quicker response to identified problems must occur. To access HACCP databases or to contribute materials, the FNIC web site is: http://www.nal.usda.gov/fnic/foodborne/foodborn.htm.

Functional Foods

Functional foods are defined as substances that may be considered food or biologically active substances that provide medical or health benefits (IFIC, web site, 1998). Isolated nutrients, dietary supplements, genetically engineered "designer food," herbal products, and specially processed soups, cereals, and beverages are included in this category (Hunt, 1994). The accompanying box, "*Focus On:* Fat Replacers and Substitutes" discusses the pros and cons of this type of change in available foods.

The philosophy that food can be health promoting beyond its nutritional value has gained acceptance within the public arena and among the scientific community as diet and food are linked to disease prevention and treatments (American Dietetic Association, 1995; Geiger, 1998; Pszczola, 1992). Table 14–7 lists functional food components and their potential benefits. See Chapter 12 for further discussion of phytochemicals.

Health Claims

The 1990 *Nutrition Labeling and Education Act (NLEA)* supported the evaluation of health claims, encouraging sufficient research before a health claim is added to a product label. Specific health claims are permitted for categories such as the role of calcium in osteoporosis, fat in cancer, or sodium in hypertension (American Dietetic Association, 1993a; FANSA, 1997; Geiger, 1998).

The FDA and USDA published final rules in 1994 defining the word *healthy* as a nutrient content claim on food labels, effective January 1, 1996 for FDA and November 10, 1995 for USDA. Table 14–8 delineates the history of health claims and their current regulatory status.

"Healthy" may be used as an implied claim if the food contains 3 g or less of fat per reference amount; 1 g or less of saturated fat per reference amount and saturated fat as 15% or less of the total kilocalories; 60 mg or less of cholesterol; at least 10% of the recommended daily allowance (RDA) or daily recommended value (DRV) of one selected micronutrient, such as vitamins A or C, protein, calcium, iron, and fiber; or 480 mg or less of sodium per reference amount. Research indicates that shorter health claims are most effective; effective messages also communicate action, contain relevant text and graphics, and are located on the front panel (Geiger, 1998).

Nutrition education, fortification of common food staples, and nutrient supplements are means of en-

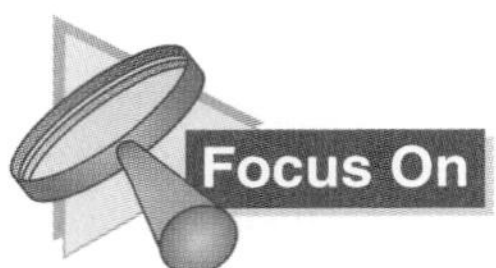

Fat Replacers and Substitutes

America's growing preference for fat-reduced diets has food manufacturers using new substances to replace most, if not all, of the fat in food. Some of these fat substitutes with trade names such as Simplesse, Olean, Avicel, and Olestra are already on the market. Fat replacers and substitutes are intended to replace the fat to reduce the calories in the food while maintaining the texture provided by fat.

Use of these fat replacements and substitutes raises questions such as: What effect do they have on the gastrointestinal system if they are not absorbed? Can they affect the absorption of fat-soluble vitamins? Can they interfere with absorption of other nutrients or drugs? What particular effects might they have in people with conditions that affect nutritional status, such as intestinal disease?

Unlike other food additives that make up only a small percent of what a person consumes, fat substitutes have the potential to make up a substantial portion of the diet because they replace fat, which is a major dietary component. This raises the concern about the unknown effect of fat substitutes. The usual method for studying negative effects, which is to give upward of 100 times the likely human intake to laboratory animals, is too impractical in this situation.

Replacing fat in the diet is not as easy as it appears. Natural fat has many natural functions in the body. Fats are a necessary nutrient for growth and development and the maintenance of cells. They carry the fat-soluble vitamins A, D, E, and K. Fat is the only source of linoleic and linolenic acids, the essential fatty acids; they are an important source of calories, particularly for infants and toddlers who have the highest energy needs per kilogram of body weight.

Fat also is important in food preparation—it gives taste, stability, and consistency to food and a feeling of satiety after a meal. However, too much is harmful. A high fat intake has been associated with certain chronic diseases such as breast, colon, and prostate cancers. A balance of fats is an important part of any dietary plan.

More information on fat replacers and substitutes is available from the International Food and Information Council Foundation at web site address http://ificinfo.health.org.

TABLE 14–7 EXAMPLES* OF FUNCTIONAL COMPONENTS

CLASS/COMPONENT	SOURCE*	POTENTIAL BENEFIT
Carotenoids		
α-carotene	Carrots	Neutralize free radicals which may cause damage to cells
β-carotene	Various fruits, vegetables	Neutralize free radicals
Lutein	Green vegetables	Contribute to maintenance of healthy vision
Lycopene	Tomatoes and tomato products (ketchup, sauces, etc.)	May reduce risk of prostate cancer
Zeaxathin	Eggs, citrus, corn	Contribute to maintenance of healthy vision
Collagen Hydrolysate	Gelatin	May help improve some symptoms associated with osteoarthritis
Dietary Fiber		
Insoluble fiber	Wheat bran	May reduce risk of breast and/or colon cancer
β-Glucan	Oats	Reduce risk of cardiovascular disease (CVD)
Soluble fiber	Psyllium	Reduce risk of CVD
Fatty Acids		
ω-3 Fatty acids—DHA/EPA	Tuna; fish and marine oils	May reduce risk of CVD & improve mental, visual functions
Conjugated linoleic acid (CLA)	Cheese, meat products	May improve body composition, may decrease risk of certain cancers
Flavonoids		
Anthocyanidins	Fruits	Neutralize free radicals, may reduce risk of cancer
Catechins	Tea	
Flavanones	Citrus	
Flavones	Fruits/vegetables	
Glucosinolates, Indoles, Isothiocyanates		
Sulphoraphane	Cruciferous vegetables (broccoli, kale), horseradish	Neutralize free radicals, may reduce risk of cancer
Phenols		
Caffeic acid	Fruits, vegetables, citrus	Antioxidant-like activities, may reduce risk of degenerative diseases; heart disease, eye disease
Ferulic acid		
Plant Sterols		
Stanol ester	Corn, soy, wheat, wood oils	Lower blood cholesterol levels by inhibiting cholesterol absorption
Prebiotics/Probiotics		
Fructo-oligosaccharides (FOS)	Jerusalem artichokes, shallots, onion powder	May improve gastrointestinal health
Lactobacillus	Yogurt, other dairy	May improve gastrointestinal health
Saponins	Soybeans, soy foods, protein-containing foods	May lower LDL cholesterol; contains anticancer enzymes
Soy Proteins, Phytoestrogens		
Isoflavones		
daidzein	Soybeans and soy-based foods	May reduce menopause symptoms, such as hot flashes
genistein		May protect against heart disease and some cancers; lower LDL cholesterol, total cholesterol and triglycerides
Lignans	Flax, rye, vegetables	
Sulfides, Thiols		
Diallyl sulfide	Onions, garlic, olives, leeks, scallions	Lower LDL cholesterol, maintain healthy immune system
Allyl methyl trisulfide, Dithiolthiones	Cruciferous vegetables	
Tannins		
Proanthocyanidins	Cranberries, cranberry products, cocoa, chocolate	May improve urinary tract health May reduce risk of cardiovascular disease

*Examples are not an all inclusive list.
(Source: IFIC @ http://ificinfo.health.org.)
CVD, cardiovascular disease; LDL, low-density lipoprotein.

hancing the intake of populations who are nutritionally at risk (Stephenson and Guthrie, 1994). The ADA supports government regulation of dietary supplements and uniform labeling of such products to ensure the safety of individuals who choose them as part of their dietary regimen.

A Gallup poll conducted in 1993 on behalf of the ADA found that 30% of consumers were aware of such nutritional information tools as the Food Pyramid and that 65% would be very likely to change their eating habits as a result of advice given by a dietitian (American Dietetic Association, 1994). Continued, appropriate advisement of the individual consumer is recommended.

TABLE 14–8 LEGISLATION MILESTONES IN HEALTH CLAIM REGULATION

NAME OF LEGISLATION	YEAR	TYPE	PRIMARY PROVISIONS
Pure Food and Drug Act	1906 (F) 1906 (E)	Law	Prohibited false and misleading statements on labels of foods and drugs.
Federal Food, Drug, and Cosmetic Act	1933 (I) 1938 (E)	Law	Regulated and defined misbranding: ". . . labeling represents, suggests, or implies that the food because of the presence or absence of certain dietary properties is adequate or effective in the prevention, cure, mitigation, or treatment of any disease or symptom." Continued prohibition of false and misleading claims in food labeling. Required "common and usual name" of food, net quantity of contents, ingredient statements, name and address of manufacturer and distributor. Required labeling of imitation and special dietary foods.
Label Statements Concerning Dietary Properties of Food Purporting to be or Represented for Special Dietary Uses	1941 (F)	Regulation	Created regulations for vitamin and mineral supplements, fortified food products, and special dietary foods.
Fair Packaging and Labeling Act	1966 (F) 1966 (E)	Law	Gave the US FDA jurisdiction over regulation of package size, provision of label information, and measurement of content.
Public Health Messages on Food Labels	1987 (I); reproposed 1990	Regulation	Proposed procedures for allowing reliable and valid consumer information on food labels. Proposed criteria for appropriate health messages. Proposed interagency health committee on health messages. Proposal was withdrawn with the passage of the National Labeling and Education Act.
Food Labeling, Advance Notice of Proposed Rule-Making	1989 (I)	Regulation	Asked for comments on the need for revision of food labels, including health messages, nutrition label format, requirements for nutrition labeling, food descriptors, and ingredient labeling. Four national public hearings convened across the nation to gather comments on ways to improve the rules.
Nutrition Labeling and Education Act	1990 (I) 1990 (F) 1990 (E)	Law	Provided for mandatory nutrition labeling of most foods under the FDA's jurisdiction. Allowed health claims for the first time, but only if consistent with the FDA final regulations. Mandated that standardized serving sizes represent amounts customarily consumed and be expressed in appropriate common household measures. Expanded list of required nutrients. Provided for consistent, defined nutrient content claims based on standardized serving sizes (reference amounts). Federal preemption for nutrient labeling. Provided for consumer education.
Food Labeling: General Requirements for Health Claims for Foods	1991 (I)	Regulation	Proposed general health claim requirements: definitions to clarify the meaning of specific terms used in the regulation; preliminary requirements a food must meet to be eligible for a health claim; a scientific standard for assessing the validity of claims for dietary supplements and for conventional foods, and general labeling requirements for health claims permitted by regulation and prohibitions on certain types of health claims; and the required content of petitions for health claims.
Food Labeling: General Requirements for Health Claims for Foods	1993 (F)	Regulation	Regulation discussed general health claim requirements: contained (a) definitions: health claim, substance, nutritive value, and disqualifying level to clarify the meaning of specific terms used in the regulation; (b) requirements a component of food must meet to be eligible for a health claim; (c) general labeling requirements for health claims permitted by regulation, and prohibitions on certain types of health claims; and (d) the required content of petitions for health claims.
Nutrition Labeling: Health Claims on Meat and Poultry Products	1994 (I)	Regulation	Proposed to permit the use of health claims and an application process for such health claims. Proposed regulations would permit health claims that are designed to parallel those issued by the FDA.
Food Labeling: Nutrient Content Claims, General Principles; Health Claims, General Requirements and Other Specific Requirements for Individual Health Claims	1995 (I)	Regulation	Proposed regulation would permit the use of shortened versions of authorized health claims under certain circumstances, would eliminate some of the required elements for health claims, would permit health claims on certain foods that do not currently qualify because they do not contain 10% of certain required nutrients, and would provide additional guidance for petitioners seeking exemption from the disqualification of some foods from bearing a health claim because they contain high levels of certain nutrients. The proposed regulations also would provide refinements to those regulations to allow additional synonyms for nutrient content claims without specific preclearance by the agency.

I, year initialized; F, year finalized; E, year enacted.

Source: Geiger C. Health claims: History, current regulatory status, and consumer research. J Am Diet Assoc 98:1313, 1998. Reprinted with permission.

FOOD TECHNOLOGY

Technology

A new relationship has developed between the food supply and the environment. Technology changes rapidly and is used to produce more food, better food with altered ingredients, and more easily distributed food to meet the demands of worldwide populations. *Biotechnology* is the word used to describe gene splicing, cell fusion, and protein purification. Food processing, food safety, pharmacology, and waste management are likely to be affected with new trends in this area.

Additives

The Federal Food, Drug and Cosmetic (FFD&C) Act of 1938 gave the FDA authority over food ingredients. **Food additives** are widely used in food processing to maintain or to improve the quality and palatability in a variety of ways (Table 14–9). The 1958 Food Additives Amendment to the FFD&C Act specified the manufacturer's responsibility of prior proof of safety to receive approval of new additives. The **Delaney Clause** prohibits approval of any food additive if it has been found to cause cancer at any level. This clause is currently under review.

The **Generally Recognized As Safe (GRAS)** list includes over 600 ingredients such as salt, sugar, and spices that need not be tested by prescribed procedures for every new food item. The GRAS list is regularly reviewed and changed as technology advances.

Irradiation

Food irradiation is one way to enhance the safety and quality of food supplies. Microbiologic hazards exist despite a relatively high level of food safety in the United States; 6.5 to 33 million cases of food borne illness occur each year, with 9000 resulting in death (American Dietetic Association 1996). Irradiation is one way to reduce potential pathogens as part of a comprehensive program.

AGRICULTURAL PRODUCTS AND CONCERNS

Pesticides

TOLERANCES AND RISK ASSESSMENT. The EPA approves the use of and establishes tolerances for pesticides at both the commodity/field level and the processed food level. The FDA monitors and enforces the tolerances. To obtain approval of a particular pesticide, the manufacturer must supply the EPA with data from toxicologic studies and residue data, and show justification of use in terms of economics and an adequate food supply.

A risk–benefit analysis leads to rejection or ac-

TABLE 14–9 FUNCTIONS AND USES OF COMMON FOOD ADDITIVES

FUNCTIONS	ADDITIVES USED	EXAMPLES OF FOODS IN WHICH ADDITIVES ARE USED
To improve nutritional value of certain foods	Thiamin, riboflavin, niacin, iron, vitamin A, vitamin D, ascorbic acid, potassium iodide	Wheat, flour, bread, rolls, biscuits, breakfast cereals, macaroni and noodle products, cornmeal, margarine, milk, iodized salt
To maintain appearance, palatability, and wholesomeness in certain foods (delaying undesirable changes in foods caused by oxidation or microbial growth; preventing food spoilage caused by molds, bacteria, yeast)	Propionic acid, calcium and sodium salts of propionic acid, ascorbic acid, butylated hydroxyanisole (BHA), butylated hydroxytoluene (BHT), propylene glycol	Bread, pie filling, cakes mixes, potato chips, crackers, cheese, syrup, fruit juices, frozen and dried fruits, margarine, shortenings, lard
To enhance flavor of certain foods	Spices (cloves, ginger, cinnamon, etc.), citrus oils, amyl acetate, carvone, benzaldehyde, monosodium glutamate, vanilla	Spice cake, gingerbread, ice cream, candy, carbonated beverages, fruit-flavored gelatins, toppings, sausage
To give characteristic color to certain foods	Annatto, carotene, cochineal, chlorophyll nitrates	Baked goods, candy, carbonated beverages, cheese, margarine, ice cream, jams, jellies, meat products
To maintain desired consistency in foods (emulsifiers and stabilizers)	Lecithin, mono- and diglycerides, gum arabic, carboxymethyl cellulose, carrageenan	Bakery products, cake mixes, salad dressings, frozen desserts, ice cream, chocolate milk, candy, beer
To control acidity or alkalinity in certain foods (leavening and neutralizing agents)	Potassium acid tartrate, tartaric acid, sodium bicarbonate, lactic acid, citric acid, adipic acid, fumaric acid	Cakes, cookies, biscuits, crackers, waffles, muffins, butter, processed cheese, cheese spreads, chocolates, carbonated beverages, confectionery
To serve as maturing and bleaching agents	Chlorine dioxide, chlorine, potassium bromate and iodate	Wheat flour (to make it white), certain cheeses
To help retain moisture (humectants), prevent caking, or act as curing agents	Glycerin, magnesium carbonate, sodium nitrate, calcium phosphate	Coconut, marshmallows, table salt, garlic and onion powder, frankfurters, sausages, dietetic foods

ceptance and establishment of a legal tolerance. Approval is granted only for the specific commodity application requested. For example, a chemical approved for use on lettuce would be considered in violation if used on cabbage or any other food.

Unfortunately, tolerances frequently cause consumer concern when they are misinterpreted to mean the levels of residue that may be expected in the marketplace (see "*Focus On:* Is It Really Organic?").

SURVEILLANCE SAMPLING. The FDA is responsible for surveillance of both imported and domestic foods. When possible, samples are collected close to the point of production so that crops in violation of tolerances can be intercepted and destroyed. Most violations are in the category of use in food crops in which tolerances have not been established for a particular pesticide/commodity combination.

TOTAL DIET STUDY (MARKET BASKET SAMPLE). The FDA also routinely surveys table-ready foods. Four times each year, 234 food items, representing the diets of American consumers are purchased in different cities around the United States. These are prepared as they would be in the home, and then analyzed for actual levels of pesticides, industrial chemicals, heavy metals, radionucleotides, and essential minerals.

The intakes for eight age-sex groups are compared with the **acceptable daily intakes (ADIs)** as established by the Food and Agriculture Organization/World Health Organization of the United Nations. The ADI is the acceptable daily intake of a chemical that, if ingested over a lifetime, appears to be without appreciable risk.

Twenty-five years of data have reported levels of pesticide residue consistently lower than the ADI. Actual pesticide intakes as determined by the Total Diet Studies are usually considerably lower than the ADI.

Antibiotics and Hormones

Subtherapeutic use of antibiotics to improve growth in food animals has been a matter of consumer concern because of the potential for the development of resistant strains of bacteria.

The Institute of Medicine of the National Academy of Sciences reported in 1989 that it was unable to find data implicating subtherapeutic amounts of antibiotics in human illness and was unable to formulate a numerical definition of risk. Except for penicillin and tetracycline, antibiotics presently added to animal feeds are not prescribed for human use.

The use of hormones in cattle feed has also been a source of concern for consumers. The use of such additives is permitted when residues do not occur in meat and milk as they arrive at the marketplace. The use of the estrogen diethylstilbestrol was discontinued when more precise analytical techniques enabled the identification of extremely small amounts in some meat products.

The use of bovine growth hormone (bovine somatotropin, BST, or gonadotropin) has resulted in sig-

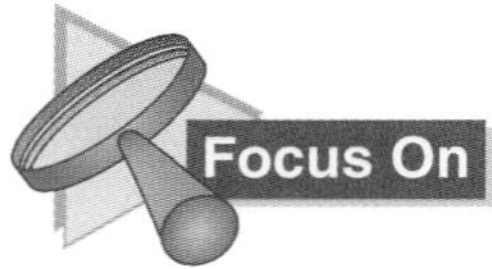

Is It Really Organic?

The popularity of organic foods has increased in recent years, in part reflecting environmental concerns as well as response to media and other pressures that have erroneously fostered lack of trust in the safety of the food supply.

Although *organic* is a somewhat ambiguous term, it generally means "free of synthetic chemicals and pesticides"and also encompasses broader concepts of environmentally sound food production (*Washington Post,* May 4, 1998). The absence of adequate definition and regulation has left the consumer without any guarantee that the produce marked *organic* is truly free of chemical additives common to modern agriculture. The grocery shopper may also be at the mercy of unscrupulous dealers who can easily substitute nonorganically grown produce without detection.

Although organically grown foods may provide psychological benefits to the user that justify the increased cost (from 20% to 100% above conventionally grown varieties), they fail to demonstrate advantages in taste, safety, or nutritive value. Pesticide residues exceed safe and acceptable levels in only 0.1% of conventionally grown foods, and then by very small margins.

Organic fertilizers may actually be a source of pathogenic bacteria. A legitimate concern of those who oppose the overuse of "chemical" fertilizers is contamination of groundwater; however, studies have shown that this is not a significant problem to date.

In December 1997, the Agricultural Marketing Service (AMS) of the USDA proposed a rule to establish a National Organic Program (NOP) under the Organic Foods Production Act of 1990. The proposed rule requires the establishment of national standards governing the marketing of certain agricultural products as "organically produced." The twofold goal is to facilitate commerce in fresh and processed food which is organically produced and to assure consumers that such products meet consistent standards.

The proposed guidelines were met with intense criticism from tens of thousands of consumers who were against various components of the proposal, which included: genetically engineered and irradiated food and crops that could be fertilized with sewage sludge; provisions for a liberal allowance for the use of antibiotics; and the use of nonorganic feed and long-term confinement of animals in the production of organic meat.

nificant increases in production of milk (by 20% to 40%) and meat (by 10% to 20%) production. Growth hormones from other species are postulated to be inactive in humans. In addition, because of its protein nature, growth hormone is inactivated and digested by enzymes in the stomach.

NUTRITIONAL PRACTICE IN THE COMMUNITY

Public health nutritionists provide medical nutrition therapy and nutrition education in community-based or public health facilities. They are employed by a wide range of employers or agencies with missions to promote health, to prevent chronic disease, or to provide primary care. To design nutrition services appropriate for a particular community, nutritionists use a wide range of data sources, guidelines, and public policies (discussed in the first section and in Chapter 15) to plan, implement, and evaluate community-based nutrition programs.

Examples of agencies that employ nutritionists in community settings include: public health agencies (state, local, or city); WIC program; elder services; long-term care facilities; community health centers; early intervention programs; Head Start; health maintenance organizations; food pantries; shelters; physician's offices; schools; and community colleges or other academic settings (Bayerl and Ries, 1995). In all of these settings, *advocacy* is a critical skill (see "*Focus On:* Legislation and Advocacy").

How an agency organizes its own nutrition services is based on the needs within the "community" in question (e.g., a nursing home, community health center, day care). The use of data as well as community input helps the health care providers to identify the areas of most concern to focus the intervention.

Nutritional problems frequently identified as a result of the assessment of nutrition indicators in the community are associated with dietary and nutritional inadequacies, excesses, or imbalances. These issues of concern (discussed in detail in other chapters) might include: risk factors for cardiovascular disease such as elevated blood cholesterol and lipids, hypertension, and stroke; diet-related cancers such as breast and colorectal cancer; obesity; diabetes; osteoporosis; teenage pregnancy; hunger and food insecurity; special health care needs in some children, including low birth weight infants.

Morbidity and mortality data on these and other illnesses are collected by the public health agency as well as other local providers such as community hospitals and health centers. This information can be particularly helpful to nutritionists in designing and implementing community-based nutrition services. The following section discusses how to assess nutrition needs and organize nutrition services within a community, and identify the types of nutrition personnel who can help address these issues.

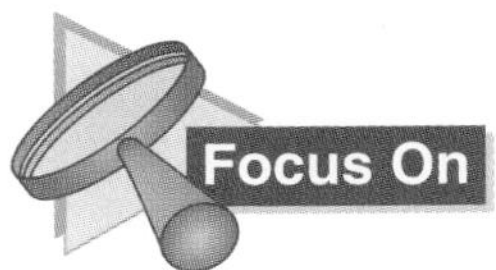

LEGISLATION AND ADVOCACY

Dietitians and other health professionals are often requested to participate in legislative activity. Many laws and regulations passed by local, state, and national officials affect the nutritional status of citizens where these health care providers work. Writing letters, serving on the work committees for a politician, donating time and money, running for office—all of these activities can favorably influence the outcomes of an election on behalf of the local community.

Many legislators do not have medical backgrounds and can benefit from visits by local dietitians or other health care professionals at their office. Encouraging students or community members who can provide honest testimony regarding the consequences of unavailable medical nutrition therapy or nutrition services can be quite influential during such a visit. Dietitians may want to invite legislators to their local agency or hospital sites to show the benefits of their work when relevant legislation is pending. Understanding how a bill becomes a law is another area where all health care providers need greater depth of knowledge. For more information, contact the American Dietetic Association at http://govaffairs@eatright.org.

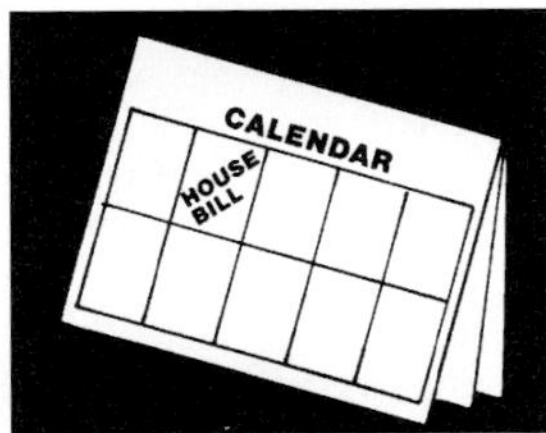

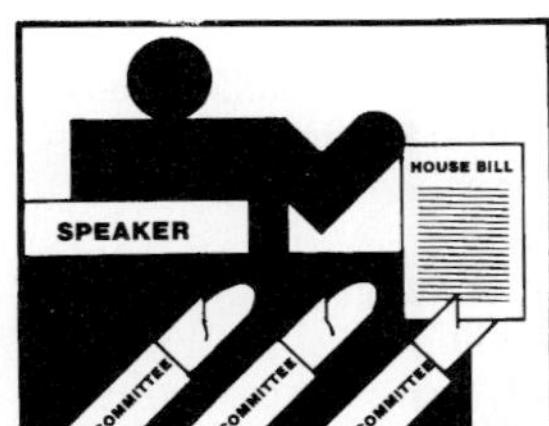

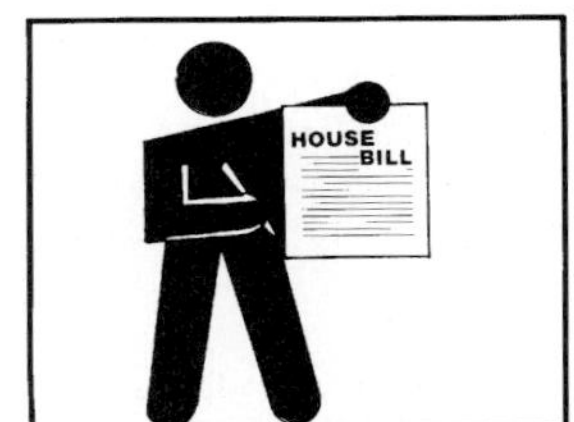

Needs Assessment for Community-Based Nutrition Services

Community generally refers to groups of people who share a common interest. In public health planning a community is usually defined by a geographical boundary. In a community-driven needs assessment process, local or state leaders and health personnel review objective health status data (e.g., numbers of low birth weight infants born in that community, deaths attributed to cancer or heart disease) as well as *subjective* observations including discussions with residents of the area or community. This is frequently referred to as a **community assessment** or *needs assessment;* the process is similar to what the business world knows as market research.

Much of the data such as number of cases of diet-related cancer gathered in this process may not relate directly to nutrition, but the experienced public health nutritionist can connect this information to nutrition- and diet-related issues. This information can be used to propose needed services, including medical nutrition therapy and nutrition counseling services as part of the strategy for improving the overall health of the community.

In addition to studying the health indicators of the community and conducting interviews with community leaders, it is important to assess the resources within that community. Persons and agencies that can help with the planning and implementation of nutrition services include: staff who provide medical nutrition therapy (screening, assessment, monitoring) within the health agency; nutrition educators; health promotion specialists who work with weight management and physical activity; agencies that enhance food security such as the Food Stamp program, food pantries and congregate meal programs; agencies that provide consumer information including homemakers skills; and the media.

The report of the Institute of Medicine, *The Future of Public Health* (Committee for the Study of Public Health, 1998), delineates the mission, roles,

TABLE 14–10 GOVERNMENT AGENCIES RELATED TO FOOD AND NUTRITION

Centers for Disease Control and Prevention
1600 Clifton Road, NE
Atlanta, GA 30333
Phone: (404) 639-3311
Internet: http://www.cdc.gov

Environmental Protection Agency
401 M Street, SW
Washington, DC 20460
Phone: (202) 260-2090
Internet: http://www.epa.gov

FDA Advisory Committees
Phone: (800) 741-8138
Food Advisory Committee x. 10564
NCTR Science Advisory Committee x. 12559
FDA Food Safety and Applied Nutrition
Phone: (800) FDA-4010

Federal Trade Commission
Public Reference
6th St. & Pennsylvania Avenue, NW
Room 130
Washington, DC 20580
Phone: (202) 326-2000
Internet: http://www.ftc.gov

Food and Agriculture Organization of the United Nations
Viale delle Terme di Caracalla,
00100 Rome,
Italy
Internet: http://www.fao.org

Food and Drug Administration
Press Office
200 C Street, SW
Washington, DC 20204
Phone: (202) 205-4144
Internet: http://www.fda.gov

National Cancer Institute
Press Office
9000 Rockville Pike
Building 31, Room 10A19
Bethesda, MD 20892-2582
Phone: (301) 496-6641
Internet: http://www.nci.nih.gov

National Health Information Center
P.O. Box 1133
Washington, DC 20013-1133
Phone: (301) 565-4167
Internet: http://www.nhic-nt.health.org

National Institutes of Health
Building 1, Room B156
1 Center Drive MSC0122
Bethesda, MD 20892-0148
Phone: (301) 496-1461
Internet: http://www.nih.gov

National Marine Fisheries Service
1315 East-West Highway
Silver Spring, MD 20910
Phone: (301) 713-2239
Internet: http://www.kingfish.ssp.nmfs.gov

U.S. Department of Agriculture Food Nutrition and Consumer Services
14th St. & Independence Avenue, SW
Room 240-E
Washington, DC 20250
Phone: (202) 720-7711
Internet: http://www.usda.gov/fcs/fcs.htm

U.S. Department of Agriculture Food Safety and Inspection Service Information and Legislative Affairs
14th St. & Independence Avenue, SW
Room 1175-South
Washington, DC 20250
Phone: (202) 720-7943
Meat and Poultry Hotline: (800) 535-4555
Internet: http://www.fsis.usda.gov

U.S. Department of Agriculture National Agricultural Library Food and Nutrition Center
National Labeling and Nutrition Information Center
10301 Baltimore Boulevard
Beltsville, MD 20705-2351
Phone: (301) 504-5719
Internet: http://www.nalusda.gov

U.S. Department of Agriculture National Agricultural Library Food and Nutrition Center
Foodborne Information and Education Information Center
10301 Baltimore Boulevard
Beltsville, MD 20705-2351
Phone: (301) 504-5414
Internet: http://www.inal.usda.gov/fnic/general

The World Health Organization
Headquarters Office in Geneva (HQ)
Avenue Appia 20
1211 Geneva 27
Switzerland
Telephone: (+41 22) 791 21 11
Facsimile (fax): (+41 22) 791 0746
Telex: 415 416
Telegraph: UNISANTE GENEVA
Internet: http://www.who.org

and responsibilities of those responsible for the public's health. The mission of public health, which is "fulfilling society's interest in assuring conditions in which people can be healthy," is addressed by public, private, and voluntary health sectors. The document identifies the three roles of public or government agencies, commonly referred to as the "core" functions of public health (community assessment, **policy development,** and **public health assurance).**

The IOM further describes various levels of government as having unique responsibilities, but it is the official state health agencies that have the primary responsibility for the three core functions. The Institute further states that those with state-level responsibility for public health nutrition must assess the capacity of their state to perform the essential functions of public health nutrition and support the attainment and monitoring of the goals and objectives of *Healthy People*.

The IOM sees the responsibility of the local health agencies as being the protection of the public's health through an effective service delivery system. The role of the federal government is to support the development and dissemination of public health knowledge, and to provide funds to strengthen the capacity to carry out the core functions. Table 14–10 lists federal agencies that are relevant to food and nutrition concern of the community.

Role of the Public Health Nutritionists

The public health/community nutritionist identifies the nutrition problems and needs within the community and proposes solutions to promote health and reduce chronic disease within that community. To do this effectively the community nutritionist must possess a range of skills including an understanding of the impact of economic, social, and political issues on health, the community, and its resources.

A national study of 7550 public health nutrition personnel by the Association of State and Territorial Public Health Nutrition Directors describes in detail the responsibilities and positions of nutritionists within public health and community nutrition as being on a *continuum,* from those who provide client-based services to those who provide population/system focused services (Haughton et al., 1998).

Client-based responsibilities are described as functions related to direct nutrition services for individuals and families, such as education, care coordination/care management, and counseling. *Population or system-focused responsibilities* are related to administration and planning for whole communities and the subpopulations within them; these responsibilities include policy-making, program planning, evaluation, and management (Gomez-Pardini, 1998).

To outline the range of skills for community nutritionists into entry and advanced level practice: the *entry level nutritionist* functions mainly as the provider of direct care nutrition services such as counseling of consumers (Fig. 14–4), educating the public, and coordinating the quality of nutrition services within the agency (Fig. 14–5).

The role of the *experienced nutritionist* combines the skills of direct care with those necessary to carry out core public functions. These skills include:

- Setting standards
- Planning
- Developing and managing services
- Implementing and evaluating services
- Ensuring quality
- Locating and maximizing resources and financing
- Providing expert consultation and educating health professional colleagues
- Participating in core functions (assessment, policy development, assurance)
- Advocating for nutrition services with state and national legislators (Fig. 14–5)
- Informing decision and policy makers of nutrition service needs
- Coordinating with other agencies.

Public health nutrition offers many exciting opportunities for employment. Many of these opportunities are based on cutting-edge studies of diet

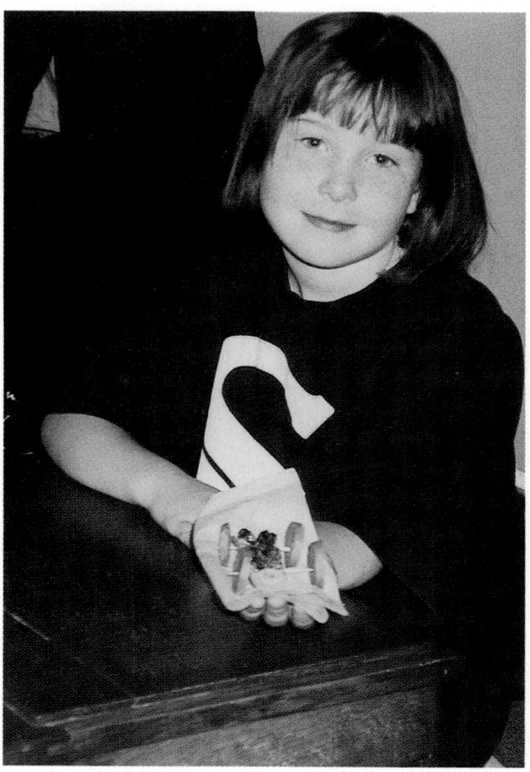

FIGURE 14–4 Community health fair—fun with Five-A-Day.

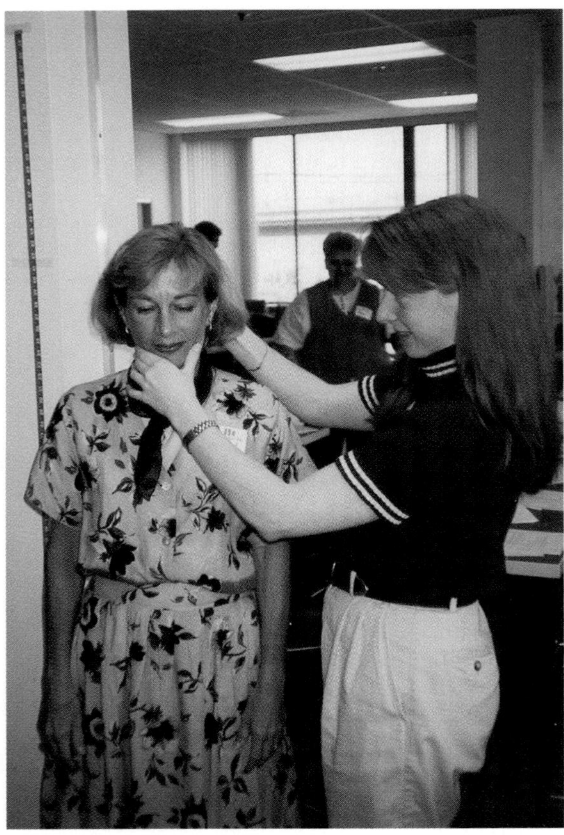

FIGURE 14–5 Primary care nutritionists learning state of the art anthropometric techniques as part of quality assurance.

CASE STUDY

Mrs. Ex has requested your help with better nutrition and reading food labels. She has type II diabetes and lives alone. She was recently screened using the Nutrition Screening Initiative Level 1 Checklist. Because she lives alone, she frequently has only toast or cereal and fruit juice for breakfast and does not seem to understand her diabetic diet. Mrs. Ex is worried as she has become more housebound due to decreased circulation in her legs, which places her into a high-risk category.

Mrs. Ex wants to choose foods that are appropriate for a diabetic diet and are easy to prepare. Because she is living alone, she needs your help to locate community resources. She has a limited income and food budget.

1. What suggestions do you have for Mrs. Ex as she reads labels and shops? Remember that her income is limited and she is relatively housebound.
2. Prepare a day's menu including three easy to prepare meals and two snacks that would be appropriate for a person on a "no concentrated sweets" diabetic diet.
3. What resources are available to Mrs. Ex in her community? Consider issues related to food and water safety, budgeting assistance, and food assistance.

and physical activity and their role in extending disease-free life (ADA, 1998b). Dietitians should participate by assisting with health promotion, research, and education programs for public awareness.

CITED REFERENCES

American Dietetic Association. Final food labeling regulations. J Am Diet Assoc 93:146, 1993.

American Dietetic Association. How are Americans making food choices? J Am Diet Assoc 94:597, 1994.

American Dietetic Association. Position of the American Dietetic Association: Phytochemicals and functional foods. J Am Diet Assoc 99:496, 1999.

American Dietetic Association. Position of the American Dietetic Association: Food irradiation. J Am Diet Assoc 96:69, 1996.

American Dietetic Association. Position of the American Dietetic Association: Domestic food and nutrition security. J Am Diet Assoc 98:337, 1998a.

American Dietetic Association. Position of the American Dietetic Association: The role of nutrition in health promotion and disease prevention programs. J Am Diet Assoc 98:205, 1998b.

Bayerl C, Ries J. EARLY START: Nutrition Services in Early Intervention. Boston: Massachusetts Department of Public Health, 1995.

Carroll MD, et al. Dietary Intake Source Data: United States, 1976–80. Vital and Health Statistics, Series 11, No. 231 (DHHS Publ No (PHS) 83-1681). Hyattsville, MD: National Center for Health Statistics, 1983.

Canadian National Institute of Nutrition. Rapport 8(4):1993, p. 1.

Committee on Diet, Nutrition and Cancer, National Research Council. Diet, nutrition and cancer. Washington, DC: National Academy Press, 1982.

Committee for the Study of Public Health. Institute of Medicine. A vision of public health in America: An attainable level. The Future of Public Health. Washington, DC: National Academy Press, 1998, p. 35–55.

Cross A, et al. Snacking patterns among 1800 adults and children. J Am Diet Assoc 94:1398, 1994.

Dollahite J, et al. Problems encountered in meeting the Recommended Dietary Allowances for menus designed according to the Dietary Guidelines for Americans. J Am Diet Assoc 95:341, 1995.

FANSA statement of dietary supplement labeling. J Am Diet Assoc 97:728, 1997.

Food and Nutrition Board, National Research Council, NAS. Recommended Dietary Allowances, 10th ed. Washington, DC: National Academy Press, 1989.

Geiger C. Health claims: History, current regulatory status, and consumer research. J Am Diet Assoc 98:1312, 1998.

Gomez-Pardini L. Community nutrition. In: King-Helm K, Samour P (eds.). Handbook of Pediatric Nutrition. Gaitherburg, MD: Aspen Publishers, 1998.

Greger JL. Food, supplements, and fortified foods: Scientific evaluations in regard to toxicology and nutrient bioavailability. J Am Diet Assoc 87:1369, 1987.

Haughton B, et al. Profile of public health nutrition personnel: Challenges for population/systems-focused roles and state-level monitoring. J Am Diet Assoc 98:664, 1998.

Healthy People. The Surgeon General's Report on Health Promotion and Disease Prevention. Washington, DC: U.S. Department of Health and Human Services, 1979.

Healthy People 2000: National Health Promotion and Disease Prevention Objectives. Washington, DC: U.S. Department of Health and Human Services, 1990.

Human Nutrition Information Service, U.S. Department of Agriculture. USDA's Food Guide Pyramid. Home Garden Bulletin 249. Washington, DC: U.S. Government Printing Office, 1992.

Hunt J. Nutritional products for specific health benefits–foods, pharmaceuticals, or something in between? J Am Diet Assoc 94:152, 1994.

Interagency Board for Nutrition Monitoring and Related Research. Third report on nutrition monitoring in the United States: Executive summary. Washington, DC: U.S. Government Printing Office, 1995.

International Food Information Council Foundation, http://ificinfo.health.org, 1998.

Joint Nutrition Monitoring Evaluation Committee Report—May, 1986. Nutritional status of the U.S. population. Nutrition Today 21(3):23, 1986.

Kant A, et al. Dietary diversity and subsequent mortality in the first NHANES epidemiological follow-up study. Am J Clin Nutr 57:434, 1993.

Kant A, Schtzkin A. Consumption of energy-dense, nutrient-poor foods by the US population: Effect on nutrient profiles. J Am Coll Nutr 13:285, 1994.

Kendall A, et al. Relationship of hunger and food insecurity to food availability and consumption. J Am Diet Assoc 96:1019, 1996.

Kuczmarski M, et al. Update on nutrition monitoring activities in the United States. J Am Diet Assoc 94:753, 1994.

McGinnis J, Lee P. Healthy People 2000 at mid decade. JAMA 273:1123, 1995.

National Center for Health Statistics. Health and Nutrition Examination Survey, 1971–74. Vital and Health Statistics, Series II, No 202 (DHEW Publ No [HRA] 77-1647). Rockville, MD: Health Resources Administration, Public Health Service, 1977.

National Cholesterol Education Program. Report of the Expert Panel on Detection, Evaluation, and Treatment of High Blood Cholesterol in Adults. NIH Publ No 88-2925, NHLBI, USDHHS, Public Health Service. Bethesda, MD: National Institutes of Health, 1988.

Nutrition and Your Health. Dietary guidelines for Americans. Home and Garden Bulletin No 232. Washington, DC: USDA and USDHHS, 1980.

Nutrition and Your Health. Dietary guidelines for Americans, 3rd ed. Home and Garden Bulletin No 232. Washington, DC: USDA and USDHHS, 1990.

Nutrition Monitoring Division, Human Nutrition Information Service. USDA nationwide food consumption survey: Continuing survey of food intakes by individuals—1985. Nutrition Today 21(3):18, 1986.

Nutrition Monitoring Division, Human Nutrition Information Service. USDA nationwide food consumption survey: Continuing survey of food intakes by individuals—1986. Nutrition Today 22(5):36, 1987.

Nutrition Monitoring Division, Human Nutrition Information Service. USDA nationwide food consumption survey: Continuing survey of food intakes by individuals—1986. Nutrition Today 24(5):35, 1989.

Ostenso G. Nutrition—policies and politics. J Am Diet Assoc 88:833, 1988.

Pennington J, Hubbard V. Derivation of daily values used for nutrition labeling. J Am Diet Assoc 97:1407, 1997.

Promoting Health/Preventing Disease. Objectives for the nation. Washington, DC: USDHHS, 1980.

Pszczola D. The nutraceutical initiative: A proposal for regulatory reform. Food Technology 46:77, 1992.

Senate Select Committee on Nutrition and Human Needs. Dietary goals for the United States. Publ No 052-070-03913-2. Washington, DC: U.S. Government Printing Office, 1977.

Senate Select Committee on Nutrition and Human Needs. Dietary goals for the United States, 2nd ed. Publ No 052-070-04376-8. Washington, DC: U.S. Government Printing Office, 1978.

Sims L. Research aspects of public policy in nutrition generating research questions to determine the impact of nutritional, agricultural and health care policy and regulation on the health and nutrition status of the public. The Research Agenda for Dietetics Conference Proceedings. Chicago: The American Dietetic Association, 1993.

Sloan, A. Food industry forecast: Consumer trends to 2020 and beyond. Food Technology 52:37, 1998.

Stephenson M, Guthrie H. Positions of the American Dietetic Association: Enrichment and fortification of foods and dietary supplements. J Am Diet Assoc 94:661, 1994.

Tauxe, R. Emerging foodborne diseases: An evolving public health challenge. Emerg Infect Dis 3(4):1, 1997.

The Surgeon General's Report on Nutrition and Health. Summary and recommendations. USDHHS (PHS) Publ No 88-50211. Washington, DC: U.S. Government Printing Office, 1988.

U.S. Department of Agriculture. Nationwide food consumption survey. Continuing survey of food intakes by individuals: Women 19–50 years and their children 1–5 years, 1 Day. Report No 85-1. Hyattsville, MD: Author, 1985.

U.S. Department of Agriculture. Continuing survey of food intakes by individuals, 1994–96. Beltsville, MD: Author, 1998.

U.S. Department of Agriculture. Nutrition program facts. http:www.usda.gov, 1999.

U.S. Department of Health and Human Services. Eat more fruits and vegetables: 5-a-day for better health. NIH Publ No 92-3248. Washington, DC: Public Health Service and National Institutes of Health, 1991.

Winslow CEA. The untilled field of public health. Modern Medicine 2:183, 1920.

Woteki C. Nutrition monitoring research. Research Agenda Conference Proceedings. Chicago: American Dietetic Association, May 14–15, 1992, p 42.

Woteki CE, et al. National Health and Nutrition Examination Survey—NHANES. Plans for NHANES III. Nutrition Today 23(1):25, 1988.

ADDITIONAL REFERENCES

Albright C, et al. Development of a curriculum to lower dietary fat intake in a multi-ethnic population with low literacy skills. J Nutr Ed 29:215, July/August 1997.

American Dietetic Association: Food labeling: Definition of the term "healthy." J Am Diet Assoc 93:404, 1993.

American Dietetic Association. Position of the American Dietetic Association: Food and water safety. J Am Diet Assoc 97:184, 1997.

Dodds JM, Kaufman M (eds.). Personnel in Public Health Nutrition for the 1990's. Washington, DC: The Public Health Foundation, 1991.

Egan M. Public health nutrition: A historical perspective. J Am Diet Assoc 94:298, 1994.

FIGHT BAC™: Keep food safe from bacteria. A National Public Education Campaign to Reduce the Risk of Foodborne Illness. Partnership for Food Safety Education. Washington, DC: USDA, 1998.

Gilmore CJ, et al. Determining educational preparation based on job competencies of entry-level dietetic practitioners. J Am Diet Assoc 97:305, 1997.

Haughton B, et al. An historical study of the underlying assumptions for U.S. food guides from 1917 through the Basic Four Food Group Guide. J Nutr Educ 19:169, 1987.

Hess AN, Haughton B. Continuing education needs for public health nutritionists. J Am Diet Assoc 96:716, 1996.

Kaufman M. Nutrition in public health: A handbook for developing programs and services. Rockville, MD: Aspen Publishers, 1990.

Kim S. Dietetics professionals and women's health research at the National Institutes of Health. J Am Diet Assoc 98:133, 1998.

Miller CA, et al. A proposed method for assessing the performance of local public health functions and practices. Am J Public Health 84:1743, 1994.

Olmstead-Schafer M, et al. Future training needs in public health nutrition: Results of a national Delphi survey. J Am Diet Assoc 96:282, 1996.

Pelletier DL, Habicht J-P. Continuing needs for food consumption data for public health policy. J Nutr 124:1846S, 1994.

Probert KL (ed.). Moving to the Future: Developing Community-Based Nutrition Services. Washington, DC: Association of State and Territorial Public Health Nutrition Directors, 1996.

Short S. Health quackery: Our role as professionals. J Am Diet Assoc 94:607, 1994.

Turnock BJ, et al. Local health department effectiveness in addressing the core functions of public health. Public Health Rep 109:653, 1994.

CHAPTER 15

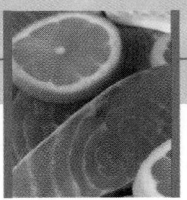

Guidelines for Dietary Planning

ROBERT EARL, MPH, RD AND SUSAN T. BORRA, RD

CHAPTER OUTLINE

- Determining Nutrient Needs
- Nutritional Status of Americans
- National Guidelines for Diet Planning
- Implementing the Guidelines
- Food Labeling
- Cultural Aspects of Dietary Planning

Key Terms

ADEQUATE INTAKE (AI)—recommended daily intake level based on observed or experimentally determined approximations of nutrient intake by a group (or groups) of healthy people; these nutrient recommendations are used when a recommended dietary allowance (RDA) cannot be determined

DAILY REFERENCE VALUES (DRVs)—a set of dietary references for food labels consisting of nutrients (except for protein) for which no set of standards previously existed; DRVs have been set for fat, saturated fatty acids, cholesterol, total carbohydrate, protein, fiber, sodium, and potassium

DAILY VALUE (DV)—dietary reference term on food labels to aid consumers in selecting a healthy diet, consisting of two sets of references, the RDIs and DRVs

DIETARY GUIDELINES FOR AMERICANS—dietary recommendations for healthy Americans age 2 years and over about food choices that promote health specifically with respect to prevention or delay of chronic diseases

DIETARY REFERENCE INTAKE (DRI)—an umbrella term designed to encompass the four specific types of nutrient recommendations featured in the DRIs (AI, EAR, RDA, and UL); the DRI will be used for nutrient recommendations for the United States and Canada

ESTIMATED AVERAGE REQUIREMENT (EAR)—nutrient intake value that is estimated to meet the requirement of half the healthy individuals in a group

ESTIMATED SAFE AND ADEQUATE DAILY DIETARY INTAKES (ESADDIs)—recommended ranges of appropriate intake of those nutrients for which not enough information is available to establish an RDA

FOOD GUIDE PYRAMID—translates the RDAs and the dietary guidelines into the kinds and amounts of food to eat each day

FOOD INSECURITY—hunger from having inadequate and insufficient access to food on a daily basis

HEALTH CLAIM—any claim on a package label or other labeling (such as an advertisement) of a food, including fish and game meats, that characterizes the relationship of any nutrient or other substance in the food to a disease or health-related condition

HEALTHY EATING INDEX (HEI)—summary measure of overall diet quality; designed to access and monitor the dietary status of Americans

NUTRITION FACTS LABEL—nutrient content information on food products designed to help consumers select foods to incorporate into a healthful diet using the food guide pyramid and the dietary guidelines

RECOMMENDED DIETARY ALLOWANCES (RDAs)—the amount of a nutrient needed to meet the requirements of nearly all (97% to 98%) of the healthy population

RECOMMENDED NUTRIENT INTAKES (RNIs)—the Canadian RDA. To be replaced by the joint U.S./Canada DRI grouping of nutrient recommendations

REFERENCE DAILY INTAKES (RDIs)—set of dietary references for food labels based on the 1968 RDAs for vitamins and minerals, this term replaces the U.S. RDA previously used with nutrition labeling on food products

TOLERABLE UPPER INTAKE LEVEL (UL)—the maximum level of daily nutrient intake that is unlikely to impose risks of adverse health effects to almost all of the individuals in the general population

This chapter is a revision of a chapter, contributed by Paul R. Thomas, EdD, RD, that appeared in the previous edition.

An appropriate diet is one that is both adequate and balanced and recognizes individual variations, such as age and stage of development, taste preferences, and food habits. It also reflects the availability of foods, socioeconomic conditions, storage and preparation facilities, and cooking skills. An adequate and balanced diet is one that meets all the nutritional needs of an individual for maintenance, repair, the living processes, and growth or development. It includes energy and all nutrients in proper amounts and proportion to each other. The presence or absence of one essential nutrient may affect the availability, absorption, metabolism, or dietary need for others. The increasing recognition of nutrient interrelationships provides further support for the principle of maintaining variety in foods to provide the most complete diet.

With increasing knowledge of the links between diet and disease (such as heart disease, some forms of cancer, osteoporosis and type II diabetes) that lead to premature disability and mortality among Americans, an appropriate diet is now considered also to be one that helps reduce the risk of developing chronic degenerative diseases and conditions.

DETERMINING NUTRIENT NEEDS

A number of standards serve as guides for planning and evaluating diets and food supplies for individuals and population groups. Many countries have issued guidelines appropriate to their individual circumstances. The Food and Agriculture Organization and the World Health Organization of the United Nations have established international standards in many areas of food quality, safety, and dietary recommendations. In the United States, the Food and Nutrition Board (FNB) of the Institute of Medicine, National Academy of Sciences (IOM/NAS) has led the development of nutrient recommendations since the 1940s. The U.S. Departments of Agriculture (USDA) and Health and Human Services (DHHS) have shared responsibility for dietary recommendations, food composition data, and nutrition information on food packages, to name a few.

Dietary Reference Intakes (Formerly Recommended Dietary Allowances)

The basic American standards for nutrient recommendations were the **recommended dietary allowances (RDAs),** established by the FNB of the IOM/NAS, first published in 1941 and most recently revised in 1989 (Food and Nutrition Board, 1989, 1994) (Table 15–1). Each revision incorporated the most recent research findings (Institute of Medicine, 1997, 1998) (see http://www2.nas.edu/fnb).

In 1993, the FNB convened a symposium to ask the question, "Should the Recommended Dietary Allowances Be Revised?" (Food and Nutrition Board, 1994). From that symposium, the FNB developed a framework for the development of future nutrient recommendations, **dietary reference intakes (DRIs).** The DRI is an umbrella term that encompasses four types of nutrient recommendations for healthy individuals—adequate intake (AI), estimated average intake (EAR), recommended dietary allowance (RDA), and tolerable upper intake level (UL). Over the next several years, the FNB's DRI committee will oversee the development of reports on interpretation and uses of DRIs, upper reference levels of nutrients, and seven groupings of related nutrients. Two reports have been completed—calcium and related nutrients, and folate and other B vitamins (Table 15–2). Reports of the subcommittees on interpretation and uses of DRIs and dietary antioxidants are in progress (Fig. 15–1).

Until all of the DRI subcommittee reports are completed, the existing RDA for a nutrient or food component not redefined by a new DRI will be retained. Thus, nutrition professionals will need to use both RDAs and DRIs for the next several years and stay abreast of new DRIs as reports are published.

Background

As scientific knowledge about diet and health has increased, technology has improved to allow measurement of small changes in individual adaptation to consumption of various levels of nutrients (Yates, 1998; Yates and Schlicker, 1998). The DRI model expands the earlier RDA, which focused on establishing adequate intakes of nutrients for healthy populations to prevent deficiency diseases. To respond to scientific advances in diet and health across the life cycle, the DRI model now includes four reference points.

The **adequate intake (AI)** is a nutrient recommendation based on observed or experimentally determined approximation of nutrient intake by a group (or groups) of healthy people when sufficient scientific evidence is not available to calculate an RDA or an EAR.

The **estimated average requirement (EAR)** is the average requirement of a nutrient for healthy individuals in which a functional or clinical assessment has been conducted and measures of adequacy have been made at a specified level of dietary intake. An EAR is the amount of intake of a nutrient at which about one half of subjects would have their needs met and one half would not. The EAR should be used for assessing nutrient adequacy of populations, *not* individuals.

The new RDA is the amount of a nutrient needed to meet the requirements of nearly all (97% to 98%) of the healthy population of individuals for whom it is developed. An RDA for a nutrient should serve as a goal for intake for individuals, *not* as a benchmark of adequacy of diets of populations.

Because of increased consumption of nutrients in concentrated form, either singly or in combination with others outside of the context of food, or from

TABLE 15–1 FOOD AND NUTRITION BOARD, NATIONAL ACADEMY OF SCIENCES—NATIONAL RESEARCH COUNCIL RECOMMENDED DIETARY ALLOWANCES,[a] Revised 1989 (Abridged) ***(Designed for the maintenance of good nutrition of practically all healthy people in the United States)***

CATEGORY	AGE (YRS) OR CONDITION	WEIGHT[b] (kg)	WEIGHT[b] (lb)	HEIGHT[b] (cm)	HEIGHT[b] (in)	PROTEIN (g)	VITAMIN A (μg RE)[c]	VITAMIN E (mg α-TE)[d]	VITAMIN K (μg)	VITAMIN C (mg)	IRON (mg)	ZINC (mg)	IODINE (μg)	SELENIUM (μg)
Infants	0.0–0.5	6	13	60	24	13	375	3	5	30	6	5	40	10
	0.5–1.0	9	20	71	28	14	375	4	10	35	10	5	50	15
Children	1–3	13	29	90	35	16	400	6	15	40	10	10	70	20
	4–6	20	44	112	44	24	500	7	20	45	10	10	90	20
	7–10	28	62	132	52	28	700	7	30	45	10	10	120	30
Males	11–14	45	99	157	62	45	1,000	10	45	50	12	15	150	40
	15–18	66	145	176	69	59	1,000	10	65	60	12	15	150	50
	19–24	72	160	177	70	58	1,000	10	70	60	10	15	150	70
	25–50	79	174	176	70	63	1,000	10	80	60	10	15	150	70
	51+	77	170	173	68	63	1,000	10	80	60	10	15	150	70
Females	11–14	46	101	157	62	46	800	8	45	50	15	12	150	45
	15–18	55	120	163	64	44	800	8	55	60	15	12	150	50
	19–24	58	128	164	65	46	800	8	60	60	15	12	150	55
	25–50	63	138	163	64	50	800	8	65	60	15	12	150	55
	51+	65	143	160	63	50	800	8	65	60	10	12	150	55
Pregnant						60	800	10	65	70	30	15	175	65
Lactating	1st 6 months					65	1,300	12	65	95	15	19	200	75
	2nd 6 months					62	1,200	11	65	90	15	16	200	75

Note: This table does not include nutrients for which Dietary Reference Intakes have recently been established (see *Dietary Reference Intakes for Calcium, Phosphorus, Magnesium, Vitamin D, and Fluoride* [1997] and *Dietary Reference Intakes for Thiamin, Riboflavin, Niacin, Vitamin* B_6*, Folate, Vitamin* B_{12}*, Pantothenic Acid, Biotin, and Choline* [1998]).

[a]The allowances, expressed as average daily intakes over time, are intended to provide for individual variations among most normal persons as they live in the United States under usual environmental stresses. Diets should be based on a variety of common foods in order to provide other nutrients for which human requirements have been less well defined.

[b]Weights and heights of Reference Adults are actual medians for the U.S. population of the designated age, as reported by NHANES II. The use of these figures does not imply that the height-to-weight ratios are ideal.

[c]Retinol equivalents. 1 retinol equivalent = 1 μg retinol or 6 μg β-carotene.

[d]α-Tocopherol equivalents. 1 mg d-α tocopherol = 1 α-TE.

TABLE 15–2 FOOD AND NUTRITION BOARD, INSTITUTE OF MEDICINE—NATIONAL ACADEMY OF SCIENCES DIETARY REFERENCE INTAKES: RECOMMENDED INTAKES FOR INDIVIDUALS

LIFE-STAGE GROUP	CALCIUM (mg/d)	PHOSPHORUS (mg/d)	MAGNESIUM (mg/d)	VITAMIN D (μg/d)[a,b]	FLOURIDE (mg/d)	THIAMIN (mg/d)	RIBOFLAVIN (mg/d)	NIACIN (mg/d)[c]	VITAMIN B_6 (mg/d)	FOLATE (μg/d)[d]	VITAMIN B_{12} (μg/d)	PANTOTHENIC ACID (mg/d)	BIOTIN (μg/d)	CHOLINE[e] (mg/d)
Infants														
0–6 mo	210*	100*	30*	5*	0.01*	0.2*	0.3*	2*	0.1*	65*	0.4*	1.7*	5*	125*
7–12 mo	270*	275*	75*	5*	0.5*	0.3*	0.4*	4*	0.3*	80*	0.5*	1.8*	6*	150*
Children														
1–3 yr	500*	**460**	**80**	5*	0.7*	**0.5**	**0.5**	**6**	**0.5**	**150**	**0.9**	2*	8*	200*
4–8 yr	800*	**500**	**130**	5*	1*	**0.6**	**0.6**	**8**	**0.6**	**200**	**1.2**	3*	12*	250*
Males														
9–13 yr	1,300*	**1.250**	**240**	5*	2*	**0.9**	**0.9**	**12**	**1.0**	**300**	**1.8**	4*	20*	375*
14–18 yr	1,300*	**1,250**	**410**	5*	3*	**1.2**	**1.3**	**16**	**1.3**	**400**	**2.4**	5*	25*	550*
19–30 yr	1,000*	**700**	**400**	5*	4*	**1.2**	**1.3**	**16**	**1.3**	**400**	**2.4**	5*	30*	550*
31–50 yr	1,000*	**700**	**420**	5*	4*	**1.2**	**1.3**	**16**	**1.3**	**400**	**2.4**	5*	30*	550*
51–70 yr	1,200*	**700**	**420**	10*	4*	**1.2**	**1.3**	**16**	**1.7**	**400**	**2.4**[f]	5*	30*	550*
> 70 yr	1,200*	**700**	**420**	15*	4*	**1.2**	**1.3**	**16**	**1.7**	**400**	**2.4**[f]	5*	30*	550*
Females														
9–13 yr	1,300*	**1,250**	**240**	5*	2*	**0.9**	**0.9**	**12**	**1.0**	**300**	**1.8**	4*	20*	375*
14–18 yr	1,300*	**1,250**	**360**	5*	3*	**1.0**	**1.0**	**14**	**1.2**	**400**[g]	**2.4**	5*	25*	400*
19–30 yr	1,000*	**700**	**310**	5*	3*	**1.1**	**1.1**	**14**	**1.3**	**400**[g]	**2.4**	5*	30*	425*
31–50 yr	1,000*	**700**	**320**	5*	3*	**1.1**	**1.1**	**14**	**1.3**	**400**[g]	**2.4**	5*	30*	425*
51–70 yr	1,200*	**700**	**320**	10*	3*	**1.1**	**1.1**	**14**	**1.5**	**400**	**2.4**[f]	5*	30*	425*
> 70 yr	1,200*	**700**	**320**	15*	3*	**1.1**	**1.1**	**14**	**1.5**	**400**	**2.4**[f]	5*	30*	425*
Pregnancy														
≤ 18 yr	1,300*	**1.250**	**400**	5*	3*	**1.4**	**1.4**	**18**	**1.9**	**600**[h]	**2.6**	6*	30*	450*
19–30 yr	1,000*	**700**	**350**	5*	3*	**1.4**	**1.4**	**18**	**1.9**	**600**[h]	**2.6**	6*	30*	450*
31–50 yr	1,000*	**700**	**360**	5*	3*	**1.4**	**1.4**	**18**	**1.9**	**600**[h]	**2.6**	6*	30*	450*
Lactation														
≤ 18 yr	1,300*	**1,250**	**360**	5*	3*	**1.5**	**1.6**	**17**	**2.0**	**500**	**2.8**	7*	35*	550*
19–30 yr	1,000*	**700**	**310**	5*	3*	**1.5**	**1.6**	**17**	**2.0**	**500**	**2.8**	7*	35*	550*
31–50 yr	1,000*	**700**	**320**	5*	3*	**1.5**	**1.6**	**17**	**2.0**	**500**	**2.8**	7*	35*	550*

Note: This table presents Recommended Dietary Allowances (RDAs) in bold type and Adequate Intakes (AIs) in ordinary type followed by an asterisk (*). RDAs and AIs may both be used as goals for individual intake. RDAs are set to meet the needs of almost all (97 or 98 percent) individuals in a group. For healthy breastfed infants, the AI is the mean intake. The AI for other life-stage and gender groups is believed to cover needs of all individuals in the group, but lack of data or uncertainty in the data prevent being able to specify with confidence the percentage of individuals covered by this intake.

[a]As cholecalciferol. 1μg cholecalciferol = 40 IU vitamin D.

[b]In the absence of adequate exposure to sunlight.

[c]As niacin equivalents (NE). 1 mg of niacin = 60 mg of tryptophan; 0–6 months = preformed niacin (not NE).

[d]As dietary folate equivalents (DFE). 1 DFE = 1 μg food folate = 0.6 μg of folic acid (from fortified food or supplement) consumed with food = 0.5 μg of synthetic (supplemental) folic acid taken on an empty stomach.

[e]Although AIs have been set for choline, there are few data to assess whether a dietary supply of choline is needed at all stages of the life cycle, and it may be that the choline requirement can be met by endogenous synthesis at some of these stages.

[f]Because 10% to 30% of older people may malabsorb food-bound B_{12}, it is advisable for those older than 50 years to meet their RDA mainly by consuming foods fortified with B_{12} or a supplement containing B_{12}.

[g]In view of evidence linking folate intake with neural tube defects in the fetus, it is recommended that all women capable of becoming pregnant consume 400 μg of synthetic folic acid from fortified foods and/or supplements in addition to intake of food folate from a varied diet.

[h]It is assumed that women will continue consuming 400 μg of folic acid until their pregnancy is confirmed and they enter prenatal care, which ordinarily occurs after the end of the periconceptional period—the critical time for formation of the neural tube.

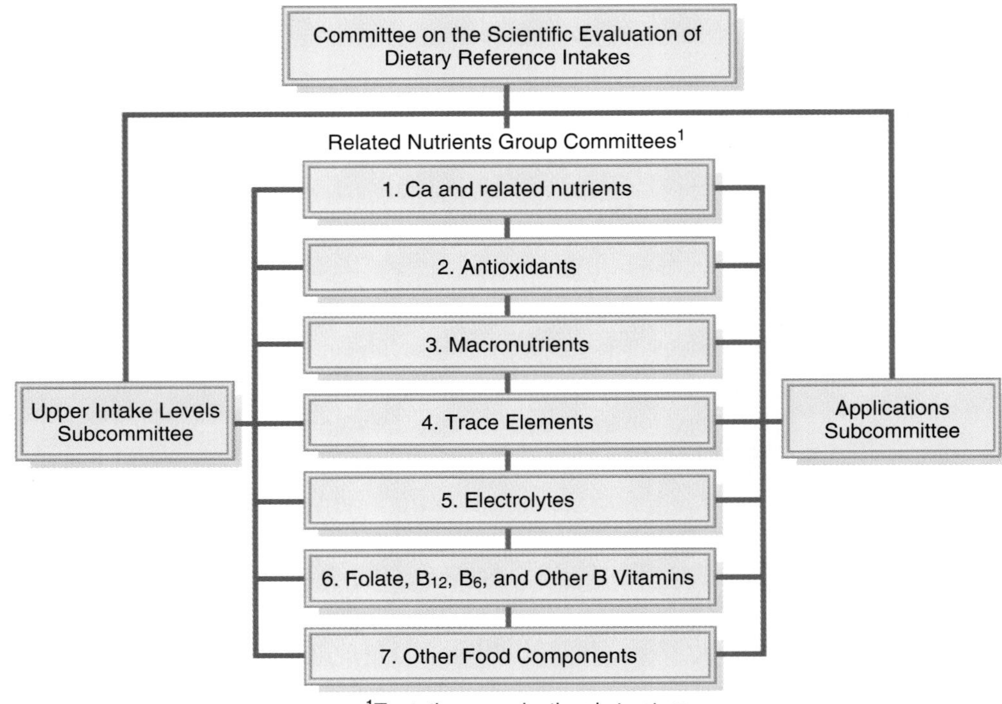

FIGURE 15–1 The organizational structure of the working subcommittee on science evaluation of dietary reference intakes.

enrichment and fortification, **tolerable upper intake levels (ULs)** will be established where adequate data are available to reduce the risk of adverse or toxic effects. A UL will be set as the maximum level of intake of a nutrient that will not cause adverse effects to almost all of the population ingesting that amount.

Target Population for DRI Recommendations

Each of the nutrient recommendation categories under the emerging DRI system is used for specific purposes among individuals or populations. The EAR is used for evaluating nutrient intake of populations. The new RDA can be used for individuals. Nutrient intakes between the RDA and the UL may further define intake that may promote health or prevent disease.

Age-Gender Groups

Because needs for nutrients are highly individualized depending on age, sexual development, and the reproductive status of women, the RDAs were listed for 15 groups based on age and gender. Beyond 10 years of age, they were divided according to gender. Recommendations for pregnancy and lactation were also included. The new DRI framework expands the age groupings to 16, adding age groupings for 51 to 70 years of age, and 70 years of age and older. It also expands the age groupings for pregnancy and lactation to three categories of each.

Reference Men and Women

Because the requirement for many nutrients is based on body weight, the RDAs are listed in terms of *reference men* and *women* of designated height and weight. These values for age-sex groups over 19 years of age are based on actual medians obtained for the American population by the third National Health and Nutrition Examination Survey (NHANES III), 1988 to 1994. Although this does not necessarily imply that these weight-for-height values are ideal, at least they make it possible to define recommended allowances appropriate for the largest number of people. Recommended energy intakes for median heights and weights are shown in Table 15–3.

Estimated Safe and Adequate Daily Dietary Intakes

A number of nutrients are known to be essential to life and health, but available data are insufficient to establish a recommended intake. These are listed as **estimated safe and adequate daily dietary intakes (ESADDIs)** in Table 15–4. Most intakes are shown as ranges, to indicate not only that spe-

TABLE 15–3 REFERENCE HEIGHTS AND WEIGHTS FOR CHILDREN AND ADULTS IN THE UNITED STATES[a]

GENDER	AGE	MEDIAN BODY MASS INDEX (kg/m^2)	REFERENCE HEIGHT (cm [in])	REFERENCE WEIGHT[b] (kg [lb])
Male, female	2–6 mo	—	64 (25)	7 (16)
	7–11 mo	—	72 (28)	9 (20)
	1–3 yr	—	91 (36)	13 (29)
	4–8 yr	15.8	118 (46)	22 (48)
Male	9–13 yr	18.5	147 (58)	40 (88)
	14–18 yr	21.3	174 (68)	64 (142)
	19–30 yr	24.4	176 (69)	76 (166)
Female	9–13 yr	18.3	148 (58)	40 (88)
	14–18 yr	21.3	163 (64)	57 (125)
	19–30 yr	22.8	163 (64)	61 (133)

[a]Based on data from the Third National Health and Nutrition Examination Survey, 1988–1994 (Briefel R., U.S. Department of Health and Human Services, 1997, personal communication).

[b]Calculated from median body mass index and median heights for ages 4–8 yr and older.

(From Institute of Medicine, 1998.)

TABLE 15–5 ESTIMATED SODIUM, CHLORIDE, AND POTASSIUM MINIMUM REQUIREMENTS OF HEALTHY PERSONS[†]

AGE	WEIGHT (kg)	SODIUM (mg)[†‡]	CHLORIDE (mg)[†‡]	POTASSIUM (mg)[§]
Months				
0–5	4.5	120	180	500
6–11	8.9	200	300	700
Years				
1	11.0	225	350	1000
2–5	16.0	300	500	1400
6–9	25.0	400	600	1600
10–18	50.0	500	750	2000
> 18[‖]	70.0	500	750	2000

(Reprinted with permission from Recommended Dietary Allowances, 10th ed., © 1989 by the National Academy of Sciences. Published by National Academy Press.)

[†]No allowance has been included for large, prolonged losses from the skin through sweat.

[‡]There is no evidence that higher intakes confer any health benefits.

[§]Desirable intakes of potassium may considerably exceed these values (~3500 mg for adults).

[‖]No allowance included for growth. Values for those below 18 years assume a growth rate at the 50th percentile reported by the National Center for Health Statistics and averaged for males and females.

cific recommendations are not justified at this time but also that at least the upper and lower limits of safety should be observed. Safe and adequate ranges for sodium, potassium, and chloride have not been included because "they are difficult to justify" (Food and Nutrition Board, 1989). Estimated minimum requirements for these electrolytes are listed in Table 15–5.

Interpretation and Uses of DRIs

Although each report of new DRIs for groupings of nutrients will contain recommendations for interpretation and uses, a separate DRI subcommittee will expand on the interpretation of new terms and concepts integral to the overall project and provide guidance for their use in dietary assessment and planning diets. These include dietary data assessment, food and nutrition assistance programs standards and evaluation, nutrition education programs and food guides, food labeling, food fortification, and medical nutrition therapy.

NUTRITIONAL STATUS OF AMERICANS

Food and Nutrient Intake Data

Twenty-two federal agencies collect information about the dietary and nutritional status of Americans and the relationship between diet and health. This effort is coordinated by the USDA and DHHS, through the National Nutrition Monitoring and Related Research Program (NNMRRP) (Haas and McGinnis, 1993). The NHANES and the Continuing Survey of Food Intakes of Individuals (CSFII) serve as the cornerstone surveys of the NNMRRP. (See Chapter 14 for a discussion of these surveys and http://www.cdc.gov/nchswww.)

TABLE 15–4 ESTIMATED SAFE AND ADEQUATE DAILY DIETARY INTAKES OF SELECTED TRACE ELEMENTS*

CATEGORY	AGE (yr)	COPPER (mg)	MANGANESE (mg)	CHROMIUM (μg)	MOLYBDENUM (μg)
Infants	0–0.5	0.4–0.6	0.3–0.6	10–40	15–30
	0.5–1	0.6–0.7	0.6–1.0	20–60	20–40
Children and adolescents	1–3	0.7–1.0	1.0–1.5	20–80	25–50
	4–6	1.0–1.5	1.5–2.0	30–120	30–75
	7–10	1.0–20	2.0–3.0	50–200	50–150
	11+	1.5–2.5	2.0–5.0	50–200	75–250
Adults		1.5–3.0	2.0–5.0	50–200	75–250

(Reprinted with permission from Recommended Dietary Allowances, 10th ed., © 1989 by the National Academy of Sciences. Published by National Academy Press.)

*Since the toxic levels for many trace elements may be only several times the usual intakes, the upper levels for the trace elements given in this table should not be habitually exceeded.

Status Report from the NNMRRP

The third report on nutrition monitoring in the United States from the NNMRRP (1995) addressed two questions:

1. What is the nutrition-related health status of Americans?
2. What is the nutritional quality of the American diet?

The nutritional quality of the American diet shows that the population is slowly changing eating patterns toward more healthful diets, although gaps exist between consumption and government recommendations among population subgroups. Intake of total fat, saturated fatty acids, and cholesterol have decreased among some portions of the population. The average consumption of servings of fruits and vegetables has risen to four per day, approaching the recommendation of five servings per day. However, on the negative side, many Americans suffer from **food insecurity,** that is, insufficiency or hunger from not getting enough to eat.

The report found that nutrition-related health measurements indicate that overweight and obesity are increasing, resulting from reported lack of physical activity. The number of people with desirable serum cholesterol levels is increasing, although some individuals still have high levels, a major risk factor for coronary heart disease. Hypertension remains a major public health problem in middle-aged and elderly people, and among non-Hispanic blacks, increasing the risk of stroke and coronary heart disease. Osteoporosis, a risk factor for broken bones and impaired mobility among women 50 years of age and older, occurs more often among non-Hispanic whites than non-Hispanic blacks or Mexican Americans.

Nutrition Monitoring Report

At the request of the DHHS and the USDA, an Expert Panel on Nutrition Monitoring was established by the Life Sciences Research Office of the Federation of American Societies for Experimental Biology (FASEB) to review the dietary and nutritional status of the American population. The report of the committee summarized the results of data from NHANES II, Hispanic HANES, and the Nationwide Food Consumption Survey (NFCS) and CSFII surveys. In general, the committee concluded that the food supply in the United States is abundant, although some may not receive an adequate share for a variety of reasons. Nutrient intakes are most likely to be low in persons living below the poverty level. Intakes of nutrients reported to be low in the general population are even lower in the poverty group.

Among the evaluations the committee undertook were categorization of various food components by the degree to which their intakes constituted public health issues (Federation of American Societies for Experimental Biology [FASEB], 1995).

Healthy Eating Index

In 1998, the Center for Nutrition Policy and Promotion, USDA, released the newly updated **healthy eating index (HEI)** (Bowman et al., 1998). The HEI is a summary measure of people's overall diet quality and is designed to assess and monitor the dietary status of Americans using data from USDA's CSFII and evaluating 10 components, each representing different aspect of a healthful diet. The dietary components used in the evaluation include grains, vegetables, fruits, milk, meat, total fat, saturated fat, cholesterol sodium, and variety (Table 15–6).

Overall, the HEI score for 1994–1996 is 63.8, which represented a slight but significant improvement since 1989 (61.5). An HEI score over 80 implies a "good" diet, an HEI score between 51 and 80 implies a diet that "needs improvement," and an HEI score less that 51 implies a "poor" diet. Scores increased for all HEI components from 1989 to 1996 except for milk, meat, and sodium. Scores improved the most for saturated fat and variety component of the index.

The results of the 1996 index shows that Americans are reducing total fat and saturated fat in their diets and eating a wider variety of foods, but still need to eat more fruit, drink more milk, and reduce sodium intake.

Food Components Constituting Current Public Health Issues

According to the NNMRRP report, the following food components were identified as current or potential public health issues. This information is summarized in Table 15–7.

TABLE 15–6 HEALTHY EATING INDEX, OVERALL AND COMPONENT MEAN SCORES, 1989 VERSUS 1996

	1989	1996
Overall	*61.5*	*63.8*
Components		
Grains	6.1	6.7
Vegetables	5.9	6.3
Fruits	3.7	3.8
Milk	6.2	5.4
Meat	7.1	6.4
Total fat	6.3	6.9
Saturated fat	5.4	6.4
Cholesterol	7.5	7.9
Sodium	6.7	6.3
Variety	6.6	7.6

Note: The overall HEI score ranges from 0–100. An HEI score over 80 implies a "good" diet, an HEI score between 51 and 80 implies a diet that "needs improvement," and an HEI score less than 51 implies a "poor" diet. HEI component scores range from 0–10. High component scores indicate intakes close to recommended ranges or amounts; low component scores indicate less compliance with recommended ranges or amounts. For 1989, scores are based on 1-day intake data.

TABLE 15–7 CLASSIFICATION OF FOOD COMPONENTS AS PUBLIC HEALTH ISSUES IN THE TRONM[1]

CURRENT PUBLIC HEALTH ISSUES	POTENTIAL PUBLIC HEALTH ISSUES FOR WHICH FURTHER STUDY IS REQUIRED	NOT CURRENT PUBLIC HEALTH ISSUES
Food energy	⇒ Total carbohydrate	Thiamin
Total fat	Dietary fiber	Riboflavin
Saturated fatty acids	Sugars‡	Niacin
Cholesterol	Polyunsaturated and monounsaturated fatty acids‡	Iodine‡
Alcohol	*Trans* fatty acids‡	
Iron	Fat substitutes‡	
Calcium	⇒ Protein	
Sodium	Vitamin A	
	Antioxidant vitamins	
	Vitamin C	
	⇒ Vitamin E	
	Carotenes	
	Folate	
	Vitamin B_6	
	⇒ Vitamin B_{12}	
	⇒ Magnesium	
	Potassium	
	Zinc	
	⇒ Copper	
	Selenium‡	
	⇒ Phosphorus	
	Fluoride	

(From Third Report on Nutrition Monitoring in the United States, Executive Summary. Prepared by the Life Sciences Research Office, Federation of American Societies for Experimental Biology, Interagency Board for Nutrition Monitoring and Related Research, 1995.)

[1]Arrows (⇒) point to components whose monitoring status has changed since the second report on nutrition monitoring was published (LSRO, 1989). Double daggers (‡) indicate components that are being evaluated for the first time for the NNMRRP.

ENERGY. Median reported energy intakes in the 1988–1991 CSFII were below recommended levels, yet approximately one fifth of adolescents and one third of adults were overweight. The high prevalence of overweight indicates that an energy imbalance exists among Americans because of physical inactivity.

TOTAL FAT, SATURATED FAT, AND CHOLESTEROL. Intakes of fat, saturated fatty acids, and cholesterol among all age groups above 2 years of age were above recommended levels (< 30% of calories for total fat and 8% to 10% of calories for saturated fatty acids). Cholesterol intakes were generally within the recommended range of 300 mg/dL or less.

ALCOHOL. Intake of alcohol is a public health concern because of displacement of food energy from food sources of nutrients more than the consequences of excessive alcohol intake.

IRON AND CALCIUM. Low intakes of iron and calcium continue to be of public health concern, particularly among infants and women of childbearing age. Prevalence of iron deficiency anemia was higher among these groups than in other age-gender groups. Low calcium intake is particularly a concern with adolescent girls and adult women for most racial and ethnic groups.

SODIUM. Sodium intake continues to exceed government recommendations of 2400 mg/day in most age-gender groups.

Food Components Considered to Be Potential Public Health Issues

Some nutrients are considered potential problems but require further study of requirements or association with risk. These include total carbohydrate and carbohydrate constituents; dietary fiber; polyunsaturated and monounsaturated fatty acids, trans fatty acids, and fat substitutes; protein; vitamin A; antioxidant vitamins (vitamin C and E, and carotenes); and in certain groups, folate, vitamins B_6 and B_{12}, and magnesium, potassium, zinc, copper, selenium, phosphorus, and fluoride.

Nutrients Not Considered to Be Potential Public Health Issues

Nutrients consumed in adequate amounts by most people, or for which there does not appear to be risk at either high or low intakes, include thiamin, riboflavin, niacin, and iodine.

NATIONAL GUIDELINES FOR DIET PLANNING

Current Health Issues

Within the last 30 years, attention has been focused increasingly on the relationship of nutrition to chronic diseases and conditions. Although this interest derives somewhat from the rapid increase in number and longevity of the elderly population, it is also prompted by the desire to prevent premature deaths from causes such as cancer and coronary heart disease.

Approximately two thirds of deaths in the United States are caused by chronic disease. Of the 10 leading causes of death, four are associated with diet (heart disease, some types of cancer, stroke, and diabetes) and three with excessive alcohol consumption (accidents, suicide, and chronic liver disease and chirrosis) (Public Health Service, 1996) (Table 15–8).

CURRENT DIETARY GUIDANCE IN THE UNITED STATES AND CANADA

Eating is one of life's greatest pleasures. People eat for enjoyment as well as to provide energy and nutrient needs. Although many genetic, environmental, behavioral, and cultural factors affect health, diet is equally important to promoting health and preventing disease.

TABLE 15–8 TEN LEADING CAUSES OF DEATH, UNITED STATES, 1996

CAUSE OF DEATH	NUMBER
Heart disease	733,834
Cancer	544,278
Stroke	160,431
Chronic obstructive pulmonary disease	106,146
Accidents	93,874
Pneumonia/influenza	82,579
Diabetes	61,559
HIV/AIDS	32,655
Suicide	30,862
Chronic liver disease and cirrhosis	25,135

(From Public Health Service. Monthly Vital Statistics Report, vol. 46, no. 1 supplement. Atlanta, GA: Centers for Disease Control and Prevention, 1996.)
AIDS, acquired immunodeficiency syndrome; HIV, human immunodeficiency virus

In 1969, President Nixon convened the White House Conference on Nutrition and Health (White House, 1970). Increased attention was being given to food security, that is, prevention of hunger and disease. The development of dietary guidelines in the United States began with the 1977 report of the U.S. Senate Select Committee on Nutrition and Human Needs, *Dietary Goals for the United States* (U.S. Senate, 1977). Although dietary recommendations have evolved over the past 30 years, the basic content of dietary guidance has not changed substantially.

Although numerous federal agencies are involved in the issuance of dietary guidance, the USDA and the DHHS lead the effort. Following the Senate's Dietary Goals report, the **Dietary Guidelines for Americans** was first published in 1980. These guidelines were revised in 1985 (2nd ed.), 1990 (3rd ed.), and 1995 (4th ed.; Nutrition and Your Health, 1995; Dietary Guidelines Alliance, 1996; see Table 15–9). With the passage of the Nutrition Monitoring Act in 1990, the dietary guidelines are now required to be reviewed every 5 years. The guidelines are currently being reviewed with either a report or revision to be completed by December 2000.

In addition to these dietary guidelines, several other important government or expert reports have addressed dietary recommendations for healthy Americans. The Surgeon General's Report on Nutrition and Health (Public Health Service, 1988) and the National Academy of Sciences Diet and Health Report (Food and Nutrition Board, 1989) provide similar and different qualitative or quantitative dietary recommendations. In Canada, dietary recommendations appear in Nutrition Recommendations for Canadians, prepared by Health Canada (National Institute of Nutrition, 1990; Minister of National Health and Welfare, 1992). See the accompanying box, "*Clinical Insight:* Nutrition Recommendations for Canadians."

The specific dietary recommendations of the Senate Select Committee and the above documents are compared in Table 15–9. Except for minor differences, they are all very much alike, and when numerical goals are specified, they are surprisingly similar to those established by the Senate Select Committee in 1977. Some, such as the Dietary Guidelines for Americans, the Surgeon General's recommendations and the Nutrition Recommendations for Canadians, are deliberately general, whereas others, such as the NAS Committee on Diet and Health recommendations, are more specific. Other differences reflect actual disagreement regarding amounts or even the need to include items such as cholesterol, sodium, sugar, or alcohol.

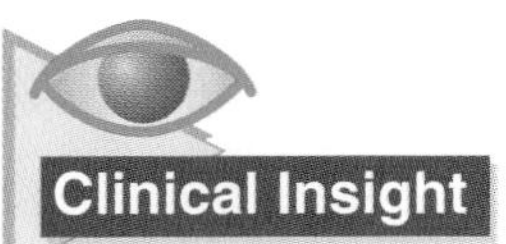

NUTRITION RECOMMENDATIONS FOR CANADIANS

In Canada, the Food Guide to Healthy Eating was released in mid-November 1992. Suggestions include 5 to 12 servings of grain products, 5 to 10 vegetables and fruits, 2 to 4 servings of milk (specified for age or for pregnancy/lactation), and 2 to 3 servings of meat or alternates. Unlike the Food Pyramid in the United States, Canada's Food Guide to Healthy Eating contains four food groups, presented in a rainbow shape, with grains representing the largest component (Minister of National Health and Welfare, 1992).

The Canadian diet should provide energy consistent with the maintenance of body weight within the recommended range.

The Canadian diet should include essential nutrients in amounts specified in the **recommended nutrients intake (RNIs).**

The Canadian diet should include no more than 30% of energy as fat (33 g/1000 kcal or 39 g/5000 kJ) and no more than 10% as saturated fat (11 g/1000 kcal or 13 g/5000 kJ).

The Canadian diet should provide 55% of energy as carbohydrates (138 g/1000 kcal or 165 g/5000 kJ) from a variety of sources. The sodium content of the Canadian diet should be reduced.

The Canadian diet should include no more than 5% of total energy as alcohol, or two drinks daily, whichever is less.

The Canadian diet should contain no more caffeine than the equivalent of four cups of regular coffee per day.

Community water supplies containing less than 1 mg/L of flouride should be fluoridated to that level.

It is believed that Canada will adopt the DRIs when they are finally established for the United States.

(From Communications/Implementation Committee, Minister of National Health and Welfare: Action towards healthy eating, Catalogue no. H39-166/199. Ottawa: Branch Publications Unit, 1990.)

TABLE 15–9 COMPARISON OF SELECTED DIETARY RECOMMENDATIONS IN THE UNITED STATES AND CANADA, 1977–1995

DIETARY GOALS, 1977	DIETARY GUIDELINES, 1st ed., 1980	SURGEON GENERAL'S REPORT ON NUTRITION AND HEALTH, 1988	NAS DIET AND HEALTH, 1989	NUTRITION RECOMMENDATIONS FOR CANADIANS, 1990	DIETARY GUIDELINES, 4th ed., 1995
To avoid overweight, consume only as much energy (calories) as is expended; if overweight, decrease energy intake and increase energy expenditure.	Eat a wide variety of foods.	Reduce consumption of fat (especially saturated fat) and cholesterol.	Reduce fat intake to 30% or less of calories; reduce saturated fatty acid intake to less than 10% of calories; and reduce the intake of cholesterol to less than 300 mg daily.	Provide energy consistent with the maintenance of body weight within the recommended range.	Eat a variety of foods.
Increase the consumption of complex carbohydrates "naturally occurring" sugars from about 28% of energy intake to about 48% of energy intake.	Maintain ideal weight.	Achieve and maintain a desirable body weight.	Every day eat five or more servings of a combination of vegetables and fruits, especially green and yellow vegetables and citrus fruits. Also, increase intake of starches and other complex carbohydrates by eating six or more daily servings of a combination of breads, cereals, and legumes.	Include essential nutrients in amounts specified in the Recommended Nutrient Intakes.	Balance the food you eat with physical activity—maintain or improve your weight.
Reduce the consumption of refined and processed sugars by about 45% to account for about 10% of total energy intake.	Avoid too much fat, saturated fat and cholesterol.	Increase consumption of whole grain foods and cereal products, vegetables, and fruits.	Maintain protein intake at moderate levels.	Include no more than 30% of energy as fat (33 g/1000 kcal or 39 g/5000 kJ) and no more than 10% as saturated fat (11g/1000 kcal or 13 g/5000 kJ)	Choose a diet with plenty of grain products, vegetables, and fruits.
Reduce overall fat consumption from approximately 40% to about 30% of energy intake.	Eat foods with adequate starch and fiber.	Reduce intake of sodium by choosing foods relatively low in sodium and limiting the amount of salt added in food preparation and at the table.	Balance food intake and physical activity to maintain appropriate body weight.	Provide 55% of energy as carbohydrates (138 g/1000 kcal or 165 g/5000 KJ) from a variety of sources.	Choose a diet low in fat, saturated fat, and cholesterol.
Reduce saturated fat consumption to account for about 10% of total energy intake; and balance that with polyunsaturated and monounsaturated fats, which should account for about 10% of energy intake each.	Avoid too much sugar.	Take alcohol only in moderation (no more than two drinks a day).	It is not recommended that you drink alcohol.	The sodium content should be reduced.	Choose a diet moderate in sugars.
Reduce cholesterol consumption to about 300 mg/d.	Avoid too much sodium.		Limit total daily intake of salt (sodium chloride) that you eat to 6 g per day or less.	Include no more than 50% of total energy as alcohol, or two drinks daily, whichever is less.	Choose a diet moderate in salt and sodium.
Limit the intake of sodium by reducing the intake of salt to about 5 g/d.	If you drink alcohol, do so in moderation.		Maintain adequate clacium intake.	Should contain no more caffeine than the equivalent of 4 cups of regular coffee per day.	If you drink alcoholic beverages, do so in moderation.
			Avoid taking dietary supplements in the excess of the RDA in any one day.	Community water supplies containing less than 1 mg/L of fluoride should be fluoridated to that level.	
			Maintain optimal intake of fluoride, particularly during the years of primary and secondary tooth formation and growth.		

Guidelines directed toward prevention of a particular disease state, such as the National Cancer Institute's Cancer Guidelines (Public Health Service, 1987), National Heart, Lung and Blood Institute's National Cholesterol Education Program Guidelines (Public Health Service, NCEP, 1993), contain recommendations unique to that condition. In addition, dietary recommendations have been published by private health organizations such as the American Heart Association and the American Cancer Society (see also http://usda.gov/cnpp).

These various guidelines can be summarized as follows:

1. The basic universal prescription for health and fitness appears to be:
   - Adjust energy intake and exercise level to achieve and maintain appropriate body weight.
   - Eat a wide variety of foods to ensure nutrient adequacy.
   - Increase total carbohydrate, increase complex carbohydrate.
   - Eat less total fat and less saturated fat.
2. To this can be added (from most, but not all, guidelines):
   - Eat more fiber.
   - Eat more fruits and vegetables.
   - Eat less cholesterol.
   - Eat less sodium.
   - Reduce intake of sugars.
   - Drink alcohol in moderation or not at all.
3. Included in a few recommendations:
   - Meet the RDA for calcium, especially adolescents and women.
   - Meet the RDA for iron, especially children, adolescents, and women of childbearing age.
   - Limit protein to no more than twice the RDA.
   - Avoid the use of dietary supplements in excess of the RDAs.
   - Drink fluoridated water.

IMPLEMENTING THE GUIDELINES

The task of planning nutritious meals centers on including the essential nutrients in sufficient amounts as outlined in the new DRIs (or previous RDAs), along with appropriate energy and amounts of protein, carbohydrate (including fiber and sugars), fat (especially saturated fat), cholesterol, and salt. Suggestions are included to assist in meeting the specifics of the recommendations. When specific numerical recommendations differ, they are presented as ranges.

The **Food Guide Pyramid** shown in Figure 15–2 offers a pattern for daily food choices based on "servings" from the five major food groups (USDA, 1992). For comparison, the Canadian Food Guide to Healthy Eating is shown in Figure 15–3. When planned to include a wide variety of foods within each food group, this pattern will result in a diet that is adequate in nutrients (see "*Focus On:* What Is a Varied Diet?"). The Food Guide Pyramid also was designed to be useful to consumers to put the dietary guidelines into action. To select an eating pattern that achieves specific health promotion or disease prevention objectives, it is necessary for the nutritionist to assist individuals in making food choices, for example, to reduce fat or to increase fiber.

By combining the dietary guidelines, the Food Guide Pyramid, and the nutrition facts panel on food labels, consumers can achieve healthful diets. Because the dietary guidelines form the basis of federal policy related to nutrition and diet as well as addressing the needs of individual consumers, the committee that prepared the fourth edition recommended a two-step process to address both dietary policy needs and those related to communicating the guidelines to the pubic.

Following this recommendation, a group of health and food professional associations in liaison with USDA and DHHS developed the Dietary Guidelines

What Is a "Varied Diet"?

Many food guides and other recommendations for Americans emphasize eating "a wide variety of foods" to achieve dietary adequacy. "Uncertainties in the knowledge base" (Food and Nutrition Board, 1989) make it impossible to establish RDAs for all the known nutrients, and there is always the possibility, albeit remote, that other essential nutrients will be discovered.

According to the Food and Nutrition Board, choosing a variety of foods to meet the RDAs should provide adequate amounts of those nutrients whose recommended levels have not been well defined. A varied diet should also ensure consuming sufficient amounts of food constituents that, though not nutrients, have biologic effects and may influence health and susceptibility to disease. Examples are the well-known dietary fiber and beta-carotene as well as lesser known phytochemicals (substances found in plant products), such as indoles and isothiocyanates in broccoli and other cruciferous vegetables. Diets rich in these phytochemicals may help reduce the risk of developing certain types of cancer.

Although it is not possible to measure the effect of a varied diet on these intangibles, it does appear that increasing the number of foods eaten over a period of time improves food choices in general. Some studies have shown that nutritional adequacy of the diet increases with a greater number of different foods. Such diets tend to include less protein, meat, and meat alternatives and more carbohydrate, fruits, and vegetables. Diets with limited food intakes, such as weight-reduction diets, have better nutritional adequacy when they include a larger number of different foods.

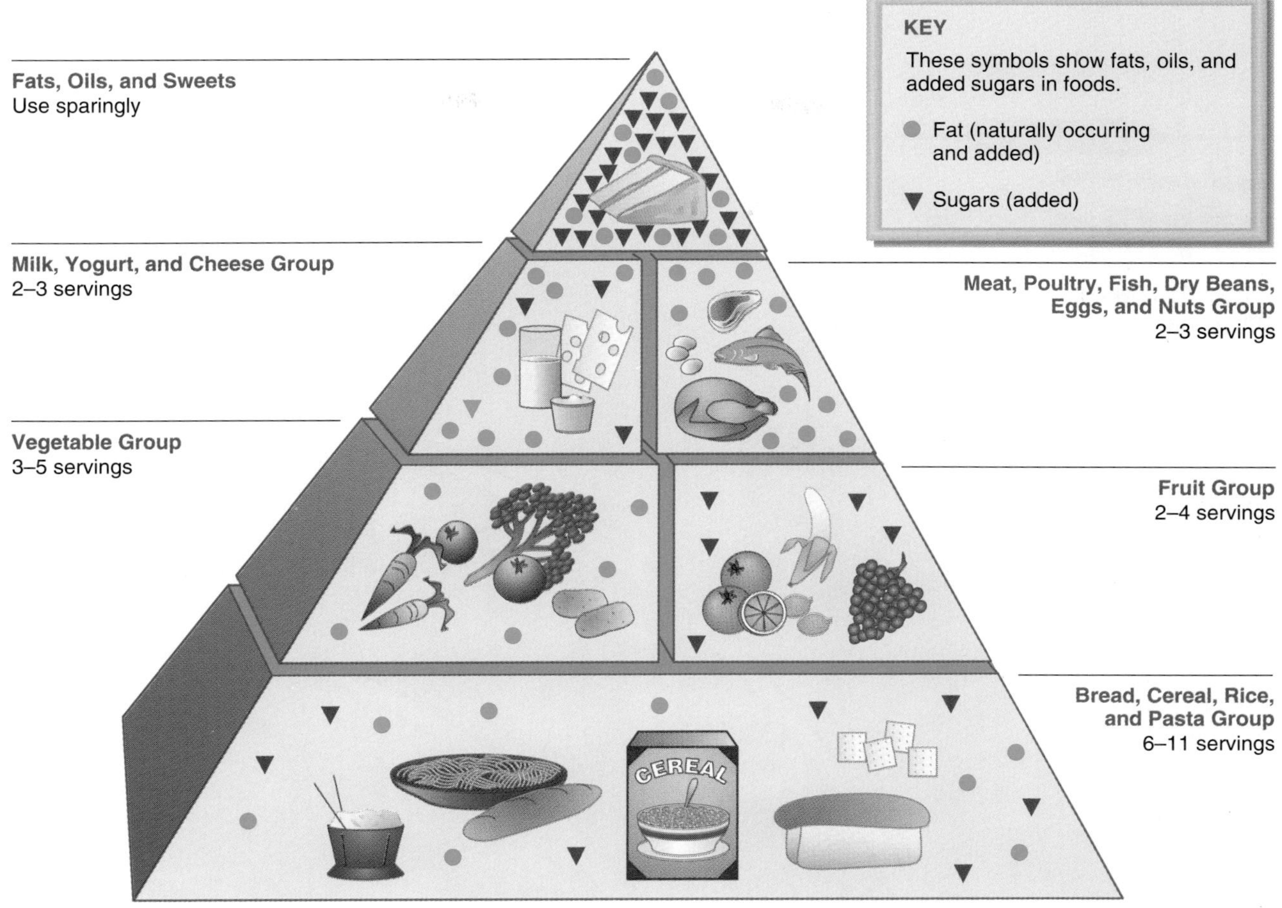
KEY
These symbols show fats, oils, and added sugars in foods.
Fat (naturally occurring and added)
Sugars (added)
Fats, Oils, and Sweets
Use sparingly
Milk, Yogurt, and Cheese Group
2–3 servings
Meat, Poultry, Fish, Dry Beans, Eggs, and Nuts Group
2–3 servings
Vegetable Group
3–5 servings
Fruit Group
2–4 servings
Bread, Cereal, Rice, and Pasta Group
6–11 servings
CEREAL
THE FOOD GUIDE PYRAMID
emphasizes foods from the five food groups shown in the three lower sections of the Pyramid.
Each of these food groups provides some, but not all, of the nutrients you need. Foods in one group can't replace those in another. No one food group is more important than another—for good health, you need them all.

FIGURE 15–2 The Food Guide Pyramid

Alliance (DGA). The mission of the DGA was to motivate consumers to change their eating and activity patterns by providing them with positive, simple messages based on the principles of the dietary guidelines. Using consumer research, the DGA developed messages that would extend the reach of the dietary guidelines to encourage consumer adoption and ultimately behavior change. The DGA messages, "It's All About You," reach out to what motivates consumers, their individual needs, and life goals and can be used in education, counseling, and communications initiatives (Fig. 15–4).

FOOD LABELING

To help consumers make choices between similar types of food products that can be incorporated into a healthful diet, the Food and Drug Administration (FDA) established a voluntary system in 1973 of providing selected nutrient information on food labels. The regulatory framework for nutrition information on food labels was revised and updated by both the USDA (which regulates meat and poultry products and eggs) and the FDA (which regulates all other foods) with enactment of the Nutrition Labeling and Education Act (NLEA) in late 1990. The new labels became mandatory in 1994 (Fig. 15–5 and Tables 15–10 through 15–12).

Mandatory Nutrition Labeling

As a result of the NLEA, nutrition labels must appear on most foods except for products that provide few nutrients (such as coffee and spices), restaurant foods, and ready-to-eat foods prepared on site, such as supermarket bakery and deli items (Food and Drug Administration, 1993).

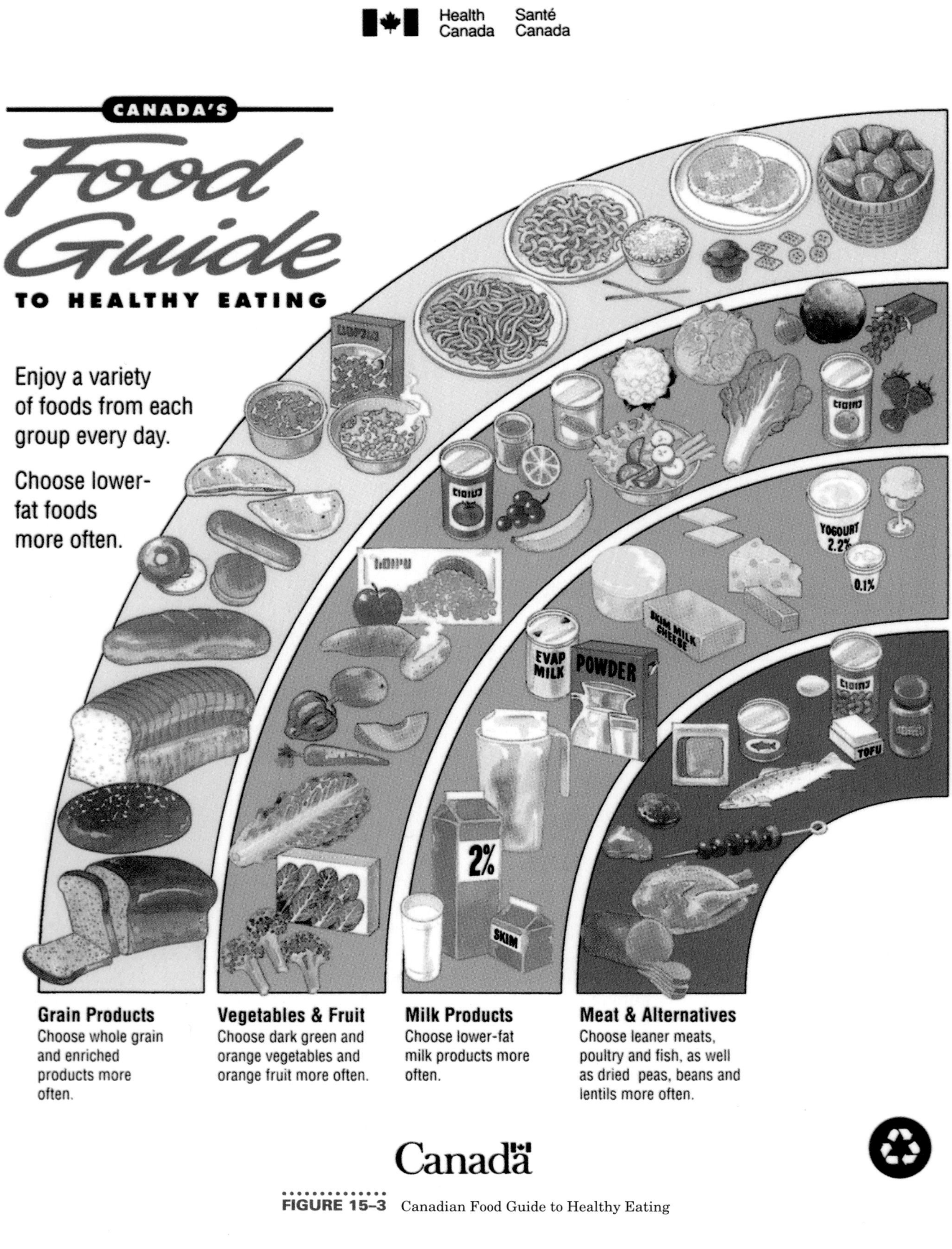

Health Canada
Santé Canada
CANADA'S
Food Guide
TO HEALTHY EATING
Enjoy a variety of foods from each group every day.
Choose lower-fat foods more often.
YOGOURT 2.2%
0.1%
SKIM MILK CHEESE
EVAP MILK
POWDER
TOFU
2%
SKIM
Grain Products
Choose whole grain and enriched products more often.
Vegetables & Fruit
Choose dark green and orange vegetables and orange fruit more often.
Milk Products
Choose lower-fat milk products more often.
Meat & Alternatives
Choose leaner meats, poultry and fish, as well as dried peas, beans and lentils more often.
Canada

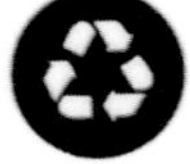

FIGURE 15–3 Canadian Food Guide to Healthy Eating

TABLE 15–10 FOOD LABEL TERMINOLOGY

1. Calories

Calorie free: fewer than 5 calories per serving

Low calorie: 40 calories or less per serving and if the serving is 30 g or less or 2 tablespoons or less, per 50 g of the food

Reduced or *fewer calories:* at least 25% fewer calories per serving than reference food

2. Fat

Fat free: less than 0.5 g of fat per serving

Saturated fat free: less than 0.5 g per serving and the level of transfatty acids does not exceed 1% of total fat

Low fat: 3 g or less per serving, and if the serving is 30 g or less or 2 tablespoons or less, per 50 g of the food

Low saturated fat: 1 g or less per serving and not more than 15% of calories from saturated fatty acids

Reduced or Less fat: at least 25% less per serving than reference food

Reduced or Less saturated fat: at least 25% less per serving than reference food

3. Cholesterol

Cholesterol free: less than 2 mg of cholesterol and 2 g or less of saturated fat per serving

Low cholesterol: 20 mg or less and 2 g or less of saturated fat per serving and, if the serving is 30 g or less or 2 tablespoons or less, per 50 g of the food

Reduced or Less cholesterol: at least 25% less and 2 g or less of saturated fat per serving than reference food

4. Sodium

Sodium free: less than 5 mg per serving

Low sodium: 140 mg or less per serving and, if the serving is 30 g or less or 2 tablespoons or less, per 50 g of the food

Very low sodium: 35 mg or less per serving and, if the serving is 30 g or less or 2 tablespoons or less, per 50 g of the food

Reduced or Less sodium: at least 25% less per serving than reference food

5. Fiber

High fiber: 5 g or more per serving. (Foods making high-fiber claims must meet the definition for low fat, or the level of total fat must appear next to the high-fiber claim.)

Good source of fiber: 2.5 g to 4.9 g per serving

More or Added fiber: at least 2.5 g more per serving than reference food

6. Sugar

Sugar free: less than 0.5 g per serving

No added sugar, Without added sugar, No sugar added:

- No sugars added during processing or packing, including ingredients that contain sugars (for example, fruit juices, applesauce, or dried fruit).
- Processing does not increase the sugar content above that amount naturally present in the ingredients. (A functionally insignificant increase in sugars is acceptable from processes used for purposes other than increasing sugar content).
- The food that resembles and for which it substitutes normally contains added sugars.
- If the food doesn't meet the requirements for a low- or reduced-calorie food, the product bears a statement that the food is not low-calorie or calorie-reduced and directs consumers' attention to the nutrition panel for further information on sugars and calorie content.

Reduced sugar: at least 25% less sugar per serving than reference food

7. Healthy

Products using the term "healthy" in the product name or as a claim on the label must contain, per serving, no more than 3 g of fat, 1 g of saturated fat, 480 mg of sodium (350 mg by the end of 1997), or 60 mg cholesterol. They must also supply at least 10% of the Daily Value for at least one of six nutrients: vitamins A and C, calcium, iron, protein, and fiber. Raw meat, poultry, and fish can be labeled "healthy" if they contain, per serving, no more than 5 g of fat, 2 g of saturated fat, and 95 mg of cholesterol.

(Adapted from Stehlin D. A little 'lite' reading. In: Food and Drug Administration: Focus on food labeling. Washington, DC: Department of Health and Human Services, 1993, p. 32, and Federal Register 59 (24219), May 10, 1994, 59 (27143), May 25, 1994.)

TABLE 15–11 DAILY REFERENCE VALUES (DRVs)[†]

FOOD COMPONENT	DRV
Fat	65 g
Saturated fatty acids	20 g
Cholesterol	300 mg
Total carbohydrate	300 g
Fiber	25 g
Sodium	2400 mg
Potassium	3500 mg
Protein[‡]	50 g

(From Kurtzweil P. "Daily values" encourage healthy diet. In: Food and Drug Administration: Focus on food labeling. Washington, DC: Department of Health and Human Services, 1993, p. 42.)

[†] Based on 2000 calories a day for adults and children over 4 only.

[‡] DRV for protein does not apply to certain populations; Reference Daily Intake (RDI) for protein has been established for these groups: children 1 to 4 years: 16 g; infants under 1 year: 14 g; pregnant women: 60 g; nursing mothers: 65 g.

TABLE 15–12 REFERENCE DAILY INTAKES (RDIs)

NUTRIENT	AMOUNT	NUTRIENT	AMOUNT
Vitamin A	5000 IU	Folic acid	0.4
Vitamin C	60 mg	Vitamin B_{12}	6 mcg
Thiamin	1.5 mg	Phosphorus	1.0 g
Riboflavin	1.7 mg	Iodine	150 mcg
Niacin	20 mg	Magnesium	400 mg
Calcium	1.0 g	Zinc	15 mg
Iron	18 mg	Copper	2 mg
Vitamin D	400 IU	Biotin	0.3 mg
Vitamin E	30 IU	Pantothenic acid	10 mg
Vitamin B_6	2.0 mg		

Based on National Academy of Sciences' 1968 Recommended Dietary Allowances. (From Kurtzweil P. "Daily values" encourage healthy diet. In: Food and Drug Administration: Focus on food labeling. Washington, DC: Department of Health and Human Services, 1993, p. 42.)

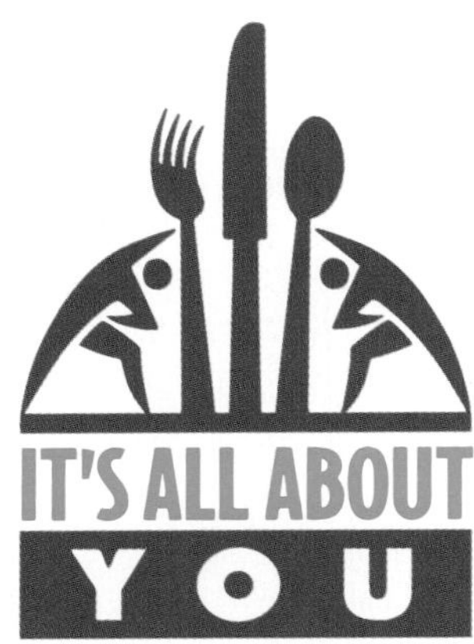

Make healthy choices that fit your lifestyle so you can do the things you want to do.

BE REALISTIC

Make small changes over time in what you eat and the level of activity you do. After all, small steps work better than giant leaps.

BE ADVENTUROUS

Expand your tastes to enjoy a variety of foods.

BE FLEXIBLE

Go ahead and balance what you eat and the physical activity you do over several days. No need to worry about just one meal or one day.

BE SENSIBLE

Enjoy all foods, just don't overdo it.

BE ACTIVE

Walk the dog, don't just watch the dog walk.

FIGURE 15–4 It's all about you. (© 1996 The Dietary Guidelines Alliance)

Providing nutrition information remains voluntary on many raw foods. The FDA and USDA, however, have called for a voluntary point-of-purchase program for nutrition information to be available in most supermarkets. Nutrition information is provided through brochures or point-of-purchase posters for the 20 most popular fruits, vegetables, and fresh fish and the 45 major cuts of fresh meat and poultry.

Standardized Serving Sizes

Serving sizes of products are set by the government based on amounts commonly consumed. For example, a serving of milk is 8 oz, and a serving of salad dressing is 2 tablespoons. Standardized serving sizes make it easier for consumers to compare the nutrient contents of similar products.

Nutrition Facts Panel

The **nutrition facts label** on a food product (see Fig. 15–5) provides information on its per-serving calories and calories from fat. The label then lists the amount (in grams) of total fat, saturated fat, cholesterol, sodium, total carbohydrate, dietary fiber, sugars, and protein. For most of these nutrients, the label also shows the percentage of the **daily value (DV)** supplied by a serving. A product's content of vitamins A and C, calcium, and iron is listed in terms of percent DV only. DVs show how the product fits into an overall diet by comparing its nutrient content to recommended intakes of those nutrients (see http://vm.cfsan.fda.gov/label.html).

It is important to remember that DVs are not recommended intakes for individuals because no one nutrient standard could apply to everyone; they are simply reference points to provide some perspective on daily nutrient needs. DVs are based on a 2000-kcal diet. However, the bottom of the nutrition label also provides the DVs for a 2500-kcal diet. Individuals who consume diets supplying more or fewer calories can still use the DVs as a rough guide to ensure that they are getting, for example, adequate amounts of vitamin C but not too much saturated fat.

The DVs exist for nutrients for which there are already RDAs (in which case they are known as **reference daily intakes [RDIs]**) and for which no RDAs exist (known as **daily reference values [DRVs]**). Food labels, however, use only the term "daily value." RDIs provide a large margin of safety; in general, the RDI for a nutrient is greater than the RDA for a specific age group. The term RDI replaces the term "US Recommended Daily Allowances" (USRDAs) used on earlier food labels (see Table 15–12).

The previously mentioned nutrients must be listed on the food label. Nutrients that a manufacturer or processor may voluntarily disclose include those for which a DV has been established, such as monounsaturated and saturated fat, potassium, vitamins such as thiamin and riboflavin, and minerals like iodine and magnesium. As new DRIs are developed in various categories (see Fig. 15–5), labeling laws will most likely be updated.

Nutrient Content Claims

Nutrient content terms such as "reduced sodium," "fat-free," "low-calorie," and "healthy" must now meet government definitions that apply to all foods (see Table 15–10). "Lean," for example, refers to a serving of meat, poultry, seafood, or game meat with less than 10 g of fat, less than 4 g of saturated fat, and less than 95 mg cholesterol per serving or per 100 g. "Extra lean" meat or poultry contains

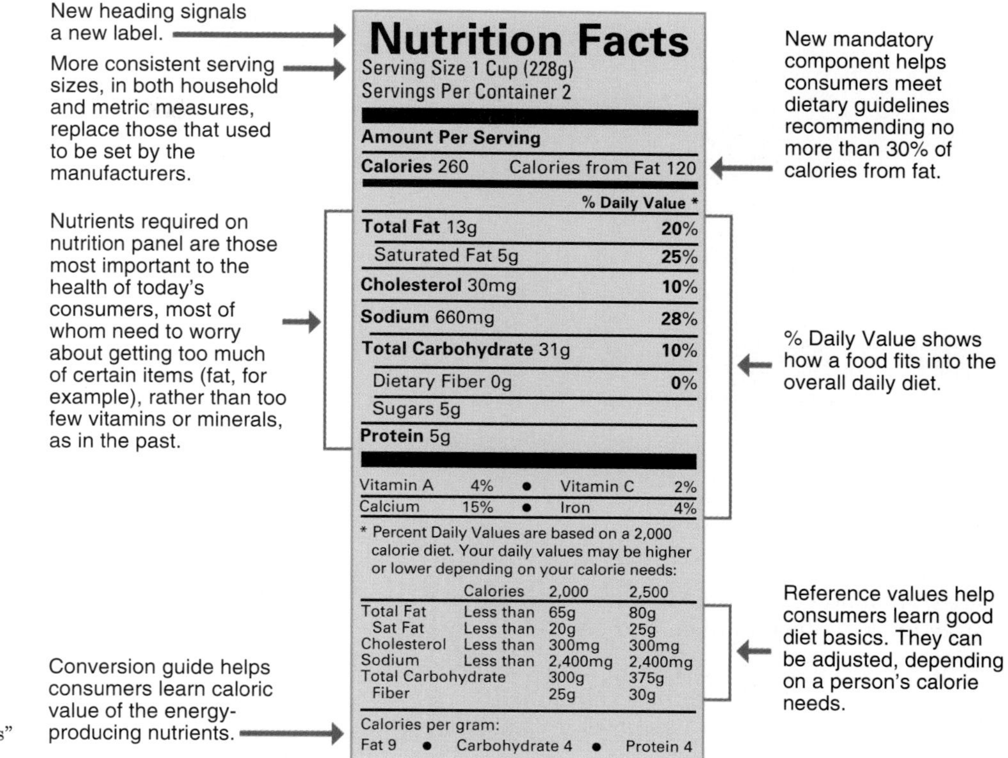
New heading signals a new label.
More consistent serving sizes, in both household and metric measures, replace those that used to be set by the manufacturers.
Nutrients required on nutrition panel are those most important to the health of today's consumers, most of whom need to worry about getting too much of certain items (fat, for example), rather than too few vitamins or minerals, as in the past.
Conversion guide helps consumers learn caloric value of the energy-producing nutrients.
Nutrition Facts
Serving Size 1 Cup (228g)
Servings Per Container 2
Amount Per Serving
Calories 260 Calories from Fat 120
% Daily Value *
Total Fat 13g 20%
Saturated Fat 5g 25%
Cholesterol 30mg 10%
Sodium 660mg 28%
Total Carbohydrate 31g 10%
Dietary Fiber 0g 0%
Sugars 5g
Protein 5g
Vitamin A 4% • Vitamin C 2%
Calcium 15% • Iron 4%
* Percent Daily Values are based on a 2,000 calorie diet. Your daily values may be higher or lower depending on your calorie needs:
Calories 2,000 2,500
Total Fat Less than 65g 80g
Sat Fat Less than 20g 25g
Cholesterol Less than 300mg 300mg
Sodium Less than 2,400mg 2,400mg
Total Carbohydrate 300g 375g
Fiber 25g 30g
Calories per gram:
Fat 9 • Carbohydrate 4 • Protein 4
New mandatory component helps consumers meet dietary guidelines recommending no more than 30% of calories from fat.
% Daily Value shows how a food fits into the overall daily diet.
Reference values help consumers learn good diet basics. They can be adjusted, depending on a person's calorie needs.

FIGURE 15–5 "Nutrition Facts" on food labels.

less than 5 g of fat, less than 2 g of saturated fat, and the same cholesterol content as "lean" per serving or per 100 g.

Health Claims

Health claims are allowed only on appropriate food products that meet specified standards. The government requires that health claims be worded in ways that are not misleading; for example, the claim must not imply the food product itself helps prevent disease. Health claims cannot appear on foods that supply more than 20% of the DV for fat, saturated fat, cholesterol, and sodium.

Manufacturers can use health claims for the following diet-disease relationships on food labels: calcium and a reduced risk of osteoporosis; dietary fat and an increased risk of cancer; dietary saturated fat and cholesterol and an increased risk of coronary heart disease; fiber-containing grain products, fruits, and vegetables and a reduced risk of cancer; fruits, vegetables, and grain products that contain fiber, particularly soluble fiber (with specific claims allowed for whole oats or psyllium seed husks), and a reduced risk of coronary heart disease; sodium and an increased risk of hypertension; fruits and vegetables and a reduced risk of cancer; and folic acid during pregnancy and a reduced risk of neural tube defects. The following is an example of a health claim for dietary fiber and cancer, "Low-fat diets rich in fiber-containing grain products, fruits, and vegetables may reduce the risk of some types of cancer, a disease associated with many factors."

CULTURAL ASPECTS OF DIETARY PLANNING

To plan diets for individuals or groups that are appropriate from a health and nutrition perspective, it is important that the nutritionist develop a cultural awareness (i.e., become culturally competent) and use resources that are targeted to the specific group. Numerous population subgroups in the United States have specific cultural, ethnic, or religious beliefs and practices that must be considered. These cultural, ethnic, or religious groups have their own set of dietary practices or beliefs that are important when considering dietary planning. Such rules can have an effect on access to food, food choices, preparation, and storage methods. The Mediterranean Diet Pyramid, for example, has been developed to represent the pattern of that culture and to propose a reasonable diet for reducing chronic disease (Fig. 15–6). (See "*Focus On:* The Mediterranean Diet—Pros and Cons.")

Cultural aspects of dietary planning include vegetarianism, ethnic heritage practices, and religious customs or rules. When considering the cultural, ethnic, and religious aspects of dietary planning, the following questions may help guide the nutri-

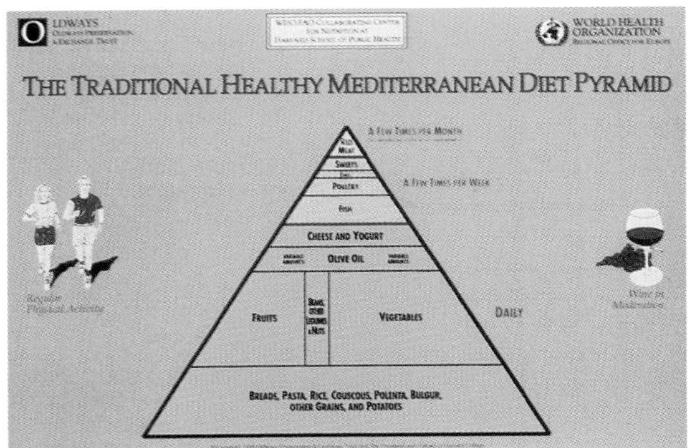

FIGURE 15–6 The traditional healthy Mediterranean diet pyramid.
(© 1998 Oldways Preservation & Exchange Trust)

tionist to blend specific food habits with dietary recommendations, food guides, and choices.

- What individual foods are the major components of the food or mixed dish to be classified?
- To what Food Guide Pyramid group(s) do the food(s) seem most related?
- What are the important nutrient sources and their contribution to overall nutrient adequacy?
- How is the food used and in what quantity is the food consumed?
- Are there any food handling, preparation or storage considerations that may compromise food safety or limit food choices?

Dietary Patterns of Southeast Asians

During the past few years, the number of Southeast Asian refugees has increased dramatically worldwide. In the United States, immigrants from Southeast Asia have become the largest ethnic group after African Americans and Hispanics. Among these immigrants are numerous groups, each with a distinct language, culture, and food habits. From Laos, Cambodia, and Vietnam come the native ethnic groups, as well as Muslims and ethnic Chinese. From Laos, Thailand, and Southern China come the nomadic hill people, the Hmong (Tripp, 1982). There are both urban and rural people whose lifestyles differ considerably, although they might come from the same country.

The traditional Hmong diet (Southeast Asian) is high in complex carbohydrates and low in refined carbohydrates, predominantly from rice, eaten at every meal (American Dietetic Association/American Diabetes Association [ADA/ADA], 1999). The Southeast Asian Hmong diet includes fruits, vegetables, soy products (mostly tofu), and smaller amounts of meat, poultry, and fish.

The Hmong value freshness as a characteristic of food and their diet. Pork is the preferred meat, along with chicken. Numerous fruits and vegetables are included in the diet with substitutions for domestically available products. Foods are boiled, grilled, steamed, and stir-fried. Lard is commonly used for frying. The most common spices used in Southeast Asian cuisine are lemon grass, coriander, chili peppers, green onion, basil, cilantro, ginger, and garlic. Lemon and lime juice often are used in place of salad dressings and salt; soy and fish sauces and monosodium glutamate are common seasonings.

Lactose intolerance has been reported to be a problem in many Southeast Asians (Anh et al., 1957). However, most children accept milk readily, and many adults are able to drink it in small amounts without any discomfort.

If the immigrants are refugees, they may be at nutritional risk for a variety of reasons. They come from countries with limited food supplies caused by long histories of war and political strife. They may have spent as much as 5 years in refugee camps where food supplies were also limited. Poor sanitation has led to an increased incidence of parasites and therefore to an increase in anemia. General malnutrition, hypertension, dental caries, and iron

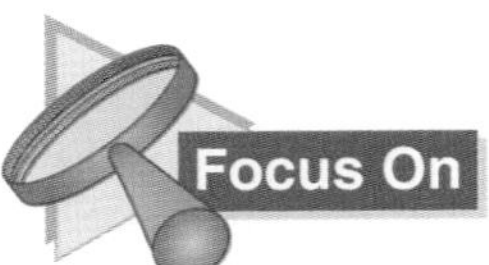

Mediterranean Diet—Pros and Cons

The Mediterranean Diet has received attention for its potential in protecting against cardiovascular disease and cancers. This meal pattern is rich in fruits, vegetables, grains, and sources of omega-3 fatty acids.

A trial was conducted as part of the Lyon Diet Heart Study; 605 patients with coronary heart disease were randomized to follow either a Mediterranean-type diet or a control diet. Those following the Mediterranean pattern ate less delicatessen food, beef, pork, butter, and cream; they used more canola-based margarine and oil, and olive oil. The control diet was similar to the step 1 AHA prudent heart diet (30% energy from fat). Follow-up occurred over a 4-year period.

The Mediterranean diet, compared with the control diet, provided higher intakes of fiber, vitamin C, oleic acid, and omega-3 fatty acids as well as lower intake of cholesterol, saturated fatty acids, and PUFA. Risk ratios were lower for cancers, cardiac death, and overall mortality rates. More use of these strategies in dietary planning may be beneficial in the U.S. Population.

(From Hakim I, et al. Mediterranean Diets and Cancer Prevention. Arch Int Med 158:1181, 1998.)

deficiency anemia have been identified as problems among incoming refugees.

Dietary Patterns of Chinese Americans

In Chinese culture, food is much more than something to eat. What is eaten, how often, in what season, and in what order are all carefully thought out (ADA/ADA, 1998a). Food is thought to play a vital role in preventing and treating diseases, as well as in addressing certain health conditions. For example, foods and herbs are frequently boiled in soup or tea for treatments of various diseases and conditions.

Most Chinese food found in the United States was created for the American palate. The traditional Chinese diet is much richer in carbohydrates (rice) with a variety of meat, poultry, and seafood, but in smaller quantities. The Chinese diet is comprised of over 80% of calories from grains, legumes, and vegetables. The remaining 20% comes from animal protein, fruits, and fats. Most typical Chinese meals include 2- to 3-cup bowls of rice. Northern Chinese cuisine may include more noodles, dumplings, and steamed buns made from wheat flour. Stir-frying, deep-fat frying, braising, roasting, smoking, and steaming are common food preparation techniques. When foods are fried, peanut or corn oil is used over lard, which is more common in Southeast Asian cuisine.

Pork is the staple meat in the Chinese diet. Poultry and eggs are also favored along with fish and shellfish. When animal products are included in traditional Chinese dishes, almost every part of an animal may be consumed—liver, kidneys, lungs, stomach, intestines, marrow, brain, feet, and tail. Other protein sources include soybeans, which may be sprouted, dried, or fermented as tofu. Dairy products are rarely used.

Fruits and vegetable are used abundantly in Chinese cuisine. Vegetables are rarely eaten raw and are most often stir-fried, steamed, or added to soups just before serving, allowing for maximum retention of nutrients.

The beverage of choice for most Chinese is clear, hot green tea. Older Chinese individuals rarely drink cold beverages. Chinese children and adults also drink a wide range of fermented beverages and juices.

Although Chinese meals are eaten communally, each region has its own set of foods, ingredients, and cooking methods. Northern cuisine is characterized by use of garlic, leeks, and scallions with noodles rather than rice. In the Western region, Hunan cuisine includes liberal use of chili peppers and hot pepper sauces. Hunan dishes are spicier and oilier. Southern Chinese cuisine is known as Cantonese, with mostly steamed and stir-fried dishes including lots of fish and shellfish. As Chinese adopt traditional American foods, their diet changes to include more sweets—cookies, chocolate, soft drinks and snacks.

Dietary Patterns of Hispanics

Hispanics are the second largest and most rapidly growing ethnic group in the United States (ADA/ADA, 1998b). Forecasts indicate that Hispanics will outnumber African Americans early in the 21st century. Mexican Americans constitute the largest subgroup of Hispanics, and older Mexican Americans constitute the fastest growing group of elderly Americans.

Hispanic cuisine, and Mexican and Latin American foods, incorporate the concept of "hot" and "cold" foods and beliefs about foods' contribution to health and well-being. "Cold" foods include most vegetables, tropical fruits, dairy products, and inexpensive cuts of meat. "Hot" foods include chili peppers, garlic, onion, most grains, expensive cuts of meat, oils, and alcohol. For example, pregnancy is considered a "hot" condition in which "hot" foods upset the stomach. Thus, chili peppers may be avoided during pregnancy for cultural reasons over any safety issues for the mother or developing fetus.

Depending on the part of the world, the main dishes of Hispanic diets may include meat (pork, veal, sausage), poultry, or fish. Rice and tortillas are mainstays of the diet, as are fruits and vegetables. Milk and cheese are used when available, but are not common in some parts of the world. Fried foods are often used and may need to be monitored where diabetes or obesity is a concern.

Hispanic cuisine often incorporates chili peppers, a rich source of vitamin C. Chili peppers can range in spiciness from mild to very hot and from small to very large. As with Chinese cuisine, Hispanic and Latin American foods often have been modified for the American palate.

Dietary Patterns of Native Americans

Native Americans (American Indian and Alaska Native) comprise more than 500 federally recognized groups that live on federal Indian reservations and in small rural communities (ADA/ADA, 1991, 1993). In Native American culture, food has great religious and social significance. It is an integral part of many celebrations, including powwows and other ceremonies. Food is more of a social or religious obligation than for nourishment alone.

Common foods may be prepared and used in different ways from region to region and by tribal organizations. Fry bread (a fried dough) is a central part of American Indian cuisine and eaten with foods such as stews, soups, and bean dishes. Fried foods are generally prepared with lard.

Corn is the carbohydrate staple of the American Indian diet along with protein-rich dried beans. Fruits and vegetables were traditionally gathered wild but also cultivated on small farms. Sheep, or mutton, and goat are used over pork or beef. Other animal food sources include game and some raised poultry.

The Alaska Native diet is changing but consists

of a mixture of traditional foods and American prepared and processed foods. The diet is high in protein and fat and is based on meat and fish versus plant foods. Meat, fish, sea mammals, and game are staple foods. Seaweed, willow leaves, and sour dock are some of the few edible plants.

The nutrition professional who works with Native Americans will be challenged with a higher prevalence of obesity and diabetes mellitus than in the general American population. It is necessary to merge cultural sensitivity with options to balance diet and health issues.

Dietary Restrictions and Patterns of Religious Groups

Jewish Food Customs and Dietary Laws

The Jewish dietary laws are biblical ordinances codified and interpreted as rules regarding food (ADA/ADA, 1989; Kaufman, 1957). The rules pertain chiefly to the selection, slaughter, and preparation of meat. Animals allowed to be eaten for food are the quadrupeds having a cloven hoof that chew a cud, specifically cattle, sheep, goats, and deer; they are considered "clean." Permissible fowl are chicken, turkey, goose, pheasant, and duck. All animals and fowl must be inspected for disease and killed by a ritual slaughterer according to specific rules. Only the forequarter of the quadruped may be used, except when the hip sinew of the thigh vein can be removed, in which case the hindquarter is also allowed.

Blood is forbidden as food because blood is synonymous with life. Thus, the traditional process of "koshering" the meat and poultry removes all blood before cooking. Koshering involves soaking the meat in water, salting it thoroughly, allowing it to drain, and then washing it three times to remove the salt.

Meat and milk cannot be combined in the same meal. Milk or milk foods may be eaten immediately before the meal but not with the meal. After meat has been eaten, 6 hours must elapse before milk products may be used. Because of the rule of separating meat and milk products, traditional orthodox Jewish homes must keep two completely separate sets of dishes, silver, and cooking equipment—one for meat meals and one for dairy meals. Only those fish having fins and scales are allowed. This bars all shellfish and eels. Fish may be eaten with either dairy or meat meals.

Eggs, too, may be used with either meat or milk. However, any egg yolk containing a drop of blood may not be used because the blood is considered a chick embryo or a sign of a new life.

Fruits, vegetables, cereal products, and all of the other foods that make up a diet may be used without restriction. Bakery products and prepared food mixtures must be produced under acceptable kosher standards.

JEWISH HOLIDAY OBSERVANCE. The most important of the holy days is the Sabbath, or day of rest, observed on Saturday. The meal on Friday night is the best of the week and usually includes both fish and chicken. No food is allowed to be cooked or heated on Saturday, thus all food eaten on the Sabbath is cooked the previous day and either kept warm in the oven or eaten cold.

The festival holidays are Rosh Hashanah, the New Year, in September; Succoth, the fall harvest holiday; Chanukah, the Feast of Lights, in midwinter; and Purim, a joyous holiday in spring. Each holiday has delicacies associated with it.

Yom Kippur, or the Day of Atonement, occurs 10 days after Rosh Hashanah and is a day of fasting, with abstinence from all food and drink, including water, from sundown on the eve of the holiday to sundown on the holiday. Pregnant women and those who are ill do not fast.

Passover, a spring commemorative festival lasting 8 days, requires special dietary consideration. During this period, leavened bread or cake is prohibited. Matzo, unleavened bread, is eaten and all cake and baked products are made from flour of ground-up matzo or potato starch, leavened only with beaten egg whites. No salt is allowed in traditional Passover matzo. Variations of fried matzo or matzo meal pancakes are prepared with generous amounts of fat.

Muslim Food Customs and Dietary Laws

Islam promotes the concept of eating to live, not living to eat (ADA/ADA, 1996). Prayers are offered before food is eaten. Muslims are advised not to eat to capacity and always to share food. Although many foods are allowed, certain codes must be observed and there are some dietary restrictions.

The flesh of animals slaughtered in a human way outlined by Islamic law is *halal*. All meat used for food must be slaughtered according to ritual letting of blood and while speaking the name of God. This may be done by anyone because there is no special person designated for this function. Muslims use kosher meat products because they know they have been slaughtered in the proper manner. Although all foods not specifically prohibited are allowed, certain foods are recommended: milk, dates, meat, seafood, sweets, honey, and vegetable oil, especially olive oil.

If the animal is not slaughtered properly, the meat becomes *haram*, or forbidden. Pork and pork products such as gelatin are prohibited, as are alcoholic beverages and alcohol products (e.g., vanilla or other alcohol-based food or flavoring extracts).

MUSLIM HOLIDAY OBSERVANCES. Fasting is practiced during the month of *Ramadan* every year, which occurs during the ninth month of the Islamic lunar calendar. Muslims fast completely from dawn to sunset and eat only twice a day—before dawn and after sunset. The end of Ramadan is marked by the Feast of Breaking the Fast (Eid-ul-Fitr).

Muslims are also encouraged to fast 3 days of every month. Menstruating, pregnant, or lactating women are not required to fast but must make up the fasting days at some other time.

Vegetarianism

Vegetarian diets of various descriptions have enjoyed increased popularity in recent years, their use motivated by philosophical, religious, and ecologic concerns as well as what some perceive to be a more healthful life-style.

Considerable evidence attests to the health benefits of a vegetarian diet. Epidemiologic data, particularly from studies of Seventh Day Adventists, indicate lower rates of non–insulin-dependent diabetes mellitus, breast and colon cancer, and cardiovascular and gallbladder disease. However, data are not sufficient to prove that an omnivorous diet, planned according to recommended guidelines and combined with a healthy life-style, is not equally beneficial (National Institute of Nutrition, 1990).

Of the 8 to 10 million people in the United States who profess to be vegetarians, most eliminate "red" meats but include fish, poultry, and dairy products ("Lessons we can learn," 1988). The *lacto-vegetarian* does not eat meat, fish, poultry, or eggs, but includes milk, cheese, and other dairy products. The *lacto-ovo-vegetarian* also uses eggs. The true vegetarian, or *vegan*, shuns all foods of animal origin. The vegan program is the only one that incorporates any real risk of inadequate nutrition, and this can be avoided by careful planning.

Vegetarian diets tend to be lower in iron than omnivorous ones, although the nonheme iron present in fruits, vegetables, and unrefined cereals is usually accompanied, either in the food or in the meal, by large amounts of ascorbic acid that aids in assimilation. Vegetarians do not have a greater risk of iron deficiency than nonvegetarians (American Dietetic Association, 1993).

Without dairy products, calcium intakes may be low, and vitamin D may be inadequate in northern latitudes. The calcium present in some vegetables is inactivated by the presence of oxalates. Phytates in unrefined cereals also can inactivate calcium; however, this is not a problem with Western vegetarians, whose diets tend to be based more on fruits and vegetables than on the unrefined cereals used in Middle Eastern cultures.

Vegans of long standing may develop megaloblastic anemia because of vitamin B_{12} deficiency, inasmuch as this vitamin occurs only in foods of animal origin. Curiously, this is less of a problem in areas where sanitation is poor because contaminating bacteria can serve as a source of this vitamin. The hazard of vegan diets is that the presence of high levels of folate may mask the neurologic damage of a B_{12} deficiency. Vegans should have a reliable source of vitamin B_{12}, such as fortified breakfast cereals or soy beverages, or take a supplement (American Dietetic Association, 1993).

Although most vegetarians meet or exceed the RDA for protein, their diets tend to be lower in this nutrient than those of omnivores. This lower intake may help vegetarians retain more calcium from their diets. Furthermore, lower protein intake usually results in reduced consumption of dietary fat because many high-protein animal products are also rich in fat (American Dietetic Association, 1993).

Well-planned vegetarian diets are safe for infants, children, and adolescents, meeting all of their nutritional requirements for growth. They are also adequate for pregnant and lactating women. The key is that the diets be well planned. Vegetarians should pay special attention to ensure they get adequate calcium, iron, zinc, and vitamins B_{12} and D. Calculated combinations of complementary protein sources do not appear to be necessary (American Dietetic Association, 1993). Vitamin B_{12} is still necessary for those persons who rely exclusively on plant foods. Although vegetarians tend to eat less protein than nonvegetarians, the total intake still exceeds the RDA in this country (Auld, 1994). Protein sources should be reasonably varied.

CASE STUDY

Marty T. is a 24-year-old vegetarian Jewish man from Israel. He follows a strict kosher dietary protocol. Recently, as an athlete, he has been taking extra calcium and magnesium capsules because he heard they will help his heart maintain its full capacity. He has no specific medical problems and is at his ideal weight for a height of 6 feet. What dietary guidance would you offer for him?

1. Discuss a dietary plan, following strict kosher protocols, that would meet his daily needs for calcium and magnesium without supplemental capsules.
2. What suggestions would you offer him about dietary guidelines for a healthy heart?
3. What special requirements does an athlete need, and do they conflict with a kosher dietary plan?
4. What impact does a vegetarian life-style have on a person following kosher guidelines? Are there any special considerations?
5. Discuss the new food label requirements as related to your client's dietary plan.

CITED REFERENCES

American Dietetic Association. Position of the American Dietetic Association: Vegetarian diets. J Am Dietet Assoc 93:1317, 1993.

American Dietetic Association and American Diabetes Association. Jewish Food Practices, Customs, and Holidays. Ethnic and Regional Food Practices Series. Chicago: American Dietetic Association, 1989.

American Dietetic Association and American Diabetes Association. Navajo Food Practices, Customs, and Holidays. Ethnic and Regional Food Practices Series. Chicago: American Dietetic Association, 1991.

American Dietetic Association and the American Diabetes Association. Hmong American Food Practices, Customs and Holidays. Ethnic and Regional Food Practices Series. Chicago: American Dietetic Association, 1999.

American Dietetic Association and American Diabetes Association. Alaska Native Food Practices, Customs, and Holidays. Ethnic and Regional Food Practices Series. Chicago: American Dietetic Association, 1993.

American Dietetic Association and American Diabetes Association. Indian and Pakistani Food Practices, Customs, and Holidays. Ethnic and Regional Food Practices Series. Chicago: American Dietetic Association, 1996.

American Dietetic Association and American Diabetes Association. Chinese American Food Practices, Customs, and Holidays. Ethnic and Regional Food Practices Series. Chicago: American Dietetic Association, 1998a.

American Dietetic Association and American Diabetes Association. Mexican American Food Practices, Customs and Holidays. Ethnic and Regional Food Practices Series. Chicago: American Dietetic Association, 1998b.

Anh NT et al. Lactose malabsorption in adult Vietnamese. Am J Clin Nutr 5:676, 1957.

Auld E. Getting to the roots of a vegetarian diet. Food Insight. Washington, DC: International Food Information Council (IFIC) Foundation, 1994.

Bowman SA et al. The Healthy Eating Index: 1994–1996. Publication CNPP-5, Center for Nutrition Policy and Promotion, U.S. Department of Agriculture. Washington, DC: U.S. Government Printing Office, 1998.

Dietary Guidelines Alliance. Reaching Consumers with Meaningful Health Messages: A Handbook for Nutrition and Food Communicators. Washington, DC: Author, 1996.

Federation of American Societies for Experimental Biology, Life Sciences Research Office. Prepared for the Interagency Board for Nutrition Monitoring and Related Research. Third Report on Nutrition Monitoring in the United States. Washington, DC: U.S. Government Printing Office, 1995.

Food and Drug Administration. Focus on Food Labeling. Special Issue of FDA Consumer Magazine, May 1993. DHHS Publication No. (FDA) 93-2262. Washington, DC: U.S. Government Printing Office, 1993.

Food and Nutrition Board, Committee on Diet and Health, National Research Council. Diet and health. Implications for Reducing Chronic disease risk. Washington, DC: National Academy Press, 1989.

Food and Nutrition Board, Institute of Medicine/National Academy of Sciences. How Should the Recommended Dietary Allowances Be Revised? Washington, DC: National Academy Press, 1994.

Food and Nutrition Board, National Research Council/National Academy of Sciences. Recommended Dietary Allowances, 10th ed. Washington, DC: National Academy Press, 1989.

Haas E, McGinnis JM. Ten-Year Comprehensive Plan for the National Nutrition Monitoring and Related Research Program. Fed Reg 58:32752, 1993.

Institute of Medicine. Dietary Reference Intakes for Calcium, Phosphorus, Magnesium, Vitamin D, and Fluoride. A Report of the Standing Committee on the Scientific Evaluation of Dietary Reference Intakes and Its Panel on Calcium and Related Nutrients and Subcommittee on Upper Reference Levels of Nutrients, Food and Nutrition Board. Washington, DC: National Academy Press, 1997.

Institute of Medicine. Dietary Reference Intakes for Thiamin, Riboflavin, Niacin, Vitamin B_6, Folate, Vitamin B_{12}, Pantothenic Acid, Biotin, and Choline. A Report of the Standing Committee on the Scientific Evaluation of Dietary Reference Intakes and Its Panel on Folate, Other B Vitamins, and Choline and Subcommittee on Upper Reference Levels of Nutrients, Food and Nutrition Board. Washington, DC: National Academy Press, 1998.

Kaufman M: Adapting therapeutic diets to Jewish food customs. Am J Clin Nutr 5:676, 1957.

Lessons we can learn from vegetarians. Tufts Univ Nutr Letter 6(5):3, 1988.

Minister of National Health and Welfare. Canada's Food Guide to Healthy Eating. Catalogue no. H39-253/1992E. Ottawa: Health and Welfare Canada, 1992.

National Institute of Nutrition (Canada). Risks and benefits of vegetarian diets. Nutrition Today 25(2):27, 1990.

National Nutrition Monitoring and Related Research Program: Third Report on Nutrition Monitoring in the United States: Executive Summary. Prepared for the Interagency Board for Nutrition Monitoring and Related Research by the Life Sciences Research Office, Federation of American Societies for Experimental Biology. Washington, DC: Government Printing Office, 1995.

Nutrition and Your Health. Dietary Guidelines for Americans, 4th ed. Home and Garden Bulletin no. 232. Hyattsville, MD: USDA, DHHS, 1995.

Public Health Service, Department of Health and Human Services, National Heart, Lung, and Blood Institute. National Cholesterol Education Program (NCEP), Second Report of the Expert Panel on Detection, Evaluation, and Treatment of High Blood Cholesterol in Adults. NIH Publication no. 93-3095. Washington, DC: U.S. Government Printing Office, 1993.

Public Health Service, Department of Health and Human Services, National Institutes of Health. Diet, Nutrition and Cancer Prevention: A Guide to Food Choices. Rev. ed. publication no. 87-2878. Washington, DC: U.S. Government Printing Office, 1987.

Public Health Service. Monthly Vital Statistics Report, vol. 46, no. 1 supplement. Atlanta, GA: Centers for Disease Control and Prevention, 1996.

Public Health Service. The Surgeon General's Report on Nutrition and Health. Summary and Recommendations. DHHS (PHS) Publication no. 88-50211. Washington, DC: U.S. Government Printing Office, 1988.

Tripp RR. World refugee survey 1982. New York: US Committee for Refugees, 1982.

U.S. Department of Agriculture. The Food Guide Pyramid. Home and Garden Bulletin no. 252. Washington, DC: U.S. Government Printing Office, 1992.

U.S. Senate. Select Committee on Nutrition and Human Needs, U.S. Senate, December 1977, 95 Congress—1st session.

White House Conference on Food, Nutrition and Health. Final report. Washington, DC: U.S. Government Printing Office, 1970.

Yates AA. Process and development of dietary reference intakes: Basis, need, and application of recommended dietary allowances. Nutr Rev 56:S5, 1998.

Yates AA, Schlicker SA. Dietary reference intakes: The new basis for recommendations for calcium and related nutrients, B vitamins, and choline. J Am Dietet Assoc 98:699, 1998.

ADDITIONAL REFERENCES

Anderson SL. A look at the Japanese dietary guidelines. J Am Dietet Assoc 90:1527, 1990.

Chang KC (ed.): Food in Chinese Culture. New Haven, CT: Yale University Press, 1977.

Communications/Implementation Committee, Minister of National Health and Welfare. Action Towards Healthy Eating. Canada's Guidelines for Healthy Eating and Recommended Strategies for Implementation. Catalogue no. H39-166/1990E. Ottawa: Minister of Supply and Services, 1990.

Duyff R et al. Food behavior and related factors of Puerto Rican American teenagers. J Nutr Educ 7:99, 1975.

Fanelli-Kuczmarski M, Wotecki CE: Monitoring the nutritional status of the Hispanic population: Selected findings for Mexican Americans, Cubans and Puerto Ricans. Nutrition Today 25(3):6, 1990.

Food and Drug Administration. The New Food Label Summaries. Washington, DC: Department of Health and Human Services, January 6, 1993.

Food Safety Information Service. Nutrition Labeling of Meat and Poultry Products. FSIS Backgrounder. Washington, DC: U.S. Department of Agriculture, 1993.

Lenfant C, Ernst N. Daily dietary fat and total food energy intakes—Third National Health and Nutrition Examination Survey, Phase 1, 1988–91. MMWR 43:116, 1994.

Monsen ER. New dietary reference intakes proposed to replace the recommended dietary allowances. J Am Dietet Assoc 96:754, 1996.

National Exchange for Food Labeling Education. Public Education Campaign on the New Food Label. FSIS Backgrounder. Washington, DC: U.S. Department of Agriculture, 1992.

Peck RE et al. Nutritional status of Southeast Asian refugee children. Am J Pub Health 71:1144, 1981.

Pennington JAT. Bowes and Church's Food Values of Portions Commonly Used, 17th ed. Philadelphia: Lippincott Williams & Wilkins, 1998.

Scientific Review Committee and Communications/Implementation Committee, Minister of National Health and Welfare. Nutrition Recommendations. A Call for Action. Catalogue no. H39-162, 1990E. Ottawa: Minister of Supply and Services, 1990.

U.S. Department of Agriculture. Report of the Dietary Guidelines Advisory Committee on the Dietary Guidelines for Americans, 1995. Washington, DC: U.S. Government Printing Office, 1995.

Welsh S, et al. Development of the food guide pyramid. Nutrition Today 27(6):12, 1992.

CHAPTER 16

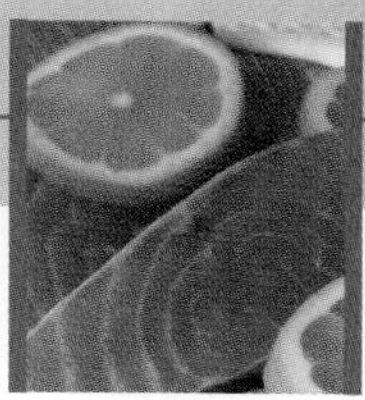

Dietary and Clinical Assessment

KATHLEEN A. HAMMOND, MS, RD, LD, CNSD, BSN, RN

Chapter Outline

- Nutritional Imbalance and Nutritional Screening
- Nutritional Screening
- Nutritional Assessment
- Classifying Malnutrition
- The Nutritional Plan of Care
- Discharge Documentation

Key Terms

ANTHROPOMETRY—the science of measuring the size, weight, and proportions of the human body

BIOELECTRICAL IMPEDANCE ANALYSIS (BIA)—a precise body composition analysis technique that utilizes a small electrical current to analyze body water and body fat; fat and bone are relatively poor conductors of electricity, whereas tissues with high fluid and electrolyte content are good conductors.

BODY MASS INDEX (BMI)—weight (kg)/height (m^2); a definition of the degree of adiposity

DIETARY HISTORY—a detailed dietary record; may include a 24-hour recall, food frequency questionnaire, and other information, such as weight history, previous diet changes, use of supplements, and food intolerances

DIETARY INTAKE DATA—data about food consumption, including information regarding appetite and intake, eating patterns, and estimations of typical nutrient intake

FOOD DIARY—a written record of the amounts of all foods and liquids consumed during a set time period, usually 3 to 7 days; often includes information on time, place, and situation of eating

FOOD FREQUENCY QUESTIONNAIRE—a method of dietary assessment in which the data collected relate to how often foods are consumed (i.e., servings per week/month/year)

KWASHIORKOR—a state of malnutrition characterized by preservation of somatic fat stores and wasting of visceral proteins

MARASMUS—a state of malnutrition characterized by gradual wasting of somatic fat and muscle stores and preservation of visceral proteins

MEDICAL NUTRITIONAL THERAPY (MNT)—the use of specific nutritional interventions to treat an illness, injury, or condition

NUTRITIONAL ASSESSMENT—the science of determining nutritional status by analyzing an individual's medical, dietary, and social history; anthropometric data; biochemical data; and drug-nutrient interactions

NUTRIENT INTAKE ANALYSIS (NIA)—a process by which food, beverage, and supplement intake is evaluated for nutrient content over a specified time period

NUTRITIONAL HEALTH HISTORY—a detailed assessment of dietary, laboratory, and clinical data to determine risk factors for developing nutrition-related problems

NUTRITIONAL SCREENING—a process used to identify nutritional problems and risk factors

NUTRITIONAL STATUS—a measurement of the extent to which the individual's physiologic need for nutrients is being met

24-HOUR RECALL—a method of dietary assessment whereby an individual is asked to remember everything eaten during the previous 24 hours

WAIST-TO-HIP RATIO (WHR)—the ratio of the waist measurement to the hip measurement; a method for assessing fat distribution

WEIGHT-FOR-LENGTH CURVE—a standard for evaluating the growth of children that gives the percentile rankings for weight according to specific heights, but disregarding age

An individual's **nutritional status** reflects the degree to which physiologic needs for nutrients are being met. The balance between nutrient intake and nutrient requirements for optimal health is shown in Figure 16–1. Nutrient intake is dependent on actual food consumption, which is influenced by many factors. These factors include economic situation, eating behavior, emotional climate, cultural influences, and the effects of various disease states on appetite and the ability to consume and absorb

This chapter is a revision of a chapter, contributed by Susan DeHoog, RD, that appeared in the previous edition.

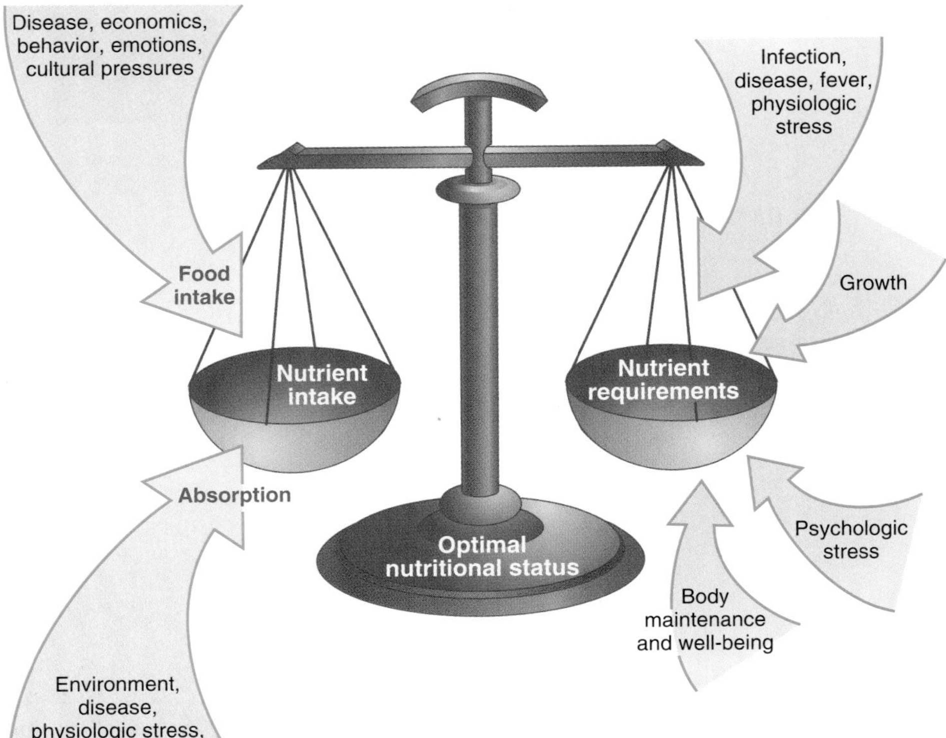

FIGURE 16–1 Optimal nutritional status viewed as a balance between nutrient intake and nutrient requirements.

adequate nutrition. On the other side of the scale are nutrient requirements, which are also influenced by many factors, including physiologic stressors, such as infection, chronic or acute disease processes, fever and/or trauma; normal anabolic states of growth and pregnancy; body maintenance and well-being; and psychological stress.

When adequate nutrients are consumed to support daily body needs, along with any increased metabolic demands, then a state of optimal nutritional status is achieved. This status promotes growth and development, maintains general health, supports activities of daily living, and assists in protection from disease and illness.

Appropriate techniques of assessment can detect nutritional deficiency in the early stages of development so that dietary intake can be improved through nutritional support and counseling before a more severe condition appears.

Assessment of nutritional status should be performed routinely in all individuals. However, the type of assessment differs for those who are basically healthy and those who are critically ill. Persons at nutritional risk can be identified on the basis of screening information that is routinely obtained at the time of admission to a hospital or nursing home. Information obtained in the nutritional assessment is used to design an individual nutritional care plan, as discussed in Chapter 20. A thorough nutritional assessment will increase the effectiveness of nutritional support and nutritional education/counseling.

NUTRITIONAL IMBALANCE AND NUTRITIONAL SCREENING

Nutrition is an important factor in the etiology and management of several major causes of death and disability in contemporary society. Atherosclerotic vascular disease, obesity, hypertension, anemia, osteoporosis, diabetes, and cancer are common diseases in which nutrition is significantly involved. Table 16–1 shows the top ten causes of death in 1996 according to the National Center for Health Statistics. Several of the leading causes of death, including coronary heart disease, stroke, diabetes, and some types of cancer, have a strong link with the type and amount of food consumed. In addition, cirrhosis of the liver, accidents, and some suicides may be associated with excessive alcohol intake. Thus, modifications in dietary intake may assist in the prevention of these diseases and events.

States of nutritional deficiency or excess occur when nutrient intake is not balanced with nutrient requirements for optimal health. Within the safe range of intake, homeostatic mechanisms of the body appear to utilize nutrients equally effectively, with no detectable advantage gained by a given level of intake. As nutritional deficiencies or excesses develop, adaptations are made to achieve a new steady state without any significant loss in physiologic function. As the intake departs further from the accepted range, the organism accommodates to the changing supply of nutrients by reduc-

TABLE 16–1 LEADING CAUSES OF DEATH IN THE UNITED STATES, 1996

CAUSE OF DEATH	RANK	NUMBER (ALL AGES) (1996 TOTAL DEATHS = 2,322,265)
Heart disease	1	733,834
Cancer	2	544,278
Stroke	3	160,431
Chronic obstructive pulmonary disease	4	106,140
Accidents	5	93,874
Pneumonia/influenza	6	82,579
Diabetes	7	61,559
HIV/AIDS	8	32,655
Suicide	9	30,862
Chronic liver disease and cirrhosis	10	25,135

(Data from National Center for Health Statistics. Leading causes of death. Monthly Vital Stat Rep 46(1), 1996.)

HIV, human immunodeficiency virus; *AIDS,* acquired immunodeficiency syndrome.

ing its function, or by changing the size or status of the affected body compartments. The nutritional status of an individual is determined by identifying the presence or absence of these adaptations. For example, before iron deficiency anemia develops, as identified by measures of hematocrit, hemoglobin, and appropriate clinical signs, a gradual diminution in iron stores can be diagnosed on the basis of increased iron absorption, decreased serum ferritin levels, or bone marrow evaluation (see Chapter 35).

When nutritional reserves are depleted, or when nutrient intake is inadequate to meet the body's daily metabolic needs, a state of undernutrition occurs. Nutrient deficiency may stem from inadequate ingestion, impaired digestion or absorption, dysfunctional metabolic processing, or increased excretion of essential nutrients. Infants, children, pregnant women, low-income individuals, hospitalized persons, and the elderly are at the greatest risk for becoming undernourished. Undernourishment may result in impaired growth and development, osteoporosis, lowered resistance to infection, poor wound healing, and poor clinical outcome with increased morbidity and mortality. Overnutrition, too, presents major nutritional problems, manifesting itself in obesity and related disease states, such as diabetes, atherosclerotic heart disease, and hypertension. These conditions may also result in poor clinical outcome, with increased morbidity and mortality.

The evaluation of nutrient deficiencies consists of a review of dietary and medical histories, physical examination, and laboratory evaluation (see Chapter 17). Figure 16–2 illustrates the general sequence of steps leading to the development of a nutritional deficiency and the points at which various components of an assessment can intervene to anticipate problems and prevent poor nutrition before it develops.

There are many different risk factors that may indicate or place one at "nutritional risk," including food and nutrient intake patterns, psychosocial factors, physical conditions associated with particular disease states and disorders, biochemical abnormalities, and medication regimens (Council on Practice Quality Management Committee, 1994). Table 16–2 elaborates on each of these categories. These risk factors can assist health professionals in screening for and assessing an individual's nutritional status.

Nutritional screening and assessment are integral parts of **medical nutrition therapy (MNT),** which is the use of specific nutritional interventions to treat an illness, injury, or condition (Council on Practice Quality Management Committee, 1994). MNT has two phases: (1) assessment of nutritional status, and (2) treatment, which may include diet therapy, counseling, or specialized nutritional supplementation.

In order to provide cost-effective MNT in today's health care environment, it is important to first identify patients who are at nutritional risk. Nutri-

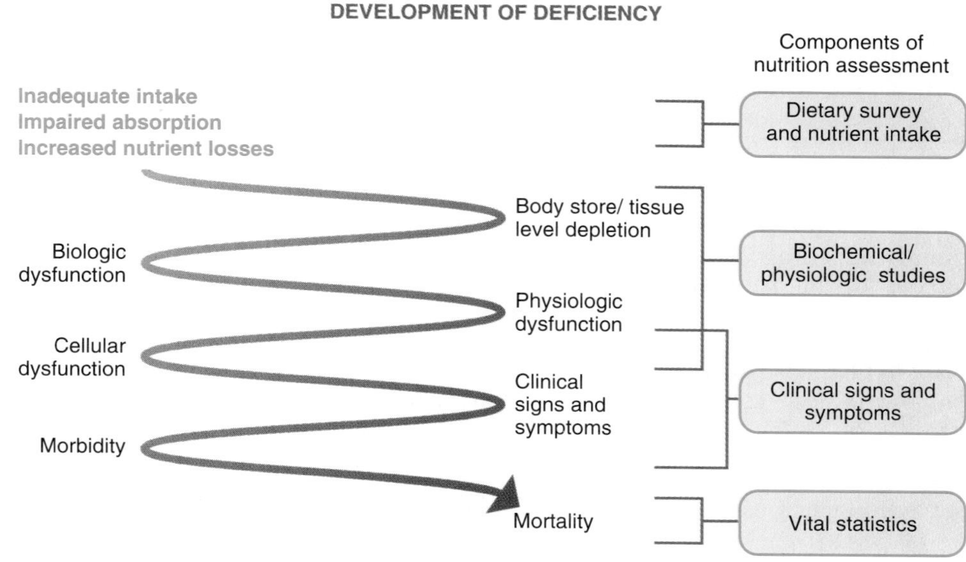

FIGURE 16–2 Development of a clinical nutritional deficiency with corresponding dietary, biochemical, and clinical evaluations.

TABLE 16–2 NUTRITIONAL RISK FACTORS

RISK CATEGORY	RISK FACTORS
Food and nutrient intake patterns	• Calorie and protein intake greater or less than that required for age and activity level • Vitamin and mineral intake greater or less than that required for age • Swallowing difficulties • Gastrointestinal disturbances • Unusual food habits (e.g., pica) • Impaired cognitive function or depression • NPO for more than 3 days • Inability or unwillingness to consume food • Increase or decrease in activities of daily living • Misuse of supplements • Inadequate transitional feeding and/or tube feeding or parenteral nutrition • Bowel irregularity (constipation, diarrhea) • Restricted diets • Feeding limitations
Psychological and/or social factors	• Low literacy • Language barriers • Cultural/religious factors • Emotional disturbances associated with feeding difficulties (depression) • Limited resources for food preparation or obtaining food and supplies • Alcohol/drug addiction • Limited/low income • Lack of or inability to communicate needs • Limited use or understanding of community resources
Physical conditions	• Extremes in age: older than 80 years of age, premature infants, very young • Pregnancy: adolescent, closely spaced, or 3 or more pregnancies • Alterations in anthropometric measurements: marked overweight or underweight for height and/or age; head circumference less than normal; depressed somatic fat and muscle stores; amputation • Fat or muscle wasting • Obesity/overweight • Chronic renal or cardiac disease and related complications • Diabetes and related complications • Pressure ulcers or altered skin integrity • Cancer and related treatments • AIDS • Gastrointestinal complications (malabsorption, diarrhea, digestive or bowel changes) • Catabolic or hypermetabolic stress (trauma, sepsis, burns, stress) • Immobility • Osteoporosis, osteomalacia • Neurologic impairment including impairment in sensory function • Visual impairment
Abnormal laboratory values	• Visceral proteins (e.g., albumin, transferrin, prealbumin) • Lipid profile (cholesterol, high-density lipoproteins, low-density lipoproteins, triglycerides) • Hemoglobin, hematocrit, and other hematologic tests • Blood urea nitrogen, creatinine, electrolytes • Fasting serum blood glucose • Other laboratory indices as indicated
Medications	• Chronic use • Multiple and concurrent administration (polypharmacy) • Drug-nutrient interactions and side effects

(Information compiled from Council on Practice, Quality Management Committee: ADA's definitions for nutrition screening and nutrition assessment. J Am Diet Assoc 94:838, 1994.)

tional screening and nutritional assessment are part of this identification process.

NUTRITIONAL SCREENING

Ideally, all persons should undergo periodic nutritional status screening and assessment throughout their lives, not just during periods of illness. Different approaches can be applied to the healthy population and to the critically ill. The assessment process involves two phases: screening and assessment. The definitions of nutritional screening and assessment may vary slightly from one setting to another. The major purpose, however, is to screen for nutritional risks and apply specific assessment techniques to determine an action plan.

Nutritional screening is defined as the process of identifying characteristics known to be associated with nutritional problems (Council on Practice,

1994). The purpose of a nutritional screen is to quickly identify individuals who are malnourished or at nutritional risk. The nutritional screen can usually be completed by a dietitian, dietetic technician, nurse, physician, or other qualified health care professional. In many settings, the nutritional screen is completed by a health professional other than the dietitian; once completed, though, patients who are at nutritional risk are usually referred to a registered dietitian. Table 16–3 outlines the characteristics of a nutritional screening tool.

The information collected during a nutritional screen depends upon (1) the particular *setting* in which the information is obtained (e.g., the home, clinic, or hospital); (2) the *disease* or *population group,* such as the elderly, pregnant women, or oncology patients; (3) the type of *data* that can easily be obtained; (4) a definition of *risk;* and (5) the *goals* of the screen. Examples of information that may be obtained using a screening tool include height, usual body weight, recent or significant loss or increase in weight; diagnosis; whether the person is receiving a therapeutic diet for a particular disease state, or is receiving parenteral or enteral nutrition, or is NPO; laboratory values, such as serum albumin, hemoglobin/hematocrit, and total lymphocyte levels; a history of gastrointestinal disturbances, such as distention, diarrhea, or nausea and vomiting; functional status, as evidenced by hand-grip dynamometry; and current medication profile.

Regardless of the information that is gathered, the goal of screening is to identify individuals who are at nutritional risk or who are likely to become at nutritional risk, as well as to identify those who need further assessment and the best source for that assessment. Several examples of screening tools can be found in the following tables. Table 16–4 is a short screening tool used for patients who are not suspected to be at risk. Table 16–5 is a nutritional questionnaire that can be used in a clinic setting, where a patient can complete it while waiting. Figure 16–3 is an example of a nutritional screen used in an acute care setting, whereas Figure 16–4 is an example of a screening tool used for a perinatal population (in this case, it is combined with a full nutrition assessment). Figure 16–5 is for Pediatrics.

TABLE 16–3 CHARACTERISTICS OF A NUTRITIONAL SCREEN

- Is simple and can be completed quickly
- Relies on data that are routinely gathered in a particular setting
- Facilitates completion of early intervention goals
- Includes collection of relevant data on risk factors and data interpretation for intervention or treatment
- Determines the need for a nutrition assessment
- Is cost-effective

(Information compiled from Council on Practice Quality Management Committee: ADA's definitions for nutrition screening and nutrition assessment. J Am Diet Assoc 94:838, 1994.)

TABLE 16–4 SHORT NUTRITION SCREEN

O: Diagnosis
Diet order
A: Per review of medical record; patient is not nutritionally compromised at this time.
P: Will reevaluate in 5–7 days or per consult.
Signature: ______________

O, objective; *A,* assessment; *P,* plan.

The *Nutrition Screening Initiative,* a joint project of the American Academy of Physicians, The American Dietetic Association, and the National Council on the Aging, Inc., was developed to focus specifically on and improve the nutritional care available to older adults (Nutrition Interventions Manual, 1991). Three tools are available that focus attention on nutrition in the elderly:

1. The *"DETERMINE Your Nutritional Health"* checklist (Fig. 16–6) is a public awareness tool designed to highlight the warning signs of poor nutritional status.
2. The *Level I Screen* (Fig. 16–7) is a tool to identify individuals who should be referred for a more comprehensive nutrition or medical follow-up, in addition to other health and community services (Barrocas et al., 1995; Nutrition Screening Initiative, 1991).
3. The *Level II Screen* (Fig. 16–8) is used when the checklist or Level I Screen identifies potentially serious nutrition or medical problems. This screen incorporates both nutritional screening and assessment measures (Barrocas et al., 1995; Nutrition Screening Initiative, 1991).

TABLE 16–5 NUTRITIONAL QUESTIONNAIRE

1. Height: _____ Usual Weight: _____ Actual Weight: _____
2. Have you had a recent weight loss of greater than 10 pounds within 30 days?
3. Have you been on a weight reduction diet? _____ yes _____ no
4. Have you had a recent change in appetite? _____ yes _____ no
5. Do you have any problems with: swallowing? _____ yes _____ no
   chewing? _____ yes _____ no
   nausea? _____ yes _____ no
   diarrhea? _____ yes _____ no
   vomiting? _____ yes _____ no
   constipation? _____ yes _____ no
6. Do you follow any special diet? _____ yes _____ no
   If yes, what type of diet? ______________
7. What foods are you allergic to?
8. Do you take any vitamin/mineral supplement? _____ yes _____ no
   If yes, please list.
9. Do you take any medications?

If yes, please list:	*Prescription*	*Over-the-counter*

NUTRITION SERVICES SCREENING ASSESSMENT FORM

ADDRESSOGRAPH

Admission Date:____________________

Medical Record Review

Diagnosis ______________________________ Age ____________

Ht. ______ Wt. ______ IBW ______ % IBW ______ UBW ______ %UBW ______

Albumin ____________ Other Labs ______________________________

Appetite: > 50% ≤ 50% Poor

Medication ______________________________

Other ______________________________

Diet Order________Date_______Diet Order________Date_______Diet Order________Date_______

Evaluation Criteria *(Check all that apply)*

- ❑ Loss of appetite > 48 hrs.
- ❑ Difficulty chewing/swallowing
- ❑ Significant food allergies/intolerances
- ❑ Malnourished appearance
- ❑ Length of stay ≥ 7 days
- ❑ > 65 years of age with a surgery this admission
- ❑ < 50% meals consumed
- ❑ Modified diet ______________________________

Pt. identified to be at nutritional risk based on meeting > 2 criteria above.

Plan

Pt. not at high nutritional risk at this time. Basic nutritional care services and follow-up will be provided per policy.

- ❑ Pt. seen for snacks/food preferences.
- ❑ Pt. to receive comfort measures only. No intervention planned unless requested/ordered by staff or pt.
- ❑ Pt./care provider familiar with dietary modifications. No education planned.
- ❑ Other ______________________________

X ______________________________

Signature Date

Nutrition Services Screening Assessment Form

3/97
Piedmont Graphics

Original - Chart
Yellow - Department

FIGURE 16–3 Nutrition screen. *IBW,* ideal body weight; *UBW,* usual body weight. (Courtesy of Northside Hospital, Atlanta, Georgia.)

These tools are simple, brief, and generic in nature and are designed to be flexible, allowing adaptation for particular patient populations (Nutrition Screening Initiative, 1991).

NUTRITIONAL ASSESSMENT

Nutritional assessment, as defined by The American Dietetic Association (Council on Practice, 1994), is a comprehensive approach, completed by a registered dietitian, for defining nutritional status using medical, social, nutritional, and medication histories; physical examination; anthropometric measurements; and laboratory data. Nutritional assessment involves interpretation of data from the nutritional screen and incorporates additional information. Once the nutritional assessment process is completed, the nutritional plan of care can be developed and implemented and then tailored for the appropriate setting (e.g., hospital, clinic, or home). (See "*Focus On:* Subjective Global Assessment.")

The goals of nutritional assessment are (1) to identify individuals who require aggressive nutritional support, (2) to restore or maintain an individual's nutritional status, (3) to identify appropriate MNTs, and (4) to monitor the efficacy of these therapies.

Studies indicate that, upon admission to acute care facilities, between 33% and 65% of all patients have some degree of malnutrition. Furthermore, in patients who are hospitalized for longer than 2 weeks, nutritional status deteriorates (see the accompanying box, "*Focus On:* Malnutrition in Hospitals"). All persons with acute or chronic illness have the potential for nutritional risk, and so should be evaluated. Malnutrition is not uncommon in obese, cachexic, elderly, and traumatized persons.

In summary, a thorough assessment of nutritional status includes (1) medical, social, medication, and nutritional histories; (2) physical exami-

Perinatal Nutrition Screening/Assessment Form

ADDRESSOGRAPH

SCREENING CRITERIA FOR POTENTIAL NUTRITIONAL RISK *(full assessment if one checked)*

SCREENING CRITERIA FOR POTENTIAL NUTRITIONAL RISK

ANTEPARTUM

- ☐ Obstetrical Condition (Multiple Gestation, PIH, IUGR, Diabetes, Hyperemesis, Anemia)
- ☐ Chronic/Systemic Condition Affecting Nutritional Status or Intake
- ☐ Adolescence (≤ 17)
- ☐ Inappropriate Weight Change
- ☐ Albumin ≤ 2.5
- ☐ Therapeutic or Limited Diet
- ☐ Lack of Knowledge re Pregnancy Diet
- ☐ Length of Stay ≥ 5 days

POSTPARTUM

☐ Gestational Diabetes this Pregnancy ☐ Albumin ≤ 2.5 ☐ Hg < 8.0

Breastfeeding mother meeting the following criteria:

- ☐ ≤ 17 Years Old
- ☐ Therapeutic or Limited Diet
- ☐ Lack of Knowledge re Lactation Diet
- ☐ Multiple Birth with Infants in Special Care Nursery

COMPREHENSIVE ASSESSMENT

SUBJECTIVE

Weight Gain/Expected Weight Gain ______

Cultural/Social Concerns ______

Activity Level ______

Plans to Breastfeed? ☐ Yes ☐ No

Other ______

OBJECTIVE

Diagnosis ______ Parity ______ EGA/EDC ______

Medical/Obstetrical History ______

Age ______ Ht ______ Pregravid Wt ______ BMI/Category ______ Current Wt ______

Medications ______ Vitamin/Mineral Supplements ______

Physical Exam ______ GI Function ______

Food Allergies/Intolerance ______ Diet Order ______

Labs ______

ASSESSMENT

Estimated Energy Needs ______ Protein ______ Other ______

Adequacy of Intake/Evaluation of Nutritional Status ______

FIGURE 16–4 Perinatal nutrition screen/assessment form. *PIH,* pregnancy-induced HPN; *IUGR,* intrauterine growth retardation; *EGA,* estimated gestational age; *EDC,* estimated date of confinement; *BMI,* body mass index; *GI,* gastrointestinal. (Courtesy of Northside Hospital, Atlanta, Georgia.)

Shriners Burns Hospital
Rehabilitation Nutrition Screening Form

DATE: ______________________ LEVEL ______________________

NAME: ______________________ UNIT# ______________________

AGE ____ __/M __/F

BIRTHDATE ______________________

REASON FOR ADMISSION ______________________

WEIGHT ____ ____%NCHS
HEIGHT ____ ____%NCHS

RECENT WEIGHT LOSS/GAIN ____Y ____N
IF YES, INTENTION ____Y ____N
HOW MUCH ____
TIME FRAME ____

RECENT: ____ NAUSEA ____ VOMITING TX: ____
____ DIARRHEA ____ CONSTIPATION
____ HX OF ANEMIA ____ CHANGE IN APPETITE
____ DENTITION CONCERNS ____ DIFFICULTY SWALLOWING

FOOD ALLERGIES ____N ____Y ______________________

DIET RESTRICTIONS ____N ____Y ______________________

COOKING FACILITIES ____STOVE ____REFRIGERATOR

DRINKS ____BOTTLE ____STRAW ____SIPPEE CUP ____CUP

VITAMIN SUPPLEMENTATION ____N ____Y TYPE ____
REASON ____

MEDICATIONS ____N ____Y TYPE(S) ____
REASON ____

CARETAKER/RELATIONSHIP ______________________

NUTRITIONAL CONCERNS STATED BY PATIENT/CARETAKER:

NUTRITIONAL INTERVENTION PROVIDED:

FIGURE 16–5 Pediatric screening form. (Courtesy of Shriners Burn Hospital, Cincinnati, Ohio.)

nation, (3) anthropometric data; and (4) laboratory data. Chapter 17 discusses biochemical assessment in greater detail. Chapter 18 provides details about potential food-drug interactions.

Histories

The information collected on individuals or populations is used as part of the nutritional status assessment. Frequently, the information is in the form of histories—medical, social, dietary, and medication histories.

Medical and Social Histories. The medical history usually includes the following information: chief complaint, present and past illness, current health, allergies, past or recent surgeries, family history of disease, psychosocial aspects, and a review of problems, by body system, from the patient's perspective (Hammond, 1998). These histories usually provide much insight into nutrition-related problems. Alcohol and drug use, increased metabolic needs, increased nutritional losses, chronic disease, recent major surgery or illness, disease or surgery of the gastrointestinal tract, and recent significant weight loss all may contribute to malnutrition. In elderly patients, further review is recommended to detect mental deterioration, constipation/incontinence, poor eyesight or hearing, slowed reactions, major organ diseases, effects of prescription and over-the-counter drugs, and physical disabilities (Table 16–6).

Social aspects of the medical history may also relate to nutritional status, such as information pertaining to socioeconomic status, the individual's ability to purchase his/her own food, living or eating alone, physical or mental handicaps, smoking, or drug and/or alcohol addiction. In the elderly, confusion secondary to environmental changes, unsuitable housing conditions, lack of socialization at meals, psychological problems, and poverty may add to the risks.

Medication History. Food and drugs interact in many ways that affect nutritional status and drug therapy effectiveness, so a medication history is an

DETERMINE YOUR NUTRITIONAL HEALTH

The Warning Signs of poor nutritional health are often overlooked. Use this checklist to find out if you or someone you know is at nutritional risk.

Read the statements below. Circle the number in the yes column for those that apply to you or someone you know. For each yes answer, score the number in the box. Total your nutrition score.

	YES
I have an illness or condition that made me change the kind and/or amount of food I eat.	2
I eat fewer than 2 meals per day.	3
I eat few fruits or vegetables, or milk products.	2
I have 3 or more drinks of beer, liquor or wine almost every day.	2
I have tooth or mouth problems that make it hard for me to eat.	2
I don't always have enough money to buy the food I need.	4
I eat alone most of the time.	1
I take 3 or more different prescribed or over-the-counter drugs a day.	1
Without wanting to, I have lost or gained 10 pounds in the last 6 months.	2
I am not physically able to shop, cook and/or feed myself.	2
TOTAL	

Total Your Nutritional Score. If it's —

0–2 **Good!** Recheck your nutritional score in 6 months.

3–5 **You are at moderate nutritional risk.** See what can be done to improve your eating habits and lifestyle. Your office on aging, senior nutrition program, senior citizens center or health department can help. Recheck your nutritional score in 3 months.

6 or more **You are at high nutritional risk.** Bring this checklist the next time you see your doctor, dietitian or other qualified health or social service professional. Talk with them about any problems you may have. Ask for help to improve your nutritional health.

Remember that warning signs suggest risk, but do not represent diagnosis of any condition.

The Nutrition Checklist is based on the Warning Signs described below.
Use the word DETERMINE to remind you of the Warning signs.

Disease Any disease, illness or chronic condition which causes you to change the way you eat, or makes it hard for you to eat, puts your nutritional health at risk. Four out of five adults have chronic diseases that are affected by diet. Confusion or memory loss that keeps getting worse is estimated to affect one out of five or more of older adults. This can make it hard to remember what, when or if you've eaten. Feeling sad or depressed, which happens to about one in eight older adults, can cause big changes in appetite, digestion, energy level, weight and well-being.

Eating Poorly Eating too little and eating too much both lead to poor health. Eating the same foods day after day or not eating fruit, vegetables, and milk products daily will also cause poor nutritional health. One in five adults skip meals daily. Only 13% of adults eat the minimum amount of fruit and vegetables needed. One in four older adults drink too much alcohol. Many health problems become worse if you drink more than one or two alcoholic beverages per day.

Tooth Loss/Mouth Pain A healthy mouth, teeth and gums are needed to eat. Missing, loose or rotten teeth, or dentures which don't fit well or cause mouth sores, make it hard to eat.

Economic Hardship As many as 40% of older Americans have incomes of less than $6,000 per year. Having less—or choosing to spend less— than $25–30 per week for food makes it very hard to get the foods you need to stay healthy.

Reduced Social Contact One-third of all older people live alone. Being with people daily has a positive effect on morale, well-being and eating.

Multiple Medicines Many older Americans must take medicines for health problems. Almost half of older Americans take multiple medicines daily. Growing old may change the way we respond to drugs. The more medicines you take, the greater the chance for side effects, such as increased or decreased appetite, change in taste, constipation, weakness, drowsiness, diarrhea, nausea, and others. Vitamins or minerals, when taken in large doses, act like drugs and can cause harm. Alert your doctor to everything you take.

Involuntary Weight Loss/Gain Losing or gaining a lot of weight when you are not trying to do so is an important warning sign that must not be ignored. Being overweight or underweight also increases your chance of poor health.

Needs Assistance in Self-Care Although most older people are able to eat, one out of every five has trouble walking, shopping, or buying and cooking food, especially as they get older.

Elder Years Above Age 80 Most older people lead full and productive lives. But as age increases, the risk of frailty and health problems increases. Checking your nutritional health regularly makes good sense.

FIGURE 16–6 "Determine Your Nutritional Health" checklist. (Reprinted with permission by the Nutrition Screening Initiative, a project of the American Academy of Family Physicians, the American Dietetic Association, and the National Council on the Aging, Inc., and funded in part by a grant from Ross Products Division, Abbott Laboratories.)

LEVEL I SCREEN

LEVEL I SCREEN — Name: — Date:

Body Weight

Measure height to the nearest inch and weigh to the nearest pound. Record the values below and mark them on the Body Mass Index (BMI) scale to the right. Then use a straight edge (ruler) to connect the two points and circle the spot where this straight ine rosses the center line (body mass index). Record the number below.

Healthy older adults should have a BMI between 24 and 27.

Height (in): ______________________

Weight (lbs): ______________________

Body Mass Index: ______________________
(number from center column)

Check any boxes that are true for the individual:

- ☐ Has lost or gained 10 pounds (or more) in the past 6 months.
- ☐ Body mass index < 24
- ☐ Body mass index > 27

A physician should be contacted if the individual has gained or lost 10 pounds unexpectedly or without intending to during the past 6 months. A physician should also be notified if the individual's body mass index is above 27 or below 24.

NOMOGRAM FOR BODY MASS INDEX

HEIGHT (IN | CM): 50–85 in; 125–210 cm

WEIGHT (LB | KG): 50–340 lb; 25–150 kg

Center column (Body Mass Index): 10, 20, 30, 40, 50, 60, 70

WOMEN		MEN
OBESE	30	OBESE
OVERWEIGHT		OVERWEIGHT
ACCEPTABLE	20	ACCEPTABLE

For the remaining sections, please ask the individual which of the statements (if any) is true for him or her and place a check by each that applies.

Eating Habits

- ☐ Does not have enough to eat each day
- ☐ Usually eats alone
- ☐ Does not eat anything on one or more days each month
- ☐ Has poor appetite
- ☐ Is on a special diet
- ☐ Eats vegetables two or fewer times daily
- ☐ Eats milk or milk products once or not at all daily
- ☐ Eats fruit or drinks fruit juice once or not at all daily
- ☐ Eats breads, cereals, pasta, rice, or other grains five or fewer times daily
- ☐ Has difficulty chewing or swallowing
- ☐ Has more than one alcoholic drink per day (if woman); more than two drinks per day (if man)
- ☐ Has pain in mouth, teeth or gums

Living Environment

- ☐ Lives on an income of less than $6000 per year (per individual in the household)
- ☐ Lives alone
- ☐ Is housebound
- ☐ Is concerned about home security
- ☐ Lives in a home with inadequate heating or cooling
- ☐ Does not have a stove and/or refrigerator
- ☐ Is unable or prefers not to spend money on food (<$25–30 per person spent on food each week)

Functional Status

Usually or always needs assistance with (check all that apply):

- ☐ Bathing
- ☐ Dressing
- ☐ Grooming
- ☐ Toileting
- ☐ Eating
- ☐ Walking or moving about
- ☐ Traveling (outside the home)
- ☐ Preparing food
- ☐ Shopping for food or other necessities

If you have checked one or more statements on this screen, the individual you have interviewed may be at risk for poor nutritional status. Please refer this individual to the appropriate health care or social service professional in your area. For example, a dietitian should be contacted for problems with selecting, preparing or eating a healthy diet, or a dentist if the individual experiences pain or difficulty when chewing or swallowing. Those individuals whose income, life-style or functional status may endanger their nutritional and overall health should be referred to available community services: home-delivered meals, congregate meal programs, transportation systems, counseling services, day care programs, etc.

Please repeat this screen at least once each year — sooner if the individual has a major change in his or her health, income, immediate family (e.g., spouse dies) or functional status.

FIGURE 16–7 Level I screen. (Reprinted with permission by the Nutrition Screening Initiative, a project of the American Academy of Family Physicians, the American Dietetic Association, and the National Council on the Aging, Inc., and funded in part by a grant from Ross Products Division, Abbott Laboratories.)

LEVEL II SCREEN

Complete the following screen by interviewing the patient directly and/or by referring to the patient chart. If you do not routinely perform all of the described tests or ask all of the listed questions, please consider including them, but do not be concerned if the entire screen is not completed. Please try to conduct a minimal screen on as many older patients as possible, and please try to collect serial measurements, which are extremely valuable in monitoring nutritional status. Please refer to the manual for additional information.

Anthropometrics

Measure height to the nearest inch and weigh to the nearest pound. Record the values below and mark them on the Body Mass Index (BMI) scale to the right. Then use a straight edge (paper, ruler) to connect the two points and circle the spot where this straight line crosses the center line (body mass index). Record the number below. Healthy older adults should have a BMI between 24 and 27; check the appropriate box to flag an abnormally high or low value.

Height (in): ____________________

Weight (lbs): ____________________

Body Mass Index: ____________________
(number from center column)

Please place a check by any statement regarding BMI and recent weight loss that is true for the patient:

- ☐ Body mass index < 24
- ☐ Body mass index > 27
- ☐ Has lost or gained 10 pounds (or more) in the past 6 months.

Record the measurement of mid-arm circumference to the nearest 0.1 centimeter and of triceps skinfold to the nearest 2 millimeters.

Mid-arm circumference (cm): ____________________

Triceps skinfold (mm): ____________________

Mid-arm muscle circumference (cm): ____________________

Refer to the table and check any abnormal values:

- ☐ Mid-arm muscle circumference < 10th percentile
- ☐ Triceps skinfold < 10th percentile
- ☐ Triceps skinfold > 95th percentile

Note: mid-arm circumference (cm) – {0.314 x triceps skinfold (mm)} = mid-arm *muscle* circumference (cm)

Percentile	Men 55–65 y	Men 65–75 y	Women 55–65 y	Women 65–75 y
Arm circumference (cm)				
10th	27.3	26.3	25.7	25.2
50th	31.7	30.7	30.3	29.9
95th	36.9	35.5	38.5	37.3
Arm muscle circumference (cm)				
10th	24.5	23.5	19.6	19.5
50th	27.8	26.8	22.5	22.5
95th	32.0	30.6	28.0	27.9
Triceps skinfold (mm)				
10th	6	6	16	14
50th	11	11	25	24
95th	22	22	22	36

For the remaining sections, please place a check by any statements that are true for the patient.

Laboratory Data

- ☐ Serum albumin below 3.5 g/dL
- ☐ Serum cholesterol below 160 mg/dL
- ☐ Serum cholesterol above 240 mg/dL

Drug Use

- ☐ Three or more prescription drugs, OTC medications, and/or vitamin/mineral supplements daily

Clinical Features

Presence of (check all that apply)

- ☐ Problems with mouth, teeth or gums
- ☐ Difficulty chewing
- ☐ Angular stomatitis
- ☐ Glossitis
- ☐ History of bone pain
- ☐ History of bone fractures
- ☐ Skin changes (dry, loose, nonspecific lesions, edema)

NOMOGRAM FOR BODY MASS INDEX

HEIGHT (IN | CM)

IN: 50, 55, 60, 65, 70, 75, 80, 85

CM: 125, 130, 135, 140, 145, 150, 155, 160, 165, 170, 175, 180, 185, 190, 195, 200, 205, 210

Body mass index (center): 70, 60, 50, 40, 30, 20, 10

WOMEN: OBESE / OVERWEIGHT / ACCEPTABLE

MEN: OBESE / OVERWEIGHT / ACCEPTABLE

WEIGHT (LB | KG)

LB: 340, 320, 300, 280, 260, 240, 220, 200, 190, 180, 170, 160, 150, 140, 130, 120, 110, 100, 95, 90, 85, 80, 75, 70, 65, 60, 55, 50

KG: 150, 140, 130, 120, 110, 100, 95, 90, 85, 80, 75, 70, 65, 60, 55, 50, 45, 40, 35, 30, 25

Eating Habits

- ☐ Does not have enough to eat each day
- ☐ Usually eats alone
- ☐ Does not eat anything on one or more days each month
- ☐ Has poor appetite
- ☐ Is on a special diet
- ☐ Eats vegetables two or fewer times daily
- ☐ Eats milk or milk products once or not at all daily
- ☐ Eats fruit or drinks fruit juice once or not at all daily
- ☐ Eats breads, cereals, pasta, rice, or other grains five or fewer times daily
- ☐ Has more than one alcoholic drink per day (if woman); more than two drinks per day (if man)

Living Environment

- ☐ Lives on an income of less than $6000 per year (per individual in the household)
- ☐ Lives alone
- ☐ Is housebound
- ☐ Is concerned about home security
- ☐ Lives in a home with inadequate heating or cooling
- ☐ Does not have a stove and/or refrigerator
- ☐ Is unable or prefers not to spend money on food (<$25–30 per person spent on food each week)

Functional Status

Usually or always needs assistance with (check all that apply)

- ☐ Bathing
- ☐ Dressing
- ☐ Grooming
- ☐ Toileting
- ☐ Eating
- ☐ Walking or moving about
- ☐ Traveling (outside the home)
- ☐ Preparing food
- ☐ Shopping for food or other necessities

Mental/Cognitive Status

- ☐ Clinical evidence of impairment (e.g., Folstein < 26)
- ☐ Clinical evidence of depressive illness (e.g., Beck Depression Inventory > 15, Geriatric Depression Scale > 5)

LEVEL II SCREEN Name: Date:

FIGURE 16–8 Level II screen. *OTC,* over-the-counter. (Reprinted with permission by the Nutrition Screening Initiative, a project of the American Academy of Family Physicians, the American Dietetic Association, and the National Council on the Aging, Inc., and funded in part by a grant from Ross Products Division, Abbott Laboratories.)

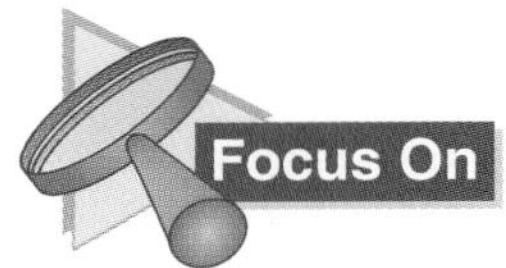

Subjective Global Assessment

In contrast to methods of assessment that employ objective biochemical and anthropometric measurements, there is a screening tool referred to as the *Subjective Global Assessment* (SGA) of nutritional status, the features of which are outlined in the following chart. This is an "eyeball" technique that requires good clinical judgment, as the information is collected by observation and interviews. Guidelines for health professionals have been set forth by the developers of this technique (Detsky et al., 1987). The correlations to clinical outcome are similar to those obtained using more objective measures. This type of evaluation has been found to be extremely useful and cost-effective (Nutritional Assessment Present and Future, 1988).

Subjective Global Assessment Summary*

HISTORY

1. Weight change

   Overall loss in past 6 months: amount = _____ kg _____%

   Change in past 2 weeks: _____ increase

   _____ no change

   _____ decrease

2. Dietary intake change (relative to normal)

   _____ no change

   _____ change

   duration: _____ weeks

   type: _____ suboptimal solid diet _____ full liquid diet

   _____ hypocaloric liquids _____ starvation

3. Gastrointestinal symptoms (persisting for >2 weeks)

   _____ none _____ nausea _____ vomiting _____ diarrhea _____ anorexia

4. Functional capacity

   _____ no dysfunction (e.g., full capacity)

   _____ dysfunction

   duration: _____ weeks

   type: _____ working suboptimally

   _____ ambulatory

   _____ bedridden

PHYSICAL EXAMINATION

For each trait, specify a rating as follows: 0 = normal, 1+ = mild, 2+ = moderate, 3+ = severe.

_____ loss of subcutaneous fat (triceps, chest)

_____ muscle wasting (quadriceps, deltoids)

_____ ankle edema

_____ sacral edema

_____ ascites

SUBJECTIVE GLOBAL ASSESSMENT RATING (Select one):

_____ A = well nourished

_____ B = moderately (or suspected of being) malnourished

_____ C = severely malnourished

*From Detsky AS, McLaughlin JR, Baker JP, et al. What is subjective global assessment? J Parent Ent Nutr 11(1):8, 1987.

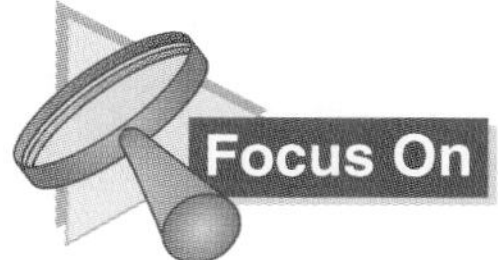

MALNUTRITION IN HOSPITALS

In a landmark article in 1974, Butterworth showed that malnutrition could indeed be found in the United States—in hospitals, where it was frequently not recognized. Over the course of the next few years, malnutrition was noted in many hospitalized patients, and attempts were made to evaluate its severity and reverse its course. Since that time, there have been periods of heightened awareness and periods of minimal awareness. With only minimal training in nutrition (defined as having nutrition courses either spread throughout the curriculum or having very few contact hours) offered in many medical schools, physicians graduate with little practical knowledge about nutrition. Not surprisingly, this results in decreased physician awareness of malnutrition. To maintain a high level of awareness, physician education programs in nutrition should be conducted regularly. The American Dietetic Association has embarked on a Physician Nutrition Education program through its strategic initiatives. In this program, physicians, dietitians, and office staff team up to help patients screen their own eating habits using the Food Guide Pyramid (see Chapter 15). if problems are identified, the practitioner then refers the patient to a dietitian, nutritionist, or qualified nutrition educator for follow-up services.

important part of any nutritional assessment. The elderly, the chronically ill, those with a history of marginal or inadequate nutritional intake, and anyone receiving multidrug therapy over a period of time are susceptible to drug-induced nutritional deficiencies. The effects of drug therapy can be altered by specific foods and by the timing of food and meals (see Chapter 18 and Appendices 33 and 34). The contents of multivitamin and mineral supplements are listed in Appendix 52 for evaluation purposes.

NUTRITION OR DIET HISTORY. Anorexia, ageusia, dysgeusia, anosmia, excess alcohol intake, poor-fitting dentures, fad dieting, chewing or swallowing problems, frequent meals away from home, adverse food and drug interactions, cultural or religious restrictions of diet, inability to eat for more than 7 to 10 days, intravenous fluid therapy for more than 5 days, taste changes, or feeding dependence can lead to inadequate nutrient intake and nutritional inadequacy. For many elderly, inability to self-feed, denture problems, changes in taste and smell, long-established poor food habits, food fads, and inadequate knowledge of nutrition are common problems.

A dietary history is perhaps the best means of obtaining this information (Table 16–7). The term **dietary history** refers to a review of an individual's usual patterns of food intake and the food selection variables that dictate food intake. Whereas a dietary assessment usually focuses on nutrient intake, a **nutritional health history** incorporates information from laboratory tests and clinical data, as well as from the diet history. **Dietary intake data** are assessed either by collecting retrospective intake data or by summarizing prospective intake data. Each method has specific purposes, strengths, and weaknesses. The choice depends on the purpose and the setting in which the assessment is completed. The goal is to determine the nutrient content of the food and the appropriateness of the intake for a particular individual. The prospective method records data at the time the food is consumed or shortly thereafter.

Nutrient Intake Analysis

Nutrient intake analysis (NIA) (also referred to as *nutrient intake record* or *calorie count* depending on the setting and information collected) is a tool used in various settings to identify nutritional inadequacies by monitoring intakes before deficiencies develop. Information about actual intake is collected by means of direct observation or an inventory of foods eaten based on observation of what remains on the individual's tray or plate.

NIAs should be recorded for a 72-hour period. Complete records for this period will usually accurately reflect an average intake for most individuals. If the record is incomplete, it may be necessary to extend the duration of the intake until a full 72-hour record can be completed.

The results of the NIA can be charted daily or at the end of the 3-day period. The patient or a family member can participate in nutritional care by recording what was eaten, either on a menu or a special form. Moreover, a graph, which can be kept in the patient's room or outside the door, can be used to record all types of dietary intake, including enteral or parental nutrition. The record of intake can then be analyzed for its nutrient content using one of several available computerized methods.

Daily Food Record/Diary

A *daily food record* or **food diary** documents dietary intake as it occurs, and is often used in outpatient clinic settings. A food record is usually most accurate if the food eaten is recorded on the same day. The individual's nutrient intake is then calculated and averaged at the end of the desired period (usually 3 to 7 days), and then compared to Recom-

TABLE 16–6 FACTORS ASSOCIATED WITH RISK OF POOR NUTRITIONAL STATUS IN OLDER AMERICANS

Inappropriate Food Intake *Meal/Snack Frequency* • Inadequate intake • Skipping of one or more meals daily • Replacement of meals by snacks that are not nutritious *Inadequate Quantity/Quality* • Milk/milk products • Meat/meat substitutes • Fruit/vegetables • Breads/cereals *Excesses of Fats or Sweets* *Dietary Modifications* • Self-imposed • Prescribed • Poor compliance • Impact on intake, appetite *Alcohol Use and/or Abuse* • Chronicity • Frequency **Dependency/Disability** *Functional Status* • Problems with daily activities • Inactivity, immobility *Disabling Conditions* • Lack of manual dexterity • Need for assistive devices **Acute/Chronic Diseases/ Conditions** *Abnormalities of Body Weight* *Cognitive or Emotional Impairment* • Depression • Dementias	*Oral Health Problems* *Pressure Ulcers* *Sensory Impairment* *Other Medical Conditions* **Chronic Medication Use** *Prescribed/Self-Administered* *Polypharmacy* *Nutritional Supplements* *Use of Unusual Remedies* **Advanced Age** • Older than 80 years of age • Older than 90 years of age • 100+ years **Poverty** *Income* • Source • Adequacy *Food Expenditures/Resources* • Food • Housing • Medical • Other • Adequacy **Social Isolation** *Support Systems* • Availability • Utilization *Living Arrangements* • Cooking/food storage • Transportation • Other

(Adapted from The Nutrition Screening Initiative: Incorporating nutrition screening and interventions into medical practice: A monograph for physicians. Washington, DC. The Nutrition Screening Initiative, June, 1994, p. 16.)

mended Dietary Allowances (RDAs) or Food Pyramid Guidelines (Fig. 16–9).

Retrospective Data

Retrospective data are collected from recollection. Two examples of this form of data collection are the food frequency questionnaire and the 24-hour recall.

Food Frequency. The **food frequency questionnaire** is a retrospective review of intake frequency—that is, by food consumed per day, per week, or per month. For ease of evaluation, the food frequency chart organizes foods into groups that have common nutrients (Table 16–8). Because the focus of the food frequency questionnaire is the frequency of usage of food groups, rather than of specific nutrients, the information obtained is general, not specific, for certain nutrients.

During illness, food consumption patterns can change with the stage of illness. It is helpful, therefore, to complete food frequency questionnaires for the period immediately prior to hospitalization, as well as the period before the illness, so as to obtain a complete and accurate history.

24-Hour Recall. The **24-hour recall** method of data collection requires that an individual list specific foods consumed in the last 24 hours, which is then analyzed by the person or professional gathering the information. Problems commonly associated with this method of data collection include (1) an inability to recall accurately the kinds and amounts of food eaten, (2) difficulty in determining whether the day being recalled represents the individual's typical intake, and (3) the tendency for persons to over-report low intakes and to under-report high intakes of foods. Concurrent use of both food frequency and 24-hour recall questionnaires—termed a *cross-check*—improves the accuracy of intake estimates.

Reliability and validity of the methods of dietary recall are important concerns (Howat, 1994). *Valid-*

TABLE 16–7 DIETARY HISTORY INFORMATION

Economics
Income—frequency and steadiness of employment
Amount of money for food each week or month and individual's perception of its adequacy for meeting food needs
Eligibility for food stamps and cost of stamps
Public aid recipient?

Physical Activity
Occupation—type, hours/week, shift, energy expenditure
Exercise—type, amount, frequency (seasonal?)
Sleep—hours/day (uninterrupted?)
Handicaps

Ethnic or Cultural Background
Influence on eating habits
Religion
Education

Home Life and Meal Patterns
Number in household (eat together?)
Person who does shopping
Person who does cooking
Food storage and cooking facilities (stove, refrigerator)
Type of housing (home, apartment, room, etc.)
Ability to shop and prepare foods

Appetite
Good, poor, any changes
Factors that affect appetite
Taste and smell perception (any changes?)

Attitude Toward Food/Eating
Disinterest in food
Irrational ideas about food, eating, or body weight
Parental interest in child's eating

Allergies, Intolerances, or Food Avoidances
Foods avoided and reason for avoidance
Length of time of avoidance
Description of problems caused by foods

Dental and Oral Health
Problems with eating
Foods that cannot be eaten
Problems with swallowing, salivation, food sticking

Gastrointestinal Factors
Problems with heartburn, bloating, gas, diarrhea, vomiting, constipation, distention
Frequency of problems
Home remedies
Antacid, laxative, or other drug use

Chronic Disease
Treatment
Length of time of treatment
Dietary modification—self-imposed or physician prescribed, date of modification, education, compliance with diet

Medication
Vitamin and/or mineral supplements—frequency of administration, type, amount
Medications—type, amount, frequency of administration, length of time on medication

Recent Weight Change
Loss or gain—how many pounds, over what length of time?
Intentional or nonvolitional

Dietary or Nutritional Problems (as Perceived by Patient)

Food Diary: DAY ____________

MEAL Foods (list)	AMOUNT EATEN	HOW PREPARED	WHERE EATEN (home, work, etc.)
Breakfast:			
Snack:			
Lunch:			
Dinner:			
Snack:			

Food Supplements Name: ____________ Cans/Day: ________
Vitamins/Mineral Supplement: ____________

FIGURE 16–9 Food diary.

TABLE 16–8 GENERAL FOOD FREQUENCY QUESTIONNAIRE*

1. Do you drink milk? If so, how much? What kind? Whole Skim Low-fat
2. Do you use fat? If so, what kind? How much?
3. How many times do you eat meat? Eggs? Cheese? Beans?
4. Do you eat snack foods? If so, which ones? How often? How much?
5. What vegetables (in each group) do you eat? How often?
   a. Broccoli green peppers cooked greens carrots sweet potato
   b. Tomatoes raw cabbage
   c. Asparagus beets cauliflower corn cooked cabbage celery peas lettuce
6. What fruits and how often?
   a. Apples or applesauce apricots bananas berries cherries grapes or grape juice peaches pears pineapple plums prunes raisins
   b. Oranges orange juice grapefruit grapefruit juice
7. Bread and cereal products
   a. How much bread do you usually eat with each meal? How much between meals?
   b. Do you eat cereal? (daily, weekly) What type? cooked dry
   c. How often do you eat foods such as macaroni, spaghetti, noodles, etc.
   d. Do you eat whole grain breads and cereals? How often?
8. Do you use salt? Do you salt your food before tasting it? Do you cook with salt? Do you crave salt or salty foods?
9. How many teaspoons of sugar do you use daily? (Be sure to remind the patient to include sugar on cereal, fruit, toast, and in coffee, tea, etc.)
10. Do you eat desserts? If so, how often?
11. Do you drink sugar-containing beverages, such as soda pop or sweetened juice drinks? How often? How much?
12. How often do you eat candy or cookies?
13. Do you drink water? How often during the day? How much each time? How much water would you say you drink each day?
14. Do you use sugar substitutes in packet form or in drinks? If so, what type do you use? How often?
15. Do you drink alcohol? How often? How much? Type: beer, wine, liquor?
16. Do you drink caffeinated beverages? How often? How much per day?

*To determine the frequency of food use, the following pattern of questions may be useful. However, questions may need to be modified based on information from the 24-hour recall. For instance, if the patient has stated that he/she drank a glass of milk yesterday, you wouldn't ask "Do you drink milk?" but rather "How much milk do you drink?" Record answers with the appropriate time frame designated (e.g., 1/day, 1/wk, 3/mo) or as accurately as possible. The frequency may need to be recorded as "occasionally" or "rarely" if the patient cannot be more specific.

ity is the degree to which the method actually reflects the usual intake. Whenever attention is directed toward an individual's diet, the person may consciously or unconsciously alter his or her intake, either to simplify recording, or to impress the interviewer, thus decreasing the information's validity. The validity of dietary recall methods in obese individuals is often questionable, as they tend to underreport their intake. The same may be true for children, patients with eating disorders, the critically ill, drug and alcohol abusers, individuals who are confused, and those whose intake may be unpredictable.

Another problem with such retrospective methods of data collection is that people tend to forget what they have actually consumed. The *reliability* of these methods refers to the consistency of the data obtained. To have significance, dietary intake data should reflect typical food patterns of the individual. Memory lapses, inaccurate knowledge of portion sizes, and overestimation or underestimation of the amounts consumed may jeopardize the reliability of any food intake method. Table 16–9 describes the advantages and disadvantages of various dietary intake methods.

Anthropometry

Anthropometry involves obtaining physical measurements of an individual and relating them to standards that reflect the growth and development of the individual. These physical measurements are another component of the nutritional assessment.

Anthropometric data are most valuable when they reflect accurate measurements and are recorded over a period of time. Common, valuable measurements are height, head circumference, weight, skinfold thicknesses, and other girth measurements. Ethnic, familial, birth weight, and environmental factors affect these parameters, and so should be taken into consideration when anthropometric measures are evaluated.

Interpretation of Height and Weight

Reference standards in current use are based on a statistical sample of the U.S. population. Therefore, an individual measurement shows how the subject's measurement compares to that of the total population, not to an absolute standard.

Height and weight measurements in children are evaluated against various norms. They are recorded as percentiles, which reflect the percentage of the total population of children of the same sex who are at or below the same height or weight at that age. This allows the child's growth at every age to be monitored by mapping data on a growth curve, also known as a **weight-for-length curve.**

Appendices 6 through 15 describe percentiles and growth charts for infants, children, and adolescents up to the age of 17 years.

TABLE 16–9 METHODS OF OBTAINING DIETARY INTAKE DATA

METHOD	ADVANTAGES	DISADVANTAGES
Nutrient intake analysis	Allows actual observation of food intake	May yield inconsistent and subjective estimates of food consumption Possible variation in portion size
Daily food record/diary	Provides daily record of food consumption Can provide information on quantity of food, how prepared, and timing of meals and snacks	Variable literacy skills of subjects Requires ability to measure/judge portion sizes Actual food intake possibly influenced by the recording process Questionable reliability of records
Food frequency	Easily standardized Can be beneficial when considered in combination with usual intake Provides overall picture of intake	Requires literacy skills Does not provide meal pattern data Requires knowledge of portion sizes
24-hour recall	Quick Easy	Relies on memory Requires knowledge of portion sizes May not represent usual intake Requires interviewing skills

(Compiled from information in Hopkins B. Assessment of nutritional status. In: Gottschlich MM, Matarese LE, Shronts EP (eds.). Nutrition Support Dietetics, 2nd ed. Silver Spring, MD: American Society for Parenteral and Enteral Nutrition, 1993, pp. 16–17.)

Height and weight are useful in determining nutritional status in adults. Both should be measured, as there is a tendency to overestimate height and underestimate weight, resulting in underestimation of the relative weight.

LENGTH AND HEIGHT. Various methods may be used to measure height and weight. Measurements of height can be obtained using a direct or indirect approach. The direct method uses a measuring rod or beam balance, and the person must be able to stand (see Table 16–10). Indirect methods, including arm span, recumbent length (tape measure) (see Appendix 17), and knee height measurements may be options for those who cannot stand or stand straight, such as individuals with scoliosis, cerebral palsy, or muscular dystrophy, or those who are elderly. Recumbent bed height measurements, using a tape measure, may be appropriate for institutionalized individuals who are comatose, critically ill, or unable to be moved. However, this method can only be used if the patient does not have musculoskeletal deformities or contractures.

Sitting heights are used for children who cannot stand, and recumbent length measurements are used for infants and children younger than 2 or 3 years of age (Fig. 16–10). In children, heights should be recorded on a growth grid, as shown in Appendices 6 through 13. This chart provides a record of a child's gain in height over time, and compares the child's height to that of other children of the same age. The rate of length or height gain reflects long-term nutritional adequacy.

WEIGHT. Weight is another measure that is easy to obtain and yet is very telling. In children, it is a more sensitive measure of nutritional adequacy than height, and it reflects recent nutritional intake.

Weight also provides a crude evaluation of overall fat and muscle stores (Hopkins, 1993). Body weight may be measured by several methods including (1) ideal weight for height, (2) usual weight, and (3) actual weight.

Ideal weight for height can be determined from reference standards, such as the Metropolitan Life Insurance Tables (1959, 1983) (see Appendix 19) and the National Health and Nutrition Examination Survey (NHANES) I and II percentiles. Ideal weight may also be determined using the Hamwi method (see the accompanying box, "*Clinical Insight:* Calculating Ideal Body Weight"):

TABLE 16–10 USING HEIGHT AND WEIGHT TO ASSESS A HOSPITALIZED PATIENT'S NUTRITIONAL STATUS

- Measure height.
- Measure weight (at admission, current, and usual).
- Determine percentage weight change over time (weight pattern).
- Determine percentage above or below usual body weight or ideal body weight.

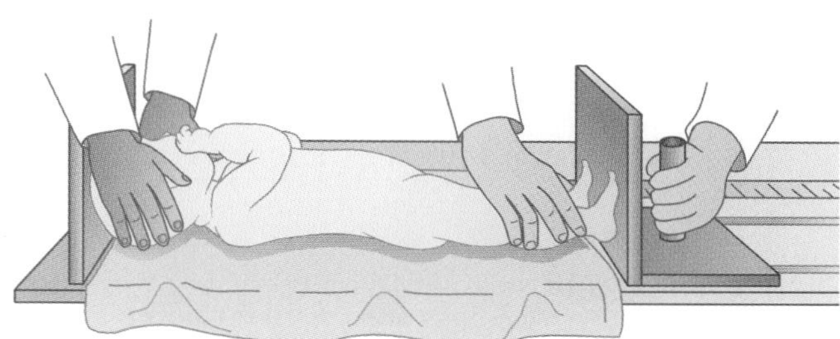

FIGURE 16–10 Measurement of the length of an infant. Crown-to-heel length should be measured in children 36 months of age and younger in the following manner: (1) The child is laid on a ruled board with an attached piece of wood at one end and a movable piece at the other. (2) The child should be stretched out on the board to give the most accurate measurement. This usually requires two people. The top of the child's head is placed against the immovable end. (3) The movable end is placed flat against the bottom of the child's foot, and the length is read from the side of the board.

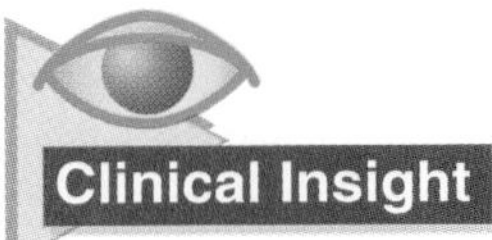

Calculating Ideal Body Weight

Ideal body weight for an individual can be calculated using the Hamwi method, as follows:

Females: 100 lb for the first 5 feet of height and 5 lb for every inch over 5 feet

Males: 106 lb for the first 5 feet of height and 5 lb for every inch over 5 feet

An adjustment is then made for a large frame (+10%) or a small frame (–10%)

Example

Thus, the ideal body weight for a small-frame woman with a height of 63 inches would be calculated as follows:

Step 1: a) 100 lb for the first 5 feet = 100 lb
b) +5 lb × 3 inches = 15 lb
c) 100 lbs + 15 lbs = 115 lb

Step 2: 10% of 115 lb = 11.5 lb

Step 3: 115 lb – 11.5 lb = 103.5 lb = ideal weight

Females: 100 lb for the first 5 feet of height and 5 lb for every inch over 5 feet

Males: 106 lb for the first 5 feet of height and 6 lb for every inch over 5 feet.

Weight is then adjusted according to whether the person has a large or small frame, as follows:

Large frame—add 10%
Small frame—subtract 10%

Frame size is determined by wrist circumference measurement or elbow breadth measurement (see Appendix 18).

Usual body weight may be a more useful parameter than ideal body weight for those who are ill. Comparing present weight to usual body weight allows changes in weight status to be assessed. One problem with usual body weight is that it is dependent on the patient's memory.

Actual body weight reflects a weight measurement obtained at the time of examination. This measurement may be influenced by changes in the individual's fluid status.

Weight loss (in lbs or kg) reflects an immediate inability to meet nutritional requirements, and thus may indicate nutritional risk. The percentage of weight loss is highly reflective of the extent and severity of an individual's illness. The following formula is useful in determining the percentage of loss:

$$\text{\% recent weight change} = \frac{\text{usual weight} - \text{actual weight}}{\text{usual weight}} \times 100$$

Significant weight loss is interpreted as a 5% loss over 1 month; a 7.5% loss over 3 months; or a 10% loss over 6 months. Severe weight loss is considered to be >5% weight loss over 1 month; >7.5% weight loss over 3 months; or >10% weight loss over 6 months (Blackburn et al., 1977). Another method for determining the percentage of weight loss is to determine an individual's current weight as a percentage of the usual weight. This percentage of usual or ideal body weight can then be used to assess the degree of malnutrition:

$$\text{\% usual body weight} = \frac{\text{actual body weight}}{\text{usual body weight}} \times 100$$

Patients whose weight is within 85% to 90% of their usual body weight are considered to be mildly malnourished. Those whose weight is within 75% to 84% of usual body weight are considered to be moderately malnourished, whereas those whose weight is <74% of usual body weight are severely malnourished. The minimum weight for survival is 48% to 55% of usual body weight (Buchman, 1997).

Reference Standards. To determine whether an adult's weight is appropriate for height, the weight is usually compared with a reference standard. The most common is the Metropolitan Life Insurance Tables (see Table 16–11 for the 1959 tables and Appendix 19 for the 1983 tables).

Body Mass Index

The **body mass index (BMI)** accounts for differences in body composition by defining the level of adiposity according to the relationship of weight to height, thus eliminating dependence on frame size (Stensland and Margolis, 1990). BMI can be calculated using the following equations:

$$\text{BMI} = \frac{\text{weight (lb)}}{\text{height (in)}^2} \times 705$$

This index has the least correlation with body height and the highest correlation with independent measures of body fatness for adults, including the elderly (Keys et al., 1972). A score of 20 to 25 is associated with the least risk of early death. Obesity is categorized by BMI according to three grades: grade I (25 to 29.9), grade II (30 to 40), and grade III (40+). In general, a BMI of 27 or more indicates obesity and an increased risk of developing health problems (Bray et al., 1976). BMI values increase with age; age-specific guidelines for BMI have, therefore, been suggested for use with the elderly (Bray, 1987; Nutrition Screening Initiative, 1991). New standards for BMI were published in 1998, but their use remains controversial at this time (see Chapter 23.)

TABLE 16–11 DESIRABLE WEIGHT FOR MEDIUM-FRAME MEN AND WOMEN, AGED 25 YEARS AND OLDER*

HEIGHT			WEIGHT	
Feet	Inches	Centimeters	Pounds	Kilograms
Men†				
5	2	157.5	121–133	55–60
5	3	160.0	124–136	56–61
5	4	162.6	127–139	57–63
5	5	165.1	130–143	59–65
5	6	167.6	134–147	60–67
5	7	170.2	138–152	62–68
5	8	172.7	142–156	64–70
5	9	175.3	146–160	66–72
5	10	177.8	150–165	68–75
5	11	180.3	154–170	70–75
6	0	182.9	158–175	71–79
6	1	185.4	162–180	73–81
6	2	188.0	167–185	75–84
6	3	190.5	172–190	78–86
6	4	193.0	175–195	80–88
Women‡				
4	10	147.3	101–113	46–51
4	11	149.9	104–116	47–53
5	0	152.4	107–119	49–54
5	1	154.9	110–122	50–56
5	2	157.5	113–126	51–57
5	3	160.0	116–130	53–59
5	4	162.6	120–135	55–62
5	5	165.1	124–139	56–63
5	6	167.6	128–143	58–65
5	7	170.2	132–147	60–67
5	8	172.7	136–151	62–69
5	9	175.3	140–155	64–71
5	10	177.8	144–159	66–72
5	11	180.3	148–163	67–74
6	0	182.8	152–167	69–76

(Adapted from the Metropolitan Life Insurance Company; data derived primarily from Build and Blood Pressure Study, 1959, Society of Actuaries. Tables correct to height without shoes.)

*Expressed in pounds according to height and frame, in indoor clothing.

†Allow ±7 lb.

‡Allow ±3 lb.

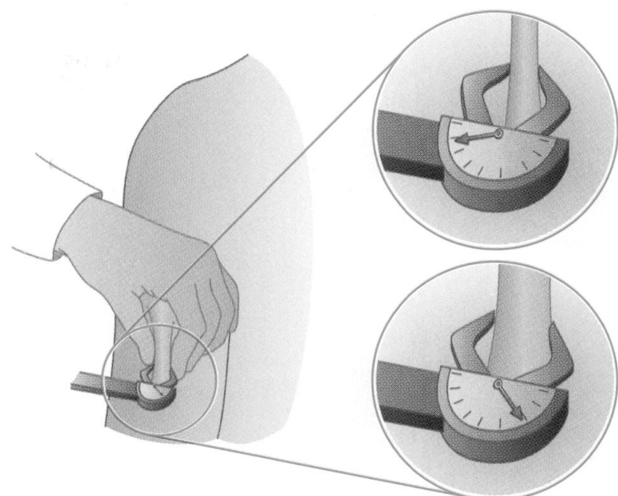

FIGURE 16–11 Skinfold calipers measure the thickness of subcutaneous fat tissue in millimeters. This gives a rough measurement of adiposity. (NOTE: Large caliper readings are read counterclockwise.) (Diagram courtesy of Dorice Czajka-Narins, PhD.)

Body Composition

Differences in skeletal size and the proportion of lean body mass can contribute to body weight variations among individuals of similar height. Muscular athletes, for example, may be classified as overweight because of excess muscle mass rather than adipose mass. Elderly persons tend to have lower bone density and may, therefore, weigh less than younger adults of the same height.

SUBCUTANEOUS FAT (SKINFOLD THICKNESS). The fatfold or skinfold thickness measurement is a means of assessing the amount of body fat an individual has. It is practical in clinical settings, although validity depends on the accuracy of the measuring technique (Fig. 16–11) and repetition of measurements over time. Changes, if they are to occur, will take 3 to 4 weeks. This measurement bases total body fat estimates on the assumption that 50% of body fat is subcutaneous. Accuracy decreases with increasing obesity. Skinfold sites identified as most reflective of body fatness are over the triceps and the biceps, below the scapula, above the iliac crest (suprailiac), and on the upper thigh. The triceps skinfold (TSF) and subscapular measurements are the most useful because the most complete standards and methods of evaluation are available for

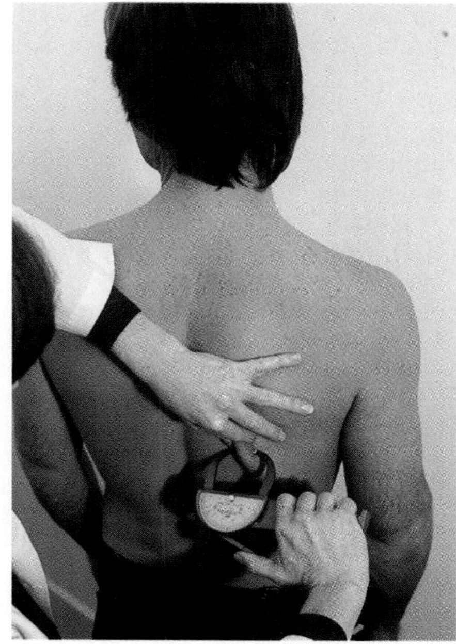

FIGURE 16–12 Measurement of the subscapular skinfold thickness.

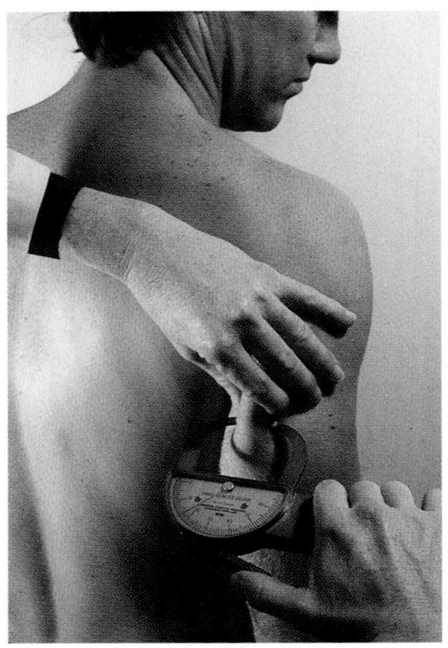

A

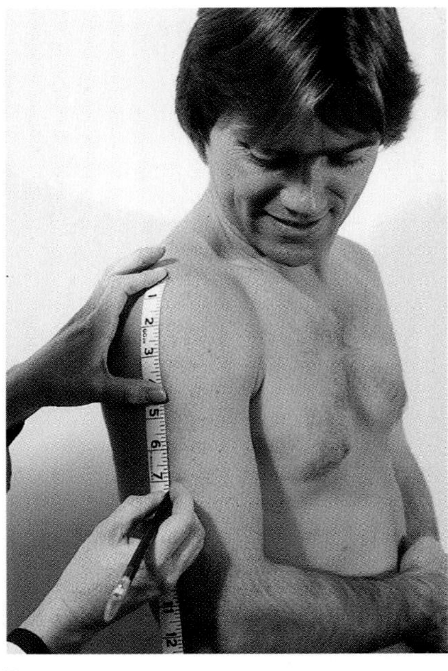

B

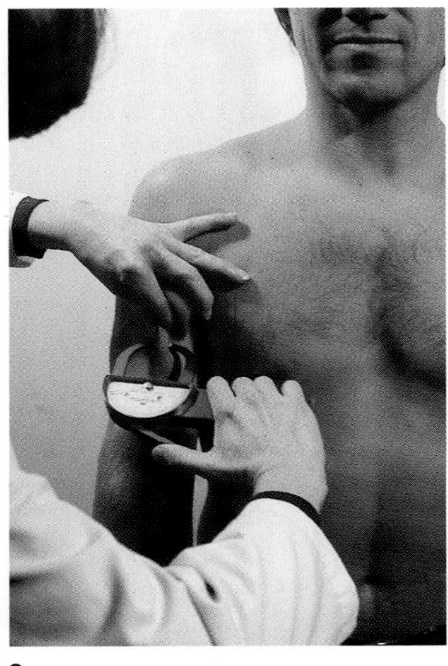

C

FIGURE 16–13 *A*, Measurement of the midpoint between the acromion process at the shoulder and the olecranon process at the elbow. *B*, Marking of the midpoint. *C*, Measurement of the arm circumference, in centimeters, at the midpoint.

these sites. Figures 16–12 and 16–13 illustrate these measurements. (See Appendices 21 through 25 for triceps skinfold percentiles for youths and adults, as well as other arm anthropometry).

Circumference Measurements

If more complete information on actual body composition is needed, additional anthropometric data can be obtained. These include additional skinfold measurements and circumference measurements (Fig. 16–14).

WAIST-TO-HIP CIRCUMFERENCE RATIO. With the recognition of fat distribution as an indicator of risk, circumferential or girth measurements have been ascribed importance. The most frequently used measure of adiposity is the **waist-to-hip ratio (WHR),** which differentiates between android and gynoid obesity (see Chapter 23). A WHR of 1.0 or greater in men or 0.8 or greater in women is indicative of android obesity and an increased risk for obesity-related diseases. This also appears to be true in children (Freedman et al., 1989). Circumferences are easy to measure with either plastic or steel measuring tapes. Difficulty in locating the waist, which moves up and down with changes in weight and muscle tone, is resolved by using the smallest circumference between the nipples and the top of the thighs. The hip circumference is defined as the largest circumference between the waist and the knees. Appendix 26 presents a nomogram for determining the WHR.

MID–UPPER ARM CIRCUMFERENCE. Mid–upper arm circumference (MAC) is measured halfway between the acromion process of the scapula and the tip of the elbow. Appendices 27 and 28 provide standards for determining the MAC. Combining the MAC with TSF measurements allows indirect determination of the *arm muscle area* (AMA) and *arm fat area*

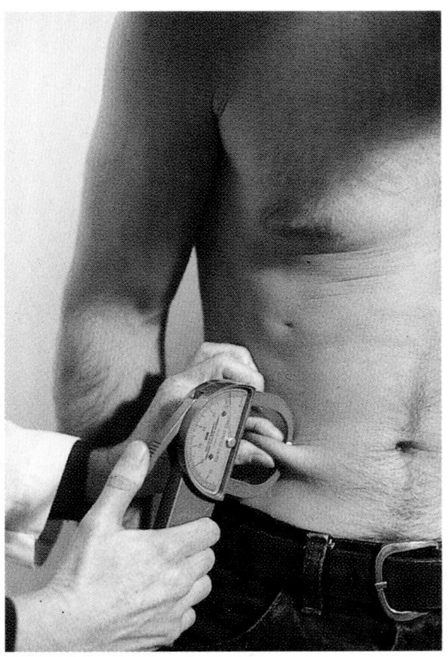

FIGURE 16–14 Waist skinfold measurement using calipers.

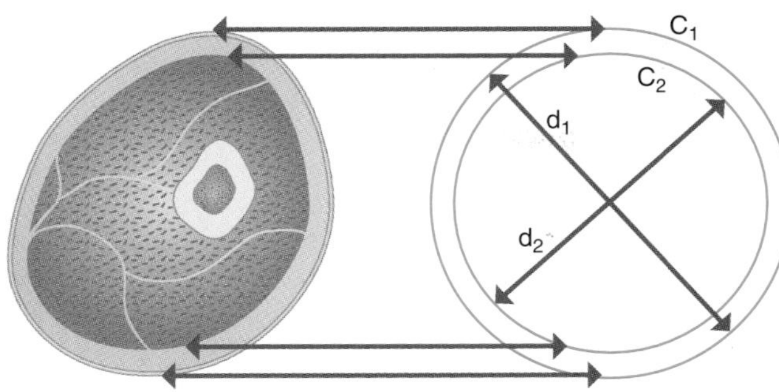

FIGURE 16–15 Upper arm area (AA), upper arm muscle area (AMA), and upper arm fat area (AFA) are derived from measurements of upper arm circumference (C_1) and triceps skinfold (T) in millimeters.

$$AA\ (mm^2 = \pi/4 \times d_1^2 \text{ where } d_1 = C_1/\pi$$
$$AMA\ (mm^2) = (C_1 - \pi T)^2/4\pi = (C_1 - \pi T)^2/12.56$$
$$AFA\ (mm^2) = AA - AMA$$
$$\text{bone-free } AMA - AMA - 10 \text{ for males}$$
$$= AMA - 6.5 \text{ for females}$$

(Arm area and muscle area can also be determined using the nomograms in Appendix Tables 27 and 28.)

(AFA). Bone-free AMA is calculated by using the formula shown in Figure 16–15; in men, a factor of 10 is subtracted from the AMA, whereas in women, a factor of 6.5 is subtracted (Frisancho, 1984).

The AMA, or bone-free muscle area, is a good indication of lean body mass and, thus, an individual's skeletal protein reserves. This is important in growing children and is especially valuable in evaluating possible protein-energy malnutrition as a result of chronic illness, stress, multiple surgeries, or inadequate diet. Norms for AFA and AMA in the elderly are given in Appendix 29.

HEAD CIRCUMFERENCE. Head circumference measurements are useful in children younger than 3 years of age, primarily as an indictor of non-nutritional abnormalities. Undernutrition must be very severe to affect head circumference (see *"Focus On:* Head Circumference").

CALF CIRCUMFERENCE. Measurements of calf circumference, combined with other anthropometric measures, can be used to estimate body weight in the elderly (Lohman et al., 1988).

BIOELECTRICAL IMPEDANCE ANALYSIS. **Bioelectrical impedance analysis (BIA)** is used for body fat analysis. It is a body composition analysis technique based on the principle that, compared to fatty tissue, lean tissue has a higher electrical conductivity and lower impedance, relative to water, based on electrolyte content. BIA involves attaching electrodes to the extremities of a patient and passing a small electrical current through the electrodes to obtain electrical and resistance measurements. Fever, electrolyte imbalance, obesity, and hydration status may impact the reliability of measurements (Shronts et al., 1998) (Fig. 16–16).

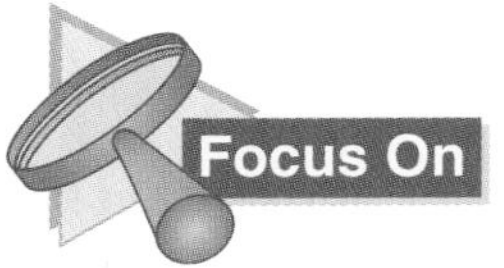

HEAD CIRCUMFERENCE

Indications

Head circumference is a standard measurement for serial assessment of growth in pediatric patients from birth to 36 months.

Equipment

Cloth tape measure

Technique

1. With the aid of an assistant, hold the subject's head completely still.
2. Place the tape measure over the most prominent part of the occiput and around the subject's forehead, just above the supraorbital ridge. *NOTE:* All measurements should be taken around fixed landmarks.
3. Tighten the tape measure and, holding it securely, note the measurement over the forehead.
4. The circumference should be read to the nearest 0.1 cm or 1/8 inch and then recorded.
5. Compare the subject's measurement with the National Center for Health Statistics' (NCHS) standard curves for head circumference.

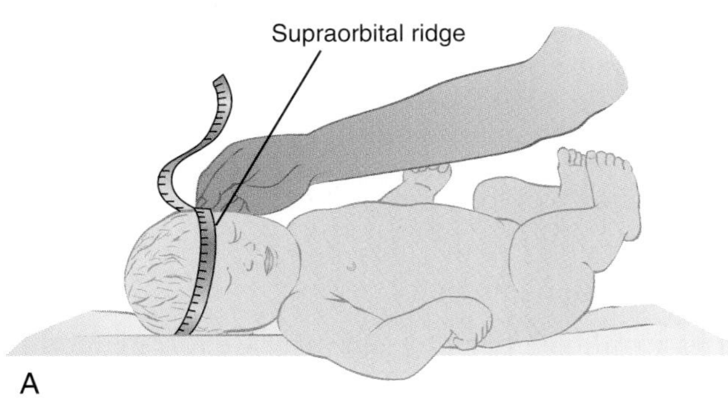

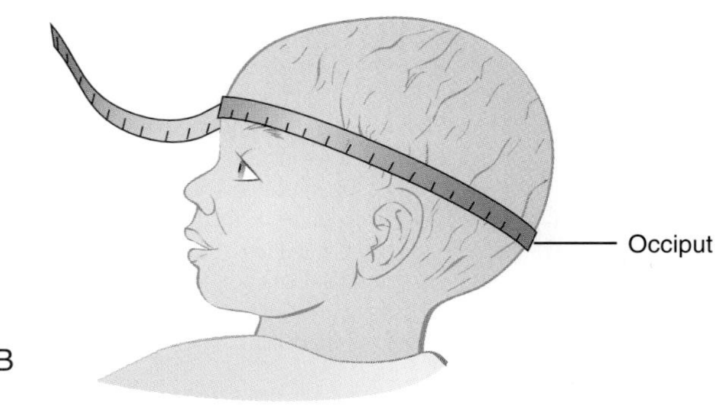

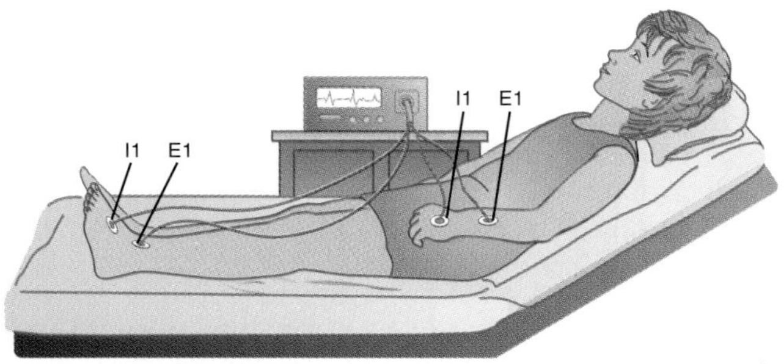

FIGURE 16–16 Bioelectrical impedance analysis.

Nutrition-Focused Physical Examination

A *nutrition-focused physical examination* is an important component of overall nutritional assessment as some nutritional deficiencies may not be identified by other assessment approaches. One must keep in mind that some signs of nutritional deficiency are nonspecific and must be distinguished from those with a non-nutritional etiology. A systems approach is applied when performing the examination, which should be conducted in an organized, logical progression from head to toe so as to ensure an efficient and complete examination. The examination moves from a global to a more defined or focused examination based on the results of the medical and nutrition histories. The nutrition-focused physical examination is tailored for each patient; that is, every body system may not have to be assessed in all cases; clinical judgment will guide this decision (Hammond, 1996, 1997, 1998).

EQUIPMENT. The extent of the nutrition-focused physical will dictate the necessary equipment. Any or all of the following may be used: stethoscope, penlight or flashlight, tongue depressor, scales, reflex hammer, calipers, tape measure, blood pressure cuff, and ophthalmoscope.

TABLE 16–12 PHYSICAL EXAMINATION TECHNIQUES

TECHNIQUE	DESCRIPTION
Inspection	General observation that progresses to a more focused observation using the senses of sight, smell, and hearing; technique most frequently used
Palpation	Tactile examination to feel pulsations and vibrations; assess body structures, including texture, size, temperature, tenderness, and mobility
Percussion	Assessment of sounds to determine body organ borders, shape, and position; not always used in a nutrition-focused physical examination
Auscultation	Use of the naked ear or a stethoscope to listen to body sounds (such as heart and lung sounds, bowel sounds, and blood vessels)

(From Hammond K. Nutrition focused physical assessment. Support Line 18(4):4, 1996.)

EXAMINATION TECHNIQUES. Four basic techniques of physical examination are used during the nutrition-focused physical examination. These techniques include inspection, palpation, percussion, and auscultation (see Table 16–12).

FINDINGS. Significant findings on physical examination include temporal wasting, proximal muscle weakness, depleted muscle bulk, and tongue atrophy. The appearance of the skin should be assessed, and pallor, scaly dermatitis, wounds, quality of wound healing, bruising, and hydration status should be noted. Membranes (conjunctiva or pharynx) should be examined for integrity, hydration, pallor, and bleeding.

Special attention should be given to the areas where signs of nutritional deficiencies appear (e.g., skin, hair, teeth, gums, lips, tongue, eyes, and, in men, the genitalia). The hair, skin, and mouth are susceptible because of the rapid cell turnover of epithelial tissue. Mucosal changes in the gastrointestinal tract are reflected by problems such as diarrhea and anorexia. Symptoms of nutrient deficiencies may or may not be apparent on the physical examination.

Many signs result from a lack of several nutrients, as well as from non-nutritional causes. Table 16–13 presents a list of physical signs suggesting malnutrition (see also Appendix 30). Potential ICD-9 codes for classifying diagnoses with a nutritional implication can be found in Appendix 3.

Skin Testing (Delayed Hypersensitivity Reactivity)

A review of results from skin testing (i.e., the intradermal injection of small amounts of antigen, most commonly tuberculin, candida, mumps, or trichophyton, just under the skin to determine reaction) has revealed a lack of supporting data and uniformity. Studies do not take into account the effects of disease (e.g., cancer and immune system diseases), infection, or therapy (e.g., irradiation, surgery, or immunosuppression), which are known to influence skin test reactivity. Evaluation of *immune competence* in relationship to nutritional status requires a precise knowledge of the patient's nutritional intake, metabolic state, current illness, recent exposure to infectious agents, and duration of the immune deficit, as well as a familiarity with genetic factors. DHR is not a useful component of the nutrition assessment in most hospitalized patients (Shronts et al., 1998). The question still remains as to whether skin testing correlates well with nutritional status; perhaps this will be answered in the next few years.

Handgrip Dynamometry

Handgrip dynamometry can provide a baseline nutritional assessment of muscle function by measuring grip strength and endurance, and it is useful in

TABLE 16–13 PHYSICAL SIGNS INDICATIVE OR SUGGESTIVE OF MALNUTRITION

	NORMAL APPEARANCE	SIGNS ASSOCIATED WITH MALNUTRITION	POSSIBLE DISORDER OR NUTRIENT DEFICIENCY	POSSIBLE NON-NUTRITIONAL PROBLEM
Hair	Shiny; firm; not easily plucked	Lack of natural shine; dull and dry Thin and sparse Dyspigmented Flag sign Easily plucked (no pain)	**Kwashiorkor** and, less commonly, **marasmus**	Excessive bleaching of hair Alopecia
Face	Uniform skin color; smooth, healthy appearance; no facial swelling	Nasolabial seborrhea (scaling of skin around the nostrils) Swollen face (moon face) Paleness	Riboflavin Kwashiorkor	Acne vulgaris
Eyes	Bright, clear, shiny; no sores at corners of eyelids; healthy, pink, and moist membranes; no prominent blood vessels or mound of tissue or sclera	Pale conjunctiva Bitot's spots Conjunctival xerosis (dryness) Corneal xerosis (dullness) Keratomalacia (corneal softening) Redness and fissuring of eyelid corners Corneal arcus (white ring around eye) Xanthelasma (small, yellowish lumps around eyes)	Anemia (e.g., iron) Vitamin A Riboflavin, pyridoxine Hyperlipidemia	Bloodshot eyes from exposure to weather, lack of sleep, smoke exposure, or alcohol
Lips	Smooth; not chapped or swollen	Angular cheilosis (white or pink lesions at corners of mouth)	Riboflavin	Excessive salivation from ill-fitting dentures
Tongue	Deep red in appearance; not swollen or smooth	Magenta tongue (purplish) Filiform papillae Atrophy or hypertrophy Red tongue	Riboflavin Folic acid Niacin	Leukoplakia
Teeth	No cavities; no pain; bright	Mottled enamel Caries (cavities) Missing teeth	Fluorosis Excessive sugar intake	Malocclusion Periodontal disease Health habits
Gums	Healthy; red; do not bleed; not swollen	Spongy, bleeding Receding gums	Vitamin C	Periodontal disease
Glands	Face not swollen	Thyroid enlargement (front of neck swollen) Parotid enlargement (swollen cheeks)	Iodine Starvation Bulimia	Allergic or inflammatory enlargement of thyroid
Nervous system	Psychological stability; normal reflexes	Psychomotor changes Mental confusion Sensory loss Motor weakness Loss of positional sense Loss of vibration Loss of ankle and knee jerks Burning and tingling of hands and feet (paresthesia) Dementia	Kwashiorkor Thiamine Niacin Vitamin B_{12}	

serial measurements. Measurements are expressed as a percentage of standard for men and women (Guenter et al., 1989).

Men: 48.8 +/– 7.0 kg
Women: 34.4 +/– 4.7 kg

Biochemical Analysis

Biochemical tests are the most objective and sensitive measures of nutritional status, but not all are appropriate. Caution must be used when interpreting results, as they can be affected by disease state and therapy. Chapter 17 provides a complete discussion of the role of laboratory data in nutritional assessment.

CLASSIFYING MALNUTRITION

Once a nutritional assessment is completed, the extent of nutritional deficiency or excess will be apparent. Malnutrition can then be classified based on several indices, including body weight, body fat, somatic and visceral protein stores, and laboratory values. Table 16–14 characterizes malnutrition using the ICD (see also Appendix 3).

Once the nutritional assessment is completed and

TABLE 16–14 CLASSIFICATION OF PROTEIN-ENERGY MALNUTRITION (PEM)

ICD-9-CM*	DIAGNOSIS/DESCRIPTION	CRITERIA/CHARACTERISTICS
260.0	Kwashiorkor—nutritional edema with dyspigmentation of skin and hair	1. Normal anthropometrics: weight >90% of standard weight for height 2. Depressed visceral protein concentrations: serum albumin < 3.0 g/dL, transferrin < 180 mg/dL 3. Caused by acute energy and protein deficiency or reflecting a metabolic response to injury 4. Characterized by edema, catabolism of muscle tissue, weakness, neurologic changes, loss of vigor, secondary infections, stunted growth in children, and changes in hair
261.0	Marasmus—nutritional atrophy; severe, chronic calorie deficiency; severe malnutrition	1. Depressed anthropometrics: weight < 80% of standard weight for height, and/or a weight loss of > 10% of usual weight in last 6 months with muscle wasting 2. Relative preservation of visceral proteins: serum albumin > 3.0 g/dL 3. Caused by chronically deficient energy intake 4. Characterized by catabolism of fat and muscle tissue, lethargy, generalized weakness, and weight loss
262.0	Other severe PEM—nutritional edema without dyspigmentation of skin and hair	1. Depressed anthropometrics: weight < 60% of standard weight for height 2. Depressed visceral protein concentration: serum albumin < 3.0 g/dL 3. Occurs when a marasmic patient is exposed to stress (e.g., trauma, surgery, or acute illness) 4. Characterized by combined symptoms of marasmus and kwashiorkor, a high risk of infection, and poor wound healing
263.0	Malnutrition of moderate degree	1. Depressed anthropometrics: weight 60% to 75% of standard weight for height 2. Relative preservation of visceral proteins: serum albumin 3.0 to 3.5 g/dL
263.1	Malnutrition of mild degree	1. Depressed anthropometrics: weight 75% to 90% of standard weight for height 2. Preservation of visceral proteins: serum albumin 3.5 to 5.0 g/dL

(From American Dietetic Association. Manual of Clinical Dietetics, 5th ed. Chicago: The American Dietetic Association, 1996, p. 18.)
*International Classification of Diseases, 9th rev. Clinical Modification.

the degree of overnutrition or undernutrition is established, a nutritional care plan can be formulated (see Chapter 20).

THE NUTRITIONAL PLAN OF CARE

Implementing a nutritional care plan (see Chapter 20) involves defining the nutritional problem to be addressed (based on assessment), identifying the therapeutic goal(s) or desired outcome(s), determining appropriate interventions to be implemented as they relate to the nutritional therapy goals, identifying the educational needs of the patient, and formulating a plan for evaluation. In many cases, the plan of care is included on the nutritional assessment form (Fig. 16–17). The plan of care is based on desired outcomes, which are observable results or measurable changes in the patient's nutritional status. If the desired outcome is not being met, then the plan of care, including interventions and goals, should be revised. The care plan can be documented by a care map or clinical pathway, as shown in Chapter 20. Chapter 20 also itemizes information to be evaluated in formulating the nutritional care plan, and provides information to include in a follow-up nutritional assessment.

DISCHARGE DOCUMENTATION

Completing a discharge nutritional summary for the next caregiver is imperative for optimal nutritional care (see Chapter 20). Appropriate discharge documentation includes a summary of nutritional therapies and outcomes; pertinent information on weights, laboratory values, and dietary intake; potential drug-nutrient interactions; expected progress or prognosis; and recommendations for follow-up services. The amount and type of instruction given, the patient's comprehension of the instruction, and the expected degree of adherence to the prescribed diet must be included. An effective discharge plan increases the likelihood of a positive outcome for the patient.

Name: ____________
Number: ____________
Date/Time: ____________
Dx: ____________

- ☐ Routine Assessment
- ☐ Comprehensive Assessment
- ☐ Nutrition Care Note: Follow-up
- ☐ Education/Instruction
- ☐ Calorie Counts

CLINICAL NUTRITION SERVICES
Medical Nutrition Therapy at Saint Joseph's Hospital of Atlanta

Subjective:

Appetite : ☐ Excellent ☐ Good ☐ Fair ☐ Poor % of meals consumed: ☐ 25% ☐ 50% ☐ 75% ☐ 100%	Food Allergies/Intolerance:
Diet Prior to Admission:	Previous Diet Counseling: ☐ Yes ☐ No
Other:	
Ethnic/Cultural:	

☐ **Write In/Type in Field:** ____________

Objective: Antropometric/Biological Indices/Nutritional Parameters

Diet Order/Feeding:					Supplements: (List all supplements – jump screen)
Ht (in/cm)	Wt (lbs/kg)	Usual Wt	Desired Wt	Frame Size: sm. med. lg.	Body Mass Index: Obese 30–40 Morbidly >40 obese
Wt change (lbs/kg) Date: ________	Time Period ______ wks	Intentional	Unintentional	Assessed Needs: BEE: ________ kcal	
Total Kcal: ________		Protein: ________ gms/day		Fluid: ________ cc/day	

Lab/Biochemical Test		Results	Lab/Biochemical Test	Results
☐ Alb	Albumin	______ g/dl	☐ Prealbumin	______ mg/dl
☐ BG	Blood Glucose	______ mg/dl	☐ HgbAlc	______ %
☐ K	Potassium	______ mmol/l	☐ SGOT	______ U/L
☐ NA	Sodium	______ mmol/l	☐ SGPT	______ U/l
☐ BUN	BUN	______ mg/dl	☐ Alk. Phos.	______ U/L
☐ HDL	HDL	______ mg/dl	☐ Lipase	______ Units
☐ LDL	LDL	______ mg/dl	☐ Amylase	______ SomU/dl
☐ CR	Creatine	______ mg/dl		
☐ TG	Triglyceride	______ mg/dl		
☐ CHO	Cholesterol	______ mg/dl		
☐ MG	Magnesium	______ mg/dl		
☐ PO4	Phosphorus	______ mg/dl		
☐ CA	Calcium	______ mg/dl		

Values may be:
☐ falsely elevated ☐ falsely decreased ☐ secondary to hydration status.
☐ Question Accuracy

Conditions That Currently Exist:

- ☐ Nausea
- ☐ Vomiting
- ☐ Diarrhea
- ☐ Chewing/Swallowing Difficulties
- ☐ Dentures/Dentition
- ☐ Skin Score ≤ 16
- ☐ Age: ______
- ☐ Activity Level: ____________

FIGURE 16–17 Assessment form. (Courtesy of Saint Joseph's Hospital, Atlanta, Georgia.)

Pertinent Medications:	
Oral Intake:	Other:
Allergies:	

❑ **Write In/Type in Field:** ______________

Assessment:

MALNUTRITION INDICATORS	DATE	VALUE	MILD	MODERATE	SEVERE
❑ Prealbumin			10–15 mg/dl	10–5 mg/dl	< 5 mg/dl
❑ Albumin			2.8–3.5 gm/dl	2.1–2.7 gm/dl	< 2.1 gm/dl
❑ Total Lymphocyte Count			1500–1800/mm^3	900–1500/mm^3	< 800/mm^3
❑ Hematocrit (%)					
❑ % Desirable Weight/Height			75–90%	60–75%	< 60%
❑ % Weight Loss				5% in 1 month	> 5% in 1 month
				10% in 6 months	> 10% in 6 months

Malnutrition indicators: ❑ Mild: ______________ ❑ Moderate: ______________ ❑ Severe: ______________

PLANS/RECOMMENDATIONS:

MD please ❑ order ❑ ordered:
❑ And
❑ Or:
Pt. at nutritional risk secondary to: ❑ age ❑ Dx
❑ wt change albumin recent surgery
❑ poor p.o. swallowing compromise.
❑ Sending diet as ordered.
❑ Please change consistency of diet to:
____
❑ Honor food preferences ❑ No preferences stated
❑ Diet counseling to be provided prior to discharge.
❑ Recommend enteral/parentral support, refer to NSS for further evaluation and follow-up.
❑ Current nutritional parameters limited, MD please order: REQUESTED
❑ Prealbumin ❑ Albumin ❑ Weight
❑ Wt 3x/wk ❑ Wt 3x/wk ❑ Ht/Wt
❑ Cholesterol ❑ Nitrogen Balance Study
❑ Swallow evaluation per SLP ❑ Check HgbAlc
❑ Accuchecks ❑ Nutrition Support Team consult from Pharmacy Dept.
❑ Assistance with feeding during meals
❑ Snacks ❑ 1000 ❑ 1500 ❑ QHS
❑ Supplements/Changes (jump screen)
❑ Calorie Count ❑ 2d ❑ 3d
❑ RD ordered:
❑ **Write In/Type in Field:** ______________

❑ Write-in list/Substitutions/Cafe options
❑ "Special" Meal
❑ Chef visit
❑ H.A. assist with menu
❑ If diet cannot be advanced within 72 hours recommend nutrition support or alternative mode of intake
❑ Will change diet to
❑ Suggest diet change to
❑ Continue with present diet managemant
❑ Referred to Op heart school
❑ Referred to OP diabetes school
❑ Referred to OP-RD for medical nutrition therapy and F/U
❑ Will F/U with diet instruction
❑ Diet education materials provided along with phone number for F/U
❑ Referred to social service, pastoral care, rehab.
❑ Will monitor progress for any status changs
❑ Changes for intolerance of supplements
❑ Poor progress noted
❑ Comfort measures only
❑ Care plan forwarded for external care facility
❑ Patient left before instructions completed
❑ Information given to setup OP visit and F/U

RD PRIORITY LISTING
Automatic Screen Flags to RD by IDX

1. NPO/CL > 3d
2. TF/TPN/PPN → NSS + FS alb.
3. Calorie Count Orders (code)
4. 80 yrs. or >
5. Albumin ≤ 2.8
6. Nutrition Score ≥ 3
7. Wt. ≤ 80% IBW or > 140%
8. All orders for consult/assessment/instruction
9. Applicable DNI medications as coded
10. Supplements specified (including nurishment and pharmacy supplemts

FIGURE 16–17 Continued

CASE STUDY 1

Mr. C. is a 32-year-old man, 5 feet, 9 inches tall, who was diagnosed as having acquired immunodeficiency syndrome (AIDS) 1 year ago. Over the past year, his weight has gradually declined from a usual weight of 175 lb to the current low of 130 lb. Visceral proteins are depleted, and a triceps skinfold measurement reveals a bodyfat value that is 55% of standard. Mr. C.'s oral intake has gradually decreased to a point that he can only take sips of an enteral supplement and occasional bites of food.

1. Is Mr. C exhibiting a degree of undernutrition? If so, classify the type of malnutrition present.
2. Mr. C's current weight is what percentage of his usual body weight?
3. What is Mr. C.'s body mass index (BMI)?
4. Develop a nutritional assessment questionnaire for Mr. C.

CASE STUDY 2

Mrs. L., a 66-year-old black woman, has contacted you to set up an outpatient nutritional screening appointment. She has a 40-year history of diabetes mellitus, a 10-year history of colon cancer, and hypertension. She is 5 feet, 8 inches tall and weighs 202 lb. Her current medications are Diabinese and a diuretic (she does not know its name).

1. What would you include in a nutrition screen for Mrs. L?
2. How would you identify her medications?
3. Should any laboratory tests be ordered?
4. If you need more details, what questions would you ask her physician?
5. What other information do you need to develop a nutritional care plan?

CITED REFERENCES

American Dietetic Association. Nutrition assessment of adults. In: Manual of Clinical Dietetics. Chicago: The American Dietetic Association, 1996, p. 3.

Barrocas A, et al. Nutrition assessment practical approaches. Clin Geriatr Med 11(4):675, 1995.

Blackburn GL, et al. Nutritional and metabolic assessment of the hospitalized patient. J Parent Ent Nutr 1(1):11, 1977.

Bray GA. Overweight is risking fate: Definition, classification, prevalence and risks. Ann NY Acad Sci 249:14, 1987.

Bray GA, et al. Evaluation of the obese patient. I: An algorithm. JAMA 235:1487, 1976.

Buchman AL. Handbook of nutritional support. Baltimore: Williams & Wilkins, 1997, pp. 1–4.

Butterworth CE. The skeleton in the hospital closet. Nutr Today March/April: 4, 1974.

Council on Practice, Quality Management Committee. ADA's definitions for nutrition screening and nutrition assessment. J Am Diet Assoc 94:838, 1994.

Detsky AS, et al. What is subjective global assessment? J Parent Ent Nutr 11:8, 1987.

Escott-Stump, S. Nutrition and Diagnosis-Related Care, 4th ed. Baltimore: Williams & Wilkins, 1998.

Freedman DS, et al. Relation of body fat patterning to lipid and lipoprotein concentrations in children and adolescents: The Bogalusa Heart Study. Am J Clin Nutr 50:930, 1989.

Frisancho AR. New standards of weight and body composition by frame size and height for assessment of nutritional status of adults and the elderly. Am J Clin Nutr 40:808, 1984.

Guenter PA, et al. Anthropometric measurements. In: Rombeau JL, Caldwell MD, Forlaw L, Guenter PA (eds.). Atlas of Nutritional Support Techniques. Boston: Little, Brown, and Company, 1989, pp. 1–35.

Hammond KA. Nutrition-focused physical assessment. Support Line 18 (4):4, 1996.

Hammond, KA. Physical assessment: A nutritional perspective. Nurs Clin North Am 32(4):779, 1997.

Hammond KA. The history and physical exam. In: Matarese LE, Gottschlich M (eds.). Contemporary Nutrition Support Practice. Philadelphia: WB Saunders Company, 1998.

Hopkins B. Assessment of nutritional status. In: Gottschlich MM, Matarese LE, Shronts EP (eds.). Nutrition Support Dietetics, 2nd ed. Silver Spring, MD: American Society for Parenteral and Enteral Nutrition, 1993.

Howat PM, et al. Validity and reliability of reported dietary intake data. J Am Diet Assoc 94:2, 1994.

Keys A, et al. Indices of relative weight and obesity. J Chronic Dis 25:329, 1972.

Lissner L, et al. Body composition and energy intake: Do overweight women overeat and underreport? Am J Clin Nutr 49:320, 1989.

Lohmann TG, et al (eds.). Anthropometric Standardization Reference Manual. Champaign, IL: Human Kinetics Publishers, 1988.

National Center for Health Statistics. Leading causes of death. Monthly Vital Stat Rep 46 (1), 1996.

Nutrition Interventions Manual for Professionals Caring for Older Americans. Executive Summary: AAFP, ADA, and National Council on Aging. Washington, DC: Nutrition Screening Initiative, 1991.

Nutrition Screening Initiative: AAFP, ADA, and National Council on Aging. Washington, DC: 1991.

Nutritional Assessment Present and Future. Nutr Support Serv 8:7, 1988.

Shronts EP, et al. Nutrition assessment. In: Nutrition Support Practice Manual. Silver Spring, MD: American Society for Parenteral and Enteral Nutrition, 1998.

Stensland SH, Margolis S. Simplifying the calculation of body mass index for quick reference. J Am Diet Assoc 90:856, 1990.

ADDITIONAL REFERENCES

Chumlea WC, et al. Estimating stature from knee height for persons 60 to 90 years of age. J Am Geriatr Soc 33:116, 1985.

Dwyer JT. Screening Older Americans' Nutritional Health: Current Practices and Future Possibilities. Washington, DC: Nutrition Screening Initiative, 1991.

Evans-Stoner N. Nutrition assessment: A practical approach. Nurs Clin North Am 32(4):637, 1997.

Falciglia G, et al. Upper arm anthropometric norms in elderly white subjects. J Am Diet Assoc 88:563, 1988.

Frisancho AR. Nutritional anthropometry. J Am Diet Assoc 88:553, 1988.

Guthrie HA. Interpretation of data on dietary intake. Nutr Rev 47:33, 1989.

Himes JH, et al. Parent-specific adjustments for assessment of recumbent length and stature. In: Monographs in Paediatrics, vol. 13. Basel: S Karger, 1981.

Jarvis, C. Physical Examination and Health Assessment. Philadelphia: WB Saunders, 1996.

Kenny JJ, et al. Applied kinesiology unreliable for assessing nutrient status. J Am Diet Assoc 88:698, 1988.

Lopes J, et al. Skeletal muscle function in malnutrition. Am J Clin Nutr 36:602, 1982.

McLaren DS. Color Atlas of Nutritional Disorders. London: Wolfe Medication Publications, 1981.

Medlin C, Skinner JD. Individual dietary intake methodology: A 50-year review of progress. J Am Diet Assoc 88:1250, 1988.

Queen P, et al. Clinical indicators for oncology, cardiovascular and surgical patients: Report of the ADA Council on Practice, Quality Management Committee. J Am Diet Assoc 93:338–344, 1993.

Segal KR. Lean body mass estimation by bioelectrical impedance analysis: A four-site cross-validation study. Am J Clin Nutr 47:7, 1988.

Subcommittee on Criteria for Dietary Evaluation, National Research Council, NAS. Nutrient Adequacy. Washington, DC: National Academy Press, 1986.

Winkler M, Lysen L (eds.). Dietitians in Nutrition Support Dietetic Practice Group: Suggested Guidelines for Nutrition and Metabolic Management of Adult Patients Receiving Nutrition Support. Chicago: American Dietetic Association, 1993.

Young CM. Subjects' estimation of food intake and calculated nutritive value of the diet. J Am Diet Assoc 29:1216, 1953.

CHAPTER 17

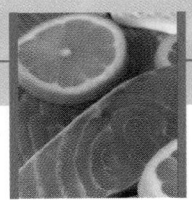

Laboratory Data in Nutrition Assessment

TIMOTHY CARLSON, PHD, RD

CHAPTER OUTLINE

- Definition and Utility of Nutrition Laboratory Data
- Specimen Types
- Types of Assays
- Laboratory Data in Protein-Energy Status
- Laboratory Data in Nutritional Anemias
- Laboratory Markers of Malabsorption
- Laboratory Data and Wellness Assessment
- Nutritional Interpretation of Routine Medical Laboratory Data

Key Terms

ALBUMIN—the most abundant (55%–65% of total) and most often measured plasma protein; a negative acute-phase respondent with a long half-life ($t_{1/2}$ = 21 d), albumin is synthesized in the liver, functions to maintain plasma oncotic pressure, and acts as a nonspecific carrier

ANEMIA OF CHRONIC DISEASE—a condition, associated with chronic inflammation, in which hemoglobin and hematocrit values fall below reference values because iron transport from storage to the sites of heme synthesis and erythrocyte production is blocked

C-REACTIVE PROTEIN (CRP)—a remarkably sensitive plasma-protein marker of inflammatory status

CREATININE—a chemical breakdown product of creatine phosphate, the high-energy phosphate storage compound found in muscle; used as a marker of renal function and muscle mass

FERRITIN—the protein that sequesters iron in a readily available form, primarily inside hepatocytes and other iron storage cells; in plasma is proportional to intracellular ferritin and can be used to assess iron status, except during inflammatory conditions

FIBRONECTIN—a large plasma protein with a short half-life (<24 hours) involved in cell adhesion and wound healing; levels decrease in acute illness, stress, and protein-energy deficit; levels increase concommitant with medical recovery

FUNCTIONAL ASSAY—the appraisal of nutrient pool size by measurement of the activity of a biochemical or physiologic function dependent on the nutrient in question

HOMOCYSTEINE—an amino acid that functions as an intermediate in the production of methionine and the methyl group donor, *S*-adenosylmethionine; because this *S*-adenosymethionine cycle is dependent on vitamin B_{12} and folate, deficiencies in these vitamins are associated with hyperhomocysteinemia, an independent risk factor for occlusive cardiovascular disease

INSULIN-LIKE GROWTH FACTOR-1 (SOMATOMEDIN C)—a peptide hormone with a half-life of about 5 hours that mediates the functions of growth hormone; responsive to protein-energy status, both in the presence and the absence of inflammation

MACROCYTIC ANEMIA—a condition marked by a mean red cell volume of <100 fL; most often caused by vitamin B_{12} or folate deficiencies

MICROCYTIC ANEMIA—a condition marked by a mean red cell volume of <80 fL; commonly associated with iron deficiency

NEGATIVE ACUTE-PHASE RESPONDENTS—a group of plasma proteins, including albumin and transthyretin, whose concentrations decrease during inflammatory states (the acute-phase reaction) because of the action of inflammatory cytokines on their synthesis

NUTRITION-SPECIFIC LABORATORY DATA—tests on body fluids (e.g., plasma, serum, and saliva), tissues (e.g., whole blood, cells, hair, and nails), and wastes (e.g., urine, feces, and sweat) that are performed by controlled physical, chemical, biochemical, molecular, diagnostic, or microscopic examination, primarily to provide information about nutrient pool status

OXIDATIVE STRESS—the balance between the formation of toxic, free radical oxidation products and the biochemical reduction reactions that convert these compounds to benign end products

POSITIVE ACUTE-PHASE RESPONDENTS—a group of plasma proteins, including CRP and alpha$_1$-acid glycoprotein (orosomucoid), whose concentrations increase during inflammatory states (the acute-phase reaction) because of the action of inflammatory cytokines on their synthesis

REACTIVE OXIDATION SPECIES (ROS)—free radical species, including hydrogen peroxide (H_2O_2), superoxide radical (O_2^-) and hydroxyl radical (OH), which are formed during metabolic processes or during metabolism of xenobiotic compounds and which degrade normal lipids, nucleic acids, and proteins

RETINOL-BINDING PROTEIN (RBP)—a negative acute-phase respondent plasma protein with a half life ($t_{\frac{1}{2}}$ = 12 h) whose concentration correlates with protein-energy status; binds and transports the vitamin A metabolite, retinol

STATIC ASSAY—appraisal of nutrient pool size by direct measurement of the nutrient in a biological fluid, tissue, or waste

TOTAL IRON-BINDING CAPACITY (TIBC)—a measurement of the potential for plasma to bind ferric acid (Fe^{3+})

TRANSFERRIN—the plasma protein synthesized in the liver that transports ferric iron from one organ to another; it is a negative acute-phase respondent that has a medium half-life ($t_{\frac{1}{2}}$ = 8 d) and is responsive to protein-energy status

TRANSTHYRETIN—a negative acute-phase respondent plasma protein, frequently called prealbumin, which binds thyroxine and retinol-binding protein and is commonly used to monitor protein-energy status; because of its relatively short half-life ($t_{\frac{1}{2}}$ = 2 d), it rapidly responds to improving protein-energy status

ZINC PROTOPORPHYRIN:HEME RATIO (ZPPH)—a measurement of the proportion of zinc protoporphyrin (a heme-like compound with a substitution of zinc for iron) to heme in red blood cells; ZPPH increases in proportion to depletion of iron stores

DEFINITION AND UTILITY OF NUTRITION LABORATORY DATA

Nutrition-specific laboratory data can be defined as information about nutrition status obtained from controlled physical, chemical (biochemical), molecular diagnostic, or microscopic examination of specimens of body tissues, fluids, and wastes. Because laboratory data can be obtained from several disciplines, including clinical biochemistry and hematology, it is incorrect to use the terms biochemical assessment and laboratory assessment synonymously. In this text, laboratory data include, but are not limited to, biochemical data. Laboratory assessment of nutrients, not discussed in this chapter, is presented in Appendix 32.

Compared to medical status, nutrition status generally changes slowly. Deteriorating nutrition status, at least initially, may not lead to a change in medical status. So, when illness occurs, it is not always clear whether nutrition contributed to the illness. However, illness or injury almost always leads to rapid deterioration in nutrition status. Because nutrition status usually changes relatively slowly, the laboratory data used to assess it must be interpreted differently than the laboratory data used to diagnose disease. Often, laboratory results are available from only a single point in time. Whereas a single laboratory result may be adequate for medical diagnosis, such data are less useful than serial results for nutrition assessment. However, one laboratory value can be very helpful in screening, or to confirm an assessment based on changing clinical, anthropometric, and dietary status. It is often very difficult to determine the exact degree of malnutrition, again because nutrition status changes slowly. The clinician who wants to obtain an accurate assessment of nutrition status must integrate data about shifts in clinical status, changes in anthropometric indices, dietary history, and, ideally, changes in laboratory indicators of nutrition status.

The great advantage of laboratory data over other kinds of objective data obtained from the body is that quality control can be stringently maintained inside the laboratory environment. This is primarily accomplished by analyzing "control" samples, which have predetermined analyte concentrations, with every batch of patient specimens. The results obtained from the control samples for a particular batch of patient samples must compare favorably with the predetermined acceptable values before the patient data are considered valid. Because of this, nutrition laboratory data used in patient screening, assessment, or monitoring generally do not include measurements made on the whole body or a portion of it. Characterization of body dimensions, density, permeability to radiation, radiation from the body, and other biophysical properties cannot be accomplished in the controlled environment that we think of as a clinical nutrition laboratory.

When data are obtained from a laboratory with a well-designed and faithfully practiced quality control program, the health practitioner can have confidence that the data are not compromised by inadequate analytical methods, or operator error or bias Fig. 17–1. Conversely, data from laboratories that do not maintain vigorous quality control may be used to confirm suppositions about nutrition status developed from clinical examination, dietary history, and anthropometric measurements, but they

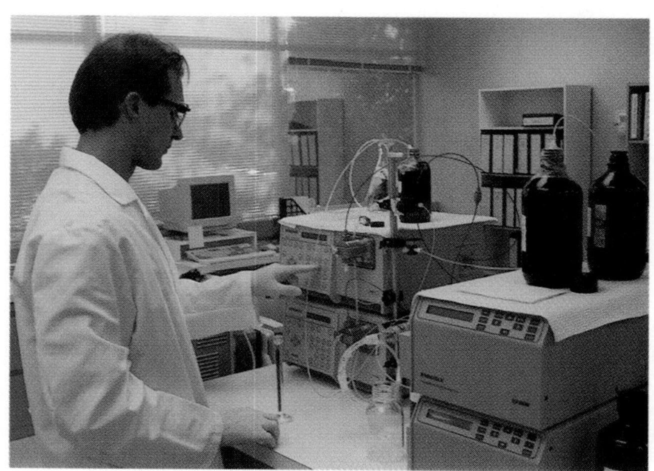

FIGURE 17–1 A technician sets up a high performance liquid chromatography (IPLC) assay to measure plasma, homocysteine, vitamins, carotenoids, etc.

lose much of their potential to be primary indicators of nutritional imbalance. The accuracy of a laboratory assessment depends not only on interpretation of the data, but also on confidence that the laboratory maintains the requisite level of quality control and quality assurance.

SPECIMEN TYPES

Several specimen types are used by laboratory personnel to test for nutrients and nutrient-related substances. Traditional specimen types include:

- Serum (the fluid obtained from blood after the blood has been clotted and then centrifuged to remove the clot and blood cells)
- Plasma (the fluid obtained after centrifugation of blood collected with anticoagulants, like ethylenediaminetetra-acetic acid [EDTA], heparin, trisodium citrate, or potassium oxalate)
- Erythrocytes (red blood cells)
- Leukocytes (white blood cells) and leukocyte fractions
- Other tissues (obtained from scrapings or biopsy samples)
- Urine (from random samples or timed collections)
- Feces (from random samples or timed collections)

Less commonly used specimens include:

- Saliva
- Hair
- Nails
- Sweat

The latter nontraditional specimens have significant drawbacks, including potential contamination from contact with the environment; lack of standardized procedures for processing, assay, and quality control; and levels of nutrient or nutrient indices that are below what can be measured accurately and precisely. (See "*Clinical Insight:* Hair Analysis.") However, because these specimens can be collected at the point of care, considerable research is being done with these kinds of specimens to improve their utility. For example, a home or a nursing home may not have phlebotomy available, but caregivers in these settings could collect a saliva sample. Because point-of-care testing saves time and money and is often more convenient for both the patient and caregiver, it is being looked upon favorably by medical economists and reimbursement officials.

TYPES OF ASSAYS

There are two fundamental types of laboratory assays of nutrient status; static assays and functional assays. The **static assay** measures the actual level of nutrient in the specimen. Examples of this kind of assay include serum iron, white blood cell ascorbic acid, and hair zinc. Although this kind of assay has the advantage of being absolutely specific for the nutrient of interest, it may not measure it correctly; that is, it may lack sensitivity. In other words, specimen nutrient concentrations do not reflect the amount of that substance stored in other, potentially more important, body pools. The other major limitation of static assays is that recent dietary intake can influence the amount of a nutrient found in serum, plasma, or any other fluid or tissue. This problem can be overcome, at least partially, by collecting the specimen when the subject is in a fasting state. An overnight (8-hour) fast is usually adequate. A **functional assay** quantitatively measures the magnitude of a biochemical activity that is dependent on the nutrient of interest. This type of assay can be very sensitive for a nutrient at its functional site. A good example of a functional test is serum ferritin (see page 389). In this case, the concentration of ferritin released into the blood is a function of the iron present in the cellular storage pool. Unfortunately, functional assays are not always specific for the nutrient of interest because many physiologic and biochemical functions are dependent on a variety of biologic factors in addition to the specific nutrient.

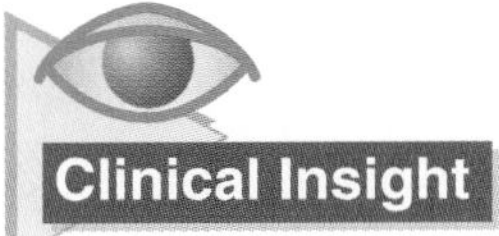

HAIR ANALYSIS

Hair analysis is not particularly useful for assessing mineral levels, such as sodium, magnesium, phosphorus, potassium, calcium, iron, and iodine, as there are already good tests for evaluating body functions related to these minerals. However, hair analysis may have a place in assessing levels of trace elements, such as zinc, copper, chromium, and manganese, for which measurements of functional status are not well developed, and levels of cadmium and lead, which have negative biologic effects.

To be clinically useful, however, hair analysis procedures must be refined and standardized, and "normal" values for hair mineral content defined and accepted. Currently, hair analysis is more useful in experimental efforts than in clinical medicine. This technique is most useful when employed to analyze levels of a single element, rather than several elements at one time, as the probability of an abnormal test result increases as the specificity of the test drops.

Even if hair analysis results were to be judged to be abnormal, it is not known whether this outcome reflects abnormal exposure to an element and, thus, a *cause* of the disease, or whether the abnormal result is an *effect* of the disease. Use of hair dyes and other chemical processes may also affect results. Lastly, there is no evidence that nutritional therapy based on hair analysis is of any benefit.

LABORATORY DATA IN PROTEIN-ENERGY STATUS

Background

Acute illness or trauma causes inflammatory stress (Chang and Bistrian, 1998), and protein-energy malnutrition often occurs simultaneously (Moldawer, 1997) (see Chapter 33). The latter results from the release of cytokines, such as interleukin-1, interleukin-6, and tumor necrosis factor, from monocytes and phagocytic cells associated with the vascular endothelium. These cytokines reorient hepatic synthesis of plasma proteins and increase the breakdown of muscle protein to meet the demand for protein and energy during the inflammatory response. Proteins that are designated **negative acute-phase respondents,** such as albumin, transferrin, transthyretin (prealbumin), and retinol-binding protein, decrease during the acute-phase response. Others, designated **positive acute-phase respondents** (and often, less correctly, called acute-phase proteins), increase to varying degrees. These include C-reactive protein, serum amyloid A, fibrinogen, haptoglobin, alpha$_1$-acid glycoprotein (orosomucoid), alpha$_1$-antitrypsin, alpha$_1$-antichymotrypsin, ceruloplasmin, and C3 and C4 proteins (Table 17–1). The change in the levels of these proteins is generally proportional to the severity of the tissue injury associated with trauma, infection, or other physiologic insult.

The decrease in the plasma levels of albumin, and in the levels of the other negative acute-phase proteins, that occurs during the acute phase is caused by (1) downregulation of gene expression and translation, (2) increases in catabolism, (3) transport to extravascular pools, and (4) a probable reduction in synthesis secondary to decreased dietary essential amino acids.

The shift of albumin (and possibly, the shift of other, similarly sized, negative acute-phase proteins) to the extravascular space during the acute inflammatory response is in contrast to what occurs during uncomplicated starvation (marasmus). In the latter, even though there is a mild decrease in albumin synthesis, plasma albumin is maintained by a shift of albumin from the extravascular space into the plasma.

TABLE 17–1 CLASSIFICATION OF SOME PLASMA PROTEINS BY FUNCTION

Immunoglobulins (Ig)
IgG, IgA, IgM, IgD, IgE

Complement Components
C1q; C1r; C1s; C2; **C3; C4;** C5; C6; C7; C8; C9; properdin; factors D, H, I, and P; C4bp; S protein; C8bp

Coagulation and Fibrinolytic Factors
Fibrinogen, prothrombin; factors V, VII, VIII, IX, XI, XII, and XIII; protein C; protein S; prekallikrein; HMW kininogen; von Willebrand factor; plasminogen

Enzyme Inhibitors
α_1-**Antitrypsin,** α_2-macroglobulin, inter-α-trypsin inhibitor, antithrombin III, C1 inhibitor, α_1-**chymotrypsin,** α_2-antiplasmin, heparin cofactor II, cystatin C, pregnancy-associated α_2-glycoprotein, tissue factor pathway inhibitor (lipoprotein-associated coagulation inhibitor [LACI])

Lipid Transport–Associated Proteins
Apoproteins A-I, A-II, B, C-I, C-II, C-III, D, and E; β_2-glycoprotein I; **serum amyloid A**

Transport Proteins
Albumin, transthyretin (prealbumin), transferrin, retinol-binding protein, thyroxin-binding protein, vitamin D–binding protein, sex hormone–binding protein, transcobalamin I, transcobalamin II, corticosteroid-binding globulin, transcortin, **hemopexin, haptoglobin, ceruloplasmin**

Proteins Having Uncertain or Other Functions
(α_1-**Acid glycoprotein,** α_1-glycoprotein, serum amyloid P component, α_1-microglobulin, Zn-α_2-glycoprotein, fibronectin, α-HS-glycoprotein, histidine-rich glycoprotein, **C-reactive protein**

Positive acute-phase proteins are shown in boldface type. Negative acute-phase proteins appear in boldface italics; proteins that are used in protein-energy assessment are underlined. Note that the positive acute-phase proteins are distributed in nearly all functional classes, whereas the main negative acute-phase proteins are transport proteins.

Nitrogen Balance

Nitrogen balance is *the* oldest biochemical technique for assessing protein status. It is also the only biochemical measurement that truly reflects both the somatic and visceral protein pools. Nitrogen balance is based on the fact that approximately 16% of the mass of proteins is nitrogen. (This varies from protein to protein, but 16% represents a good average estimate for dietary protein.) Therefore, if daily protein intake can be determined accurately, measurements of nitrogen excretion, along with corrections for insensible losses (e.g., from skin and gastrointestinal (GI) sloughing, hair loss, and sweat), allow determination of nitrogen balance. In healthy adults, nitrogen balance is zero. Nitrogen balance is negative during starvation and in several forms of protein-energy malnutrition (in which nitrogen loss exceeds intake), and it is positive in growing children, pregnant women, and adults who are adding mass (weight) or recovering from injury or illness. Nitrogen balance may be calculated as:

$$\text{Nitrogen balance} = \text{N intake (g/24 h)} - (\text{urinary N [g/24 h]} + 2\text{ g/24 h})$$

If urinary nitrogen is replaced by urinary urea measurement, the correction factor becomes +4 g/24 h to account for nitrogenous compounds, like uric acid, ammonia, creatinine, and amino acids, in the urine.

Total urinary nitrogen can be measured by Kjeldahl analysis, which is laborious and generally not suitable for clinical purposes, or by pyrochemiluminescence. The latter method can be done more easily and cheaply than the old Kjeldahl determination. Furthermore, it is superior to urinary urea values for determining nitrogen balance because although urinary non–urea nitrogen averages about 4 g/day, it ranges from 0 to about 6 g/day in normal persons, and may exceed 10 g/day in the critically ill.

The chief difficulty with nitrogen balance measurements is that it may not be possible to estimate protein intake in subjects who are consuming an oral diet. However, these measurements are extremely valuable for monitoring the appropriateness of a completely defined intake, as in parenteral nutrition or enteral tube feeding. Nitrogen balance should be measured at least weekly during short-term nutrition support, perhaps more often in the initial stages. (See Chapter 22.) These measurements allow the dietitian, pharmacist, and physician to assess not only if the patient is in nitrogen balance, but whether the patient is able to utilize the amount of protein that a total parenteral nutrition regimen (TPN) or enteral prescription is providing. Thus, even if the balance is positive, it may be appropriate to lower the protein given in order to prevent large-scale deamination of amino acids that cannot be utilized in de novo protein synthesis. The appropriate amount of protein will result in a decrease in energy expenditure for amino acid deamination and urea formation.

Visceral (Plasma) Protein Indicators

Proteins in plasma and extravascular fluids represent approximately 3% of the total body protein, whereas visceral organ protein constitutes about 10%. Because albumin and many other plasma proteins are synthesized in the liver, plasma proteins can be thought of as functional indices of hepatic protein status. Of course, the proteins in visceral organs and somatic tissues do not function independently, so the total body protein status is, to some extent, reflected by measurements of certain plasma proteins. Unlike nitrogen balance that assesses only short-term changes in whole body protein status, plasma protein levels (and measurements of muscle mass) integrate protein synthesis and degradation over longer periods of time. As compared to other methods of assessing changing protein-energy status, plasma protein measurements are quicker, more precise, and less expansive. Furthermore, proper interpretation of plasma protein data can make these data very valuable to the nutrition professional, especially in an institutional care environment.

More than 300 proteins have been identified in human plasma. Table 17–1 shows where acute-phase respondent proteins, and proteins that have been studied as indicators of protein nutrition status, fit into a functional classification of plasma proteins.

Albumin

Because **albumin** is abundant in serum, simple to prepare, stable, highly soluble in water, and easily purified, it has been one of the most intensively studied of all proteins. Because it has been studied so intensively and for so long,* some of the diagnostic uses of serum albumin values are based on old, out-of-date data. This is especially true in the area of nutrition assessment and monitoring. In truth, albumin probably only reflects protein intake in specialized experimental conditions, such as when animals, housed in stressful facilities, are fed diets deficient only in protein. Studies in which albumin levels in total starvation have been compared to protein-limited diets have shown that albumin levels decrease dramatically in protein-free diets, but are more preserved in total starvation. These results are similar to the effect of marasmus and kwashiorkor on albumin. Because inflammation is an almost universal finding in cases of kwashiorkor (protein deficiency), in many hospitalized patients with low albumin levels, it is probable that inflammation (e.g., infection, trauma, or another physiologic stress) is necessary for a decline in albumin levels.

In addition to this limitation is another; albumin is a negative acute-phase reactant and it has a long half-life (~20 d). This means that plasma albumin concentration increases slowly in patients recovering from stress and in those receiving nutrition intervention. Another shortcoming of albumin in monitoring changes in protein-energy malnutrition (PEM) is related to the large extravascular albumin pool. Albumin outside of the bloodstream (extravascular albumin) represents 1.5 to 2.0 times that in the blood. Some of this large pool returns to the circulation when blood concentrations decrease, and this tends to blunt changes in plasma albumin concentration. So, when synthesis decreases, large amounts of albumin can return to the circulation; when synthesis increases, albumin leaves to replenish the extravascular pool. These considerations indicate that albumin is, at best, a poor index of PEM.

Transferrin

Transferrin is the first of several proteins that function exclusively in the transport of other essential compounds and are being used in the assessment of PEM. It, like albumin, is a negative acute-phase respondent, but it has a shorter half-life (8 d) (Table 17–2).

In addition to being responsive to dietary protein and energy, the plasma transferrin level is controlled by the size of the iron storage pool. When iron stores are depleted, transferrin synthesis increases. Therefore, its level may reflect iron status, instead of PEM status.

---

*Albumin has been studied for at least 150 years. In 1839, Ancell wrote in *The Lancet*, "Albumin . . . is found not only in the serum of the blood, but in lymph, chyle, in the exhilations from surfaces, in the fluid of cellular tissue, in the aqueous and vitreous humus of the eye, [and] in many other animal fluids. . . ." (Ancell H. Lancet 1:222, 1839–1840, as quoted in Am J Dig Dis 14:711, 1969).

TABLE 17–2 PROPERTIES OF PROTEINS COMMONLY USED IN PROTEIN-ENERGY ASSESSMENT

PROTEIN	APPROXIMATE HALF-LIFE	MOLECULAR WEIGHT	REFERENCE RANGE
Albumin	3 weeks	65,000	3.5–5.2 g/dL
Transferrin	1 week	80,000	200–400 mg/dL
Transthyretin	2 days	55,000	19–43 mg/dL
Retinol-binding protein	12 hours	21,000	2.1–6.4 mg/DL

Although the half-life of transferrin is shorter than that of albumin, it still does not respond rapidly enough to protein-energy status to be useful in acute care settings. This factor, along with its nonspecificity, makes transferrin only slightly more useful than albumin as a marker of protein-energy status.

Transthyretin

During the last two decades, there has been interest in the use of **transthyretin** (TTHY) for the assessment of protein-energy status (Mears, 1996). TTHY is a transport protein that binds retinol-binding protein. As indicated by its name (it is also called thyroxin-binding prealbumin, or simply *prealbumin*), transthyretin also binds thyroxin. Apparently, TTHY, like albumin, has multiple physiologic roles.

TTHY levels have been shown to correlate with short-term changes in PEM status. However, the use of TTHY in the assessment of PEM is associated with some of the same problems that plague the use of albumin and transferrin. Most importantly, it is a negative acute-phase protein. Hence, its use in screening for PEM is limited because a low level could result from either inadequate nutrition or inflammatory stress. On the other hand, because TTHY has a half-life of just 2 days, it is very useful in monitoring improvements in protein-energy status (see Table 17–2). If a baseline value is obtained at or near its nadir—the time when the hypermetabolic period of the inflammatory response wanes—subsequent increases in TTHY values correlate with positive nitrogen balance. Thus, the short half-life of TTHY allows a short-term and sensitive assessment of improving status.

One drawback to the use of TTHY is that zinc deficiency affects hepatic TTHY synthesis and secretion. Therefore, zinc status, in addition to inflammatory status, should be taken into account when interpreting a low plasma TTHY level.

Retinol-Binding Protein

Another protein with a short half-life that has been used to assess PEM is **retinol-binding protein** (RBP). This protein has a half-life of about 12 hours. It is small for a plasma protein, but does not pass through the renal glomerulus because it circulates in a complex with TTHY. As implied by its name, RBP binds retinol, and transport of this metabolite of vitamin A seems to be its exclusive function. RBP is synthesized in the liver and then released in combination with retinol. After RBP releases retinol in peripheral tissue, its affinity for TTHY decreases, leading to dissociation of the TTHY-RBP complex, and filtration of apo-RBP by the glomerulus. The protein is catabolized in the renal tubule.

Plasma RBP concentration has been shown to be correlated with protein-energy status in uncomplicated PEM. However, confounding the interpretation of RBP level is its behavior during inflammatory stress. Like albumin, transferrin, and TTHY, RBP is a negative acute-phase protein. This means that RBP, like the other plasma protein indicators of PEM discussed to this point, does not reflect protein-energy status in acutely stressed patients.

The simultaneous secretion of RBP and retinol from the liver means that retinol status also complicates the interpretation of reduced RBP values. RBP cannot reliably be used to assess protein-energy status when vitamin A status is compromised.

Another problem associated with the use of RBP in assessing PEM is related to the catabolism of apo-RBP by the kidney. Patients with renal failure are likely to have elevated RBP levels, regardless of their protein-energy status, because the RBP must reach the renal tubule to be catabolized.

C-Reactive Protein

When used as indicators of protein-energy status, the major difficulty associated with each of the four plasma proteins discussed thus far is their behavior during inflammatory stress. Indeed, most patients in acute care settings experience some degree of inflammation, making it difficult to interpret accurately any decreases in levels of albumin, transferrin, transthyretin, or retinol-binding protein. Perhaps the best way to circumvent this shortcoming is not to utilize them for protein-energy assessment during the ebb-and-flow phases of the inflammatory response. Determining the optimal time for initiating aggressive nutrition intervention during the resolution of inflammation is difficult.

One approach to the standardization of nutrition therapy during the inflammatory response is to use an objective indicator of the acute phase. An approach that is increasingly employed is to use one of the positive acute-phase respondent proteins to monitor the progress of the stress reactions, and to begin more aggressive nutritional intervention when this indicator shows that the inflammatory reactions are subsiding. Probably the best protein for this purpose is **C-reactive protein (CRP).** Although the exact function of this protein is not entirely clear, CRP increases early in acute stress, usually within 4 to 6 hours of surgery or other trauma. Furthermore, its level increases as much as 1000-fold, depending on the intensity of the stress response (Thompson et al., 1992). Experience indicates that when the CRP level begins to recede, the patient has entered the anabolic period of the inflammatory response, and more intensive nutrition therapy will be beneficial. Because TTHY levels begin to increase at about the same time that CRP starts to decline, and because increasing levels of TTHY correlate well with improving protein-energy status, the beginning of nutrition intervention can be tied to changes in both of these plasma proteins.

Insulin-Like Growth Factor 1

An alternative approach to using two proteins—like CRP and TTHY or RBP—to monitor inflammation and nutrition states separately would be to find one protein that would assess protein-energy status even during the acute-phase response. Such a protein could be used both in screening and monitoring of nutrition status. A candidate for this role is **insulin-like growth factor-1 (IGF-1, or somatomedin C).** This peptide hormone mediates at least some of the effects of growth hormone. It has a half-life of approximately 4 hours, rapidly responds to changes in protein-energy status independent of inflammatory status, and appears to be particularly sensitive to protein intake. Its concentration is affected by hepatic, renal, and some autoimmune diseases. Unfortunately, cost-effective and rapid IGF-1 assays are only now beginning to become available.

Fibronectin

One other protein that deserves mention as a candidate for screening and monitoring of protein-energy status is **fibronectin.** Fibronectin is a large plasma protein that is involved in cell adhesion and differentiation, wound healing, and opsonizing functions. The fibronectin level decreases when there is physiologic consumption in acute illness or injury.

Protein-energy deficit is associated with decreasing levels of fibronectin; levels return to normal during repletion. Fibronectin differs from the other proteins that have been used to assess protein-energy status because increasing levels appear to participate directly in the patient's medical recovery. This phenomenon has been illustrated by studies showing that the infusion of fibronectin concentrates enhances the rate of survival of children with kwashiorkor.

Two theoretical advantages of fibronectin are its relatively short half-life ($t_{\frac{1}{2}} = 24$ h) and its high molecular weight. The latter attribute prevents massive leakage of fibronectin from the plasma compartment during the increased capillary leakage associated with acute inflammation; furthermore, a relatively small extravascular pool prevents vascular return of fibronectin from masking response to nutritional intervention. Despite its potential to remain undiluted during leakage of other proteins from the vascular system, the consumption of fibronectin in unrelenting inflammatory states, such as occur with sepsis and post-traumatic injury, significantly decreases its plasma concentration. Therefore, a decreased level is difficult to interpret in an acutely ill patient. Additional research is needed to differentiate the response of fibronectin to illness and injury and to protein-energy status.

Somatic Indicators of PEM

Urinary Creatinine and Creatinine-Height Ratio

Creatinine is formed from creatine, a compound found almost exclusively in muscle tissue. Creatine is synthesized from the amino acids glycine and arginine, with addition of a methyl group from the folate- and cobalamin-dependent methionine-*S*-adenosylmethionine-homocysteine cycle. It functions as a high-energy phosphate buffer, to maintain a constant supply of adenosine triphosphate (ATP) for muscle contraction. When creatine is dephosphorylated, some of it is spontaneously converted to creatinine in an irreversible, nonenzymatic reaction. Creatinine has no specific biologic function; it is continuously released from the muscle cell and excreted by the kidneys with very little reabsorption. When a patient is consuming a meat-restricted diet, the size of the patient's somatic (muscle) protein pool is directly proportional to the amount of creatinine excreted. This means that men generally excrete larger amounts of creatinine than women do, and that individuals with greater muscular development excrete larger amounts than those who are less muscular. (Total body weight is not proportional to creatinine excretion, but muscle mass is. Creatinine excretion rate is related to muscle mass, as reflected by the following equation:

$$\text{muscle} = k + k' \text{ (urinary creatinine)}$$

where k and kí are empirical constants. Using computed tomography as a gold standard, the following equation has been developed:

$$\text{skeletal muscle mass (kg)} = 4.1 + 18.9 \times \text{24-h creatinine excretion in g/d}$$

This relationship works well for normal individuals, but not body builders, and it has not been tested in sick or injured patients.

An approach formerly used to assess somatic protein status involves the use of the creatinine-height index (CHI):

$$\text{CHI} = \frac{\text{24-h urine volume (dL)} \times \text{urinary creatinine concentration (mg/dL)}}{\text{expected 24-h urine creatinine excretion (mg)}}$$

The expected 24-hour creatinine excretion is related to the patient's height, and tables have been constructed that contain the expected values.

Clearly, muscle mass is not entirely dependent on height, so the CHI must be used with caution in tall, thin, or muscular individuals. The use of creatinine and CHI to assess somatic protein status is also confounded by consumption of an omnivorous diet because, as already mentioned, creatine is stored in muscle, muscle meats are rich in creatine. Creatinine that is derived from dietary sources cannot be distinguished from endogenously produced creatinine. Another factor confounding interpretation of urinary creatinine data is that there is significant intraindividual variability in daily creatinine excretion, probably because of sweat losses. In addition, the test is based on 24-hour urine collections, and it is often difficult to obtain quantitative urine collections. Because of these limitations, the use of urinary creatinine as a marker of muscle mass is primarily semi-quantitative.

3-Methylhistidine Excretion

Muscle mass is also related to the excretion of the amino acid *3-methylhistidine.* This amino acid is found only in the actin and myosin of muscle tissue, and is produced by modification of the histidine residues of these proteins, after synthesis is complete. During the normal turnover of muscle proteins, 3-methylhistidine is released and cannot be recycled. Therefore, its level in urine is related to somatic protein mass. 3-methylhistidine is not often used in protein-energy assessment because it requires labor-intensive assay procedures. In addition, like creatinine, the amount supplied by the diet (i.e., through consumption of muscle meats) is difficult to estimate accurately, and 24-hour urine collections are required.

LABORATORY DATA IN NUTRITIONAL ANEMIAS

Anemia is a condition characterized by a reduction in the number of erythrocytes per unit of blood volume, or a decrease in hemoglobin content of blood below the level of physiologic need. By convention, anemia is defined as a hemoglobin concentration below the 95th percentile for healthy reference populations of men, women, or age-grouped children. Anemia is not a disease, but a symptom of a variety of situations, including extensive blood loss, excessive blood cell destruction, or decreased blood cell formation. Clinical nutritionists are primarily concerned with differentiating nutritional anemias secondary to nutritional inadequacies from anemia due to other causes (see Chapter 35).

Classification of Anemia

Nutritional deficits are the major causes of decreased hemoglobin and erythrocyte production. However, because blood loss or excessive red cell destruction can also cause anemia, it is necessary to determine the potential cause. The initial, descriptive classification of anemia is derived from the hematocrit value or complete blood count (CBC) and associated calculations. Anemias associated with a mean red blood cell volume of less than 80 fL (femtoliters) are termed microcytic, whereas those with values of 80 to 99 fL are termed normocytic, and those associated with values of greater than 100 fL are macrocytic (Massey et al., 1992).

Data from the complete blood count are helpful in differentiating nutritional causes for anemia. **Microcytic anemia** is most often associated with iron deficiency, whereas **macrocytic anemia** is generally caused by either folate- or vitamin B_{12}–deficient erythropoiesis. However, because of the low specificity of these indices, additional data are needed to distinguish between the various nutritional causes of microcytic and macrocytic anemias and their non-nutritional causes, such as thalassemia trait and chronic renal insufficiency. Microcystosis can also be associated with inadequate iron utilization, most commonly in the anemia of chronic disease. This type of anemia is associated with rheumatic diseases, chronic infection, cancer, severe tissue injury, multiple fractures, and Hodgkin's disease. Hence, anemia with microcytosis is not sufficient cause for recommending iron supplementation.

Other information from the CBC that helps to differentiate the non-nutritional causes of anemia include leukocyte and platelet counts. When these are low, marrow failure is indicated; high counts are associated with anemia caused by leukemia or infection. If anemia is associated with normal-sized red cells, it is most likely caused by acute blood loss. However, in hemolytic anemias and early iron deficiency anemia, the red blood cell size may also be normal. (See Fig. 35–1.)

To further rule out non-nutritional causes of anemia, the reticulocyte count can be evaluated. Reticulocytes are large, nucleated, immature red blood cells that are released in small numbers with mature cells. When red blood cell production rates increase, reticulocyte counts also increase. Any time anemia is accompanied by a high reticulocyte count, elevated erythropoietic activity in response to bleeding should be considered. In such cases, stool specimens can be tested for occult blood to rule out chronic gastrointestinal blood loss. Other causes of a high reticulocyte count include intravascular hemolysis syndromes and an erythropoietic response to therapy for iron, vitamin B_{12}, or folic acid deficiencies.

Laboratory Tests for Iron Deficiency Anemias

Several laboratory tests are available that can identify iron deficiency anemias (Worwood, 1997).

SERUM IRON. To establish iron deficiency in microcytic anemia, serum iron and total iron-binding capacity are often determined. Although it is widely available and a relatively easy test to perform, serum iron is a relatively poor indicator of iron status because of large day-to-day changes, even in healthy persons. There is also a diurnal variation, with the highest concentrations occurring mid-morning (6 AM to 10 AM), and a nadir, averaging 30% less than the morning level, occurring mid-afternoon. Hence, other tests are needed to assess iron status.

TOTAL IRON-BINDING CAPACITY AND TRANSFERRIN SATURATION. **Total iron-binding capacity (TIBC)** depends on the number of free binding sites on the plasma iron-transport protein, transferrin. Each transferrin molecule binds ferric ions (Fe(III)) at each of two binding sites and two bicarbonate ions at separate sites.

Intracellular iron availability regulates the synthesis and secretion of transferrin. Therefore, the plasma transferrin concentration (usually stated as TIBC) increases in iron deficiency. In addition, when the amount of stored iron available for release to transferrin decreases, and when dietary iron intake is low, saturation of transferrin decreases.

In iron-replete persons, the normal plasma transferrin concentration is 200 to 400 mg/dL (25 to 50 mol/L). Therefore, because transferrin has two iron binding sites and an atomic weight of 56 daltons, the expected TIBC would be 2800 to 5600 μg/L (280 to 560 μg/dL). However, the range of normal TIBC values is 270 to 400 μg/dL, indicating that full occupation of all transferrin binding sites does not occur. Because bicarbonate binding by transferrin is required to activate iron binding fully, loss of this ion from the serum upon standing in a tube, or intrinsically inadequate amounts of it, could explain the incomplete saturation of transferrin, even in the presence of excess iron. Because of this discrepancy, direct correlation of TIBC with transferrin level cannot be interpreted as a 1:1 relationship.

There are several exceptions to the general rule that transferrin saturation decreases and TIBC increases in iron-depleted patients. For example, hepatitis increases TIBC. This value also increases in hypoxia, pregnancy, and with oral contraceptive usage or estrogen replacement. On the other hand, TIBC decreases in the presence of malignant disease, nephrosis, acute and chronic inflammatory diseases, megaloblastic anemias (discussed later in this chapter), and hemolytic anemias. Furthermore, the plasma level of transferrin may be decreased during protein-energy malnutrition, fluid overload, and liver disease. Thus, although TIBC and transferrin saturation are more specific then hematocrit or hemoglobin values, they are not perfect indicators of iron status.

An additional concern with the use of serum iron, TIBC, and transferrin saturation values is that normal values persist until frank deficiency actually occurs. Thus, they cannot detect decreasing iron stores and pre-anemic iron deficiency.

Although TIBC and transferrin saturation are not definitive tests for the assessment of iron deficiency, transferrin saturation is useful in screening for hemochromatosis. Hemochromatosis, a hereditary disease that results from failure of the body to regulate iron absorption, is the most common genetic disease in individuals of Northern European ancestry, and its expression results in elevated transferrin saturation. Normal transferrin saturation is in the range of 20% to 40%, but individuals who are homozygous for the hemochromatosis gene may have values exceeding 60%, and many have a transferrin saturation level in the 80% to 100% range. Diagnosis of hemochromatosis is usually confirmed by genetic analysis, or by determination of the hepatic iron index, a test that requires analysis of the iron stored in a liver biopsy specimen. Although genetic analysis only confirms that a person is at risk for the disease, high transferrin saturation, accompanied by elevation of serum ferritin levels (discussed in a later section), confirms expression of the disease (see Chapter 35). Once the diagnosis of hemochromatosis has been confirmed, serum ferritin levels may be used to monitor changes in patient status.

ZINC PROTOPORPHYRIN:HEME RATIO AND FREE-ERYTHROCYTE PROTOPORPHYRIN. A simple, cost-effective test for iron status is the **zinc protoporphyrin heme ratio (ZPPH):** (Wong et al., 1996). This test, which can be performed using a single drop of blood, is based on the finding that protoporphyrin IX, the molecule that binds iron to form the heme portion of the hemoglobin molecule, may also bind zinc. In iron-replete individuals, through a nonenzymatic process, 1 out of approximately 20,000 hemoglobin molecules contains protoporphyrin IX bound to Zn^{2+} rather than Fe^{2+}. As the iron available for erythropoiesis declines, the fraction of zinc protoporphyrin increases. Iron stores are considered to be depleted when the ratio of zinc protoporphyrin in red blood cells to heme molecules increases to less than 1 in 12,000. The conventional way of reporting these data is as a ratio of the μmol of zinc protoporphyrin per mol heme in red blood cells. This ratio is easily measured by a portable and relatively inexpensive instrument called a hematofluorometer. Abnormal ZPPH ratios are 80 μmol/mol and above. Because the ZPPH measurement is a ratio of intracellular porphyrin species, it has the advantage over concentration-based measurements of being unaffected by hydration status or recent blood loss.

Unlike TIBC and transferrin saturation, the ZPPH ratio is very stable in iron-replete individuals, and it is minimally affected by the many physiologic and pathophysiologic factors that influence many other tests of iron. In addition, depletion of the storage pool can be monitored by the ZPPH ratio. Factors other than iron deficiency that increase the ZPPH ratio are limited to lead poisoning, protoporphyria (rare), and chronic inflammation (common).

A test that is analogous to the ZPPH ratio is free-erythrocyte protoporphyrin (FEP). This test does not actually measure an iron-free protoporphyrin, as the name suggests. Rather, it measures a chemically derived product of zinc protophorphyrin. Therefore, even though measurement of this compound is much more laborious, it measures essentially the same phenomenon gauged by direct measurement of ZPPH. In addition to being a less costly procedure, the ZPPH ratio is a preferred screening test because, as indicated earlier, it is independent of hematocrit, hydration status does not affect it, and recent blood loss or causes of anemia not related to iron deficiency do not alter it.

RED CELL DISTRIBUTION WIDTH. Another sensitive screening test for iron deficiency that can be derived from CBC results is the red cell distribution width (RDW). This index measures abnormalities in red cell size and shape. RDW is a percentage related to the coefficient of variation of the red cell volumes, and it increases as the variation in the range of red cell volumes increases. Normal values of RDW are usually considered to be less than 16%. Microcytic anemia with an RDW of 16% or more indicates iron deficiency. Although RDW is a sensitive iron indicator and can be calculated with other red cell indices, it is usually not reported as part of the CBC results. The reason for not reporting RDW is that many hospitalized patients have been transfused with red blood cells, so the RDW becomes an uninterpretable average of cells from endogenous and exogenous sources. Of course, this argument does not apply to individuals with simple iron deficiency, and RDW would be a helpful and inexpensive addition to the complete blood count report.

FERRITIN. To obtain laboratory confirmation of iron deficiency anemia after screening for ZPPH ratio, FEP, or RDW, the serum **ferritin** level, an indicator of iron storage, is often measured (Ponka et al., 1998). The only tests currently available for this purpose are serum ferritin level or staining of a bone marrow aspirate for iron. Because collection of a marrow aspirate is a very involved procedure and is unpleasant for the patient, it is not practical for routine assessment of iron status. Serum ferritin levels, however, are used routinely for this purpose.

Ferritin is the storage protein that sequesters the iron that is normally gathered in the liver (reticuloendothelial system), spleen, and marrow. As the iron supply increases, the intracellular level of ferritin increases to accommodate iron storage. A small amount of this ferritin leaks into the circulation. This ferritin can be measured by a variety of immunologic assays that are available in most clinical laboratories. Serum ferritin concentration is directly proportional to the amount of ferritin inside storage cells, and indirectly proportional to the amount of iron in those cells. Therefore, measurement of ferritin that has leaked into the serum is an excellent indicator of the size of the body's iron storage pool.

Effect of Inflammation on Anemia

Unfortunately, ferritin levels may, under some circumstances, give a skewed representation of iron status. This occurs because the ferritin level increases during inflammation. Cytokines and other inflammatory mediators can increase ferritin synthesis or ferritin leakage from cells, or both. This means that patients with iron deficiency could have a normal or elevated serum ferritin level if they have a chronic or acute inflammatory condition.

Anemia of chronic disease (ACD) is the primary condition in which ferritin fails to correlate with iron stores (Krantz, 1994). ACD, probably the most common form of anemia in hospitalized patients, occurs in inflammatory, infectious, and neoplastic disorders. It occurs during inflammation because red cell production decreases as the result of inadequate mobilization of iron from its storage sites. This is apparently caused by the release of cytokines, like interleukin-1 and tumor necrosis factor (TNF), which also inhibit division of erythroid progenitors and may inhibit erythropoietin production. In arthritis, depletion of stored iron occurs, in part, because of reduced absorption of iron from the gut. On the other hand, the regular use of nonsteroidal anti-inflammatory drugs can cause occult GI blood loss. This form of anemia is usually mild and normocytic (not microcytic or macrocytic). In 30% to 50% of patients, however, hypochromic (having inadequate amounts of hemoglobin), microcytic red cells are made, serum iron levels and TIBC are low, and iron stores are normal or elevated. Because iron stores are not decreased, normal amounts of ferritin should be present in the plasma. In some cases, however, iron stores may be depleted but inflammatory mediators may cause normal ferritin levels. In complicated clinical conditions, such as in some patients with rheumatoid arthritis, reduced or deficient stores are often part of the picture. Thus, ACD has many possible faces, and it is necessary to distinguish it from iron deficiency anemia so that inappropriate iron supplementation is not initiated.

The inflammatory blockage of iron transport seen in the acute-phase response, which lingers on in ACD, may be a nonspecific defense mechanism preventing the growth of pathogenic microorganisms or cancers. Because plasma iron enhances the growth of many bacteria and tumors, it may not be appropriate to attempt to treat ACD with iron supplementation.

SERUM TRANSFERRIN RECEPTOR (sTfR) TEST FOR IRON DEFICIENCY. Several tests for iron deficiency are currently being developed. Some of these are not affected by inflammatory status. The most promising of these—serum transferrin receptor (sTfR)—is now finding its way into clinical laboratories (Ahluwalia, 1998). This receptor protein binds holotransferrin (transferrin + Fe(III)) during cellular iron uptake. When cellular iron levels decrease, synthesis of sTfR increases. sTfR reflects the amount of this protein on the surface of cells, and an increase in serum levels correlates with iron deficiency. It appears that sTfR effectively monitors iron status in the normal state, in inflammatory conditions, and in iron overload. It is possible that sTfR will someday replace ferritin in confirming iron deficiency.

Laboratory Assessment of Macrocytic Anemias Associated with B Vitamin Deficiencies

The nutritional causes of macrocytic anemia (also referred to as megaloblastic anemia because of the presence of giant red cell precursors in the blood) are related to the availability of folate and vitamin B_{12} (cobalamin) in the marrow. What must be determined is which vitamin is associated with this condition and, if vitamin B_{12} deficiency is the cause, what is the etiology of this deficit.

Static Test for Folate and Vitamin B_{12} Status

Usually, patients with macrocytic anemia are tested for both folate and vitamin B_{12} deficiency by static measurement of these vitamins in blood. These can be assayed by testing the ability of the patient's blood specimen to support the growth of microbes that require either folate or vitamin B_{12}. However, nowadays, radiobinding assays and various kinds of immunoassays are more commonly used.

Folate is most often simultaneously measured in whole blood (plasma + blood cells), and in the serum alone. The difference between whole blood folate and serum folate is then used to calculate the red blood cell folate concentration. It is generally thought that the level of folate in red blood cells better reflects the size of the total folate pool than does the serum level. However, there is considerable evidence that a serum sample obtained after scrupulous fasting is as good for assessing folate status as red blood cell folate. The advantage of the serum measurement is that it is considerably less laborious and, thus, less expensive.

Vitamin B_{12} is usually measured in the serum, and all indications are that the serum level gives as much information about vitamin B_{12} status as does the red blood cell level.

Functional Tests to Determine the Causes of Macrocytic Anemias

HOMOCYSTEINE. Folate and vitamin B_{12} are required for the synthesis of *S*-adenosylmethionine (SAM), the biochemical precursor involved in the transfer of one-carbon (methyl) groups during many biochemical syntheses. SAM is synthesized from the amino acid methionine by a reaction that includes the addition of a methyl group and the purine base adenine (from ATP). When SAM donates to a methyl group for the synthesis of, for example, thymine, choline, creatine, epinephrine, and protein (e.g., 3-methylhistidine formation), and DNA methylation, it is converted to *S*-adenosyl homocysteine. After loss of the adenosyl group, the remaining **homocysteine** can either be converted to cysteine by the vitamin B_6–dependent transsulfuration pathway or converted back to methionine in a reaction that is dependent on folate and vitamin B_{12}. (See Fig. 35–7 and Chapters 4 and 26).

When either folate or vitamin B_{12} is lacking, the homocysteine-to-methionine reaction is virtually blocked. This means that homocysteine will build up in the affected tissue, "spilling" into the circulation. On the other hand, the vitamin B_6–dependent transsulfuration pathway can metabolize excess homocysteine. Therefore, an elevated homocysteine level would be expected to be indicative of either genetic defects involved in the enzymes that catalyze these reactions, or a deficiency in folate, vitamin B_{12}, or vitamin B_6. Indeed, homocysteine has been shown to be very sensitive to folate and vitamin B_{12} deficiency (Savage et al., 1994). Unfortunately, with only an elevated plasma homocysteine concentration, it is not possible to tell which of these B vitamins is deficient and is causing the hyperhomocysteinemia.

METHYLMALONIC ACID. Once a genetic cause is ruled out, the most straightforward biochemical method for differentiating folate and vitamin B_{12} deficiencies is to follow up on the hyperhomocysteinemia with a serum or urinary methylmalonic acid measurement. This metabolite is formed during the degradation of the amino acid valine and odd-chain fatty acids. Methylmalonic acid is a side product in this metabolic pathway that increases when the conversion of methylmalonyl CoA to succinyl CoA is blocked by lack of vitamin B_{12}, a coenzyme for this reaction. Deficiency, therefore, leads to an increase in the methylmalonic acid pool, and this is reflected by the serum or urinary methylmalonic acid level. The advantage of homocysteine testing over assaying serum vitamin B_{12} levels or serum and red cell folate levels is that it tends to detect impending vitamin deficiencies better than the static assays. This is especially important in assessing the status of certain patients, like vegans and the elderly, who could have vitamin B_{12} deficiency associated with central nervous system (CNS) impairment.

Although plasma homocysteine measurements will likely soon be routine in many clinical laboratories because elevated plasma homocysteine is a risk factor for cardiovascular disease (see Chapter 26), methylmalonic acid measurements to determine B_{12} deficiency will almost certainly still be done in only a few specialized laboratories. Hence, it is recommended that individuals with a risk of folate or vitamin B_{12} deficiency be screened by plasma homocysteine measurements, and those individuals with positive test results be further tested for folate and vitamin B_{12} levels, or just the latter.

VITAMIN B_{12} MALABSORPTION. If serum vitamin B_{12} status is compromised, the Schilling test may be used to detect defects in B_{12} absorption. In this test, the subject is given an oral dose of radiolabeled cobalamin and an injection of unlabeled vitamin. The latter saturates vitamin B_{12} storage sites so that all of the radiolabeled vitamin that is absorbed is excreted in the urine within approximately 24 hours. If less than the expected amount of radioactivity appears in the urine, vitamin B_{12} malabsorption is confirmed. The test can then be repeated with administration of a combination of radiolabeled cobalamin and intrinsic factor. If urinary radioactivity reaches the expected levels, intrinsic factor deficiency is the cause of the malabsorption. The term *pernicious anemia* is commonly applied to vitamin B_{12} deficiency resulting from lack of intrinsic factor (see Chapter 35).

This syndrome appears to have genetic and autoimmune causes, but it may be defined more broadly to include inadequate intrinsic factor secretion arising from such causes as gastric atrophy, gastrectomy, some endocrine disorders, and achlorhydria. In addition to these causes, vitamin B_{12} deficiency can be associated with diseases that affect the ability of the distal ileum to absorb it. These include:

- The presence of competitive organisms as a result of bacteria associated with intestinal blind loop syndrome and some tapeworms
- Chronic pancreatic disease, as occurs in some patients with cystic fibrosis
- Crohn's disease
- Ileal resection
- Radiation-induced ileitis
- Celiac disease or gluten-sensitive enteropathy
- Drug-induced malabsorption

Folate malabsorption may also occur. Folate is absorbed by the jejunum, and there are several causes of malabsorption, but a specific test for folate absorption has not been developed. The possibility and extent of deficiency, however, should be assessed in patients with celiac disease, or in those with a history of chronic use of certain drugs, including anticonvulsants and sulfasalazine. Ethanol, on the other hand, interferes with folate utilization.

LABORATORY MARKERS OF MALABSORPTION

The malabsorption syndrome refers to a condition in which several nutrients and other dietary compounds are not normally absorbed (see Chapter 31). In nearly all such disorders, fat fails to be absorbed normally. These disorders are also associated with decreased absorption of fat-soluble substances, including vitamins A, E, D, and K. Malabsorption results from such diverse causes as pancreatic exocrine insufficiency, gastric surgery, reduced bile salt secretion, a wide variety of conditions associated with abnormal intestinal mucosa, short-gut syndrome, infection, lymphatic obstruction, some cardiovascular diseases, certain drugs, and unexplained causes associated with diseases not commonly considered to affect the GI tract. Table 17–3 provides a list of common tests that can be useful in screening for malabsorption. Several of these tests lack sensitivity and are nonspecific, but if clinical symptoms are consistent with a diagnosis of malabsorption, and if several of these tests are positive, a microscopic stool fat test is warranted. If that test is positive, more sophisticated and disease-specific tests are in order. However, because all of these tests lack specificity, individuals with persistent symptoms may require additional, more specific tests, even though screening tests may be negative.

TABLE 17–3 SCREENING TESTS FOR MALABSORPTION SYNDROMES

TEST	REFERENCE RANGE	COMMENTS
Serum carotene	60–200 μg/dL	A good test if fruit and vegetable intakes are normal; constitutes a mixture of several fat-soluble substances, of which β-carotene is only a fraction
Prothrombin time	11–15 sec	Quite sensitive test, but not specific
Serum calcium	8.5–10.5 mg/dL	Not very sensitive or specific
Serum magnesium	1.6–2.6 mg/dL	Not very sensitive or specific
Serum albumin	3.5–5.0 mg/dL	Not sensitive or specific
Serum cholesterol	>150 mg/dL	Not sensitive or specific
Qualitative stool fat	No fat globules in microscopic field	Numerous stained globules are seen in various syndromes; serves as an inexpensive follow-up test in cases involving nonspecific indicators, but is not completely specific

LABORATORY DATA AND WELLNESS ASSESSMENT

Lipid Indices of Cardiovascular Risk

Early in the 1990s, more than 600,000 Americans died of cardiovascular disease (CVD) annually (see Chapter 26). About 75% of these deaths resulted from coronary heart disease. The underlying cause of the most prevalent forms of CVD is atherosclerosis, a process that usually begins in childhood or adolescence and slowly continues during maturity. The risk of CVD is related to both unmodifiable factors, such as heredity, gender, and age, and modifiable factors, such as life-style, exercise patterns, and diet (see Chapter 26 and Table 26–7). Through proper assessment and alteration of the modifiable factors, risk for CVD can be reduced. All of these intermediary risk factors are quantitatively determined using objective measurement methods, and diagnosis and treatment are related to cutoff values obtained from epidemiologic research relating risk to these quantitative indices. In addition to understanding how the modifiable factors—diet, exercise, and life-style (such as use of tobacco)—influence

TABLE 17–4 SERUM LIPID CUTOFF VALUES FOR ESTIMATING RISK OF CHD ACCORDING TO NATIONAL CHOLESTEROL EDUCATION PROGRAM (NCEP) GUIDELINES

SERUM INDEX	DESIRABLE	BORDERLINE RISK	HIGH RISK
Total cholesterol	<200 mg/dL (5.2 mmol/L)	200–239 mg/dL (5.2–6.2 mmol/L)	≥240 mg/dL (6.2 mmol/L)
LDL cholesterol	<130 mg/dL (≥3.4 mmol/L)	130–159 mg/dL (3.4–4.1 mmol/L)	≥160 mg/dL (≥4.1 mmol/L)
HDL cholesterol	>60 mg/dL (>1.6 mmol/L)	—	<35 mg/dL (<0.9 mmol/L)
Triglycerides*	<200 mg/dL (<2.3 mmol/L)	200–400 mg/dL (2.3–4.5 mmol/L)	>1000 mg/dL (>4.5 mg/dL)

LDL, low-density lipoprotein; *HDL*, high-density lipoprotein.
*Elevated triglycerides have not unequivocally been established as an independent risk factor for CHD.

CVD resulting from atherosclerosis, the skilled nutrition professional must be able to independently interpret how a patient's nutritional patterns and interventions affect lipid indices.

The National Cholesterol Education Program (NCEP) Adult Treatment Panel has established guidelines for serum levels of total cholesterol, low-density lipoprotein (LDL) cholesterol, and high-density lipoprotein (HDL) cholesterol that are associated with risk of coronary heart disease (CHD) or CVD (Table 17–4). In the presence of two or more CHD risk factors, the target value for LDL cholesterol decreases from less than 160 mg/dL to less than 130 mg/dL. When CHD is present, a target of less than 100 mg/dL is recommended (see Chapter 26 for risk factors that modify basic NCEP recommendations). The NCEP recommendations are based on the assumption that the laboratory responsible for the lipid measurements will produce precise (coefficients of variation, 3%) and unbiased (bias, 3%) results (Meyers et al., 1997). To be confident of the validity of their recommendations, health professionals must be confident that laboratories performing these analyses meets these requirements.

Patients undergoing lipid assessment should be fasting (a 12-hour fasting period is recommended) at the time of blood sampling. This is primarily because triglyceride levels rise and fall dramatically in the postprandial state, and LDL cholesterol values are calculated from measured total serum cholesterol and HDL cholesterol concentrations. This calculation, based on a formula called the *Friedewald equation,* is most accurate for triglyceride concentrations below 400 mg/dL. One should be aware that the Friedewald equation gives an estimate of fasting LDL cholesterol levels that is generally within 4 mg/dL when triglyceride concentrations are less than 400 mg/dL.

New methods for directly measuring serum LDL cholesterol levels are being developed. When the accuracy and precision, as well as the cost of these assays, become acceptable, laboratories may no longer use the Friedewald equation for LDL cholesterol measurement. However, triglyceride concentrations will still need to be assayed when a lipid profile is determined, so fasting will still be necessary.

Beside the standard serum lipid risk factors, recent research has linked other lipid and lipoprotein indices to CHD. All of these are measured in the laboratory, but most have either not been studied enough to demonstrate a clear link to CHD risk, or they are too costly to measure except in rare cases. Some of these new lipid-related risk factors are listed in Table 17–5. It is not yet known how nutrition and the other modifiable risk factors for CHD will affect these indices.

Beside CVD, dietary lipids are apparently linked to other chronic diseases, including cancer and diabetes. However, unlike CVD, the risk of these diseases is not known to be related to serum lipid indices. This suggests that there are multiple intermediary steps between the development of these diseases and lipid-rich dietary patterns.

Indices of Oxidative Stress

Current research indicates that many chronic diseases, including CVD and at least some forms of cancer, are initiated by free-radical oxidation of lipids, nucleic acids, or proteins. For example, the underlying mechanism for the development of atherosclerosis is now thought to be mediated by free-radical compounds called **reactive oxidation species (ROS).** These products include the superoxide radial (O_2^-), hydroxyl radical (OH), and hydrogen peroxide (H_2O_2). The formation of ROS is sometimes, but not always, mediated by certain essential trace elements (e.g., iron, copper, chromium, and nickel), and once formed, ROS react with unsaturated fatty acids in LDLs, creating lipid peroxides, another free-radical species. Like all free radicals, lipid peroxides initiate the oxidation of other compounds, including the proteins (apoproteins) present in lipoproteins. This leads to the formation of free-radical products throughout the large, heterogeneous lipoprotein particle (Fig. 17–2). Cells asso-

TABLE 17–5 "NEW" LIPID AND LIPOPROTEIN CORONARY HEART DISEASE RISK FACTORS

Small (more dense) low-density lipoprotein particles
Increased apoprotein B concentration
Decreased apoprotein A-1 concentration
Increased lipoprotein a (Lp(a)) concentration
Increased remnant lipoprotein cholesterol and triglyceride concentrations

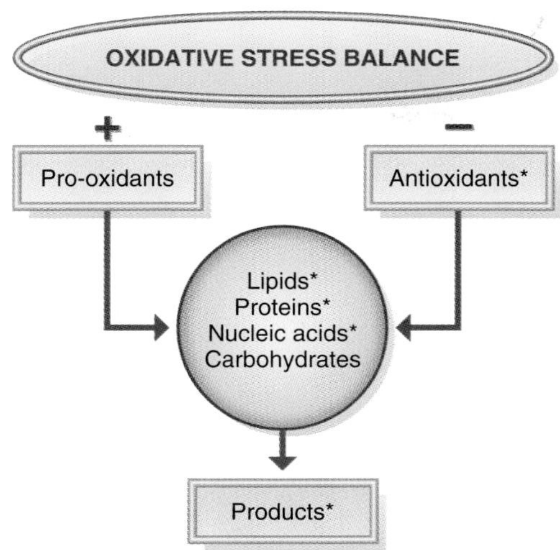

FIGURE 17–2 The balance between pro-oxidants (reactive oxygen species) and antioxidants used as markers of oxidative stress balance.
*Indicates compounds that are markers of oxidative stress.

ciated with the arterial wall ingest the resulting oxidized lipoproteins. Once present in these cells, further metabolism of this modified complex does not seem to occur. Over time, other pathophysiologic responses stabilize the deposited oxidized lipoprotein as atherosclerotic plaque (Anderson, 1977).

In addition to the oxidized compounds within lipoproteins, oxidized products of lipids, proteins, and carbohydrates are also present in body fluids. These compounds can be measured in the laboratory, and some of these tests are now being done in clinical laboratories. There is some evidence that nutritional supplements can decrease the level of some of these markers, and a few research studies have shown that diet alone affects these markers. Additional research is needed, however, to show if and how diet and nutrition affect current or yet-to-be-developed markers. Until additional research becomes available, these tests may not help the nutrition professional to counsel clients definitively as to how and to what degree these markers relate to their risk of chronic diseases, or as to the effect of nutritional intervention on risk. On the other hand, if these potential markers of oxidative stress are ignored completely, there is the risk that clients will not receive information that could help them decrease their risk of chronic disease. It may be better to use these imperfect tests in good faith than to do nothing at all. With their use, our understanding of the relationships between chronic disease and oxidative stress is likely to increase, allowing new and better tests to emerge.

Antioxidant Status

An indirect way of assessing the level of **oxidative stress** is to measure the levels of antioxidant compounds present in body fluids (Reaven and Witztum, 1996). This can be done because oxidative stress is related to levels of:

- antioxidant vitamins (tocopherols and ascorbic acid)
- minerals with antioxidant roles (e.g., selenium)
- dietary phytochemicals with antioxidant properties (e.g., carotenes and lycopene)
- endogenous antioxidant compounds and enzymes (e.g., superoxide dismutase and glutathione)

More precisely, the concentration of these compounds is correlated with the balance between their intake or production and their use during the inhibition of free-radical compounds (Halliwell, 1999).

Markers of Oxidative Stress

The most commonly used chemical markers of oxidative stress are presented in Table 17–6. Some tests measure the presence of one class of free-radical products. Others measure the global antioxidant capacity of plasma or a plasma fraction (Halliwell, 1999). These tests have been promoted on the assumption that knowledge of the individual concentrations of free-radical markers or antioxidants might be less useful than the total antioxidant potency of the medium concerned (e.g., plasma). This total antioxidant activity is determined by a test that assesses the combined antioxidant capacities of its constituents. Unfortunately, the results of these tests include the antioxidant capacities of compounds like uric acid and albumin, and so are not specific for the compounds of interest. This means that no one type of assay is likely to provide a global picture of the oxidative stress to which an individual is exposed.

Despite this lack of correlation or specificity of assays of oxidative stress, there are two assays that seem promising. The first of these is the immunoassay of oxidatively modified LDL particles (see Table 17–6). Because it measures a product that may directly participate in atherogenesis, this assay, which may be available in many clinical laboratories in the next few years, may allow a specific correlation of CVD risk with dietary and supplemental antioxidant consumption. The second assay is the measurement of the compound isoprostane $F_{2\alpha}$ (Patrono and Fitzgerald, 1997). This test is already available in some clinical nutrition laboratories. It measures the presence of a continuously formed free-radical compound that is produced by free-radical oxidation of specific polyunsaturated fatty acids (Basu, 1998). Isoprostane $F_{2\alpha}$ has a structure similar to that of the prostaglandins, and has already been shown to reflect the oxidative stress status of infants receiving therapeutic levels of oxygen (see Table 17–6).

Homocysteine

Many individuals who die of atherosclerotic disease do not have lipoprotein cholesterol and triglyceride concentrations that would place them in an at-risk

TABLE 17–6 MARKERS OF OXIDATIVE STRESS

	FUNCTION(S)	COMMENTS
Class I—Antioxidant Markers		
Vitamin C (plasma or leukocyte)	Specific inhibitor of water-soluble radicals	Measured by chromatography, capillary electrophoresis, or an automated enzymatic assay
α-Tocopherol	An inhibitor of lipid peroxidation	Measured by chromatography or capillary electrophoresis
γ-Tocopherol	An inhibitor of the nitrous oxide radical	Measured by chromatography or capillary electrophoresis
Carotenoids	Primary inhibitors of lipid peroxidation	Measured by chromatography; includes α- and β-carotene, lycopene, cryptoxanthin, zeaxanthin, and lutein
Class II—Endogenous Systems		
Glutathione assays	Detoxification of ROS and hydrogen peroxide (H_2O_2)	Plasma or erythrocyte glutathione or ratio of reduced to oxidized glutathione
Class III—Global Tests of Antioxidant Capacity		
LDL oxidative susceptibility	Reflects the concentration of antioxidants in LDL	In vitro determination of the rate of formation of LDL oxidation products—conjugated dienes
ORAC (oxygen radical absorbance capacity)	Measures decline in fluorescence over time and reflects the total antioxidant capacity of the specimen	
TRAP (total peroxyl radical trapping parameter)	Measures total antioxidant capacity; also reflects uric acid and albumin levels	
ABTS (2,2′-azino-bis3-ethyl benzythiazolinesulfonic acid)		ABTS assay, commercial kit available; also called total antioxidant status (TAS)
Class IV—Products of Free-Radical Reactions		
Modified LDL	May directly reflect risk of atherosclerosis	Immunoassay of oxidized LDL proteins; may become commercially available
Isoprostane	No known function	Primary form, isoprostane $F_{2\alpha}$, measured by chromatography or immunoassay Immunoassay is available commercially and results can be determined rapidly.
TBARS (Thiobarbituric acid–reactive substances)	Used to measure products of lipid peroxidation called aldehydes (malondialdehyde)	A colorimetric assay that is easy to perform, but not specific for oxidation products.

LDL, low-density lipoprotein; ROS, reactive oxidation species.

group. One possible explanation for this is that more than one mechanism may be involved in the development of atherosclerosis. Recent research strongly supports the hypothesis that an elevated plasma concentration of the sulfur-containing amino acid, homocysteine, is an independent risk factor for CVD (see page 390 and Chapter 26.)

Although homocysteine plays an important role in the synthesis of methionine, the bulk of the current evidence suggests that when cellular homocysteine leaks into the circulation, even in slightly elevated amounts, the risk of CHD, stroke, peripheral vascular disease, and venous thrombosis and pulmonary embolism increases significantly (Stein and McBride, 1998). In addition, there is preliminary evidence that hyperhomocysteinemia is a risk factor for the development of some forms of cancer. Just as the mechanism for the effect of plasma lipoproteins on the development of atherosclerosis was not initially clear, the mechanism of the effect of homocysteine in atherogenesis is not yet known. However, there is evidence that homocysteine damages the endothelial lining of vessels, contributing either to ongoing development of atherosclerotic plaque, or to the initiation of procoagulant reactions that trigger acute disease events (e.g., myocardial infarction, thrombotic stroke, or deep-venous thrombosis).

TABLE 17–7 CARDIOVASCULAR DISEASE RISK AND PLASMA HOMOCYSTEINE CONCENTRATION

RANGE TYPE	CONCENTRATION (μMOL/L)	COMMENTS
Usual reference ("normal") range	5–15	This range is consistently quoted in the literature, but is higher than the ranges established by recent studies.
Updated reference range	6–12	Reference range for healthy, well-nourished adults.
Moderate-risk range	12–30	The upper and lower limits of this range are not well established. Homocysteine concentrations increase with age and with onset of menopause.
High-risk range	>30	Usually associated with extreme nutrient deficiency or genetic defects in homocysteine metabolism
Target levels	<9	Below this level, risk appears to be minimal.
Optimal levels	<7	Associated with the lowest risk of coronary heart disease

TABLE 17–8 SUMMARY OF KNOWLEDGE ABOUT HOMOCYSTEINE AND CARDIOVASCULAR DISEASE (CVD)

Known Facts

- Homocysteine is an independent risk factor for the development of CVD.
- Most studies suggest that individuals with plasma homocysteine levels of about 15 μmol/L or higher have an increased risk for the development of CVD.
- A "normal" homocysteine level, much like a "normal" serum cholesterol level, may still be associated with increased CVD risk.
- Supplementation with folate, vitamin B_{12}, and vitamin B_6 reduces the level of homocysteine in nearly all individuals.

Persisting Questions

- What is the mechanism of the effect of homocysteine on atherosclerosis or CVD-related events?
- What are the appropriate serum homocysteine levels that result in a reduced risk of CVD?
- Does lowering serum homocysteine by vitamin supplementation decrease the risk of CVD?
- Can reasonable dietary changes decrease homocysteine concentration?
- Is homocysteine associated with the risk of any chronic diseases other than CVD?

Table 17–7 presents data relating to the association of risk of CVD with plasma homocysteine concentrations. Because the study of homocysteine is a new undertaking, these values must be considered to be rough guidelines. It is important to point out that even individuals with a plasma homocysteine that is within the population reference (normal) range may be at increased risk of CVD. In addition, almost all individuals can reduce their homocysteine levels by adding vitamin B supplements to their diet, and there is now some evidence suggesting that replacing fat intake with fruits and vegetables can also produce a significant decrease. (See Table 17–8 for a summary of related current knowledge.)

NUTRITIONAL INTERPRETATION OF ROUTINE MEDICAL LABORATORY DATA

From routine laboratory screening of patients with medical complaints or from routine laboratory monitoring of patients during medical treatment, a variety of data are generated that can be helpful in screening for nutritional deficiencies. Although the

TABLE 17–9 CONSTITUENTS OF COMMON SERUM CHEMISTRY PANELS

ANALYTES	REFERENCE RANGE*	SIGNIFICANCE
Serum Electrolytes		Of general use in monitoring many medical populations, such as those receiving TPN or those with renal disease, COPD, uncontrolled DM, certain endocrine disorders, ascitic and edematous conditions, or acidosis/alkalosis
Na^+	135–145 mEq/L†	
K^+	3.6–5.0 mEq/L†	Decreased K^+ levels are associated with diarrhea, vomiting, or nasogastric aspiration, in addition to use of certain drugs, licorice ingestion, and use of diuretics.
Cl^-	101–111 mEq/L†	K^+ levels are increased in renal disease, crush injury, infection, and hemolyzed blood specimens.
HCO_3^- (or total CO_2)	21–31 mEq/L†	
Glucose	70–110 mg/dL (fasting)	A fasting glucose value of >125 mg/dL is diagnostic for DM (thus obviating the need to perform oral glucose tolerance tests). A value of > 110 mg/dL is a marker of insulin resistance. Patients receiving TPN with triglycerides should be monitored for glucose intolerance.
Creatinine	0.8–1.4 mg/dL (males) 0.6–1.2 mg/dL (females)	Levels are increased in renal disease and decreased in protein-energy malnutrition (i.e., BUN:creatinine ratio >15:1).
BUN or urea	5–20 mg urea nitrogen/dL (1.8–7.0 mmol/L)	Values are increased in renal disease and excessive protein catabolism, but decreased in liver failure, negative nitrogen balance, and pregnancy.
Albumin	3.5–5.0 mg/dL	Levels are decreased in liver disease or acute inflammatory disease. Prognostic index
Serum Enzymes		Values are increased in a variety of malignant, muscle, bone, intestinal, and liver diseases and injuries. AST and ALT are useful in monitoring liver function in patients receiving TPN or certain medications.
Alkaline phosphatase	25–140 U/L	
AST (SGOT)	1–40 U/L	
ALT (SGPT)	0–45 U/L	
Bilirubin, total	0.1–1.0 mg/dL	Values are elevated by certain drugs and by gallstones and other biliary duct diseases, intravascular hemolysis, and hepatic immaturity; levels are decreased in some anemias.
Calcium, total	8.5–10.5 mg/dL	Hypercalcemia is associated with endocrine disorders, malignant disease, and hypervitaminosis D. Hypocalcemia occurs in vitamin D deficiency, inadequate hepatic or renal activation of vitamin D, hypoparathyroidism, magnesium deficiency, renal failure, and nephrotic syndrome.
Phosphorous (phosphate)	2.5–4.5 mg/dL	Hypophosphatemia occurs in hypoparathyroidism. Hyperphosphatemia is associated with hyperparathyroidism, chronic antacid ingestion, and renal failure.
Cholesterol, total	>150 mg/dL	Values decrease in protein-calorie malnutrition, liver disease, and hyperthyroidism.
Triglycerides	40–300 mg/dL (age- and sex-dependent)	Levels are increased in cases of glucose intolerance and combined hyperlipidemia, as well as in unfasted plasma specimens.

COPD, chronic obstructive pulmonary disease; *DM,* diabetes mellitus; *TPN,* total parenteral nutrition; *BUN,* blood urea nitrogen; *AST,* aspartate aminotransferase; *SGOT,* serum glutamic-oxaloacetic transaminase; *ALT,* alanine aminotransferase; *SGPT,* serum glutamic-pyruvic transaminase.

*Reference ranges may vary slightly from laboratory to laboratory.

†1 mEq/L = 1 mmol/L.

abundance of this kind of nonspecific data has decreased as the result of attempts to decrease the cost of medical diagnosis and treatment, much information is still available.

Clinical Chemistry Panels

Until recently, panels of medical tests were extremely common. In part, this is because the autoanalyzers that were initially developed for the determination of routine blood chemistry and hematology analytes could perform panels of tests on the same blood or serum sample for only a slightly higher cost than one or two tests. One of these panels—called the "Chem 7" or "Minipanel"—still exists. The components of this panel, now designated the "Basic Metabolic Panel" by the Health Care Financing Administration Common Procedure Coding System (HCPCS), are discussed in Table 17–9.

A panel that is often run in routine screening, now called the "Comprehensive Metabolic Panel" by the HCPCS, includes all the tests in the Basic Metabolic Panel except CO_2, plus all the remaining tests profiled in Table 17–9 except phosphorous, cholesterol, and triglycerides. These last three tests are often ordered along with the comprehensive metabolic panel, so they are included in the table. Well-informed nutritionists can use their understanding of the nutritional, as well as the basic medical, significance of these tests to support their nutrition assessment. The information provided in Table 17–9 is not exhaustive, so the interested reader is advised to consult textbooks that present more detailed information than can be provided here (see also Appendix 32).

TABLE 17–10 CONSTITUENTS OF THE HEMOGRAM (COMPLETE BLOOD COUNT [CBC] AND DIFFERENTIAL)

ANALYTES	REFERENCE RANGE*	SIGNIFICANCE
Red blood cell (RBC) count	4.3–5.9 × 10^6/mm^3 (men) 3.5–5.9 × 10^6/mm^3 (women)	In addition to nutrition deficits (see text), RBC values may be decreased in cases of hemorrhage, hemolysis, genetic aberrations, marrow failure, renal disease, or the use of some drugs. Not a sensitive test for iron, vitamin B_{12}, or folate deficiencies.
Hemoglobin concentration	14–17 g/dL (men) 12–15 g/dL (women) <11g/dL (pregnant women) 14–24 g/dL (neonates)	See RBC count
Hematocrit	39%–49% (men) 33%–43% (women) <33% (pregnant women) 44%–64% (neonates)	See RBC count
Mean cell volume (MCV)	80–95 fL 96–108 fL (neonates)	Decreased (microcytic) values are associated with iron deficiency, thalassemia trait, and chronic renal anemia or anemia of chronic disease. Increased (macrocytic) values occur in vitamin B_{12} or folate deficiency and in genetic defects in DNA synthesis. Neither microcytosis nor macrocytosis is sensitive to marginal nutrient deficiencies.
Mean cell hemoglobin (MCH)	27–31 pg 23–34 pg (neonates)	The causes of abnormal MCH values are essentially the same as those of MCV.
Mean cell hemoglobin concentration (MCHC)	32–36 g/dL 32–33 g/dL (neonates)	Decreased values are associated with iron deficiency and thalassemia trait. Not sensitive to marginal nutrient deficiencies.
White blood cell (WBC) count	5–10 × 103/mm^3 (>2 yr of age) 6–17 × 103/mm^3 (<2 yr of age) 9–30 × 103/mm^3 (neonates)	Values are increased (leukocytosis) in infection, neoplasia, and stress. Decreased values (leukopenia) are associated with protein-energy malnutrition, overwhelming infection, chemotherapy or radiation therapy, and autoimmune diseases.
Differential	55%–70% neutrophils 40%–60% lymphocytes 4%–8% monocytes 1%–4% eosinophils 0.5%–1% basophils	Neutrophilia is associated with ketoacidosis, trauma, stress, pus-forming infections, and leukemia. Neutropenia occurs in protein-energy malnutrition, aplastic anemia, chemotherapy, and overwhelming infection. Lymphocytosis arises in the presence of infection, leukemia, myeloma, and mononucleosis. Lymphocytopenia is associated with leukemia, chemotherapy, sepsis, and AIDS. Eosinophilia occurs in parasitic infestation, allergy, eczema, leukemia, or autoimmune disease, whereas eosinopenia is associated with increased steroid production.

AIDS, autoimmune deficiency syndrome.
*Reference ranges may vary slightly from laboratory to laboratory.

The Complete Blood Count

Another panel of tests that is commonly available for review by nutritionists is the CBC. The CBC is often accompanied by a differential count (often called a differential or diff), which enumerates each of the specific classes of leukocytes. Table 17–10 provides a list of the basic elements of the CBC and differential (collectively termed the hemogram), with reference ranges and some interpretative comments.

Urinalysis

A panel of tests that is routinely performed on urine is the urinalysis (UA). This test can be done in medical facilities that are not licensed to do more complex laboratory testing, so it is often part of a patient's medical record. Because it is so commonly available, it is advisable that the nutritionist become familiar with its components and be able to interpret them. UA data are qualitative or semiquantitative, and much of the data reflect the function of urinary tract status. However, some UA data has broader medical and nutritional significance. The full UA includes a record of (1) the urine's appearance, (2) the results of basic tests done with chemically impregnated reagent strips (often called dipsticks) that can be read visually or by an automated reader, and (3) the microscopic examination of urine sediment. Table 17–11 provides a list of the chemical tests performed in a UA, and their significance.

In summary, laboratory data can be used to assess specific nutrient deficiencies, as in determining the causes of nutritional anemia, or they may be primarily useful for screening and monitoring, as in assessing the risk of cardiovascular disease. In the case of protein-calorie status, tests are available that can be used in screening, assessment, and monitoring. Because laboratory data are currently increasing our knowledge of the mechanisms involved in the development of chronic disease, new laboratory tests are consistently being developed. For example, there are many new tests that have potential for use in the assessment of oxidative stress. Although the efficacy of these tests has not been proven, it is expected that eventually it will be. When to start using these tests in nutrition and dietetic practice is a subjective and, often, philosophical decision. Finally, a wealth of laboratory data may be suggestive of, but not specific for, nutritional deficiency. These data, which are ubiquitous in patients' medical records, can be used by informed practitioners to confirm and strengthen nutrition assessments.

TABLE 17–11 CHEMICAL TESTS INCLUDED IN A URINALYSIS

ANALYTE	EXPECTED VALUE	SIGNIFICANCE
Specific gravity	1.010–1.025 mg/mL	Can be used to monitor the concentrating and diluting abilities of the kidney. Values are low in diabetes insipidus, glomerulonephritis, and pyelonephritis, and high in the presence of vomiting, diarrhea, sweating, fever, adrenal insufficiency, hepatic diseases, and heart failure.
pH	6.0–8.0 (normal diet)	Acidic in the presence of a high-protein diet or acidosis (e.g., uncontrolled diabetes mellitus or starvation), during administration of some drugs, and in association with uric acid, cystine, and calcium oxalate kidney stones. Alkaline in individuals consuming diets rich in vegetables or dairy products, in urinary tract infection, immediately after meals, with administration of certain drugs, and with phosphate and calcium carbonate kidney stones.
Protein	2–8 mg/dL	Marked proteinuria in nephrotic syndrome, severe glomerulonephritis, and congestive heart failure; moderate proteinuria in most renal diseases, preeclampsia, and urinary tract inflammation; minimal proteinuria in some renal diseases and in disorders of the lower urinary tract
Glucose	Not detected (2–10 g/dL in individuals with diabetes mellitus)	Positive in individuals with diabetes mellitus; rare in benign conditions
Ketones	Negative	Positive in uncontrolled diabetes mellitus (more often in type 1); also positive in fever, anorexia, fasting, or starvation, some GI disturbances, persistent vomiting, and cachexia
Blood	Negative	Indicative of urinary tract infection, neoplasm, or trauma; also positive in cases of traumatic muscle injury and hemolytic anemia
Bilirubin	Not detected	Index of unconjugated bilirubin; increased levels associated with certain liver diseases (e.g., gallstones)
Urobilinogen	0.1–1.0 U/dL	Index of conjugated bilirubin; increased in hemolytic conditions; used to distinguish hepatic diseases
Nitrite	Negative	Index of bacteriuria
Leukocyte esterase	Negative	Indirect test for bacteriuria; detects leukocytes

CASE STUDY

Leanne K. is the 18-month-old daughter of immigrant parents. She has two older siblings (brothers) and has been enrolled in the Women, Infants and Children (WIC) program since the age of 6 months. During a recent visit to the WIC clinic, Leanne appeared pallid and listless, and she was found to have a hematocrit value of 34.0%. The clinic staff was evaluating the use of the hemato-fluorometer (zinc protoporphyrin:heme [ZPPH] ratio) in their clinic, and found that Leanne's ZPPH ratio was 135 μmol/mol. Her head circumference was 45 cm (compared to 44.5 at 12 months of age), she was 30 inches tall (compared to 28.5 inches at 12 months of age); and she weighed 21 lb (compared to 19 lb at the age of 12 months).

Her mother reports that Leanne has been increasingly less active in the last 3 months. She began to walk at 13 months, but now prefers to play in her bed or sit on the floor or sofa. During the last 2 months, Leanne has had at least three colds, and now has a nasal discharge, but no fever or other symptoms. Leanne's mother reports that her daughter usually consumes 5 to 6 6-oz bottles of cow's milk (whole milk) each day, and that she eats a small amount of solid food (primarily, polished rice).

A complete blood count (CBC) was ordered and the following results were obtained:

Hct = 33.5%
Hb = 11.0 g/dL
RBC = ⅜ million/mm^3
MCV = 80 fL
Platelet count = $195 \times 10^3/mm^3$
WBC = 16,000/mm^3
MCH = 27 pg
MCHC = 33g/dL
Reticulocytes = 0.8%

1. Comment on Leanne's growth and development. Is there a problem?
2. How would you interpret her CBC?
3. What does the ZPPH ratio indicate? Why was it fortunate that a ZPPH ratio just happened to be available to the clinic on the day that Leanne was evaluated?
4. Why was a serum ferritin level done?
5. What nutritional inadequacies would you consider, given Leanne's diet?

CITED REFERENCES

Ahluwalia N. Diagnostic utility of serum transferrin receptors measurement in assessing iron status. Nutr Rev 56:133, 1998.

Anderson TJ. Oxidative stress, endothelial function and coronary atherosclerosis. Cardiologia 42:701, 1997.

Basu S. Metabolism of 8-isoprostaglandin $F_{2\alpha}$. Fed Exp Biol Soc Lett 428:32, 1998.

Chang HR, Bistrian B. The role of cytokines in the catabolic consequences of infection and injury. J Parenter Enteral Nutr 22:156, 1998.

Halliwell B. Establishing the significance and optimal intake of dietary antioxidants: The biomarker concept. Nutr Rev 57:104, 1999.

Krantz SB. Pathogenesis and treatment of the anemia of chronic disease. Am J Med Sci 307:353, 1994.

Massey AC. Microcytic anemia, differential diagnosis and management of iron deficiency anemia. Med Clin North Am 76:549, 1992.

Mears E. Outcomes of continuous process involvement of a nutritional care program incorporating serum prealbumin measurements. Nutrition 12:479, 1996.

Meyers GL, et al. Standardization of lipid and lipoprotein measurements. In: Rifai N, Warnick GR, Sominiczak MH (eds.). Handbook of Lipoprotein Testing. Washington, DC: AACC Press, 1997, pp. 223–250.

Moldawer LL, Copeland EM III. Proinflammatory cytokines, nutritional support, and the cachexia syndrome: Interactions and therapeutic options. Cancer 79:1828, 1997.

Patrono C, Fitzgerald GA. Isoprostanes: Potential markers of oxidant stress in atherothrombotic disease. Arterioscler Thromb Vasc Biol 17:2309, 1997.

Ponka P, et al. Function and regulation of transferrin and ferritin. Semin Hematol 35:35, 1998.

Reaven PD, Witztum JL. Oxidized low density lipoproteins in atherogenesis: Role of dietary modification. Ann Rev Nutr 16:51, 1996.

Savage DG, et al. Sensitivity of serum methylmalonic acid and total homocysteine determinations for diagnosing cobalamin and folate deficiencies. Am J Med 96:239, 1994.

Stein JH, McBride PE. Hyperhomocysteinemia and atherosclerotic vascular disease: Pathology, screening and treatment. Arch Intern Med 158:1301, 1998.

Thompson D, et al. The value of acute phase protein measurements in clinical practice. Ann Clin Biochem 29:123, 1992.

Wong SS, et al. Detection of iron-deficiency anemia in hospitalized patients by zinc protoporphyrin. Clin Chim Acta 244:91, 1996.

Worwood M. The laboratory assessment of iron status—An update. Clin Chim Acta 259:3, 1997.

ADDITIONAL REFERENCES

Bernstein LH. Relationship of nutritional markers to length of hospital stay. Nutrition. Mar–Apr; 11 (2 Suppl):205, 1995.

Fernandez-Ortiz A, Fuster V. Evolution of atheroscleroitic plaque. In: Rifkind BM (ed.). Lowering Cholesterol in High-Risk Individuals and Populations. Marcel Dekker, New York, 1995, pp. 69–98.

Halliwell B, Gutteridge JMC. Free radicals in biology and medicine, 3rd ed. Oxford: Oxford University Press, 1999.

Hoffbrand V, Procan D. ABC of clinical haematology. Macrocytic anemias. Br Med J 314:430, 1997.

Jacobsen DW. Homocysteine and vitamins in cardiovascular disease. Clin Chem 44: 1833, 1998.

Lee RD, Nieman DC. Nutritional Assessment. Mosby-Year Book, St. Louis, 1996.

Siegel RM, LaGrone DH. The use of zinc protoporphyrin in screening young children for iron deficiency. Clin Pediatr 33:473, 1994.

Summary of the Second Report of the National Cholesterol Education Program (NCEP) Expert Panel on Detection, Evaluation, and Treatment of High Blood Cholesterol in Adults. JAMA 269:3015, 1993.

Veldee MS. Nutritional assessment, therapy, and monitoring. In: Burtis CA and Ashwood ER (eds.). Tietz Textbook of Clinical Chemistry, 3rd edition. W.B. Saunders, Philadelphia, 1998, pp. 1359–1394.

CHAPTER 18

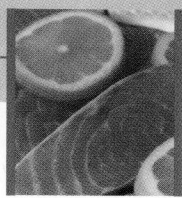

Interactions Between Drugs and Nutrients

VICTORIA HAKEN, MS, RD, CNSD

Chapter Outline

- Basic Pharmacology: Nutritional Aspects
- Phases of Drug Actions
- Risk Factors for Drug-Nutrient Interactions
- Effects of Drugs on Nutritional Status and Requirements
- Effect of Food and Nutrition on Drug Therapy
- Medication and Enteral Nutrition Incompatibility

Key Terms

AGONIST—a chemical substance capable of activating a receptor to induce a pharmacologic response

ANTAGONIST—a drug that counteracts the effects of another drug

ANTIVITAMIN—substances that inactivate a vitamin or inhibit its synthesis

BIOAVAILABILITY—the degree to which a drug or other substance becomes available to the target tissue

BIOTRANSFORMATION—hepatic metabolism of drugs by oxidation, reduction, hydrolysis, acetylation, and sulfuration reactions

DRUG-NUTRIENT INTERACTIONS—the results of the action between a drug and a nutrient that would not happen with the nutrient or the drug alone

LUMINAL EFFECTS—actions of drugs that take place in the lumen of the intestine

MIXED-FUNCTION OXIDASE SYSTEM (MFOS)—a multi-enzyme system in the liver responsible for the metabolism of a variety of foreign compounds and drugs

NARINGENIN—a flavonoid in grapefruit juice thought to be responsible for the inhibition of the oxidation of drugs that occurs with concomitant grapefruit juice ingestion

PHARMACODYNAMICS—the study of the physiologic and biochemical effects of a drug or a combination of drugs and the mechanisms of their actions

PHARMACOKINETICS—the action of a drug in the body, including absorption, distribution, metabolism, and elimination

TYRAMINE—a vasoactive amine found in decayed animal tissue, ripe cheese, and other foods

VASOACTIVE (PRESSOR) AMINES—organic compounds containing nitrogen that cause vasodilation and an increase in small vessel permeability

The management of many diseases requires long-term care and drug therapy, frequently involving the use of multiple drugs. **Drug-nutrient interactions** are a commonly overlooked aspect of the prescribing practices of physicians. Therapeutic effects or side effects of medications may ultimately diminish nutritional status; alternatively, the nutritional status of the patient may decrease a drug's efficacy or increase its toxicity.

Loss of therapeutic efficacy occurs when a food substance retards or impairs drug absorption, accelerates the rate of drug metabolism, or blocks the drug effect through some pharmacodynamic interaction. Acute toxic reactions, including food-drug incompatibilities and the effects of vitamin antagonism, have significant clinical outcomes. There are also long-term effects of drugs in relation to nutrition resulting in changes in appetite, taste, maldigestion and malabsorption, and mineral and vitamin depletion from urinary losses and the effects of drugs on nutrient catabolism. All of these mechanisms can lead to impaired nutrition status.

Situations that typically lead to serious drug-nutrition interactions occur when:

1. Drugs are taken with food.
2. Drugs are taken with nutrient supplements.
3. Drugs are taken with alcohol.
4. Drugs are used to achieve specific drug-nutrient interactions.
5. Drugs are taken in multiple-drug regimens in

which more than one drug produces an adverse effect because of drug and diet interactions.

6. Drugs that cause nutrient depletion are taken for long periods of time.

The Joint Commission on Accreditation of Healthcare Organizations (JCAHO) clearly defined the significance of drug-nutrient interactions in the publication, *1997 Comprehensive Accreditation Manual for Hospitals*. Included in the Education section is Standard PF.1.5: "Patients are educated about potential drug-food interactions and provided counseling on nutrition and modified diets." Thus, it is important for dietitians and nurses to monitor in-hospital drug therapy, as well as discharge medications, and to provide appropriate interventions. See www.fda.gov for the Food and Drug Administration website.

BASIC PHARMACOLOGY: NUTRITIONAL ASPECTS

A drug is defined as any chemical used to prevent or treat disease. To understand the interaction between diet and drugs, it is necessary to define the parameters involved in determining the effect of drugs and how they are influenced by diet. Drug action occurs in three stages: (1) the *pharmaceutical stage* (dissolution or disintegration of the drug); (2) the *pharmacokinetic stage* (absorption, distribution, metabolism, and elimination of the drug); and (3) the *pharmacodynamic stage* (the body's physiologic or psychologic response to a drug or combination of drugs). Because they are more difficult to study, food-drug pharmacodynamic interactions have been examined less extensively than pharmacokinetic interactions.

PHASES OF DRUG ACTIONS

Many factors influence the **pharmacokinetics** of a drug. Absorption of a drug can be altered by the dosage form, the solubility at the site of absorption, the degree of ionization, and the route of administration (oral, tube-fed, or intravenous). Drug distribution in the body usually delivers the highest concentrations to the heart, liver, kidney, and brain. The remainder of the drug is distributed to the muscle, skin, and fat tissues. Drug entry into the central nervous system is usually restricted. The **biotransformation** of drugs depends on enzyme systems, such as the **mixed-function oxidase system** (MFOS). (See Fig. 12–1.) The components of this system (cytochrome P-450, nicotinamide-adenine-dinucleotide-phosphate [NADPH]-cytochrome P-450 reductase, and phosphatidylcholine) use NADPH and oxygen to catalyze the oxidation of a variety of substances. The function of these enzyme systems depends on many nutrients and can be decreased by deficiencies in protein, essential amino acids, ascorbic acid, tocopherol, and retinol. Excretory organs, such as the kidney and lungs, eliminate drugs unchanged or as metabolites. Drug metabolites, formed in the liver, may also be excreted via bile or feces. Many factors affect drug excretion, such as the protein or fiber content of the diet and the urinary pH.

The **pharmacodynamics,** or mechanism of action of a drug can affect the rate of action or magnitude of any body function. A drug may exert **agonist** or **antagonist** activity, meaning it may enhance or interfere with normal metabolism and physiologic function. Usually, a drug exerts its action by combining with a specific receptor at the cellular level. Drugs do not usually produce only a single effect, but a wide variety of desirable or undesirable effects. The ultimate potency of the drug is determined by its absorption, distribution, biotransformation, excretion, and ability to combine with receptors.

RISK FACTORS FOR DRUG-NUTRIENT INTERACTIONS

Drug-induced malnutrition occurs most commonly during long-term treatment for chronic disease. The elderly are at a particularly high risk because of increased exposure to drugs for chronic health conditions, decreased efficiency of nutrient absorption, and an increased risk of consumption of marginal diets deficient in nutrients. Poor patient compliance and physicians' prescribing patterns further complicate the risk. The developing fetus, infant, and pregnant woman are also at high risk for drug-nutrient interactions, since their requirements for many nutrients are elevated.

Existing malnutrition also places people at risk for drug-nutrient interactions. Drugs are frequently administered to patients who are malnourished, including those with active neoplastic disease with significant anorexia and wasting. Moreover, drug disposition can be affected by alterations in the gastrointestinal tract, such as vomiting, diarrhea, hypochlorhydria, mucosal atrophy, and motility changes. Protein alterations and changes in body composition secondary to malnutrition may affect drug disposition by altering protein binding and the volume of distribution. The rate of drug oxidation is often normal or increased in mild to moderate malnutrition, but is usually impaired when edema or other signs of severe malnutrition are present. For highly protein-bound drugs that undergo renal excretion, the half-life may be shorter when hypoalbuminemia is severe because the drug is eliminated more rapidly owing to lack of protein-binding in the plasma.

Specific nutrient deficiencies can affect drug metabolism by influencing the MFOS. Iron deficiency increases the activity of the cytochrome P-450–dependent MFOS, whereas magnesium deficiency decreases it (Strobel et al., 1983). Selenium and chromium are involved in the mechanisms by which glutathione detoxifies foreign compounds (Relling, 1989). Zinc may also be important to the proper function of specific enzymes associated with drug biotransformation.

Body composition is an important consideration in determining drug response. Distribution of fat-soluble drugs is increased in the obese and the elderly, in whom the proportion of adipose tissue to lean body mass is increased. Excessive accumulation of a drug and its metabolites in adipose tissue may result in prolonged clearance and increased toxicity.

EFFECTS OF DRUGS ON NUTRITIONAL STATUS AND REQUIREMENTS

The status of almost every nutrient is potentially affected by drugs. Calcium, folate, pyridoxine, and vitamin A are particularly important because, in addition to being affected by drugs in common use, their intake is often marginal.

Drugs That Affect Dietary Intake

Decreased nutrient intake as either a primary or secondary effect of drug intake, can be desirable or undesirable (Table 18–1). Numerous drugs, such as *methylphenidate (Ritalin)*, which acts on the central nervous system, decrease appetite. These compounds are prescribed because of their calming effect in hyperactive children. Long-term use can result in growth retardation, followed by "catch-up growth" when the medication is discontinued (see Chapter 10).

Cancer patients have the highest prevalence of malnutrition of any group of hospitalized patients. The presence of the tumor alone may lead to reduced intake of different nutrients, and treatment modalities, such as chemotherapy and radiation, may further exacerbate nutritional disturbances (Henriksson et al., 1991). *Cisplatin* and other cytotoxic agents commonly cause nausea, vomiting, and reduced food intake. Cancer specialists, however, are experimenting with diet modifications, such as colorless, odorless meals (cottage cheese, applesauce, ice cream) to increase overall food intake and decrease nausea and vomiting (Menashran et al., 1992).

TABLE 18–1 EXAMPLES OF DRUGS THAT MAY CAUSE LOSS OF APPETITE

Sulfasalazine (Azulfidine)	Diabinese
Colchicine	Furosemide (Lasix)
Temazepam (Restoril)	Hydrochlorothiazide (HydroDIURIL)
Tylenol with Codeine	Hydralazine (Apresoline)
Tamoxifen	Fluphenazine (Prolixin)
Digitalis	Carbamazepine (Tegretol)
Amphogel	

TABLE 18–2 EXAMPLES OF MEDICATIONS THAT ALTER OR DIMINISH TASTE PERCEPTION

Acetyl sulfasalicylic acid	Griseofulvin
Allopurinol	Lidocaine
Amphetamines	Lithium carbonate
Amphotericin B	Meprobamate
Ampicillin	Methicillin sodium
Amylocaine	Methylthiouracil
Benzocaine	Metronidazole
Captopril	Nifedipine
Chlorpheniramine maleate	D-Penicillamine
Clofibrate	Phenindione
Diltiazem	Phenytoin
Dinitrophenol	Probucol
5-Fluorouracil	Sulfasalazine
Flurazepam (Dalmane)	Triazolam (Halcion)

In addition to causing anorexia, *penicillamine,* a metal chelating agent, leads to reduced levels of zinc and copper, which can cause hypogeusia and dysgeusia. Patients who are deficient or potentially deficient in these minerals should be given supplements.

The taste and smell of food also play a major role in maintaining adequate nutritional status. Drugs can cause an alteration in taste sensation (dysgeusia), reduced acuity of taste sensation (hypogeusia), or an unpleasant aftertaste, any of which may affect food intake (Table 18–2). The mechanisms by which drugs alter the chemical senses are not well understood. They may alter turnover of taste cells or interfere with transduction mechanisms inside taste cells. They may also alter neurotransmitters in the central nervous system that process chemosensory information (Schiffman, 1994). Common drugs that cause dysgeusia include the antimicrobials *amphotericin B* and *ampicillin,* the hypoglycemic agent *glipizide,* and the antiepileptic *phenytoin.*

Anorectic agents used to treat obesity have the desirable effect of reducing appetite. The two main categories of obesity drugs are centrally active adrenergic and serotoninergic agents. These drugs reduce appetite, enhance satiety, and increase energy expenditure. Amphetamines are adrenergic agents that stimulate secretion of norepinephrine from central nervous system (CNS) nerve terminals and reduce food intake. Because of their abuse potential, they are not routinely prescribed by responsible physicians (Atkinson, 1997).

Serotoninergic drugs, such as *fenfluramine* and *dexfenfluramine,* offer another approach. These drugs act by inhibiting the reuptake of serotonin, thereby increasing satiation and reducing food intake. However, these drugs are associated with adverse events of major concern, including changes in brain biochemistry (Atkinson et al., 1995) and primary pulmonary hypertension (Abenhaim et al., 1996). New findings suggest that approximately

30% of the patients taking these drugs also exhibit abnormal echocardiogram results, indicating heart valve problems. In 1997, the Food and Drug Administration (FDA) asked the manufacturers of fenfluramine and dexfenfluramine to voluntarily withdraw the drugs from the market. The FDA did not request the withdrawal of *phentermine*, another medication widely used for obesity.

Sibutramine and *orlistat* are two new drugs that are currently approved or under consideration for obesity treatment by the FDA. Sibutramine is a monoamine antidepressant that blocks reuptake of both norepinephrine and serotonin. Clinical trials show weight losses of about 10 kg (Bray et al., 1996). Adverse effects of this drug include increased heart rate and blood pressure. Orlistat reduces absorption of fat by binding to lipase in the intestine and by inhibiting its action (Drent and van der Veen, 1995). Consequently, fecal fat excretion is increased, a factor which contributes to the gastrointestinal complaints associated with the drug. Orlistat has an advantage over centrally active adrenergic and serotoninergic agents, however, because it acts peripherally and so is not expected to have any adverse effects on cardiovascular function. Currently, innovative approaches to influencing leptin and its receptors are in development. Obesity research is also focusing on biological substances thought to influence satiety, such as bombesin, cholecystokinin, and neuropeptide Y (see Chapters 1 and 23).

Increased caloric intake as a result of drug therapy can have the undesirable effect of promoting weight gain (Table 18–3). Some antidepressant drugs can induce weight gain amounting to 20 kg over several months of treatment. Monoamine oxidase inhibitors appear to cause less body weight change than tricyclic antidepressants (Pijl and Meinders, 1996). Anticonvulsants, such as valproic acid, cause weight gain in a considerable percentage of patients. It is also well documented that treatment with corticosteroids is associated with dose-dependent body weight gain in many patients.

TABLE 18–3 SOME COMMONLY USED DRUGS THAT INCREASE APPETITE

Anticonvulsants
Carbamazepine
Valproic acid
Antihistamines
Cyproheptadine hydrochloride (Periactin)
Psychotropic Drugs
Chlordiazepoxide hydrochloride (Librium)
Diazepam (Valium)
Chlorpromazine hydrochloride (Thorazine)
Meprobamate (Equanil)
Amitriptyline hydrochloride (Elavil)
Trifluoperazine
Corticosteroids
Cortisone
Prednisone

Propofal has recently been introduced as a sedative agent in acutely ill patients. Its formulation includes 10% soybean oil (lipid emulsion), so it contributes 1.1 kcal/mL. When infused at doses up to 9 mg/kg/hr in a patient weighing 70 kg, for instance, it may contribute an additional 1663 kcal/day solely as lipid emulsion. *Lorazepam, morphine,* and *pancuronium* may decrease energy expenditure but do not provide calories (Mirenda and Broyles, 1995).

Recently, pharmacologic options for the treatment of cachexia in patients with acquired immunodeficiency syndrome (AIDS) and cancer have gained popularity. Wasting syndrome contributes to both the morbidity and mortality of AIDS and cancer (see Chapter 39). Cachexia occurs before death in most patients with cancer, and is one of the most frequently occurring AIDS-related clinical conditions (see Chapter 40).

Therapeutic approaches for cancer-related cachexia have included anabolic steroids, corticosteroids, *cyproheptadine,* dronabinol, *hydrazine sulfate,* medroxyprogesterone acetate, megestrol acetate, and *pentoxifylline* (Herrington et al., 1997). The anabolic steroid *nandrolone decanoate* was tested in a sarcoma mouse model and shown to increase weight, yet 85% of the gain was attributed to water retention (Lyden et al., 1995). Both corticosteroids and cyproheptadine have undergone several controlled trials and have failed to produce significant weight gain. *Dronabinol* is currently FDA-approved for the treatment of chemotherapy-induced nausea, but placebo-controlled trials documenting its benefit in specific patient populations are lacking.

Medroxyprogesterone acetate, also called *megestrol acetate,* is a synthetic derivative of progesterone that is useful for the treatment of hormone-sensitive breast and endometrial carcinomas. It is associated with increased appetite and food intake, as well as weight gain. A randomized study comparing doses in patients with cancer showed that approximately 45% of the patients being treated with the drug experienced weight gain after 35 days (Gebbia et al., 1996). When the drug was tested in children with solid tumors, the authors noted that the weight gain experienced by study participants was primarily adipose tissue, rather than fat-free mass (Azcona et al., 1996). Controversy still persists as to which dose of medroxyprogesterone acetate is the safest and most efficacious.

Megestrol acetate also has been shown to promote weight gain in patients with AIDS. In a study of 100 patients with AIDS who had experienced a weight loss of 10% or more, the average daily caloric intake was increased by 608 kcal (Oster et al., 1994).

Treatment regimens that merely increase energy intake do not consistently restore body cell mass in patients with AIDS-related wasting syndrome. Because treatment with human growth hormone has induced nitrogen retention in catabolic patients following surgery and burns, it is now being used experimentally in patients with AIDS. Short-term growth hormone treatment increases both protein anabolism and protein-sparing lipid oxidation, effects that should increase body cell mass (Schambelan et al., 1996). However, controversy still persists as to whether quality of life can be improved.

Oxandrolone, an anabolic agent similar to testosterone, that is being used to promote weight gain after surgery, trauma, or in AIDS-related wasting. Studies show a significant increase in body weight with a dose of 15 mg/day (Berger et al., 1996).

Drugs That Affect Nutrient Absorption

Because most drugs and nutrients are absorbed in the small intestine and drug-nutrient interactions are common in this area. The specific effects reflect complicated interrelationships that depend on the drug dosage, type and amount of food, timing, and the presence of disease or malnutrition.

In general, drugs can cause malabsorption either by exerting an effect in the intestinal lumen, or by impairing the absorptive ability of the gastrointestinal mucosa. Many drugs cause malabsorption by more than one mechanism.

Luminal Effects

Drugs can reduce nutrient absorption by exerting **luminal effects.** Such effects include influencing the transit time of food and nutrients in the gut. Cathartic agents and laxatives reduce transit time and may cause steatorrhea, both of which lead to losses of calcium and potassium. Osmotic diarrhea may also decrease transit time and absorption. This may be induced by many drugs containing sorbitol, such as theophylline solutions used in critically ill patients (Hill et al., 1991).

A number of drugs affect bile acid activity, thus affecting the absorption of fat, fat-soluble vitamins, carotene, and cholesterol. *Cholestyramine,* used to reduce cholesterol absorption, and neomycin, used to reduce gut flora, both sequester bile acids and inhibit fat digestion and absorption. Fortunately, cholestyramine shows no effect on vitamin D, calcium, or phosphorus plasma levels, even after long-term administration (7 to 10 years) (Hoogwerf et al., 1992).

Chronic use of mineral oil as a laxative does not appear to interfere with absorption of the fat-soluble vitamins A and E, but does decrease levels of serum beta-carotene (Clark et al., 1987).

A drug may also prevent nutrient absorption by changing the gastrointestinal environment. *Cimetidine,* used for ulcer disease, inhibits gastric acid secretion and impairs absorption of vitamin B_{12} by reducing cleavage from its dietary sources. Cimetidine is a histamine H_2-receptor antagonist that also reduces intrinsic factor secretion; this can be a problem for vitamin B_{12} absorption after use over several years (Force and Nahata, 1992).

Antacids also change the gastrointestinal environment by changing the pH of the stomach and chelating with minerals to prevent their absorption. Raising gastric pH to a more alkaline state decreases the absorption of calcium, iron, magnesium, and zinc.

Some drugs are used to inhibit small intestinal enzymes, such as the antihyperglycemic agent *acarbose.* Such action leads to a delayed and reduced rise in postprandial blood glucose levels and plasma insulin responses (Coniff et al., 1995). The major adverse effect of alpha-glucosidase inhibitors, such as acarbose, is gastrointestinal intolerance secondary to both osmotic effect and bacterial fermentation of undigested carbohydrates in the distal bowel.

Mucosal Effects

The drugs with the greatest effect on nutrient absorption are those that damage the intestinal mucosa. Damage to the structure of the villi and microvilli inhibits the brush border enzymes and intestinal transport systems involved in nutrient absorption. The result is general or specific malabsorption of varying degrees. Chronic laxative abuse often has this effect, causing a mild steatorrhea. Within 6 hours of administration, *neomycin* causes histologic changes in the gut mucosa that lead to reversible malabsorption of fat, protein, sodium, potassium, and calcium. An example of drug-induced mucosal damage is that which may be caused by aspirin and other acidic drugs, which are capable of altering the gastrointestinal tract's ability to absorb minerals, especially iron and calcium. Damage to the gut mucosa also commonly results from chemotherapeutic agents and long-term antibiotic therapy.

Nonsteroidal anti-inflammatory drugs (NSAIDs) may adversely affect the colon by causing a nonspecific colitis or by exacerbating a preexisting colonic disease (Faucheron and Parc, 1996). Patients with NSAID-induced colitis present with bloody diarrhea, weight loss, and iron deficiency anemia. The pathogenesis of this colitis is still controversial. Local or systemic effects of NSAIDs on mucosal cells may lead to an increased intestinal permeability.

Drugs that affect intestinal transport mechanisms include (1) *colchicine,* an anti-inflammatory agent used to treat gout; (2) *para-aminosalicylic acid (PASA),* an antituberculosis drug; (3) *sulfasalazine,* an agent used for ulcerative colitis; and (4) *trimethoprim* and pyrimethamine, which are antibacterial and antiprotozoal agents. The first two impair absorption of vitamin B_{12}; the others are competitive inhibitors of folate transport mechanisms.

Drugs That Affect Nutrient Metabolism and Excretion

Antivitamins

Some drugs, termed **antivitamins,** inhibit synthesis of specific enzymes by competing for the vitamins or vitamin metabolites necessary to their structure. Cancer chemotherapeutic agents operate on this principle. Two common antivitamins are the folate antagonists *methotrexate (MTX),* used in treating leukemia and rheumatoid arthritis, and *pyrimethamine,* used in treating malaria and ocular toxoplasmosis. Folic acid is displaced from the enzyme dihydrofolate reductase by these drugs, and the unbound folic acid is then excreted. Without folic acid, DNA synthesis is inhibited, cell replication stops, and the cell dies.

Recent studies show that administration of daily folic acid supplements can lower toxicity without affecting efficacy in patients with rheumatoid arthritis who are receiving low-dose methotrexate therapy (Morgan et al., 1990).

A drug may also form a complex with a nutrient, making it unavailable for use by the body. *Isoniazid* (isonicotinic acid hydrazide, or INH) functions in this manner. This drug, used in the long-term treatment of tuberculosis, forms a complex with pyridoxine, interfering with its metabolism at several points and leading to vitamin B_6 deficiency in some patients. Some other drugs that function as vitamin B_6 antagonists are *hydralazine, penicillamine, L-dopa,* and *cycloserine.*

Other drugs that function as antivitamins are the *coumarin* anticoagulants, used as intentional vitamin K antagonists. Because they create a partial deficiency of the active form of the vitamin K, they reduce the risk of abnormal blood clotting. Many patients are advised to avoid vitamin K–containing foods, which greatly limits their vegetable intake. A more reasonable approach to patient management would be to estimate the vitamin K content of the patient's diet at the time of initiation of therapy and to caution the patient against allowing daily intake to fluctuate more than 250 μg. Then the amount of anticoagulant needed should be balanced with the vitamin K intake (Harris, 1995). This translates into avoiding kale and parsley and limiting spinach, broccoli, and brussel sprouts to a ½ cup per day. All other foods may be consumed according to the patient's usual pattern. The patient should also be advised to avoid high-dose supplements of vitamin A, D, and E, which may increase the risk for abnormal bleeding. Chronic, heavy ingestion of alcohol can also have effects on the liver that adversely affect coagulation.

Monoamine Oxidase Inhibitors

A well-known example of drug-food interaction involves monoamine oxidase inhibitors (MAOIs) and the pressor amines in foods. The two classes of biologically active amines are (1) the psychoactive amines (neurotransmitters), including norepinephrine and dopamine, and (2) the **vasoactive (pressor) amines,** which include **tyramine,** serotonin, and histamine. Biologically active amines are normally present in many foods, but they rarely constitute a hazard because they are deaminated very rapidly by monoamine and diamine oxidases. However, action of these oxidases is inhibited by antidepressant, antimicrobial, antihypertensive, and antineoplastic drugs (Table 18–4). Thus, the tolerance for vasoactive amines (principally, tyramine) in food is lowered. Presence of the unoxidized pressor amines causes constriction of blood vessels and elevation of blood pressure. Symptoms include tachycardia, chest pains, and severe occipital headache. In severe cases, the crisis can result in intracranial hemorrhage, cardiac arrhythmias, and cardiac failure. Avoidance of tyramine-containing foods is beneficial (Table 18–5).

A survey conducted among psychiatric patients showed the most frequently consumed high-risk food item was hard cheese (Sweet et al., 1995). Ninety percent of patients reported daily or weekly consumption of some foods containing cheese; yeast products, aged meat, broad beans, and sauerkraut were consumed only monthly by 50% of the patients. Individually targeted dietary assessment and education remain important components in the treatment of these patients.

Another class of antidepressants with considerable therapeutic effect consists of reversible inhibitors of monoamine oxidase (RIMA). *Moclobemide* is an example of an RIMA. It is free of hepatotoxicity and produces a much weaker potentiation of the tyramine pressor effect than the classic irreversible MAO inhibitor (DaPrada et al., 1990). The mean dose of oral tyramine required to increase systolic blood pressure by 30 mm Hg is 15 mg. The mean dose of tyramine that produced a clinical response in subjects treated with moclobemide was 240 mg (Simpson and Gratz, 1992). Although these

TABLE 18–4 DRUGS THAT INHIBIT THE ACTION OF MONOAMINE AND DIAMINE OXIDASES

Antidepressants
- Phenelzine sulfate (Nardil)
- Tranylcypromine sulfate
- Isocarboxazid (Marplan)
- Moclobemide (Aurorix)
- Selegiline (Deprenyl)
- Clorgiline
- Toloxatone

Antimicrobials
- Furazolidone (Furoxone)

Antineoplastics
- Procarbazine (Matulane)
- Isoniazid (INH)

TABLE 18–5 THE TYRAMINE-RESTRICTED DIET

FOODS THAT MUST BE AVOIDED	FOODS THAT MAY BE USED WITH CAUTION	FOODS WITH INSUFFICIENT EVIDENCE FOR RESTRICTION
Cheese	Avocado	Fresh fish
Smoked or pickled fish	Raspberries	Canned figs
Nonfresh meats, livers	Soy sauce	Mushrooms
Chianti and vermouth wines	Chocolate	Cucumber
Broad beans	Red and white wines, port wines	Sweet corn
Banana peels	Distilled spirits	Fresh pineapple
Meat extracts	Peanuts	Worcestershire sauce
Yeast extracts/ brewers' yeast	Yogurt and cream from unpasteurized milk	Salad dressings
Dry sausage		Yeast bread
Sauerkraut		Raisins
Beer and ale		Tomato juice
		Curry powder
		Beet root
		Junket
		Boiled egg
		Coca Cola
		Cookies (English biscuits)
		Cottage cheese
		Cream cheese

drugs are less likely to induce hypertensive reactions with the concomitant consumption of tyramine-rich foodstuffs, it still seems wise to advocate a degree of caution with regard to the dietary intake of food likely to contain high levels of tyramine (Livingston and Livingston, 1996).

Excretion of Nutrients

Drugs act to increase the excretion of a nutrient by displacing the vitamin from its binding site on a plasma protein. An unbound vitamin is filtered through the kidneys and excreted. *D-penicillamine* is used to treat heavy metal poisoning, Wilson's disease, cysteinuria, or rheumatoid arthritis by chelating with the intended metal. At the same time, it may also chelate with other metals (e.g., zinc) and increase their excretion in the urine. *Ethylenediaminetetra-acetic acid (EDTA),* administered intravenously to treat lead poisoning, may also lead to excessive urinary excretion of zinc.

Vitamin K may be depleted by administration of certain antibiotics, such as cephalosporins (cefotetan, cephalexin), causing prolonged prothrombin times. Intravenous vitamin K may be needed to correct the deficiency associated with this type of therapy.

Drug-Induced Electrolyte Alterations

Drugs can also increase the excretion of a nutrient by interfering with its reabsorption by the kidneys. Oral diuretics, such as *furosemide, ethacrynic acid,* and *triamterene,* can produce hypercalciuria by reducing calcium reabsorption; indeed, furosemide administration has actually been used as a temporary means of controlling symptoms of hypercalcemia. Because diuretics increase renal excretion of potassium, magnesium, and zinc, chronic use may result in the depletion of these minerals.

The addition of a thiazide to a loop diuretic regimen enhances the loss of sodium in the urine. Potassium-sparing diuretics augment the sodium loss in the urine induced by loop or thiazide diuretics, but limit or prevent urinary potassium or magnesium loss (Nicholls, 1990). Serum levels of electrolytes must be monitored closely during therapy, and often, potassium must still be supplemented.

Another well-recognized complication associated with the use of chemotherapeutic agents is the development of acute hypomagnesemia following *cisplatin* administration. Magnesium is mainly an intracellular cation. Its availability is not represented reliably by plasma levels; therefore, erythrocyte concentrations are used for assessment in research settings. An actual depletion is usually manifested after the third course of chemotherapy. Besides renal magnesium wasting, magnesium metabolism is influenced by cisplatin at the cellular level. Oral magnesium supplements taken between chemotherapeutic courses may be a means of preventing magnesium depletion without exposing the patient to hypermagnesemia, as may occur in cisplatin-induced acute renal failure (Sartori et al., 1993). Appendices 33 and 34 list other effects of drugs on nutrient status.

Drugs of Abuse

Drugs of abuse is a general term that includes legal compounds, such as coffee, tobacco, and alcohol, as well as illegal compounds, such as marijuana, cocaine, and crack. It also includes substances with recognized medical uses that are used for nonmedical purposes (e.g., barbiturates and amphetamines used for mind-altering effects or pleasure). Although the major effects of street drugs are not nutritional, their use can induce nutritional problems, either directly by reducing food intake during periods of altered state, or indirectly by depleting the financial resources needed for food (Table 18–6).

TABLE 18–6 EFFECTS OF SELECTED DRUGS OF ABUSE ON APPETITE

Amphetamines	Decreased appetite, delayed onset of hunger (although tolerance eventually develops); mechanism involves blocking of catecholamine uptake
Cocaine	Loss of appetite
Codeine	Loss of appetite with chronic use
Marijuana	Reported to enhance appetite, but not all studies agree; users appear to be more likely to lose appetite and weight
Methadone	Loss of appetite with chronic use

(Adapted from Enig MG. Pharmacologic basis of drug-nutrient interaction related to drug abuse during pregnancy. Clin Nutr 6:235, 1987.)

The Nutrition-Related Actions of Some Common Drugs

Anticonvulsants

Anticonvulsants, such as *phenytoin, phenobarbital,* and *primidone,* have been shown to induce biochemical or clinical deficiencies of folate, biotin, or vitamin D. In the latter case, the mechanism is thought to be interference with the hepatic conversion of cholecalciferol to 25-OHD_3. Clinical rickets and osteomalacia are uncommon complications of anticonvulsants, however, and usually result from factors present prior to anticonvulsant treatment, such as highly pigmented skin and inadequate exposure to sunlight.

Chronic phenytoin treatment has long been associated with folate deficiency, and megaloblastic anemia has been seen in a small percentage of patients who take anticonvulsants. It has been suggested that the pH changes in the gut associated with phenytoin ingestion may be responsible for decreased folate uptake, either by direct inhibition of folate transport into the intestinal mucosa, or by inhibition of folate conjugase activity.

Folic acid and phenytoin are structurally similar and may also compete with each other for the same surface receptors. Controversy exists as to the recommendation for folate supplementation, as competition on brain cell surface receptors may compromise seizure control. Supplementation with folic acid prevents deficiency, but also changes phenytoin pharmacokinetics. A recent study demonstrated an interdependence between the two (Berg, 1995). Phenytoin reduced serum folate levels whereas folic acid supplements improved phenytoin pharmacokinetics. Folate supplementation during initial phenytoin therapy may prevent possible teratogenicity, such as neural tube defects, and should be considered in women of childbearing age with epilepsy.

Dermatitis and ataxia—clinical manifestations of biotin deficiency—are also among the side effects of anticonvulsant therapy. Circulating concentrations of vitamin A, retinol-binding protein, copper, and ceruloplasmin are higher than average in patients taking anticonvulsants. The clinical significance of these changes is not known.

Oral Contraceptives

Low-estrogen oral contraceptives now in general use do not alter nutritional status as did the high-estrogen forms used in the past. Previously, it was thought that women taking oral contraceptives had significantly increased requirements for vitamin B_6, but this is generally not the case. Some women who take oral contraceptives have decreased serum and red blood cell folate levels, with increased excretion of formiminoglutamic acid (FIGLU), a urinary metabolite of folic acid. Supplementation, however, during oral contraceptive use cannot be justified for healthy young women (Mooij et al., 1992). In the case of women with poor dietary habits or increased folate requirements, or those anticipating getting pregnant, a multivitamin supplement that contains folic acid is recommended (see Appendix 51).

Women who take estrogen-containing oral contraceptives have elevated blood concentrations of vitamin A. In laboratory animals, estrogen-containing oral contraceptives stimulate hepatic synthesis of several nutrient-specific transport proteins, resulting in high circulating concentrations of the nutrients. These higher concentrations of circulating vitamin A could lead to depletion of vitamin A stores, particularly in women who are chronically malnourished. Serum iron levels in oral contraceptive users are also higher than in nonusers, whereas no difference is noted in other hematologic parameters (Mooij et al., 1992).

Anti-Inflammatory Drugs

Glucocorticoids are useful therapeutic agents for a wide variety of clinical disorders because of their anti-inflammatory, immunosuppressive, and cytotoxic properties. They may be prescribed for eczema, asthma, systemic lupus erythematosus, and rheumatoid arthritis. Unfortunately, they cause an array of undesired side effects that greatly limit their clinical utility. These include obesity, hyperglycemia, hypertension, impaired wound healing, and bone loss. The development of osteoporosis is critical, and occurs in at least 50% of persons who require long-term glucocorticoid therapy (Lukert and Raisz, 1990). Calcium absorption is reduced, and calcium excretion is increased within 8 to 10 days of starting drug therapy. Long-term administration leads to reduced bone mass in adults and growth retardation in children. The problem is compounded by the low calcium intake that is typical of many women, beginning at the age of 10 to 11 years (see Chapter 28).

Various vitamin D metabolites are currently under investigation to prevent glucocorticoid-induced osteopenia. The best results in experimental animals have been obtained by a combination of 1-alpha-(OH)-D_3 (which increases calcium absorption in the gut) and 24,25$(OH)_2D_3$ (which acts on bone to enhance bone formation and mineralization) (Turnquist et al., 1992). Reasonable recommendations for patients include the use of a glucocorticoid with a short half-life in the lowest dose possible, maintenance of physical activity, adequate calcium and vitamin D intake, and sodium restriction.

In one study, calcitriol and calcium were used prophylactically to prevent cortiocosteroid-induced osteoporosis (Sambrook et al., 1993). Bone loss leading to fractures is common with the use of these medications, especially at the spine, hip, and rib. With prophylactic calcitriol and calcium, with or without calcitonin, bone loss at the lumbar spine was significantly reduced. This addition of calcium therapy may be beneficial to patients who must continue a regimen of high-dose corticosteroids.

Antihypertensives

Patients with hypertension frequently take diuretics that can adversely affect mineral metabolism. Potassium deficiency is a risk in these patients, especially in those who also have low intakes of potassium and are regular laxative users. Calcium, magnesium, and zinc depletion may also be seen in patients receiving long-term diuretic therapy.

Fifty percent of patients taking *glucothiazide* diuretics experience hypokalemia, and all patients should be monitored for the condition. However, 50% of all those with hypokalemia are also hypomagnesemic. Because magnesium has an important role in keeping potassium within cells, it is impossible to replenish potassium in the presence of a magnesium deficiency. *Therefore, patients receiving these drugs should be treated with magnesium as well as with potassium.*

Prolonged use of sodium-free, tube-feeding formulas by elderly patients receiving diuretics can cause sodium depletion. Hyponatremia may be overlooked in the elderly, because the mental confusion that is symptomatic of sodium depletion may be thought to be caused by organic brain syndrome or senility.

Beta-adrenergic blocking drugs (beta-blockers) used to lower blood pressure may cause increased serum triglyceride levels and decreased concentrations of high-density lipoproteins (HDLs). Beta-blockers may also impair glucose tolerance and reduce the response of diabetic patients to oral hypoglycemic agents.

Medications Used in Human Immunodeficiency Virus (HIV) Infection

Since 1981, when the Centers for Disease Control (CDC) first described AIDS, many drugs have been employed to fight human immunodeficiency virus (HIV) and AIDS-related opportunistic infections. Nutritional debilitation is often a major component of AIDS and can have a major impact on a patient's clinical course (see Chapter 40). Some of the causes of protein-calorie malnutrition are increased metabolic needs, decreased food intake (secondary to anorexia, nausea, vomiting), and diarrhea, often accompanied by malabsorption. Many drugs used in the treatment of AIDS-related infections and cancers have side effects that actually exacerbate these problems and further deplete nutritional status.

Azidothymidine (zidovudine, Retrovir), which is used to inhibit HIV replication, commonly causes nausea, vomiting, and severe (non-nutritional) megaloblastic anemia secondary to reduced erythropoiesis. Clinical studies have shown recombinant human erythropoietin to be effective in correcting the anemia of zidovudine-treated patients by producing increased hematocrit levels, thus decreasing the need for blood transfusions (Phair et al., 1993). *Bactrim*, used to treat *Pneumocystis carinii* pneumonia, often produces nausea, vomiting, anorexia, and megaloblastic anemia related to folate deficiency. If megaloblastic anemia is present, supplementation with folic acid should be considered. *Pentamidine*, also used to treat *P. carinii* pneumonia, often produces hypocalcemia and hypomagnesemia with renal magnesium wasting (Shah et al., 1990). Serum levels of these nutrients should be monitored and supplementation offered as needed. Drugs used to treat toxoplasmosis, such as *pyrimethamine*, produce megaloblastic anemia by inhibiting dihydrofolate reductase. Researchers recommend administration of folic acid (5 to 20 mg/day) as soon as cytopenia is noted (Niyongabo et al., 1991). *Amphotericin B*, an antifungal medication used to treat cryptococcosis, histoplasmosis, and candidiasis, is very nephrotoxic and produces increased creatinine levels and hypokalemia in 60% to 80% of patients (Cruz et al., 1992). Serum levels of electrolytes should be monitored closely and supplements administered if necessary.

EFFECT OF FOOD AND NUTRITION ON DRUG THERAPY

Effect on Drug Absorption and Availability

The presence of food and nutrients in the lumen may reduce the therapeutic dosage of a drug by slowing and thus reducing absorption. As a result, the drug may never reach effective levels in the blood, or effects may be prolonged, with the slow absorption acting to sustain drug release.

The effect of food and fluid volume on the route and extent to which oral drugs are absorbed has only been under investigation for a short time. Absorption is probably the most common mechanism responsible for food-drug interactions because most drugs are taken by mouth. Depending on the type and degree of interaction, absorption of drugs can be decreased, delayed, increased, or unaffected by the physiologic changes that occur in the gastrointestinal tract when food is present. Drug absorption may be influenced by stomach and intestinal pH, motility, the presence of material in the lumen of the bowel, the absorptive capacity of the cells, and the rate of splanchnic blood flow.

The rate of gastric emptying is influenced by the presence and type of meal or food ingested. Gastric emptying may be retarded by the consumption of high fiber meals, meals containing fats, foods that have been heated, and high-viscosity solutions (Roe, 1986). Basic drugs are better absorbed when gastric emptying is delayed because they have a longer exposure to the acidic contents of the stomach. *Nitrofurantoin* and *hydralazine* are examples of such drugs. However, acid-labile drugs, with extended time in the stomach, are degraded and inactivated before reaching absorption sites in the small intestine. *L-dopa, penicillin G,* and *digoxin* are examples of drugs whose effectiveness is reduced by delayed gastric emptying.

Although active transport, pinocytosis, and lymphatic absorption are all possible drug absorption routes, most drugs are transported across the gastrointestinal epithelium into the bloodstream by passive diffusion. This process depends on gastrointestinal pH and the resultant ionizational status of the drug. Because pH is such an important factor, any situations resulting in changes in gastric acid pH, such as achlorhydria or hypochlorhydria, may reduce drug absorption. An example of such an interaction is the failure of ketoconazole to clear candidal infection in patients with HIV due to the high prevalence of achlorhydria in this population and the resultant impaired drug absorption (Welage et al., 1995). *Saquinavir* is a protease inhibitor used to treat HIV that has the opposite reaction. Indeed, maximum plasma concentrations increased twofold following the consumption of a heavy breakfast (Muirhead et al., 1992). The increased **bioavailability** of *saquinavir* following a meal has been attributed in part to the increased solubilization induced by increased gastric pH.

Certain nutrients can affect the absorption of drugs. Because calcium chelates *tetracycline*, thus preventing its absorption, tetracycline derivatives should be taken without milk, milk products, or calcium supplements. Milk can also affect absorption by raising stomach pH, causing enteric-coated tablets to dissolve in the stomach, with the potential for producing gastric irritation.

Other minerals in foods can form complexes with drugs, altering the gastrointestinal environment in such a way as to affect the normal absorption of drugs and minerals. Iron is one such mineral now under investigation. Concurrent ingestion of iron causes marked decreases in the bioavailability of a number of drugs, including *tetracycline, penicillamine, methyldopa, carbidopa, captopril, and thyroxine* (Sartori, 1993). The major mechanism of these drug interactions is the formation of iron-drug complexes. Table 18–7 lists the effects of food on the absorption and serum levels of some drugs.

Phenytoin has a high affinity for protein, so its absorption decreases in the presence of food proteins. In contrast, a high-fat intake increases absorption of *griseofulvin*, which is highly lipid-soluble, possibly by stimulating the secretion of bile.

Suspensions and solutions are much less affected by food and nutrients: This is because they do not depend on the rate of dissolution and can move from the stomach to the small intestine with relative ease.

Recently, the consequences of following a sodium-restricted diet while taking certain medications have received some attention (Bennett, 1997). These adverse effects are particularly common in elderly patients with impaired sodium conservation mechanisms. Dietary sodium restriction in animals enhances the chronic nephrotoxicity of the immunosuppressive agent *cyclosporine.* Sodium restriction can enhance the renal tubular absorption of certain drugs, such as the antipsychotic *lithium,* leading to toxic blood levels. Certain calcium antagonists may also have improved efficacy when prescribed to patients with a normal sodium intake and a blunted effect when patients are restricting sodium. So although sodium restriction potentiates the antihypertensive action of diuretics, beta-blockers, and angiotensin-converting enzyme (ACE) inhibitors, it may have the opposite effect in patients taking calcium antagonists, such as *nifedipine* and *verapamil.* It is the responsibility of the health care team to identify and evaluate the potential effects of sodium restriction on a patient's response to prescribed medications.

Some drugs demonstrate a significantly greater bioavailability when administered with grapefruit juice. The predominant mechanism for this enhanced bioavailability is the inhibition of oxidative drug metabolism in the small intestine (Ameer and Weintraub, 1997). The components of citrus juice that are responsible for this phenomena have not been fully identified. Based on the flavonoid **naringenin's** abundance in grapefruit and its ability to inhibit metabolic enzymes, it is likely to be a key component. Recently, quercetin (also found in strawberries) and other components that have been isolated from grapefruit juice have been found to inhibit human drug oxidation (Fukuda et al., 1997). The structures of these compounds have been identified as furocoumarin derivatives. To date, citrus juice interactions with *cyclosporine* have been studied more extensively than any other drug. A warning to avoid grapefruit juice when taking oral formulations of cyclosporine has already been issued to minimize toxicity. The other main drugs of concern include calcium channel blockers, such as *felodipine, nifedipine,* and *verapamil,* whose mean bioavailability increased 1.2-fold to 2.8-fold. The antihistamine *terfenadine,* the hormone *ethinyl estradiol*, the sedative *medazolam*, the antiviral agent *saquinavir,* and the immunosuppressant *cyclosporine* are also affected (Feldman, 1997). Given the variability in the degree of enhancement by grapefruit juice, it is difficult to predict significant clinical interactions at this point. Presently, there is no consensus that patients should avoid grapefruit juice while taking these medications.

Effect on Drug Metabolism

Drug metabolism may be altered in states of nutritional deficiency or nutritional manipulation because the activity of the hepatic MFOS is influenced by the specific quantities of protein, carbohydrate, and lipid. Research results suggest that manipulation of major dietary components could be of particular clinical significance in certain situations, such as protein increase in some weight-reduction programs, body building regimens, or postoperative therapy using only intravenous glucose. Deficiencies of nutrients (protein, tocopherol, retinol, essential fatty acids, zinc, copper, selenium, and potas-

TABLE 18–7 EFFECTS OF VARIOUS FOODS AND BEVERAGES ON DRUG ACTION

FOOD OR BEVERAGE	DRUG	EFFECT
Beverages		
Coffee, tea, and other caffeine-containing beverages	Theophylline	Increased intake may enhance drug side effects (nervousness, insomnia).
	Neuroleptic agents (fluphenazine, haloperidol)	Increased intake may result in wide variations in plasma concentrations of drug and may reduce its clinical effectiveness.
Citrus juices	Quinidine	Excessive intake may increase blood levels of drug (alkalinization of urine).
Fiber		
Bran	Digoxin	May reduce drug absorption
Pectin	Acetaminophen	May depress rate of drug absorption
Food (in general)	Chlorothiazide	May increase drug absorption
	Propranolol	May increase drug absorption
	Nitrofurantoin	Increases bioavailability of the drug
	Cimetidine	Delayed absorption may benefit patient by maintaining blood concentrations of drug between meals.
	Aspirin	May decrease drug absorption and absorptive rate
	Antimicrobial agents (celphalexin, penicillin G, erythromycin stearate, penicillin V, tetracycline)	May reduce drug absorption
High-fat meal	Griseofulvin	Increases drug absorption
High-protein diet	Levodopa, methyldopa	Amino acids from dietary protein inhibit absorption of drugs.
Licorice	Antihypertensive agents diuretics	The glycyrrhizic acid in natural licorice tends to induce hypokalemia and sodium retention; ingestion in large amounts may complicate antihypertensive drug therapy.
	Digoxin	Licorice-induced hypokalemia may enhance the action of digitalis and result in drug toxicity.
Milk and milk products	Tetracycline	Calcium inhibits drug absorption.
Protein or charcoal-broiled meats	Theophylline	High-protein or low-carbohydrate diet, or ingestion of charcoal-broiled meats, may decrease the plasma half-life of this drug.
Salty foods, sodium (salt)	Lithium	Increased intake of sodium may reduce therapeutic response to this drug. Low-salt diets may enhance drug activity.
Vegetables		
Boiled or fried onions	Warfarin	May increase fibrinolytic activity of drug
Broccoli, turnip greens, lettuce, cabbage	Warfarin	Vegetables rich in vitamin K may inhibit hypoprothrombinemic response to oral anticoagulants.

(Adapted from Nelson JK, et al. Mayo Clinic Diet Manual: A Handbook of Nutrition Practices, 7th ed. St. Louis: Mosby-YearBook, 1994.

sium) can make the drug metabolizing systems less effective, thus reducing the biotransformation of drugs. Increased biotransformation requires excess energy, thiamin, and iron; therefore, these nutrients may become depleted. Excessive intake of other vitamins can adversely affect drug actions. For example, increased pyridoxine intake during treatment with *levodopa* may increase its metabolism and decrease its therapeutic effect.

Albumin is the primary protein to which drugs are bound; however, it is the unbound form of the drug that can diffuse through the capillary wall and exert a pharmacologic effect. In certain conditions, such as malnutrition or liver disease, the serum albumin level is decreased, leading to increased serum levels of the drug and heightened pharmacologic action. Highly protein-bound drugs, such as *phenytoin* and *warfarin,* are most affected. Other situations that can affect the binding of a drug to serum albumin are high-fat meals and fasting, both of which lead to high serum levels of free fatty acids that compete with the drug for albumin-binding sites. The net effect is more free drug, greater pharmacologic effect, and potential toxicity.

There are other examples of drug absorption and metabolism being affected by the composition of a meal. Bioavailability of *propranolol* is enhanced when taken with a high-protein meal. High-protein diets can accelerate the metabolism of drugs by increasing the MFOS activity. The metabolism of *theophylline*, a bronchodilator used in the treatment of asthma, is also accelerated in the presence of a high-protein diet, but this can also have the negative effect of clearing the drug from the blood too rapidly (Anderson, 1982).

Recently, attention has been focused on *levodopa* therapy, used to treat Parkinson's disease. It significantly reduces disability and extends the life expectancies of patients with this disease. However, motor response fluctuations frequently appear in patients after long-term treatment with levodopa. Now, exciting results have been reported with concomitant use of a protein-restricted or protein-redistributed diet (Duarte et al., 1993). The diet typically entails a total protein restriction to 50 to 60 g/day, with most of the protein consumed at the dinner meal and very little consumed at breakfast and lunch (8 g/meal). Most patients have shown improvement in motor response, thus delaying the need to increase the doses of L-dopa. Additional large-scale studies are needed before the diet can be recommended to all patients on L-dopa therapy. A diet rich in insoluble fiber is also being investigated in relation to its positive effect on L-dopa concentration and motor function in Parkinson's disease (Astarloa et al., 1992). The mechanism behind fiber intake and higher bioavailability of L-dopa is not completely understood.

A number of compounds increase the activity of the MFOS, resulting in amplified metabolism of drugs. Polycyclic aromatic hydrocarbons in the environment and charcoal-broiled foods, as well as compounds in certain vegetables, such as Brussels sprouts and cabbage, induce MFOS activity in the liver and intestine and reduce the active time of drugs.

Other factors that influence the metabolism of drugs include the rate of intestinal absorption and delivery of the drug to the liver; the presence of other disease, including malnutrition; the status of liver function; and the concomitant administration of other drugs that either increase or decrease the metabolism of the first drug.

Effect on Drug Excretion

Food and nutrient intake can affect drug excretion by changing the urinary pH. Drugs that require an acid medium are excreted more rapidly in an alkaline urine (see Chapter 38 for foods that acidify urine). Mineral drugs, such as *lithium carbonate,* are affected by body levels of other minerals. Sodium depletion provokes increased reabsorption of both sodium and lithium carbonate and increased potential for lithium toxicity. Lithium excretion increases with sodium supplementation or increased fluid intake. Nutritional effects on renal excretion of drugs are most prominent in drugs with a narrow therapeutic range.

General dietary factors that affect drug excretion include the ability of a high-protein diet to promote increased renal excretion of *barbiturates, theophylline,* and *phenytoin* (Lamy, 1982). High fiber intake can increase the excretion of fat-soluble compounds. Foods that result in an acid urine cause increased clearance of alkaline drugs, such as *amphetamines.* Foods causing an alkaline urine increase excretion of acidic drugs, such as *phenobarbital.*

Alcohol Interactions

Alcohol is classified as a drug, but it is widely used as a beverage. Interactions of ethyl alcohol with various drugs are common. The consequences vary, depending on the pharmacologic effects of the drugs, the doses and the mode of administration of drugs, and the amount of alcohol consumed. Acute, substantial doses of alcohol consumed over a short period of time tend to inhibit drug metabolism, thus enhancing its effects. However, chronic consumption of alcohol may accelerate the metabolism of certain drugs because chronic alcohol ingestion induces the microsomal ethanol oxidizing system, which in turn, affects the drug-metabolozing systems in hepatic microsomes, leading to acceleration of drug metabolism. Alcoholics often exhibit a metabolic drug tolerance, thus reducing drug action (Mattila, 1990). An example of this paradoxical situation is with the drug *phenytoin*. Acute alcohol ingestion reduces clearance of phenytoin because both drugs compete for the same hepatic oxidase system; however, in chronic drinkers, the rate of phenytoin clearance is enhanced during periods of abstinence.

The action of several different classes of drugs have combined effects with alcohol (Lieber, 1994). Concurrent ingestion of ethanol and sedatives for example, leads to greater psychomotor impairment than ingestion of the drug alone. This effect is caused by a combination of CNS depressant action, impairment of degradation processes of the sedative, and drug metabolism that is altered by ethanol. An internet site for the Alcohol and Drug Clearinghouse is www.health.org.

Disulfiram (Antabuse) reactions occur when alcoholic beverages are consumed by persons taking this drug. Symptoms, such as flushing, headache, and nausea appear within 15 minutes of the time of alcohol ingestion. Because these symptoms are unpleasant, the drug is used as an aid in preventing alcoholics from returning to drinking. The signs and symptoms are attributable to an increase in acetaldehyde in the body. Other drugs that cause the acetaldehyde syndrome include *metroniadazole, griseofulvin,* and *procarbazine*.

MEDICATION AND ENTERAL NUTRITION INCOMPATIBILITY

Physical Incompatibility

Continuous enteral feeding is an effective method of providing nutrients to patients who are unable to eat adequately (see Chapter 22). However, the use of the feeding tube to administer medication can cause problems. When liquid medications are mixed with enteral feeding formulas, incompatibilities may occur. Types of physical incompatibility include granulation, gel formation, and separation. This frequently results in clogged feeding tubes and can interrupt delivery of nutrition to the patient. Examples of drugs that can cause granulation and gel formation are *Mellaril, Thorazine, Feosol, Dimetapp Elixir, Robitussin* expectorant, and *pseudoephedrine* (Sudafed Cough Syrup). Emulsion breakage also commonly occurs when acidic pharmaceutical syrups are added to enteral formulas. This reaction is more common in enteral formulas with intact protein and less common with hydrolyzed protein or free amino acids (Burns et al., 1988; Thomson and Rollins, 1991). Two drugs that produce this effect are *Kaopectate* and *Robitussin*.

Pharmaceutical Incompatibility

Pharmaceutical incompatibilities can occur as a result of either a change in the drug administered or a change in the feeding formula, resulting in altered potency or efficacy. Drug preparations with the potential for such alterations include enteric-coated tablets, sustained-release preparations, and sublingual medications that should not be crushed. To avoid pharmaceutical incompatibilities, use liquid dosage forms or select an alternative route of administration. Dosages may need to be changed if the drug action differs with drug form (e.g., solid versus liquid), especially for drugs such as *theophylline* or *phenytoin*. Feeding tubes should be flushed with 15 to 30 mL of water prior to medication administration (Miller and Miller, 1995). Irritating or viscous liquids should be diluted with 15 to 100 mL of water; tablets should be crushed to fine powder and mixed with 15 to 100 mL of water. Medications should not be combined, although they may be given separately if the tube is flushed with water between administrations.

Physiologic Incompatibility

Physiologic incompatibilities are defined as nonpharmacologic actions of a medication that alter tolerance to nutritional support. Administration of hypertonic medications is commonly associated with enteral feeding intolerance. Deposition of hyperosmolar solutions into the small bowel results in a tremendous flux of electrolytes and water into the intestinal lumen. When the absorptive capacity of the small bowel is overwhelmed, the result is osmotically triggered diarrhea (Dickerson and Melnick, 1988). The average osmolalities of commercial preparations available as liquid formulations range from 450 to 10,950 mOsm/kg. To prevent diarrhea, the medication should be diluted with water prior to administration, and the tube should be irrigated before and after delivery. The sorbitol in some medications can also produce diarrhea in tube-fed patients.

Recently, the osmolality of medications commonly used in neonatal intensive care units was studied (Jew, 1997). Most of the medications analyzed had an osmolality in excess of 2000 mOsm/kg. Most infant formulas had an osmolality within the American Academy of Pediatrics recommendations (400 mOsm/L). Final osmolality of infant feedings should

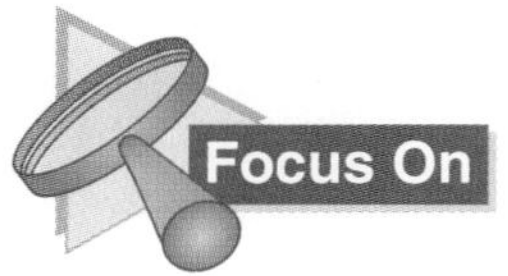

NUTRIENTS, DRUG INTERACTIONS, AND THE ELDERLY

Many factors contribute to nutrient-drug interactions, although all patients do not have the same degree of risk for nutrient-drug interactions. The elderly are at increased risk owing to pathophysiologic changes related to aging, endocrine dysfunction, and the common ingestion of restricted diets. As a result of the various illnesses associated with aging, the elderly commonly take many more drugs than do younger people. Older people also consume more over-the-counter drug products, such as laxatives and antacids. Drug-induced adverse outcomes can compromise the therapeutic outcome by affecting the nutritional status of the geriatric patient.

Care must be taken to monitor levels of vitamin A (in the oral diet, supplements, or tube feedings) when aluminum hydroxide, cholestyramine, mineral oil, or warfarin are being used. Phenytoin alters serum levels of folic acid, calcium, and vitamin B_6 over time. Alcohol, used in many syrups and elixirs, reduces absorption of magnesium, potassium, and zinc. Concurrent high protein intake with levodopa medications may reduce the drug's effectiveness.

All of these factors make treatment of the elderly, who often take several medications each day, challenging. The interdisciplinary team, which includes physician, pharmacist, nurse, and dietitian, must work together to plan and coordinate the medication regimen to ensure the highest possible level of nutrition without jeopardizing the patient treatment goals. Drugs whose usefulness is limited for the elderly should be reviewed and reduced when possible, even if just for a "drug holiday."

be measured or calculated when medications are added and when calories are concentrated in excess of 24 kcal/oz. The equation for calculating final osmolality of a mixture of drug and formula is as follows (Ernst et al., 1983):

$$\text{Osm} = \frac{\text{Od (Vd)} + \text{Of (Vf)}}{\text{Vd} + \text{Vf}}$$

where *Osm* is the osmolality of the drug and formula; *Od* is the osmolality of the drug; *Of* is the osmolality of the formula; *Vd* is the volume of the drug expressed in liters; and *Vf* is the volume of the formula expressed in liters (see Chapter 6).

Pharmacokinetic Incompatibility

Pharmacokinetic incompatibility occurs when the enteral formula alters the bioavailability, distribution, metabolism, or elimination of the medication. Alterations in dietary protein and lipid have been shown to affect both hepatic and intestinal drug metabolism in humans and animals. Therefore, investigators are now looking into the effect of varying the protein, fat, and carbohydrate content of enteral formulas. Findings suggest that the composition of feeding formulas may have a significant impact on hepatic function; specifically, the presence of lipid in such preparations may be important in maintaining normal levels of hepatic drug metabolism (Knodell, 1990).

Perhaps the most studied drug in terms of enteral feedings is the anticonvulsant *phenytoin*. Numerous reports describing its interaction with enteral feedings have been published since 1982. Because of phenytoin's narrow therapeutic range, these interactions present significant difficulties. A number of factors have been reported to affect phenytoin's absorption, including (1) dosage size, (2) antacid therapy, and (3) concurrent food or enteral feedings. However, the role of these factors is the subject of much controversy. In studies in which phenytoin has been administered to healthy volunteers, results have often shown no interference of enteral formulas with phenytoin absorption (Marvell and Bertino, 1991; O'Hagan et al., 1994). The possibility must be considered that other factors cause low serum concentrations, such as binding of the drug to nasogastric tubes, hypoalbuminemia, or uremia. Some studies indicate that the reaction is pH-dependent. There appears to be a physical entrapment of the large suspension particles when protein in the enteral solution denatures at a lower pH (Splinter et al., 1990). Also, irreversible loss of phenytoin has been observed at low pH levels as a result of the nasogastric tubing, leading to decreased phenytoin absorption (Fleischer et al., 1990). A prudent approach to administering phenytoin to patients who are receiving enteral feeding is to stop the enteral feeds 1 to 2 hours before and after administration of the drug, and to flush the tubing well with sterile water. Another alternative is to administer the drug intravenously.

Nutrition Counseling

Before patients are counseled about food-drug interactions, all medications should be reviewed for potential effects (see the accompanying box, "*Focus On:* Nutrients, Drug Interactions, and the Elderly"). A diet history in relation to medications should also be obtained, to ascertain the use of alcohol, vitamin and mineral supplements, and other supplements. The patient should be asked about altered taste, weight changes, appetite, nausea, diarrhea, and the presence of dry mouth as well. When determining the extent of drug-nutrient interactions, it is also important to consider the patient's age, drug dose, and duration of therapy on certain medications (Fig. 18–1).

Various strategies have been undertaken at health care facilities to meet the JCAHO's requirements for food-drug interaction counseling. A policy addressing this issue and a procedure describing the steps to be taken to conform to the policy should be on record. An example of a policy statement is: "Patients discharged on modified diets receive written instructions and individualized counseling before discharge, including drug-nutrient interaction counseling if appropriate." Educational materials on food-drug interactions should be developed at each facility by a collaborative team of pharmacists and dietitians for distribution to patients. Documentation in the medical record is also required when instruction has been given, including assessment of the patient's comprehension and ability to follow instructions.

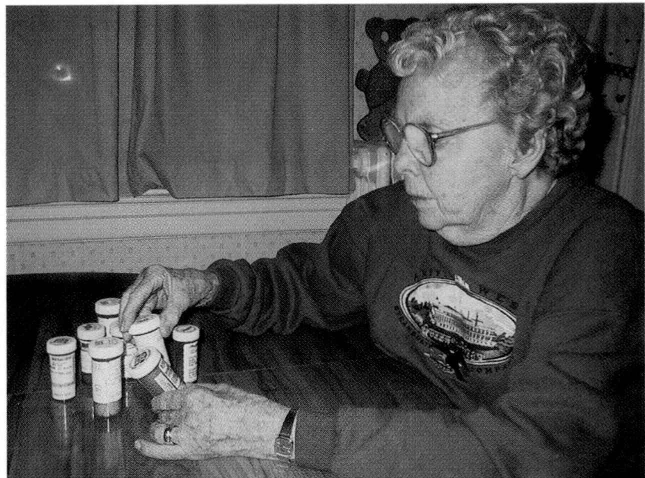

FIGURE 18–1 As a result of the increased potential for illness with aging, the elderly often take multiple drugs, both prescription and over-the-counter preparations. This places them at increased risk for drug-drug and drug-nutrient interactions.

CASE STUDY

Jennifer V. is a 24-year-old woman who was admitted to the hospital through the emergency room for evaluation of dehydration. Her medical history is significant for epilepsy and ulcerative colitis. The patient reports an increased incidence of diarrhea and abdominal pain for the past 6 months.

Data Obtained from the Medical Record

Lab values:	Elevated MCH, elevated MCV, depressed Hgb, serum Alb = 3.0 mg/dL
Medications:	Phenytoin and sulfasalazine started
Diet order:	Regular diet, low residue
Anthropometric data:	Height, 63 inches; current weight, 104 lb (down from 119 lb 6 months ago)
Physical examination:	Glossitis present; pale conjunctiva noted by MD

Data Obtained from the Patient Interview

A short-term diet recall reveals that Jennifer V. has been skipping breakfast and drinking coffee instead. Lunch usually consists of a cup of soup, and dinner is usually fast food. Lately, the patient has been unable to eat a full meal owing to stomach pains.

A food frequency questionnaire reveals that Jennifer consumes a diet that is relatively high in fat, with poor intake of fruits, vegetables, and milk. Caloric intake has been less than 1200 kcal/day, and daily protein intake has been approximately 20 g.

The patient reports that her doctor advised her to take a multivitamin, but she has not complied in the past year. However, she is now considering purchasing some vitamins because she and her husband are trying to start a family.

1. What type of anemia is characterized by an elevated MCH and MCV? Which nutrient and which medication may be involved?
2. How do Ms. V.'s dietary habits contribute to her anemia?
3. How would you evaluate the adequacy of Ms. V.'s vitamin D intake? What factors influence her requirements for vitamin D ?
4. How do low serum albumin levels affect drug disposition?
5. What are the implications of the physical findings?
6. What are the risks for Jennifer if she becomes pregnant?
7. What nutritional care would you recommend for the patient? Be sure to include educational needs.

MCH, mean corpuscular hemoglobin; *MCV,* mean corpuscular volume; *Hgb,* hemoglobin; *Alb,* albumin.

CITED REFERENCES

Abenhaim L, et al. Appetite suppressant drugs and the risk of primary pulmonary hypertension. N Engl J Med 335:609, 1996.

Ameer B, Weintraub RA. Drug interactions with grapefruit juice. Clin Pharmacokinet 33:103, 1997.

Anderson KE, et al. Nutritional influences on chemical biotransformation in humans. Nutr Rev 40:161, 1982.

Astarloa R, et al. Clinical and pharmacokinetic effects of a diet rich in insoluble fiber on Parkinson disease. Clin Neuropharmacol 15:375, 1992.

Atkinson RL. Use of drugs in the treatment of obesity. Annu Rev Nutr 17:383, 1997.

Atkinson RL, et al. Combined treatment of obesity. Obes Res 3(suppl4):497, 1995.

Azcona C, et al. Megestrol acetate therapy for anorexia and weight loss in children with malignant solid tumors. Aliment Pharmacol Ther 10:577, 1996.

Bennett WM. Drug interactions and consequences of sodium restriction. Am J Clin Nutr 65(suppl 2): 678s, 1997.

Berg MJ, et al. Folic acid improves phenytoin pharmacokinetics. J Am Diet Assoc 95:352, 1995.

Berger, et al. Oxandrolone in AIDS wasting/myopathy. J NeuroVirol 2:32, 1996.

Bray GA, et al. A double-blind randomized placebo-controlled trial of sibutramine. Obes Res 4:263, 1996.

Burns P, et al. Physical compatability of enteral formulas with various common medications. J Am Diet Assoc 88:1094, 1988.

Clark JH, et al. Serum beta-carotene, retinol, and alpha-tocopherol levels during mineral oil therapy for constipation. Am J Dis Child 141:1210, 1987.

Coniff RF, et al. Multi-center, placebo controlled trial comparing acarbose with placebo, tolbutamide, and tolbutamide-plus-acarbose in NIDDM. Am J Med 98:443, 1995.

Cruz JM, et al. Rapid infusion of amphotericin B: A pilot study. Am J Med 93:123, 1992.

DaPrada M, et al. Some basic aspects of reversible inhibitors of monoamine oxidase-A. Acta Psychiatr Scand (supplementum)360:7, 1990.

Dickerson RN, Melnick G. Osmolality of oral drug solutions and suspensions. Am J Hosp Pharm 45:832, 1988.

Drent ML, van der Veen EA. First clinical studies with orlistat. Obes Res 3:623, 1995.

Duarte J, et al. Efficiency of the protein redistribution diet in the antiparkinsonian effect of L-dopa. Neurologia 8:248, 1993.

Ernst JA, et al. Osmolality of substances used in the intensive care nursery. Pediatrics 72:347, 1983.

Faucheron JL, Parc R. Non-steroidal anti-inflammatory drug induced colitis. Int J Colorectal Dis 11:99, 1996.

Feldman EB. How grapefruit juice potentiates drug bioavailability. Nutr Rev 55:398, 1997.

Fleisher D, et al. Phenytoin interaction with enteral feedings administered through nasogastric tubes. J Parent Ent Nutr 14:513, 1990.

Force RW, Nahata MC. Effect of histamine H-2 receptor antagonists on vitamin B_{12} absorption. Ann Pharmacother 26:1283, 1992.

Fukuda K, et al. Specific CYP3A4 inhibitors in grapefruit juice: Furocoumarin dimers as components of drug interaction. Pharmacogenetics 7:391, 1997.

Gebbia V, et al. Prospective randomized trial of two dose levels of megestrol acetate in the management of anorexia-cachexia syndrome in patients with metastatic cancer. Br J Cancer 73:1576, 1996.

Harris J. Interaction of dietary factors with oral anticoagulants: Review and applications. J Am Diet Assoc 95:580, 1995.

Henriksson R, et al. Interaction between cytostatics and nutrients. Med Oncol Tumor Pharmacother 8:79, 1991.

Herrington AM, et al. Pharmacologic options for the treatment of cachexia. Nutr Clin Prac 12(3):101, 1997.

Hill DB, et al. Osmotic diarrhea induced by sugar-free theophyline solution in critically ill patients. J Parent Ent Nutr 15:332, 1991.

Hoogwerf B, Hibbard DM, Hunninghake DB. Effects of long-term cholestyramine administration on vitamin D and parathormone levels in middle-aged men with hypercholesterolemia. J Lab Clin Med 119:407, 1992.

Howard PA, Hannaman KN. Warfarin resistance linked to enteral nutrition products. J Am Diet Assoc 85:713, 1985.

Jew RK, et al. Osmolality of commonly used medications and formulas in the neonatal intensive care unit. Nutr Clin Prac 12(3):158, 1997.

Knodell RG. Effects of formula composition on hepatic and intestinal drug metabolism during enteral nutrition. J Parent Ent Nutr 14:34, 1990.

Lieber CS. Mechanisms of ethanol-drug interactions. Clin Toxicol 32:631, 1994.

Livingston MG, Livingston HM. Monoamine oxidase inhibitors. Drug Safety 14:219, 1996.

Lukert BP, Raisz LG. Glucocorticoid-induced osteoporosis: Pathogenesis and management. Ann Intern Med 112:353, 1990.

Lyden E, et al. Effects of nandrolone propionate on experimental tumors and cancer cachexia. Metabolism 44:445, 1995.

Marvel ME, Bertino JS. Comparative effects of an elemental and a complex enteral feeding formulation on the absorption of phenytoin suspension. J Parent Ent Nutr 15:316, 1991.

Mattila MJ. Alcohol and drug interactions. Ann Med 22:363, 1990.

Menashran L, et al. Improved food intake and reduced nausea and vomiting in patients given a restricted diet while receiving cisplatin chemotherapy. J Am Diet Assoc 92:58, 1992.

Miller D, Miller H. Giving meds through the tube. RN 85(1):44, 1995.

Mirenda J, Broyles G. Propofol as used for sedation in the ICU. Chest 108:539, 1995.

Mooij PN, et al. The effects of oral contraceptives and multivitamin sup-

plementation on serum ferritin and hematological parameters. Int J Clin Pharmacol Ther Toxicol 30:57, 1992.
Morgan SL, et al. The effect of folic acid supplementation on the toxicity of low-dose methotrexate in patients with rheumatoid arthritis. Arthritis Rheum 33:9, 1990.
Muirhead GJ, et al. Pharmacokinetics of the HIV-protease inhibitor, RO 318959, after single and multiple doses in healthy volunteers. Br J Pharmacol 34:170, 1992.
Nicholls MG. Interaction of diuretics and electrolytes in congestive heart failure. Am J Cardiol 65:17E, 1990.
Niyongabo T, et al. Usefulness of folinic acid in cytopenia induced by antiparasitic drugs in AIDS patients. Presse Med 20:1677, 1991.
O'Hagan M, et al. Enteral formula feeds interfere with phenytoin absorption. Brain Dev 16(2):165, 1994.
Oster MH, et al. Megestrol acetate in patients with AIDS and cachexia. Ann Intern Med 121:400, 1994.
Phair JP, et al. Recombinant human erythropoietin treatment: Investigational new drug protocol for the anemia of the acquired immunodeficiency syndrome. Arch Intern Med 153:2669, 1993.
Pijl H, Meinders AE. Bodyweight change as an adverse effect of drug treatment. Drug Experience 14:329, 1996.
Relling MV. Polymorphic drug metabolism. Clin Pharmacol 8:852, 1989.
Roe DA. Drug-food and drug-nutrient interactions. J Envir Pathol Toxicol Oncol 5:115, 1986.
Sambrook P, et al. Prevention of corticosteroid osteoporosis. N Engl J Med 328:1747, 1993.
Sartori S, et al. Changes in intracellular magnesium concentrations during cisplatin chemotherapy. Oncology 50:230, 1993.
Schambelan M, et al. Recombinant human growth hormone in patients with HIV-associated wasting. Ann Intern Med 125:873, 1996.
Schiffman S. Changes in taste and smell: Drug interactions and food preferences. Nutr Rev 52(suppl 8):S11, 1994.
Shah GM, et al. Symptomatic hypocalcemia and hypomagnesemia with renal magnesium wasting associated with pentamidine therapy in a patient with AIDS. Am J Med 89:380, 1990.
Simpson GM, Gratz SS. Comparison of the pressor effect of tyramine after treatment with phenelzine and moclobemide in healthy volunteers. Clin Pharmacol Therap 52:286, 1992.
Splinter MY, et al. Effect of pH on the equilibrium dialysis of phenytoin suspension with and without enteral feeding formula. J Parent Ent Nutr 14:275, 1990.
Strobel HN, et al. Cytochrome P-450 reductase interactions. Drug Metab Rev 20:519, 1983.
Sweet RA, et al. Monoamine oxidase inhibitor dietary restrictions: What are we asking patients to give up? J Clin Psychiatry 56:196, 1995.
Thomson C, Rollins C. Enteral feeding and medication incompatabilities. Support Line 13(3):9, 1991.
Turnquist J, et al. Effects of 1-alpha-(OH)-vitamin D_3 and 24,25$(OH)_2$-vitamin D_3 on long bones of glucocorticoid-treated rats. Acta Anatom 145:61, 1992.
Welage LS, et al. Alterations in gastric acidity in patients infected with HIV. Clin Infect Dis 21:1431, 1995.

ADDITIONAL REFERENCES

Campbell NR, Hasinoff B. Iron supplement: A common cause of drug interactions. Br J Clin Pharmacol 31:251, 1991.
Carl GF, Smith ML. Phenytoin-folate interactions: Differing effects of the sodium salt and the free acid of phenytoin. Epilepsia 33:372, 1992.
Cook MC, Tarren DL. Nutritional implications of medication use and misuse in elderly. J Fla Med Assoc 77:606, 1990.
Kuehl AK, et al. Recombinant erythropoietin for zidovudine-induced anemia in AIDS. Ann Pharmocother 29:778, 1995.
Marvel ME, Bertino JS. Comparative effects of an elemental and a complex enteral feeding formulation on the absorption of phenytoin suspension. J Parent Ent Nutr 15:316,1991.
McCabe BJ. Dietary tyramine and other pressor amines in MAOI regimens: A review. J Am Diet Assoc 86:1059, 1986.
Murray JS, Healy MD. Drug-mineral interactions: A new responsibility for the hospital dietitian. J Am Diet Assoc 91:66, 1991.
Nagai H, et al. Vitamin A, a useful biochemical modulator capable of preventing intestinal damage during methotrexate treatment. Pharmacol Toxicol 73:69, 1993.
Nielson H. Hypomagnesaemia asssociated with pentamidine therapy. AIDS 8:561, 1994.
Pathak A, et al. Amphotericin B use in a community hospital, with special emphasis on side effects. Clin Infect Dis 26:334, 1998.
Roe DA. Handbook on Drug and Nutrient Interactions: A Problem-Oriented Reference Guide. Chicago: American Dietetic Association, 1989.
Thomas JA. Drug-nutrient interactions. Nutr Rev 53:271, 1995.
Williams L, et al. The influence of food on the absorption and metabolism of drugs. Med Clin North Am 77:815, 1993.

CHAPTER 19

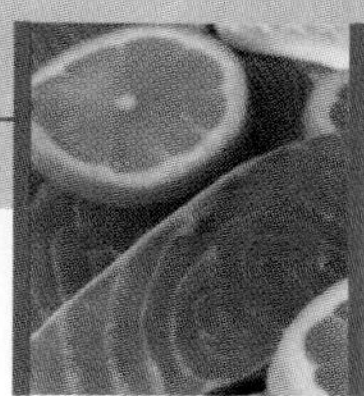

Integrative Medicine and Herbal Therapy

KIMBERLY MATHAI, MS, RD

Chapter Outline

- Complementary and Adjunctive Therapies
- Assessment
- Regulation
- Commonly Used Botanicals or Phytomedicines
- Consumer Advice

Key Terms

ACUPUNCTURE—use of thin needles inserted into points on the meridians to stimulate the body's vital energy

ALLICIN—a sulfur compound contained in garlic, which is responsible for garlic's odor; acts as an antibacterial agent

BOTANICALS—plants (including their leaves, flower, stems, or roots) that are used for medicinal purposes

CHI (QI)—a term in traditional Chinese medicine that means life force energy; the center of the body's functions

COMMISSION E MONOGRAPHS—therapeutic monographs on phytomedicines developed in Germany by an expert commission of health care professionals

DIETARY SUPPLEMENT HEALTH AND EDUCATION ACT OF 1994 (DSHEA)—a law that defines dietary supplements with provisions related to the marketing of these products

ECHINACEA—a botanical that may be used to strengthen the immune system and that has adjunctive application for reducing the duration and severity of symptoms of colds and influenza

FEVERFEW—a botanical that may relieve symptoms of migraine headache by a suggested action of relaxing smooth muscle and reducing platelet aggregation

GARLIC—a botanical that acts on the cardiovascular system and appears to lower serum lipid levels

GINGER—a botanical that has adjunctive therapeutic use as an antiemetic

GINKGO BILOBA EXTRACT—a botanical from an ancient tree used as an adjunctive treatment for cerebral insufficiency and dementia

GINSENG—a botanical that has a normalizing effect, affecting the whole organism in a positive way

HAWTHORN—a botanical that has a concentration of flavonoids, particularly oligomeric procyanidins, which affect the cardiovascular system

HOLISTIC THERAPIES—treatments that emphasize the healing force of nature and the body's ability to self-heal

HOMEOPATHY—a school of medicine based on the theory that substances in large doses that produce symptoms of a disease in healthy people, will cure the same symptoms when administered in very dilute amounts

MERIDIAN—a concept in traditional Chinese medicine relating to channels of energy

MILK THISTLE—a botanical that has silymarin as its principle active constituent and is known for its hepatoprotective characteristics

MOXIBUSTION—the application of heat along meridian acupuncture points to affect Qi and blood to balance the substances and organs

NATUROPATHY—a therapeutic system that uses natural methods of healing (i.e., light, heat, air, water, and massage); modalities of naturopathy include phytomedicines, nutrition, nutritional supplements, and natural forces

PHAMACOGNOSY—the science of natural drugs and their physical, botanical, and biochemical properties and applications

PHYTOTHERAPY—the science of using plant-based medicines to treat illness

SAW PALMETTO—a plant from which lipophilic extracts of berries are used as an adjunctive treatment for benign prostatic hyperplasia

SILYMARIN—a bioflavonoid compound that is the active constituent in milk thistle and is derived from the seeds of the dried flower; used as an adjunctive therapy for chronic inflammatory liver conditions and cirrhosis

ST. JOHN'S WORT—a botanical that is sometimes used as an antidepressant, with applications for mild to moderate depression

VALERIAN—a botanical that has adjunctive therapeutic application as a sleep aid and that acts on the central nervous system

COMPLEMENTARY AND ADJUNCTIVE THERAPIES

The use of complementary and adjunctive therapies to enhance conventional medical practices has been increasing in the United States since the 1960s. These therapies are now common in the United States, and increasingly, health care providers are including some forms of alternative and complementary therapies in their practices. Two national surveys conducted by physicians at Harvard Medical School in 1990 and 1997 found that significant numbers of Americans visit providers of complementary and alternative therapies. In 1997, more than 40% of Americans used some form of alternative or complementary therapy. In both survey years, more Americans visited complementary care providers than U.S. primary care physicians (Eisenberg et al., 1998).

Complementary and alternative therapies, which include naturopathy, homeopathy, acupuncture, and phytotherapy, are not new. In fact, their roots can be traced to early Greek and Chinese cultures. Although natural therapies are often described as being "cutting edge," they are actually much older than conventional Western interventions. Experts estimate that herbal remedies and ayurveda, the traditional medicine of India, are more than 5000 years old.

As a result of the increased interest in complementary and alternative therapies, the Office of Alternative Medicine of the National Institutes of Health was created in 1992 to evaluate these modalities. As of 1998, the Office had grown significantly from an original budget of $2 million to a budget of $50 million. It was given increased status when it was renamed the National Center for Complementary and Alternative Medicine (NCCAM). The mandate of this federally funded agency is to investigate and evaluate alternative therapies and their effectiveness. Although the NCCAM does not operate as a referral service, it does serve as a public information clearing house as well as a research training program. Table 19–1 provides an overview of the institution-affiliated centers of research on alternative medicine that exist throughout the United States.

Complementary and adjunctive therapies are considered to be holistic. **Holistic therapies,** derived from the Greek word *holos,* meaning a "whole," are based on the theory that health is a vital dynamic state, reflecting a profound will and wisdom to maintain wellness, rather than simply being the absence of disease. *Vis mediatrix naturae*, the healing force of nature, is the underlying precept of holistic medicine. According to this precept, all living things can self-heal; organisms have inherent self-defense mechanisms against illness. When they are properly stimulated, these mechanisms will heal. Naturopathy, homeopathy, traditional Chinese medicine, acupuncture, and phytotherapy are based on these concepts. See the Office of Alternative Medicine web site at www.nih.gov.

Naturopathy

The first precept of **naturopathy,** one of the disciplines of holistic medicine, is based on the concept of the healing force of nature, which emphasizes the prevention of disease and the maintenance of health. A second principle of naturopathy is derived from the Hippocratic precept, "First do no harm." Naturopathic doctors avoid therapies that weaken the body's innate ability to self-heal, or take over a function of the body. Instead, naturopathic practice emphasizes the concepts of wellness, prevention, and the role of the health care provider as a teacher.

As defined by the Department of Labor, naturopathic physicians diagnose and treat patients based on natural laws. Naturopaths are trained to diagnose and treat at the primary care level and may prescribe some drugs and do minor surgery. Their modalities include phytotherapy (treatment with plant-based medicines), electrotherapy, physiotherapy, minor orificial surgery, mechanotherapy, and naturopathic corrections and manipulation. Other treatments used by naturopathic doctors include nutrition, with an emphasis on whole foods and nutritional supplements used for the prevention of disease. Naturopathic doctors do not perform major surgery or use x-ray or radium modalities therapeutically.

Training for a degree in naturopathic medicine is conducted in 4-year, postgraduate institutions. Classes in medical sciences include pathology, microbiology, histology, physical and clinical diagnosis, and **pharmacognosy** (the science of natural drugs and their physical, botanical and chemical properties). Clinical training in botanical medicine, pharmacognosy, hydrotherapy, physiotherapy, therapeutic nutrition, and homeopathy are also included in the curriculum of naturopathic medical schools.

States with naturopathic licensure laws (doctor of naturopathy, N.D.) require a resident course of study in naturopathic medicine of at least 4 years duration, as well as 4100 hours study in a college or university recognized by the state examining board. Licensure examinations test students in the areas of basic sciences, diagnostic and therapeutic subjects, and clinical sciences. States that currently license naturopathic doctors include Alaska, Arizona, Connecticut, Hawaii, Maine, Montana, New Hampshire, Oregon, Utah, Vermont, and Washington.

Homeopathy

The root words of homeopathy are derived from the Greek *"homios,"* meaning like and *"pathos,"* meaning suffering. Homeopathy is a medical theory and practice that was advanced to counter the conven-

TABLE 19–1 INSTITUTION-AFFILIATED CENTERS OF RESEARCH ON ALTERNATIVE MEDICINE

INSTITUTION AND LOCATION	NAME OF CENTER	SPECIALTY OF CENTER
Bastyr University Bothell, WA	Bastyr University AIDS Research Center	HIV/AIDS
Columbia University New York, NY	Center for Complementary and Alternative Medicine Research in Women's Health	Women's health issues
Harvard Medical School, Beth Israel Hospital Deaconess Medical Center Boston, MA	Center for Alternative Medicine Research	General medical conditions
Kessler Institute for Rehabilitation West Orange, NJ	Center for Research in Complementary and Alternative Medicine for Stroke and Neurological Disorders	Stroke and neurologic conditions
Palmer Center for Chiropractic Research Davenport, IA	Consortial Center for Chiropractic Research	Chiropractic
Stanford University Palo Alto, CA	Complementary and Alternative Medicine Program at Stanford	Aging
University of Arizona Health Sciences Center Tucson, AZ	Program in Integrative Medicine	Pediatric conditions
University of California, Davis Davis, CA	Center for Alternative Medicine Research in Asthma and Immunology	Asthma, allergy, and immunology
University of Maryland School of Medicine Baltimore, MD	Center for Alternative Medicine Pain Research and Evaluation	Pain
University of Michigan Ann Arbor, MI	University of Michigan Complementary and Alternative Medicine Research Center for Cardiovascular Diseases	Cardiovascular diseases
University of Minnesota Medical School Minneapolis, MN	Center for Addiction and Alternative Medicine Research	Addiction
University of Texas Health Science Center Houston, TX	University of Texas Center for Alternative Medicine	Cancer
University of Virginia Charlottesville, VA	University of Virginia Center for the Study of Complementary and Alternative Therapies	Pain

HIV/AIDS, human immunodeficiency virus/acquired immunodeficiency syndrome.

tional medical practices of 200 years ago; it endeavors to help the body heal itself by treating like with like, commonly known as the law of similars. The law of similars is based on the theory that if a large amount of a substance causes symptoms in a healthy volunteer, a smaller amount of the same substance can be used to treat an ill patient.

Samual Hahnemann, an 18th century German physician, is credited with founding homeopathy. The law of similars is the concept that Hahnemann devised based on his own experience with quinine as a remedy for malaria. He observed that the remedy produced symptoms of the disease itself. Hahnemann called these tests, performed on himself and others, "provings."

The amounts of the remedies used in homeopathic medicines are extremely diluted. According to homeopathic principles, the remedies are potentiated; that is, they become more powerful through shaking. The healing power of the remedy is ascribed to the transfer of the remedy's vibrational pattern into a substrate of water, alcohol, or lactose. A tincture is made directly from the source material. One drop of the tincture is then mixed with 99 drops of water or alcohol to make the first potency. The mixture is vigorously shaken more than 100 times, a process called *succussion*. One drop of the succussion mixture is then combined with 99 drops of water or alcohol and the process is repeated; succussion makes the remedy more potent. Potentized remedies are used to make pills and creams; alternatively, they may be taken as a tincture. The minimum-dose principle means that many homeopathic remedies are so dilute that no actual molecules of the healing substance can be detected by chemical tests.

Homeopathic practitioners emphasize that assessment of all aspects of the physical, mental, and emotional life of a patient is essential for the prescription of appropriate remedies. The goal of homeopathy is to select a remedy that will bring about a sense of well-being on all levels—physical, mental, and emotional—and that will alleviate physical symptoms and restore the patient to a state of wellness and creative energy. Homeopathy is practiced by a wide range of health care providers, including medical doctors, naturopathic physicians, nurses, and dentists.

Clinical evidence on the efficacy of homeopathy is highly contradictory, yet for some conditions, it appears to be more efficacious than conventional medicine. A review of 107 controlled trials of homeopathy revealed 81 studies in which homeopathic treatments were superior to control therapies; however, authors of this review noted that definite conclusions on the effectiveness of homeopathy could not be made (Ernst and Kaptchuck, 1996).

Homeopathic treatment of acute childhood diarrhea with oral rehydration therapy (ORT) as an adjunctive treatment shortened the course of diarrhea in children in one clinical trial involving pediatric patients in Nicaragua (Jacobs et al., 1994). In another study, undertaken to determine whether homeopathy affected pain and inflammation following surgery, homeopathic remedies were found to have no positive effects. Measurement outcomes, such as postoperative pain and swelling, did not prove the efficacy of homeopathic remedies for relieving pain or inflammation. However, the physicians conducting the study did note the "remarkably" low pain scores after operations, and the patients' persistent strong confidence in homeopathy, regardless of outcome. The low pain scores and patient satisfaction with the homeopathic remedies were attributed in part to the clinical skill of the homeopaths involved (Lokken et al., 1995).

Many homeopathic remedies are considered to be relatively safe. Several reports to the Federal Drug Administration (FDA) on reports of illness caused by homeopathic remedies have been discounted (FDA Consumer, 1996). The homeopathic products involved were judged not to be the cause of the adverse reaction, as the homeopathic remedies contained little or no active ingredients. However, homeopathic remedies have been reported by health care providers to potentiate the effects of pharmaceutical drugs (De Schepper, 1998).

Traditional Chinese Medicine (TCM)

Traditional Chinese medicine is based on the concept that energy, also termed **Chi (Qi)** or life force energy, is the center of body functions. Chi is the intangible force that animates life and enlivens all activity. Wellness is a function of the balanced and harmonious flow of chi, whereas illness or disease results from disturbances in its flow. Wellness also requires preserving an equilibrium between the contrasting states of yin and yang (dual nature of all things). The underlying principle of traditional Chinese medicine is preventive in nature, and the body is viewed as a reflection of the natural world.

Four substances—blood, *jing* (essence, substance of all life), *shen* (spirit), and fluids (body fluids other than blood)—constitute the fundamentals of oriental medicine. The nutritional modality of Chinese medicine has several components: food as a means of obtaining nutrition, food as a tonic or medicine, and the abstention from food or fasting. Foods are classified according to taste (sour, bitter, sweet, spicy, and salty) and property (cool, cold, warm, hot, and plain) in order to regulate yin, yang, chi, and blood.

Within this framework of traditional Chinese medicine, the **meridians** are channels that carry Qi and blood throughout the body. These are not channels per se, but rather invisible vertical networks that act as energy circuits, unifying all parts of the body and connecting the inner and the outer body. In traditional Chinese medicine, organs are not viewed as anatomic concepts, but as energetic fields.

Acupuncture is the use of thin needles, inserted into points on the meridians, to stimulate the body's chi or vital energy. This therapy is used to treat disharmony in the body, which leads to disease. Disharmony, or loss of balance, is caused by a weakening of the ying force in the body, which preserves and nurtures life, and the yang force, which generates and activates life. Related to the concept of acupuncture is **moxibustion,** or the application of heat along meridian acupuncture points for the purpose of affecting Qi and blood so as to balance substances and organs.

Acupuncture has also been used to produce regional anesthesia. Its method of action appears to be through needle stimulation, which triggers the release of opioids (natural, morphine-like substances) into the body. In 1997, a National Institute of Health panel found that, although there have been many studies of the potential usefulness of acupuncture, many of these studies have yielded equivocal results because of design, sample size, or other factors. One problem in designing appropriate studies is related to the issue of controls (e.g., placebo or sham acupuncture). Areas in which acupuncture has been shown to be efficacious include adult postoperative management, chemotherapy-induced nausea and vomiting, and postoperative dental pain. The panel also found that acupuncture may be useful as a complementary or alternative therapy for the treatment of other conditions, including addiction, stroke rehabilitation, headache, menstrual cramps, tennis elbow, fibromyalgia, myofascial pain, osteoarthritis, low back pain, carpal tunnel syndrome, and asthma (NIH Consensus Conference, 1998).

The use of Chinese herbs is integral to the practice of Oriental medicine. The Chinese pharmacopeias, published as early as the third century B.C., contain herbs and minerals as well as animal products. Typically, a Chinese medicinal formula incorporates three to five different substances. Chinese herbs, in a formulation which includes ginseng, ginger, and other herbs, were given in conjunction with chemotherapy to patients with cirrhosis and liver cancer in a clinical trial. Patients who received the Chinese herbs in addition to chemotherapy had a higher survival rate than patients who received only chemotherapy (Oka et al., 1995). In another clinical trial, patients who were treated with a standard Chinese herbal medicine for irritable bowel syndrome (IBS) showed significant improvement in bowel symptom scores, and the degree of interference in life caused by IBS symptoms was significantly reduced (Bensoussan et al., 1998).

Phytotherapy

Phytotherapy (from *phyto,* the Greek word for plant) is the science of using plant-based medicines to treat illness. Plants—including their leaves, flowers, stems, and roots—when used medicinally, are technically called **botanicals,** but the terms herb and botanical are often used interchangeably. Herb technically refers only to a plant with a non-woody stem that dies back in the winter.

Phytomedicines are therapeutic agents derived from plants, parts of plants, or the preparations made from them. In Europe, phytomedicines have a significant history of research and clinical use. As mentioned, Chinese herbs are an integral part of Oriental medicine.

For many botanical medicines, the active ingredients and the mode of action have been defined; others are still being researched. The scientific basis for botanical medicine is investigated with the same scientific tools, such as double-blind, placebo-controlled clinical trials, as other drugs. Research information on phytotherapy as a modality of complementary medicine is burgeoning. Medline, the National Institute of Health's data base on health sciences topics, listed more than 30,000 peer-reviewed journal articles in the category of medicinal plants in the data base for 1990 to 1997. See www.herbalgram.org.

Popular interest in phytomedicines is widespread in the United States. One survey of patients presenting to an emergency room in an urban teaching hospital revealed that more than 20% of these patients use herbal preparations, with more women than men using herbs. Asians had significantly higher use of herbs than other ethnic groups, but 37.8% of these patients did not tell their physicians they used herbal medicines. The most commonly used preparations include garlic, ginseng, and peppermint tea (Hung et al., 1997). Patients typically do not inform their health care practitioners about the use of phytomedicines or other complementary therapies. Researchers who documented the enormous presence of complementary therapies in the U.S. noted that virtually all conventional medical health care professionals see patients who routinely use complementary or adjunctive therapies. Only 3 in 10 of these patients discuss complementary therapies with their doctors (Eisenberg et al., 1998).

ASSESSMENT

In 1997, an estimated 15 million adults were taking herbal remedies and prescription drugs concurrently (Eisenberg et al., 1998). An important assessment tool for health care providers is a directed history, with questions to determine the use of phytomedicines, herbs, or other complementary treatments, including naturopathic treatments, homeopathic remedies, Chinese herbs, or acupuncture. Health care providers should ask the following types of questions about the use of herbal products:

- What allergies, if any, do you have to plant materials?
- Are you currently pregnant or breast-feeding?
- What prescriptions or over-the-counter (OTC) drugs are you currently taking?

Intake and follow-up information on these therapies may provide relevant pharmacologic and treatment information for the health care provider.

REGULATION

Botanical medicines are regulated in the United States as dietary supplements. The **Dietary Supplement Health and Education Act of 1994 (DSHEA)** is a law that clarifies marketing regulations for herbal medicines and reclassifies them as dietary supplements, distinct from food or drugs. Under DSHEA, dietary supplements, which include plant extracts, enzymes, vitamins, minerals, and hormonal products that are available to consumers without prescription, may carry "structure/function" claims. That is, the physiologic effects of a product can be noted, but no claims about prevention or cure of specific conditions can be made. For example, a product manufacturer cannot claim that a dietary supplement "prevents heart disease;" however, it can be said that a product "helps to increase blood flow to the heart." Products must display the following disclaimer: "This statement has not been evaluated by the Food and Drug Administration. This product is not intended to diagnose, treat, cure, or prevent any disease." DSHEA does allow supplement manufacturers to use third-party literature in connection with sales, as this literature can help customers become better informed about the product without promoting a specific company or brand of supplement. This law does not require (1) premarket testing of the safety or efficacy of a dietary supplement or (2) standardization codes for manufacture.

Selected botanicals are approved as OTC medications; these can carry more specific therapeutic claims and can also be sold as dietary supplements. Table 19–2 lists botanicals currently in this category.

Currently, there are no government regulatory standards for proper identification of or appropriate

TABLE 19–2 BOTANICALS APPROVED AS OVER-THE-COUNTER DRUG INGREDIENTS

HERB	APPROVED USE
Aloe (*Aloe ferox*)	Stimulant laxative
Cascara sagrada (*Rhanmus purshiana*)	Stimulant laxative
Peppermint oil (*Menthax piperita*)	Antitussive
Psyllium (*Plantago afra*)	Bulk laxative
Red pepper (*Capsicum* spp.)	Counterirritant
Senna (Alexandrian) (*Cassia senna*)	Stimulant laxative
Slippery elm (*Ulmus fulva*)	Demulcent*
Witch hazel (*Hamamelis virginiana*)	Astringent

(From Food and Drug Administration. OTC Drug Review Ingredient Status Report. Rockville, MD: Food and Drug Administration, September, 1994.)

*An agent that soothes irritated tissue, especially mucous membranes.

quality for herbal medicines in the United States. In the late 1800s, the United States Pharmacopeia (USP) and the National Formulary (NF) established legal standards of identity and quality of herbal medicines, but these standards are not now recognized. Herbal monographs, with information covering use, dosage, side effects, and contraindications, are being developed by the USP, but they do not have the force of law.

The regulation of herbal medicines in Europe is distinctly different. In Germany, an Expert Commission for Phytopharmaceuticals at the Federal Health Agency in Germany was established in 1978. Phytomedicines were reviewed by this expert commission of professionals, drawn from a variety of health care disciplines. This group, known as the Commission E, developed 330 therapeutic monographs on phytomedicines until it was disbanded in 1993, with 77 of the monographs supporting therapeutic recommendations. These **Commission E monographs** include information on the pharmacologic properties and toxicology of herbal drugs, and outline their uses, contraindications, side effects, dosages, and administration, in addition to noting any special warnings for use (Blumenthal et al., 1998). Phytomedicines in the European market, especially in Germany, are considered to be drugs, and are prescribed by physicians and dispensed by pharmacists.

The lack of regulation in herbal medicines may lead to problems, such as misrepresentation of the potency of products, inadequate information about how a company's herbs are grown and processed, or poor standards of quality, product safety, or active ingredients (Edzard, 1998). Although rare, herb contamination and misidentification do occur (Slifman et al., 1998). Because herbs are not regulated in the United States at this time, and because no standards for manufacture have been established by any government agency, formulations may vary in potency and recommended dosages. Selected guidelines and resources for evaluating herbal products are listed in Table 19–3.

Phytomedicines are available in a number of forms, for example, as bulk herbs, extracts, tinctures, and capsules or tablets with powdered or freeze-dried herbs or extracts. Table 19–4 describes the modes of delivery of phytomedicines. Herbal medicines should be taken exactly as identified on the package label. The adage "If a little is good, more is better" does not apply to these medicines or any others. Moreover, since botanicals are not regulated, every effort should be made to obtain the highest quality product available. Table 19–5 pre-

TABLE 19–3 HERBAL PRODUCTS: GUIDELINES AND INFORMATION RESOURCES

Guidelines

- Investigate various companies that sell the product.
- Contact companies for information on how the herbs are grown and processed.
- Choose organically grown herbs when possible.
- Check product for batch control number, safety seal, and expiration date.

Resources (Organizations)

- American Botanical Council, PO Box 1444345, Austin, TX 78714-4345; (512) 926-4900. Web site: www.herbalgram.org. Nonprofit organization; produces the quarterly journal *Herbalgram*, herb information packets, and mail-order books.
- Herb Research Foundation, 1007 Pearl Street, Suite 200, Boulder, CO 80302 (303) 449-2265. Web site: www.herbs.org. Nonprofit organization; offers monographs on individual herbs.
- United States Pharmacopeia, 12601 Twinbrook Parkway, Rockville, MD 20852 (301) 816-8223. Web site: www.usp.org. Offers selected herbal monographs available free of charge.

TABLE 19–4 TYPES OF HERBAL FORMULATIONS

TYPE	FORM
Bulk herbs	Sold loose to be used as teas; rapidly lose potency; should be stored in opaque containers, away from light
Extracts	Made by pressing herbs with a heavy hydraulic press and soaking in alcohol or water; excess alcohol or water is then allowed to evaporate to yield a concentrated extract.
Tinctures	Liquid extracts of plants, often in an alcohol base; taken by dropperful in a small amount of juice or water
Capsules/ Tablets	Contain freeze-dried or powdered herbs or extracts; may be the preferred form for herbs with an unpleasant taste Freeze-drying preserves potency better than powdering. Both forms may contain binders and fillers.
Teas	Water-based extraction brewed using 1 oz (25 g) of dried herb or 2 oz (50 g) of fresh herb and 500 mL of boiling water Boiling water is poured over the herb and allowed to brew (1 to 3 minutes for flowers; 2 to 4 minutes for leaves; 4 to 10 minutes for bark, roots, or hard seeds)
Decoctions	Water-based extraction brewed from seeds, bark, and roots using the same quantities as for tea (above) The mixture of water and herb is brought to a boil, then simmered for 20 to 30 minutes, after which the mixture is strained and water is added to a volume of 500 mL.

TABLE 19–5 POTENTIAL PROBLEMS OF SOME HERBAL EXTRACTS

HERB	ACTIVE/TOXIC INGREDIENT	POTENTIAL ADVERSE/TOXIC EFFECTS
Arnica*	Extracts contain choline plus two unidentified substances.	Arnica, an active irritant can produce violent gastroenteritis, CNS disturbances, change in pulse rate, intense muscular weakness, collapse and death.
Belladona* (Deadly nightshade)	Extracts contain the toxic salnaceous alkaloids, hyoscyamine, atropine and hyoscine.	Typical atropine-like poisoning, dilated pupils, blurred vision, increased heart rate, urinary retention, fever, convulsions and coma.
Camomile	Tiglic acid esters	Contact dermatitis, anaphylaxis, diarrhea. Use with caution in asthmatics. Anaphylaxis may occur in persons who are sensitive to other members of the *Compositae* family, e.g. chrysanthemums.
Coltsfoot*	Pyrrolizidine alkaloids	Hepatotoxicity and carcinogenicity. Avoid use in pregnancy.
Comfrey	Pyrrolizidine alkaloids. Presence of the alkaloids is controversial. However, long-term internal use of comfrey should best be avoided.	Hepatotoxicity and carcinogenicity.
Ginseng	Complex mixture of sugars, steroids and saponin glycosides.	Excessive use (>15 g/day) may lead to hypertension, estrogenic effects, swollen and painful breasts and vaginal bleeding. Various side-effects such as insomnia, nervousness, excitation, amenorrhea and hypertension have been termed a "ginseng abuse syndrome."
Hemlock*	Poisonous plants of the parsley family. Contains the poisonous alkaloid coniine and four other closely related alkaloids.	Peripheral muscular paralysis. Nicotine-like ganglionic blockade also occurs. Main manifestations are convulsions and respiratory failure.
Lily of the valley*	Contains toxic cardiac glycosides.	Digitalis-like toxicity
Licorice	Glycyrrhizinic acid	Licorice may produce sufficient sodium retention and potassium loss by its mineralocorticoid action to produce hypertension or severe hypokalemia
Mistletoe*	Complex mixture of toxic amines and proteins.	Vomiting, diarrhea and slowed pulse.
Pennyroyal	The oil contains pulegone.	Abortifacient and may cause hepatotoxicity. Avoid in pregnancy.
Sassafrass*	Contains safrole	Has been shown to be hepatotoxic and carcinogenic.
Vitamin B17* (laetrile, amygdalin) Found in apricot, peach and plum kernels	Contains cyanogenic glycosides.	Cyanide poisoning especially after oral administration.

(Adapted from A glance at herbal remedies. Nurs RSA 7(2):40, 1992.

sents potential adverse effects of some medicinal herbs and lists unsafe herbs that are not used medicinally.

COMMONLY USED BOTANICALS OR PHYTOMEDICINES

Echinacea

Echinacea is a genus of plants, related to the daisy family native to Kansas, Nebraska, and Missouri, which are also known as purple coneflower, Sampson root, or hedgehog (Fig. 19–1A). It was the most commonly used herb of the Plains Native Americans, who used the root of the plant externally for healing wounds, burns, and insect bites. Infections, toothache, joint pains, and rattlesnake bites were treated internally with echinacea. Introduced to American medicine by a physician in Nebraska in the late 1800s, by 1920, echinacea as a plant drug was widely used as an anti-infective. However, with the subsequent introduction of antibiotics, echinacea's use as a botanical medicine waned.

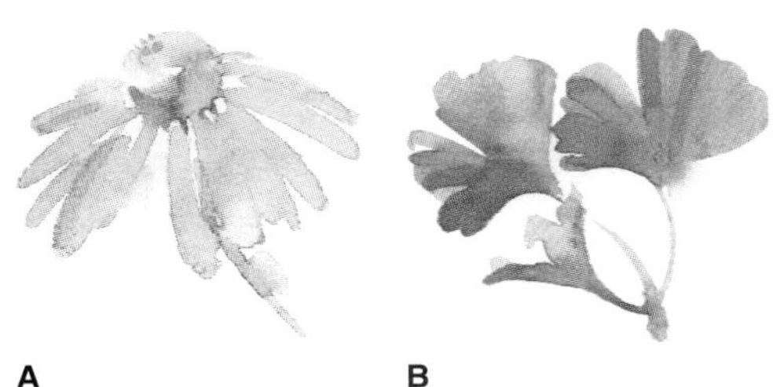

FIGURE 19–1 (A) Echinacea. (B) Gingko biloba. (Courtesy of Pharmanex, Provo, Utah.)

Echinacea purpurea, Echinacea angustifolia, and *Echinacea pallida* are the most commonly used of the nine species of the plant. The medicinal properties of *Echinacea purpurea* have been the subject of the most research, and *E. purpurea* is the most widely cultivated species.

Indications and Common Uses

At present, the most common adjunctive use of echinacea is for the prevention or moderation of the symptoms of colds and flus. In Germany, *E. purpurea* has been approved by the Commission E as supportive therapy for colds and chronic infections of the upper respiratory tract (Blumenthal et al., 1998). Clinical trials in Europe using the expressed juice of *E. purpurea* have shown that patients with colds who received the preparation had a longer interval between infections and less severe infections (Hoheisel et al., 1997). However, echinacea's effect on healthy volunteers in another clinical trial showed no prophylactic effect (Melchart et al., 1998). *E. purpurea* is approved in Germany for topical application for hard-to-heal superficial wounds, eczema, burns, psoriasis, and herpes simplex (Brown, 1995).

Mechanisms of Action and Active Constituents

Echinacea's effect as a nonspecific immune system stimulant has been extensively researched (Tyler, 1994) and may be attributable to the plant's high-molecular-weight polysaccharides. Arabinogalactan, one of the plant's polysaccharides, has been shown to be effective in activating macrophages to produce tumor necrosis factor and other immune potentiators, such as interferon (Stimpel et al., 1984). Other constituents in echinacea, including flavonoids and caffeic acid derivatives, may also contribute to echinacea's immune-stimulating effect (Murray, 1995). No single compound, however, may be said to be responsible for the plant's pharmacologic actions (Echinacea, The Lawrence Review of Natural Products, 1996).

Echinacea may help protect the body from infection by stabilizing hyaluronic acid (Tyler, 1994). The latter is a mucopolysaccharide that is one component of the ground substance in connective tissue that protects cells and connective tissue from invasion by microorganisms.

Contraindications, Side Effects, and Toxicity

When used at the recommended doses, echinacea has been termed essentially nontoxic when taken orally (Murray, 1995). Because of its impact on the immune system, echinacea should not be taken by persons with systemic illnesses, including lupus erythematosus, tuberculosis, leukosis, or multiple sclerosis, or by individuals with allergies to the sunflower family (Tyler, 1994).

Echinacea products are available in many different forms: crude plant in either ground or powdered form; freeze-dried; alcohol-based tinctures and liquid extracts; aqueous tinctures and liquid extracts; and dry powdered alcoholic or aqueous extracts. The dosage of echinacea depends on the potency of the particular formulation. Safe dosages for long-term use are ½ to 1 tsp of the liquid (expressed juice of the herb stabilized at 22% alcohol) or one capsule of dried juice (88.5 mg/capsule) three times daily. Other dosage forms for echinacea include: dried root (1–2 g), tincture (0.75 to 1 tsp), fluid extract (0.25 to 0.5 tsp), and solid (dry powdered) extract (3.5% echinacoside [compounds in the plant used as chemicals markers for standardization], 300 mg). Cycled use of echinacea (an 8-week course of therapy followed by 1 week's rest) is recommended owing to its possible weakened effect with continual use (Brown, 1995).

Feverfew

Feverfew (*Tanacetum parthenium)* is a short, bushy perennial, a member of the daisy family. Its yellow flowers and yellow-green leaves resemble those of chamomile. Its name is a corruption of the Latin term, *febrifugia,* or fever reducer. Historically, the plant was used as an antipyretic.

Indications and Common Uses

Feverfew has become a popular prophylactic for migraine headaches and in Canada, it is sanctioned as a preventive therapy for migraine headache. Other uses for feverfew in folk history include treatment of other inflammatory conditions, such as arthritis.

Mechanisms of Action and Active Constituents

Feverfew may act to mitigate the symptoms of migraines by acting on platelets. During a migraine attack, one theory suggests that platelets release serotonin, which constricts blood vessels. In addition, the platelets appear to aggregate, and inflammatory substances are released. Parthenolide, one of feverfew's sesquiterpene lactones, is the active constituent in feverfew, which apparently acts to reduce serotonin production, inhibit platelet aggregation, and reduce inflammatory processes.

Studies examining the efficacy of feverfew in the treatment of migraines have yielded mixed results. Comparison of results from various trials is difficult because different preparations of feverfew have been used, and methodologies are flawed (Foster, 1990). A recent clinical trial that showed feverfew to be effective in migraine prevention used the form of feverfew that has been shown to be most effective—a dried preparation of the leaves with 0.2 percent of parthenolide (Palevitch et al., 1997).

The Canadian regulatory agency that approves feverfew's use for migraine headache recommends preparations with 125 mg of dried feverfew leaf, and these products are required to have a standard content of 0.2% parthenolide (Foster, 1990). A 4- to 6-week course of continual use of the herbal drug is suggested to impact migraines (Brown, 1995).

The quality of feverfew products can vary greatly. Analyses of the parthenolide content of more than 35 different commercial preparations indicated wide variation in the amounts of parthenolide. Only traces of this active principle were found in most of the products (Heptinstall et al., 1992).

Contraindications, Side Effects, and Toxicity

Long-term studies on the toxicity of feverfew have not been conducted. No reports of toxic reactions have been reported in short-term (6-month) migraine studies (Foster, 1990). Side effects associated with chewing feverfew leaves included minor ulceration of the oral mucosa and tongue inflammation, but these effects can be avoided by using dried, encapsulated forms of feverfew (Feverfew, Lawrence Review of Natural Products, 1994). Feverfew should not be used by pregnant or lactating women or children younger than 2 years of age, nor by persons who are sensitive to ragweed, as feverfew is a potential allergen. Feverfew is contraindicated for persons receiving anticoagulant therapy (Wyandt and Williamson, 1998).

Garlic

Garlic, *Allium sativum,* is a member of the botanical family *Lilliaceace,* and it belongs to the same genus as the onion, leek, and shallot. Garlic, which is creamy white and composed of a number of small bulbs or cloves, grows wild almost everywhere in the world. As a medicinal herb, garlic has been used since the earliest days of recorded history; for the Greek physician, Galen (130–200 A.D.), it was known as the great panacea.

Indications and Common Uses

Garlic is the fourth best selling botanical in the U.S. mass market and one of the most researched herbal medicines, with more than 1000 articles on the therapeutic effects of garlic published in the past 20 years (Foster, 1991). The most frequent uses of garlic are to treat hyperlipoproteinemia (i.e., to lower total serum cholesterol and triglyceride levels) and as an antibiotic (Tyler, 1994).

Mechanisms of Action and Active Constituents

A medium-sized clove of garlic contains about 0.2 g of protein, 0.01 g of fat, approximately 0.001 mg of carbohydrate, 0.05 g of fiber, and vitamins A, B_1, B_2, B_3, and C. Minerals in garlic include potassium, phosphorus, calcium, sodium, iron, manganese, and zinc. Selenium and germanium may be present in the garlic if it is grown in the proper soil. Garlic contains a high amount of sulfur, and may be the highest plant source of this mineral. The chemical constituents of garlic are sulfur-containing compounds, including allicin, diallyl disulfide, and diallyl trisulfide, all volatile oils, and S-allyl cysteine (SAC), a water-soluble amino acid (Murray, 1995).

Whole garlic bulbs or cloves, before they are crushed or macerated, contain an odorless, sulfur-containing amino acid derivative know as alliin. When garlic is crushed or macerated, alliin comes into contact with the enzyme alliinase and is converted to **allicin.** Allicin (the compound responsible for garlic's characteristic odor), in turn, yields a variety of other compounds, including diallyl disulfides, methyl allyl sulfides, and dimethyl sulfides, dithiins, and ajoenes.

One measure of garlic's total activity is its allicin formation, which in fresh garlic, is developed when the garlic is chewed in the mouth. Most dried dietary supplements of garlic contain allicin potential; that is, they contain alliin and the enzyme alliinase, but alliinase is inactivated by stomach acids so no allicin is developed in the stomach. Therefore, dried garlic preparations are most effective if they are enteric-coated. Many commercial garlic products are standardized for allicin content; however, dietary supplements of garlic standardized for SAC are also available. At recommended doses of garlic, a commercial preparation should deliver a minimum of 10 mg of alliin or a total allicin potential of 5000 μg in an enteric-coated form. Suggested raw garlic dosage is one clove, equal to 4 gms (Brown, 1995).

The health benefits attributed to garlic include moderate reductions in blood pressure, decreased blood cholesterol levels, inhibition of platelet aggregation, and antibacterial properties. Ajoene, one of the breakdown products of allicin, is the compound in garlic that has been purported to act as an antithrombotic agent (Tyler, 1994). Ajoene also apparently increases fibrinolysis, the process by which breakdown of fibrin occurs, which slows down blood coagulation (Murray, 1995). The antibacterial properties of garlic are attributable to the activity of allicin (Tyler, 1993).

In a meta-analysis of studies on patients with cholesterol levels exceeding 200 mg/dL, ingestion of a garlic supplement of 900 mg/day (equivalent to 0.5 to 1 clove of garlic per day) decreased total serum cholesterol levels by about 9% (Warshafsky et al., 1993). However, because there may be considerable differences in the composition of commercial garlic preparations, comparisons between studies, or extrapolation of clinical results obtained from one product to another, may be difficult. For example, evidence of garlic's suggested health benefit of lowering blood pressure was examined by researchers who combined the results of eight different studies that used the same dried garlic preparation. These researchers concluded that garlic may be of some clinical use in subjects with mild hypertension (Silagy and Neil, 1994). However, another well-designed study using the same garlic preparation failed to show a significant effect on lowering cholesterol (Isaacsohn et al., 1998). Yet another study questioned the tablet quality and allicin release efficiency of the garlic preparations used in trials that failed to show garlic's cholesterol-lowering effect (Lawson, 1998b). Garlic oil preparations in another study showed no significant cholesterol-lowering activity (Berthold et al., 1998); unlike allicin-standardized garlic powder tablets, the allyl sulfides in the garlic oil preparation are apparently less active (Lawson, 1998a).

Contraindications, Side Effects, and Toxicity

No health risk has been reported for normal persons who consume moderate amounts of garlic (Murray, 1995). Consumption of garlic in amounts of five or more cloves per day may produce heartburn or flatulence. Other side effects of garlic ingestion may include mild allergic reactions, dermatitis, and gastrointestinal symptoms (Tyler, 1994). Garlic reduces clotting time and should be used with caution when using aspirin or other anticoagulant drugs, such as warfarin (Rose et al., 1990). Garlic therapy should not automatically be recommended for treatment of hypercholesterolemia (Berthold et al., 1998).

Ginger

Ginger (*Zingiber officinale*) is a rhizome (underground stem) native to the orient. The plant has green-purple flowers, resembles an orchid, and is also known as Jamaica ginger, African ginger, Cochin ginger, black ginger, and race ginger.

Indications and Common Uses

Ginger's most popular therapeutic application is as a prophylactic treatment for digestive system problems, especially nausea, motion sickness, and hyperemesis gravidarum (excessive vomiting during pregnancy). Because it suppresses inflammatory substances, including leukotrienes and prostaglandins (Kuchi et al., 1992), other possible beneficial applications of ginger include the treatment of arthritis, both rheumatoid and osteoarthritis, and muscular pain (Tyler, 1993).

The Commission E monograph on ginger recommends ginger for both indigestion and the prevention of symptoms of motion sickness (Blumenthal et al., 1998). One study found ginger to be as effective as Dramamine in reducing symptoms of motion sickness (Mowrey and Clayson, 1982), but other studies have not confirmed the same effect. Poor-quality ginger may have been used in the studies that reported negative results (Tyler, 1994).

Ginger has also traditionally been used as a remedy for nausea and vomiting in the first trimester of pregnancy. In a review of drug therapy during pregnancy, ginger and vitamin B_6 have both been recognized as effective treatments for nausea and vomiting in early pregnancy. Adjunctive use of ginger to reduce nausea and vomiting after surgery, particularly for day surgery, has shown promising results (Phillips et al., 1993).

Ginger is usually taken in the form of capsules, each containing 500 mg of powdered ginger (Tyler, 1994). When used as an antiemetic, 1 to 2 g of ginger are taken in two divided doses. For maximum effect on motion sickness, ginger should be used several days before travel, with continuous usage during the trip (Brown, 1995).

Contraindications, Side Effects, and Toxicity

Ginger may be used briefly during pregnancy in dosages not exceeding 1 g of the powdered product daily. However, long-term use during pregnancy is not recommended (Niebyl, 1992). Persons with gallstones are advised not to use ginger unless under the supervision of a health care practitioner, and ginger to control postsurgical nausea should only be used with the advice of a physician (Brown, 1995).

High doses—greater than 6 g of dried ginger powder—have been shown to increase exfoliation of human gastric epithelial cells. Also, ingestion of such excessive amounts of ginger may result in gastric distress and, potentially, ulcer formation (Murray, 1995). Concomitant use of pharmacologic doses of ginger and anticoagulants is contraindicated (Verma et al., 1994).

Ginkgo

Ginkgo, or *Ginkgo biloba,* is the oldest living species of trees and can be traced back more than 200 million years to the fossils of the Permian period (see Fig. 19–1B on page 421). It was used medically in China for hundreds of years and is now a popular ornamental tree in parks and gardens throughout the world. **Ginkgo biloba extract (GBE)** is the term for standardized preparations of ginkgo.

Indications and Common Uses

Ginkgo apparently has a wide range of physiologic actions, including vasodilation, inhibition of platelet aggregation, increased oxygen and glucose utilization, and action to improve peripheral circulation (Blumenthal et al., 1998).

GBE is widely used in Europe, particularly in Germany, for the treatment of cardiovascular disease, peripheral vascular disease, and intermittent claudication (Tyler, 1994). GBE has been found to be useful for treating age-related decline in mental function secondary to cerebrovascular insufficiency (short-term memory loss, poor concentration, tinnitus, possibly dementia) (Kleijnen and Knipschild, 1992), and early stage senility of the Alzheimer's type may also be improved by the use of GBE (LeBars et al., 1997).

Mechanisms of Action and Active Constituents

The herbal extract of gingko, GBE, is derived from green-picked ginkgo leaves that have been developed specifically for pharmaceutical purposes. The leaves are extracted with an acetone-water mixture, the organic solvent is removed, and the extract is processed, dried, and standardized. Standardized preparations of ginkgo typically contain 24% ginkgo flavone glycosides (including bioflavonoids, such as quercetin, kaempferol, and isorhammnetin) and 6% terpene lactones (ginkgolides and bilobalide, compounds unique to ginkgo) (Blumenthal et al., 1998).

The flavone glycosides in the standardized extract exert antioxidant activity and protect cells against free radical damage, particularly damage to the lipid layer of the cell membrane (Blumenthal et al., 1998). The flavone glycosides also inhibit platelet aggregation. The ginkgolides act as platelet activating factor (PAF) antagonists. PAF promotes aggregation of blood platelets and is involved in many of the effects of allergic response. The ginkgolides apparently block these actions and, in addition, increase blood fluidity to enhance circulation (Tyler, 1994).

Ginkgo leaves are used in the form of concentrated, standardized GBE. The product is marketed in both solid and liquid form, with each tablet and capsule containing 40 mg of GBE. The normal adult dose of GBE is 120 to 160 mg daily (Tyler, 1994). The recommended dosage for cerebrovascular insufficiency and early-stage Alzheimer's disease is 240 mg daily. A 6- to 8-week course is advised to determine GBE's therapeutic effect (Brown, 1995).

Good clinical and scientific research on ginkgo utilizes an extract, produced in Germany, named EGb 761 by Schwabe GmbH and Company. The efficacy of other products is not known.

Contraindications, Side Effects, and Toxicity

Mild side effects reported with GBE use include mild gastrointestinal complaints, headache, and allergic skin reactions, but these reactions are rare (Kleijnen and Knipschild, 1992). Whole ginkgo plant, particularly the plant pulp, however, has been associated with severe allergic reactions (Ginkgo, Lawrence Review of Natural Products, 1994). Ginkgo extract should be used with caution by persons who are taking anticoagulants or acetominophen, as GBE has a blood thinning effect (Rowin and Lewis, 1996).

Ginseng

Ginseng is a yellowish, radish-like herb and a slow-growing and exacting plant that takes at least 6 years of cultivation to produce a marketable product. Ginseng has a rich history in Eastern medicine; in China, ginseng has been in continuous use for more than 4000 years.

There are numerous varieties of ginseng, and almost all are cultivated. The most common is *Panax* ginseng, also called Korean, Chinese, or Asian ginseng, and it is the form that has been researched most extensively. The American variety of ginseng, *P. quinquifolium,* has been declared an endangered species, and is subject to stringent requirements governing its collection and sale (see "*Focus On:* Phytomedicines: Will We Run Out?"). A related species of the ginseng family is commonly known as Siberian ginseng, but is actually *Eleutherococcus sentiocosus* and contains different active constituents than either *Panax* or *P. quinquifolium*.

The colors of ginseng indicate how the herb has been processed. Red ginseng means that the ginseng root has been sterilized and preserved through steam treatment, hence its red color. White ginseng

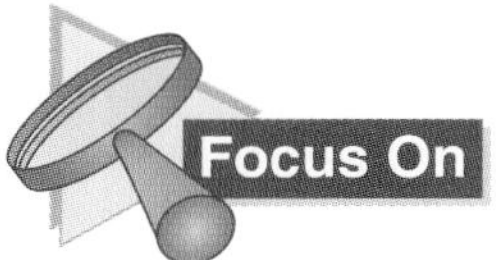

Phytomedicines—Will We Run Out?

The U.S. botanical market is burgeoning, with the US market for medicinal botanicals in 1998 estimated at nearly 4 billion dollars. (Brevoort, 1998). With this tremendous growth in interest and sales of botanical products, what are some of the trends for the future of herbs?

One of the most significant factors affecting both producers and consumers of herbal products is the stress on the supply of raw materials. For some plants, like St. John's wort, demand for the phytomedicine is already exceeding the supply. Other plants take years to grow, and quality plants may soon become unavailable. The danger with limited plant supply is that poor quality, low-grade materials may be used for medicinal products.

The threatened extinction of many plants will also mean that their potential medicinal uses will never be realized. Scientists find that in in every 1,000 plants, one plant has significant medical use. A recent report by the World Conservation Union found more than 34,000 plant species have become so rare that they may disappear, thus 34 medicinal plants may be lost. Already entire plant families of some species are threatened with extinction, including the yew family which is used to produce the anti-cancer drug taxol. (Johnston, 1998)

In the United States, 29 percent of the country's 16,000 plants are threatened with extinction. Especially in eastern North American deciduous forests, this decimation of native habitat from residential and commercial building, mining, and timber operations is threatening the populations of many wild botanicals used to make herbal preparations. To protect the dwindling number of these plants, certain species are now protected, including American ginseng, but widespread collection of the plant and threats to its habitat continue. (Robbins, 1998)

Another issue confronting the future of the growth of herbal medicines is how to compensate indigenous peoples for their knowledge in the use of these botanicals. Scientists are going into areas rich in flora and fauna and interviewing traditional healers about the medicinal uses of these plants. For example, two ethnobotanists working in Samoa recognized that they should return as much to the traditional healers as they were getting in exchange. (Balick and Cox, 1996) Their efforts resulted in a payment back to the community for every sale of the product which incorporates the botanical knowledge of the healers who collaborated with the scientists.

The challenge, therefore, for the future of quality herbal products lies both with producers and consumers. Producers of herbal products must ensure that only high quality plant products from reputable sources are used, and consumers should choose only those products whose companies are mindful of the environment of the plants and the community with the knowledge of their use.

is the dried root. There is no chemical difference between the two varieties, simply a color variation.

Indications and Common Uses

The name *Panax,* from a Greek word meaning "all healing," implies the many suggested uses for ginseng, including antifatigue and antistress actions, mental performance improvements, immune system enhancement, cardiovascular effects, and supportive therapy for diabetes.

In Chinese medicine, gingseng's traditional use is as a tonic to help the body cope with stress of all types. Ginseng is also known as an *adaptogen,* a substance that reduces excesses, stimulates deficient states, exerts a balancing action, and is nontoxic. Ginseng's effect, in improving physical or mental performance, or countering physical or mental fatigue, has been shown primarily in animal studies (Tyler, 1994).

Ginseng may be beneficial for persons with type II (non–insulin-dependent) diabetes. One study showed reduced fasting blood glucose levels and improvements in glycated hemoglobin (HbA1C) in persons with diabetes who received 200-mg doses of Asian ginseng (Sotaniemi et al., 1995).

Immune system enhancement may be a benefit of consistent use (for 8 weeks). Healthy volunteers who received 100 mg of a standardized extract of ginseng in a clinical study showed enhanced natural killer cell activity, interferon production, and macrophage activity (Scaglione et al.,1990).

Mechanisms of Action and Active Constituents

Ginseng species differ in their composition and mechanisms of action. *Panax* ginseng is the most complex, with 13 identified ginsenosides, which are steroid-like compounds known as saponin glycosides. Because of the interaction of the ginsenosides, which are all in the root of the plant and occur in small amounts, the whole root is used in herbal preparations. The interaction of the ginsenosides is evidenced by the actions of ginsenosides Rb1 and Rg1, which exert different yet harmonizing influences on the body. Rb1 has a hypoactive effect on blood pressure and a mildly sedative effect, whereas Rg1 is thought to exert a mildly stimulatory action on the central nervous system (Murray, 1995).

Contraindications, Side Effects, and Toxicity

At the recommended dosage of 100 mg once or twice daily, using a preparation of 4% to 7% ginsenosides, ginseng is generally regarded as safe (Ginseng, Lawrence Review of Natural Products, 1990). Cycled use of ginseng in 2- to 3-week intervals with 1- to 2-week rest periods is advised. Reported side effects of ginseng use include overstimulation and possible insomnia, which may diminish after continual use or after dosage reduction. However, ginseng consumption with caffeine may cause overstimulation and gastrointestinal distress. Individuals with hypertension are advised not to use ginseng.

Long-term consumption of ginseng is reported to have adverse effects, including hypertension, nervousness, insomnia, and morning diarrhea, known as "Ginseng abuse syndrome." Reports of ginseng abuse syndrome are often associated with the ingestion of inordinate amounts of the herb, up to 15 g daily, with concurrent use of other stimulants, like caffeine (Tyler, 1994). According to the American Botanical Council, ginseng should generally not be used by individuals undergoing steroid therapy or using monoamine oxidase (MAO) inhibitors, or by those with cardiac disorders or diabetes.

Hawthorn

Hawthorn (*Crataegus oxyacantha*) is a small to medium-sized tree native to Europe; other species include *C. monogyna* and *C. pentagyna*. The leaves, blossoms, and fruits are used in modern standardized extracts. Only the leaf and blossom formulations are approved for use in Germany, where much research on hawthorn has been conducted using proprietary formulas.

Indications and Common Uses

Hawthorn is used in Europe for the treatment of atherosclerosis and angina pectoris and, sometimes, early stage congestive heart failure. It is not used, however, for acute angina because the drug action is slow (Hawthorn, Lawrence Review of Natural Products, 1994).

Mechanisms of Action and Active Constituents

Hawthorn leaves, berries, and blossoms contain oligomeric procyanidins and other flavonoids. Hawthorn appears to act on the cardiovascular system in two ways: (1) hawthorn directly dilates the coronary vessels to lower blood pressure; and (2) hawthorn improves the metabolic processes of the heart through its inotropic (strength of contraction) and chronotropic (heart rate) effects, increasing nerve conductivity and heart muscle contractability (Hamon, 1988). Hawthorn apparently inhibits angiotensin converting enzyme (ACE), which converts angiotensin I to angiotensin II, a powerful blood vessel constrictor. In a clinical trial, a hawthorn extract preparation (900 mg of a proprietary product) compared favorably to the ACE inhibitor captopril, a pharmaceutical drug, in increasing capacity to withstand exercise-induced stress, reducing postexercise shortness of breath, and reducing fatigue in study participants (Tauchert et al., 1994).

The best quality hawthorn extracts are standardized to 20% procyanidins or 2.2% flavonoid content, with typical daily doses of 160 mg (Murray, 1994). Higher doses of hawthorn should not be self-prescribed (Tyler, 1994).

Contraindications, Side Effects, and Toxicity

Side effects of hawthorn are not well documented (Murray, 1995). However, individuals with heart disease should be advised to consult health care professionals for appropriate treatment.

Milk Thistle

Milk thistle (*Silybum marianum*) is a tall plant with prickly leaves and a milky sap. It is a member of the daisy family and is also known as St. Mary's thistle, blessed thistle, and Our Lady's thistle. It is native to the Mediterranean region and is naturalized to the eastern United States, California, and other parts of North America (Fig. 19–2A). Since the 16th century, milk thistle has been used to enhance liver function.

Indications and Common Uses

Milk thistle is known as the liver herb because of its apparent hepatoprotective characteristics. In Europe, intravenous preparations of the active constituent in milk thistle—silymarin—are used clinically to counter the overdose effects of the death cap mushroom (*Amanita phalloides*), primarily because it protects the liver cells from damage secondary to the action of phalloidine, a toxic liver poison in the mushroom (Milk Thistle, Lawrence Review of Natural Products, 1997).

Adjunctive uses for silymarin, approved by the German Commission E, include treatment of inflammatory liver damage secondary to cirrhosis, hepatitis, or fatty infiltration caused by alcohol or other toxins (Blumenthal et al., 1998). Silymarin has also been shown to regenerate hepatocytes in individuals with chronic viral hepatitis B (Berenguer and Barrasco, 1977) or alcoholic cirrhosis, provided the liver cells have not been damaged irreversibly (Deak et al., 1990).

Mechanisms of Action and Active Constituents

The active constituent of milk thistle is **silymarin,** found in highest concentrations in the seeds of the plant. Silymarin consists of flavonolignins, unique forms of flavonoids, and silibinin, considered to be the most important component of silymarin. Silymarin appears to act on the liver and kidneys, moving along the cycle from blood plasma to liver bile, concentrating in hepatocytes. Silymarin supports the liver by protecting hepatocytes from toxins, and increasing the ability of liver cells to regenerate by stimulating protein synthesis (Hobbs, 1992). Additionally, silymarin has antioxidant and free-radical scavenging properties (Tyler, 1994).

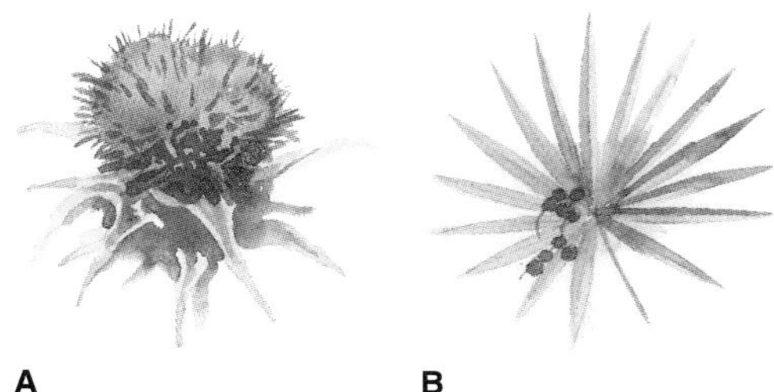

FIGURE 19–2 (A) Milk thistle. (B) Saw palmetto. (Courtesy of Pharmanex, Provo, Utah.)

Silymarin is very poorly soluble in water, making water-based extractions (e.g., tea) less effective than other preparations. Milk thistle extracts, standardized to 70% to 80% silymarin, are apparently the most effective form (Brown, 1995). In the United States, the botanical is available in capsule form, usually containing 200 mg of concentrated extract equal to 140 mg of silymarin.

Contraindications, Side Effects, and Toxicity

There are no known contraindications to the use of milk thistle extract at recommended doses (Tyler, 1994). In rare cases, milk thistle is reported to cause loose stools and diarrhea (Brown, 1995). The Commission E monograph indicates that those with gallstones should be cautious with its use (Blumenthal et al., 1998).

Saw Palmetto

Saw palmetto *(Serenoa repens, Sabal serrulata)* is a shrub-like palm tree that is native to the southeastern portion of the United States. It is found in Florida, Georgia, Louisiana, and South Carolina (see Fig. 19–2B). Its fruits were used during the early 1900s as a mild diuretic and for enlarged prostate.

Indications and Common Uses

Saw palmetto acts to reduce the incidence of benign prostatic hyperplasia (BPH), which is a nonmalignant abnormal growth of the prostate gland. This condition affects 50% to 60% of men aged 40 to 60 years, and more than 90% of men older than 80 years of age. BPH has a significant impact on lifestyle owing to its irritative symptoms and obstruction to urinary flow.

Saw palmetto extract has been found to compare favorably with the pharmaceutical drug finasteride (Proscar) in the management of BPH. In a clinical trial that compared the efficacy of a commercial saw palmetto extract to finasteride, both products relieved symptoms in two-thirds of the men. The saw palmetto extract, however, had fewer adverse side effects, such as impotence and decreased libido, than finasteride. Saw palmetto reduced the symptoms of BPH; it did not significantly reduce the size of the prostate (Carraro et al., 1996).

Mechanisms of Action and Active Constituents

The active constituents of saw palmetto are derived from the herb's red-brown-black berries that contain free fatty acids and sterols. The berries contain approximately 1.5% of an oil (beta-sitosterol) that contains saturated and unsaturated fatty acids and sterols. A purified fat-soluble extract of the berries containing the fatty acids and sterols is used medicinally.

As a phytomedicine, saw palmetto appears to act as a weak antiandrogen to reduce the action of 5-alpha-reductase (5-AR). The 5-AR enzyme converts testosterone to dihydrotestosterone (DHT). DHT fosters changes in prostatic cell growth by binding to androgen receptor sites in prostate cells and increasing cell growth and division. 5-AR activity increases as men age. The lipophilic extract of saw palmetto apparently blocks the action of the 5-AR enzyme and inhibits binding of DHT to prostate cells, thus limiting overproduction of cells and prostatic enlargement.

For stage I or II BPH, a dosage of 160 mg of the lipophilic extract (standardized to 85% to 95% fatty acids and sterols) twice a day has been used in clinical trials. To assess efficacy, 6 to 8 weeks of continuous use is advised; however, to assess clinical efficacy, a minimum 6-month trial is required (*Serenoa repens,* 1998). Tea made with saw palmetto is of little value because few of the active ingredients are water-soluble.

Contraindications, Side Effects, and Toxicity

The Commission E monograph on saw palmetto lists rare cases of stomach problems as a side effect, but lists no contraindications (Blumenthal et al., 1998). There is no current evidence that saw palmetto has any effect on prostate-specific antigens (PSA), and so does not mask prostate carcinoma (Braeckman J et al., 1997).

St. John's Wort

St. John's wort (*Hypericum perforatum*), an aromatic perennial with small, five-petaled flowers, has gained much popular attention as an antidepressant. St. John's wort is also known as goat weed, Johnswort, and Klamath weed. The plant's name is derived from the yellow flower it produces at St. John's Tide, June 24th (the summer solstice), the day traditionally celebrated as the birthday of John the Baptist.

Indications and Common Uses

St. John's wort appears to have benefit as an antidepressant for persons experiencing mild to moderate depression (Tyler, 1994). The limited research that has been conducted on its application for severe depression supports its beneficial effects (Vorbach et al., 1997), but additional research in this area is needed.

Mechanisms of Action and Active Constituents

Not all active principles in St. John's wort are currently known. Of the identified constituents, hyperforin may be the most active; other known constituents include hypericin and pseudohypericin, flavonoids, xanthones, and essential oils.

The mechanism of action of St. John's wort is not understood completely, but a number of actions have been proposed, including inhibition of reuptake of serotonin, norepinephrine, and dopamine, with weak inhibition of MAO-A and MAO-B activity (Muller et al., 1997). Another proposed action of St. John's wort is that the hypericin in St. John's wort may act to increase light utilization to help modulate depressive moods (Gruenwald, 1997).

Clinical trials have confirmed the efficacy of St. John's wort as an antidepressant, including one study in which patients receiving 900 mg of St. John's wort reported fewer depressive symptoms after 4 weeks of therapy (Harrar et al., 1994). In studies that have compared St. John's wort with prescription antidepressants, St. John's wort has been found to have similar efficacy with significantly fewer side effects. In one study, patients who were given imipramine, a tricyclic antidepressant, at a dosage of 75 mg/day showed a 45% improvement according to the Hamilton Depression scale; 16% of the patients reported side effects. By comparison, patients receiving St. John's wort (900 mg/day) showed a 56% improvement according to the depression scale, and only 12% noted side effects (Vorbach et al., 1994).

The recommended daily dosage for St. John's wort based on clinical studies involving the management of mild to moderate depression, is 900 mg, given with meals in three divided doses of 300 mg (Brown, 1995).

Contraindications, Side Effects, and Toxicity

Reported side effects of St. John's wort include emotional vulnerability, fatigue, pruritis, and weight increase. Although the side effects of St. John's wort are reported to be milder and less frequent than those associated with prescription antidepressant drugs, patients taking St. John's wort may experience side effects in the first 2 to 4 weeks of use (Bastyr University, 1995). Photosensitivity is possible, particularly for persons with fair skin, so caution is advised if exposure to the sun is anticipated.

Concomitant use of prescription antidepressants, including fluoxetine and MAO inhibitors, such as phenelzine and tranylcypromine, is not currently advised. Other medications that should not be taken concurrently with St. John's wort include narcotics, amphetamines, and over-the-counter flu and cold preparations (Bastyr University, 1995).

Valerian

Valerian, *Valeriana officinalis,* also know as wild valerian and garden heliotrope, is a tall perennial herb whose hollow stem bears leaves with white or reddish flowers. Valerian consists of the dried rhizome and roots; the vertical rhizome and its numerous rootlets are harvested in the autumn in the second year of growth. It is these parts that possess the volatile, essential oil that contains the distinctive odor of valerian.

Indications and Common Uses

Valerian has a 1000-year history of use as a minor tranquilizer and sleep aid. Nervous system disorders, including anxiety and insomnia, are conditions for which valerian may be useful.

Mechanisms of Action and Active Constituents

At the present time, the specific ingredients responsible for the sedative effects of valerian remain unknown. However, the identified chemical components, which include the monoterpenes in the volatile oil (primarily, sesquiterpene derivatives including valerenic acid), may account for valerian's action (Reichert, 1998). The mechanism of action of valerian appears to be similar to that of benzodiazepines and barbiturates, which bind gamma-aminobutyric acid-A (GABA-A) receptor sites to depress central nervous system activity. Valerian weakly binds these receptor sites, so sedation results without adverse effects, such as addiction or dependence. However, valerian may also have other actions not related to GABA binding (Reichert, 1998).

Clinical studies with valerian have demonstrated that this phytomedicine appears to improve the quality of sleep time and reduces the time required to fall asleep, even in older persons and in poor or irregular sleepers, without producing morning sleepiness. In a study that compared the efficacy of a combination valerian and lemon balm preparation to benzodiazepine in shortening sleep latency and increasing sleep quality, the valerian combination (160 mg of valerian combined with 80 mg of lemon balm [*Mellissa officinalis*]) compared favorably to 0.125 mg of triazolam (Halcion). Patients treated with the phytomedicines experienced no daytime sedation or loss of concentration (Dressing et al., 1992).

The recommended dosage of valerian for treatment of insomnia is 300 to 400 mg of standardized valerian root extract (containing not less than 0.5% essential oil), administered 1 hour before bedtime. Persons suffering from anxiety may also benefit from an added morning dose of 200 to 300 mg (Brown, 1995). The Commission E monograph notes that 100 g of valerian may be used externally as a bath (Blumenthal et al., 1998), but its effectiveness in this form may be limited (Tyler, 1994).

Contraindications, Side Effects, and Toxicity

At recommended dosages, use of valerian has not been associated with side effects or contraindications. Alcohol use does not increase valerian's sedative properties, and although valerian can be used safely while operating a car or other machinery, caution is still advised (Reichert, 1998). Valerian should not be used concurrently with other sedative-hypnotics, antianxiety, or antidepressant drugs.

CASE STUDY

Ellen Y. is 66 years old and has been diagnosed as having hypertension, hypercholesterolemia, and type II diabetes (non–insulin-dependent diabetes mellitus). She has been referred by her physician for nutritional counseling, with a specific request from the referring physician that you evaluate any herbal preparations she is taking. At the initial consult, Ellen Y. tells you that she is taking the following dietary supplements: garlic pills, ginseng, ginkgo, and St. John's wort, along with the following medications: warfarin, tricyclic antidepressant, and blood pressure–lowering medication.

1. What additional questions would you ask regarding Ellen's supplements?
2. List potential drug/drug interactions between the botanicals and the prescription drugs.
3. What recommendations would you make about Ellen's diet?

CONSUMER ADVICE

Complementary and alternative medicine, along with related modalities, such as acupuncture, moxibustion, and naturopathy, is commonly practiced in the United States. These holistic therapies emphasize the healing force of nature and the body's ability to heal itself. Phytotherapy with the use of botanical medicines is growing in popularity, but self-treatment with botanicals is generally appropriate only for minor, self-limiting conditions or as preventive measures against certain chronic diseases.

CITED REFERENCES

A glance at herbal remedies. Nurs RSA (7(2):40, 1992.

Balick M, Cox P. Plants, People, and Culture. The Science of Ethnobotany. New York, WH Freeman and Company, 1996.

Bastyr University, Continuing Professional Education Program. Herbal Medicine: An Introduction for Pharmacists. Seattle, WA: Bastyr University, 1995.

Bensoussan A, et al. Treatment of irritable bowel syndrome with Chinese herbal medicine: A randomized controlled trial. JAMA 280:1585, 1998.

Berenguer J, Barrasco D. Double–blind trial of silymarin versus placebo in the treatment of chronic hepatitis. Munch Med Wochenschr 119:240, 1977.

Berthold HK, et al. Effect of a garlic oil preparation on serum lipoproteins and cholesterol metabolism: A randomized controlled trial. JAMA 279:1900, 1998.

Blumenthal M, et al. (eds.). The Complete German Commission E Monographs—Therapeutic Guide to Herbal Medicines. (Klein S, Rister RS, Trans.). Austin, TX: American Botanical Council, Integrative Medicine Communications, 1998.

Braeckman J, et al. Efficacy and safety of the extract of *Serenoa repens* in the treatment of benign prostatic hyperplasia: Therapeutic equivalence between twice and once daily dosage forms. Phytother Res 11:558, 1997.

Brevoort P. The booming U.S. botanical market. A new overview. HerbalGram 44:33, 1998.

Brown DJ. Herbal Prescriptions for Better Health. Rocklin, CA: Prima Publishing Co., 1995.

Carraro JC, et al. Comparison of phytotherapy (Permixon) with finasteride in the treatment of benign prostate hyperplasia: A randomized international study of 1,098 patients. Prostate 29:231, 1996.

De Schepper L. The People's Repertory. Santa Fe, NM: Full of Life Publishing, 1998.

Deak G, et al. Immunomodulator effect of silymarin therapy in chronic alcoholic liver diseases. Orv Hetil 131:1291, 1990.
Dressing H, et al. Insomnia: Are valerian/lemon balm combinations of equal value to benzodiazepine? Therapiewoche 42:726, 1992.
Echinacea. The Lawrence Review of Natural Products. Facts and Comparisons. ISSN 0734–4961, December, 1996.
Edzard E. Harmless herbs? A review of the recent literature. Am J Med 104:170, 1998.
Eisenberg DM, et al. Trends in alternative medicine use in the United States 1990–1997: Results of a follow-up national survey. JAMA 280:1569, 1998.
Ernst E, Kaptchuk TJ. Homeopathy revisited. Arch Intern Med 19:2612, 1996.
FDA Consumer. Homeopathy: Real medicine or empty promises? 30:15, 1996.
Feverfew. Lawrence Review of Natural Products: Facts and Comparisons. ISSN 0734–4961, December, 1994.
Food and Drug Administration. OTC Drug Review Ingredient Status Report. Rockville, MD: Government Printing Office. September, 1994.
Foster S. Feverfew (*Tanacetum parthenium*). Botanical Series No. 310. Austin, TX: American Botanical Council, 1990.
Foster S. Garlic (*Allium sativum*). Botanical Series No. 131. Austin, TX: American Botanical Council, 1991, p. 7.
Ginkgo. Lawrence Review of Natural Products: Facts and Comparisons. ISSN 0734–4961, February, 1994.
Ginseng. Lawrence Review of Natural Products: Facts and Comparisons. ISSN 0734–4961, September, 1990.
Gruenwald J. Standardized St. John's Wort extract clinical monograph. Q Rev Natl Med Winter: 289, 1997.
Hamon NW. Hawthorns. Can Pharm J Nov:708, 724, 1988.
Harrar G, Sommer H. Treatment of mild to moderate depressions with Hypericum. Phytomedicine 1:3, 1994.
Hawthorn. Lawrence Review of Natural Products: Facts and Comparisons. ISSN 0734–4961, January, 1994.
Heptinstall S, et al. Parthenolide content and bioactivity of feverfew (*Tanactetum parthenium* (L.) Schultz-Bip.) Estimation of commercial and authenticated feverfew products. J Pharm Pharmacol 44:391, 1992.
Hobbs C. Milk Thistle: The Liver Herb, 2nd ed. Capitola, CA: Botanica Press, 1992.
Hoheisel O, et al. Echinagard treatment shortens the course of the common cold: A double-blind, placebo-controlled clinical trial. Eur J Clin Res 9:261, 1997.
Hung O, et al. Herbal preparation use among urban emergency department patients. Acad Emerg Med 4:209, 1997.
Isaacsohn JL, et al. Garlic powder and plasma lipids and lipoproteins. Arch Intern Med 158:1189, 1998.
Jacobs J, et al. Treatment of acute childhood diarrhea with homeopathic medicine: A randomized clinical trial in Nicaragua. Pediatrics 93:719, 1994.
Johnston B. Major diversity loss: 1 in 8 plants in global study threatened. HerbalGram 43:54, 1998.
Kleijnen J, Knipschild P. Drug Profile: Ginkgo biloba. Lancet 340:1136, 1992.
Kuchi F, et al. Inhibition of prostaglandin and leukotriene biosynthesis by gingerols and diarylheptanoids. Chem Pharm Bull 40:387, 1992.
Lawson L. Garlic powder for hyperlipidemia. Analysis of recent negative results. Q Rev Natl Med Fall: 187, 1998a.
Lawson L. Effect of garlic on serum lipids. JAMA 280:1568, 1998b.
LeBars PL, et al. A placebo-controlled, double-blind, randomized trial of an extract of *Ginkgo biloba* for dementia. JAMA 278:1327, 1997.
Lokken P, et al. Effect of homeopathy on pain and other events after acute trauma: Placebo-controlled trial with bilateral oral surgery. Br Med J 310:1439, 1995.
Melchart D, et al. Echinacea root extracts for the prevention of upper respiratory tract infections: A double-blind, placebo-controlled randomized trial. Arch Fam Med 7:541, 1998.
Milk Thistle. Lawrence Review of Natural Products: Facts and Comparisons. ISSN 0734–4961, 1997.
Mowrey D, Clayson DL. Motion sickness, ginger, and psychophysics. Lancet 1:655, 1982.
Muller WE, et al. Effects of hypericum extract (LI 160) in biochemical models of antidepressant activity. Pharmacopsychiatry 30(suppl):102, 1997.
Murray M. The Healing Power of Herbs, 2nd ed. Rocklin, CA: Prima Publishing Co., 1995.
National Institutes of Health Consensus Conference. Acupuncture. JAMA 280:1518, 1998.
Niebyl J. Drug therapy during pregnancy. Curr Opin Obstet Gynecol 4:43, 1992.
Oka H, et al. Prospective study of chemoprevention of hepatocellular carcinoma with Sho-saiko-to(TJ-9). Cancer 76:743, 1995.
Palevitch D, et al. Feverfew (*Tanacetum parthenium*) as a prophylactic treatment for migraine: A double-blind placebo-controlled study. Phytother Res 11:508, 1997.
Phillips S, et al. *Zingiber officinale* (ginger)—An antiemetic for day case surgery. Anaesthesia 48:715, 1993.
Reichert RG. Valerian clinical monograph. Q Rev Natl Med Fall:207, 1998.
Robbins C. Medicinal plant conservation—A priority at TRAFFIC. HerbalGram 44:52, 1998.
Rose KD, et al. Spontaneous spinal epidural hematoma with associated platelet dysfunction from excessive garlic ingestion: A case report. Neurosurgery 26:880, 1990.
Rowin J, Lewis S. Spontaneous bilateral subdural hematomas associated with chronic *Ginkgo biloba* ingestion. Neurology 46:1775, 1996.
Scaglione F, et al. Immunomodulatory effects of two extracts of *Panax* ginseng (C.A. Meyer). Drugs Exp Clin Res 16:537, 1990.
Serenoa repens. Monograph. Alt Med Rev 3:227, 1998.
Silagy CA, Neil HA. A meta-analysis of the effect of garlic on blood pressure. J Hypertens 12:463, 1994.
Slifman N, et al. Contamination of botanical dietary supplements by *Digitalis lanata*. N Engl J Med 339:806, 1998.
Sotaniemi E, et al. Ginseng therapy in non–insulin-dependent diabetic patients. Diabetes Care 8:1373, 1995.
Stimpel M, et al. Macrophage activation and induction of macrophage cytotoxicity by purified polysacccharide fractions from the plant *Echinacea purpurea*. Infect Immun 46:845, 1984.
Tauchert M, et al. Effectiveness of hawthorn extract LI 132 compared with the ACE inhibitor captopril: Multicenter double-blind study with 132 NYHA stage II. Muench Med Wochenschr 136 (suppl):S27, 1994.
Tyler VE. Herbs of Choice: The Therapeutic Use of Phytomedicinals. New York: Haworth Press, 1994.
Tyler VE. The Honest Herbal, 3rd ed. Binghamton, NY: Pharmaceutical Products Press, 1993.
Verma SK, et al. Effect of ginger on platelet aggregation in man. Indian J Med Res 98:240, 1994.
Vorbach EU, et al. Effectiveness and tolerance of the hypericum extract LI 160 in comparison with imipramine: Randomized double-blind study with 135 outpatients. J Geriatr Psychiatry Neurol 7(1 suppl):S19, 1994.
Vorbach EU, et al. Efficacy and tolerability of St. John's Wort extract LI160 versus imipramine in patients with severe depressive episodes according to ICDE-10. Pharmacopsychiatria 30:S81, 1997.
Warshafsky S, et al. Effect of garlic on total serum cholesterol. A meta-analysis. Ann Intern Med 119:599, 1993.
Wyandt M, Williamson J. An herbal update. Pharmacists training to prescribe herb remedies. Drug Top 142:66, 1998.

ADDITIONAL REFERENCES

Block E. The chemistry of garlic and onions. Sci Am 151:118, 1985.
Bone ME, et al. Ginger root—A new antiemetic. The effect of ginger root on postoperative nausea and vomiting after major gynecological surgery. Anaesthesia 45:669, 1990.
Cassileth BR. The Alternative Medicine Handbook: The Complete Reference Guide to Alternative and Complementary Medicines. New York: WW Norton, 1998.
de Weerdt JJ, et al. Herbal medicines in migraine prevention: Randomized, double-blind, placebo-controlled crossover trial of feverfew preparation. Phytomedicine 3:225, 1996.
Eisenberg D. Unconventional medicine in the U.S. N Engl J Med 328:246, 1993.
Pizzorno JP, Murray M. Encyclopedia of Natural Medicine. Rocklin, CA: Prima Publishing, 1991.
Schoenberger D. The influence of immune-stimulating effects of pressed juice from *Echinacea purpurea* on the course and severity of colds. Forum Immunol 8:2, 1992.
Weiner M. The Complete Book of Homeopathy. Garden City Park, NY: Avery Publishing, 1989.
Weiss RF. Herbal Medicine, 6th ed. Sweden: Ab Arcanum, 1988.
Wren RC. Potter's New Cyclopaedia of Botanical Drugs and Preparations. Saffron Walden: CW Daniel Co., 1985.

CHAPTER 20

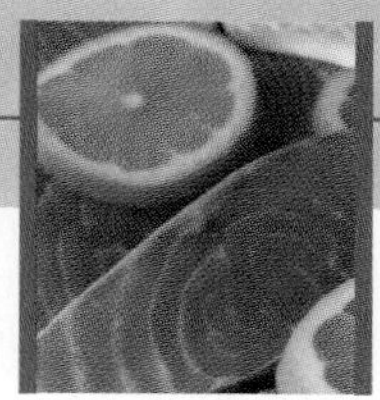

The Nutritional Care Process

CYNTHIA BRYLINSKY, MS, RD

Chapter Outline

- Nutritional Care Process
- Charting and Documentation
- Nutritional Intervention and Diet Modification
- Nutritional Care for the Hospitalized Patient

Key Terms

ADVANCE DIRECTIVES—guidelines established by a patient allowing a designated person(s) to make medical decisions if the patient loses decision-making capabilities; may include items such as use of mechanical ventilation or feeding tubes
CASE MANAGEMENT—process of achieving patient care goals in a timely, efficient, cost-effective manner
CLEAR LIQUID DIET—a diet consisting of clear liquids that should be used only for a short time as it is generally nutritionally inadequate; usually used in preparation for surgery or during periods of nausea or vomiting
DIET PRESCRIPTION—designates the type, amount, and frequency of feeding; may include amounts and forms of protein, carbohydrate, fat, fluid, vitamins, and minerals
DISCHARGE PLANNING—team planning for necessary education, counseling, and resources needed by the patient
DISEASE MANAGEMENT—a disease-specific approach to patient care, primarily in outpatient settings
FULL LIQUID DIET—a diet composed of foods that are liquid at room or body temperature; used when solid foods are not tolerated
JOINT COMMISSION ON ACCREDITATION OF HEALTHCARE ORGANIZATIONS (JCAHO)—a peer review organization that evaluates health care institutions and ranks their compliance with established standards
MEDICAL NUTRITIONAL THERAPY PROTOCOLS—preestablished, standardized guidelines that provide step-by-step instructions for providing nutritional care
NUTRITIONAL ASSESSMENT—the process by which the nutritional status of an individual is determined; usually includes dietary history and intake data, laboratory data, clinical examination and health history, anthropometric data, and psychosocial data
NUTRITIONAL CARE PROCESS—the process of planning for and meeting the nutritional needs of an individual
NUTRITIONAL CARE RECORD—written documentation of the nutritional care process, including the interventions and activities used to meet the nutritional objectives
PATIENT-CENTERED OBJECTIVE—a goal that is stated in terms of what the patient will achieve or be able to do when the objective is met
PATIENT-FOCUSED CARE—care that is rendered with the patient as the central figure of the team, the "customer" of health services
PREFERRED PROVIDER ORGANIZATION (PPO)—an organization that has negotiated a contract that specifies health care services for a specific population group
SOFT DIET—an adequate diet that is moderately low in cellulose, connective tissue, and residue; usually prescribed for conditions in which mechanical ease in eating or digestion is desired
STANDARDS OF CARE—practice guidelines that are established by a facility to ensure that, at a minimum, reasonable care is rendered
UTILIZATION MANAGEMENT—cost-efficient patient care management with a focus on reducing excessive use of diagnostic or therapeutic tests, procedures, or services

NUTRITIONAL CARE PROCESS

Nutritional care is an organized group of activities allowing identification of nutritional needs and provision of care to meet these needs. The **nutritional care process** consists of (1) assessing nutritional status, (2) analyzing data to identify nutritional needs or problems, (3) planning and prioritizing objectives of nutritional care to meet these needs, (4) implementing strategies necessary to meet the objectives, and (5) evaluating the nutritional care outcomes (American Dietetic Association, 1994).

Nutritional care for a healthy person differs from the care provided for an ill or hospitalized patient. The type of care provided depends on the presence of disease or potential disease, the environment, the state of growth and development of the individual, and socioeconomic issues. It may include an assessment of the adequacy of nutritional intake, manipulation of the diet, provision of enteral or parenteral support, and intervention in the form of counseling or education. In most cases, institutions will have established standards of care or practice guidelines that describe recommended steps in the nutritional care process (see Fig. 20–1). These standards often serve as a basis for assessing the quality of care provided to the patient.

Thorough nutritional care involves many disciplines; the physician, dietitian, nurse, pharmacist, social worker, case manager, and other care providers may all be integral in achieving desired outcomes depending on the care setting. A collaborative approach helps to ensure that care is coordinated and that all team members are aware of patient care goals and priorities. Coordinating the activities of health care professionals requires documentation of the process, as well as regular discussions to allow for the communication and interaction necessary for complete nutritional care (Fig. 20–2). Patients benefit from interdisciplinary decision making regarding nutritional and medical concerns. Team conferences, formal or informal, are useful in many settings, such as home care, nursing homes, or hospitals.

Identification of Nutritional Risk

Both overnutrition and undernutrition have been shown to impact negatively on the response of a patient to medical treatment. Malnutrition has been shown to increase morbidity, length of hospital stay, and mortality. To facilitate identification of patients at nutritional risk, *nutritional screening* is used. Nutritional screening can be done for patients regardless of the setting (hospital, nursing home, or clinic) or the age of the individual (infant, adolescent, or geriatric). Nutritional screening involves using simple assessment techniques to identify patients who would benefit from more intensive nutritional assessment. Screening should be repeated during the course of the patient's stay, as nutritional risk increases in patients who are hospitalized for 2 weeks or longer. Reassessment helps to determine whether changes in diagnosis or condition have occurred that place the patient at risk nutritionally.

Nutritional screening should be quick and efficient and be able to be performed by a member of the health care team. The person(s) administering

STANDARDS OF CARE FOR THE GENERAL PATIENT

Threshold	Data Base	Plan	Documentation	Exceptions
	1. Review medical record within 3 days			
95%	a) Diet order 1. Diet prior to admission 2. Appetite or % intake	a1) Assess appropriateness of diet order a2) Evaluate adequacy of intake/acceptance of diet if appropriate	a) Document if diet order inappropriate	Data Unavailable Weekend or Holiday
	b) Physical Data 1. Height 2. Weight History 3 Usual Weight c) Diagnosis-med history d) Lab values 1. Albumin 2. Others as appropriate e) Medications impacting nutritional status	b-e) Evaluate appropriate data in terms of patients nutrition status	b-e) Document evaluation of data if needed for intervention	
100%	2. Determine need for intervention		Request Consult	No Consult Received
	a) Education	a) Nutrition Counseling Service referral	a-c) Document intervention and outcome	
	b) Poor Intake	Recommend if appropriate: b1) Supplementation b2) Calorie Count b3) Alternate	(Refer to calorie count and TF/TPN policies)	
	c) No intervention needed	c) Rescreen in 7 days		
100%	3. Review patient's nutritional status and response to changes in data and/or patient condition	Evaluate and adjust accordingly	Document evaluation and adjustments in care plan	

FIGURE 20–1 Sample standards of care for a general patient population. The threshold is the level below which services are considered to be substandard. (Courtesy of Barnes Hospital, St. Louis, MO.)
IF, intravenous fluid; *TPN,* total parenteral nutrition; *IBW,* ideal body weight; *PMH,* past medical history.

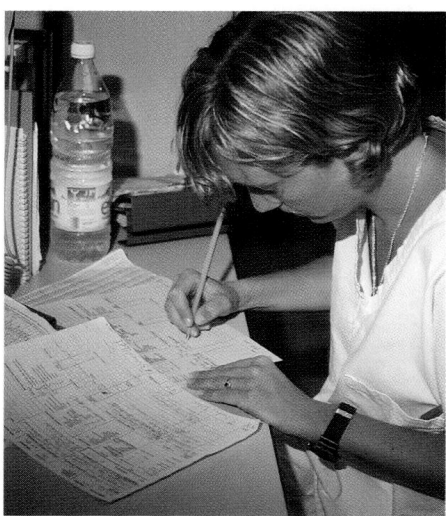

FIGURE 20–2 Dietitian documenting nutritional care. (From Leahy J, Kisilay P. Foundations of Nursing Practice: A Nursing Process Approach. Philadelphia: WB Saunders, 1998.)

the screen will vary depending on the setting in which the screening is taking place. Patients identified as being "at risk" during the initial screening process should have their nutritional status reviewed by a registered dietitian. Table 20–1 lists information that is frequently included in a nutritional screen. Information included on the screen will vary according to the nature of the individual being screened, but it is information that is easy to gather at the facility conducting the screen. Chapter 16 provides additional information about the screening process. A good screening program can be a valuable tool in providing cost-effective and appropriate care to patients.

Nutritional Care Plan

The *nutritional care plan* consists of a nutritional assessment; identification of nutritional problems; development of a plan with specific objectives, including education and other interventions; implementation of the plan; and determination of a means for evaluating the results. Documentation is important in all aspects of the care plan; it assures communication to all disciplines involved in the care of the patient.

TABLE 20–1 NUTRITIONAL SCREENING INFORMATION

Age
Height
Usual weight
Ideal weight
Present weight
Percentage weight change from the ideal or usual weight
Change in appetite
Dysphagia or difficulty with chewing
Presence of nausea, vomiting, or diarrhea
Serum albumin level
Hemoglobin and hematocrit values
Total lymphocyte count

Assessment

Assessment involves the gathering and evaluation of information. The identification of nutritional problems (present and potential) evolves naturally from a thorough **nutritional assessment.** Table 20–2 defines nutritional screening and assessment according to categories of risk. A complete discussion of nutritional assessment techniques appears in Chapter 16 and Chapter 17.

An assessment of nutritional status is made from these data, and any problems or needs are identified, prioritized, and documented in the medical record. Many facilities utilize standardized formats to facilitate communication of this information (see Figure 20–3).

The following is an example of a nutritional assessment with identification of nutritional problems:

Case Presentation

DA is a 20-year-old white woman with diabetes. A review of the patient's health record, laboratory data, anthropometric data, and nutritional history reveals the need for further nutritional management.

Laboratory Data

- Elevated fasting blood glucose level: 193 mg/dL
- Glycosylated hemoglobin: 9.6% ($HgbA_1C$)—elevated
- Episodes of hypoglycemia; blood glucose levels of 50–60 mg/dL

Anthropometric Data

- Height: 65″
- Weight: 108 lb (down 10% from usual weight of 118 lb in 3 months)
- Triceps skinfold thickness: 12 mm (below standard)

Dietary Data

- Caloric intake: 1400 kcal/day (less than energy needs)
- Meals: irregular throughout the day; drinks coffee frequently

Medical History

- Diagnosed 1 year ago as having Type 1 diabetes mellitus; was given little instruction about nutri-

TABLE 20–2 DEFINITIONS FOR NUTRITIONAL SCREENING AND ASSESSMENT*

FOOD AND NUTRIENT INTAKE PATTERNS	PSYCHOLOGICAL AND/OR SOCIAL FACTORS	LABORATORY VALUES	MEDICATIONS	PHYSICAL CONDITIONS AND DISEASES/ DISORDERS
The potential risk category involving food and nutrient intake patterns is based on a history of or evidence of the following risk factors: Intake less than or greater than the standard, for age and activity level, for caloric intake and protein intake Intake less than or greater than the standard for age for nutrients (e.g., vitamins and minerals, such as zinc, iron, folate, and vitamin B_{12}) Dysphagia Changes in sensory perceptions, such as taste and smell Dental problems (e.g., difficulty chewing, ill-fitting dentures, refusal to wear dentures, missing teeth) Nausea/vomiting Cultural factors or religious food habits that` result in limited intake of desired nutrients Unusual food habits (e.g., pica, faddism, meal skipping) Physician's order of nothing by mouth or a clear liquid diet for more than 5 days without tube feeding or total parenteral nutrition/peripheral parenteral nutrition Problems with the oral cavity (e.g., lesions on the gums or in the mouth) Unwillingness or inability to ingest food (e.g., impaired feeding skills or lack of ability to feed self) Changes in functional status (i.e., an increase or decrease in ADL) Inappropriate supplement use (e.g., vitamins, minerals, and/or fortified food products) Inadequate transitional feeding and/or tube feeding or total parenteral nutrition	The potential risk category involving psychological and/or social factors is based on a history of or evidence of the following risk factors: Literacy level or language barriers Cultural factors that alter intake of desired nutrients, calories, or food groups Religious beliefs that alter intake of desired nutrients, calories, or food groups Emotional disturbances (e.g., depression, stress) with associated feeding problems Inadequate or absent caregiver/social support system Social isolation (motivational level for self-care) Eating or feeding disorders (e.g., bulimia, early satiety, autism, rapid pace of eating) Limited resources for food preparation or limited access to transportation to obtain food Substance/alcohol abuse Limited or low income (i.e., below poverty level) Limited ability/use/knowledge of normal nutrition, food preparation, food safety and/or community resources Lack of ability to communicate needs (e.g., dyspraxia)	The potential risk category involving abnormal laboratory values should be considered in terms of age-specific norms (pediatric, adult, and geriatric). It is based on a history of or evidence of the following risk factors: Abnormal serum albumin, transferrin, or lipid levels (i.e., cholesterol, high-density lipoproteins, low-density lipoproteins) or abnormal triglyceride values Abnormal phosphorus Abnormal hemoglobin, hematocrit, iron values (where appropriate) Abnormal blood urea nitrogen, creatinine, electrolyte levels Abnormal fasting blood glucose levels Other abnormal laboratory values depending upon the condition	The potential risk category involving medications is based on a history of or evidence of the following risk factors: Chronic use of medications (e.g., laxatives) Multiple and concurrent medication use (i.e., polypharmacy) Drug-nutrient interactions and side effects (e.g., affecting food intake or causing anorexia or nausea)	The potential risk category involving physical conditions and diseases/disorders is based on a history of or evidence of the following risk factors: Pressure ulcers or altered skin integrity Excessive activity level Immobility (due to dependency, disability, or impairment in performance of activities of daily living [ADL]) Cancer and its treatments AIDS or human immunodeficiency virus (HIV) infection Gastrointestinal complications (e.g., malabsorption, diarrhea, digestion, bowel changes) Catabolic or hypermetabolic conditions (e.g., burns, surgery) Physical signs (e.g., alopecia) Food allergies Alterations in anthropometric measures, weight, or body mass index, including recent significant changes; marked overweight or underweight for height and age; midarm muscle circumference/triceps skinfold measurements as appropriate; amputation; length, height, and head circumference measurements Declining sensory function (e.g., loss of smell, taste, vision) Fat or muscle wasting (including cachexia) Obesity/overweight Chronic renal or cardiac problems, diabetes and related complications, hypertension Osteoporosis or osteomalacia Fluid and/or electrolyte imbalance

(continued)

TABLE 20–2 DEFINITIONS FOR NUTRITIONAL SCREENING AND ASSESSMENT* (continued)

FOOD AND NUTRIENT INTAKE PATTERNS	PSYCHOLOGICAL AND/OR SOCIAL FACTORS	LABORATORY VALUES	MEDICATIONS	PHYSICAL CONDITIONS AND DISEASES/ DISORDERS
Minimal or no intake of foods from a major food group				Neurologic impairment
Constipation or diarrhea				Visual impairment
Restricted diets				Other acute and chronic disorders
Literacy level which limits planning				Extremes in age (e.g., older than 80 years of age, very young, premature infant)
Fluid intake less than output				Adolescent pregnancy, closely spaced pregnancies, or three or more pregnancies
Feeding limitations (e.g., inability to drink from a cup, need for special utensils)				

Reprinted by permission from the American Dietetic Association, the Journal of The American Dietetic Association, 94:838, 1994.

*Nutritional screening is the process of identifying risk factors known to be associated with nutritional problems. Nutritional assessment is a comprehensive approach, used by the registered dietitian, to define the nutritional status of an individual. The screening and risk assessments may include any or all of the parameters in this table.

tional management of diabetes; has hypoglycemic episodes

- Taking two injections of insulin daily: 28 units NPH and 4 units regular in the morning, and 6 units NPH and 4 units regular in the evening

Psychosocial Data

DA lives at home, attends college, and has a part-time job. She rarely eats a meal per se.

NUTRITIONAL ASSESSMENT

DA, although diagnosed 1 year ago as having type 1 diabetes mellitus, is not in good control, does not completely understand the influence of diet on her disease, and does not take much interest in it because of her numerous other activities. She has been consuming fewer calories than she requires, and does not follow a regular meal plan. Her medical problem can be described as type 1 diabetes mellitus in poor control. More specifically, her nutritional problems consist of (1) hyperglycemic and hypoglycemic episodes related to poor control of diabetes mellitus, (2) weight loss, and (3) inadequate knowledge or understanding of appropriate nutritional management of diabetes.

Development of a Plan/Objectives for Nutritional Care

Identification of nutritional problems leads to formulating a plan for dealing with each of the problems individually, with greatest attention being paid to the problem(s) of highest priority. If the nutritional information is not complete, the first objective is to collect the necessary data. To facilitate change, goals must be agreeable to those involved. In the case of a patient being tube-fed, the dietitian and physician should discuss the amount of fluid that can be provided by the tube feeding. If the dietitian were to establish this goal without consulting with the physician, a recommendation might be made which would not be acceptable. In the education process, goals must be established mutually by both the client and the counselor, and they must be achievable. For example, one objective in the case above might be to find out when DA's hypoglycemic episodes occur and the frequency of their occurrence, then setting a goal to manage them.

The objectives should be in behavioral form and stated in terms of what the patient will achieve if the objectives are met. For example, a **patient-centered objective** would be: "DA will be able to identify carbohydrate-containing foods and plan meals with consistent carbohydrate content after instruction." This is more appropriately stated than "I will teach DA how to identify carbohydrate-containing foods and plan meals with consistent carbohydrate content." In the latter form, the objective identifies what needs to be done, but does not make the counselor or DA responsible for learning.

Objectives should be realistic and appropriate. They should consider the educational level and the economic and social resources of the patient and or family. They should also be stated in quantifiable terms to facilitate evaluation.

The objectives for the three nutritional problems identified for DA might be stated as follows:

PROBLEM 1. Hypoglycemic episodes

Objectives: (1) The timing and cause of hypoglycemic episodes will be identified by DA and the nutrition counselor. (2) DA will demonstrate an understanding of hypoglycemia through a verbal explanation of why it happens, what her body needs

CLINIC NOTES
NUTRITION SERVICES
Penn State Geisinger Health System

☐ Geisinger Medical Center Danville, PA 17822 ☐ Penn State Geisinger Wyoming Valley Medical Center

☐ Penn State Geisinger Health Group

Date: ____________

Referring Physician: ____________ Service: ____________

Primary Care Physician (if different): ____________

S: ____________

Weight Hx: ____________ Weight Goal: ____________

Activity: ____________ Supplements: ____________

Prior Nutrition Counseling: ____________

O: Age/Sex: ______ Height: ______ Weight: ______ Body Mass Index: ______

Ideal Body Weight: ______ % Ideal Body Weight: ______

Energy needs: ____________

Diagnosis: ____________ PMH: ____________

Medications: ____________ Other Significant Information: ____________

Labs: ____________

Diet Instruction: ____________ Videos: ____________

Handouts: ____________

A: ____________

Patient's Comprehension:
☐ Poor: Demonstrated limited understanding.
☐ Basic: Can explain rationale of diet; can identify foods to limit.
☐ Comprehensive: Can plan sample menus using diet modifications; Can effectively evaluate how to incorporate changes into lifestyle.

Expected Outcome:
☐ Demonstrated no interest in learning; expect minimal changes.
☐ Expect attempts at changing eating habits.
☐ Patient very motivated. Expect adherence to diet.

Patient Goals: ____________

P: Nutrition Services phone number was made available to patient.
☐ Return appointment recommended but patient declined.
☐ No return appointment necessary.
☐ Return in ______ to review ____________
☐ Other ____________

Signature/Title: ____________

#A-260-179-FMR Rev. 8/97js Approved MRPC: 8/97 *White - Medical Record* *Yellow - Physician*

FIGURE 20–3 Sample form to simplify charting. (Reprinted by permission of Geisinger Medical Center, Danville, PA.)

when it does happen, and how it can be prevented. (3) DA will modify her diet and/or insulin in such a manner as to avoid hypoglycemia.

PROBLEM 2. Weight loss

Objectives: (1) DA will stop losing weight, and begin to slowly gain weight up to 118 lb. (2) DA will demonstrate continued weight maintenance/gain at check-ups.

PROBLEM 3. Lack of knowledge about proper eating patterns for blood glucose control

Objectives: (1) DA will demonstrate knowledge of the relationship of food intake and insulin to blood glucose level by verbal review with the counselor. (2) DA will demonstrate an understanding of the principles of her eating plan by writing several days of sample menus.

Implementation of Nutritional Care

Implementation can begin once the objectives are determined. Implementation is the part of the nutritional care process that translates assessment data into strategies, activities, or interventions that will enable the patient or client to meet the objectives established. This might include changing the diet prescription, counseling the patient, providing food or nutritional supplements, implementing a tube feeding for a patient who cannot eat, or providing information on financial or food resources. The care process is a continuous one; the initial plan may change as the condition of the patient changes or as new needs are identified.

Interventions should be specific; they are the

"what, where, when and how" of the care plan. For example, in a patient with anorexia, an objective might be an increase in caloric intake. This would be implemented through provision of high-calorie, high-protein foods via small, frequent meals and snacks; or through provision of a supplement or milkshake between meals. Intervention plans must be communicated with the entire health care team and the patient to ensure that optimal care is being provided. In this role as an "intervention specialist" (Insull, 1992), the dietitian increases the likelihood of adherence to the plan. See Chapter 21 for information regarding counseling intervention strategies.

Referring again to DA, the nutritional interventions for each objective might be stated as follows:

FOR HYPOGLYCEMIA. The timing and cause of hypoglycemic episodes will be identified by DA and by the nutrition counselor.

Intervention: DA will learn and be able to conduct self–blood glucose monitoring (SBGM) and perform it at least four times per day, especially when she feels "shaky."

Intervention: DA will keep a log of the results of her SBGM to help pinpoint causes of the hypoglycemic episodes.

FOR UNDERWEIGHT. DA will maintain her weight and slowly regain her usual weight of 118 lb.

Intervention: DA will increase her energy intake to 2000 kcal/day, and complete a 3-day food record for analysis of adequacy.

FOR DIET COUNSELING. DA will demonstrate an understanding of the principles of her meal plan.

Intervention: DA will be taught how to select a diet appropriate in calories and carbohydrates using carbohydrate counting.

Intervention: DA will complete a 3-day food record, which will be analyzed by the counselor.

This process of defining interventions is continued for every objective of each problem. In the case being discussed, care must be taken not to overwhelm the patient, but rather to implement changes incrementally as success is achieved. Focusing on high-priority objectives and formulating short-term and long-term goals can help to make the problem list more manageable. The interventions just described would be implemented over several counseling sessions to allow the patient to focus her efforts on the items of highest priority. Once a high-priority intervention has been successfully accomplished, additional changes would be pursued.

Evaluation of Nutritional Care

The last step in the nutritional care process is to evaluate the care provided. This step makes the nutritional care plan dynamic and responsive to the patient's needs. If objectives have been written in measurable behavioral terms, evaluation is relatively easy, as new behavior is being measured against a behavior that has already been defined. For example, an evaluation might be: "DA was not able to conduct self–blood glucose monitoring four times a day because she was unable to purchase supplies due to their expense." A revision in the care plan at this point might include the following: "DA will be provided with supplies for a 1-week period to enable her to complete self–blood glucose monitoring; other sources of funding for supplies will be pursued." This new intervention is then implemented and evaluated to determine whether the objective was met.

The goal of nutritional care is to meet the nutritional requirements of the patient; thus, the objectives must be reviewed frequently to ensure that unmet objectives are addressed and that care is evaluated and modified as needed. When the evaluation reveals that objectives are not being met or that new needs have arisen, the process begins again with reassessment, identification of new needs, and formulation of a new nutritional care plan.

EXAMPLE. For a patient with anorexia, supplements have been provided. Evaluation of this intervention reveals that the patient has developed a dislike of the current supplement and has stopped drinking it. A taste test of products available in the facility is conducted and the patient agrees to change to a different supplement and to receive smaller, more frequent portions. Further review will be needed to ascertain if the change in supplement/method of delivery improves intake.

Table 20–3 summarizes the nutritional care process, including the criteria necessary for each step.

Nutritional Care Record

The nutritional care process, as applied to an individual in either a hospital or an outpatient setting, must be documented in the health or medical record. The medical record is a legal document; if it is not recorded, it "was not done." Documentation has the following advantages:

1. It helps to ensure that nutritional care will be relevant, complete, and effective by providing a record that identifies the problems and sets criteria for evaluating the care.
2. It allows the entire health care team to understand the rationale for nutritional care, the means by which it will be provided, and what each team member's role is in its success.
3. It allows the health care team to participate in the nutritional care and to reinforce the plan whenever there is an opportunity.
4. Notes in the medical record serve as a communication tool, verifying important information for evaluation of health care delivery, as well as for accreditation and peer review (see "*Focus On:* Joint Commission on Accreditation of Healthcare Organizations").

Much of the information needed to develop a nutritional care plan is collected routinely by various

TABLE 20–3 NUTRITIONAL CARE PROCESS

STEPS	COMPONENTS	FACTORS TO CONSIDER
1. Assessment of Nutritional Status Collect information (database). Identify problems.	Diet history Biochemical data Clinical examination findings Medical history Anthropometric data Psychosocial data	The information should be accurate, pertinent to the patient, and appropriately interpreted. The problems identified should be the same as those in the medical record, given priority ratings in the order of their importance, related to assessment data, and should include present and potential problems.
2. Analysis of Data to Identify Nutritional Needs	Organize and evaluate available information.	Professional judgment must be used to analyze information.
3. Planning for Nutritional Care Set objectives.	Collect additional necessary information. Identify available resources. Assess the educational level of the patient and family. Modify dietary intake. Supplement nutrient intake. Institute measures to enable patient to meet nutritional requirements. Treat medical problems affecting nutritional status.	Objectives should be patient-centered, stated in behavioral terms, realistic, measurable, and designated as short- or long-term.
4. Implementation of Nutritional Care Determine nutritional interventions.	Modify intake, as required, to make it acceptable to the patient. Teach the patient and family about the nutritional care plan. Provide necessary nutritional supplements and alternative forms of nutritional support. Resolve health problems. Provide assistance in obtaining food.	Interventions should specifically relate to the problem and objective, be individualized for each patient, and be specific in describing what, how, why, when, and where.
5. Evaluation of Nutritional Care Determine the effectiveness of nutritional care and change the nutritional care plan if necessary.	Monitor food and fluid intake; evaluate intake for adequacy in meeting patient's nutritional needs. Assess nutritional knowledge of the patient/family as reflected by behavioral (food choice) change. Monitor biochemical data related to nutritional status. Monitor anthropometric data. Monitor the patient's clinical condition.	Evaluation should include a comparison between observed behavior and expected behavior, a determination of the effectiveness of intervention in meeting objectives, an explanation of the effectiveness or ineffectiveness of intervention, and suggestions for revising the care plan based on evaluation.

health professionals, including physicians, nurses, dietitians, pharmacists, case managers, and social workers. For example, a physician completes a medical history, including information about the gastrointestinal tract, medications, weight loss, and other relevant factors; and a nurse usually weighs and measures the patient and asks about food allergies. Social workers may ask about the economic issues related to food and the patient's living conditions. The **nutritional care record** ensures that all aspects of nutritional care are summarized in one place as part of the total health record. Parts of this information may be incorporated into the nursing care plan, which is a detailed record kept by the nurse, and summarized periodically for inclusion in the medical record.

A detailed care record may be kept by the clinical dietitian, but if this is the case, the information it contains should be summarized periodically in the permanent health record, as shown in Figure 20–2. The detailed information may be important for hospital care audits, professional standards reviews, patient education, and other efforts to maintain quality health care. Figure 20–4 is an example of a nutritional care record.

CHARTING AND DOCUMENTATION*

The purpose of the medical record is to serve as a tool for communication among members of the health care team. It is a continuous account of hospitalizations and clinic visits and typically includes sections on physician orders, medical history and physical examinations, laboratory test results, consults, and progress and prognosis of the patient. It also serves as the basis for evaluating the care that

*This section was previously contributed by Susan DeHoog, RD.

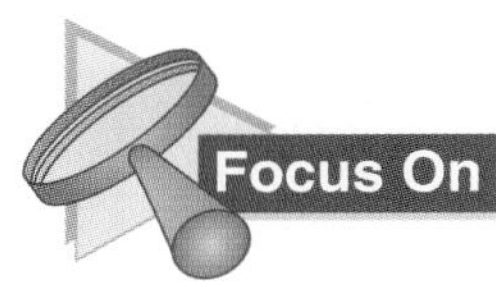

Joint Commission on Accreditation of Healthcare Organizations (JCAHO)

The Joint Commission on Accreditation of Healthcare Organizations (JCAHO) is a large health care accrediting organization. It seeks to improve the quality of patient care in various health settings, such as hospitals, long-term care organizations, home care organizations, ambulatory care organizations, and organizations that offer mental health services. This is accomplished through a set of standards, to which adherence is measured by a formal survey and evaluation of a facility. Accreditation by JCAHO is voluntary, but is highly regarded in terms of its impact on third-party payment and its effect on confidence rating by the community, physician recruitment, and fulfillment of portions of state/federal licensure/certification requirements.

Accreditation focuses on the actual facility's performance of important governance, managerial, clinical, and support functions (i.e., those functions that directly affect the delivery of quality patient care). It also focuses on the continual improvement in an organization's performance of these functions. Standards are provided in an "Accreditation Manual for Hospitals" document, which is updated and revised on a yearly basis. This document consists of three sections: (1) Care of the Patient, (2) Organizational Functions, and (3) Structures with Important Functions. Its approach is a functional one, and all departments and disciplines need to be familiar with relevant issues found in applicable chapters. Most chapters contain standards that affect the care provided by a dietitian.

The section on "Care of the Patient" contains standards that apply specifically to medication use, rehabilitation, anesthesia, operative and other invasive procedures, and special treatments, and it includes nutritional care standards. The focus of nutritional care standards is the provision of appropriate nutritional care in a timely and effective manner using an interdisciplinary approach (i.e., with the involvement of physicians, registered dietitians, nurses, pharmacists, and other disciplines as appropriate). Appropriate care is considered to include screening of patients for nutritional need, assessment and reassessment of patient needs, development of a nutritional care plan, ordering and communication of the diet order, preparation and distribution of the diet order, monitoring of the process, and continual reassessment and improvement of the nutritional care process. A facility can define who, when, where, and how the process is accomplished, but JCAHO does specify that a qualified dietitian must be involved in establishing this process. A plan for the delivery of nutritional care may be as simple as providing a regular diet for a patient who is not at nutritional risk, or as complex as managing tube feedings in a ventilator-dependent patient, which involves the collaboration of multiple disciplines.

The accreditation process typically involves a survey process that lasts for several days. During this survey, adherence to standards is ascertained through interviews, review of documents (including patient medical records) and visits to patient care and other areas. Dietitians are actively involved in the survey process. Standards set by JCAHO play a large role in influencing the standards of care delivered to patients in all health care disciplines.

For more information, see website www.jcaho.org.

is delivered. The dietitian provides written communication on nutritional status, assessment regarding nutrition support or education for patients and family, and communication about goals of nutritional therapy as information for other professionals. The following are guidelines for documentation:

1. Medical records are permanent legal documents; therefore, all entries should be written in black pen or typewritten. No soft felt pens, multicolored pens, or pencils should be used.
2. Documentation should be complete, clear, concise, legible, and accurate.
3. Entries should be documented by service, date, and time. Each medical record page should be identified by the patient's stamp or written name and hospital number.
4. Entries should be in chronological order and on consecutive lines.
5. The first word of every statement should be capitalized, with periods placed at the end of each thought. Complete sentences are not necessary, but grammar and spelling should be correct.
6. All entries should be consistent and noncontradictory.
7. Abbreviations with multiple meanings should be avoided. Institutions generally have a document defining acceptable use of abbreviations.
8. All entries must be signed at the end of the chart note.
9. No one should ever chart or sign the medical record for another individual.
10. Charting must be objective.
11. Charting must be specific. Many words can have different meanings.
12. Personal opinions and comments criticizing or casting doubt on the professionalism of others should never be included in the chart.
13. Documentation must be done at the time of the actual procedure or service. The frequency depends on the patient's degree of illness, the therapies administered, and standards of care.
14. Late entries should be identified as such, including the actual date and time of the entry and the date and time it should have been recorded.

NUTRITIONAL CARE RECORD

Rm. No. ____
Name ____
Address and Phone No. ____

Age ____ Sex ____

Problem List

ASSESSMENT—Data Base

Diet HX ____ Date
24 Hr. Recall

Allergies:
Use of sugar: ☐ salt: ☐
Use of alcohol: ☐ none ___ occas. ___ oz. ___ often
Fluid intake ____

Feeding and G.I. Habits
Consistency of food:
Appetite:
Bowel habits:
Recent changes in eating habits:
Recent wgt. chngs.:
Dental condition:

Evaluation of Intake
P ____
F ____
C ____

Cal. ____ ____ ____
____ ____ ____
____ ____ ____

Medications/Vits. & Mins./Supplements

	Date		Date	

Medical HX & Clinical Findings

Biochemical Findings

Social HX

Activities
Occup.: ____
Exercise ____ hr./wk.

Anthropometry
Triceps skinfold thickness
Arm circumf.: %Body fat:
Arm muscle circumf.:

Frame type: S M L
IBW: Surface area:

Hgt.: Wgt.:

Patient's Wgt. goal:

Usual wgt.: % Usual wgt.:

Nutritional Care Flow Sheet: Weights, Lab Values, I & O

	Dates									
Serum transferrin or serum pre-albumin or serum retinol-binding protein										
Wgt.										
Cal:N ratio										
Intake–tray pro./kcal.										
Intake–Supps. pro./kcal.										
Intake–P. Vein pro./kcal.										
Intake–C. Vein pro./kcal.										
Urine cc./24 hr.										
Stools Avg./24 hr.										

NUTRITIONAL CARE PLAN

Basal Energy Expenditure: ____ kcal.
Anabolic Req.: ____ kcal. ____ gm. pro. ____ gm. N
Maintenance Req.: ____ kcal. ____ gm. pro. ____ gm. N

Diet Calculation ____ kcal.
CHO = Pro = Fat = Na^+ =

Time					
Milk					
Meat					
Bread					
Fruit					
Fat					
Veg.					
Misc. CHO					
Total P F C	P F C	P F C	P F C	P F C	P F C

EVALUATION OF NUTRITIONAL CARE—PROGRESS NOTES

Date

RECOMMENDATIONS FOR FOLLOW-UP

FIGURE 20–4 The nutritional care record shows assessment data, the nutritional care plan, intervention strategies, and monitoring and evaluation data.
I&O, intake and output; *IBW,* ideal body weight; *cal.,* calories; *Req.,* requirement; *PFC,* patient focused care; *DTR,* Dietetic Technician Registered; *RD,* registered dietitian; *TF,* tube feeding; *TPN,* total parenteral nutrition; *NPO,* nothing by mouth.

NUTRITION RISK ASSESSMENT

Date ____________
Time ____________

O. Admit date ____________ Diagnosis ____________
Ht. ________ Wt. ________ Sex: F M %IBW ____________
Albumin (date) ____________ Other pertinent labs: ____________
Diet order ____________

A. Nutritional Status
________ Insufficient data to complete risk assessment.
________ No detectable risk at this time.
________ At risk based on available data.
________ Potential for nutritional risk 2° to ____________.
________ ____________.

P. ________ Will reattempt reassessment within the next five days.
________ No identified need for nutrition intervention at this time. Patient will be reassessed in 7-10 days.
________ Patient will be assessed according to department standards (see below) and care plan recommendations and goals will be placed in the progress notes. (See Progress Notes Section.)
________ ____________
________ ____________, R.D.

Followup Risk Assessment (See P. above)

Date	Not at Risk	At Risk	Comments	R.D.	Date	Not at Risk	At Risk	Comments	R.D.

COMPREHENSIVE NUTRITION ASSESSMENT

Date ____________
Time ____________

S. Usual wt. ____________ % Wt. change/time ____________
Diet PTA ____________ Previous diet educ. ____________
Eating/Digestive related problems: ____________
Other: ____________

O. PMH ____________
Pertinent labs ____________
Pertinent meds ____________
Other ____________

A. Assessment of visceral protein stores:
adequate ________ unable to assess ________
mild depletion ________ moderate depletion ________
severe depletion ________
Estimate needs: KCAL = HB (   ) x SF (   ) = ____________
protein = ____________
other nutrients ____________
Additional Comments ____________
____
____

P. **See Nutrition Note in Progress Notes Section**
____________, R.D.

CAROLINAS
MEDICAL CENTER

DEPARTMENT OF DIETETICS
ADULT NUTRITION ASSESSMENT/REASSESSMENT
DO NOT THIN

2888
D(0195)CS

ADDRESSOGRAPH PLATE

FIGURE 20–5 A nutritional chart format that includes both screening and assessment information. PTA, prior to admission; PMH, past medical history; HB, Harris-Benedict; SF, stress factor. (Courtesy of Carolinas Medical Center.)

Medical record entries should always be legible. If an error is made, apply the following guidelines:

I. When making a correction, NEVER
   - A. Use White-Out, correction tape, or self-adhesive labels.
   - B. Obliterate an entry by use of a thick marker or pen strokes.
   - C. Add notes after the fact without accurately authenticating, dating, and referencing the original entry.
   - D. Remove the original and replace it with a copy.

II. When performing corrections at the time an entry is in progress
   - A. Minor errors in transcription, spelling, one word, etc.
     1. The person who made the initial entry should correct the error.
     2. A single line should be drawn through the correction; the correction should then be entered, initialed, and dated.
   - B. Other errors (e.g., an entry in the wrong chart)
     1. One line should be drawn through the entry, or an X made through the paragraph or page in error.
     2. Note "error" plus the date and time. Initial the correction.
        Example: error 04/24/99 0900 S.D.
        ~~The patient would not respond to questions regarding self-induced vomiting.~~
        (Continue entry and sign.)
   - C. Omitted information
     1. Beside the original entry, note "See addendum," enter the date, and initial.
     2. Write the addendum in chart sequence. Identify it as an addendum and reference the original entry (e.g., "4/29/99 0900 Addendum to (progress) note of 4/28/99"). Continue entry and sign.

III. Corrections performed some time since the original entry (e.g., because an interval of time has elapsed during which the chart has been out of the recorder's possession)
   - A. Minor errors in transcription, spelling, one word, etc.
     1. Errors should be corrected by the person who made the error.
     2. A single line should be drawn through the error, followed by the correction, date, time, and signature.
   - B. Other errors, test results, misquoted orders, entry in wrong chart, etc.
     1. An error should be corrected by the person who made the error.
     2. One line should be drawn through the entry or an X through the section or page.
     3. Note "error" plus the date and time. Sign the correction.

A format frequently used for medical record documentation is the problem-oriented record. This record is organized according to the patient's primary problems. Entries into the medical record can be done in many styles. One of the most common forms is the SOAP note (Subjective, Objective, Assessment, and Plan), an example of which follows.

SUBJECTIVE

- Information provided by patient, family, or significant other
- Significant nutritional history
- Pertinent socioeconomic, cultural information
- Level of physical activity
- Current dietary intake (in terms of nutrients)

OBJECTIVE

- Factual, reproducible observations (i.e., anthropometric and laboratory data)
- Height, weight, or weight gain patterns, and age
- Desirable weight or a realistic goal
- Pertinent laboratory data
- Diet order
- Pertinent medications
- Calculation of nutrient needs

ASSESSMENT

- Interpretation of the patient's status based on subjective and objective data
- Evaluation of the nutritional history as it pertains to medical condition
- Assessment of laboratory data as they apply to nutrition/hydration status
- Assessment of patient's comprehension and motivation, if appropriate
- Assessment of the diet order and/or feeding modality
- Anticipated problems and/or difficulties for patient compliance or adherence

PLAN

- Diagnostic studies needed
- Suggestions for gaining further pertinent data
- Further work-up, data gathering, consultations, etc.
- Medical nutrition therapy goal
- Recommendations for nutritional care
- Referrals to other health care providers

An example of a SOAP note follows:

S—Patient states that she "never eats fish and is allergic to milk."

O—45-year-old white female; hx type 1 diabetes mellitus for 20 years. Hospitalized for gastroparesis and GI discomfort. Ht. 65″, Wt. 125 lb, fasting blood glucose—122 mg/dL; BUN 16. No other labs.

A—Pt. is at IBW. Demonstrates strong knowledge of diet related to diabetes and to milk allergy;

uses nondairy sources of calcium. Some questions regarding eating at restaurants and traveling and sick days.

P—Review foods appropriate at restaurants or when traveling and on sick days.

Other documentation styles include *DAR* (diagnosis, assessment, recommendations), *PIE* (problem, intervention, evaluation), *HOAP* (history, observation, assessment, plan), *SAP* (screen, assess, plan), *focus/DAR charting* (a positive instead of negative perspective on a problem with data, action, response), and *diagnostic charting* (a clinical judgment about an individual that describes an actual or potential nutritional problem, but not a diagnosis of a disease.) The important factor is the content of the documentation, not necessarily the style. It should address the issues of nutritional status and needs. The accompanying box, "*Focus On:* Coding for Malnutrition" highlights key information that should be included to ensure that malnutrition is adequately addressed in the patient's medical record (see also Appendix 3).

Even though electronic charting has been in existence for some time, its use is expected to increase. Computer documentation can reduce duplication and repetition of information, save time, and offer new tools for decision making, such as providing alerts or reminders for care providers. Brevity in charting, regardless of the style used, is important. In one study of the use of abbreviated charting style, physicians were found to more readily implement brief dietitian recommendations than lengthy ones (Grace-Farfaglia and Rosow, 1995). Figure 20–5 shows a format that documents both screening and assessment notes in an abbreviated style. Medical record charting is often less time-consuming when protocol-driven care is implemented.

Managed Care Organizations

Changes in the delivery of health care over the past several years have resulted in additional parameters affecting the provision of medical nutritional therapy. Health care providers, consumers, payors, and the government have all emphasized the need to contain health care costs. Managed care organizations (MCOs), preferred provider organizations (PPOs) and health maintenance organizations (HMOs) have changed the face of health care in recent years.

Strategies used by MCOs and HMOs aim to contain health care costs while providing efficient and effective care that is of consistent quality. To accomplish this, practice guidelines (or **standards of care**) are often used. These guidelines are a set of recommendations that serve as a guide for defining appropriate care for a patient with a specific diagnosis or problem. They help to ensure consistency and quality for both providers and clients in a health care system, and as such, are usually specific to an institution or health care organization.

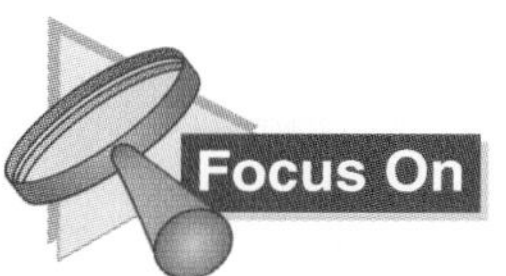

Coding for Malnutrition

Malnourished patients require nutritional attention to improve their medical outcomes and responsiveness to other therapies. Previous studies have suggested that post-discharge nutritional care may be warranted to reduce the need for rehospitalization, to speed wound healing, and to enhance well-being (Weddle et al., 1991).

When a dietitian or other health professional documents malnutrition in the medical record, the dietitian can point out potential nutritional deficits or complications that may help the physician decide how, when, and where to intervene. The use of ICD-9 codes, an international classification system for disease, allows multiple practitioners to gather data and to conclude which diagnoses and conditions will be addressed in the overall plan of care. Commonly, pulmonary, gastrointestinal, endocrine, and mental disorders, and cancer, may lead to malnutrition as a comorbidity factor. Codes frequently used to classify malnutrition include:*

- 260—kwashiorkor (nutritional edema with dyspigmentation of skin and hair)
- 261—nutritional marasmus (nutritional atrophy or severe energy deficiency)
- 262—other severe protein-calorie malnutrition (nutritional edema without dyspigmentation of skin and hair)
- 263—other and unspecified protein-calorie malnutrition
- 263.0—moderate malnutrition (weight for age 60% to 75% of standard)
- 263.1—mild malnutrition (weight for age 75% to 90% of standard)
- 263.2—arrested development following protein-calorie malnutrition (nutritional dwarfism; physical retardation from malnutrition)
- 263.8—other protein-calorie malnutrition
- 263.9—unspecified protein-calorie malnutrition (other dystrophy)

Coordinated nutritional care and coding for malnutrition are important elements in patient services. Use of **medical nutrition therapy protocols,** established by The American Dietetic Association (1998), may improve client outcomes. By shortening the time delays between *identification* of nutritional risks or documented malnutrition and *interventions* by a qualified nutrition professionals, positive outcomes are more easily achieved.

*Adapted from International Classification of Diseases, Clinical Modification Tabular List, 9th ed. Washington, DC: U.S. Department of Health and Human Services, 1980.

Care Management Strategies

Case management is a process that strives to promote the achievement of patient care goals in a cost-effective, efficient manner. The process is a key component in MCO and HMO efforts at delivering care in a manner that provides a positive experience for the patient and ensures that clinical outcomes are achieved while making wise use of resources. Case management involves assessing, evaluating, planning, implementing, coordinating, and monitoring care, especially in patients with chronic disease or those who are at high risk; it typically occurs in an inpatient setting. Case management is most appropriate for patients who present a complex picture in terms of their health, economic status, and social, emotional, and psychological care, not necessarily in terms of the acuity or severity of their condition (Laramee, 1995). Critical pathways are a key component in case management systems. They identify key elements that should occur in the patient's care, and define a time frame in which the activity should occur to maximize patient outcomes.

Disease management is a disease-specific approach to patient care that focuses on the outpatient setting (Biesemeier, 1997). The goal is to prevent disease progression or exacerbations and to reduce the frequency and severity of disease symptoms and complications. Education is a key component, as are other strategies that maximize compliance with disease treatment. Provision of education to a patient with Type 1 diabetes regarding control of blood glucose levels would be an example of a disease management strategy; it is aimed at decreasing the complications associated with the disease (nephropathy, neuropathy, and retinopathy) and the frequency with which the client needs to access the care provider, especially on an emergent basis. Decreasing the number of emergency room visits related to hyperglycemic episodes would be a sample goal.

Utilization management is a system that strives for cost-efficiency by eliminating or reducing unnecessary tests, procedures, and services. A manager is usually assigned to a group of patients and is responsible for ensuring that preestablished criteria are followed.

Patient-Focused Care

Patient-focused care (PFC) represents a fundamental change in how care is delivered to a patient. It focuses on the patient's needs and perspective, rather than on the caregiver's perspective. It drastically reduces the number of individuals with whom the patient comes in contact by decentralizing services and cross-training personnel in efforts to increase the continuity and quality of care provided. Hospitals have moved to PFC to overcome the fragmentation in care that has occurred as health care has become more specialized.

How PFC is delivered varies from institution to institution, but its basic elements focus on the patient's needs, cost-effectiveness of care, reduction in work steps, and more direct patient care. Team membership varies, but usually includes both skilled (licensed) and unskilled (unlicensed) personnel. Cross-training is important in making the model work. Typically, only patient care services that require highly specialized expertise remain centralized. Clinical dietitians may be centralized or decentralized depending on the model adopted by a specific institution. Certain departments, such as food service, accounting, and human resources, remain centralized in most models because some of the functions for which these departments are responsible are not directly related to patient care. Dietitians should be involved in the planning and instituting of PFC to ensure that quality medical nutrition therapy is considered as part of any redesign of patient care.

NUTRITIONAL INTERVENTION AND DIET MODIFICATION

Therapeutic diets are based on a normal, adequate diet which has been modified as necessary to provide for individual requirements, such as digestive and absorptive capacity, alleviation or arrest of a disease process, and psychosocial factors. In general, the therapeutic diet should vary as little as possible from the individual's normal diet. Personal eating patterns and food preferences should be recognized, along with socioeconomic conditions, religious practices, and any environmental factors that influence food intake, such as where the meals are eaten and who prepares them (see Chapter 15, Cultural Aspects of Dietary Planning).

A nutritious and adequate diet can be planned in many ways. One foundation of such a diet is the Food Guide Pyramid (see Chapter 15). This is a basic plan; additional foods or more of the foods listed are included to provide additional energy and increase the intake of required nutrients for the individual. The Dietary Guidelines for Americans may also be used in meal planning and to promote wellness. The latest revision was released in 1990 and includes seven key components related to health maintenance (see Chapter 15). The Recommended Dietary Allowances (RDAs), although formulated for healthy persons, are also often used as a basis for evaluating the adequacy of therapeutic diets. Nutrient requirements specific to a particular disease state or disorder must always be kept in mind during diet planning.

The Diet Prescription

The **diet prescription** designates the type, amount, and frequency of feeding based on the individual's disease process and disease management goals. The prescription may specify a caloric level or other restriction to be implemented. It may also limit or increase various components of the diet, such as carbohydrate, protein, fat, vitamins, minerals, fiber, phytonutrients, or water.

Energy Allowance

Appetite regulates weight with surprising accuracy in most normally active people. However, it is not always valid or reliable in disease. Energy needs may be calculated by a variety of methods. When necessary, actual measurement of the basal or resting metabolic rate using a metabolic cart and indirect calorimetry can be very useful (see Chapter 2).

An individual's energy requirement can be calculated by either (1) calculating the required number of kcal/kg/day or (2) calculating the percentage increase over basal metabolic demands. To make these determinations, the patient's desirable weight, based on sex, age, height, and body build (frame), is determined. The weight that should be used for calculating nutritional needs is often debated and variable. Desirable weight is generally used, rather than actual current weight, which may be abnormal as a result of undernutrition or overnutrition. An exception is made, however, for very malnourished patients. In these cases, actual weight is used, as overfeeding could occur if desirable weight is used.

The basal energy expenditure (BEE) is calculated by using one of the methods described in Chapter 2. An additional factor is added depending on the activity level of the patient. Another factor may be added if the patient is under physiologic stress (see Chapter 33).

Patients with mild stress, such as those undergoing uncomplicated surgery, may require additional energy, up to 20% over their BEE. Those with multiple fractures or trauma are considered to be under moderate stress and may need an additional increase. Acute major infections or burns may increase the need for energy intake to 100% over basal requirements. When calculating needs, it is helpful to remember that even the most hypermetabolic patients usually do not require more than 35 to 40 kcal/kg ideal body weight for anabolism. Table 20–4 presents the energy RDAs for unstressed patients, but the actual energy requirement should be determined based on an assessment of the individual and his or her medical condition.

Determination of the energy requirement is illustrated by the following example:

EXAMPLE. Suppose that DA (the patient referred to earlier in this chapter) is a 20-year-old student with a height of 165 cm (5 ft, 5 in) and a medium body build. Her weight is appropriate at 53.6 kg (118 lb). Her activity level is light. According to Table 20–4, she requires 38 kcal/kg/day. Thus, her average caloric allowance would be 38 kcal × 53.6 kg, or about 2036 kcal/day.

TABLE 20–4 RECOMMENDED ENERGY INTAKES FOR CHILDREN AND ADULTS

AGE (YEARS), CATEGORY, OR CONDITION		WEIGHT		HEIGHT		REE	MULTIPLES OF REE	AVERAGE ENERGY ALLOWANCE (KCAL)*	
		kg	lb	cm	in	(kcal/day)		Per kg	Per day†
Infants	0–0.5	6	13	60	24	320		108	650
	0.5–1.0	9	20	71	28	500		98	850
Children	1–3	13	29	90	35	740		102	1300
	4–6	20	44	112	44	950		90	1800
	7–10	28	62	132	52	1130		70	2000
Males	11–14	45	99	157	62	1440	1.70	55	2500
	15–18	66	145	176	69	1760	1.67	45	3000
	19–24	72	160	177	70	1780	1.67	40	2900
	25–50	79	174	176	70	1800	1.60	37	2900
	51+	77	170	173	68	1530	1.50	30	2300
Females	11–14	46	101	157	62	1310	1.67	47	2200
	15–18	55	120	163	64	1370	1.60	40	2200
	19–24	58	128	164	65	1350	1.60	38	2200
	25–50	63	138	163	64	1380	1.55	36	2200
	51+	65	143	160	63	1280	1.50	30	1900
Pregnant	1st trimester								+0
	2nd trimester								+300
	3rd trimester								+300
Lactatation	1st 6 months								+500
	2nd 6 months								+500

(Reprinted with permission from Recommended Dietary Allowances, 10th ed. © 1989 by the National Academy of Sciences. Published by National Academy Press.)

REE, resting energy expenditure.

*In the range of light to moderate activity, the coefficient of variation is 620%.

†Figure is rounded.

Protein Allowance

The RDA for protein is 0.8 g/kg of body weight for adults (see Chapter 3). The RDA level is usually considered adequate for previously well-nourished individuals who are ambulatory, or who require only brief periods of hospitalization. The actual minimum need to maintain nitrogen balance in healthy adults is 0.5 g/kg.

In the presence of malabsorption or protein loss from burns, exudates, ascites, or renal disease, an increase in protein allowance is required. Infection, fever, trauma, burns, and surgery also increase protein catabolism, so the patient should be given additional protein. Chapter 33 discusses the protein allowance in relationship to the energy:nitrogen ratio (kcal:N_2). Sections of this text dealing with specific disease states review protein needs related to specific conditions or illnesses.

Minerals and Vitamins

Appropriate levels of vitamins and minerals are difficult to determine for stressed individuals. In times of stress, inadequacies of nutrients may be countered with mobilization of body stores, decreased losses, increased absorption, or improved utilization. Individual responses vary, and true deficiencies with clinical signs and symptoms may take weeks, months, or even years to develop. Biochemical measurements capable of identifying inadequacies at early stages are still being developed (see Chapter 17).

To determine an appropriate vitamin and mineral intake, the following should be considered: (1) requirements for healthy individuals, (2) nature of the disease or injury, (3) body stores of specific nutrients, (4) normal and abnormal losses through the skin, urine, or intestinal tract, and (5) drug-nutrient interactions (see Chapter 18). These factors are discussed further in the chapters relating to nutritional care for various disease states.

Fluids

A normal healthy adult at rest and not perspiring needs 1800 to 2500 mL/day (about 2 to 2½ quarts) of water (or approximately 1 mL per kcal consumed) to provide for urinary excretion and replace insensible fluid losses. Optimal convalescence demands adequate tissue hydration. Additional fluids must be added to replace water lost by excessive perspiration, vomiting, diarrhea, tube drainage, or other conditions marked by increased water loss. If sufficient water is not obtained through fluid intake and food, it must be supplied parenterally, usually along with electrolytes.

Modifications of the Normal Diet

Normal nutrition is the foundation upon which therapeutic diet modifications are based. Regardless of the type of diet prescribed, the purpose of the diet is to supply needed nutrients to the body in a form that it can handle. Adjustment of the diet may take any of the following forms:

1. Change in consistency of foods (liquid diet, soft diet, low-fiber diet, high-fiber diet)
2. Increase or decrease in energy value of diet (weight-reduction diet, high-calorie diet)
3. Increase or decrease in the type of foods consumed (sodium-restricted diet, lactose-restricted diet, high-fiber diet, high-potassium diet)
4. Omission of specific foods (allergy diet, gluten-free diet)
5. Adjustment in the ratio and balance of proteins, fats, and carbohydrates (diabetic diet, ketogenic diet, renal diet, cholesterol-lowering diet)
6. Rearrangement of the number and frequency of meals (diabetic diet, postgastrectomy diet)
7. Change in route of delivery of nutrients, such as enteral or parenteral nutrition

Foods as Nutrient Sources

Correct evaluation of normal and therapeutic diets requires a knowledge of the nutrients contained in different foods. In particular, it is helpful to be aware of the nutrient-dense foods that contribute in a major way to dietary adequacy. Chapters 4 and 5 provide more detailed information on specific minerals and vitamins and the foods that contain them. Often, a vitamin-mineral supplement is necessary to meet the patient's needs.

NUTRITIONAL CARE FOR THE HOSPITALIZED PATIENT

Food is an important part of nutritional support. Attempts should be made to honor patient preferences, provide a pleasant atmosphere, and arrange for assistance with eating when needed. Imagination and ingenuity in menu planning are essential when designing foods acceptable to a varied patient population. Attention to color, texture, composition, and temperature of the foods, coupled with a sound knowledge of therapeutic diets, is required for menu planning. To the patient, however, good taste and attractive presentation are the most important elements. When possible, patient selection of menus results in the delivery of food that will most likely be consumed. The ability to make food selections gives the patient an option in an otherwise limiting environment.

Standard Hospital Diets

All hospitals and institutions have some specific, basic, routine diets designed for uniformity and convenience of service. These standard diets are based on the foundation of an adequate diet pattern, which is derived from the RDAs. Hospital diets should be as flexible as possible, yet allow the nutritional needs of patients to be met. In many facilities, the diet focuses on providing foods that the patient is willing and able to eat, which is the most important consideration of the diet offered. With the trend toward shortened lengths of stay in all health care settings, optimizing intake of calories and protein during hospitalization, especially when therapeutic restrictions may compromise intake and subsequent recovery from surgery, stress, or illness, often translates into a relatively liberal approach to therapeutic diets.

Types of standard diets vary, but can generally be classified as either general, soft, or liquid. These diets are used routinely for patients and serve as a foundation for more diversified therapeutic diets. Table 20–5 summarizes the basic hospital diets and their components.

General or Normal Diet

In some hospitals, the general diet is also known as the "regular" or "house" diet. It is used when the patient's medical condition does not warrant a restriction. The general diet is a basic, adequate, normal diet of approximately 1600 to 2200 kcal; it usually contains 60 to 80 g of protein, 80 to 100 g of fat, and 180 to 300 g of carbohydrate. Although there are no particular food restrictions, some hospitals have instituted general diets that are low in fat, saturated fat, cholesterol, sugar, and salt to follow the dietary recommendations for the general population (Singer et al., 1996). In other facilities, the diet focuses on providing foods the patient is willing and able to eat, with less focus on restriction of nutrients. Many hospitals have a selective menu that allows the patient certain choices; the adequacy of the diet will vary based on the patient's selection.

TABLE 20–5 SUMMARY OF BASIC HOSPITAL DIETS

FOOD	GENERAL, ADEQUATE, OR "HOUSE" DIET	SOFT DIET	FULL LIQUID DIET	CLEAR LIQUID DIET
Milk, cream, buttermilk	Included	Included	Included	Not included
Eggs	Pasteurized or cooked	Included	In beverages (eggnog)	Not included
Cheese	All varieties	Cottage, cream, mildly flavored cheeses	Not included	Not included
Fats	All kinds	Butter, margarine, oil, mayonnaise, and mildly seasoned dressing	Butter, margarine, oil	Not included
Meat, fish, poultry	All included	Tender beef, lamb, veal; liver, bacon, fish and poultry	Not included	Not included
Vegetables	All included	Cooked or canned vegetables of low fiber; tender lettuce; vegetable juices	Vegetable juices, vegetable purée used in soups	
Fruits	All included	Fruit juices, ripe bananas, cooked fruit without skin or seeds	Fruit juices, fruitades	Strained fruit juices, fruitades
Breads	All varieties	Refined grain products, rye without seeds, refined crackers	Not included	Not included
Cereals	All varieties	Refined	Cooked, refined cereals	Not included
Cereal products	All varieties	Cooked macaroni, spaghetti, noodles, white rice	Not included	Not included
Soups	All varieties	Clear broth, and consommé; cream and vegetable soups containing allowed items	Clear broth, and consommé; strained vegetable and cream soups	Clear broth and consommé
Beverages	All kinds	All kinds	Tea, decaffeinated or regular coffee, carbonated beverages, eggnog	Tea, decaffeinated coffee, carbonated beverages
Desserts	All kinds	Plain puddings, yogurt, simple cakes and cookies, frozen desserts without nuts, custard, gelatin	Plain gelatin dessert, ice cream or yogurt without nuts and seeds, ices, sherbets, soft custard, pudding	Plain gelatin desserts and ices
Other			Liquid supplements listed in Appendices 35-40	Elemental liquids, such as shown in Appendices 35–40

Soft Diet

The **soft diet,** as described in Table 20–6, is used as a transition diet between a liquid and general diet. It is moderately low in cellulose and connective tissue and low in residue. The soft diet is often prescribed for patients postoperatively or for those with gastrointestinal problems. It is not appropriate for patients whose dentition is poor; these patients require a change in consistency, such as the mechanical soft diet. The soft diet is most useful when the selection of food is guided by the patient's tolerance.

The average composition of the soft diet is 1800 to 2000 kcal. However, energy levels, as well as protein, fat, and carbohydrate levels, will vary, based on menu selection, patient preferences, and other restrictions that may be imposed.

Liquid Diets

Liquid diets are commonly ordered for patients with conditions whose treatment requires nourishment that is easily digested and consumed, or that has minimal residue. Such diets are often ordered for a brief period for patients undergoing diagnostic tests or following surgery. Chewing or swallowing difficulties or dental wiring may also necessitate a liquid diet.

The two varieties of oral liquid diets are the clear liquid diet and the full liquid diet.

TABLE 20–6 SOFT DIET

MEAL PLAN	SAMPLE MENU	SERVING SIZE
Breakfast		
Fruit	Orange juice	½ cup
Cereal	Cooked farina	½ cup (cooked weight)
Egg	Poached egg	1
Bread	Toast	1 slice
Butter	Butter or margarine	1 pat
Milk	Milk (2%)	1 cup
Sugar	Sugar	3 tsp
Coffee	Coffee	2 cups
Lunch		
Soup	Tomato consommé	½ cup
Entrée	Baked macaroni and cheese	1 cup
Vegetables	Cooked asparagus tips	½ cup
Bread	White bread	1 slice
Butter	Butter or margarine	1 pat
Fruit	Applesauce	½ cup
Milk	Milk (2%)	1 cup
Dinner		
Meat	Chicken breast	3 oz
Potato	Mashed potato	½ cup
Vegetable	Buttered spinach	½ cup
Bread	White bread	1 slice
Butter	Butter or margarine	1 pat
Dessert	Chocolate ice cream, ice milk, or frozen yogurt	½ cup
Milk	Milk (2%)	1 cup

TABLE 20–7 CLEAR LIQUID DIET

MEAL PLAN	SAMPLE MENU	SERVING SIZE
Breakfast		
Fruit juice	Apple juice	½ cup
Beverage	Coffee (decaffeinated)	2 cups
Sugar	Sugar	2 tsp
AM Snack		
Fruitade	Lemonade	1 cup
Lunch		
Soup	Beef broth	½ cup
Fruit juice	Grape juice	½ cup
Tea	Tea	2 cups
Sugar	Sugar	2 tsp
Fruit ice	Cherry fruit ice	½ cup
PM Snack		
Carbonated beverage	Gingerale	1 cup
Dinner		
Fruit juice	Fruit punch	½ cup
Soup	Chicken broth	½ cup
Gelatin	Raspberry gelatin	¼ cup
Tea	Tea	2 cups
Sugar	Sugar	2 tsp
Evening (h.s.) Snack		
Fruit juice	Cranberry juice	1 cup

CLEAR LIQUID DIET. The **clear liquid diet,** such as that listed in Table 20–7, is frequently ordered for postoperative patients to furnish fluids, some electrolytes, and small amounts of energy before gastrointestinal function returns. It is composed chiefly of water and carbohydrates and is inadequate in calories and essential nutrients. The average clear liquid diet contains 500 to 600 kcal, 5 to 10 g of protein, minimal fat, 120 to 130 g of carbohydrate, and has small amounts of sodium and potassium. As it is inadequate in calories, fiber, and all other essential nutrients, it should be used only for short periods of time.

The clear liquid diet cannot replace the electrolytes lost in vomitus and diarrheal fluid. Electrolytes are often replaced via intravenous fluids until the diet can be advanced to a more nutritionally adequate one. Clear liquids should be served at frequent intervals to supply the tissues with fluid and relieve thirst.

As the name indicates, the diet consists of clear liquids, such as tea, broth, carbonated beverages, clear fruit juices, and gelatin. Milk and liquids prepared with milk are omitted, as are fruit juices that contain pulp. Carbonated beverages, especially gingerale, are usually well tolerated.

When a nutritious clear liquid is needed, an appropriate liquid elemental or defined formula diet can be selected from the formulas presented in Appendices 36 to 40.

FULL LIQUID DIET. The full liquid diet, such as that presented in Table 20–8, is made up of foods that are liquid or semi-liquid at room or body tempera-

TABLE 20–8 FULL LIQUID DIET—SAMPLE MENU

MEAL PLAN	SAMPLE MENU	SERVING SIZE
Breakfast		
Fruit	Orange juice	½ cup
Cereal	Cooked farina	1 cup (cooked weight)
Supplement	Commercial eggnog	1 cup
Butter	Butter or margarine	2 tsp
Milk	Milk (2%)	1 cup
Sugar	Sugar	2 tsp
Coffee or tea	Coffee or tea	1 cup
AM Snack		
Supplement	Commercial milkshake (chocolate)	1 cup
Lunch		
Soup	Cream of potato soup (strained) with margarine/butter	1 cup
Fruit	Pineapple juice	½ cup
Milk	Milk (2%)	1 cup
	Vanilla pudding	½ cup
Coffee or tea	Coffee or tea	1 cup
Sugar	Sugar	2 tsp
PM Snack		
Supplement	Commercial milkshake (strawberry)	1 cup
Dinner		
Fruit	Apple juice	½ cup
Soup	Cream of mushroom (strained) with margarine/butter	1 cup
Supplement	Commercial milkshake	1 cup
Milk	Ice cream	½ cup
Coffee or tea	Coffee or tea	1 cup
Sugar	Sugar	2 tsp
Bedtime (h.s.) Snack		
Gelatin	Gelatin, strawberry	½ cup
Supplement	Commercial milkshake (vanilla)	1 cup

ture. For example, ice cream and gelatin are both included in a full liquid diet. The diet is used for patients unable to chew, swallow, or digest solid foods, as it is easily consumed and digested. With proper design, the diet can be adequate for maintenance requirements except for fiber. The average full liquid diet contains 1000 to 1500 kcal, with 45 to 50 g of protein, 50 to 65 g of fat, and 150 to 170 g of carbohydrate. With careful planning, the diet can be increased in protein and caloric value to approach a regular diet, or even a high-calorie diet. These changes are necessary when the diet must be continued for a prolonged period. Protein and vitamin supplements (see Appendix 51) can be added to increase the nutrient content. Because this diet is inadequate in fiber, constipation may result from its prolonged use. A canned fiber-containing formula or a fiber supplement may be useful in some patients.

Full liquid diets can be planned to meet the needs of a patient with diabetes, renal disease, or any other disorder. A lactose-free product can be used in place of milk as the protein source when planning a lactose-free liquid diet.

Food Intake

Food served does not necessarily represent the actual intake of the patient. Prevention of iatrogenic malnutrition requires observation and monitoring of the adequacy of patient intake. If the diet consumed is inadequate, measures can be taken to provide foods or supplements that may be better accepted or tolerated. Regardless of the type of diet prescribed, both the food served and the amount actually eaten must be considered to obtain an accurate indication of the patient's energy and nutrient intake. Nourishments and calorie-containing beverages consumed between meals must also be considered in the overall intake. Calorie counts are often ordered in hospitalized patients to quantify the actual intake of the patient. Good records of intake require a systemized data collection procedure that typically involves both nursing and nutrition and food service personnel.

Psychological Factors

Meals and between-meal nourishments are often highlights of the day and are anticipated with pleasure by the patient. Mealtime should be as positive an experience as possible. Food intake is encouraged in a draft-free room at a comfortable temperature, with the patient in a comfortable eating position in bed or sitting in a chair located away from unpleasant sights or unpleasant odors. Many patients prefer to wash before eating and to eat at a table free of other objects.

Arrangement of the tray should reflect consideration of the patient's needs. Dishes and utensils should be in a convenient location. Independence should be encouraged in those who require assistance in eating. The caregiver can accomplish this by asking patients to specify the sequence of foods to be eaten and having them participate in eating, if only by holding their bread. Even visually impaired persons can eat unassisted if they are told where to find foods on the tray. Patients who require feeding assistance should be fed when the foods are still at an optimal temperature. The feeding process requires about 20 minutes as a general rule.

Rejection of meals or the prescribed diet frequently reflects a negative patient attitude toward the illness and hospitalization. Other reasons for poor acceptance may be unfamiliar foods, a change in eating schedule, improper food temperatures, or the effects of medical therapy. Food acceptance is also improved when personal selection of menus is encouraged. Patients should be given the opportunity to share concerns regarding meals, which may improve acceptance and intake.

In encouraging acceptance of a therapeutic diet, the attitude of the caregiver is important. The nurse who understands that the diet contributes to the restoration of the patient's health will communicate this conviction by actions, facial expressions, and conversation. Patients who understand that the diet is important to the success of their medical or surgical therapy usually accept it more willingly.

When the patient must adhere to a therapeutic dietary program indefinitely, an interdisciplinary approach will help the patient achieve nutritional goals. Because they have frequent contact with patients, nurses have an important role in a patient's acceptance of nutritional care.

Nutritional Counseling

Nutritional counseling is an important part of the medical nutrition therapy provided to many patients. The goal of counseling is to help the patient acquire the knowledge and skills needed to make changes, including modifying behavior to facilitate sustained change. Nutritional counseling and resultant dietary changes implemented by the patient result in many benefits. One of the most important benefits is the control of the disease or symptoms, but others, such as improved health status, improved quality of life, and decreased health care costs, may also result when dietary changes are successful. As the average length of hospital stay has decreased, the role of the dietitian in counseling patients in the hospital has changed to providing only "survival" skills. These survival skills include basic types of foods to limit, timing of meals, and portion sizes. Follow-up outpatient counseling regarding details of the diet should reinforce the basic counseling given during hospitalization. See Chapter 21 for more information on counseling for change.

DISCHARGE SUMMARY

Name ____________________ Discharge date ____________________

Hospital Number ____________________ Admission date ____________________

Age ________ Sex ________ Diagnosis ____________________

Anthropometrics: Ht. ________ Wt.: ________ Admit Wt.: ________ DC Wt.: ________

Usual Wt. ________ Activity level ____________________

Laboratory Albumin: ________ Prealbumin: ____________________

Other ____________________

Diet: Estimated Needs: ________ Kcal ________ gm pro

________ Kcal/kg ________ gm/kg

Current diet: ____________________ Nutritional supplements ____________________

Major Nutritional Problems:

ongoing: follow-up recommendations:

resolved:

FIGURE 20–6 Discharge summary. (Courtesy of University of Washington Medical Centers, Seattle, WA.)

Discharge Planning and Home Care

Nutritional care continues as a part of **discharge planning** when the patient returns home or goes to a long-term care facility or rehabilitation center. Education, counseling, and mobilization of resources to provide home care and nutritional support are included as part of discharge procedures. Home health care agencies are available to provide a variety of services related to nutrition, including enteral or parenteral nutrition at home. Follow-up monitoring may be needed to provide continuity of care in the new setting, or to ensure a smooth transition back to the original health care site, should readmission be necessary. Effective discharge planning begins on day 1 of a hospital or nursing home stay and continues throughout the institutionalization. Appropriate discharge documentation includes a summary of nutritional therapies and outcomes; pertinent information on weights, laboratory values, and dietary intake; expected progress or prognosis; and recommendations for follow-up services (Fig. 20–6). Level of educational instruction given, including expected adherence to prescribed diet and comprehension of instructions, must be included. Potential drug-nutrient interactions and expected outcome or goal are also important. The patient must be included in every step of the planning process.

Care of the Terminally Ill or Hospice Patient

Maintenance of comfort and quality of life are the goals of nutritional care for the terminally ill patient. Dietary restrictions are rarely appropriate. Nutritional care should include techniques that facilitate symptom and pain control. Recognition of the various phases of dying—denial, anger, bargaining, depression, and acceptance—will help the health care practitioner understand the patient's response to food and nutritional support. Constant communication and explanations to the family are important.

The decision as to when life support should be terminated often involves the issue of whether to continue enteral or parenteral nutrition. Nutritional support should be continued as long as the patient is competent to make this choice, and as long as it is adding to the possibility of meaningful remaining days of life. The primary consideration should be the wishes of the competent, informed patient, or the surrogate decision-maker (King and Maillet, 1992).

With **advance directives,** the patient can advise family and health care team members of his or her individual preferences with regard to heroic measures. Ordinary food and hydration issues may also be discussed, such as whether or not tube feeding should be initiated, and under what circumstances.

Palliative care encourages the alleviation of physical symptoms, anxiety, and fear while attempting to maintain the patient's ability to function independently. Hospice home care programs allow the patient to stay at home as long as possible before hospital admission. Quality of life is the critical component. Services by a registered dietitian, although not mandatory, can benefit the patient and family members as efforts are made to help them adjust to approaching death (Sloan, 1992). The physician, nurse, dietitian, social worker, and other team members should document any discussions held with the patient or family members.

CITED REFERENCES

American Dietetic Association. Identifying patients at risk: ADA's definitions for nutrition screening and nutrition assessment. J Am Diet Assoc 94:838, 1994.

American Dietetic Association. Medical Nutrition Therapy Protocols. Chicago: American Dietetic Association, 2nd ed., 1998.

Biesemeier C. Case manager/registered dietitian partnerships: Teaming up to achieve positive patient outcomes. J Care Mgmt 3:72, 1997.

Grace-Farfaglia P, Rosow P. Automating clinical dietetics documentation. J Am Diet Assoc 95:688, 1995.

Insull W. Dietitians as intervention specialists: A continuing challenge for the 1990s. J Am Diet Assoc 92:551, 1992.

International Classification of Diseases. Clinical Modification Tabular List, 9th ed. Washington, DC: U.S. Department of Health and Human Services, 1980.

King D, Maillet JO. Position of the American Dietetic Association: Issues in feeding the terminally ill adult. J Am Diet Assoc 92:996, 1992.

Laramee S. Case management: An overview. Clin Nutr Mgmt Newslett 14(4):1, 1995.

Singer AJ, et al. The nutritional value of university-hospital diets (letter). N Engl J Med, 335:1466, 1996.

Sloan SL. The hospice movement: A study in the diffusion of innovative palliative care. Am J Hospice Palliative Care 9:24, 1992.

Weddle D, et al. In-patient and post-discharge course of the malnourished patient. J Am Diet Assoc 91:307, 1991.

ADDITIONAL REFERENCES

American Dietetic Association. Position on management of health care food and nutrition services. J Am Diet Assoc 97:1427, 1997.

Chicago Dietetic Association and The South Suburban Dietetic Association. Manual of Clinical Dietetics, 5th ed. Chicago: The American Dietetic Association, 1996.

Escott-Stump S. Nutrition and Diagnosis-Related Care, 4th ed. Philadelphia: Williams & Wilkins, 1998.

Mittleman L. The legal implications of withholding and withdrawing nutrition support. Newsletter of Dietitians in Nutrition Support, Vol. 14, p. 1. Chicago: The American Dietetic Association, 1992.

Nelson J, et al. Mayo Clinic Diet Manual, 7th ed. St. Louis: CV Mosby, 1994.

Ouslander J, et al. Decisions about enteral tube feeding among the elderly. J Am Geriat Soc 41:70, 1993.

Page G, et al. Developing key-feature problems and examinations to assess clinical decision-making skills. Acad Med 70:194, 1995.

Parks S. Impact of health care reform on career opportunities in the profession. Top Clin Nutr 10:1, 1995.

Simko MD, et al. Nutrition Assessment: A Comprehensive Guide for Planning Intervention, 2nd ed. Gaithersburg, MD: Aspen Publishers, 1995.

CHAPTER 21

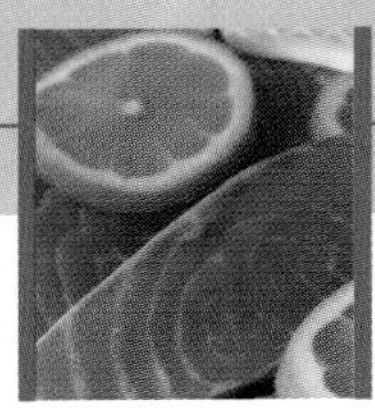

Counseling for Change

LINDA SNETSELAAR, PhD, RD

Chapter Outline

- Stages of Change
- Activities That Facilitate Behavior Change
- Intervention Model
- Resistance Behaviors and Potential Strategies to Modify Them

Key Terms

AFFIRMING—when a counselor tells a patient that what he or she is doing is normal and understandable given the circumstances; supporting the patient's efforts in change

ALIGNMENT—supportive statement telling a patient that the counselor understands and is with him or her in difficult times

AMBIVALENCE—when a patient has mixed feelings about change modifying behaviors that are difficult

DISCREPANCY—when change results in positive and negative consequences; this strategy identifies conflicting feelings

DOUBLE-SIDED REFLECTION—statement from the counselor describing a discrepancy between the patient's current and previous words that provides ideas for open discussion to facilitate change

EMPATHY—a technique by which the counselor accepts a patient's feelings of turmoil about making changes

MOTIVATIONAL INTERVIEWING—counseling style designed to achieve the willingness to change within a patient

NEGOTIATION—strategy where the patient and counselor interaction allows for a compromise designed to achieve a specific goal

NORMALIZATION—statement indicating that the patient's behavior is perfectly within reason and normal, which validates the patient's reaction to a given situation

REFLECTIVE LISTENING—guessing at what a patient feels and stating that feeling; promotes understanding on the part of the counselor

REFRAMING—strategy in which the counselor changes the patient's interpretation of the same basic data that he or she has given and offers a new viewpoint

SELF-EFFICACY—when a patient believes in his or her ability to carry out change

SELF-MANAGEMENT—strategy where the counselor facilitates the ability to change through the patient's decisions

SELF-MONITORING—recording by the patient of changes in behavior

STAGES OF CHANGE MODEL OR TRANSTHEORETICAL MODEL—describes behavior change as a process in which individuals progress through a series of six distinct stages: precontemplation, contemplation, preparation, action, maintenance, and relapse

People are motivated to change through their ability to self-manage behaviors. The nutrition counselor sets up an environment that is a transient support system to prepare the patient to handle social and personal demands more effectively while providing favorable conditions for change.

The following concepts are important to consider in facilitating dietary changes:

- People make behavioral changes only when they are ready to change.
- The nutrition intervention, including both the content and nutritionist's style, is a powerful determinant of resistance and denial, as well as motivation, in persons who want to make changes in their diet.
- People cycle through different phases of changing and maintaining their dietary modifications.
- Different interventions are needed for people in different phases of motivation.
- Ambivalence is a key blocker to motivation and can be resolved through intervention.
- Resistance and denial get in the way of meeting behavioral goals.

STAGES OF CHANGE

The **Transtheoretical Model,** also referred to as the **Stages of Change Model,** describes behavior change as a process in which individuals progress

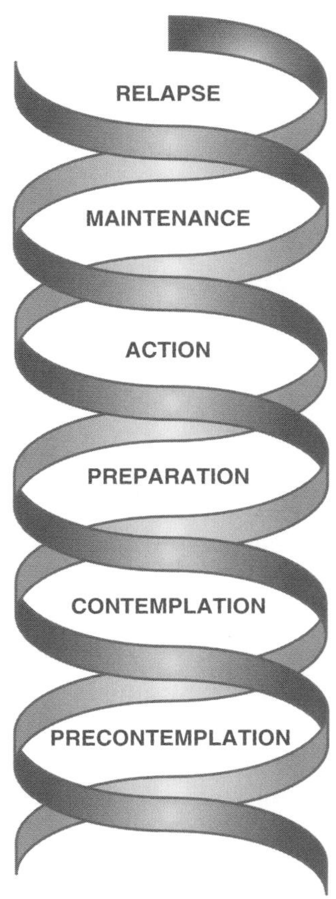

FIGURE 21–1 A spiral model of the stages of change. In changing, a person moves up this spiral to maintenance. If relapse occurs, he or she must re-enter the spiral again at any point.

through a series of six distinct stages of change, as shown in Figure 21–1: (1) precontemplation, (2) contemplation, (3) preparation, (4) action, (5) maintenance, (6) relapse (Prochaska and DiClemente, 1982, 1984; Sigman-Grant, 1996). See "*Focus On:* Stages of Change."

Research data have shown that the value of the Transtheoretical Model is in determining which stage an individual is in and then using change processes matched to that stage (Prochaska et al., 1992). Behavior change is more successfully facilitated using this approach rather than the traditional approach of assigning the same intervention techniques to everyone, regardless of the readiness or stage of change (Prochaska et al., 1994).

Traditional nutrition counseling focuses on the change process matched to the action and maintenance stages. This works well for persons who are actively trying to make behavior change. However, the majority of individuals with a problem dietary behavior are in a pre-action stage that includes one of the following: precontemplation, contemplation, or preparation. These individuals are not yet ready to change (Sandoval et al., 1994; Sporny and Contento, 1995). The traditional approach, which assumes that the patient is already in the action or maintenance stage, does not meet the needs of many and may be one of the reasons for lack of success in long-term maintenance of many intervention programs (Brownell, 1982; National Cholesterol Education Program, 1993; Ockene et al., 1988; Prochaska et al., 1994).

ACTIVITIES THAT FACILITATE BEHAVIOR CHANGE

A variety of principles are important when determining what facilitates behavior change. The following are important when working with individuals who struggle with behavior change:

1. Expressing **empathy**
2. Developing **discrepancy**
3. Avoiding arguments or defensiveness
4. Rolling with resistance
5. Supporting **self-efficacy**

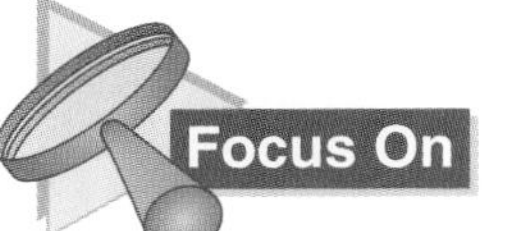

STAGES OF CHANGE

Precontemplation: This is the point at which the patient has not even contemplated having a problem or needing to make a change. A person in the precontemplative stage needs information and feedback to raise his or her awareness of the problem and possibility of change. Nutrition advice for eating changes is counterproductive at this point.

Contemplation: Once some awareness of the problem arises, the person enters a period of ambivalence: the contemplation stage. The contemplator seesaws between reasons to change and reasons to stay the same. At this stage, the counselor works with the patient on advantages and disadvantages of making dietary changes.

Preparation: The preparation stage is a window of opportunity that either allows the patient to move forward or fall back into contemplation. At this point, the patient needs help in finding a change strategy or goal that is acceptable, achievable, and appropriate.

Action: The patient engages in actions that bring about change. At this point, the goal is to produce a change in the problem area.

Maintenance: During this stage, the challenge is to sustain the change accomplished by previous action and to prevent relapse.

Relapse: If relapse occurs, the individual's task is to start the change process again rather than become stuck in this stage. Slips and relapses are normal, expected occurrences as a person seeks to change any long-standing pattern of behavior. The goal is to resume action efforts.

Expressing Empathy

Counselor acceptance of what a patient feels in times of turmoil can often result in change. Acceptance facilitates change. A woman wrote a letter to her nutritionist saying that she wanted to stop working on her dietary changes. Life was too complicated and the dietary changes were more than she could master. The nutritionist reviewed several scenarios for approaching this problem. One certainly is to take the woman's word seriously and allow her to drop out of the diet intervention. Another is to immediately call the woman to discuss the letter, always indicating acceptance of the woman's concerns.

Beyond this acceptance is a skillful form of **reflective listening,** which allows the woman to describe her thoughts and feelings, while the nutritionist reflects back understanding. Many people have no one to talk to about problems in their lives. This opportunity to have someone listen and really try to understand the emotions behind the words is crucial to eventual dietary change.

As most people talk about their lives and a lack of time for dietary changes, the counselor will hear **ambivalence.** On the one hand, patients want to make changes; on the other hand, they want to pretend that change is not important. Ambivalence is normal.

Developing Discrepancy

An awareness of consequences is important. Identifying the advantages and disadvantages of modifying a behavior is a crucial process in making changes.

Avoiding Arguments or Defensiveness

Arguments are counterproductive. A counselor's urges may lead in the direction of defending one's own ideas, but the result is frequently defensiveness on the part of the patient. When a patient resists, this is the signal to the counselor to change strategies.

Rolling with Resistance

Invite new perspectives without imposing them. The patient is a valuable resource in finding solutions to problems. Perceptions can be shifted, and the counselor's role is to help with this process.

Supporting Self-Efficacy

Belief in the possibility of change is an important motivator. The patient is responsible for choosing and carrying out personal change. Hope exists when there are alternative approaches to a problem.

These concepts along with other intervention models shape the content of each contract described below in the motivational intervention model. This model is made up of an integration of the following theories: stages of change (Prochaska and DiClemente, 1982, 1986), **motivational interviewing** (Miller and Rollnick, 1991), brief **negotiation** (Watson and Tharp, 1989), and behavioral **self-management.**

INTERVENTION MODEL

First Session

The first session is an important time to establish the counseling relationship. The environment should be conducive to privacy, and there should be a plan for reduction of interruptions (no telephone calls, staff or other patients knocking on the door, etc.). The counselor should be seated in a manner that reflects interest in the client, such as sitting directly across from one another in chairs, without a desk as a barrier. Communication skills and body language are also important (see *"Clinical Insight:* Body Language and Communication Skills").

In an *initial visit* the counselor introduces the subject of the session. The following are samples:

- "The purpose of this visit is to see how you are doing in covering your dietary carbohydrate intake with insulin."
- "In looking at your monitoring tools, it seems that you have had excellent progress at some times and at other times it may have been more difficult."
- "Could we talk about your diet records, to identify problems which we could solve?"

The following approaches might be used during a *follow-up contact*:

- "I talked to you about a month ago to see how you were doing with your carbohydrate levels for each meal and insulin doses."
- "I'd like to see if you have made any changes or had any further thoughts on meeting your fat intake goals."

To make the stages of change model less complicated, an alternative is to view the stages in terms of three phases: Stage 1—not ready to change; Stage 2—considering meeting goals; Stage 3—ready to change. To identify which of these three stages a patient is in, it is important to assess the patient's situation (Fig. 21–2).

Assessment

The purpose of assessment is to identify the patient's stage of change phase and to provide appropriate help in facilitating change. The assessment should be completed in the first visit, if possible. If conversation extends beyond the designated time for the session, the assessment steps should be completed at the next session. The stage of readiness for the change should be assessed and documented.

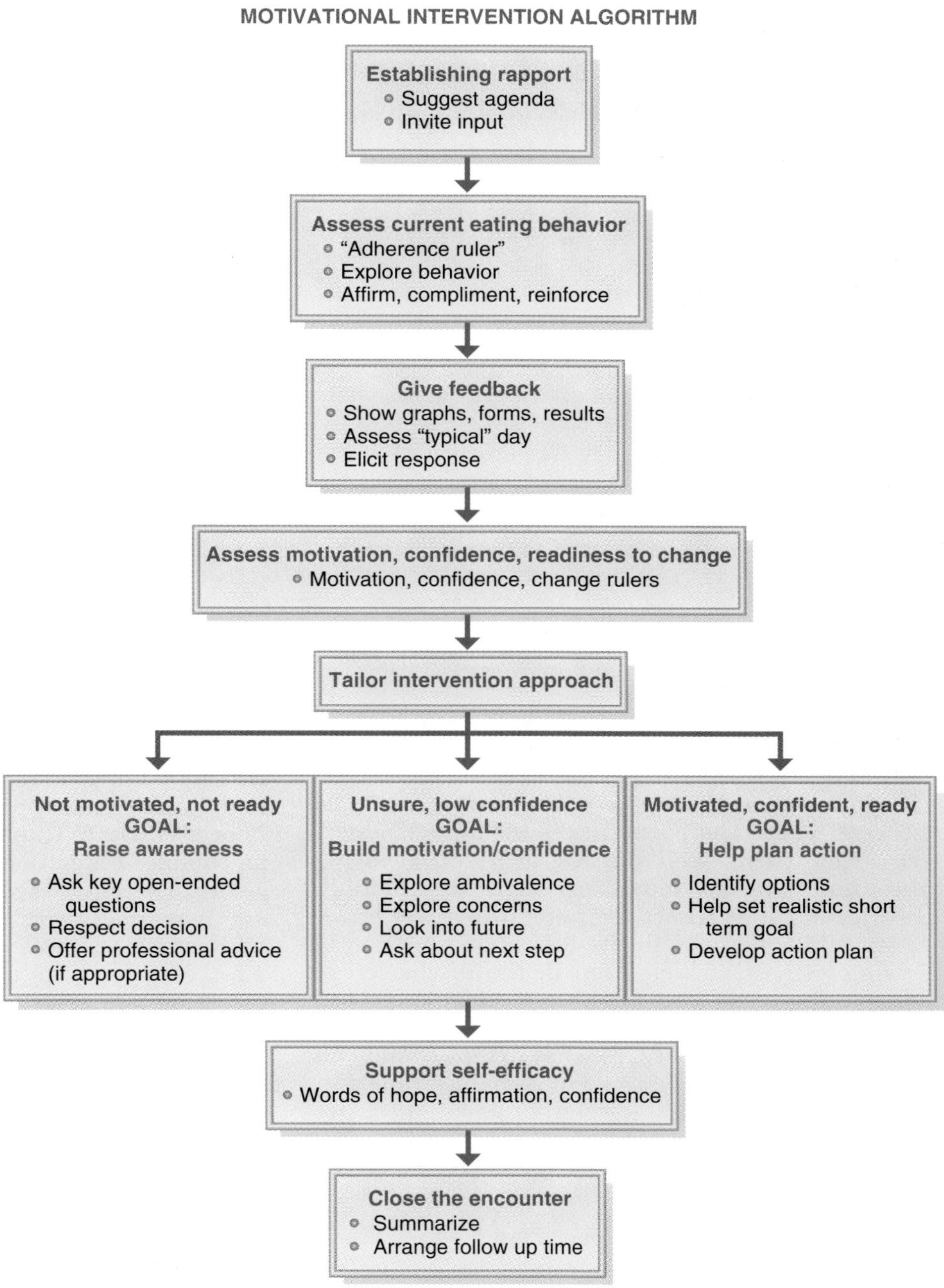

MOTIVATIONAL INTERVENTION ALGORITHM

Establishing rapport
- Suggest agenda
- Invite input

↓

Assess current eating behavior
- "Adherence ruler"
- Explore behavior
- Affirm, compliment, reinforce

↓

Give feedback
- Show graphs, forms, results
- Assess "typical" day
- Elicit response

↓

Assess motivation, confidence, readiness to change
- Motivation, confidence, change rulers

↓

Tailor intervention approach

↓

Not motivated, not ready GOAL: Raise awareness	Unsure, low confidence GOAL: Build motivation/confidence	Motivated, confident, ready GOAL: Help plan action
• Ask key open-ended questions • Respect decision • Offer professional advice (if appropriate)	• Explore ambivalence • Explore concerns • Look into future • Ask about next step	• Identify options • Help set realistic short term goal • Develop action plan

↓

Support self-efficacy
- Words of hope, affirmation, confidence

↓

Close the encounter
- Summarize
- Arrange follow up time

FIGURE 21–2 Algorithm of motivational intervention. (Data from Miller WR and Rollnick S (eds.). Motivational Interviewing: Preparing People to Change Addictive Behavior. New York: Guilford Press, 1991; and Berg-Smith SM, et al. A brief motivational intervention to improve dietary adherence in adolescents. Health Education Research, 1999 (accepted for publication).

Contact Opening

To build rapport, one begins by asking one or two questions that are relevant to important aspects of the participant's life.

- "How's it going?"
- "Tell me about how _________ (e.g., hobby or interest) is going?"
- "We have about _____ minutes to meet today. I thought we might talk about how you're doing with your dietary changes. How does this sound to you?"

Assessment of Current Eating Behavior

Determining present eating habits provides ideas on how to change in the future. Below are a few questions used to assess current eating behavior.

- "How do you limit the amount of saturated fat in your diet now?"
- "Would you say you are now eating a low-fat diet?"
- "During the past 6 months, have you thought about changes that you could make to reduce the amount of saturated fat in your diet?"

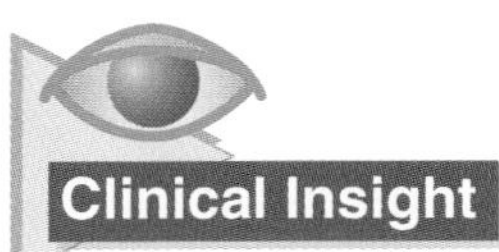

Body Language and Communication Skills

Active listening forms the basis for effective nutrition counseling. Two components are involved in effective listening, nonverbal and verbal. *Nonverbal listening skills* consist of varied eye contact, attentive body language, a respectful but close space, adequate silence, and encouragers. Eye contact would be direct, yet varied. Lack of eye contact implies that the counselor is too busy to spend time with the client. When the counselor leans forward slightly and has a relaxed posture and avoids fidgeting and gesturing, the client will be more at ease. Showing the client respectful but close space is another important nonverbal message. Silence can give the client time to think and provide positive time for the counselor to contemplate what the client has said. Shaking one's head in agreement can be a positive encourager leading to more conversation. Moving forward slightly toward the client is an encourager that allows for more positive interaction.

Verbal components of listening include keeping the focus on the client by demonstrating a willingness to listen. Often the nutritionist feels obligated to solve a problem or give advice. These two desires can decrease the time left for active listening. Emphasize questions that are open to detailed descriptions. Use questions that begin with "what," "how," "why," and "could."

Two types of *encouragers* are important in counseling, paraphrasing and summarizing. *Paraphrasing* is a brief repeat of the essence of what the speaker has said using fresh and concise wording. It is not parroting or word-swapping. Paraphrasing is not easy and requires careful listening and caring. *Summarizing* is more lengthy than paraphrasing because it uses more information and summarizes what has been said over a period of time.

In general it is important to accomplish these as the basis for the interactive relationship before beginning the actual process of nutrition counseling.

- "In the next month, do you plan to make any changes to reduce the amount of fat in your diet?"

It is important to review **self-monitoring** tools or assess where the patient sees his or her adherence level. Using food diaries to identify eating habits and potential modifications is very helpful. Using a ruler that allows the patient to select his or her level of adherence to the diet is one method of allowing patient participation in the discussion of dietary adherence. You might say, "The ruler will help us see where you are in terms of changing your diet. On a scale of 1 to 12, to what extent would you say you are meeting your goal of changing your diet in the past month? (1 = absolutely never; 12 = absolutely always)."

Explore eating behaviors by using the following statements:

- "Tell me about your progress so far."
- "Why did you choose that number on the ruler? Why did you not choose '1'? Why did you not choose '12'?"
- "How do you generally feel about following this new eating pattern?"

Always provide positive confidence-building statements:

- "It is great that you ____________."
- "You've worked really hard at this."

To elicit responses from the patient on ideas about where changes in the diet need to occur, it is helpful to provide feedback on the patient's progress toward a goal. Show the patient an example of his or her progress. Indicate what the goal is and what the average score for the targeted nutrient is. Then ask, "What do you think about this?"

Assessment of Readiness to Change

At this point it is important to assess readiness to make additional changes. A ruler works very well here also. Up to this point discussions have focused on changes the patient has already made. The counselor then asks the patient, "On a scale of 1 to 12, how ready are you right now to make any new changes to eat less fat? (1 = not ready to change; 12 = very ready to change)." Figure 21–3 shows a nutrition counselor assessing readiness to change.

At this point the intervention becomes very specific to the readiness to change. Three possibilities for readiness exist: (1) not ready to change; (2) unsure about change; (3) ready to change.

There are many concepts to remember when working with patients where readiness to change is

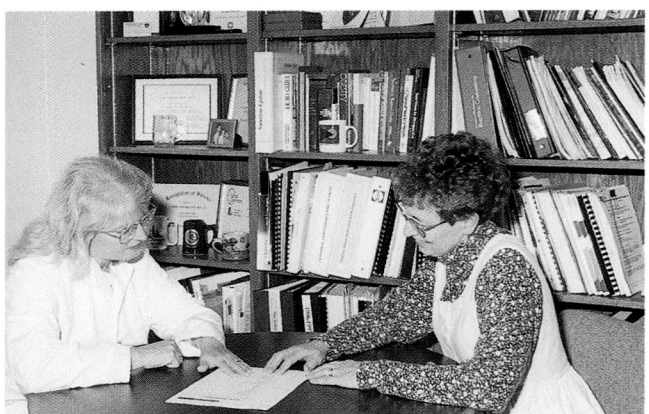

FIGURE 21–3 This nutrition counselor is using reflective listening techniques with her patient.

an issue. Readiness to change may fluctuate during the course of the discussion. The counselor must be ready to move back and forth between the phase-specific strategies. If the patient seems confused, detached, or resistant during the discussion, the counselor should return and ask about readiness to change. If readiness has lessened, tailoring the intervention is necessary. Every counseling session does not have to end with patient agreement to change; even a decision to think about change can be a useful conclusion.

Not-Ready-to-Change Counseling Sessions

To approach the not-ready-to-change stage of intervention, three goals are the focus: (1) to facilitate the patient's ability to consider change, (2) to identify and reduce the patient's resistance and barriers to change, and (3) to identify behavioral steps toward change that are tailored to each patient's needs.

To achieve these goals, several communication skills are important to master: asking open-ended questions, listening reflectively, affirming, summarizing, and eliciting self-motivational statements.

Asking Open-Ended Questions

The counselor asks questions that must be answered by explaining and discussing, not by one-word answers. The following statements and questions are examples that create an atmosphere for discussion:

- "We are here to talk about your dietary change experiences up to this point. Could you start at the beginning and tell me how it has been for you?"
- "What are some things you would like to discuss about your dietary changes so far? What do you like about them? What don't you like about them?"

Reflective Listening

Nutrition counselors not only listen but also try to tag those feelings that surface as a patient is describing difficulties with an eating pattern. Listening is not simply hearing the words spoken by the patient and paraphrasing them back. Reflective listening involves a guess at what the person feels and is phrased as a statement not a question. By stating a feeling the counselor communicates understanding. One also more fully understands the patient by labeling a feeling. The following are examples of listening reflectively.

EXAMPLE #1:

Patient: "I really do try, but I am retired and my husband always wants to eat out. How can I stay on the right path when that happens?"

Nutrition Counselor: "You feel frustrated because you want to follow the diet, but at the same time you want to be spontaneous with your husband."

EXAMPLE #2:

Patient: "I feel like I let you down every time I come in to see you. We always discuss plans and I never follow them. I almost hate to come in."

Nutrition Counselor: "You are feeling like giving up. You haven't been able to modify your diet, and it is difficult for you to come into our visits when you haven't met the goals we set."

EXAMPLE #3:

Patient: "Some days I just give up. It is on those days that I do very badly in following my diet."

Nutrition Counselor: "You just lose the desire to try to eat well on some days and that is very depressing for you."

EXAMPLE #4:

Patient: "I just don't want to do this any more!"

Nutrition Counselor: "You sound hassled by other priorities, and feel that the changes in your eating habits just get in the way."

Affirming

We often understand the idea of supporting a patient's efforts at following a new eating style, but do not put those thoughts into words. When the counselor is **affirming** someone, there is alignment and normalization of the patient's issues. **Alignment** involves the counselor telling the patient that he or she understands and is with him or her in understanding difficult times. **Normalization** means telling the patient that he or she is perfectly within reason and very normal to have such reactions and feelings. Below are some statements that indicate affirmation:

- "I know that it is hard for you to tell me this. But, thank you."
- "You have had amazing competing priorities. I feel that you have done extremely well, given your circumstances."
- "Many people I talk with express the same problems. I can understand why you are having difficulty."

Summarizing

The counselor tries to periodically summarize the content of what the patient has said by covering all the key points. Simple and straightforward statements are most effective, even if they involve negative feelings. If conflicting ideas arise, the counselor can use the strategy "on the one hand you . . . and on the other hand you . . ."; this reminds both individuals about the issues and ensures greater clarity.

Eliciting Self-Motivational Statements

The four communication strategies (to ask open-ended questions, listen reflectively, affirm, and summarize) are important to the final strategy of eliciting *self-motivation statements.* In this step the goal is for the patient to realize that a problem exists, that concern exists about it, and that positive steps in the future can be taken to correct the problem. The goal is to use these realizations to set the stage for later efforts at dietary change. Below are examples of questions to use in eliciting the self-motivational feeling statements.

PROBLEM RECOGNITION:

- "What things make you think that eating out is a problem?"
- "In what ways has following your diet been a problem?"

CONCERN:

- "How do you feel when you can't follow your diet?"
- "In what ways does not being able to follow your diet concern you?"
- "What do you think will happen if you don't make a change?"

INTENTION TO CHANGE:

- "The fact that you're here indicates that at least a part of you thinks it's time to do something. What are the reasons you see for making a change?"
- "If you were 100% successful and things worked out exactly as you would like, what would be different?"
- "What things make you think that you should keep on eating the way you have been? And what about the other side? What makes you think it is time for a change?"
- "What would be the advantages of making a change?"

OPTIMISM:

- "What makes you think that if you decide to make a change you could do it?"
- "What encourages you that you can change if you want to?"
- "What do you think would work for you, if you decided to change?"

Patients in this "not-ready-to-change" category have already told the counselor they are not doing well at making changes. Usually if a tentative approach is used by asking permission to approach the problem, the patient will not refuse. One asks permission by saying, "Would you be willing to continue our discussion and talk about the possibility of change?"

At this point, it is helpful to discuss thoughts and feelings about the current status of dietary change by asking open-ended questions:

- "Tell me why you picked _____ on the ruler." (Refer to previous discussion on the use of a ruler.)
- "What would have to happen for you to move from a _____ to a _____ (referring to a number on the ruler). How could I help get you there?"
- "What would need to be different for you to consider making new or additional changes in your eating?"
- "If you did start to think about changing, what would be your main concern?"

To show real understanding about what the patient is saying, summarizing the statements about his or her progress, difficulties, possible reasons for change, and what would need to be different to move forward, is beneficial. This form of paraphrasing will allow the patient to rethink his or her reasoning about readiness to change. This mental processing provides new ideas that can promote actual change.

Counselors often expect a decision and at least a goal-setting session when working with a patient. However, it is important in this stage to realize that traditional goal setting will result in feelings of failure on both the part of the patient and the nutritionist. If the patient is not ready to change, respectful acknowledgment of this decision is important. The counselor might say, "I can understand why making a change right now would be very hard for you. The fact that you are able to indicate this as a problem is very important, and I respect your decision. Our lives do change and if you feel differently later on, I will always be available to talk with you. I know when the time is right for you to make a change, you will find a way to do it."

When the session ends, the counselor will let the patient know that the issues will be revised after he or she has a time to think. Expression of hope and confidence in the patient's ability to make changes in the future, when the time is right, will be beneficial. Arrangements for follow-up contact can be made at this time.

With a patient who is not ready to change it is easy to become defensive and authoritarian. At this point, it is important to avoid pushing, persuading, confronting, coaxing, or telling the patient what to do. It is reassuring to a nutritionist to know that change at this level will often occur outside the office. The patient is not expected to be ready to do something during the visit.

Unsure-about-Change Counseling Sessions

The only goal in this stage of change is to build readiness to change. This is the point at which big changes can occur. This "unsure" stage is a transition from not being ready to deal with a problem eating behavior to preparing to continue the change. It involves summarizing the patient's perceptions of what is going on, including self-motivational statements that the participant has made. It includes the process of identifying the participant's ambivalence. The counselor can restate any statements that the participant has made about intentions or plans to change or do better in the future.

One crucial aspect of this stage is the process of discussing thoughts and feelings about current status. Use of open-ended questions as shown on page 457 will help the participant discuss dietary change progress and difficulties, and will help him or her discuss possible reasons for change; that is, what would need to be different to move forward.

This stage is characterized by feelings of ambivalence. The counselor should encourage the patient to explore ambivalence to change by thinking about "pros" and "cons." Some questions to ask are:

- "What are some of the things you like about your current eating habits?"
- "What concerns you about your current eating habits?"
- "What are some of the good things about making a new or additional change?"
- "What are some of the things that are not so good about making a new or additional change?"

By trying to look into the future, one can help patients see new and often positive scenarios. The counselor helps to tip the balance away from being ambivalent about change toward considering change, by guiding the patient to talk about what life might be like after a change, anticipating the difficulties as well as the advantages. An opening to generate discussion with the patient might go like this: "I can see why you're unsure about making new or additional changes in your eating. Imagine that you decided to change. What would that be like? What would you want to do?" The counselor then summarizes the patient's statements about the "pros" and "cons" of making a change, and includes any statements about wanting, intending or planning to change.

The next step is to *negotiate a change*. There are three parts to the negotiation process. The first is setting goals. Set broad goals at first, and hold more specific nutritional goals until later. "How would you like things to be different from the way they are?" and "What is it that you would like to change?"

The second step is to *consider options*. The counselor asks about alternative strategies and options, and then asks the patient to choose from among them. This is effective because if the first one does not work, the patient has other choices.

The third step is to *arrive at a plan*. This should be a plan that has been devised by the patient. The counselor touches on the key points and the problems, then writes down the plan.

To end the session, the counselor asks about the next step, allowing the patient to bring up the topic. The following questions provide some ideas for questions that might promote discussion:

- "Where do you think you will go from here?"
- "What do you plan to do between now and the next visit?"
- "Where does this leave you now?"

Arrange for the next contact.

Clinicians always want to jump ahead. Instead, the counselor must take this process slowly and not assume that the patient is ready to change. In a rush to help, counselors often give advice too soon. An astute counselor will avoid giving advice about change and will not feel badly if the patient does not agree to change. One might say the following: "You say you're unsure about what to do. I will not push you into a decision. It is up to you. Take your time to think about it. Let me know if you want to talk about it again. You have made changes in the past, and you are the best judge of when it is the best time to consider change."

Ready-to-Change Counseling Sessions

The major goal in this stage of change is to collaborate with the patient to set goals for change that include a plan of action. The nutrition counselor provides the patient with the tools to use in meeting nutritional goals.

This is the stage of change that is most often assumed when a counseling session begins. To erroneously assume this stage means that all of the strategies used to make a change are misused. The assumption of this stage often results in lack of adherence on the part of the patient and discouragement on the part of the nutritionist.

Initially, it is important to discuss thoughts and feelings about where the patient stands relative to current dietary change status. Use of open-ended questions helps the patient confirm and justify the decision to make a change. The following questions may elicit information about feelings toward change:

- "Tell me why you picked _____ on the ruler."
- "Why did you pick _____ instead of '1' or '12'?"
- "Give me some ideas for why you think you are ready to change."

Helping the patient to identify change options by asking if he or she would like to change and what a first step might be is an effective method. The following questions might help the patient identify options:

- "What could you do to change your eating habits?"
- "Is this feasible?"
- "How do you see things turning out if you make these changes?"

This is the stage where goal setting is extremely important. Here the counselor helps the patient to set a realistic and achievable short-term goal. "Let's do things gradually. What is a reasonable first step?"

Following goal setting, an action plan is set to help the patient map out the specifics of what must be done to achieve a goal. Having supportive people around to help with dietary adherence is important. What can others do to help? Early identification of barriers to adherence is important. If barriers are identified, plans can be formed to help eliminate those roadblocks to adherence.

Many patients fail to notice when a plan is working. Make sure that the patient knows when an action plan is a success by asking the patient to summarize the plan. The counselor then documents the plan for discussion at future sessions and assures that the patient has the plan in writing too.

The session should be closed with an encouraging statement and reflection about how the patient identified this plan by himself or herself. Indicate that each person is the expert on his or her own behavior. Compliment the patient on carrying out the plan. Below are ways of expressing these ideas to patients:

- "You are working very hard at this, and it's clear that you're the expert on what is best for you. You can do this!"
- "Keep in mind that change is gradual and takes time. If this plan doesn't work, there will be other plans to try."

Arrange for the next contact.

The key point to remember for this stage is to avoid telling the patient what to do. Clinicians often want to provide advice. However, it is critical that the patient express ideas of what will work best. "There are a number of things you could do, but what do you think will work best for you?"

RESISTANCE BEHAVIORS AND POTENTIAL STRATEGIES TO MODIFY THEM

Resistance to change is the most consistent emotion or state that will be faced when dealing with poor performers. Following are examples of resistance to change. In one type of resistance the patient contests the accuracy, expertise, or integrity of the nutrition counselor. In another type, the patient directly challenges the accuracy of what the nutrition counselor has said. In a third way, the patient discounts the nutrition counselor by questioning the therapist's personal authority and expertise. Finally, the nutrition counselor may be confronted with a hostile patient.

Resistance may also surface as interrupting, when the patient breaks in during a conversation in a defensive manner. The patient speaks while the nutrition counselor is still talking without waiting for an appropriate pause or silence. The patient may also break in with words obviously intended to cut off the nutrition counselor's discussion.

When patients express an unwillingness to recognize problems, cooperate, accept responsibility, or take advice they may be denying a problem. Some patients blame other people for problems; a wife may blame her husband for her inability to follow a diet.

Patients may disagree with the nutrition counselor when a suggestion is offered, but they frequently provide no constructive alternative. This includes the familiar "Yes but . . . ," which explains what is wrong with the suggestions.

Patients try to excuse their behavior. They may say, "I want to do better, but my life is always in a turmoil since my husband died 3 years ago." An excuse that was once acceptable, is reused beyond the point of it actually being a factor in the woman's life.

Some patients will make pessimistic statements about themselves or others. "My husband will never help me." "I have never been good at sticking with a goal. I'm sure I won't do well with it now."

Some patients are reluctant to accept advice. They express reservations about information or advice given. "I just don't think that will work for me."

Some patients will express a lack of willingness to change or an intention not to change. They make it very clear that they want to stop the dietary regimen.

Often patients show evidence of not following the nutrition counselor's advice. Clues that this is happening include using a response that does not answer the question, providing no response to a question, or changing the direction of the conversation.

A variety of strategies are available to assist the nutrition counselor in dealing with these problem situations. These strategies include: reflecting, double-sided reflecting, shifting focus, agreeing with a twist, emphasizing personal choice, and reframing. Each of these options will be described below.

Reflecting

In reflecting, the counselor identifies the patient's emotion or feeling and reflects it back. This allows the patient to stop and think about what was said. An example of this type of counseling skill is: "You seem to be very frustrated by what your husband says about your food choices."

Double-Sided Reflection

In **double-sided reflection,** the counselor will use ideas that the patient has expressed previously, to show the discrepancy between the patient's current words and the previous ones. For example:

Patient: "I am doing the best I can." (Previously this patient stated that she sometimes just gives up and doesn't care about following the diet.)

Nutrition Counselor: "On the one hand you say you

are doing your best, but on the other hand I believe I recall a time when you said you just felt like giving up and didn't care about following the diet. Do you remember that? Was that point in time different than now?"

Shifting Focus

Patients may hold onto an idea that they feel is getting in the way of their progress. If this really isn't the problem, the counselor should state that. For example:

Patient: "I will never be able to follow this low-fat diet as long as my grandchildren come to my house and want snacks."
Nutrition Counselor: "Are you sure that this is really the problem? Is part of the problem that you like those same snacks?"
Patient: "Oh, you are right. I love them too."
Nutrition Counselor: "Could you compromise? Ask your grandchildren which of this long list of low-fat snacks they like and buy them."

Agreeing with a Twist

This strategy involves offering agreement, but then moving the discussion in a different direction. The counselor agrees with a piece of what the patient says, but then offers another perspective on her problems. This allows the opportunity to agree with her statement and her feeling, but then to redirect the conversation onto a key topic. For example:

Patient: "I really like eating out, but I always eat too much and my blood sugars go sky high."
Nutrition Counselor: "You are in the majority when you say that you like eating out. Now that you are retired it is easier to eat out than to cook. I can understand that. What can we do to make you feel great about eating out, because you can still follow your eating plan and keep your blood glucose values in normal range?"

Emphasizing Personal Choice

Counselors should always emphasize that any future action belongs to the patient. Any advice given can be taken or avoided. This emphasis on personal choice helps patients avoid feeling trapped and confined by the discussion.

Reframing

With **reframing** the counselor changes the patient's interpretation of the same basic data, by offering a new one from another person's perspective. The counselor repeats the basic observation that the participant has provided, and then offers a new hypothesis for interpreting the data. For example:

Patient: "I gave up trying to meet my dietary goals because I was having some difficulties when my

CASE STUDY

Jane S. has struggled with changing her dietary fat intake and keeping her carbohydrate intake consistent over the past several months. She is concerned that she hasn't been doing well and wants to stop following the new style of eating and forget that she has non–insulin-dependent diabetes

Patient: "I feel so guilty when I come to talk with you because I haven't done any of the things to change my diet that we've talked about. I can hardly come to visits any more."
Nutrition Counselor: "You are feeling like giving up. You haven't been able to meet the goals we set and that makes it hard to come to visits."

Reword this statement to indicate your own thoughts about the patient's statement above.

Patient: "Yes, that is right."
Nutrition Counselor: "Please don't feel that you are alone. I talk to others who have your same feelings. I don't want you to feel guilty. In fact, I am the one who may have been missing signals from you. We were proceeding too quickly."
Patient: "You make me feel so much better."
Nutrition Counselor: "That's great! To summarize what we have said, you are hoping to eliminate some of those guilty feelings by just giving up on the new eating patterns. Let's try to look at other options. Would that work for you?"

What are other summarization statements that you might say?

Patient: "Yes, I would like to explore other ideas."
Nutrition Counselor: "If you were 100% successful and things worked out exactly as you would like them to, what would be different?" (This statement is getting at intention to change.)

What other open-ended questions could you ask to determine intention to change?

Patient: "I would feel comfortable being spontaneous and would still be able to eat less fat and keep my carbohydrate intake consistent."
Nutrition Counselor: "Great! Now, in which situations are you most often spontaneous?"
Patient: "Eating out is most often a problem."
Nutrition Counselor: "Wonderful. Let's talk about specifics. For example, what restaurants do you eat out in most often and what plans can we make so that you have control over spontaneous situations?"

This is just one example of a means toward eliciting self-motivational statements. It sends the counseling session in a positive direction with focus on a specific type of problem.

1. What does the patient's initial statement indicate about her stage of change?
2. Which of the counselor's statements are affirming ones?
3. What are other directions you might take this interview to elicit self-motivational statements?
4. What are some problem recognition questions?
5. What questions would you ask to elicit patient concerns?
6. What questions might you ask to determine the patient's optimism relative to change?

husband died, and I have decided now that I just cannot meet those strict goals."

Nutrition Counselor: "I remember how devastated you were when he died and how just cooking meals was an effort. Do you think that this happened as a kind of immediate response to his death and that you might have just at that time decided that all of the goals were too strict?" (Pause)

Patient: "Well, you are probably right."

Nutrition Counselor: "Could we look at where you are now and try to find things that will work for you now to help you in following the goals we have set?"

In summary, facilitating dietary self-management in patients involves knowledge of where they are in regard to their willingness to change. In facilitating change, nutrition counselors should tailor strategies to each stage of change. Successful change interventions lead to satisfying outcomes for both counselor and client.

REFERENCES

Brownell KD. Obesity: Understanding and treating a serious, prevalent, and refractory disorder. J Consult Clin Psychol 50:829, 1982.

Miller W, Rollnick S. Motivational Interviewing: Preparing People to Change Addictive Behaviors. New York: Guilford Press, 1991.

National Cholesterol Education Program. Hearty Habits Don't Eat Your Heart Out. NIH Publication no. 93-3102. Washington, DC: National Heart, Lung, and Blood Institute, 1993.

Ockene J, et al. The Coronary Artery Smoking Intervention Study. Worcester, MA: National Heart, Lung, and Blood Institute, 1988.

Prochaska J, DiClemente C. Toward a comprehensive model of change. In: Miller WR, Heather N (eds.): Treating Addictive Behaviors: Processes of Change. New York: Plenum, 1986, p. 3.

Prochaska JO, DiClemente CC. Transtheoretical therapy: Toward a more integrative model of change. Psychotherapy: Theory, Research, and Practice 20:161, 1982.

Prochaska JO, DiClemente CC. The Transtheoretical Approach: Crossing Traditional Boundaries of Change. Homewood, IL: Dorsey Press, 1984.

Prochaska JO, et al. In search of how people change. Am Psychol 47:1102, 1992.

Prochaska JO, et al. Changing for Good. New York: William Morrow, 1994.

Sandoval WM et al. Stages of change: A model for nutrition counseling. Topics in Clinical Nutrition 9:64, 1994.

Sigman-Grant M. Stages of change: A framework for nutrition interventions. Nutrition Today 31:162, 1996.

Sporny LA, Contento IR. Stages of change in dietary fat reduction: social psychological correlates. Journal of Nutrition Education 27:191, 1995.

Watson DL, Tharp RG. Self-directed Behavior: Self-Modification for Personal Adjustment, 5th ed. Pacific Grove, CA: Brooks/Cole, 1989.

ADDITIONAL REFERENCES

AbuSha R, Achterberg C. Review of self-efficacy and locus of control for nutrition- and health-related behavior. J Am Dietet Assoc 10:1122, 1997.

Baldwin T, Falciglia G. Application of cognitive behavioral theories to dietary change in clients. J Am Dietet Assoc 95:1315, 1995.

Bowen DJ, et al. Preliminary evaluation of the processes of changing to a low-fat diet. Health Ed Res 9:85, 1994.

Danish S, et al. The anatomy of a dietetic counseling interview. J Am Dietet Assoc 75:626, 1979.

DiClemente CC, et al. The process of smoking cessation: An analysis of precontemplation, contemplation, and preparation stages of change. J Consult Clin Psychol 59:295, 1991.

Fitzgerald RE, Prochaska JO. Nonprogressing profiles in smoking cessation: What keeps people refractory to self-change? J Subst Abuse 2:87, 1990.

Greene G, Rossi S. Stages of change for reducing dietary fat over 18 months. J Am Dietet Assoc 98:529, 1998.

Marcus BH, et al. Using the stages of change model to increase the adoption of physical activity among community participants. American Journal of Health Promotion 6:424, 1992.

Marlatt GA. Mindfulness and metaphor in relapse prevention: An interview with G. Alan Marlatt. J Am Dietet Assoc 94:846, 1994.

Pallonen UE, et al. A 2-year self-help smoking cessation manual intervention among middle-aged Finnish men: An application of transtheoretical model. Prev Med 23:507, 1994.

Prochaska JO, et al. Predicting change in smoking status for self-changers. Addict Behav 17:35, 1985.

Prochaska JO, et al. Standardized, individualized, interactive, and personalized self-help programs for smoking cessation. Health Psychol 12:399, 1993.

Rollnick S, et al. Negotiating behavior change in medical settings: The development of brief motivational interviewing. Journal of Mental Health 1:25, 1992.

Snetselaar L. Nutrition Counseling Skills, 3rd ed. Baltimore: Aspen Publishers, 1997.

Warpeha A, Harris J. Combining traditional and nontraditional approaches to nutrition counseling. J Am Dietet Assoc 93:797,1993.

Wilcox N, et al. Client characteristics as predictors of self-change in smoking cessation. Addict Behav 40:407, 1985.

CHAPTER 22

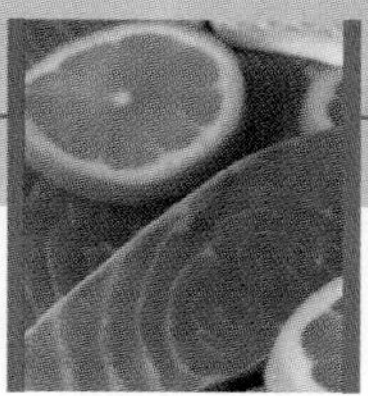

Enteral and Parenteral Nutrition Support

ABBY S. BLOCH, PhD, RD, FADA
AND CHARLES MUELLER, MS, RD, CNSD

Chapter Outline

- Rationale and Criteria for Appropriate Nutrition Support
- Enteral Nutrition
- Parenteral Nutrition
- Transitional Feeding
- Nutritional Support in Long-Term and Home Care
- Ethical Issues
- Interdisciplinary Nutrition Support Services
- Pharmacologic Use of Nutrients
- Research Trends

Key Terms

ASPIRATION OF RESIDUALS—withdrawal of the stomach's fluid volume to check for adequate gastric emptying

BACTERIAL TRANSLOCATION—the potential for passage of enteric pathogens or endotoxin through the epithelial mucosa of an impaired gastrointestinal tract into the blood or lymphatic system

BOLUS FEEDING—infusion of up to 500 cc of enteral formula into the stomach over 5 to 20 minutes, usually with a large-bore syringe

CATHETER—a very fine tube that can be threaded into the lumen of a blood vessel for infusion of fluids or withdrawal of blood

CONTINUOUS DRIP FEEDING—enteral formula administration into the gastrointestinal tract via pump usually over 8 to 24 hours per day

CYCLIC TOTAL PARENTERAL NUTRITION—administration of total parenteral nutrition solution for 12 to 18 consecutive hours, usually at night, followed by a 6- to 12-hour period of no infusion

ELEMENTAL OR DEFINED FORMULA DIET—nutritionally adequate liquid formula that leaves minimal residue in the bowel; can be fed orally or enterally

ENTERAL NUTRITION—provision of nutrients to the gastrointestinal tract through a tube or catheter when oral intake is inadequate

GASTRIC DECOMPRESSION—prevention of gaseous inflation (distention) of the gastrointestinal tract by the application of intermittent or continuous negative pressure (suction) through a nasogastric tube

This chapter is a revision of a chapter, contributed by Susan Bradford, MS, RD, CNSD, that appeared in the previous edition.

GASTROPARESIS—paralysis of the stomach resulting in impeded gastric emptying

HEMODYNAMIC STABILITY—the ability of a patient to maintain adequate blood volume and pressure

INTERMITTENT DRIP FEEDING—enteral formula administered at specified time periods throughout the day, generally in smaller volume and at a slower rate than a bolus feeding but in larger and faster volume than continuous feedings

LUMEN—the interior area of a tube, catheter, or blood vessel

MONOMERIC—when referring to protein and carbohydrate, the form in which the nutrient has been hydrolyzed into its smaller parts

NASOENTERIC TUBE—a tube inserted through the nasal passage into the stomach, duodenum, or jejunum

NEEDLE CATHETER JEJUNOSTOMY—feeding tube used to provide small-bore needle insertion into the jejunum at time of surgery

PARENTERAL NUTRITION—provision of nutrients directly into the bloodstream intravenously

PERCUTANEOUS ENDOSCOPIC GASTROSTOMY (PEG)—feeding tube whose insertion into the stomach involves using an endoscope and pulling the tube through a small incision in the abdominal wall

PERCUTANEOUS ENDOSCOPIC JEJUNOSTOMY (PEJ)—feeding tube inserted into the jejunum by use of endoscopic technique

PERIPHERAL PARENTERAL NUTRITION (PPN)—delivery of nutrients into a peripheral vein

POLYMERIC—when referring to protein and carbohydrate, the form in which the molecules appear intact or as an isolate

PULMONARY ASPIRATION—inadvertent inspiration into

the lungs of body fluids such as reflux contents from the stomach

REBOUND HYPOGLYCEMIA—low blood sugar resulting from abrupt cessation of total parenteral nutrition solutions

STOMA—artificially created opening between a body cavity and the body's surface that has healed

TOTAL NUTRIENT OR "THREE-IN-ONE" ADMIXTURES—referring to a parenteral nutrition mixture in which all three nutrients (amino acids, lipid, and glucose) are included in the same container

TOTAL PARENTERAL NUTRITION—delivery of nutrients into a large central vein, usually the superior vena cava

TRANSITIONAL FEEDING—the process of progressing from one method of nutrition support to another or to oral feeding

VILLOUS ATROPHY—erosion of the intestinal epithelial cell projections resulting in reduced absorptive or digestive capacity

---

Nutrition support is the delivery of formulated enteral or parenteral nutrients to appropriate patients for the purpose of maintaining or restoring nutritional status. **Enteral nutrition** refers to the provision of nutrients into the gastrointestinal tract through a tube or catheter when oral intake is inadequate. In certain instances, enteral nutrition may include the use of formulas as oral supplements or meal replacements. In this chapter, enteral nutrition will refer to the delivery of nutrients via a tube or **catheter** into the gastrointestinal tract. **Parenteral nutrition** is the provision of nutrients intravenously.

The origins of enteral and parenteral nutrition support trace back to the beginnings of medical care. Ancient Egyptians and Greeks used rectal feeding. President Garfield was fed in this manner after he was shot by an assassin. Forced feeding of the upper gastrointestinal tract and gastrointestinal decompression via relatively large tubes were first practiced in the 18th century. These early attempts at enteral nutrition used broths, wine, spirits, and milk as nutrient sources. Saline solutions given intravenously were used in the cholera epidemic of 1831. In the middle of the 19th century attempts to inject milk and broths subcutaneously met with little success. The first time that blood was transfused from one person to another by Blundell in 1891 marks the beginning of intravenous or parenteral therapy.

Modern techniques for enteral nutrition began with forced feeding of the upper gastrointestinal tract and gastrointestinal decompression as mentioned above. In 1919, Einhorn fed a patient through the small bowel. In 1938, Abbott and Rawson decompressed postoperative patients gastrically while simultaneously feeding into the jejunum. In the 1930s, mixtures of protein hydrolysates with glucose, levulose, invert sugar, casein gelatin, and ethyl alcohol were given to patients undergoing surgery, with limited success. The first commercially available enteral product was a hypoallergenic formula used to feed infants. In the late 1950s, a hydrolyzed enteral formula was developed for oral consumption by astronauts to, theoretically, minimize in-flight waste. This later became the first **monomeric** or **elemental** or **defined formula** for medical nutrition therapy (McCamish et al., 1997; Rhodes and Dudrick, 1993).

In 1953, Seldinger described a technique for placing an intravenous catheter into a (large) central vein that continues to be the standard method for accessing large central veins (Seldinger, 1953). This type of access made parenteral feeding of concentrated nutrients possible. A seminal report in 1968 described the growth of an infant with intestinal atresia maintained by central vein feeding (Wilmore and Dudrick, 1968). Throughout the 1970s and 1980s parenteral nutrition use expanded as access technology improved, intravenous macro- and micronutrient requirements were established, and complications were recognized and minimized. Enthusiasm for parenteral nutrition led to overzealous use in some instances. By the late 1980s, evidence suggested that there were advantages to using enteral as opposed to parenteral nutrition. Enteral access technology improved dramatically in the 1980s and the commercial enteral formula market expanded rapidly.

Historically, the use of enteral nutrition for acutely ill, postoperative, or post-trauma patients rested on evidence of bowel function as indicated by bowel sounds and flatus. These signs verify colonic motility. However, small bowel motility returns much sooner, within hours of surgery and trauma (Catchpole, 1989), and is the primary site of nutrient absorption. The feeding technique described by Abbott and Rawson (1939) requires small bowel motility but not colonic and gastric motility. Using this technique, which requires gastric decompression with concomitant small bowel feeding, enteral nutrition is now implemented in patients with small bowel function who previously were supported parenterally because their gastrointestinal function was assumed to be inadequate. Most practitioners agree that enteral nutrition presents fewer risks than parenteral nutrition and provides advantages to the patient that parenteral nutrition does not.

RATIONALE AND CRITERIA FOR APPROPRIATE NUTRITION SUPPORT

The theory that enteral nutrition is better for a patient than parenteral nutrition provides the rationale for justifying its use whenever feasible. This theory is based on the hypothesis that parenteral nutrition or bowel rest, rather than enteral nutrition during critical illness, causes a breakdown of the gastrointestinal mucosal barrier and increases its permeability to bacteria and endotoxins (**bacte-**

rial translocation) (see Fig. 33–6). This in turn causes or contributes to sepsis syndrome and multiple organ dysfunction syndrome (Alexander, 1990; Deitch, 1992). A major component of the gastrointestinal mucosa, *gut associated lymphoid tissue* or *GALT* is also compromised by bowel rest or parenteral nutrition. GALT comprises 50% of total body immunity, and 70% to 80% of total body immunoglobulin production is secreted across the gastrointestinal mucosa to defend against pathogenic substances in the gastrointestinal **lumen** (Langkamp-Henken et al., 1992).

Most research reports that form the basis for evidence that parenteral feeding can compromise gastrointestinal barrier and immune function have used animal models not human trials. Additionally, studies that have investigated gastrointestinal permeability in humans, have not tested the ability of bacteria and endotoxins to move across the gastrointestinal mucosa, but only harmless substances such as lactose and mannitol. These substances are not comparable to bacteria and endotoxins because their mechanism for crossing gastrointestinal mucosa is different. Nevertheless, compelling indirect data indicate that parenteral feeding or bowel rest in trauma and surgical populations is associated with higher infection rates (Moore et al., 1992). There is no evidence to suggest that stable individuals who are dependent on parenteral nutrition automatically translocate bacteria, become septic, or develop organ dysfunction. Such individuals usually have less than 2 to 3 feet (60 to 100 cm) of functioning small bowel available for absorption of nutrients. For these individuals, parenteral nutrition is life-sustaining therapy.

The following criteria can be applied to select appropriate candidates for nutrition support (Table 22–1). Enteral nutrition should be used in patients

TABLE 22–1 CONDITIONS THAT OFTEN REQUIRE NUTRITIONAL SUPPORT

CONDITION	RECOMMENDED ROUTE OF FEEDING	TYPICAL DISORDERS
Impaired nutrient ingestion	Enteral nutrition	Neurologic disorders HIV/AIDS Facial trauma Oral or esophageal trauma Congenital anomalies Respiratory ailments such COPD Cystic fibrosis Traumatic brain injury
Inability to consume adequate nutrition orally	Enteral nutrition	Hyperemesis of pregnancy Hypermetabolic states such as with burns Comatose states Anorexia in congestive heart failure, cancer Impaired intake after orofacial surgery or injury Spinal cord injury
Impaired digestion, absorption, metabolism	Enteral nutrition	Severe gastroparesis Inborn errors of metabolism Crohn's disease Short bowel syndrome with minimal resection
Severe wasting or depressed growth	Enteral nutrition	Cystic fibrosis Failure to thrive Cancer Congenital heart disease Burns or trauma Cerebral palsy Myasthenia gravis
Gastrointestinal incompetency	Parenteral nutrition	Short bowel syndrome—major resection Severe acute pancreatitis Severe inflammatory bowel disease Small bowel ischemia Intestinal atresia Severe liver failure Major gastrointestinal surgery
Hypermetabolic state with poor enteral tolerance or accessibility	Parenteral nutrition	Multiorgan system failure Major trauma or burns Bone marrow transplantation Acute respiratory failure with ventilator dependency and gastrointestinal malfunction Severe wasting in renal failure with dialysis Small bowel transplantation, immediate postoperatively

AIDS, acquired immunodeficiency syndrome; COPD, chronic obstructive pulmonary disease; HIV, human immunodeficiency virus.

who have at least 2 to 3 feet of functional gastrointestinal tract, who are or will become malnourished, and in whom oral intake is inadequate to restore or maintain nutritional status. Parenteral nutrition should be used in patients who are or will become malnourished and who do not have sufficient gastrointestinal function to be able to restore or maintain nutritional status (Matarese and Gottschlich, 1998). Figure 22–1 presents an algorithm for selecting enteral and parenteral nutrition routes.

These guidelines would seem to make the selection of the best type of nutrition support an easy decision; however, this is not always the case. For example, not all access methods reviewed in this chapter are universally available in all health care settings. Therefore, if a specific type of small bowel access is not available for enteral nutrition then parenteral nutrition may be the only realistic option. Often parenteral nutrition is used temporarily until adequate gastrointestinal function can support either enteral nutrition or oral intake. In this situation, a combination of feeding methods is used toward the goal of total reliance on the gastrointestinal tract for maintenance of nutritional status (see Transitional Feeding in this chapter).

Although nutrition support methodology can be standardized for the course of certain disease states or treatments, it is important to note that every patient presents an individual challenge, and nutrition support must often be adapted to unanticipated developments or complications. The optimal treatment plan requires interdisciplinary input and is closely aligned with the overall patient care plan. In a few instances, nutrition support may be warranted, but may be physically impossible to implement within the overall care plan. Conversely, nutrition support may be achievable, but may not be warranted because of the prognosis, unacceptable risk, or the patient's right to self-determination.

ENTERAL NUTRITION

By definition, enteral means "within or by the way of the gastrointestinal tract." In practice, enteral nutrition is generally considered as tube feeding. The consensus of nutrition experts is that the gastrointestinal tract is more physiologically and metabolically effective than the intravenous route for nutrient utilization (Klein et al., 1997; Lord et al., 1998). Once the patient has been assessed and found to be a good candidate for enteral nutrition, the clinician selects the appropriate tube and route of access for tube placement (Fig. 22–1). Enteral access selection depends on several factors: (1) anticipated length of time enteral feeding will be required, (2) degree of risk for aspiration or tube displacement, (3) presence or absence of normal digestion and absorption, (4) whether or not there is a planned surgical intervention, and (5) administration issues such as formula viscosity and volume.

Enteral Access

NASOGASTRIC ROUTE. For short-term enteral nutrition of 3 to 4 weeks, a **nasogastric tube** passed through the nose into the stomach is appropriate. Patients with normal gastrointestinal function and gag reflex tolerate this method, which takes advantage of normal digestive, hormonal, and bactericidal processes in the stomach. Feedings can be administered by bolus injection or intermittent or continuous infusions (see section on Administration). Soft, flexible, and well-tolerated polyurethane or silicone tubes of various diameters, lengths, and design features may be used, depending on formula characteristics and feeding requirements. For a more complete description of feeding tube characteristics, many resources are available (Guenter et al., 1997; Kirby et al., 1998). Tube placement is verified by aspirating gastric contents in combination with auscultation of air insufflation into the stomach or radiographic confirmation of the tube tip location. Techniques for placement verification have been described elsewhere (Levy, 1998). When soft, small-bore tubes are used, aspiration of gastric contents must be cautious to prevent the tube from collapsing.

NASODUODENAL OR NASOJEJUNAL ROUTE. For short-term enteral nutrition support of 3 to 4 weeks in patients at high risk for aspiration, esophageal reflux, delayed gastric emptying, or persistent nausea and vomiting, nasoenteric tubes placed postpylorically (into the small bowel) are appropriate. These tubes have various design features, such as weighted or nonweighted tips and stylets to guide placement. The tube is passed through the nose and esophagus and inserted into the stomach. The tip of the tube migrates into the small bowel via peristaltic activity. In critically ill patients, tube migration can take several days causing feeding delays. Radiologic verification of tube placement is the preferred method of confirmation to ensure safety. Tubes can also be placed with endoscopic or fluoroscopic guidance (Metheny, 1996; Shike and Bloch, 1998).

PERCUTANEOUS ENDOSCOPIC GASTROSTOMY (PEG) OR JEJUNOSTOMY (PEJ). The **percutaneous endoscopic gastrostomy (PEG)** is a nonsurgical technique for placing a tube directly into the stomach through the abdominal wall, performed under local anesthesia using an endoscope. Tubes are endoscopically guided into the stomach or the jejunum and then brought out through the abdominal wall to provide the access route for enteral feedings. The PEG is the preferred access route for patients requiring tube feeding for more than 3 to 4 weeks due to its short procedural time required for insertion, limited need for anesthesia, and minimal wound complications. After the initial PEG tube has been used successfully and the abdominal **stoma** site healed, it can be replaced with a "low-profile" device that allows the patient more freedom of movement and convenience such as ease in showering or wearing tight clothing. It is also possible to place a je-

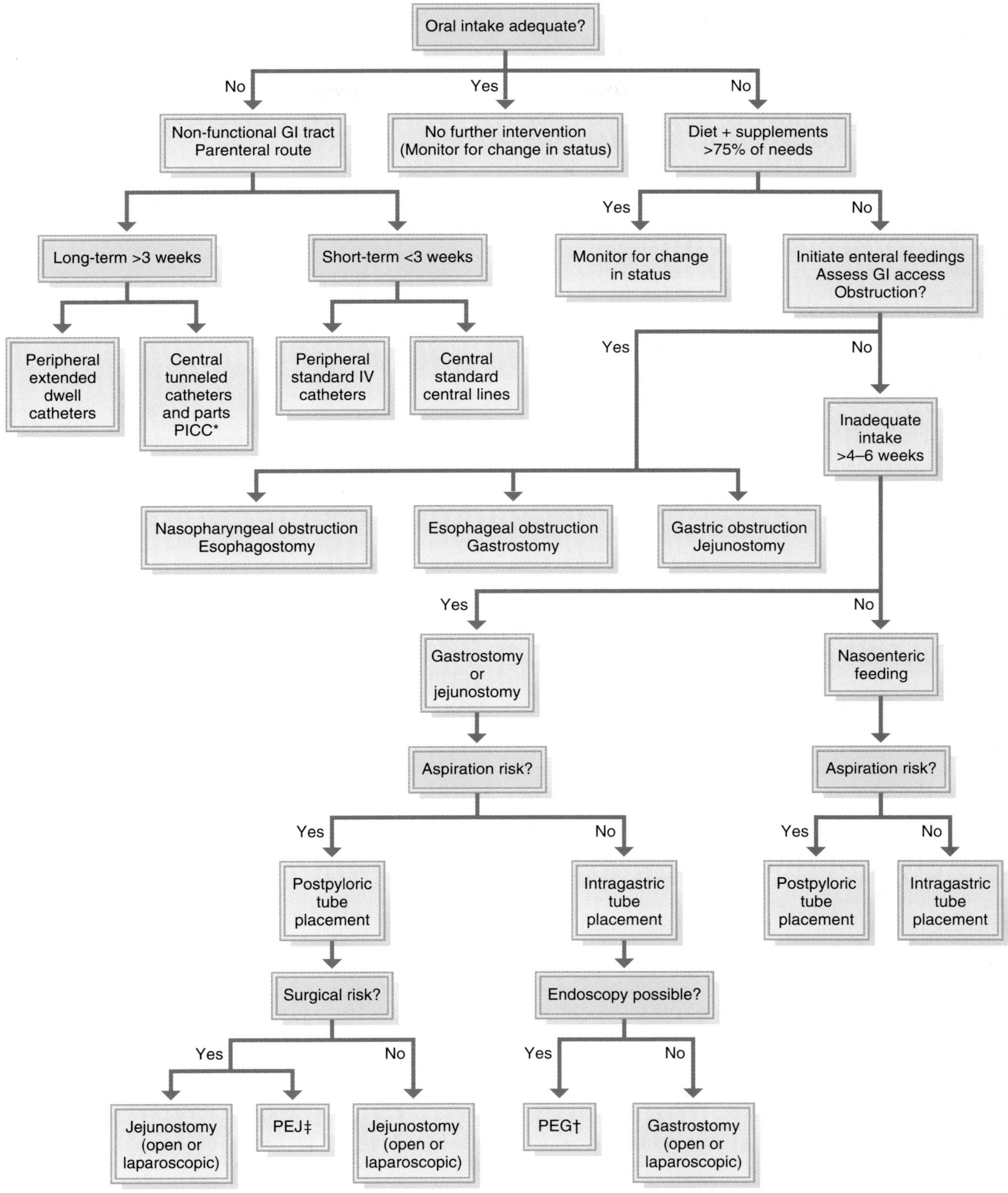

FIGURE 22–1 Algorithm for route selection. (Modified and adapted from: Gorman RC, Morris JB. Minimally invasive access to the gastrointestinal tract. In: Rombeau JL, Rolandelli RH (eds.). Clinical Nutrition: Enteral and Tube Feeding. Philadelphia: WB Saunders, 1997, p. 174; Ali A et al., 1988.)

junostomy tube percutaneously (PEJ). However, this procedure carries a higher degree of risk (Gorman and Morris, 1997; Kirby et al., 1998; Shike and Bloch, 1998).

OTHER MINIMALLY INVASIVE TECHNIQUES. High-resolution video cameras have made percutaneous radiologic and laparoscopic gastrostomy and jejunostomy enteral access an option for patients in whom endoscopic procedures are contraindicated. Using fluoroscopy, a radiologic technique, tubes can be visually guided into the stomach or the jejunum and then brought out through the abdominal wall to provide the access route for enteral feedings (Georgeson and Owings, 1998). Neither laparoscopic nor fluoroscopic techniques are widely used at this time but offer potential options for enteral access in the future (Gorman and Morris, 1997; Shike and Bloch, 1998).

SURGICALLY PLACED ENTEROSTOMIES. Surgical gastrostomies and jejunostomies are placed in patients requiring enteral support who are undergoing a surgical procedure or in whom endoscopic and radiologic techniques are not possible. The simplest surgical procedures for placing a gastrostomy tube are the Stamm and Witzel techniques. A more permanent method is the Janeway procedure. Surgical gastrostomy tubes have virtually the same use as PEGs (Ideno, 1992; Kirby et al., 1998; Shike and Bloch, 1998).

The Witzel jejunostomy and **needle-catheter jejunostomy** are short-term small bowel access methods. They are usually used for early postoperative enteral nutrition in combination with **gastric decompression.** The small lumen size of the needle-catheter jejunostomy can be problematic because it is easily dislodged and not all formulas flow readily through the catheter. Surgical jejunostomies provide the same decreased risk of pulmonary aspiration as nasojejunal and PEJ feeding techniques.

MULTIPLE LUMEN TUBES. Gastrojejunal dual tubes are available for either endoscopic or surgical placement. These tubes are designed for patients in whom prolonged gastric decompression is anticipated. The tube has one lumen for decompression and the other lumen is used to feed into the small bowel. These tubes are used for early postoperative feeding. For a summary of access sites, see Figure 22–2.

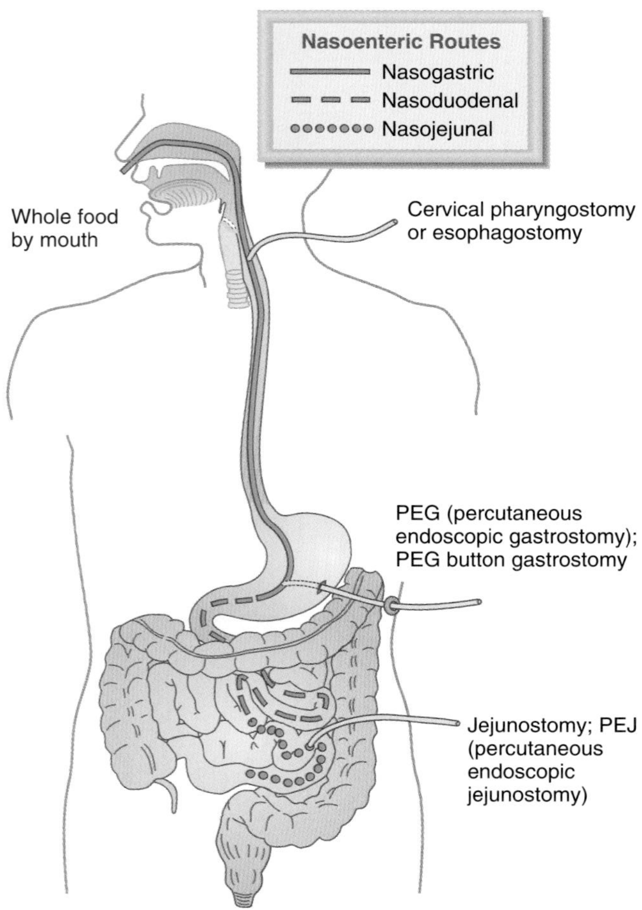

FIGURE 22–2 Diagram of enteral tube placement.

Enteral Formula Composition

A wide variety of enteral feeding products are commercially available. Evaluation of the suitability and efficacy of products, whether for individual use or for institutional use, is increasingly complex. As more products become available, with claims for pharmacologic effects, clinical trial evidence for each new product must be carefully evaluated by the clinician before a decision to use a product is reached (Matarese, 1998).

The suitability of a feeding formula for a patient should be evaluated based on the following characteristics: (1) functional status of the patient's gastrointestinal tract, (2) physical characteristics of the formula such as, osmolality, fiber content, caloric density, and viscosity, (3) macronutrient ratios, (4) digestion and absorption capability of the patient, (5) specific metabolic needs, (6) contribution of the feeding to fluid and electrolyte needs or restrictions, and (7) cost effectiveness. Small bowel feeding requires careful selection of formula because of sensitivity to osmolality and absorptive function of the small bowel. Figure 22–3 presents an algorithm for formula selection. See Chapter 9 for a similar discussion related to feeding infants.

Formulas are classified in a variety of ways usually based on protein or overall macronutrient composition. Table 22–2 presents one method of categorizing enteral formulas (see Appendices 35–40 also). General purpose formulas are tolerated by most patients, and most of these formulas provide 1.0 kcal/mL. General formulas that provide 1.5 to 2.0 kcal/mL are used when it is necessary to restrict fluid for patients with cardiopulmonary, renal, and hepatic failure. High-nitrogen formulas are used for patients with increased protein re-

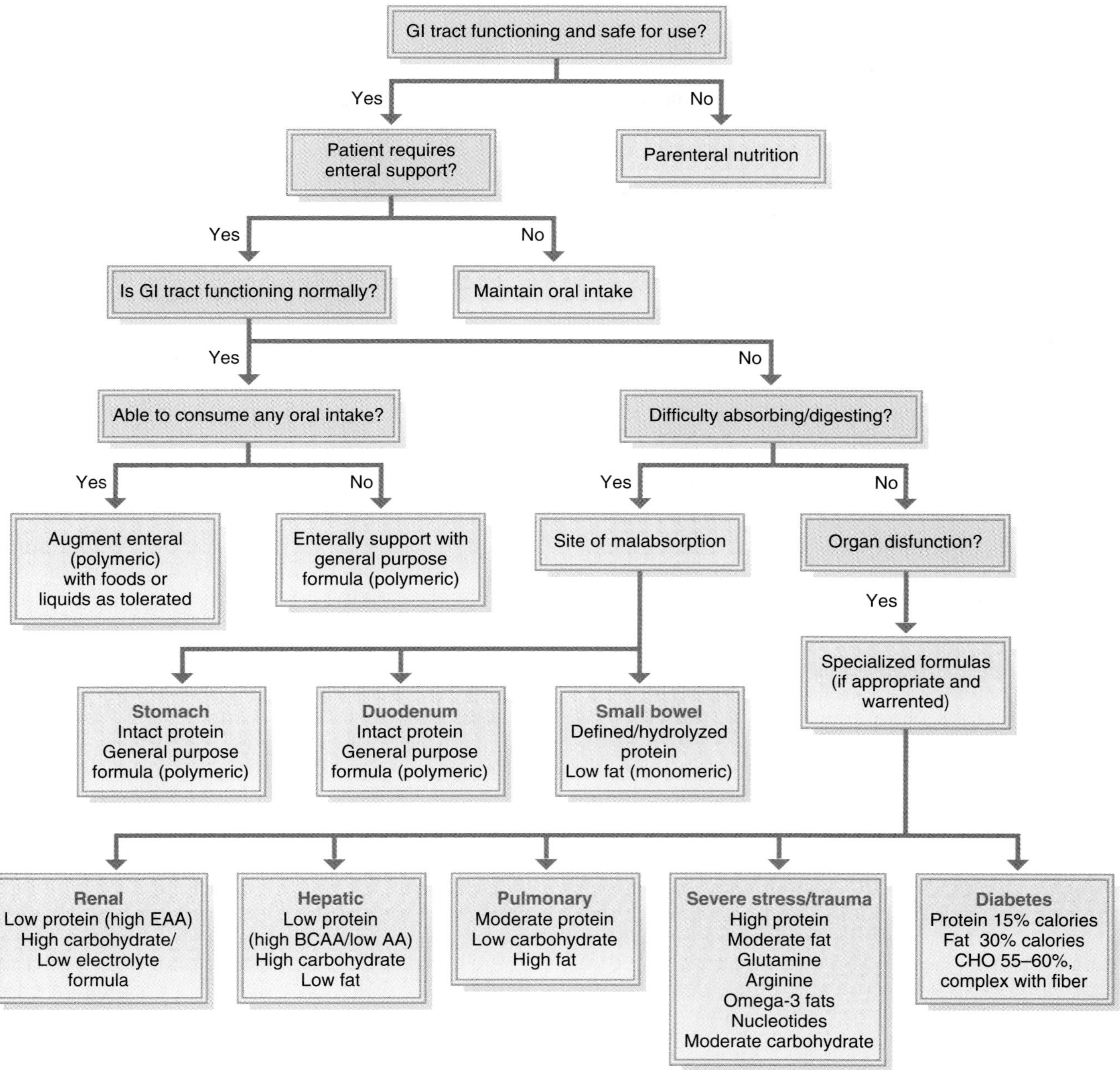

FIGURE 22–3 Algorithm for enteral formula selection. (Modified and adapted from Ali et al., 1988.)

quirements such as those with burns, fistulas, sepsis, and trauma. Disease-specific formulas are available for patients who have renal, hepatic, and cardiopulmonary disease, metabolic stress, immunosuppression, or glucose intolerance. The efficacy of disease-specific formulas is controversial (Gottschlich et al., 1997).

PROTEIN. Protein in enteral formulas provides 4% to 32% of total kilocalories (Olree et al., 1998). **Polymeric** formulas contain biologically complete, intact proteins such as caseinate, lactalbumin, beef, and soy protein isolate. Formulas containing peptide fragments (di- or tri- or oligopeptides) and amino acids derived from hydrolysis of casein, whey, lactalbumin, or soy, are available for patients with maldigestion and malabsorption. These formulas have higher osmolalities because of the hydrolyzed protein. The form of protein (intact or hydrolyzed) that is most efficiently digested and absorbed by the gastrointestinal tract remains controversial (Olree et al., 1998). High-protein formulas increase nitrogenous waste excretion by the kidneys. This process requires adequate amounts of fluid for efficient excretion, which is particularly

TABLE 22–2 **ENTERAL FORMULA CATEGORIES**

General Purpose/ Intact (Polymeric)	For use in patients with normal or minimally impaired digestion; absorption required; contains intact protein; can be instituted at full strength; low viscosity; 300–500 mOsm/kg; 1–1.2 kcal; lactose-free; 30–40 protein/L; inexpensive; also known as "house," general, meal replacement.
Defined/ Hydrolyzed (Monomeric)	For patients with GI compromise who require hydrolyzed nutrients for improved digestion; osmolality depends on hydrolysis; 1–1.2 kcal/cc; lactose free; 30–45 g protein/L; is more expensive than general purpose formula; also known as chemically defined, peptide-based, elemental formula.
Semielemental	For use in patients with limited GI function; contains free amino acids; minimal fat; minimal residue; hyperosmolar; low viscosity; 1 kcal/cc, 40 g protein/L; expensive; also known as free amino acid formula.
Disease-Specific	Designed for specific organ dysfunction or metabolic abnormality; may not be nutritionally complete; most are hyperosmolar; products specific for hepatic, renal, and pulmonary diseases, glucose intolerance, impaired immune function, and trauma (BCAA); expensive, available data should be evaluated carefully for efficacy and benefits.
Rehydration	For patients requiring an optimal ratio of simple carbohydrates to electrolytes for the purpose of maximizing fluid and electrolyte absorption and rehydration.
Modular	Formula providing protein, fat, or carbohydrate as single nutrients to alter the nutrient composition of commercial formulas or food; may also contribute electrolytes and increase osmotic or renal solute load; increase cost, require labor and safe mixing technique; also known as modular formulas.

(Developed from Olree K. et al. Enteral formulations. In: ASPEN (ed.). The ASPEN Nutrition Support Manual. Silver Spring, MD: American Society for Parenteral and Enteral Nutrition, 1998, p. 4–1; Gottschlich MM et al. Defined formula diets. In: Rombeau JR, Rolandelli RH (eds.). Clinical Nutrition: Enteral and Tube Feeding. Philadelphia: WB Saunders, 1997, p. 207; Ideno KT. Enteral nutrition. In: Gottschlich MM et al. Nutrition Support Dietetics Core Curriculum. Silver Spring, MD: American Society for Parenteral and Enteral Nutrition, 1992, p. 71.)

important in patients who cannot communicate thirst.

CARBOHYDRATE. Carbohydrate contributes 40% to 90% of total kilocalories in enteral formulas. Carbohydrate sources used in formulas are pureed fruits and vegetables, corn syrup solids, corn and tapioca starch hydrolysates, maltodextrins, sucrose, fructose, and glucose. Similar to protein, the carbohydrate source and degree of hydrolysis affect osmolality. Lactose is not used as a carbohydrate source in most formulas because lactase deficiency is common among acutely ill patients.

LIPID. Lipid provides 1.5% to 55% of total kilocalories of enteral formulas. General purpose formulas have between 30% to 40% of their total kilocalories provided by lipids, usually from corn, soy, sunflower, or safflower oils. Defined or monomeric formulas usually have minimal amounts of lipid. Approximately 2% to 4% of the daily calories in the form of linoleic acid is necessary to prevent essential fatty acid deficiency. Research suggests that high dosages of linoleic acid may suppress immune function. Short-chain and medium-chain saturated fatty acids, monounsaturated fatty acids, and omega-3 polyunsaturated fatty acids have been included in disease-specific formulas as alternatives to the high linoleic acid-containing vegetable oil formulas. Formulas high in lipid that are intended to prevent excess carbon dioxide retention and facilitate weaning from mechanical ventilation are also available (Gottschlich et al., 1997).

VITAMINS, MINERALS, AND ELECTROLYTES. Most, but not all, available formulas are designed to meet the recommended dietary allowances (RDAs) for vitamins and minerals if a sufficient volume is taken. It should be noted that these recommendations are for healthy populations, not acute or chronically ill populations. Electrolytes are provided in relatively modest amounts compared with oral diets and may require supplementation when diarrhea or drainage losses occur. Patients with compromised cardiopulmonary, renal, or hepatic function often require electrolyte restriction.

FLUID. Fluid needs for adults can be estimated at 1 mL of water/kcal, or 30 to 35 mL/kg of usual body weight (Lord et al., 1998). Without an additional source of fluid, tube-fed patients may not get enough free water to meet their needs, particularly when nutrient-dense formulas are used. Standard formulas contain 80% to 85% free water. Calorically dense formulas may have as little as 60% free water. All sources of fluid being given to a patient receiving enteral nutrition including feeding tube flushes, medications, and intravenous fluids should be considered when determining a patient's needs. Additional water can be provided through the feeding tube as needed.

OSMOLALITY. The size and number of the nutrient particles in a solution defines its osmolality (see Chapter 6). General purpose formulas have osmolalities between 300 to 500 mOsm/kg, which is close to the osmolality of body fluids. Osmolalities of nutrient-dense formulas are higher, ranging from 400 to 700 mOsm/kg. Hydrolyzed formulas are as high as 900 mOsm/kg water. Table 22–3 summarizes factors to consider when selecting an enteral formula.

Administration

The three common methods of tube feeding administration are bolus feeding, intermittent drip, and continuous drip. Method selection is based on a patient's clinical status and quality of life considerations. One method can serve as a transition to another method as the patient's status changes.

BOLUS. The feeding modality of choice when patients are clinically stable with a functional stomach is the syringe **bolus method.** Syringe bolus feedings are more convenient and less expensive than pump or gravity bolus feedings and should be

TABLE 22–3 FACTORS TO CONSIDER WHEN CHOOSING AN ENTERAL FORMULA

Gastrointestinal function
The type of protein, fat, carbohydrate, and fiber in the formula as related to the patient's digestive and absorptive capacity
Caloric and protein density of the formula (i.e., kcal/mL, g protein/mL, and kcal: nitrogen ratio)
Ability of the formula, taken in the amounts tolerated, to meet the patient's nutritional requirements
Sodium, potassium, magnesium, and phosphorus content of the formula, especially for patients with cardiopulmonary, renal, or hepatic failure
Viscosity of the formula related to tube size and method of feeding

encouraged when tolerated. A 60-mL syringe is used to infuse the formula. If bloating or abdominal discomfort develops, the patient is encouraged to wait 10 to 15 minutes before proceeding with the remainder of formula allocated for that feeding. The patient with normal gastric function can usually tolerate 500 mL of formula at each feeding. Three or four bolus feedings per day can provide the daily nutritional requirements for most patients (Lord et al., 1998).

INTERMITTENT DRIP. Quality of life issues are often the reason for the initiation of **intermittent drip feeding** regimens, which allow mobile patients more free time and autonomy as compared with continuous drip infusions. These feedings can be given by pump or gravity drip. A schedule is based on four to six feedings per day administered for 20 to 60 minutes. Formula administration is initiated at 100 to 150 mL per feeding, and increased incrementally as tolerated. Success with this method of feeding depends largely on the degree of mobility, alertness, and motivation of the patient to tolerate the regimen. Intermittent feedings as well as bolus feedings should not be used with patients at high risk for **pulmonary aspiration.**

CONTINUOUS DRIP. **Continuous drip** infusion of formula requires a pump. This method is appropriate for patients who do not tolerate large volume infusions such as occur with bolus or intermittent methods. Patients with compromised gastrointestinal function because of disease, surgery, antineoplastic therapy, and other physiologic impediments are candidates for continuous drip infusion. Patients with jejunostomies should also be fed by continuous drip infusion. The goal feeding rate, in milliliters per hour, is set by dividing the total daily volume by the number of hours per day of administration (usually 18 to 24 hours). Feeding is started at one quarter to one half the goal rate and advanced every 8 to 12 hours to the final volume. Formulas with osmolalities between 300 to 500 mOsm/kg can be started at full strength. Hyperosmolar formulas should be advanced conservatively to ensure tolerance. Dilution of formulas is not necessary (Lord et al., 1998).

Modern enteral pumps are small and easy to handle. Many pumps are battery operated for up to 8 hours in addition to being electrically powered, allowing flexibility and mobility for the patient. Most pumps have a complete delivery system available, including bags and tubing compatible with proper pump operation.

Monitoring and Complications

COMPLICATIONS. Table 22–4 provides a comprehensive list of complications associated with enteral nutrition and possible solutions. Aspiration of formula into the airway is a major concern for patients receiving enteral nutrition. To prevent aspiration patients should be positioned with their head and shoulders above their chest during and immediately after feeding. There is confusion in the literature as to the efficacy of checking *gastric residuals*. Stable patients, especially those on long-term feeding, do not need residuals checked regularly. Also, it is very difficult to aspirate the stomach contents and the residual may contain more secretions and gastric fluids than feeding. **Aspiration of gastric residual** is most relevant in critically ill patients and others at risk for **gastroparesis.** In these pa-

TABLE 22–4 COMPLICATIONS OF ENTERAL NUTRITION

Access Problems
Pressure necrosis/ulceration/stenosis
Tube displacement/migration
Tube obstruction
Leakage from ostomy/stoma site

Administration Problems
Regurgitation
Aspiration
Microbial contamination

Gastrointestinal Complications
Nausea/vomiting
Distention/bloating/cramping
Delayed gastric emptying
Constipation
High gastric residuals
Diarrhea
- Osmotic
- Secretory
- Drugs/medications
- Treatment/therapies
- Hypoalbuminemia
- Maldigestion/malabsorption
- Formula choice/rate

Metabolic Complications
Refeeding syndrome
Drug–nutrient interactions
Glucose intolerance/hyperglycemia/hypoglycemia
Hydration status—dehydration/overhydration
Hyponatremia
Hyperkalemia/hypokalemia
Hyperphosphatemia/hypophosphatemia
Micronutrient deficiencies

(Adapted from Hamaoui E, Kodsi R. Complications of enteral feeding and their prevention. In: Rombeau JL, Rolandelli RH (eds.). Clinical Nutrition: Enteral Tube Feeding. Philadelphia: Saunders, 1997; p. 554; Ideno KT. Enteral nutrition. In: Gottschlich MM et al. Nutrition Support Dietetics Core Curriculum. Silver Spring, MD: American Society for Parenteral and Enteral Nutrition, 1992.)

tients, residuals are usually checked every 4 hours, or as needed (Catchpole, 1989; Lord et al., 1998).

Abdominal leakage of gastric contents from a gastrostomy site can cause skin erosion and skin breakdown leading to infection and peritonitis. However, fewer than 10% of patients experience serious complications. The remainder of complications are minor and can be prevented with careful patient monitoring (Gorman and Morris, 1997; Hamaoui and Kodsi, 1997).

Diarrhea is a common complication frequently associated with enteral nutrition. The most likely causes of diarrhea among enterally fed patients are bacterial overgrowth, hypoalbuminemia, antibiotic therapy, and gastrointestinal motility disorders associated with acute and critical illness. Hyperosmolar medications such as magnesium-containing antacids, sorbitol-containing elixirs, and electrolyte replacement supplements can also contribute to diarrhea. Adjustment of medications or administration methods can frequently correct the diarrhea. The addition of soy polysaccharide, pectin, and other fibers, bulking agents, and antidiarrheal medications can also help.

Among stable patients receiving enteral nutrition, constipation may be a problem. Fiber-containing formulas or stool-bulking medication may be helpful, and adequate fluid must be provided. Gastrointestinal motility should be assessed. Diarrhea can coexist with constipation, usually when a patient is impacted.

MONITORING. Once enteral nutrition is initiated, frequent monitoring of the patient's actual intake and tolerance is necessary to ensure that nutritional goals are achieved and maintained. During routine patient care, actual feeding time is commonly lost from the patient's prescribed feeding schedule. One study has shown that less than half of tube-fed patients receive their entire prescribed intake on any given day. The most common reasons are (1) tube dislodged, (2) gastrointestinal intolerance, (3) medical procedures that required discontinuation of feeding, and (4) difficulties with the feeding tube position (Abernathy et al., 1989).

Monitoring of metabolic and gastrointestinal tolerance, hydration status, and nutritional status is extremely important. Table 22–5 gives guidelines for monitoring the tube-fed patient. Practice guidelines, institutional protocols, and standardized ordering procedures are helpful to ensure optimal, safe provision of enteral nutrition support. Figure 22–4 displays an enteral nutrition order form.

TABLE 22–5 ENTERAL NUTRITION MONITORING

Weight (at least 3 times/wk)
Signs and symptoms of edema (daily)
Signs and symptoms of dehydration (daily)
Fluid intake and output (daily)
Adequacy of enteral intake (at least 2 times/wk)
Nitrogen balance (24-h urine urea nitrogen) (weekly), if appropriate
Gastric residuals (every 4 h) if appropriate
Serum electrolytes, blood urea nitrogen (BUN), creatinine, (2–3 times weekly)
Serum glucose, calcium, magnesium, phosphorus, (weekly or as ordered)
Stool output and consistency (daily)

PARENTERAL NUTRITION

Assuming a patient is an appropriate candidate for parenteral nutrition, the next decision is to select the most appropriate type of venous access. First, it is necessary to choose between central and peripheral access (see Figure 22–1). *Central access* refers to catheter tip placement in a large, high blood flow vein such as the superior vena cava. *Peripheral access* refers to catheter tip placement in a small vein typically in the arm. Many clinicians do not use **peripheral parenteral nutrition (PPN)** because they argue that it is short-term therapy with minimal impact on nutritional status. Therefore, they feel that central access is required for effective parenteral nutrition. However, newer peripheral devices have made it possible to infuse PPN with a single catheter placed for up to a month. Others argue that PPN can be used as a supplemental feeding or in a transitional phase to enteral or oral feeding. Peripheral veins cannot tolerate concentrated solutions; therefore, diluted larger volume infusions are often necessary to meet nutritional requirements. Volume-sensitive patients such as those with cardiopulmonary, renal, or hepatic failure are not good candidates for PPN.

Additional helpful information for appropriate access selection is previous access history, edema or skin damage at the access site, medical and medication history, coagulation time, need for additional infusions, peripheral vein condition, functional status, and lifestyle (Krzysda and Edmiston, 1998). See Chapter 9 for similar discussion related to feeding low birthweight infants.

Parenteral Access

PERIPHERAL ACCESS. Nutrient solutions not exceeding 800 to 900 mOsm/kg can be infused through a routine peripheral intravenous catheter placed in a vein in good condition. Protocols for dressing changes and rotation of the site are used to prevent the principle complication of peripheral catheters—thrombophlebitis.

A more recent development in peripheral catheter technology is the *extended dwell catheter*. These catheters are sometimes called midline or midclavicular catheters, depending on their position. Extended dwell catheters require a vein large enough to advance the catheter 5 to 7 inches into the vein. These catheters can remain at the original site for 3 to 6 weeks and have made PPN a more feasible option in patients with veins that are large enough to tolerate the catheter (Krzysda and Edmiston, 1998).

ENTERAL NUTRITION SUPPORT ORDER
Date: ____________Time: ______________________________
DX: ____
Reason for TF: ______________________________________

ENTERAL NUTRITION SUPPORT ORDERS:

1. ROUTE: Check tube type
   ( ) NGT ( ) PEG/G-TUBE ( ) PEG/JTUBE

2. FORMULA: Check the desired formula

Formula	kcal/cc	Formula	kcal/cc
( ) general purpose	1.0	( ) fiber enriched	1.0
( ) general purpose Hi Nitrogen	1.2-1.4	( ) monomeric	1.0

3. METHOD OF FEEDING: Check the desired schedule

( ) Schedule A: Bolus Feeding Via Syringe/Gravity Bag
1. 8:00 am 240 cc formula
   12:00 pm 240 cc formula
   4:00 pm 240 cc formula
   8:00 pm 240 cc formula
2. Water can be added to gravity bag pending hydration needs.
3. As tolerated, Registered Dietitian to advance feeding and adjust water to meet goal rates.
4. Formula progression to goal: ____________
   ____
   ____
   ____

( ) Schedule B: Pump
1. Begin Full Strength 30cc/hr X 8 hrs.
2. If tolerated after 8 hrs., advance to 50cc/hr X 24 hrs.
3. As tolerated, Registered Dietitian to advance feeding and adjust water to meet goal rates.
4. Formula progression to goal:
   ____
   ____
   ____
   ____
   ____

( ) Schedule C: Tube Feeding Protocol Via Gravity Bag
1. Schedule: 6:00 am 2:00 pm
   10:00 am 6:00 pm
   10:00 pm
2. Initial Feeding - 240 cc water
   At next scheduled time - 240 cc Formula + 240 cc water
3. As tolerated, Registered Dietitian to advance feeding and adjust water to meet goal rates.
4. Formula progression to goal:

4. ( ) ALTERNATE ORDERS:
   CONSULT REGISTERED DIETITIAN TO DETERMINE FORMULA AND SCHEDULE:
   1. Formula ______________________
   2. Schedule: ______________________
      ____
      ____
      ____

REGISTERED DIETITIAN:

1. NUTRITIONAL GOAL:

Formula: ______________________
Calories: ______________________
Protein: ______________________
Vitamins/Minerals: ______________________
____
____
____

2. RECOMMENDATIONS:
____
____
____

Registered Dietitian: ______________________

ENTERAL NUTRITION SUPPORT GUIDELINES:
PHYSICIAN:
1. PLACEMENT: Confirm placement of NGT by abdominal x-ray.
2. MEDICATIONS: Identify Via enternal feeding tube:
   A. consult pharmacist to verify appropriate form of medication.
   B. 30 cc water flush before and after each medication.
   C. Administer each medication separately.
3. FLUID BALANCE: Patient fluid needs should be assessed, include IV, water flush and water available from tube feeding (formula is approximately 80% free water).
4. LABORATORY WORK-UP:
   A. Initial: Na, K, CO_2, C1, Bun, Creat, Mg, Ca, Phos
   B. Thereafter, as needed.

FIGURE 22–4 Enteral nutrition order form. (Courtesy of Memorial Sloan-Kettering Cancer Center.)

SHORT-TERM CENTRAL ACCESS. Catheters used for central or **total parenteral nutrition (TPN)** ideally consist of a single lumen. If central access is needed for other reasons, such as hemodynamic monitoring, drawing blood samples, or giving medications, multiple-lumen catheters are available. To reduce the risk of infection, the catheter lumen used to infuse TPN should be reserved for only that purpose. A central venous catheter is the most commonly used access for TPN. The line is inserted into the subclavian vein and advanced until the catheter tip is in the superior vena cava, using strict aseptic technique. Alternatively, an internal or external jugular vein catheter can be used with the same catheter tip placement. The motion of the neck, however, makes this site much more difficult for maintaining the integrity of a sterile dressing. Radiologic verification of tip site is necessary before infusion of nutrients can begin. Strict infection control protocols should be used for catheter placement and maintenance (Krzysda and Edmiston, 1998). Figure 22–5 shows alternative venous access sites for TPN.

LONG-TERM CENTRAL ACCESS. The most commonly used long-term catheter is a *"tunneled" catheter*. These single- or multiple-lumen catheters are placed in the cephalic, subclavian, or internal jugular veins and fed into the superior vena cava. A subcutaneous tunnel is created so that the catheter exits the skin several inches away from its venous entry site. Another type of long-term catheter is a port device that is implanted under the skin where the catheter would normally exit at the end of the subcutaneous tunnel. The entrance port must be accessed by a special needle. Ports can be single or double with an individual port being equivalent to a lumen. The latest development in long-term catheter technology is a *peripherally inserted central catheter* or *PICC*. This catheter is inserted into a vein in the antecubital area of the arm and threaded into the subclavian vein with the catheter tip placed in the superior vena cava. PICCs can be placed by trained professionals in the home setting, whereas placement of a tunneled catheter is a surgical procedure (Krzysda and Edmiston, 1998).

Long-term catheters are used for extended therapy in the hospital and are frequently used for home infusion therapy. Their greatest advantage for patients is better mobility and time away from infusion, which can be cycled at intervals. They also minimize risk of infection because the tunnel creates a barrier between the entry of the catheter into the skin and into the vein. Care of long-term catheters requires knowledgeable specialized handling and extensive patient education (see section on Home Care).

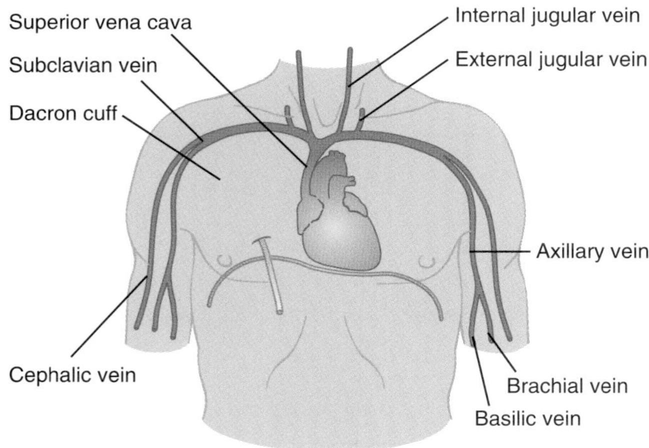

FIGURE 22–5 Venous sites from which the superior vena cava may be accessed.

Parenteral Nutrition Solutions

PROTEIN. Commercially available standard solutions are composed of both essential and nonessential crystalline amino acids. Specialized solutions with adjusted amino acid content are available for patients with hypermetabolism or renal or liver disease. These products are used on a limited basis because of their expense and the lack of conclusive research data supporting the efficacy of their use.

The concentration of amino acids in these solutions ranges from 3% to 15%. Thus, a 10% solution of amino acids supplies 100 g of protein per liter. The percentage of a solution is usually expressed at its final concentration after dilution with other nutrient solutions, but it is sometimes described by initial concentration. The caloric content of amino acid solutions is approximately 4 kcal/g protein provided. Approximately 15% to 20% of total energy intake should come from protein. Some practitioners calculate only nonprotein calories as the energy content of TPN, applying the theory that the protein will be used for anabolic processes rather than as a energy source (Strausburg, 1998).

CARBOHYDRATE. Carbohydrate is supplied as dextrose monohydrate in concentrations ranging from 5% to 70%. The dextrose monohydrate yields 3.4 calories/g. As with amino acids, a 10% solution yields 100 g of carbohydrate per liter of solution. The use of carbohydrate (100 g/day for a 70-kg individual) ensures that protein is not catabolized for energy. Maximal rates of carbohydrate administration should not exceed 5 mg/kg/min. Excessive administration can lead to hyperglycemia, hepatic abnormalities, and increased ventilatory drive. Calculation of osmolarity of a parenteral solution may be useful to ensure venous tolerance (Strausburg, 1998). See the accompanying box, "*Clinical Insight:* Calculating the Osmolarity of a Parenteral Nutrition Solution."

LIPID. Lipid emulsions, available in 10% and 20% concentrations, are composed of aqueous suspensions of soybean or safflower oil with egg yolk phospholipid as the emulsifier. The three-carbon molecule, glycerol, which is water soluble, is added to the emulsion to provide osmolarity. Glycerol is oxi-

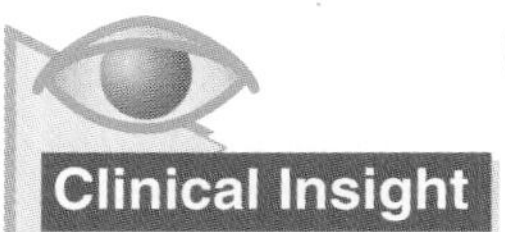

Clinical Insight: Calculating the Osmolarity of a Parenteral Nutrition Solution

1. Multiply the grams of dextrose per liter by 5. Example: 50 g of dextrose x 5 = 250 mOsm/L
2. Multiply the grams of protein per liter by 10. Example: 30 g of protein x 10 = 300 mOsm/L
3. Fat is isotonic and does not contribute to osmolarity.
4. Electrolytes further add to osmolarity. Total osmolarity = 250 + 300 = 550 mOsm/lL

(See also Chapter 6, Water and Electrolytes.)

dized and yields 4.3 kcal/g. A 10% emulsion provides 1.1 kcal/mL; a 20% emulsion provides 2.0 kcal/mL. Approximately 10% of calories per day from fat emulsions provides the 2% to 4% of calories from linoleic acid required to prevent essential fatty acid deficiency. Linoleic acid alters prostaglandin metabolism when it is a major source of energy and therefore can decrease immune function (Bell et al., 1991). Because soybean and safflower oils are a rich source of linoleic acid, lipid infusions that provide significantly more than 30% of total calories may be immunosuppressive. However, sometimes clinicians will provide more than 30% of total calories as lipid to help hyperglycemic patients control serum glucose levels or pulmonary-compromised patients to decrease carbon dioxide production and to improve respiratory function. Maximal dosage of lipid should not exceed 2.0 g/kg/day.

Electrolytes, Vitamins, and Trace Elements. General guidelines for daily requirements are given for electrolytes (Table 22–6), vitamins (Table 22–7), and trace elements (Table 22–8). Because parenterally administered vitamins and trace elements do not go through the digestive and absorptive processes, these recommendations are lower than the RDAs. Parenteral solutions also represent a significant portion of total daily fluid and electrolyte intake. Once a solution is prescribed and initiated, minor to major adjustments for proper fluid and electrolyte balance may be necessary, depending on the relative stability of the patient. The choice of the salt form of electrolytes (e.g., chloride, acetate) has an impact on acid–base balance. Vitamin K is usually not included in parenteral vitamin preparations in the hospital. If it is not contraindicated due to coagulopathy, it can be given by injection on a weekly basis. In the outpatient setting for long-term management, vitamin K may be added to the solution. Iron is also not normally part of parenteral infusions. It is given as needed to stable home care patients as iron dextran.

Fluid Needs. Fluid needs for parenteral and enteral nutrition are calculated similarly. Maximum volumes of TPN rarely exceed 3 liters, with typical prescriptions of 1.5 to 3 L/day. In critically ill patients, volumes of prescribed TPN should be closely coordinated with the overall care plan. The administration of other medical therapies requiring fluid administration such as intravenous medications and blood products necessitates careful monitoring. Patients with cardiopulmonary, renal, and hepatic failure are especially sensitive to fluid administration.

Compounding Methods. Parenteral nutrition prescriptions require preparation or compounding by

TABLE 22–6 DAILY ELECTROLYTE REQUIREMENTS DURING TOTAL PARENTERAL NUTRITION—ADULTS

ELECTROLYTE	PARENTERAL EQUIVALENT OF RDA	STANDARD INTAKE
Calcium	10 mEq	10–15 mEq
Magnesium	10 mEq	8–20 mEq
Phosphate	30 mmol	20–40 mmol
Sodium	N/A	1–2 mEq/kg + replacement
Potassium	N/A	1–2 mEq/kg
Acetate	N/A	As needed to maintain acid–base balance
Chloride	N/A	As needed to maintain acid–base balance

(From National Advisory Group on Standards and Practice Guidelines for Parenteral Nutrition, ASPEN: Safe practices for parenteral nutrition formulations. J Parenter Enteral Nutr, 22(2):49, 1998, with permission.)

TABLE 22–7 DAILY VITAMIN SUPPLEMENTATION TO ADULT PARENTERAL NUTRITION FORMULATIONS*†

VITAMINS	INTAKE
Thiamin (B_1)	3.0 mg
Riboflavin (B_2)	3.6 mg
Niacin (B_3)	40.0 mg
Folic acid	400.0 μg
Pantothenic acid	15.0 mg
Pyridoxine (B_6)	4.0 mg
Cyanocobalamin (B_{12})	5.0 μg
Biotin	60.0 μg
Ascorbic acid (C)	100.0 mg
Vitamin A	3300.0 IU
Vitamin D	200.0 IU
Vitamin E	10.0 IU

(From National Advisory Group on Standards and Practice Guidelines for Parenteral Nutrition, ASPEN: Safe practices for parenteral nutrition formulations. J Parenter Enteral Nutr 22(2):49, 1998, with permission.)

*Assumes normal organ function.

†Vitamin K supplementation 2–4 mg/wk in TPN patients not receiving oral anticoagulation therapy.

TABLE 22–8 DAILY TRACE ELEMENT SUPPLEMENTATION TO ADULT TOTAL PARENTERAL NUTRITION FORMULATIONS*

TRACE ELEMENT	INTAKE
Chromium	10–15 μg
Copper	0.3–0.5 mg
Manganese	60–100 μg
Zinc	2.5–5.0 mg

(From National Advisory Group on Standards and Practice Guidelines for Parenteral Nutrition, ASPEN: Safe practices for parenteral nutrition formulations. J Parenter Enteral Nutr 22(2): 49, 1998, with permission.)
*Assumes normal organ function.

competent pharmacy personnel under laminar airflow hoods using aseptic techniques. Prescriptions are compounded in two general ways. One method compounds all components except the fat emulsion, which is infused separately. Solutions are usually mixed in one bag at a 1:1 dextrose-to-amino acid volume ratio. The second method combines the lipid emulsion with the dextrose and amino acid solution and is referred to as a **total nutrient admixture** or **3-in-1 solution.** Standard solutions that can be compounded in batches save labor and lower costs. However, flexibility for individualized compounding should be available when warranted (Anderson, 1993; Strausburg, 1998). Standard order forms are often useful (Table 22–9).

It is possible to include medications with TPN, including antibiotics, vasopressors, narcotics, diuretics, and many other commonly administered drugs. In fact, this occurs infrequently, because it requires specialized knowledge of physical compatibility or incompatibility of the solution contents. The most common drug additives are insulin for persistent hyperglycemia and antacids to avoid gastroduodenal stress ulceration (Klang, 1998). Other drug additives, which are controversial, include heparin and exogenous albumin (Foley et al., 1990).

Administration

CONTINUOUS INFUSION. Parenteral solutions are usually initiated at 42 mL/h or 1000 mL/day via a volumetric pump, then increased incrementally over a 2- or 3-day period to attain the prescribed final volume. Some practitioners start parenteral nutrition based on the amount of dextrose with initial prescriptions containing 100 to 200 g/day and advancing over a 2- or 3-day period to a final goal. With high dextrose concentrations, abrupt cessation of TPN should be avoided, particularly if the patient's glucose tolerance is abnormal. If TPN is interrupted, infusion of a 10% dextrose solution will prevent **rebound hypoglycemia.** If TPN is to be stopped, it is prudent to taper the rate of infusion in an unstable patient to prevent rebound hypoglycemia. For most stable patients, however, this is not necessary.

TABLE 22–9 SAMPLE PARENTERAL NUTRITION FORMULATIONS

Adult Patient*
Institution/Pharmacy Name, Address and Pharmacy Phone Number

Name	Dosing weight: 70 kg	Location
Administration Date/Time		Expiration Date/Time
Basic formula	Amount/day	(Amount/L)
Dextrose	400 g	(166.7 g/L)
Amino acids [a]	100 g	(41.7 g/L)
Lipid [a]	65 g	(27.1 g/L)
Electrolytes		
Sodium chloride	80 mEq	(33.3 mEq/L)
Sodium acetate	80 mEq	(33.3 mEq/L)
Potassium chloride	40 mEq	(16.7 mEq/L)
Potassium phosphate	30 mmol of P	(12.5 mmol/L)
	(45 mEq of K)	(18.8 mEq/L)
Calcium gluconate	10 mEq	(4.2 mEq/L)
Magnesium sulfate		
Vitamins, trace elements, and medications		
Multiple vitamins [a]	10 mL	
Multiple trace elements [a]	1–3 mL [b]	
Infusion rate 100 mL/h	Volume 2400 mL	Infuse over 24 h

Admixture contains 2400 mL plus 100 mL overfill

*****Central Line Use Only*****

*(From National Advisory Group on Standards and Practice Guidelines for Parenteral Nutrition, ASPEN: Safe practices for parenteral nutrition formulations. J Parenter Enteral Nutr 22(2):56, 1998, with permission.)
[a] Specify product name.
[b] Volume dependent on specific product used.

Cyclic Infusion. **Cyclic TPN** can be infused for 8- to 12-hour periods usually at night, to improve quality of life. This permits a free period of 12 to 16 hours each day. The goal cycle for infusion time is established incrementally because a higher rate of infusion or a more concentrated solution is required. Cycled infusions should not be attempted if glucose intolerance or fluid tolerance is a problem.

Monitoring and Complications

As with enteral feeding, routine monitoring of actual intake is necessary to ensure compliance with the treatment plan. Administration time may be decreased due to patient ambulation and bathing, tests or other treatments, intravenous administration of medications, or other therapies.

Table 22–10 lists complications that can occur with parenteral nutrition. The primary associated complication is infection. Therefore, strict adherence to protocols and monitoring for signs of infection such as chills, fever, tachycardia, sudden hyperglycemia, or elevated white blood cell count are necessary to prevent infection. Monitoring of metabolic tolerance is critical to parenteral nutrition therapy. Electrolytes, acid–base balance, glucose tolerance, renal function, and cardiopulmonary and **hemodynamic stability** can be affected by parenteral nutrition and should be monitored carefully. Table 22–11 lists parameters that should be monitored routinely.

Catheter Care. The TPN catheter site is a potential source for introduction of microorganisms into a major vein. Protocols to prevent infection include dressing change at the catheter site every 48 to 72 hours and tubing change every 24 to 72 hours. With signs of infection, the catheter should be removed and the catheter tip cultured.

Refeeding Syndrome. Patients who require parenteral nutrition therapy are frequently moderately to severely malnourished. Aggressive administration of nutrition, particularly via the intravenous route, can precipitate the complication known as *refeeding syndrome* with severe, potentially dangerous electrolyte fluctuations leading to metabolic, neuromuscular, and hematologic problems. Refeeding syndrome occurs when energy substrates, particularly carbohydrate, are introduced into the plasma of anabolic patients. Proliferation of new tissue requires increased amounts of glucose, potassium, phosphorus, magnesium, and other nutrients essential for tissue growth. If intracellular electrolytes are not supplied in sufficient quantity to keep up with tissue growth, low serum levels of potassium, phosphorus, and magnesium develop. Low levels of these electrolytes are the hallmark of refeeding syndrome. Carbohydrate metabolism by cells also causes a shift of electrolytes to the intracellular space as glucose moves into cells for oxidation. Rapid infusion of carbohydrate stimulates insulin, which reduces salt and water excretion and increases the chance of cardiac and pulmonary complications from fluid overload.

TABLE 22–10 PARENTERAL NUTRITION COMPLICATIONS

Mechanical Complications
Pneumothorax
Hemothorax
Hydrothorax
Tension pneumothorax
Subcutaneous emphysema
Brachial plexus injury
Subclavian artery injury
Subclavian hematoma
Central vein thrombophlebitis
Arteriovenous fistula
Thoracic duct injury
Hydromediastinum
Air embolism
Catheter fragment embolism
Catheter misplacement
Cardiac perforation
Endocarditis
Infection and Sepsis
Catheter entrance site
Contamination during insertion
Long-term catheter placement
Catheter seeding from blood-borne or distant infection
Solution contamination
Metabolic Complications
Dehydration from osmotic diuresis
Hyperosmolar, nonketotic, hyperglycemic coma
Rebound hypoglycemia on sudden cessation of parenteral nutrition
Hypomagnesemia
Hypocalcemia
Hypercalcemia
Hyperphosphatemia and hypophosphatemia
Hyperchloremic metabolic acidosis
Uremia
Hyperammonemia
Electrolyte imbalance
Trace mineral deficiencies
Essential fatty acid deficiency
Hyperlipidemia
Gastrointestinal Complications
Cholestasis
Hepatic abnormalities
Gastrointestinal villous atrophy

Patients just starting parenteral nutrition who have received no form of nutrition for a significant period of time should be monitored for electrolyte fluctuation and fluid overload. They should receive conservative amounts of carbohydrate and be given adequate amounts of intracellular electrolytes. The syndrome may also be seen, and should be closely monitored, in enterally fed patients. However, the digestive and absorptive processes somewhat mediate a rapid impact from refeeding syndrome. In the early phase of refeeding, nutrient prescriptions should be moderate in carbohydrate, lactose-free, and supplemented with phosphorus, potassium, and magnesium (Hamaoui and Kodsi, 1997).

TABLE 22–11 THE PARENTERAL NUTRITION MONITORING*

VARIABLE TO BE MONITORED	SUGGESTED FREQUENCY	
	Initial Period*	Later Period*
Weight	Daily	Daily
Serum electrolytes	Daily	3/wk
Blood urea nitrogen	3/wk	1/wk
Serum total calcium or ionized Ca^{++}, inorganic phosphorus, Magnesium	3/wk	1/wk
Serum glucose	Daily	3/wk
Serum triglycerides	Weekly	Weekly
Liver function enzymes	3/wk	1/wk
Hemoglobin, hematocrit	Weekly	Weekly
Prothrombin time	Weekly	Weekly
Platelets	Weekly	Weekly
WBC count	As indicated	As indicated
Clinical status	Daily	Daily
Catheter site	Daily	Daily
Temperature	Daily	Daily
I & O	Daily	Daily

*Initial period refers to that period in which a full glucose intake is being achieved. Later period implies that the patient has achieved a steady metabolic state. In the presence of metabolic instability, the more intensive monitoring outlined under initial period should be followed.

I & O, intake and output, refers to all fluids going into the patient: oral, intravenous, medication; and all fluid coming out: urine, surgical drains, suctioning, vomitus, diarrhea.

WBC, white blood cells.

TRANSITIONAL FEEDING

All nutrition support care plans strive to use the gastrointestinal tract when possible whether with enteral nutrition or by a total or partial return to oral intake. Therefore, care plans frequently involve **transitional feeding,** moving from one type of feeding to another with multiple feeding methods being used simultaneously. The challenge to clinicians is to maintain adequate feeding to meet nutritional requirements throughout the transition period. This requires careful monitoring of patient tolerance and quantification of intake by parenteral, enteral, and oral routes. Most experts advise that oral diets to initially be low fat, lactose free, and low in other simple carbohydrates. These provisions will make digestion easier and minimize the possibility of an osmotic-type diarrhea. Attention to individual tolerance and food preferences will help maximize intake.

Parenteral to Enteral Feeding. To begin the transition from parenteral to enteral feeding, the initial step is to introduce a minimal amount of enteral feeding at a low rate of 30 to 40 mL/h to establish gastrointestinal tolerance. Once this has been established over a period of hours, the parenteral rate can be decreased to keep the nutrient levels at the same prescribed amount. As the enteral rate is increased by 25- to 30-mL/h increments every 8 to 24 hours, the parenteral prescription is reduced accordingly. Once it is established that the patient tolerates approximately 75% of nutrient needs by the enteral route, the parenteral solution can be discontinued. This process ideally takes 2 to 3 days. However, it may become more complicated, depending on the degree of gastrointestinal function. At times, this weaning process may not be practical and parenteral therapy can be stopped sooner. This will depend on overall treatment decisions and likelihood for tolerance of enteral feeding.

Parenteral to Oral Feeding. Once again, this transition is ideally accomplished by monitoring oral intake and concomitantly decreasing the parenteral infusion to maintain a stable nutrient intake until approximately 75% of the nutrient needs can be met consistently by oral intake. This process is often less predictable than the transition to enteral feeding, and depends on the patient's appetite, motivation, and general well-being. It is important to continue monitoring the patient for adequate oral intake once parenteral nutrition has been stopped and to initiate alternate nutrition support if necessary.

Enteral to Oral Feeding. A stepwise decrease is also used in the transition from tube feeding to oral feeding. It is usually more effective to move from continuous feeding to a 12- and then an 8-hour formula administration cycle during the night. This reestablishes hunger and satiety cues during daytime oral intakes. In practice, oral diets are often tried after inadvertent or deliberate removal of a nasoenteric tube. This type of interrupted transition should be monitored closely for adequate oral intake. Patients receiving enteral nutrition who desire to eat, and for whom it is safe to eat, can be encouraged to do so. Patients who cannot meet their needs by the oral route can be maintained by a combination of enteral nutrition and oral intake. Often oral supplements are useful.

Oral Supplements. The most common type of oral supplements are commercially available formulas meant primarily to augment the intake of solid foods. They generally provide approximately 250 kcal/8-oz or 240-mL portion, and approximately 8 to 14 g of intact protein. Fat sources are most commonly long-chain triglycerides although some contain medium-chain triglycerides. More concentrated, and thus more nutrient-dense formulas are also available, as well as a variety of flavors, consistencies, and modifications of nutrients for various disease states. Some oral supplements, theoretically, provide a nutritionally complete diet if taken in sufficient volume.

The form of carbohydrate is a key factor to patient acceptance and tolerance. The greater the amount of simple carbohydrate, the sweeter the taste and the higher the osmolality, which may contribute to gastrointestinal intolerance. Individual taste preferences vary widely, and normal taste is altered by certain drug therapies, most commonly chemotherapy. More concentrated formulas or greater volumes can contribute to taste, fatigue, and satiety. It is wise to monitor the intake of food as well as the actual intake of prescribed supplement. Oral supplements that contain hydrolyzed protein and free amino acids such as those developed for renal, liver, and malabsorptive diseases tend to be mildly to markedly unpalatable, and acceptance by the patient depends on motivation. Some of these formulas also lack sufficient vitamins and minerals.

Although commercially available supplements are most commonly used for convenience, modules of protein, carbohydrate, or fat or commonly available food items can produce highly palatable additions to a diet that needs nutritional bolstering. As examples, liquid or powdered milk, yogurt, tofu, or protein powders can be used to enrich cereals, casseroles, soups, or milk shakes. Thickening agents are now used to add variety, texture, and aesthetics to pureed foods which are used when swallowing ability is limited (see chapters on cancer, AIDS, and swallowing disorders). Imagination and individual tailoring can sometimes do much to increase oral intake, avoiding the necessity for more complex forms of nutrition support.

TABLE 22–12 SELECTING APPROPRIATE CANDIDATES FOR HOME NUTRITION SUPPORT

Considerations:

1. Potential improvement in the patient's quality of life
2. Benefit of long-term nutrition support for the patient's nutritional status
3. Patient's or family's ability to handle the financial commitment
4. Patient's or caretaker's ability to learn the protocol for administration
5. Ability to comply with the standards for safety
6. Patient's or caretaker's physical limitations that influence the ability to administer nutrition support safely

(Data from Matarese L. Nutrition support: Enteral nutrition. In: Lysen LK (ed.). Quick Reference to Clinical Dietetics. Gaithersburg, MD: Aspen Publishers, 1997, p. 177; Weckwerth J et al. Home nutrition support. In: Gottschlich MM et al. Nutrition Support Dietetic Core Curriculum. Silver Spring, MD: American Society for Parenteral and Enteral Nutrition, 1993, p. 467.)

NUTRITIONAL SUPPORT IN LONG-TERM AND HOME CARE

Long-Term Care. Long-term care generally refers to the nursing home setting and health care provided to the large proportion of elderly residents who reside in these facilities. Health care provided to long-term care residents focuses on quality of life and self-determination in addition to the management of acute and chronic disease. Indications for enteral and parenteral nutrition are generally the same for the elderly as they are for younger adults. Legal documents that state resident preferences about aspects of care, including those regarding the use of nutrition support, are important to help guide interventions on behalf of long-term care residents when they are no longer able to participate in decision-making. Finally, advanced age and end-stage dementia often blur distinctions between malnutrition and frailty. Differentiation between the effects of advanced age and malnutrition in this population is beginning to receive research attention, as is the influence that nutrition support has on the quality of life among long-term care residents (Karkeck, 1993).

Home Care. Resources and technology for safe and effective management of long-term enteral or parenteral therapy are now widely available for the home care setting (Ireton-Jones, 1997; Ireton-Jones et al., 1997; Nelson et al., 1998; Nutrition Intervention, 1998). The elements needed to implement home nutrition successfully include identification of appropriate candidates, choice of a suitable nutrition support regimen, training of the patient and family, and a plan for medical and nutritional follow-ups. These objectives are achieved through coordinated efforts of an interdisciplinary group of health care professionals.

Home nutrition therapy providers are organizations that provide nutrients, medications, supplies, equipment, and professional clinical services to patients at home in accordance with standards developed by professional organizations (American Society for Parenteral and Enteral Nutrition, 1992). Commercial companies manage nutrition support therapy alone or in combination with other home therapies, and may be affiliated with acute care facilities or private subcontractors. Criteria for selecting a home care company to provide nutrition support should be based on the company's ability to provide ongoing nutritional assessment, monitoring, and care plan revision (American Dietetic Association, 1994).

Although home management has been available for over 20 years, little outcome data have been generated. Mandatory reporting requirements do not exist in the United States for patients receiving home nutrition support. Therefore, the exact number of patients receiving home nutrition support is unknown (Howard et al., 1998).

The key factors in successful home nutrition support therapy are careful and coordinated discharge planning as well as patient and caregiver education (Evans and Czopek, 1995). Table 22–12 presents criteria to be considered when selecting candidates for home nutrition support. Patients can successfully manage their home care with the support of their families, an interdisciplinary team consisting of the physician, nurse, dietitian, pharmacist, social worker or discharge planner or case manager, working in conjunction with the home care provider (Nelson et al., 1998; Nutrition Intervention, 1998).

ETHICAL ISSUES

Whether to provide or withhold nutrition support is often a central issue in "end of life" decision-making. For patients who are terminally ill or in a persistent vegetative state, nutrition support can extend life to the point that issues of quality of life and the patient's right to self-determination come into play. Often, surrogate decision-makers are involved in treatment decisions. It is the responsibility of the nutrition support practitioner to know if documentation, such as a living will regarding the patient's wishes for nutrition support, is in the medical record, and, whether counseling and support resources for legal and ethical aspects of patient care are available to the patient and significant others (American Dietetic Association, 1992).

INTERDISCIPLINARY NUTRITION SUPPORT SERVICES

Optimal nutrition support requires the dedication and involvement of multiple disciplines. Organizational structure at the institutional level is necessary for the quality, safety, and cost effectiveness of nutrition support. Often, this structure begins with a nutrition committee charged with setting or suggesting policy and standards of care. Historically, in institutions where patients required complex and sophisticated nutrition support, nutrition support teams or services were often developed with patient care provided by a team consisting of physician, dietitian, pharmacist, and nurse specialist. These teams became models for interdisciplinary care. In fact, the Joint Commission on Accreditation of Healthcare Organizations (JCAHO) and the Health Care Financing Administration (HCFA) both emphasize effective, efficient, collaborative and consistent action from an interdisciplinary team (Comprehensive Accreditation Manual for Hospitals, 1998; Health Care Financing Administration, 1998).

Some experts believe standards of care and practice guidelines for optimal nutrition support have reduced the need for nutrition support teams and services (American Society for Parenteral and Enteral Nutrition, 1998). Cost containment has resulted in the dismantlement of teams, although conversely, institutions have justified the interdisciplinary team approach to help control costs (ChrisAnderson et al., 1996; Wesley, 1994). This apparent contradiction highlights the importance of documenting outcomes affected by health care interventions such as nutrition support.

PHARMACOLOGIC USE OF NUTRIENTS

Nutrition is entering an era in which ongoing research suggests a therapeutic role for specific nutrients and other food substances. This research shows promise for the future as researchers learn more about specific metabolic pathways in disease, stress, and trauma and begin to be able to manipulate these pathways with the use of specific nutrients.

Nutrients that have been supplemented in commercially available nutrition support products for a therapeutic effect have been limited primarily to adult enteral nutrition formulas. In the United States these formulas are the equivalent to medical foods. Parenteral solutions are regulated as drugs and therefore must undergo prior approval for demonstration of safety and efficacy before becoming clinically available.

Some of these nutrients and substances are recognized by the government as dietary supplements and have relatively flexible regulations governing product claims for health and well-being (Mueller and Nestle, 1995). In 1994, Congress passed the Dietary Supplement Health and Education Act. This legislation provides flexible guidelines for health claims and exempts dietary supplements from premarket approval regulations such as those that exist for food additives (Bartels and Miller, 1998). Table 22–13 presents nutrients and substances that are being investigated for their potential therapeu-

TABLE 22–13 SUBSTANCES BEING INVESTIGATED FOR POTENTIAL THERAPEUTIC EFFECTS IN ENTERAL OR PARENTERAL SOLUTIONS

Antioxidants such as beta-carotene, vitamin C, vitamin E, vitamin A, zinc, copper, manganese, and selenium have specific roles in deactivating free radicals.

Arginine is an amino acid that may enhance nitrogen retention, wound healing, and immune function.

Carnitine is a nitrogenous compound synthesized from lysine and methionine that is required for oxidation of long-chain fatty acids.

Choline is an amine that is required for phospholipid synthesis and very-low-density lipoprotein production; choline deficiency has been associated with hepatic abnormalities in patients receiving parenteral nutrition.

Glutamine is an amino acid that plays a pivotal role in metabolic processes; it is utilized by intestinal and immune cells as fuel.

Medium-chain triglycerides (MCT) do not require bile acids for digestion and are absorbed directly into hepatic portal circulation; they also do not require carnitine for oxidation.

Omega-3 fatty acids are precursors of prostaglandins that may enhance immune function and decrease the risk of cardiovascular disease.

Phytochemicals are active chemical compounds found in foods of plant origin which play a potential beneficial role in the prevention and treatment of disease. Some classes of phytochemicals include organosulfur compounds (allium), polyphenols including flavonoids and isoflavones, and terpenes, which include carotenoids.

Short-chain fatty acids are derived from dietary fiber after digestion by colonic bacteria and provide fuel for intestinal cells and maintaining healthy gastrointestinal mucosa.

Structured lipids are artificially produced lipids comprised of both long-chain and medium-chain fatty acids on the same glycerol moiety.

Taurine is an amino acid synthesized from cysteine that may be conditionally essential in metabolic stress.

tic effects. Some of them are classified as dietary supplements.

RESEARCH TRENDS

Health care outcomes and outcome research represent a significant trend in nutrition support research. Indeed, the JCAHO and HCFA have made outcomes the standard by which all health care is evaluated. The goal of this type of research is to identify medical care that is effective, and there is tremendous pressure on nutrition support clinicians to prove that enteral and parenteral nutrition are effective interventions (August, 1996). Research investigating the metabolic and physiologic differences between parenteral and enteral nutrition, as mentioned in the introduction, is ongoing. Another important area of research focuses on the use of nutrients and other substances normally occurring in foods as pharmacologic or preventive agents for specific diseases and conditions.

CASE STUDY

Jerome W. is a 44-year-old man admitted to the emergency room after a motor vehicle accident. After being stabilized, he was transferred to the operating room where he underwent a splenectomy, Whipple procedure, ascending colectomy including the ileocecal valve, and a needle catheter jejunostomy as a result of blunt abdominal trauma. He also underwent a left thoracotomy for chest tube placement because of a perforated lung and placement of a triple lumen right internal jugular (IJ) catheter for central venous access. After stabilization in the postanesthesia care unit Jerome was transferred to the intensive care unit (ICU) with an endotrachial tube in place for mechanical ventilation. He had a nasogastric tube in place for gastric decompression and bilateral Jackson Pratt tubes in place for postoperative abdominal wound drainage.

Jerome had an unremarkable medical history. He was 5 ft, 10 in. tall and 180 lbs on admission to the ICU. He had +1 pitting edema in his arms and legs on admission to the ICU.

Parenteral nutrition was started on postoperative day 2 in the ICU via the IJ catheter because the surgeons were concerned that the small bowel was not yet functional, although there was no abdominal distention. On postoperative day 4, 20 mL/h of enteral formula was started via the needle catheter jejunostomy with concomitant intermittent nasogastric decompression. By postoperative day 8, the jejunostomy enteral nutrition infusion was at 40 mL/h, providing close to half the amount of protein and energy that Jerome required. The parenteral nutrition infusion was decreased by half. On postoperative day 11 the parenteral nutrition was stopped because the jejunostomy infusion had been advanced to 80 mL/h. On postoperative day 12 the endotracheal tube was removed because Jerome had been successfully weaned from mechanical ventilation. An antiaspiration pureed diet was started.

Self-Assessment Questions

1. What were Jerome's fluid and electrolyte requirements in the first 5 days postoperatively?
2. What was the rationale for starting enteral nutrition through the needle catheter jejunostomy even though Jerome was on gastric decompression?
3. What kind of enteral formula would you recommend for Jerome and why?
4. At what point in the transition from enteral nutrition to an oral diet would you recommend stopping the enteral nutrition?
5. What is the nutritional significance of Jerome's resection of the ascending colon and ileocecal valve?

CITED REFERENCES

Abbott WO, Rawson AJ. Tube for use in postoperative care of gastroenterostomy patients. JAMA, 112:2414, 1939.

Abernathy GB, et al. Efficacy of tube feeding in supplying energy requirements of hospitalized patients. J Parenter Enteral Nutr 13(4):387-391, 1989.

Alexander JW. Nutrition and translocation. J Parenter Enteral Nutr 14:170s, 1990.

Ali A, et al. Nutrition Support Algorithms. Nutritional Support Services, vol. 8, #7: July, 1988, p. 13.

American Dietetic Association. Position of the American Dietetic Association: Issues in feeding the terminally ill adult. J Am Diet Assoc 92: 996, 1992.

American Dietetic Association. Position of the American Dietetic Association: Nutrition monitoring of the home parenteral and enteral patient. J Am Diet Assoc 94:664, 1994.

American Society for Parenteral and Enteral Nutrition. Standards of practice: Standards for home nutrition support. Nutr Clin Pract 7:65, 1992.

American Society for Parenteral and Enteral Nutrition. The A.S.P.E.N. Nutrition Support Practice Manual. Silver Spring, MD: Author, 1998.

Anderson JD. Components and compounding of total parenteral nutrition. Support Line 15:12, 1993.

August DA. Creation of a specialized nutrition support outcomes research consortium: If not now, when? J Parenter Enteral Nutr 20:394, 1996.

Bartels CL, Miller SJ. Herbal and related remedies. Nutr Clin Pract 5:211, 1998.

Bell SJ, et al. Alternative lipid sources for enteral and parenteral nutrition: Long- and medium-chain triglycerides, structured triglycerides and fish oils. J Am Diet Assoc 91(1):74, 1991.

Catchpole BN. Smooth muscle and the surgeon. Aust N Z J Surg 59:199, 1989.

ChrisAnderson D, et al. Metabolic complications of total parenteral nutrition: Effects of a nutrition support service. J Parenter Enteral Nutr 20(3):206, 1996.

Comprehensive Accreditation Manual for Hospitals. The Official Handbook. Oakbrook Terrace, IL: Joint Commission on Accreditation of Healthcare Organizations, 1998.

Deitch EA. Multiple organ failure. Ann Surg 216:117, 1992.

Dudrick SJ, et al. Management of the short bowel syndrome. Surg Clin North Am 71:625, 1991.

Evans MA, Czopek S. Home nutrition support materials. Nutr Clin Pract 10:37, 1995.

Foley EF, et al. Albumin supplementation in the critically ill. Arch Surg 125:739, 1990.

Georgeson K, Owings E. Surgical and laparoscopic techniques for feeding tube placement. In: Shike M, Bloch AS (eds.). Gastrointestinal Endoscopy Clinics of North America. Philadelphia: WB Saunders, 1998, p. 581.

Gorman RC, Morris JB. Minimally invasive access to the gastrointestinal tract. In: Rombeau JL, Rolandelli RH (eds.). Clinical Nutrition: Enteral and Tube Feeding. Philadelphia: WB Saunders, 1997, p. 174.

Gottschlich MM, et al. Defined formula diets. In: Rombeau JL, Rolandelli RH (eds.). Clinical Nutrition: Enteral and Tube Feeding. Philadelphia: WB Saunders, 1997, p. 207.

Guenter P, et al. Delivery systems and administration of enteral nutrition. In: Rombeau JL, Rolandelli RH (eds.). Clinical Nutrition: Enteral and Tube Feeding. Philadelphia: WB Saunders, 1997, p. 240.

Hamaoui E, Kodsi R. Complications of enteral feeding and their prevention. In: Rombeau JL, Rolandelli RH (eds.). Clinical Nutrition: Enteral and Tube Feeding. Philadelphia: WB Saunders, 1997, p. 554.

Health Care Financing Administration (HCFA). Medicare and Medicaid Programs; Hospital Conditions of Participation; Provider Agreements and Supplier Approval: Proposed Rule. Federal Register, 62:66726, 1998.

Howard L, et al. Outcome of long-term enteral feeding. In: Shike M, Bloch AS (eds.). Gastrointestinal Endoscopy Clinics of North America. Philadelphia: WB Saunders, 1998, p. 705.

Ideno KT. Enteral nutrition. In: Gottschlich MM, (eds.). Nutrition Support Dietetics Core Curriculum. Silver Spring, MD: American Society of Parenteral and Enteral Nutrition, 1992, p. 71.
Ireton-Jones C. Nutrition management of the patient outside the hospital setting. In: Lysen L (ed.). Quick Reference to Clinical Dietetics. Gaitherburg, MD: Aspen Publishers, 1997, p. 199.
Ireton-Jones C, et al. Clinical pathways in home nutrition support. J Am Diet Assoc 97:1003, 1997.
Karkeck JM. Nutrition support for the elderly. Nutr Clin Pract 5:211, 1987.
Kirby DF, et al. Enteral access and infusion equipment. In: ASPEN (ed.). The ASPEN Nutrition Support Practice Manual. Silver Spring, MD: American Society for Parenteral and Enteral Nutrition, 1998, p. 3-1.
Klang MC. Drug-nutrient considerations-parenteral nutrition. In: ASPEN (ed.). The ASPEN Nutrition Support Practice Manual. Silver Spring, MD: American Society for Parenteral and Enteral Nutrition, 1998.
Klein S, et al. Nutrition support in clinical practice: Review of published data and recommendations for future research directions. J Parenter Enteral Nutr 21(3):133, 1997.
Krzysda EA, Edmiston CE. Parenteral access and equipment. In: ASPEN (ed.). The ASPEN Nutrition Support Practice Manual. Silver Spring, MD: American Society for Parenteral and Enteral Nutrition, 1998.
Langkamp-Henken B, et al. Immunologic structure and function of the gastrointestinal tract. Nutr Clin Pract 7:100, 1992.
Levy H. Nasogastric and nasoenteric feeding tubes. In: Shike M, Bloch AS (eds.). Gastrointestinal Endoscopy Clinics of North America. Philadelphia: WB Saunders, 1998, p. 529.
Lord L, et al. Enteral nutrition implementation and management. In: ASPEN (ed.). The ASPEN Nutrition Support Practice Manual. Silver Spring, MD: American Society for Parenteral and Enteral Nutrition, 1998, p. 5-1.
Matarese L. Nutrition support: Enteral nutrition. In: Lysen LK (ed.). Quick Reference to Clinical Dietetics. Gaithersburg, MD: Aspen Publishers, 1997, p. 177.
Matarese LE. Enteral feeding solutions. In: Shike M, Bloch AS (eds.). Gastrointestinal Endoscopy Clinics of North America. Philadelphia: WB Saunders, 1998, p. 593.
Matarese LE, Gottschlich MM. Contemporary Nutrition Support Practice. Philadelphia: WB Saunders, 1998.
McCamish MA, et al. History of enteral feeding: Past and present perspectives. In: Rombeau JL, Rolandelli RH (eds.). Clinical Nutrition: Enteral and Tube Feeding. Philadelphia: WB Saunders, 1997, p. 1.
Metheny N. Verification of feeding tube placement. In: Ross Current Issues in Enteral Nutrition Support. Report of the First Ross Conference on Enteral Devices. Columbus, OH: Ross Products Division, Abbott Laboratories, 1996, p. 34.
Moore FA, et al. Early enteral feeding compared with parenteral reduces postoperative septic complications. Ann Surg 216:172, 1992.
Mueller C, Nestle M. Regulation of medical foods: Toward a rational policy. Nutr Clin Pract 10:8, 1995.
National Advisory Group on Standards and Practice Guidelines for Parenteral Nutrition, ASPEN: Safe practices for parenteral nutrition formulations. J Parenter Enteral Nutr 22(2):49, 1998.
Nelson JK, et al. Considerations for home nutrition support. In: ASPEN (ed.). The ASPEN Nutrition Support Practice Manual. Silver Spring, MD: American Society for Parenteral and Enteral Nutrition, 1998, p. 35-1.
Nutrition Intervention in Home Care; New Paradigms for Quality Patient Care. In: Ross Roundtables on Medical Issues, vol. 18. Columbus, OH: Ross Products Division, Abbott Laboratories Inc, 1998.
Olree K, et al. Enteral formulations. In: ASPEN (ed.). The ASPEN Nutrition Support Practice Manual. Silver Spring, MD: American Society for Parenteral and Enteral Nutrition, 1998, p. 4-1.
Rhodes JE, Dudrick SJ. History of intravenous nutrition. In: Rombeau JL, Caldwell MD (eds.). Parenteral Nutrition. Philadelphia: WB Saunders, 1993, p. 1-10.
Seldinger SI. Catheter replacement of needle in percutaneous arteriography: A new technique. Acta Radiol 39:368, 1953.
Shike M, Bloch AS. Enteral nutrition. Gastrointestinal Endoscopy Clinics of North America 8(3):529, 1998.
Strausburg KM. Parenteral nutrition admixture. In: ASPEN (ed.). ASPEN Nutrition Support Practice Manual. Silver Spring, MD: American Society for Parenteral and Enteral Nutrition, 1998, p. 8-1.
Weckwerth J, et al. Home nutrition support. In: Gottschlich MM et al. (eds.). Nutrition Support Dietetics Core Curriculum. Silver Spring, MD: American Society for Parenteral and Enteral Nutrition, 1993, p. 467.
Wesley JR. Nutrition support teams: Past, present, and future. Nutr Clin Pract 9:165, 1994.
Wilmore DW, Dudrick SJ. Growth and development of an infant receiving all nutrients exclusively by vein. JAMA 203:869, 1968.

ADDITIONAL REFERENCES

Abushufa R, et al. Essential fatty acid status in patients on long-term home parenteral nutrition. J Parenter Enteral Nutr 19:286, 1995.
ASPEN Board of Directors. Guidelines for the use of parenteral and enteral nutrition in adult and pediatric patients. J Parenter Enteral Nutr 17(suppl): 1SA-52SA, 1993.
ASPEN Board of Directors. Definition of terms used in ASPEN guidelines and standards. Nutr Clin Pract 10:1, 1995.
Berseth C. Minimal enteral feedings. Clin Perinatol 22:195, 1995.
Bower R, et al. Early enteral administration of a formula (Impact) supplemented with arginine, nucleotides, and fish oil in intensive care unit patients: Results of a multicenter, prospective, randomized clinical trial. Crit Care Med 23:436, 1995.
Brinson RR, et al. Hypoalbuminemia-associated diarrhea in critically ill patients. J Crit Illness 2:9, 1987.
Chima C, et al. Relationship of nutritional status to length of stay, hospital costs, and discharge status of patients hospitalized in the medicine service. J Am Diet Assoc 97:975, 1997.
Choban P, et al. Hypoenergetic nutrition support in hospitalized obese patients: A simplified method for clinical application. Am J Clin Nutr 66:546, 1997.
DeMeo MT. Current Issues in Enteral Nutrition Support, Report of the First Ross Enteral Device Conference. Columbus, OH: Ross Products Division, Abbott Laboratories, 1996.
Dietscher JE, et al. Nutritional response of patients in an intensive care unit to an elemental formula vs. a standard enteral formula. J Am Diet Assoc 98:335, 1998.
Dorner B, et al. To "feed or not to feed" dilemma. J Am Diet Assoc 97:S172, 1997.
Gogos C, et al. Total parenteral nutrition and immune system activity: A review. Nutrition 11:339, 1995.
Hebuterne X, et al. Acute renutrition by cyclic enteral nutrition in elderly and younger patients. JAMA 273:638, 1995.
Hester D, et al. Evaluation of the appropriate use of parenteral nutrition in an acute care setting. J Am Diet Assoc 96:602, 1996.
Metheny N, et al. PH concentrations of pepsin and trypsin in feeding tube aspirates as predictors of tube placement. JPEN J Parenter Enteral Nutr 21:279, 1997.
Mitchell S, et al. The risk factors and impact on survival of feeding tube placement in nursing home residents with severe cognitive impairment. Arch Intern Med 157:327, 1997.
Mizock B, Troglia S. Nutritional support of the hospitalized patient. Disease-a-Month 43(6), 1997.
Mueller C, et al. Order writing for parenteral nutrition by registered dietiticians. J Am Diet Assoc 96:764, 1996.
Quan-Yang Duh. Decision tree for route of enteral nutrition support: Placement techniques. In: Current Issues in Enteral Nutrition Support: Report of the First Ross Conference on Enteral Devices. Columbus, OH: Ross Products Division, Abbott Laboratories, 1996.
Reynolds J, et al. Does the role of feeding modify gut barrier function and clinical outcome in patients after major upper gastrointestinal surgery? J Parenter Enteral Nutr 21:196, 1997.
Schloerb P, Henning J. Patterns and problems of adult total parenteral nutrition use in US academic medical centers. Arch Surg 133:7, 1998.
Shronts E. Essential nature of choline with implications for total parentral nutrition. J Am Diet Assoc 97:639, 1997.
Swails W, et al. Effect of a fish oil structured lipid-based diet on prostaglandin release from mononuclear cells in cancer patients after surgery. J Parenter Enteral Nutr 21:266, 1997.
Winkler MF, Lysen LK. Suggested Guidelines for Nutrition and Metabolic Management of Adult Patients Receiving Nutrition Support, 2nd ed. Chicago: American Dietetic Association, 1993.

PART 4

Nutrition for Health and Fitness

The chapters in this section reflect the evolution of nutritional science, from the identification of nutrient requirements and the practical application of this knowledge to the more recent concepts that relate nutrition to the prevention of degenerative disease.

The relationship between nutrition and dental disease has long been recognized. In more recent decades, the possibility for reducing the incidence of cancer, atherosclerotic heart disease, hypertension, and osteoporosis by emphasizing appropriate nutrition has continued to accumulate supportive evidence.

Government agencies have traditionally assumed responsibility for ensuring the safety of the food supply and for making adequate nutrients available to high-risk segments of the population. The recommended dietary allowances have been a part of the nutrition scene for almost 50 years; new revision are being expanded and called reference dietary intakes. However, the setting of nutritional goals appropriate to health and fitness and specifically to prevention of degenerative diseases is a new role for government. The first federal guidelines on the identification, evaluation and treatment of overweight and obesity in adults were released in the summer of 1998. The opportunities for an affluent society to choose from a great variety of foods may easily lead to an overabundant intake of energy, and efforts to reduce body weight, widely pursued with varying degrees of enthusiasm and diligence, are seldom successful.

The prevention, or at least postponement, of various degenerative diseases is closely associated with physical fitness and is achieved in part through exercise and management of body weight.

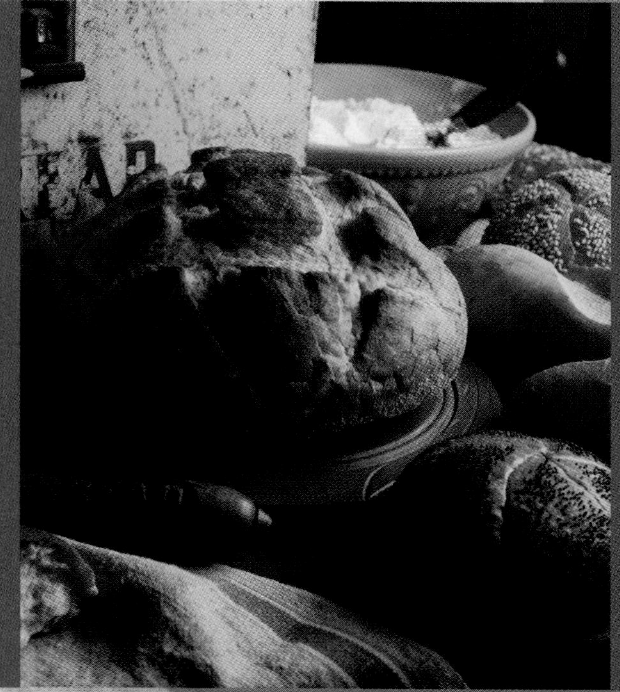

CHAPTER 23

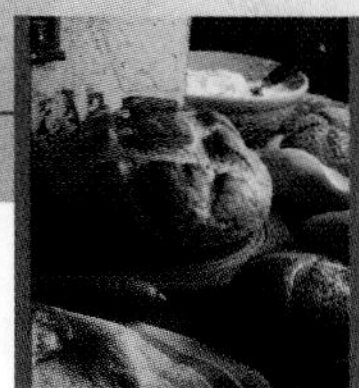

Nutrition for Weight Management

IDA LAQUATRA, PhD, RD

Chapter Outline

- Components of Body Weight
- Adipose Tissue: The Fat Depot
- Regulation of Body Weight
- Weight Imbalance: Obesity
- Tissue Adaptation to Weight Loss
- Management of Obesity
- Weight Imbalance: Excessive Leanness

Key Terms

ANDROID FAT DEPOSITION—deposition of fat around the waist and upper abdomen; "apple-shape" fat distribution
BARIATRICS—branch of medicine concerned with weight control, including gastroplasty and other types of surgical procedures
BROWN ADIPOSE TISSUE (BAT)—fat located in the scapular area that is involved in heat production for cold adaptation and possibly burning off excess energy
COMORBIDITY—any condition associated with obesity that usually worsens as the degree of obesity increases and often improves as the obesity is successfully treated
ESSENTIAL FAT—the body fat located in specific sites that is necessary for survival; about 3% to 12% of body weight
GASTRIC BYPASS—a surgical procedure in which the size of the stomach is reduced by a stapling procedure, and the small intestine is connected to the smaller stomach pouch through a new opening
GASTROPLASTY—a surgical procedure in which the size of the stomach is reduced with a row of staples across the top half of the stomach with a small opening left into the distal stomach
GYNOID FAT DISTRIBUTION—deposition of fat in the thighs and buttocks; "pear-shape" fat distribution
HORMONE-SENSITIVE LIPASE (HSL)—an enzyme in the adipose cell that is responsible for the hydrolysis of triglyceride into fatty acids and glycerol, which then leave the adipose cell and enter the circulation
HYPERPHAGIA—a period of overeating
HYPERPLASIA—increase in tissue size by an increase in the number of cells
HYPERTROPHY—increase in tissue size by an increase in cell size
HYPOPHAGIA—a period of undereating
LEAN BODY MASS (LBM)—the total of all body components except storage lipid and bone
LIFE-STYLE MODIFICATION—the examination of antecedents, behaviors, and consequences associated with eating habits, exercise, or thinking patterns
LIPOGENESIS—fat formation
LIPOPROTEIN LIPASE (LPL)—an enzyme on the luminal side of the capillary that facilitates transport of lipid from the blood and into the adipose cell
LIPOSUCTION—aspiration of fat deposits by means of a small incision through which a tube is fanned out into the adipose tissue
MORBID OBESITY—a state of adiposity in which body weight is 100% above the ideal body weight; a body mass index of 45 or greater
OBESITY—a state of adiposity in which body fatness is above the ideal; a body mass index of 30–30.9
OVERWEIGHT—a state in which weight exceeds a standard based on height; having a body mass index of 25–29.9 or greater
SENSORY SPECIFIC SATIETY—a decline in the pleasantness of a food as it is consumed
STORAGE FAT—the fat that accumulates under the skin and around internal organs
SYNDROME X—a condition associated with glucose intolerance, insulin resistance, hyperlipidemia, and hypertension; strongly linked to visceral obesity (fat accumulation predominantly in the intra-abdominal cavity)
UNDERWEIGHT—a body weight 15% to 20% below the accepted weight standard; a body mass index of less than 20
VERY LOW CALORIE DIET (VLCD)—a diet providing 800 kcal or less per day
WHITE ADIPOSE TISSUE—repository for triglycerides; a cushion to protect body organs and an insulator to preserve body heat
YO-YO EFFECT—the process of losing and gaining weight several times throughout a lifetime; often characterized by increased fatness with each cycle

Most adults maintain a constant body weight, due to a complex system of neural, hormonal, and chemical mechanisms that keeps the balance between energy intake and energy expenditure within fairly precise limits. Abnormalities of these mechanisms, many of which are not completely understood, result in exaggerated weight fluctuations. Of these, the most common are overweight and obesity. The inability to gain weight can be a problem, although this is usually secondary to another disease state.

Although the total energy intake in the United States decreased by 10% between 1900 and the 1980s, the extent of obesity doubled (Pi-Sunyer, 1988). The 1971 to 1974 National Health and Nutrition Examination Surveys (NHANES) reported 28.8 million obese individuals in the United States, of whom 8.4 million were classified as severely obese. According to NHANES II, these numbers had increased between 1976 and 1980 to 34 million obese, of whom 13 million were severely obese. According to NHANES III (1988–1991), 33% of Americans, translating to one in eight or 58 million people, are obese (Kuczmarski et al., 1994). The Federal Obesity Clinical Guidelines state that 97 million American adults (55%) are either overweight or obese (NIH, 1998). "Obese" is defined as being 20% above desirable body weight and "severely obese" as being 40% above desirable body weight.

Obesity is more common in women than in men; in non-Hispanic black and Mexican American women than in white women; in middle-aged black men than in white men of the same age; in women in poverty than in well-to-do women; and in affluent men than in men in lower income brackets. In children, poverty and neglect are important factors; a study in Denmark of 9- to 10-year-old children found that those who had poor hygiene and were neglected were more likely to be obese 10 years later (Lissau and Sorensen, 1994). The percentages of overweight for age, sex, and race categories are shown in Figure 23–1.

Obesity has been directly linked with mortality and many chronic ailments (NIH, 1998; Manson et al., 1995; Sjostrom et al., 1992). Mortality rates are one and one-half to two times higher among obese women compared to the leanest women enrolled in the Nurses' Health Study, a prospective study established in 1976, which follows the health of registered nurses in 11 states (Colditz, 1990). Furthermore, a weight gain of 10 kg (22 lb) or more since age 18 years was a predictor for increased mortality (Manson et al., 1995). Chronic diseases such as heart disease, type 2 diabetes, hypertension, stroke, gallbladder disease, sleep apnea, certain cancers, and osteoarthritis are associated with obesity and tend to worsen as the degree of obesity increases (NIH, 1998; Pi-Sunyer, 1993a; Shape Up America! and American Obesity Association, 1998).

The costs of obesity are staggering. Health economists, using prospective studies and national health statistics, pegged the cost for obesity at $99.2 billion in 1995 (Wolf and Colditz, 1998). Perhaps equally devastating is its negative image in current society, which fosters the widespread attitude that obesity is a disgrace. Young children, 6 to 9 years of age, have already adopted the disparaging attitudes of their parents toward the obese (Feldman et al., 1988).

Although society is gradually being exposed to the concept that fatness is a more complex issue than a matter of self-control, the obese—particularly women, adolescent girls, and the morbidly obese—continue to encounter discrimination in areas such as college placement, employment, and social opportunities. Victims typically are caught up in a vicious cycle of low self-esteem, depression, overeating for consolation, increased fatness, social

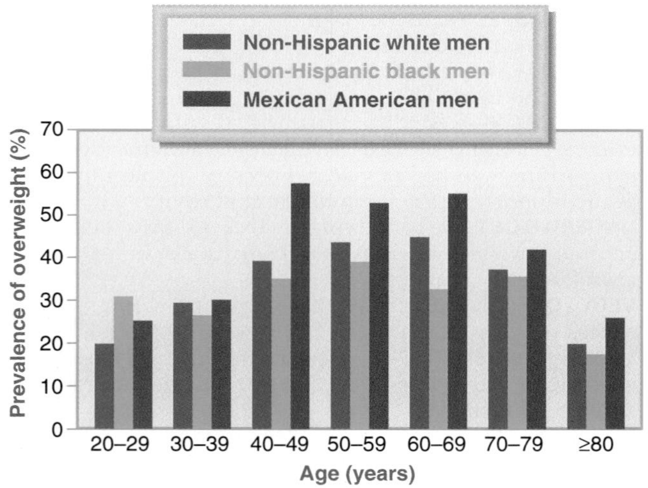

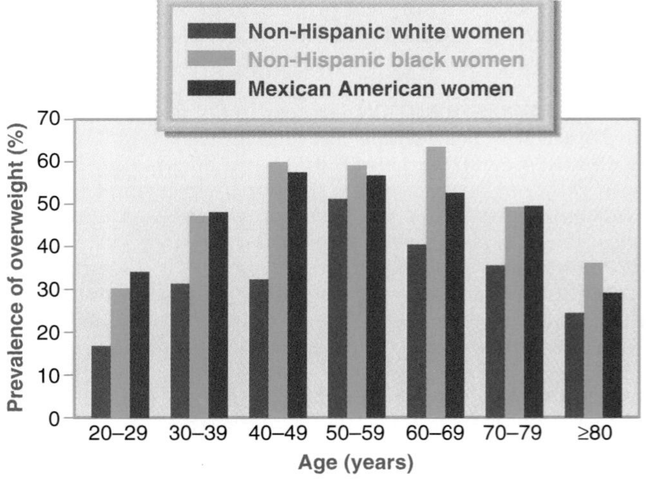

FIGURE 23–1 Unadjusted prevalence of overweight by age and race/ethnicity for men and women, US population 20 years of age or older, 1988 to 1991. (Redrawn from Kuczmarski RJ, et al. Increasing prevalence of overweight among US adults. The National Health and Nutrition Examination Surveys, 1960 to 1991. JAMA 272:205, 1994.)

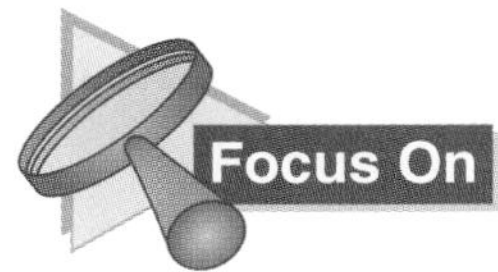

FAT DISCRIMINATION

Obese people, particularly women, are socially stigmatized. This negative perception adversely affects their educational, socioeconomic, marital and employment status (Enzi, 1994). Obese high school students, despite comparable grades, test scores, attendance, and extracurricular activities as their nonobese counterparts, were found to be less likely to be accepted into college (Wing and Greeno, 1994). Overweight women were found to have lower household incomes, a higher incidence of household poverty, and were less likely to be married (Enzi, 1994). Too many employers are unwilling to hire overweight individuals. Research confirms diverse groups, including children, adults, and medical personnel hold negative stereotypes of the obese (Wing and Greeno, 1994). These negative attitudes may stem from the belief that lack of willpower is a cause of obesity and that obese persons are weak-willed and self-indulgent (Stunkard, 1996).

The Council on Size & Weight Discrimination is working to end discrimination based on standards for body size and weight or shape, through public policy and opinions. The Council is interested in eliminating weight-loss surgeries, which can be life-threatening and disabling; enacting laws banning size and weight discrimination in employment, housing, and education; initiating sensitivity training for health care professionals and physicians; and tightening regulation of the diet industry to prevent erroneous claims.

Another organization working to overcome the stigma attached to obesity is the American Obesity Association. Founded in 1995, this nonprofit corporation is dedicated to encouraging individuals with obesity to obtain the best possible medical care for their condition; achieving greater research of obesity as a disease; and urging health insurance companies and government agencies (such as Medicare) responsible for programs to treat obesity as they do other diseases.

(Sources: Council on Size & Weight Discrimination, PO Box 305, Mt. Marion, NY 12456 (www.cswd.org); American Obesity Association, 1250 24th St NW, Suite 300, Washington, DC 20037.)

rejection, and further self-defeating actions (see "*Focus On:* Fat Discrimination").

Among health professionals at least, the simplistic view of obesity as a reflection of excessive intake or inadequate physical activity is gradually being abandoned in favor of recognizing the complex interaction among the physiologic, metabolic, and genetic factors that lead to an undesirable physical state.

The government has recognized that obesity is a public health concern. *Healthy People 2000* included a goal for reducing obesity prevalence in the United States to less than 20% (US Department of Health and Human Services, 1991). The 1995 Dietary Guidelines for Americans include a guideline for maintaining or improving body weight. The explanatory text addresses the increasing prevalence of obesity in the United States and the need to balance intake and output (Kennedy et al., 1996). The new Federal guidelines are a result of evidence-based principles for management of obesity (NIH, 1998).

There is no biologic reason to suggest that persons should increase their body weight as they age; there is more evidence to the contrary (Langseth, 1991). Energy restriction in genetically obese animals greatly increases longevity and slows signs of aging even when animals remain obese. Typically, a 40% reduction in food intake below that of animals eating freely increases the length of life in rodents by 50% (Masoro, 1994). Studies on rhesus monkeys suggest that the antiaging effects of calorie restriction in rodents can also occur in longer-lived species (Lane et al., 1997). These studies strengthen the possibility that calorie restriction will also prove beneficial in humans. Strong evidence suggests that longevity is affected by energy intake, not necessarily just fat calories. Plasma glucose and insulin levels are markedly lower when energy intake is reduced, and stress-protective glucocorticoids are higher.

Standard height–weight tables (see Appendix 19) have little meaning for individuals and may do more harm than good by categorizing individuals too simply. More emphasis should be placed on healthy life-styles and less on body weight alone (Abernathy and Black, 1994).

COMPONENTS OF BODY WEIGHT

Body weight is the sum of bone, muscle, organs, body fluids, and adipose tissue. Some or all of these components are subject to normal change as a reflection of growth, reproductive status, variation in exercise levels, and the effects of aging. Water, which makes up 60% to 65% of body weight, is the most variable component, and the state of hydration can induce fluctuations of several pounds. Muscle and even skeletal mass adjust to some extent to support the changing burden of adipose tissue. However, true weight loss and excessive weight gain are associated primarily with a change in the size of the fat depots.

Nonadipose tissue is frequently described in terms of **lean body mass (LBM).** Measures of *fat-free mass (FFM)*, or tissue devoid of all extractable fat, are available only by direct carcass analysis, whereas LBM can be determined clinically. LBM is higher in men, increases with exercise, and is lower in women and in the elderly; it is the major determinant of the resting metabolic rate (see Chapter 2).

ADIPOSE TISSUE: THE FAT DEPOT

Fat, the primary energy reserve of the body, is stored as triglyceride in depots made up of adipose tissue. Appropriate body fatness for an adult woman ranges from 20% to 25% of body weight with about 12% as **essential fat** (Fig. 23–2). In women, the essential fat includes an extra 5% to 9% *sex-specific body fat* in the breasts, pelvic regions, and thighs. It is not clear whether this fat is expendable or a reserve store. In men, appropriate body fatness is 12% to 15% of body weight, and approximately 3% is essential fat. This essential fat in both sexes includes fat stored in bone marrow, heart, lung, liver, spleen, kidneys, intestines, muscles, and lipid-rich tissues in the nervous system and is necessary for normal physiologic functioning. **Storage fat** is the fat that accumulates in the adipose tissue under the skin and around internal organs, to protect them from trauma. Body fatness below the level of essential fat appears to be incompatible with good health.

The totality of fat stores in *adipocytes* is capable of extensive variation, thus allowing for changing requirements of growth, reproduction, and aging, as well as fluctuations in environmental and physiologic circumstances such as the availability of food and the demands of physical exercise.

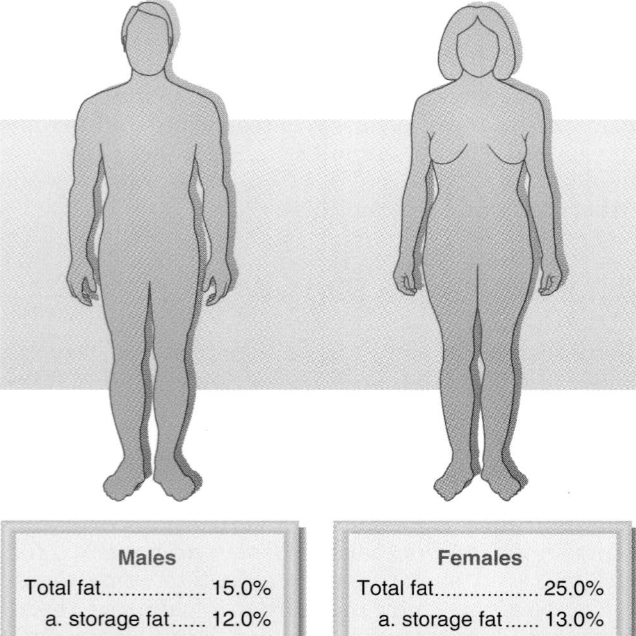

Males	
Total fat	15.0%
a. storage fat	12.0%
b. essential fat	3.0%
Muscle	44.8%
Bone	14.9%
Remainder	25.3%

Females	
Total fat	25.0%
a. storage fat	13.0%
b. essential fat	12.0%
Muscle	38.0%
Bone	12.0%
Remainder	25.0%

FIGURE 23–2 Behnke's theoretical body composition model for a man and woman.

Structure

Adipose tissue is located primarily under the skin, in the mesenteries and omentum, and behind the peritoneum. **White adipose tissue** serves as a repository for triglycerides, a cushion to protect abdominal organs, and an insulator to preserve body heat. Carotene gives it a slight yellow color. **Brown adipose tissue (BAT),** seen in infants and in very small amounts in adults, occurs primarily in the scapular and subscapular areas. The brown color is due to extensive vascularization. It has been studied most extensively in animals, where it appears to be involved in heat production as a means of adapting to cold and possibly of dissipating excess energy. Its function in adults remains controversial.

Regional Distribution

Interest in the genetics and phenotype of obesity is strong, because variability between individuals has been noted. Regional patterns of fat deposit are controlled genetically and differ between and among men and women. Four types of obesity have been recognized (Bouchard, 1991):

Type I	Excess body mass or percentage fat
Type II	Excess subcutaneous truncal-abdominal fat (android)
Type III	Excess abdominal visceral fat
Type IV	Excess gluteofemoral fat (gynoid)

Type I refers to an overall predominance of body fat, sometimes called "ovoid" shape (Egger, 1992). In this type, there is no particular concentration of fat in any given area of the body. Type II is defined as excess subcutaneous fat on the trunk, particularly in the abdominal area. Called **android fat deposition,** or "apple shape," this type of obesity is more common among men. Studies indicate that this type of obesity is highly correlated with insulin resistance (National Institutes of Health, 1998).

Type III is characterized by an excessive amount of fat in the abdominal visceral area (abdominal cavity). Studies suggest that the visceral fat component is strongly correlated with risk factors such as glucose intolerance, hyperlipidemia, and hypertension (Matsuzawa et al., 1994). Although type III obesity is not identical to the android type of obesity, the abdominal visceral fat accumulation is more prevalent in men than in women. Aging is also an important factor in visceral fat accumulation.

Type IV, **gynoid fat distribution,** is characterized by the "pear shape" created by heavier deposits of fat around the thighs and buttocks. Gynoid obesity is more common in women, and the fat deposits are presumably energy reserves to support the demands of pregnancy and lactation. Women with the gynoid type of obesity do not develop the impairments of glucose metabolism seen in obese women of the same weight who carry their fat in the abdominal area.

Postmenopausal women more closely follow the male pattern of abdominal fat stores. As a result, these women are at increased risk for blood glucose, lipid, and pressure abnormalities. Combinations of abdominal fat accumulation and gluteofemoral fat accumulation are also seen, particularly in women. Regional fat distribution defines risk of hyperlipidemia in obese children as it does in adults (Freedman et al., 1989). In both men and women who were obese during adolescence, rates of cardiovascular disease and diabetes are increased (Dietz, 1998).

Adipocytes

The mature adipocyte consists of a large central lipid droplet surrounded by a thin rim of cytoplasm, which contains the nucleus and the mitochondria. Adipocytes store fat in quantities equal to 80% to 95% of their volume.

Hypertrophy and Hyperplasia

Adipose tissue increases either by increasing the size of cells already present when lipid is added (**hypertrophy**) or by increasing the number of cells (**hyperplasia**). Weight gain may be the result of hypertrophy, hyperplasia, or a combination of the two. Obesity is always characterized by hypertrophy, but only some forms of obesity also involve hyperplasia (Bray, 1990).

The fat depots can expand as much as 1000 times through hypertrophy alone, a process that can occur at any time as long as space is available in the adipocytes. Hyperplasia occurs primarily as a part of the growth process during infancy and adolescence, but it can also occur in adulthood when the fat content of existing cells has reached the limit of their capacity. When weight is reduced due to trauma, illness, starvation, or changes in diet and exercise, fat cell size decreases.

Contrary to theories developed in the 1970s, it is now well accepted that the number of fat cells can increase throughout life. Cell numbers do not increase until maximal cell size is reached. The number of cells does not decrease with weight loss. Prevention is the key because once fat is gained and maintained over time, it is more difficult to lose.

Fat Cell Development

The greatest level of fatness in normal growth (approximately 25%) occurs at the age of 6 months. In lean children, fat cell size then decreases; however, this decrease does not occur in obese children. At the age of 6 years in lean children, increase in fatness occurs ("adiposity rebound"), with the increase being greater in girls than in boys. An early adiposity rebound occurring before 5.5 years is predictive of a higher level of adiposity at 16 years of age and in adulthood, a relationship that appears to occur regardless of the child's adiposity at 1 year of age. A later rebound is correlated with normal adult weight (Rolland-Cachera et al., 1984, 1990).

Cell number increases in both lean and obese children throughout childhood into adolescence, but the number increases faster in obese than in lean children. After adolescence, increases in body fat occur primarily by an increase in fat cell size.

Fat Storage

Source of Lipid in Fat Cells

Most depot fat comes directly from dietary triglycerides, as is evidenced by the fact that fatty acid composition of adipose tissue mirrors the fatty acid composition of the diet. Excess dietary carbohydrate and protein are also converted to fatty acids in the liver by means of a comparatively inefficient process, **lipogenesis.**

Composition of the diet has been the focus of intense study. Dietary fat provides a metabolizable energy value often greater than 9 kcal/g, in a range of 10.9 to 11.2 kcal/g (Dattilo, 1992). Under normal feeding conditions, little dietary carbohydrate is used to produce adipose tissue, and it requires approximately three times as much energy to convert excess energy from carbohydrate to fat storage as it does from dietary fat. However, when high carbohydrate diets are fed, and in particular, when the carbohydrate is simple sugars, lipogenesis from carbohydrate does occur (Hirsch, 1995). Additionally, data from several sources indicate that Americans eat too many calories, even though they eat less fat than consumed 30 years ago (Foreyt and Poston, 1997). Therefore, recommendations to simply reduce dietary fat are inappropriate. The type of carbohydrate recommended and total calories are critical variables (see "*Focus On*: Do Americans Understand Weight Management?").

Role of Lipoprotein Lipase

Dietary triglyceride is transported to the liver as a part of chylomicrons and removed from the blood by the enzyme **lipoprotein lipase (LPL),** which sits on the luminal side of the capillary and facilitates removal of lipid from the blood and its entry through the capillary wall into the adipose cell. Triglyceride, synthesized in the liver from free fatty acids, travels as part of *very-low-density lipoprotein (VLDL)* particles and is removed from the blood in the periphery by LPL. This enzyme hydrolyzes triglyceride into free fatty acids and glycerol. Glycerol proceeds to the liver; fatty acids enter the adipocyte, where they are re-esterified into triglyceride. When needed by other cells, the latter are hy-

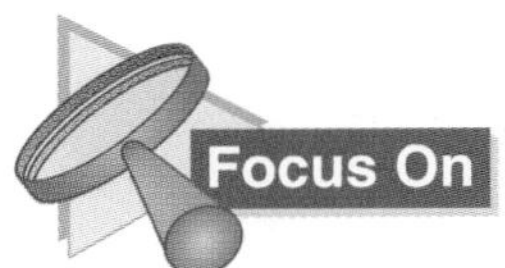

Do Americans Understand Weight Management?

For years, the media, health organizations and the government have been carrying an important message to American consumers: "fat intake should be reduced to 30% or less of calories." The Surgeon General, the National Academy of Sciences, the American Heart Association, and the American Dietetic Association all advocate this reduction in dietary fat. The new food nutrition labels implemented in early 1994 are predicated on the 30% fat intake level.

Recently, research has begun to suggest that the message is taking hold—at least somewhat. A survey conducted by the National Center for Health Statistics (NCHS) shows that in 1990, the average American diet contained 34% of total calories from fat, down 2% from 36% in 1978. Although this still does not meet the standards set by the government, it is an encouraging decrease from the 40% level of the 1960s.

But now Americans are faced with a new dilemma, one that will continually challenge food manufacturers—Americans are getting heavier. NCHS research found that the proportion of US adults who are overweight increased by 8%—to 33%—in the past decade.

Other studies support this. The National Institutes of Health (NIH) conducted a study indicating that in 1992–1993, the average body weight of Americans 25 to 30 years of age, was 171 lb. In 1985–1986, the average weight was 161 lb for the same age group (Figure 23–3). If the percentage of fat in the diet is decreasing, why are Americans getting heavier? The answer may not be simple. Experts believe a number of factors contribute to the increase in body weight. Americans' continued lack of exercise, for example, has been cited by a number of researchers.

The 1996 Surgeon General's Report on Physical Activity and Health confirms the sedentary life-style of the US population. According to this report,

- Only about 15% of US adults engage regularly in vigorous activity during leisure time.
- Approximately 22% of adults engage regularly in sustained physical activity of any intensity during leisure time.
- About 25% of adults report no physical activity at all in their leisure time.

Excess energy intake is also a factor. According to the latest National Health and Nutrition Examination Survey (NHANES III), total average energy intake by adults increased from 1969 calories in 1978 to 2200 calories in 1990. Merely controlling grams of fat consumed, which is popular nutrition advice, does not necessarily result in a reduction in calories, and therefore does not lead to weight control.

The American Dietetic Association's 1997 position on weight management for adults states that it "requires a lifelong commitment to healthful lifestyle behaviors emphasizing eating practices and daily physical activity that are sustainable and enjoyable." Although Americans often hear they need to balance food intake with output, is the message really understood? Do Americans have the knowledge and skills necessary to manage their weight? Is it a problem of wanting instant gratification rather than future rewards?: "I want that piece of food now" versus lower weight and improved health and cardiovascular fitness? Is it a belief that an effortless solution exists (a pill, cream, drink, new diet)? Is it a combination of factors? What can health professionals do to stem the tide of increasing weight and decreasing physical activity? (Pfizer, 1994).

drolyzed once again to fatty acids and glycerol through the action of **hormone-sensitive lipase (HSL)** and they re-enter the circulation.

Hormones affect LPL activity in different adipose tissue regions. *Estrogens* appear to stimulate LPL activity in the gluteofemoral adipocytes and thus promote fat storage in this area, an effect that is seldom seen in obese men. This may be for the specific purpose of providing for childbearing and lactation. However, in the abdominal region, estrogen appears to stimulate lipolysis. The "postmenopausal stomach" may thus have a hormonal association (Egger, 1992; Ley et al., 1992).

Lipoprotein lipase increases during periods of weight gain in both the obese and nonobese (Pi-Sunyer, 1994). After weight is lost, LPL returns to normal levels in the nonobese; however, in the reduced-obese (obese individuals who lost weight), the LPL does not decrease but in fact increases. This increase is one of the factors contributing to the rapid weight regain that is so common.

An increase in LPL activity is reported after cessation of cigarette smoking (Carney and Goldberg, 1984). Indeed, smoking is associated with lower body weight and the cessation of smoking is associated with weight gain. In fact, during 10 years of follow-up, a weight gain of 4.4 kg (about 10 lb) for men and 5.0 kg (11 lb) for women was observed after smoking cessation (Flegal et al., 1995). Still, the physiologic mechanisms by which cigarette smoking reduces body weight and smoking cessation increases body weight are uncertain. Some research indicates smoking cessation has no metabolic effects favoring fat deposition (Hellerstein et al., 1994). Despite the weight gain that occurs after an individual stops smoking, the health benefits of smoking cessation are greater and well-documented (U.S. Department of Health and Human Services, 1990).

REGULATION OF BODY WEIGHT

A variety of regulatory systems exist to maintain body weight at some predetermined point. Neurochemicals, body fat stores, protein mass, hormones and postingestive factors all play a role in regulating intake and also weight. Some evidence suggests that regulation takes place on both a short-term and long-term basis. *Short-term regulation* governs consumption of food from meal to meal; *long-term regulation* is controlled by the availability of adipose stores (Bray, 1987). Total calories are more important than any singular nutrient alone (Fig. 23–3).

Short-Term Regulation

Short-term controls are concerned primarily with factors governing hunger, appetite, and satiety. *Satiety* is associated with the postprandial state when excess food is being stored. *Hunger* is associated with the postabsorptive state when those stores are being mobilized. Physical triggers for hunger are much stronger than those for satiety, and it is easier to override the signals for satiety (Blundell et al., 1993).

A study investigated the effects of aging on mechanisms of body energy regulation, trying to determine the causes of unexplained weight loss in older persons (Roberts et al., 1994). Healthy younger and older men of normal weight consumed a typical diet and performed usual activities. When either overfeeding or underfeeding interventions were made, the younger men exhibited spontaneous **hypophagia** or **hyperphagia** to alter body weight accordingly. The older men did not have the same responsiveness to changes in caloric intake. Findings from this study suggest that older persons are more vulnerable to unexplained weight losses and gains because of their inability to control spontaneous short-term changes in food intake. Age alone should not preclude weight loss treatment in older adults; careful evaluation of risks and benefits is needed (NIH, 1998).

Long-Term Regulation

A feedback mechanism has been proposed involving a signal from the *adipose mass* that is released when "normal" body composition is disturbed, possibly when weight loss occurs. This factor may play a bigger role in younger persons than in the elderly.

Set-Point Theory

Fat storage in nonobese adults appears to be regulated in a manner that preserves a specific body weight. In both animals and humans, deliberate efforts to starve or overfeed are followed by a rapid return to the original body weight, as though the latter constituted a "set point" that is amenable to physiologic influences. If this is true, then some forms of obesity could be the result of an abnormally established set point.

Body weight remains remarkably stable despite variations, possibly from internal regulatory mechanisms that are genetically determined (Rosencrans, 1994). An animal has normal metabolism only at its normally maintained body weight. In a study of obese and nonobese subjects, a 10% increase or decrease in usual body weight was accompanied by a 16% increase or 15% decrease in 24-hour total energy expenditure corrected for body composition (Leibel et al., 1995). Some recent studies suggest that body weight can only be displaced temporarily and that resting metabolic rate changes until body weight returns to normal. The set point adjusts to a new level when it is maintained over time, and regulation may be disturbed by overeating, exercise, brain lesions, and drugs (Rosencrans, 1994). Unless the set point or normal weight is lowered, dieting is generally futile.

An important aspect of counseling with regard to the set-point theory is that reaching a plateau in weight loss is common, and if calorie control is maintained, additional weight loss should occur. It appears to be especially difficult to lose those last few pounds before the healthy body weight is reached.

Factors Regulating Energy Intake and Body Weight

THERMOGENESIS AND THE THERMOGENIC EFFECT OF FOOD (TEF)

The components of energy expenditure are the *resting energy expenditure (REE)* expressed as *resting metabolic rate (RMR),* the energy expended in

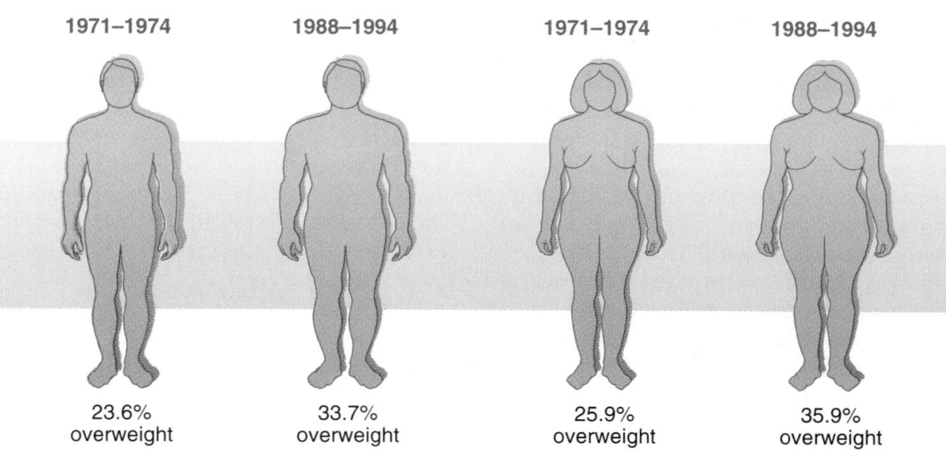

FIGURE 23–3 Americans are learning that total calories, not just calories from fat, are important in weight control.

voluntary activity, and the *thermogenic effect of food (TEF)* or *diet-induced thermogenesis.* These concepts are discussed in detail in Chapter 2.

Meal size, meal composition, the nature of the previous diet, insulin resistance, physical activity, and aging influence TEF. The TEF is made up of an obligatory component related to the energy value of the food consumed and an additional adaptive component that presumably responds to overeating by eliminating the excessive energy in the form of heat (see Chapter 2). The existence of the adaptive component has been demonstrated in animals, primarily in the BAT. However, the amount of BAT in adults is not sufficient to account for this adaptive thermogenesis. Whether a blunting of the adaptive component is a significant factor in the obese is controversial; nonetheless, it is an attractive theory to account for the ability of the nonobese to adjust without effort to excessive intakes and the failure of obese persons to maintain leaner weight levels. There is support for the hypothesis of a defect in TEF in those with obesity, but it is not clear whether this defect causes the obesity or results from the obesity (de Jonge and Bray, 1997).

Workers who work at night and eat snacks that provide about 20% of daily kilocalorie intake during their shifts may have a different metabolic efficiency. Diet-induced thermogenesis is higher after a morning snack than after afternoon or night snacks, suggesting that the effect of thermogenesis declines as the evening progresses (Romon et al., 1993).

RESTING METABOLIC RATE (RMR)

When the body is suddenly deprived of adequate energy, such as with involuntary or deliberate starvation or semistarvation, the RMR adapts to conserve energy against an unpredictable future by dropping rapidly, by as much as 15% in 2 weeks. When adequate food intake is restored, the RMR returns to baseline levels (Ravussin and Swinburn, 1992).

BRAIN NEUROTRANSMITTERS

Regulatory systems involving neurotransmitters in the brain govern feeding activities in response to signals originating in affected body tissues. The catecholamines *norepinephrine* and *dopamine* are released by the sympathetic nervous system (SNS) in response to dietary intake. These neurotransmitters mediate the activity of areas in the hypothalamus that govern feeding behavior. Fasting and semistarvation lead to decreased SNS activity and increased adrenal medullary activity with a consequent increase in epinephrine, which fosters substrate mobilization (Katzeff et al., 1986; Vasselli and Maggio, 1988). Dopaminergic pathways in the brain are thought to play a role in the reinforcement properties associated with food.

Serotonin, neuropeptide Y, and *endorphins* are other neurochemicals that are thought to be involved in feeding behaviors. Decreases in serotonin and increases in neuropeptide Y have been associated with an increase in carbohydrate appetite. The level of neuropeptide Y increases during food deprivation, suggesting that it may be a factor leading to an increase in appetite after dieting. Preferences and cravings for sweet high-fat foods observed among obese and bulimic patients may involve the endorphin system (Drewnowski et al., 1992).

Corticotropin-releasing factor (CRF) is produced in the brain and is involved in controlling adrenocorticotropic hormone release from the pituitary gland. CRF is a potent anorexic agent. It decreases food intake on its own and weakens the feeding response produced by norepinephrine and neuropeptide Y. CRF is released during exercise and increased levels of CRF have been noted in depressed patients and during starvation (Morley et al., 1992; Richard, 1989).

GUT PEPTIDES

Mechanical contact of food with the mucosa of the stomach and small intestine muscles stimulates secretion of gut peptides, which have an immediate effect on satiety (see Chapter 1). Among those that have been identified is *cholecystokinin (CCK).* CCK is released by the intestinal tract when fats and proteins reach the small intestine. Receptors for CCK have been found in the gastrointestinal tract and the brain. CCK causes the gallbladder to contract and stimulates the pancreas to release enzymes. At the brain level, CCK inhibits food intake.

Released by the nerve cells of the gut, *bombesin* is another gut peptide. Bombesin reduces food intake and enhances the release of CCK.

Apolipoprotein A-IV is synthesized and secreted by the intestine in the process of the lymphatic secretion of chylomicrons. After entering the circulation, a small portion of apoliprotein A-IV enters the central nervous system (CNS) and suppresses food consumption.

Another peptide produced by the intestine is *enterostatin,* which seems to be involved specifically with the satiety following the consumption of fat.

THYROID HORMONES

Thyroid hormones modulate the tissue responsiveness to the catecholamines secreted by the SNS. A decrease in triiodothyronine lowers the response to SNS activity and consequently diminishes adaptive thermogenesis. Such a subtle defect could be one of the factors predisposing some obese persons to excessive weight gain.

INSULIN

Peripheral administration of *insulin* leads to an acute increase in food intake. This response is attributed to peripheral hypoglycemia, which is a potent stimulus for eating. Impaired insulin activity may lead to reduced SNS activity and thus to impaired thermogenesis. It is possible that obese persons with insulin resistance or deficiency have a defective glucose disposal system and a depressed level of thermogenesis (Pi-Sunyer, 1994). Additionally, the greater the insulin resistance, the lower the TEF.

Fasting insulin levels increase proportionately with the degree of obesity. However, many obese individuals demonstrate insulin resistance due to a lack of response by insulin receptors, impaired glucose tolerance, and associated hyperlipidemia. These sequelae can usually be corrected with weight loss.

LEPTIN

Leptin is a hormone secreted by the adipose tissue that seems to inform the brain about the amount of adipose tissue in the body. Animal studies support a role for leptin in increasing satiety and energy expenditure (Flier and Maratos-Flier, 1998; Pelleymounter et al., 1995). Mice deficient in leptin develop severe obesity. When leptin is administered to these mice, their weight drops and metabolism increases. Unlike the obese mouse, obese humans produce significant amounts of leptin. Its concentration is correlated with the percentage of body fat and is elevated in obese individuals (Considine et al., 1996). The finding of increased serum leptin concentrations in obese individuals suggests a "leptin resistance." Two mechanisms have been explored to explain this resistance. The first is a defect in the blood–brain barrier transport system; that is, the leptin cannot cross the barrier to act on the brain. The second proposed mechanism involves defects in the sites of leptin action within the CNS (Flier and Maratos-Flier, 1998).

Weight loss is associated with a reduction in leptin. During the maintenance period, serum leptin concentrations increased slightly despite no changes in body weight. This finding suggests that leptin secretion is regulated by other factors in addition to adipose tissue size. Factors proposed include energy intake and insulin levels (Considine et al., 1996).

WEIGHT IMBALANCE: OBESITY

Overweight is a state in which weight exceeds a standard based on height; **obesity** is a condition of excessive fatness, either generalized or localized. It is possible to be obese at a weight within normal limits according to standard tables, just as it is possible to be overweight without being obese. However, in most people, overweight and obesity tend to parallel each other.

Assessment

Underweight and obesity are assessed in a variety of ways, depending on the necessity for accuracy. The tables of the Metropolitan Life Insurance Company are widely used to establish a standard of *ideal body weight (IBW)*. The more preferred methods include *body mass index (BMI)*, or Quetelet Index (W/H^2) in which W is weight in kilograms and H is height in meters), waist circumference, and *waist–hip ratio (WHR)*, which compares the circumference measurements of waist and hip to identify abdominal and gluteofemoral body fat. Excess abdominal fat is an independent risk factor of disease risk. Waist circumference over 40 in men and over 35 in women signifies increased risk in those with BMIs of 25 to 34.9 (NIH, 1998). These and other body fatness assessment methods are discussed in detail in Chapter 16. Tables for determining BMI and WHR are presented in Appendix 20 and 26, respectively. The IBW tables appear in Appendix 19.

Overweight and obesity as defined by the National Institutes of Health (NIH) are shown in Table 23–1. NIH clinical guidelines have been met with some controversy. Not all scientists support classifying individuals with a BMI of 25 as overweight. Although the risk for some comorbidities increases at BMIs less than 25, mortality does not significantly increase until BMI reaches 27 (Manson et al., 1995). Furthermore, when a BMI of 25 is used as a cutoff point, approximately half of US adults fall into the category of overweight or obese!

Risk

Obese adults are considered at risk for developing **comorbidities,** that is, developing other chronic diseases. A 20% increase in body weight substantially increases the risk for hypertension, coronary artery disease, lipid disorders, and non–insulin-dependent diabetes mellitus. Obesity is also considered a risk factor for joint disease, gallstones, obstructive sleep apnea, and other respiratory conditions (NIH, 1998).

Following the initial NHANES Survey, 1971–1975, women who had a high body mass index at enrollment (BMI over 27 for women aged 45 to 59 years and BMI over 28 in women aged 60 to 74 years) doubled their risk of disability and mobility problems over a period of 15 years (Launer et al., 1994).

TABLE 23–1 CLASSIFICATION OF OVERWEIGHT AND OBESITY

CLASSIFICATION	BMI kg/m^2
Underweight	<18.5
Normal	18.5–24.9
Overweight	25.0–29.9
Obesity, class I	30.0–34.9
Obesity, class II	35.0–39.9
Extreme obesity, class III	≥40

(From National Institutes of Health, National Heart, Lung, and Blood Institute. Clinical guidelines on the identification, evaluation, and treatment of overweight and obesity in adults—the evidence report. Obes Res 6(suppl 2):51S, 1998.)
BMI, body mass index.

Genetically obese experimental animals show reductions in various aspects of cell-mediated immunity and decreased resistance to bacterial and viral infections (Stallone, 1994). Obesity is also a risk factor for cancer, poor wound healing, and poor antibody response to hepatitis B vaccine.

A study from the Harvard School of Public Health surveyed 19,297 healthy men who filled out questionnaires in 1962 and 1966. By 1988, 4370 of these individuals had died. The lowest mortality was among those weighing an average of 20% below the U.S. average for men of comparable age and height. Current or former smokers and persons with cancer that was undetected at the time of the surveys were excluded from the findings (Lee et al., 1993). Figure 23–4 shows mortality risks at various body mass indices.

Some chronic disorders have been linked together as **syndrome X.** These include glucose intolerance, insulin resistance, hyperlipidemia, and hypertension (Reaven, 1988). Risks are linked strongly with visceral or intra-abdominal obesity, with waist-to-hip measures often being more conclusive than BMI (see Chapter 12).

Etiology

The nature and causes of obesity are the subject of intensive and continuing research. Both environmental and genetic factors are involved in a complex interaction of variables, which include psychological and cultural influences as well as physiologic regulatory mechanisms.

Over the years many hypotheses have evolved to explain why some people become fat while others remain lean, and why it is so difficult for the reduced-obese to maintain the weight loss so painstakingly achieved. The fact that no single theory can completely explain all manifestations of obesity, or apply consistently to all individuals, underscores the complex nature of this condition. Theories suggesting imbalances of energy input are generally related to factors influencing hunger and appetite or satiety. Theories relating to imbalances of energy output are concerned primarily with TEF, physical activity, and RMR. Heredity and environment influence both the input and output of energy.

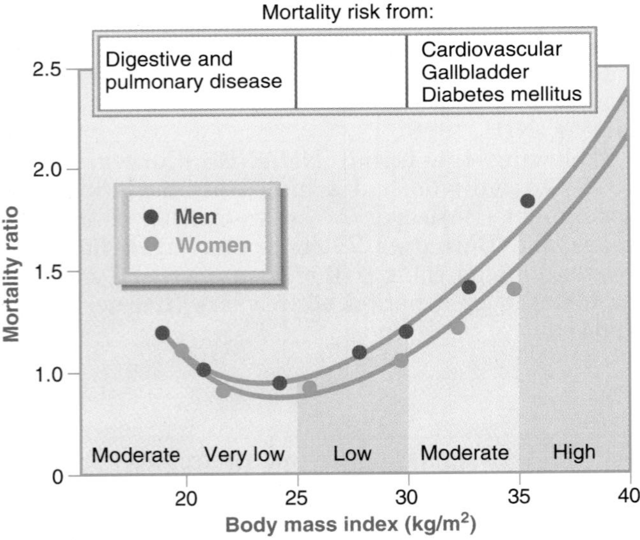

FIGURE 23–4 Body mass index and mortality risk. Data from the American Cancer Society study have been plotted for men and women to show the relationship of BMI to overall mortality risk. At a BMI below 20 kg/m^2, and above 30 kg/m^2, there is an increase in relative mortality. The major causes for this increased mortality are listed, along with a division of body mass index groupings into various levels of risk. (Adapted from Bray GA, Gray DS. Obesity, part I: Pathogenesis. West J Med 149:429, 1988; and Lew EA, Garfinkle L: Variations in mortality by weight among 750,000 men and women. J Clin Epidemiol 32:563, 1979.)

Heredity

Many of the hormonal and neural factors involved in normal weight regulation are determined genetically. These include the short- and long-term signals that determine satiety and feeding activity. Small defects in their expression or interaction could contribute significantly to weight gain. Number and size of fat cells, regional distribution of body fat, and RMR are also determined genetically.

The first studies of the role of inheritance in obesity estimated it to be from 66% to 80%. There is a growing consensus that these studies overestimated the influence of genetics. A more reasonable estimate now accepted is a heritability of the BMI of about 33% (Stunkard, 1996). The number of genes and other markers associated or linked with obesity has increased over the years. In fact, the 1997 human obesity gene map includes genes on every chromosome except the Y chromosome (Chagnon et al., 1998). Still remaining is the task of identifying the combination of genes and mutations that contribute to human obesity and defining the environmental circumstances that result in obesity when these genes and mutations are present (Foreyt and Poston, 1997).

Although numerous genes are involved in obesity, two have received much attention recently—the *ob* gene and the *β_3-adrenoreceptor* gene. The *ob* gene produces leptin, and mutations in the mouse *ob* gene result in obesity. Mechanisms are being explored to explain leptin activities in humans but some scientists believe that it is unlikely that the *ob* gene plays a major role in human obesity (Foreyt and Poston, 1997).

The *β_3-adrenoreceptor* gene, located primarily in the adipose tissue, is thought to regulate RMR and fat oxidation in humans. It was hypothesized that individuals with a mutation of the gene for the β_3-adrenergic receptor may have an increased capacity to gain weight (Clement et al., 1995); however, there is no evidence that the mutation is more frequent among obese subjects. Therefore, the gene is not likely to be a major determinant of obesity, but may contribute to weight gain in some individuals.

Recent findings suggest that genes provide the susceptibility for obesity but are not the actual cause. This means that although genes appear to increase vulnerability to obesity, other determinants must be present for obesity to occur (Foreyt and Poston, 1997). A major factor is the environment.

Factors Affecting Weight Gain

Evidence strongly suggests that dietary and activity patterns are the primary causes of weight problems in industrial societies and that there is a mismatch between how we live and our genetic makeup (Foreyt and Poston, 1997). Excessive energy intake appears to be the result of hyperphagia; however, many studies indicate that the obese do not eat more than the nonobese; they often eat less. In the process of becoming obese, however, hyperphagia is indeed a factor. Animal studies demonstrating excessive eating in response to foods high in fat or sugar or to "cafeteria diets" apply to humans. In one study of 23 lean men, 23 obese men, 17 lean women, and 15 obese women, no differences were found in energy or total sugar intake, but obese individuals derived a greater portion of their energy intake from fat and added sugars and dietary fiber was lower in the obese groups (Miller et al., 1994).

Research supports that food and its taste elements evoke pleasure responses (Van Horn et al., 1998). The endless variety of food available at any time at a reasonable cost can contribute to higher calorie intake, because people eat more when offered a variety of choices than when a single food is available. Normally, as foods are consumed, they become less pleasant. This decline is known as **sensory-specific satiety** and is associated with a shift to other food choices during the meal (Rolls and Drewnowski, 1996). An example of this principle in action is an all-you-can-eat buffet. Although sensory-specific satiety can promote the intake of a more varied and nutritionally balanced diet, it can also lead to overconsumption of calories.

The effect of eating more calories than needed is worsened when few calories are expended. The sedentary nature of the American society is a contributory factor to the growing problem of obesity. Fewer Americans are exercising and more time is being spent in low-energy activities such as watching television and working on the computer.

To summarize, energy needs of individuals differ based on genetic makeup, and a growing portion of the U.S. population is consuming more calories than are being expended. To increase the awareness of the need to balance energy intake with energy output, Dr. C. Everett Koop, the former U.S. Surgeon General, mounted an antiobesity initiative called "Shape Up America!" The nonprofit corporation was launched in 1994 to focus attention on healthy weight as a priority. With the ultimate goal of behavior change, Shape Up America! is conducting a broad-based educational effort to encourage better nutritional habits and increased physical activity among all individuals.

TISSUE ADAPTATION TO WEIGHT LOSS

Tissue response to starvation, or even semistarvation of the kind encountered in most weight loss programs, is one of adaptation to an anticipated period of deprivation. The classic starvation studies done by Keys (1950) found that during the first 10 days of a fast and after utilization of glycogen stores, approximately 8% to 12% of the energy expenditure is from protein with the balance from fat. As starvation progresses, up to 97% of energy expenditure is from stored triglyceride. Use of fat, with more than twice the kilocalories of protein, is not only more efficient but also spares vital protein tissues. However, even when the body has adjusted completely, 5% of weight loss is still from protein in muscle supporting adipose tissue (Bray and Gray, 1988a). Metabolic aberrations that occur during starvation cause a host of negative effects including bradycardia, hypotension, dry skin and hair, easy fatigue, constipation, nervous system abnormalities, depression, and death (Callaway, 1988) (see Chapters 24 and 33).

Plateau Effect

A common experience in weight reduction programs is arrival at a weight plateau, when weight remains at the same level for a period of time. Eventually, weight loss halts completely. One theory is that interim plateaus reflect a reduction of lipid in individual adipocytes to some signal that demands metabolic adjustment and weight maintenance.

Any weight loss, whether fast or slow, results in a loss of the extra muscle that has developed to support the excess adipose tissue. Because this extra LBM has contributed to an increased metabolic rate, RMR decreases as LBM is lost. The fact that RMR decreases very rapidly at the onset of a weight reduction diet, by as much as 15% within 2 weeks, indicates that other adaptations to the lower weight as well as to the threat of deprivation are taking place.

Other factors join to decrease RMR and limit effectiveness of the restricted energy intake. A decrease in the total kilocalories ingested results in a decrease in TEF. Because a body that weighs less requires less energy expenditure to move around, the cost of physical activity is also less. A state of equilibrium is eventually reached at which the energy intake is equal to energy expenditure. Unless a change is made in either nutritional intake or physical activity, weight loss stops at this point.

Weight Cycling

Many obese people lose and gain weight several times over their lifetimes (i.e., the **yo-yo effect**). With each turn of the cycle, it takes longer to lose the same amount of weight and, conversely, less time to regain it. The Framingham Study (Lissner et al., 1991) suggests that variability in weight contributes to health risks, but other studies have not shown the same results (Jeffrey et al., 1992; Wing, 1992). Moderate weight loss followed by weight gain does not increase visceral fat accumulation compared with body fatness before the loss. There is a slight tendency for accumulation of subcutaneous fat at the expense of visceral fat. Weight cycling should still not be viewed as free from consequences because other cardiac risks seem to be involved (Van der Kooy et al., 1993). Furthermore, the psychological effects of repeatedly regaining weight are usually discouraging.

MANAGEMENT OF OBESITY

In 1992, 33% to 40% of American women and 20% to 24% of American men were dieting (NIH, 1992). A chronic disease prevention model that involves both life-style interventions and interdisciplinary team therapies from physicians, dietitions, exercise specialists and behavior therapists offers the best treatment opportunity (Rippe et al., 1998). Weight reduction programs with the most promise of success integrate healthier food choices, exercise, and life-style modification. Pharmacologic treatment and surgical intervention are appropriate in some circumstances, but are not a substitute for the necessary changes in eating and physical activity patterns. Figure 23–5 presents an algorithm for the management of obesity.

Goals of Treatment

The American Dietetic Association (ADA) has taken the position that the goal of obesity treatment should be refocused from weight loss alone to weight management, defined as attaining the best weight possible in the context of overall health (ADA, 1997). Achieving ideal body weight or percentage of body fat is not always realistic or desirable, and under some circumstances it may not be appropriate at all.

Although achieving a desirable body weight can be an appropriate end point for many of the mildly obese, a program of management that promotes a modest weight loss or maintains present body weight without further gain may be the best one. Depending on the type and severity of the existing obesity and on the age and life-style of the individual, successfully reducing body weight varies from a relatively simple matter to being virtually impossible. Maintaining present body weight or achieving a moderate loss is beneficial. Obese individuals who lose even small amounts of weight (5% to 10% of initial body weight) are likely to improve their health in the short run by reducing the severity of the comorbidities associated with obesity (NIH, 1998). A review of studies in which patients experienced approximately a 10% or less weight reduction showed that they also had improved glycemic control, reduced blood pressure, and reduced cholesterol levels. Weight loss of 10% of initial weight in one study resulted in significant improvements in serum lipids even though patients remained more than 20 kg overweight (Andersen et al., 1995). In addition, it also appears to increase longevity (Goldstein, 1992).

The critical question of whether modest weight losses, if maintained, would have a long-term impact is beginning to be answered. A study of obese patients with diabetes mellitus, who experienced more than a 5% reduction in body weight and maintained the loss, showed that they had significant improvements in glycosylated hemoglobin values at 1 year compared to patients losing less weight and those who gained weight (Wing et al., 1987). The study showed, however, that the initial effects on glycemic control were greater than the long-term effects. This suggests that improvement may be due to a combination of energy restriction and weight reduction per se. The maintenance of improvements at 1 year supported the prediction that long-term improvements in body weight could have a long-term effect on glycemic control. Medical nutrition therapy and weight loss are useful adjunctive therapies for diabetes management (Franz, 1998).

Despite the recognition that modest weight loss is beneficial and may be more achievable, it has been found that obese individuals have self-defined goal weights that are very different from goals suggested by professionals (Foster et al., 1997). Their personal weight loss goals and expectations are often unrealistic and not achievable. Health professionals must therefore intervene to help patients accept more modest weight loss. They must also help patients understand what can realistically be achieved with current treatment methods.

In addition to developing realistic goals, a comprehensive assessment is needed for any patient who is 40% or more above ideal body weight; medical evaluation is also warranted (Rippe et al., 1998; Brownell and Wadden, 1991). Psychosocial, behavioral, and biologic factors should also be assessed in the plan.

Rate and Extent of Weight Loss

Reduction of body weight involves loss of both protein and fat, in amounts determined to some degree by the rate of weight reduction. Steady weight loss over a longer period favors reduction of fat stores, limits the loss of vital protein tissues, and avoids the sharp decline in RMR that accompanies rapid weight reduction. One approach designed to minimize the decrease in RMR recommends loss of ½ to 1½ lb/wk, leading to a weight reduction at the end of the first year of 10% to 15% of body weight. After a period of adjustment to the lower weight, the year-long program can be repeated.

Final goals should be individualized and chosen

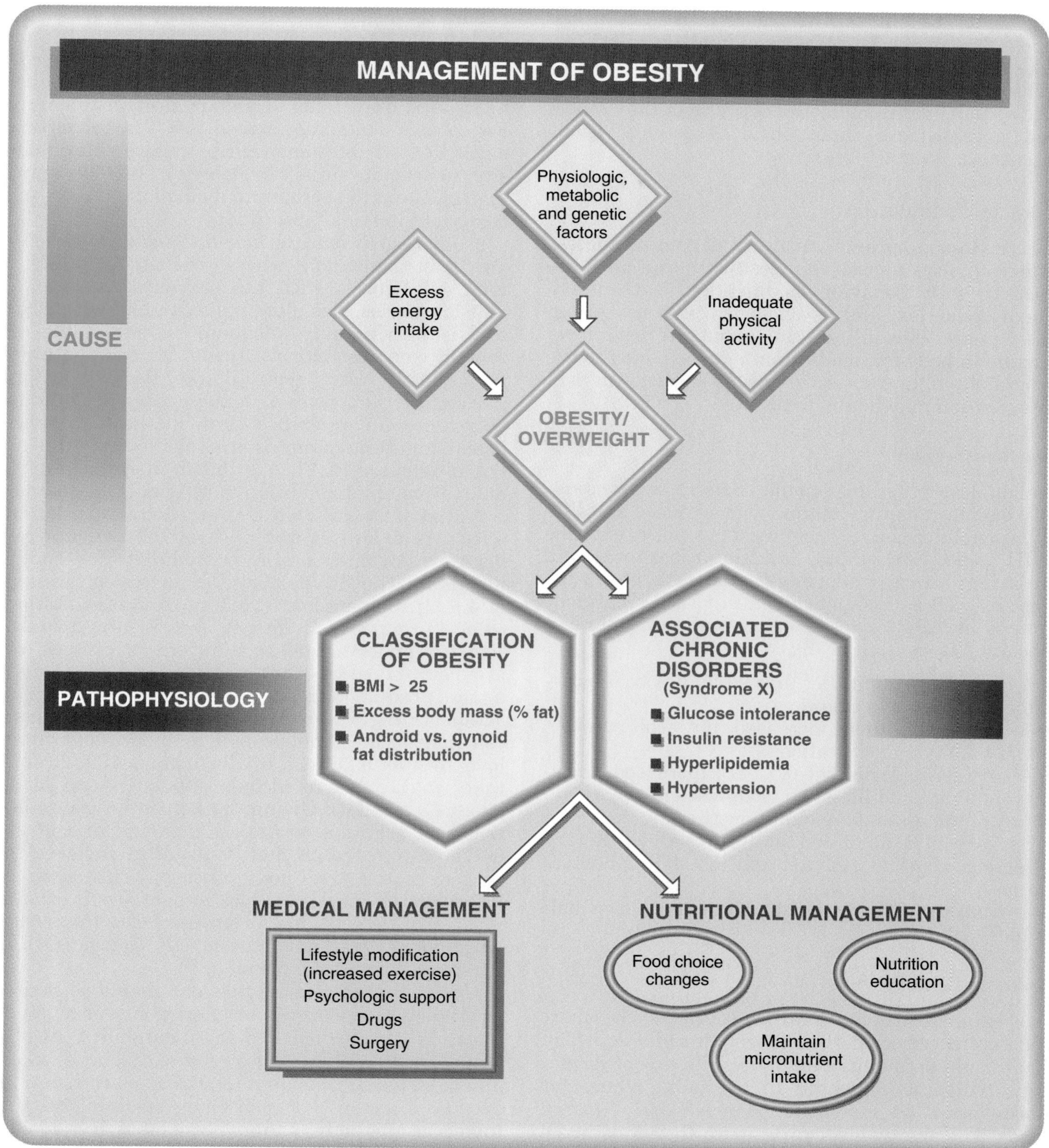

FIGURE 23–5 Pathology algorithm—management of obesity. (Algorithm content developed by John Anderson, Ph.D., and Sanford C. Garner, Ph.D., 2000.)

realistically with reduction of body fat as the focus. For example, neither the hyperplastic obese nor the gynoid types will be able to maintain a large weight loss. Female role models of dress sizes 6 to 10 and male models with 30-inch to 34-inch waists "may not be appropriate to the obese population," and in fact even BMIs of 25 are unreasonable goals for many dieters (Blackburn, 1988).

Even with the same caloric intake, rates of weight reduction vary. Men reduce weight faster than women of similar size because of their higher LBM and RMR. The heavier person, who because of the higher weight expends more energy than one who is less obese, loses faster on a given calorie intake than a lighter person. Some obese persons who fail to lose weight on a diet they state is low in calories actually consume more energy than they report and overestimate their physical activity levels (Lichtman, 1992).

Dietary Modification

Weight loss programs with any degree of success integrate food choice changes with exercise, frequently with behavior modification, with nutritional education, and psychological support. When these approaches fail to bring about the desired reduction in body fat, medication may be added to the program and, in the case of morbid obesity, surgical intervention may be required.

Recommendations

Weight loss programs should combine a nutritionally balanced dietary regime with exercise and life-style modification at the least possible expense (NIH, 1998; NIH, 1992). Selecting the appropriate treatment strategy depends on the goals of the patient as well as his or her health risks. Treatment options include (Shape Up America! and American Obesity Association, 1996):

- A moderate deficit diet, increased physical activity, and life-style modification
- A low-calorie diet, increased physical activity, and life-style modification
- A very-low-calorie diet (VLCD), increased physical activity, and life-style modification
- Any of the above plus pharmacotherapy
- Surgery plus an individually prescribed dietary regime, physical activity, and life-style modification
- Prevention of weight gain through energy balance

Restricted-Energy Diets

A balanced energy-controlled diet is the most widely prescribed method of weight reduction. The diet should be nutritionally adequate except for energy, which is decreased to the point where fat stores must be mobilized to meet daily energy needs. The energy level varies with the individual's size and activities and falls into three main categories: a moderate deficit diet containing 1200 calories daily for women, 1400+ calories daily for men; a low-calorie diet containing 800 to 1200 calories/day for women and 800 to 1400 calories/day for men; and a VLCD containing 800 calories or less daily. Regardless of the level of calorie restriction, healthful eating should be taught and emphasized and recommendations for increasing physical activity should be included (Shape Up America! and American Obesity Association, 1996).

Both the moderate deficit diet and the low-calorie diet should be relatively high in carbohydrates, primarily starch (50% to 55% of total kilocalories) with generous protein, about 15% to 25% of kilocalories, to prevent conversion of dietary protein to energy. Fat content should not exceed 30%. The inclusion of extra fiber is recommended to reduce caloric density, to promote satiety by delaying stomach emptying time, and to decrease to a small degree the efficiency of intestinal absorption.

A *high-carbohydrate, low-fat diet*, proposed by Dr. Dean Ornish and others, restricts fat to 10% of total kilocalories with the carbohydrate level at 80% of calories. The diet produces rapid weight loss and is nutritionally adequate as formulated, although very restrictive. A popular variation limits fat to 20% of total energy intake. Because fat provides more than twice as much energy per gram as either protein or carbohydrate (9 kcals versus 4 kcals), an effective diet is one that controls this nutrient extensively. Fat also has a lipogenic quality, apart from and in addition to its energy content.

A study at Vanderbilt University investigated the effects of a low-fat diet with ad lib carbohydrate versus a low-fat/calorie-restricted diet (Schlundt et al., 1993). The "low-fat only" group lost an average of 4.6 kg compared with 8.3 kg in the low-fat/low-calorie group. Although not as dramatic a loss, a "low-fat" program may be sufficient for persons who are discouraged by other programs and do not mind a more gradual loss.

Calculating fat grams has become a trend in recent years. One simple rule is to divide ideal calorie level by 4 for a 25% fat intake (e.g., an 1800-kcal intake would need to include 450 kcal from fat or about 63 g of fat). Giving the person license to distribute fat grams as desired throughout the day makes the approach more appealing, involves the person in the treatment process, and results in lower energy intake without hunger. Total calories must also be considered, however (see the earlier box, "*Focus On:* Controversies: Do Americans Understand Weight Management?").

Alcohol and foods high in sugar should be limited as unnecessary sources of energy; however, small amounts can be included for palatability. Alcohol makes up 10% of the diet for many regular drinkers and contributes 7 kcal/g. Alcohol behaves like a fat because it spares fat from being oxidized. Ethanol increases 24-hour energy expenditure and decreases lipid oxidation when added to the diet or substituted for other foods (Suter et al., 1992).

Heavy drinkers (who consume 50% or more of daily calories from alcohol) may have a depressed appetite to the point of weight loss, emaciation, and even malnutrition, but moderate users tend to gain weight with the alcohol calories added to their usual diet. Habitual use of ethanol in excess of energy requirements most likely favors lipid storage and weight gain and should be considered a risk factor for obesity.

Artificial sweeteners (discussed in Chapter 34) and fat substitutes (discussed in Chapter 3) may improve the acceptability of limited food intakes for some people. However, there is no evidence that using artificial sweeteners reduces food intake or results in weight loss. Noncaloric sweeteners do not seem to increase hunger or food intake (Canty and Chan, 1991). In a rigorous study, researchers found that use of aspartame or saccharin did not increase hunger; in fact, hunger-related ratings tested 15 to 45 minutes later were highest after consumption of water, then artificial sweeteners, then sucrose.

Vitamin and mineral supplements that meet age-related recommended dietary allowances (RDA) are usually recommended with weight reduction programs that provide less than 1200 kcal for women or 1800 kcal for men.

EXCHANGE SYSTEM DIETS

A popular and easily manipulated method for planning a diet program tailored to the individual is the exchange system, which is described in Appendix 53. A 1200-kcal diet based on this system is shown in Table 23–2. The energy content of the diet can be increased by adding midafternoon and evening snacks, or by increasing the number of servings from various groups. Nonnutritious, high-energy foods, such as sweets, desserts, or alcohol, can be added sparingly.

TABLE 23–2 1200-KCAL DIET—22% OF KILOCALORIES FROM FAT

FOOD	FOOD EXCHANGES* (NO.)	CARBOHYDRATE (G)	PROTEIN (G)	FAT (G)
Milk, skim	2	24	16	—
Vegetables	3	15	6	
Fruits	4	60		
Bread	5	75	10	
Meat,[†] lean	5		35	15
Fat	3			15
	Totals	174	67	30

SAMPLE MEAL PLAN

Breakfast
Fruit, 1 exchange
Bread, 2 exchanges
Milk, skim, 1 exchange

Lunch or Supper
Vegetables, 1 exchange
Bread, 2 exchanges
Meat, lean, 2 exchanges
Fruit, 1 exchange
Milk, skim, 1 exchange

Dinner or Supper
Meat, lean, 3 exchanges
Vegetable, 2 exchanges
Bread, 1 exchange
Fat, 1 exchange
Fruit, 2 exchanges

SAMPLE MENU

Breakfast
½ grapefruit
1 slice of whole-wheat toast
1 glass (8 oz) of skim milk
¾ cup of dry cereal
Coffee or tea as desired

Lunch
Sandwich:
2 slices of rye bread
2 oz of sliced turkey
2 stalks of celery
1 carrot
1 peach (medium)
1 glass (8 oz) of skim buttermilk

Dinner
Bouillon
1 parsley potato (2-in. in diameter)
3 oz of roast veal, lean
½ cup of peas and carrots
1 green salad
2 tsp salad dressing
½ cup applesauce (unsweetened)
1 small banana
Tea or coffee as desired

*From exchange lists, see Appendix 53.
[†]Lean meat with visible fat removed is used, reducing the fat content from 5 to 3 mg per Meat Exchange.

FORMULA DIETS OR MEAL REPLACEMENT PROGRAMS

Formula diets or meal replacement programs come in a variety of forms. The good ones contain high-quality protein, sugar as fructose and a moderate amount of monounsaturated fat. Total calories range from 1000 to 1600 calories daily with the meal replacement drink or bars replacing one or two meals each day. The recommended daily quantity of the drink or powder supplies approximately 900 kcal distributed as 20% protein, 30% fat, and 50% carbohydrate. At this energy level, and with vitamins and minerals to meet the RDAs, these formulas are considered to be safe. Quantities of the meal replacement equivalent to a single meal are used successfully as substitutes for a meal at times when it is difficult to obtain foods appropriate to a weight reduction program. Negative aspects of these diets include dependence on a particular product, failure to develop appropriate long-term eating habits, and boredom.

COMMERCIAL PROGRAMS

Millions of Americans use commercial weight loss programs to lose weight and new programs enter the marketplace regularly (Table 23–3). Most offer diets that are balanced. Programs can be evaluated by comparing them to sound nutritional practices.

Currently, data to support the long-term effectiveness of these programs is lacking; however, due to pressures from the government and advocacy organizations, a number of programs have begun to collect data on the effects of treatment including dropout rates, success rates, and maintenance data. As Table 23–3 illustrates, the programs vary considerably. Some require the use of proprietary prepackaged low-fat meals. Some provide classes on self-introspection, behavior modification, and nutrition. Prepackaged diets appeal to some people because they allow them to avoid making choices about food. However, even though such programs are effective for weight reduction, they may actually limit long-term success at weight maintenance.

EXTREME ENERGY RESTRICTION

Extreme energy-restricted diets provide fewer than 800 kcal/day, and starvation or fasting diets provide fewer than 200 kcal/day.

Fasting. Fasting is seldom prescribed as a treatment for obesity. However, it is frequently invoked by individuals as a part of religious or protest regimes or in a personal effort to lose weight. Under these circumstances, it is seldom continued long enough to produce the serious neurologic, hormonal, and other side effects that accompany prolonged starvation. Over 50% of the rapid weight reduction is fluid, which often leads to serious hypotension problems. Accumulation of uric acid can precipitate episodes of gout; gallstones can also occur.

TABLE 23–3 POPULAR COMMERCIAL DIET PROGRAMS

NAME	FOODS OR PRODUCTS	EDUCATION	TEACHERS/COUNSELORS	MAINTENANCE
VLCD Programs				
Health Management Resources (HMR)	Special drink, multidisciplinary team	1½-h weekly group meetings w/RD	Physicians, health educators, registed nurses, registered dietitians, exercise physiologists	Weekly meetings for 18 mo
Medifast	Special drink; physician supervised	Weekly individual sessions Weekly group meetings	Supervised by physicians	Weekly meetings for 5 mo
New Direction	Special drink; physician supervised	Weekly session with one-on-one interaction	Health professionals	6–12 mo
Optifast	Special drink; physician supervised	Weekly individual sessions w/MD 1½-h weekly group meetings 1 meeting w/RD	Physicians, registered nurses, registered dietitians, and psychologists at most locations	No time limit
Diet Programs				
Diet Center	Regular food	Daily individual sessions	Trained staff	Maintenance—weekly meetings for the first 3 mo; biweekly for mos 4–6; monthly for months 6–12
Jenny Craig	Prepackaged foods	14 1-h video group classes; weekly individual sessions	Registered dietitians and psychologists	Monthly meetings for 6 mo or 1 year
Nutri/System	Prepackaged foods	30-min weekly group meetings; 10-min weekly individual sessions	College graduates	1-y transition diet—program and regular foods
Weight Watchers	Regular food	45-min weekly group meetings	Program graduates	Weekly meetings for 6 wk; free meetings if maintain goal weight
The Solution	Regular food	Weekly 2-hr group meetings	Registered dietitians and psychologists certified by the program	Continuation with weekly meetings as necessary; no time limit

VLCD, very low calorie diet.

VERY-LOW-CALORIE DIETS. Diets providing 200 to 800 kcal are classified as **very-low-calorie diets (VLCDs).** Little evidence suggests that intakes of fewer than 800 calories daily are of any advantage (NIH, 1993). Most VLCDs have the following characteristics: they are hypocaloric, but are relatively rich in protein (0.8 to 1.5 g/kg IBW per day); they are designed to include a full complement of the RDAs for vitamins, minerals, electrolytes, and essential fatty acids, but not for calories; they are given in a form that completely replaces usual food intake; and they are usually given for a period of 12 to 16 weeks (NIH, 1993). Their major advantage is rapid weight loss. Because of potential side effects, prescription of these diets is reserved for individuals with a BMI above 30 for whom other diet programs with psychotherapy have been unsuccessful. Occasionally, VLCDs may be indicated for individuals with a BMI of 27 to 30 who have comorbidities or other risk factors.

The VLCD that first became popular in the early 1970s resulted in several deaths. However, improved formulation with respect to protein quality has led to acceptability for those whose obesity is potentially life-threatening.

Currently most VLCDs are in one of two forms. The *protein-sparing modified fast (PSMF)* contains 1.5 g protein/kg IBW in the form of lean meat, fish and poultry, no carbohydrate, and only the fat contained in the protein sources. In PSMF, nitrogen excretion is high, at 11 to 23 g/day, declining steeply in the first few days to obligate levels; simply adding 100 g carbohydrate to the diet may prevent further losses of nitrogen (Pi-Sunyer, 1994) (see "*Focus On:* History of Protein-Sparing Modified Fast Diets").

The second and most common form of the VLCD uses *commercially formulated liquid diets* based on milk or egg protein. These typically contain 33 to 70 g protein, 30 to 45 g carbohydrate, and a small amount of fat.

Proper use of VLCDs requires careful instruction and follow-up. Long-term effectiveness is improved when they are combined with life-style modification, increased exercise, and nutritional counseling to facilitate maintenance of weight loss. Used alone, their long-term effectiveness is no greater than that of other diet programs. One study compared three treatment programs—a VLCD, life-style modification, and a combined approach using both treatments. The group with the combination approach achieved significantly greater weight loss, but at the end of 1 year had regained one third of the lost weight. However, this was considerably better than the two thirds regained by the diet-only group (Wadden, 1993).

Patients who follow a VLCD (400 to 800 kcal/day) lose 20 kg in 12 to 16 weeks and maintain 33% to 50% of this loss in the following year (Wadden, 1993). Cardiac complications, including risk of sudden death, are a concern. Risks include potassium loss as well as loss of body protein, which is proportionately greater (20 g/kg of weight lost) in the less obese than in the more obese (Forbes, 1987). Serum electrolytes need to be monitored and supplemented when necessary. VLCDs can lead to an increase of urinary ketones that interfere with the renal clearance of uric acid, resulting in increased serum uric

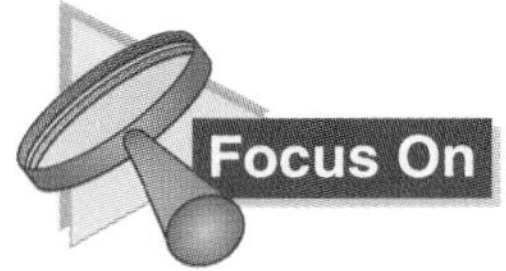

History of Protein-Sparing Modified Fast Diets

The first protein-sparing modified fast (PSMF) diets were developed after observing that during total fasts, popular for weight reduction in the late 1950s and early 1960s, dieters lost large amounts of potassium and protein. The first PSMF diets were developed to add protein to the fasting regime. Protein in the early formulas was exclusively in the form of hydrolyzed collagen, a protein lacking the essential amino acid tryptophan. The formulas were not supplemented with vitamins, minerals, or electrolytes and were not necessarily supported by medical supervision. The products were used by more than 100,000 people, among whom 60 diet-related deaths had been reported to the Centers for Disease Control and Prevention by the end of 1977.

The diet was directly implicated as the basis for the cardiac dysrhythmia causing 17 deaths (Isner et al., 1979). Of these 17 deaths, those with the highest percentage of body fat before the diet began were better able to preserve body protein, especially that in the myocardium (Van Itallie and Yang, 1984).

Sudden death during dieting continues with a classic prolonged QT interval on the electrocardiogram. The highest risk for sudden death syndrome is during weight loss with total fasting, with very-low-calorie diets, or following obesity surgery (Berg, 1994). Suggested theories of cause include nutritional inadequacies, depletion of myocardial proteins, excessive β-adrenergic sensitivity of the myocardium, electrolyte abnormalities leading to ventricular fibrillation, ingestion of medications, or predisposition to aggravation of cardiac dysrhythmia. The heart is usually small in children or adults who die from protein-energy malnutrition or anorexia, although it may be enlarged in some patients who are starving. Patients should be made aware of the risks for sudden death syndrome with restrictive dieting.

These hazardous products were removed from the market. PSMF formulas currently contain complete protein and some carbohydrate, are supplemented with vitamins, minerals, and electrolytes, and are usually included as part of a complete multidisciplinary program. Patients must be carefully screened before they start these programs and then closely monitored.

acid levels, often manifested in gout. Higher serum cholesterol levels resulting from mobilization of adipose stores pose a risk of gallstones. Additional adverse reactions that are common include cold intolerance, fatigue, light-headedness, nervousness, euphoria, constipation or diarrhea, dry skin, thinning reddened hair, anemia, and menstrual irregularities. Some of these are typical of triiodothyronine deficiency.

The American Dietetic Association has outlined the criteria that should be followed in using the VLCD for weight management (ADA, 1990) (see "*Clinical Insight:* American Dietetic Association Criteria for Use of Very-Low-Calorie Diets").

FAD DIETS AND PRACTICES

A continuous supply of new and often bizarre approaches to weight reduction is available to the consumer through the popular press. Although some of the programs are sensible and appropriate, most emphasize fast results with minimal effort. Often the proposed diets would lead to nutritional deficiencies over an extended period; however, the potential health risks are seldom realized because the diets are usually abandoned after a few weeks. On the other hand, fad diets encourage unrealistic expectations, setting the dieter up for failure, subsequent guilt, and feelings of helplessness at ever managing the weight problem.

Variations of a low-carbohydrate, high-fat diet are popular. Carbohydrate was severely restricted, but protein and fat intakes were unlimited. Protein obtained from animal sources meant that fat, saturated fat, and cholesterol intakes were also high. Although these diets featured high ketone production, they suppressed appetite to only a minor degree. Even with total fasting, converting fats to ketones lowers the energy value of the diet by only 100 kcal/day. The initial rapid weight loss from diuresis was secondary to the carbohydrate restriction.

Another popular regimen (often referred to as the "Zone" diet) restricts carbohydrate to no more than 40% of total calories, with fat and protein providing 30% of calories each. This particular diet composition is claimed to keep insulin in check, which is blamed for fat storage. The diet includes generous amounts of fiber and fresh fruits and vegetables. Weight loss ensues not because insulin is kept in a narrow range, but because calories are restricted. Calculations have shown that at most, the diet provides 1700 calories daily (Gladwell, 1998).

Table 23–4 provides some guidelines for evaluating fad diets. Although hypnosis and acupuncture are popular with some, there is no definitive support for these practices.

To help consumers find their way through the maze of programs available for weight loss, several initiatives have been undertaken. In 1995, the Institute of Medicine published *Weighing the Options,* a report designed to develop a set of criteria that could be used by others to evaluate and treat the problems of overweight and obesity. The report defined the approaches to treatment and created a model of the decision-making process regarding treatment and outcome. In 1996, Shape Up America! and the

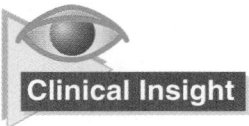

AMERICAN DIETETIC ASSOCIATION CRITERIA FOR USE OF VERY-LOW-CALORIE DIETS

Although VLCDs promote rapid weight reduction and may benefit certain individuals, such diets have health risks and should be undertaken only with the supervision of a multidisciplinary health team with monitoring by a physician and nutrition counseling by a registered dietitian (American Dietetic Association, 1990).

The VLCD is only one part of a weight reduction program and, to be most effective, should be combined with nutrition education, psychological counseling, exercise, and behavior therapy. The following criteria should be used in selecting candidates for a VLCD program:

1. At least 30% overweight with a minimum BMI of 32
2. Free from contraindicated medical conditions: pregnancy or lactation, active cancer, hepatic disease, renal failure, active cardiac dysfunction, or severe psychologic disturbances
3. Committed to establishing new eating and life-style behaviors that will assist the maintenance of weight loss
4. Committed to taking the time to complete both the treatment and the maintenance components of a program

The VLCD should be preceded by 2 to 4 weeks on a well-balanced 1200-kcal diet that allows time for the body to adjust to the caloric deprivation and promotes a gradual diuresis.

The VLCD should be limited to 12 to 16 weeks to reduce the risk of adverse complications related to body protein losses, in particular cardiac problems. Dieters should be closely monitored.

The VLCD should be followed by a gradual refeeding period of 2 to 4 weeks during which time food, especially simple sugars, is reintroduced slowly to prevent a rapid fluid weight gain.

Dieters should continue a follow-up or maintenance program for at least 12 months, or until they can demonstrate voluntary restriction of eating, particularly during times of stress, a normal eating pattern, and a sense of well-being.

Some dieters will require ongoing support even after the maintenance program has ended, and all dieters will need to continue with regular exercise (aerobic and weight training) for long-term weight reduction success.

TABLE 23–4 TIPS FOR EVALUATING FAD DIETS AND PRACTICES

1. Stay current in the medical and nutrition literature. Read professional journals regularly to stay on the cutting edge; read more than one reliable reference.
2. Teach consumers to make healthy choices wherever they are—at home, at a restaurant, in other homes for holidays and special events.
3. Think first before advancing the latest diet trend; review the content of the proposed diet first.
4. Stick to logical nutrition principles, such as maintaining an intake of 15–20% protein and ≤30% fat. Calculate the individual's needs accordingly.
5. Keep language simple for the consumer's benefit.
6. Evaluate fads and trends using the following principles:
   - Does the diet exclude any major food groups (using the Food Guide Pyramid as a guideline)? For example, a high-meat diet would be too low in breads/cereals. A high-fat diet would be higher than recommended amounts to match current standards (i.e., ≤30% calories from fat).
   - Does the diet propose use of supplements, pills, or drugs to the exclusion of normal foods? This may be a dangerous practice.
   - Does the diet suggest avoiding certain foods because they "cause" certain diseases (such as cancer, arthritis, heart disease)? No individual food has been verified as the cause of disease at this time.
   - Does the diet suggest including certain foods because they "cure" certain diseases? No singular food cures disease. Foods and nutrients in combination have been suggested as being beneficial in preventing some forms of cancer, but focusing on any given food should not exclude other foods or food groups.
   - Food forms (frozen versus fresh, etc.) should not be highlighted. It is not necessary to use only raw fruits and vegetables to the exclusion of canned and frozen foods.
   - Beware of sweeping statements—"salty foods cause weight gain in everyone." Not everyone is sensitive to sodium.
   - More is not always better. Too much of one food to the exclusion of others is a tip-off that a diet is unbalanced.
7. Analyze for total content, including a balance of vitamins, minerals, protein, carbohydrate, and fat, using current guidelines.

American Obesity Association released the first edition of *Guidance for Treatment of Adult Obesity,* an educational resource for physicians. It provides the tools needed to identify and intervene as appropriate and gives treatment guidance and support for patients. The website is www.shapeup.org.

In 1997, the Federal Trade Commission (FTC) convened a conference to better understand the problem of obesity and to explore ways to improve the information that consumers routinely receive about the nature of obesity and weight loss products and programs. It marked the first time that representatives of the weight loss industry, members of the scientific and academic community, agencies from state and federal government, and public interest and consumer groups met together to explore voluntary approaches and to address issues regarding weight loss products and programs (Gross and Daynard, 1997).

In 1998, the NIH released *Clinical Guidelines on the Identification, Evaluation, and Treatment of Overweight and Obesity in Adults—The Evidence Report.* The intent of the guidelines is to provide evidence for the effects of treatment on overweight and obesity. The guidelines are directed to physicians and associated health professionals in clinical practice, health care policy makers, and clinical investigators (NIH, 1998). Expert recommendations for managing obesity in children and adolescents are found in *"Clinical Insight:* Evaluation and Treatment of Childhood and Adolescent Obesity: Expert Committee Recommendations."

Life-Style Modification

Life-style modification or behavior modification interventions rely on analyzing behavior to identify events that are associated with inappropriate as well as appropriate eating, exercise, or thinking habits (Wadden and Sarwer, 1998). Antecedents, behaviors, and consequences are analyzed to determine how to modify the situation. For example, if an individual finds that he or she overeats when angry, steps are taken to help the person deal with anger in more constructive ways. In addition to nutrition and exercise, the principal components of treatment include self-monitoring, problem-solving, stimulus control, slowing of eating, and cognitive restructuring (Wadden and Sarwer, 1998).

Self-monitoring with daily records of place and time of food intake, as well as accompanying thoughts and feelings, helps identify the physical and emotional settings in which eating occurs. It also provides feedback on progress and places the responsibility for change and accomplishment on the patient. Self-monitoring also gives clues to the occurrence of relapses and consequent guilt and how they can be prevented.

Problem-solving is a process for defining the eating or weight problem, generating possible solutions, evaluating the solutions and choosing the best one, implementing the new behavior, evaluating the outcome, and re-evaluating alternative solutions if the one selected is not successful.

Stimulus control involves modification of (1) the settings or the chain of events that precede eating, (2) the kinds of foods consumed when eating does occur, and (3) the consequences of eating. Patients are taught to slow their rate of eating to become mindful of satiety cues and reduce food intake. Strategies such as putting down the utensils between bites, pausing during meals, and chewing for a minimum number of times are some of the ways to slow the eating process.

Cognitive restructuring teaches patients to identify, challenge, and correct the negative thoughts that frequently undermine their efforts. For example, excessive self-criticism in response to a dietary lapse could lead to total abandonment of effort. Positive self-talk, such as "I had a piece of cake. One slice is not going to increase my weight. I will continue eating in a healthful way" can sometimes help patients more constructively deal with such incidents. Some life-style modification strategies are listed in Table 23–5. A program of this type that ap-

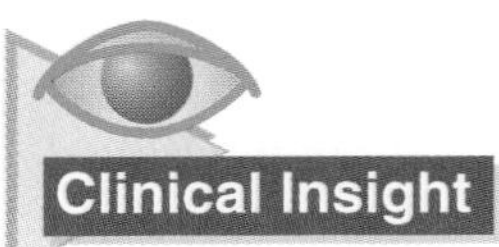

Evaluation and Treatment of Childhood and Adolescent Obesity: Expert Committee Recommendations

To develop guidance for health professionals who care for obese children, the Maternal and Child Health Bureau, Health Resources and Services Administration, and the Department of Health and Human Services convened a committee of pediatric obesity experts in 1997. The committee issued recommendations for identifying obese children, evaluating them medically, and treating them. Because so few studies exist in this area, the recommendations represented a consensus of professionals who treat obese children and adolescents rather than a distillation of research studies.

The Committee identified the following cut-off points for evaluation and possible treatment: children with a body mass index (BMI) greater than or equal to the 85th percentile with complications of obesity, or with a BMI greater than or equal to the 95th percentile with or without complications. The pediatric obesity experts made clear that these children should be carefully assessed for any underlying syndromes (genetic, endocrinologic, or psychologic) or secondary complications such as hypertension, dyslipidemias, sleep apnea, and orthopedic problems. If the complications are found to cause serious morbidity and require rapid weight loss, referral to a pediatric obesity specialist is recommended. Otherwise, parent and child readiness to make changes should be evaluated along with a careful assessment of eating and activity patterns. Once assessment is complete, treatment can begin.

The Committee felt strongly that the primary goal of treatment is to achieve healthy eating and activity, not to achieve an ideal body weight. The group outlined the use of weight maintenance versus weight loss depending on the patient's age, baseline BMI percentile, and presence of medical complications. The following guidelines were issued: For children ≤ 7 years of age, prolonged weight maintenance, which allows for a gradual decline in BMI as children grow in height, is an appropriate goal in the absence of any secondary complications of obesity. However, if secondary complications are present, children in this age group may benefit from weight loss if their BMI is at the 95th percentile or higher. For children older than 7 years, prolonged weight maintenance is appropriate if their BMI is between the 85th and 95th percentile and if they have no secondary complications. If a secondary complication is present, or if BMI is at the 95th percentile or above, weight loss (approximately 1 pound per month) is advised.

Treatment recommendations called for family involvement and gradual changes in activity and eating patterns. Also family support was highlighted, since obesity is a chronic problem requiring lifelong attention.

(Source: Barlow SE, Dietz WH. Obesity evaluation and treatment: Expert committee recommendations. Pediatrics 102:3, 1998.)

pears to be successful is *The Solution* (see Table 23–3).

Comprehensive life-style modification in weight control appears to be most effective for the mildly obese (20% to 40% overweight). The low attrition rate averages 13.5% compared with 25% to 75% in most other programs (Bray and Gray, 1988b). Patients can lose 20 to 25 lb and successfully maintain the weight loss if they continue to practice the techniques and exercise regularly. It also appears that the longer programs are the most successful (Buckmaster and Brownell, 1988). Most programs usually last for 15 weeks and result in an average weight loss of 1.2 lb/wk. Average weight reduction at the end of the program is 20 lb.

A review of life-style modification studies from 1985 to 1995 indicated that patients treated by behavior therapy combined with a 1200 calories/day diet regained 30% to 35% of their weight loss in the year following treatment. Five years after treatment, subjects had, on average, returned to their baseline weight (Wadden and Sarwer, 1998). Weight regain is a problem regardless of the type of program.

Exercise

Exercise is an extremely important part of a weight management program. By increasing LBM in proportion to fat, exercise helps to balance the loss of LBM and reduction of RMR that inevitably accompany even a well-managed weight reduction program. By lowering glycogen stores, *aerobic exercise* promotes the use of fat for fuel. Numerous positive side effects include strengthening cardiovascular integrity as well as increasing sensitivity to insulin. Possibly the most valuable contributions of exercise are the relief of boredom, increased sense of control, and improved sense of well-being (Fig. 23–6). A combination of aerobic and resistance training is optimal. *Resistance training* increases LBM, adding to the resting metabolic rate and the ability to utilize more of the energy intake (see Chapter 25). Resistance training also increases bone mineral density, especially important for women (see Chapter 28).

Increased exercise can result in an energy deficit, and even without diet, exercise alone can be expected to lower weight around 2 to 3 kg depending on the intensity, duration, and type of exercise (Blair, 1993; NIH Technology Assessment Conference Panel, 1992). Dieters with hypertrophic obesity lose more fat during an exercise program than the very obese with hyperplastic obesity (Bjorntorp, 1983). This may account for the observation that although the moderately obese lose body fat during physical training, it is difficult to demonstrate this result in the massively obese.

Some studies of programs combining diet and ex-

TABLE 23–5 LIFE-STYLE MODIFICATION STRATEGIES*

Elimination of Eating Cues
Eat only sitting down at one designated place.
Sit in a different seat at the table.
Leave the table as soon as eating is done.
Do not combine eating with other activities, such as reading or watching television.
Do not put bowls of food on the table.
At a restaurant, limit intake from the bread basket to one roll with no or a small amount of butter.
Stock home with healthier food choices.
Keep all food in cupboards where it cannot be seen.
Shop for groceries from a list after a full meal.
Limit the amount of money taken when shopping.
Plan meals and snacks.
Plan for special events, parties, and dinners.
Immediately place leftovers in storage containers and refrigerate or freeze them for another meal.
Negotiate with the family to eat healthier foods when around.
Ask others to monitor eating patterns and provide positive feedback.
Substitute other activities for snacking.
Snack on fresh vegetables and fruit.
Behaviors to Prolong Eating and Reduce the Amount of Food Eaten
Eat slowly and savor each mouthful.
Put down the fork between bites.
Delay eating for 2 to 3 min and converse with others.
Postpone a desired snack for 10 min.
Serve food on a smaller plate.
Leave 1 or 2 bites of food on the plate.
Divide portions in half so that another portion can be permitted.

*(Adapted from Holli BB. Using behavior modification in nutrition counseling. J Am Diet Assoc 88:1530, 1988.)

ercise have shown that although there is no increase in weight loss in the exercising group over diet alone, an increased loss of body fat does occur (Hill et al., 1987; Van Dale et al., 1987). A decrease in body fat does not necessarily mean a decrease in body weight. Initially, physical exercise increases muscle mass, and because LBM is denser than the fat it replaces, body weight may not change. With continued exercise, the limited capacity of muscle mass to increase is overcome by the decrease in fat, resulting in a net decrease in body weight. A minimum of 2 months is needed to obtain any reduction of adipose tissue with training programs.

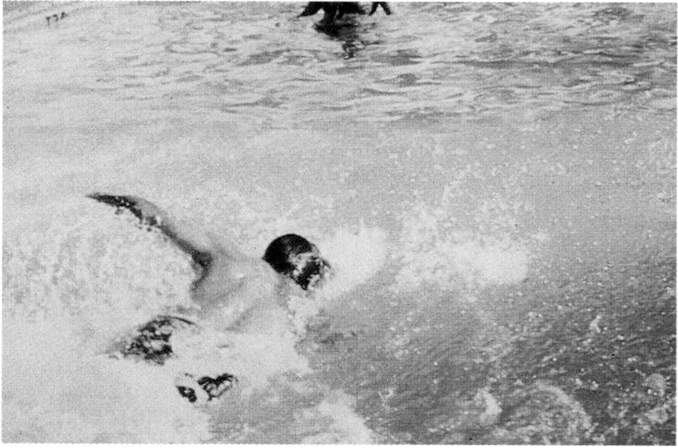

FIGURE 23–6 Swimming is an excellent aerobic activity to include in a weight reduction program.

The RMR is elevated during aerobic exercise. Except after fairly high levels of intensity or large amounts of exercise, RMR returns to resting levels within an hour or so following exercise (Brehm and Keller, 1990). Energy expenditure during this period represents replacement of muscle glycogen as well as the effects of hormonal changes and the increase in metabolic processing of fuel stores. Whether or not exercise has an effect on TEF remains unresolved. Increases in lean body mass result in 8% to 14% higher daily energy expenditures in moderately and highly active men compared with sedentary men (Horton and Geissler, 1994). However, this study did not find that habitual exercise leads to prolonged stimulation of metabolic rate per unit of active tissue.

One study monitored the effects of television watching on children age 8 to 12 years. Measurements of energy expenditure were lower during television watching than during rest, especially in obese children (Klesges et al., 1993). The conclusion that television watching has a profound effect on energy expenditure and obesity in children is significant for nutrition counselors and physicians working with pediatric populations.

Contrary to popular belief, spot reduction, that is, reducing fat in one area of the body, is not possible with exercise; fat is burned from the largest concentrations of adipose tissue. Another misconception is that exercise is counterproductive because it increases the desire to eat. Although lean individuals usually compensate for energy expended in physical activity by increasing their food intake, obese persons do not, possibly because the exercise level is less strenuous (Pi-Sunyer, 1988).

Consistency is key to realizing the benefits of exercise. Previous exercise recommendations usually called for 20 to 60 minutes of moderate- to high-intensity endurance exercise performed three or more times weekly. It now appears that the majority of health benefits can be gained by physical activity of moderate intensity (enough to expend 200 kcals daily) accumulated in intermittent short bouts. The current recommendation is: "Every U.S. adult should accumulate 30 minutes or more of moderate-intensity physical activity on most, preferably all, days of the week" (Pate et al., 1995).

Programs that involve supervision or regular participation within a social group appear to be more successful in the long term. Socioeconomic circumstances can be an important factor. Many exercise programs are expensive, and it is not always possible, or even safe, to indulge in brisk walking in some neighborhoods.

Only 10% of Americans meet exercise requirements thought to be needed to reduce disease risks. In one recent study, 82% of overweight adults believed that they failed to maintain healthy weight because they did not exercise, even though they were aware of the benefits (Miller, 1994). This society tends to view the barriers to exercise as outweighing its benefits.

Whatever the selected exercise, it should be readily available, pleasant, affordable, and easy to do. Exercise contributes to well-being and self-esteem, even if weight loss is not achieved. Exercise also helps the individual maintain weight loss. It has been demonstrated that weight regain is significantly less likely to occur when physical activity is combined with any other weight reduction method (Blair, 1993).

Pharmaceutical Management

In patients with BMIs of 30 and above, or 27 and above with other risks, pharmaceutical agents can be a helpful addition to a diet and exercise program. They cause an energy deficit through a number of mechanisms, including acting on the brain to suppress appetite; producing bulk to fill the stomach, thereby suppressing appetite; possibly increasing thermogenesis; increasing metabolism; and selectively interfering with fat absorption. However, medications have side effects, and the benefits and risks must be weighed carefully for each individual.

Medications currently available can be categorized as CNS-acting agents and non-CNS acting agents. The CNS-acting agents fall into the categories of catecholaminergic agents, serotoninergic agents, and combination catecholaminergic-serotoninergic agents. Common side effects of CNS-acting agents are dry mouth, headache, insomnia, and constipation.

Catecholaminergic drugs act on the brain, increasing the availability of norepinephrine. Table 23–6 lists catecholaminergic agents. Drug Enforcement Agency (DEA) Schedule II anorexic agents, such as amphetamines, have a high potential for abuse and are not recommended for obesity treatment. DEA Schedule III agents also pose abuse potential that should be carefully considered. Commonly used DEA Schedule IV catecholaminergic agents such as *phentermine,* have a low potential for abuse. Because of its effects on blood pressure, phentermine is prescribed with caution in patients with even mild hypertension. The over-the-counter medication, *phenypropanolamine,* has been shown to be safe and effective for early weight loss. Its efficacy after 4 weeks is lower than the prescription medications (Greenway, 1992).

Serotoninergic agents act by increasing serotonin levels in the brain. Two drugs in this category, *fenfluramine HCL* and *dexfenfluramine HCL,* were re-

TABLE 23–6 AVAILABLE CATECHOLAMINERGIC AGENTS

AGENT	TRADE NAME	DAILY DOSAGE (mg)*
Schedule II Agents		
amphetamine	Biphetamine	10–15
phenmetrazine HCl	Preludin	75
Schedule III Agents		
benzphetamine HCl	Didrex	25–50 to 75–150
phendimetrazine tartrate	Bontril	105
	Slow-Release Bontril	105
	Prelu-2	105
	Plegine	105
	X-Trozine	105
	Extended Release X-Trozine	105
Schedule IV Agents		
diethypropion HCl (amfepramone)	Tenuate	75
	Tenuate Dospan	75
mazindol HCl	Sanorex	1–3
	Mazanor	1–3
phentermine HCl	Adipex-P	37.5*
	Fastin	30
	Obenix	37.5
	Oby-Cap	30
	Oby-Trim	30
	Zantryl	30
phentermine resin	Ionamin	30†
Unscheduled (OTC) Agents		
phenylpropanolamine	Dexatrim	75
	Acutrim	

(From Shape Up America! and the American Obesity Association. Guidance for Treatment of Adult Obesity, 2nd ed. Bethesda, MD: Authors, 1998.)

OTC, over the counter.

*Represents recommended daily intake. Ranges represent initial dose to maximum dose. Titration may be indicated depending on each patient's therapeutic response.

†Usual dosage. Some patients may respond to half this dosage.

moved from the market on September 15, 1997 after concerns were raised regarding the possible side effect of cardiac valvulopathy and regurgitation (Connolly et al., 1997). In this disease, the heart valves have a glistening white appearance that is plaquelike, and regurgitation is present. These drugs had also been associated with primary pulmonary hypertension, a rare, often fatal disease (Abenhaim et al., 1996). Further studies clarified the relationship between fenfluramine and dexfenfluramine and valvular abnormalities (Jick et al., 1998; Khan et al., 1998; Weissman et al., 1998).

Combination catecholaminergic-serotoninergic agents include *sibutramine* (Meridia), which inhibits the reuptake of serotonin and norepinephrine. The drug was initially developed to counteract depression. Classified as a DEA Schedule IV agent, it has a low potential for abuse; however, careful observation of blood pressure and heart rate of patients using sibutramine has been recommended (Lean, 1997). Caution is needed in patients with hypertension; use is not recommended for patients with coronary heart disease, arrhythmias, stroke, or congestive heart failure (Aronne, 1998).

Orlistat, a non-CNS acting agent, is not an appetite suppressant. It acts directly on the gastrointestinal tract to inhibit fat absorption (Guerciolini, 1997). Orlistat (Xenical) is taken with mildly hypocaloric meals resulting in a 30% reduction in fat absorption. Inhibiting fat absorption raises concern about fat-soluble vitamins. However, fat-soluble vitamins generally remain within the normal range in patients treated with orlistat (James et al., 1997). A small percentage of patients showed reductions in blood levels of vitamins D and E and β-carotene, which were corrected with vitamin supplementation (James et al., 1997). Side effects are gastrointestinal in nature: oily spotting, fecal urgency, and flatus with discharge. Health benefits include reduced LDL cholesterol and elevated HDL cholesterol, improved glycemic control, and reduced blood pressure (Aronne, 1998).

Not all individuals respond to pharmacotherapy, but for patients who do respond, a weight loss of about 1 lb/wk can be expected. Most studies conducted for less than 24 weeks show continued weight loss for the duration of the study. Long-term studies show most weight loss occurs during the first 6 months of therapy. Significant maintenance of loss has been shown at 1 year or more as long as the drug treatment is continued. After medication is stopped, the majority of patients regain weight.

Natural weight loss aids are now commonly available and hold varying degrees of promise for weight loss results (see "*Focus On:* Natural Weight Loss Aids").

Surgical Procedures

Morbid obesity is sometimes treated surgically. Surgery should be considered adjuvant therapy. This treatment is preferably reserved for those with a BMI of 40 or higher, or a BMI of 35 or higher with other risk factors (NIH, 1998; Shape Up America! and American Obesity Association, 1998). Various surgical procedures have been used to decrease the amount of food entering or being absorbed from the gastrointestinal tract. These include esophageal banding, gastric restrictive surgery, and jejunoileal bypass. Gastric restrictive surgery is currently the surgery of choice.

Before any morbidly obese person is considered for surgery, failure of a comprehensive program including calorie restriction, exercise, life-style modification, psychological counseling, and family involvement should be demonstrated. Failure is defined as an inability of the patient to reduce body weight by one third and body fat by one half, and an inability to maintain any weight loss achieved. Such patients have *intractable morbid obesity* and should be considered for surgery. Before surgery the patient should be evaluated extensively with respect to physiologic and medical complications, psychological problems such as depression and poor self-esteem, and the extent of motivation.

Postoperative follow-up includes evaluation at regular intervals by the surgical team and a registered dietitian. In addition, behavioral or psychological support is necessary. Lifelong follow-up on the part of the patient and surgeon, including involvement of the patient's primary physician, is essential (NIH, 1998; Choban et al., 1996).

GASTRIC RESTRICTION (GASTRIC BYPASS AND GASTROPLASTY)

Gastric restriction, which surgically reduces the reservoir capacity of the stomach by closing off a part of it, is successful in achieving weight reduction in people who are morbidly obese, and at present is the only well-accepted **bariatric** surgery for that purpose (Consensus Development Conference Panel, 1991). Of the two common procedures, the gastric bypass appears to be slightly more effective in achieving weight loss. Although gastroplasty may be minimally safer in terms of operative morbidity and mortality, long-term results appear to be more consistent with the bypass surgery (Bray and Gray, 1988b). In addition to the greater absolute weight loss observed, the gastric bypass tended to have fewer long-term mechanical complications with fewer revisional surgeries required (Benotti and Forse, 1995).

Gastroplasty reduces the size of the stomach by applying rows of stainless-steel staples across the top of the stomach in a manner that leaves only a small opening (0.8 to 1 cm) into the distal stomach. This opening may be banded by a piece of mesh to prevent it from enlarging during the years after surgery. **Gastric bypass** involves reducing the size of the stomach with the stapling procedure, but then connecting a small opening in the upper portion of the stomach to the small intestine by means of an intestinal loop (Fig. 23–7). Both procedures

NATURAL WEIGHT LOSS AIDS

Americans are constantly being told that "diets don't work." Furthermore, the lure of a quick and easy solution to the challenge of weight management is strong. As a result, the market for natural weight loss aids is booming. Some of the more popular weight loss aids include one or more of the following ingredients: chromium picolinate or some other form of chromium, dihydroepiandrosterone (DHEA), ma huang, and senna. What are the claims? What are the facts?

According to the claims, **chromium** should promote fat loss and increase lean body mass. We know that chromium potentiates the action of insulin in carbohydrate, lipid, and protein metabolism, although the exact mechanism is not known. Dietary surveys indicate that most individuals consume less than recommended amounts of chromium (Anderson and Kozlovsky, 1985). Also, participating in strenuous physical activity results in increased acute losses of chromium (Anderson et al., 1988).

Findings suggest that indiscriminate use of chromium supplements has no effect on body composition. When sensitive methods of human body composition are used, data indicate that chromium supplementation during strength training does not promote an increase in muscle mass and fat loss in men (Clancy et al., 1994; Lukaski et al., 1996).

Chromium competes with iron for binding on transferrin. Researchers hypothesized that significant increases in serum chromium concentration as a result of chromium supplementation, particularly as chromium picolinate, may adversely affect iron transport and distribution (Lukaski et al., 1996). A recent study examined the effects of chromium picolinate supplementation on iron status in older men who participated in resistance training. The results showed that chromium did not affect changes in iron transport and did not compromise iron status in the men (Campbell et al., 1997). The toxicity of trivalent chromium, the chemical form in diets, is very low, with a substantial margin of safety.

Among other claims, **DHEA** (dehydroepiandrosterone) is supposed to promote weight loss. Unfortunately, only animal work has been completed for testing the effects of DHEA on weight loss. Problems noted with DHEA include liver cancer that occurred in rats. Additionally, supplementation can lead to increased insulin resistance, the growth of unwanted hair, and a drop in high-density lipoprotein cholesterol, increasing the risk for heart disease (see Chapter 25).

Ma huang (ephedra) promoters claim benefits such as weight loss, increased energy, performance enhancement, and increased LBM. Studies demonstrated that ma huang given alone does not result in weight loss; however, when combined with caffeine plus a calorie-restricted diet, greater weight loss can be achieved than with calorie-restricted diets alone (Astrup et al., 1992; Breum, et al., 1994; Daly et al., 1993).

Ma huang is a CNS stimulant, and it does have side effects. It increases blood pressure and heart rate. The increase in blood pressure was offset by the decrease in blood pressure that occurred with weight loss in the studies. Ma huang is hazardous to those with heart ailments, diabetes, hypertension, and thyroid conditions. When combined with caffeine-containing herbs (kola nut, guarana, and mat), ma huang can be especially hazardous. The Food and Drug Administration received more than 100 reports of adverse reactions ranging from heart attacks to hepatitis and several deaths among people who used supplements containing a ma huang-kola nut combination. Common, less severe side effects of ma huang-caffeine combinations are insomnia, dizziness, and tremor. When individuals discontinue treatment, they can experience headache and fatigue.

Senna or senna leaves are the dried leaflets of plants found in Egypt and India. Senna is a potent cathartic (Tyler, 1993). Use of this herb, which induces diarrhea, can lead to low potassium levels. Three deaths have been associated with senna use.

have the effect of reducing the amount of food that can be eaten at one time and producing early satiety. The new stomach capacity may be as small as 30 mL.

The most frequent complications of gastric restriction are bloating of the pouch, nausea, and vomiting. A postsurgical food record noting the tolerance for specific foods in particular amounts helps in devising a program to avoid these episodes. A careful postoperative 6-week feeding regimen of pureed or liquid foods is followed by a regimen consisting of frequent small meals of high nutrient-density foods. Attention to protein intake and vitamin and mineral supplementation, particularly vitamin B_{12}, folate, and iron, is advised. Patients should be counseled to eat slowly, chew food well, and avoid swallowing chunks of meat or other food that cannot be completely liquefied and that could block the pouch opening. Frequent small meals are important. Patients tend to choose liquids; however, weight loss can be deterred by drinking too much calorically dense liquid, such as milk shakes and soft drinks. Eventually, the pouch expands to accommodate 4 to 5 oz at a time.

Because use of the lower part of the stomach is omitted, the gastric bypass patient may also have *dumping syndrome* (see Chapter 30). The symptoms of tachycardia, sweating, and abdominal pain are so negative that they can further motivate the patient to make the appropriate behavior changes and refrain from overeating.

Completion of the surgery does not end the obesity treatment; in fact, consent to the procedure is considered an agreement to lifelong follow-up and regular monitoring by a multidisciplinary team of health care professionals. Monitoring should include an assessment of body fat loss, potential anemia, and deficiencies of potassium, magnesium, fo-

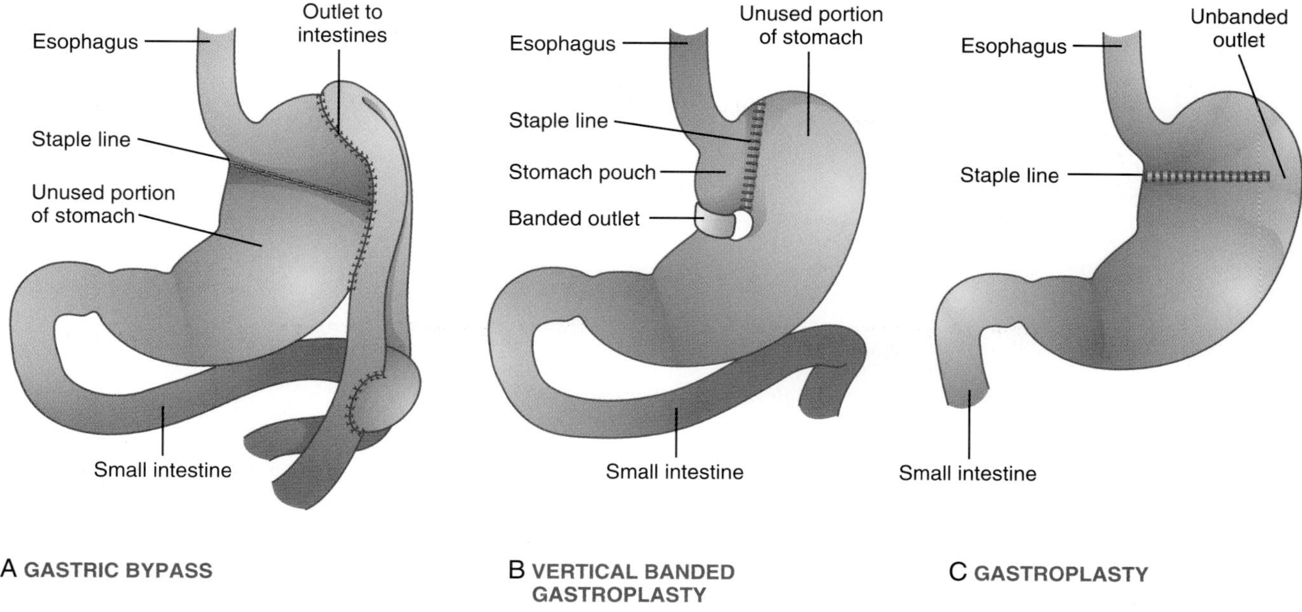

FIGURE 23–7 Gastric surgeries for obesity.

late, and vitamin B_{12}, especially in patients with gastric bypass. The results of gastric surgery are favorable and are attended by fewer complications than with the intestinal bypass surgery practiced during the 1970s. On average, the reduction of excess body weight after gastric restriction surgery is 40% to 75%. This correlates to about 30% to 40% of initial body weight (Brolin et al., 1994; Sugerman et al., 1987; Sugerman et al., 1989).

A review of more than 5000 patients from 12 centers showed a mortality rate after gastric restriction surgery one fourth that of morbidly obese patients and equivalent to normal-weight patients of the same age (Forse et al., 1989). In addition, most patients report positive psychological results—improved self-esteem and feeling more attractive and less depressed.

JAW WIRING (MAXILLOMANDIBULAR FIXATION)

Wiring the jaws closed restricts eating to liquids that can be taken through a straw. Dental attention before wiring as well as oral hygiene and nutritional care while the jaws are wired are important. Counseling should include recommendations for combinations of liquids and supplements that will provide adequate nutrients. The patient should also be taught how to cut the wires if necessary and how to deal with any episode of vomiting.

This technique has been effective in producing weight reduction; however, without education and ongoing support, body weight generally returns to pretreatment levels after the wires are removed. New behaviors need to be internalized, and a sense of control must be established if weight reduction is to be maintained.

LIPOSUCTION

Liposuction involves aspiration of fat deposits by means of a 1- to 2-cm incision through which a tube is fanned out into the adipose tissue. The most successful operations are performed on younger persons with only small amounts of fat to be removed, where the elastic properties of the skin are able to allow tightening over the aspirated areas. It is not a weight reduction technique but rather a cosmetic surgery, because only 5 lb of fat can be removed at a time; not all cases provide the anticipated outcome.

Weight Management in Children

Approximately 25% of children and adolescents 6 to 17 years of age are overweight or obese. Obese children are often the targets of discrimination. Childhood obesity increases the risk of obesity in adulthood. For the child who is obese, after 6 years of age, the probability of obesity in adulthood exceeds 50% and the risks are significantly greater if either the mother or the father is obese (Whitaker et al., 1997). New BMI tables for determining childhood obesity are available for use by health care practitioners.

Children should not be put on "diets." The treatment goal for the child who is overweight should be weight maintenance or a slowing of the rate of weight gain. This gives the child time to "grow into" his or her weight. If the weight appropriate for the child's anticipated adult height has already been reached, then maintenance at that weight should be the lifetime goal (see "*Clinical Insight:* Determining Appropriate Rate of Weight Gain in the Obese Child").

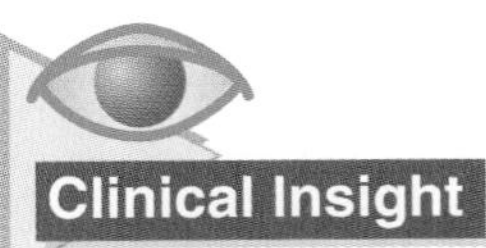

Determining Appropriate Rate of Weight Gain in the Obese Child

From the history of family growth patterns and review of the prior growth pattern of the obese child, determine the predicted adult height of the child. He or she will probably maintain his or her present height growth channel. For example, an 8-year-old girl on the 75th percentile for height will probably maintain that growth channel and will achieve 67 in. as an adult height.

Determine a rough estimation of the appropriate weight for the anticipated adult height. Using the Hamwi equation, for women, the rule is 100 lb for the first 5 ft of height and an additional 5 lb for each inch in height over 5 ft. For men, it is 106 lb for the first 5 ft and an additional 6 lb for each inch over 5 ft. An appropriate range is 10% on either side of this weight.

Subtract the child's present weight from the calculated appropriate adult weight. The remainder is the number of pounds that the child should gain throughout the rest of his or her growth period. This amount, divided by the number of years remaining of linear growth, is the appropriate yearly rate of weight gain for the child to achieve a normal adult weight. The number of years of growth remaining is based on the parental report of their own growth patterns and assessment of the present channel of height gain and the Tanner stage of adolescent development (see Chapter 11). In the case of the 8-year-old girl, if her mother reports reaching adult height at age 15, then probably her daughter will do the same. Thus, the daughter has 7 years of growth remaining.

Example: An 8-year-old girl who presently weighs 90 lb (over 95th percentile) and is 52 in. tall (75th to 90th percentile).

Eventual adult height = 67 in.
Appropriate weight for adult height = 100 lb + 35 lb = 135 lb (+ or – 13 lb)
Number of years of growth remaining = 15 years (age when the mother reached adult height) – 8 years (present age) = 7 years
(125 lb to 145 lb) - 90 lb (present weight) = 35 lb to 55 lb to be gained over next 7 years
Approximate rate of weight gain = 5 to 8 lb per year for the next 7 years

The child who already exceeds his or her optimal adult weight can safely experience a slow weight loss of 10 to 12 lb/y until the optimal adult weight is reached. Obviously, the child who needs to reduce weight is going to require more attention from family and health professionals, and effort on his or her part, than the child able to still gain weight, even if at a slower rate. This attention should be directed to all the areas mentioned previously with family modification of eating habits and increased physical activity. The program should be long term over the entire growth period and perhaps longer (Mahan, 1987).

Increased physical activity is extremely important in weight management program for children. Inactivity usually coupled with excessive TV watching must be changed in order for the child to eventually reach the long-term weight goal.

Maintenance of Reduced Body Weight

Prognosis for maintaining the status of the reduced-obese is poor. Of those who do reduce weight, only 5% manage to keep from gaining weight by the end of 5 years. This population may not be representative of those who reduce weight because the successful weight reducers do not present themselves to a medical program and are not available for follow-up and inclusion in the statistics. The typical picture, however, is one of recidivism. Continued dieting, with repeated ups and downs, leads gradually to a net increase in body fat and thus to a health risk for hyperlipidemia, hypertension, and diabetes.

Energy requirements for weight maintenance after weight reduction appear to be 25% lower than at the original weight. The net effect is that the reduced-obese are faced with the necessity of maintaining a reduced energy intake even after the desired weight has been lost. Whether this reduced intake must be maintained for an indefinite period is not known.

Life-style modification appears to be a key to weight maintenance. This may be related to the fact that, because obesity is a chronic disease, its management requires continuous treatment (modification of unacceptable behaviors) as with other chronic diseases (e.g., insulin for diabetes or medication for hypertension). A shift from the medical model to empowerment of the individual (healthy living) encourages choice and positive expressions and self-awareness (Dalton, 1998).

Regular, planned *physical activity* may be even more important in maintaining the reduced obese state over the long term (Bray and Gray, 1988b). The data strongly support the addition of exercise for improved long-term maintenance of lowered body weight. A 3-year follow-up study of men who were previously 22% overweight showed that to be effective, exercise must be carried out at least three times per week with a 1500-kcal/wk expenditure (Pavlou et al., 1989). Maintenance of reduced body weight of those in the study who continued to exercise was almost 100%.

Support groups are invaluable for the obese who are trying to lose weight and for the reduced-obese who are maintaining a new lower weight. They help individuals facing similar problems to learn ways of staying with their programs. Two large networks of self-help support groups are Overeaters Anonymous and Take Off Pounds Sensibly (TOPS). These groups are very inexpensive, continuous, include a "buddy system," and encourage participation on a regular basis or as often as needed. The Weight Watchers program offers free life-long maintenance classes for those who have reached and are maintaining their goal weights. The website address is www.weightwatchers.com.

WEIGHT IMBALANCE: EXCESSIVE LEANNESS

Almost eclipsed by the attention focused on obesity is the effort of some people to gain weight. The term **underweight** is applicable to those who are 15% to 20% or more below accepted weight standards. Because underweight is often a symptom of a disease, it should be assessed medically (Egbert, 1996). A low BMI is associated with greater mortality risk (Bray and Gray, 1988b).

Undernutrition itself may lead to underfunction of the pituitary, thyroid, gonads, and adrenals. Other risk factors include loss of energy and susceptibility to injury and infection, as well as distorted body image and other psychological problems.

Etiology

Underweight may be caused by (1) an intake insufficient in quantity to meet activity needs; (2) excessive activity, such as in the case of compulsive athletes in training; (3) poor absorption and utilization of the food consumed; (4) a wasting disease, such as cancer or hyperthyroidism, that increases the metabolic rate and energy needs; and (5) psychological or emotional stress.

Assessment

Assessing the cause and extent of underweight before starting a treatment program is important. A thorough history and pertinent medical tests usually determine whether underlying disorders are causing the underweight. From anthropometric data such as arm muscle and fat areas, it is possible to determine whether health-endangering underweight really exists. Biochemical measurements will indicate whether malnutrition accompanies the underweight.

Assessment of body fatness is useful, especially in dealing with the patient who has an eating disorder and needs to begin the body acceptance process (see Chapter 24).

Management

Any underlying cause of underweight must be dealt with as a first priority. A wasting disease or malabsorption requires treatment. Activity should be modified, and psychological counseling should be started if necessary. Nutritional support and dietary change are effective along with or after treatment of the underlying disorder, or when the cause of the underweight is merely inappropriate or inadequate food intake.

TABLE 23–7 SUGGESTIONS FOR INCREASING ENERGY INTAKE

ADDITIONAL FOODS	KCAL	PROTEIN (G)
Plus 500 kcal (Served Between Meals)		
1. 1 cup dry cereal	110	2
1 banana	80	
1 cup whole milk	159	8
1 slice toast	60	2
1 T peanut butter	86	4
	495	16
2. 8 saltine crackers	99	3
1 oz cheese	113	7
1 cup ice cream	290	6
	502	16
3. 6 graham cracker squares	165	3
2 T peanut butter	172	8
1 cup orange juice	122	
2 T raisins	52	
	511	11
Plus 1000 kcal (Served Between Meals)		
1. 8 oz fruit flavored yogurt	240	9
1 slice bread	60	2
2 oz cheese	226	14
1 apple	87	
¼ of 14″ cheese pizza	306	16
1 small banana	81	1
	1000	42
2. Instant Breakfast with whole milk	280	15
1 cup cottage cheese	239	31
½ cup pineapple	95	
1 cup apple juice	117	
6 graham cracker squares	165	3
1 pear	100	1
	996	50
Plus 1500 kcal (Served Between Meals)		
1. 2 slices bread	120	4
2 T peanut butter	172	8
1 T jam	110	
4 graham cracker squares	110	2
8 oz fruit flavored yogurt	240	9
¾ cup roasted peanuts	628	28
1 cup apricot nectar	143	1
	1523	52
2. 1 baked custard	285	13
Instant Breakfast with whole milk	280	15
1 cup dry cereal	110	2
1 banana	80	
1 cup whole milk	159	8
1 cup orange juice	122	
4 T raisins	104	
1 bagel	165	6
2 T cream cheese	99	2
2 T jam	110	
	1514	46

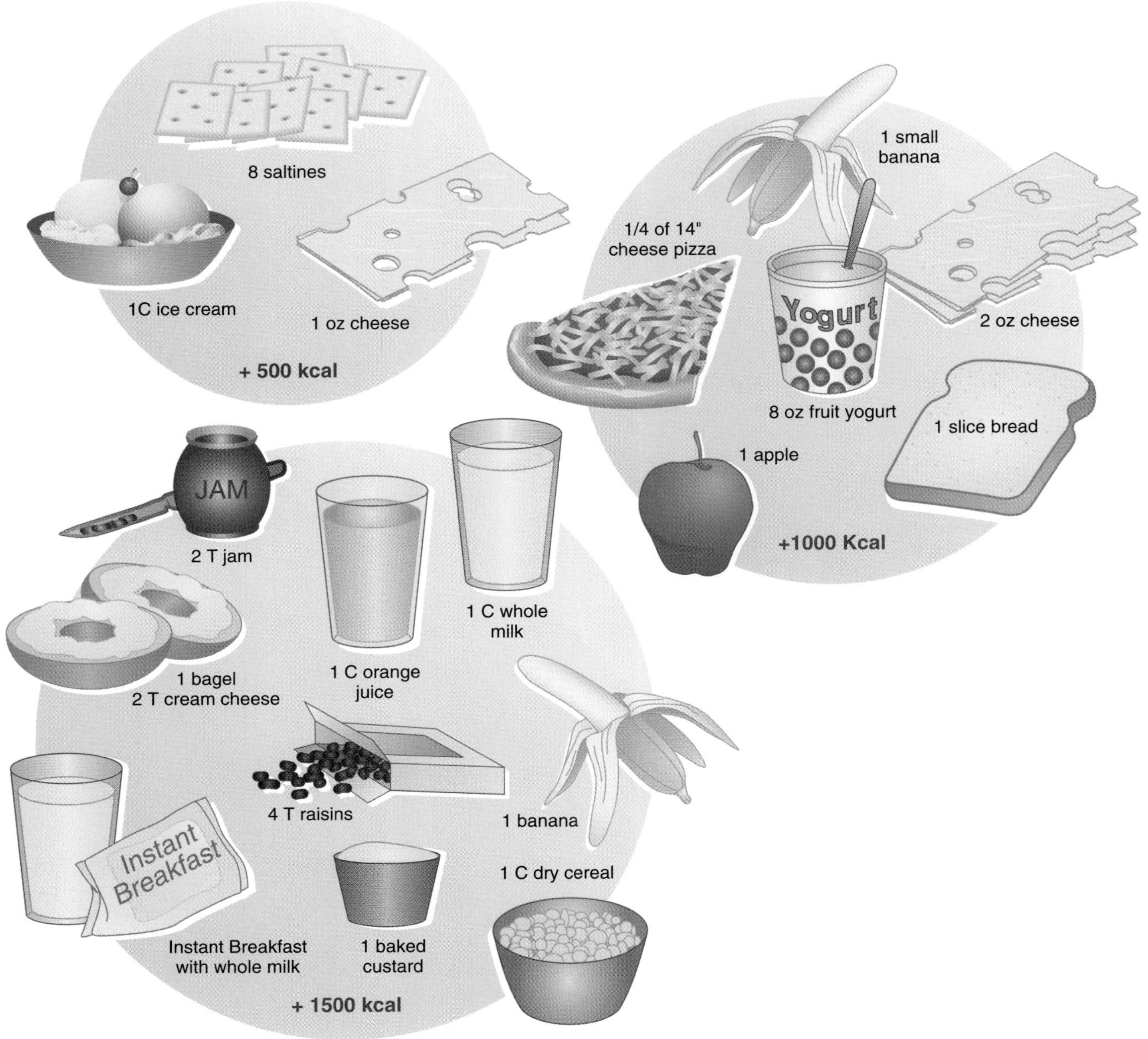
8 saltines
1C ice cream
1 oz cheese
+ 500 kcal
1 small banana
1/4 of 14" cheese pizza
Yogurt
2 oz cheese
8 oz fruit yogurt
1 slice bread
1 apple
+1000 Kcal
JAM
2 T jam
1 C whole milk
1 bagel
2 T cream cheese
1 C orange juice
4 T raisins
1 banana
Instant Breakfast
1 C dry cereal
Instant Breakfast with whole milk
1 baked custard
+ 1500 kcal

FIGURE 23–8 Each circle illustrates the total amount of food that can be added to the diet to increase the intake by either 500 kcal, 1000 kcal, or 1500 kcal.

High-Energy Diets for Weight Gain

A careful dietary history prior to planning a dietary program may reveal inadequacies in dietary habits and nutritional intakes. Meals at scheduled hours instead of hastily planned, quickly eaten meals are advised. Because nervous tension often contributes to underweight in some individuals, mealtimes should be relaxed.

In addition to the kilocalories needed to meet total energy requirements, an allowance of 500 to 1000 extra kilocalories per day should be planned. Daily energy requirements can be calculated on the basis of the individual's present weight. If 2400 kcals are normally needed to maintain present weight, 2900 to 3400 kcal would be required to achieve weight gain. The intake should be increased gradually to these levels to avoid gastric discomfort and periods of discouragement and more seriously, electrolyte imbalances and heart dysfunction. A 500-kcal step-up program is outlined in Table 23–7 and Figure 23–8.

The energy distribution of the diet should be about 30% of the kilocalories from fat; the majority unsaturated from mono- or polyunsaturated sources, with at least 12% to 15% of the kilocalories from protein. A basic vitamin and mineral supplement may be necessary depending on nutritional status revealed by the initial assessment.

CASE STUDY

Weight Management

Maria L. is a 45-year-old white woman who has tried numerous weight loss programs. She has followed very strict diets and has never exercised in previous weight loss attempts. She takes several cardiac medications, none of which she can remember. Her blood pressure is 160/90 and she is 5 ft 4 in. and weighs 195 lb. Her lowest body weight has been 130 lb at age 30, maintained for 2 years. Maria mentioned that she tried numerous diets while a teenager, when she weighed 170 lb for 3 years. What guidelines would you offer to Maria at this time?

1. How would you address the concern about medications?
2. What types of exercise would you be likely to discuss?
3. Which nutrients would you discuss with Maria, for example, total fat, saturated fat, sodium, potassium, calcium?
4. How would you bring up exercise and what would you recommend for Maria?
5. What would be the goals of her treatment?

The underweight person frequently must be encouraged to eat, even when not hungry. The secret is to individualize the program with readily available foods that the individual really enjoys and with a plan for regular eating times throughout the day. In addition to larger meals, snacks are usually necessary to adequately increase the energy intake. Often a liquid supplement taken with meals or between meals is effective because it is easy to prepare and consume. This is important when it is necessary to overcome a lack of interest in food and eating.

CITED REFERENCES

Abenhaim L, et al. Appetite-suppressant drugs and the risk of primary pulmonary hypertension. N Engl J Med 335:609, 1996.

Abernathy R, Black D. Is adipose tissue oversold as a health risk? J Am Diet Assoc 94:641, 1994.

American Dietetic Association. Position of the American Dietetic Association: Very-low-calorie weight loss diets. J Am Diet Assoc 90:722, 1990.

American Dietetic Association. Position of the American Dietetic Association: Weight management. J Am Diet Assoc 97:71, 1997.

Andersen RE, et al. Relation of weight loss to changes in serum lipids and lipoproteins in obese women. Am J Clin Nutr 62:350, 1995.

Anderson RA, Kozlovsky AS. Chromium intake, absorption, and excretion of subjects consuming self-selected diets. Am J Clin Nutr 41:1177, 1985.

Anderson RA, et al. Exercise effects on chromium excretion of trained and untrained men consuming a constant diet. J Appl Physiol 64:249, 1988.

Aronne L. Modern medical management of obesity: The role of pharmaceutical management. J Am Diet Assoc 98:23, 1998.

Astrup A, et al. The effect and safety of an ephedrine/caffeine compound compared with ephedrine, caffeine and placebo in obese subjects on an energy restricted diet. A double blind trial. Int J Obes 16:269, 1992.

Barlow SE, Dietz WH. Obesity evaluation and treatment: Expert committee recommendations. Pediatrics 102:3, 1998.

Benotti PN, Forse A. The role of gastric surgery in the multidisciplinary management of severe obesity. Am J Surg 169:361, 1995.

Berg F. Sudden death syndrome continues to chill treatment centers. Healthy Weight J 8(3):51, 1994.

Bjorntorp P. Physiological and clinical aspects of exercise in obese persons. Exerc Sport Sci Rev 11:159, 1983.

Blackburn GL. Weight management. Presentation at the American Dietetic Association Annual Meeting, 1988, San Francisco.

Blair SN. Evidence for success of exercise in weight loss and control. Ann Intern Med 119(7 pt 2):702, 1993.

Blundell JE, et al. Mechanisms of appetite control and their abnormalities in obese patients. Horm Res 39(suppl 3):72, 1993.

Bouchard C. Current understanding of the etiology of obesity: Genetic and nongenetic factors. Am J Clin Nutr 53:1561S, 1991.

Bray GA. Obesity: A disease of nutrient or energy balance? Nutr Rev 45:33, 1987.

Bray GA. Obesity. In: Brown ML (ed.). Present Knowledge in Nutrition, 6th ed. Washington, DC: International Life Sciences Institute, Nutrition Foundation, 1990.

Bray GA, Gray DS. Obesity, part I: Pathogenesis. West J Med 149:429, 1988a.

Bray GA, Gray DS. Obesity, part II: Treatment. West J Med 149:555, 1988b.

Brehm BA, Keller BA. Diet and exercise factors that influence weight and fat loss. Idea Today October:33, 1990.

Breum L, et al. Comparison of an ephedrine/caffeine combination and dexfenfluramine in the treatment of obesity. A double-blind multicentre trial in general practice. Int J Obesity Rel Metab Dis 18:99, 1994.

Brolin RE, et al. Weight loss and dietary intake after vertical banded gastroplasty and Roux-en-Y bypass. Ann Surg 220:782, 1994.

Brownell K, Wadden T. Matching weight control programs to individuals: How to find the best fit. Weight Control Dig 1(5):65, 1991.

Buckmaster L, Brownell KD. Behavior modification: The state of the art. In: Frankle RT, Yang M-U (eds.). Obesity and Weight Control. Rockville, MD: Aspen Publishers, 1988.

Callaway CW. Biologic adaptations to starvation and semistarvation. In: Frankle RT, Yang M-U (eds.). Obesity and Weight Control. Rockvile, MD: Aspen Publishers, 1988.

Campbell WW, et al. Chromium picolinate supplementation and resistive training by older men: Effects on iron-status and hematologic indexes. Am J Clin Nutr 66:944, 1997.

Canty D, Chan M. Effects of consumption of caloric and noncaloric sweet drinks on indices of hunger and food consumption in normal adults. Am J Clin Nutr 53:1159, 1991.

Carney RM, Goldberg AP. Weight gain after cessation of cigarette smoking: A possible role of adipose-tissue lipoprotein lipase. N Engl J Med 310:614, 1984.

Chagnon YC, et al. The human obesity gene map. The 1997 update. Obes Res 6:76, 1998.

Choban PS, et al. Obesity treatment: The role of surgery. Medical Update for Psychiatrists 1:21, 1996.

Clancy SP, et al. Effects of chromium picolinate supplementation on body composition, strength and urinary chromium loss in football players. Int J Sports Nutr 4:142, 1994.

Clement K, et al. Genetic variation in the β_3-adrenergic receptor and an increased capacity to gain weight in patients with morbid obesity. N Engl J Med 333:352, 1995.

Colditz GA. The Nurses' Health Study: Findings during 10 years of follow-up of a cohort of U.S. women. Curr Probl Obstet Gynecol Fertil 13:131, 1990.

Connolly H, et al. Valvular heart disease associated with fenfluramine-phentermine. N Engl J Med 337:581, 1997.

Consensus Development Conference Panel. Gastrointestinal surgery for severe obesity: Consensus development conference statement. Ann Intern Med 115:956, 1991.

Considine RV, et al. Serum immunoreactive-leptin concentrations in normal-weight and obese humans. N Engl J Med 334:292, 1996.

Dalton S. The dietitians' philosophy and practice in multidisciplinary weight management. J Am Diet Assoc 98:49, 1998.

Daly PA, et al. Ephedrine, caffeine and aspirin: Safety and efficacy for treatment of human obesity. Int J Obes Relat Metab Disord 17(suppl 1):S73, 1993.

Datillo A. Dietary fat and its relationship to body weight? Nutr Today 27(1):13, 1992.

de Jonge L, Bray GA. The thermic effect of food and obesity: A critical review. Obes Res 5:622, 1997.

Dietz WH. Childhood weight affects adult morbidity and mortality. J Nutr 128(25):411, 1998.

Drewnowski A, et al. Taste responses and preferences for sweet high-fat foods: Evidence for opioid involvement. Phys Behav 51:371, 1992.

Egbert A. The dwindles: Failure to thrive in older patients. Nutr Rev 54(1):S25, 1996.

Egger G. The case for using waist to hip ratio measurements in routine medical checks. Med J Aust 156:280, 1992.

Enzi G. The socioeconomic consequences of obesity. The effect of obesity on the individual. Pharm Econ 5(suppl 1):54, 1994.

Feldman W, et al. Culture vs. biology: Children's attitudes toward thinness and fatness. Pediatrics 81:190, 1988.

Flegal KM, et al. The influence of smoking cessation on the prevalence of overweight in the United States. N Engl J Med 333:1165, 1995.

Flier JS, Maratos-Flier E. Obesity and the hypothalamus: Novel peptides for new pathways. Cell 92:437, 1998.

Forbes GB. Lean body mass-body fat interrelationships in humans. Nutr Rev 45:225, 1987.

Foreyt JP, Poston WSC II. Diet, genetics, and obesity. Food Tech 51:70, 1997.

Forse A, et al. Morbid obesity: Weighing the treatment options-surgical options. Nutr Today 24(5):10, 1989.

Foster GD, et al. What is a reasonable weight loss? Patients' expectations and evaluations of obesity treatment outcomes. J Consult Clin Psychol 65:79, 1997.

Franz M. Managing obesity in patients with comorbidities. J Am Diet Assoc 98:39, 1998.

Freedman DS, et al. Relation of body fat patterning to lipid and lipoprotein concentrations in children and adolescents: The Bogalusa Heart Study. Am J Clin Nutr 50:930, 1989.

Gladwell M. The Pima paradox. The New Yorker, Feb 2:44, 1998.

Goldstein DJ. Beneficial health effects of modest weight loss. Int J Obes 16:397, 1992.

Greenway FL. Clinical studies with phenylpropanoloamine: A meta-analysis. Am J Clin Nutr 55:203S, 1992.

Gross WC, Daynard MD (eds.). Commercial weight loss products and programs. What consumers stand to gain and lose. Report of the Presiding Panel, Federal Trade Commission, Washington, DC, 1997.

Guerciolini R. Mode of action of orlistat. Int J Obes 21(suppl 3):S12, 1997.

Hellerstein MK, et al. Effects of cigarette smoking and its cessation on lipid metabolism and energy expenditure in heavy smokers. J Clin Invest 93:265, 1994.

Hill JO, et al. Effects of exercise and food restriction on body composition and metabolic rate in obese women. Am J Clin Nutr 46:622, 1987.

Hirsch J. Role and benefits of carbohydrate in the diet: Key issues for future dietary guidelines. Am J Clin Nutr 61:996S, 1995.

Hoebel BG, et al. Microdialysis studies of brain norepinephrine, serotonin, and dopamine release during ingestive behavior. Theoretical and clinical implications. Ann N Y Acad Sci 575:171, 1989.

Holli BB. Using behavior modification in nutrition counseling. J Am Diet Assoc 88:1530, 1988.

Horton T, Geissler C. Effect of habitual exercise on daily energy expenditure and metabolic rate during standardized activity. Am J Clin Nutr 59:13, 1994.

Isner JM, et al. Sudden, unexpected death in avid dieters using the liquid-protein-modified-fast diet. Circulation 60:1401, 1979.

James WPT, et al. A one-year trial to assess the value of orlistat in the management of obesity. Int J Obes 21(suppl 3):S24, 1997.

Jeffery R, et al. Weight cycling and cardiovascular risk factors in obese men and women. Am J Clin Nutr 55:641, 1992.

Jick H, et al. A population-based study of appetite-suppressant drugs and the risk of cardiac valve regurgitation. N Engl J Med 339:719, 1998.

Katzeff HL, et al. Metabolic studies in human obesity during overnutrition and undernutrition: Thermogenic and hormonal responses to norepinephrine. Metabolism 35:166, 1986.

Kennedy E, et al. The 1995 Dietary Guidelines for Americans: An overview. J Am Diet Assoc 96:234, 1996.

Keys A. The Biology of Human Starvation. Minneapolis: University of Minnesota Press, 1950.

Khan MA, et al. The prevalence of cardiac valvular insufficiency assessed by transthoracic echocardiography in obese patients treated with appetite-suppressant drugs. N Engl J Med 339:713, 1998.

Klesges R, et al. Effects of television on metabolic rate: Potential implications for childhood obesity. Pediatrics 91:281, 1993.

Kuczmarski R, et al. Increasing prevalence of overweight among U.S. adults. JAMA 272:205, 1994.

Lane MA, et al. Beyond the rodent model: Calorie restriction in rhesus monkeys. Age & Aging 20:45, 1997.

Langseth L (ed.). Body weight: Editorial condemns new weight guidelines. Nutr Res Newsletter X(6):63, 1991.

Launer L, et al. Body mass index, weight change, and risk of mobility disability in middle-aged and older women. JAMA 271:1093, 1994.

Lean MEJ. Sibutramine—a review of clinical efficacy. Int J Obes 21(suppl 1):S30, 1997.

Lee I, et al. Body weight and mortality: A 27-year follow-up of middle-aged men. JAMA 270:2823, 1993.

Leibel RL, et al. Changes in energy expenditure resulting from altered body weight. N Engl J Med 332:621, 1995.

Lew EA, Garfinkle L. Variations in mortality by weight among 750,000 men and women. J Chronic Dis 32:563, 1979.

Ley CJ, et al. Sex- and menopause-associated changes in body-fat distribution. Am J Clin Nutr 55:950, 1992.

Lissau I, Sorensen T. Parental neglect during childhood and increased risk of obesity in young adulthood. Lancet 343:324, 1994.

Lissner L, et al. Variability of body weight and health outcomes in the Framingham population. N Engl J Med 324:1839, 1991.

Lukaski HC, et al. Chromium supplementation and resistance training: Effects on body composition, strength, and trace element status of men. Am J Clin Nutr 63:954, 1996.

Mahan LK. Family-focused behavioral approach to weight control in children. Pediatr Clin North Am 34:983, 1987.

Manson JE, et al. Body weight and mortality among women. N Engl J Med 333:677, 1995.

Masoro E. Energy intake and the aging process: Clues from the laboratory. Nutr and the MD 20:1, 1994.

Matsuzawa Y, et al. Pathophysiology and pathogenesis of visceral fat obesity. Diabetes Res Clin Prac 24(suppl):S111, 1994.

Miller W, et al. Dietary fat, sugar and fiber predict body fat content. J Am Diet Assoc 94:612, 1994.

Miller W. Exercise: Americans don't think it's worth it! Obesity and Health 8(2):29, 1994.

Morley JE, et al. Effects of peripheral hormones on memory and ingestive behaviors. Psychoneuroendocrinology 17:391, 1992.

National Institutes of Health. Methods for voluntary weight loss and control. Technology Assessment Conference. Bethesda, MD: 1992.

National Institutes of Health, National Task Force on Prevention and Treatment of Obesity. Very low calorie diets. JAMA 270:967, 1993.

National Institutes of Health, National Heart, Lung, and Blood Institute. Clinical guidelines on the identification, evaluation, and treatment of overweight and obesity in adults—the evidence report. Obes Res 6(suppl 2):51S, 1998.

Pate RR, et al. Physical activity and public health. A recommendation from the Centers for Disease Control and Prevention and the American College of Sports Medicine. JAMA 273:402, 1995.

Pavlou KN, et al. Exercise as an adjunct to weight loss and maintenance in moderately obese subjects. Am J Clin Nutr 49:1115, 1989.

Pelleymounter MA, et al. Effects of the obese gene product on body weight regulation in *ob/ob* mice. Science 269:540, 1995.

Pfizer Food Science Group. Americans are getting the message on fat. Food Forum 4(4):2, 1994.

Pi-Sunyer FX. Exercise in treatment of obesity. In: Frankle RT, Yang M-U (eds.). Obesity and Weight Control. Rockville, MD: Aspen Publishers, 1988.

Pi-Sunyer FX. Medical hazards of obesity. Ann Intern Med 119:655, 1993a.

Pi-Sunyer FX. Short-term medical benefits and adverse effects of weight loss. Ann Intern Med 119:722, 1993b.

Pi-Sunyer FX, et al. Obesity. In: Shils ME, et al. (eds.). Modern Nutrition in Health and Disease. Philadelphia: Lea & Febiger, 1994, p. 994.

Ravussin E, Swinburn BA. Effect of caloric restriction and weight loss on energy expenditure. In: Wadden TA, Van Itallie TB (eds.). Treatment of the Seriously Obese Patient. New York: Guilford Press, 1992.

Reaven GM. Role of insulin resistance in human disease. Diabetes 37:1595, 1988.

Richard D. Involvement of corticotropin-releasing factor in the control of food intake and energy expenditure. Ann N Y Acad Sci 575:155, 1989.

Rippe J, et al. Obesity as a chronic disease. Modern medical and lifestyle management. J Am Diet Assoc 98:9, 1998.

Roberts S, et al. Control of food intake in older men. JAMA 272:1601, 1994.

Rolland-Cachera M-F, Bellisle F. Letter to the editor. Lancet 335:918, 1990.

Rolland-Cachera M-F, et al. Adiposity rebound in children: A simple indicator for predicting obesity. Am J Clin Nutr 39:129, 1984.

Rolls BJ, Drewnowski A. Diet and nutrition. Encyclopedia of Gerontology 1:429, 1996.

Romon M, et al. Circadian variation of diet-induced thermogenesis. Am J Clin Nutr 57:476, 1993.

Rosencrans K. Does the body defend weight at a set-point? Healthy Weight J 8(3):47, 1994.

Schlundt D, et al. Randomized evaluation of a low fat ad libitum carbohydrate diet for weight reduction. Int J Obes Relat Metab Disord 17:623, 1993.

Shape Up America! and the American Obesity Association. Guidance for treatment of adult obesity, 2nd ed. Bethesda, MD: Authors, 1998.

Sjostrom L, et al. Swedish obese subjects (SOS). Recruitment for an intervention study and a selected description of the obese state. Int J Obes 16:465, 1992.

Stallone D. The influence of obesity and its treatment on the immune system. Nutr Rev 52(2 part 1):37, 1994.

Stunkard AJ. Current views on obesity. Am J Med 100:230, 1996.

Sugerman HJ, et al. Randomized prospective trial of gastric bypass versus vertical banded gastroplasty for morbid obesity and their effects on sweets versus non-sweets eaters. Ann Surg 205:613, 1987.

Sugerman HJ, et al. Weight loss with vertical banded gastroplasty and Roux-Y gastric bypass of morbid obesity with selective versus random assignment. Am J Surg 157:93, 1989.

Suter P, et al. The effect of ethanol on fat storage in healthy subject. N Engl J Med 326:983, 1992.

Tyler VE. The honest herbal. New York: Pharmaceutical Products Press, 1993.

U.S. Department Health and Human Services. The health benefits of smoking cessation: A report of the Surgeon General, 1990. Washington, DC: US Government Printing Office, 1990.

U.S. Department Health and Human Services. Healthy People 2000: National health promotion and disease prevention objectives. Publication

PHS 91-50212. Washington, DC: US Government Printing Office, 1991.

Van Dale D, et al. Does exercise give an additional effect in weight reduction regimens? Int J Obes 11:367, 1987.

Van der Kooy K, et al. Effect of a weight cycle on visceral fat accumulation. Am J Clin Nutr 58:853, 1993.

Van Horn L, et al. The dietitian's role in developing and implementing the first federal obesity guidelines. J Am Diet Assoc 98:1115, 1998.

Van Itallie TB, Yang M. Cardiac dysfunction in obese dieters: A potentially lethal complication of rapid, massive weight loss. Am J Clin Nutr 39:695, 1984.

Vasselli JR, Maggio CA. Mechanisms of appetite and body-weight regulation. In: Frankle RT, Yang M (eds.). Obesity and Weight Control. Rockville, MD: Aspen Publishers, 1988.

Wadden T. Treatment of obesity by moderate and severe caloric restriction: Results of clinical research trial. Ann Intern Med 119:688, 1993.

Wadden T, Sarwer DB. Behavioral treatment of obesity: New approaches to an old disorder. In: Goldstein D (ed.). The Management of Eating Disorders. Totowa, NJ: Humana Press, 1998.

Weissman NJ, et al. An assessment of heart valve abnormalities in obese patients taking dexfenfluramine, sustained-release dexfenfluramine, or placebo. N Engl J Med 339:725, 1998.

Whitaker RC, et al. Predicting obesity in young adulthood from childhood and parental obesity. N Engl J Med 337:869, 1997.

Wing R. Weight cycling in humans: A review of the literature. Ann Behav Med 14:113, 1992.

Wing RR, Greeno GC. Behavioural and psychosocial aspects of obesity and its treatment. Bailliere's Clin Endocrinol Metab 8:689, 1994.

Wing RR, et al. Long-term effects of modest weight loss in type II diabetic patients. Arch Intern Med 147:1749, 1987.

Wolf AM, Colditz GA. Current estimates of the economic cost of obesity in the United States. Obes Res 6:97, 1998.

ADDITIONAL REFERENCES

Abdallah L. Cephalic phase responses to sweet taste. Am J Clin Nutr 65:737, 1997.

AbuSabha R, Achterberg C. Review of self-efficacy and locus of control for nutrition and health-related behavior. J Am Diet Assoc 97:1122, 1997.

American Dietetic Association. Position of the ADA: Fat replacements. J Am Diet Assoc 91:1285, 1991.

Behnke AR, Wilmore JH. Evaluation and Regulation of Body Build and Composition. Englewood Cliffs, NJ: Prentice-Hall, 1974.

Blackburn G, et al. The effect of aspartame as part of a multidisciplinary weight-control program on short- and long-term control of body weight. Am J Clin Nutr 65:409, 1997.

Bouchard C, et al. The response to long-term overfeeding in identical twins. N Engl J Med 322:1477, 1990.

Dulloo A, et al. Poststarvation hyperphagia and body fat overshooting in humans: A role for feedback signals from lean and fat tissues. Am J Clin Nutr 65:717, 1997.

Galuska D, et al. Trends in overweight among US adults from 1987 to 1993: A multistate telephone survey. Am J Public Health 86:1729, 1996.

Kue Young T, Gelskey D. Is noncentral obesity metabolically benign? JAMA 274:1939, 1995.

Loube D, et al. Continuous positive airway pressure treatment results in weight loss in obese and overweight patients and obstructive sleep apnea. J Am Diet Assoc 97:896, 1997.

Naslund E, et al. Reduced food intake after jejunoileal bypass: A possible association with prolonged gastric emptying and altered gut hormone patterns. Am J Clin Nutr 66:26, 1997.

National Institutes of Health. First federal obesity clinical guidelines released. Press release. June 17, 1998. Internet site: http://www.nhlbi.nih.gov/nhlbi/news/obere14f.htm.

National Task Force on the Prevention and Treatment of Obesity. Long term pharmacotherapy in the management of obesity (Review). JAMA 276:1907, 1996.

Pekkarinen T, Mustajoki P. Comparison of behavior therapy with and without very-low-energy diet in the treatment of morbid obesity. Arch Intern Med 157:1581, 1997.

Ronnemaa T, et al. Relation between plasma leptin levels and measures of body fat in identical twins discordant for obesity. Ann Intern Med 126:26, 1997.

Schwartz M, Seeley R. The new biology of weight reduction. J Am Diet Assoc 97:54, 1997.

St Jeor S. New trends in weight management. J Am Diet Assoc 97:1096, 1997.

St Jeor S, et al. A classification system to evaluate weight maintainers, gainers and losers. J Am Diet Assoc 97:481, 1997.

U.S. Department of Health and Human Services. Physical activity and health: A report of the Surgeon General. Atlanta, GA: US Department of Health and Human Services, Centers for Disease Control and Prevention, National Centers for Chronic Disease Prevention and Health Promotion, 1996.

Van Itallie T, Simopoulos A. Summary of the National Obesity and Weight Control Symposium. Nutr Today 28(4):33, 1993.

CHAPTER 24

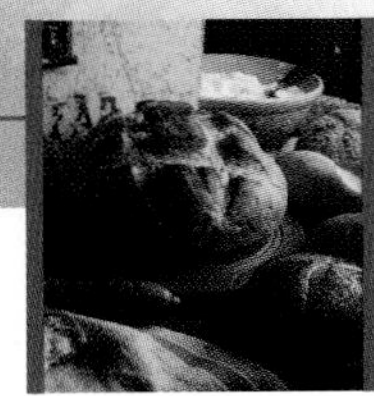

Nutrition in Eating Disorders

JANET SCHEBENDACH, MA, RD AND
PAMELA REICHERT-ANDERSON, MA, RD

Chapter Outline

- Diagnostic Criteria
- Epidemiology
- Pathophysiologic Consequences of Eating Disorders
- Psychological Management
- Nutritional Assessment
- Nutrition Management
- Nutrition Education
- Prognosis

Key Terms

AMENORRHEA—absence of three consecutive menstrual periods when otherwise expected to occur

ANOREXIA NERVOSA (AN)—a disease characterized by: (1) refusal to maintain a minimally normal body weight; (2) intense fear of gaining weight; (3) body image distortion; and (4) amenorrhea in postmenarcheal females; may be one of two subtypes: restricting or binge eating/purging

BINGE—an episode of eating marked by three particular features: (1) the amount of food eaten is larger than most individuals would eat under similar circumstances; (2) the excessive eating occurs in a discrete period of time, usually less than 2 hours; and (3) the eating is accompanied by a subjective sense of loss of control

BINGE EATING DISORDER (BED)—a disorder characterized by the occurrence of binge eating episodes at least twice a week for a 6-month period

BODY IMAGE DISTORTION—a significant disturbance in the perception of body shape or size

BULIMIA NERVOSA (BN)—an illness characterized by repeated episodes of binge eating followed by inappropriate compensatory methods such as purging including self-induced vomiting or misuse of laxatives, diuretics, or enemas, or nonpurging including fasting or engaging in excessive exercise

EDNOS (EATING DISORDER NOT OTHERWISE SPECIFIED)—a diagnostic category for eating disorders that fail to meet full criteria for either anorexia nervosa or bulimia nervosa

HYPERCAROTENEMIA—an elevation of serum carotene, frequently encountered in patients with eating disorders; most likely an acquired defect in carotene metabolism, secondary to semistarvation

MARASMUS—a starvation state characterized by maintenance of the circulatory pool of visceral proteins at the expense of somatic protein stores

PURGING—methods intended to reverse the effects of binge eating; self-induced vomiting is the most common purging method, but additional methods include laxative, enema, and diuretic abuse

Anorexia nervosa and bulimia nervosa are eating disorders primarily affecting adolescents and young adult women. Weight preoccupation is a primary symptom in both disorders.

Anorexia nervosa (AN) is a condition characterized by voluntary self-starvation and emaciation. Weight loss is viewed as a sign of extraordinary achievement and self-discipline, whereas weight gain is perceived as an unacceptable loss of self-control (American Psychiatric Association [APA], 1994). Although the incidence rates over the past 50 years in older women and men have been relatively constant, over the past decade the rates have increased among 10- to 19-year-old girls (Lucas et al., 1991). Prevalence studies among women in late adolescence and early adulthood have reported rates of 0.5% to 1.0% for presentations that meet full criteria and a higher prevalence for the subthreshold diagnosis of an eating disorder not otherwise specified (APA, 1994). **Bulimia nervosa (BN)** is a disorder characterized by recurrent episodes of binge eating followed by one or more inappropriate compensatory behaviors to prevent weight gain. These behaviors include self-induced vomiting, laxative abuse, diuretic abuse, excessive fasting, or compulsive exercise. The prevalence of BN among adolescent and young adult women is 1% to 3%, and the rate of occurrence in men is approximately one tenth that seen in women (APA, 1994) (see Eating Disorders Awareness and Prevention at http://members.aol.com/edapinc/or The Anorexia/Bulimia Association at www.aabainc.org).

DIAGNOSTIC CRITERIA

At the end of the 17th century, Morton described a condition that would later be defined as AN. One hundred seventy years later Gull in England and Laseque in France gave the condition its current name (Russell, 1985). Criteria for establishment of a diagnosis of AN were first published in 1972 by Feighner. In 1980, the American Psychiatric Association (APA, 1980) published criteria for diagnosis of AN, but it was not until 1987 that the association recognized AN and BN as two separate and distinct clinical entities.

The most current diagnostic criteria for AN and BN were published by the APA in 1994 and are listed in Table 24–1. In addition to the diagnoses of AN and BN, the table also includes the criteria for the diagnosis of an *eating disorder not otherwise specified (EDNOS)* and binge eating disorder.

Anorexia Nervosa

Essential to the diagnosis of AN is a refusal to maintain a minimally normal body weight. Although the Feighner and DSM-III criteria required a weight loss of at least 25% of original body weight, both the revised DSM-III and DSM-IV specify a body weight less than 85% of that expected. The weight deficit is often computed using Metropolitan Life Insurance tables (see Appendix 19), but the APA encourages clinicians to consider the patient's body build and weight history as well. If AN develops during childhood or early adolescence, there may be failure to make expected weight gains (while growing in height) instead of weight loss. Stunting may also occur in prepubertal children afflicted with this disorder, and it is essential that growth records be obtained. If stunting has occurred, the weight deficit should be calculated using the patient's height percentile before the illness.

TABLE 24–1 AMERICAN PSYCHIATRIC ASSOCIATION DIAGNOSTIC CRITERIA

Anorexia Nervosa (AN)

A. Refusal to maintain body weight at or above a minimally normal weight for age and height (e.g., weight loss leading to maintenance of body weight less than 85% of that expected; or failure to make expected weight gain during period of growth, leading to body weight less than 85% of that expected.
B. Intense fear of gaining weight or becoming fat, even though underweight.
C. Disturbance in the way in which one's body weight or shape is experienced, undue influence of body weight or shape on self-evaluation; or denial of the seriousness of the current low body weight.
D. In postmenarcheal females, amenorrhea, i.e., the absence of at least three consecutive menstrual cycles.
   1. *Restricting type:* During the current episode of AN, the person has not regularly engaged in binge eating or purging behavior.
   2. *Binge eating/purging type:* During the current episode of AN, the person has regularly engaged in binge eating and purging behavior.

Bulimia Nervosa (BN)

A. Recurrent episodes of binge eating. An episode of binge eating is characterized by both of the following:
   1. Eating, in a discrete period of time (e.g., within any 2-hour period), an amount of food that is definitely larger than most people would eat during a similar period of time and under similar circumstances.
   2. A sense of lack of control over eating during the episode (e.g., a feeling that one cannot stop eating or control what or how much one is eating).
B. Recurrent inappropriate compensatory behavior in order to prevent weight gain, such as self-induced vomiting, misuse of laxatives, diuretics, enemas, or other medications, fasting, or excessive exercise.
C. The binge eating and inappropriate compensatory behaviors both occur, on average, at least twice a week for 3 months.
D. Self-evaluation is unduly influenced by body shape and weight.
E. The disturbance does not occur exclusively during episodes of AN.
   1. *Purging type:* During the current episode of BN, the person has regularly engaged in self-induced vomiting or the misuse of laxatives, diuretics, or enemas.
   2. *Nonpurging type:* During the current episode of BN, the person has used other inappropriate compensatory behaviors, such as fasting or excessive exercise, but has not regularly engaged in self-induced vomiting or the misuse of laxatives, diuretics, or enemas.

Eating Disorder Not Otherwise Specified (EDNOS)

This category is for disorders of eating that do not meet criteria for any specific eating disorder. For example:
   1. For females, all of the criteria for AN are met except that the individual has regular menses.
   2. All of the criteria for AN are met except that, despite significant weight loss, the individual's current weight is in the normal range.
   3. All of the criteria for BN are met except that the binge eating and inappropriate compensatory mechanisms occur at a frequency of less than twice a week or for a duration of less than 3 months.
   4. The regular use of inappropriate compensatory behavior by an individual of normal body weight after eating small amounts of food.
   5. Repeatedly chewing and spitting out, but not swallowing, large amounts of food.

Binge Eating Disorder (BED)

Recurrent episodes of binge eating in the absence of the regular use of inappropriate compensatory behaviors characteristic of BN.

(From American Psychiatric Association. Diagnostic and Statistical Manual of Mental Disorders, 4th ed. Washington, DC: Author, 1994.)
This manual is referred to in the text as DSM-IV. The 1980 edition is DSM-III.

Patients with AN have **body image distortion,** causing them to feel fat despite their often cachectic state. Some individuals feel overweight all over, whereas others are overly concerned about the fatness of a specific body part, such as the abdomen, buttocks, or thighs.

The DSM-IV criterion of **amenorrhea** is defined as the absence of at least three consecutive menstrual cycles in postmenarcheal women, but this criterion may not be useful for diagnosis in younger patients. If AN develops before early puberty, sexual maturation may be arrested and menarche may be delayed. Furthermore, even healthy adolescent girls have periods of amenorrhea during the first 1 to 2 years after menarche (Fisher et al.,1995).

Patients with AN manifest symptoms of depression that may be due, in part, to the psychological stress of starvation. In a study of physical and psychological effects of semistarvation conducted in the 1940s, healthy male volunteers developed symptoms of psychological deterioration and depression during a 6-month period of restricted caloric intake (50% of maintenance energy requirements). Patients with AN exhibit obsessive-compulsive features, particularly with regard to food. Participants in the Minnesota Study also developed obsessional behaviors during the semistarvation period, and many of these did not reverse immediately on refeeding (Keys et al., 1950). This suggests that food-related obsessive-compulsive behaviors may be caused or exacerbated by malnutrition. The APA recommends that in AN: (1) depressive symptoms should be reassessed after partial or complete weight restoration and (2) patients exhibiting non-food-related obsessive-compulsive behaviors should be evaluated for a comorbid diagnosis of obsessive-compulsive disorder (APA, 1994).

Bulimia Nervosa

Essential features of BN are the existence of binge eating and one or more inappropriate compensatory behaviors intended to prevent weight gain. Unlike AN patients with binge eating/purging subtype, patients with BN are typically within the normal weight range, although some may be slightly under- or overweight. Like their AN counterparts, these individuals place considerable importance on body shape and size, and they are often frustrated by their inability to attain an underweight state.

It is commonly thought that vomiting is the predominant feature of BN; however, it is the binge eating behavior that is central to the diagnosis. A **binge** is an unusually large amount of food eaten in a discrete period of time (usually less than 2 hours). There is a sense of lack of control over the eating episode. A binge may start in one setting and continue in another. Although continuous ingestion of small amounts of food throughout the day may result in excessive caloric intake, this would not constitute a binge.

The most commonly used compensatory behavior is self-induced vomiting, seen in 80% to 90% of individuals with BN. Patients stimulate the gag reflex with a finger or instrument (i.e., toothbrush, eating utensil), and some individuals can vomit at will. Syrup of ipecac is frequently used to induce vomiting. This dangerous practice can result in cardiomyopathies and sudden death. Approximately one third of patients will abuse laxatives and some will also abuse enemas (APA, 1994). Compulsive exercise is described as that which significantly interferes with life activities or occurs at inappropriate times or in inappropriate settings. Despite injury or other medical complications, these individuals will often continue to exercise compulsively.

An increased frequency of depressive symptoms and mood disorders is seen in patients with BN, and their onset may occur before the development of the eating disorder. Among patients with BN, increased rates have been reported for anxiety disorders, chemical dependency, bipolar disorder, and personality disorders (Yager et al., 1993). Mood and anxiety disorders may remit during successful treatment of BN.

Although patients with AN typically reject intervention, patients with BN are more distressed by their symptoms and seek relief from their disorder. One of the chief psychological characteristics is guilt over the cycle of binge eating and purging that is carried out in secret, even while their lives may seem ideal to those around them.

Eating Disorders Not Otherwise Specified (EDNOS)

Patients diagnosed with an **eating disorder not otherwise specified (EDNOS)** comprise approximately 50% of the population with eating disorders. These individuals have partial symptoms of either AN or BN. For example, this may be the patient who meets all criteria for AN except amenorrhea. Another example would be an individual of normal weight who does not binge but self-induces vomiting after an average-size meal. If left untreated patients with EDNOS may develop eating disorders that meet the full criteria for AN or BN.

Binge Eating Disorder

Binge eating disorder (BED) has been described and proposed as a new eating disorder. Research criteria for BED are listed in Table 24–1. Binge eating, similar to that seen in BN, is characteristic of BED; however, there are no inappropriate compensatory behaviors after the binge. Binge episodes must occur at least 2 days per week for a period of 6 months. Individuals with BED experience similar feelings of powerlessness over their eating as do BN patients. Significant emotional distress, characterized by feelings of disgust, guilt, and depression, occurs after the binge. The onset of BED generally occurs in late adolescence or the early twenties, with women 1.5 times more likely to develop this disorder than men. Community samples suggest that most patients with this disorder are overweight, with a 15% to 50% prevalence among participants in weight control programs.

EPIDEMIOLOGY

The etiology of AN is multifactorial with biologic, genetic, intrapersonal, familial, and sociocultural precipitants to the development and maintenance of the disorder.

Onset of AN, most common during adolescence, is often viewed as biopsychological developmental arrest. Pubertal changes in body habitus heighten concern about body shape and size. Patients are typically introverted, obsessional, and perfectionistic in nature. They are overachievers but feel ineffective. Low self-esteem is common. Family pathology is characterized by enmeshment, overprotectiveness, rigidity, and lack of conflict resolution. Development of the disorder may be viewed as an attempt to gain control and autonomy. Comorbid anxiety and depressive disorders are common in this population. There is an increased risk of AN among first-degree biologic relatives of individuals with the disorder and a higher concordance in monozygotic twins compared with dizygotic twins.

Several etiologic models have been proposed for the development of BN. These include addiction, family, sociocultural, cognitive-behavioral, and psychodynamic. The addiction model suggests food and behavioral addiction with treatment similar to that used in alcohol and substance abuse patients (i.e., 12-step programs). The family model focuses on the identification and treatment of family dysfunction. The sociocultural model attributes development of BN to cultural pressures for thinness. Because this body type is not naturally attained in all individuals, susceptible individuals resort to bulimic behaviors when conventional methods of dieting fail. The cognitive-behavioral model attributes the development of BN to irrational thoughts and beliefs concerning body weight, dieting, and self-esteem. Treatment is aimed at identification and behavioral treatment of dysfunctional beliefs. The psychodynamic model is one of the stongest etiologic models. Here BN represents the patient's attempt to control, avoid, or minimize the impact of distressful feelings, impulses, and anxieties. Comorbidity for mood disorders, anxiety disorders, personality disorders, and substance abuse is common in the BN population.

PATHOPHYSIOLOGIC CONSEQUENCES OF EATING DISORDERS

Although eating disorders are classified as psychiatric illnesses, they are associated with significant medical complications, morbidity, and mortality rates between 5% to 15%. Although the primary dysfunction is related to deficiencies in the sense of self, identity, and autonomy, the physical and psychological consequences of malnutrition dominate the clinical picture.

Numerous physiologic changes result from the weight control habits of patients with AN and BN (Table 24–2). Some are minor changes that occur secondarily to a reduced energy intake; some are pathologic alterations that may have long-term consequences; and a few represent potentially life-threatening conditions.

Clinical Characteristics and Medical Complications: Anorexia Nervosa

Patients with AN have a typical and distinctive appearance. Their cachectic and prepubescent body habitus often makes them look younger than their age. Common physical characteristics include lanugo, brittle listless hair, cyanosis of the extremities, and dry skin that may have a yellow cast due to **hypercarotenemia.** Bradycardia below 60 beats/min and hypotension below 70 mm Hg (systolic) are frequently present. Patients with AN will often ascribe their low heart rates and low blood pressures to their exercise regimen and proclaim physical fitness. However, cardiovascular testing has shown altered cardiovascular response to exercise in AN (Nudel et al., 1984). Patients are hypothermic and often wear more clothing than is environmentally appropriate (Fig. 24–1).

Cardiovascular complications have been associated with death in AN. Reduction in heart mass is associated with reduced blood pressure and pulse rate. Mitral valve prolapse may be related to hypovolemia or cardiomyopathy. Unlike chronically ill adults with AN, adolescents have relatively well-preserved cardiac output; however, death from congestive heart failure may occur in AN patients of any age (Fisher et al., 1995).

The gastrointestinal tract may be profoundly affected in AN. Complications secondary to starvation include delayed gastric emptying, decreased small bowel motility, and constipation. These complications may result in complaints of abdominal bloating and a prolonged sensation of abdominal fullness, which can last several hours after eating.

Major changes in the central nervous system occur in AN. Although controlled studies provide evidence of structural abnormalities in the brains of adults, less is known about the long-term effect of these structural changes in adolescents with AN (Fisher et al., 1995).

Bone marrow hypoplasia, found in 50% of AN patients, results in varying degrees of leukopenia, anemia, and rarely thrombocytopenia (Hardoff et al., 1991). The cause of this bone marrow dysfunction is unknown, but depletion of bone marrow fat has been documented. It may be that this depletion adversely affects the local environment for normal hematopoiesis (Lambert et al., 1997). The low

TABLE 24–2 MEDICAL COMPLICATIONS OF EATING DISORDERS

	AN		BN	
	RESTRICTING	BINGE-EATING PURGING	PURGING	NON-PURGING
Fluid and Electrolyte Imbalance				
Hypokalemia		✓	✓	
Hyponatremia		✓	✓	
Hypochloremic alkalosis		✓	✓	
Elevated BUN	✓	✓	✓	✓
Inability to concentrate urine	✓	✓		
Decreased glomerular filtration rate	✓	✓		
Ketonuria	✓	✓	✓	✓
Cardiovascular				
Bradycardia	✓	✓		
Orthostatic hypotension	✓	✓	✓	✓
Dysrhythmias	✓	✓	✓	✓
Electrocardiographic abnormalities				
Prolonged QT interval	✓	✓	✓	
T wave abnormalities	✓	✓	✓	
Conduction defects	✓	✓	✓	
Ipecac cardiomyopathy		✓	✓	
Mitral valve prolapse	✓	✓		
Congestive cardiac failure	✓	✓		
Pericardial effusion	✓	✓		
Gastrointestinal				
Parotid hypertrophy		✓	✓	
Perimolysis and increased incidence of dental caries		✓	✓	
Constipation	✓	✓	✓	✓
Bloody diarrhea		✓	✓	
Delayed gastric emptying	✓	✓	✓	✓
Intestinal atony	✓	✓	✓	✓
Esophagitis		✓	✓	
Mallory-Weiss tears		✓	✓	
Esophageal or gastric rupture		✓	✓	
Perforation/rupture of stomach		✓	✓	
Barrett esophagus		✓	✓	
Fatty infiltration and focal necrosis of liver	✓	✓		
Superior mesenteric artery syndrome	✓	✓		
Gallstones	✓	✓	✓	✓
Skeletal				
Osteopenia	✓	✓	?	?
Fractures	✓	✓	?	?
Dermatologic				
Acrocyanosis	✓	✓		
Yellow dry skin (hypercarotenemia)	✓	✓		
Brittle hair and nails	✓	✓		
Lanugo	✓	✓		
Russell sign (calluses over the knuckles)		✓	✓	
Pitting edema	✓	✓	✓	✓
Endocrine				
Growth retardation and short stature	✓	✓		
Delayed puberty	✓	✓		
Amenorrhea	✓	✓		
Low T3 syndrome	✓	✓		
Decreased capacity to concentrate urine 2° to	✓	✓		
↓ vassopressin secretion	✓	✓		
Hypercortisolism	✓	✓		
Hematologic				
Bone marrow supression				
Mild anemia	✓	✓		
Leukopenia	✓	✓		
Thrombocytopenia	✓	✓		
Low sedimentation rate	✓	✓		
Impaired cell-mediated immunity	✓	✓		
Neurologic				
Seizures	✓	✓	✓	✓
Myopathy	✓	✓	✓	
Peripheral neuropathy	✓	✓		
Cortical atrophy	✓	✓		

(From Fisher M et al. Eating disorders in adolescents: A background paper. J Adolesc Health 16:424, 1995, with permission.)

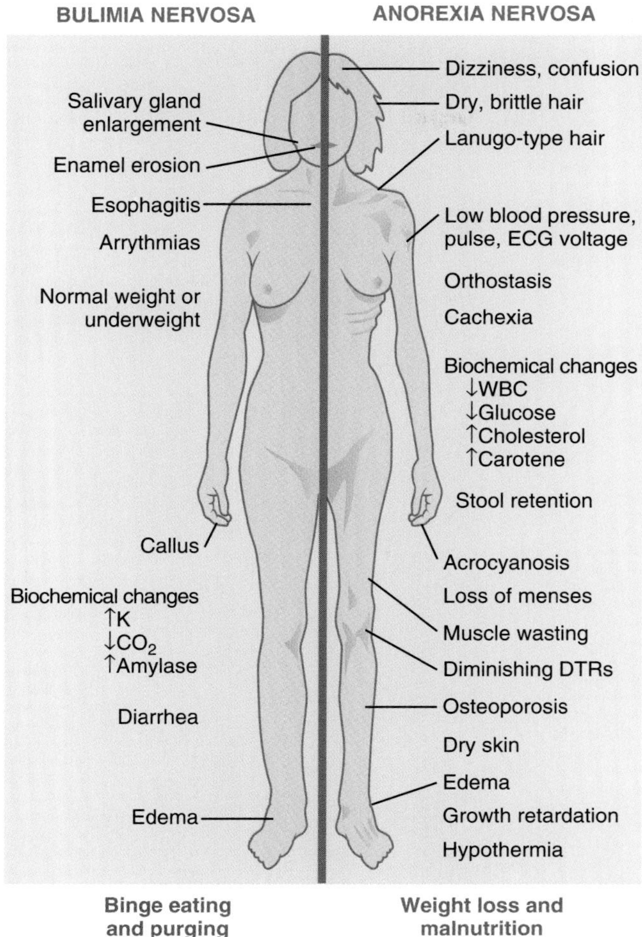

FIGURE 24–1 Physical signs and symptoms of anorexia nervosa and bulimia nervosa. DTRs, deep tendon reflexes; ECG, electrocardiographic; WBC, white blood cell.

erythrocyte sedimentation rates may result from decreased fibrinogen production by the malnourished liver (Fisher et al., 1995).

Osteopenia, which may result in vertebral compression and pathologic fractures, is one of the most serious medical complications of AN. Estrogen deficiency, elevated glucocorticoid levels, malnutrition, and reduced body mass may all contribute to this state.

Children and adolescents with AN develop unique medical complications that affect normal growth and development. Complications include pubertal delay or interruption, reduction in peak bone mass, and structural abnormalities in the brain (Katzman and Zipursky, 1997).

Clinical Characteristics and Medical Complications: Bulimia Nervosa

Clinical signs and symptoms of BN are more difficult to detect because patients are usually of normal weight and are secretive in behavior. When vomiting occurs there may be clinical evidence such as: (1) scarring of the dorsum of the hand used to stimulate the gag reflex, known as Russell's sign; (2) parotid gland enlargement; and (3) erosion of dental enamel with increased dental caries.

Chronic vomiting can result in dehydration, alkalosis, and hypokalemia. Common clinical manifestations include sore throat, esophagitis, mild hematemesis, abdominal pain, and subconjunctival hemorrhage. More serious gastrointestinal complications include Mallory-Weiss esophageal tears, rare occurrence of esophageal rupture, and acute gastric dilatation or rupture. Laxative abuse may lead to dehydration, elevation of serum aldosterone and vasopressin levels, rectal bleeding, intestinal atony, and abdominal cramps. Diuretic abuse may lead to dehydration and hypokalemia. Cardiac arrhythmias can occur secondary to electrolyte and acid–base imbalance caused by vomiting, laxative, and diuretic abuse. Ipecac, used to induce vomiting, may cause irreversible myocardial damage and sudden death. Although the profound amenorrhea associated with AN is uncommon in BN, menstrual irregularities may occur (see Figure 24–1).

PSYCHOLOGICAL MANAGEMENT

Management of patients with eating disorders is best performed by a multidisciplinary team consisting of physicians, nutritionists, and psychotherapists experienced in working with this patient population. Treatment settings vary and include inpatient medical or psychiatric units, day treatment programs, or outpatient programs. Treatment guidelines, published by the Society for Adolescent Medicine (Kreipe et al., 1995) and the APA (Yager et al., 1993), state that nutritional rehabilitation must be an early goal of treatment, because until severe malnutrition has been corrected, psychotherapy will have limited effectiveness. As stated by Hilde Bruch, "The fact is that no true picture of the psychological problems can be formulated, nor can psychotherapy be effective, until the worst malnutrition is corrected . . ." (Bruch, 1982). Nutrition professionals should not, however, take on the care of these patients outside of a multidisciplinary team. Severe malnutrition seen in AN is associated with serious psychological problems. Refeeding may precipitate both increased psychological stress and potentially life-threatening medical complications attributed to the refeeding syndrome (Kohn et al., 1998).

Nutritional rehabilitation includes a nutritional assessment, diet therapy, and nutrition education (Fig. 24–2). Although AN and BN are distinct illnesses, there are similarities in both the nutritional consequences and nutritional management of the two disorders.

NUTRITIONAL ASSESSMENT

Nutritional assessment routinely includes a diet history, as well as the assessment of biochemical, metabolic, and anthropometric indices of nutri-

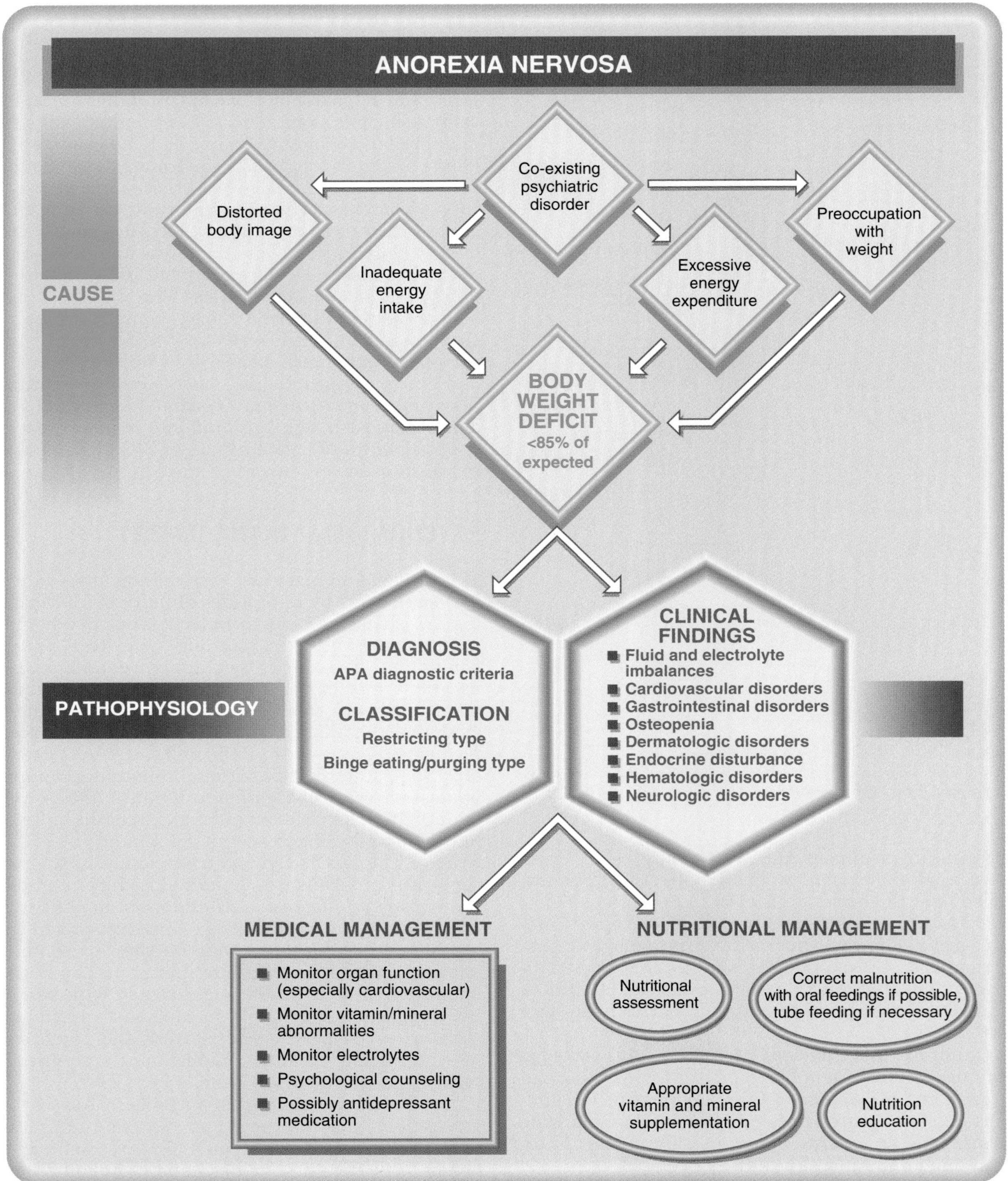

FIGURE 24–2 Pathophysiology algorithm—anorexia nervosa. (Algorithm content developed by John Anderson, Ph.D., and Sanford C. Garner, Ph.D., 2000.)

EATING DISORDER ASSESSMENT

Date of birth: ______________________________

DIAGNOSIS:
- ❑ Anorexia Nervosa
- ❑ Bulimia Nervosa
- ❑ Eating Disorder NOS

Hospitalizations for eating disorder:
- ❑ In-patient
- ❑ Day patient
- ❑ Out-patient

WEIGHT HISTORY
Wt. loss: #lb ________From ________To ________
Minimum weight at current height ______________
Maximum weight at current height ______________
IBW:______ %IBW:______ %Wt loss:______ BMI:______

ANTHROPOMETRIC PROFILE
Skinfolds (mm): ______________________________
Triceps:________ Biceps:________ Subscapular:________
Suprailiac:________
Sum of sites (mm):______ % Body fat:______ TSF%:______
MAC (cm):______ MAMC (cm):______ MAMC%:______

BODY IMAGE: ______________________________

FOOD ALLERGIES: ______________________________

24-HOUR RECALL: ______________________________

FLUID INTAKE: ______________________________

VITAMIN/MINERAL SUPPLEMENTS: ______________________________

OTHER SUPPLEMENTS: ______________________________

SUGAR AND FAT SUBSTITUTES: ______________________________

MISCELLANEOUS: Chewing gum: ______________
Hard candy: ______________
Condiments: ______________

BINGES: # per day # per week
Duration per episode: ______________________________
Binge foods: ______________________________
Approximate kcal/binge: ______________________________

SELF-INDUCED VOMITING:
Times per day:________ Method: ______________

LAXATIVES:
Type/brand:______________ Amount:______________
Duration of use:______________ Frequency of use:______________

DIURETICS:
Type:______________ Amount:______________
Duration of use:______________ Frequency of use:______________

EXERCISE:
Type:______________________________
Minutes/day:__________ Times/week:______________
Purpose of exercise:______________________________

MENSTRUAL HISTORY:
Age of menarche: ______________________________
Last menstrual period: ______________________________

MEDICATIONS (prescription and over-the-counter):

BOWEL FUNCTION: ______________________________

FIGURE 24–3 Sample nutritional assessment form for eating disorders.

tional status (see Chapters 16 and 17 and Fig. 24–3).

Diet History

Guidelines for assessment of nutrient intake are indicated in Table 24–3 (see also Chapter 16). Inadequate energy consumption is seen in AN, and reported intakes are generally less than 1000 kcal/day (Fernstrom et al., 1994; Rock and Yager, 1987). Total energy consumption in BN patients is more unpredictable due to variability in the energy content of a binge, residual energy after a purge, and the degree of restrained eating between binge episodes. Indeed, Mitchell et al. (1981) reported binges in the range of 1200 to 11,500 kcal per episode. In a study of 54 female BN patients, Weltzin et al. (1991) reported a mean 24-hour intake of 4446 (±584) kcal, but also noted a wide range of caloric intake, with 44% overeating and

TABLE 24–3 ASSESSMENT OF NUTRIENT INTAKE

1. Calories
   A. Compare intake to RDA
   B. Estimate typical caloric intake
   C. Determine range of intake in BN
   D. Determine hidden sources: gum, hard candy, etc.
2. Macronutrients
   A. Carbohydrate
      1. Determine percent kcal intake
      2. Simple
      3. Complex
      4. Fiber: water soluble versus insoluble
   B. Protein
      1. Determine percent kcal intake
      2. Compare intake to RDA
      3. Evaluate vegetarian diet for high biologic value sources
   C. Fat
      1. Determine percent kcal intake
      2. Source of essential fatty acid
3. Micronutrients
   A. Vitamins
      1. Water soluble
      2. Fat soluble
      3. Identify supplements
   B. Minerals
      1. Calcium
      2. Iron
      3. Zinc
      4. Identify supplements
4. Fluid
   A. Determine total daily consumption
   B. Identify sources
5. Miscellaneous
   A. Alcohol
   B. Caffeine
   C. Amount and type of nonnutritive sweeteners and fat substitutes
   D. Other nutritional supplements, i.e., herbal supplements

(Adapted from Luder E, Schebendach J. Nutrition management of eating disorders. Topics in Clinical Nutrition 8:53, 1993, with permission.)
RDA, recommended dietary allowance

19% undereating compared to controls. Bulimic patients assume that vomiting is an efficient mechanism for eliminating calories consumed during binge episodes. However, study of the caloric content of food ingested and purged in a feeding laboratory revealed that, as a group, 17 BN subjects consumed a mean of 2131 (±1154) kcal during a binge and vomited only 979 (±1003) kcal afterward (Kaye et al., 1993). There was, however, an apparent ceiling on caloric retention, regardless of whether binges were smaller or larger. (See "*Clinical Insight:* Can Dieting Cause Eating Disorders?").

Inadequate energy intake results in decreased consumption of carbohydrate, protein, and fat. Patients with AN were historically described as carbohydrate avoiders (Crisp, 1965; Hurst et al., 1977), but now appear to preferentially restrict dietary fat (Drewnowski et al., 1988; Fernstrom et al., 1994; Moreiras-Varela et al., 1989; Schebendach et al., 1997). Limited carbohydrate consumption is often evident in bulimics during periods of restrained eating, and it has been suggested that this restriction may impede normal brain serotonin metabolism, thereby triggering binge eating episodes (Wurtman and Wurtman, 1984). Dietary fat avoidance is also apparent in BN. In a study of eating behavior, Walsh et al. (1989) found that the bulimic group consumed a smaller percentage of total fat calories at a nonbinge meal than the control group. Severe restrictions of dietary fat will increase the risk for essential fatty acid deficiency, which has been reported in the AN population (Langan and Farrell, 1985; Holman et al., 1995). Percent of calories contributed by protein may be in the average to above average range, but the adequacy of intake will be relative to total caloric consumption. For example, one study revealed that although the mean percentage of calories provided by protein was 22% in early

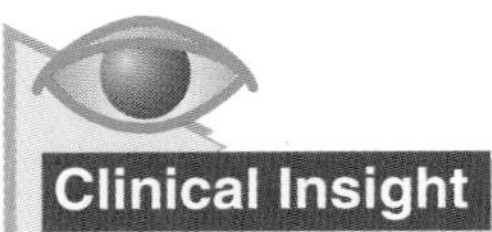

Can Dieting Cause Eating Disorders?

In a review of five studies with 3037 participants, Hsu (1997) concluded that . . ."longitudinal studies point unanimously to the role of dieting behavior in the pathogenesis of an eating disorder." In bulimia nervosa, patients may diet in response to a binge; however, current research suggests that dieting may actually precipitate binge eating in biologically predisposed individuals.

Animal and human studies suggest that serotonin, a central nervous system neurotransmitter, is involved in the control of feeding. Serotonin contributes to satiety after eating and research suggests that decreased serotonin function may lead to impaired satiety and weight gain. The synthesis of serotonin in the brain is dependent on the availability of its amino acid precursor, tryptophan, in plasma. When the effect of a liquid diet devoid of the serotonin precursor tryptophan was compared in 10 recovered female subjects with a history of BN and 12 healthy controls, the recovered bulimic subjects exhibited a significant decrease in mood and increase in body image concern, as well as subjective loss of control of eating, 7 hours after the ingestion of the tryptophan free formula. An occurrence not noted in the healthy subjects (Smith et al., 1999). A 1000 kcal, low-carbohydrate diet has been shown to decrease plasma tryptophan levels and alter brain serotonin function in healthy women (Smith et al., 1997). The authors suggest that persistent dieting may result in chronic depletion of plasma tryptophan and brain serotonin and subsequent development of eating disorder symptoms in a biologically vulnerable individual.

Hsu LKG. Can dieting cause an eating disorder? Psycol Med 27:509, 1997.

Smith KA, et al. Relapse of depression after rapid depletion of tryptophan. Lancet 349:915, 1997.

Smith KA, et al. Symptomatic relapse in bulimia nervosa following acute tryptophan depletion. Arch Gen Psychiatry 56:171, 1999.

illness and 21% in late illness, actual protein intake was only 38 and 17 g/day, respectively, in patients with AN (Beaumont et al., 1981). Many patients with eating disorders are vegetarians (Bakan et al., 1993). This appears to be a means of eliminating animal fats. A recent school-based survey of 12- to 20-year-olds indicated an increased frequency of dieting, self-induced vomiting, and laxative abuse among vegetarian students (Neumark-Sztainer et al., 1997). Clearly, teenagers and young adults on vegetarian diets should be evaluated for covert eating disorders.

An inadequate energy intake, limited variety, and poor food group representation all increase the risk for inadequate vitamin and mineral intake. Deficient vitamin intake is well documented in AN, but clinical and biochemical evidence is more variable. Vitamin supplements may be used, and patients should be queried regarding this.

When obtaining a diet history, typical fluid intake should also be determined. Some patients severely restrict intake, being intolerant of the feeling of fullness after fluid ingestion. Others drink excessive amounts, attempting to stave off hunger. Abnormalities in fluid balance are prevalent in this population. Extremes in fluid restriction or consumption may require monitoring of urine specific gravity and serum electrolytes.

Eating Behavior

Characteristic attitudes, behaviors, and eating habits seen in AN and BN are shown in Table 24–4. Food aversions, common in this population, are typically to energy-dense foods with a high fat content.

TABLE 24–4 ASSESSMENT OF EATING ATTITUDES, BEHAVIORS, AND HABITS

1. Eating attitudes
   - Food aversions
   - "Safe" foods
   - Magical thinking
   - Binge trigger foods
   - Ideas on appropriate amounts of food
2. Eating behaviors
   - Ritualistic behaviors
   - Unusual food combinations
   - Atypical seasoning of food
   - Atypical use of eating utensils
3. Eating habits
   - Intake pattern
     - Number of meals and snacks
     - Time of day meals and snacks are consumed
     - Duration of feedings
     - Eating environment: where and with whom
     - How consumed: sitting or standing
   - Avoidance of particular food groups
   - Variety of foods consumed
   - Fluid intake: restricted or excessive

(Adapted from Schebendach J, Nussbaum M. Nutrition management in adolescents with eating disorders. Adolescent Medicine: State of the Art Reviews 3(3):545, 1992 with permission.)

Common food aversions include red meat, baked goods, desserts, added fats, and fried foods. Patients with eating disorders often regard specific foods or groups of foods as absolutely "good" or absolutely "bad" for them. Irrational beliefs and dichotomous thinking about food choices should be identified and challenged throughout the treatment process.

In the assessment, it is important to determine unusual or ritualistic behaviors, which may include the ingestion of food in an atypical manner or with nontraditional utensils, unusual food combinations, or the excessive use of spices, vinegar, or lemon juice. Meal spacing and length of time allocated for a meal should also be determined. Many patients will save their self-allotted food ration until late in the day, yet others are fearful of eating past a certain time of day. Setting time limits for completion of meals and snacks is important. Many BN patients eat very quickly, reflecting their difficulties with satiety cues. Many AN patients eat in an excessively slow manner, often playing with their food and cutting it into small pieces. This is sometimes regarded as a tactic to avoid food intake, yet it may also represent a starvation effect (Keys et al., 1950). The establishment of specific mealtimes of reasonable duration is helpful for strengthening hunger and satiety cues in both AN and BN patients. Lastly, BN patients may identify foods they fear will trigger a binge eating episode. The patient may have an all-or-nothing approach to "trigger" foods. Although the patient may prefer avoidance, assistance with reintroduction of controlled amounts of these foods may be helpful.

Laboratory Data

The often marked cachexia of AN may lead one to expect biochemical indices of malnutrition, but this is rarely the case. Compensatory mechanisms are remarkable, and laboratory abnormalities may not be observed until the illness is far advanced.

In AN, serum albumin levels are generally within normal limits. Although true levels may be masked by dehydration in early treatment, significant alterations in visceral protein status are not common. Indeed, adaptive phenomena that occur in chronic starvation are aimed at the maintenance of visceral protein metabolism at the expense of the somatic compartment.

Despite the eating of low-fat, low-cholesterol diets, patients with AN often have elevated serum cholesterol levels and abnormal lipoprotein profiles. This is distinct from the low serum cholesterol observed in protein energy malnutrition from other causes. Although the exact nature of the lipoprotein dysfunction is unknown, several mechanisms have been postulated. These include mild hepatic dysfunction, decreased bile acid secretion, hypothalamic dysfunction, and abnormal eating patterns (Arden et al., 1990). Obviously, elevated lipids do not warrant continuation of a low-fat, low-cholesterol diet by the AN patient. In a study of 126 women with BN, 67% were found to have elevated serum cholesterol levels, and this was attributed to the high fat and cholesterol intake during binge eating episodes (Sullivan et al., 1998).

Serum glucose tends to be low because of a deficit of precursors for gluconeogenesis and glucose production. Thyroid hormone production tends to be normal, but the peripheral deiodination of thyroxine favors formation of the less metabolically active reduced triiodothyronine (rT_3) rather than T_3. This metabolic state, known as the low T_3 syndrome, is characteristic of AN but resolves with refeeding (Fisher et al., 1995).

Vitamin and Mineral Abnormalities

The incidence of hypercarotenemia is well documented in AN, and its etiology is attributed to mobilization of lipid stores, catabolic changes due to weight loss, and metabolic stress, not to an excessive carotene intake. Normalization of serum carotene is seen as soon as refeeding occurs.

Despite apparent dietary deficiencies, the existence of vitamin deficiency states is rarely seen in AN (Comerci, 1988). This has been attributed to a decreased metabolic need for micronutrients in a catabolic state, the use of vitamin supplements (Rock and Yager, 1987), and the judicious selection of micronutrient-rich foods despite a low caloric intake. Observed vitamin deficiencies may include riboflavin and vitamin B_6, thiamin, γ-tocopherol, and α-tocopherol (Langan and Farrell, 1985; Rock and Vasantharajan, 1995; and Rock and Yager, 1987). These deficiencies were more likely to occur in AN and BN patients who were at a lower relative body weight.

Despite a deficient iron intake, iron deficiency anemia is uncommon in AN perhaps because of reduced iron requirements secondary to amenorrhea, as well as to decreased iron needs in a catabolic state. The hematologic picture is variable because of altered states of hydration, and abnormalities of laboratory indices may be masked by hemoconcentration in early treatment (Lucas, 1977).

Zinc deficiency due to suboptimal intake (7 to 8 mg/day) has been documented in both AN and BN (Bakan et al., 1993) and its etiology attributed to inadequate energy intake, avoidance of red meat, and the adoption of vegetarian food choices. Zinc's relationship to altered taste and poor appetite have led some to investigate whether zinc deficiency perpetuates poor food intake in this population (Casper et al., 1980).

Although inadequate calcium intake is common, blood values are neither specific nor sensitive markers of a deficiency state. A calcium intake significantly less than the recommended dietary allowance (RDA) has been reported in patients with AN (Schebendach et al., 1997). Inadequate calcium intake in amenorrheic AN female patients will contribute to the development of osteopenia and osteoporosis. Dual x-ray absorptiometry (DXA) must be performed to determine the degree of impaired bone mineralization (see Chapter 28).

Fluid and Electrolyte Abnormalities

Vomiting and laxative and diuretic use can result in significant fluid and electrolyte imbalances in patients with eating disorders. Laxative use may result in hypokalemia, and diuretic use can lead to dehydration and hypokalemia. Vomiting may result in dehydration, hypokalemia, and alkalosis with hypochloremia. Hyponatremia is a serious complication that is seen less frequently.

Urine concentration is decreased and urine output increased in semistarvation. Starvation edema may present initially, and refeeding edema may develop during nutritional rehabilitation (Barbosa-Saldivar and Van Itallie, 1979). Fluid consumption varies from restricted to excessive intake. Depletion of glycogen and lean tissue is accompanied by obligatory water loss that reflects characteristic hydration ratios. For example, the obligatory water loss associated with glycogen depletion may be in the range of 600 to 800 mL.

Metabolic Assessment

Many patients with AN and BN have below normal metabolic rates (Devlin et al., 1990; Kaye et al., 1986; Melchior et al., 1989; Schebendach et al., 1995). This adaptive response occurs secondary to weight loss and in response to restricted caloric intake.

For example, 21 AN patients measured by indirect calorimetry on admission to an inpatient medical unit were found to have a mean resting energy expenditure (REE) of 62% (±18%) of Harris-Benedict (Harris and Benedict, 1919) predicted values (Schebendach et al., 1995). A revised equation for calculation of fasting REE and basal energy expenditure (BEE) is recommended (Schebendach et al., 1998). (See Table 24–7.) Eleven BN patients had a mean measured REE of 83% (±17%) of Harris-Benedict predicted values; however, the range of metabolic rates was extremely variable (55% to 118% of predicted values), and no correlation between measured and predicted values was apparent (Schebendach et al., 1995).

In addition to changes in fasting metabolic rate, variation in the postprandial metabolic rate must also be considered. Stordy et al. (1977) measured metabolic response to 100 g glucose and found an average increase of 16% in the AN group versus 6 % in matched controls. In a recent study of the effects of nutritional rehabilitation on both fasting and postprandial energy expenditure in 50 AN patients, postprandial energy expenditure increased from a mean of 17.5% (±18.2%) to 27.9% (±15.9%) above fasting during the first 2 weeks of hospitalization (Schebendach et al., 1997). Other investigators have reported similar increases in postprandial energy expenditure in AN (Green and Miller, 1975; Moukaddem et al., 1997; Vaisman et al., 1991).

Although changes in fasting and postprandial metabolic rates can be anticipated, premorbid weight history may alert the clinician to a patient's potential for metabolic response. Indeed, Stordy et al. (1977) found that previously obese subjects gained weight more rapidly on the same food intake and had lower postprandial metabolic responses than AN subjects who were of normal weight before their illness began. Likewise, Walker et al. (1979) reported that previously obese AN patients gained weight faster because of a smaller increase in both basal and postprandial energy expenditure.

Cardiac atrophy and the subsequent inability to handle a sudden increase in the metabolic rate during refeeding have been described in malnutrition (Keys et al., 1950). Congestive heart failure secondary to refeeding has been reported in AN (Powers, 1982). Both the potential for a hypometabolic rate and the dangers of vigorous refeeding must be acknowledged in the treatment of patients with eating disorders (see Chapter 33).

Anthropometric Assessment

Patients with AN have protein energy malnutrition characterized by significantly depleted adipose and somatic protein stores but a relatively intact visceral protein compartment. These patients meet the criteria for a diagnosis of **marasmus** (see Appendix 30). During nutritional rehabilitation, fat and lean stores regenerate but do so at varying rates.

An accurate body fat percentage can be obtained from underwater weighing or bone mineral densitometry (DXA) equipped with body composition software; however, these methods are not generally available in an office or clinic setting (Chapter 16). Another method, bioelectrical impedance analysis (BIA), is more available, but is unreliable in AN due to changes in intracellular and extracellular fluid compartments (Birmingham et al., 1996; Scalfi et al., 1993). Percent body fat can also be estimated from the sum of four skinfolds measurements (triceps, biceps, subscapular, and suprailiac crest) using the calculations of Durnin (Durnin and Rahaman, 1967; Durnin and Wormersley, 1974) (see Appendix 25). This method has been validated against underwater weighing in adolescent girls with AN (Probst et al., 1996).

Changes in the lean compartment can be assessed from the midarm muscle circumference, which is derived from the midarm circumference and triceps skinfolds and compared to sex- and age-matched population standards (see Appendices 23 and 24). A laboratory evaluation of somatic protein depletion can be obtained from the creatinine height index (see Appendix 32). Although this is a reliable method for estimation of lean body mass, its validity depends on an accurate urine collection, which is difficult to obtain.

Body weight is assessed and routinely monitored in patients with eating disorders. In AN, weight gain is necessary. In BN the short-term goal should be weight maintenance. Although weight loss may be warranted, this cannot be addressed until chaotic eating patterns are stabilized. Weight change in eating disorders may be affected by the state of hydration, glycogen stores, metabolic factors, and changes in body composition (Table 24–5).

Rehydration and replenished glycogen stores contribute to weight gain in early treatment of AN, but further gains in weight require increases in lean and fat stores. It is generalized that one needs to increase or decrease caloric intake by 3500 kcal to affect a 1-lb change in body weight; however, the true energy cost depends on the type of tissue gained. More energy is required to gain fat versus lean tissue, and actual weight gain may be a mix of tissues. In a study of 9 AN patients, Forbes et al. (1982) found that those in the early stage of recovery gained significantly more weight per excess unit of energy consumed because the tissue gained had a larger portion of lean. The energy cost of weight gain increases as more fat is laid down during late treatment (Walker et al., 1979).

The anthropometric status of patients with eating disorders should be assessed and monitored regularly (see Chapter 16 and Table 24–7). The patient's goal weight can be determined by various methods, none of which are perfect. The National Center for Health Statistics (NCHS) height–weight tables should be used to assess boys and girls up to 18 years of age (see Appendix Tables 8 and 12) and Metropolitan Life Insurance Company (1983) tables (see Appendix 19) can be used in young adults. A bone age may be obtained in adolescents with stunted height to determine catch-up growth potential.

TABLE 24–5 FACTORS AFFECTING RATE OF WEIGHT GAIN IN ANOREXIA NERVOSA

1. Fluid balance
   a. Polyuria seen in semistarvation
   b. Edema
      1. Starvation
      2. Refeeding
   c. Hydration ratios in tissues
      1. Glycogen: 3–4:1
      2. Protein: 3–4:1
2. Metabolic rate
   a. Resting energy expenditure
   b. Postprandial energy expenditure
3. Energy cost of tissue gained
   a. Adipose tissue
   b. Lean body mass
4. Previous obesity
5. Physical activity

(Adapted from Schebendach J, Nussbaum M. Nutrition management in adolescents with eating disorders. Adolescent Medicine: State of the Art Reviews 3(3):548, 1992, with permission.)

If a patient is hospitalized, a daily preprandial, early morning weight should be obtained. On an outpatient basis, a gowned weight should be obtained on the same scale, at approximately the same time of day, at least once a week in early treatment. Prior to weigh-in, the patient should void, and urine specific gravity should be checked for dehydration or fluid loading. If the patient claims to be unable to provide a urine specimen, a physician should examine the patient to see if the bladder is full. Patients may resort to deceptive tactics (water loading, hiding heavy objects on their person, and withholding urine and bowel movements) to make a mandated weight goal (Ammerman et al., 1996).

NUTRITION MANAGEMENT

Anorexia Nervosa

Patients with AN often require hospitalization to begin the refeeding process. Although the use of a nasogastric tube feeding for primary or supplemental nourishment is occasionally needed, the majority of patients with AN can be fed by mouth. The treatment goal will be to increase the intake gradually while energy output is decreased, to achieve a positive balance (Table 24–6). For this reason, "privileges" such as being out of bed, using the telephone, or visiting with friends and family may be combined with weight gain as contingencies in a behavior modification program. A genuine change in attitude is as important as a gain to weight appropriate for height as a basis for discharge from the hospital.

A total daily energy intake of 130% of either measured or predicted energy expenditure should be prescribed in AN (Schebendach et al., 1995). Generally speaking, the initial prescription is in the range of 1200 to 1400 kcal/day. Daily intake is increased in 100- to 200-kcal increments every few days to promote a consistent rate of weight gain. The desired rate of weight gain will vary among treatment programs and treatment settings. For example, the rate of weight gain may be 2 to 3 lb/wk on an inpatient unit, but 1 lb/wk in an outpatient program.

During the course of refeeding, the number of calories needed to gain weight increases. Changes in metabolic rate, postprandial energy expenditure, and type of tissue gained are all factors. In addition, energy cost of physical activity must be considered. Even though they are markedly underweight and hypometabolic, the total daily energy expenditure of AN patients may be similar to that of normal weight controls (1972 versus 1985 kcal/day). This is attributed to the fact that AN patients expend more energy in physical activity than do control subjects, and they also require more calories for weight maintenance, a mean of 2899 in one study (Pirke et al., 1991), again due to excessive activity levels (Casper et al., 1991; Kaye et al., 1988).

TABLE 24–6 GUIDELINES FOR DIET THERAPY IN ANOREXIA NERVOSA

1. Caloric prescription: weight gain
   A. 1.3 × measured REE for sedentary male or female
   or
   B. 1.3 × adjusted Harris-Benedict predicted REE in females as follows:
      1. Calculate Harris-Benedict Equation: 655 + (9.6 × wt in kg) + (1.85 × ht in cm) – (4.7 × age in yrs)
      2. Adjust for hypometabolic rate as follows: (1.84 × Harris-Benedict calculated REE) – 1435
         1.3 (1.84 × Harris-Benedict calculated REE – 1435)
   C. Initial prescriptions generally in the range of 1200 to 1400 kcal/day
   D. Additional calories may be needed for increased activity levels
   E. Increase caloric prescription in 100 to 200 kcal increments
2. Macronutrients
   A. Protein
      1. Minimum intake = RDA in g/kg ideal body weight
      2. 15–20% kcal
      3. High biological value sources
   B. Carbohydrate
      1. 50–55% kcal
      2. Encourage water insoluble fiber for treatment of constipation
   C. Fat
      1. 25–30% kcal
      2. Encourage small increases in fat intake until goal can be attained
      3. Provide source of essential fatty acid
3. Micronutrients
   A. 100% RDA multivitamin tablet with minerals
   B. Note that iron-containing preparations may aggravate constipation

(Adapted from Luder E, Schendenbach J. Nutrition management of eating disorders. Top Clin Nutr 8:59, 1993, with permission.)

Anorectics required 8301 ± 2272 kcal (mean ± SD) to gain 1 kg body weight, and 73% of AN patients had higher levels of physical activity compared to normal volunteers (Kaye et al., 1988). These levels of activity tend to continue after recovery and dictate the need for more calories to maintain the new weight at least in the first few weeks after recovery (Kaye et al., 1988).

Once the initial caloric prescription is written, a reasonable distribution among macronutrients can be prescribed. Patients may express multiple aversions, fat being the primary one. However, persistent avoidance of dietary fat can make gaining and maintaining weight difficult. Although the promotion of a high-fat diet is unnecessary, a dietary fat intake in the range of 25% to 30% of calories is recommended. Some patients will accept small amounts of added fat, such as salad dressing or butter. Others do better when the fat source is less obvious, such as in whole milk or peanut butter. Protein intake in the range of 15% to 20% of total calories is recommended, and to ensure adequacy, the minimum protein prescription should equal the RDA for age and sex in grams per kilogram of ideal body weight (see Table 15–1). Vegetarian diets are discouraged during nutritional rehabilitation. Carbohydrate intake in the range of 50% to 55% of calories is well tolerated. Sources of insoluble fiber should be included to offset the constipation frequently seen in this population.

Although vitamin and mineral supplements are not universally prescribed, the potential for increased needs during anabolic processes must be considered. A vitamin and mineral supplement providing 100% of the RDA can be prescibed; however, iron-containing preparations may aggravate constipation in some patients. Care must be taken throughout the refeeding process to ensure a reasonable variety of intake. Particular attention to the inclusion of calcium-rich foods is recommended due to increased risk of osteopenia and osteoporosis.

Delayed gastric emptying with complaints of abdominal distention and discomfort after eating are common in AN. In early treatment, caloric intake is generally low and can be tolerated in a three-meal setting. Snacking may relieve some physical discomfort but may result in guilt feelings for indulging between meals. As the caloric prescription increases in late treatment, multiple feedings become unavoidable. At this point defined formula liquid supplements may be useful (see Appendices 35 through 40) and products containing 30 to 45 calories per fluid ounce may be prescribed once or twice a day. Because patients are fearful that they will become accustomed to the large amount of food required to fulfill late treatment caloric requirements, liquid feeding is appealing because it can easily be discontinued when goal weight is attained.

Bulimia Nervosa

Bulimia nervosa is described as a state of dietary chaos, characterized by periods of uncontrolled, poorly structured eating, often followed by a period of restrained food intake. The nutritionist's role is to help develop a plan for controlled eating while assessing the patient's need and tolerance for structure.

In bulimia, much of the patient's eating and purging behavior is aimed at weight loss, and she will often ask for help in attaining this goal. Although long-term weight loss may be reasonable, the immediate goal should be interruption of the binge–purge cycle with stabilization of body weight. Unlike the AN population, patients with BN are hospitalized less frequently, and when hospitalization does occur, it may be a brief admission for the purpose of correcting dehydration and electrolyte imbalance.

Although most patients with bulimia are normal to overweight, they are often hypometabolic, and this must be considered when prescribing the caloric intake. A study of Harris-Benedict predicted REE versus indirect calorimetry measurement of REE revealed good correlation between predicted and measured values in the AN group but poor correlation in the BN group (Schebendach et al., 1995). The Harris-Benedict equation could be adjusted to reflect the predictably low metabolic state of AN, but this was not so in BN. If indirect calorimetry measurement of REE can be obtained, then maintenance calories at 120% to 130% of measured REE can be prescribed. If the patient engages in bouts of compulsive exercise, more moderate daily exercise should be encouraged so that the caloric prescription better reflects daily energy expenditure.

When indirect calorimetry is not available, the nutritionist must assess for the possibility of a low metabolic rate. The range of caloric intake in relation to change in weight status, dieting history, and cold intolerance may give clues to the patient's metabolic status. If a low metabolism is suspected, then an initial caloric prescription may be equal to 100% of the Harris-Benedict predicted REE. This would cover basal metabolic requirements plus sedentary activity. Typically, this is in the range of 1200 to 1500 kcal daily.

Body weight should be monitored with a goal of stabilization. If the patient's weight is stabilized on a lower than average caloric intake, then small but consistent increases in the caloric prescription should be attempted over time. This may tease up the metabolic rate to a more appropriate level. BN patients need a great deal of encouragement to follow weight maintenance versus weight loss diets. They must be reminded that attempts to significantly restrict caloric intake may only increase the risk of binge eating and that their pattern of restrained intake followed by binge eating has not facilitated weight loss in the past (Table 24–7).

A balanced macronutrient intake should be encouraged in patients with BN. This should include sufficient carbohydrate to prevent craving and adequate protein and fat to promote satiety. In general, a balanced diet providing 50% to 55% of the calories from carbohydrate, 15% to 20% from protein, and 25% to 30% from fat is reasonable. Small amounts of dietary fat should be encouraged at each meal. As is the case with AN, this may be better tolerated when provided in a less obvious manner, such as in peanut butter, cheese, or whole milk.

Bulimic patients are likely to remain on low calorie intakes for longer periods of time than their anoretic counterparts. Adequacy of micronutrient intake relative to the caloric prescription and variety of intake should be assessed. A multivitamin, multimineral preparation may be prescribed to ensure adequacy, particularly in the initial phase of treatment.

Bingeing, purging, and restrained intake often impair recognition of hunger and satiety cues in bulimic individuals. The cessation of purging behavior, coupled with a reasonable daily distribution of calories at three meals and prescribed snacks, can be instrumental in strengthening these biologic cues. However, many patients with BN are afraid to eat earlier in the day, fearful that these calories will only contribute to caloric excess if they binge later. Patients may also digress from their meal plan after a binge, attempting to restrict intake to balance out the binge calories. Patience and support

TABLE 24–7 GUIDELINES FOR NUTRITION MANAGEMENT OF BULIMIA NERVOSA

1. Caloric prescription: weight maintenance
   - A. 1.2 × measured REE for sedentary activity
     1.3 × measured REE for moderate activity
   - B. If indirect calorimetry measurement is not available, prescribe diet at 100% Harris-Benedict predicted REE as follows:
     Females: 655 + (9.6 × wt in kg) + (1.85 × ht in cm) – (4.7 × age in y)
     Males: 66 + (13.7 × wt in kg) + (5.0 × ht in cm) – (6.8 × age in y)
   - C. Monitor anthropometric status and adjust caloric prescription for weight maintenance.
   - D. Avoid weight reduction diets until eating patterns and body weight are stabilized.
   - E. Initial prescriptions are generally in the range of 1200 to 1500 kcal/day.
2. Macronutrients
   - A. Protein
     1. Minimum intake = RDA in g/kg ideal body weight
     2. 15–20% kcal
     3. High biologic value sources
   - B. Carbohydrate
     1. 50–55% kcal
     2. Encourage water-insoluble fiber for treatment of constipation.
   - C. Fat
     1. 25–30% kcal
     2. Provide source of essential fatty acids.
3. Micronutrients
   - A. 100% RDA multivitamin tablet with minerals
   - B. Note that iron-containing preparation may aggravate constipation.

(Adapted from Luder E, Schebendenbach J: Nutrition management of eating disorders. Topics in Clinical Nutrition 8:59, 1993 with permission.)
RDA, recommended dietary allowance; REE, resting energy expenditure

are essential in the process of helping bulimic individuals make positive changes in their eating habits.

Monitoring

Guidelines for monitoring the nutritional management of patients with eating disorders are indicated in Table 24–8. The treatment team, patient, and family must be realistic about treatment, which is often a long-term process. Care may be provided in inpatient, day hospital, or outpatient settings. Although outcomes may be favorable, the course of treatment is rarely a smooth one and the clinician must be prepared to monitor progress carefully.

NUTRITION EDUCATION

Patients with eating disorders appear quite knowledgeable about nutrition. Despite this, nutrition education is an essential component of their treatment plan. Indeed, some patients spend significant amounts of time reading nutrition-related information, but their source may be unreliable and their interpretation potentially distorted by their illness. Malnutrition may impair the patient's ability to as-

TABLE 24–8 PATIENT MONITORING

1. Body weight
   - A. Establish goal weight
   - B. Determine
     1. Acceptable rate of weight gain in AN
     2. Maintenance weight range in BN
   - C. Monitor
     1. Inpatient
        - a. Daily
        - b. Gowned
        - c. Preprandial
        - d. Postvoid
        - e. Obtain urine specific gravity
        - f. Obtain additional, random, afternoon, or evening weight if fluid loading is suspected
     2. Day treatment
        - a. May vary depending on diagnosis, age of patient, and treatment setting, i.e., daily; several times per week; once per week
        - b. Gowned
        - c. Postvoid
        - d. Same time of day
        - e. Same scale
        - f. Obtain urine specific gravity
     3. Outpatient
        - a. Once every 1–2 wk in early treatment, less frequently in mid- to late treatment
        - b. Gowned
        - c. Postvoid
        - d. Same time of day
        - e. Same scale
        - f. Obtain urine specific gravity
2. Height
   - A. Obtain baseline: (NCHS percentile for children and adolescents)
   - B. Monitor: every 1–2 mo in patients with growth potential
3. Anthropometric measurements
   - A. Obtain baseline
     1. Skinfolds: triceps, biceps, subscapula, suprailiac
     2. Midarm circumference
     3. Midarm muscle circumference
   - B. Monitor
     1. Inpatient: every 2 wk
     2. Outpatient: every month or as medically indicated
4. Resting and postprandial energy expenditure
   - A. Obtain baseline indirect calorimetry if available
   - B. Monitor
     1. Inpatient: every 2 wk
     2. Outpatient: as medically indicated
5. Outpatient diet monitoring
   - A. Anorexia nervosa
     Daily food record to include:
     1. Food
     2. Fluid: caloric and noncaloric, alcohol
     3. Artificial sweeteners and fat substitutes
     4. Eating behavior: time, place, how eaten, with whom
     5. Exercise
   - B. Bulimia nervosa
     Daily food record to include:
     1. Food
     2. Fluid: caloric and noncaloric, alcohol
     3. Artificial sweeteners and fat substitutes
     4. Eating behavior: time, place, how eaten, with whom
     5. Emotions/feelings when eating
     6. Foods eaten at a binge
     7. Time and method of purge
     8. Exercise

(Adapted from Luder E, Schebendenbach J: Nutrition management of eating disorders. Topics in Clinical Nutrition 8:62, 1993, with permission.)

TABLE 24–9 TOPICS FOR NUTRITION EDUCATION

1. Impact of malnutrition on growth and development
2. Impact of malnutrition on behavior
3. Set-point theory
4. Metabolic adaptation to dieting
5. Restrained eating and disinhibition
6. Causes of bingeing and purging
7. What does "weight gain" mean?
   Glycogen storage
   Fluid balance
   Lean body mass
   Adipose tissue
8. Impact of exercise on caloric expenditure
9. Ineffectiveness of vomiting, laxatives, and diuretics in long-term weight control
10. Portion control
11. Food exchange system
12. Social dining and holiday dining
13. Food Guide Pyramid
14. Hunger and satiety cues
15. Interpreting food labels
16. Nutrition misinformation

(Adapted from Schebendach J, Nussbaum MP. Nutrition management in adolescents with eating disorders. Adolescent Medicine: State of the Art Reviews 3(3):556, 1992, with permission.)

similate and process new information. Early and mid-adolescent development is characterized by the transition from concrete to abstract operations in problem-solving and directed thinking, and normal developmental issues must be considered when teaching adolescents with eating disorders (see Chapter 11).

Although the interactive process of a group setting may have advantages, these topics can be effectively incorporated into individual counseling sessions as well. Topics for nutrition education are suggested in Table 24–9.

PROGNOSIS

Early and more knowledgeable treatment of AN has led to a decline in mortality from around 10% to .56%. However, only 50% will have full recovery after treatment, 30% will have a partial recovery, and 20% will have life-long problems with irrational dieting and food fears (Becker et al., 1999). The present emphasis on the broad range of treatment issues should contribute to a similar improvement in the other outcomes of the disorder. Outcome criteria encompass weight and dietary habits (including food intake, weight and shape ideation, and weight-for-height proportion), menstruation, and adjustment of sexual, psychologic, and social attitudes. These must be assessed for several years after a crisis to identify true outcome.

Nutrition management must promote health, support growth and development, and decrease food conflicts in patients with eating disorders. Although correction of some pathophysiologic consequences (i.e., hypometabolic rate) is well documented, less is known about restoration of others (i.e., loss of brain tissue, osteopenia). Hopefully, nutritional rehabilitation will restore complete health.

When refeeding occurs in an outpatient setting, the treatment team (psychotherapist, nutritionist, physician) should advise both the patient and family on the appropriate degree of parental or spousal involvement. This is critical for maintenance of appropriate boundaries, the containment of manipulative behaviors, and the avoidance of power struggles and control issues. During treatment both the patient and family benefit from education on all aspects of the disease. Nutrition education may help the patient make more rational and scientifically based decisions regarding food choices. Develop-

CASE STUDY 1

Anorexia Nervosa

Sara T. is a 13-year-old girl. She presents at a height of 61 in. and a weight of 72 lb. Sara began menstruating at age 12 but has not menstruated for the past 5 months.

Laboratory Status: glucose: 62 mg/dL; albumin: 4.6 g/dL; cholesterol: 240 mg/dL; phosphorus: 2.3 mg/dL; T_3-RIA (radioimmune assay): 78 ng/dL; ESR: 2 mm/h

Anthropometric Status: Skinfolds: triceps: 4 mm; biceps: 2 mm; subscapular: 5 mm; suprailiac: 4 mm; midarm circumference: 18.0 cm; midarm muscle circumference: 16.7 cm.

Sara's maximum weight was 103 lb 8 months ago. She was concerned that her hips and thighs were fat and started to eliminate snacks and desserts from her diet. Sara was pleased with her "willpower." She then decided to eat heart healthy, and excluded all sources of dietary fat. About 5 months ago, Sara eliminated red meat, poultry, and seafood claiming that a vegetarian diet was a healthier option. As she lost weight, Sara became increasingly more concerned about her body shape and size. Her diet became more restricted in the amount and variety of intake, providing about 650 kcal/day. Sara's family expressed concern about her eating behaviors. She would ritualistically cut small portions of food into many pieces and spend up to an hour consuming one small meal. After eating, Sara expressed considerable guilt about overeating and often cried. Some days she barely ate at all, consuming only large amounts of water and diet soda. Despite her limited caloric intake, Sara's parents were amazed at her energy level. She continued to play soccer (1 to 2 h/day, 5 days a week), did regular calisthenics (leg lifts and situps, 30 minutes daily), and went running each morning (5 to 7 miles).

1. What are some possible medical complications that Sara may develop secondary to self-starvation?
2. Discuss laboratory values and what you might expect to happen to these indices during refeeding.
3. Determine Sara's ideal body weight, goal weight for treatment, and recommended rate of weight gain.
4. Calculate Sara's initial caloric prescription and discuss how you arrived at this. How might this change over time and why?
5. Plan a sample menu.

CASE STUDY 2

Bulimia Nervosa

Jennifer A. is a 19-year-old woman. She presents at a height of 65 in. and a weight of 138 lb.

Laboratory Status: glucose 82 mg/dL; albumin: 4.2 g/dL; cholesterol: 180 mg/dL; potassium: 2.7 mmol/L; serum CO_2: 31 mmol/L

Anthropometric Status: Skinfolds: triceps: 20 mm; biceps: 7 mm; subscapular: 10 mm; suprailiac: 13 mm; midarm circumference: 26.7 cm; midarm muscle circumference: 20.4 cm.

Jennifer has always been unhappy with her weight. She went on every fad diet throughout high school and lost some weight but always regained it. About 1 year ago, Jennifer began binge eating. Binge episodes now occur three to four times per week. During these binges, Jennifer consumes about 1500 to 2000 kcal in a 2-hour period. Binge foods include ice cream, cookies, potato chips, and other foods Jennifer describes as "fattening and unhealthy." After binge eating Jennifer feels extremely guilty and vomiting is immediately self-induced. Jennifer always tries to eat as little as possible the next day, sometimes consuming only 700 or 800 kcal. Three months ago, Jennifer started to overdose on laxatives about three times a week. She occasionally uses over-the-counter diet pills but they never really help. Jennifer feels fat in her abdomen, buttocks, and thighs. Her physical activity includes 100 situps and 100 leg lifts three or four times per week.

1. What are some possible medical complications that Jennifer may develop secondary to binge eating and her compensatory behaviors?
2. Discuss her laboratory values and what you might expect to happen to these indices during rehabilitation.
3. Determine Jennifer's ideal body weight and goal weight for short-term and long-term treatment.
4. Calculate Jennifer's initial caloric prescription and discuss how you arrived at this.
5. Plan a sample menu.
6. Discuss how you would handle those foods Jennifer considers binge "trigger" foods.
7. What would you suggest for Jennifer to help control her episodes of vomiting, laxative use, and diet pill use?

mental issues, cognitive abilities, and psychological readiness must all be considered in the design of nutrition education programs.

Early intervention and improved treatment modalities have contributed to the decline in mortality from AN and BN. However, both AN and BN must be understood and appreciated to be chronic disorders. Family expectation of a quick cure should be dispelled. Likewise, professional staff can also become frustrated by the patient's lack of progress, relapse, and seemingly self-destructive behaviors. Learning to anticipate and accept relapse in the natural course of treatment and recovery may enable the patient, family, and treatment team to maintain a unified effort and optimistic attitude. Hopefully, this will improve outcome.

CITED REFERENCES

American Psychiatric Association. Diagnostic and Statistical Manual of Mental Disorders, 3rd ed. Washington, DC, 1980.

American Psychiatric Association. Diagnostic and Statistical Manual of Mental Disorders, 4th ed. Washington, DC, 1994.

Ammerman S, et al. Unique considerations for treating eating disorders in adolescents and preventive intervention. Topics in Clinical Nutrition 12(1):79, 1996.

Arden MR, et al. Effect of weight restoration on the dyslipoproteinemia of anorexia nervosa. J Adolesc Health 11:199, 1990.

Bakan R, et al. EM: Dietary zinc intake of vegetarian and nonvegetarian patients with anorexia nervosa. Int J Eating Disord 13:229, 1993.

Barbosa-Saldivar JL, Van Itallie TB. Semistarvation: An overview of an old problem. Bull N Y Acad Med 55:774, 1979.

Beaumont PJ, et al. The diet composition and nutritional knowledge of patients with anorexia nervosa. Journal of Human Nutrition 35:265, 1981.

Becker AE, et al. Eating disorders. N Engl J Med 340:1092, 1999.

Birmingham CL, et al. The reliability of bioelectrical impedance analysis for measuring changes in the body composition of patients with anorexia nervosa. Int J Eating Disord 19:311, 1996.

Bruch H: Anorexia nervosa: Therapy and theory. Am J Psych 139:1531, 1982.

Casper RC, et al. An evaluation of trace metals, vitamins, and taste function in anorexia nervosa. Am J Clin Nutr 33:1810, 1980.

Casper RC, et al. Total daily energy expenditure and activity level in anorexia nervosa. Am J Clin Nutr 53:1143, 1991.

Crisp AH. Some aspects of the evolution, presentation and follow-up of anorexia nervosa. Proc R Soc Med 58:814, 1965.

Devlin MJ, et al. Metabolic abnormalities in bulimia nervosa. Arch Gen Psychiatry 47:144, 1990.

Drewnowski A, et al. Fat aversion in eating disorders. Appetite 10:119, 1988.

Durnin JVGA, Rahaman MM. The assessment of the amount of the amount of body fat in the human body from measurements of skinfold thickness. Br J Nutr 21:681, 1967.

Durnin JVGA, Womersley J. Body fat assessed from total body density and its estimation from skinfolds thickness: Measurements of 481 men and women aged from 16 to 72 years. Br J Nutr 32:77, 1974.

Feighner JP, et al. Diagnostic criteria for use in psychiatric research. Arch Gen Psychiat 26:57, 1972.

Fernstrom MH, et al. Twenty-four hour intake in patients with anorexia nervosa and in healthy control subjects. Biol Psychiatry 36:696, 1994.

Fisher M, et al. Eating disorders in adolescents: A background paper. J Adolesc Health 16:420, 1995.

Forbes GB, et al. Body composition and the energy cost of weight gain. Hum Nutr: Clin Nutr 36c:485, 1982.

Green E, Miller DS. Oxygen consumption of obese and anorectic patients. Proc Nutr Soc 34:14A, 1975.

Hardoff D, et al. Pathological consequences of eating disorders. Children's Hospital Quarterly 3:17, 1991.

Harris JA, Benedict FG. A Biometric Study of Basal Metabolism in Man. Washington, DC: Carnegie Institute, 1919, p. 266.

Holman RT, et al. Patients with anorexia nervosa demonstrate deficiencies of selected fatty acids, compensatory changes in nonessential fatty acids and decreased fluidity of plasma lipids. J Nutr 125:901, 1995.

Hurst PS, et al. Teeth, vomiting and diet: A study of the dental characteristics of seventeen anorexia nervosa patients. Postgrad Med J 53:298, 1977.

Katzman DK, Zipursky RB. Adolescents with anorexia nervosa: The impact of the disorder on bones and brains. In: Jacobson MS, Rees JM, Golden NH (eds.). Adolescent Nutritional Disorders. New York: Ann N Y Acad Sci 817:127, 1997.

Kaye WH, et al. Caloric intake necessary for weight maintenance in anorexia nervosa: Nonbulimics require greater caloric intake than bulimics. Am J Clin Nutr 44:435, 1986.

Kaye WH, et al. Relative importance of calorie intake needed to gain weight and level of physical activity in anorexia nervosa. Am J Clin Nutr 47:989, 1988.

Kaye WH, et al. Amounts of calories retained after binge eating and vomiting. Am J Psychiatry 150:969, 1993.

Keys A, et al. The Biology of Human Starvation, vols. 1-2. Minneapolis: University of Minnesota Press, 1950.

Kohn MR, et al. Cardiac arrest and delirium: Presentations of the refeeding syndrome in severely malnourished adolescents with anorexia nervosa. J Adolesc Health 22:239, 1998.

Kreipe R, et al. Eating disorders in adolescents: A position paper of the Society for Adolescent Medicine. J Adolesc Health 16:475, 1995.

Lambert M, et al. Hematological changes in anorexia nervosa are correlated with total body fat mass depletion. Int J Eating Disord 21:329, 1997.

Langan SM, Farrell PM. Vitamin E, vitamin A and essential fatty acid status of patients hospitalized for anorexia nervosa. Am J Clin Nutr 41:1054, 1985.

Lucas A. On the meaning of laboratory values in anorexia nervosa. Mayo Clin Proc 52:748, 1977.

Lucas AR, et al. 50-year trends in the incidence of anorexia nervosa in Rochester, Minn: A population-based study. Am J Psychiatry 148:917, 1991.

Luder E, Schebendach J. Nutrition management of eating disorders. Topics in Clinical Nutrition 8(3):48, 1993.

Melchior JC, et al. Energy expenditure economy induced by decrease in lean body mass in anorexia nervosa. Eur J Clin Nutr 43:793, 1989.

Mitchell JE, et al. Frequency and duration of binge eating episodes in patients with bulimia. Am J Psych 138:835, 1981.

Moreiras-Varela O, et al. Nutritional status and food habits assessed by dietary intake and anthropometrical parameters in anorexia nervosa. Int J Vitam Nutr Res 60:267, 1989.

Moukaddem M, et al. Increase in diet-induced thermogenesis at the start of refeeding in severely malnourished anorexia nervosa patients. Am J Clin Nutr 66:133, 1997.

Neumark-Sztainer D, et al. Adolescent vegetarians: A behavioral profile of a school-based population in Minnesota. Arch Pediatr Adolesc Med 151:833, 1997.

Nudel DB, et al. Altered exercise performance in patients with anorexia nervosa. J Pediatr 105:34, 1984.

Pirke KM, et al. Average total energy expenditure in anorexia nervosa, bulimia nervosa, and healthy young women. Biol Psychiatry 30:711, 1991.

Powers PS. Heart failure during treatment of anorexia nervosa. Am J Psych 139:1167, 1982.

Probst M, et al. Body composition in female anorexia nervosa patients. Br J Nutr 76:639, 1996.

Rock C, Yager J. Nutrition and eating disorders: A primer for clinicians. Int J Eating Dis 6:267, 1987.

Rock CL, Vasantharajan S. Vitamin status of eating disorder patients: Relationship to clinical indices and effect of treatment. Int J Eating Disord 18:257, 1995.

Russell GFM. The changing nature of anorexia nervosa. J Psychiatric Res 19:101, 1985.

Scalfi L, et al. Bioimpedance and resting energy expenditure in undernourished and refed anorectic patients. Eur J Clin Nutr 47:61, 1993.

Schebendach J, Nussbaum M. Nutrition management in adolescents with eating disorders. Adolescent Medicine: State of the Art Reviews 3(3):545, 1992.

Schebendach J, et al. Use of indirect calorimetry in the nutritional management of eating disorders. Int J Eating Disord 1:59, 1995.

Schebendach J, et al. Nutrient quality of diets of adolescents with anorexia nervosa (Abstract). J Adolesc Health 20:151, 1997.

Schebendach J, et al. Validation of an equation for calculation of resting energy expenditure in anorexia nervosa. J Psychosom Res, accepted for publication, 1998.

Stordy BJ, et al. Weight gain, thermic effect of glucose and resting metabolic rate during recovery from anorexia nervosa. Am J Clin Nutr 30:138, 1977.

Sullivan PF, et al. Elevated total cholesterol in bulimia nervosa. Int J Eating Disord 23:425, 1998.

Vaisman N, et al. Effect of refeeding on the energy metabolism of adolescent girls who have anorexia nervosa. Eur J Clin Nutr 45:527, 1991.

Walker J, et al. Caloric requirements for weight gain in anorexia nervosa. Am J Clin Nutr 32:1396, 1979.

Walsh BT, et al. Eating behavior of women with bulimia. Arch Gen Psychiatry 46:54, 1989.

Weltzin TE, et al. Feeding patterns in bulimia nervosa. Biol Psychiatry 30:1093, 1991.

Wurtman RJ, Wurtman JJ. Nutrients, neurotransmitter synthesis, and control of food intake. In: Stunkard AJ, Stellar E (eds.). Eating and Its Disorders. New York: Raven Press, 1984.

Yager J, et al. American Psychiatric Association practice guidelines for eating disorders. Am J Psychiatry 150:207, 1993.

ADDITIONAL REFERENCES

American Dietetic Association. Position Paper: Nutrition intervention in the treatment of anorexia nervosa, bulimia nervosa, and binge eating. J Am Diet Assoc 94:902, 1994.

Bhanji S, Mattingly D. Anorexia nervosa: Some observations on dieters and vomiters, cholesterol and carotene. Br J Psych 139:238, 1981.

Brownell KD, Fairburn CG. Eating Disorders and Obesity. New York: Gilford, 1995.

Forbes GB, et al. Body composition changes during recovery from anorexia nervosa: Comparison of two dietary regimens: Am J Clin Nutr 40:1137, 1984.

Gwirtsman HE, et al. Energy intake and dietary macro nutrient content in women with anorexia nervosa and volunteers. J Am Diet Assoc 89:54, 1989.

Gwirtsman H, et al. Decreased caloric intake in normal weight patients with bulimia: Comparison with female volunteers. Am J Clin Nutr 49:86, 1989.

Keel PK, et al. Long-term outcome of bulimia nervosa. Arch Gen Psychiat 56:63, 1999.

Kensiger G. Binge eating, psychopathology and maladaptive eating behaviors. Dietetics in Developmental and Psychiatric Disorders Newsletter 95:1109, 1995.

Krahn DD, et al. Changes in resting energy expenditure and body composition in AN patients during refeeding. J Am Diet Assoc 93:434, 1993.

Kratina K, King N. Disordered eating treatment strategies: Focusing on a food/feeling journal. Scan's Pulse 14(4):8, 1995.

Melve KK, Baerheim A. Signs of subclinical eating disorders in teenagers. Scand J Prim Health Care 12:197, 1994.

Mordasini R, et al. Secondary type II hyperlipoproteinemia in patients with anorexia nervosa. Metabolism 27:71, 1978.

Moyano D, et al. Plasma total-homocysteine in anorexia nervosa. Eur J Clin Nutr 52:172, 1998.

Newman MM, et al. Relationship of clinical factors to caloric requirements in subtypes of eating disorders. Biol Psychiatry 22:1253, 1987.

Piaget J, Inhelder B. The Growth of Logical Thinking from Childhood to Adolescence. New York: Basic Books, 1958.

Reiff D, Reiff K. Eating disorders: Nutrition therapy in the recovery process. Rockville, MD: Aspen Publishers, 1992.

Schebendach J, et al. The metabolic responses to starvation and refeeding in adolescents with anorexia nervosa. In: Jacobson MS, Rees JM, Golden NH (eds.). Adolescent Nutritional Disorders. New York: Ann N Y Acad Sci 817:110, 1997.

Sedlet KJ, Ireton-Jones CS. Energy expenditure and the abnormal eating pattern of a bulimic: A case report. J Am Diet Assoc 89:74, 1989.

Thibault L, Roberge AG. The nutritional status of subjects with anorexia nervosa. Int J Vitam Nutr Res 57:447, 1987.

Vaisman N, et al. Energy expenditure and body composition in patients with anorexia nervosa. J Pediatr 113:919, 1988.

Viteri F. Primary protein-calorie malnutrition—clinical, biochemical, and metabolic changes. In: Suskind RM (ed.). Textbook of Pediatric Nutrition. New York: Raven Press, 1981.

Whisenant SL, Smith BA. Eating disorders: Current nutrition therapy and perceived needs in dietetic education and research. J Am Diet Assoc 95:1109, 1995.

Woodruff PWR, et al. Neuromyopathic complications in a patient with anorexia nervosa and vitamin C deficiency. Int J Eating Disord 16:205, 1994.

CHAPTER 25

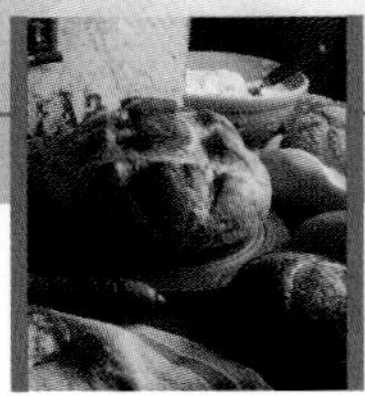

Nutrition for Exercise and Sports Performance

JACQUELINE R. BERNING, PhD, RD

Chapter Outline

- Energy Production
- Nutritional Requirements of Exercise
- Other Considerations
- Ergogenic Aids
- Weight Gain or Loss

Key Terms

ACTOMYOSIN—a complex of the proteins actin and myosin occurring in muscle

ADENOSINE DIPHOSPHATE (ADP)—a nucleotide involved in energy metabolism; it is produced by the hydrolysis of ATP and converted back to ATP by the processes of oxidative phosphorylation

ADENOSINE TRIPHOSPHATE (ATP)—a nucleotide occurring in all cells; is involved in energy transfer

AEROBIC METABOLISM—the transfer of usable energy through oxidative phosphorylation in the respiratory chain in the presence of oxygen

ANAEROBIC METABOLISM—the production of energy from glucose without the presence of oxygen

CREATINE PHOSPHATE (CP)—an important temporary storage form of high-energy phosphate in muscle cells

ERGOGENIC AID—a substance or practice that increases energy or work output

FEMALE ATHLETE TRIAD—a pattern in strenuously exercising athletes of estrogen deficiency and athletic amenorrhea, disordered eating and low body fat, and loss of bone mass

GLYCOGEN—the form of carbohydrate storage in animals

GLYCOGEN LOADING (GLYCOGEN SUPERCOMPENSATION)—a combination of exercise and high-carbohydrate diet that enables muscles to store glycogen beyond their normal capacity

GLYCOGENOLYSIS—the hydrolysis of glycogen to yield glucose

GLYCOLYSIS—the breaking down of glucose with or without the presence of oxygen into simpler compounds, chiefly pyruvate or lactate

LACTIC ACID—a product of anaerobic glucose metabolism

MITOCHONDRIA—spherical components in the cytoplasm of cells, which are the principal sites of the generation of energy in the form of ATP; they contain the enzymes of the Kreb's and fatty acid cycles and the respiratory pathway

MYOGLOBIN—a ferrous protoporphyrin protein similar to hemoglobin but with only one iron atom per molecule instead of four; contributes to the color of muscle and acts as a store of oxygen

OXYGEN DEBT—recovery oxygen consumption; the difference between O_2 consumption during the recovery period following exercise and the O_2 consumption at rest

RESPIRATORY EXCHANGE RATIO (RER)—the amount of CO_2 produced by the body divided by the amount of O_2 consumed by the body in metabolizing the dietary intake

SPORTS ANEMIA—a transient anemia seen in heavily training athletes characterized by a decrease in the red blood cell count, hemoglobin concentration, and packed cell volume, but with normal red blood cell morphology

THERMOREGULATION—the body's system for maintaining appropriate temperatures by transferring heat from the body core to the skin where it is dissipated through convection, radiation, sweat production and evaporation

V_{O_2}MAX—a measure of maximal oxygen uptake; liters of O_2 consumed per kilogram of body weight per minute

The past two decades have seen an incredible interest in physical fitness and sport among Americans. Nutrition is an important complement of any physical fitness program and it is generally accepted that a balanced eating style is an integral part of any fitness or sports program. The main dietary goal for active individuals is to obtain adequate nutrition to optimize health and fitness or sports performance. Unfortunately, there is much misinformation regarding a proper diet for physically active individuals. In the quest for success many health- and fitness-conscious individuals will try any dietary regimen or nutritional supplement in the hope of reaching a new level of wellness or physical performance. It is important for professionals in the field of nutrition to have a good working knowledge and understanding of exercise science and sports nutrition so that they may help their clients perform closer to their potential (website: www.fitnesslink.com/govcouncil).

ENERGY PRODUCTION

The human body must continuously be supplied with energy to perform its many complex functions. As an individual's energy demands increase with exercise, the body must provide additional energy or the exercise will cease. Two metabolic systems supply energy for the body—one dependent on oxygen (**aerobic metabolism**) and the other able to function without oxygen **(anaerobic metabolism).** Both of these systems provide energy; however, the use of one system over the other depends on the duration, intensity, and type of physical activity.

ATP

The body obtains its continuous supply of fuel through an energy-rich compound called **adenosine triphosphate** or simply **ATP.** ATP is the fuel used for all the energy-requiring processes found within the cells of the body. ATP has been called the *energy currency* of the cell.

The energy produced from the breakdown of ATP activates the energy-requiring processes of muscle contraction. The energy from ATP is transferred to the contractile filaments (myosin and actin) in the muscle, which form an attachment of actin to the cross-bridges on the myosin molecule, thus forming **actomyosin.** Once activated the myofibrils slide past each other and cause the muscle to contract.

ATP-CP

Although ATP is the main currency for energy in the body, it is stored in limited amounts. In fact, only about 3 oz of ATP is stored in the body at any one time. This provides only enough energy for several seconds of exercise. ATP must constantly be resynthesized to provide a constant energy source during exercise. As ATP is split, releasing energy, the resulting **adenosine diphosphate (ADP)** is combined with enzymatically released high-energy phosphate from **creatine phosphate (CP)** to resynthesize ATP. The concentration of high-energy CP in the muscle is five times that of ATP.

Creatine kinase catalyzes the reaction of CP with ADP and inorganic phosphate to produce creatine and regenerate ATP. It is the fastest and most immediate means of replenishing ATP, and it does so without the use of oxygen (anaerobic). Although this system has great power, it is limited due to the concentration of CP found in the muscles (see creatine on page 552).

The energy released from this ATP-CP system will sustain an all-out exercise effort for about 5 to 8 seconds such as in a powerlift, tennis serve, or sprint. If the all-out effort continues for longer than 8 seconds, or if moderate exercise is to proceed for longer periods, an additional source of energy, derived from the energy-providing nutrients, must be provided for the resynthesis of ATP (Fig. 25–1). The production of ATP carries on within the muscle cells through two important pathways . . . anaerobic or aerobic metabolism.

Anaerobic or Lactic Acid Pathway

The most rapidly available mechanism for supplying ATP for more than a few seconds is the process of anaerobic **glycolysis.** In this pathway the energy in glucose is released without the presence of oxygen. **Lactic acid** is the end product of anaerobic glycolysis. With the transference of two hydrogen atoms to pyruvic acid, thus converting it to lactic acid, a vital coenzyme (nicotinic acid dehydrogenase) is freed to participate in further ATP synthesis. The amount of ATP furnished is relatively small (the process is only 30% efficient). This pathway contributes energy during an all-out effort lasting up to 60 to 120 seconds. Examples would be a 440-yard sprint and many sprint swimming events.

Although the production of ATP is rapid during glycolysis, it is limited and it does produce lactic acid. Lactic acid is rapidly removed from the muscle and transported into the bloodstream. It is eventually converted to energy, in either muscle, liver, or brain, or it is converted to **glycogen.** This con-

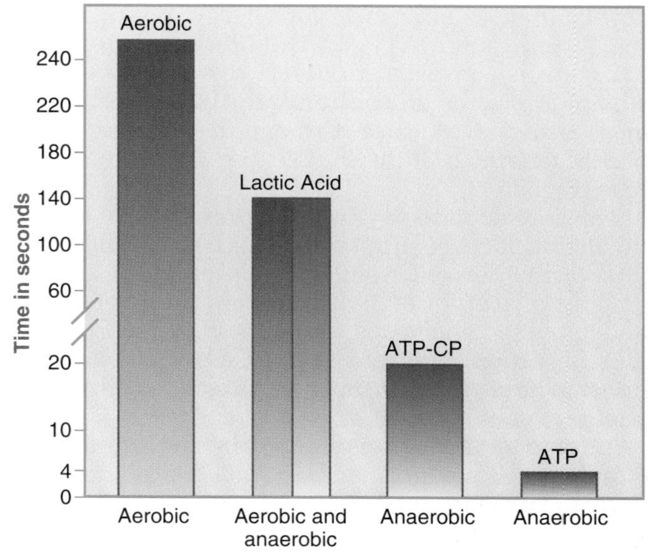

FIGURE 25–1 Classification of activities based on duration of performance and the predominant pathways of energy production.

version to glycogen occurs in the liver and to some extent in muscle, particularly among trained athletes.

Although this process provides immediate protection from the consequences of insufficient oxygen, it cannot continue indefinitely. When exercise continues at intensities beyond the body's ability to supply oxygen and convert lactic acid to fuel, lactic acid accumulates in the blood, eventually lowering the pH to a level that interferes with enzymatic action, leading to fatigue. An **oxygen debt** can develop. Also, the amount of ATP produced through glycolysis is very small compared with that available through aerobic pathways. Substrate for this reaction is limited to glucose from blood sugar or the glycogen stored in the muscle. Liver glycogen contributes but is limited in amount.

Aerobic Pathway

Production of ATP in amounts sufficient to support continued muscle activity for longer than 90 to 120 seconds requires the input of oxygen. Energy stored in nutrients is transferred to the high-energy phosphate bonds in ATP through a complex series of enzymatically guided reactions, involving separation of hydrogen atoms from the parent compounds. Vital to the continuation of these reactions is the presence of coenzymes, which act as hydrogen acceptors until the process of oxidative phosphorylation culminates with the formation of ATP.

Ultimately, hydrogen is combined with oxygen to form water, and the coenzymes are thus freed to accept more hydrogen in a continuation of the process. If sufficient oxygen is not present to combine with the hydrogen, no further ATP is forthcoming. Therefore, the oxygen furnished through the process of respiration is of vital importance.

In the aerobic pathway, glucose can be broken down far more efficiently for energy, producing 18 to 19 times more ATP. In the presence of oxygen, pyruvate is converted to acetyl coenzyme A (CoA), which enters the **mitochondria.** In the mitochondria, acetyl CoA goes through the Krebs cycle, which generates 36 to 38 ATP per molecule of glucose (Fig. 25–2).

The aerobic pathway can also provide ATP by metabolizing fats and proteins. The beta oxidation of fatty acids derived from lipolysis provides a large amount of acetyl CoA, which enters the Krebs cycle and provides enormous amounts of ATP. Proteins may be catabolized into acetyl CoA or Krebs cycle intermediates or they may be directly oxidized as another source of ATP.

Aerobic metabolism is limited by the availability of substrate, a continuous and adequate supply of oxygen and the availability of coenzymes. At the onset of exercise and with the increase of exercise intensity, the capability of the cardiovascular system to supply adequate oxygen becomes a limiting factor, and this is largely due to the level of conditioning.

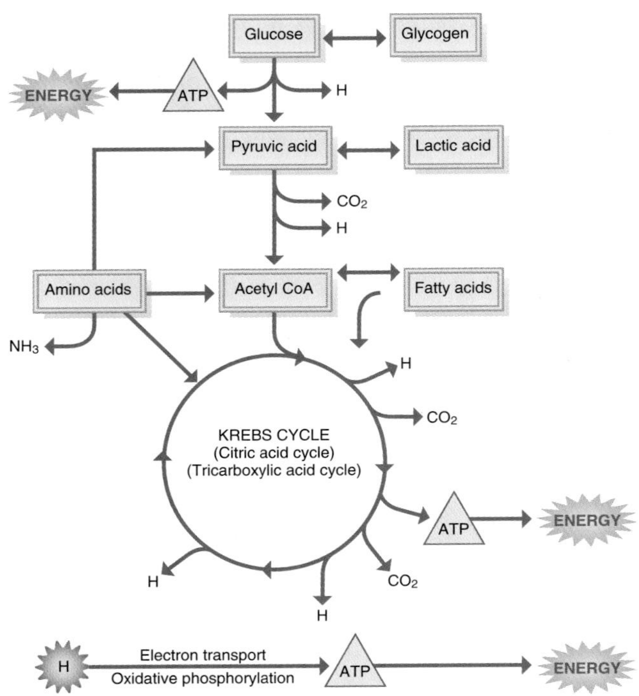

FIGURE 25–2 Pathways of energy production. H, hydrogen atoms; ATP, adenosine triphosphate; CoA, coenzyme A.

Energy Continuum

Although each of the systems above produce ATP for the exercising muscle, an individual who is exercising may use one or more energy pathways for the physical activity. For example, at the beginning of any physical activity ATP is produced anaerobically. As exercise continues, the lactic acid system is producing ATP for exercise. If the individual continues to exercise and does so at a moderate intensity for a prolonged period, then the aerobic pathway will become the dominant pathway for fuel. On the other hand, the anaerobic pathway provides most of the energy for short-duration, high-intensity exercise such as sprinting, the 200-meter swim, or high-power, high-intensity moves in basketball, football, or soccer.

The production of ATP for exercise is on a continuum that depends on the availability of oxygen. Other factors that influence oxygen capabilities and thus energy pathways, are the capacity for intense exercise and its duration. These two factors are inversely related. For example, an athlete cannot perform high-power, high-intensity moves over a prolonged period. To do this he or she would have to decrease the intensity of the exercise in order to increase the duration (Fig. 25–3).

The aerobic pathway cannot tolerate the same level of intensity as the duration increases, due to the decreased availability of oxygen and accumulation of lactic acid. As the duration of exercise increases, power output decreases. The contribution

Duration of maximal exercise									
	Seconds			Minutes					
	10	30	60	2	4	10	30	60	120
Anaerobic (%)	90	80	70	50	35	15	5	2	1
Aerobic (%)	10	20	30	50	65	85	95	98	99

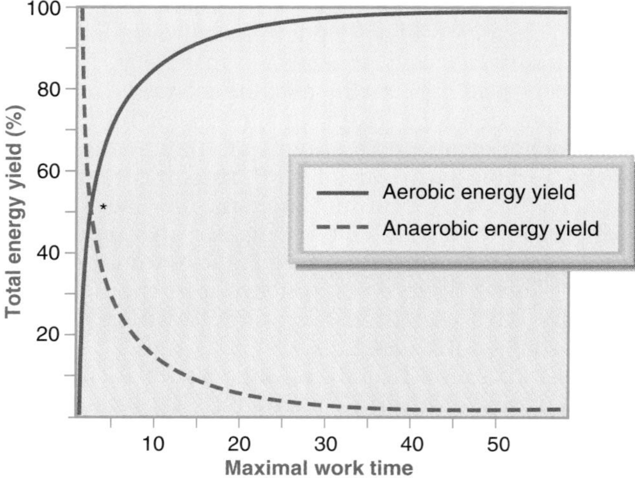

FIGURE 25–3 Relative contribution of aerobic and anaerobic energy during maximal physical activity of various durations. Note that 90 to 120 seconds of maximal effort requires 50% of the energy from each of the aerobic and anaerobic processes. This will also be the point when the lactic acid pathway for energy production will be at its maximum.

of energy-yielding nutrients must be considered also. As the duration of exercise lengthens, the contribution of fats as an energy source becomes greater. The opposite is true for high-intensity exercise. As intensity increases, the body relies more on carbohydrate as its fuel source.

Fuel of Muscle Contraction

Sources of Fuel

Proteins, fats, and carbohydrates are all possible sources of fuel for muscle contraction. The glycolytic pathway is restricted to glucose, which can originate in dietary carbohydrates or can be synthesized from the carbon skeletons of certain amino acids through the process of *gluconeogenesis*. The Krebs cycle is fueled by three-carbon fragments of glucose, two-carbon fragments of fatty acids, and carbon skeletons of specific amino acids, primarily alanine. All of these substrates are used most of the time during exercise. However, the intensity and duration of the exercise determine the relative rates of substrate utilization.

Substrate Choice

A variety of factors determine which type of fuel the muscle will use during exercise. These include intensity, duration, fitness level of the individual, and dietary intake.

INTENSITY

The intensity of the exercise is particularly important in determining what fuel will be used by the body. High-intensity, short-duration exercise has to rely on anaerobic production of ATP because not enough oxygen can be drawn into the body during the activity. Because oxygen is not available for aerobic pathways, only glucose stored in the form of glycogen can be broken down anaerobically for fuel. When glucose is broken down anaerobically, muscle glycogen is used 18 to 19 times faster than when glucose is broken down aerobically. When individuals are performing in high-intensity workouts or competitive races, muscle glycogen is broken down at a very rapid rate and the athlete runs the risk of running out of muscle glycogen before the event or exercise is done.

Sports that use both the anaerobic and aerobic pathways also require a higher glycogen utilization rate and the athlete also runs the risk of running out of fuel before the race or exercise is finished. Sports like basketball, football, soccer, and swimming are good examples of activities where athletes have a higher glycogen utilization rate due to their intermittent bursts of high-intensity sprints and running drills. In moderate-intensity sports or exercise like jogging, hiking, aerobic dance, gymnastics, cycling, and recreational swimming, about half of the energy for these activities comes from the aerobic breakdown of muscle glycogen (Fig. 25–4). The other half comes from circulating blood glucose and fatty acids.

Moderate- to low-intensity exercise, such as walking, is entirely fueled by the aerobic pathway, thus a greater proportion of fat can be used to create ATP for energy. Fatty acids cannot supply ATP during high-intensity exercise because fat cannot be

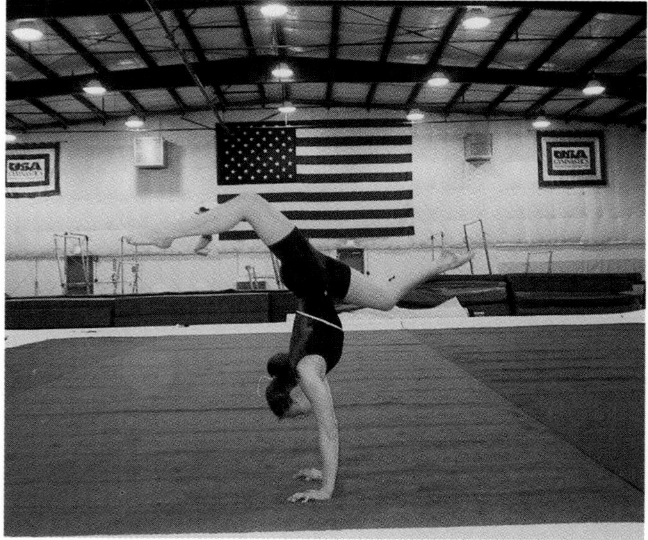

FIGURE 25–4 Gymnastics, a moderate form of exercise, requires a moderate amount of energy.

broken down fast enough to provide the energy. Also, fat provides less energy per liter of oxygen consumed than does glucose (4.65 kcal/L of O_2 versus 5.01 kcal/L of O_2). Therefore, when less oxygen is available at high-intensity activities, there is a definite advantage for the muscles to be able to use glycogen because less oxygen is required to produce energy from glycogen.

In general, both glucose and fatty acids provide fuel for exercise, in proportions depending on the intensity and duration of the exercise and the fitness of the athlete. Exertion of very high intensity and short duration draws primarily on reserves of ATP and CP. High-intensity exercise that continues for more than a few seconds depends on anaerobic glycolysis. During exercise of low to moderate intensity (< 60% **Vo_2max**), energy is derived mainly from fatty acids. Carbohydrate becomes a larger fraction of the energy source as intensity increases until, at an intensity level of 85% to 90% Vo_2max, carbohydrate from glycogen is the principal energy source and the duration of activity is limited (Fig. 25–5).

DURATION

How long the activity lasts also determines what substrate is used during the exercise bout. For example, the longer the time spent exercising the greater the contribution of fat as the fuel. Fat can supply up to 60% to 70% of the energy needs for ultra-endurance events lasting 6 to 10 hours. As the duration of exercise increases the reliance on aerobic metabolism becomes greater and a greater amount of ATP can be produced from fatty acids. However, it must be noted that fat cannot be metabolized unless carbohydrate is available. Therefore, muscle glycogen and blood glucose are the limiting factors in human performance of any type of intensity or duration.

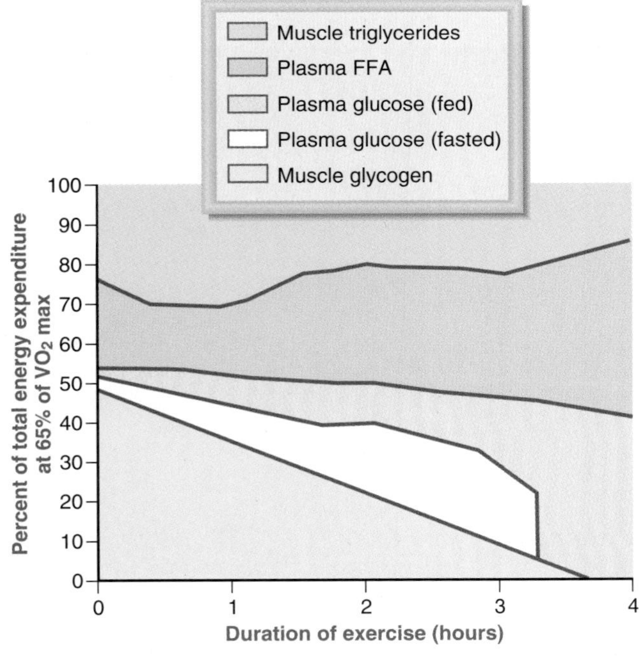

FIGURE 25–5 Sources of energy during 4 hours of exercise.

EFFECT OF TRAINING

The length of time that an athlete can oxidize fatty acids as a fuel source is related to the athlete's conditioning as well as exercise intensity. In addition to improving cardiovascular systems involved in oxygen delivery, training increases the number of mitochondria and the levels of enzymes involved in the aerobic synthesis of ATP, thus increasing the capacity for fatty acid metabolism. Increases in mitochondria with aerobic training are seen mainly in the type IIA (intermediate fast-twitch) muscle fibers. These fibers very quickly lose their aerobic capacity with cessation of aerobic training, reverting to the genetic baseline.

These changes from training result in a lower **respiratory exchange ratio (RER),** lower blood lactate and catecholamine levels, and a lower net muscle glycogen breakdown at a certain power output. These metabolic adaptations enhance the ability of muscle to oxidize all fuels, but especially fat.

DIET

The makeup of the exercising individual's diet will also determine which substrate is used during an exercise bout. If an athlete is consuming a high-carbohydrate diet then he or she will use more glycogen as fuel for the exercise. If the diet is high in fat, then more fat will be oxidized as a fuel source. This does not mean that the athlete or exercising individual should consume a high-fat diet. Even the leanest athlete has more than enough fat stored in his body to fuel any long or endurance exercise. (See "*Focus On:* The 40-30-30 Diet.")

Eating more fat, especially saturated fat, can increase the athlete's risk for heart disease and other life-style diseases associated with high-fat diets. The goal is to increase the availability of fat as a fuel during exercise. The proper way to do that is by training, not consuming a high-fat diet. Athletes who have tried to perform on high-fat diets find that their performance suffers due to lower glycogen stores. Glycogen stores are limited because the amount of carbohydrate consumed in the diet is limited. Low muscle glycogen stores limit endurance and the ability of the athlete to perform high-intensity exercise, which may occur during a competition.

NUTRITIONAL REQUIREMENTS OF EXERCISE

Fluid

Proper fluid balance maintains blood volume, which, in turn, supplies blood to the skin for body temperature regulation. Because exercise produces

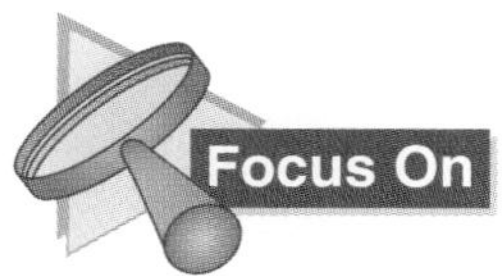

The 40-30-30 Diet by Ellen Coleman, MS, MPH, RD

A popular sports nutrition dietary fad revolves around the myth that high-carbohydrate diets impair athletic performance and make athletes fat. Proponents of this dietary regimen believe that food has a tremendous impact on the complex hormonal systems that help control physiologic processes within the body—processes such as cellular oxygen transfer, maintenance of blood glucose, and regulation of body fat.

Athletes must supposedly eat the perfect ratio of protein, carbohydrate, and fat at each meal and snack to control these hormonal systems and thus reach their maximum performance and ideal weight. This "perfect ratio" consists of 40% carbohydrate, 30% protein, and 30% fat at each meal and snack. Proponents claim that this diet promotes optimal athletic performance and health by altering the production of eicosanoids so that the body makes more "good" eicosanoids than "bad" ones. A balanced production of eicosanoids regulates the local tissue response to stimulatory events. (See Chapters 3 and 43 for a discussion of eicosanoids.)

The carbohydrate/protein/fat ratio of the 40-30-30 diet allegedly maintains the proper balance between the hormones insulin and glucagon. The correct insulin-glucagon balance in turn supposedly increases the production of "good" eicosanoids that inhibit platelet aggregation, promote vasodilation, and are anti-inflammatory. Proponents of the diet recommend limiting carbohydrate to keep the body from producing too much insulin, because high insulin levels allegedly increase the production of "bad" eicosanoids. Prostaglandin-E_2, thromboxanes, and leukotrienes are supposedly "bad" eicosanoids because they promote platelet aggregation, vasoconstriction, and are proinflammatory. "Bad" eicosanoids and high insulin levels purportedly impair athletic performance by reducing oxygen transfer to the cells, lowering blood glucose levels, and interfering with body fat utilization.

Proponents of the 40-30-30 diet also claim that insulin makes it hard for people to stay or become thin. Basically, insulin is treated as the "monster" hormone that makes people fat. Insulin supposedly does this by taking carbohydrate and storing it as fat, rather than allowing the body to use it for energy.

Protein supposedly increases glucagon levels, and glucagon helps to increase the production of "good" eicosanoids by opposing the effect of insulin. Protein then, along with carbohydrate in a meal or snack, promotes this "glucagon favorable diet," which supposedly maintains blood glucose, increases endurance by increasing fatty acid utilization, and reduces body fat by increasing the utilization of stored fat.

The scientific basis for this diet for athletes can be faulted on many fronts, beginning with the claim that high-carbohydrate diets increase insulin levels, thereby causing low blood glucose and suppressing fat mobilization. During exercise, serum glucose levels increase while serum insulin levels fall. This occurs due to the exercise-induced rise in the catacholamines (epinephrine and norepinephrine) and growth hormone, which inhibit the release of insulin from the pancreas. This enhances liver glucose output by making the liver more sensitive to the effects of glucagon and epinephrine. The hormonal changes that occur during exercise prompt greater fat oxidation.

Endurance training also causes several major adaptations in the muscles that increase fat utilization. First, endurance training increases the number of capillaries in the trained muscles, so that the muscles receive more blood and oxygen. Second, endurance training increases the activity of the specific muscle enzymes that are responsible for burning fat. Third, endurance training increases tissue insulin sensitivity, resulting in lower plasma insulin levels.

The claim that a high-carbohydrate diet promotes greater body fat storage is also unfounded. Insulin is not a "monster" hormone—it is required for the transport of glucose into the body's cells, where it is used to fuel all activities. Insulin-mediated glucose uptake is also necessary for muscle and liver glycogen synthesis—the primary fuel for endurance exercise.

The 40-30-30 diet does not improve access to the body's fat stores so that more fat is burned during exercise. Carbohydrate, not fat, is the preferred energy source during exercise at or above 70% of Vo_2max—the intensity at which most endurance athletes train and compete. Athletes do not usually work out long enough to burn significant amounts of fat during exercise. Rather, it is the caloric deficit resulting from the exercise session that promotes body fat utilization. And, as for gradual loss of body fat, that comes from burning more calories than are consumed at the table, not from some special dietary ratio. Because endurance training already creates a metabolic milieu favorable for fat metabolism, the best way to crank up the body's fat-burning ability is to keep working out.

heat, which must be eliminated from the body to maintain appropriate body temperatures, regular fluid intake is essential for maintaining a body temperature that maximizes performance.

The human body is not efficient at converting potential energy from oxygen and nutrients into mechanical energy. During exercise only about one fourth of this potential energy is converted into mechanical energy, resulting in about 75% of the energy turnover generated as heat. Most of the heat generated by exercising muscle transfers to the blood, circulating through the body and raising core temperature. The amount of heat produced during exercise, even in physically fit individuals, is enough to raise core body temperatures by 1°C every 5 to 8 minutes. Without effective means to dissipate this heat, moderate-intensity exercise could raise body temperatures to lethal levels in 15 to 30 minutes.

The body maintains appropriate temperatures by a means of a system referred to as **thermoregulation.** As heat is generated in the muscles during exercise it is transferred via the blood to the body's core. Increased core temperature results in increased blood flow to the skin, where, in cool to moderate ambient temperatures, heat is transferred to the environment by convection, radiation, and evaporation.

Environmental conditions have a large impact on thermoregulation. When ambient temperatures range from warm to hot, the body must dissipate the heat generated from exercise as well as the heat absorbed from the environment. When this occurs, the body relies solely on the evaporation of sweat to maintain appropriate body temperatures. Thus, maintaining hydration becomes crucial when ambient temperatures reach or exceed 36°C. The hotter the temperature, the more important sweating is for body heat dissipation.

Humidity also affects the body's ability to dissipate heat to a greater extent than air temperatures. As humidity increases, the rate at which sweat evaporates decreases, which means more sweat drips off the body without transferring heat from the body to the environment. Combining the effects of a hot, humid environment with a large metabolic heat load produced during exercise taxes the thermoregulatory system to its maximum. Ensuring proper and adequate fluid intake is key to reducing the risk of heat stress.

Fluid Balance

The body fluid of healthy individuals is conserved on a daily basis by factors that control intake and output of both water and electrolytes. Antidiuretic hormone (vasopressin; ADH) and the renin–angiotensin–aldosterone system are hormonal control mechanisms that maintain the osmolality, sodium content, and volume of extracellular fluids and play a major role in the regulation of fluid balance.

There is a continuous loss of water from the skin and respiratory tract plus intermittent losses from the kidneys and gastrointestinal tract. When fluid is lost from the body in the form of sweat, plasma volume decreases and plasma osmolality increases. The kidneys, under hormonal control, regulate water and solute excretion in excess of the obligatory urine loss. However, when the body is subjected to hot environments, whether the heat load is imposed internally or externally, certain hormonal adjustments occur to maintain body function. The body begins by trying to conserve both water and sodium. The pituitary gland releases ADH to increase water absorption from the kidneys, which causes the urine to become more concentrated, thus conserving fluid and making the urine a dark gold color.

This feedback process helps to conserve body water and blood volume. At the same time, *aldosterone* is released from the adrenal cortex and acts on the renal tubules to increase the reabsorption of sodium, which helps maintain the correct osmotic pressure. These reactions also activate thirst mechanisms in the body; however, in situations where water losses are increased acutely, such as in athletic workouts or competition, the thirst response can be delayed, making it difficult for athletes to trust their thirsts to ingest enough fluid to offset the volume of fluid that is lost during training and competition. A loss of 1.5 to 2 liters of fluid is necessary before the thirst mechanism kicks in, and this level of water loss already has a serious impact on temperature control. Athletes need to rehydrate on a timed basis rather than as a reaction to thirst, and it should be enough to maintain the pre-exercise weight.

It appears that plain water is not the best beverage to consume following exercise to replace the water lost as sweat. The replacement of electrolytes, particularly sodium, as well as water is essential for effective rehydration. If sufficient amounts of sodium and water are ingested, plasma osmolality and sodium concentration do not decline, as may occur if plain water is ingested. As a result, the circulating levels of vasopressin and aldosterone are maintained, and the excess urine output that would otherwise occur, even though the body is still in net negative fluid balance, is prevented.

Also, when there are no restrictions on fluid intake, maintenance of the plasma osmolality and the circulating sodium concentration plays an important role in maintaining the drive to drink, thus ensuring that an adequate volume of fluid is consumed. Several researchers (Costill and Sparks, 1973; Gonzalez-Alonso et al., 1992; Nose et al., 1988) have found that rehydration with water alone dilutes the blood rapidly, increases its volume, and stimulates urine output. Blood dilution lowers both sodium and the volume-dependent part of the thirst drive, thus removing much of the drive to drink and replace fluid losses.

Another electrolyte that is involved with maintaining body fluids is potassium. Potassium is the major ion of the intracellular fluid. As the major electrolyte inside the body cells, potassium works in close association with sodium and chloride in the maintenance of body fluids and in the generation of electrical impulses in the nerves and the muscles, including the heart. Potassium balance, like sodium balance, is also regulated by aldosterone. Potassium regulation in the body is precise and deficiencies are rare although they may occur during fasting, episodes of diarrhea, and diuretic use.

Most researchers agree that there is little loss of potassium through sweat. Nevertheless, Nadel et al. (1990) suggest that inclusion of potassium in beverages consumed after sweat loss may aid in the movement of water into the intracellular spaces in rehydration.

Fluid Absorption

Most athletes believe that as soon as they ingest a fluid it is rehydrating their system. However, the speed at which fluid is absorbed depends on a number of different factors, including the amount, type and osmolality of the fluid consumed, and the rate of gastric emptying.

The proximal small intestine (duodenum and jejunum) is the primary site of fluid absorption where about 50% to 60% of any given fluid load is absorbed. The colon absorbs approximately 80% to 90% of the fluid it receives, but accounts for only about 15% of the total fluid load. Intestinal fluid absorption is a passive process and can occur against an osmotic gradient. The intestinal mucosa is a semipermeable membrane with relatively large aqueous channels. Thus, in the presence of an osmotic gradient there is a large and rapid movement of water across the duodenojejunum, compared with only a modest water flux across the colon (Gisolfi, 1990).

Water-soluble electrolytes such as sodium can also rapidly move across the proximal intestines. Water movement occurs passively and generally depends on solute absorption. For example, if solute absorption is zero then water absorption is zero. However, Leiper and Maughan (1986b) found that the perfusion of a hypotonic solution through the jejunum increases water absorption with increasing solute absorption. This suggests that the greater osmotic gradient the greater the water movement from the intestinal lumen to the blood. It is also true that, although water movement is usually passive, water can be absorbed against a concentration gradient.

FACTORS ENHANCING FLUID ABSORPTION

Glucose and Sodium. Because glucose is actively absorbed in the intestines, it can markedly increase both sodium and water absorption. It has been known for over 70 years that the small intestine absorbs certain hexoses faster than others. The first suggestion of selectivity of the intestinal membrane for simple sugars was made by Cori (1925), who found that sugars disappeared from the intestine at strikingly different rates galactose > glucose > fructose > mannose > xylose > arabinose.

It was established that galactose and glucose were actively absorbed against a concentration gradient and that fructose, mannose, xylose, and arabinose were not. According to Crane (1965) the glucose and sodium associate with a carrier in the microvilli on the intestinal cell. The complex travels to the inner side of the membrane where it disassociates, releasing the glucose and sodium. The sodium is then actively transported out of the cell, while the glucose is emptied into the bloodstream. It appears that the sodium ion attaches to the carrier first, changing the configuration of the carrier and allowing the glucose molecule to attach for transfer across the membrane, and then it assumes another shape when the site accommodates potassium going out of the cell.

Early studies indicate that water absorption is maximized when luminal glucose concentrations range from 1% to 3% (55–140 mM) (Malawer, 1965). However, most sports drinks contain two to three times this quantity without causing adverse gastrointestinal symptoms. If the concentration of glucose in the lumen reaches 10% (550 mOsm), it can cause fluid secretions and gastrointestinal distress (Gisolfi et al., 1990).

A recent comparison of the rates of absorption of popular sports drinks with water showed that fluid absorption rates for water and a 6% carbohydrate sports drink were similar (Ryan et al., 1998). Sports drinks with higher concentrations of carbohydrate (8% or 9%) had slower absorption rates and should not be used. To determine the concentration of carbohydrate in a sports drink, the grams of carbohydrate in a serving is divided by the weight of a serving of the drink, which is usually 240 g, the approximate weight of 1 cup of water (Table 25–1).

OSMOLALITY

Sports drinks are either hypertonic, isotonic, or hypotonic. Some evidence indicates that hypotonic solutions are more efficacious in maximizing water absorption than isotonic solutions (Leiper and Maughn, 1986a and 1986b). Although exercise produces a condition of hypertonic dehydration that may favor fluid absorption from a hypotonic solution, this concept requires further investigation in human subjects.

Fluid Requirements

SHORT-DURATION EVENTS

Athletes who participate in short-duration events often believe that they are not exposed to the heat stress that endurance athletes are exposed to, and that they do not need to worry about fluid consumption or hydration. However, athletes who participate in short-duration activities, such as sprint running in track and field, or stop-and-go sports like basketball, volleyball, or baseball, are just as likely to develop dehydration as are distance runners or ultra-marathoners. Although many athletes, like sprinters, have short-duration events, they may have to run several heats before making a championship event, thus exposing themselves to both environmental and internal heat stresses. All individuals who participate in physical activity or sports should be educated about the guidelines of drinking fluids to prevent dehydration.

It was once thought that if the physical activity was less than an hour, water would be the best choice for fluid replacement. However, researchers (Jackson et al., 1995) are finding that using a sports drink during high-intensity stop-and-go sports like basketball, volleyball, and sprint cycling helps delay fatigue and maintains hydration. Unfortunately, athletes who just consume water as a fluid replacement, even for short-term exercise, risk the chance of diluting the blood and increasing urine output, thus shutting off the drive to drink and becoming dehydrated.

Young children are more likely to participate in physical activities that are less than 60 minutes in

TABLE 25–1 SPORTS DRINK COMPARISON CHART

BEVERAGE	CHO SOURCE	% CHO	SODIUM (mg/8 oz)	POTASSIUM (mg/8 oz)	OTHER VITAMINS AND MINERALS
Gatorade Thirst Quencher (The Gatorade Company)	**Powder:** sucrose and glucose **Liquid:** sucrose & glucose/syrup solids	6	110 mg	25 mg	Chloride Phosphorus
Power-Ade (Coca-Cola)	High fructose corn syrup Maltodextrin	7.9	73 mg or less	33 mg	Chloride
All Sport (Pepsico)	High fructose corn syrup Maltodextrin	8–9	55 mg	55 mg	Chloride Phosphorus Calcium
Sportalyte (IDN/Pharmanex)	Glucose Fructose Maltodextrin	7	150 mg	70 mg	Magnesium Calcium Chloride Phosphorus Vitamins C, E
XLR8 (Advanced Nutritional)	Glucose Fructose Glucose polymers Maltose Glycerol	5.2	40 mg	30 mg	Calcium Magnesium
Quickick (Cramer Products)	Fructose Sucrose	4.7	116 mg	23 mg	Calcium Chloride Phosphorus
Hydra Fuel (Twin Labs)	Glucose polymers Glucose Fructose	7	25 mg	50 mg	Chloride Magnesium Chromium Phosphorus Vitamin C
10K (Suntry Water Group)	Sucrose Glucose Fructose	6	55 mg	30 mg	—
Everlast	Sucrose Fructose	6	100 mg	20 mg	—
Cytomax (Champion Nutrition)	Fructose corn syrup Sucrose	5	53 mg	100 mg	Chromium Magnesium
Coca-cola	High fructose corn syrup Sucrose	11	9.2 mg	Trace	Phosphorus
Diet Soft Drinks	None	0	0–25 mg	Low	Phosphorus
Orange Juice	Fructose Sucrose	11–15	2.7 mg	510 mg	Vitamins A, C Niacin Thiamin Riboflavin
Water	0	0	Low	Low	Low

(Compiled from product labels and sources provided by The Gatorade Company and from Burke ER, Berning JR. Training nutrition: The diet and nutrition guide for peak performance. Carmel, IN: Cooper Publishing, 1996.)

duration. Many youth soccer, t-ball, and basketball games are less than 60 minutes in duration. Children, like adults, do not drink enough when offered fluids ad libitum during exercise in hot and humid climates. But children are different from adults in that for any given level of dehydration, children's core temperatures rise faster than those of adults, putting them at far greater risk for heat stress. Children who participate in sports activities must be taught to prevent dehydration by drinking above and beyond thirst and drinking at frequent intervals, for example, every 20 minutes (Bar-Or et al., 1992).

A rule of thumb is that a child 10 years of age or younger should drink until he or she does not feel thirsty, and then should drink an additional half a glass (⅓ cup to ½ cup). Older children and adolescents should follow the same guidelines; however, they should consume an additional cup of fluid (8 oz). When relevant, regulations for competition should be modified to allow children to leave the playing field periodically in order to drink.

Other concerns with children are the palatability of the drink and its ability to stimulate further thirst. Prepubertal and early pubertal girls and boys prefer grape flavor to apple and orange flavors in sports drinks. This preference is apparent at rest, following a maximal exercise bout, and during rehydration after prolonged exercise in hot, dry conditions (Meyer et al., 1994). One of the hurdles to getting children to consume fluids is to provide fluids they like. Providing them a sports drink that will maintain the drive to drink and rehydrate them is the key to preventing active children from becoming dehydrated.

Table 25–2 gives the American College of Sports Medicine (ACSM, 1996) recommendations for fluid replacement during exercise. These guidelines emphasize the importance of an aggressive fluid-replacement plan designed to prevent even slight dehydration during training and competition (Murray, 1998).

ENDURANCE EVENTS

Marathoners talk of "hitting the wall." Cyclists speak of "bonking." Both groups attribute their fatigue in long events to drained fuel stores. Along with replacing fluids, athletes who participate in activities that last longer than an hour also need to be concerned about supplying the brain and muscles with a continuous supply of carbohydrate for energy.

When exercise lasts longer than an hour, blood glucose levels start to dwindle. After 1 to 3 hours of continuous cycling, running, or swimming at 65% to 80% of maximum effort, or after repeated bouts of intense sprinting at 85% plus of maximum effort, muscle glycogen stores may become depleted. In addition if only water is being consumed, blood glucose levels may be very low (hypoglycemia) and this will result in higher use of muscle glycogen. When muscle glycogen levels are low and blood glucose levels have dropped, no matter how fast an athlete wants to go, the body cannot respond, and the athlete "hits the wall" or runs out of available fuel.

The liver generally supplies glucose to maintain blood sugar for proper functioning of the central nervous system. As muscles run out of glycogen, they begin to take up glucose that is available in the blood, placing a drain on the liver glycogen stores. The longer the exercise bout, the greater the utilization of blood glucose by the muscles for energy. It appears that carbohydrate feedings improve performance by maintaining blood glucose levels at a time when muscle glycogen stores are diminished. This allows carbohydrate utilization and energy production to continue at high rates.

Athletes can help maintain the supply of energy by consuming about 25 to 30 g carbohydrate every half-hour during exercise. Most 8- to 12-oz servings of sport drinks provide about 15 to 20 g carbohydrate, so drinking 8 to 12 oz every 15 minutes should help to fight off the fatigue that occurs when the muscles and liver run out of glycogen.

TABLE 25–2 GUIDELINES FOR PROPER HYDRATION

Weigh in before and after exercise, especially during hot weather.
For each pound of body weight lost during exercise, drink 2 cups of fluid.
Do not restrict fluids before or during an event.
Drink at least 8–16 oz (1–2 cups) of fluid 2 h before practice or competition.
Drink at least 4–8 oz of fluid immediately before exercise.
Drink at least 4–8 oz of fluid every 15–20 min during training and competition.
Drink at least 8–16 oz of fluid after exercise.
Drink at least 8 oz of fluid with each meal.
Drink at least 8 oz of fluid between meals.
The replacement drink should contain 80–120 mg sodium per 8 oz.
The replacement drink should contain 6–8% carbohydrate either as glucose, glucose polymers, or fructose.
The drink should be cool.

Nutrients

An athlete's energy and nutrient requirements vary with weight, height, age, sex, and metabolic rate and with the type, frequency, intensity, and duration of training. Because the emotional and physical stress of training and competition, combined with hectic travel schedules, affect dietary intake, adequate caloric and essential nutrient intake must be planned carefully to meet requirements for training and fitness.

Depending on the training regimen, athletes need to consume at least 50%, but ideally 60% to 70% of their total calories from carbohydrate. The remaining calories should be obtained from protein (10–15%) and fat (20–30%). Calories and nutrients should come from a wide variety of foods on a daily basis.

Carbohydrate

The first source of glucose for the exercising muscle is its own glycogen store. When this is depleted, **glycogenolysis** and then gluconeogenesis (both in the liver) maintain the glucose supply. During endurance exercise that exceeds 90 minutes, such as marathon running, muscle glycogen stores become progressively lower. When they drop to critically low levels, high-intensity exercise cannot be maintained. In practical terms, the athlete is exhausted and must either stop exercising or drastically reduce the pace.

Glycogen depletion may also be a gradual process, occurring over repeated days of heavy training, in which muscle glycogen breakdown exceeds its replacement as well as during high-intensity exercise that is repeated several times during competition or training. For example, a distance runner who averages 10 miles per day, but does not take the time to consume enough carbohydrates in his diet, or the swimmer who completes several interval sets at above her maximal oxygen consumption can both deplete glycogen stores rapidly.

In a classic study Costill and associates (1977b) compared glycogen synthesis on a 40% carbohydrate diet to that on a 70% carbohydrate diet during repeated days of 2-hour workouts. On the low-carbohydrate diet, the muscle glycogen stores dropped lower with each successive day of training. After several days of the diet and exercise regimen, the athletes had low muscle glycogen stores and could not exercise at even a moderate intensity. The high-carbohydrate diet provided nearly maximal repletion of the muscle glycogen stores after the strenuous training. The high-carbohydrate or *glycogen loading* diet provided the athletes with muscle glycogen values that remained above the 100 mmol/kg and they were able to continue the heavy training. This study and others suggest that athletes who fail to consume enough carbohydrate on a daily basis while training, will possibly decrease endurance as well as exercise performance.

It is suggested that athletes in heavy training should consume a carbohydrate intake of 7 to 10 g/kg body weight per day to help prevent daily carbohydrate and glycogen depletion. This means that a 70-kg (154 lb) athlete would consume 350 to 700 g carbohydrate per day. Table 25–3 lists several products that could be consumed during or after exercise for the maintenance of blood glucose or for glycogen resynthesis.

Types of Carbohydrate

The optimal type of carbohydrate for the athlete is still debatable. One study by Costill et al. (1981) compared the effects of simple and complex carbohydrate consumption during a 48-hour period after a glycogen-depleting exercise. During the first 24 hours, no differences were found in muscle glycogen synthesis; however, at 48 hours, the complex carbohydrates resulted in significantly greater muscle glycogen synthesis than the simple carbohydrates. However, Kiens et al. (1990) reported that increases in muscle glycogen content were significantly greater during the first 6 hours after exercise with simple rather than complex carbohydrate and that plasma insulin levels were greater after the intake of simple carbohydrates.

The question of which type of carbohydrate is better for athletic performance may be better understood if the carbohydrate is classified by its physiologic reaction in the body, by its glycemic index, rather than by its structure. *Glycemic index* represents the ratio of the area under the blood glucose curve resulting from the ingestion of a given quantity of carbohydrate and the area under the glucose curve resulting from the ingestion of the same quantity of white bread or glucose. Coyle and Hargreaves both recommend that carbohydrates with a moderate to high glycemic index be consumed after exercise. (Coyle, 1991; Hargreaves, 1991) Indeed, preliminary work (Burke et al., 1993) has demon-

TABLE 25–3 RECOMMENDATIONS FOR USE OF SPORTS FOODS

		GUIDELINES FOR CONSUMPTION IN EXERCISE		
SPORT FOOD	CHARACTERISTICS	Before	During	After
Sport drink	*CHO: 5–7% by volume (about 14 g/8 oz) *Sodium: 20–30 mEq/L (110–165 mg/8 oz) *Multiple CHO with high glycemic index	0.5 L (16 oz) 1 h prior to exercise	150–300 mL every 15–20 min (20–40 oz/h)	0.75 L/0.5 lb body weight lost (24 oz/1 lb lost)
High CHO energy drink	*CHO: >13% by volume (more than 100 g/8 oz) *Optional B vitamins: thiamin, niacin, and riboflavin at 10–40% of RDA	0.5 L (16 oz) 2–5 h prior to exercise	Typically used as part of a high-carbohydrate diet rather than during the event	Immediately after and at 1-h intervals to deliver 1 g CHO/kg body weight
Sports bar	*CHO: >70% of total kcal *High glycemic index *Fat: low (1–2 g/bar) or absent *Vitamins and minerals not critical components	One bar 2 h prior to exercise	Usually not advised except for those desiring solid foods during long-duration events	One to two bars immediately after exercise and with daily meals as desired
Sport shake	*CHO: >65% of total kcal (>18 g/100 mL) *High glycemic index *Fat: not to exceed 25% of total kcal *Protein: 15–20% of total kcal *Vitamins and minerals: optional at low levels (10–40% of RDA)	0.5 L (16 oz) 2–5 h before exercise	Not recommended	Immediately after to deliver 1 g CHO/kg body weight and as a supplement to daily meals
Energy gel	*CHO: >50% by volume (>50 g/100 mL or 15 g/oz) *Vitamins and minerals: trace or absent *Avoid those with herbs	1 packet prior to exercise; consume adequate fluid to promote absorption	If overall fluid intake is adequate, enough to supply 30–60 g CHO/h	Immediately after exercise and at 1-h intervals to deliver 1 g CHO/kg body weight

(From Gatorade Sports Science Exchange Roundtable. Sport foods for athletes: What works? Vol. 9 No. 2, 1998 [with permission]).

strated that a diet based on high glycemic carbohydrate foods promoted greater glycogen storage in the first 24 hours of recovery after strenuous exercise than an equal amount of carbohydrate eaten in the form of low glycemic index foods. Table 25–4 and Appendix 54 list the glycemic indexes of foods.

Carbohydrate Intake Before, During, and After Exercise

PRE-EXERCISE MEAL

The pre-event or pretraining meal serves two purposes. It keeps the athlete from feeling hungry before and during the exercise bout, and it maintains optimal levels of blood glucose for the exercising muscles during training and competition. Athletes who train early in the morning before eating or drinking risk developing low liver glycogen stores, and this can impair performance, particularly if the exercise regimen involves endurance training.

Carbohydrate feedings before exercise can help restore suboptimal liver glycogen stores, which may be called on during prolonged training and high-intensity competition. While allowing for personal preferences and psychological factors, the pre-event meal should be high in carbohydrate, nongreasy, and readily digested. Fat should be limited because it delays stomach emptying time and takes longer to digest. A meal eaten 3½ to 4 hours before competition can have as much as 25% of the kilocalories from fat. Closer to the event the fat content should be less than 25% of the kilocalories. Exercising with a full stomach also may cause indigestion, nausea, and vomiting.

The pregame meal should be eaten 3 to 4 hours before an event and should provide 200 to 350 g carbohydrate (4 g/kg). Evidence indicates that eating within 4 hours of an event benefits performance over competing on an empty stomach (Jandrain et al., 1984). Allowing time for partial digestion and absorption provides for a final addition to muscle glycogen, additional blood sugar, and also relatively complete emptying of the stomach. To avoid gastrointestinal distress, the carbohydrate content of the meal should be reduced the closer the meal is to the exercise. For example, 4 hours before the event it is suggested that the athlete consume 4 g carbohydrates/kg body weight, whereas 1 hour before the competition the athlete would consume 1 g carbohydrate/kg body weight (Coleman, 1998).

Commercial liquid formulas providing an easily digested fluid, high-carbohydrate meal are popular with athletes and probably do leave the stomach faster. Other appropriate pregame meals are toast with jelly, a baked potato, spaghetti with tomato sauce, cereal with skim milk, or low-fat yogurt with fruit-sugar flavorings.

Within 15 minutes before a long event, the athlete should drink 4 to 8 oz of water or fluid. This prehydration allows for maximal absorption of fluid without urination. After exercise begins, the kidney slows down urine production to compensate for water loss. Table 25–5 suggests pre-event meals based on time of competition.

Fifteen years ago, Costill et al. (1977a) suggested that preexercise glucose intake could be associated with hypoglycemia and increased muscle glycogen utilization during exercise. A study by Hargreaves (1991) contradicts this earlier finding. Cyclists consumed 75 g glucose or water 45 minutes before cycling to exhaustion. Although the sugar feedings caused high blood insulin and low blood glucose levels, there were no differences in the exercise time to exhaustion between the two trials. Does this mean

TABLE 25–4 CARBOHYDRATES GROUPED BY GLYCEMIC INDEX*

LOW GLYCEMIC INDEX (<60)	MEDIUM GLYCEMIC INDEX (60–85)	HIGH GLYCEMIC INDEX (>85)
Fructose	All-bran cereal	Glucose
Apple	Banana	Sucrose
Applesauce	Grapes	Maple syrup
Cherries	Oatmeal	Corn syrup
Kidney beans	Orange juice	Honey
Navy beans	Pasta	Bagel
Garbanzo beans	Rice	Candy
Lentils	Whole-grain rye bread	Corn flakes
Dates	Yams	Carrots
Figs	Corn	Crackers
Peaches	Baked beans	Molasses
Plums	Potato chips	Potatoes
Ice cream	Macaroni	Raisins
Milk	Peas	White/wheat bread
Yogurt		Soda pop
Tomato soup		Sports drinks with glucose polymers
Peanuts		Sports drinks with sugar

(From Williams, LMH. Nutrition for health and fitness and sport. New York: McGraw Hill, 1999.)

*The glycemic index is a measure of the rate of digestion and absorption of carbohydrate foods and the resultant effect on the blood glucose levels.

TABLE 25–5 EXAMPLES OF PRE-EVENT MEALS

For athletes who compete in events all day such as with track or swimming meets or soccer, basketball, volleyball, and wrestling tournaments, nutritious food choices may be a problem. The athlete should consider the amount of time between eating and performance when choosing foods during all-day events. Suggested precompetition menus include the following:

1 h or Less Before Competition

Fresh fruit such as apples, watermelon, peaches, grapes, oranges, or a sports energy bar

and/or

1½ cups of a commercial sport drink

2–3 h Before Competition

Fresh fruit and fruit and vegetable juices

and/or

Breads, bagels, English muffins with limited amounts of butter or margarine or cream cheese or low-fat yogurt, oatmeal, pancakes with limited amounts of butter and syrup, or a sports bar

and/or

4 cups of a commercial sport drink or 1 can of a sports nutritional supplement

3–4 h Before Competition

Fresh fruit and fruit and vegetable juices

and

Breads, bagels, baked potatoes, cereal with low-fat milk, low-fat yogurt, sandwiches with a small amount of peanut butter or lean meat, or low-fat cheese, spaghetti with a tomato sauce,

and/or

7½ cups of a commercial sport drink or 1–2 cans of a sports nutritional supplement

that endurance athletes should load up on soft drinks and candy before their events? Comparison of the results of the old and new studies suggests that individuals differ in their susceptibility to a lowering of blood glucose from sugar consumption before exercise. The physiologic and biochemical bases for these differences have not been determined. At this time, therefore, exercising individuals should be advised that consuming sugar 30 to 45 minutes before exercise could harm their performance if they are sensitive to a lowering of their blood glucose level.

CARBOHYDRATE INTAKE DURING EXERCISE

Carbohydrate consumed during endurance exercise lasting longer than 1 hour ensures the availability of sufficient amounts of energy during the later stages of exercise. Consuming a sports drink with carbohydrate during exercise offers an advantage over water alone in that blood glucose levels are maintained throughout the exercise bout, allowing the individual to perform closer to potential. The rate of carbohydrate ingestion should be about 25 to 30 g/30 min, an amount equivalent to 1 cup of a 6% to 8% carbohydrate solution taken every 15 to 20 minutes (Harkins et al., 1993). This ensures that 1 g carbohydrate will be delivered to the tissues per minute at the time fatigue sets in (Butterfield and Gates, 1994). It is unlikely that a carbohydrate concentration of less than 5% is enough to help performance, but solutions with a concentration greater than 10% are often associated with abdominal cramps, nausea, and diarrhea.

The improved performance associated with carbohydrate feedings probably results from the maintenance of blood glucose levels. The dietary carbohydrate supplies glucose for the muscles at a time when their glycogen stores are diminished. Thus, carbohydrate utilization (and therefore ATP production) can continue at a high rate, and endurance is enhanced.

Fatigue is not prevented by carbohydrate feeding, it is simply delayed. During the final portions of exercise, when muscle glycogen is low and athletes rely heavily on blood glucose for energy, their muscles feel heavy and they must concentrate to maintain exercise at intensities that are ordinarily not stressful when muscle glycogen stores are filled.

CARBOHYDRATES AFTER EXERCISE

On average only 5% of the muscle glycogen used during exercise is resynthesized each hour following exercise. Accordingly, at least 20 hours will be required for complete restoration after exhaustive exercise, provided approximately 600 g carbohydrate is consumed. When carbohydrate at 2 g/kg is consumed immediately after exercise, muscle glycogen synthesis is 15 mmol/kg. When the carbohydrate feeding is delayed for 2 hours after exercise, muscle glycogen synthesis is cut by 66% to 5 mmol/kg. By 4 hours after exercise, total muscle glycogen synthesis for the delayed feeding is still 45% slower than for the feeding given immediately after exercise (Ivy et al., 1988).

This means that delaying carbohydrate intake for too long after exercise will reduce muscle glycogen resynthesis. Resynthesis is promoted when carbohydrates are consumed immediately after exercise, and the current recommendations are to consume around 100 g carbohydrate within 30 minutes after exercise to maximize muscle glycogen synthesis.

Many athletes find it difficult to consume food immediately after exercise. Usually when body or core temperature is elevated appetite is depressed and it is difficult to consume carbohydrate-rich foods. Many athletes find it easier and simpler to drink their carbohydrates rather than eat them. For them a sports drink rich in carbohydrates after a hard practice will not only provide the necessary carbohydrate for glycogen synthesis, but will also help with rehydration.

Not only does consuming carbohydrates immediately after exercise help restore muscle glycogen stores faster, but adding about 5 to 9 g of protein with every 100 g of carbohydrate will further increase the glycogen resynthesis rate (Zawadski et al., 1992). It appears that this small amount of protein with 100 g of carbohydrate illicits a greater insulin response and therefore activates glycogen synthase, the enzyme responsible for glycogen storage. Table 25–6 lists some examples of foods that contain about 100 g carbohydrate and about 5 to 9 g protein that could be used immediately after exercise.

Protein

Although it has long been a popular belief among athletes that additional protein increases strength and enhances performance, nutritionists and some exercise physiologists generally hold that data are not available to support this thesis. Noting that the small amount of protein required for muscle development during training is easily met by the average diet, the 1989 recommended daily allowances (RDAs) for protein do not specify intakes different for work or training from those indicated for adults. This recommendation is 12% to 15% of energy intake (Food and Nutrition Board, 1989).

Protein Needs for Endurance Athletes

Early research showed a decrease in nitrogen balance in response to initiation of a moderate endurance exercise program, suggesting an increased need for protein under these conditions (Gontzea et al., 1974; Yoshimura, 1961). However, this decline corrected itself within 2 weeks of the start of exercise without dietary intervention. Nitrogen balance was more positive after adaptation to the exercise than before, suggesting that the protein intake required for nitrogen equilibrium in individuals performing moderate endurance exercise may actually be lower than that of a sedentary population, provided energy intake is adequate (Butterfield and Tremblay, 1994).

More recent work suggests that individuals who exercise at a higher intensity have protein needs that might be greater (Meredith et al., 1981; Tarnopolsky et al., 1988, 1992). A classic nitrogen balance regression assessment of trained male runners exercising daily at 75% of their Vo_2max estimated protein requirements of 0.94 g/kg body weight per day (Meredith et al., 1981).

Protein need in exercise depends on energy intake. Butterfield (1987) demonstrated that feeding as much as 2 g protein/kg body weight per day to men running 5 or 10 miles a day at 65% to 75% of their Vo_2max is insufficient to maintain nitrogen balance when energy intake is inadequate by as little as 100 kcal/day. Delvin et al. (1990) observed an increase in whole body protein degradation during 2 hours of 75% of Vo_2max exercise, returning to baseline levels within 2 hours after exercise.

Another indicator that endurance athletes may require higher protein intake than the recommended intake is that muscle contractile proteins are broken down during prolonged exercise (Dohm et al., 1987; Snyder et al., 1984). These studies point out the important role that calories play in sparing protein. Protein will be used as an energy source if calories are insufficient.

TABLE 25–6 FOODS OR COMBINATION OF FOODS TO EQUAL 100 g CARBOHYDRATE WITH 5 TO 9 g PROTEIN

One bagel with 2 tablespoons of peanut butter and ⅔ cup raisins
One cup low-fat yogurt, one banana, and 1 cup of orange juice
One turkey sandwich on whole-wheat bread with 1 cup applesauce
One cup spaghetti with meat sauce and 2 slices of garlic bread
8 oz of skim milk, one apple, one orange, two slices of bread, and three pancakes
One serving of a protein and carbohydrate drink and one bagel

Protein Needs for Resistance Exercise

For body builders or individuals who are interested in increasing body mass, the mythology of increased protein needs is rampant. Weight lifters consume anywhere from 1.2 to 3.4 g of protein/kg body weight per day, and most of this protein is in the form of supplements. The basis for this practice is word of mouth and traditions that have not been substantiated by scientific studies. The traditional thinking among body builders and weight lifters is the more protein consumed, the bigger the muscles.

There is now sufficient data that the study of protein needs with resistance exercise is divided into two areas: the need for maintenance (minimum protein required to accomplish nitrogen equilibrium) and the need for increasing lean tissue (positive nitrogen balance).

Experienced body builders can maintain nitrogen equilibrium on intakes similar to those required by sedentary controls (Tarnopolsky et al., 1991). However, the requirements for maintenance of nitrogen balance under circumstances of initiation of a resistance exercise program may depend on the intensity of the exercise. Protein requirements in young novice male body builders exercising 6 days a week for 1.5 hours a day were estimated to be 1.5 g/kg body weight per day (Tarnopolsky et al., 1988). But, energy intake was not reported. In another study Tarnopolsky et al. (1992) found that whole body protein synthesis was increased in strength athletes consuming 1.4 g protein/kg body weight per day when compared to those consuming 0.9 g protein/kg body weight per day. When intake was increased to 2.4 g protein/kg body weight per day, protein synthesis did not increase above that which was achieved when consuming the 1.4 g protein/kg body weight per day.

On the other hand, Hickson et al. (1990) found no change in nitrogen excretion with the initiation of a program of 30 minutes of lifting three times a week at an intensity of about 50% of maximum capacity, when subjects were consuming 0.8 g protein/kg body weight per day, the RDA for protein for adults.

In an attempt to establish the relevance of added protein in the accretion of lean tissue in recreational weight lifters, it was observed that when energy intake exceeded the need by 400 kcal/day, increasing the nitrogen intake from the requirement (mean = 10 g N/day) to 1.5 times requirement (mean = 15 g N/day) had no significant effect on nitrogen retention. Any improvement in nitrogen balance seen with increased energy and protein intake was explained by the energy contribution of the protein (Butterfield, 1991).

Nutritional Implications

If the need for protein during exercise is slightly elevated above that for sedentary individuals, the usual protein intake of the population will more than meet these needs. Reports of food intake in athletes and nonathletes consistently indicate that protein represents from 12% to 20% of total energy intake or 1.2 to 2 g protein/kg body weight per day. The exception to the rule will be small active women who may consume a low-energy intake in conjunction with an exercise or training program. These women may consume close to the RDA for protein, and if the data of Butterfield are correct, this value in conjunction with the restricted energy intake may be inadequate to maintain lean body mass.

Consuming more protein than the body can use is not necessary and should be avoided. When athletes consume diets that are high in protein, they compromise their carbohydrate status and may therefore affect their ability to train and compete at peak levels. High-protein intakes can also result in diuresis and potential dehydration. Protein foods are often also high in fat, and consumption of excess protein can create difficulty in maintaining a low-fat diet. In addition, the hypercalciuric effect of high-protein diets is still considered by some a significant factor in calcium balance, and until the controversy is settled, a conservative approach is advised.

Amino Acid Supplementation

Protein or amino acid supplementation in the form of powders or pills is not necessary and should be discouraged. Taking large amounts of protein or amino acid supplements can lead to dehydration, loss of urinary calcium, weight gain, and stress on the kidney and liver (Snyder and Naik, 1998). Taking single amino acids or in combination, such as arginine and lysine, may interfere with the absorption of certain other essential amino acids (Wardlaw, 1999). An additional concern is that substituting amino acid supplements for food may cause deficiencies of other nutrients found in protein-rich foods such as iron, niacin, and thiamin.

Athletes and coaches need to realize that amino acid supplements taken in large doses have not been tested in human subjects and no margin of safety is available. It is important for the health professional to develop a strategy to effectively approach and discuss supplement use with both athletes and coaches (Berning, 1998).

Table 25–7 estimates the requirements of the athlete whose protein needs are greatest—a growing male adolescent in rigorous training in a warm climate. This very liberal allowance is for about 104 g/day of protein or 1.5 g/kg body weight. Although greater than the RDA of 0.85 g/kg for the male adolescent, this is still easily within the range of intake of most male teenagers and athletes. Many studies of athletes' diets indicate that their protein intakes are two to three times higher than the RDA. In meeting his energy needs, the athlete described would probably be consuming at least 3500 kcal. Considering the usual composition of diets in the United States, this would provide 10% to 15% protein, or 87 to 131 g/day. Thus, there is generally no need to recommend additional protein unless this nutrient makes up less than 12% of adequate energy intake for weight maintenance.

In the case of young or small female athletes, protein needs calculated as a percentage of energy intake may be inadequate; a better calculation is based on 1 to 1.5 g/kg. The same is true for athletes with exceptionally high energy requirements. Protein needs based on 12% to 15% of energy results in an excessive protein intake.

Fat

Even though maximal performance is impossible without muscle glycogen, fat also provides energy for exercise. Fat is the most concentrated source of food energy and supplies more than twice as many calories (9 kcal/g) by weight as protein (4 kcal/g) or carbohydrate (4 kcal/g). Fat provides essential fatty acids that are necessary for cell membranes, skin, hormones, and transport of fat-soluble vitamins. The body has total glycogen stores (both muscle and liver) equalling about 2500 calories, whereas each

TABLE 25–7 LIBERAL ESTIMATE OF PROTEIN REQUIREMENT FOR A 70-kg MALE ADOLESCENT ATHLETE*

28.7 g	Replacement of obligatory nitrogen loss in urine, feces, skin, and other sites assuming largest loss
8.6 g	30% allowance for individual variation
4.8 g	Allowance for growth assuming most rapid growth
7.5 g	Replacement of nitrogen lost in sweat during 4 h of vigorous exercise in the heat
6.3 g	Allowance for increased muscle mass, as during some kinds of training
8.6 g	Allowance for loss of efficiency of standard protein
39.5 g	Allowance for use of protein for energy during rigorous exercise[†]
104 g	Total estimated protein requirement = 1.5 g/kg

(*Data from Report of Joint FAO/WHO Ad Hoc Expert Committee. Energy and protein requirements. WHO, Tech. Sys. Series, No. 522. Geneva, Switzerland: WHO, 1973 and Durnin JVGA. Nutrition, physical fitness, and health. Baltimore: University Press, 1978.)

[†]Determined using an energy expenditure during activity of an average of 12 kcal/min and exercising time daily of 240 min, and the assumption that 5.5% of the total energy expenditure during exercise is from protein.

pound of body fat supplies 3500 calories. This means that an athlete weighing 74 kg (163 lb) with 10% body fat has 16.3 lb of fat, which equals 57,000 calories.

Fat is the major, if not most important, fuel for light- to moderate-intensity exercise. Although fat is a valuable metabolic fuel for muscle activity during longer aerobic exercise, and performs many important functions in the body, no attempt should be made to consume more fat over the usual amount, unless the athlete is eating less than 15% of calories from fat. In addition, athletes who consume a high-fat diet typically consume fewer calories from carbohydrate.

Simonsen et al. (1991) had elite rowers consume either 40% of their calories from fat or 20% of their calories from fat, and then compared the power output and speed of the rowers. After biopsying the muscle, they found that the rowers who consumed the low-fat, high-carbohydrate diet had more muscle glycogen. Rowers on the high-fat, low-carbohydrate diet had moderate levels of muscle glycogen and actually were able to complete the workout sets. However, when it came to power output and faster speeds those athletes who consumed the lower fat, higher carbohydrate diets had significantly higher power and speed. This has big implications for athletes in muscular endurance sports where they need a burst of power, such as rowing, swimming, gymnastics, figure skating, judo, or boxing, or any sport that will need to have some energy generated by the anaerobic pathway. Following a low-fat, high-carbohydrate diet is also important for health reasons, because a high-fat diet is associated with cardiovascular disease, obesity, diabetes, and some types of cancers.

Athletes should consume 20% to 30% of their calories from fat. Aside from decreasing overall calories, limiting consumption of dietary fat is the first step toward losing excess body fat. Doing so eliminates excess calories, but not nutrients. However, severe fat restriction (< 15% of energy intake) may limit performance by hindering intramuscular triglyceride storage, which provides a significant proportion of energy at all intensities of exercise (Butterfield and Tremblay, 1994).

Vitamins and Minerals

It has usually been assumed that if the athlete meets requirements for increased energy, the vitamin and mineral requirements will also be satisfied. Although this may be true in most cases, one study of triathletes indicates low intakes of selenium, molybdenum, iron, copper, and biotin even though the athletes were consuming energy at levels two to three times the RDA (Green et al., 1989). The authors speculate that because of training and work schedules, athletes seldom eat three balanced meals, but rely heavily on snacking to maintain their energy levels, and these snacks may be less nutrient dense than the meals they replace. The poor nutritional status of some athletes may be due to their training and work schedules.

The need for vitamins and minerals in exercise has been reviewed recently by Haymes and Clarkson (1998), with the consensus that unless an individual is deficient in a given nutrient, supplementation with that nutrient does not have a major effect on performance. However, several nutrients are of concern in athletes, including folate, the B vitamins, calcium, and zinc. Because many women athletes are also vegetarians, iron and specifically vitamin B_{12} may be of concern in this subgroup.

Iron

Iron performs several functions vital to muscle activity. As a component of hemoglobin, it is instrumental in transporting oxygen from the lungs to the tissues. It performs a similar role in **myoglobin,** which acts within the muscle as an oxygen acceptor to hold a supply of oxygen readily available for use by the mitochondria. Iron is also a vital component of the cytochrome enzymes involved in the production of ATP.

It thus follows that iron deficiency anemia limits aerobic endurance and the capacity for work. However, partial depletion of iron stores in the liver, spleen, and bone marrow, as evidenced by low serum ferritin levels, can have a detrimental effect on exercise performance, even when anemia is not present.

Although iron deficiency anemia is not frequently seen among athletes, suboptimal iron stores as assessed by serum ferritin levels are relatively common. Early screening for serum ferritin levels is recommended (American Dietetic Association and Canadian Dietetic Association, 1993). Athletes at risk for developing low iron stores are the rapidly growing male adolescent, the female athlete with heavy menstrual losses, the athlete with an energy-restricted diet, distance runners who may have increased gastrointestinal iron loss, and those training heavily in hot climates with heavy sweating.

SPORTS ANEMIA

Heavy training can cause a transient **sports anemia,** which is characterized by a significant decrease in red blood cell count, hemoglobin concentration, and packed cell volume. However, the erythrocyte morphology remains normal, and performance does not appear to deteriorate. Possible causes include a hemodilution effect of expanded blood volume and an increased rate of red cell destruction due to intravascular hemolysis. Excessive iron losses can also occur through the gastrointestinal tract or sweating.

Some athletes, especially long distance runners, experience gastrointestinal bleeding. Iron loss through gastrointestinal bleeding can be detected by fecal hemoglobin assays. The percentage of runners who experience gastrointestinal bleeding ranges from 8% to more than 80% (Stewart et al., 1984).

The iron concentration of sweat during exercise ranges from 0.13 to 0.42 mg/L. Waller and Haymes (1996) observed that the iron concentration in sweat was lower in a hot environment (35°C) than in a thermoneutral environment (25°C). Because sweating was greater in the heat, the same amount of sweat iron was lost during 1 hour of exercise in both environments with male athletes losing three times as much sweat iron as female athletes. They also found that as the exercise time went on less iron was lost in the sweat. Sweat iron concentration decreased significantly from 30 to 60 minutes. This suggests that much of the iron lost in sweat is done early in the exercise bout.

Iron supplementation can be beneficial in improving iron stores of athletes who are iron depleted, but the effects on aerobic performance of nonanemic athletes are equivocal. Because large doses of iron (≥ 75 mg/day) may be toxic in persons with the genetic disorder hemochromatosis (see Chapter 35), such supplements should be used only by those diagnosed as iron depleted or anemic (Haymes and Clarkson, 1998). At present the data do not support the value of iron supplementation for either treating or preventing sports anemia. However, testing serum ferritin may be useful in assessing iron stores in athletes. If true iron depletion is present, iron supplementation along with vitamin C to enhance its absorption is appropriate. Oral iron therapy is effective and maintains performance in runners who are deficient in iron but not anemic.

Calcium

Osteoporosis is a major health concern, especially for women. Although the disease has been regarded as a problem of elderly women, young women, especially those who have had interrupted menstrual function, may be at risk for decreased bone mass. Although there is still much to be discovered about the cause of osteoporosis, three major risk factors have been identified: hormonal status, particularly estrogen deficiency; deficient calcium consumption; and physical inactivity.

Bone mass is attained until the age of 35 to 40 years; however, peak rate of bone mass accumulation is between the ages of 14 and 24 years. The amount of bone mass a woman has by age 35 strongly influences her susceptibility to fractures in later years. Therefore, it is important that young women consume calcium throughout the peak bone mass years and throughout early adulthood. Unfortunately, the National Health and Nutrition Examination Survey (NHANES) found that 50% of all women age 15 and over consume less than 75% of the RDA of 1200 mg, and that three fourths of women over age 35 consume less than the RDA of 800 mg (see Chapter 28).

ATHLETIC AMENORRHEA/FEMALE ATHLETE TRIAD

In 1997, the ACSM identified the **female athlete triad** as a disturbing pattern emerging in women's athletics (Otis et al., 1997). It is characterized by estrogen deficiency, evidenced as athletic amenorrhea, disordered eating and low body fat, and loss of bone mass. Some women who exercise strenuously stop menstruating, a condition known as *athletic amenorrhea*. Unfortunately, the exact cause of amenorrhea has not been fully determined, but probably many factors are involved. The two most current theories are that the excessive exercise is an "energy drain" that may lead to a hypothalamic dysfunction or that excess cortisol levels inhibit the release of gonadotropins (Loucks, 1990). Regardless of the cause, the lack of estrogen has a negative impact on bone and if the estrogen deficiency persists, bone loss may be substantial and bone may never be regained (Drinkwater et al., 1986; Jonnavithula et al., 1993).

Strategies to promote the resumption of menses include estrogen replacement therapy; weight gain; dietary modification to include more calcium, vitamin D, and magnesium; and reduced training. Regardless of menstrual history, most female athletes need to increase their calcium intake to meet the RDA for calcium. Low-fat and nonfat dairy products, calcium-fortified fruit juices, calcium-fortified soy milk, and tofu made with calcium sulfate are all good sources. Amenorrheic athletes who need 1500 mg calcium daily may require supplementation with calcium and vitamin D (see Chapter 28).

Antioxidant Vitamins and β-Carotene

As a result of exercise the oxidative processes in the muscle increase, leading to increased generation of lipid peroxides and free radicals. In animals it has been shown that there is a two- to threefold increase in free radical concentrations in the muscle and liver following exercise to exhaustion (Davies et al., 1982). However, Kanter (1993) questions the fact that this study was published over 15 years ago and that these results have never been replicated.

Most studies that investigate free radical formation during exercise actually determine indirect measures of lipid peroxidation and not free radical production. Despite the lack of specificity, sensitivity, and reproducibility (Halliwell and Gutteridgen 1985; Wong et al., 1987), much of our understanding about exercise and free radicals is based on these methodologies. A few recent studies have looked at the effect of exercise on the susceptibility of low-density lipoprotein to oxidation. The results suggest that strenuous exercise does indeed promote free radical formation (Sanchez-Quesada et al., 1995).

Vitamins with antioxidant activity, particularly vitamin C, vitamin E, and β-carotene, neutralize free radicals, and the question is whether they enhance recovery from exercise. Results from studies in humans show that when 10 mg (33,333 IU) β-carotene, 800 IU vitamin E, and 1000 mg vitamin C were added to the diets of moderately trained runners for 3 to 4 weeks, levels of creatine phosphokinase and lactic dehydrogenase (both indices of muscle damage) were significantly lower, plasma glutathione did not increase, and recovery after exercise was faster (Viguie et al., 1989). Another study showed that these same three nutrients, when given in high amounts, decreased elevated serum malondialdehyde and breath pentane (measures of lipid oxidation) in individuals at rest and during exercise (Singh, 1992).

Antioxidant nutrients may have a role in enhancing recovery from exercise and maintaining optimal immune response, but there is no consistent evidence that they improve performance per se. The available evidence suggests that antioxidant supplementation has favorable effects on markers of lipid peroxidation after exercise. Although the physiologic implications of this effect remain to be elucidated, the prudent use of an antioxidant supplement may provide insurance against a suboptimal diet and the increased demand of physical activity.

Athletes need to understand that more is not always better. The National Academy of Sciences has established the Dietary Reference Intakes (DRIs) for vitamins and minerals as a guide for determining nutritional needs. The RDA is the daily amount of a nutrient recommended for practically all healthy individuals to promote optimal health (see Chapter 15). Although it has been shown that a severely inadequate intake of certain vitamins can impair performance, it is unusual for an athlete to have such deficiencies. Even marginal deficiencies do not appear to markedly affect the ability to exercise efficiently.

B Vitamins

Increased energy metabolism creates a need for more of the B vitamins that serve as part of coenzymes involved in the energy cycles (see Chapters 2, 3, and 4). However, when dietary intakes are expanded to meet increased energy needs, the extra foods consumed usually provide enough B vitamins to enable the release of that energy. There is no evidence that supplementing the well-nourished athlete with B vitamins will increase performance (Keith, 1989).

Studies have shown, however, that athletes can become depleted in some B vitamins, and in these athletes, dietary change or supplementation will improve exercise performance (Belko et al., 1983). A deficiency of vitamin B_{12}, found only in animal foods, could develop in a vegetarian athlete after several years of a strict vegan intake (see Chapter 35); a vitamin B_{12} supplement warranted for these individuals. Vitamin B_{12} metabolism may also be altered in ultra-endurance athletes (Singh et al., 1993).

The intake of folic acid is marginal for a large portion of the U.S. population, and could be low in an athlete whose consumption of whole fruits and vegetables is low. If diets of athletes reflect those of the general population, they could easily not contain the recommended number of fruits and vegetables. The NHANES studies have found that 90% of the study participants fail to ingest the recommended minimum of five servings of fruits and vegetables daily (Patterson, 1990). A folate supplement to meet the RDA is recommended for such athletes. For some athletes such as wrestlers, gymnasts, or rowers who consume low-calorie diets for long periods of time, a B-vitamin supplement to meet the RDA may be appropriate (Williams, 1989).

Vitamin C

The effect of vitamin C supplementation on performance has received considerable attention, mainly because athletes consume vitamin C in large quantities, often because of the volume of food they consume. In studies where athletes were deficient in vitamin C, supplementation improved physical performance, but a thorough analysis of these studies supports the general conclusion that vitamin C supplementation does not increase physical performance capacity in subjects with normal body levels of vitamin C (Keith, 1994). On the other hand, because exercise is a stressor to the body, some nutritionists recommend that the active individual may need slightly more vitamin C than the RDA. Keith suggests vitamin C supplementation may be beneficial for heat acclimation, an idea that merits more research.

Vitamin E

Vitamin E is used widely as a supplement by athletes who hope to improve performance. Recent research is showing vitamin E to have a protective effect against exercise-induced oxidative injury and the acute immune response changes that exercise produces. Researchers found that supplementation with vitamin E enhances the immune response, preventing changes similar to those of infectious disease seen after exercise (Cannon et al., 1990; Ismail et al., 1983; Meydani et al., 1993). Over the course of an exercise season with intense workouts and competition, vitamin E supplementation at the level of 200 to 450 IU/day may help prevent oxidative injury (Cooper, 1994). However, further studies are recommended.

Whether this vitamin has a protective effect during exercise in polluted environmental conditions is unclear (Dillard et al., 1978). The positive effect of vitamin E may be due to protection against oxidative injury caused by inhalation of pollutants.

OTHER CONSIDERATIONS

Alcohol

Alcohol consumption has a detrimental effect on athletic performance, even though by reducing feelings of insecurity, tension, and discomfort it may cause the athlete to feel that he or she is performing better. Perceptual motor performance is affected; however, except for some deleterious effects on prolonged endurance performance, alcohol has no effect on the physiologic processes of maximal exercise. Light social drinking (1 or 2 drinks) during the day before a competition will probably not influence athletic performance the following day.

Caffeine

Caffeine contributes to endurance performance, apparently because of its ability to enhance mobilization of fatty acids and thus conserve glycogen stores. Caffeine may also directly affect muscle contractility, possibly by facilitating calcium transport. It could reduce fatigue as well, by reducing plasma K^+ accumulation, which contributes to fatigue (Lindinger et al., 1993). There are probably some ergogenic effects at doses of 6.5 mg/kg taken before endurance exercise; however, caffeine does not seem to offer any benefits before high-intensity exercise (Tarnopolsky, 1994).

Presently caffeine is listed as a restricted drug by the International Olympic Committee (IOC) and is considered a doping agent if the intake results in urine concentrations above 12 mg/L. To have ergogenic benefits, caffeine must therefore be taken at doses (about 6.5 mg/kg) that do not exceed the IOC urine limit (Tarnopolsky, 1994). In a 70-kg man, this would be 455 mg caffeine, the amount in 4 to 5 cups of coffee.

Caffeine's diuretic action could be a negative effect for athletes with excessive water needs, or for those in long-distance events who do not want to have to urinate during the event.

ERGOGENIC AIDS

Many athletes use nutritional **ergogenic aids** because they are bombarded with advertisements and testimonials from other athletes and coaches about their effects on performance. Many believe that ergogenic aids will improve their performance and assist in recovery. As in the past, and probably in the future, many of these ergogenic aids are not supported by scientific studies. In fact many only act as placebos.

The increased visibility has occurred primarily because of the passage of the Dietary Supplement Health and Education Act (DSHEA) in 1994 (Bass and Young, 1996); see Chapter 14. Under this act the Food and Drug Administration (FDA) no longer has regulatory control of supplements including vitamin, mineral, amino acid, herbal, and other botanical preparations. This has led to an increased number of nutritional ergogenic aids on the market (Table 25–8).

Nutritional supplements are now classified as foods and not as food additives or drugs. Another interesting and somewhat controversial section of the act allows manufacturers to publish limited information about the benefits of dietary supplements in the form of statements of support as well as so-called structure and function claims. The result is a great deal of printed material at the points of sale of nutritional products.

β-HYDROXY-β-METHYLBUTYRATE

β-Hydroxy-β-methylbutyrate (HMB) is an important compound made in the body and is a metabolite of the essential amino acid leucine. Several studies done with both animals and humans have found that subjects supplemented with HMB have less stress-induced muscle protein breakdown (Abumrad and Flakoll, 1991; Nissen et al., 1996). In one study, the volunteers supplemented with HMB had greater strength gains when compared to the control group (Nissen et al., 1996). However, it is interesting to point out that the control group started out much stronger than the HMB-supplemented group and, therefore, it is not surprising that the control group, who were more highly trained, had lesser strength gains from the same exercise protocol than the lesser trained experimental HMB group.

CREATINE

Creatine, in the form of phosphocreatine and ATP, supplies most of the energy for short-term, maximal exercise like base running and stealing, swinging the bat, and throwing. When creatine stores in the muscles are depleted, ATP synthesis is prevented and energy can no longer be supplied at the rate required by the working muscle. Creatine is a naturally occurring compound that can be found in considerable amounts in meat and fish. In normal healthy individuals, muscle creatine is broken down to creatinine and excreted by the kidneys. For meat eaters, dietary intake of creatine is about 1 g/day. The body also synthesizes about 1 g creatine per day for a total production of about 2 g/day. The normal daily excretion of creatine is about 2 g for most individuals. It appears that vegetarians may be at the highest risk of not having enough creatine. Vegetarian athletes with lower stores of creatine demonstrate a greater uptake of creatine after supplementation than athletes with higher stores.

Creatine supplementation elevates muscle creatine levels and facilitates the regeneration of phosphocreatine, which in turn helps regenerate ATP. Ingesting 20 g/day (four 5-g doses per day) for 5 days can produce a 20% increase in muscle creatine levels (Greenhaff et al., 1994). Human muscle ap-

TABLE 25–8 UNPROVEN ERGOGENIC AIDS FOR ATHLETES

ERGOGENIC AID	DESCRIPTION	CLAIM	ADVERSE SIDE EFFECTS/CAUTION
Amino acid supplements	Arginine, ornithine, glycine plus lysine, predigested amino acids, branch-chain amino acids	Promotes muscle development	
Bee pollen	Mixture of bee saliva, plant nectar, and pollen	Increases energy levels, enhances physical fitness	Reports anecdotal; not proven; allergic reactions in bee-sensitive individuals most common adverse side effect; because of content of nucleic acids, should be avoided by those with gout
Boron	Nonmetallic trace element that influences calcium and magnesium metabolism	Increases testosterone	Intakes of 50 mg/day may be toxic
Brewer's yeast	By-product of beer brewing; rich source of B vitamins and bioavailable chromium	Increases energy levels	Claims of blood glucose improvement due to chromium content are documented (see Chapters 5 and 34)
Carnitine	A compound synthesized in the body from lysine and methionine	Improves cardiovascular function and muscle strength; delays fatigue; decreases muscle pain; decreases body fat	Although necessary for fat metabolism (see Chapter 4), appears that body synthesizes adequate amounts
Choline	Precursor of the neurotransmitter acetylcholine	Improves performance	Should be avoided by athletes with gout
Chromium	Essential component of the glucose tolerance factor	Improves insulin sensitivity and carbohydrate metabolism during exercise	Prolonged or excessive supplementation may lead to chromium accumulation in the body to levels at which chromosomal damage has been observed in animals and in vitro
Conjugated linoleic acid (CLA)	Structured lipid	Antioxidant; addition of lean body mass and reduction of body fat; immune stimulation	No human studies have been published in peer-reviewed journals
Creatine	A nitrogen-containing compound known as an amine	Improves performance by enhancing the body's pool of creatine phosphate	Weight gain; safety and efficacy of chronic use not known. Anecdotal reports of muscle cramping and muscle tears
DNA/RNA	Deoxyribonucleic acid, ribonucleic acid	Tissue regeneration	
Gelatin	Obtained from collagen	Improves muscle contraction	
Ginseng	Extract of ginseng root	Protects against tissue damage	Ginseng products (teas, powders, extracts) are of variable quality and strength because of expense of the authentic product
Glycine	An amino acid that is a phosphocreatine precursor	Improves muscle contraction	
Kelp	Seaweed	Vitamin/mineral source	
Lecithin	Phosphatidylcholine	Decreases triglyceride and cholesterol levels	
Medium-chain triglycerides	Fatty acids with shorter carbon chain lengths (8–12)	Improves performance by sparing muscle glycogen; promotes muscularity and lower body fat	Gastric distress in some subjects
Octacosanol	Alcohol isolate extracted from wheat germ oil	Supplies energy and improves performance	
Pangamic acid	Also referred to as vitamin B_{15}; varied composition depending on the supplier	Increases delivery of oxygen	
Royal jelly	Substance produced by worker bees and fed to the queen bee	Increases strength	
Spirulina	Microscopic blue-green algae; excellent source of beta-carotene	Protein source	Probably does not function as protein source, but supplies β-carotene, a powerful antioxidant for which athletes may have increased need
Superoxide dimutase	Antioxidant enzyme system	Protects body against oxidative cell damage incurred from aerobic metabolism	Antioxidant protection provided may affect recovery from athletic endeavors

pears to have an upper limit of creatine storage; thus, creatine will presumably be of little benefit to someone with an already high concentration of muscle creatine, or to an individual who has been ingesting high doses of creatine for many weeks. Once creatine is taken up by the muscles, it is trapped within the muscle tissue. It is estimated that muscle creatine stores will decline very slowly and will still be elevated 2 to 3 months after ingestion of 20 g for 5 days. Recent evidence shows that muscle creatine stores can be maintained at a high level if the regimen of 20 g for 5 days is followed by continual supplementation at a lower dose of 2 g/day.

Creatine supplementation does not enhance endurance activities. But it is associated with an increase in body weight and lean body mass of around 2 to 6 lb, which is either due to fluid retention or enhanced skeletal muscle synthesis. This weight gain might interfere with the performance of some athletes. Although there are no scientific reports of dangerous side effects, there have been anecdotal descriptions of athletes who have had muscle strains and pulls as well as dehydration problems while taking creatine supplements. This is a bigger problem in athletes who play in hot humid environments.

Because the safety of long-term creatine use has not been studied, and because excess creatine cannot be stored in the muscles and must be excreted by the kidneys, a maintenance dose of no more than 5 g/day is recommended.

DHEA

Dehydroepiandrosterone (DHEA) is a product of dehydroandrosterone-3-sulfate (DHEAS) and is a precursor of at least two hormones, testosterone and estradiol. Although DHEAS is the most abundant circulating adrenal hormone in humans, its physiologic role and that of DHEA are poorly understood.

Dehydroepiandrosterone has been labeled as the "youth hormone" because its levels peak during early adulthood. Several studies have suggested a positive correlation between increased plasma levels of DHEA and improved vigor, health, and well-being in individuals who ranged in age from 40 to 80 years (Morales et al., 1994). Is DHEA anabolic? By modifying cortisol output, DHEA may indeed exert an anabolic effect. Scientists originally thought that DHEA may competitively bind to cortisol cell receptors in a manner analogous to anabolic steroids, but studies failed to prove this hypothesis (Regelson and Kalimi, 1994). Other studies involving DHEA and liver cortisol receptors show that the DHEA directly decreases cortisol in the liver by 50% (Regelson et al., 1994). If this were to occur in muscle tissue as well, the anabolic effect would be comparable to that of anabolic steroids. However, no proof of this currently exists. Yet, DHEA is a precursor to testosterone and estrogen.

Because DHEA can take several different hormonal pathways, the one that it follows depends on several factors, including existing levels of other hormones. It can take several routes in the body and interact with certain enzymes along the sex-steroid pathway. Thus, it can turn into less desirable by-products of testosterone including dehydrotestosterone, which is associated with male pattern baldness, prostate enlargement, and acne.

Until recently, DHEA was a prescription drug. Because of the 1994 DSHEA, it is now sold over the counter. The benefits of taking DHEA for sports performance have not been clearly established and the effects of chronic DHEA ingestion are not known. Long-term safety has not been established. DHEA is not recommended for athletic use and has been banned by the U.S. Olympic Committee, the National Football League (NFL), and the National Collegiate Athletic Association (NCAA).

Recently a "safe" alternative to DHEA has been touted—Mexican yam. Although Mexican yams contain a DHEA precursor (a plant sterol used in the semisynthetic production of DHEA in the laboratory), the idea that the body can convert this plant sterol to testosterone is a complete scam.

ANDRO

Androstenedione (andro) has about one seventh the activity of testosterone and is directly converted to testosterone by a single reaction. It is naturally produced in the body either from DHEA or 17-α-hydroxyprogesterone. Researchers have found that taking androstenedione elevates testosterone more than DHEA does; however, the induced increase lasts only several hours and remains at peak levels for just a few minutes (Mahesh and Greenblatt, 1962). The results of this single, 38-year-old study remain the basis for marketing androstenedione as a muscle-building supplement for athletes, and there is no scientific evidence to support using androstenedione to improve athletic performance.

Andro was used by the athletes in the former East Germany as an anabolic energy-enhancing supplement, but very few details are available on its use and dosages. Because of its short half-life, athletes would need to take androstenedione several times a day or on nearly a continual basis to maintain a substantial blood level. To get around this several companies are now marketing time-release forms of androstenedione. However, there is no scientific proof that these formulations are effective or safe. If it does in fact increase testosterone levels, it has the potential to cause the same side effects as androgenic anabolic supplements such as steroids and growth hormones. Details of the doping program in the former East Germany reveal a litany of adverse reactions in male and female athletes including muscle tightness and cramps, increased body weight, acne, gastrointestinal problems, changes in libido, amenorrhea, liver damage, and stunted growth in adolescents (Franke and Berendonk, 1997).

Weindruch of the University of Wisconsin-Madison states "epidemiological data suggest that diet and serum androstenedione levels may influence the progression of latent forms of prostate cancer into more aggressive prostate cancer." He adds that one prospective study linked high androstenedione levels with later development of prostate cancer. Selling androstenedione may be irresponsible because of the potential risks associated with long-term use (Weindruch, 1997).

Until there is scientific support for its use, androstenedione should not be sold under the assumption that it is either an effective or safe athletic ergogenic aid. Clearly, it should not be used by adolescents or women of childbearing age. In 1998, androstenedione was added to the list of banned substances by the IOC and several amateur and professional organizations including the NFL and the NCAA.

WEIGHT GAIN OR LOSS

In efforts to maximize performance, many athletes alter normal energy intake to either gain or lose weight. For example, 41% of college wrestlers surveyed have weight fluctuations of 11 to 20 lb every week during the competitive season (Steen and Brownell, 1990). Although such efforts are sometimes appropriate, weight reduction programs may involve elements of risk. For some young athletes, achievement of unrealistically light weights may jeopardize growth and development (Pugliese et al., 1983; Strauss et al., 1985). Chronic dieting of female athletes, many of whom are dancers and gymnasts, can lead to eating disorders, delayed menarche, amenorrhea, and potential osteoporosis (see Chapters 24 and 28).

The goal weight of an athlete should be based on body fatness (see Chapters 16 and 23). Adequate time should be allowed for a slow, steady weight loss of about ¼ to 1 lb/week over several weeks. Weight loss should be achieved before the competitive season begins to ensure maximal strength. In addition, the exercise should be of moderate intensity because at this level a greater proportion of energy is derived from fat than carbohydrate, and the exercise can be sustained for a longer period of time.

Weight gain should be achieved through a gradual increase in energy intake combined with a strength training program to maximize muscle weight gain over fat gain. A realistic goal is ½ to 1 lb/week (Hoffman, 1994). Fat intake should not exceed 30% of kilocalories from fat, and protein should be 1 to 1.5 g/kg body weight.

Appropriate programs for modifying weight of athletes and others are discussed in Chapter 23. Because pressure to have the perfect body for a sport, which for many sports (e.g., gymnastics, track, swimming, diving, rowing, dancing, and figure skating) means leanness for both performance and appearance, unrealistic dieting and eating disorders are common (Beals and Manore, 1994). The pursuit of thinness leading to calorie restriction is especially evident in women involved in college athletics where the pressure to perform, contribute to the team, and maintain scholarships is great (Lindeman, 1994). The professional working with an elite athlete with an eating disorder must remember the tremendous motivation supplied by the desire to perform well in the sport (see Chapter 24).

CASE STUDY

Lisa H, is a 35-year-old single mother of two children who is a dedicated marathon runner. Her daily 3:30 AM workout during the week includes 1 hour of running 7 to 8 miles on her treadmill, and 15 to 20 minutes of stretching and strength building with free weights. On weekends, when her children are with their father, she does a long run of 10 to 15 miles. She has a marathon coming up in 2 months.

Lisa works as a stockbroker, and because she lives on the West Coast, she must be in her office at least by 6:00 AM. She is a vegetarian. She often skips breakfast and eats lunch at her desk. Dinner is hurried between her children's sports, homework, and housework.

Within the past 6 months Lisa has had a weight gain of 8 lb that she would like to lose before the marathon. She is not sure why she gained the weight because she claims to eat a low-fat diet (10–15% of kilocalories from fat). She has come to you for a nutritional program to accompany her training for this event.

1. Is it reasonable to expect Lisa to meet her weight goal before the marathon? Explain.
2. What would you recommend for fat intake for Lisa and why?
3. Is calcium a concern for Lisa? How could you find out, and if it is, what would you advise?
4. What protein intake would you recommend and how would you find out if Lisa is getting enough?
5. What vitamins might be of concern, and how would you advise Lisa to optimize her intake?
6. Lisa has asked you specifically about her premarathon diet, both right before and a few days ahead. What would you recommend?

CITED REFERENCES

Abumrad N, Flakoll P. The efficacy and safety of CaHMB (beta-hydroxy-beta-methylbutyrate) in humans. Memphis, TN: Vanderbilt University Medical Center, Annual Report: MTI, 1991.

American College of Sports Medicine. Position on exercise and fluid replacement. Med Sci Sports Exerc 28:i, 1996.

American Dietetic Association and Canadian Dietetic Association. Position statement: Nutrition for physical fitness and athletic performance for adults. J Am Diet Assoc 93:691, 1993.

Bar-Or O, et al. Voluntary dehydration and heat intolerance in patients with cystic fibrosis. Lancet 339:696, 1992.

Bass IS, Young AL. The Dietary Supplement Health and Education Act: A legislative history and analysis. Washington DC: Food and Drug Law Institute, 1996, pp. 5–100.

Beals KA, Manore MM. The prevalence and consequences of subclinical eating disorders. Internal J Sports Nutr 4:175, 1994.

Belko AZ, et al. Effects of exercise on riboflavin requirements of young women. Am J Clin Nutr 37:509, 1983.

Berning JR. Eating while traveling. In: Berning JR, Steen S (eds.). Nutrition for sport and exercise. Gaithersburg, MD: Aspen Publishers, 1998.

Burke LM, et al. Muscle glycogen storage after prolonged exercise: Effect of the glycemic index of carbohydrate feedings. J Appl Physiol 75:1019, 1993.

Butterfield GE. Whole body protein utilization in humans. Med Sci Sports Exerc 19:S157, 1987.
Butterfield GE. Amino acids and high protein diets. In: Lamb DR, Williams MH (eds.). Perspectives in exercise science and sports medicine, Vol 4: Ergogenic enhancement of performance in exercise and sport. Ann Arbor, MI: Brown and Benchmark, 1991.
Butterfield GE, Gates JE. Fueling Activity: Current Concepts. Topics in Nutrition and Food Safety. Hershey, PA: Hershey Foods Corporation, Fall, 1994, pp. 1–6.
Butterfield GE, Tremblay A: Physical activity and nutrition in the context of fitness and health. In: Bouchard C et al. (eds.). Physical Activity, Fitness and Health, International Proceedings and Consensus Statement. Champaign, IL: Human Kinetics Publishers, 1994, pp. 257–269.
Cannon JG, et al. Acute phase response in exercise: Interaction of age and vitamin E on neutrophils and muscle enzyme release. Am J Physiol (Regulatory Integ Comp Physiol) 259(28):R1214, 1990.
Coleman E. Carbohydrate—the master fuel. In: Berning JR, Steen SN (eds.). Nutrition for sport and exercise. Gaithersburg, MD: Aspen Publishers, 1998.
Cooper K. Cooper's antioxidant revolution. Nashville, TN: Thomas Nelson Publishers, 1994.
Cori CF. The fate of sugar in the animal body. I. The rate of absorption of hexoses and pentoses from the intestinal tract. J Biol Chem 66:7691, 1925.
Costill DL, et al. Effects of elevated plasma FFA and insulin on muscle glycogen usage during exercise. J Appl Physiol 43:695, 1977a.
Costill DL, et al. Muscle glycogen utilization during prolonged exercise on successive days. J Appl Physiol 31:834, 1977b.
Costill DL, et al. The role of dietary carbohydrate in muscle glycogen resynthesis after strenuous running. Am J Clin Nutr 34:1831, 1981.
Costill DL, Sparks KE. Rapid fluid replacement following thermal dehydration. J Appl Physiol 34:299, 1973.
Coyle EF. Timing and method of increased carbohydrate intake to cope with heavy training, competition, and recovery. J Sport Sci 9:29, 1991.
Crane RK. Na-dependent transport in the intestine and other animal tissues. Fed Proc 24:1000, 1965.
Davies KJA, et al. Free radical and tissue damage produced by exercise. Biochem Biophys Res Commun 107:1198, 1982.
Delvin J, et al. Amino acid metabolism after intense exercise. Am J Physiol 258:E249, 1990.
Dillard CJ, et al. Effects of exercise, vitamin E, and ozone on pulmonary function and lipid peroxidation. J Appl Physiol Respir Environ Exerc Physiol 45:927, 1978.
Dohm G, et al. Protein degradation during endurance exercise and recovery. Med Sci Sports Exerc 19:5166, 1987.
Drinkwater BL, et al. Bone mineral density after resumption of menses in amenorrheic athletes. JAMA 256:380, 1986.
Food and Nutrition Board, National Research Council. Recommended Dietary Allowances. 10th ed., Washington, D.C.: National Academy Press, 1989.
Franke WW, Berendonk B. Hormonal doping and androgenization of athletes: A secret program of the German Democratic Republic government. Clin Chem 43:1262, 1997.
Gisolfi CV, et al. Human intestinal water absorption: Direct vs. indirect measurements. Am J Physiol 258:G216, 1990.
Gontzea I, et al. The influence of muscular activity on nitrogen balance and on the need of man for protein. Nutr Rep Int 10:35, 1974.
Gonzalez-Alonso J, Heaps CL, Coyle EF. Rehydration after exercise with common beverages and water. Int J Sports Med 13:399, 1992.
Green DR et al. An evaluation of dietary intakes of triathletes: Are RDAs being met? J Am Diet Assoc 89:1653, 1989.
Greenhaff PL, et al. The effect of oral creatine supplementation on skeletal muscle ATP degradation during repeated bouts of maximal voluntary exercise in man. Am J Physiol 266(SPTI):E725, 1994.
Halliwell B, Gutteridge JMC. Free radicals in biology and medicine. Oxford: Clarendon Press, 1985, pp. 162–164.
Hargreaves M. Carbohydrate and exercise. J Sport Sci 9:17, 1991.
Harkins C, et al. Protocols for developing dietary prescriptions. In: Benardot D (ed.). Sports Nutrition. A Guide for the Professional Working with Active People, 2nd ed. Chicago: Am Diet Assoc, 1993.
Haymes EM, Clarkson PM. Minerals and trace minerals. In: Berning JR, Steen SN (eds.). Nutrition for sport and exercise. Gaithersburg, MD: Aspen Publishers, 1998, pp. 77–107.
Hickson JF, et al. Repeated days of body building exercise do not enhance urinary excretions from untrained young adult males. Nutr Res 10:723, 1990.
Hoffman CJ, et al. Weight change concerns of collegiate athletes. Top Clin Nutr 10(1):38, 1994.
Ismail AH, et al. Dietary supplementation with vitamin E and vitamin D in fit and nonfit adults: Biochemical and immunological changes. Fed Proc 42:335, 1983.
Ivy JL, et al. Muscle glycogen synthesis after exercise: Effect of time of carbohydrate ingestion. J Appl Physiol 64:1480, 1988.
Jackson D, et al. Effects of carbohydrate feedings on fatigue during intermittent high-intensity exercise in males and females. Med Sci Sports Exer 27:S223, 1995.
Jandrain B, et al. Metabolic availability of glucose ingested three hours before prolonged exercise in humans. J Appl Physiol 56:1314, 1984.
Jonnavithula S, et al. Bone density is compromised in amenorrheic women despite return of menses: A 2 year study. Obstet Gynecol 81:669, 1993.
Kanter M. Antioxidant supplementation for persons who are physically active. In: Berning JR, Steen SN (eds.). Nutrition for sport and exercise. Gaithersburg, MD: Aspen Publishers, 1998, pp. 109–115.
Keith RE. Vitamins and physical activity. In: Wolinsky I, Hickson JF (eds.). Nutrition in exercise and sport. Boca Raton, FL: CRC Press, 1994.
Kiens B, et al. Benefit of dietary simple carbohydrates on the early post exercise muscle glycogen repletion in athletes. Med Sci Sports Exerc 22(S4):88, 1990.
Leiper JB, Maughn RJ. Absorption of water and electrolytes from hypotonic, isotonic and hypertonic solutions. J Physiol 373:90P, 1986a.
Leiper JB, Maughn RJ. The effect of luminal tonicity on water absorption from a segment of the intact human jejunum. J Physiol 378:95P, 1986b.
Lindeman AK. Body image and college women athletes. Top Clin Nutr 10(1):58, 1994.
Lindinger MI, et al. Caffeine attenuates the exercise-induced increase in plasma [K+] in humans. J Appl Phys 74:1149, 1993.
Loucks AB. Effects of exercise training on the menstrual cycle: Existence and mechanism. Med Sci Sports Exerc 22:275, 1990.
Mahesh VB, Greenblatt RB. The in vivo conversion of dehydroepiandrosteron and andtrostenedione to testosterone in the human. Acta Endocrinol 41:400, 1962.
Malawer SJ. Interrelationship between jejunal absorption of sodium, glucose, and water in man. Am Soc Clin Invest 44:1072, 1965.
Meredith CN, et al. Dietary protein requirements and body protein metabolism in endurance trained men. J Appl Physiol 66:2850, 1981.
Meydani M, et al. Protective effect of vitamin E on exercise-induced oxidative damage in young and older adults. Am J Physiol 264:R992, 1993.
Meyer FO, et al. Hypohydration during exercise in children: Effect on thirst, drink preferences and rehydration. Int J Sports Nutr 1:22, 1994.
Morales AJ, et al. Effects of replacement dose of DHEA in men and women of advancing age. J Endocrinol Metab 78:1360, 1994.
Murray R. Fluid replacement: The American College of Sports Medicine Position. Sports Science Exchange 9:4, 1996.
Murray R. Fluid needs of athletes. In: Berning JR, Steen SN (eds.). Nutrition for sport and exercise. Gaithersburg, MD: Aspen Publishing, 1998.
Nadel ER, et al. Influence of fluid replacement beverages on body fluid homeostasis during exercise and recovery. In: Gisolfi CV, Lamb DR (eds.). Perspectives in exercise science and sports medicine, Vol. 3: Fluid homeostasis during exercise. Indianapolis, IN: Benchmark Press, 1990, pp. 1181–1205.
Nissen S, et al. Effect of leucine metabolite beta hydroxy beta methylbutyrate on muscle metabolism during resistance training. J Appl Physiol 81:2095, 1996.
Nose H, et al. Role of osmolality and plasma volume during rehydration in humans. J Appl Physiol 65:325, 1988.
Otis CL, et al. American College of Sports Medicine position stand on the female athlete triad. Med Sci Sports Exerc 29(5):i, 1997.
Patterson BH, et al. Fruit and vegetables in the American diet: data from the NHANES II Survey. Am J Publ Hlth 80: 1443, 1990.
Pugliese MT, et al. Fear of obesity: A cause of short stature and delayed puberty. N Engl J Med 309:513, 1983.
Regelson W, Kalimi M. Dehydroepiandrosterone (DHEA)—the multifunctional steroid. II. Effects on the CNS, cell proliferation, metabolic and vascular, clinical, and other effects. Ann N Y Acad Sci 719:564, 1994.
Regelson W, et al. Dehydroepiandrosterone (DHEA)—the mother steroid I. Immunological action. Ann N Y Acad Sci 719:553, 1994.
Ryan AJ, et al. Effect of hypohydration on gastric emptying and intestinal absorption during exercise. J Appl Physiol 84:1581, 1998.
Sanchez-Quesada JL, et al. Increase of LDL susceptibility to oxidation occurring after intense, long duration aerobic exercise. Athero, 118:297, 1995.
Simonsen JC, et al. Dietary carbohydrate, muscle glycogen, and power output during rowing training. J Appl Physiol 70:1500, 1991.
Singh A, et al. Dietary intakes and biochemical profiles of nutritional status of ultramarathoners. Med Sci Sport Exerc 25:328, 1993.
Singh VN. A current perspective on nutrition and exercise. J Nutr 122:760, 1992.
Steen SN, Brownell KD: Patterns of weight loss and regain in wrestlers: Has the tradition changed? Med Sci Sports Exerc 22:762, 1990.
Stewart JG, et al. Gastrointestinal blood loss and anemia in runners. Ann Intern Med 100:843, 1984.
Strauss RH, et al. Weight loss in amateur wrestlers and its effect on serum testosterone levels. JAMA 254:3337, 1985.
Synder AC, et al. Myofibrillar protein degradation after eccentric exercise. Experientia 40:69, 1984.
Synder AC, Naik J. Protein requirement of athletes. In: Berning JR, Steen

SN (eds.). Nutrition for sport and exercise. Gaithersburg, MD: Aspen Publishers, 1998.
Tarnopolsky MA. Caffeine and endurance performance. Sports Med 18:109, 1994.
Tarnopolsky MA, et al. Effect of body building exercise on protein requirements. Can J Sports Sci 15:225, 1991.
Tarnopolsky M, et al. Evaluation of protein requirements for trained strength athletes. J Appl Physiol 73:1986, 1992.
Tarnopolsky MA, et al. Influence of protein intake and training status on nitrogen balance and lean body mass. J Appl Physiol 64:187, 1988.
Viguie CA, et al. Antioxidant supplementation affects indices of muscle trauma and oxidant stress in human blood during exercise. Med Sci Sports Exerc 21:S16, 1989.
Wardlaw GM. Perspectives in Nutrition, 4th ed. New York: WCB–McGraw Hill, 1999, p. 174.
Waller MF, Haymes EM. The effects of heat and exercise on sweat iron loss. Med Sci Sport Exerc 28:197, 1996.
Weindruch R. National Institute of Aging Grant Number 5RC1AG10536-05 CRISP, 1997.
Williams MH. Nutritional ergogenic aids and athletic performance. Nutr Today 24(1):7, 1989.
Wong SHY, et al. Lipoperoxide in plasma as measured by liquid-chromatographic separation of malondialdehyde-thiobarbituric acid adduct. Clin Chem 33(2) 214, 1987.
Yoshimura H. Adult protein requirements. Fed Proc 20:103, 1961.
Zawadski KM, et al. Carbohydrate-protein complex increases the rate of muscle glycogen storage after exercise. J Appl Physiol 72:1854, 1992.

ADDITIONAL REFERENCES

American Dietetic Association. Timely statement of the American Dietetic Association. Nutrition guidance for child athletes in organized sports. J Am Diet Assoc 96:610, 1996.
Beals K, Manore M. Nutritional status of female athletes with subclinical eating disorders. J Am Diet Assoc 98:419, 1998.
Below PR, et al. Fluid and carbohydrate ingestion independently improve performance during 1 hour of intense exercise. Med Sci Sports Exerc 27:200, 1994.
Bosch A, et al. Fuel substrate kinetics of carbohydrate loading differs from that of carbohydrate ingestion during prolonged exercise. Metabolism 45:415, 1996.
Clarkson P. Antioxidants and physical performance. Crit Rev Food Sci Nutr 35(1&2):131, 1995.
Feldman EB. Creatine: A dietary supplement and ergogenic aid. Nutr Rev, 57:45, 1999.
Haymes EM. Vitamin and mineral supplementation to athletes. Int J Sport Med 1:146, 1991.
Kirschner E, et al. Bone mineral density and dietary intake of female college gymnasts. Med Sci Sports Exerc 27:543, 1995.
Leddy J, et al. Effect of a high or a low fat diet on cardiovascular risk factors in male and female runners. Med Sci Sports Exerc 29:17, 1997.
Maughan R, et al. Rehydration and recovery after exercise. Sports Science Exchange 9:1, 1996.
Oppliger R, et al. The Wisconsin wrestling minimum weight project: A model for weight control among high school wrestlers. Med Sci Sports Exerc 27:1220, 1995.
Ryan M. Sports drinks: Research asks for reevaluation of current recommendations. J Am Diet Assoc 97:S197, 1997.
Sanborn CF, et al. Athletic amenorrhea, lack of association with body fat. Med Sci Sports Exerc 19:207, 1987.
Tegelman R, et al. Influence of a diet regimen on glucose homeostasis and serum lipid levels in male elite athletes. Metabolism 45:435, 1996.
Thompson J, Manore M. Predicted and measured resting metabolic rate of male and female endurance athletes. J Am Diet Assoc 96:30, 1996.
Volek J, et al. Creatine supplementation enhances muscular performance during high-intensity resistance exercise. J Am Diet Assoc 97:765, 1997.

CHAPTER 26

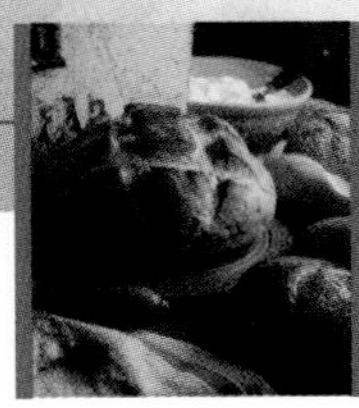

Nutrition in Cardiovascular Disease

DEBRA KRUMMEL, PhD, RD

CHAPTER OUTLINE

- Prevalence and Incidence
- Mortality
- Pathophysiology and Etiology
- Risk Factors for Coronary Heart Disease
- Genetic Hyperlipidemias: Classification and Diagnosis
- Dietary Factors
- Prevention of Coronary Heart Disease
- Treatment

Key Terms

ANGINA—chest pain resulting from impaired blood flow to the heart (ischemia)
APOLIPOPROTEIN—protein component of lipoproteins that provides structure and controls the metabolic fate of lipoproteins
ARTERIOSCLEROSIS—sclerosis (hardening) and thickening of the arterial wall, with loss of elasticity
ATHEROMA—Any of the lesions of atherosclerosis; another name for plaque
ATHEROSCLEROSIS—a form of arteriosclerosis; a complex process of thickening and narrowing of the arterial walls caused by the accumulation of lipids, primarily oxidized cholesterol, in the intimal or inner layer in combination with connective tissue and calcification
BILE ACID SEQUESTRANTS—drugs that adsorb bile acids and, by preventing their absorption back into the bloodstream, lower blood cholesterol levels
CHYLOMICRONS—lipoproteins that transport dietary fat from the gut to the periphery
CORONARY HEART DISEASE (CHD) OR CORONARY ARTERY DISEASE (CAD)—disease involving the network of blood vessels surrounding and serving the heart; manifested in clinical end points of myocardial infarction and sudden death
FAMILIAL COMBINED HYPERLIPIDEMIA (FCHL)—a common lipid disorder characterized by elevated plasma low-density lipoprotein cholesterol or a triglyceride level above the 90th percentile in at least two family members; the result of overproduction of lipoproteins by the liver
FAMILIAL DYSBETALIPOPROTEINEMIA—a rare lipoproteinemia characterized by elevated serum total cholesterol and triglycerides and apo E-2 allele
FAMILIAL DYSLIPIDEMIA—a common lipid disorder in which at least two family members have fasting triglyceride levels above the 90th percentile
FAMILIAL HYPERCHOLESTEROLEMIA (FH)—a genetic defect in the ability to metabolize low-density lipoprotein cholesterol; characterized by hypercholesterolemia (>300 mg/dL), xanthomas, advanced atherosclerosis, and premature death
FATTY STREAKS—earliest lesions in atherosclerosis; characterized by lipid-rich macrophages and smooth muscle cells
HIGH-DENSITY LIPOPROTEIN (HDL)—a plasma lipoprotein containing mostly protein and less cholesterol and triglyceride, high levels of which are associated with a decreased risk of coronary heart disease, probably because it removes cholesterol from the arterial intima
HMG CoA REDUCTASE INHIBITORS—cholesterol-lowering drugs that inhibit the rate-limiting enzyme (HMG CoA reductase) in cholesterol synthesis
HYPERCHOLESTEROLEMIA—elevated cholesterol level in the blood
HYPERTRIGLYCERIDEMIA—elevated blood triglyceride level
INTERMEDIATE-DENSITY LIPOPROTEINS (IDLs)—lipoproteins that are formed during catabolism; precursors of low-density lipoproteins
ISCHEMIA—insufficient blood flow in a tissue due to functional constriction or actual obstruction of a blood vessel
LIPOPROTEINS—a diverse class of particles, containing varying amounts of triglyceride, cholesterol, phospholipids, and protein, that solubilize lipids for blood transport
LOW-DENSITY LIPOPROTEINS (LDLs)—lipoproteins that are the major cholesterol carriers in the blood; high levels are associated with increased risk of coronary heart disease; main target for interventions
MYOCARDIAL INFARCTION (MI)—ischemia in the coronary arteries resulting in necrosis, tissue damage, and sometimes, sudden death
PLAQUE—part of the lesions seen in atherosclerosis; composed of lipids, cholesterol, calcium, and fibrin
RISK FACTORS—characteristics that increase the likelihood of a person developing a disease; for coronary heart disease, major risk factors are hypercholesterolemia, hypertension, and cigarette smoking
THROMBUS—an aggregation of blood factors, primarily

platelets and fibrin which, if small, can contribute to growth of plaque; if large, it can obstruct a blood vessel, resulting in angina, myocardial infarction, or sudden death

VERY LOW-DENSITY LIPOPROTEINS (VLDLs)—lipoproteins that contain more triglyceride than cholesterol; they transport lipid from the liver to the periphery

XANTHOMA—cholesterol deposits (from low-density lipoproteins) seen on tendons and elbows

Cardiovascular disease (CVD) kills more people yearly than the next seven causes of death combined (American Heart Association, 1997). Coronary heart disease (CHD), also known as coronary artery disease (CAD) or ischemic heart disease (IHD), is the most deadly of cardiovascular diseases; 50% of all cardiac deaths result from CHD. The morbidity and mortality associated with CVD make it a major public health problem, with costs exceeding $274 billion a year.

Although most CHD deaths occur in people older than 65 years of age, the large number of premature deaths has led to extensive research into prevention. Epidemiologic studies (observational studies, such as cohort and cross-sectional studies) and experimental studies (clinical or community trials) have delineated the risk factors associated with CHD development, which constitutes a major breakthrough for CHD prevention. For more information, the American Heart Association website is: www.amhrt.org.

PREVALENCE AND INCIDENCE

More than 58 million Americans have at least one form of CVD (i.e., hypertension, CHD, stroke, or rheumatic heart disease). Fourteen million have symptomatic CHD. One in nine women and one in six men aged 45 to 64 years have some form of heart disease. After the age of 65, one in three women and one in eight men are afflicted.

The United States ranks 17th among industrialized nations for the incidence of CVD (Fig. 26–1). Within the United States, the incidence of CHD in the Framingham population (see the accompanying box, "*Focus On:* Framingham Heart Study") shows marked gender differences. For women, there is a 40-fold difference in the incidence of CHD between the youngest and the oldest age groups (Fig. 26–2) (Lerner and Kannel, 1986). Most women are diagnosed with CHD after the age of 55. Many studies have shown a 10-year lag between the incidence of CHD in women and men. For men, a sixfold difference in the incidence of CHD between the youngest and oldest groups exists, with a peak occurring at about the age of 45, after which there is a leveling off.

MORTALITY

CHD, expressed as myocardial infarction, is the leading cause of death in American men and women (American Heart Association, 1997); about 482,000 people died from CHD in 1995. Mortality from all heart diseases increases with age in all races (Table 26–1). In 45- to 64-year-olds, premature death rates are approximately 1.7 times higher in blacks than in whites, approximately 10% lower in Native Americans than in whites, and much lower (30% to 60%) in Asian and Hispanic adults (Health, United States, 1991). Beyond 65 years of age, blacks still have the lowest mortality from heart disease of all ethnic groups. Among immigrants who migrate from countries with low rates of death from CHD, the death rate is more similar to that of their adoptive country after acculturation than to that of their native country.

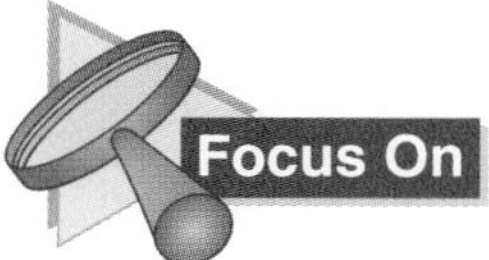

FRAMINGHAM HEART STUDY

Of the many extensive studies to identify the risk factors leading to coronary heart disease (CHD), a unique and most productive one is the Framingham Heart Study. This prospective and noninvasive study, which was initiated in 1949 under the direction of Dr. William Castelli, involves every other adult between the ages of 30 and 62 years living in the manufacturing town of Framingham, Massachusetts. Of the original 5,209 participants, all of whom agreed to return for check-ups and data collection at regular intervals for the rest of their lives, 2,500 were still living in 1985 (NIH, 1985).

Among the CHD risk factors positively identified by this study for the first time were high blood pressure, elevated cholesterol level, and cigarette smoking. Also associated were obesity and the protective effect of exercise. Later, the relationships of the different cholesterol fractions were clarified. The study was also the first to identify high blood pressure as the major cause of stroke.

In 1972, a companion study was initiated to measure the influence of heredity and environment on the offspring of the original participants (Wilson et al., 1989). Dietary practices, which were not followed in the initial study, were included along with more sophisticated measurements of physical status. This cohort of 5,000, which also includes spouses of the offspring, appears to date to be more health conscious that the older generation as reflected in less smoking, lower blood pressure, and lower cholesterol levels than seen in their parents at the same age. It will be interesting to see what this means in terms of CHD morbidity and mortality in this second generation.

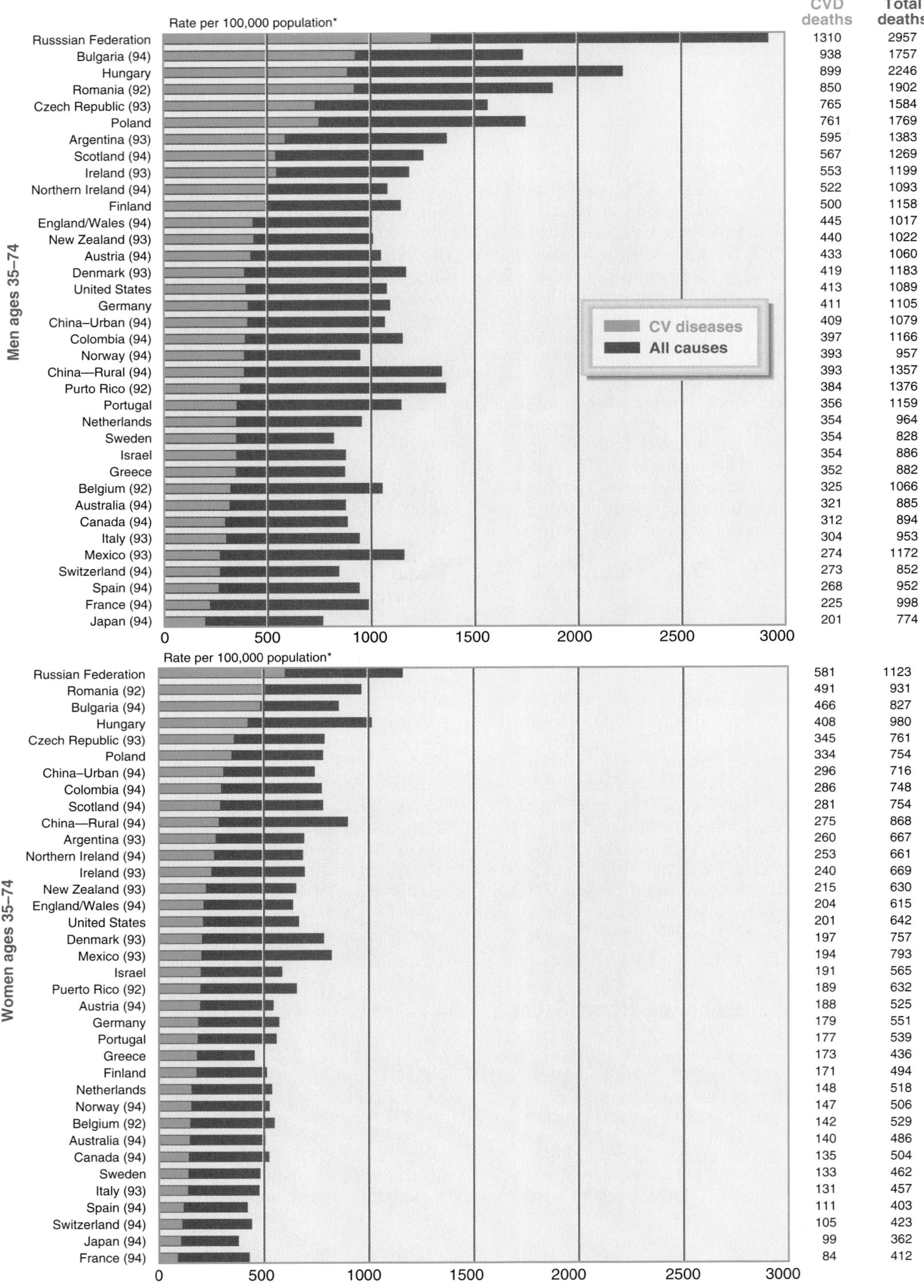

* ICD/9 390–459 for cardiovascular disease. Rates adjusted to the European Standard population.

FIGURE 26–1 1999 Heart and stroke statistical update. (Adapted from the 1999 Heart and Stroke Statistical Update, American Heart Association.) (*CV*, cardiovascular; *CVD*, cardiovascular disease.)

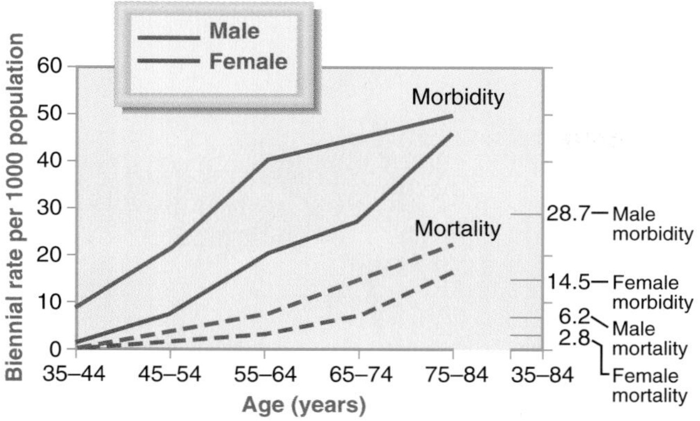

FIGURE 26–2 Incidence of coronary heart disease morbidity and mortality by age and sex: 26-year follow-up Framingham Study. (Redrawn with permission from Lerner DJ, Kannel SB. Patterns of coronary heart disease morbidity and mortality in the sexes: A 26-year follow-up of the Framingham population. Am Heart J 111:383, 1986, © Mosby Yearbook.)

Epidemic levels of CVD began around 1920 when CHD became a major cause of death in the United States. Mortality (from diseases of the heart) increased until the mid-1960s, when it began to drop abruptly from an age-adjusted rate of 286 deaths per 100,000 people to 152 per 100,000 in 1990, a decrease of 47% (Health, United States, 1991). This decrease started slowing in the late 1980s. All age, sex, ethnic, and population groups have experienced a decline in heart disease–related mortality. Reasons for the decrease in mortality include better treatment and primary prevention efforts, such as life-style changes to modify risk factors (discussed later in this chapter). Computer modeling studies have shown that 25% of the decline in CHD is attributable to primary prevention and 70% to behavioral changes affecting risk factors or improvements in treatment (Hunink et al., 1997).

PATHOPHYSIOLOGY AND ETIOLOGY

Coronary heart disease (CHD) results from a lack of blood flow to the network of blood vessels surrounding the heart and serving the myocardium (Fig. 26–3). The major underlying cause of CHD is atherosclerosis, which involves structural and compositional changes in the innermost or intimal layer of the large arteries. Atherosclerosis is thus the main cause of heart attack, stroke, and gangrene of the extremities. Hence, the arteries most often affected are the abdominal aorta and the coronary and cerebral arteries.

TABLE 26–1 MORTALITY FROM DISEASES OF THE HEART BY RACE/ETHNICITY*

AGE (YEARS)	RACE/ETHNICITY				
	Hispanic	Asian	Native American	Black	White
25–44	12	7	20	44	17
45–64	166	99	224	426	244
>65	1336	870	1128	2181	2079

(From the National Center for Health Statistics, 1990. Hyattsville, MD: Public Health Service, 1991.)

*Deaths per 100,000 population.

Atherosclerosis

Atherosclerosis is a slow, progressive disease that begins in childhood and takes decades to advance. It is now known that the pathogenesis of atherosclerosis is multifactorial. The lesions that develop are the result of (1) proliferation of smooth muscle cells, macrophages, and lymphocytes (cells involved in the inflammatory response); (2) formation of smooth muscle cells into a connective tissue matrix; and (3) accumulation of lipid and cholesterol in the matrix around the cells. The lipid deposits and other materials (cellular waste products, calcium, fibrin) that build up in the intimal layer are called **plaque** or **atheroma.** Plaque forms in response to injuries to the endothelium in the artery wall. Some of the factors that cause injury are hypercholesterolemia, oxidized low-density lipoprotein (LDL), hypertension, cigarette smoking, diabetes, obesity, homocysteine, and diets high in cholesterol and saturated fat. After injury, platelets adhere to the arterial wall and release growth factors that promote lesion development. Thus, atherosclerosis is an inflammatory and proliferative response to arterial wall injuries.

Pathophysiology

The lesions of atherosclerosis are classified as fatty streaks, intermediate lesions, fibrous plaques, and complicated lesions. There are five phases of *atherogenesis,* with characteristic lesions and symptoms at each phase (Fuster et al., 1996). Phase 1, an asymptomatic phase, consists of fatty streaks, which are often seen in people younger than 30 years of age. **Fatty streaks** are nonobstructive, lipid-filled cells (macrophages and smooth muscle cells) that form at bends in the artery in response to chronic injury to the arterial endothelium. Not all fatty streaks progress to advanced lesions.

Phase 2 is characterized by plaque with a high lipid content that may be prone to rupture. The lipid is derived from plasma LDLs that enter the injured endothelial wall. Because of the instability of the intermediate lesions in phase 2, these lesions can progress to phase 3 (acute, complicated lesions with rupture and nonocclusive thrombus) or phase 4 (acute, complicated lesions with occlusive thrombus), which are associated with angina or **myocardial infarction** and sudden death. Phase 3 lesions can progress to phase 5 (fibrotic or occlusive) lesions with similar clinical outcomes. Risk factors strongly influence and accelerate progression to more complicated lesions. Oxidized LDL converts macro-

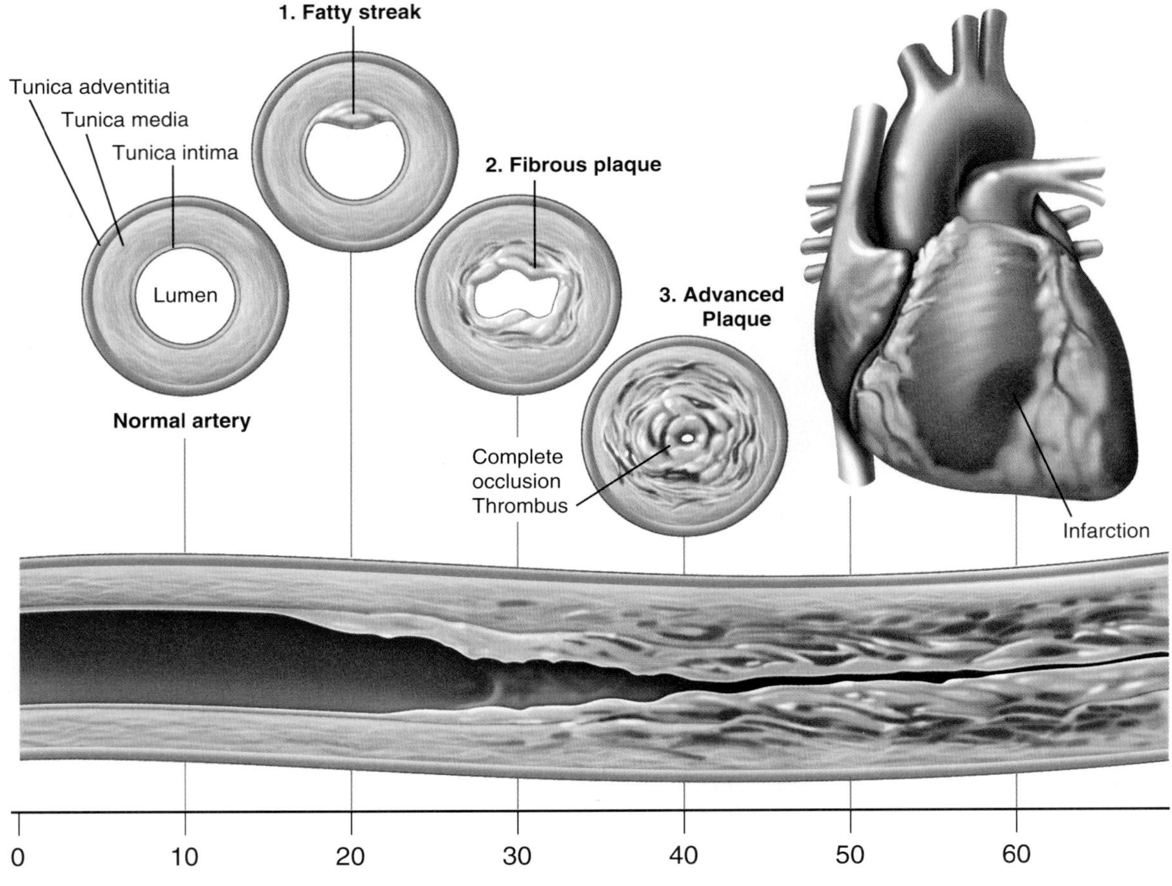

FIGURE 26–3 Natural progression of atherosclerosis. (From Harkreader H. Fundamentals. Philadelphia: W.B. Saunders, 2000.)

phages into foam cells. High-density lipoprotein (HDL) prevents lipid accumulation in the arterial wall by inhibiting LDL oxidation and by transporting cholesterol to the liver. Most sudden deaths after myocardial infarction result from ruptures in the fibrous cap of complicated lesions, leading to hemorrhage in the plaque, thrombosis, and blockage of the artery. Small thrombi help plaque grow, whereas large thrombi can cause acute clinical events. The progression of atherosclerotic lesions is not linear or predictable. Lesions can appear in arteries that were judged to be "normal" on angiography months earlier (Fuster et al., 1996) (see Fig. 24–4A and B).

Clinical Determination

Noninvasive tests, such as electrocardiograms, treadmill exercise tests, thallium scans, and echocardiography, are used initially to establish a diagnosis of CHD. However, the most definitive, widely available test is invasive *angiography (cardiac catheterization),* in which a dye is injected into the arteries and radiographic images of the heart are obtained. Narrowing and blockages from atherosclerosis are readily apparent on *angiograms.* However, smaller phase 2 lesions are often not visible on angiography, but can cause acute ischemic events. Thus, angiography cannot determine which lesions will rupture or where future occlusion will occur (Fuster et al., 1996).

Intravascular ultrasound detects plaque more frequently than angiography and can provide information about plaque composition, which in the future, may affect treatment modalities (Hausmann et al., 1996). Mild coronary lesions have been associated with significant progression to severe stenosis or total occlusion in as many as two thirds of patients with unstable angina or acute coronary syndromes. Thus, early detection is critical.

Other indicators of CHD are evidence of myocardial infarction, clinically significant myocardial **ischemia,** history of coronary artery surgery, and coronary angioplasty (National Cholesterol Education Program [NCEP], 1993). Although no blood tests are specific for atherosclerosis, white blood cell count and fibrinogen in the normal range of values both appear to indicate active lesions that may be unstable (Kannel, 1992). For the men participating in the Framingham study, each standard deviation increase in white blood cell count correlated with a 42% increase in CHD incidence. Men with high normal fibrinogen levels were 1.8 times more likely to have developed CHD after 16 years of fol-

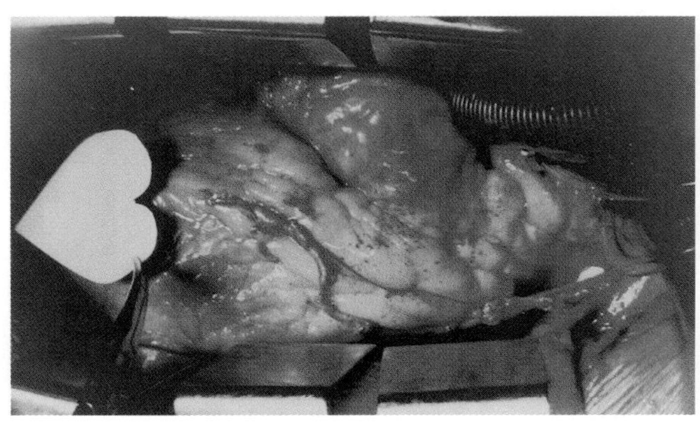

A

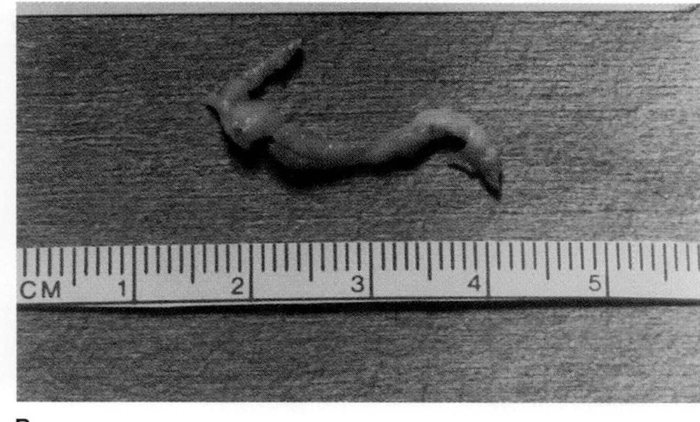

B

FIGURE 26–4 (**A, B**) Plaque that has been surgically removed from coronary artery. (Photographs courtesy of Ronald D. Gregory and John Riley, MD.)

low-up; women were 1.7 times more likely to have CHD. This magnitude of risk is similar to that for other risk factors.

End Points

When the occlusion of the arteries is significant, acute clinical events, such as unstable **angina,** myocardial infarction, and sudden death, can occur. When ischemia causes an infarction, the myocardium (or other tissue) is deprived of oxygen and nourishment. Whether the heart is able to continue beating depends on the extent of the musculature involved, the presence of collateral circulation, and the oxygen requirement.

Thrombosis

Thrombus formation and platelet activation are critical to plaque progression and the manifestations of acute angina or myocardial infarction (Fuster et al., 1992b). Thrombogenic risk factors include local factors, such as the degree of plaque disruption, the degree of stenosis, and vasoconstriction, as well as systemic factors, such as cigarette smoking, stress, elevated cholesterol and lipoprotein(a) levels, homocysteinemia, diabetes, and impaired fibrinolysis (Fuster et al., 1996). The role of diet in thrombosis and hemostasis is controversial and needs further research (Knapp, 1997).

RISK FACTORS FOR CORONARY HEART DISEASE

A landmark achievement of epidemiologic research has been the identification of **risk factors** for CHD. These risk factors were found to be particularly prevalent in persons who later developed CHD. Once the prospective studies identified risk factors, prevention and intervention studies were undertaken to test how strong these factors were, either alone or in combination, as disease predictors. An individual with one risk factor was found to be at greater risk of developing CHD than an individual with no risk factors.

Many risk factors occur together, and risk increases markedly with the addition of each risk factor. Most of the risk factors that were identified in the 1940s to the 1960s were found to be very strong predictors of subsequent CHD in healthy persons. These risk factors, along with others that have been identified subsequently, have been tested, and mechanisms have been elucidated for their role in CHD development. The primary prevention of CHD involves the assessment and management of these risk factors in asymptomatic individuals.

Blood Lipids and Lipoproteins

Cross-population, within-population, clinical, and pathologic studies have consistently shown that a high serum cholesterol level causes CHD, and is, therefore, associated with the incidence of CHD and associated mortality. In the last 30 years, the carriers of blood lipids—lipoproteins—have come to the forefront as predictors of risk.

Definitions

Blood lipids (cholesterol, triglycerides, and phospholipids) are transported in the blood bound to proteins. These complex particles, called **lipoproteins,** vary in composition, size, and density (Table 26–2). The five classes of lipoproteins—chylomicrons, very low-density lipoproteins (VLDLs), intermediate-density lipoproteins (IDLs), low-density lipoproteins (LDLs), and high-density lipoproteins (HDLs)—consist of varying amounts of triglyceride, cholesterol, phospholipid, and protein.

Each class of lipoproteins actually represents a continuum of particles. The protein:fat ratio determines the density; thus, particles with more protein are denser (e.g., HDLs have more protein than

TABLE 26–2 CHARACTERISTICS AND FUNCTIONS OF THE PLASMA LIPOPROTEINS

	CLASSES OF LIPOPROTEINS				
CHARACTERISTICS	**Chylomicron**	**VLDL**	**IDL**	**LDL**	**HDL**
Density, g/mL	<0.95	0.95–1.006	1.006–1.019	1.019–1.063	1.063–1.210
Electrophoretic mobility		Pre-β	Pre-β to β	β	α
Origin	Intestine	Liver and intestine	In circulation secondary to catabolism of other lipoproteins Liver	Liver	Liver and intestine
Physiologic role	Transport of dietary triglyceride	Transport of endogenous triglyceride	LDL precursor	Major cholesterol transport lipoprotein	Reverse cholesterol transport
Relative atherogenicity	0	+	+++	++++	Negatively correlated with atherosclerosis
Composition (%)					
Triglyceride	90	60	40	10	5
Cholesterol	5	10	30	50	20
Phospholipid	3	18	20	15	25
Protein	2	10	10	25	50
Major apolipoproteins	A-1 A-IV B-48 CI CII CIII	B-100 CI CII CIII E	B-100 E	B-100	A-I A-II

(From Kris-Etherton PM, et al. The effect of diet on plasma lipids, lipoproteins, and coronary heart disease. J Am Diet Assoc 88:1373, 1988. Reprinted with permission.)
VLDL, very low-density lipoprotein; *IDL*, intermediate-density lipoprotein; *LDL*, low-density lipoprotein; *HDL*, high-density lipoprotein.

LDLs. The physiologic role of lipoproteins includes transporting lipid to cells for energy or storage and serving as a substrate for prostaglandins, thromboxanes, and leukotrienes (see Chapters 3 and 43). Because of different metabolic roles, the lipoproteins also vary in atherogenicity.

Some of the protein components, known as **apolipoproteins (apo),** are specific to a class of lipoproteins; for example, apo B-48 is found only in chylomicrons, whereas others (e.g., apo E) transfer between the lipoproteins during metabolism. The main apolipoprotein in LDL is apo B-100; the primary apolipoproteins in HDL are apo A-I and A-II. These three apolipoproteins are affected by diet. Another apolipoprotein, apo E, affects blood cholesterol levels but is not affected by diet.

Total Cholesterol

A total cholesterol measurement is the cholesterol contained in all lipoprotein fractions. Sixty percent to 70% of the total is carried on LDL, 20% to 30% on HDL, and 10% to 15% on VLDL. Because of its ease of measurement, total cholesterol in both older epidemiologic research and present-day screening is the first blood lipid measured to assess risk. Total blood cholesterol is measured because earlier prospective studies established a direct, positive relationship between total serum cholesterol and CHD. Populations that consume diets high in saturated fatty acids have increased blood cholesterol levels and CHD risk. Within populations, the blood cholesterol level, particularly when high, is a strong predictor of CHD mortality (Fig. 26–5).

Increased levels of serum cholesterol, measured in individuals in their 20s, are strongly associated with later incidence of CHD (follow-up after 40 years), when the mean level at entry into the study was in the desirable range (Klag et al., 1993). The Second Report of the Expert Panel on Detection, Evaluation, and Treatment of High Blood Cholesterol in Adults (Adult Treatment Panel II, or ATP-II) reaffirms that, "increased blood cholesterol level, specifically LDL-cholesterol, increases risk for CHD. Conversely, lowering total cholesterol and LDL-C reduces CHD risk" (NCEP, 1993).

For screening purposes, blood cholesterol can be measured using a nonfasting blood sample. A blood cholesterol level of less than 200 mg/dL is considered desirable; 200 to 239 mg/dL is borderline high, and 240 mg/dL is a high blood cholesterol level, or **hypercholesterolemia.** Forty percent of the U.S. population surveyed in the third National Health and Examination Survey (NHANES III) required further lipoprotein analyses because (1) they had a desirable blood cholesterol level, but low HDL cholesterol; (2) they had borderline high blood cholesterol, normal HDL cholesterol, and two other risk factors; (3) they had borderline high blood cholesterol and low HDL cholesterol; or (4) they had high blood cholesterol levels (Sempos et al., 1993). Numerous factors affect serum cholesterol levels, including age; diets high in fat, saturated fat, and cholesterol; genetics; endogenous sex hormones (ab-

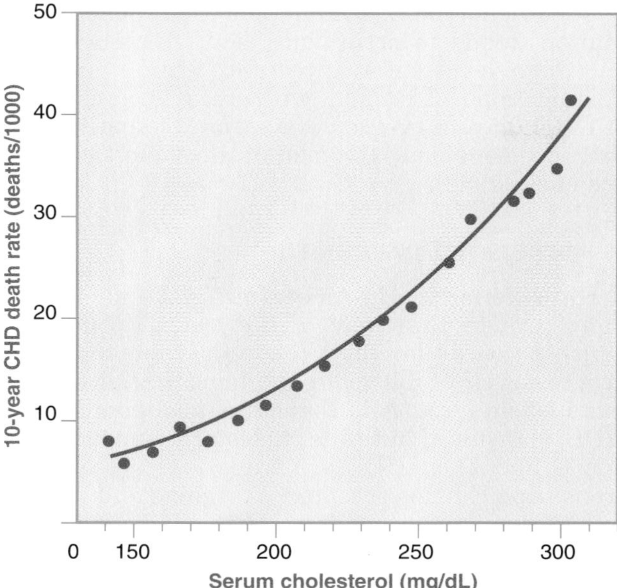

FIGURE 26–5 Relationship between serum cholesterol level and coronary heart disease (CHD) rate. (From National Cholesterol Education Program. Report of the Expert Panel on Population Strategies for Blood Cholesterol Reduction. U.S. Department of Health and Human Services, Public Health Service, National Institutes of Health, NIH Publication No. 90-3046. Bethesda, MD: National Heart, Lung, and Blood Institute, 1990.)

sence in postmenopausal women or presence during menstrual cycle); exogenous steroids (anabolic or sex hormones); drugs (beta-blockers, thiazide diuretics); body weight; glucose tolerance; physical activity level; diseases (diabetes, thyroid, liver); and season of the year.

Serum cholesterol levels in the United States population have been declining since 1960; more than half of that decline occurred between 1976 and 1991, after national preventive education efforts (Johnson, 1993). Since HDL cholesterol and VLDL cholesterol did not change during this period, the decline in total cholesterol levels is due to decreased LDL cholesterol. The greatest declines were seen in white women (–18 mg/dL), followed by white men (–13 mg/dL), black women (–11 mg/dL), and black men (–10 mg/dL). CHD mortality rates fell concurrently. Based on the Coronary Primary Prevention Trial, for every 1% decline in serum cholesterol level, a 2% decline in CHD incidence is predicted (NCEP, 1990).

Total Triglycerides

The triglyceride-rich lipoproteins include chylomicrons, VLDL, and any remnants or intermediary products formed in catabolism. Of these triglyceride-rich lipoproteins, IDL and chylomicron and VLDL remnants are known to be atherogenic. Some research suggests that postprandial triglyceride measurements may be more predictive of CHD risk than fasting levels (Ginsberg, 1994).

Triglyceride levels are classified as normal (<200 mg/dL), borderline high (200 to 400 mg/dL), high (400 to 1000 mg/dL), and very high (>1000 mg/dL) (NCEP, 1993). Patients with familial dyslipidemias will have triglyceride levels in the borderline high or high range. Triglycerides in the very high range place the patient at risk for pancreatitis. These patients usually have hyperchylomicronemia and require very low-fat diets (10% to 20% of calories derived from fat). Patients with a deficiency of lipoprotein lipase (LPL) will also have very high triglyceride levels and will require 10%-fat diets. Drugs are often necessary to lower triglyceride levels in these patients.

Lipoproteins and Metabolism

CHYLOMICRONS

The largest particles, the **chylomicrons,** transport dietary fat and cholesterol from the small intestine to the periphery (see Chapter 1). Once in the bloodstream, the triglycerides in the chylomicrons are hydrolyzed by LPL, located on the endothelial cell surface in muscle and adipose tissue. Apo C-II, one of the apolipoproteins in chylomicrons, is a cofactor for LPL. When approximately 90% of the triglyceride is hydrolyzed, the particle is released back into the blood as a remnant. These chylomicron remnants are metabolized by the liver, but some deliver cholesterol to the arterial wall and thus are considered atherogenic. Consumption of high-fat meals produces more chylomicrons and remnants. When fasting plasma studies are done, chylomicrons are normally absent.

VERY LOW-DENSITY LIPOPROTEINS

Very low-density lipoproteins (VLDLs) are synthesized in the liver to transport endogenous triglyceride and cholesterol. Sixty percent of the VLDL particle is triglyceride (see Table 26–2). VLDL particles are very heterogeneous. The large, buoyant VLDL particle is believed to be nonatherogenic (NIH Consensus Conference, 1993). Vegetarian diets and estrogen increase the formation of these large VLDLs. Smaller VLDL particles (i.e., remnants) are formed from triglyceride hydrolysis by LPL. Normally, these remnants, called VLDL remnants or IDL, are taken up by receptors on the liver or converted to LDL.

About 50% of the remnants lose apo E and apo C and become LDL. LDL itself is not atherogenic; there are different particle sizes. Some of the smaller particles stay in the blood and become atherogenic when oxidized. These intermediary particles are formed at high rates with excessive cholesterol feeding in animals and in dysbetalipoproteinemia in humans. At present, concentrations of remnants can be determined only by methods (e.g., analytical ultracentrifuge) that are not commonly available in most laboratories. Clinically, a total triglyceride level is a measurement of the triglyceride in VLDL, remnants, and IDL.

INTERMEDIATE-DENSITY LIPOPROTEINS

Intermediate-density lipoproteins (IDLs) are formed with the catabolism of VLDL and are a precursor of LDL. They are rich in cholesterol and apo E (see Table 26–2). High concentrations of IDL and VLDL remnants have been directly related to lesion progression and subsequent coronary events in men and women (Phillips et al., 1993). As with VLDL remnants, IDL can be measured only by using density-gradient ultracentrifugation, which is not widely available.

LOW-DENSITY LIPOPROTEINS

Low-density lipoproteins (LDLs) are the primary transporters of cholesterol in the blood (see Table 26–2); consequently, total cholesterol levels and LDL cholesterol levels are highly correlated. Ninety-five percent of the apolipoproteins in LDL are apo B-100, known as apo B. Apo B is also present in smaller amounts in VLDL and IDL. After LDL is formed in VLDL catabolism, 60% is taken up by LDL receptors on the liver, adrenals, and other tissues. The remainder is catabolized via nonreceptor pathways. Both the number and activity of these LDL receptors are major determinants of LDL cholesterol levels in the blood.

Both LDL cholesterol and apo B are risk factors for atherogenesis and CHD. The atherogenic effect of LDL cholesterol is readily apparent in genetic disease, such as familial hypercholesterolemia, which is characterized by high levels of LDL cholesterol and few or no LDL receptors, resulting in defective LDL metabolism and severe, premature atherosclerosis and CHD. Without LDL receptors, LDL is metabolized via alternative pathways.

Some LDL can be oxidized and taken up by endothelial cells and macrophages in the arterial wall, leading to the first stages of atherosclerosis. Because of this oxidation, antioxidants are now being investigated in clinical trials exploring prevention and treatment of CHD.

The effects of other dietary changes, such as replacement of monounsaturates, which would be less susceptible to oxidation than polyunsaturates, are also being investigated. Estrogen has been shown to inhibit LDL oxidation, which may help to explain the lower rates of CHD seen in premenopausal women (Rifici and Khachadurian, 1992).

Like other lipoproteins, LDLs are also heterogeneous in size, density, and lipid components. With the use of sophisticated methods, two LDL subclasses, with different risks, have been identified. *Phenotype A* is indicated by very large LDL particles, which are not associated with risk of disease. By contrast, *phenotype B* is typified by small, dense LDL particles that are triglyceride-rich and cholesterol-depleted and that are predictive of CHD risk in both men and women (Austin and Hokanson, 1994). Phenotype B, seen in 30% of the general population, tends to occur with low HDL cholesterol and high levels of triglyceride, VLDL, and IDL. Postmenopausal women, who are at increased risk of CHD, have a greater prevalence of smaller LDL than premenopausal women of the same age (Campos et al., 1988).

HIGH-DENSITY LIPOPROTEINS

High-density lipoproteins (HDLs) contain more protein than any of the other lipoproteins, which accounts for their theoretical metabolic role as a reservoir of the apolipoproteins that direct lipid metabolism. Apo A-I, the main apolipoprotein in HDL, is involved in tissue cholesterol removal. Both apo C and E on HDL are transferred to chylomicrons. Apo E helps receptors recognize and metabolize chylomicron remnants. High HDL levels are, therefore, associated with low levels of chylomicrons, VLDL remnants, and small, dense LDL. Of the several classes of HDL, HDL-2, which is relatively large and lipid-rich, and HDL-3, which is small and relatively dense, predominate in human plasma. The use of these subfractions as predictors of risk has been debated, but total HDL cholesterol remains the best predictor.

Lipoprotein Assessment

Adult reference percentiles for total cholesterol, LDL cholesterol, and HDL cholesterol are shown in Tables 26–3 to 26–5. Corresponding levels of lipids, expressed in mmol/L, are given. Total cholesterol and LDL cholesterol increase with aging. Over the 45-year period from age 20 to 65, total cholesterol levels in men increase by 13%. In women, over the same period, the increase is 21%.

Reference plasma lipid levels for children and adolescents are presented in the "*Clinical Insight:* NCEP Recommendations for Detection and Management of Hypercholesterolemia in Children and Adults." Children of both sexes have similar levels of HDL cholesterol until puberty, after which the levels in females consistently run about 10 mg/dL higher than those in males throughout life. Black men have slightly higher levels of HDL than white men.

Adults older than 20 years of age should have their serum cholesterol level measured at least once every 5 years, and HDL cholesterol should be measured at the same time, if possible (NCEP, 1993). Because LDL cholesterol and total cholesterol are highly correlated, total cholesterol levels are used for initial screening to detect high LDL cholesterol levels. The advantages of using total cholesterol as the first assessment of risk include (1) low cost, (2) wide availability, and (3) no required fasting. The initial classification for primary prevention based on total cholesterol and HDL cholesterol levels is shown in Table 26–6.

A desirable blood lipid profile is a total cholesterol level of less than 200 mg/dL and an HDL cholesterol level greater than 35 mg/dL. People whose

TABLE 26–3 TOTAL SERUM CHOLESTEROL LEVELS (MG/DL) FOR PERSONS 20 YEARS OF AGE AND OLDER BY RACE/ETHNICITY, SEX, AND AGE: UNITED STATES, 1988–91

RACE/ETHNICITY, SEX, AND AGE	NUMBER OF EXAMINED PERSONS	MEAN	SELECTED PERCENTILE 5th	10th	15th	25th	50th	75th	85th	90th	95th
Men 20 Years and Older	3953	205	143	153	162	176	201	231	247	260	276
20–34 years	1186	189	134	145	151	162	186	211	225	236	260
35–44 years	653	207	144	155	167	182	205	231	245	258	269
45–54 years	508	218	152	170	180	191	215	242	257	268	283
55–64 years	535	221	154	169	180	195	221	245	264	274	285
65–74 years	557	218	157	173	179	190	214	241	256	270	286
75 years and older	514	205	145	156	164	175	202	232	248	257	275
Women 20 Years and Older	3885	207	143	154	162	175	202	233	252	269	287
20–34 years	1177	185	134	143	150	160	182	204	218	229	254
35–44 years	709	195	142	152	159	170	193	215	232	242	254
45–54 years	464	217	158	165	171	187	212	240	264	279	297
55–64 years	503	237	168	184	191	204	228	264	280	291	323
65–74 years	493	234	168	180	186	205	232	261	278	290	308
75 years and older	539	230	163	175	184	198	227	263	279	287	316
Mexican-American											
Men	1092	202	140	151	159	172	199	225	245	257	277
Women	1046	200	139	149	158	169	195	224	241	258	279
Non-Hispanic Black											
Men	922	199	136	149	156	170	195	224	242	252	276
Women	985	203	137	150	159	172	200	227	248	262	286
Non-Hispanic White											
Men	1816	206	144	154	163	177	203	232	247	260	276
Women	1734	208	144	155	163	176	202	234	254	271	288

(Data from National Cholesterol Education Program [NCEP]. Second Report of the Expert Panel on Detection, Evaluation, and Treatment of High Blood Cholesterol in Adults [Adult Treatment Panel II]. NIH Publication No. 93-3095. Bethesda, MD: National Institutes of Health. National Heart, Lung, and Blood Institute, 1993.)

TABLE 26–4 LOW-DENSITY LIPOPROTEIN CHOLESTEROL LEVELS (MG/DL) FOR PERSONS 20 YEARS OF AGE AND OLDER BY RACE/ETHNICITY, SEX, AND AGE: UNITED STATES, 1988–91

RACE/ETHNICITY, SEX, AND AGE	NUMBER OF EXAMINED PERSONS	MEAN	SELECTED PERCENTILE 5th	10th	15th	25th	50th	75th	85th	90th	95th
Men 20 Years and Older	1669	131	75	87	95	106	129	154	167	179	194
20–34 years	487	120	67	78	86	97	121	139	152	165	186
35–44 years	274	134	85	92	98	111	131	156	166	176	192
45–54 years	224	138	78	91	100	118	136	163	174	187	195
55–64 years	228	142	78	90	104	117	143	165	175	194	205
65–74 years	259	141	93	104	109	119	134	163	177	185	199
75 years and older	197	132	83	88	93	106	130	154	170	186	196
Women 20 Years and Older	1673	126	69	81	88	99	122	150	165	175	191
20–34 years	525	110	59	70	75	88	108	129	142	155	173
35–44 years	316	117	67	85	88	97	116	138	146	155	165
45–54 years	214	132	70	87	93	107	130	157	173	182	198
55–64 years	213	145	79	90	101	122	145	170	184	189	209
65–74 years	202	147	92	97	109	119	148	169	185	192	206
75 years and older	203	147	90	102	109	121	143	168	189	197	209
Mexican-American											
Men	448	124	70	77	85	96	120	148	161	172	188
Women	471	122	67	80	86	95	118	144	158	166	189
Non-Hispanic Black											
Men	393	126	69	76	82	96	123	146	168	186	206
Women	422	126	67	76	86	100	124	147	162	174	192
Non-Hispanic White											
Men	773	132	76	88	97	108	129	154	168	179	194
Women	729	126	69	82	89	99	122	151	166	176	192

(Data from National Cholesterol Education Program [NCEP]. Second Report of the Expert Panel on Detection, Evaluation, and Treatment of High Blood Cholesterol in Adults [Adult Treatment Panel II]. NIH Publication No. 93-3095. Bethesda, MD: National Institutes of Health. National Heart, Lung, and Blood Institute, 1993.)

TABLE 26–5 HIGH-DENSITY LIPOPROTEIN CHOLESTEROL LEVELS (MG/DL) FOR PERSONS 20 YEARS OF AGE AND OLDER BY RACE/ETHNICITY, SEX, AND AGE: UNITED STATES, 1988–91

RACE/ETHNICITY, SEX, AND AGE	NUMBER OF EXAMINED PERSONS	MEAN	SELECTED PERCENTILE								
			5th	10th	15th	25th	50th	75th	85th	90th	95th
Men 20 Years and Older	3920	46.5	28.0	31.0	34.0	37.0	44.1	53.1	59.1	64.0	73.0
20–34 years	1178	47.1	30.0	34.0	35.1	38.0	46.0	54.0	60.1	64.0	71.0
35–44 years	642	46.3	28.0	30.0	33.0	37.0	44.0	53.0	58.1	63.0	73.0
45–54 years	502	46.6	28.0	30.0	33.0	36.0	43.1	53.0	61.0	66.1	77.1
55–64 years	533	45.6	29.0	31.0	33.0	36.1	43.0	53.0	59.0	62.0	72.0
65–74 years	553	45.3	28.0	31.0	32.0	36.0	43.0	53.0	58.0	62.1	71.0
75 years and older	512	47.2	28.0	32.0	34.0	38.0	45.0	54.0	62.0	67.0	75.1
Women 20 Years and Older	3855	55.7	34.0	38.0	41.0	44.1	54.0	65.0	71.0	76.1	83.0
20–34 years	1167	55.7	34.0	38.0	41.0	44.1	54.0	64.1	70.1	75.1	83.1
35–44 years	701	54.3	33.0	37.0	40.0	44.0	53.0	64.1	69.1	72.1	79.0
45–54 years	459	56.7	37.0	38.1	41.0	46.0	56.0	65.0	72.1	77.1	84.1
55–64 years	500	56.1	33.0	37.0	40.0	44.0	53.0	66.0	73.0	79.0	87.1
65–74 years	492	55.7	34.0	37.0	40.0	44.1	54.0	65.1	73.0	78.0	83.1
75 years and older	536	57.1	33.0	39.0	41.0	44.1	56.0	66.1	73.1	78.1	87.0
Mexican-American											
Men	1077	46.9	30.0	33.0	34.1	38.0	45.0	54.0	59.0	64.0	69.0
Women	1040	53.3	34.0	37.0	40.0	44.0	52.0	61.0	68.0	72.1	78.0
Non-Hispanic Black											
Men	918	53.3	30.0	35.0	38.0	42.0	51.0	62.0	69.1	75.1	86.1
Women	978	57.8	37.0	40.0	43.0	47.0	55.1	67.1	74.0	78.1	86.0
Non-Hispanic White											
Men	1803	45.5	28.0	30.0	33.1	36.1	44.0	52.1	58.0	62.0	71.1
Women	1717	55.7	33.1	37.0	40.0	44.0	54.0	65.1	71.1	77.0	83.1

(Data from National Cholesterol Education Program [NCEP]. Second Report of the Expert Panel on Detection, Evaluation, and Treatment of High Blood Cholesterol in Adults [Adult Treatment Panel II]. NIH Publication No. 93-3095. Bethesda, MD: National Institutes of Health. National Heart, Lung, and Blood Institute, 1993.)

profiles fall within these parameters should receive dietary information and be advised to have their levels rechecked in 5 years. All others should undergo fasting lipoprotein analysis.

Lipoprotein Profile

A complete lipoprotein profile includes measurement of total cholesterol, LDL cholesterol, HDL cholesterol, and triglyceride level after fasting. Most clinical laboratories cannot quantify LDL cholesterol directly. Therefore, determination of LDL cholesterol requires measurement of total cholesterol, triglyceride, and HDL cholesterol. Although cholesterol levels can be determined in the nonfasting state, triglycerides must be measured after an 8- to 12-hour fast to allow time for chylomicrons to clear.

The Friedewald formula for calculating LDL-C is as follows:

$$\text{LDL-C} = (\text{TC}) - (\text{HDL-C}) - (\text{TG}/5)$$

where LDL-C is low-density lipoprotein cholesterol; TC is total cholesterol; HDL-C is high-density lipoprotein cholesterol; and TG is triglyceride. Calculating the LDL cholesterol level by difference can be done only when triglyceride levels are less than 400 mg/dL.

A desirable lipoprotein profile would be a total cholesterol level of less than 200 mg/dL, LDL cholesterol less than 130 mg/dL, HDL cholesterol greater than 35 mg/dL, and triglyceride level less than 200 mg/dL (NCEP, 1993). However, one major study shows that this HDL cholesterol level is too low as a cut-off point for women. In the Lipid Research Clinics' Follow-up Study, an HDL cholesterol of less than 50 mg/dL was strongly predictive of CVD-related death in women aged 50 to 69 years (Bass, 1993); that is, women with desirable total cholesterol and LDL cholesterol levels were at increased risk if their HDL cholesterol level was less than 50 mg/dL.

TABLE 26–6 INITIAL CLASSIFICATION BASED ON TOTAL CHOLESTEROL AND HDL CHOLESTEROL

Total Cholesterol	
<200 mg/dL	Desirable blood cholesterol
200–239 mg/dL	Borderline high blood cholesterol
≥240 mg/dL	High blood cholesterol
HDL-Cholesterol	
<35 mg/dL	Low HDL cholesterol

(Data from National Cholesterol Education Program [NCEP]. Second Report of the Expert Panel on Detection, Evaluation, and Treatment of High Blood Cholesterol in Adults [Adult Treatment Panel II]. NIH Publication No. 93-3095. Bethesda, MD: National Institutes of Health. National Heart, Lung, and Blood Institute, 1993.)

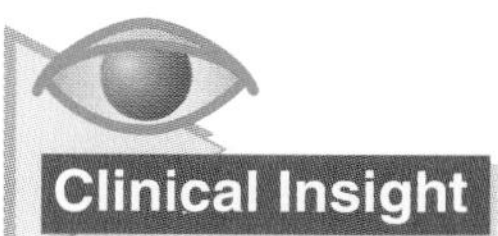

NCEP Recommendations for Detection and Management of Hypercholesterolemia in Children and Adolescents

In 1991, the National Cholesterol Education Program (NCEP) made recommendations for the management of hypercholesterolemia to be applied to adolescents and children older than 2 years of age (National Heart, Lung, and Blood Institute, 1991). This is the first time there has been consensus among pediatric experts, lipid researchers, and nutrition and health care communities on this subject.

For the general population of children and adolescents in the United States, NCEP recommended adoption of eating patterns to meet the following criteria:

- Nutritionally adequate, varied diet
- Adequate energy intake to support growth and development and maintain appropriate body weight
- Saturated fat—less than 10% of total calories
- Total fat—an average of no more than 30% of total calories
- Dietary cholesterol—less than 300 mg/day

Implementation of these dietary patterns requires involvement of the entire community—parents, in selecting and preparing foods; schools, in modifying school food service; health care clinics, in health education; government, in improvement of food labeling; and the food industry, in developing low saturated fat, low fat foods that are appealing to children.

NCEP also aims to identify and treat individual children and adolescents who have hypercholesterolemia and a family history of premature cardiovascular disease, or whose parents have hypercholesterolemia. For this group, the NCEP recommends:

1. Blood cholesterol screening of children and adolescents whose parents or grandparents, at 55 years or younger, were found to have coronary atherosclerosis; suffered myocardial infarction, peripheral vascular disease, cerebrovascular disease, or sudden death; or underwent invasive cardiac therapy (balloon angioplasty or coronary artery bypass surgery).
2. Blood cholesterol screening of offspring of a parent with a blood cholesterol of 240 mg/dL or greater.

For children with an elevated blood cholesterol level, the Step I Diet is used for 3 months, after which the blood cholesterol level is reassessed. If the desired cholesterol level has not been reached, the Step II Diet is implemented for at least another 6 months. If after 6 months to 1 year of dietary therapy blood lipid lowering is insufficient, drug therapy can be considered in children older than 10 years of age.

Visit the website http://rover.nhlbi.nih.gov/chd for more information.

LEVELS OF BLOOD TOTAL AND LDL CHOLESTEROL IN CHILDREN AND ADOLESCENTS

CATEGORY	TOTAL CHOLESTEROL, mg/dL	LDL CHOLESTEROL, mg/dL
Acceptable	<170	<110
Borderline	170–199	110–129
High	≥200	≥130

The greatest risk was assigned women with HDL cholesterol levels of less than 50 mg/dL and triglyceride levels greater than 400 mg/dL. Because women have higher HDL cholesterol than men, and 35 mg/dL is about the 5th percentile for women, a higher HDL cholesterol level is recommended to properly assess risk in women.

Ratios of various lipoproteins have been used to assess risk. A high risk of CHD is associated with a total cholesterol:HDL ratio of 5.6 or greater in women or 6.4 or greater in men followed over a 10-year period (Kinosian et al., 1994). A total cholesterol:HDL ratio of 7 in men or 6 in women is considered the target for beginning intervention (Schaefer, 1994b). Although many different ratios have been used to assess CHD risk, the Adult Treatment Panel II discourages their use as assessment parameters because each of the lipoproteins is an independent risk factor for CHD.

Assessing Risk

The American College of Cardiology has proposed four risk factor categories that match the intensity of risk factor management with the evidence for an association with CVD, clinical usefulness, and response to therapy (Pasternak, 1996) (Table 26–7). Category I risk factors are those for which interventions have been proven to lower CVD risk. Category II risk factors are those for which interventions are likely to lower CVD risk. Category III risk factors are those for which additional evidence is needed to determine if interventions can lower risk. Category IV risk factors are those that cannot be modified.

It is known that diet is the predominant environmental cause of coronary atherosclerosis, and that diet modification unequivocally can reduce risk of CHD. Thus, if diet were listed as a separate risk factor, it would be a Category I risk factor.

Category I Risk Factors

CIGARETTE SMOKING

The increased risk of CVD from smoking has been recognized for more than 30 years. The 1964 Surgeon General's Report, which outlined the health hazards of smoking, impacted the prevalence of smoking in adults; 42% of all adults in 1965 declining to 26% in 1994 (Giovino et al., 1994). Among

TABLE 26–7 CARDIOVASCULAR RISK FACTORS: EVIDENCE TO SUPPORT INTERVENTIONS

	EVIDENCE FOR ASSOCIATION WITH CVD		CLINICAL MEASUREMENT	RESPONSE TO:	
RISK FACTOR	Epidemiologic	Clinical Trials	Usefulness	Nonpharmacologic Therapy	Pharmacologic Therapy
Category I (Risk Factors for Which Interventions Have Been Proven to Lower CVD Risk)					
Cigarette smoking	+++	++	+++	+++	++
LDL cholesterol	+++	+++	+++	++	+++
High-fat/cholesterol diet	+++	++	++	++	–
Hypertension	+++	+++ (stroke)	+++	+	+++
Left ventricular hypertrophy	+++	+	++	–	++
Thrombogenic factors	+++ (fibrinogen)	+++ (aspirin, warfarin)	+ (fibrinogen)	+	+++ (aspirin, warfarin)
Category II (Risk Factors for Which Interventions Are Likely to Lower CVD Risk)					
Diabetes mellitus	+++	+	+++	++	+++
Physical inactivity	+++	++	++	++	–
HDL cholesterol	+++	+	+++	++	+
Triglycerides; small, dense LDL	++	++	+++	++	+++
Obesity	+++	–	+++	++	+
Postmenopausal status (women)	+++	–	+++	–	+++
Category III (Risk Factors Associated With Increased CVD Risk That, if Modified, Might Lower Risk)					
Psychosocial factors	++	+	+++	+	–
Lipoprotein (a)	+	–	+	–	+
Homocysteine	++	–	+	++	++
Oxidative stress	+	–	–	+	++
No alcohol consumption	+++	–	++	++	–
Category IV (Risk Factors Associated With Increased CVD Risk Which Cannot Be Modified)					
Age	+++	–	+++	–	–
Male gender	+++	–	+++	–	–
Low socioeconomic status	+++	–	+++	–	–
Family history of early-onset CVD	+++	–	+++	–	–

(From Davidson MH, Maki KC. Cardiovascular risk factors: Evaluation and treatment goals. In: Kris-Etherton PM, Burns JH [eds.]. Cardiovascular nutrition: Strategies and tools for disease management and prevention. Chicago: American Dietetic Association, 1998; and Califf RM, et al. Task force 5. J Am Coll Cardiol 27:1007, 1996. Reprinted with permission from the American College of Cardiology.)

CVD, cardiovascular disease; *HDL*, high-density lipoprotein; +, weak, somewhat consistent evidence; ++, moderately strong, rather consistent evidence; +++, very strong, consistent evidence; –, evidence poor or nonexistent.

races, more blacks smoke than whites, and fewer Hispanics smoke than non-Hispanics. Because of the high prevalence of smoking and the reversibility of its effects, smoking is a major risk factor for the progression of atherosclerosis (Howard et al., 1998). The 1989 Surgeon General's Report summarized definitive evidence that smoking increases cardiovascular mortality by 50% and doubles the incidence of CVD. Over time, smoking increases the risk for carotid stenosis in older patients who also have high levels of cholesterol and high systolic blood pressure (Wilson et al., 1997).

Smoking is synergistic with other risk factors (i.e., the risk of CHD is much higher with multiple risk factors) and directly influences acute coronary events, including thrombus formation, plaque instability, and arrhythmias. For example, women who smoke and use oral contraceptives have 10 times greater risk of CHD than nonusers. Risk also increases with the number of cigarettes smoked each day; low-tar brands do not reduce the risk. Nicotine and by-products of smoking are involved in the initiation and progression of atherosclerosis. Consequently, any exposure, including passive smoking, increases the risk of the nonsmoker (Steenland, 1992). Second-hand smoke is the third leading cause of preventable death in the United States (Glantz and Parmley, 1995). Clinically, smoking decreases HDL cholesterol (by an average of 6 to 8 mg/dL) and increases VLDL cholesterol and blood glucose levels.

Smoking cessation has been attainable for some smokers; 50% of the smoking population from 1965 to 1991 was able to quit. In younger men and women who stop smoking, CHD risk falls precipitously 2 to 3 years after smoking ceases, approaching that of nonsmokers. Older smokers who may already have established disease will experience a reduced risk of CHD at this point, but it may not be as low as that for nonsmokers for many years (McBride, 1992).

LDL CHOLESTEROL

As discussed earlier, LDL cholesterol is conclusively linked to CHD development and acute events. Consequently, LDL cholesterol is the primary blood lipid target for intervention efforts. A decrease of 1 mg/dL in LDL cholesterol results in about a 1% to 2% decrease in the relative risk for CHD. Factors that increase LDL cholesterol include aging, genetics, diet, reduced estrogen levels (as occurs in postmenopausal women), progestins, diabetes, hypothyroidism, nephrotic syndrome, obstructive liver disease, obesity, and some steroid and antihypertensive drugs.

Of these factors, an imprudent diet and obesity are the most prevalent. Diets high in saturated fat and cholesterol elevate LDL by downregulating the LDL receptors in the liver (Woollett et al., 1992). With suppression of LDL receptor activity, less LDL is cleared from the plasma; hence, levels rise. Obesity increases production of apo B–containing lipoproteins—VLDL and, consequently, LDL. For individuals without disease, LDL levels are classified as desirable (<130 mg/dL), borderline high risk (130 to 159 mg/dL), or high risk (>160 mg/dL).

Lowering LDL cholesterol has been shown to regress lesions, delay progression of atherogenesis, and reduce events, morbidity, and mortality in both primary and secondary prevention trials (Pasternak et al., 1996). The target LDL cholesterol level for persons with disease is less than 100 mg/dL (see Table 26–8).

HYPERTENSION

Hypertension is a risk factor for CHD, stroke, and congestive heart failure. About 30% of Americans have hypertension, defined as an average blood pressure of 140/90 mmHg, or use antihypertensive medication (Pasternak et al., 1996). The prevalence increases with age, and is seen more often in blacks than non-Hispanic whites. Hypertension contributes to disease development by causing vascular injury and stresses to the myocardium. The higher the blood pressure, the greater the risk of CHD. Hypertension is frequently present with other risk factors, such as hypercholesterolemia and obesity (see Hypertension, Chapter 27). Treating hypertension decreases the incidence of stroke, CHD, and congestive heart failure.

TABLE 26–8 PHENOTYPE CLASSIFICATION OF HYPERLIPIDEMIAS

PHENOTYPE	LIPOPROTEIN ABNORMALITY	BLOOD LIPIDS
Type I	↑↑ Chylomicrons	↑↑↑ Triglycerides ↑ Cholesterol
Type IIa	↑↑ LDL	↑↑ Cholesterol
Type IIb	↑↑ LDL, ↑ IDL, ↑↑ VLDL	↑↑ Cholesterol ↑↑ Triglycerides
Type III	↑ IDL, ↑ VLDL, ↑ remnants	↑↑ Cholesterol ↑↑ Triglycerides
Type IV	↑ VLDL	↑ Cholesterol ↑↑ Triglycerides
Type V	↑↑ Chylomicrons, ↑ VLDL	↑↑ Triglycerides ↑ Cholesterol

(Data from Naito HK. The clinical significance of apolipoprotein measurements. J Clin Immunoassay 9:11, 1986; and Schonfeld G. The genetic dyslipoproteinemias—nosology update 1990. Atherosclerosis 81:81, 1990.)

LDL, low-density lipoproteins; *IDL*, intermediate-density lipoproteins; *VLDL*, very low-density lipoproteins.

LEFT VENTRICULAR HYPERTROPHY

The left ventricle increases in size in response to high blood pressure and increased workload secondary to obesity. In the Framingham study, left ventricular hypertrophy (LVH) was found to be a strong risk factor for CVD, congestive heart failure, and sudden death. LVH is a risk factor in all age, gender, and ethnic groups. Intervention trials are being conducted to determine whether regressing LVH will improve the clinical course. In the meantime, the presence of LVH necessitates more intensive risk factor management.

THROMBOGENIC FACTORS

Most myocardial infarctions are the result of an intracoronary thrombosis. To date, the most widely studied preventive factor for thrombogenesis is the use of aspirin. Daily use of 80 to 325 mg of aspirin is recommended for patients with CHD. Depending on the risk factor profile, aspirin may be recommended for primary prevention also.

Category II Risk Factors

DIABETES

Diabetes, like hypertension, is both a disease and a risk factor. It is less prevalent than hypertension, affecting 16 million people in the United States compared to 50 million. Both type 1 insulin-dependent and type 2 non–insulin-dependent diabetes increase the risk for CHD, with occurrence at younger ages. Eighty percent of deaths in persons with diabetes are attributable to atherosclerosis (Pasternak et al., 1996). In women, diabetes increases the risk of early CHD to levels of similarly aged men (Barrett-Connor et al., 1991; Liao et al., 1993). Some of the increased risk for CHD seen in patients with diabetes is attributable to the concurrent presence of other risk factors, such as dyslipidemia, hypertension, and obesity (see Chapter 34). Because of multiple risk factors, the LDL cholesterol treatment goal for diabetics is 100 mg/dL. Strict blood glucose control lessens microvascular complications in patients with type 1 and type 2 diabetes.

PHYSICAL INACTIVITY

Physical inactivity or a low level of fitness is an independent risk factor for CHD. Twelve percent of all mortality in the United States is related to a sedentary life-style, and sedentary people have twice the risk of developing CHD as people who are active (Powell et al., 1987). This magnitude of risk is similar to that associated with high blood cholesterol or smoking. Despite public health recommendations to increase activity levels, 60% of respondents surveyed in the 1994 Behavioral Risk Factor Surveillance System were sedentary (Physical Activity and Health, 1996).

The least active groups are women, blacks, Hispanics, older adults, and the less affluent (American Heart Association, 1997). Physical inactivity is the most prevalent modifiable risk factor. The Healthy People 2000 goal was for no more than 15% of the population older than 6 years of age to be inactive (Public Health Service, 1991). Thirty minutes of daily activity of moderate intensity is now recommended (Pate et al., 1995). Moderate-intensity activities include walking at 3 to 4 mph, climbing stairs, gardening, and housecleaning.

Physical activity lessens CHD risk by retarding atherogenesis, increasing the vascularity of the myocardium, increasing fibrinolysis, and modifying other risk factors, such as increasing HDL cholesterol, improving glucose tolerance and insulin sensitivity, aiding in weight management, and reducing blood pressure.

HIGH-DENSITY LIPOPROTEIN CHOLESTEROL

Many population studies have shown that HDL cholesterol is a strong, negative, independent predictor of CHD incidence and mortality in men and women. HDL cholesterol is a more powerful predictor of asymptomatic disease observed by intravascular ultrasound than other lipoproteins (Hausmann et al., 1996). In patients with CHD, HDL cholesterol is also inversely related to coronary artery stenosis in both genders. This protective effect of HDL has been confirmed by intervention studies in which HDL cholesterol level was raised.

Increasing HDL cholesterol level by hormone replacement therapy in women decreased CVD mortality (Bush et al., 1987). In the Helsinki Heart Study, simultaneous increases in HDL cholesterol and decreases in LDL cholesterol during gemfibrozil therapy were accompanied by a 34% reduction in CHD events in middle-aged men (Huttunen et al., 1991). After controlling for other risk factors, a 1 mg/dL increase in HDL cholesterol has been shown to reduce CHD risk by 2% to 3% (NIH Consensus Conference, 1993). Because of the inverse relationship between HDL and CHD risk, a high HDL cholesterol level (>60 mg/dL) is now considered to be a negative risk factor, and a low HDL cholesterol level (<35 mg/dL) is considered to be a positive risk factor (NCEP, 1993).

The exact mechanism of HDL's antiatherogenic effect is unknown. The most widely accepted theory is that HDL is involved in transporting excess cholesterol from membranes to triglyceride-rich lipoproteins, which are then removed by receptors on the liver (Patsch, 1994). This process, known as reverse cholesterol transport, helps rid the body of cholesterol, and prevents lipid accumulation in the arterial wall. A high HDL cholesterol level would mean the system is operating at a high capacity.

It has also been suggested that HDL cholesterol may just be a marker for efficient metabolism of triglyceride-rich lipoproteins with fewer atherogenic remnants being formed (Patsch, 1994). Although the cholesterol involved in lipoprotein metabolism is popularly referred to as "good" or "bad" cholesterol, it is, of course, the lipoprotein form, rather than the cholesterol being transported, that is associated with CHD.

Major factors that increase HDL cholesterol level are exogenous estrogen, exercise, loss of excess body fat, and moderate consumption of alcohol. HDL cholesterol is lowered by obesity, inactivity, cigarette smoking, androgenic and related steroids (anabolic steroids, progesterone-dominant oral contraceptives), beta-adrenergic blocking agents, hypertriglyceridemia, and genetic factors. Dietary factors, discussed in the section on diet and serum lipids, also affect HDL cholesterol levels.

Because interventions often affect all lipoproteins, the effectiveness of raising HDL cholesterol levels alone, in terms of CHD mortality, is not known. Studies are being conducted to investigate this question.

OBESITY

Recently, the NIH revised the definitions of obesity (NIH, 1998). Overweight is now defined as a body mass index (BMI) of 25 to 29.9 and obesity is defined as a BMI greater than 30. Fifty-five percent of U.S. adults (over the age of 20 years) are overweight or obese, with 33% classified as overweight and 22% as obese. While the prevalence of overweight has remained stable in the United States, the prevalence of obesity rose markedly between NHANES II and NHANES III. BMI and CHD are positively related; as BMI goes up, the risk of CHD also increases. Seventy percent of the cases of CHD in women are attributable to increased adiposity.

How obesity affects atherogenesis is not clear, but it is probably related to the coexisting risk factors seen in obese individuals—specifically, glucose intolerance and diabetes, hypertension, and dyslipidemia. Dyslipidemia is directly related to BMI. In women, higher BMIs are associated with triglyceride levels that are 35 to 48 mg/dL higher than average, and HDL cholesterol levels that are 5 to 9 mg/dL lower (Denke et al., 1994).

Weight distribution (upper-body or abdominal versus lower-body) is also predictive of CHD risk and affects glucose tolerance and serum lipid levels. A waist-to-hip ratio of less than 0.8 for women and 0.9 for men is recommended. A 0.15-unit increase in the waist-to-hip ratio has been correlated with a 60% higher risk of death from all causes (Folsom et al., 1993). However, the appropriateness of using one waist-to-hip ratio for all ages and races has been challenged (Croft et al., 1995).

In a study in which abdominal adipose tissue was

measured by computed tomography, waist circumferences (>100 cm) or abdominal sagittal diameter values (>25 cm) were better indicators of risk than waist-to-hip ratios (Pouliot et al., 1994). Small weight losses (5 to 20 lb) can improve risk factors even if an ideal BMI is not achieved. Although there have not been many studies that have explored whether weight loss has any effect on coronary events (Pasternak et al., 1996), predictions indicate that compliance with current NIH recommendations to lower calorie intakes and to increase exercise can help obese persons to achieve and sustain weight loss goals (Carmichael et al., 1998). Obesity is discussed in greater detail in Chapter 23.

MENOPAUSAL STATUS

Endogenous estrogen confers protection against CVD in premenopausal women, probably by preventing vascular injury. Loss of estrogen following natural or surgical menopause is associated with increased CVD risk. *Premature menopause* without hormone replacement therapy is now considered to be a risk factor for CHD (NCEP, 1993). Rates of CHD in premenopausal women are low except in women with multiple risk factors. During the menopausal period, total cholesterol, LDL cholesterol, and triglyceride levels increase and HDL cholesterol level decreases, especially in women who gain weight (Krummel, 1996).

In a longitudinal study of women going through menopause, average serum cholesterol levels increased by 19% in the perimenopausal period (van Beresteijn et al., 1993). Hormone replacement therapy can correct these negative changes in lipid levels. Whether hormone replacement therapy definitively reduces cardiac events, however, will not be known until the Women's Health Initiative study is completed in the year 2005.

Category III Risk Factors

PSYCHOSOCIAL FACTORS

Psychosocial factors, such as type A personality (time-urgent, impatient, and compulsive), stress, depression, and education level (less than high school) are all associated with increased CVD risk. However, interventions for those factors that may be amenable to intervention (i.e., stress) have not demonstrated a decrease in risk. More research is needed.

TRIGLYCERIDES

Data associating high levels of plasma triglycerides with coronary heart disease are conflicting. In studies analyzing just triglyceride and CHD incidence or mortality, **hypertriglyceridemia** is associated with increased frequency of disease. However, in prospective studies in which HDL cholesterol levels are controlled, the association is not significant.

Because of their roles in metabolism, triglyceride and HDL cholesterol levels are inversely related; that is, when a patient has high triglyceride levels, the HDL cholesterol levels are usually low. Hence, HDL cholesterol levels, not triglyceride levels, explain the variance in risk. In the Framingham data, it was the combination of high triglyceride and low HDL cholesterol, independent of other risk factors, that predicted CHD (Castelli, 1992). Overall, triglycerides appear to be a stronger risk factor in women than in men (Austin and Hokanson, 1994), and they are also a risk factor for older adults (Corti et al., 1997).

Reasons for the discrepancies in the literature include (1) the heterogeneity in triglyceride-containing lipoproteins and (2) the large biological variability (<20%) in triglyceride measurements, which means a single sample analyzed for blood triglyceride may not reflect true levels. The NIH Consensus Conference recommends taking at least two fasting samples 1 week apart before treatment decisions are made (NIH Consensus Conference, 1993).

Factors that increase triglyceride levels are diet (vegetarian, low-fat, refined carbohydrate), estrogens, alcohol, obesity, untreated diabetes, untreated hypothyroidism, chronic renal disease, and liver disease. Treatment of hypertriglyceridemia includes (1) weight loss for overweight patients, (2) consumption of a low–saturated fat/low-cholesterol diet, (3) increased physical activity, (4) smoking cessation, (5) management of diabetes if present, and (6) restricted alcohol use. Drug therapy is indicated for hypertriglyceridemia when it coexists with established CHD, a positive family history, or concurrent high cholesterol and low HDL cholesterol levels, and when the genetic disease form is present.

LIPOPROTEIN (A)

Lipoprotein (a) [Lp(a)] is a unique lipoprotein that has been a controversial analyte for over 30 years. In addition to apo B, Lp(a) has the protein apo (a), which is very similar to plasminogen, a proenzyme involved in the breakdown of fibrin. Many early studies showed that Lp(a) was a strong, independent risk factor for premature CHD. However, large prospective studies have yielded mixed results. The incongruity is due to methodologic differences and the heterogeneity of this particle.

Until further data are available, routine screening of Lp(a) is not recommended. Lp(a) levels are skewed to lower values, and within a given population, the levels can vary by 1000-fold (Pasternak, 1996). The 75th and 90th percentiles for Lp(a) are 25 mg/dL and 40 mg/dL, respectively. Lp(a) is a category III risk factor because data are lacking on intervention trials. Estrogens, anabolic steroids, and niacin are known to lower Lp(a).

HOMOCYSTEINE

The amino acid homocysteine is positively associated with an increased risk of CHD and peripheral artery disease (Graham et al., 1997; Welch and Loscalzo, 1998) (see Chapter 17). Children who were deficient in cystathionine B synthase, the essential catabolic enzyme for homocysteine, were found to have premature atherosclerosis and mortality.

Similarly, adults with hyperhomocysteinemia (>10 μmol/L) are 30 times more likely to have premature disease (Clarke et al., 1991). Reduced enzyme activity occurs in 5% to 7% of the population; severe deficiency is rare (Welch and Loscalzo, 1998). At any given time, from 25% to 45% of patients with CHD may have high serum homocysteine levels.

In patients with angiographically documented disease, the 4-year mortality rate was 25% in patients with high homocysteine levels (>15 μmol/L), compared to 4% in patients with levels less than 9 μmol/L (Nygard et al., 1997). Atherogenic mechanics for homocysteine include procoagulant activity or endothelial injury (Woo et al., 1997). Inadequate dietary intake of folate and vitamins B_{12} and B_6 increases plasma homocysteine levels. Thus, assuring appropriate dietary intake of these B vitamins will reduce plasma homocysteine.

Low dietary folate intake, lack of exercise, male sex, older age, smoking, and coffee consumption (>1 cup/day) were associated with higher levels of homocysteine in a large population study. Of these factors, smoking, coffee consumption, and folate intake were the strongest predictors of homocysteine levels. Nonsmokers with high folate intakes and minimal coffee consumption (<1 cup/day) had homocysteine levels 3 to 4 μmol/L lower than smokers who drank coffee and had low dietary folate intake (Nygard et al., 1998).

Increasing folate intake by 200 μg/day reduces homocysteine levels by 4 μmol/L (Bousney et al., 1995). A 1 μmol/L rise in homocysteine level is associated with a 10% increase in CVD risk (Blom, 1998). Intervention trials have not been conducted to determine whether lowering the homocysteine level will reduce CVD risk.

OXIDATIVE STRESS

Oxidation of LDL in the vessel wall hastens the atherogenic process by recruiting macrophages, stimulating autoantibodies, increasing LDL uptake, and increasing vascular tone and coagulability (Pasternak, 1996). Dietary factors that can decrease LDL oxidation include vitamin C, vitamin E, beta-carotene, selenium, flavonoids, magnesium, and monounsaturated fat. Although these factors have the potential to reduce LDL oxidation, conclusive data from intervention trials are lacking (Jha et al., 1995). In this regard, the strongest interest has been associated with vitamin E (Meydani et al., 1997), but final results from randomized clinical trials are not yet available.

In contrast, iron, copper, zinc, and saturated fat increase LDL oxidation. Consumption of foods high in nutrients that theoretically could reduce the oxidant potential is prudent. The effectiveness of vitamin suplementation has not been definitively established (Mandel et al., 1997).

ALCOHOL CONSUMPTION

Moderate alcohol consumption (1 to 2 drinks/day) is associated with a 40% to 50% reduction in CHD risk (Gaziano et al., 1993), but the use of alcohol is not recommended as an intervention strategy (see the section entitled "Dietary Factors").

Category IV Risk Factors

Age is a nonmodifiable risk factor for CHD. With increasing age, higher mortality rates from CHD are seen in all races and both genders (see Table 26–1). Gender, however, is a factor for the assessment of risk. The incidence of premature disease in men 35 to 44 years old is three times as high as the incidence in women of the same age. Therefore, being older than 45 years of age is considered a risk factor for men (NCEP, 1993). For women, the increased risk comes after the age of 55 years, which is after menopause for most women. Overall, the risk of CHD increases markedly as one ages.

A family history of premature disease is a strong risk factor, even when other risk factors are considered. A family history is considered to be positive when myocardial infarction or sudden death occurs before the age of 55 years in a male first-degree relative, or the age of 65 in a female first-degree relative (parents, siblings, offspring). Numerous hyperlipidemias are inheritable and lead to premature atherosclerosis and CHD. The presence of a positive family history, although not modifiable, will influence the intensity of risk factor management.

GENETIC HYPERLIPIDEMIAS: CLASSIFICATION AND DIAGNOSIS

Several relatively rare forms of hyperlipidemia have strong genetic components. Originally, hyperlipidemias were classified according to the predominant aberrant lipoprotein (see Table 26–8). For example, type I was defined by the presence of chylomicrons after an individual had fasted; type IIa was evidenced by an abnormal LDL level and a normal VLDL level. Although this system does describe the lipoprotein alteration, it does not provide information about the etiology of the disorder; nor is HDL considered in any of the types. Consequently, this method of classification is being used less often.

Familial Hypercholesterolemia

Familial hypercholesterolemia (FH, type IIa; or high LDL cholesterol, normal triglyceride) is a heritable disease in which a genetic defect occurs in the

LDL receptor function. The LDL receptors are either absent or nonfunctional in these patients. A person is heterozygous if only one defective gene is inherited, and homozygous if both defective genes are inherited. The heterozygous form (affecting 1 in 500 people in the United States) is much more prevalent than the homozygous form (affecting 1 in 1 million people). Hypercholesterolemia (250 to 500 mg/dL, with an average of 360 mg/dL) is present at birth. Early detection with aggressive therapy can prevent or delay CHD.

Homozygotes have more severe hypercholesterolemia and atherosclerosis, expressed as myocardial infarction or death in the first or second decade of life. In heterozygotes, the average age of CHD onset is 45 years in men and 55 years in women (Schaefer, 1994a). Clinically, tendon **xanthomas,** corneal arcus, premature CHD, and a strong family history of hypercholesterolemia are common. Diagnosis is based on LDL cholesterol levels that lie above the 90th percentile in two or more family members, and the presence of tendon xanthomas in members within the family tree.

Treatment for homozygotes involves extreme measures, such as biweekly plasmaphoresis to remove LDL. Liver transplant, gene therapy, and portacaval shunts are experimental modes of treatment. For heterozygotes, Step II Diets with combination drug therapy are usually needed to achieve the goals for LDL levels (see Table 26–12).

Polygenic Familial Hypercholesterolemia

Polygenic familial hypercholesterolemia is the result of multiple gene defects that have yet to be identified. The diagnosis is based on LDL cholesterol levels above the 90th percentile and the absence of tendon xanthomas in two or more family members. Usually, these patients have lower LDL cholesterol levels than patients with the nonpolygenic form, but they remain at high risk for premature disease. The apo E-4 allele is common in polygenic familial hypercholesterolemia. The treatment is similar to that for heterozygous familial hypercholesterolemia—that is, the Step II Diet in conjunction with cholesterol-lowering drugs.

Familial Combined Hyperlipidemia

Familial combined hyperlipidemia (FCHL) is a disorder characterized by serum LDL cholesterol and/or triglyceride levels above the 90th percentile in at least two family members, with both abnormalities seen in the kindred. Several lipoprotein patterns may be seen in patients with FCHL. These patients can have (1) elevated LDL levels with normal triglyceride levels (type IIa); (2) elevated LDL levels with elevated triglyceride levels (type IIb); or (3) elevated VLDL levels (type IV). Often, these patients have the small, dense LDL associated with CHD. Consequently, all forms of FCHL cause premature disease; about 15% of patients who have a myocardial infarction before the age of 60 have FCHL. The defect in FCHL is hepatic overproduction of apo B-100 and, thus, VLDL.

Patients with FCHL usually have a constellation of other risk factors—namely, obesity, hypertension, diabetes, and gout. Treatment includes Step II Diet, weight reduction, diabetes control, increased activity, and medication if life-style measures are ineffective. Patients with elevated triglyceride levels also need to avoid alcohol.

Familial Dyslipidemia

Familial dyslipidemia is a combination of familial hypertriglyceridemia, defined as at least two persons in a family having a triglyceride level above the 90th percentile, and a low HDL cholesterol level, defined as less than the 10th percentile (Schaefer, 1994a). Fifteen percent of patients with CHD have familial dyslipidemia. Other risk factors common in these patients are android obesity, insulin resistance, type 2 diabetes, and hypertension. No specific treatment exists except for life-style interventions to modify all risk factors.

Familial Dysbetalipoproteinemia

Familial dysbetalipoproteinemia (type III hyperlipoproteinemia) is relatively uncommon (affecting 1 in 5000 persons in the United States). Catabolism of VLDL remnants, IDL, and chylomicron remnants is delayed owing to a basic abnormality in the structure of apolipoprotein E (apo E-2 is present, instead of apo E-3 and E-4). For dysbetalipoproteinemia to be seen, other risk factors, such as age, hypothyroidism, obesity, or diabetes, or other dyslipidemias, such as FCHL, must be present. Total cholesterol levels range from 300 to 600 mg/dL, and triglyceride levels range from 400 to 800 mg/dL.

This condition creates increased risk of premature CHD and peripheral vascular disease. Diagnosis is based on determining isoforms of apo E. Treatment involves weight reduction, control of hyperglycemia and diabetes, and dietary restriction of cholesterol and saturated fat. If the dietary regimen is not effective, drug therapy is recommended.

DIETARY FACTORS

For more than 40 years, epidemiologic studies, experimental studies, and clinical trials have shown that numerous dietary risk factors affect serum lipids, atherogenesis, and CHD. The classic Seven Countries Study was the first to show that a population's intake of saturated fatty acids (SFAs) was strongly correlated with serum cholesterol levels in the population. Countries with the highest SFA intake (>15% of total kilocalories) and the highest serum cholesterol levels had the highest CHD mortality.

Fat quantity, fat quality, cholesterol, and numerous other dietary substances have been investigated to see how they affect serum lipids and lipoproteins. When studying the effects of fatty acids on serum lipids, two points of comparison are made. First, how do the fatty acids compare to carbohydrate substitution, which is considered neutral? Second, how do they compare when they replace saturated fatty acids?

Fatty Acids

Saturated Fatty Acids

In general, SFAs tend to elevate blood cholesterol in all lipoprotein fractions (i.e., both LDL and HDL cholesterol) when substituted for carbohydrate or other fatty acids. The most hypercholesterolemic or atherogenic SFAs are lauric (C12:0), myristic (C14:0), and palmitic (C16:0) acids (see Chapter 3). Myristic acid is the most potent, followed by palmitic, and then lauric acid. Although an SFA, *stearic acid (C18:0)* has no effect on blood lipoproteins and is considered to be neutral, like carbohydrate (Kris-Etherton and Yu, 1997). *Palmitic acid* is the most prevalent hypercholesterolemic SFA in the American diet, comprising 60% of total SFA intake. Although palmitate is present in plant sources, most dietary palmitate comes from animal foods. *Myristic acid* is found mostly in butterfat and coconut and palm kernel oils. It is less prevalent in the American diet than palmitic acid. Lauric acid, the only medium-chain SFA, is found in palm kernel and coconut oils. Of all the added fats in the diet, the most hypercholesterolemic are palm kernel, coconut and palm oils and butter. In the NHANES III, the mean consumption of SFA was 12% of kilocalories, and this figure did not vary by ethnic group (McDowell et al., 1994).

In their classic metabolic ward studies, Keys and colleagues developed equations to predict the blood cholesterol response for changes in SFA, polyunsaturated fatty acid (PUFA), and cholesterol intake. For every 1% increase in total energy intake from saturated fatty acids, a 2.7 mg/dL increase in plasma cholesterol level is predicted. For example, raising consumption of SFA (as a percentage of kilocalories) from 7% to 17% increases plasma cholesterol levels by 27 mg/dL. Although SFAs are extremely hypercholesterolemic, not all people respond the same way. People with the apo E-4 phenotype have the greatest blood cholesterol responses to SFA (Grundy, 1994). SFAs raise LDL cholesterol by decreasing LDL receptor synthesis and activity. All fatty acids will lower fasting triglycerides if they replace carbohydrate in the diet (Katan, 1994a).

Dietary fatty acids have also been associated with the progression of coronary artery disease in men. After controlling for other risk factors, atherosclerosis progressed most in men consuming more stearic and elaidic acids over a 39-month period (Watts et al., 1996). Palmitic and palmitoleic acids were also associated with disease progression, but not when other risk factors were controlled. The food sources of these fatty acids are milk, cheese, butter, and lamb. Trans-fatty acids in the lamb were correlated with disease progression, whereas trans-fatty acids from margarine were not (Watts, 1996). Lesions stabilized in men who restricted these foods. Thus, fatty acids affect disease progression through lipids and other mechanisms, possibly thrombosis.

Polyunsaturated Fatty Acids

OMEGA-6 POLYUNSATURATED FATTY ACIDS

If carbohydrate is replaced by *linoleic acid (C18:2),* the predominant dietary omega-6 PUFA, LDL cholesterol is lowered and HDL cholesterol is raised. When SFAs are replaced with PUFA in a low fat diet, LDL and HDL cholesterol levels will be lowered (Nydahl et al., 1994). Overall, eliminating SFA is twice as effective in lowering serum cholesterol levels as is increasing PUFA (Grande et al., 1972; Kris-Etherton et al., 1988). A 1% increase in omega-6 PUFA would lower total cholesterol by 1.4 mg/dL. PUFAs have been shown to decrease VLDL, apo B, and HDL synthesis. In the past, a polyunsaturated:saturated ratio (P:S ratio) was used to assess fatty acid composition of foods and diets. However, this ratio is not recommended because it does not separate the cholesterol-raising SFAs from the neutral SFAs (Denke et al., 1994).

Omega-6 (n-6) PUFAs are widespread in foods, but their major source is vegetable oils. Current U.S. population intake is at 7% of total kilocalories (McDowell et al., 1994). Because linoleic acid is not consumed in large amounts in any population, and experimental feeding of large amounts increases LDL oxidation (Abbey et al., 1993), an increase in linoleic acid is not recommended above current intakes. At this level of intake, with the current recommendation for fat consumption set at less than 30% of total kilocalories, PUFAs would lower total cholesterol, LDL cholesterol, and HDL cholesterol. The clinical significance of diets that lower HDL cholesterol is open to debate. At present, it is believed that an HDL cholesterol level that is lowered by diet does not carry the risk of a low HDL cholesterol level before intervention, especially since the rest of the lipoprotein profile will be altered favorably by diet (NIH Consensus, 1993).

OMEGA-3 POLYUNSATURATED FATTY ACIDS

The main omega-3 (n-3) fatty acids—*eicosapentaenoic acid (EPA)* and *docosahexaenoic acid (DHA)*—are high in fish oils, fish oil capsules, and ocean fish. Most studies have shown that omega-3 fatty acids do not affect total cholesterol; however, they do increase LDL cholesterol (5% to 10%) and decrease triglycerides (25% to 30%) (Harris, 1997). LDL cholesterol tends to be raised in patients with hypertriglyceridemia and lowered or unchanged in normal subjects fed concentrated sources of omega-3 fatty acids. Omega-3 fatty acids lower triglycerides by inhibiting VLDL and apo B-100 synthesis and by decreasing postprandial lipemia.

The effects of n-3 fatty acids on triglyceride level are dose-dependent; that is, higher doses produce greater effects. Their greatest clinical utility, therefore, is for the hyperlipoproteinemias in which triglyceride level is also elevated (types II-b, III, IV, and V) (Connor, 1991). Omega-3 fatty acids affect many other steps in atherogenesis; most notably, they are precursors of the prostaglandins that interfere with blood clotting. Therefore, high intakes prolong bleeding times, a condition that is common in Eskimo populations with high dietary intakes and low incidence of CHD. It is now postulated that consumption of fish and fish oils rich in EPA and DHA will lower cholesterol, LDL, and triglyceride levels with a subsequent reduction in sudden cardiac death rates (Albert et al., 1998; Daviglus et al., 1997) (see Chapter 3).

Monounsaturated Fatty Acids

CIS-MONOUNSATURATED FATTY ACIDS

Oleic acid (C18:1) is the most prevalent cis-monounsaturated fatty acid (MUFA) in the American diet. Substituting oleic acid for carbohydrate has almost no appreciable effect on blood lipids. However, replacing SFA with MUFA lowers serum cholesterol levels, LDL cholesterol levels, and triglyceride levels to about the same extent as PUFA. The effects of MUFA on HDL cholesterol depend on the total fat content of the diet. When intake of both MUFA (>15% of total kilocalories) and total fat (>35% of kilocalories) is high, HDL cholesterol does not change or increases slightly compared to what it is with a lower fat diet. At the recommended fat levels (<30% of total kilocalories from fat and 15% from MUFA), HDL cholesterol levels would be decreased.

In epidemiologic studies, high-fat diets of people in Mediterranean countries have been associated with low blood cholesterol levels and CHD incidence. Among other factors, the main fat source is olive oil, which is high in MUFA. This observation led to many studies on the benefits of high-fat/high-MUFA diets. A Step I Diet (30% total fat, 10% SFAs, 10% MUFAs) and a high-MUFA diet (38% total fat, 10% SFAs, 18% MUFAs) were equally effective in lowering total cholesterol and LDL cholesterol without changing the HDL cholesterol level (Ginsberg et al., 1990). Although higher fat diets (low in SFA, with MUFA as the predominant fat) can lower blood cholesterol, they should be used with caution owing to the caloric density of high-fat diets and the results of clinical trials, which have shown new atherosclerotic lesions in men who consume higher fat diets (Blankenhorn et al., 1990).

The negative association between the Mediterranean diet and CHD could be due to factors other than MUFA intake. For example, these populations consume more fruits and vegetables than many populations. Current MUFA intake in the U.S. population averages about 12.5% of kilocalories (McDowell et al., 1994).

TRANS-FATTY ACIDS

Stereoisomers (trans form) of the naturally occurring cis-linoleic acid are produced in the hydrogenation process widely used in the food industry to harden unsaturated oils (see Chapter 3). Harder fats, such as stick margarine, contain more trans-fatty acids than do soft margarines. Trans-fatty acids are also present in beef, butter, and milk fats. Cookies and crackers made from partially hydrogenated vegetable oil contain 3% to 9% trans-fatty acids, and many snack foods contain 8% to 10% (Denke et al., 1994). Fifty percent of trans-fatty acid intake comes from animal foods; the other 50% comes from hydrogenated vegetable oils. The major food sources of trans-fatty acids in the U.S. diet are stick margarine, shortening, commercial frying fats, and high-fat baked goods (Food and Nutrition Science Alliance, 1994).

Elaidic acid, the trans isomer of oleic acid, is hypercholesterolemic when compared to PUFA, but hypocholesterolemic when compared to myristic and lauric acids (Kris-Etherton and Yu, 1997). Consuming trans-fatty acids at levels typical of American diets (3% of kilocalories) will raise LDL cholesterol levels, but to a lesser extent than SFAs, including butter (Judd et al., 1994). Increased trans-fatty acid intakes (6% of energy) also lower HDL cholesterol. Press releases from these and other studies (Willett et al., 1993) led some consumers to switch from margarine to butter. However, margarine contains only 11% of cholesterol-raising saturates plus 1% trans, whereas butter contains 40% saturates plus 5% trans (Katan, 1994a and 1994b); hence, soft or spray or liquid margarine is the preferred spread. The average intake of trans-fatty acids is estimated to be 7% to 8% of total fat intake (Emken, 1995).

Consuming appropriately homemade low fat desserts, low fat dairy products, and low fat meats will lower trans-fatty acid intakes. Decreasing the intake of total fat and SFAs will also reduce trans-fatty acids.

Amount of Dietary Fat

Total fat intakes are related to obesity, which affects many of the major risk factors for atherosclerosis. Also, high-fat diets increase postprandial lipemia and chylomicron remnants, both of which are associated with increased risk of CHD. When fat is reduced in the diet, and carbohydrate is the replacement source of kilocalories, VLDL and HDL levels are affected. Low-fat diets (<25% of total kilocalories from fat) raise triglyceride levels (30 to 100 mg/dL) and lower HDL cholesterol levels (3 to 8 mg/dL) (Denke, 1994). Although these changes appear to be negative, they are not associated with CHD risk because (1) LDL cholesterol levels are low in persons consuming low-fat diets, and (2) the VLDL that are produced are large, triglyceride-rich VLDL, which are not associated with risk.

Lower fat diets (<30% of total kilocalories from fat) that are high in SFAs (14% of kilocalories) will not lower LDL cholesterol compared with higher fat diets (37% of kilocalories from fat) (Barr et al., 1992). Low-fat diets, therefore, lower LDL cholesterol levels only when accompanied by a decrease in SFA.

Total fat intake increases the relative risk of new coronary lesions (Kwiterovich, 1997). Persons consuming a diet with less than 23% of calories derived from fat had a relative risk of 1 of developing new lesions, compared to 12.3 for those consuming more than 34% of calories from fat (Blankenhorn, 1990).

Dietary Cholesterol

Dietary cholesterol raises total cholesterol and LDL cholesterol, but to a lesser extent than SFAs. A 25 mg increase in dietary cholesterol would raise serum cholesterol by 1 mg/dL (Denke et al., 1994). When cholesterol intakes reach 500 mg per day, even smaller increments in blood cholesterol occur. Thus, there appears to be a threshold for a plasma cholesterol response to dietary cholesterol, which is why experiments that involve feeding eggs to subjects already on the typical American diet fail to affect serum cholesterol levels.

Cholesterol responsiveness also varies widely among individuals. Some people are hyporesponders (i.e., their plasma cholesterol level does not increase after dietary cholesterol challenge), whereas others are hyperresponders (i.e., their plasma cholesterol level responds to a cholesterol challenge more strongly than expected). It has been suggested that hyperresponders may have poor rates of conversion of cholesterol to bile acids or the apo E-4 allele, which causes elevated LDL cholesterol. Feeding cholesterol to animals enriches lipoproteins, which are atherogenic beyond just the rise in serum cholesterol.

Dietary cholesterol intakes in the United States have been declining since the 1960s. Between 1988 and 1991, the average cholesterol intake for the total population was 270 mg (McDowell et al., 1994). Non-Hispanic blacks and Mexican-Americans had higher intakes—301 and 324 mg/day, respectively.

In addition to the effects of dietary cholesterol alone on serum lipids, dietary saturated fatty acids and cholesterol have a synergistic effect on LDL cholesterol level. Together, they decrease LDL receptor synthesis and activity, increase VLDL enriched with apo E, increase all lipoproteins, and decrease chylomicron size (which is associated with CHD risk) (Kris-Etherton et al., 1988). The intake of cholesterol has generally been positively related to the risk of CHD after adjusting for other risk factors, such as age, blood pressure, serum cholesterol level, and cigarette smoking.

Other Dietary Factors

Fiber

Soluble fibers—pectins, gums, mucilages, algal polysaccharides, and some hemicelluloses—in legumes, oats, fruits, and psyllium lower serum cholesterol and LDL cholesterol. The quantity of fiber needed to produce the lipid-lowering effect varies by food source; higher quantities of legumes are needed than pectin or gums (Table 26–9).

The average decline in LDL cholesterol was 14% for hypercholesterolemics and 10% for normocholesterolemics when soluble fiber was added to a low-fat diet (Glore et al., 1994). Proposed mechanisms for the hypocholesterolemic effect of soluble fiber include the following: (1) the fiber binds bile acids, which lowers serum cholesterol to replete the bile acid pool, and (2) bacteria in the colon ferment the fiber to compound acetate, propionate, and butyrate, which inhibit cholesterol synthesis.

Insoluble fibers, such as cellulose and lignin, have no effect on serum cholesterol levels. Of the total recommended fiber intake (25 to 30 g daily for adults), approximately 6 to 10 g should be from soluble fiber. This level is easy to achieve with the recommended five or more servings of fruits and/or vegetables per day and six or more servings of grains (if whole grains and high fiber cereals are chosen).

Alcohol

Alcohol affects both total triglyceride and HDL cholesterol levels. The effects of alcohol on triglyceride levels are dose-dependent and are greater in persons with triglyceride levels exceeding 150 mg/dL. In population studies, moderate levels of alcohol consumption have been associated with decreased risk of myocardial infarction and CHD mortality (in white men only) (Gaziano et al., 1993; Coate, 1993).

TABLE 26–9 QUANTITY OF SOLUBLE FIBER NEEDED DAILY TO PRODUCE LIPID-LOWERING EFFECT

SOURCE	QUANTITY (g)
Pectin	6–40
Gums	8–36
Dried beans or legumes	100–150
Dry oat bran	25–100
Oatmeal	57–140
Psyllium	10–30

(Data from Glore SR, et al. Soluble fiber and serum lipids: A literature review. J Am Diet Assoc 94:425, 1994.)

Alcohol raises both the HDL_2 and HDL_3 cholesterol subfractions of HDL cholesterol. Current alcohol intake among the U.S. population is 2% of total kilocalories (McDowell et al., 1994), and no increase is recommended to decrease CHD risk.

Wine contains *resveratrol,* an antifungal compound in grape skins that increases HDL cholesterol and inhibits LDL oxidation. The French may experience lower rates of CVD, despite a high-fat diet, due to red wine consumption.

Coffee

Mixed results have been shown in studies investigating the effects of coffee on serum lipids. Heavy consumption of regular coffee (720 mL/day) causes minor increases in total cholesterol (9 mg/dL), LDL cholesterol (6 mg/dL), and HDL cholesterol (4 mg/dL) (Fried et al., 1992). Boiled coffee (European method) produces even greater elevations in plasma lipids than filtered coffee (American method) (Bak and Grobbee, 1989).

Most large population studies have failed to find associations between coffee consumption and CHD incidence or mortality. Any associations found are thought to be related to a constellation of risk factors seen in coffee drinkers. The coffee drinkers consumed more saturated fat and cholesterol, smoked more cigarettes, and were less likely to exercise than non–coffee drinkers (Puccio et al., 1990).

Antioxidants

Two dietary components that affect the oxidation potential of LDL cholesterol are the level of linoleic acid in the particle and the availability of antioxidants. Vitamins C, E, and β-carotene, at physiologic levels, have antioxidant roles in the body. At supplement levels, they can be either pro-oxidant or antioxidant, depending on concentrations of other metal ions (Herbert, 1994b). Epidemiologic studies suggest that antioxidant vitamins reduce CVD, but randomized trials have not supported this theory (Jha et al., 1995).

Data is strongest for vitamin E, but as indicated, randomized clinical trial data are inconclusive. Vitamin E is the most concentrated antioxidant carried on LDL, the amount being 20 to 300 times greater than any other antioxidant (Kwiterovich, 1997). A major function of vitamin E is to prevent oxidation of PUFA in the cell membrane.

In vitro, vitamin E inhibits LDL oxidation, and it is superior to combined supplementation with vitamins C, E, and β-carotene (Jialal and Grundy, 1993; Witzum et al., 1993). Associations are not proof of a causal effect; however, they support further investigation. Double-blind, placebo-controlled trials are necessary to determine (1) whether antioxidant supplementation will decrease the risk of CHD; (2) whether antioxidant supplements have a positive role and what the level of intake should be; (3) whether there are any negative side effects from supplementation; (4) whether supplementation offers any benefit against the progression of the disease, and (5) which of the vitamins have a protective role (Steinberg, 1993a, 1993b; Herbert, 1994a, 1994b).

Several clinical trials are in progress, and a definitive answer will soon be available (Manson et al., 1993). Until then, the American Heart Association recommends that vitamin E be obtained from a diet low in saturated fat (Krauss et al., 1996).

Thus, evidence for vitamin E affecting CVD is stronger than that for beta-carotene or vitamin C. Carotenoid studies suggest that these nutrients play a role later, rather than early, in the atherosclerotic process by preventing arterial plaque formation (Kritchevsky et al., 1998). Studies are continuing.

Calcium

Calcium supplementation produces small decreases in LDL cholesterol in hypercholesterolemic men. In a double-blind, placebo-controlled trial, 1200 mg of calcium carbonate was reported to lower LDL cholesterol by 4.4% and increase HDL cholesterol by 4.1% in men on a Step I Diet (Bell et al., 1992). Along with current recommendations to increase calcium intakes to prevent osteoporosis, there may be an additional positive lipid-lowering benefit.

PREVENTION OF CORONARY HEART DISEASE

To prevent CHD, two strategies are necessary: the clinical or patient-based strategy, in which those individuals at highest risk are identified and treated; and the population strategy, involving facilitating life-style changes, such as diet, to lower blood cholesterol levels and thus reduce CHD prevalence. *Primary prevention* involves clinical management, including diet, exercise, and other life-style changes that will lower the risk of CHD in patients who have no evidence of CHD but who have risk factors. *Secondary prevention* is the treatment of hypercholesterolemia in patients who already have CHD.

Primary Prevention

National Cholesterol Education Program (NCEP) Adult Treatment Panel-II

In 1985, the *National Cholesterol Education Program (NCEP),* of the National Heart, Lung, and Blood Institute, began a mission to reduce the prevalence of hypercholesterolemia in the United States. Four reports have been issued from NCEP, the most recent being the Second Report on Detection, Evaluation, and Treatment of High Blood Cholesterol in Adults, known as ATP-II (NCEP, 1993).

Like ATP-I, ATP-II focuses on LDL cholesterol as the target lipoprotein. ATP-II also focuses on (1) the use of CHD risk status to guide the intensity of therapy so that patients at increased risk of developing CHD in the short term will receive more intensive interventions than those at lower risk; (2) increased emphasis on secondary prevention; (3) increased emphasis on HDL cholesterol as a risk factor; and (4) management issues for young adults, women, and the elderly.

The recommended treatment program is based on monitoring LDL and HDL cholesterol levels, instituting life-style interventions (diets that progressively reduce SFA and cholesterol, weight reduction, physical activity, smoking cessation), and prescribing medication. Levels of LDL cholesterol, as well as the presence or absence of CHD risk factors, determine the appropriate measurement frequency, dietary requirements, and necessity for medication. Regardless of initial classification, medical nutrition therapy is the cornerstone to lowering blood cholesterol. Recommendations for children and adolescents are presented in the earlier *"Clinical Insight"* box.

RATIONALE

The rationale for the NCEP guidelines stems from extensive data accumulated over a number of years that (1) identify LDL cholesterol as a major constituent of atherosclerotic plaque, (2) show, via epidemiologic, clinical, and prospective studies, that

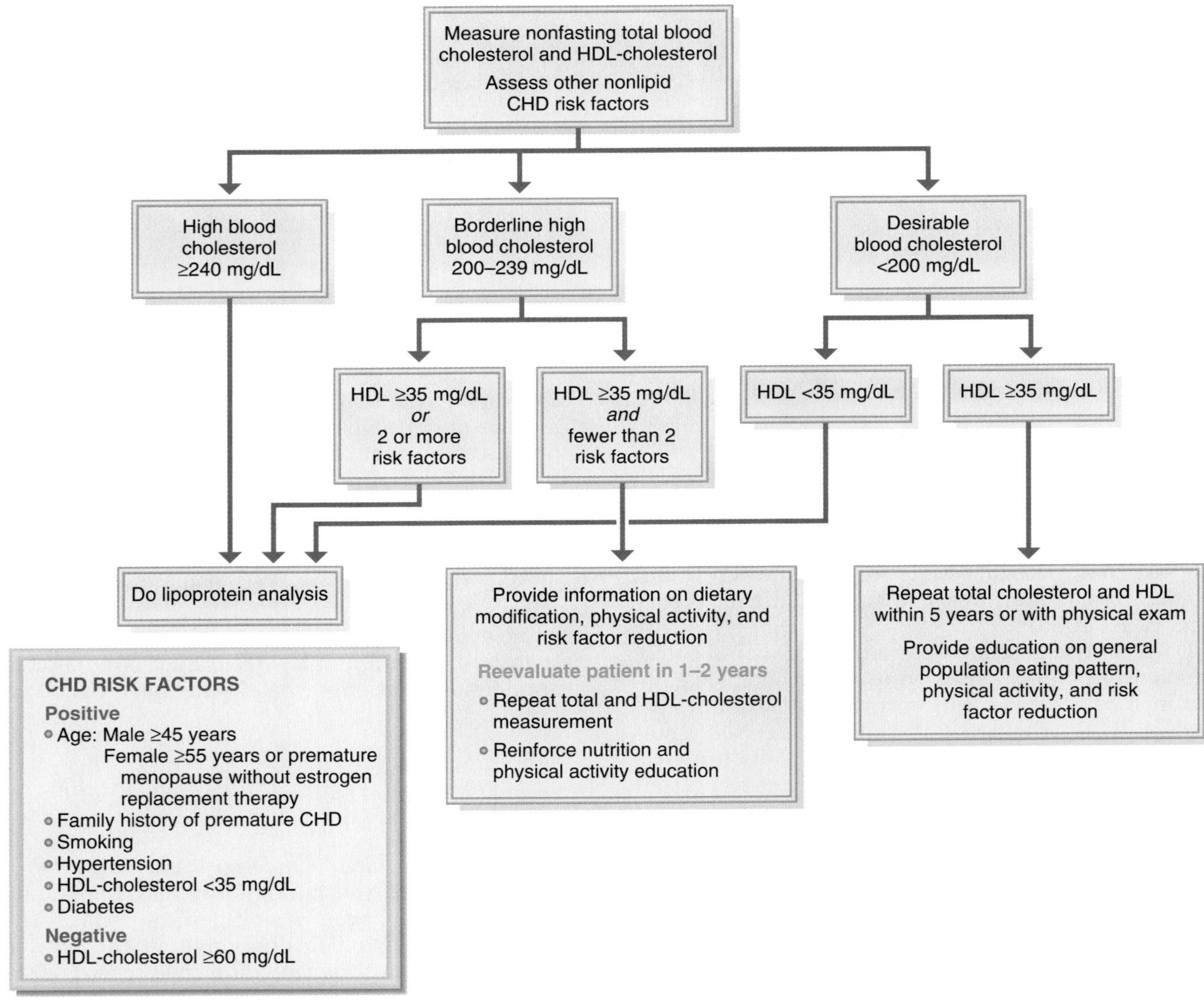

FIGURE 26–6 Primary prevention in adults without evidence of coronary heart disease (CHD). (From National Cholesterol Education Program: Second Report of the Expert Panel on Detection, Evaluation, and Treatment of High Blood Cholesterol in Adults (Adult Treatment Panel II). National Institutes of Health, NIH Publication No. 93-3095. Bethesda, MD: National Heart, Lung, and Blood Institute, 1993.) *HDL*, high-density lipoprotein.

serum cholesterol levels are positively associated with CHD morbidity and mortality, and (3) demonstrate, via primary and secondary intervention trials, that lowering LDL cholesterol reduces the risk of CHD.

ASSESSMENT OF RISK

The objective of the NCEP is to reduce CHD by identifying and reducing elevated levels of LDL cholesterol. The initial classification is based on total cholesterol and HDL cholesterol testing of a nonfasting blood sample (Fig. 26–6). Diet and physical activity information is given to individuals with normal lipid levels. In patients with a total cholesterol level of greater than 200 mg/dL or an HDL cholesterol level of less than 35 mg/dL, a fasting lipoprotein profile is needed, and treatment decisions are based on the LDL cholesterol level (Fig. 26–7).

Initiation of diet therapy begins when LDL cholesterol is greater than 160 mg/dL in people with fewer than two risk factors, and at lower levels in those with two or more risk factors (Table 26–10). Twenty-nine percent of all adults participating in the NHANES III survey were candidates for diet therapy, based on their LDL cholesterol levels (Sempos, 1993). The three nutrition factors that have a major effect on LDL cholesterol are high SFA intake, high cholesterol intake, and obesity. Diet changes for primary prevention must be permanent and lifelong. The diets recommended for prevention and treatment are the Step I and Step II Diets.

STEP I AND STEP II DIETS

NCEP-specified diet modifications consist of recommendations for lowering total fat, saturated fat, and cholesterol and adjusting energy intake to achieve appropriate weight (Table 26–11). In the *Step I Diet,* less than 30% of total kilocalories are derived from fat, 8% to 10% of kilocalories are from SFAs, and cholesterol intake is limited to less than 300 mg/day. The *Step II Diet* contains the same percentage of total kilocalories from fat, but SFAs are reduced to less than 7% of kilocalories and cholesterol to less than 200 mg/day. A variety of foods from all food groups, within the constraints of the diet, ensures that these diets are nutritionally adequate.

Reducing fat intake to 30% of kilocalories de-

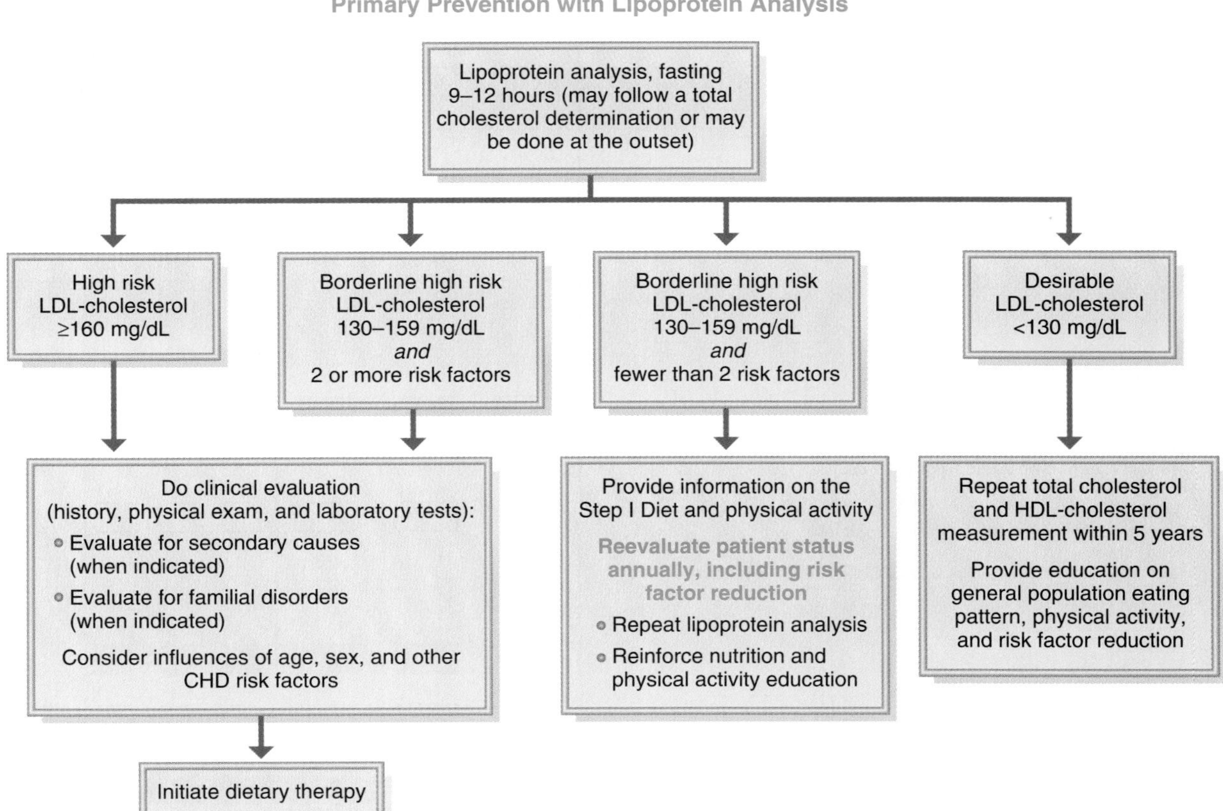

FIGURE 26–7 Primary prevention algorithm based on low-density lipoprotein (LDL) cholesterol. (From National Cholesterol Education Program: Second Report of the Expert Panel on Detection, Evaluation, and Treatment of High Blood Cholesterol in Adults (Adult Treatment Panel II). National Institutes of Health, NIH Publication No. 93-3095. Bethesda, MD: National Heart, Lung, and Blood Institute, 1993.)

Quick Method of Diet Assessment

MEDFICTS: Dietary Assessment Questionnaire

(**M**eats, **E**ggs, **D**airy, **F**ried foods, **I**n baked goods, **C**onvenience foods, **T**able fats, **S**nacks)

Directions: For each food category for both Group 1 and Group 2 listings: Please check a box in the "Weekly Consumption" column and in the "Serving Size" column. If patient rarely or never eats the food listed, please check only the "Weekly Consumption" box.

FOOD CATEGORY	WEEKLY CONSUMPTION: Rarely/ Never	WEEKLY CONSUMPTION: 3 or less serv/wk	WEEKLY CONSUMPTION: 4 or more serv/wk	SERVING SIZE: Small	SERVING SIZE: Average	SERVING SIZE: Large	SCORE: For office use
M Meats • Average amount per day: 6 oz (equal in size to 2 decks of playing cards) • Base your estimate on the food you consume the most of							
Group 1 **Beef**: Ribs, Steak, Chuck blade, Brisket, Ground Beef, Meatloaf, Corned Beef **Processed meats**: Regular hamburger, Fast food hamburger, Bacon, Lunchmeat, Sausage, Hot dogs, Knockworst **Pork & Others**: Pork shoulder, Pork chops, roast, Pork ribs, Ground pork, Regular ham, Lamb steaks, ribs, chops, Organ meats, Poultry with skin	☐	3 pts	7 pts	x 1 pts	2 pts	3 pts =	____
Group 2 **Lean Cuts of Beef**: Sirloin tip, Flank steak, Round steak, Rump roast, Chuck arm roast **Low-fat Processed Meats**: Low-fat lunchmeat, Low-fat hot dogs, Canadian bacon **Poultry, Fish, Meat**: Poultry without skin, Fish, seafood, Lamb flank, leg-shank, sirloin, roast, Lean ham cured and fresh, Pork loin chops, tenderloin, Veal chops, cutlets, roast, Venison	☐	☐	☐	☐	☐	+ 6 pts =	____
E Eggs • Weekly consumption is expressed as times/week				How many eggs do you eat each time?			
Group 1 Whole eggs, Yolks	☐	3 pts	7 pts	x ≤1 1 pts	2 2 pts	≥3 3 pts =	____
Group 2 Egg whites, Egg substitutes (1/2 cup = 2 eggs)	☐	☐	☐	≤1	2	≥3	
D Dairy							
Milk • Average serving: 1 cup							
Group 1 Whole milk, 2% milk, 2% buttermilk, Yogurt (whole milk)	☐	3 pts	7 pts	x 1 pts	2 pts	3 pts =	____
Group 2 Skim milk, 1% milk, Skim milk-buttermilk Yogurt (nonfat & low-fat)	☐	☐	☐	☐	☐	☐	
Cheese • Average serving: 1 oz.							
Group 1 Cream cheese, Cheddar, Monterey Jack, Colby, Swiss, American processed, Blue cheese Regular cottage cheese and Ricotta (1/2 cup)	☐	3 pts	7 pts	x 1 pts	2 pts	3 pts =	____
Group 2 Low-fat & fat-free cheeses, Skim milk mozzarella String cheese Low-fat & fat-free cottage cheese, and Skim milk ricotta (1/2 C)	☐	☐	☐	☐	☐	☐	
Frozen Desserts • Average serving: 1/2 cup							
Group 1 Ice cream, Milk shakes	☐	3 pts	7 pts	x 1 pts	2 pts	3 pts =	____
Group 2 Ice Milk, Frozen yogurt	☐	☐	☐	☐	☐	☐	

+Score 6 points if this box is checked.

Comments: ______________________________ Total ______

FIGURE 26–8 Quick method of diet assessment. (From National Cholesterol Education Program: Second Report of the Expert Panel on Detection, Evaluation, and Treatment of High Blood Cholesterol in Adults (Adult Treatment Panel II). National Institutes of Health, NIH Publication No. 93-3095. Bethesda, MD: National Heart, Lung, and Blood Institute, 1993.)

MEDFICTS

FOOD CATEGORY	WEEKLY CONSUMPTION			SERVING SIZE			SCORE
	Rarely/ Never	3 or less serv/wk	4 or more serv/wk	Small	Average	Large	For office use
F Fried Foods • Average serving: see below							
Group 1 French fries, Fried vegetables: (1/2 cup) *Fried chicken, fish, and meat: (3 oz.) *Check meat category also	☐	■ 3 pts	■ 7 pts	x ■ 1 pts	■ 2 pts	■ 3 pts =	____
Group 2 Vegetables, - not deep fried Meat, Poultry, or fish - prepared by baking, broiling, grilling, poaching, roasting, stewing	☐	☐	☐	☐	☐	☐	
I In Baked Goods • Average serving: 1 serving							
Group 1 Doughnuts, Biscuits, Butter rolls, Muffins, Croissants, Sweet rolls, Danish, Cakes, Pies, Coffee cakes, Cookies	☐	■ 3 pts	■ 7 pts	x ■ 1 pts	■ 2 pts	■ 3 pts =	____
Group 2 Fruit bars, Low-fat cookies/cakes/pastries, Angel food cake, Homemade baked goods with vegetable oils	☐	☐	☐	☐	☐	☐	
C Convenience Foods • Average serving: see below							
Group 1 Canned, Packaged, or Frozen dinners: e.g., Pizza (1 slice), Macaroni & cheese (about 1 cup), Pot pie (1), Cream soups (1 cup)	☐	■ 3 pts	■ 7 pts	x ■ 1 pts	■ 2 pts	■ 3 pts =	____
Group 2 Diet/Reduced calorie or reduced fat dinners (1 dinner)	☐	☐	☐	☐	☐	☐	
T Table Fats • Average serving: see below							
Group 1 Butter, Stick margarine: 1 pat Regular salad dressing or mayonnaise, Sour cream: 1-2 Tbsp	☐	■ 3 pts	■ 7 pts	x ■ 1 pts	■ 2 pts	■ 3 pts =	____
Group 2 Diet and tub margarine, Low-fat & fat-free salad dressings Low-fat & fat-free mayonnaise	☐	☐	☐	☐	☐	☐	
S Snacks • Average serving: see below							
Group 1 Chips (potato, corn, taco), Cheese puffs, Snack mix, Nuts, Regular crackers, Regular popcorn, Candy (milk chocolate, caramel, coconut)	☐	■ 3 pts	■ 7 pts	x ■ 1 pts	■ 2 pts	■ 3 pts =	____
Group 2 Air-popped or low-fat popcorn, Low-fat crackers, Hard candy, Licorice, Fruit rolls, Bread sticks, Pretzels, Fat-free chips Fruit	☐	☐	☐	☐	☐	☐	

Directions for scoring:
Multiply Weekly Consumption points (3 or 7) by Serving Size points (1, 2, 3) for Group 1 foods only except for a large serving of Group 2 meats

Example: ■ 3 pts ■✓ 7 pts ■ 1 pts ■ 2 pts ■✓ 3 pts

3 x 7 = 21 points

Add score on page 1 and page 2 to get Final Score

Key

40 - 70	- Step I Diet
less than 40	- Step II Diet

■ - Foods high in fat, saturated fat, and/or cholesterol

Total ____

Score from page 1 + ____

Final Score ____

FIGURE 26–8 *Continued*

TABLE 26–10 TARGET LDL CHOLESTEROL LEVEL FOR INITIATING DIET THERAPY

	DIETARY THERAPY		DRUG TREATMENT	
	Initiation Level (mg/dL)	LDL Goal (mg/dL)	Consideration Level (mg/dL)	LDL Goal (mg/dL)
Without CHD and with fewer than 2 risk factors	≥160	<160	≥190*	<160
Without CHD and with 2 or more risk factors	≥130	<130	≥160	<130
With CHD	>100	≤100	≥130†	≤100

(Data from National Cholesterol Education Program [NCEP]. Second Report of the Expert Panel on Detection, Evaluation, and Treatment of High Blood Cholesterol in Adults [Adult Treatment Panel II]. NIH Publication No. 93-3095. Bethesda, MD: National Institutes of Health. National Heart, Lung, and Blood Institute, 1993.)

CHD, coronary heart disease; *LDL*, low-density lipoprotein.

*In men younger than 35 years of age and premenopausal women with LDL cholesterol levels of 190 to 219 mg/dL, drug therapy should be delayed except in high-risk patients, such as those with diabetes.

†In patients with CHD and LDL cholesterol levels of 100 to 129 mg/dL, the physician should exercise clinical judgment in deciding whether to initiate drug treatment.

creases the caloric content of the diet and helps facilitate weight reduction for those patients who need it. For those who do not need to lose weight, high-carbohydrate foods can be substituted for fat. Emphasizing whole-grain breads and cereals, vegetables, and fruits for the carbohydrate replacement also increases the fiber content of the diet.

When the Step I Diet is followed, the serum cholesterol level is lowered 3% to 14%. It should be measured first after 6 weeks on the diet and again at 3 months. Dietary compliance must be monitored during this period. A quick method of assessment can be used (Fig. 26–8), or more labor-intensive methods (24-hour recall, 3-day food records, food frequency questionnaires) may be used if greater accuracy is desired (see Chapter 16). If blood lipid goals are not achieved by a compliant patient after 3 months on the Step I Diet, then the patient progresses to the Step II Diet. The Step II Diet may lower serum cholesterol another 3% to 7%. Individuals with baseline high-fat diets who lose weight may reduce their total cholesterol by up to 25% with good adherence.

Based on NHANES III data, the average American needs to reduce fat intake from 34% to 30% of the total kilocalories, and to reduce the SFA level from 12% to 10% of total kilocalories. Data from several national surveys show that only about 20% of American women, or 23% of the total population, consume diets with less then 30% of energy derived from fat (Kris-Etherton and Krummel, 1993; Lewis et al., 1994). Furthermore, only 2% of women have diets that meet total fat goals and two thirds of the RDA for all nutrients (Murphy et al., 1992). Clearly, nutrition education is needed for diet optimization.

Medical nutrition therapy for compliant patients should be tried for a minimum of 6 months before drug therapy is started. Medical nutrition therapy, with 3 to 4 visits of 50 minutes duration with a dietitian over several months, has been found to be associated with a significant reduction in serum cholesterol levels, and with a savings in health care costs (Sikand et al., 1998).

Secondary Prevention

Patients with established CHD have a fivefold to sevenfold higher risk of subsequent myocardial infarction; therefore, LDL cholesterol goals are lower (100 mg/dL). Diet therapy is critical for secondary prevention, as SFA levels have been shown to be related to disease progression in men (Watts et al., 1996). Usually, to attain these lower LDL cholesterol levels, aggressive diet therapy is needed (see the following sections). Major life-style interventions can slow lesion development or promote regression of existing lesions.

TABLE 26–11 DIET THERAPY FOR HIGH BLOOD CHOLESTEROL

NUTRIENT		RECOMMENDED INTAKE Step I Diet	Step II Diet
Total fat	≤30% of total calories		
Saturated fatty acids		8%–10% of total calories	<7% of total calories
Polyunsaturated fatty acids	Up to 10% of total calories		
Monounsaturated fatty acids	Up to 15% of total calories		
Carbohydrates	55% or more of total calories		
Protein	Approximately 15% of total calories		
Cholesterol		<300 mg/day	<200 mg/day
Total calories*	To achieve and maintain desirable weight		

(Data from National Cholesterol Education Program [NCEP]. Second Report of the Expert Panel on Detection, Evaluation, and Treatment of High Blood Cholesterol in Adults [Adult Treatment Panel II]. NIH Publication No. 93-3095. Bethesda, MD: National Institutes of Health. National Heart, Lung, and Blood Institute, 1993.)

*Calories from alcohol not included.

In the Lifestyle Trial, the intervention was a very low-fat, nearly vegetarian diet (egg whites and nonfat milk allowed; total fat comprising 10% of kilocalories), coupled with exercise, weight reduction, smoking cessation, and stress reduction (Ornish and Brown, 1993). After 1 year, these patients had a 37% reduction in LDL cholesterol, and 82% had overall regression of coronary atherosclerosis. These patients were able to meet the LDL goals without drugs. (The average final LDL cholesterol level was 95 mg/dL.)

In a second study, the intervention involved a less rigorous diet (<20% of kilocalories derived from fat) and exercise. The latter intervention slowed progression of disease and promoted regression in more intervention patients than in the usual care group (Schuler et al., 1992). The American Heart Association recommends that a lower level of calories be derived from fat. If LDL cholesterol goals are unattainable by diet alone, drug therapy may be indicated.

TREATMENT

Treatment of CHD involves modification of all the risk factors. Smoking cessation, weight control, normalization of blood lipids, active life-style, and Step I Diet are key factors for treatment. Dietary modifications for the prevention and control of hypertension are outlined in Chapter 27, and information on sodium restriction appears in Chapter 36.

Medical Nutrition Therapy and Life-Style Changes

Medical nutrition therapy is the primary intervention for patients with elevated LDL cholesterol. With diet, exercise, and weight reduction, patients can often reach lipid goals. Consequently, these interventions are tried before drug therapy. The Step I Diet is recommended for populations older than 2 years of age, as well as for the first level of primary intervention. Behavior modification and goal-setting are key strategies used by the dietitian to help patients adopt the Step I and Step II Diets for a lifetime. Behavior modification and weight-reduction programs are discussed in Chapter 23.

Step I and II Diets

The Step I and Step II Diets emphasize grains, cereals, legumes, vegetables, fruits, lean meats, poultry, fish, and nonfat dairy products (Table 26–12). Some different strategies to reduce fat and SFA are (1) avoiding fats as spreads or for flavoring, (2) avoiding or reducing the consumption of meat, (3) using specially manufactured low-fat foods (e.g., fat-free salad dressings), (4) modifying common foods to be lower in fat (e.g., removing skin from chicken), and (5) replacing high-fat foods with low-fat foods (e.g., substituting skim milk for whole milk).

Because animal fats provide about two thirds of the SFA in the American diet, these foods are restricted. High-fat choices are omitted, but low-fat choices can be included. Meat is limited to 5 to 6 oz/day and eggs to 4/week. The fat, SFA, and cholesterol content of meat, fish, and poultry are listed in Table 26–13. Lean meats are high in protein, zinc, and iron; hence, if patients wish to consume meat, a 6-oz portion or less is allowed per day. Similarly, with dairy products, nonfat choices are recommended. Neither food group has to be omitted; it is a matter of choice. For lower-fat diets, meats are further restricted.

Some patients, particularly those who need to reduce weight, like to use the exchange system for their Step I or Step II Diets (Table 26–14). These plans should be individualized to facilitate long-term compliance. Although some patients prefer the exchange method, others prefer counting grams of fat (Table 26–15).

The nutrition labels on foods will help patients who want to count fat grams. Labeling terms that relate to diet modifications for CHD are shown in Table 26–16. The limitation of this method is that only fat, SFA, or cholesterol is counted, without attention to calories or to including adequate levels of other nutrients. Many new low-fat products are lacking in essential nutrients, and a diet based on these products without basic foods may be nutritionally incomplete. Both the Step I and Step II Diets can be designed using foods from many cultures. Tables 26–17 through 26–19 illustrate menus for the Step I and Step II Diets that feature different ethnic cuisines.

With the Step I and Step II Diets, increased soluble fiber intake should be encouraged. This can be achieved with frequent use of legumes, oatmeal or oat bran, fresh fruits, and fibrous vegetables. For women in a low-fat diet trial (intensive intervention on a 20% fat diet), increasing the consumption of grains, fruits, and vegetables was the most difficult change to make (Burrows et al., 1993). Nutrition education efforts are needed in this area.

Meeting sodium guidelines (2400 mg/day) on a Step I or Step II Diet can be a challenge, as lower-fat processed foods often contain salt to increase palatability. Patients may need to limit convenience and processed foods.

Aggressive Diets

For highly motivated patients who want to avoid drug therapy, sometimes very low-fat diets are effective for reaching blood lipid goals. These diets can also be used as an adjunct to drug therapy for secondary prevention and possible regression of lesions. Such diets contain minimal amounts of animal products; hence, SFA (<3%), cholesterol (<5 mg), and total fat (<10%) intakes are very low. The emphasis is on low-fat grains, legumes, fruits, veg-

TABLE 26–12 FOOD CHOICES FOR STEP I AND STEP II DIETS

FOOD GROUP	CHOOSE	DECREASE
Lean meat, poultry, and fish ≤5–6 oz per day	Beef, pork, lamb—lean cuts, well trimmed before cooking	Beef, pork, lamb—regular ground beef, fatty cuts, spare ribs, organ meats
	Poultry without skin	Poultry with skin, fried chicken
	Fish, shellfish	Fried fish, fried shellfish
	Processed meat—prepared from lean meat (e.g., lean ham, lean frankfurters, lean meat with soy protein or carrageenan)	Regular luncheon meat (e.g., bologna, salami, sausage, frankfurters)
Eggs ≤4 yolks per week, Step I ≤2 yolks per week, Step II	Egg whites (two whites can be substituted for one whole egg in recipes), cholesterol-free egg substitute	Egg yolks (if more than 4 per week on Step I or if more than 2 per week on Step II); includes eggs used in cooking and baking
Low-fat dairy products 2–3 servings per day	Milk—skim, ½%, or 1% fat (fluid, powdered, evaporated), buttermilk	Whole milk (fluid, evaporated, condensed), 2% fat milk (low-fat milk), imitation milk
	Yogurt—nonfat or low-fat yogurt or yogurt beverages	Whole-milk yogurt, whole-milk yogurt beverages
	Cheese—low-fat natural or processed cheese	Regular cheeses (American, blue, Brie, cheddar, Colby, Edam, Monterey Jack, whole-milk mozzarella, Parmesan, Swiss), cream cheese, Neufchatel cheese
	Low-fat or nonfat varieties, such as cottage cheese—low-fat, nonfat, or dry curd (0 to 2% fat)	Cottage cheese (4% fat)
	Frozen dairy dessert—ice milk, frozen yogurt (low-fat or nonfat)	Ice cream
	Low-fat coffee creamer Low-fat or nonfat sour cream	Cream, half & half, whipping cream, nondairy creamer, whipped topping, sour cream
Fats and oils ≤6–8 tsp per day	Unsaturated oils—safflower, sunflower, corn, soybean, cottonseed, canola, olive, peanut	Coconut oil, palm kernel oil, palm oil
	Margarine—made from unsaturated oils listed above; light or diet margarine, especially soft or liquid forms	Butter, lard, shortening, bacon fat, hard margarine
	Salad dressings—made with unsaturated oils listed above; low-fat or fat free	Dressings made with egg yolk, cheese, sour cream, whole milk
	Seeds and nuts—peanut butter, other nut butters	Coconut
	Cocoa powder	Milk chocolate
Breads and cereals ≥6 servings per day	Breads—whole-grain bread, English muffins, bagels, buns, corn or flour tortilla	Bread in which eggs, fat, and/or butter are a major ingredient; croissants
	Cereals—oat, wheat, corn, multigrain	Most granolas
	Pasta	
	Rice	
	Dried beans and peas	
	Crackers, low-fat—animal type, graham, soda crackers, breadsticks, melba toast	High-fat crackers
	Homemade baked goods using unsaturated oil, skim or 1% milk, and egg substitute—quick breads, biscuits, cornbread muffins, bran muffins, pancakes, waffles	Commercial baked pastries, muffins, biscuits
Soups	Reduced- or low-fat and reduced-sodium varieties (e.g., chicken or beef noodle, minestrone, tomato, vegetable, potato), reduced-fat soups made with skim milk	Soups containing whole milk, cream, meat fat, poultry fat, or poultry skin
Vegetables 3–5 servings per day	Fresh, frozen, or canned, without added fat or sauce	Vegetables fried or prepared with butter, cheese, or cream sauce
Fruits 2–4 servings per day	Fruits—fresh, frozen, canned, or dried	Fried fruit or fruit served with butter or cream sauce
	Fruit juice—fresh, frozen, or canned	
Sweets and modified-fat desserts	Beverages—fruit-flavored drinks, lemonade, fruit punch	
	Sweets—sugar, syrup, honey, jam, preserves, candy made without fat (candy corn, gumdrops, hard candy), fruit-flavored gelatin	Candy made with milk chocolate, coconut oil, palm kernel oil, palm oil
	Frozen desserts—low-fat and nonfat yogurt, ice milk, sherbet, sorbet, fruit ice, popsicles	Ice cream and frozen treats made with ice cream
	Cookies, cake, pie, pudding—prepared with egg whites, egg substitute, skim milk or 1% milk, and unsaturated oil or margarine; ginger snaps; fig and other fruit bar cookies, fat-free cookies; angel food cake	Commercial baked pies, cakes, doughnuts, high-fat cookies, cream pies

(Data from National Cholesterol Education Program [NCEP]. Second Report of the Expert Panel on Detection, Evaluation, and Treatment of High Blood Cholesterol in Adults [Adult Treatment Panel II]. NIH Publication No. 93-3095. Bethesda, MD: National Institutes of Health. National Heart, Lung, and Blood Institute, 1993.)

TABLE 26–13 FAT, SFA, CHOLESTEROL AND IRON CONTENT OF MEAT, POULTRY, AND FISH (3-OZ PORTIONS) COOKED WITHOUT ADDED FAT

SOURCE	TOTAL FAT (g/3 oz)	SATURATED FAT (g/3 oz)	CHOLESTEROL (mg/3 oz)	IRON (mg/3 oz)
Lean red meats				
Beef (rump roast, shank, bottom round, sirloin)	4.2	1.4	71	2.5
Lamb (shank roast, sirloin roast, shoulder roast, loin chops, sirloin chops, center leg chop)	7.8	2.8	78	1.9
Pork (sirloin cutlet, loin roast, sirloin roast, center roast, butterfly chops, loin chops)	11.8	4.1	77	1.0
Veal (blade roast, sirloin chops, shoulder roast, loin chops, rump roast, shank)	4.9	2.0	93	1.0
Organ meats				
Liver				
Beef	4.2	1.6	331	5.8
Calf	5.9	2.2	477	2.2
Chicken	4.6	1.6	537	7.2
Sweetbread	21.3	7.3	250	1.3
Kidney	2.9	0.9	329	6.2
Brains	10.7	2.5	1747	1.9
Heart	4.8	1.4	164	6.4
Poultry				
Chicken (without skin)				
Light (roasted)	3.8	1.1	72	0.9
Dark (roasted)	8.3	2.3	79	1.1
Turkey (without skin)				
Light (roasted)	2.7	0.9	59	1.1
Dark (roasted)	6.1	2.0	72	2.0
Fish				
Haddock	0.8	0.1	63	1.1
Flounder	1.3	0.3	58	0.3
Salmon	7.0	1.7	54	0.3
Tuna, light, canned in water	0.7	0.2	25	1.3
Shellfish				
Crustaceans				
Lobster	0.5	0.1	61	0.3
Crab meat				
Alaskan King Crab	1.3	0.1	45	0.6
Blue Crab	1.5	0.2	85	0.8
Shrimp	0.9	0.2	166	2.6
Mollusks				
Abalone	1.3	0.3	144	5.4
Clams	1.7	0.2	57	23.8
Mussels	3.8	0.7	48	5.7
Oysters	4.2	1.3	93	10.2
Scallops	1.2	0.1	27	2.6
Squid	2.4	0.6	400	1.2

(Data from National Cholesterol Education Program [NCEP]. Second Report of the Expert Panel on Detection, Evaluation, and Treatment of High Blood Cholesterol in Adults [Adult Treatment Panel II]. NIH Publication No. 93-3095. Bethesda, MD: National Institutes of Health. National Heart, Lung, and Blood Institute, 1993.)
SFA, saturated fatty acid.

TABLE 26–14 EATING PLANS FOR STEP I AND STEP II DIETS

FOOD GROUP	DAILY PORTIONS—STEP I DIET				DAILY PORTIONS—STEP II DIET			
	1200 kcal	1600 kcal	2000 kcal	2500 kcal	1200 kcal	1600 kcal	2000 kcal	2500 kcal
Fats and oils	3	4	6	8	3	5	7	8
Fish, poultry, meat	6 oz	6 oz	6 oz	6 oz	6 oz	6 oz	6 oz	6 oz
Egg yolks	3/wk	3/wk	3/wk	3/wk	1/wk	1/wk	1/wk	1/wk
Dairy foods	2	3	3	4	2	2	2	3
Bread, beans, grains, and starches	3	4	7	10	4	5	8	10
Fruit	3	3	3	5	3	3	4	7
Vegetables	4	4	4	4	4	4	4	5
Sugars, sweets, alcohol	0	2	2	2	0	2	2	2

(Data from National Cholesterol Education Program [NCEP]. Second Report of the Expert Panel on Detection, Evaluation, and Treatment of High Blood Cholesterol in Adults [Adult Treatment Panel II]. NIH Publication No. 93-3095. Bethesda, MD: National Institutes of Health. National Heart, Lung, and Blood Institute, 1993.)
*The average daily intake for women is about 1800 kcal; for men, it is about 2500 kcal.

TABLE 26–15 MAXIMAL FAT AND SFA IN STEP I AND STEP II DIETS*

	TOTAL CALORIE LEVEL (KCAL)							
	1600	1800	2000	2200	2400	2600	2800	3000
Total fat (g)[†]	53	60	67	73	80	87	93	100
Saturated fat (g)—Step I[‡]	18	20	22	24	27	29	31	33
Saturated fat (g)—Step II[‡]	12	14	16	17	19	20	22	23

(Data from National Cholesterol Education Program [NCEP]. Second Report of the Expert Panel on Detection, Evaluation, and Treatment of High Blood Cholesterol in Adults [Adult Treatment Panel II]. NIH Publication No. 93-3095. Bethesda, MD: National Institutes of Health. National Heart, Lung, and Blood Institute, 1993.)

SFA, saturated fatty acid.

*The average daily intake for women is about 1800 kcal; for men, it is about 2500 kcal.

[†]Total fat content of both diets is 30% of total calories consumed (estimated by multiplying the caloric level of the diet by 0.3 and dividing the product by 9 kcal/g).

[‡]The recommended intake of saturated fat on the Step I Diet is 8% to 10% of total calories; saturated fat content is less than 7% for the Step II Diet.

etables, and nonfat dairy foods. Because egg whites are allowed, the plan is a lacto-ovovegetarian regimen. To ensure nutritional adequacy, a food plan, such as that shown in Table 26–20, should be followed. Quick tips are summarized in Table 26–21.

Pharmacologic Management

Patients requiring drug therapy should already be following a Step II Diet. A regimen combining diet and drugs enables more patients to achieve blood lipid goals than a drug-only regimen (Cobb et al., 1992). A Step II Diet with drugs can reduce serum cholesterol levels by up to 40%. More restrictive diets with drugs have not been investigated. The classes of drugs include (1) **bile acid sequestrants** (cholestyramine), (2) nicotinic acid, (3) **HMG CoA reductase inhibitors** (lovastatin, pravastatin), (4) fibric acid derivatives (clofibrate, gemfibrozil), and (5) probucol. Classes 1, 2, and 3 are the first choices for treatment (Larsen and Illingworth, 1994).

TABLE 26–16 NUTRITION LABELING TERMS RELATED TO MODIFIED DIETS FOR CORONARY HEART DISEASE

NUTRIENT	FREE	LOW	REDUCED/LESS/FEWER	OTHER
All	Synonyms for "Free": "Free of," "No," "Zero," "Without," "Trivial Source of," "Negligible Source of," "Dietary Insignificant Source of"	Synonyms for "Low": "Contains a Small Amount of," "Low Source of," "Low in"	Synonyms for "Reduced/Less/Fewer": "Reduced in," "Lower," "Low"	
Kilocalories	<5 kcal/reference serving	<40 kcal/reference serving	Reduced by at least 25%	
Total fat	<0.5 g/reference serving	≤3 g/reference serving Meal and main dish products: ≤3 g/100 g and 30% or less calories from fat	Reduced by at least 25%	"__% Fat Free," "__% Lean," must meet requirements for "Low Fat"
Saturated fat	<0.5 g/reference serving; levels of trans-fatty acids must be 1% or less of total fat	≤1 g/reference serving and 15% or less of calories from saturated fatty acids Meal and main dish products: ≤1 g/100g and less than 10% of calories from saturated fat	Reduced by at least 25%	
Cholesterol	<2 mg/reference serving; saturated fat content must be 2 g or less	≤20 mg/reference serving; saturated fat content must be 2 g or less per serving Meal and main dish products: ≤20 mg/100 g, with saturated fat content less than 2 g/100g	Reduced by at least 25% Contains 2 g or less of saturated fat per reference serving	
Sodium	<5 mg/reference serving	≤140 mg/reference serving Meal and main dish products: ≤140 mg/100 g of food	Reduced by at least 25%	"Very Low Sodium," "Very Low in Sodium": ≤35 mg/reference serving

(Data from National Cholesterol Education Program [NCEP]. Second Report of the Expert Panel on Detection, Evaluation, and Treatment of High Blood Cholesterol in Adults [Adult Treatment Panel II]. NIH Publication No. 93-3095. Bethesda, MD: National Institutes of Health. National Heart, Lung, and Blood Institute, 1993.)

TABLE 26–17 SAMPLE AMERICAN MENUS FOR STEP I AND STEP II DIETS

STEP I: SAMPLE MENUS—TRADITIONAL AMERICAN CUISINE FEMALES 25–49 YEARS*	STEP II: SAMPLE MENUS—TRADITIONAL AMERICAN CUISINE FEMALES 25–49 YEARS*
Breakfast	**Breakfast**
Bagel, plain (½ medium)	Bagel, plain (½ medium)
Cream cheese, low-fat[†] (1 tsp)	**Margarine** (1 tsp)
	Jelly (1 tsp)
Cereal, shredded wheat (1 cup)	Cereal, shredded wheat (1 cup)
Banana (1 small)	Banana (1 small)
Milk, **1%** (1 cup)	Milk, **skim** (1 cup)
Orange juice (¾ cup)	Orange juice (**1 cup**)
Coffee (1 cup)	Coffee (1 cup)
Milk, **1%** (1 oz)	Milk, **skim** (1 oz)
Lunch	**Lunch**
Minestrone soup, canned, low sodium (½ cup)	Minestrone soup, canned, low sodium (½ cup)
Roast beef sandwich	Roast beef sandwich
Whole wheat bread (2 slices)	Whole wheat bread (2 slices)
‡ Lean roast beef, unseasoned (**3 oz**)	‡ Lean roast beef, unseasoned (**2 oz**)
American cheese, low-fat and low-sodium (¾ oz)	American cheese, low-fat and low-sodium (¾ oz)
Lettuce (1 leaf)	Lettuce (1 leaf)
Tomato (3 slices)	Tomato (3 slices)
Mayonnaise, low-fat and low-sodium (2 tsp)	**Margarine** (2 tsp)
Apple (1 medium)	Apple (1 medium)
Water (1 cup)	Water (1 cup)
Dinner	**Dinner**
‡ **Salmon** (3 oz)	‡ **Flounder** (3 oz)
Vegetable oil (1 tsp)	Vegetable oil (1 tsp)
‡ Baked potato (½ medium)	‡ Baked potato (½ medium)
Margarine (1 tsp)	Margarine (1 tsp)
‡ Green beans (½ cup), seasoned with margarine (½ tsp)	‡ Green beans (½ cup), seasoned with margarine (½ tsp)
‡ Carrots (½ cup), seasoned with margarine (½ tsp)	‡ Carrots (½ cup), seasoned with margarine (½ tsp)
White dinner roll (1 medium)	White dinner roll (1 medium)
Margarine (1 tsp)	Margarine (1 tsp)
Ice milk (½ cup)	**Frozen yogurt** (½ cup)
Iced tea, unsweetened (1 cup)	Iced tea, unsweetened (1 cup)
Snack	**Snack**
‡ Popcorn (2 cups)	‡ Popcorn (3 cups)
Margarine (**1 tsp**)	Margarine (**2 tsp**)

Totals

	Step I		Step I		Step II		Step II
Calories:	1831	Total carb, % kcal:	52	Calories:	1867	Total carb, % kcal:	55
Total fat, % kcal:	30	Simple carb, % carb:	37	Total fat, % kcal:	29	Simple carb, % carb:	38
SFA, % kcal:	8.7	Complex carb, % carb:	63	SFA, % kcal:	6.8	Complex carb, % carb:	62
Cholesterol, mg:	156	‡Sodium, mg:	1415	Cholesterol, mg:	134	‡Sodium, mg:	1417
Protein, % kcal:	18			Protein, % kcal:	16		

(Data from National Cholesterol Education Program [NCEP]. Second Report of the Expert Panel on Detection, Evaluation, and Treatment of High Blood Cholesterol in Adults [Adult Treatment Panel II]. NIH Publication No. 93-3095. Bethesda, MD: National Institutes of Health. National Heart, Lung, and Blood Institute, 1993.)

SFA, saturated fatty acid; *carb*, carbohydrates.

*100% RDA met for all nutrients except zinc (90%).

[†]Boldface food items represent differences between the Step I and Step II Diets.

[‡]No salt is added in recipe preparation or as seasoning. All margarine is low-sodium.

Most patients can reach lipid goals with diet and a bile acid sequestrant. All of these drugs affect nutritional status, which needs to be monitored (Table 26–22). Lipid-lowering drugs, once initiated, are required for life. Although most patients will achieve lipid goals with one drug, some require double or triple combination therapy. With multiple drugs, a 60% reduction in LDL cholesterol can be achieved.

Medical Intervention

Coronary Angioplasty

Percutaneous transluminal coronary angioplasty (PTCA) is a procedure that uses a balloon to break up plaque deposits in an occluded artery. Because the procedure is performed under local anesthesia in a cardiac catheterization laboratory, recovery is

(Text continues on page 593.)

TABLE 26–18 SAMPLE MEXICAN-AMERICAN MENUS FOR STEP I AND STEP II DIETS

STEP I: SAMPLE MENUS—MEXICAN-AMERICAN CUISINE MALES 25–49 YEARS*

Breakfast

- Cantaloupe (½ cup)
- ‡ Farina, prepared with **1%**[†] milk (1 cup)
- White bread (2 slices)
  - Margarine (2 tsp)
  - Jelly (2 tsp)
- Orange juice (¾ cup)
- Hot cocoa, prepared with **1%** milk (1 cup)

Lunch

- Beef enchilada
  - Tortilla, corn (2 tortillas)
  - ‡ Lean roast beef (**3 oz**)
  - Vegetable oil (**1 tsp**)
  - Cheddar cheese, low-fat and low-sodium (1 oz)
  - Onion (⅛ cup)
  - Tomato (⅛ cup)
  - Lettuce (¼ cup)
  - Chili peppers (2 tsp)
- ‡ Refried beans (¾ cup), prepared with vegetable oil
- Carrots (6 sticks), Celery (6 sticks)
- Milk, **1%** (½ cup)

Dinner

- Chicken taco
  - Tortilla, corn (2 tortillas)
  - ‡ Chicken breast, without skin (3 oz)
  - Vegetable oil (**1 tsp**)
  - Cheddar cheese, low-fat and low-sodium (1 oz)
  - Guacamole (2 T)
  - Salsa (2 T)
- ‡ Corn (**½ cup**), seasoned with margarine (**½ tsp**)
- ‡ Spanish rice (1 cup), prepared with margarine
- Banana (1 medium)
- Coffee (1 cup)
  - Milk, **1%** (1 oz)

Snack

- **Ice Milk** (¾ cup)

Totals

Calories:	2557	Total carb, % kcal:	52
Total fat, % kcal:	29	Simple carb, % carb:	40
SFA, % kcal:	8.3	Complex carb, % carb:	60
Cholesterol, mg:	185	‡Sodium, mg:	1801
Protein, % kcal:	19		

STEP II: SAMPLE MENUS—MEXICAN-AMERICAN CUISINE MALES 25–49 YEARS*

Breakfast

- Cantaloupe (½ cup)
- ‡ Farina, prepared with **skim** milk (1 cup)
- White bread (2 slices)
  - Margarine (2 tsp)
  - Jelly (2 tsp)
- Orange juice (¾ cup)
- Hot cocoa, prepared with **skim** milk (1 cup)

Lunch

- Beef enchilada
  - Tortilla, corn (2 tortillas)
  - ‡ Lean roast beef (**2 oz**)
  - Vegetable oil (**½ tsp**)
  - Cheddar cheese, low-fat and low-sodium (1 oz)
  - Onion (⅛ cup)
  - Tomato (⅛ cup)
  - Lettuce (¼ cup)
  - Chili peppers (2 tsp)
- ‡ Refried beans (¾ cup), prepared with vegetable oil
- Carrots (6 sticks), Celery (6 sticks)
- Milk, **skim** (½ cup)

Dinner

- Chicken taco
  - Tortilla, corn flour (2 tortillas)
  - ‡ Chicken breast, without skin (3 oz)
  - Vegetable oil (**½ tsp**)
  - Cheddar cheese, low-fat and low-sodium (1 oz)
  - Guacamole (2 T)
- ‡ Corn (**1 cup**), seasoned with margarine (**1 tsp**)
- ‡ Spanish rice (1 cup), prepared with margarine
- Banana (1 medium)
- Coffee (1 cup)
  - Milk, **skim** (1 oz)

Snack

- **Popcorn** (3 cups)
  - **Margarine** (1 T)

Totals

Calories	2574	Total carb, % kcal:	55
Total fat, % kcal:	28	Simple carb, % carb:	36
SFA, % kcal:	6.2	Complex carb, % carb:	64
Cholesterol, mg:	136	‡Sodium, mg:	1921
Protein, % kcal:	17		

(Data from National Cholesterol Education Program [NCEP]. Second Report of the Expert Panel on Detection, Evaluation, and Treatment of High Blood Cholesterol in Adults [Adult Treatment Panel II]. NIH Publication No. 93-3095. Bethesda, MD: National Institutes of Health. National Heart, Lung, and Blood Institute, 1993.)

SFA, saturated fatty acid; *carb*, carbohydrates.

*100% RDA met for all nutrients except zinc (90%).

†Boldface food items represent differences between the Step I and Step II Diets.

‡No salt added in recipe preparation or as seasoning. All margarine is low-sodium.

TABLE 26–19 SAMPLE ASIAN-AMERICAN MENUS FOR STEP I AND STEP II DIETS

STEP I: SAMPLE MENUS—ASIAN-AMERICAN CUISINE MALES 25–49 YEARS*

Breakfast

- Banana (1 medium)
- Whole wheat bread (2 slices)
  - Margarine (2 tsp)
- Orange juice (¾ cup)
- Milk, **1%**† (1 cup)

Lunch

- Beef noodle soup, canned, low-sodium (1 cup)
- Chinese noodle and beef salad
  - ‡ **Lean Roast Beef** (3 oz)
  - Peanut oil (**2 tsp**)
  - Soy sauce, low-sodium (1 tsp)
  - Peanuts, unsalted (**1 T**)
  - Carrots (½ cup)
  - Squash (½ cup)
  - Onion (½ cup)
  - Chinese noodles, soft type (¼ cup)
- ‡ Steamed white rice (1 cup)
- Apple (1 medium)
- Tea, unsweetened (1 cup)

Dinner

- Pork stirfry with vegetables
  - Pork cutlet (**3 oz**)
  - Peanut oil (**2 tsp**)
  - Soy sauce, low-sodium (1 tsp)
  - Peanuts, unsalted (**1 T**)
  - Broccoli (½ cup)
  - Carrots (½ cup)
  - Mushrooms (¼ cup)
- ‡ Steamed white rice (1 cup)
- ‡ Wonton soup, prepared with low-sodium broth (½ cup)
- Milk, **1%** (1 cup)
- Tea, unsweetened (1 cup)

Snack

- Egg roll, vegetarian, baked with peanut oil and low-sodium soy sauce (1 medium)
  - Chinese mustard (1 tsp)
  - Sweet and sour sauce (1 tsp)
- Tea, unsweetened (1 cup)

Totals

Calories:	2494	Total carb, % kcal:	53
Total fat, % kcal:	30	Simple carb, % carb:	30
SFA, % kcal:	8.1	Complex carb, % carb:	70
Cholesterol, mg:	238	‡Sodium, mg:	1663
Protein, % kcal:	17		

STEP II: SAMPLE MENUS—ASIAN-AMERICAN CUISINE FEMALES 25–49 YEARS*

Breakfast

- Banana (**½ medium**)
- Whole wheat bread (2 slices)
  - Margarine (2 tsp)
- Orange juice (¾ cup)
- Milk, **skim** (1 cup)

Lunch

- Beef noodle soup, canned, low-sodium (½ cup)
- ‡ Chinese noodle and beef salad
  - **Sirloin steak** (3 oz)
  - Peanut oil (**1 tsp**)
  - Soy sauce, low-sodium (1 tsp)
  - Carrots (½ cup)
  - Squash (½ cup)
  - Onion (¼ cup)
  - Chinese noodles, soft type (¼ cup)
- ‡ Steamed white rice (½ cup)
- Apple (1 medium)
- Tea, unsweetened (1 cup)

Dinner

- Pork stirfry with vegetables
  - Pork cutlet (**2 oz**)
  - Peanut oil (**1 tsp**)
  - Soy sauce, low-sodium (1 tsp)
  - Broccoli (½ cup)
  - Carrots (½ cup)
  - Mushrooms (¼ cup)
- ‡ Steamed white rice (½ cup)
- Milk, **skim** (¾ cup)
- Tea, unsweetened (1 cup)

Snack

- ‡ Wonton soup, prepared with low-sodium broth (½ cup)
- Tea, unsweetened (1 cup)

Totals

Calories:	1815	Total carb, % kcal:	52
Total fat, % kcal:	39	Simple carb, % carb:	33
SFA, % kcal:	6.8	Complex carb, % carb:	67
Cholesterol, mg:	176	‡Sodium, mg:	1300
Protein, % kcal:	19		

(Data from National Cholesterol Education Program [NCEP]. Second Report of the Expert Panel on Detection, Evaluation, and Treatment of High Blood Cholesterol in Adults [Adult Treatment Panel II]. NIH Publication No. 93-3095. Bethesda, MD: National Institutes of Health. National Heart, Lung, and Blood Institute, 1993.)

SFA, saturated fatty acid; *carb,* carbohydrates.

*100% RDA met for all nutrients except zinc (90%).

†Boldface food items represent differences between the Step I and Step II Diets.

‡No salt is added in recipe preparation or as seasoning. All margarine is low-sodium.

TABLE 26–20 FOOD PLAN FOR AN AGGRESSIVE LOW-FAT DIET (<10% KCAL FROM FAT)

SERVING SIZE	RECOMMENDED DAILY INTAKE
Nonfat Dairy	2 servings
1 cup skim milk	
1 cup nonfat yogurt	
1 oz nonfat cheese*	
½ cup nonfat cottage cheese*	
½ cup nonfat ricotta	
2 tablespoons nonfat cream cheese*	
Protein	4–8 oz
Dried beans, cooked (4 oz)	
4 egg whites (4 oz)	
½ cup nonfat egg substitute (4 oz)	
Fat-free gluten meat substitute (4 oz)	
Reduced-fat tofu or soy protein (4 oz)	
Vegetables	≥5 servings
1 cup raw	
½ cup cooked	
½ cup vegetable juice*	
Fruits	≥2 (limit of 2/day with elevated triglyceride level)
1 medium raw fruit	
½ large fruit	
1 cup fresh fruit	
½ cup fruit sauce or juice	
¼ cup dried fruit	
Breads/Cereals/Starches	≥6
1 slice bread	
1 medium potato	
1 cup pasta, rice, or cereal	
6 crackers	
½ bagel or English muffin	
Nonfat Sweets and Treats	Rarely

(Reprinted with permission from Reversal Eating Plan, © 1996 Gerry Krag, MA, RD, Grosse Pte. Park, MI.)

*Higher sodium food.

TABLE 26–21 QUICK TIPS FOR AGGRESSIVE LIPID-LOWERING DIETS

ABCs of the Reversal Eating Plan:

A. Fat intake of 12–14 g/day
B. Vegetarian eating—no meat, poultry, fish
C. No added fats—fat or oil is not added to any food
D. Higher fat foods are not used—e.g., nuts, seeds, avocado, olives
E. No "fat-free" foods with fat in the ingredient list (e.g., whipped topping mix, dairy creamers, etc.)

Use These Foods Daily:

A. Nonfat dairy foods
B. Nonfat egg substitutes and egg whites
C. Nonfat egg substitutes, such as preformed fat-free soy burgers, textured soy nuggets, and wheat gluten
D. Fat-reduced tofu
E. Dried beans and peas
F. Breads, cereals, pasta, starches, rice, and grains
G. Vegetables and fruits

To Make Foods Taste Good: Use for Sauces, Gravies, and Seasonings:

A. Nonfat vegetable broth
B. Fat-free, meat-based broth
C. Herbs and seasonings
D. Nonfat butter-flavored sprinkles and liquids

Also use but in very small quantity: vegetable cooking spray

(Reprinted with permission from Reversal Eating Plan, © 1996 Gerry Krag, MA, RD, Grosse Pte. Park, MI.)

TABLE 26–22 EFFECTS OF SELECTED CHOLESTEROL-LOWERING MEDICATIONS ON NUTRITIONAL STATUS

DRUG CLASS/GENERIC NAME*	NUTRITIONAL IMPACT/COMMON SIDE EFFECTS
Bile Acid Sequestrants	
Cholestyramine	Decreases absorption of calcium, fat, fat-soluble vitamins, folate, MCT, and glucose In healthy patients, supplementation is not necessary. Side effects: nausea/vomiting, belching, dyspepsia, pain, constipation
Nicotinic Acid	Take with food or milk to decrease GI upset. Side effects: nausea/vomiting, peptic ulcer, cramps, diarrhea, flatulence
HMG-CoA Reductase Inhibitors	
Lovastatin	Take with meals. GI side effects: nausea, dyspepsia, abdominal pain, change in bowel function
Fibrates	
Gemfibrozil	Take ½ hour before meals. GI side effects: dyspepsia, abdominal pain, diarrhea, epigastric distress, constipation, flatulence
Probucol	Side effects: abdominal pain, changes in bowel function, nausea

(Data from National Cholesterol Education Program [NCEP]. Second Report of the Expert Panel on Detection, Evaluation, and Treatment of High Blood Cholesterol in Adults [Adult Treatment Panel II]. NIH Publication No. 93-3095. Bethesda, MD: National Institutes of Health. National Heart, Lung, and Blood Institute, 1993.)

MCT, medium-chain triglyceride; *GI*, gastrointestinal.

*Compiled from Larson ML, Illingworth R. Drug treatment of dyslipoproteinemia. Med Clin North Am 78:225, 1994; and Pronsky ZM. Powers and Moore's Food Medication Interactions, 8th ed. Pottstown, PA; Food Medication Interactions, 1993.

quicker than with bypass surgery. PTCA is being done more and more frequently every year; 419,000 angioplasty surgeries were performed in 1995. Usually, patients with no more than two occluded arteries are candidates for PTCA. The most common problem with PTCA is restenosis of the artery. Nutrition medical therapy would include the Step II Diet, or perhaps more aggressive diet therapy in motivated patients.

Coronary Bypass Surgery

In coronary artery bypass graft (CABG) surgery, a vein (or veins) from the leg or an artery from the chest is used to redirect blood flow around a diseased vessel. Candidates for CABG usually have more than two occluded arteries. CABG is the most frequently performed surgical procedure, with 573,000 operations performed in 1995. These surgeries improve survival time, relieve symptoms, and markedly improve the quality of life for patients with CHD. However, CABG does not cure atherosclerosis; the new grafts are also susceptible to atherogenesis. Consequently, restenosis is common. Risk factor modification, including, at a minimum, a Step II Diet and probably a more aggressive diet, are needed to stop progression.

In the postoperative period, post-CABG patients, like others undergoing major surgery, are in a catabolic state; adequate nutritional intake via oral routes is, therefore, essential. Patients with complications may be at risk for developing cardiac cachexia, which is often associated with heart failure (see Chapter 36). If oral intake is inadequate, either tube-feeding or total parenteral nutrition is indicated to meet increased energy, protein, and nutrient needs (see Chapter 22).

In some facilities, after either cardiac surgery or an acute myocardial infarction, the dietary regimen starts with a "cardiac liquid" diet (i.e., full liquids/no added salt with the omission of caffeine and restricted in cholesterol). For example, eggnog, high-fat cream soups, caffeinated soda pop, coffee, and chocolate are excluded. A salt substitute is generally used unless the patient has renal complications.

Once the patient is stabilized and ready to progress to a more complex diet, he or she may choose selections from the appropriate menu. The doctor will often recommend a weight loss regimen in addition to cardiac restrictions. Caffeine may still be limited, and the NCEP Step II Diet is generally ordered.

Because of high hospital costs, efforts to standardize patient care have led to the use of clinical pathways or care maps, which indicate the timing, activities, and services that are provided for the patient. In cardiac units, the clinical pathway designates when patient education will be offered by all disciplines. In many facilities, special group classes are offered to patients after their cardiac event or surgical procedure, to encourage them to make permanent life-style changes. Diet plays an important role in this process.

CASE STUDY

Lenora W. is a 60-year-old black woman with non–insulin-dependent diabetes mellitus, hypertension, and obesity. She lives with her husband of 40 years and maintains a moderate amount of activity. Because their children are grown, many meals are consumed at restaurants. In the past, she has been unsuccessful in maintaining any weight losses. Her family history for coronary heart disease (CHD) is positive. Her height is 5′4″ and her weight is 250 lb. Her medications are Diabinase, Diazide, Enalapril, and Premarin. At her last check-up, the laboratory tests revealed:

TG: 400 mg/dL	Total cholesterol: 253 mg/dL
HDL cholesterol: 37 mg/dL	LDL cholesterol: 185 mg/dL
Fasting blood glucose: 178 mg/dL	

1. What are Lenora's risk factors for CHD?
2. What type of diet would you recommend for Lenora? What additional information needs to be obtained before teaching her about a new eating plan?
3. What suggestions for restaurant eating will help Lenora adhere to the new eating plan?
4. What dietary factors could optimize Lenora's lipid profile?

TG, triglyceride; *HDL,* high-density lipoprotein; *LDL,* low-density lipoprotein

CITED REFERENCES

Abbey M, et al. Oxidation of low-density lipoproteins: Intraindividual variability and the effect of dietary linoleate supplementation. Am J Clin Nutr 57:391, 1993.

Albert C, et al. Fish consumption and risk of sudden cardiac death. JAMA 279:23, 1998.

American Heart Association. 1998 Heart and Stroke Statistical Update. Dallas, TX: American Heart Association, 1997.

Austin MA, Hokanson JE. Epidemiology of triglycerides, small dense-low-density lipoprotein, and lipoprotein (a) as risk factors for coronary heart disease. Med Clin North Am 78:99, 1994.

Bak AA, Grobbee DE. The effect on serum cholesterol levels of coffee brewed by filtering or boiling. N Engl J Med 321:1432, 1989.

Barr SL, et al. Reducing total dietary fat without reducing saturated fatty acids does not significantly lower total plasma cholesterol concentrations in normal males. Am J Clin Nutr 55:675, 1992.

Barrett-Connor E, et al. Why is diabetes mellitus a stronger risk factor for fatal ischemic heart disease in women than in men? JAMA 265:627, 1991.

Bass KM, et al. Plasma lipoprotein levels as predictors of cardiovascular death in women. Arch Intern Med 153:2209, 1993.

Bell L, et al. Cholesterol-lowering effects of calcium carbonate in patients with mild to moderate hypercholesterolemia. Arch Intern Med 152:2441, 1992.

Blankenhorn DH, et al. The influence of diet on the appearance of new lesions in human coronary arteries. JAMA 263:1646, 1990.

Blom HJ. Determinants of plasma homocysteine. Am J Clin Nutr 67:188, 1998.

Bousney C, et al. A quantitative assessment of plasma homocysteine as a risk factor for vascular disease. JAMA 274:1049, 1995.

Burrows ER, et al. Nutritional applications of a clinical low fat dietary intervention to public health change. J Nutr Ed 25:167, 1993.

Bush TL, et al. Cardiovascular mortality and noncontraceptive use of estrogen in women: Results from the Lipid Research Clinics Program Follow-Up Study. Circulation 75:1102, 1987.

Campos H, et al. Differences in low density lipoprotein subfractions and apolipoproteins in premenopausal and postmenopausal women. J Clin Endocrinol Metab 67:30, 1988.

Carmichael H, et al. Lower fat intake as a predictor of initial and sustained weight loss in obese subjects consuming an otherwise ad libitum diet. J Am Diet Assoc 98:35, 1998.
Castelli WP. Epidemiology of triglycerides: A view from Framingham. Am J Cardiol 70:3H, 1992.
Clarke R, et al. Hyperhomocysteinemia: An independent risk factor for vascular disease. N Engl J Med 3324:1149, 1991.
Coate D. Moderate drinking and coronary artery heart disease mortality: Evidence from NHANES I and NHANES I Follow-up. Am J Public Health 83:888, 1993.
Cobb MM, et al. Lovastatin efficacy in reducing low-density lipoprotein cholesterol levels on high- vs. low-fat diets. JAMA 265:997, 1992.
Connor WE. The decisive influence of diet on the progression and reversibility of coronary heart disease. Am J Clin Nutr 64:253, 1996.
Connor WE. Evaluation of publicly available scientific evidence regarding certain nutrient-disease relationships: Omega-3 fatty acids and heart disease. Washington, DC: Life Sciences Review Office, 1991.
Corti M, et al. Clarifying the direct relation between total cholesterol levels and death from coronary heart disease in older persons. Ann Intern Med 126:753, 1997.
Croft JB, et al. Waist-to-hip ratio in a biracial population: Measurement, implications, and cautions for using guidelines to define high risk for cardiovascular disease. J Am Diet Assoc 95:60, 1995.
Daviglus M, et al. Fish consumption and the 30-year risk of fatal myocardial infarction. N Engl J Med 336:1046, 1997.
Denke MA, et al. Excess body weight. An under-recognized contributor to dyslipidemia in white American women. Arch Intern Med 154:401, 1994.
Emken EA. Physiochemical properties, intake, and metabolism of trans fatty acids. Am J Clin Nutr 62(suppl):659S, 1995.
Folsom AR, et al. Body fat distribution and 5-year risk of death in older women. JAMA 269:483, 1993.
Food and Nutrition Science Alliance: Statement on trans fatty acids. J Am Diet Assoc 94:1098, 1994.
Fried RE, et al. The effect of filtered-coffee consumption on plasma lipid levels. JAMA 267:811, 1992.
Fuster V, et al. Task Force 1. Pathogenesis of coronary disease: The biologic role of risk factors. J Am Coll Cardiol 27:964, 1996.
Gaziano JM, et al. Moderate alcohol intake, increased levels of high-density lipoprotein and its subfractions and decreased risk of myocardial infarction. N Engl J Med 329:1829, 1993.
Ginsberg HN. Lipoprotein metabolism and its relationship to atherosclerosis. Med Clin North Am 78:1, 1994.
Ginsberg HN, et al. Reduction of plasma cholesterol levels in normal men on an American Heart Association Step I Diet or a Step I Diet with added monounsaturated fat. N Engl J Med 322:574, 1990.
Giovino GA, et al. Surveillance for selected tobacco-use behaviors—United States, 1900–1994. MMWR 43:1, 1994.
Glantz SA, Parmley WW. Passive smoking and heart disease. Mechanisms and risk. JAMA 273:1047, 1995.
Glore SR, et al. Soluble fiber and serum lipids: A literature review. J Am Diet Assoc 94:425, 1994.
Graham I, et al. The European concerted action project. JAMA 277:1775, 1997.
Grande F, et al. Diets of different fatty acid composition producing identical serum cholesterol levels in man. Am J Clin Nutr 25:53, 1972.
Grundy SM. Influence of stearic acid on cholesterol metabolism relative to other long-chain fatty acids. Am J Clin Nutr 60(suppl):986S, 1994.
Harris WS. N-3 fatty acids and serum lipoproteins: Human studies. Am J Clin Nutr 65(suppl):1645S, 1997.
Hausmann D, et al. Angiographically silent atherosclerosis detected by intravascular ultrasound in patients with familial hypercholesterolemia and familial combined hyperlipidemia: Correlation with high density lipoprotein. J Am Coll Cardiol 27:1562, 1996.
Health, United States, 1990. National Center for Health Statistics. Hyattsville, MD: Public Health Service, 1991.
Herbert V. The antioxidant supplement myth. Am J Clin Nutr 60:157, 1994a.
Herbert V. Antioxidants, pro-oxidants, and their effects. JAMA 272:1659, 1994b.
Howard G, et al. Cigarette smoking and progression of atherosclerosis. JAMA 279:119, 1998.
Hunink MG, et al. The recent decline in mortality from coronary heart disease, 1980–1990: The effect of secular trends in risk factors and treatment. JAMA 277:535, 1997.
Huttunen JK, et al. The Helsinki Heart Study: Central findings and clinical implications. Ann Intern Med 23:155, 1991.
Jha P, et al. The antioxidant vitamins and cardiovascular disease. A critical review of epidemiologic and clinical trial data. Ann Intern Med 23:860, 1995.
Jialal I, Grundy S. Effect of combined supplementation with α-tocopherol, ascorbate, and β-carotene on low-density lipoprotein oxidation. Circulation 88:2780, 1993.
Johnson CL, et al. Declining serum total cholesterol levels among U.S. adults. The National Health and Nutrition Examination Surveys. JAMA 269:3002, 1993.
Judd JT, et al. Dietary trans fatty acids: Effects on plasma lipids and lipoproteins of healthy men and women. Am J Clin Nutr 59:861, 1994.
Kannel WB. The Framingham experience. In: Marmot M, Elliott P (eds.). Coronary Heart Disease Epidemiology. Oxford: Oxford University Press, 1992.
Katan MB, et al. Effects of fats and fatty acids on blood lipids in humans: An overview. Am J Clin Nutr 60(suppl):1017s, 1994a.
Katan MB. European researcher calls for reconsideration of trans fatty acids [Letter to editor]. J Am Diet Assoc 94:1097, 1994b.
Kinosian B, et al. Cholesterol and coronary heart disease: Predicting risk by levels and ratios. Ann Intern Med 121:641, 1994.
Klag MJ, et al. Serum cholesterol in young men and subsequent cardiovascular disease. N Engl J Med 328:313, 1993.
Knapp HR. Dietary fatty acids in human thrombosis and hemostasis. Am J Clin Nutr 65(suppl):1687s, 1997.
Kris-Etherton PM, et al. The effect of diet on plasma lipids, lipoproteins, and coronary heart disease. J Am Diet Assoc 88:1373, 1988.
Kris-Etherton PM, Krummel DA. Role of nutrition in the prevention and treatment of coronary heart disease in women. J Am Diet Assoc 93:987, 1993.
Kris-Etherton PM, Yu S. Individual fatty acid effects on plasma lipids and lipoproteins: Human studies. Am J Clin Nutr 65(suppl):1628S, 1997.
Kritchevsky S, et al. Provitamin A carotenoid intake and carotid artery plaques: The Atherosclerosis Risk in Communities Study. Am J Clin Nutr 68:726, 1998.
Krummel DA. Cardiovascular disease. In: Krummel DA, Kris-Etherton PM (eds.). Nutrition and Women's Health, Gaithersburg, MD: Aspen Publishers, 1996.
Kuczmarski RJ, et al. Increasing prevalence of overweight among U.S. adults. The National Health and Nutrition Examination Surveys, 1960 to 1991. JAMA 272:205, 1994.
Kwiterovich PO. The effect of dietary fat, antioxidants, and pro-oxidants on blood lipids, lipoproteins, and atherosclerosis. J Am Diet Assoc 97 (suppl):S31, 1997.
Larsen ML, Illingworth R. Drug treatment of dyslipoproteinemia. Med Clin North Am 78:255, 1994.
Lerner DJ, Kannel WB. Patterns of coronary heart disease morbidity and mortality in the sexes: A 26-year follow-up of the Framingham population. Am Heart J 111:383, 1986.
Lewis CJ, et al. Healthy People 2000. Report on the 1994 Nutrition Progress Review. Nutr Today 29:6, 1994.
Liao Y, et al. Sex differences in the impact of coexistent diabetes on survival in patients with coronary heart disease. Diabetes Care 16:708, 1993.
Mandel C, et al. Dietary intake and plasma concentrations of vitamin E, vitamin C, and beta-carotene in patients with coronary artery disease. J Am Diet Assoc 97:655, 1997.
Manson JE, et al. Antioxidants and cardiovascular disease: A review. J Am Coll Nutr 12:426, 1993.
Manson JE, et al. A prospective study of obesity and risk of coronary heart disease in women. N Engl J Med 322:882, 1990.
McBride PE. The health consequences of smoking. Cardiovascular diseases. Med Clin North Am 76:333, 1992.
McDowell MA, et al. Energy and macronutrient intakes of persons ages 2 months and over in the United States: Third National Health and Nutrition Examination Survey, Phase 1, 1988–1991. Advance data from Vital and Health Statistics; No. 225. Hyattsville, MD: National Center for Health Statistics, 1994.
Meydani S, et al. Vitamin E supplementation and in vivo immune response in healthy elderly subjects: A randomized, controlled trial. JAMA 277:1380, 1997.
Murphy SM, et al. Demographic and economic factors associated with dietary quality for adults in the 1987–88 Nationwide Food Consumption Survey. J Am Diet Assoc 92:1352, 1992.
National Cholesterol Education Program (NCEP). Report of the Expert Panel on Blood Cholesterol in Children and Adolescents. NHLBI, USDHHS. National Institute of Health (NIH) Publication. Bethesda, MD: NIH 1991.
National Cholesterol Education Program (NCEP). Report of the Expert Panel on Population Strategies from Blood Cholesterol Reduction. Bethesda, MD: U.S. Department of Health & Human Services, NIH Publication No. 90-3046, 1990.
National Cholesterol Education Program (NCEP). Second Report of the Expert Panel on Detection, Evaluation, and Treatment of High Blood Cholesterol in Adults (ATP-11). NIH Publication No. 93–3095. Bethesda, MD: National Institute of Health, 1993.
National Heart, Lung, and Blood Institute. Report of the Expert Panel on Blood Cholesterol Levels in Children and Adolescents. U.S. Dept. of Health and Human Services, Publication No. 91-2732. September, 1991.
National Institutes of Health (NIH). NHLBI Obesity Education Initiative Expert Panel on the Identification, Evaluation, and Treatment of Overweight and Obesity in Adults. The Evidence Report, 1998.

NIH Consensus Conference: Triglyceride, high-density lipoprotein, and coronary heart disease. JAMA 269:505, 1993.
Nydahl MC, et al. Lipid-lowering diets enriched with monounsaturated or polyunsaturated fatty acids but low in saturated fatty acids have similar effects on serum lipid concentrations in hyperlipidemic patients. Am J Clin Nutr 59:115, 1994.
Nygard O, et al. Major lifestyle determinants of plasma total homocysteine distribution: The Hordland Homocysteine Study. Am J Clin Nutr 67:263, 1998.
Nygard O, et al. Plasma homocysteine levels and mortality in patients with coronary artery disease. N Engl J Med 337:230, 1997.
Ornish D, Brown SE. Treatment of screening for hyperlipidemia [Letter to editor]. N Engl J Med 329:1124, 1993.
Pasternak RC, et al. Task Force 3. Spectrum of risk factors for coronary heart disease. J Am Coll Cardiol 27:978, 1996.
Pate R, et al. Physical activity and public health: A recommendation from the Centers for Disease Control and Prevention with the American College of Medicine. JAMA 273:402, 1995.
Patsch JR. Triglyceride-rich lipoproteins and atherosclerosis. Atherosclerosis 110:S23, 1994.
Physical Activity and Health: A Report of the Surgeon General, United States Department of Health and Human Services. Bethesda, MD: DHHS, 1996.
Pouliot M-C, et al. Waist circumference and abdominal sagittal diameter: Best simple anthropometric indexes of abdominal visceral adipose tissue accumulation and related cardiovascular risk in men and women. Am J Cardiol 73:460, 1994.
Powell KE, et al. Physical activity and the incidence of coronary heart disease. Ann Rev Public Health 8:243, 1987.
Public Health Service. Healthy People 2000: National health promotion and disease prevention objectives. Full report with commentary. USDHHS Publication No. (PHS) 91-50212. Washington, DC: U.S. Department of Health and Human Services, 1991.
Puccio EM, et al. Clustering of atherogenic behaviors in coffee drinkers. Am J Public Health 80:1310, 1990.
Rifici VA, Khachadurian AK. The inhibition of low-density lipoprotein oxidation by 17-b estradiol. Metabolism 41:1110, 1992.
Schaefer EJ. Familial lipoprotein disorders and premature coronary artery disease. Med Clin North Am 78:21, 1994a.
Schaefer EJ, et al. Lipoprotein (a) levels and risk of coronary heart disease in men. The Lipid Research Clinics Coronary Primary Prevention Trial. JAMA 271:999, 1994b.
Schuler G, et al. Regular physical exercise and low-fat diet. Effects of progression on coronary artery disease. Circulation 86:1, 1992.
Sempos CT, et al. Prevalence of high blood cholesterol among U.S. adults. An update based on guidelines from the second report of the National Cholesterol Education Program Adult Treatment Panel. JAMA 269: 3009, 1993.
Sikand G, et al. Medical nutrition therapy lowers serum cholesterol and saves medication costs in men with hypercholesterolemia. J Am Diet Assoc 98:889, 1998.
Steenland K. Passive smoking and the risk of heart disease. JAMA 267:94, 1992.
Steinberg D. Antioxidant vitamins and coronary heart disease. N Engl J Med 328:1487, 1993a.
Steinberg D. Letter to the Editor. N Engl J Med 329:1426, 1993b.
van Beresteijn ECH, et al. Perimenopausal increase in serum cholesterol: A 10-year longitudinal study. Am J Epidemiol 137:383, 1993.
Watts GF, et al. Dietary fatty acids and progression of coronary artery disease in men. Am J Clin Nutr 64:202, 1996.
Welch G, Loscalzo J. Homocysteine and atherosclerosis. N Engl J Med 338:1042, 1998.
Willett WC, et al. Intake of trans fatty acids and risk of coronary heart disease among women. Lancet 341:581, 1993.
Wilson P, et al. Cumulative effects of high cholesterol levels, high blood pressure, and cigarette smoking on carotid stenosis. N Engl J Med 337:516, 1997.
Witzum JL, et al. Studies on the ability of dietary supplementation with β-carotene to protect low-density lipoprotein from oxidative modification. Ann NY Acad Sci 691:200, 1993.
Woo KS, et al. Hyperhomocysteinemia is a risk factor for arterial endothelial dysfunction in humans. Circulation 96:2542, 1997.
Woollett LA, et al. Saturated and unsaturated fatty acids independently regulate low density lipoprotein receptor activity and production rate. J Lipid Res 33:77, 1992.

ADDITIONAL REFERENCES

Adler A, Holub B. Effect of garlic and fish-oil supplementation on serum lipid and lipoprotein concentrations in hypercholesterolemic men. Am J Clin Nutr 65:445, 1997.
Darling G, et al. Estrogen and progestin compared with simvastatin for hypercholesterolemia in postmenopausal women. N Engl J Med 337: 595, 1997.
Grimsgaard S, et al. Highly purified eicosapentaenoic acid and docosahexaenoic acid in humans have similar triacylglycerol-lowering effects but divergent effects on serum fatty acids. Am J Clin Nutr 66:649, 1997.
Howell W, et al. Plasma lipid and lipoprotein responses to dietary fat and cholesterol: A meta-analysis. Am J Clin Nutr 65:1747, 1997.
Ingster L, Feinleib M. Could salicylates in food have contributed to the decline in cardiovascular disease mortality? Am J Public Health 87:1554, 1997.
Jeppesen J, et al. Effects of low-fat, high-carbohydrate diets on risk factors for ischemic heart disease in postmenopausal women. Am J Clin Nutr 65:1027, 1997.
Markus R, et al. Influence of lifestyle modification on atherosclerotic progression determined by ultrasonographic change in the common carotid intima-media thickness. Am J Clin Nutr 65:1000, 1997.
Mayer-Davis E, et al. Vitamin C intake and cardiovascular disease risk factors in persons with non–insulin-dependent diabetes mellitus: From the Insulin Resistance Atherosclerosis Study and the San Luis Valley Diabetes Study. Prevent Med 26:277, 1997.
Pieper R, et al. Trends in cholesterol knowledge and screening and hypercholesterolemia awareness and treatment, 1980–1992. Arch Intern Med 157:232, 1997.
Plotnick G, et al. Effect of antioxidant vitamins on the transient impairment of endothelium-dependent brachial artery vasoactivity following a single high-fat meal. JAMA 278:1682, 1997.
Retzlaff B, et al. Iron and zinc status of women and men who followed cholesterol-lowering diets. J Am Diet Assoc 98:149, 1998.
Rexrode K, et al. A prospective study of body mass index, weight change, and risk of stroke in women. JAMA 277:1539, 1997.
Rimm E, et al. Folate and vitamin B-6 from diet and supplements in relation to risk of coronary heart disease among women. JAMA 279:359, 1998.
Romon M, et al. Circadian variation of postprandial lipemia. Am J Clin Nutr 65:934, 1997.
Schrott H, et al. Adherence to National Cholesterol Education Program Treatment goals in postmenopausal women with heart disease. JAMA 277:1281, 1997.

CHAPTER 27

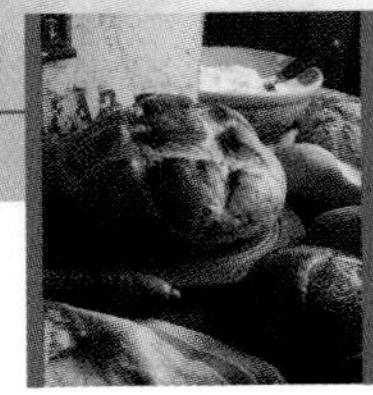

Nutrition in Hypertension

DEBRA KRUMMEL, PH D, RD

CHAPTER OUTLINE

- Definition and Classification
- Prevalence
- Morbidity and Mortality
- Pathophysiology
- Primary Prevention
- Management

Key Terms

DASH DIET (Dietary Approaches to Stop Hypertension)—eating plan that is high in fruits, vegetables, and low-fat dairy foods; shown to reduce hypertension

DIASTOLIC BLOOD PRESSURE (DBP)—blood pressure during the relaxation phase of the cardiac cycle; 80 mm Hg is optimal

ESSENTIAL HYPERTENSION—hypertension of unknown etiology; also known as primary hypertension

NORMOTENSIVE—relating to a normal blood pressure, which is a systolic blood pressure of 130 mm Hg and a diastolic blood pressure of 85 mm Hg; read as a blood pressure of 130/85

HYPERTENSION—persistently high arterial blood pressure, defined as systolic blood pressure above 140 mm Hg and/or diastolic blood pressure above 90 mm Hg

SALT-RESISTANT HYPERTENSION—blood pressure that is not affected by salt intake

SALT-SENSITIVE HYPERTENSION—blood pressure that rises or falls with corresponding changes in salt intake

SECONDARY HYPERTENSION—hypertension secondary to another disease

SYSTOLIC BLOOD PRESSURE (SBP)—blood pressure during the contraction phase of the cardiac cycle; 120 mm Hg is optimal

Hypertension is the most common public health problem in developed countries. Untreated hypertension leads to many degenerative diseases including congestive heart failure, end-stage renal disease, and peripheral vascular disease. It is often called a silent killer because people with hypertension can be asymptomatic for years and then have a fatal stroke or heart attack. Although no cure is available, prevention and management decrease the incidence of hypertension and disease sequelae. Some of the decline in cardiovascular disease (CVD) mortality over the last two decades has been attributed to the increased detection and control of hypertension. The emphasis on life-style modifications has given diet a prominent role for both the primary prevention and management of hypertension.

Ninety to 95% of those with high blood pressure have **essential** or **primary hypertension,** for which the cause cannot be determined. Although the cause is probably multifactorial, it is now known that renal dysfunction accompanies the development of hypertension (Cowley and Roman, 1996). In a small group, hypertension is caused by another disease, usually endocrine, and thus is referred to as **secondary hypertension.** Depending on the extent of the underlying disease, secondary hypertension can be cured.

DEFINITION AND CLASSIFICATION

A general definition of hypertension is a **systolic blood pressure (SBP)** of 140 mm Hg or higher or a **diastolic blood pressure (DBP)** of 90 mm Hg or higher or both. In the Sixth Report of the Joint National Committee on Detection, Evaluation, and Treatment of High Blood Pressure (Joint National Committee, 1997), hypertension is classified in stages based on the risk of developing CVD (Table 27–1). A high-normal category is included because these people are at high risk of developing essential hypertension and CVD. Stage 1 (140 to 159/90 to 99 mm Hg) is the most prevalent level seen in adults. In other words, this is the group most likely to have a myocardial infarction or stroke. The defining point for hypertension is arbitrary because any

TABLE 27–1 CLASSIFICATION OF BLOOD PRESSURE FOR ADULTS AGED 18 YEARS AND OLDER*

	BLOOD PRESSURE, mm Hg		
CATEGORY	Systolic		Diastolic
Optimal†	<120	and	<80
Normal	<130	and	<85
High-normal	130–139	or	85–89
Hypertension‡			
Stage 1	140–159	or	90–99
Stage 2	160–179	or	100–109
Stage 3	≥180	or	N≥110

(From the Joint National Committee on Prevention, Detection, Evaluation, and Treatment of High Blood Pressure. Sixth Report (NNCVI). Arch Intern Med 157:2413, 1997.)

*Not taking antihypertensive drugs and not acutely ill. When systolic and diastolic blood pressures fall into different categories, the higher category should be selected to classify the individual's blood pressure status. For example, 160/92 mm Hg should be classified as stage 2 hypertension, and 174/120 mm Hg should be classified as stage 3 hypertension. Isolated systolic hypertension is defined as systolic blood pressure 140 mm Hg or greater and diastolic blood pressure less than 90 mm Hg and staged appropriately (eg, 170/82 mm Hg is defined as stage 2 isolated systolic hypertension). In addition to classifying stages of hypertension on the basis of average blood pressure levels, clinicians should specify presence or absence of target organ disease and additional risk factors. This specificity is important for risk classification and treatment.

†Optimal blood pressure with respect to cardiovascular risk is less than 120/80 mm Hg. However, unusually low readings should be evaluated for clinical significance.

‡Based on the average of two or more readings taken at each of two or more visits after an initial screening.

level of elevated blood pressure is associated with increased incidence of CVD and renal disease. Therefore, normalization of blood pressure is important for all stages of hypertension.

PREVALENCE

Approximately 24% or 43 million adult, civilian, noninstitutionalized Americans have hypertension (Burt et al., 1995). Slightly more men (26%) than women (22%) have hypertension. Despite improvements in detection, there has not been any decline in the prevalence of hypertension (Kannel, 1996). As many as 7 million children also have high blood pressure (American Heart Association, 1997). In children, hypertension is defined as blood pressure readings greater than the 95th percentile for a given height on at least three separate occasions (National Heart, Lung, and Blood Institute, 1997).

African Americans have a higher prevalence of hypertension (30% of men; 27% of women) than non-Hispanic whites (26% of men; 24% of women) or Mexican Americans (15% of men; 14% of women) (Burt et al., 1995). Because the prevalence of hypertension rises with increasing age, over half the adult population older than 60 years has hypertension (Table 27–2). For every age-race group, hypertension is seen more often in men until the age of 59. Hypertension is more prevalent in women after age 60 for non-Hispanic blacks and Mexican Americans and age 70 for non-Hispanic whites (Burt et al., 1995). The age-related risk for high blood pressure is a function of life-style variables, rather than just aging, and is believed to be preventable (Stamler et al., 1993).

TABLE 27–2 PREVALENCE OF HYPERTENSION BY AGE*†

AGE	% HYPERTENSIVE
18–29	4
30–39	11
40–49	21
50–59	44
60–69	54
70–79	64
80+	65

*Source: Centers for Disease Control and Prevention, National Center for Health Statistics, National Health and Nutrition Examination Survey III (1989–91). National High Blood Pressure Education Program Working Group Report on Primary Prevention of Hypertension. Arch Intern Med 153:186, 1993.

†Hypertension is defined as three blood pressure measurements averaging 140/90 mm Hg or more on a single occasion in a patient taking antihypertensive medication.

Population awareness of hypertension, treatment, and control improved over the last three decades leveled off since 1993 (Joint National Committee, 1997). In the third National Health and Nutrition Examination Survey (NHANES III), 69% of hypertensives were aware, 53% treated, and 24% controlled (Burt et al., 1995). Women with hypertension were more likely to be aware, treated, and controlled than men.

MORBIDITY AND MORTALITY

Although hypertensive patients are often asymptomatic, hypertension is not a benign disease. Cardiac, cerebrovascular, and renal systems are affected by chronically elevated blood pressure (Table 27–3). Atherosclerosis, the underlying cause of much CVD, is a direct result of hypertension-in-

TABLE 27–3 MANIFESTATIONS OF TARGET ORGAN DISEASE FROM HYPERTENSION

ORGAN SYSTEM	MANIFESTATIONS
Cardiac	Clinical, electrocardiographic, or radiologic evidence of coronary artery disease; left ventricular hypertrophy; left ventricular function or cardiac failure
Cerebrovascular	Transient ischemic attack or stroke
Peripheral	Absence of one or more pulses in extremities (except for dorsalis pedis) with or without intermittent claudication; aneurysm
Renal	Serum creatinine > 130 µmol/L (1.5 mg/dL); proteinuria (1 + or greater); microalbuminuria
Retinopathy	Hemorrhages or exudates, with or without papilledema

(From the Joint National Committee on Detection, Evaluation, and Treatment of High Blood Pressure. Fifth report (JNC V). Arch Intern Med 153:154, 1993.)

TABLE 27–4 FACTORS INDICATING POOR PROGNOSIS IN HYPERTENSION

Black race
Youth
Male
Persistent diastolic pressure > 115 mm Hg
Smoking
Diabetes mellitus
Hypercholesterolemia
Obesity
Excessive alcohol intake
Evidence of target organ disease

(From Williams GH. Hypertensive vascular disease. In: Issilbacher K, et al. (eds.). Harrison's principles of internal medicine, 13th ed. New York: McGraw-Hill, 1994.)

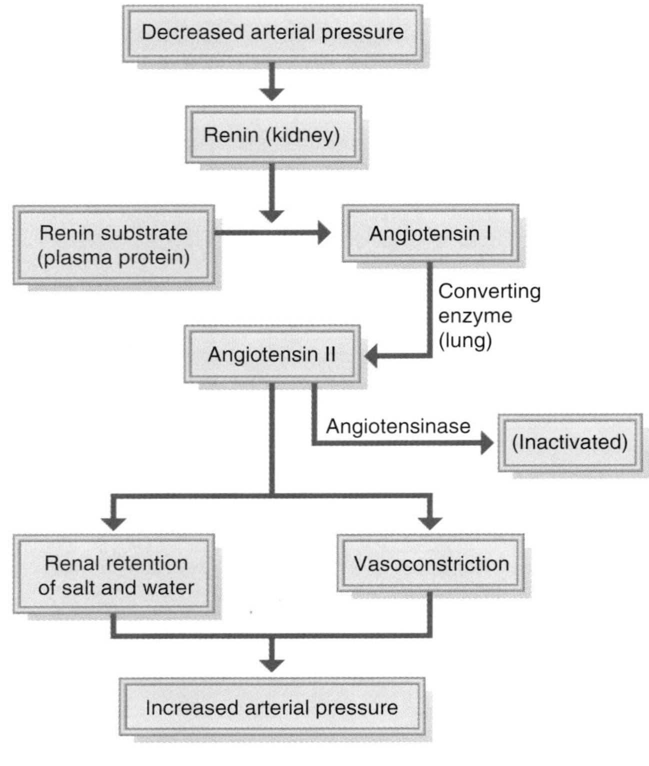

FIGURE 27–1 Renin–angiotensin cascade.

duced end-organ damage (Schwartz et al., 1994). In middle-aged men, a 20 mm Hg increase in SBP results in 60% higher mortality from CVD (Poulter and Sever, 1992). Consequently, 50% of patients with hypertension die from coronary heart disease or congestive heart failure, 33% from stroke, and 10% to 15% from renal failure (Kaplan, 1992). Stroke and myocardial infarction also are major contributors to morbidity; between 500,000 and a million people have nonfatal events each year. The factors associated with a poor prognosis in hypertension are shown in Table 27–4.

PATHOPHYSIOLOGY

Blood pressure is a function of cardiac output multiplied by the peripheral resistance (the resistance in the blood vessels to the flow of blood). The diameter of the blood vessel markedly affects blood flow. When the diameter is decreased (as in atherosclerosis), resistance and blood pressure increase. Conversely, when the diameter is increased (as with vasodilator drug therapy), resistance decreases and blood pressure is lowered.

Many systems maintain homeostatic control of blood pressure. The major regulators are the sympathetic nervous system (for short-term control) and the kidney (for long-term control). In response to a fall in blood pressure, the sympathetic nervous system secretes *norepinephrine,* a vasoconstrictor, which acts on small arteries and arterioles to increase peripheral resistance and raise blood pressure. The kidney regulates blood pressure by controlling the extracellular fluid volume and secreting renin, which activates the renin–angiotensin system (Fig. 27–1). When the regulatory mechanisms falter, hypertension develops. There are probably many neurohormonal and intrarenal causes of abnormal blood pressure.

In most cases of hypertension, peripheral resistance increases. This resistance forces the left ventricle of the heart to increase effort in pumping blood through the system. With time, left ventricular hypertrophy and eventually congestive heart failure can develop (see Chapter 36).

PRIMARY PREVENTION

Primary prevention of hypertension could have a major impact on the population for improving quality of life and costs associated with medical management of hypertension and its complications. A population strategy would be to reduce blood pressure in those with higher than optimal levels (above 120/80), but below the cut points for diagnosis. A downward shift of 3 mm Hg in SBP would decrease the mortality from stroke by 8% and from CHD by 5% (Joint National Committee, 1993). Individuals at highest risk (Table 27–5) should be strongly encouraged to adopt healthier life-styles. Several life-style changes are essential for both prevention and management of hypertension (Table 27–6).

Diet-Related Factors

Changing four modifiable factors has documented efficacy in the primary prevention and control of hypertension. These are overweight, high salt intake, alcohol consumption, and physical inactivity (National High Blood Pressure Education Program, 1993). A 5-year intervention trial in **normotensive** men and women demonstrated that life-style changes could lessen the incidence of hypertension.

TABLE 27–5 RISK FACTORS FOR DEVELOPING HYPERTENSION

High-normal blood pressure
Family history of hypertension
African American ancestry
Overweight
Excessive salt consumption
Physical inactivity
Alcohol consumption

(Adapted from National High Blood Pressure Education Program Working Group report on primary prevention of hypertension. Arch Intern Med 153:186, 1993. Copyright 1993, American Medical Association. Reprinted with permission.)

Intervention goals were to (1) lose 4.5 kg or 5% of body weight (whichever was greater), (2) follow an American Heart Association fat-modified diet, (3) reduce sodium intake to 1800 mg/day or less, (4) limit alcohol to no more than two drinks per day, and (5) increase physical activity to 30 minutes three times per week. The incidence of hypertension was 8% in the intervention group and 19% in the control group (Stamler et al., 1989).

More recently, the Trials of Hypertension Prevention (TOHP) (Trials, 1997) and DASH studies (Appel et al., 1997) showed that nutritional interventions prevented hypertension or lowered blood pressure in individuals with high-normal pressures. In the TOHP, weight loss (goal 4.5 kg loss) alone or in combination with sodium restriction (goal 80 mmol/day) lowered the incidence of hypertension. However, behavior changes were not sustained over time, thus diminishing the positive effects on blood pressure. The **DASH (Dietary Approaches to Stop Hypertension)** study showed that a diet high in fruits, vegetables, and nonfat dairy foods and low in saturated fat and total fat decreased systolic blood pressure an average of 6 to 11 mm Hg (Appel et al., 1997). The DASH diet (Tables 27–7 and 27–8) is used both for preventing and controlling high blood pressure. Because this diet contains substantially more fruits and vegetables (8–10 servings) than the amount the average American consumes, or what is recommended by several national organizations, patient adherence could be challenging outside the clinical setting. Other interventions with limited or unproven efficacy include stress management; potassium, calcium, magnesium, or fish oil supplementation; and changes in percentages of macronutrients.

TABLE 27–6 LIFE-STYLE MODIFICATIONS FOR HYPERTENSION PREVENTION AND MANAGEMENT

Lose weight if overweight
Limit alcohol intake to no more than 1 oz (30 mL) of ethanol (e.g., 24 oz [720 mL] of beer, 10 oz [300 mL] of wine, or 2 oz [60 mL] of 100-proof whiskey) per day or 0.5 oz (15 mL) of ethanol per day for women and lighter weight people
Increase aerobic physical activity (30–45 min most days of the week)
Reduce sodium intake to no more than 100 mmol/day (2.4 g sodium or 6 g sodium chloride)
Maintain adequate intake of dietary potassium (approximately 90 mmol/day)
Maintain adequate intake of dietary calcium and magnesium for general health
Stop smoking and reduce intake of dietary saturated fat and cholesterol for overall cardiovascular health

(From the Joint National Committee on Prevention, Detection, Evaluation, and Treatment of High Blood Pressure. Sixth report (JNC VI). Arch Intern Med 157:2413, 1997.)

Overweight

Body weight is a determinant of blood pressure in most ethnic groups at all ages. A *body mass index (BMI)* of greater than 27 is correlated with increased blood pressure (Joint National Committee, 1997). Excess abdominal fat (waist circumference > 34 inches in women and 39 inches in men) is associated with increased risk for hypertension and other CVD risk factors (Pouliot et al., 1994). The risk of developing elevated blood pressure is two to six times higher in overweight than in normal-weight individuals (National High Blood Pressure Education Program, 1993). Twenty to 30% of the hypertension seen in this country is attributable to the high prevalence of overweight.

Weight gain during adult life is responsible for much of the rise in blood pressure seen with aging. In the Framingham study, an increase in relative weight of 10% was predictive of a rise in blood pressure of 7 mm Hg.

Some of the physiologic changes proposed to explain the relationship between overweight and blood pressure are insulin resistance and hyperinsulinemia (see Chapter 12), activation of the sympathetic nervous and renin–angiotensin systems, and physical changes in the kidney (Hall, 1994). Increased energy intake is also associated with elevated plasma insulin, which is a potent natriuretic factor causing increased renal sodium reabsorption and consequent blood pressure elevation.

As evidenced by the increasing prevalence of overweight in this country, weight management is a major effort for many individuals, especially women. Interventions to prevent weight gain should target groups before they reach midlife. In African American women, adolescence is the critical period for intervention (Melnyk and Weinstein, 1994). BMI is recommended as a screening tool for all adolescents (Himes and Dietz, 1994). A BMI above 30 is the cut-off point for obesity, and referral for follow-up is warranted. With a large percentage of the population obese and hypertensive, better strategies are needed to prevent excess weight gain and improve compliance with treatment (St. Jeor et al., 1993) (see Chapter 23).

Early identification of children as potential hypertensives has been recommended and a flow chart for identifying hypertensive children is shown in Figure 27–2 (Strong et al., 1992). Body fatness

TABLE 27–7 THE DASH DIET

FOOD GROUP	DAILY SERVINGS	ONE SERVING EQUALS:	EXAMPLES AND NOTES	SIGNIFICANCE OF EACH FOOD GROUP TO THE DASH DIET PATTERN
Grains and grain products	7–8	1 slice bread ½ C dry cereal ½ C cooked rice, pasta, or cereal	Whole-wheat breads, English muffin, pita bread, bagel, cereals, grits, oatmeal	Major sources of energy and fiber
Vegetables	4–5	1 C raw leafy vegetable ½ C cooked vegetable 6 oz vegetable juice	Tomatoes, potatoes, carrots, peas, squash, broccoli, turnip greens, collards, kale, spinach, artichokes, beans, sweet potatoes	Rich sources of potassium, magnesium, and fiber
Fruits	4–5	6 oz fruit juice 1 medium fruit ¼ C dried fruit ½ C fresh, frozen, or canned fruit	Apricots, bananas, dates, grapes, oranges, orange juice, grapefruit, grapefruit juice, mangoes, melons, peaches, pineapples, prunes, raisins, strawberries, tangerines	Important sources of potassium, magnesium, and fiber
Low-fat or nonfat dairy foods	2–3	8 oz milk 1 C yogurt 1.5 oz cheese	Skim or 1% milk, skim or low-fat buttermilk, nonfat or low-fat yogurt, part-skim mozzarella cheese, nonfat cheese	Major sources of calcium and protein
Meats, poultry, fish	2 or less	3 oz cooked meats, poultry, or fish	Select only lean; trim away visible fats; broil, roast, or boil, instead of frying; remove skin from poultry	Rich sources of protein and magnesium
Nuts	1–2	1.5 oz or 1/3 C or 2 Tbsp seeds ½ C cooked legumes	Almonds, filberts, mixed nuts, peanuts, walnuts, sunflower seeds, kidney beans, lentils	Rich sources of energy, magnesium, potassium, protein, and fiber

(Appel LJ, et al. A clinical trial of the effects of dietary patterns on blood pressure. N Engl J Med 336:1117, 1997.)

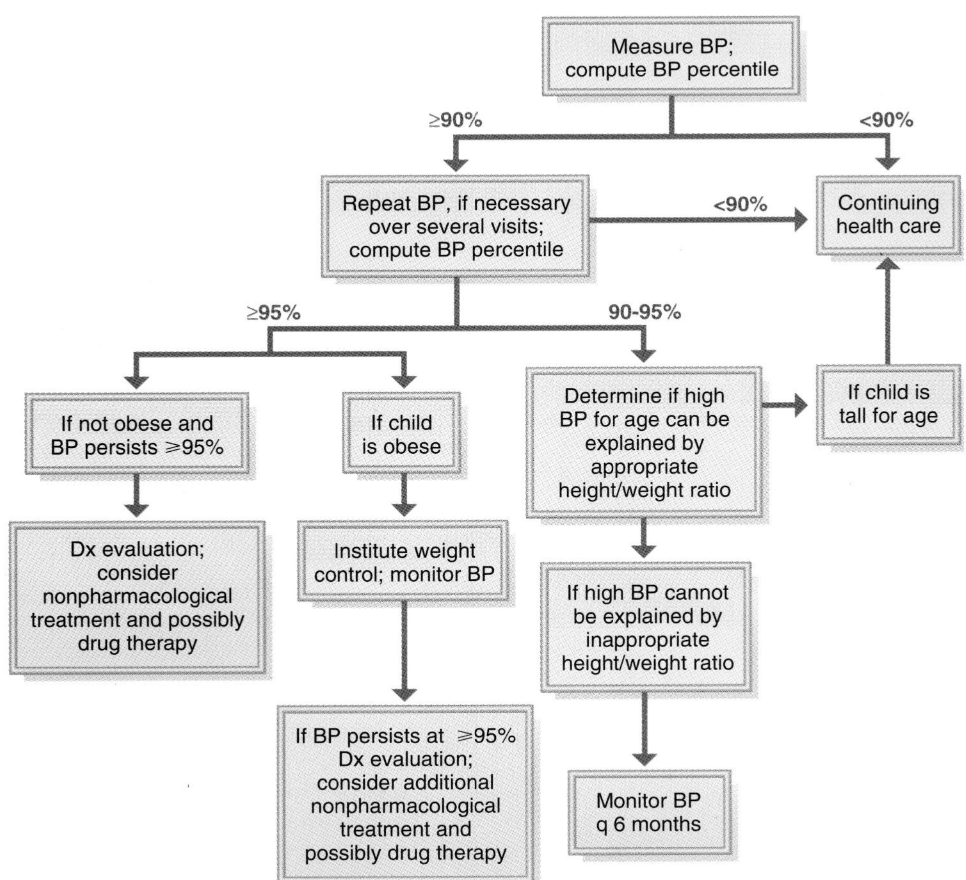

FIGURE 27–2 Flow chart for identifying children with high blood pressure (BP).

TABLE 27–8 SAMPLE MENU FOR THE DASH DIET

FOOD	AMOUNT	SERVINGS PROVIDED
Breakfast		
orange juice	6 oz	1 fruit
1% low-fat milk	8 oz (1 C)	1 dairy
corn flakes (with 1 tsp sugar)	1 C	2 grains
banana	1 medium	1 fruit
whole-wheat bread (with 1 Tbsp jelly)	1 slice	1 grain
soft margarine	1 tsp	1 fat
Lunch		
chicken salad	¾ C	1 poultry
pita bread	½ slice, large	1 grain
raw vegetable medley:		
carrot & celery sticks	3–4 sticks each	1 vegetable
radishes	2	
loose-leaf lettuce	2 leaves	
part-skim mozzarella cheese	1.5 slice (1.5 oz)	1 dairy
1% low-fat milk	8 oz	1 dairy
fruit cocktail in light syrup	½ C	1 fruit
Dinner		
herbed baked cod	3 oz	1 fish
scallion rice	1 C	2 grains
steamed broccoli	½ C	1 vegetable
stewed tomatoes	½ C	1 vegetable
spinach salad:		
raw spinach	½ C	1 vegetable
cherry tomatoes	2	
cucumber	2 slices	
light Italian salad dressing	1 tbsp	½ fat
whole-wheat dinner roll	1 small	1 grain
soft margarine	1 tsp	1 fat
melon balls	½ C	1 fruit
Snacks		
dried apricots	1 oz (1/4 C)	1 fruit
mini-pretzels	1 oz (3/4 C)	1 grain
mixed nuts	1.5 oz (1/3 C)	1 nuts
diet ginger ale	12 oz	0

(Appel LJ, et al. A clinical trial of the effects of dietary patterns on blood pressure. N Engl J Med 336:1117, 1997.)

above 25% in boys and 30% in girls increases the risk of elevated blood pressure (Williams et al., 1992). The goal in children is to prevent the adoption of life-style factors (overweight, high salt intake, and sedentary patterns) that are related to the development of hypertension. Strategies for the prevention of obesity and hypertension in children are shown in Table 27–9.

TABLE 27–9 STRATEGIES FOR PREVENTING OBESITY AND HYPERTENSION IN CHILDREN

Encourage planned activities instead of food as part of the family reward system.
Limit the amount of sedentary activities; encourage a time for physical activity.
Emphasize the benefits of regular physical activity: improved cardiovascular risk factor profile, increased energy expenditure, improved weight control, a general sense of well-being, improved interpersonal skills, and an outlet for psychological tension.
Encourage participation in active games, noncompetitive activities, and organized sports; emphasize sports that can be enjoyed throughout life; encourage participation in summer camp and school physical education programs.
Choose a low-fat (no more than 30% of energy), high complex carbohydrate (fruits and vegetables) diet.
Use moderation (no more than once or twice per week), not restriction, as a rule of thumb.
Have first helpings, not seconds.
Limit snacking and concentrate on low-calorie, healthy snacks.
Encourage parents to be role models for food intake and physical activity.
Encourage moderate salt intake.

(Adapted from Strong WB, et al. Integrated cardiovascular health promotion in childhood. A statement for health professionals from the Subcommittee on Atherosclerosis and Hypertension in Childhood of the Council on Cardiovascular Disease in the Young. Circulation 85:1638, 1992.)

Excessive Consumption of Sodium Chloride

Epidemiologic studies of populations support an etiologic role for salt in hypertension development. Primitive societies in which the intake of sodium is low (70 mEq/day) experience very little hypertension, and the blood pressure increase with age, common in industrialized societies, does not occur (Stamler, 1992). Hypertension is prevalent and stroke is the leading cause of death in countries with very high salt consumption (9–12 g/day or 150–200 mEq sodium/day).

The relationship between dietary electrolytes and blood pressure was investigated in the large INTERSALT study (Elliot et al., 1996). This cross-sectional study involved 52 centers worldwide and more than 10,000 subjects. SBP was found to be significantly related to dietary sodium intake **(salt-sensitive hypertension).** Excreting a 100 mmol difference in sodium in the urine (170 mmol sodium versus 70 mmol) was associated with an increase of 3 to 6 mm Hg in SBP (see "*Focus On:* Sodium Equivalents"). In another population study of 24

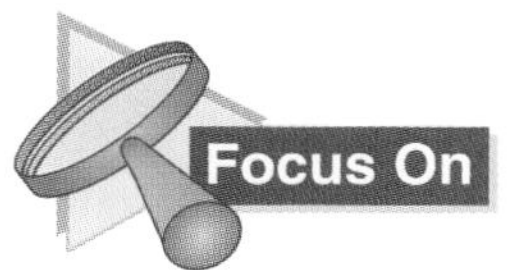

SODIUM EQUIVALENTS

Molecular weight and equivalent weight of atoms with single charges are the same. Therefore, 140 mEq of Na per liter of serum equals 140 mmol of Na per liter. 4.0 mEq of K per liter equals 4.0 mmol K per liter.

communities, a difference in sodium intake of 100 mEq/24 hours was associated with a 10 mm Hg fall in SBP in 60- to 69-year-olds. The rise in SBP seen with aging over a 30-year period would be 9 mm Hg less and the rise in DBP 4.5 mm Hg less if the average sodium intake were lowered by 100 mEq/day.

Not everyone reacts to salt intake with an increase in blood pressure **(salt-resistant hypertension).** Salt-sensitive people experience a 10 mm Hg decrease in blood pressure when following a low-salt diet after salt loading or a more than 5% increase in blood pressure during salt repletion after restriction (Kotchen, 1991). Currently, methods are lacking for identifying these "salt-sensitive" individuals (see "*New Directions:* Method for Determining Salt Sensitivity"). Approximately 30% to 50% of hypertensives and 15% to 25% of normotensives are salt-sensitive. Groups most likely to be salt-sensitive are stage 4 hypertensives, obese hypertensives, African Americans, persons with diabetes, and the elderly (Kotchen, 1991). However, in a recent study, all racial and ethnic groups were equally salt sensitive (Chrysant et al., 1997).

A high salt intake has also been implicated in hypertensive target organ disease (Messerli et al., 1997). Nine studies showed that 24-hour urinary sodium excretion was an independent determinant of left ventricular mass and other studies have found that salt intake affects hypertensive renal disease and cerebrovascular disease especially in salt-sensitive individuals. Because one cannot readily determine salt sensitivity, and Americans consume salt in great excess of physiologic requirements, a reduction in salt intake to no more than 6 g/day (100 mEq or 2400 mg Na/day) is recommended to prevent hypertension. This level can be achieved by cooking with as little salt as possible, refraining from adding salt at the table, and avoiding highly salted, processed foods (see Chapter 36).

Alcohol Consumption

Five to 7% of the hypertension in the population is due to alcohol consumption. Three drinks per day (a total of 3 oz of alcohol) is the threshold for raising blood pressure and is associated with a 3 mm Hg rise. For preventing high blood pressure, alcohol intake should be less than two drinks per day (24 oz beer, 10 oz wine, or 2 oz 100-proof whiskey). In women and lighter weight individuals, no more than one drink a day is recommended.

Physical Activity

Less active individuals are 30% to 50% more likely to develop hypertension than their active counterparts. In the Framingham study, medium to high levels of physical activity were protective against developing stroke (Kiely et al., 1994). Despite the benefits of activity and exercise in reducing disease, many Americans remain inactive. Twenty-eight percent of the total population, 37% of the low-income population, and 42% of the elderly (> 65 years) population reported no leisure-time physical activity during the previous month (Special Focus Behavioral Risk . . . , 1993). Intervention trials show that more physical activity produces a fall in SBP and DBP of about 6 to 7 mm Hg. Thus, increasing physical activity of low to moderate intensity to 30 to 45 minutes most days of the week is an important adjunct to other strategies for the primary prevention of hypertension.

Other Dietary Factors

Potassium. In population studies, dietary potassium and blood pressure are inversely related, that is, higher potassium intakes are associated with lower blood pressures. More often, the sodium/po-

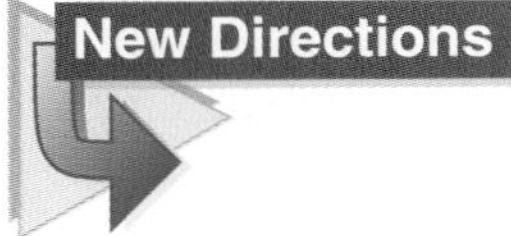

Method for Determining Salt Sensitivity

A Salt Step Test was developed to help determine which hypertensive patients are sensitive to salt. The three phases of the test are:

Phase 1 Consume a normal diet to establish baseline salt intake
Measure blood pressure
Determine urinary salt excretion

Phase 2 Consume a 2-g (34 mmol/day equivalent to 745 mg Na/day) salt-restricted diet for 2 weeks
Measure blood pressure
- If DBP <90 mmHg, the patient is salt-sensitive and needs a 24-hr urine collection
- After 1 month, if DBP is >90 mmHg, with a urinary NaCl of <34 mmol/24 hr, then patient is salt-resistant

Phase 3 Consume a 2 g salt diet, but add 1 g of salt/day
Each 1 g increase in salt is consumed for 3 days
Blood pressure is measured at each step
- When DBP is >90 mmHg, then 24-hr urine is collected

A threshold for salt intake is established

Data from Espinel C: The salt step test: Its usage in the diagnosis of salt sensitive hypertension and in the detection of the salt hypertension threshold. J Am Coll Nutr 11:526, 1992.

tassium ratio of the diet is related to blood pressure. With a dietary sodium intake of 100 mmol less than normal, and a potassium consumption up to 70 mmol/day for a sodium/potassium ratio of about 1.0, a 3.4 mm Hg decrease in SBP is predicted. Effects of potassium intake on blood pressure include reduced peripheral vascular resistance by direct arteriolar dilatation, increased loss of water and sodium from the body, suppression of renin and angiotensin secretion, decrease of adrenergic tone, and stimulation of the sodium–potassium pump activity. A meta-analysis found that high dietary potassium may help prevent and control hypertension (Whelton et al., 1997).

Potassium intake has also been related to stroke mortality. In a large population-based cohort, a 10 mEq/day (10 mmol/day) increase in potassium intake—the equivalent of one or two extra servings of fruit, citrus juice, vegetable, or potato—was related to a 40% decrease in the incidence of stroke-related deaths. This effect appeared to be unrelated to any change in blood pressure (Khaw and Barrett-Connor, 1988).

The Joint National Committee recommends a potassium intake of approximately 90 mmol/day (90 mEq/day) from fresh fruits and vegetables (Joint National Committee, 1997).

CALCIUM. Most population studies have found no significant relationship between dietary calcium and the prevalence of hypertension. Where a relationship existed, it appeared more often in African Americans and women. In the large, prospective Nurse's Health Study, consuming the recommended daily allowance (RDA) for calcium (800 mg/day) resulted in lower risk of developing hypertension than consuming only 400 mg/day (Witteman et al., 1989). However, clinical trials showed minimal hypotensive effects of high dietary calcium intakes from foods or supplements. Increasing dairy product consumption (for a total calcium intake of 1500 mg/day) had no effect on blood pressure in hypertensive men (Kynast-Gales and Massey, 1992). Thus, the role of calcium supplementation in preventing hypertension is yet unproven. Calcium from dietary sources to meet the adequate intake of 1200 mg/day is recommended.

MAGNESIUM. Magnesium is a potent inhibitor of vascular smooth muscle contraction and may play a role in blood pressure regulation as a vasodilator. An inverse relationship has been reported between dietary magnesium and blood pressure (National High Blood Pressure Education Program, 1993). In most clinical studies, however, magnesium supplementation has been ineffective in altering blood pressure, possibly because of the confounding effects of antihypertensive medications and the short duration of the studies. Overall, adequate data are lacking to recommend routine supplementation with magnesium to prevent hypertension.

LIPIDS. Fewer vegans have hypertension than omnivores even though their salt intake is not significantly different. The vegan diet tends to be higher in polyunsaturated fatty acids (PUFAs), among other nutrients, and lower in total fat, saturated fatty acids, and cholesterol. PUFAs are precursors of prostaglandins, whose actions affect renal sodium excretion and relax vascular musculature. Thus, an effect on blood pressure is plausible.

Both the amount and type of fat have been studied with respect to blood pressure. In two large cohort studies of female nurses (Witteman et al., 1989) and male health professionals (Ascherio et al., 1992), neither total fat nor specific fatty acids were related to baseline blood pressure or incidence of hypertension over a 4-year period. The majority of other studies have found no hypotensive effect of PUFAs, which led the National High Blood Pressure Working Group (1994) to conclude that "macronutrient alteration has limited or unproven efficacy in the primary prevention of hypertension." Factors other than dietary fat, such as increased potassium levels, appear to lower blood pressure in vegans. Although dietary lipids do not seem to affect blood pressure, they strongly affect CVD risk; thus, the Step I Diet is recommended for preventing complications from hypertension and CVD (see Chapter 26).

Large doses of fish oils (50 mL daily with 15 g ω-3 fatty acids) have lowered blood pressure in mildly hypertensive men (Knapp and Fitzgerald, 1989). Smaller doses (6–20 g fish oil/day) had no effect on blood pressure in hypertensive men (Lofgren et al., 1993) or normotensive subjects (Sacks et al., 1994). Because even small doses affect bleeding time, weight gain, glycemic control, and low-density lipoprotein cholesterol, supplementation with large doses of ω-3 fatty acids is not recommended for preventing hypertension.

Combination of Risk Factors for Cardiovascular Disease

Hypertension often occurs with other risk factors for CVD. In the NHANES III survey (National Education Programs, 1991) 40% of persons with hypertension had high blood cholesterol levels (> 240 mg/dL). Fifty-five percent of overweight men have hypertension compared to 27% of normal-weight men. Having a combination of risk factors markedly increases the risk for CVD. A nonsmoker with normal blood cholesterol and blood pressure has one tenth the risk of developing CVD of a person with hypertension and hypercholesterolemia.

Researchers have noted a larger than normal clustering of three risk factors—hypertension, insulin resistance, and central body fat distribution. Along with elevated blood pressure, these patients have hypertriglyceridemia, low high-density lipoprotein (HDL) cholesterol, obesity and central or truncal adiposity, glucose intolerance, insulin resistance, and often full-blown diabetes. Many names, most frequently *syndrome X* or *dyslipidemic hypertension* have been used for this constellation of risk

TABLE 27–10 COMPONENTS OF CARDIOVASCULAR RISK STRATIFICATION IN PATIENTS WITH HYPERTENSION

Major Risk Factors
Smoking
Dyslipidemia
Diabetes mellitus
Age >60 y
Sex (men and postmenopausal women)
Family history of cardiovascular disease: women <65 y or men <55 y
Target Organ Damage/Clinical Cardiovascular Disease
Heart diseases
Left ventricular hypertrophy
Angina or prior myocardial infarction
Prior coronary revascularization
Heart failure
Stroke or transient ischemic attack
Nephropathy
Peripheral arterial disease
Retinopathy

(From The Joint National Committee on Prevention, Detection, Evaluation, and Treatment of High Blood Pressure. Sixth report (JNC VI). Arch Intern Med 157:2413, 1997.)

factors. In a large New England sample, the prevalence of dyslipidemic hypertension was 15%, or 1.5 times the expected number if the diseases were independent (Eaton et al., 1993). Life-style modifications can prevent syndrome X from developing (see Chapters 12 and 23).

Medications

A number of medications either raise blood pressure or interfere with the effectiveness of antihypertensive drugs. These include oral contraceptives, steroids, nonsteroidal anti-inflammatory drugs (NSAIDS), nasal decongestants and other cold remedies, appetite suppressants, cyclosporin, tricyclic antidepressants, and monoamine oxidase inhibitors (see Chapter 18).

MANAGEMENT

The goal of hypertension management is to reduce morbidity and mortality from stroke, hypertension-associated heart disease, and renal disease. Three objectives for evaluating patients with hypertension are (1) to identify the possible causes, (2) to assess the presence or absence of target organ disease and clinical cardiovascular disease, and (3) to identify other CVD risk factors that will help guide treatment (Joint National Committee, 1997). Weight history, leisure-time physical activity, and dietary assessment of sodium, alcohol, saturated fat, and caffeine are components of the medical history (Fig. 27–3). The presence of risk factors and target organ damage (Table 27–10) determines treatment aggressiveness. As shown in Table 27–11, life-style changes are primary therapy in four of the nine risk groups and adjunctive therapy in all other groups.

The *Healthy People 2000* objective for blood pressure management was to increase to at least 50% the number of people with hypertension whose blood pressure is reduced to less than 140/90 mm Hg. Control must be achieved with the fewest number of side effects and at the lowest cost. In NHANES III, only 24% of hypertensive patients had achieved the blood pressure goal of less than 140/90 mm Hg (Burt et al., 1995). Of all treated hypertensives, 45% were adequately controlled.

Life-Style Modifications

Life-style modifications are definitive therapy for some and adjunctive therapy for all persons with hypertension (Joint National Committee, 1997). Depending on the risk group, 6 to 12 months of compliant life-style modifications should be tried before drug therapy is begun. Even if life-style modifications cannot completely correct the blood pressure, they will help increase the efficacy of pharmacologic agents and improve other CVD risk factors. Management of hypertension requires a life-long commitment. The American Heart Association website has more information at http://www.amhrt.org/.

TABLE 27–11 RISK STRATIFICATION AND TREATMENT

BLOOD PRESSURE STAGES (MM HG)*	LOW RISK GROUP (NO RISK FACTORS; NO TOD/CCD†)	MEDIUM RISK GROUP (AT LEAST 1 RISK FACTOR, NOT INCLUDING DIABETES; NO TOD/CCD)	HIGH RISK GROUP (TOD/CCD AND/OR DIABETES, WITH OR WITHOUT OTHER RISK FACTORS)
High-normal (130–139/85–89)	Life-style modification	Life-style modification	Drug therapy§
Stage 1 (140–159/90–99)	Life-style modification (up to 12 mo)	Life-style modification‡ (up to 6 mo)	Drug therapy
Stages 2 and 3 (≥160/≥100)	Drug therapy	Drug therapy	Drug therapy

(Adapted from the Joint National Committee on Prevention, Detection, Evaluation, and Treatment of High Blood Pressure. Sixth report (JNC VI). Arch Intern Med 157:2413, 1997.)

*Note: For example, a patient with diabetes and a blood pressure of 142/94 mm Hg plus left ventricular hypertrophy should be classified as having stage 1 hypertension with target organ disease (left ventricular hypertrophy) and with another major risk factor (diabetes). This patient would be categorized as "Stage 1, Risk Group C," and recommended for immediate initiation of pharmacologic treatment. Life-style modification should be adjunctive therapy for all patients recommended for pharmacologic therapy.

†TOD/CCD indicates target organ disease/clinical cardiovascular disease.

‡For patients with multiple risk factors, clinicians should consider drugs as initial therapy plus life-style modifications.

§For those with heart failure, renal insufficiency, or diabetes.

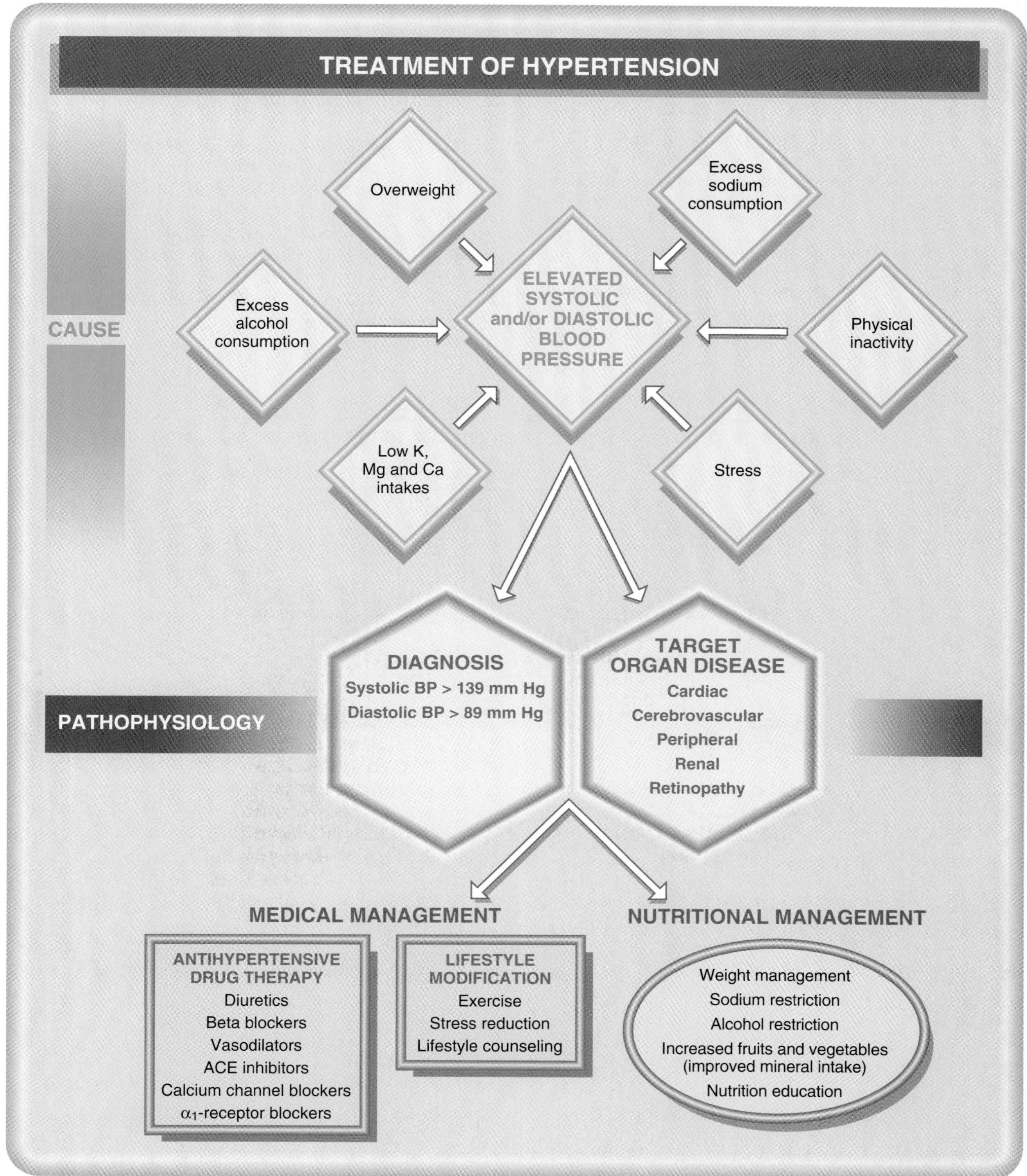

FIGURE 27–3 Pathophysiology algorithm—treatment of hypertension. ACE, angiotensin-converting enzyme; BP, blood pressure. (Algorithm content developed by John Anderson, Ph.D., and Sanford C. Garner, Ph.D., 2000.)

Weight Management

The effectiveness of weight reduction has been well documented in both mild and severe hypertensives. Hypertensive patients who weigh more than 115% of ideal body weight should be placed on an individualized weight reduction program that focuses on both hypocaloric dietary intake and exercise. Themes for a weight reduction program are shown in Table 27–12 (also see Chapter 23). In the Trial of Antihypertensive Intervention and Management, the goal for energy intake to facilitate weight loss was 25 kcal/kg minus 500 to 1000 kcal daily to produce a 0.5- to 1-kg/week deficit (Wylie-Rosett et al., 1993). An initial target should be to achieve a weight loss of at least 4.5 kg. This modest loss will not only lower blood pressure, but often will normalize blood lipids and glucose. The greater the weight loss, the greater the blood pressure reduction (Stevens et al., 1993). Some stage 1 hypertensives achieve normal blood pressure by weight loss alone.

Another benefit of weight loss on blood pressure is the synergistic effect with drug therapy. In subjects who lost weight and were taking one antihypertensive drug, lowering blood pressure was greater than in those taking the drug alone (Wylie-Rosett et al., 1993). Therefore, weight loss should be an adjunct to drug therapy because it may decrease the dose or number of drugs necessary to control blood pressure. Furthermore, weight loss lowers blood pressure significantly more than a low-

TABLE 27–12 PROGRAMS FOR INTENSIVE INTERVENTIONS FOR HYPERTENSION MANAGEMENT

WEIGHT CONTROL INTERVENTION	LOW-SODIUM/HIGH-POTASSIUM INTERVENTION
Session 1 • Introduction to program, process, and monitoring • Establishing weight and energy intake goals	**Session 1** • Introduction to program, process, and monitoring • Rationale for low-sodium/high-potassium modification
Session 2 • Assessing life-style factors that influence eating • Reading labels focusing on ingredients, kilocalorie information, and serving size (introduction to the concept of caloric density)	**Session 2** • Establishing goals for sodium and potassium intake • Reading labels and identifying foods low in sodium and high in potassium
Session 3 • Identifying and changing eating cues	**Session 3** • Identifying sources of sodium and potassium from diaries
Session 4 • Food shopping, preparation, and restaurant eating	**Session 4** • Changing shopping habits (e.g., reducing number of processed foods) • Selecting low-sodium/high-potassium items from restaurant menus
Session 5 • Assessing social supports and self-reinforcement and establishing control over situations that involve eating	**Session 5** • Examining problem foods that are high in sodium (cue and response analysis)
Session 6 • Identifying low-calorie snack foods, fast foods, and beverages • Establishing routine physical activities	**Session 6** • Preparing foods to maintain maximal potassium content (e.g., steaming, using a minimum amount of water, or consuming raw)
Session 7 • Setting realistic goals • Coping with feelings and behavioral lapses • Evaluating the Trial of Antihypertensive Intervention and Management cookbook	**Session 7** • Learning to use spices and herbs as alternatives to high-sodium seasonings • Evaluating the Trial of Antihypertensive Intervention and Management cookbook
Session 8 • Evaluating and promoting personal motivation and commitment • Evaluating changes in preparation and food selection	**Session 8** • Modifying recipes to lower sodium content • Reviewing low-sodium cookbooks • Preparing low-sodium, high-potassium snacks and desserts
Session 9 • Planning food for a party and for special occasions • Modifying favorite recipes	**Session 9** • Sharing low-sodium and high-potassium recipes • Planning food for special party occasions
Session 10 • Learning how to maintain weight loss and behavioral changes • Reviewing accomplishments (knowledge and skill acquired) • Assessing long-term commitment to new behavior and to follow-up program	**Session 10** • Learning how to maintain changes (e.g., in shopping and food preparation) • Reviewing accomplishments • Assessing long-term commitment and follow-up

Themes for the 10 group sessions during intensive intervention. The first 15 to 30 minutes of each session is devoted to reviewing (by use of diaries) progress on goals established the previous week. Each session ends with behavioral goal setting.

(From Wylie-Rosett J, et al. Trial of antihypertensive intervention and management: Greater efficacy with weight reduction than with a sodium-potassium intervention. J Am Diet Assoc 93:408, 1993. Reprinted with permission.)

sodium/high-potassium diet. Because weight loss and exercise increase insulin sensitivity, lower levels of triglycerides, and raise HDL-cholesterol, this combined intervention is also recommended for treating dyslipidemic hypertension (Eaton et al., 1993).

Once weight is lost, maintenance is critical. Unfortunately, relapse and weight gain are common following weight loss. Two modifiable factors associated with weight gain are a high fat intake and a low level of physical activity (Haus et al., 1994; Klesges et al., 1992). Weight maintenance goals for life are: (1) not to gain more than 10 to 15 lb after the age of 21 and (2) not to have more than a 2- to 3-in. increase in waist circumference after age 21 (Report of the American Institute of Nutrition, 1994). Some factors associated with effective weight maintenance are exercise, positive self-statements related to weight reduction efforts, self-monitoring activities (use of a food diary, goal setting, early attention to weight regain), and problem-solving skills in lieu of eating during stressful times (Kayman et al., 1990) (see Chapter 23).

Salt Restriction

Moderate salt restriction (6 g salt, 100 mEq or 2400 mg Na/day) is recommended for treatment of hypertension. The restriction is for salt because the chloride ion with sodium raises blood pressure. In stage 1 hypertension, this level of salt restriction may be sufficient to normalize blood pressure. Patients who require drug therapy also need salt restriction for enhanced drug efficacy. Adherence is better for less restrictive salt reductions. Therefore, more severe salt restrictions are not necessary unless congestive heart failure is present (see Chapter 36). To assess dietary salt intake, 3 days of diet records and three overnight urine collections provide the best estimate (Dubbert et al., 1992).

Because most dietary salt comes from processed foods, changes in food processing will help patients reach the sodium goal. A sensory study showed that commercial processing could develop and revise recipes using lower sodium concentrations (0.15–0.30% sodium concentration as the baseline for initial acceptance testing), and reduce added sodium by 30% to 50% without affecting consumer acceptance (Adams et al., 1994).

Other Dietary Modifications

MINERALS. Although some data suggest a benefit with increased intakes of potassium, calcium, and magnesium, the information available at this time is insufficient to support a specific recommendation for increased levels of intake, including the use of supplements, except to meet the AI for calcium and the RDA for magnesium and to increase intakes of fruits and vegetables when possible. Sodium and potassium goals based on body weight are shown in Table 27–13.

TABLE 27–13 GOALS FOR SODIUM AND POTASSIUM INTAKES BASED ON BODY WEIGHT

WEIGHT (kg)	SODIUM (mEq)	POTASSIUM (mEq)
≤50.0	52.2	61.5
50.5–60.0	60.1	71.8
60.5–70.0	70.0	82.1
70.5–80.0	78.3	92.3
80.5–90.0	87.5	102.6
≥90.5	100.0	115.4

(From Wylie-Rosett J, et al. Trial of antihypertensive intervention and management: Greater efficacy with weight reduction than with a sodium-potassium intervention. J Am Diet Assoc 93:408, 1993. Reprinted with permission.)

LIPIDS. Current recommendations for lipid composition of the diet are those of the Step I or Step II Diet (see Chapter 26) to help control weight and decrease the risk of CVD.

ALCOHOL. The diet history should contain information about alcohol consumption. As discussed earlier, alcohol intake should be limited to not more than 1 oz of ethanol/day in men, which is equivalent to 2 oz of 100-proof whiskey, 8 oz of wine, or 24 oz of beer. Women or lighter weight men should consume half this amount (.5 oz of ethanol/day).

Exercise

Moderate physical activity, defined as 30 to 45 minutes of brisk walking on most days of the week, is recommended as an adjunct therapy in hypertension. Because exercise is strongly associated with success in weight reduction and maintenance programs, any increase in activity level should be encouraged.

Pharmacologic Treatment

If blood pressure remains elevated after 6 to 12 months of life-style changes, antihypertensive medications are started. Most patients with more severe than stage 1 hypertension require drug treatment. However, life-style modifications are still a part of therapy even when drugs are used. The standard treatment for hypertension includes diuretics and β-blockers, although other drugs (angiotensin-converting enzyme inhibitors, α_1-receptor blockers, and calcium antagonists) are equally effective. All of these drugs can affect nutritional status (Table 27–14) and other CVD risk factors (Table 27–15).

Diuretics lower blood pressure in some patients by promoting volume depletion and sodium loss. However, thiazide diuretics increase urinary potassium excretion, especially in the presence of a high salt intake, thus leading to potassium loss and possibly hypokalemia. Except in the case of a potassium-sparing diuretic such as spironolactone or triamterene, additional potassium is usually required.

TABLE 27–14 EFFECTS OF SOME ANTIHYPERTENSIVE MEDICATIONS ON NUTRITIONAL STATUS

DRUG CLASS/GENERIC NAME*	NUTRITIONAL IMPACT†
Diuretics	
Thiazides	
Hydrochlorothiazide	Avoid taking with natural licorice. Caution if taken with calcium supplements. GI side effects: anorexia, increased thirst, dry mouth, nausea/vomiting, GI irritation, diarrhea, constipation.
Loop diuretics	
Furosemide	Avoid taking with natural licorice. GI side effects: anorexia, increased thirst.
Potassium-sparing diuretics	
Spironolactone	Avoid taking with salt substitutes, potassium substitutes, or natural licorice. GI side effects: anorexia, increased thirst, nausea/vomiting, diarrhea.
β-blockers	
Propranolol	Avoid natural licorice. GI side effects: anorexia, dry mouth, nausea/vomiting, epigastric distress, diarrhea, constipation, flatulence.
α-β-blockers	
Labetalol	Avoid natural licorice. GI side effects: taste changes, dry mouth, nausea/vomiting, diarrhea, indigestion.
α_1-Receptor blockers	
Prazosin	Avoid natural licorice. GI side effects: dry mouth, nausea/vomiting, diarrhea, constipation.
ACE inhibitor	
Enalapril	Avoid taking with salt substitutes, potassium substitutes, or natural licorice. GI side effects: anorexia, taste loss, dry mouth, glossitis, stomatitis, nausea/vomiting, abdominal pain, diarrhea, constipation.
Calcium antagonists	
Verapimil	GI side effects: nausea, constipation.
Direct vasodilator	
Hydralazine HCl	Avoid taking with natural licorice. GI side effects: anorexia, increased thirst, dry mouth, unpleasant taste, nausea/vomiting, GI distress, diarrhea, constipation.

*Drugs are those from the Joint National Committee on Detection, Evaluation, and Treatment of High Blood Pressure. Fifth report (JNC V). Arch Intern Med 153:154, 1993.
†Data from Pronsky ZM. Powers and Moore's food medication interactions, 8th ed. Pottstown, PA: Food Medication Interactions, 1993.
ACE, angiotensin-converting enzyme; GI, gastrointestinal.

Treatment of Blood Pressure in the Elderly

Over half of the elderly population has hypertension, but this is not a normal consequence of aging. CVD risk in the elderly is two to three times higher than in the middle-aged population. The life-style modifications discussed earlier are the first step in treatment of the elderly, as with younger populations. Recently, the Trial of Nonpharmacologic Interventions in the Elderly study found that losing weight (8–10 lb) and reducing salt intake (1800 mg/day) can lessen or eliminate the need for drugs in obese, hypertensive elderly (60–80 years of age) (Whelton et al., 1998). At the end of the 30-month study, 31% of the sodium reduction alone group, 36% of the weight reduction alone group, and 53% of the combination group were off medications. Although this study showed that losing weight and decreasing sodium in the elderly were very effective in lowering blood pressure, how to facilitate these changes and promote adherence remains an obstacle for health professionals. Only 38% were able to reach the sodium intake goals. Care should be taken to ensure that severe sodium restrictions are not adopted because these could lead to volume depletion in elderly patients with renal damage (National High Blood Pressure Education Program, 1994).

TABLE 27–15 IMPACT OF ANTIHYPERTENSIVE DRUGS ON CARDIOVASCULAR RISK FACTORS

	DIURETIC	β-BLOCKER	CALCIUM BLOCKER	ACE INHIBITOR	α-BLOCKER
Blood pressure	+	+	+	+	+
Cholesterol	–	+/–	0	0	+
HDL-cholesterol	0	–	0	0	+
Triglycerides	–	–	0	0	+
Glucose intolerance	–	–	0	+	+
Hyperinsulinemia	–	–	0	+	+
Physical activity	0	–	0	0	0
Left-ventricular hypertrophy	0	+/0	+	+	+

(From Poulter NR, Sever PS. Intervention in high risk groups: Blood pressure. In: Marmot M, Elliott P (eds). Coronary heart disease epidemiology. New York: Oxford University Press, 1992. Reprinted by permission of Oxford University Press.)
+, beneficial; –, adverse; 0, neutral.

CASE STUDY

Bob G. is a 56-year-old white man who works as a truck driver. He is on the road every week, and recently saw his doctor about headaches, dizziness, and insomnia. He was diagnosed as having hypertension, with three BP tests of 160/90, 175/95, and 177/92. His doctor gave him a diuretic, Lasix, and a β-blocker, Inderal. Bob was also given a diet sheet with a brief overview of a No Added Salt diet. Bob has contacted you for assistance in planning menus he can follow.

1. Write a week's set of menus which Bob can follow, starting with a meal at home for breakfast, at a restaurant for lunch, and from a carry-out deli late at night.
2. Bob generally consumes one or two beers before bedtime and is willing to give up that habit. What healthy snack habits might Bob have in the evening?
3. Because Bob is on the road so much, food safety might be a problem. What tips would you suggest for meals and snacks that he can keep in his truck?

Adherence

The major reason for inadequate control of high blood pressure is poor adherence to therapy. The *Healthy People 2000* objective was to increase to at least 90% the number of people with hypertension who are trying to normalize their blood pressure. This goal has not yet been achieved. Thirty-one percent of subjects in NHANES III with high blood pressure were not even aware they had hypertension (Burt et al., 1995). Barriers to adherence need to be investigated and remedied. A combined effort by physicians, nurses, and dietitians is needed to help more patients achieve optimal blood pressure (Second Report of the Expert Panel on Detection, Evaluation and Treatment of High Blood Cholesterol in Adults, 1993).

CITED REFERENCES

Adams SO, et al. Sodium and potassium mixtures can reduce sodium levels. J Am Diet Assoc 94:1313, 1994.

American Heart Association. 1998 Heart and stroke statistical update. Dallas, TX: AHA, 1997.

Appel LJ, et al. A clinical trial of the effects of dietary patterns on blood pressure. N Engl J Med 336:1117, 1997.

Ascherio A, et al. A prospective study of nutritional factors and hypertension among US men. Circulation 86:1475, 1992.

Burt VL, et al. Prevalence of hypertension in the US adult population. Results from the Third National Health and Nutrition Examination Survey, 1988–91. Hypertension 25:305, 1995.

Chrysant SG, et al. There are no racial, age, sex or weight differences in the effect of salt on blood pressure in salt-sensitive hypertensive patients. Arch Intern Med 157:2489, 1997.

Cowley AW, Roman RJ. The role of the kidney in hypertension. JAMA 275:1581, 1996.

Dubbert P, et al. Estimation of sodium intake by analyzing food records with augmented nutrition software and by overnight urine collections. J Am Diet Assoc 92:87, 1992.

Eaton CB, et al. Prevalence of hypertension, dyslipidemia, and dyslipidemic hypertension. J Fam Pract 36:17, 1993.

Elliott P, et al. INTERSALT revisited: Further analyses of 24 hour sodium excretion and blood pressure within and across populations. BMJ 312:1249, 1996.

Hall JE. Renal and cardiovascular mechanisms of hypertension in obesity. Hypertension 23:381, 1994.

Haus G, et al. Key modifiable factors in weight maintenance: Fat intake, exercise, and weight cycling. J Am Diet Assoc 94:409, 1994.

Himes JH, Dietz WH. Guidelines for overweight in adolescent preventive services: Recommendations from an expert committee. Am J Clin Nutr 59:307, 1994.

Joint National Committee on the Prevention, Detection, Evaluation and Treatment of High Blood Pressure. Fifth report (JNC V). Arch Intern Med 153:149, 1993.

Joint National Committee on the Prevention, Detection, Evaluation and Treatment of High Blood Pressure. Sixth report (JNC VI). Arch Intern Med 157:2413, 1997.

Kannel WB. Blood pressure as a cardiovascular risk factor. JAMA 275:1571, 1996.

Kaplan NM. Systemic hypertension: Mechanisms and diagnosis. In: Braunwald E (ed): Heart disease. Philadelphia: WB Saunders, 1992.

Kayman S, et al. Maintenance and relapse after weight loss in women: Behavioral aspects. Am J Clin Nutr 52:800, 1990.

Khaw K-T, Barrett-Connor E. The association between blood pressure, age, and dietary sodium and potassium: A population study. Circulation 77:53, 1988.

Kiely DK, et al. Physical activity and stroke risk: The Framingham study. Am J Epidemiol 140:608, 1994.

Knapp HR, Fitzgerald GA. The antihypertensive effects of fish oil. N Engl J Med 320:1037, 1989.

Klesges RC, et al. A longitudinal analysis of the impact of dietary intake and physical activity on weight change in adults. Am J Clin Nutr 55:818, 1992.

Kotchen T. Evaluation of publicly available scientific evidence regarding certain nutrient-disease relationships: Sodium and hypertension. Bethesda, MD: Life Sciences Research Office, Federation of American Societies for Experimental Biology, 1991.

Kynast-Gales SA, Massey LK. Effects of dietary calcium from dairy products on ambulatory blood pressure in hypertensive men. J Am Diet Assoc 92:1497, 1992.

Lofgren RP, et al. The effect of fish oil supplements on blood pressure. Am J Public Health 83:267, 1993.

Melnyk MG, Weinstein E. Prevention of obesity in black women by targeting adolescents: A literature review. J Am Diet Assoc 94:536, 1994.

Messerli F, et al. Salt. A perpetrator of hypertensive target organ disease. Arch Intern Med 157:2449, 1997.

National Education Programs Working Group Report on the Management of Patients with Hypertension and High Blood Cholesterol. Ann Intern Med 114:224, 1991.

National Heart, Lung, and Blood Institute. National Institutes of Health. Update on the Task Force report (1987) on high blood pressure in children and adolescents: A working group report from the National High Blood Pressure Program. NIH Publ No 97-3790, 1997.

National High Blood Pressure Education Program (NHBPEP) Working Group report on primary prevention of hypertension. Arch Intern Med 153:186, 1993.

National High Blood Pressure Education Program (NHBPEP) Working Group report on hypertension in the elderly. Hypertension 23:275, 1994.

Pouliot MC, et al. Waist circumference and abdominal saggital diameter: Best simple anthropometric indexes of abdominal visceral adipose tissue accumulation and related cardiovascular risk in men and women. Am J Cardiol 73: 460, 1994.

Poulter NR, Sever PS. Intervention in high risk groups: Blood pressure. In: Marmot M, Elliot P (eds.). Coronary heart disease epidemiology. New York: Oxford Medical Publications, 1992.

Report of the American Institute of Nutrition (AIN) Steering Committee on Healthy Weight. J Nutr 124:2240, 1994.

Sacks FM, et al. Short report: The effect of fish oil on blood pressure and high-density lipoprotein cholesterol levels in phase I of the Trials of Hypertension Prevention. J Hypertens 12:209, 1994.

Schwartz CJ, et al. Prevention of atherosclerosis and end-organ damage: A basis for antihypertensive interventional strategies. J Hypertens 12 (suppl):S3, 1994.

Second Report of the Expert Panel on Detection, Evaluation, and Treatment of High Blood Cholesterol in Adults. NIH Publ No 93-3095, 1993.

Special Focus: Behavioral Risk Factor Surveillance—United States, 1991. MMWR 42:1, 1993.

Stamler J, et al. Blood pressure, systolic and diastolic, and cardiovascular risks. Arch Intern Med 153:598, 1993.

Stamler R. The primary prevention of hypertension. In: Marmot M, Elliot P (eds.). Coronary heart disease epidemiology. New York: Oxford Medical Publications, 1992.

Stamler R, et al. Primary prevention of hypertension by nutritional-hygienic means. JAMA 262:1801, 1989.

Stevens V, et al. Weight loss intervention in phase I of the Trials of Hypertension Prevention. Arch Intern Med 153:849, 1993.

St. Jeor ST, et al. Obesity. Circulation 88:1391, 1993.

Strong WB, et al. Integrated cardiovascular health promotion in childhood. A statement of health professionals from the Subcommittee on Atherosclerosis and Hypertension in Childhood of the Council on Cardiovascular Disease in the Young. Circulation 85:1638, 1992.

Trials of Hypertension Prevention Collaborative Research Group (TOHP). Effects of weight loss and sodium reduction intervention on blood pressure and hypertension incidence in overweight people with high-normal blood pressure. Arch Intern Med 157:657, 1997.
Whelton PK, et al. Effects of oral potassium on blood pressure: Meta-analysis of randomized controlled clinical trials. JAMA 277:1624, 1997.
Whelton PK, et al. Sodium reduction and weight loss in the treatment of hypertension in older persons. A randomized controlled Trial of Nonpharmacologic Interventions in the Elderly (TONE). JAMA 279:839, 1998.
Williams DP, et al. Body fatness and risk for elevated blood pressure, total cholesterol, and serum lipoprotein ratios in children and adolescents. Am J Public Health 82:358, 1992.
Witteman JCM, et al. A prospective study of nutritional factors and hypertension among U.S. women. Circulation 80:1320, 1989.
Wylie-Rosett J, et al. Trial of antihypertensive intervention and management: Greater efficiency with weight reduction than with a sodium-potassium intervention. J Am Diet Assoc 93:408, 1993.

ADDITIONAL REFERENCES

Appel L, et al. Does supplementation of diet with fish oil reduce blood pressure? A meta-analysis of controlled clinical trials. Arch Intern Med 153:1429, 1993.
Davis B, et al. Reduction in long-term antihypertensive medication requirements: Effects of weight reduction by dietary intervention in overweight persons with mild hypertension. Arch Intern Med 153:1773, 1993.
Espinel C. The salt step test: Its usage in the diagnosis of salt-sensitive hypertension and in the detection of the salt hypertension threshold. J Am Coll Nutr 11:526, 1992.
Feldman R. A low-sodium diet corrects the defect in β-adrenergic response in older subjects. Circulation 85:612, 1992.
Lewis C, et al. Inconsistent associations of caffeine-containing beverages with blood pressure and with lipoproteins. Am J Epidemiol 138:502, 1993.
McCarron DA. Dietary patterns and blood pressure. N Engl J Med 337:636, 1997.
Morris M, et al. Does fish oil lower blood pressure? Circulation 88:523, 1993.
Obarzanek E, et al. Dietary protein and blood pressure. JAMA 275:1598, 1996.
Sabate J, et al. Effects of walnuts on serum lipid levels and blood pressure in normal men. N Engl J Med 328:603, 1993.
Singer D, et al. Blood pressure and endocrine responses to changes in dietary sodium in cardiac transplant recipients: Implications for the control of sodium balance. Circulation 89:1153, 1994.
Volpe M, et al. Abnormalities of sodium handling and of cardiovascular adaptations during high salt diet in patients with mild heart failure. Circulation 88:1620, 1993.

CHAPTER 28

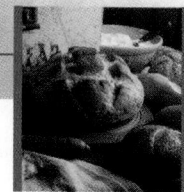

Nutrition for Bone Health

JOHN J. B. ANDERSON, PhD

Chapter Outline

- Bone Structure and Physiology
- Bone Mass
- Nutrition and Bone
- Osteoporosis

Key Terms

AGE-ASSOCIATED OSTEOPOROSIS (TYPE II)—loss of bone mineral density in both cortical and trabecular bone that occurs in elderly of both sexes after age 70; characterized by hip and vertebral fractures

BISPHOSPHONATES—drugs that act on osteoclasts to inhibit their resorption of bone tissue; examples include etidronate, alendronate, and pamidronate

BONE DENSITOMETRY—measurement of bone using tissue absorption of x-rays (photons) by instrument called a dual energy x-radiographic absorptiometer (DXA)

BONE MARKERS—molecules or portions of molecules derived from bone tissue that can be measured in blood serum or urine; matrix markers include portions of collagen molecules, whereas bone cell markers include enzymes such as alkaline phosphatase

BONE MINERAL CONTENT (BMC)—a measurement of bone mass expressed as the content of mineral per centimeter of bone; used to assess the amount of bone accumulated prior to cessation of growth

BONE MINERAL DENSITY (BMD)—a measure of bone density expressed in grams per centimeter squared (area density); used to assess the amount of bone after the developmental period is complete

BONE MODELING—the process by which bones grow in size and change their longitudinal and cross-sectional dimensions; formation and resorption are usually spatially separated

BONE REMODELING—the process by which bone is continually dismantled and reformed to repair itself, grow, adapt to external strains, and furnish calcium for other body needs; resorption and formation involve the same bone space

BONE TISSUE—the tissue that exists in all bones and contains both organic matrix (osteoid) and mineral (hydroxyapatite) components

CALCITRIOL—the hormonal form of vitamin D

CALCIUM HOMEOSTASIS—the process of maintenance of a constant serum calcium concentration (i.e., at a set level)

CORTICAL BONE—the compact bone of the shaft that surrounds the medullary cavity of the long bones

ESTROGEN RECEPTOR (ER)—cellular molecule that binds to estrogens, selective estrogen receptor modulators, and phytoestrogens before delivering these molecules to the nuclear DNA for the initiation of the events typical of estrogen stimulation of the cell

ESTROGEN REPLACEMENT THERAPY (ERT)—administration of estrogen molecules to replace the natural hormone, which declines drastically after menopause; similar to hormone replacement therapy (HRT)

HYDROXYAPATITE—a crystalline structure composed of calcium phosphate and calcium carbonate in an organic collagen matrix that gives strength and rigidity to bones and teeth

MATRIX (OSTEOID)—the organic component of bone that consists mainly of collagen, but also several other molecules, such as osteocalcin and osteopontin, that have essential roles; provides both strength and flexibility to bones

OSTEOBLAST—a bone cell responsible for the formation of bone

OSTEOCALCIN—a vitamin K-dependent bone-specified protein that is released into blood from the resorbed matrix as well as from the osteoblast cells that make it

OSTEOCLAST—bone cell responsible for the resorption and removal of bone

OSTEOCYTE—bone cell derived from an osteoblast that gets buried in mineralized bone after the bone forms; it maintains communication with osteoblasts on bone surfaces by cell processes passing through canaliculi

OSTEOMALACIA—condition of impaired mineralization caused by vitamin D and calcium deficiency

OSTEOPENIA—too little bone mass at any stage of the life cycle; a specific definition of bone conditions that is based on bone densitometry

OSTEOPOROSIS—loss of bone tissue to the point that the specific skeletal site is unable to sustain ordinary strains; a specific definition that is based on bone densitometry

PEAK BONE MASS (PBM)—the greatest amount of bone accumulated at any age; typically occurs by approximately 30 years of age

PHYTOESTROGENS—estrogen-like molecules derived from soybeans, clover, and other plant sources; act on estrogen receptors more like SERMs than true estrogens

POSTMENOPAUSAL OSTEOPOROSIS (TYPE I)—loss of bone mineral density involving primarily the trabecular bone tissue and characterized by fractures of the distal radius and ulna, and crush fractures of the lumbar vertebrae

PRIMARY IDIOPATHIC OSTEOPOROSIS—loss of bone density that affects premenopausal women and young or middle-aged men
SECONDARY OSTEOPOROSIS—loss of bone density secondary to another disease, such as liver disease or renal disease
SELECTIVE ESTROGEN RECEPTOR MODULATOR (SERM)—molecule, including a specific class of drugs, that acts on estrogen receptors in osteoblasts to promote the maintenance of bone tissue, but without having the undesirable effects on reproductive tissues that lead to breast or uterine cancers; examples include tamoxifen and raloxifene
TRABECULAR BONE (CANCELLOUS BONE)—the spongy bone in the knobby ends of the long bones, the iliac crest, scapula, and vertebrae

Adequate nutrition is essential for the development and maintenance of the skeleton, that is, bone health. Although diseases of the bone, such as **osteoporosis** and **osteomalacia,** have complex etiologies, the development of these diseases can be minimized by providing adequate nutrients at appropriate periods during the life cycle. Of these diseases, osteoporosis is the most common and the most destructive of productivity and quality of life. The number of elderly (over 65 years) in the United States is projected to reach almost 25% by 2020, a doubling since 1988 (Schneider and Guralnik, 1990), greatly increasing the numbers in the population at risk for osteoporosis. The average life expectancy in the United States in 1995 was almost 80 years for women and 73 for men. As a result of the increasing numbers of elderly, this disease, as manifested by hip fractures, will become more significant in both morbidity and mortality, as well as in cost. Because the provision of bone-building nutrients is necessary even after the onset of osteoporosis, the benefits of adequate intakes of calcium and other nutrients during adulthood and the elderly period remain as significant as during the early life period of bone growth and development.

BONE STRUCTURE AND PHYSIOLOGY

Bone is a term used to mean both an organ, such as the femur, and a tissue, such as trabecular bone tissue. Each bone (organ) contains **bone tissues** of two major types, trabecular and cortical (Fig. 28–1). These tissues undergo bone modeling during growth (height) and bone remodeling after growth ceases.

Composition of Bone

Bone consists of an organic **matrix** or *osteoid,* primarily collagen fibers, in which salts of calcium and phosphate are deposited in combination with hydroxyl ions in crystals of **hydroxyapatite.** The tensile capacity of collagen and the hardness of hydroxyapatite combine to give bone its great strength. Other components of the bone matrix include osteocalcin, osteopontin, and several other matrix proteins.

Types of Bone Tissue

Approximately 80% of the skeleton consists of compact or **cortical bone** tissue. Shafts of the large bones are primarily cortical bone. The remaining 20% of the skeleton is **trabecular,** or **cancellous bone** tissue, which exists in the knobby ends of the long bones, the iliac crest of the pelvis, the wrists, scapulas, vertebrae, and in the regions of bones that line the marrow. Trabecular bone is less dense than cortical bone tissue as a result of its open structure of interconnecting bony spicules that resemble a sponge in appearance. Thus, trabecular bone is also called *spongy bone* or *spongiosa*. The elaborate interconnecting components (columns and struts) of trabecular bone tissue add support to the cortical bone tissue shell of the long bones as well as provide a large surface area that is exposed to circulating fluids from the marrow and that is lined by a disproportionately larger number of cells than cortical bone tissue. Trabecular bone tissue is, therefore, much more responsive to estrogens or the lack of estrogens than is cortical bone tissue (see Fig. 28–1). The loss of trabecular bone tissue late in life is largely responsible for the occurrence of fractures.

Bone Cells

Two cells are primarily responsible for the formation or production of bone tissue, **osteoblasts,** and the resorption or breakdown of bone, **osteoclasts.** (Also see below under Bone Modeling and Bone Remodeling.) The functions of these two cell types are listed in Table 28–1. The other important cell types also exist in bone tissue, **osteocytes** and bone-lining cells, both of which are derived from osteoblasts. The origin of the osteoblasts and osteoclasts is from primitive precursor cells found in bone marrow.

TABLE 28–1 FUNCTIONS OF OSTEOBLASTS AND OSTEOCLASTS

OSTEOBLASTS	OSTEOCLASTS
Bone Formation	**Bone Resorption**
Synthesis of matrix proteins	Degradation of bone tissue via enzymes and acid (H^+) secretion
Collagen type 1 (90%)	Communication via secretion of cytokines that act on osteoblasts
Osteocalcin and others (10%)	
Mineralization	
Communication via secretion of cytokines that act on osteoclasts	

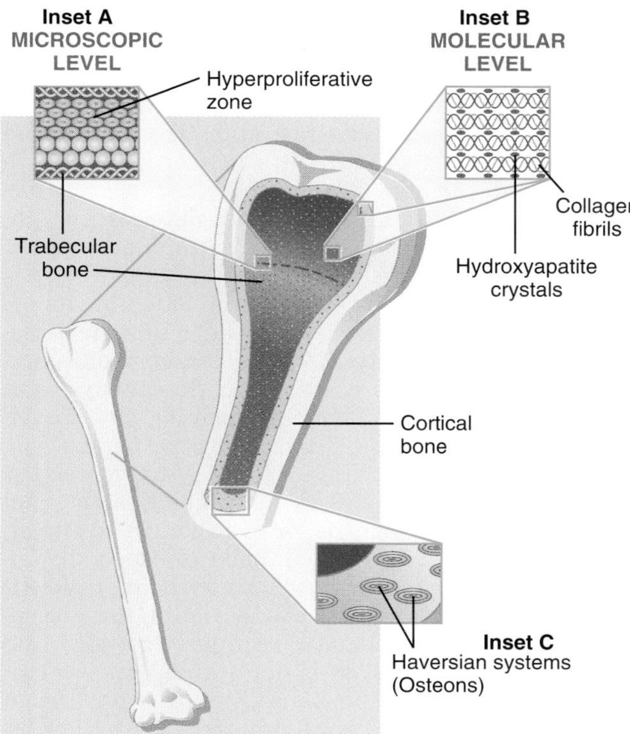

FIGURE 28–1 Schematic diagram of the structure of a long bone (hemisection of a long bone, such as the tibia). The ends of the long bones contain high percentages of trabecular (cancellous) bone tissue, whereas the shaft contains predominantly cortical bone tissue. **Inset A** includes an enlarged section (approximately 100-fold) of the growth plate (epiphysis) and the subjacent hyperproliferative zone containing cartilage cells stacked like coins. Mineralization in this zone produces the primary spongiosa that is subsequently modeled by osteoblasts and osteoclasts to form the mature trabecular bone tissue. (Cartilage is replaced by bone in this region.) **Inset B** includes a section of collagen molecules (triple helices) surrounded by mineralized deposits (dark spheroids) at a magnification of approximately one million-fold. These collagen–mineral complexes exist in both trabecular and cortical bone tissues in association with other matrix proteins (not shown). **Inset C** shows the cross-section of half of the mid-shaft of long bone (magnification approximately 10-fold). This section of cortical bone tissue contains vertical haversian systems (osteons) that run in parallel with the shaft axis (many are required to extend this system from one end of the shaft to the other). At the center of each osteon is a canal that contains an artery that supplies bone tissues with nutrients and oxygen, a vein for removing wastes, and a nerve for returning afferent relays to the brain. The lamellar structure of haversian systems not only adds strength to the bone, but these units also undergo remodeling, which permits both repair of microfractures and adaptation to loads (strains) of the body bearing on the bone.

Calcium Homeostasis

Bone tissue serves as a reservoir of calcium and other minerals that are used by other tissues of the body. **Calcium homeostasis** is almost totally reliant on this source of calcium when the diet is inadequate. Bone tissue is also dynamic—although a slow dynamic—because it undergoes both modeling early in life and remodeling after skeletal growth or height gain ceases.

Although 99% of the body calcium is found in the skeleton, the remaining 1% is critical to a great variety of indispensable life processes. The concentration of calcium in blood and other extracellular fluids is regulated by complex mechanisms that balance calcium intake and excretion with bodily needs. When calcium intake is not adequate, homeostasis is maintained by drawing on mineral from the bone to keep the serum calcium ion concentration at its set level of approximately 10 mg/dL or 2.5 mmol. Depending on the amount of calcium required, homeostasis can be accomplished by drawing from two major skeletal sources: readily mobilizable calcium ions in the bone fluid or, through the process of osteoclastic resorption, from the bone tissue itself.

Adaptation of the homeostatic mechanism regulating blood calcium concentration is achieved through two calcium-regulating hormones, *parathyroid hormone (PTH)* and *1,25-dihydroxyvitamin D* (**calcitriol**). (See Chapter 5.) This calcium-regulatory system works more efficiently early in life, especially during the first few decades, but the efficiency undergoes a gradual decline in later life. For example, within a few years following the menopause, urinary calcium losses from the body increase, but intestinal absorption of calcium does not increase sufficiently to balance the losses. PTH activity, which directly contributes to bone loss, increases in most individuals during the seventh decade of life, even though PTH measurements typically remain within the normal range but at the high end.

The hormonal form of vitamin D, calcitriol, also plays an adaptational role by increasing the efficiency of intestinal calcium absorption in the lower half of the small bowel when dietary calcium is inadequate. This hormone is especially critical in the pre- and postpubertal growth years of girls and boys who have less than optimal intakes of calcium. Calcitriol, however, is much less effective in improving intestinal calcium absorption by women a decade or so after the onset of the menopause, even though calcitriol levels are elevated (Ebeling et al., 1992).

Bone Modeling

Bone modeling is the term applied to the growth of the skeleton until mature height is achieved. For example, during bone modeling long bones elongate and widen by undergoing great internal changes as well as external expansions in their structures. In modeling, the process of formation of new bone tissue occurs first and it is followed by the resorption of old tissue. Growth occurs at the epiphyses (growth plates that undergo hyperproliferation) and circumferentially; cells undergo division and contribute to the formation of new bone tissue (see Fig. 28–1).

Bone modeling is typically completed in girls by 16 to 18 years of age and in boys by 18 to 20 years. After growth in height ceases, gains in bone tissue

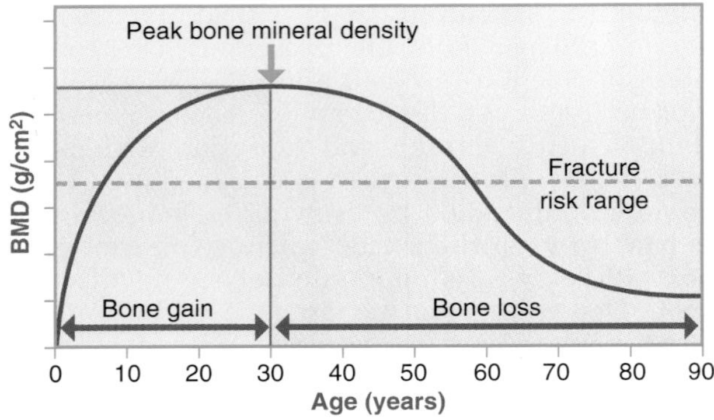

FIGURE 28–2 The early gain and later loss of bone in females. Peak bone mineral density (BMD) is typically achieved by age 30. Menopause occurs at approximately age 50. Postmenopausal women typically enter the fracture risk range after age 60. Men have a more gradual decline in BMD starting at age 50.

may continue by the process known as bone consolidation (see below under Peak Bone Mass). The major activity of the skeleton in early life is growth and gain in bone, whereas in later life it is the loss of bone (Fig. 28–2). This concept underlines the inevitable decline of bone mass in the late stages of life.

Bone Remodeling

After skeletal growth is completed, bone continuously undergoes remodeling in response to strains on the skeletons, adapts to changes in life style factors and dietary intakes, maintains the set calcium concentration in extracellular fluids, and repairs microscopic fractures that occur over time. About 4% of the total bone surface is involved in remodeling at any given time as new bone is renewed continually at specific sites throughout the skeleton. Even in the mature skeleton, bone remains a dynamic tissue. Normal bone turnover is illustrated in Figure 28–3.

Both types of bone tissue are subject to the remodeling process, although the greater proportion occurs in the trabecular bone, especially at those sites located in areas subject to the greatest weight-bearing strains. Remodeling of both cortical and trabecular bone tissues occurs in response to both strains and the microscopic fractures that result from the gradual strain-related deterioration of bone tissue (see "*Clinical Insight:* Jumping Bones").

Bone remodeling is a process in which bone is continuously resorbed through the action of the osteoclasts and reformed through the action of the osteoblasts. After activation by specific hormones and cytokines, osteoclasts resorb both the mineral and organic components of bone by forming small cavities on bone surfaces. The resorptive process is rapid and completed within a few days, whereas the refilling of these cavities by osteoblasts is slow, on the order of 3 to 6 months, or even longer in the elderly. The loss of trabecular bone is especially increased following menopause, but without sufficient bone formation. In normal young adults, the resorption and formation phases are tightly coupled and the amount of bone mass is maintained at zero balance. In the elderly, bone loss involves an uncoupling of the phases of bone remodeling with an increase of resorption over formation. As a result of the uncoupled bone remodeling, bone loss occurs.

The remodeling process is initiated by the *activation* of pre-osteoclastic cells in the bone marrow. Interleukin-1 and other cytokines released from bone-lining cells (i.e., inactive osteoblasts) are considered to act as the triggers in the activation process. The pre-osteoclast cells migrate to the surfaces of bone while differentiating into mature osteoclasts. The osteoclasts then cover a specific area of trabecular or cortical bone tissue, and begin excavating the surface to a fairly uniform depth and width. Acids and proteolytic enzymes released by the osteoclasts *resorb* both bone mineral and matrix on the surface of trabecular bone or cortical bone. The *rebuilding*

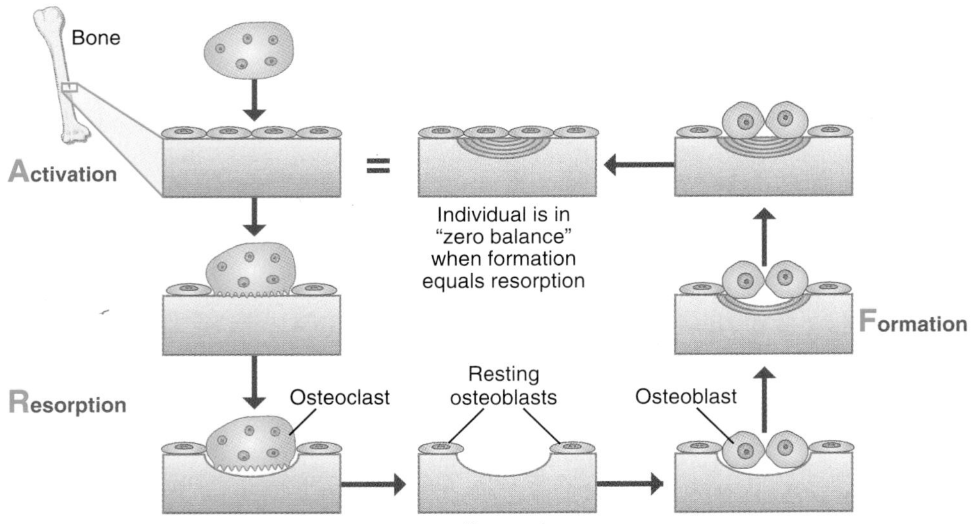

FIGURE 28–3 Bone turnover in healthy adults.

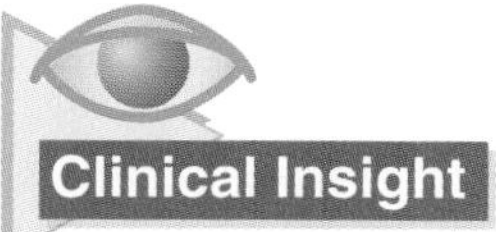

Jumping Bones

It has long been thought and repeated by health professionals that any weight-bearing exercise was good for building bones. It was assumed that activities such as walking and running would be better for building bones than swimming or cycling. However, weight-bearing exercise is not as effective as thought. NASA found that even when the astronauts walked on treadmills daily while weighted down, they could not prevent bone loss.

What Dr. Snow at the University of Oregon Bone Research Laboratory realized is that the skeleton needs to be shocked or surprised to build and maintain density in hip bones, for example. It wasn't enough to be just pounding the pavement as a marathon runner might; it needed to be an activity that resulted in the equivalent of 12 times the body weight hitting the ground. Yes, jumping! When Dr. Snow compared the hip bone density of marathon runners to that of gymnasts (who hit the ground in jumps all the time), she found that the gymnasts had 30% more bone than the runners (Bassey and Ramsdale, 1994). An 18-month trial of high-impact exercise in premenopausal women showed a greater increase in BMD at weight-bearing sites than in controls. The high-impact exercises three times per week included 20 minutes of jump or step training (Heinonen et al., 1996).

or *formation* stage involves secretion of collagen (type I) and other matrix proteins by the osteoblasts. Collagen polymerizes to form mature triple-stranded fibers. In a few days, salts of calcium and phosphate begin to precipitate on the collagen fibers, developing into crystals of hydroxyapatite. When the resorption and formation phases are in balance, the same amount of bone tissue exists at the completion of the formation phase (see Fig. 28–3). The benefit to the skeleton of this remodeling is the renewal of bone without any microfractures. When dietary calcium intake is low, however, osteoclastic resorption becomes greater than formation by osteoblasts, because of a persistently elevated PTH concentration in blood (Fig. 28–4).

The action of PTH in promoting activity of the osteoclasts is countered by estrogen, which reduces the response of osteoblasts to PTH. PTH acts directly on osteoblasts, which increase the production of interleukin-6 and other cytokines that in turn stimulate osteoclasts to resorb bone. Estrogen helps to block the production of PTH-stimulated interleukin-6 and other cytokines. These steps of bone remodeling are illustrated in Figure 28–5. *Calcitonin* directly inhibits osteoclast activity (i.e., resorption), but the significance of its physiologic role in humans is not clear. Impaired production of this hormone could occur in the elderly, which could contribute to age-related bone loss, but no data have been published to support this possibility.

Bone Markers

Bone markers exist for both bone formation and bone resorption. Plasma bone-specific alkaline phosphatase is a marker of bone formation, although total plasma alkaline phosphatase may also be used. Markers of bone resorption include plasma cross-linked *collagen telopeptides, urinary N-telopeptides,* and *plasma tartrate-resistant acid phosphatase.* **Osteocalcin,** considered a bone formation marker, is also released from resorbed bone matrix, and therefore interpretation of its blood values is not clear under most conditions.

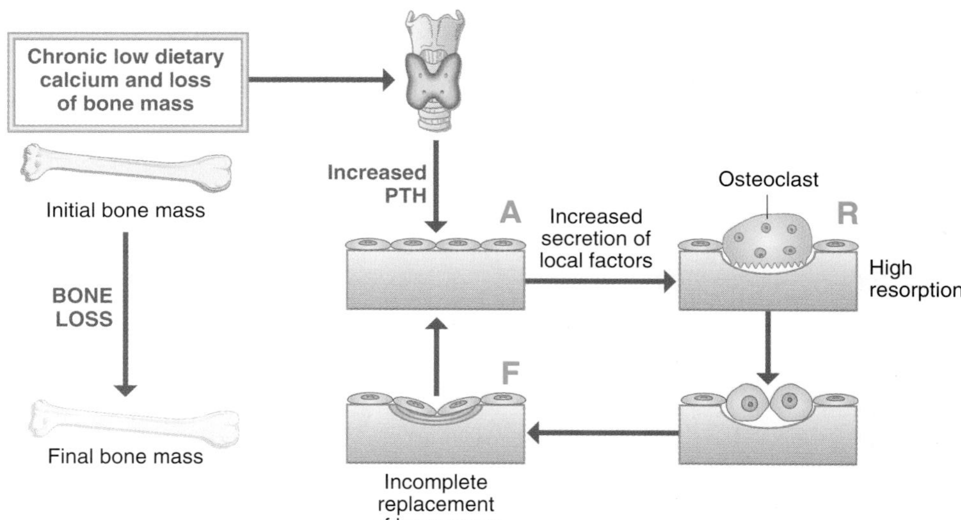

FIGURE 28–4 Effects of persistently elevated parathyroid hormone (PTH) on bone mass. A, activation; F, formation; R, reabsorption.

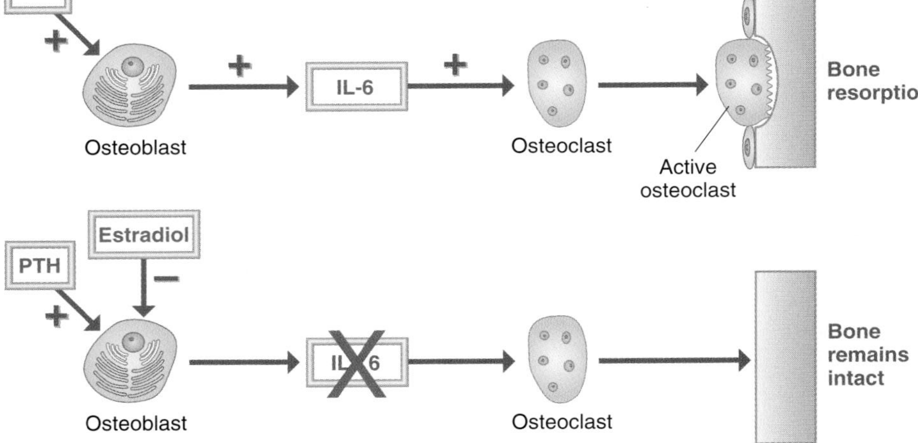

FIGURE 28–5 Interaction between osteoblasts and osteoclasts in bone remodeling. The role of parathyroid hormone (PTH) in stimulating osteoclasts to resorb bone (upper) is contrasted with the inhibitory action of estrogens on osteoblasts that negate the action of PTH (lower).

BONE MASS

Bone mass is a generic term that refers to **bone mineral content (BMC)**, but not to **bone mineral density (BMD).** BMC is more appropriate in assessing the amount of bone accumulated before the cessation of growth or height gain, whereas BMD is used to describe bone after the developmental period is completed. These measurements are often used interchangeably, but BMD is more useful in studies of adults.

Measurement of Bone Mineral Content and Bone Mineral Density

Bone densitometry measures bone mass on the basis of tissue absorption of photons produced by one or two monoenergetic x-ray tubes. *Dual energy x-ray absorptiometry (DXA)* is available in most hospitals and many clinics for the measurement of the total body and regional skeletal sites of interest, such as the lumbar vertebrae and the proximal femur (hip). Results of BMC measurements are expressed as grams of mineral per centimeter of bone. BMD is expressed as grams per centimeter squared and is calculated from the BMC divided by the width of the bone at the measurement site.

Computed tomography may also be used to measure BMD (a true volumetric density) of the spine, and this technique has now been developed to measure the limbs.

Ultrasound Measurements of Bone

Quantitative ultrasound measurements of the heel bone (calcaneus) and the kneecap are now possible. Measurements by ultrasound machines provide information on two properties, the elasticity and strength of bone, that cannot be assessed by DXA. The ultrasound values are not equivalent to the BMD measurements because ultrasound assesses the properties of collagen in the organic matrix rather than the mineral phase of bone tissue. Ultrasound instruments actually measure the velocity of sound waves transmitted through bone and *broadband ultrasound attenuation (BUA)*. Measurements at the calcaneus correlate well with BMD measurements at this same skeletal site, meaning that low values by DXA are typically mirrored by low values of BUA. Therefore, ultrasound is about as good as DXA in predicting the risk of fracture (Baran et al., 1991).

Accumulation of Bone

During the growth periods of childhood and puberty and into adulthood, formation exceeds the resorption of bone. **Peak bone mass** is reached around the age of 35 years (see Fig. 28–2). The long bones stop growing in length before age 18 in girls and age 20 in boys, but bone mass continues to accumulate for a few more years by a process known as *consolidation*. The age when BMD acquisition ceases varies, depending not only on diet but also on physical activity and strain on the skeleton (Recker et al., 1993). In women who have children, the loading related to lifting and carrying of children may improve skeletal mass and density (Anderson and Rondano, 1996).

Peak Bone Mass (PBM)

Peak bone mass (PBM) is greater in men than in women because of their larger frame size. Both BMC and BMD levels are normally lower in women. One study demonstrated a 15% lower BMD and a 30% lower BMC in women than in men after skeletal growth (height) was complete (Mazess, 1982).

Bone mineral density is also greater in African Americans and Hispanics than in whites and Asians, a factor that may be related to larger muscle mass. A comparative study of subjects from three different ethnic groups demonstrated the differences in near PBM attainment (20 years of age) at the mid-radial shaft that can be attributed in part to hereditary factors. In order of greatest PBM: African American females > white Americans > Japanese (Anderson and Pollitzer, 1994). A strong *hereditary component* is also related to the development of bone mass (Pocock et al., 1987; Pollitzer and Anderson, 1989). The contribution of hereditable factors to bone is estimated to be approximately 70%, which means the estimated contribution from environmental factors is only about 30% (Johnston, Slemenda, and Melton, 1992). Premenopausal daughters of osteoporotic mothers have demonstrated reduced bone mass in the spine and femoral neck compared with daughters of normal mothers within the normal range of bone measurements (Seeman et al., 1989).

Peak bone mass is related to both dietary calcium intakes and weight-bearing physical activity. Calcium intake appears to be a critical factor in the postmenarcheal growth of girls (Jackman et al., 1997; Matkovic et al., 1994). The contribution of weight-bearing exercise to PBM during the growth and development period may be greater than that of calcium (Tylavsky et al., 1992). Whether an interaction exists between these two variables is not yet clear, but a positive interaction between them appears to favorably affect measurements of BMD (Specker, 1996).

Physical activity and dietary calcium appear to play a large role in supporting gains in bone mass in the third decade of life in women, as do oral contraceptives (Recker et al., 1993). Women who used oral contraceptives for several years during early adulthood may benefit after menopause by having larger bone mass, especially in the lumbar spine and femoral neck (Kritz-Silverstein and Barrett-Connor, 1993).

Finally, total weight is a good indicator of greater BMC and BMD. Studies that adjust for other factors report that body weight is the most consistent factor related to bone mass, both in elderly women (Edelstein and Barrett-Connor, 1993) and in young adult women (Halioua and Anderson, 1990).

Loss of Bone Mass

Age is an important determinant of BMD. If the age of a woman is known, her vertebral bone mass can often be predicted within 10% (see "*Clinical Insight:* Women, BMD, and Osteoporosis" and Fig. 28–2).

At approximately age 40, BMD begins to diminish gradually in both sexes, but bone loss increases greatly in women after age 50, or the time of menopause. A continuous loss thereafter in postmenopausal women occurs at a rate of 1.2% per year over the next decade. Men continue to have bone loss also, but at a much slower rate than for women of the same age, until age 70, when the loss rates are about the same for both genders. Loss of bone mass is the result of changes in the hormone-directed mechanisms that govern bone remodeling. The processes of resorption and formation are uncoupled to a degree that interferes with the ability of osteoblastic activity to keep pace with the resorptive activities of osteoclasts to maintain balance. In the elderly, the bone mass may get so low that indi-

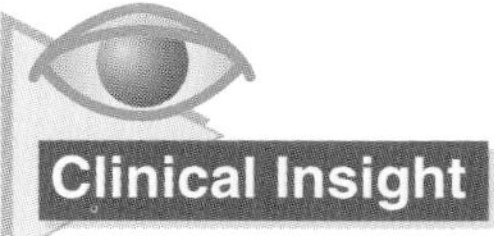

Women, BMD, and Osteoporosis

At present, safe and effective treatment is not readily available to replace bone that is already lost. It is, nevertheless, important to identify women who are at risk of developing osteoporosis as early as possible, so that measures can be taken to prevent further bone loss. Because low BMD is a major risk factor for osteoporosis, its assessment is clinically useful.

Assessment of bone status based on the existence of one or more risk factors, such as age, height, weight, smoking status, alcohol consumption, calcium intake, exercise, frame size, and selected bone markers, is not sufficiently accurate. BMD, as measured by bone densitometry, is more clinically useful. The machines that make these measurements are now readily available. Fees for the measurements are reasonable, and the procedure is safe, providing very low radiation exposure. In addition, the measurements are both precise and accurate. Low BMD itself is a risk factor for osteoporotic fractures.

A committee of the National Osteoporosis Foundation has recommended several situations in which bone densitometry is appropriate, two of which are (1) estrogen deficiency and (2) long-term glucocorticosteroid therapy (Johnston et al., 1991). A BMD measurement of an at-risk woman entering menopause, that is, prior to becoming estrogen deficient, serves as a baseline for subsequent measurements as the individual becomes increasingly estrogen deficient and develops low bone mass, especially osteoporosis according to the World Health Organization (WHO) definition. This information helps physicians and patients make decisions about the need for drug therapy, such as estrogen replacement therapy, bisphosphonates, and selective estrogen receptor modulators. In individuals on long-term glucocorticosteroid therapy, a BMD measurement can indicate the need for treatment with a bone-preserving medication, such as those listed and also calcitonin.

Typically total body BMD is measured, as well as regional sites, such as the proximal femur and lumbar vertebrae. In addition, an evaluation of the skeletal status of a woman at age 50 may also include the measurement of bone markers and the assessment of dietary intakes of calcium and other bone-enhancing nutrients.

viduals are at greatly increased risk of fragility fractures that result from minimal trauma.

Cortical bone tissue and trabecular bone undergo different patterns of aging. Loss of cortical bone eventually plateaus and may even cease late in life. Trabecular bone begins to diminish in both sexes as early as 40 years of age. Premenopausal loss of trabecular bone in women is much greater than of cortical bone. Loss of both kinds of bone accelerates in women after menopause, although trabecular bone is lost at a much higher rate (Fig. 28–6).

The accelerated bone loss rate of 2% to 3% per year continues for 5 to 10 years after menopause, and then the rate declines gradually to 0.5% to 1% per year thereafter. However, a subgroup of postmenopausal women lose bone at an even faster rate (Christiansen et al., 1987) (Fig. 28–7). A woman who reaches age 80 will have lost up to 45% to 50% of her PBM, and a similarly aged man will have lost approximately 30% of his PBM (Riggs and Melton, 1986).

The typical bone loss in elderly women amounts to approximately 300 mg calcium per day that is lost in both the urine and the stool. If calcium balance is to be maintained, this amount must be replaced by the diet each day. Older women without estrogen lose more calcium in their urine than premenopausal women, as much as 100 mg more per day. Calcium absorption from the gut is governed to a large extent by need, so that the body can theoretically adapt to reduced intakes of calcium and increase absorption and maintain calcium balance. The vitamin D adaptive mechanisms, however, typically become less efficient with age. Therefore, calcium homeostasis is maintained, but at the expense of a loss of bone tissue. In the elderly not on estrogen replacement therapy (ERT) or other drug therapy, the achievement of calcium balance seldom occurs, even though calcium homeostasis can be maintained.

The normal bone loss that occurs with aging in both sexes is related to the decline of osteoblastic function, such as the reduced production of type I collagen, osteocalcin, osteopontin, and other matrix proteins. As a result of the uncoupling of the remodeling process, resorption exceeds formation with an increasing differential. Bone loss in men may accelerate in later years, typically 10 years later than in women, as other body functions begin to decline as well. The reason for bone loss in men has not yet been established, but it may be related to the decline in androgen production by the gonads or the adrenal cortex.

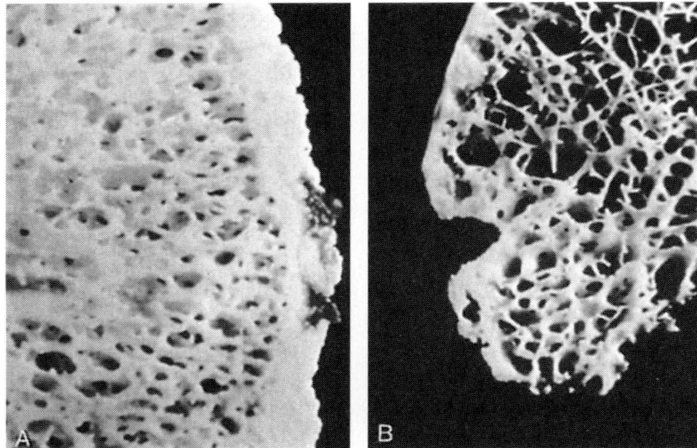

FIGURE 28–6 Difference between normal bone (A) and osteoporotic bone (B). (From Maher AB, Salmond SW, Pellino TA. Orthopaedic nursing. Philadelphia: WB Saunders, 1994, p. 469.)

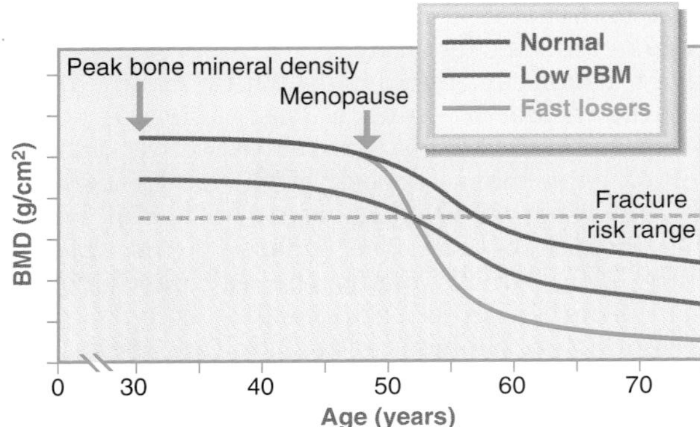

FIGURE 28–7 Variable patterns of bone loss in women after the onset of menopause at approximately 50 years of age. The rapid loss of BMD in some women, referred to as fast losers, is contrasted to the loss of slow losers. Women who start with low peak BMD have less bone mass than women with normal BMD, but they also can lose BMD either as slow or fast losers.

Age-related changes leading to type II osteoporosis in both men and women are not well understood. Impaired calcitriol activity in target tissues, such as the small intestine, is certainly one important factor, and decreased levels of local growth factors, such as insulin-like growth factor 1, that stimulate osteoblasts to increase bone formation, is another (Ebeling et al., 1992; Wakisaka et al., 1998). In addition, some evidence suggests that the loss of estrogens at menopause also permits an increase in the loss of urinary calcium, which continues into late adulthood (Nordin et al., 1991). Information on menopause is available from websites: http://www.menopause.org/ and from the National Osteoporosis Foundation at http://www.nof.org.

NUTRITION AND BONE

Calcium, phosphate, and vitamin D are essential for normal bone structure and function, but several other micronutrients also have essential roles in bone. Nonnutrients such as **phytoestrogens** may also improve the status of bone tissues (see Chapter 12).

Calcium

Calcium from Foods

Calcium intake in the primary prevention of osteoporosis has received much attention. Recommendations for the intakes of calcium and several bone-related nutrients were made in 1998 by the Institute of Medicine (Food and Nutrition Board, 1998). These recommendations are given in Table 28–2. Instead of recommended dietary allowances (RDAs), the new recommendations for calcium and a few other nutrients are given as adequate intakes (AIs), because the Board did not think that the requirements for calcium during the stages of the life cycle were firmly established. The Board expressed its concern that maximizing bone mass during the adolescent growth period was extremely important, by increasing the AI from preadolescence (age 11 years) through adolescence (up to 19 years) to 1300 mg/day (Food and Nutrition Board, 1998), which exceeds the previous RDA of 1200 mg/day (Food and Nutrition Board, 1989).

Calcium intakes often do not meet the desired AI for age, especially for females. According to the U.S. Department of Agriculture (USDA) Household Food Consumption Survey (USDA, 1994), teen and adult women consume considerably less than the current AIs; men are more likely to consume somewhat greater amounts than women, but they do not meet the recommended levels either. These deficits translate, on average, into the need for an additional 500 mg/day for teenage girls and adult women. Although it is recommended that calcium should be supplied by foods because of the coingestion of other essential nutrients, many individuals, especially elderly women, may need to increase their intakes of calcium by using supplements.

A major concern among nutritionists is that a large percentage of girls beyond age 11 are not consuming sufficient amounts of calcium. The importance to adolescents of an adequate calcium intake is unquestioned, even though the precise requirements may not be known with certainty. Reaching AI levels of calcium should be the first goal. In one study, the goal of increasing daily calcium intake from 80% of the RDA to 110% through supplementation with calcium citrate malate resulted in significant increases in spinal and total body bone density in adolescent girls, which may translate into later protection against osteoporosis (Lloyd et al., 1993).

Calcium consumption during childhood and adolescence is beneficial for the acquisition of PBM. An 18-month double-blind study was conducted on BMD of 70 pairs of identical twins to determine the impact of additional calcium from supplements (Johnston et al., 1992). The twins who were given calcium supplements had significantly greater BMD at all sites after 18 months than those given placebo. Mean daily calcium intakes were 908 mg for those taking placebo, and 1612 mg for those taking the supplement. The gain in BMD of the supplemented group, however, did not persist after an additional period of 12 months without supplementation.

Low *calcium bioavailability* from selected foods may adversely affect calcium status. For example, spinach and a few other high oxalate-containing vegetables that contain calcium have low calcium bioavailability (Weaver et al., 1991). Dairy products have high amounts of calcium in a well-absorbed form. Wheat bread may be a good source of calcium for those who consume a lot of bread; green, leafy vegetables such as broccoli, kale, and bok choy have good calcium bioavailability; and calcium from soybeans is also very well absorbed. The amount of calcium in major food sources is listed in Table 28–3. An additional benefit of meeting calcium requirements from foods alone is that the foods containing calcium are also rich in several other nutrients needed for health in general, and for bone health in particular, and that the consumption of a calcium-rich diet from foods is also a marker of a balanced intake with respect to practically all micronutrients (Barger-Lux et al., 1992). Calcium fortification of foods is another way to increase the consumption of

TABLE 28–2 RECOMMENDED INTAKES OF BONE-RELATED NUTRIENTS

AGE (y)	CALCIUM (mg/day)	PHOSPHORUS (mg/day)	MAGNESIUM (mg/day)		VITAMIN D (μg/day)	FLUORIDE (mg/day)	
	AI	RDA	RDA		AI	AI	
1–3	500	460	80		5	0.7	
4–8	800	500	130		5	1.1	
			M	F		M	F
9–13	1300	1250	240	240	5	2.0	2.0
14–18	1300	1250	410	360	5	3.2	3.9
19–30	1000	700	400	310	5	3.8	3.1
31–50	1000	700	420	320	5	3.8	3.1
51–70	1200	700	420	320	10	3.8	3.1
>70	1200	700	420	320	15	3.8	3.1

(From the Food and Nutrition Board, Institute of Medicine, National Academy of Sciences. Dietary reference intakes. Washington, DC: National Academy Press, 1998.)
AI, Adequate intake; RDA, recommended dietary allowance.

TABLE 28–3 CALCIUM IN SELECTED FOODS

FOOD/PORTION	CALCIUM (mg)
Yogurt, part skim, 1 C	415
Sardines, in oil, drained, 3 oz	372
Collard greens, cooked, 1 C	357
Ricotta cheese, ½ C	337
Nonfat milk, 1 C	302
Pudding, vanilla 1 C	298
Whole milk, 1 C	291
Custard, 1 C	297
Buttermilk, 1 C	286
Ice milk, soft serve, 1 C	274
Swiss cheese, 1 oz	272
Turnip greens, cooked 1 C	249
Rhubarb, cooked, 1 C	212
Cheddar cheese, 1 oz	204
Spinach, cooked, 1 C	200
Pumpkin pie, 4 inch section	166
Refried beans, canned, 1 C	141

(Source: Home and Garden Bulletin #72. Human Nutrition Information Service, USDA, 1985.)

calcium by women. Calcium is currently being added to some brands of orange juice at about 300 mg/cup of juice and some brands of soy milk at 200 to 300 mg/cup. It is also added to some breads and other foods.

Although increasing calcium intake for the first several years after menopause has little effect in slowing the high rate of BMD loss of 1% to 2% per year, it remains important to maintain an adequate calcium intake for even a potentially small benefit (Dawson-Hughes et al., 1990). Beyond these early postmenopausal years, however, BMD has been shown to be retained when calcium supplements are taken (Reid et al., 1993). One major benefit of the additional calcium from supplements is the suppression of PTH secretion and, hence, the retention of bone (McKane et al., 1996). Men are thought to respond to adequate intakes of calcium in a similar way as women. Recommendations to meet the current AIs seem reasonable at all ages, including the elderly years, to try to match calcium losses as best as possible and to suppress PTH.

Calcium from Supplements

The bioavailability of calcium supplements depends on the anion used with calcium and many calcium-containing supplements on the market today have good bioavailability. Calcium citrate malate supplements appear to be absorbed slightly more efficiently than calcium carbonate and other calcium supplements, but the difference is typically only a couple of percentage points (Weaver et al., 1991). Calcium carbonate can have a constipating effect that may be minimized by dividing the dose and taking more fluids and fiber. High-dose calcium supplements may reduce the absorption of nonheme iron, and possibly zinc, magnesium, and other divalent cations, but additional evidence is needed to substantiate these potentially adverse interactions. Table 28–4 lists potential risks of calcium supplementation.

Evidence indicates that those with a lifetime history of adequate calcium intake will be at a lower risk of osteoporosis when they are older (Nieves et al., 1995), and it is apparently never too late to start taking calcium supplements.

Achlorhydria is fairly common in elderly subjects, and they have increased difficulty absorbing several specific nutrients that require gastric acid for digestion or release of nutrients from binding molecules within foods, or a more acidic pH in the upper part of the small bowel. For the elderly, it is generally recommended that they take calcium supplements with meals when gastric acid secretion is at its highest, and the same is recommended for iron supplements. Because calcium may interfere with the absorption of the nonheme iron in supplements, it is preferable to take calcium supplements with one meal (e.g., breakfast) and iron supplements with another meal (e.g., dinner or supper).

Phosphate

Phosphates are available in practically all foods, whereas calcium is not so available in the food supply. The simple act of eating foods provides a rather constant amount of phosphate, roughly 1000 to 1200 mg/day for adult women and 1200 to 1400 mg/day for men. Proportionate amounts of calcium are not consumed unless a conscious effort is made to select enough servings of the few calcium-rich foods, but both calcium and phosphate ions in proportionate amounts are needed for the mineralization of bone. Excessive phosphorus intake as phosphates can greatly alter the calcium/phosphate ratio, especially if calcium intakes are low (Calvo and Park, 1996). Too much phosphate compared to calcium stimulates PTH, and, if this pattern of intake is chronic, bone loss follows (see Fig. 28–4).

Vitamin D

Adequate vitamin D intake is important, but excess above the AI should be avoided. Use of excessive vitamin D supplementation may be toxic because high doses induce hypercalcemia and raise the risk

TABLE 28–4 POTENTIAL RISKS ASSOCIATED WITH EXCESSIVE CALCIUM INTAKE*

Contamination of bone meal or dolomite supplements with cadmium, mercury, arsenic, or lead
Urinary tract stones in susceptible individuals
Hypercalcemia from extremely high intakes (4000 mg/day or more)
Milk alkali syndrome from extremely high intakes (4000 mg/day or more)
Deficiency of iron and other mineral divalent cations resulting from decreased absorption
Constipation

(From Committee on Dietary Guidelines, Institute of Medicine, National Academy of Sciences, 1998.)

*2000 mg calcium is safe upper limit (UL) from both foods and supplements.

of soft tissue calcification, especially in the kidneys (see Chapter 4). The AIs for vitamin D across the life cycle are given in Chapter 15. See Appendix 48 for food sources.

Sunlight exposure for skin biosynthesis of vitamin D may be a useful source for persons who commonly obtain little vitamin D from their food intake. However, the skin of older individuals is less efficient in producing vitamin D following exposure to ultraviolet (UV) light (MacLaughlin and Holick, 1985). In addition, elderly subjects living in nursing homes and similar institutions typically have little exposure to sunlight. (See "*Focus On:* Sunshine and Vitamin D" in Chapter 4.) Those who live at northerly latitudes in the United States and Canada may also be at increased risk of osteomalacia and osteoporosis during the winter and spring months because of limited UV light during these seasons (Holick, 1996; Rosen et al., 1994). The elderly may benefit from supplementation in addition to sunlight.

Vitamin D deficiency is associated with secondary hyperparathyroidism and increased bone turnover (Ooms et al., 1995). Low levels of 25-hydroxyvitamin D have been found in free-living elderly women as well as those living in nursing homes (Kinyamu et al., 1997). One report has shown that supplementation of elderly subjects with vitamin D, without a supplement of calcium, contributes to increased BMD or reductions in fractures (Heikinheimo et al., 1991). A study of general medical patients less than 65 years of age and with no known risk factors for hypovitaminosis D admitted to a Boston hospital showed that 42% were vitamin D deficient based on a serum vitamin D analysis, and 22% were severely deficient (Thomas et al., 1998). This suggests that many more people have inadequate intakes than previously thought.

Calcium and vitamin D supplements are often given together to elderly people to reduce the circulating concentration of PTH when it is at the upper end of the normal range (or possibly beyond this limit in a small percentage of elderly hyperparathyroid subjects). The effects of supplements of both calcium and vitamin D on hip fractures were studied in 3270 healthy women aged 78 to 90 years over an 18-month period, using tricalcium phosphate (1200 mg elemental calcium) and 800 IU vitamin D. Half the group received the supplements and half received a placebo. Among the women who completed the study, significant reductions in the loss of BMD and in the rate of hip fractures were found in those who received the supplements (Chapuy et al., 1992). Both calcium (500 mg) and vitamin D (700 IU) supplementation to older women and men for 3 years result in significantly improved BMD and reduced fracture rates (Dawson-Hughes et al., 1997).

Magnesium

More than half of the magnesium in the body is found in bone tissue, but the role of this mineral in bone functions is poorly understood. The largest percentage of the magnesium ions in bone exist in the bone fluids, but a smaller fraction of these ions is bound in the bone crystals, probably at the surfaces only. A small percentage of the magnesium ions is located within bone cells where they serve as enzyme cofactors, as in all other cells (Rude, 1998). The AIs for magnesium across the life cycle are given in Table 28–2.

Vitamin K

Vitamin K is an essential micronutrient for bone health. Its role in post-translational modification of several matrix proteins, including osteocalcin, is now well established. **Osteocalcin,** a bone-specific protein made by osteoblasts, requires vitamin K for its post-translational carboxylation (i.e., maturation). This molecule is secreted into the bone matrix where it appears to be involved in the mineralization process, perhaps acting to stop the formation of crystals to prevent overmineralization. Some osteocalcin is also secreted by osteoblasts directly into the circulating blood. A second way that osteocalcin enters blood is following bone resorption and the release of these molecules, and, in this way, osteocalcin serves as a serum bone marker for predicting the risk of a fracture. For example, elderly women were found to have a significant increase in risk of hip fracture when they had low intakes of vitamin K and undercarboxylation of osteocalcin (Liu and Peacock, 1998; Szulc et al., 1996). Individuals on long-term hemodialysis who consume suboptimal amounts of vitamin K are also at increased risk of fractures (Kohlmeier et al., 1997a).

Many elderly individuals, perhaps as high as 50%, have inadequate intakes of vitamin K, primarily because their consumption of dark green leafy vegetables is so low (Kohlmeier et al., 1997b). The elderly may also be taking medications that reduce vitamin K intake. Antibiotic therapy often depletes vitamin K-producing bacteria and replacement supplementation may be warranted. Others taking coumadin or anticoagulants may have been told by their physicians to avoid dark-green leafy vegetables and supplements containing vitamin K.

Trace Minerals

Trace minerals, especially fluoride, iron, zinc, copper, manganese, and boron, function in bone metabolism, but their roles in preventing bone loss are not well established. In one study, the administration of several trace elements (copper, fluoride, manganese, and zinc) along with calcium for 1 year resulted in a smaller loss of lumbar BMD compared to a control group that received calcium only (Strause et al., 1994).

FLUORIDE. Fluoride enters the hydroxyapatite crystals of bone and, within narrow limits, increases the hardness of bone mineral without any adverse effects. However, at intakes of 2 ppm or greater, fluoride is considered to produce bone that is subject to increased microfractures because of the change in the properties of the hydroxyapatite crystals. Studies regarding use of fluoride in preventing or treating osteoporosis are not yet definitive but warrant review. The AIs for fluoride across the life cycle are given in Table 28–2.

COPPER. Copper is needed for the cross-linking of collagen and elastic molecules, and it may have roles with other enzymes of bone cells.

MANGANESE. Manganese is required for the biosynthesis of mucopolysaccharides in bone matrix formation and as a cofactor in energy-generating reactions.

IRON. Iron serves as a catalytic cofactor for the vitamin C-dependent hydroxylations of proline and lysine in collagen maturation. Iron also has other roles in mitochondrial oxidative phosphorylation in osteoblasts and osteoclasts, as well as in other enzymes, similar to the needs of other cells in the body.

ZINC. Zinc is essential for enzymes in osteoblasts that are responsible for collagen synthesis. In addition, an important enzyme in osteoblasts, alkaline phosphatase, requires zinc for its activity.

BORON. Boron appears to be used by osteoblasts for bone formation, as demonstrated in both rodent and human studies (Nielsen et al., 1992), but whether boron is absolutely required for human bone formation has not yet been settled. It appears that boron is related to magnesium in its effects on bone (Hunt et al., 1997).

Other Dietary Factors

Several other dietary factors associated with bone health have been identified. It is not yet clear how quantitatively important any of these factors is in the typical North American diet.

DIETARY FIBER. Excessive dietary fiber intake may interfere with calcium absorption, but any interference is considered extremely small in the typical U.S. low-fiber diet. Vegans who may consume as much as 50 g of fiber a day would be the individuals most likely to have a significant depression in intestinal calcium absorption.

When consumed in large daily quantities, such as 40 to 50 g, as is common in many vegans, dietary fiber has a modest inhibitory effect on intestinal calcium absorption (Kelsey et al., 1979). In long-term studies, however, the differences in calcium absorption or balance between the high-fiber and control groups were quite small, even though they may have been significantly different. Whether these small differences have an important adverse effect on calcium status among high-fiber consumers is not known with certainty, but most investigators are in agreement that dietary fiber does have a modest effect on calcium bioavailability (Heaney, 1993b; O'Brien et al., 1993). Whether elderly vegans who are postulated to have greater prevalence rates of osteoporosis than omnivores are at a disadvantage from high-fiber diets has not been established; rather it is thought that vegans may be more at risk of developing osteoporosis because of a lower lifetime exposure to physiologic estrogens than omnivores (Anderson and Miller, 1998).

PROTEIN. Excessive protein consumption may lead to increased urinary calcium excretion (Kerstetter and Allen, 1990; Schuette and Linkswiler, 1982). Although high calcium intakes are not significantly affected by a high protein intake, low calcium intakes are generally not sufficient to offset a high protein intake (Heaney, 1993a). Also important is total protein in the diet. Low levels of serum albumin negatively affect transport of serum calcium. Fracture patients may be especially vulnerable to the relationship between low calcium and high protein intakes.

Animal protein increases urinary losses of calcium acutely, that is, with each meal containing large amounts of animal protein, while soy protein has little effect on urinary calcium losses (Anderson et al., 1987). The effects of high levels of protein have not yet been confirmed. See the accompanying box, "*Focus On:* Does a High Animal Protein Diet Increase Urinary Calcium Excretion?"

VEGETARIAN DIETS. Vegetarian diets may be more beneficial than animal protein diets in many respects (Messina, 1994), but they may also contribute to a lower lifetime exposure to estrogens,

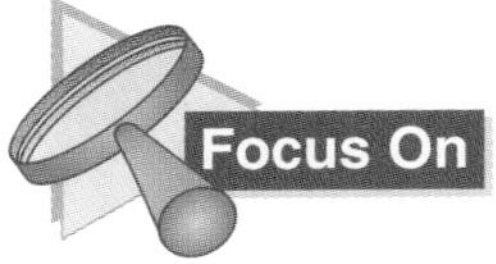

DOES A HIGH ANIMAL PROTEIN DIET INCREASE URINARY CALCIUM EXCRETION?

Two views of the hypercalciuric effect of animal protein exist. One side, supported by most investigators, holds that a good amount of animal protein in a single meal or in the usual dietary pattern induces an additional loss of calcium ions in urine beyond the amount lost on a diet containing minimal amounts of animal protein (Anderson et al., 1987; Kerstetter and Allen, 1990). The mechanisms attributed to the increased loss of calcium include increased acid or hydrogen ion (sulfuric and phosphoric acids) generation from the amino acids that are rich in animal proteins, or the increased secretion of glucose-regulating hormones, including both insulin and glucagon, following the consumption of a protein-rich meal. On the other hand, one investigator has reported data that show little long-term effect of a high-protein (red meat) regimen on urinary calcium excretion (Spencer et al., 1988). These investigators hold that an adaptation to a high-meat diet follows after several days on such a regimen. These two opposing views have not been resolved.

which could increase the risk of osteoporotic fractures in vulnerable individuals (Anderson and Miller, 1998).

SODIUM. High sodium intakes, particularly in association with low calcium intakes, can contribute to osteoporosis because they result in an increase in calcium excretion (Nordin, 1993). Data from one study suggest that reducing daily sodium excretion by 50% (from 3450 to 1725 mg/day) can reduce bone loss to the same extent as increasing daily calcium intake by 891 mg (Devine et al., 1995).

POTASSIUM BICARBONATE. In postmenopausal women, an oral dose of potassium bicarbonate sufficient to neutralize endogenous acid improves calcium balance and bone. Decreased bone resorption and an increased rate of bone formation result. The skeleton serves as a buffer to help regulate acid–base balance, and a high-acid diet may contribute to the progressive decline in bone mass and osteoporosis (Barzel, 1995; Kraut and Coburn, 1994; Sebastian, 1994).

PHYTOESTROGENS. The isoflavones in soybeans, which function both as phytoestrogens and antioxidants, may result in the inhibition of bone resorption (Anderson and Garner, 1997). Populations with low calcium intakes from dairy products, such as the Japanese, may have some protection against osteoporosis and hip fractures when the intake of soy foods is high. Phytoestrogens are similar to selective estrogen receptor modulators (SERMs) (see below), because they appear to promote bone health without stimulating proliferation of reproductive tissues.

CAFFEINE. The relationship of moderate consumption of caffeine to osteoporosis has not been clearly established. One study suggests that excessive caffeine intake may have a deleterious effect on BMD of women, even if they consume adequate amounts of calcium (Massey and Whiting, 1993). Excessive intakes are considered to be 2 or more cups of caffeinated coffee a day over the adult decades (20 years and older). Caffeine may have an adverse effect on calcium balance in older women who do not compensate for their less effective intestinal absorption of calcium, with sufficient amounts of calcium-rich dairy products (Harris and Dawson-Hughes, 1994). Another study, however, showed that BMD was not affected by lifetime coffee intake if the subjects drank at least one glass of milk daily during adulthood (Barrett-Connor, 1994). More recently it was shown that caffeine does not appear to influence bone loss in healthy postmenopausal women (Lloyd et al., 1997).

ALCOHOL. Alcohol (ethanol) intake generally has adverse effects on the skeleton. Several reports have implicated alcohol as a major contributor to bone loss (Moniz, 1994). Heavy alcohol consumption of over two drinks per day, however, is often accompanied by poor dietary intake and cigarette smoking, especially in women. This confounds the effect of alcohol because many nutrients are also missing.

OSTEOPOROSIS

Osteoporosis, a disease that generally manifests itself late in life, may have its origin in early life during the period of skeletal growth and PBM accumulation. Although women have almost twice the hip fracture rate as men, the rate in men will increase as the average life span continues to lengthen. Practically everyone over 80 years of age can be said to be osteoporotic and at risk for a hip fracture.

The bone loss that begins in mid-adult life, that is, after age 40, and continues into old age is a normal process. Bone composition is unchanged, but both the BMC and BMD decrease with age. **Osteoporosis** occurs when the bone mineral density becomes so low that the skeleton is unable to sustain ordinary strains, a condition marked by the occurrence of fractures. Deterioration of bone tissue, especially trabecular bone tissue, results in microfractures, another essential feature of osteoporosis.

The World Health Organization (WHO) definitions are based on measurements of BMD by DXA (Kanis et al., 1994). The standard BMD values for comparison are the mean values for 20 to 29 year olds because this age group is considered to represent the healthiest adults who have essentially achieved peak bone density. **Osteopenia,** low BMD, is a precursor state to the more severe osteoporosis. The definitions of osteopenia and osteoporosis are given in Table 28–5.

Prevalence of Osteoporotic Fractures

In the early 1990s, approximately 25 million Americans were affected by osteoporosis, and 1.5 million fractures occur annually as a result, at a cost of over $10 billion in health care. Half of these osteoporosis-related fractures involve the vertebrae; 200,000 are fractures of the hip, which result in incapacitation, long-term nursing care, and frequently death. Although incidence rates of fractures in the United States are not expected to increase substantially, the actual numbers (prevalence) are predicted to increase greatly until 2030 (Melton, 1997). Statistics indicate that women are about four times more likely than men to develop osteoporosis, although with aging, all people gradually lose bone mass and become more vulnerable. Recent data on low femoral BMD for men and women in the United States have been compiled from analyses of National Health and Nutrition Examination Survey (NHANES III) findings (Looker et al., 1995, 1997).

TABLE 28–5 WORLD HEALTH ORGANIZATION DEFINITIONS OF OSTEOPENIA AND OSTEOPOROSIS

	EXTENT BELOW MEAN BMD OF 20–29 YEAR OLDS
Osteopenia	1–2.5 standard deviations
Osteoporosis	> 2.5 standard deviations

(From Kanis JA, et al. The diagnosis of osteoporosis. J Bone Miner Res 9:1137, 1994.)

TABLE 28–6 CHARACTERISTICS OF PRIMARY OSTEOPOROSIS: TYPES I AND II

	TYPE I	TYPE II
Gender	Females; rare in males	Female and male
Age/Period of life cycle	Menopause (~50 y)	Beyond 65 years of age
Bone tissue	Trabecular	Trabecular and cortical
Fracture sites	Lumbar vertebrae and wrists	Hips and vertebrae; any other bone in the skeleton
Etiology	Loss of estrogens or androgens	Aging—otherwise poorly understood

(Adapted from data published in Riggs BL, Melton LJ III: Involutional osteoporosis. N Engl J Med 314:1676, 1986.)

Types of Osteoporosis

The two types of **primary** or **idiopathic osteoporosis** are distinguished by the sex of the individuals, the age at which fractures occur, and the kinds of bone involved. Table 28–6 lists the characteristics of these two types of osteoporosis. Osteoporosis should be considered, however, to be a disease with a broad spectrum of variant forms of the disorder. Only for simplicity is the classification of the two types used here.

Type I, postmenopausal osteoporosis, occurs in women within a few years of menopause, and it primarily involves loss of trabecular bone tissue because of a cessation of ovarian production of estrogens. Men may also develop type I osteoporosis during adulthood if they have a significant decline in androgen production. Type I osteoporosis is characterized by fractures of the distal radius (Colles' fractures) and crush fractures of the lumbar vertebrae that are often painful and deforming. Acceleration of the process that occurs in women after menopause is directly related to the lack of estrogen. BMC and BMD of the lumbar spine of women with postmenopausal osteoporosis have been measured at levels 33% lower than in age-matched nonosteoporotic controls (Seeman et al., 1989). Other areas with a preponderance of trabecular bone, such as the pelvis and the proximal femur, are also typically affected in postmenopausal osteoporosis.

Type II, or **age-associated osteoporosis,** occurs around age 65 and beyond, and it affects both sexes. Both types of bone tissue, cortical and trabecular, undergo remodeling, but the greater degree of remodeling occurs in trabecular tissue. In the elderly period, the processes of bone resorption and bone formation become uncoupled. Fractures of the hips characterize type II osteoporosis, but vertebral fractures continue to increase with age. A dramatic increase in hip fractures occurs late in life, and almost all women beyond 80 years of age are at risk for hip fractures. Wedge fractures of vertebrae typically lead to back pain, loss of height, spinal deformity, and kyphosis, or "dowager's hump" (Fig. 28–8). Many women lose several inches in height between 50 and 80 years of age. Fractures may occur during ordinary activities, such as lifting a sack of groceries or stepping over a shower opening, but a large percentage of the hip fractures result from a fall.

Although age-associated osteoporosis affects both sexes, women are more severely affected because they have a smaller skeletal mass than men, and they live longer. Hip fractures affect nearly 20% of postmenopausal women up to age 80 and almost 50% of those beyond that age (Anderson, 1990).

Secondary osteoporosis results when an identifiable drug (Table 28–7) or disease process (Table 28–8) causes loss of bone tissue.

Etiology and Pathophysiology

Osteoporosis is a complex heterogeneous disorder of unknown etiology. Why otherwise normal processes lead to bone density inadequate to support the body in some people is not known. Although the fracture-precipitating condition of inadequate bone mass is common to all types of osteoporosis, the processes by which this end is reached probably result from etiologies distinctive to each of the types or the many forms of the disease.

Loss of bone mass to a degree that produces frac-

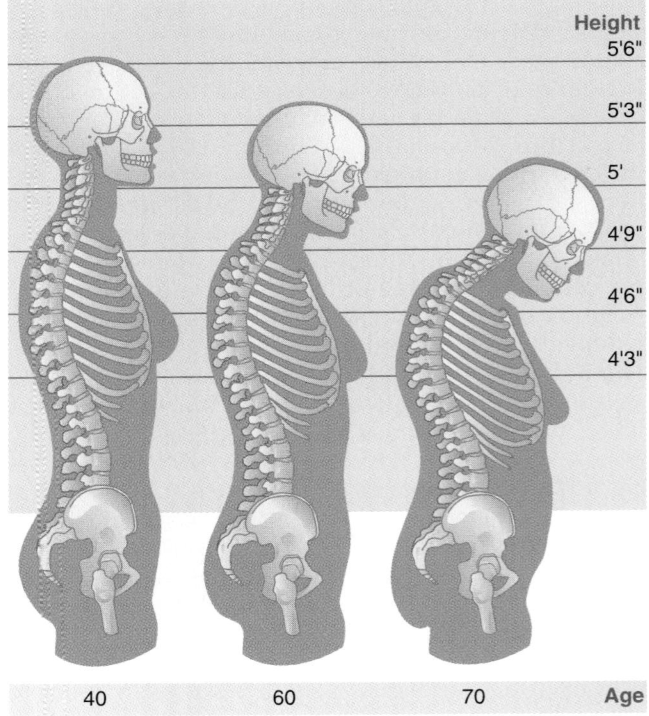

FIGURE 28–8 Normal spine at age 40 and osteoporotic changes at ages 60 and 70. These changes can cause a loss of as much as 6 to 9 inches in height and result in the so-called dowager's hump (far right) in the upper thoracic vertebrae.

TABLE 28–7 COMMON DRUGS THAT INCREASE CALCIUM LOSS

Phenytoin (Dilantin)	Lithium
Phenobarbital	Tetracycline
Thyroid hormone	Aluminum-containing antacids
Corticosteroids	Heparin
Methotrexate	Phenothiazine derivatives
Cyclosporin	

tures can result from (1) an excessive acceleration of loss, especially after menopause, or (2) a peak bone mass so low that after enough normal wearing down, the bones become fragile and susceptible to fracture (see Fig. 28–9).

Risk Factors

Risk factors for osteoporosis include age, race, sex, body weight, family history, premature menopause, nulliparity, number of lactations, dietary factors, limited exercise, use of cigarettes, excessive alcohol consumption, and prolonged use of medications (Table 28–9).

RACE AND ETHNICITY. Whites and Asians suffer more osteoporotic fractures than blacks and Hispanics, who have a greater bone density. Data now suggest that differences exist between blacks and whites in bone metabolism (Perry et al., 1993), but more studies are needed to explain the differences, especially for the intake of lactose, vitamin D, and calcium. Hypovitaminosis D with secondary hyperparathyroidism (Fig. 28–9) occurs more often in the black population. Petite or thin women, particularly of northern European extraction, are more susceptible to osteoporosis (Edelstein and Barrett-Conner, 1993).

MENSTRUAL STATUS. Loss of menses at any age is a major determinant of osteoporosis risk in women. Acceleration of bone loss coincides with menopause, either natural or surgical, at which time the ovaries stop producing estrogen. Estrogen and hormone replacement therapy have been shown to conserve BMD and reduce the risk following menopause, but young amenorrheic women may also benefit from the use of oral contraceptive agents to promote a normal menstrual cycle (Lindsay et al., 1986).

TABLE 28–8 DISEASES OR CONDITIONS THAT RESULT IN NEGATIVE CALCIUM BALANCE AND RISK FOR DEVELOPING OSTEOPOROSIS

Hyperthyroidism
Diabetes
Chronic renal failure
Chronic diarrhea or malabsorption
Hyperparathyroid disease
Chronic obstructive lung disease
Subtotal gastrectomy
Hemiplegia

TABLE 28–9 RISK FACTORS FOR DEVELOPING OSTEOPOROSIS

Family history of osteoporosis
Female
White or Asian
Slight body build
Estrogen depletion
Menopause
Early oophorectomy in women
Hypogonadism in men
Hypogonadism in women with excessive exercise
Age: especially after age 60
Lack of exercise
Prolonged use of certain medications (see Table 28–7)
Diseases or conditions that affect calcium and bone metabolism (see Table 28–8)
Underweight or underfat
Cigarette smoking
Excessive alcohol consumption
Very excessive fiber consumption
Excessive caffeine consumption
Inadequate calcium or vitamin D intake

Any interruption of menstruation for an extended period results in bone loss. The amenorrhea that accompanies excessive weight loss seen in patients with anorexia nervosa or in individuals who participate in high-intensity sports, dance, or other forms of exercise has the same adverse effect on bones as menopause. BMD in amenorrheic athletes has been measured at levels 25% to 40% below control levels. When menses were resumed in these athletes, bone mass increased, but eventually plateaued at a level lower than that of sedentary women (Drinkwater et al., 1986). Young women with the athlete triad of disordered eating, amenorrhea, and low BMD are at increased risk for having fractures while involved in athletics (Anderson et al., 1997) (see Chapter 25).

LACTATION. A striking but transient bone loss, especially from the femoral neck and lumbar spine, occurs in women who breast-feed for 6 months or longer (Sowers et al., 1993). Sufficient calcium and vitamin D intake are essential during this time for the mother to replete her own serum and storage levels, but repletion typically does not occur until several months after peak lactation (Kalkwarf et al., 1997). Many lactations over a few years may contribute to significant bone loss by the end of the period of childbearing, and nursing twins or triplets presumably results in a significant loss of bone mass because of the significant elevation of PTH (Greer et al., 1984) (see Chapter 7).

LIMITED EXERCISE. Immobility in varying degrees is well recognized as a cause of bone loss (Fig. 28–10). Maintenance of healthy bone requires exposure to weight-bearing pressures. Stresses from muscle contraction and maintaining the body in an upright position against the pull of gravity stimulate osteoblast function. Bones not subjected to normal use rapidly lose mass. Persons confined to bed

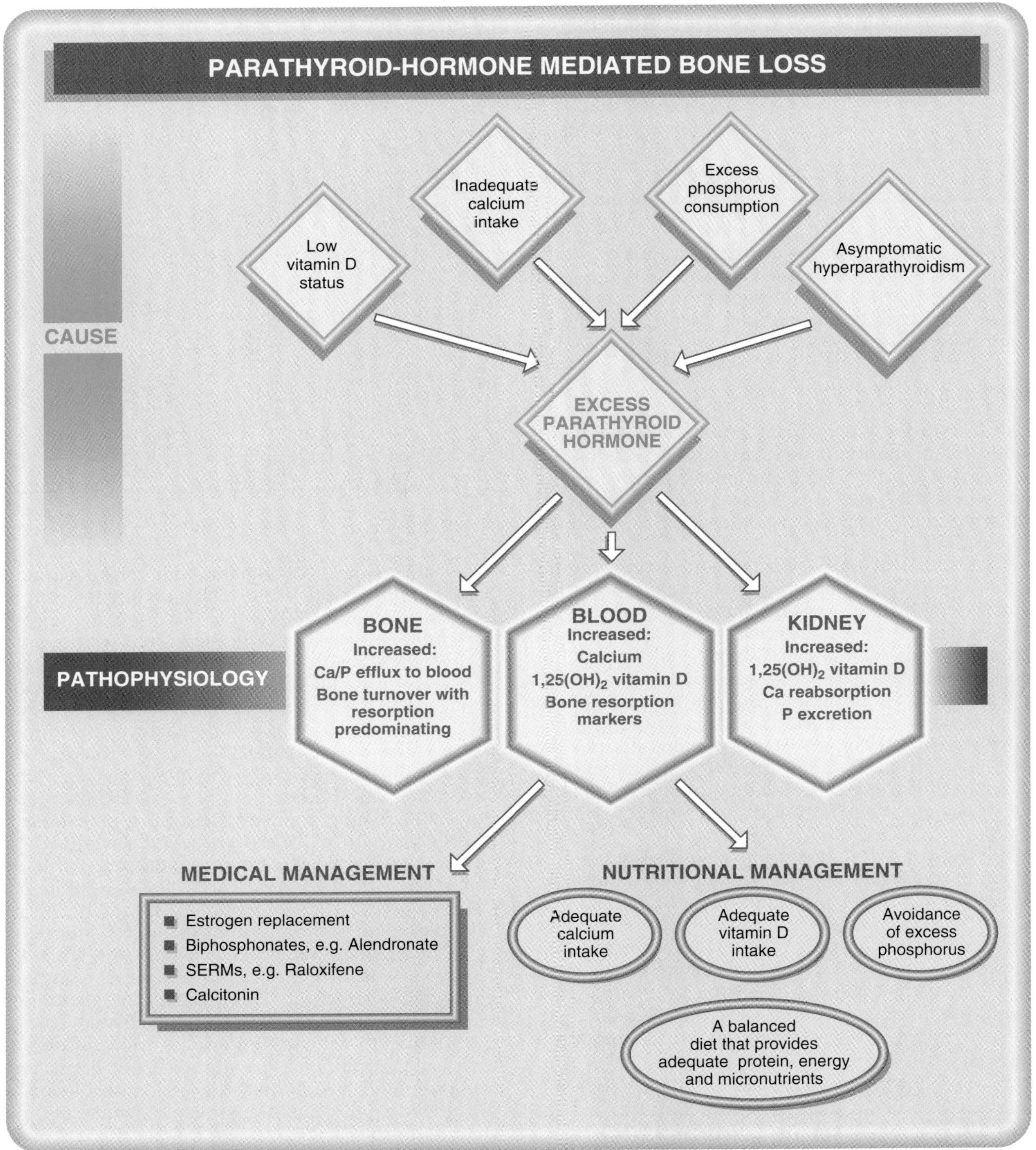

FIGURE 28–9 Pathophysiology algorithm—parathyroid hormone-mediated bone loss. SERMs, selective estrogen receptor modulators. (Algorithm content developed by John Anderson, PhD, and Sanford C. Garner, PhD., 2000.)

and those unable to move freely are commonly affected. Astronauts living in conditions of zero gravity for only a few days experience so much bone loss that appropriate exercise is a feature of their daily routines. To a lesser degree, lack of exercise and a sedentary mode of living that continue over a lifetime also contribute significantly to bone loss, although their most important influence is probably on inadequate accumulation of bone mass (Fig. 28–10).

Physical activity, especially upper body activities, may also contribute to an increase in bone mass or

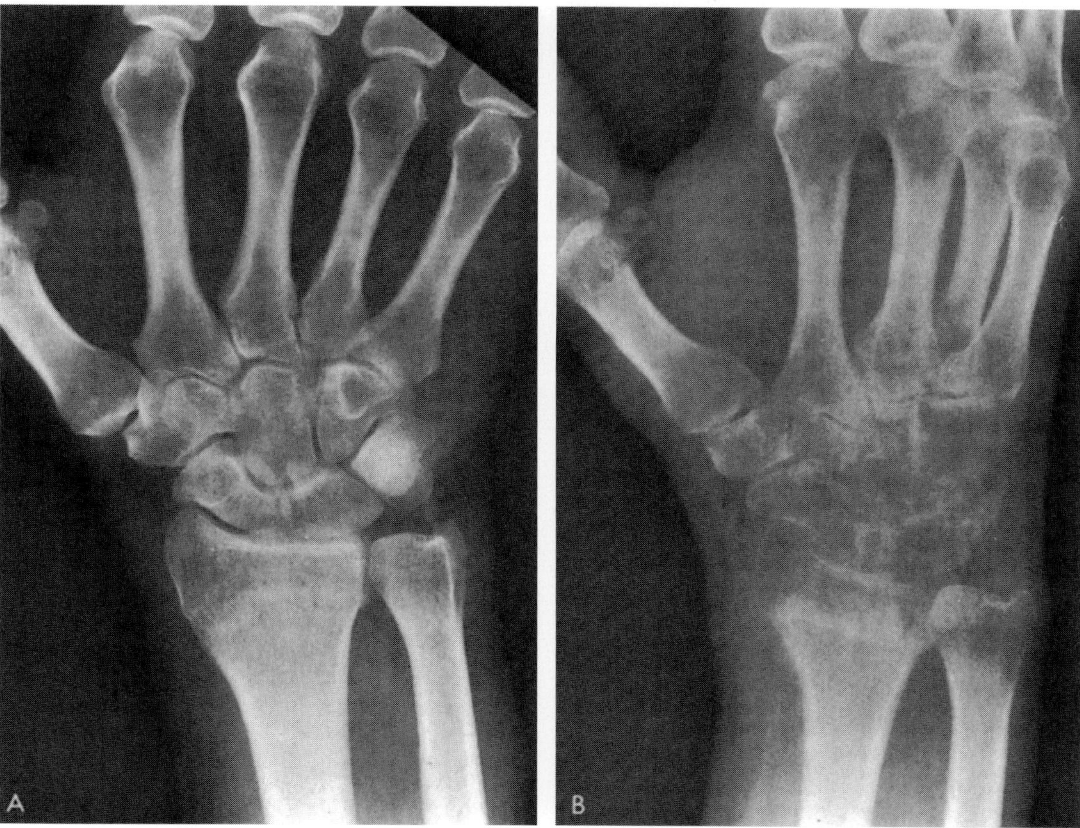

FIGURE 28–10 (A) Roentgenogram of the carpal area shortly after fracture of the distal radius. The part was immobilized by a plaster cast. (B) Roentgenogram of the same area several weeks after immobilization. Note the disuse atrophy of the carpal bones. (From Aegerter EE, Kirkpatrick JA. Orthopedic diseases: Physiology, pathology, radiology, 4th ed. Philadelphia: WB Saunders, 1975, p. 32.)

density. A few studies of postmenopausal women have shown that a shift from relative inactivity to a high-activity regimen may increase bone measurements by a significant amount, whether a woman is on ERT or not (Fig. 28–11).

BODY WEIGHT. Body weight (mass) is an important factor that affects BMC and BMD. The greater the body mass, the greater the BMD; and the converse is also true, the lower the body mass, the lower the BMD. For example, young girls who are typically premenarcheal may incur fractures with minimal trauma, in part because of low BMC and BMD related to rapid growth in height that is not accompanied with a proportionate increase in weight (Goulding et al., 1998). Weight loss in dieting subjects is also typically associated with bone loss. The reason for the greater BMD in heavier individuals relates largely to the load (weight) that is borne by the different skeletal sites. The non–weight-bearing bones of the arms are less affected by body weight than they are by repetitive use in physical activities.

DIETARY FACTORS. Many nutrients and several nonnutrients have been implicated as etiologic risk factors for osteoporosis. Several of these nutrients have been covered in the previous section. The nonnutrients like dietary fiber, phytoestrogens, and many other plant molecules may also play important roles in either maintaining bone or contributing to bone loss. Exposure to a few nonnutrients in some vegan diets may have adverse effects on lifetime estrogen exposure of the skeleton. This may, therefore, contribute to lower bone mass and possi-

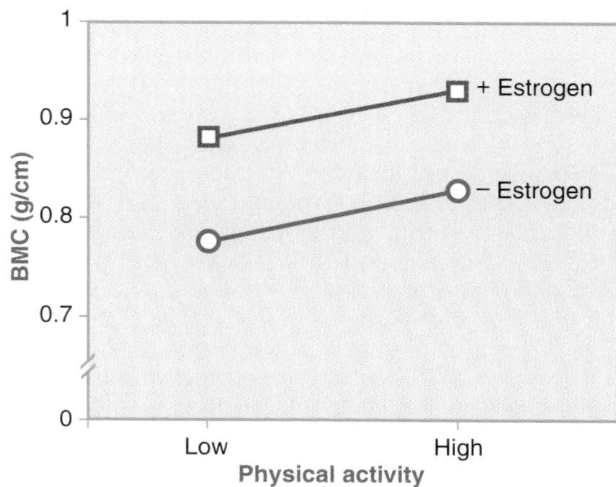

FIGURE 28–11 Effects of physical activity and estrogen treatment on trabecular bone mineral content (BMC) of postmenopausal women. Estrogen improves BMC whether women are exercising at a high or low level.

bly increase the risk of osteoporosis compared to that in omnivores (Anderson and Miller, 1998).

MEDICATIONS. A number of medications contribute to osteoporosis, either by interfering with calcium absorption or by actively promoting calcium loss from bone (see Table 28–7). Steroids, for example, affect vitamin D metabolism and can lead to bone loss. Excessive amounts of exogenous thyroid hormone, even in very low amounts, can promote loss of bone mass over time (Schneider et al., 1994).

ALCOHOL AND CIGARETTES. Cigarette smoking and excessive alcohol consumption are risk factors for developing osteoporosis, probably because of toxic effects on the osteoblasts. However, occasional social drinking was found to be associated with higher bone density after adjusting for age, sex, body mass index, smoking, exercise, and estrogen replacement (in women) (Holbrook and Barrett-Connor, 1993). However, daily excesses over two drinks should be avoided (see "*Focus On:* The Impact of Alcohol and Cigarettes on the Skeleton—A Double Whammy!!").

Prevention and Treatment

Because virtually all elderly are affected by osteoporosis, the increasing longevity of the population emphasizes the need for prevention of osteoporosis, especially after menopause and later in life. Secondary prevention is a form of treatment following the development of osteoporosis, either type I or type II. Primary prevention applies to individuals who have no osteoporotic disease, typically adults under age 50.

Because bone health is influenced by the three major interacting factors of diet, exercise, and estrogen, it is never too early or too late to prevent or lessen the onset and severity of osteoporosis. Ensuring adequate intakes of calcium from foods (and supplements), engaging in regular weight-bearing exercises, and, if necessary, taking bone-conserving drugs, such as ERT, bisphosphonates, or SERMs may be beneficial. The weight-bearing exercises and estrogens may have additive effects on the BMD of older women (Kohrt et al., 1995).

Estrogen Replacement Therapy

Estrogen replacement therapy (ERT) is one method for reducing bone resorption and arresting postmenopausal bone loss in women. It is most effective when used during the first 5 to 15 years after menopause, but even if estrogen is started a few years after menopause, it can still reduce the fracture rate. Some evidence suggests that ERT, combined with high calcium supplementation, may result in increased BMD (Aloia et al., 1994). A smaller dose of estrogen may be as effective as the standard dose in women who are also consuming 1500 mg calcium daily (Ettinger et al., 1987). However, a high calcium intake alone will not substitute for ERT in blunting postmenopausal bone loss.

Hazards of ERT include the possible risk of endometrial cancer; however, adding progestin lowers that risk. Return of the menses, however, discourages its use for some women. Serious concerns about breast cancer remain and it has been reported that breast cancer rates are higher in ERT or hormone replacement users than nonusers. Some evidence suggests that women who use estrogen long-term and who consume two or more drinks of

THE IMPACT OF ALCOHOL AND CIGARETTES ON THE SKELETON—A DOUBLE WHAMMY!!

Cigarette smoking is a risk factor for vertebral, forearm, and hip fractures, especially in slender women. In a cross-sectional study of bone density at the lumbar spine and the femoral neck and shaft in 41 pairs of twins, bone density was 0.9% to 2% lower for every 10 pack-years of smoking (Hopper and Seeman, 1994). Smoking was also associated with higher follicle-stimulating hormone (FSH) and luteinizing hormone (LH) and lower serum parathyroid hormone levels, serum calcium, and urinary pyridinoline concentrations, a marker for bone resorption. Conclusions of this study suggest that women who smoke about one pack of cigarettes daily will have an average deficit of 5% to 10% in bone density, which increases the risk of fracture. A meta-analysis of 48 studies of smokers and nonsmokers showed that by age 85 the estimated cumulative risk for hip fracture was 19% in smokers and 12% in nonsmokers. There was a dose response—the more the woman smoked, the greater the risk of fracture (Law and Hackshaw, 1997).

The strong correlation between reproductive function and bone mass and density appears to be affected by smoking through a decrease in estrogens. Women who smoke enter menopause 1 to 2 years earlier and lose bone more rapidly than nonsmokers (Slemenda, 1994). Females who smoke need to be educated about the risk of a decrease in BMD, which may lead to an increase in fractures.

Alcohol, especially excessive consumption (more than two drinks a day) for an extended period of time, results in bone loss because the metabolism of alcohol generates additional acid that is buffered in part by the skeleton. One research group in Finland suggests that alcohol consumption is a major risk factor for osteoporosis in young and middle-aged women (Laitinen et al., 1993). The combination of smoking and alcohol, so common among young women, places them at increased risk for osteoporosis, because both these risk factors operate to reduce BMD. Men are affected in a similar way.

alcohol a day are at increased risk of breast cancer (Colditz et al., 1995).

Bisphosphonates

The **bisphosphonates** act on osteoclasts to reduce their resorptive activities. Examples include etidronate and alendronate.

ETIDRONATE. Etidronate is a bisphosphonate, chemically related to pyrophosphate. Its effect is to inhibit osteoclast-mediated bone resorption. After 3 years, cyclic administration of etidronate to women with postmenopausal osteoporosis provides greatly increased vertebral bone mineral content and reduced fractures. Seven years of treatment has demonstrated long-term beneficial effects on the maintenance of BMD (Miller et al., 1997).

ALENDRONATE. The skeletal benefits of alendronate have been similar to those of etidronate, but alendronate has been somewhat more effective in fracture reduction (Lieberman et al., 1995). This drug has become widely accepted in the United States and other nations, but it may result in esophageal reflux, a side effect that makes it difficult for a small subset of the population to continue this oral therapy every day. This drug may also be used in combination with a SERM (see below) or another bone-conserving drug in an effort to protect the skeleton.

Selective Estrogen Receptor Modulators (SERMs)

Drugs that positively affect **estrogen receptors** in bone tissue, but have little effect on reproductive tissues of the breast or uterus, are known as **selective estrogen receptor modulators (SERMs).** Two examples of these drugs in the marketplace are *tamoxifen* and *raloxifene*. *Genistein*, a phytoestrogen found in soy foods, may act as a SERM (see Chapter 12).

TAMOXIFEN. Tamoxifen was developed as an antiestrogen to help prevent breast cancer, and it was found by chance to conserve bone. This drug is not prescribed, however, for preventing bone loss.

RALOXIFENE. Raloxifene is the most recent drug approved by the Food and Drug Administration (FDA) for the express purpose of maintaining bone and reducing fractures. The first report on this drug supports its efficacy (Delmas et al., 1998), and additional studies are anticipated.

Other Drug Treatments

CALCITONIN. Calcitonin, a hormone, is used as a drug to inhibit osteoclastic bone resorption by blocking the stimulatory effects of PTH on these cells. Calcitonin therapy decreases the rate of bone loss in osteoporotic women; however, it is most effective if given early after menopause. Calcitonin was previously administered by subcutaneous injection, but now there is an effective nasal spray. Calcitonin treatment improves BMD, especially of the lumbar spine, and it may reduce the recurrence of fractures in patients with osteoporosis.

SODIUM FLUORIDE. Dramatic increases in bone mass, especially in trabecular bone, follow treatment with sodium fluoride. However, incorporating fluoride into hydroxyapatite alters the size and structure of the crystals and may decrease the mechanical competence of the bone. Fluoride clearly increases bone mass in patients with osteoporosis, but can alter the structural integrity of the new bone, even to the point of increasing fractures (Pak et al., 1994). Side effects include irritation of the gastric mucosa and lower extremity pain. Fluoride therapy has so far not been approved by the FDA and must still be regarded as experimental.

VITAMIN D. The AI for vitamin D intakes of the elderly have been greatly increased (see Table 28–2), but supplements are most likely necessary because it is almost impossible for the elderly to consume this amount from foods. Maintenance of an adequate dietary intake of vitamin D (200 IU or 5 μg cholecalciferol) is important for healthy younger adults, but it is inadequate for the many housebound elderly who fail to get adequate exposure to sunlight.

CALCITRIOL. Calcitriol, or 1,25-dihydroxyvitamin D without calcium, has had little use in the treatment of osteoporosis because of its potential toxicity. In elderly women with high PTH levels, calcitriol levels were similar to those seen in people with secondary hyperparathyroidism (Ledger et al., 1994). Calcium plus calcitriol may be useful, however, with high-dose corticosteroid therapy, during which vertebral fractures are common. In one study patients who were given 1000 mg calcium and calcitriol (0.5 to 1.0 μg) were found to lose less lumbar BMD after 1 year (Sambrook et al., 1993). Other investigators have also shown the benefits of countering the adverse effects of glucocorticoids on bone with calcium or calcitriol or both (Reid et al., 1994).

Dietary Treatment

A novel approach to the dietary treatment of patients who are recovering from hip fractures, however, has been shown to be effective. Elderly patients with hip fractures were found to benefit from protein supplements coupled with adequate amounts of micronutrients. In one study, clinical outcomes and BMD were improved in patients who were given 250 mL daily of a liquid supplement containing 20 g protein, 525 mg calcium, 750 IU vitamin A, and 25 IU vitamin D for an average of 38 days (Tkatch et al., 1992).

Other Treatment Modalities

Several approaches to preventing fractures have been examined. These approaches include exercise, strength activities, falls prevention education, ultraviolet lamps, and special hip padding from girdles.

EXERCISE. Physical activities, such as regular walking and swimming, appear to have little or no skeletal benefits for older individuals, but more active participation, such as weight-bearing exercises and intensive walking, have positive effects on BMD (Dalsky et al., 1988; Notelovitz et al., 1991; Prince et al., 1991). A recent study of over 9000 mostly white women over age 64 and living in the community showed that the active women had 36% lower risk for a hip fracture (Gregg et al., 1998).

STRENGTH ACTIVITIES. Upper-body strength activities have been shown to improve bone measurements of the proximal femur (Snow-Harter et al., 1990). In terms of prevention, these types of activities have been underutilized. In very old men strength exercises of the thigh muscles resulted in significant improvement of strength, and possibly of BMD of the femur, although the latter was not measured (Fiatarone et al., 1990).

PREVENTION OF FALLS. Fractures of the humerus, wrist, pelvis, and hip are considered to be age-related, resulting from a combination of osteoporosis and falling. Although only 5% of falls result in fractures, preventing falls through education and attention to the living environment of the very old is an important measure (Cummings, 1995).

HIP PROTECTOR GIRDLES. The wearing of girdles with built-in pads to protect the hips during a fall has been demonstrated in Denmark to significantly reduce the rate of fractures in a well-controlled investigation (Lauritzen et al., 1993).

UV LAMPS. The development of new UV lamps, with built-in safety against excessive skin damage, may be a potential way to improve vitamin D status of elderly individuals, especially those living in nursing homes and similar institutions.

CASE STUDY

Annie B., a 70-year-old white woman of Northern European ancestry, developed lactose intolerance during her early sixties when she had a serious gastrointestinal infection. She currently is retired, lives alone with her cat, and stays indoors most of each day watching television. Approximately 3 years earlier at age 67, she had DXA measurements, which showed that she had low BMD values of her proximal femur and lumbar vertebrae (both values would be classified as osteoporotic according to WHO definitions). Her physician recommended that she start taking supplements of calcium (1000 mg/day) and vitamin D (600 IU/day) because of her lactose intolerance and her lack of consumption of all dairy products.

Annie took the supplements regularly for a year when a second set of DXA measurements revealed that she maintained her BMD values of 1 year earlier rather than having any loss. The continuing low measurements, however, concerned her physician, and he ordered laboratory tests of calcium-regulatory hormones to see if she had any hormonal complications. These tests showed that her PTH and 25-hydroxyvitamin D concentrations fell in the upper half of the normal range for each variable. Other routine measurements, such as serum calcium and phosphate, were normal. Her physician, in consultation with Annie, decided to place her on a bisphosphonate (alendronate), because she refused to consider taking estrogen. After 1 year on the new therapy plus continuing the calcium and vitamin D, her BMD values (her third set of DXA measurements) actually increased a few percentage points, even though they remained within the classification of osteoporosis. Her physician instructed her to continue on this therapeutic regimen.

1. How would you classify Annie's calcium intake at the initial visit with her physician (who did not take a diet history or estimate her calcium intake)? Her vitamin D intake? Her exposure to sunlight?
2. What would you have recommended to improve her calcium intake from foods so that she could reduce her supplemental calcium to 500 mg/day? Why would you recommend foods to provide calcium rather than supplements?
3. Design a set (3 days minimum) of daily menus that provide approximately 800 mg calcium from foods alone that coupled with a 500-mg supplement would provide a total of 1300 mg, the current AI for calcium.

CITED REFERENCES

Aloia J, et al. Calcium supplementation with and without hormone replacement therapy to prevent postmenopausal bone loss. Ann Intern Med 120:97, 1994.

Anderson JJB, Garner SC. The effects of phytoestrogens on bone. Nutr Res 17:1617, 1997.

Anderson JJB, Miller C. Lower lifetime estrogen exposure among vegetarians as a possible risk factor for osteoporosis: A hypothesis. Vegetarian Nutr 2:4, 1998.

Anderson JJB, Pollitzer WS. Ethnic and genetic differences in susceptibility to osteoporotic fractures. In: Draper HH (ed.). Advances in Nutritional Research, vol. 9. New York: Plenum Press, 1994, p. 129.

Anderson JJB, Rondano PA. Peak bone mass development of females: Can young adult women improve their peak bone mass? J Am Coll Nutr 15:570, 1996.

Baran DT, et al. Broadband ultrasound attenuation of the calcaneus predicts lumbar and femoral neck density in Caucasian women: A preliminary study. Osteoporosis Int 1:110, 1991.

Barger-Lux MJ, et al. Nutritional correlates of low calcium intake. Clin Appl Nutr 2(4):39, 1992.

Barrett-Connor E. Coffee-associated osteoporosis offset by daily milk consumption: The Rancho Bernardo Study. JAMA 271:280, 1994.

Barzel US. The skeleton as an ion exchange system: Implications for the role of acid–base imbalance in the genesis of osteoporosis. J Bone Miner Res 10:1431, 1995.

Bassey EJ, Ramsdale SJ. Increase in femoral bone density in young women following high impact exercises. Osteoporosis Int 4:72, 1994.

Calvo MS, Park YK. Changing phosphorus content of the US diet: Potential for adverse effects on bone. J Nutr 126:1168S, 1996.

Chapuy M, et al. Vitamin D and calcium to prevent hip fractures in elderly women. N Engl J Med 327:1637, 1992.

Christiansen C, et al. Prediction of rapid bone loss in postmenopausal women. Lancet 1:1105, 1987.

Colditz GA, et al. The use of estrogens and progestins and the risk of breast cancer in postmenopausal women. N Engl J Med 332:1589, 1995.

Cummings SR, et al. Risk factors for hip fractures in white women. N Engl J Med 332:767, 1995.

Dalsky G, et al. Weight-bearing exercise training and lumbar bone mineral content in postmenopausal women. Ann Intern Med 108:824, 1988.

Dawson-Hughes B, et al. A controlled trial of the effect of calcium supplementation on bone density in postmenopausal women. N Engl J Med 323:878, 1990.

Dawson-Hughes B, et al. Effect of calcium and vitamin D supplementation on bone density in men and women 65 years of age or older. N Engl J Med 337:670, 1997.

Delmas PD, et al. Effects of raloxifene on bone mineral density, serum cholesterol concentrations, and uterine endometrium in postmenopausal women. N Engl J Med 337:1641, 1997.

Devine A, et al. A longitudinal study of the effect of sodium and calcium intakes on regional bone density in postmenopausal women. Am J Clin Nutr 62:740, 1995.

Drinkwater BL, et al. Bone mineral density after resumption of menses in amenorrheic athletes. JAMA 256:380, 1986.

Ebeling PR, et al. Evidence of an age-related decrease in intestinal responsiveness to vitamin D: Relationship between serum 1,25-dihydroxyvitamin D_3 and intestinal vitamin D receptor concentrations in normal women. J Clin Endocrinol Metab 75:176, 1992.

Edelstein S, Barrett-Connor E. Relation between body size and bone mineral density in elderly men and women. Am J Epidemiol 138:160, 1993.

Ettinger B, et al. Postmenopausal bone loss is prevented by treatment with low-dosage estrogen with calcium. Ann Intern Med 106:40, 1987.

Fiatarone MA, et al. High-intensity strength training in nonagenarians. JAMA 263:3029, 1990.

Food and Nutrition Board, National Research Council. Recommended Dietary Allowances, 10th ed. Washington, DC: National Academy Press, 1989.

Food and Nutrition Board, Institute of Medicine, National Academy of Sciences. Dietary Reference Intakes. Washington, DC: National Academy Press, 1998.

Goulding A, et al. Bone mineral density in girls with forearm fractures. J Bone Miner Res 13:143, 1998.

Greer FR, et al. Elevated serum parathyroid hormone, calcitonin, and 1,25-dihydroxyvitamin D in lactating women nursing twins. Am J Clin Nutr 40:562, 1984.

Gregg EW, et al. Physical activity and osteoporotic fracture risk in older women. Ann Intern Med, 129:81, 1998.

Halioua L, Anderson JJB. Lifetime calcium intake and physical activity habits: Independent and combined effects on the radial bone of healthy premenopausal Caucasian women. Am J Clin Nutr 49:534, 1989.

Harris S, Dawson-Hughes B. Caffeine and bone loss in healthy postmenopausal women. Am J Clin Nutr 60:573, 1994.

Heaney RP. Protein intake and the calcium economy. J Am Diet Assoc 93:1259, 1993a.

Heaney RP. Nutritonal factors in osteoporosis. Annu Rev Nutr 13:287, 1993b.

Heikinheimo RJ, et al. Serum vitamin D level afer annual intramuscular injection of ergocalciferol. Calcif Tissue Int 49:S87, 1991.

Heinonen A, et al. Randomized controlled trial of the effect of high-impact exercise in selected risk factors for osteoporotic fractures. Lancet 348:1343, 1996.

Holbrook T, Barrett-Connor E. A prospective study of alcohol consumption and bone mineral density. BMJ 306:1506, 1993.

Holick M. Vitamin D and bone health. J Nutr 126:1159S, 1996.

Hopper J, Seeman E. The bone density of female twins discordant for tobacco use. N Engl J Med 330:387, 1994.

Hunt CD, et al. Metabolic responses of postmenopausal women to supplemental dietary boron and aluminum during usual and low magnesium intake: Boron, calcium and magnesium absorption and retention and blood mineral concentrations. Am J Clin Nutr 65:803, 1997.

Jackman LA, et al. Calcium retention in relation to calcium intake and postmenarcheal age in adolescent females. Am J Clin Nutr 66:327, 1997.

Johnston CC, et al. Clinical use of bone densitometry. N Engl J Med 324:1105, 1991.

Johnston CC, et al. Calcium supplementation and increases in bone mineral density in children. N Engl J Med 327:82, 1992.

Johnston CC, et al. Changes in skeletal tissue during the aging process. Nutr Rev 50:385, 1992.

Kalkwarf H, et al. The effect of calcium supplementation on bone density during lactation and after weaning. N Engl J Med 337:523, 1997.

Kanis JA, et al. The diagnosis of osteoporosis. J Bone Miner Res 9:1137, 1994.

Kelsey JL, et al. Effect of fiber from fruits and vegetables on metabolic responses of human subjects. II. Calcium, magnesium, iron, and silicon balances. Am J Clin Nutr 32:1876, 1979.

Kerstetter JE, Allen LH. Dietary protein increases urinary calcium. J Nutr 120:134, 1990.

Kinyamu HK, et al. Serum vitamin D metabolites and calcium absorption in normal young and elderly free-living women and in women living in nursing homes. Am J Clin Nutr 65:790, 1997.

Kohlmeier M, et al. Bone health of adult hemodialysis patients is related to vitamin K status. Kidney Int 51:1218, 1997a.

Kohlmeier M, et al. Vitamin K: A vegetarian promoter of bone health. Vegetarian Nutr 1:53, 1997b.

Kohrt WM, et al. Additive effects of weight-bearing exercise and estrogen on bone mineral density in older women. J Bone Miner Res 10:1303, 1995.

Kraut J, Coburn J. Bone, acid and osteoporosis. N Engl J Med 330:1821, 1994.

Kritz-Silverstein D, Barrett-Connor E. Bone mineral density in postmenopausal women as determined by prior oral contraceptive use. Am J Public Health 83:100, 1993.

Laitinen K, et al. Is alcohol an osteoporosis-inducing agent for young and middle-aged women? Metabolism 42:875, 1993.

Lauritzen JB, et al. Effect of external hip protectors on hip fractures. Lancet 341:11, 1993.

Law MR, Hackshaw AK. A meta-analysis of smoking, bone mineral density and risk of hip fracture: Recognition of a major effect. BMJ 315:841, 1997.

Ledger GA, et al. Abnormalities of parathyroid hormone secretion in elderly women that are reversible by short-term therapy with 1,25-dihydroxyvitamin D_3. J Clin Endocrinol Metab 79:211, 1994.

Lieberman U, et al. Effect of oral alendronte on bone mineral density and the incidence of fractures in postmenopausal osteoporosis. N Engl J Med 333:1437, 1995.

Lindsay R, et al. The effect of oral contraceptive use on vertebral bone mass in pre- and post-menopausal women. Contraception 34:333, 1986.

Liu G, Peacock M. Age-related changes in serum undercarboxylated osteocalcin and its relationship with bone density, bone quality, and hip fracture. Calcif Tissue Int 62:286, 1998.

Lloyd T, et al. Calcium supplementation and bone mineral density in adolescent girls. JAMA 270:841, 1993.

Lloyd T, et al. Dietary caffeine intake and bone status of postmenopausal women. Am J Clin Nutr 65:1826, 1997.

Looker AC, et al. Prevalence of low femoral bone density in older US women from NHANES III. J Bone Miner Res 10:796, 1995.

Looker AC, et al. Prevalence of low femoral bone density in older US adults from NHANES III. J Bone Miner Res 12:1761, 1997.

MacLaughlin J, Holick MF. Aging decreases capacity of human skin to produce vitamin D. J Clin Invest 76:1536, 1985.

Massey L, Whiting S. Caffeine, urinary calcium, calcium metabolism and bone. J Nutr 123:1611, 1993.

Matkovic V, et al. Timing of peak bone mass in Caucasian females and its implication for the prevention of osteoporosis. J Clin Invest 93:799, 1994.

Mazess RB. On aging bone loss. Clin Orthop 165:239, 1982.

McKane WR, et al. Role of calcium intake in modulating age-related increases in parathyroid function and bone resorption. J Clin Endocrinol Metab 81:1699, 1996.

Melton LJ III. The prevalence of osteoporosis (Editorial). J Bone Miner Res 12:1769, 1997.

Messina M. Osteoporosis—Not just a deficiency disease. The Soy Connection 2:(2):1, 1994, Chesterfield, MO: United Soybean Board.

Miller PD, et al. Cyclical etidronate in the treatment of postmenopausal women: Efficacy and safety after seven years of treatment. Am J Med 103:468, 1997.

Moniz C. Alcohol and bone. Brit Med Bull 50:67, 1994.

Nielsen FH, et al. Boron enhances and mimics some effects of estrogen therapy in postmenopausal women. J Trace Elements Exp Med 5:237, 1992.

Nieves JW, et al. Teenage and current calcium intake are related to bone mineral density of the hip and forearm in women aged 30–39. Am J Epidemiol 141:342, 1995.

Nordin BEC, et al. Evidence for a renal calcium leak in postmenopausal women. J Clin Endocrinol Metab 72:401, 1991.

Nordin BEC, et al. The nature and significance of the relationship between urinary sodium and urinary calcium in women. J Nutr 123: 1615, 1993.

Notelovitz M, et al. Estrogen therapy and variable-resistance weight training increase bone mineral in surgically menopausal women. J Bone Miner Res 6:583, 1991.

O'Brien KO, et al. High fiber diets slow bone turnover in young men but have no effect on efficiency of intestinal calcium absorption. J Nutr 123:2122, 1993.

Ooms ME, et al. Vitamin D status and sex hormone binding globulin: Determinants of bone turnover and bone mineral density in elderly women. J Bone Miner Res 10:1177, 1995.

Pak C, et al. Slow-release sodium fluoride in the management of postmenopausal osteoporosis: A randomized controlled trial. Ann Intern Med 120:625, 1994.

Perry H, et al. A preliminary report of vitamin D and calcium metabolism in older African Americans. J Am Geriatr Soc 41:612, 1993.

Pocock NA, et al. Genetic determinants of bone mass in adults: A twin study. J Clin Invest 80:706, 1987.

Pollitzer WS, Anderson JJB. Ethnic and genetic differences in bone mass: A review with an hereditary vs. environmental perspective. Am J Clin Nutr 50:1244, 1989.

Prince RL, et al. Prevention of postmenopausal osteoporosis. N Engl J Med 325:1189, 1991.

Recker R, et al. Bone gain in young adult women. JAMA 268:2403, 1993.

Reid I, et al. Effect of calcium supplementation on bone loss in postmenopausal women. N Engl J Med 328:460, 1993.

Reid IR, et al. Glucocorticoid osteoporosis. J Asthma 31:7, 1994.

Riggs BL, Melton LJ III. Involutional osteoporosis. N Engl J Med 314:1676, 1986.

Rosen CJ, et al. Elderly women in Northern New England exhibit seasonal changes in bone mineral density and calciotropic hormones. J Bone Miner Res 25:83, 1994.

Rude RK. Magnesium deficiency: A cause of heterogenous diseases in humans. J Bone Miner Res 13:749, 1998.

Sambrook P, et al. Prevention of corticosteroid osteoporosis—A comparison of calcium, calcitriol, and calcitonin. N Engl J Med 328:1747, 1993.
Schneider D, et al. Thyroid hormone use and bone mineral density in elderly women—Effects of estrogen. JAMA 271:1245, 1994.
Schneider EL, Guralnik JM. The aging of America: Impact on health care costs. JAMA 263:2335, 1990.
Schuette SA, Linkswiler HM. Effects on Ca and P metabolism in humans by adding meat, meat plus milk, or purified proteins plus Ca and P to a low protein diet. J Nutr 112:338, 1982.
Sebastian A. Improved mineral balance and skeletal metabolism in postmenopausal women treated with potassium bicarbonate. N Engl J Med 330:1776, 1994.
Seeman E, et al. Reduced bone mass in daughters of women with osteoporosis. N Engl J Med 320:554, 1989.
Slemenda C. Cigarettes and the skeleton (Editorial). N Engl J Med 330:430, 1994.
Snow-Harter C, et al. Muscle strength as a predictor of bone mineral density in young women. J Bone Miner Res 5:589, 1990.
Sowers M, et al. Changes in bone density with lactation. JAMA 269:3130, 1993.
Specker B. Evidence for an interaction between calcium intake and physical activity on changes in bone mineral density. J Bone Miner Res 11:1539, 1996.
Spencer H, et al. Do protein and phosphorus cause calcium loss? J Nutr 118:657, 1988.
Strause L, et al. Spinal bone loss in postmenopausal women supplemented with calcium and trace minerals. J Nutr 124:1060, 1994.
Szulc P, et al. Serum uncarboxylated osteocalcin is a marker of the risk of hip fracture: A three year follow-up study. Bone 18:487, 1996.
Thomas MK, et al. Hypovitaminosis D in medical patients. N Engl J Med 338:777, 1998.
Tkatch L, et al. Benefits of oral protein supplementation in elderly patients with fracture of the proximal femur. J Am Coll Nutr 11:519, 1992.
Tylavsky F, et al. Are calcium intakes and physical activity paterns during adolescence related to radial bone mass of white college-age females? Osteoporosis Int 2:232, 1992.
US Department of Agriculture. Continuing Survey of Food Intake by Individuals (CSFIII): Diet and Health Knowledge Survey 1991. Springfield, VA: National Technical Information Service, 1994.
Wakisaka A, et al. Effect of locally infused IGF-1 on femoral gene expression and bone turnover activity in old rats. J Bone Miner Res 13:13, 1998.
Weaver CM, et al. Calcium absorption from foods. In: Burckhardt P, Heaney RP (eds.). Nutritional aspects of osteoporosis, Serono Symposium No. 85. New York: Raven Press, 1991, p. 133.

ADDITIONAL REFERENCES

Adachi J, et al. Intermittent etidronate therapy to prevent corticosteroid-induced osteoporosis. N Engl J Med 337:382, 1997.
Anderson JJB, et al. Biphasic effects of genistein on bone tissue in the ovariectomized, lactating rat model. Proc Soc Exp Biol Med 217:345, 1998.
Anderson JJB, Garner SC. Calcium and phosphorus in health and disease. Boca Raton, FL: CRC Press, 1996.
Felson D, et al. Alcohol intake and bone mineral density in elderly men and women: The Framingham study. Am J Epidemiol 142:485, 1995.
Greendale G, et al. Lifestyle factors and bone mineral density: The Postmenopausal Estrogen/Progestins Intervention Study. J Women's Health 4:231, 1995.
Heaney RP. Protein intake and the calcium economy. J Am Diet Assoc 93:1259, 1993.
Heaney RP. Nutritional factors in osteoporosis. Annu Rev Nutr 13:287, 1993.
Nordin BEC. Calcium and osteoporosis. Nutrition 13:664, 1997.
Orwoll E, et al. Axial bone mass in older women. Ann Intern Med 124:197, 1996.
Pacifici R. Estrogen, cytokines, and pathogenesis of postmenopausal osteoporosis. J Bone Miner Res 11:1043, 1996.
Sowers MF. Pregnancy and lactation as risk factors for subsequent bone loss and osteoporosis. J Bone Miner Res 11:1052, 1996.
Speroff L, et al. The comparative effect on bone density, endometrium, and lipids of continuous hormones as replacement therapy (CHART study). JAMA 276:1397, 1996.
Ulrich C, et al. Bone mineral density in mother-daughter pairs: Relations to lifetime exercise, lifetime milk consumption, and calcium supplements. Am J Clin Nutr 63:72, 1996.
Writing Group for the PEPI Trial. Effects of hormone therapy on bone mineral density: Results from the postmenopausal estrogen/progestin interventions (PEPI) trial. JAMA 276:1389, 1996.

CHAPTER 29

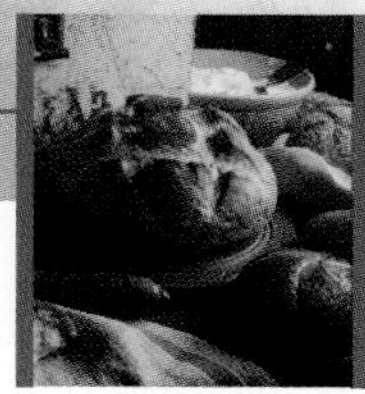

Nutrition for Oral and Dental Health

RIVA TOUGER-DECKER, PHD, RD, FADA

Chapter Outline

- Nutritional Factors in Tooth Development
- Dental Caries
- Fluoride
- Preventive Care
- Periodontal Disease
- Maxillary Anterior Caries or Baby Bottle Tooth Decay
- Tooth Loss and Dentures
- Oral Manifestations of Systemic Disease
- Polypharmacy

Key Terms

ANTICARIOGENIC—suppressing the development of caries by preventing plaque from recognizing an acidogenic food

BABY BOTTLE TOOTH DECAY (BBTD)—caries pattern in infants or children, also known as maxillary anterior caries (MAC) generally caused by prolonged exposure to sweetened beverages

CALCULUS—a hard, stone-like concretion that forms on the teeth as a result of calcification of dental plaque

CANDIDIASIS—an infection caused by the yeast-like fungus Candida, usually *Candida albicans*

CARIOGENIC—containing fermentable carbohydrates that can cause a decrease in salivary pH to <5.5 and demineralization when in contact with microorganisms in the mouth; promoting caries development

CARIOGENICITY—caries-promoting properties of a food

CARIOSTATIC—having the characteristic of not being metabolized by microorganisms in plaque to cause a drop in salivary pH to <5.5

DENTAL CARIES—an oral infectious disease in which acid produced by bacterial metabolism of fermentable carbohydrates leads to bacterial invasion, causing demineralization of enamel and destruction of the tooth structure

DENTIN—the chief organic tissue of the tooth that surrounds the pulp and is covered by enamel on the crown and by cementum on the roots

EDENTULISM—partial or complete loss of natural teeth

ENAMEL—an inorganic, white, crystalline, compact, and very hard substance that covers and protects the dentin of the tooth

FLUOROAPATITE—the form in which the fluoride ion, along with calcium and phosphorus, is incorporated into dentin and enamel

FLUOROSIS—a condition caused by exposure of the tooth enamel to excessive amounts of fluoride; characterized by white, chalky spots on the enamel surface that progress to brown stains and, in the extreme, are manifested as mottling

GINGIVAE—the part of the oral mucosa overlying the crowns of unerupted teeth and encircling the necks of those that have erupted; the gums

GINGIVAL SULCUS—a shallow, V-shaped space around the tooth that is bounded by the tooth surface on one side and the epithelium lining the gingiva on the other

OCCLUSION—the relationship of opposing teeth in opposing jaws; complete occlusion is when anterior (front) and posterior (back) maxillary (upper) and mandibular (lower) teeth come together

ODYNOPHAGIA—pain with swallowing

PERIODONTAL DISEASE—oral infectious disease characterized by inflammation and destruction of the attachment apparatus of the teeth, including the ligamentous attachment of the tooth to the surrounding alveolar bone

PLAQUE—a sticky, colorless film of microorganisms, salivary proteins, inorganic components, and polysaccharides that adheres to teeth and gums

STOMATITIS—inflammation of the oral mucosa

STREPTOCOCCUS MUTANS—an oral bacteria implicated in the formation of dental caries

XEROSTOMIA—mouth dryness secondary to insufficiency or lack of saliva

Diet and nutrition play a major role in tooth development, gingival and oral tissue integrity, bone strength, and the prevention and management of diseases of the oral cavity. Diet is differentiated from nutrition in that diet has a local effect on tooth integrity; that is, the type, form, and frequency of foods and beverages consumed have a direct effect on teeth. Nutrition, by contrast, has a systemic effect. The impact of nutrient intake systemically affects development, maintenance, and repair of the teeth and oral tissues. Nutrient deficiencies of the B vitamins riboflavin, folate, and B_{12}, along with vitamin C and iron and other nutrients, are often detected of the mouth due to the rapid tissue turnover rate in the oral mucosa.

While nutrition and diet affect the oral cavity, the reverse is also true. That is, the status of the oral cavity affects one's ability to consume an adequate diet and, thus, to achieve nutrient balance. Oral diseases extend beyond dental caries. Tooth loss, or **edentulism,** is common in individuals older than 65 years of age and can have a significant impact on intake. According to the Center for Disease Control's Oral Health Program (1996–97), about 44% of the elderly have lost their natural teeth (US-DHHS 1997) (see *"Clinical Insight:* "Bacteremias, Endocarditis, and Preventive Dentistry"). Periodontal disease damages the gingiva and periodontium and may affect tooth stability. Dental caries occur in varying patterns in different age groups.

Oral cancer, often secondary to tobacco and alcohol abuse, can have a significant impact on eating ability and nutritional status. This is compounded by the increased caloric and nutrient needs of individuals with oral carcinomas. Surgery, radiation therapy, and chemotherapy are modalities used to treat oral cancer that can also affect dietary intake, appetite, and integrity of the oral cavity.

In addition to these primary diseases of the oral cavity, several chronic and acute diseases have oral sequelae that affect eating ability. Poorly controlled diabetes can result in burning tongue syndrome, candidiasis, and xerostomia, which in turn compromise an individual's eating ability and appetite. Oral manifestations of immunosuppressive diseases, such as acquired immunodeficiency syndrome (AIDS), also have an impact on appetite, intake, and nutrient needs (see Chapter 40).

NUTRITIONAL FACTORS IN TOOTH DEVELOPMENT

Primary tooth development begins at 2 to 3 months of gestation. Mineralization begins at about 4 months' gestation and continues through the preteen years. Maternal nutrients must, therefore, supply the pre-eruptive teeth with the appropriate building materials. Table 29–1 details the effects of nutrient deficiencies on tooth development. Figure 29–1 shows the parts of a tooth.

Teeth are formed by the mineralization of a protein matrix. In **dentin,** protein is present as collagen, which depends on vitamin C for normal synthesis. Vitamin D is essential to the process by which calcium and phosphorus are deposited in crystals of *hydroxyapatite*. Fluoride, added to the hydroxyapatite, provides unique caries-resistant properties in both prenatal and postnatal developmental periods.

Diet and nutrition are important in all phases of tooth development, eruption, and maintenance. Posteruption, diet and nutrient intake continue to affect tooth development and mineralization, enamel development and strength, as well as eruption patterns of the remaining teeth. The local effects of diet, particularly fermentable carbohydrates and eating frequency, affect the production

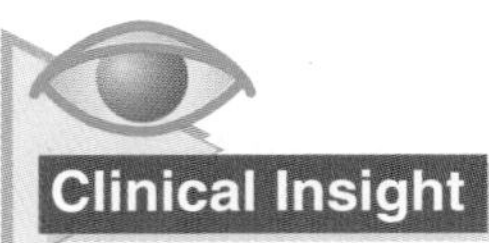

BACTEREMIAS, ENDOCARDITIS, AND PREVENTIVE DENTISTRY

Bacteremia is a serious condition of bacteria in the bloodstream. Bacteria can move or translocate into the blood from the gastrointestinal tract at any point along the tract, including the oral cavity. Poor oral hygiene and periodontal infections put people at risk for this translocation during common activities such as tooth brushing and chewing. Some surgical or dental procedures involving mucosal surfaces of the mouth can cause transient bacteremia. Edentulous patients may develop bacteremia from ulcers caused by ill-fitting dentures.

When these blood-borne pathogens lodge on damaged or abnormal heart valves, an uncommon but life-threatening endocarditis can result. Bacterial endocarditis usually develops in individuals with underlying cardiac defects as from rheumatic heart disease or it may complicate an infection such as an improperly treated urinary tract infection or pneumonia.

Treatment of bacterial endocarditis requires constant antimicrobial therapy. Prevention in susceptible patients also entails antimicrobial therapy, but the potential adverse reactions to these prophylactic measures, the cost benefit ratio, and the patient risk should all be considered before antimicrobial therapy is instituted. Antiseptic rinses applied immediately before dental procedures can be helpful.

Health care providers must be aware of the importance of maintenance of a clean, well-nourished and intact oral cavity and related mucosal surfaces for optimal health, and should always make this part of their assessment.

Source: Website: *www.ada.org/adapco/jada/9708/endo-03/.html*

TABLE 29–1 EFFECTS OF NUTRIENT DEFICIENCIES ON TOOTH DEVELOPMENT

NUTRIENT	EFFECT ON TISSUE	EFFECT ON CARIES	HUMAN DATA
Protein/calorie malnutrition	Delayed tooth eruption Decreased tooth size Decreased enamel solubility Salivary gland dysfunction	Yes	Yes
Vitamin A	Decreased epithelial tissue development Tooth morphogenesis dysfunction Decreased odontoblast differentiation Increased enamel hypoplasia	Yes	Yes
Vitamin D/calcium/phosphorus	Lowered plasma calcium levels Hypomineralization (hypoplastic defects) Compromised tooth integrity (decreased mineral concentration) Delayed eruption patterns	Yes	Yes
Ascorbic acid	Dental pulpal alterations Odontoblastic degeneration Aberrant dentin	No	No
Fluoride	Increased stability of enamel crystal (enamel formation) Inhibition of demineralization Stimulation of remineralization Mottled enamel (excess) Inhibition of bacterial growth	Yes	Yes
Iodine	Delayed tooth eruption Altered growth patterns Malocclusions?	No	Yes
Iron	Slow growth Salivary gland dysfunction	Yes	No

(From DePaola D, Faine MP, Vogel RI. Nutrition in relation to dental medicine. In: Shils ME, Olson JA, Shike M (eds.). Modern Nutrition in Health and Disease, vol. 2, 8th ed. Philadelphia: Lea & Febiger, 1994. Reprinted with permission.)

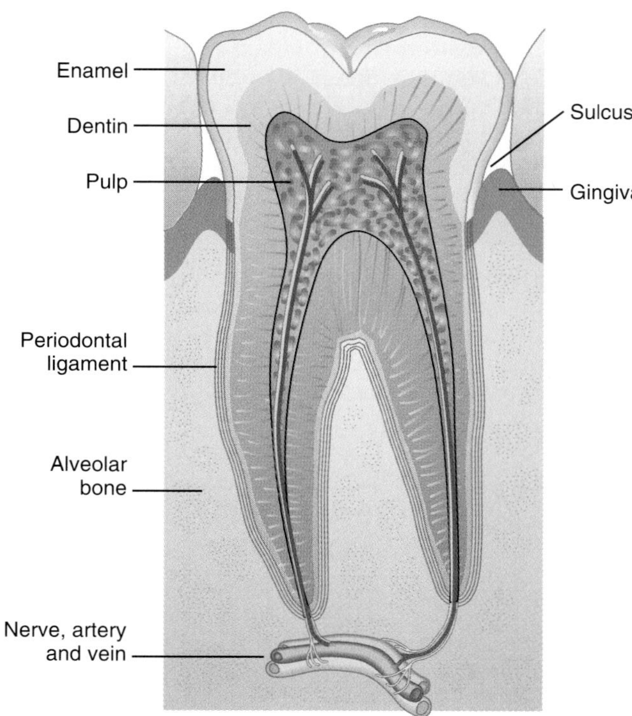

FIGURE 29–1 Anatomy of a tooth.

of organic acids by oral bacteria and the rate of decay. Throughout the life span, diet and nutrition continue to affect tooth, bone, and oral mucosal integrity, resistance to infection, and tooth longevity. The website for the American Dental Association is www.ada.org, where more information is available.

DENTAL CARIES

Pathophysiology

Dental caries is an oral infectious disease in which organic acid metabolites produced by the metabolism of oral microorganisms lead to gradual demineralization of tooth **enamel,** followed by rapid proteolytic destruction of the tooth structure (Figure 29–2). Caries can occur on any tooth surface.

The etiology of dental caries is multifactorial. Four factors must be present simultaneously: (1) a susceptible host or tooth surface; (2) microorganisms, such as ***Streptococcus mutans*** in the dental plaque or oral environment; (3) fermentable carbohydrates in the diet, which serve as the substrate for bacterial metabolism; and (4) time (duration) in the mouth for bacteria to metabolize the fermentable carbohydrates, produce acids, and cause a

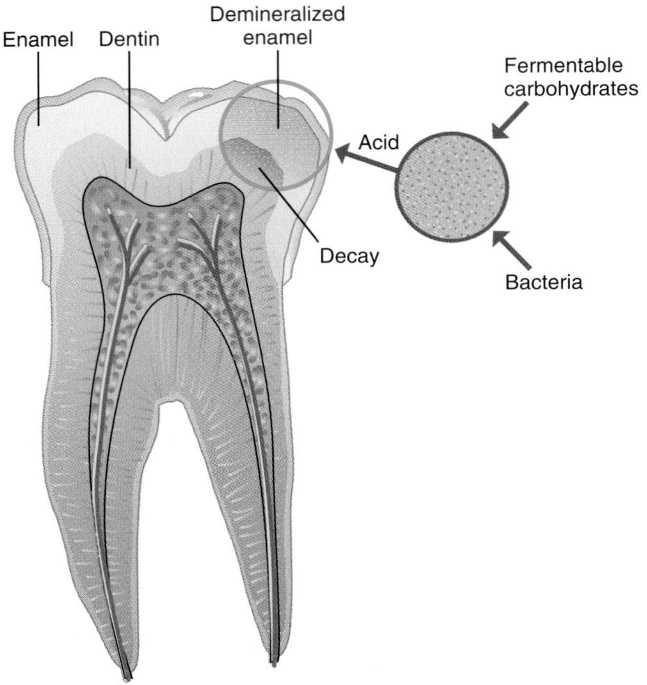

FIGURE 29–2 Formation of dental caries.

drop in salivary pH to less than 5.5. Once the pH falls below 5.5, oral bacteria can initiate the caries process.

Susceptible Tooth

The development of dental caries requires the presence of a tooth that is vulnerable to attack. The composition of enamel and dentin, location of teeth, quality and quantity of saliva, and the presence and extent of pits and fissures in the tooth crown are some of the factors that govern susceptibility. Composition of the saliva is also important. Alkaline saliva may have a protective effect, whereas an acidic saliva increases susceptibility to decay. It is difficult to separate the effects of family factors of food selection, eating patterns, and oral hygiene from possible genetic influences.

Microorganisms

Bacteria are an essential part of the decay process. Several microorganisms are capable of fermenting dietary carbohydrate. *Streptococcus mutans* is the most prevalent, followed by *Lactobacillus casein* and *Streptococcus sanguis*. All three contribute to the process, as they metabolize carbohydrates and produce acid at levels sufficient to cause decay.

Substrate

Fermentable carbohydrates are the ideal substrate for bacterial metabolism. The acids produced by their metabolism cause a drop in salivary pH to less than 5.5, creating the environment for decay. In light of The Dietary Guidelines and the Food Guide Pyramid, both of which recommend a diet high in carbohydrate, it is important to be aware of the myriad factors affecting the potential for bacterial action on fermentable carbohydrates and to guide individuals in integrating positive diet and oral hygiene habits to improve oral health status. Factors affecting cariogenicity of substrates are listed in Table 29–2.

Fermentable carbohydrates are found in four of the six food guide pyramid food groups: grains, fruits, dairy products, and the added sugar and fats/sweets. Although a few of the vegetables may contain fermentable carbohydrate, little has been reported as to the cariogenicity of vegetables. Examples of grains and starches include crackers, chips, pretzels, hot and cold cereals, and breads. All fruits (fresh, dried, and canned) and fruit juices may be cariogenic. Fruits with high water content, such as melons, have a lower cariogenicity than others, such as bananas and dried fruits. Fruit drinks, sodas, ice teas and other sugar-sweetened beverages, desserts, cookies, candies, and cake products may be cariogenic. Dairy products sweetened with fructose, sucrose, or other sugars can also be cariogenic because of the added sugars.

Sucrose, like other sugars (glucose, fructose, maltose, and lactose), stimulates bacterial activity. All dietary forms of sugar, including honey, molasses, brown sugar, and corn syrup solids, have cariogenic potential, and can be used by bacteria to produce organic acid by-products of metabolism.

The five-carbon sugar alcohol, xylitol, is considered anticariogenic. It is not broken down by salivary amylase and is not subject to bacterial degradation. Noncarbohydrate sweeteners, such as saccharin, cyclamate, and aspartame, are cariostatic. There is some evidence to support the idea that aspartame and saccharin may inhibit bacterial action, as neither provides a usable substrate for streptococcus bacteria (Grenby et al., 1989).

Cariogenicity of Individual Foods

It is important to differentiate between cariogenic, cariostatic, and anticariogenic foods. **Cariogenic** foods are those that contain fermentable carbohydrates which, when in contact with microorganisms in the mouth, can cause a drop in salivary pH to 5.5

TABLE 29–2 FACTORS AFFECTING FOOD CARIOGENICITY

Frequency of consumption of fermentable carbohydrates
Food form (e.g., liquid, solid, slowly dissolving)
Sequence of eating foods and beverages
Combination of foods
Nutrient composition of foods and beverages
Duration of exposure of teeth to food and beverages

or less and stimulate the caries process. **Cariostatic** foods, or foods that do not contribute to decay, are not metabolized by microorganisms in plaque and so do not cause a drop in salivary pH to 5.5 or less within 30 minutes. Examples of cariostatic foods are protein foods, such as eggs, fish, meat, and poultry, many vegetables, fats, and sugarless gums. **Anticariogenic** foods are those that prevent plaque from recognizing an acidogenic food when it is eaten first (acidogenic = cariogenic). Sources include xylitol gums and cheeses, such as aged cheddar, Monterey jack, and Swiss cheese.

Sophisticated testing methods have enabled an evaluation of the cariogenicity of specific foods. Results of such studies have demonstrated that the amount of acid formed from a food as a result of fermentation by salivary bacteria is not proportional to its sugar content. Nor does the amount of demineralization necessarily parallel the amount of acid produced from the food. These observations may reflect the formation of different types of fermentation products, or the presence of substances in the food that reduce, reverse, or accentuate a sugar's caries-producing action. Cariogenicity is also influenced by the volume and quality of saliva an individual produces; the sequence, consistency, and nutrient composition of the foods eaten; plaque build-up; and the genetic predisposition of the host to decay.

Factors Affecting Cariogenicity of Food

Foods containing fermentable carbohydrate are the basis for bacterial action, which, in turn, stimulates caries development. **Cariogenicity** refers to the caries-promoting properties of a diet or food. However, individual cariogenicity of a food varies depending on the form in which it occurs, the nutrient composition, the sequence in which it is eaten in conjunction with other foods and fluids, the duration of exposure of the tooth to the food, and the frequency of eating (see Table 29–2).

A food's form and consistency have a significant impact on its cariogenic potential and pH-lowering or buffering capacity. Food form determines the *duration of exposure* or *retention time* of a food in the mouth, which, in turn, affects how long the decrease in pH or the acid-producing activity will last. Liquids are rapidly cleared from the mouth and have low adherence (or retentiveness) capabilities. Solid foods, such as crackers, chips, and cookies, can stick between the teeth (in the interproximal spaces) and have high adherence (or retention) capability. Consumption of hard candies results in prolonged sugar exposure in the mouth.

Consistency also affects adherence. Chewy foods, such as gum drops and marshmallows, although high in sugar content, stimulate saliva production and have a lower adherence potential than solid, sticky foods, such as pretzels or potato chips. The latter, although lower in sucrose, have a longer duration of exposure. Sugar-free chewing gum, which causes an increase in saliva, may help reduce decay potential due to the cleansing effect of the saliva. This is why sugarless gum is recommended after meals and snacks to reduce caries potential. High-fiber foods with little fermentable carbohydrate, such as popcorn, also have a low caries potential.

Duration of exposure may be best explained with starchy foods, which are fermentable carbohydrates subject to the action of salivary amylase. The longer starches are retained in the mouth, the greater their cariogenic potential (Kashket et al., 1996). Given sufficient time, such as when food particles become lodged between the teeth, salivary amylase makes additional substrate available as it hydrolyzes starch to simple sugars. Processing techniques make some starches rapidly fermentable, either by partial hydrolysis or by reducing particle size, thus increasing availability for enzyme action. Although sugar-containing candies cause a rapid increase in the amount of sugars available in the oral cavity to be hydrolyzed by bacteria, their effect is short-lived. By comparison, starch-based snacks and dessert foods (e.g., potato chips, pretzels, cookies, cakes, and doughnuts) provide gradually increasing oral sugar concentrations for a longer time duration, as these foods often adhere to the tooth surfaces and are retained for longer periods of time than candies (Kashket et al, 1996).

Nutrient composition contributes to the substrate's ability to produce acid and the duration of the acid exposure. Dairy products, by virtue of their calcium and phosphorus buffering potential, are considered to have low cariogenic potential. Studies have shown that cheese and milk, when taken with cariogenic foods, provide some protection against the cariogenic agent. Cheeses—in particular, cheddar cheese—have anticariogenic properties and stimulate an alkaline saliva, which reduces plaque bacteria (Jenkins and Hargreaves, 1989). Eating cheese with a fermentable carbohydrate, such as dessert at the end of a meal, may decrease the cariogenicity of the meal. Nuts, which do not contain a significant amount of fermentable carbohydrates and are high in fat and dietary fiber, are cariostatic. Protein foods, such as seafood, fish, meats, eggs, and poultry, along with other fats, such as oils, margarine, butter, and seeds, are also cariostatic.

Eating sequence and *combination of foods* also affect the caries potential of the substrate. Bananas, which are cariogenic due to their fermentable carbohydrate content and adherence capability, have less potential to contribute to decay when eaten with cereal and milk than when eaten alone as a snack. Milk, as a liquid, reduces the adherence capability of the fruit. Crackers eaten with cheese carry a lower caries-promoting risk than when eaten alone. The buffering capacity of cheese and milk makes them desirable foods to eat at the end of a meal or in combination with other fermentable carbohydrates to reduce potential cariogenicity.

The *frequency* with which a cariogenic food or beverage is consumed determines the number of opportunities for acid production. Every time a fermentable carbohydrate is consumed, a decline in pH, causing caries-promoting activity, is initiated within 5 to 15 minutes and lasts about 20 to 30 minutes. Small, frequent meals and snacks, often high in fermentable carbohydrate, increase the cariogenicity of a diet considerably more than a diet consisting of three meals and minimal snacks. Eating several cookies at once, followed by brushing or rinsing the mouth with water, is less cariogenic than eating one cookie several times throughout a day.

The Decay Process

The carious process begins with the production of acids as a by-product of bacterial metabolism taking place in the dental plaque. Decalcification of the surface enamel continues until the buffering action of the saliva is able to raise the pH above the critical level (see Fig. 29–2).

Plaque Formation

Plaque is a sticky, colorless mass of microorganisms, salivary proteins, and polysaccharides that adheres to teeth and gums. It harbors acid-forming bacteria and keeps the organic products of their metabolism in close contact with the enamel surface. As a cavity develops, the plaque shields the tooth, to some extent, from the buffering and remineralization action of the saliva. In time, the plaque combines with calcium and hardens to form **calculus.** In this state, it becomes a local irritant to the gingiva and is a significant factor in the development of periodontal disease.

Acid Production

In the absence of foods, beverages, or medications containing fermentable carbohydrates, the pH of plaque stays relatively constant. When food or drink containing fermentable carbohydrate is ingested, however, the pH of the plaque is reduced. At a pH of less than 5.5 (the critical pH), acid begins to dissolve tooth enamel. This process continues for 20 or 30 minutes until the buffering effect of saliva neutralizes plaque acidity.

Saliva Function

Salivary flow clears food from around the teeth. By means of the bicarbonate-carbonic acid and phosphate buffer system, it also provides buffering action to neutralize bacterial acid metabolism. Chewing promotes saliva production, and may account for the reduced cariogenicity of fermentable carbohydrates consumed with a meal.

Saliva is supersaturated with calcium and phosphorus. Once buffering action has restored plaque pH above the critical point, remineralization can occur. If fluoride is present in the saliva, the minerals are deposited in the form of **fluoroapatite,** which is resistant to erosion. However, constant or frequent acid challenges (such as sucking on a lemon or self-induced vomiting) cause enamel decalcification, demineralization, and erosion.

Salivary production decreases during sleep, as a result of diseases affecting salivary gland function (e.g., Sjögren's syndrome), as a side effect of fasting, as a result of radiation therapy to the head and neck, or with the use of certain medications. Medications associated with reduced salivary flow are listed by category in Table 29–3.

Caries Patterns

Caries patterns describe the location and surfaces of the teeth affected. Although the overall incidence of decay in the United States has declined, up to 17% of children between the ages of 2 and 4 years of age have tooth decay (U.S. Department of Health and Human Services, 1997). However, dental examiners in the nutrition and health survey known as NHANES III found that only 55% of children and adolescents between the ages of 5 and 17 years of age had no caries in their permanent dentition (National Institute of Dental Health, 1996). Most adults (94%) older than 18 years of age had untreated decay and/or filled teeth.

Root caries, occurring on the root surfaces of teeth secondary to gingival recession, affect a large portion of the elderly population. Josti et al. (1994) reported a 52% incidence of root caries in New England elderly. In a study of 196 Dutch elderly (mean age of 79 years), root caries was reported in 52% of men and 35% of women (Narhi et al., 1998). A primary factor in the development of root decay is gingival recession, often secondary to periodontal disease, which results in exposure of root surfaces to the oral environment. These surfaces lack an enamel layer and are, therefore, more vulnerable to rapid decay. Other factors related to the increased incidence of this decay pattern are age, lack of fluoridated water, and frequent eating of fermentable carbohydrates. Management of root caries includes dental restoration, as well as diet counseling. Root caries is a dental infectious disease that is increasing in older adults, partly because this population is

TABLE 29–3 MEDICATIONS THAT MAY CAUSE XEROSTOMIA

Antianxiety agents
Anticonvulsants
Antidepressants
Antihistamines
Antihypertensives
Diuretics
Narcotics
Sedatives
Serotonin uptake inhibitors
Tranquilizers

retaining their natural teeth for a longer period (Shay, 1997).

Lingual caries, or caries on the lingual side (surface next to or toward the tongue) of the anterior teeth, are seen in individuals with bulimia or anorexia-bulimia (see Chapter 24). Frequent intake of fermentable carbohydrates, combined with repeated episodes of induced vomiting of acidic stomach contents, results in a constant influx of acids into the oral cavity. The caries are the end result of tooth erosion characterized by erosion of the palatal and buccal surfaces of the maxillary anterior teeth and the lingual surfaces of the palatal surface of the maxillary posterior teeth (Robb and Geidrys-Leeper, 1995).

FLUORIDE

Fluoride is the most effective anticaries agent available. Water fluoridation alone led to a 40% to 60% decline in caries prevalence from 1946 to 1979 in individuals consuming fluoridated water from birth through adolescence. Fluoridation contributed to a 30% decline in caries incidence from 1979 to 1989 (Newbrun, 1989). The impact of fluoride on caries prevention continues with water fluoridation, fluoridated toothpastes, oral rinses, and dentrifices, as well as beverages made with fluoridated water.

Mechanism of Action

Fluoride contributes to decay-resistant teeth by three primary mechanisms. First, when incorporated into enamel and dentin along with calcium and phosphorus, it forms fluoroapatite, a compound more resistant to acid challenge than hydroxyapatite. Fluoride also promotes repair and remineralization of tooth surfaces with early carious lesions. It helps reverse the decay process while promoting the development of a tooth surface that has increased resistance to decay. Finally, fluoride may also help deter the harmful effects of bacteria in the oral cavity by interfering with acid production by the bacterial cell.

Fluoride can be used topically and systemically. Fluoride, consumed in food and drink, enters the systemic circulation and is deposited in bones and teeth. Systemic sources have a topical benefit as well, as they provide fluoride to the saliva. A very small amount of fluoride enters soft tissues; the remainder is excreted. The primary source of systemic fluoride is fluoridated water; food and beverages supply a smaller amount. Topical fluoride sources include toothpastes, gels, and rinses used by consumers daily, along with more concentrated forms applied by dental professionals in the form of gels, foams, and rinses. Frequent fluoride exposure via topical fluorides, fluoridated toothpastes, rinses, and fluoridated water is important in maintaining a high concentration of fluoride on the tooth enamel (see the accompanying box, "*Focus on:* Water Fluoridation").

Other Sources of Fluoride

Most foods, unless prepared with fluoridated water, contain minimal amounts of fluoride. Brewed tea (approximately 1.4 ppm) is the most significant fluid source of fluoride (Kiritsky et al., 1997). Fluoride may be unintentionally added to the diet in a number of ways, including the use of fluoridated water in the processing of foods and beverages. Fruit juices and drinks, particularly white grape juice produced in cities with fluoridated water, may have increased fluoride content; however, due to the wide variation in fluoride content, it is difficult to estimate amounts consumed. It is prudent for health professionals to consider a child's fluid intake, as well as sources and the availability of fluoridated water in the community, before prescribing fluoride supplements. Because bones are repositories of fluoride, bone meal, fish meal, and gelatin made from bones are potent sources of the mineral.

In communities without fluoridated water, dietary fluoride supplements are recommended for children aged 6 months to 16 years (Table 29–4). Causes of mild fluorosis include misuse of dietary fluoride supplements, ingestion of fluoridated toothpastes and rinses, and the "halo" effect (i.e., excessive fluoride intake secondary to fluoride in foods and beverages processed in fluoridated areas and transported to other areas) (American Dietetic Association, 1994). Supplementation is now recom-

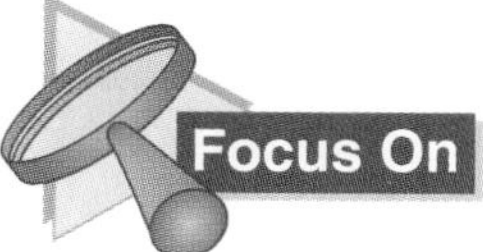

WATER FLUORIDATION

Water fluoridation in the United States is the most cost-effective means of caries prevention available. It has the added benefit of being able to reach significant portions of the population, independent of age or economic level, and to reduce the costs of dental care. The American Dental Association reports (1996) indicate that approximately 145 million people in the United States (about 58%) have fluoridated water. The Health Objectives for the Year 2000 included a plan to increase this percentage to 75% of the population. Fluoride intake at optimal levels (0.7 to 1.2 ppm) has not been shown to cause skeletal fluorosis or other bone-related disorders (American Dietetic Association, 1996).

TABLE 29–4 1994 RECOMMENDATIONS FOR FLUORIDE SUPPLEMENTATION

AGE	CONCENTRATION OF FLUORIDE IN DRINKING WATER*		
	< 0.3 ppm	0.3–0.6 ppm	>.0.6 ppm
Birth–6 months	0	0	0
6 months–3 yrs	0.25 mg	0	0
3–6 yrs	0.50 mg	0.25 mg	0
6–16 yrs	1.0 mg	0.50 mg	0

(Data from American Dietetic Association: Position of ADA: The impact of fluoride on dental health. J Am Diet Assoc 94:1428, 1994.)

*Milligrams of supplemental fluoride recommended according to fluoride concentration in drinking water.

mended to start at the age of 6 months if the level of fluoride in the water supply is less than 0.6 ppm (not 0.7 ppm as previously designated). Fluoride supplements are no longer recommended on a routine basis for breast-fed infants living in fluoridated communities if these infants receive drinking water between feedings.

Topical fluorides, available as fluoridated toothpaste and mouthwashes, are effective sources of fluoride that can be used in the home, school, or dental office. The fluoride rinse programs recently initiated in schools have resulted in up to a 20% decrease in caries incidence. Children younger than 6 years of age should not use fluoridated mouthwashes. Older children should be instructed to rinse, but not swallow, mouthwash. No more than a pea-sized amount of toothpaste should be placed on a child's toothbrush to reduce the risk of accidental fluoride ingestion. Topical fluorides may also be administered in the dental office.

Fluoride gels are often prescribed for adults and older individuals. Such gels have been shown to be effective in reducing the risk of coronal and root decay and tooth loss.

Fluorosis, or mottling of the enamel, can occur secondary to excessive fluoride intake from diet and supplements, excessive topical fluoride, or ingestion of fluoridated toothpastes, rinses, or dentrifices. Starting with white patchy spots, fluorosis progresses to dark brown stains on the teeth as it becomes severe. *Mottling*, which occurs in severe fluorosis, results in pitting of the enamel surface of the tooth.

Fluoride supplementation has been endorsed as a public health measure by the American Dental Association and American Dietetic Association (American Dietetic Association, 1994). The 1989 Diet and Health Report by the National Research Council and the 1988 U.S. Surgeon General's Report also stressed the value of fluoridation in dental disease prevention and tooth protection. Despite this support, however, the widespread use of fluoride has been challenged by "antifluoridationists" who claim that fluoridation restricts individual freedom of choice and increases the risk of AIDS and cancer. Disease-associated risks of fluoride are unfounded. No epidemiologic studies have demonstrated any link between fluoride and cancer or AIDS. Fluoride has no adverse health effects, and the risk of toxicity is negligible (American Dietetic Association, 1994).

PREVENTIVE CARE

Caries prevention programs focus on a balanced diet, modification of the sources and quantities of fermentable carbohydrates, and the integration of oral hygiene practices into individual life-styles. Meals and snacks should be followed by brushing, rinsing the mouth with water, or chewing sugarless gum for 15 to 20 minutes. Positive habits should be encouraged, including snacking on anticariogenic or cariostatic foods, chewing sugarless gum after eating or drinking cariogenic items, and having sweets with meals rather than as snacks. Despite the potential for a diet that is based on the Food Guide Pyramid to be cariogenic, with proper planning and good oral hygiene, a balanced diet low in cariogenic risk can be planned (Figure 29–3). Practices to avoid include sipping carbonated beverages over extended periods, snacking frequently, and harboring candy, sugared breath mints, or hard candies in the mouth for extended periods. Over-the-counter chewable or liquid medications and vitamin preparations may also contain sugar. Chewable vitamin C is one example of a sugar-containing acid product that may contribute to tooth decay. Careful label reading is important to avoid or minimize use of such products. Table 29–5 provides caries prevention guidelines.

Fermentable carbohydrates, such as candy, crackers, cookies, pastries, pretzels, and chips, should be eaten with meals. A piece of cheese at the end of a meal or with a snack is an example of a caries reduction strategy. Although fruits and fruit juices are fermentable carbohydrates, oral hygiene practices, such as toothbrushing, rinsing with water, or chewing sugarless gum following these foods, can reduce potential caries risk. Combining fruits with cheese and juices with meals helps reduce the cariogenic potential of these foods.

Growing evidence supports the use of xylitol-sweetened gum as an anticaries agent after meals

TABLE 29–5 CARIES PREVENTION GUIDELINES

Brush at least twice daily, preferably after meals.
Rinse mouth after meals and snacks when brushing is not possible.
Chew sugarless gum for 15 to 20 minutes after meals and snacks.
Floss twice daily.
Use fluoridated toothpastes.
Pair cariogenic foods with cariostatic foods.
Snack on cariostatic and anticariogenic foods, such as cheese, nuts, popcorn, and vegetables.
Limit between-meal eating and drinking of fermentable carbohydrates.

Breakfast:	1 1/2 cups toasted oat cereal + 1 cup low fat milk or 2 slices wheat toast with 1 oz melted cheese 1 cup fresh berries coffee + low-fat milk BRUSH TEETH
Lunch:	2 slices of mushroom pizza small salad with 2 TB Italian dressing 16 oz spring water banana FOLLOW WITH 2 pieces xylitol gum
Afternoon snack:	1 cup pretzels + 1 oz cheese FOLLOW WITH 2 pieces xylitol gum
Dinner:	tossed salad with 2 TB grated cheese 1 1/2 cups spaghetti + 1 cup marinara sauce + 1/2 cup sauteed peppers 1 cup fresh fruit salad 1 slice Italian bread with 1 pat of margarine 1/2 cup ice cream 1 cup low fat milk
Snack:	4 cups popcorn BRUSH TEETH BEFORE BED

FIGURE 29–3 A balanced diet plan with low cariogenic risk.

and snacks (Steinberg et al, 1992). Xylitol is a five-carbon sugar that cannot be metabolized by oral bacteria. Research has documented its ability to reduce caries incidence by reducing the levels of *S. mutans* in saliva. The current recommended dose is two pieces after each meal or snack containing fermentable carbohydrates. Twenty minutes of chewing appears to cause a rise in salivary pH to a level greater than 5.5. Xylitol is considered to be anticariogenic because it is not hydrolyzed by salivary amylase, and because it raises salivary pH, promoting remineralization.

PERIODONTAL DISEASE

Pathophysiology

Periodontal disease is an inflammation of the gingiva with destruction of the tooth attachment apparatus. *Gingivitis*, an early form of periodontal disease, is an inflammation and infection of the **gingiva,** the oral tissue component of the periodontium. Both are the result of infections caused by oral bacteria in the plaque. Periodontitis results in a gradual loss of tooth attachment to the bone. Progression is influenced by the overall health of the host and the integrity of the immune system.

The primary etiologic factor in the development of periodontal disease is plaque. Plaque in the **gingival sulcus** produces toxins that destroy tissue and permit loosening of the teeth. Several host factors are also important, including age, faulty tooth restorations, poor tooth alignment, and traumatic **occlusion** of the teeth.

Important factors in the defense of the gingiva to bacterial invasion are (1) oral hygiene, (2) integrity of the immune system, and (3) optimal nutrition. The defense mechanisms of the gingival tissue, epithelial barrier, and saliva are affected by nutritional intake and status. Healthy epithelial tissue prevents the penetration of bacterial endotoxins into subgingival tissue. Deficiencies of vitamin C, folate, and zinc increase the permeability of the gingival barrier at the gingival sulcus, increasing susceptibility to periodontal disease. Severe deterioration of the gingiva is seen in individuals with scurvy or vitamin C deficiency.

Diet and nutrition may be seen as having distinct relationships to periodontal disease. Diet contributes to plaque build-up in the gingival crevice between teeth. Food that is retained around the teeth is metabolized by oral bacteria and contributes to plaque accumulation. Although individual nutrients, including vitamins A, E, and C, beta-carotene, folate, and protein, have a role in maintaining gingival and immune system integrity, there is little scientific data to support supplemental uses of any of these nutrients to treat periodontal disease.

Numerous studies have attempted to link nutrient deficits to periodontal disease. However, in societies where malnutrition and periodontal disease are prevalent, poor oral hygiene is also usually evident. In such instances, it is difficult to determine whether malnutrition is the cause of the disease or one of many contributing factors that include poor oral hygiene, heavy plaque build-up, insufficient saliva, or coexisting illness.

Nutritional Care

Nutritional and dietary management of the patient with periodontal disease follows many of the guidelines listed in Table 29–5. Beginning with a diet evaluation, including a multi-day food diary or diet recall to determine eating frequency, food intake, and oral hygiene habits, a dental or dietetic professional can evaluate the overall nutritional adequacy and eating pattern of the diet. Individual dental nutrition risk factors that may contribute to oral disease are areas that can then be addressed in counseling the patient about diet and oral health.

Diet adequacy is particularly important prior to and following periodontal surgery, when adequate nutrients are needed to regenerate tissue and maintain an immune response to prevent infection. Adequacy of calories, protein, and micronutrients should be ensured. If the ability to consume one's regular diet will be altered, a diet modified in consistency can be individually designed for each patient. Oral supplements can be used, when necessary, to augment calories, protein, and other nutrients derived from meals.

MAXILLARY ANTERIOR CARIES OR BABY BOTTLE TOOTH DECAY

Maxillary anterior caries, often called **baby bottle tooth decay** (BBTD), is a term used to describe a caries pattern in the maxillary anterior teeth of infants and young children. Known characteristics include rapidly developing carious lesions in the primary anterior teeth and the presence of lesions on tooth surfaces not associated with a high caries risk. This condition often occurs secondary to prolonged bottle-feeding, especially at night, of juice, milk, formula, or other sweetened beverages. The extended contact time with the fermentable carbohydrate-containing beverages, coupled with the position of the tongue against the nipple, which causes pooling of the liquid around the maxillary incisors, particularly during sleep, contribute to the decay process. The lower front teeth are usually spared as a result of the protective position of the lip and tongue (see Figure 29–4).

BBTD is particularly prevalent in Native American and Native Alaskan communities. A study of 3- to 5-year-old children in Head Start programs in five southwestern states demonstrated a 24% incidence of BBTD (Barnes et al., 1992). Native Americans had the highest incidence of BBTD (35.1%), followed by Hispanics (23.8%), caucasians (22.2%), and blacks (20.5%). Rural children had more BBTD than city children, independent of water fluoridation.

A 1989 survey of five Alaskan regions included 708 Head Start children, aged 3 to 5 years, of which 70% were Native Alaskans and 51% lived in urban areas. BBTD was found in 40% of the Native Alaskans and 8% of the non-Native Alaskan children. Incidence was higher in the rural villages and varied significantly on a statewide basis. Overall, oral health was related to race, community, employment, and educational level of the mother.

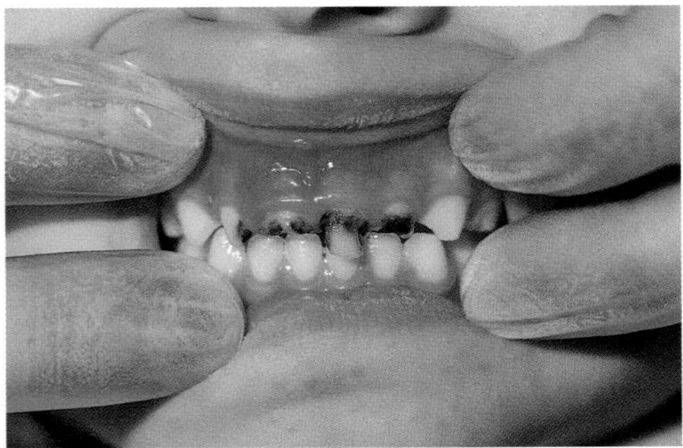

FIGURE 29–4 Baby bottle tooth decay. (From Swartz MH. Textbook of Physical Diagnosis, History, and Examination, 3rd ed. Philadelphia: WB Saunders, 1998.)

Low-income, undereducated groups are also at high risk for BBTD, as well as other dental diseases. In a 1994 study of the nutrition and oral health habits of infants and young children at several urban, low-income day care centers, a 24% incidence of BBTD was noted (Koenigsberg et al., 1994). Health habits that contributed to this high percentage included poor oral hygiene, failure to brush a child's teeth at least daily, frequent use of bottles filled with sweetened beverages, lack of fluoridated water, low literacy, and lack of parent understanding of the relationship between diet and oral health (Koenigsberg et al., 1994).

In a study of the incidence of BBTD in Texas multicultural children, 72.2% of Hispanics and 37% of black children were found to have BBTD. Those children who were weaned from a bottle after 14 months of age had a greater incidence of BBTD than those who were weaned at a younger age (Febres et al., 1997). Children with maxillary anterior caries at ages 3 to 4 years had a greater incidence of future caries than those who were caries-free at an earlier age (O'Sullilvan and Tinanoff, 1996).

Management of BBTD

Management of BBTD includes diet and oral hygiene education for parents, guardians, and caregivers. Dietary guidelines include removal of the bedtime bottle and modification of the frequency and content of the daytime bottles. Bottle contents should be limited to water, formula, milk, and diluted fruit juice. Infants and young children should not be put to bed with a bottle. Teeth and gums should be cleaned with a gauze pad or washcloth after all bottle-feedings. All efforts should be made to wean children from a bottle by the age of 2 years.

Educational efforts should be positive and simple, focusing on oral hygiene habits and promotion of a balanced, healthy diet. Parents and caregivers need to understand the causes of BBTD and how it can be avoided.

TOOTH LOSS AND DENTURES

Tooth loss, edentulism, and removable prostheses can have a significant impact on dietary habits and adequacy, masticatory function, and olfaction. Typically, the intake of fruits, vegetables, and whole grains are inadequate in edentulous individuals or those individuals with maxillary and mandibular dentures. This results in an inadequate intake of dietary fiber and vitamins A and C, as well as other vitamins and minerals (Touger-Decker et al., 1997; Joshipura et al., 1996). Poor diet quality can have a negative impact on nutritional and overall health status in dentate, as well as edentulous, individuals (U.S. Department of Health and Human Services, 1994). This problem is more pronounced in the elderly person, whose appetite and intake may be compromised further by chronic disease, social isolation, and use of multiple medications. An inverse relationship between the number of natural teeth and fruit and vegetable intake was identified in a study of free-living subjects aged 40 to 80 years old (Joshipura and Willet, 1994).

Unfortunately, dentures do not fully solve the problem. As demonstrated in a longitudinal study of individuals both before and after denture placement, many individuals continued to experience eating difficulty (biting and chewing) after denture insertion (Touger-Decker et al., 1997). The foods that were found to cause the greatest difficulty for individuals wearing complete dentures included fresh whole fruits and vegetables (e.g., apples and carrots), corn on the cob, hard-crusted breads, and steak.

Dietary assessment and counseling as it relates to oral health should be provided to the denture-wearer. Simple guidelines should be provided for cutting and preparing fruits and vegetables to minimize the need for biting and reduce the amount of chewing. Changing the dentition of an individual does not consistently result in improved eating habits. Studies have shown that, despite improving objective and subjective chewing ability, significant changes in eating habits may be difficult to produce (Touger-Decker et al., 1997; Ettinger, 1998). The importance of positive eating habits needs to be stressed as a component of preventive health. Overall, health guidelines that reinforce the importance of a balanced diet based on the food guide pyramid should be part of the routine health counseling given to all patients.

ORAL MANIFESTATIONS OF SYSTEMIC DISEASE

Acute systemic diseases, such as cancer and AIDS, as well as chronic diseases, such as diabetes mellitus, autoimmune diseases, and end-stage renal disease, are characterized by oral manifestations that may alter diet and nutritional status. Cancer therapies, including irradiation of the head and neck region, chemotherapy, and oral surgery, have a significant impact on the integrity of the oral cavity and on an individual's eating ability, and, consequently, can affect nutritional status.

Viral and fungal infections, stomatitis, xerostomia, periodontal disease, and Kaposi's sarcoma are oral manifestations of human immunodeficiency virus (HIV) that can cause limitations in nutrient intake and result in weight loss and compromised nutritional status. The infections are often compounded by a compromised immune response, pre-existing malnutrition, and gastrointestinal sequelae of HIV infection. Viral diseases, including herpes simplex and cytomegalovirus, result in painful ulcerations of the mucosa. **Candidiasis** on the tongue, palate, or esophagus can make chewing, sucking, and swallowing painful **(odynophagia),** thus compromising intake. Table 29–6 outlines the impact of HIV infection in the uppermost portion of the gastrointestinal tract.

Oropharyngeal fungal infections may cause a burning, painful mouth and dysphagia. The ulcers that accompany viral infections, such as herpes simplex and cytomegalovirus, cause pain and reduced oral intake. Kaposi's sarcoma compromises oral intake and increases nutrient needs. Very hot and cold foods or beverages, spices, and sour/tart foods also may be painful and should be avoided. Consumption of temperate, moist foods without added spices should be encouraged. Small, frequent meals followed by rinsing with lukewarm water or brushing to reduce the risk of dental caries are helpful. Once the type and extent of oral manifestations are identified, a nutrition care plan can be developed. Oral calorie supplements in liquid or pudding form may be needed to meet calorie requirements (see Chapter 40).

Stomatitis, or inflammation of the oral mucosa, causes severe pain and ulceration of the gingiva, oral mucosa, and palate, which makes eating painful. **Xerostomia**, or dry mouth, is seen in poorly controlled diabetes mellitus, Sjögren's syn-

TABLE 29–6 IMPACT OF ORAL INFECTIONS

LOCATION	PROBLEM	EFFECT	DIET MANAGEMENT
Oral cavity	Candidiasis, KS, herpes, stomatitis	Pain, infection, lesions, altered ability to eat; dysgeusia	Increase kcal and protein intake. Administer oral supplements. Provide caries risk reduction education.
	Xerostomia	Increased caries risk, pain, no moistening power, tendency of food to stick, dysgeusia	Moist, soft, nonspicy foods; "smooth" cool/warm foods and fluids; caries risk reduction education
Esophagus	Candidiasis, herpes, KS, cryptosporidiosis	Dysphagia, odynophagia	Try oral supplementation first. If that is unsuccessful, initiate NG feedings using silastic feeding tube or PEG.
	CMV CMV + ulceration	Dysphagia, food accumulation	PEG

KS, Kaposi's sarcoma; *CMV,* cytomegalovirus; *NG,* nasogastric; *PEG,* percutaneous endoscopic gastrostomy.

drome, several autoimmune diseases, and as a consequence of radiation therapy and certain medications (see Table 29–3). Xerostoma from radiation therapy may be more permanent than that from other causes (Garg and Malo, 1997). Efforts to stimulate saliva production using pilocarpine and citrus-flavored, sugar-free candies may ease eating difficulty. Individuals without any saliva at all have the most difficulty eating; artificial salivary agents may not offer relief. Lack of saliva impedes all aspects of eating, including chewing, swallowing, and the sensation of taste; causes pain; and increases the risk of dental caries and infections. Dietary guidelines focus on the use of moist foods without added spices, and use of lemon glycerine or liquids with all meals and snacks. Problems with chewy (steak), crumbly (cake, crackers), dry (chips), and sticky (peanut butter) foods are common in individuals with severe xerostomia, and avoiding these foods may help a great deal with eating. Good oral hygiene habits are important to reduce the risk of tooth decay.

Diabetes is associated with several oral manifestations, many of which occur only in periods of poor control. These include burning mouth syndrome, periodontal disease, candidiasis, dental caries, and xerostomia (Finney et al., 1997; Touger-Decker and Sirois, 1995). The microangiopathies seen in diabetes, along with altered responses to infection, contribute to periodontal disease risk in affected individuals. Besides blood glucose control, dietary management of the individual with diabetes following any surgical procedures and or placement of dentures should include modifications in the consistency, temperature, and texture of food to increase eating comfort, reduce oral pain, and prevent infections or decay.

Surgery

Head and neck and oral cancers can alter eating ability and nutrition status by virtue of the surgeries and therapies used to treat these cancers. Surgery, depending on the location and extent, may alter eating and/or swallowing ability, as well as the capacity of the individual to produce saliva. Radiation therapy of the head and neck area, as well as chemotherapeutic agents, can affect the quantity and quality of saliva and the integrity of the oral mucosa. A thick, ropey saliva is often the result of radiation therapy to the head and neck area causing xerostomia. Dietary management focuses on the recommendations described earlier for xerostomia, along with modifications in food consistency postsurgery.

POLYPHARMACY

Several categories of medications can alter the integrity of the oral mucosa, taste sensation, and salivary production. Table 29–3 lists medications associated with xerostomia. Dilantin may cause severe gingivitis. Many of the protease inhibitor drugs used to treat AIDS are associated with altered taste and dry mouth. Care should be taken to assess the effects of medication on the oral cavity and how these effects can be minimized by alterations in diet or drug therapy.

In planning nutrition care, the dietetics professional is encouraged to incorporate questions on the patient's oral health status as a component of nutritional screening and assessment, including problems with biting, chewing or swallowing, dry mouth, or the presence of sores in the mouth that interfere with eating comfort.

CASE STUDY

Nathan C., a 3-year-old black boy, is brought to the local health clinic by his grandmother because his front teeth are "turning black." Nathan seems small for his age; his height is measured at 35.5 in., and his weight is 25 lb. According to the growth charts, he is in the 10th percentile for height, the 5th percentile for weight, and below the 5th percentile in terms of weight for height for his age.

Upon examination by the dentist, the child is found to have eight decayed surfaces on his four anterior teeth (the two central incisors and the two lateral incisors). The dentist recommends that Nathan have metal crowns put on the decayed teeth. She also recommends that the grandmother have the child's diet and nutritional status evaluated by the clinic's registered dietitian.

The grandmother agrees, and the dietary history taken by the dietitian reveals the following:

- A diet high in simple sugar with small, frequent meals
- Continued use of a bottle filled with fruit drink, soda, or strawberry-flavored milk three times a day, including naptime
- Suboptimal calorie and protein intake (70% and 75% of estimated needs, respectively)
- Lack of vitamin–mineral and fluoride supplements
- Nonrenewal of WIC checks within the last 6 months because the grandmother does not like traveling to the area in which the clinic is located
- Inconsistent toothbrushing (The grandmother reports brushing the child's teeth three to four times per week. She does not think care of baby teeth is important, as "they fall out anyway.")

1. What are the cultural, educational, and environmental influences that are impacting the dental and nutritional health of Nathan?
2. What type of dental condition does Nathan have? What are the diet counseling recommendations for this condition?
3. What are the nutritional and dietary risk factors?
4. Design a nutrition care plan to improve this youngster's dental health and growth.

CITED REFERENCES

American Dietetic Association: Position of the ADA: The impact of fluoride on dental health. J Am Diet Assoc 94:1428, 1994.

American Dietetic Association: Position of the American Dietetic Association (ADA): Oral health and nutrition. J Am Diet Assoc 96:184, 1996.

Barnes GP, et al. Ethnicity, location, age and fluoridation factors in baby bottle tooth decay and caries prevalence of Head Start children. Public Health Rep 107(2):167, 1992.

Ettinger RL. Changing dietary patterns with changing dentition: How do people cope? Spec Care Dentistry 18(1):33, 1998.
Febres C, et al. Parental awareness, habits, and social factors and their relationship to baby bottle tooth decay. Pediatr Dentistry 19(1):22, 1997.
Finney LS, et al. What the mouth has to say about diabetes. Careful examinations can avert serious complications. Postgrad Med 102:117, 1997.
Garg AK, Malo M. Manifestations and treatment of xerostomia and associated oral effects secondary to head and neck radiation therapy. J Am Dental Assoc 97:1128, 1997.
Grenby TH, et al. Laboratory studies of the dental properties of soft drinks. Br J Nutr 62:451, 1989.
Jenkins GN, Hargreaves JA. Effect of eating cheese on Ca and P concentrations of whole mouth saliva and plaque. Caries Res 23:159, 1989.
Joshipura KJ, Willet WC. Effect of edentulousness on diet and nutrition. J Dent Res 73 (IADR Abstr):207, 1994.
Joshipura KJ, et al. The impact of edentulousness on food and nutrient intake. J Am Dent Assoc 127:459, 1996.
Josti A, et al. The distribution of root caries in community dwelling elders in New England. J Publ Health Dent 54:15, 1994.
Kashket S, et al. Accumulation of fermentable sugars and metabolic acids in food particles that become entrapped on the dentition. J Dent Res 75:1885, 1996.
Kiritsky MC, et al. Assessing fluoride concentration of juices and juice-flavored drinks. J Am Dent Assoc 127:895, 1997.
Koenigsberg S, et al. Incidence of baby bottle tooth decay in young inner city children. Unpublished report, 1994.
Narhi TO, et al. Salivary findings, daily medication and root caries in the elderly. Caries Res 32(1):5, 1998.
National Institute of Dental Health. Results of National Oral Health Survey Released. Available: www.nidr.nih.gov/news; March 12, 1996.
Newbrun E. Effectiveness of water fluoridation. J Pub Health Dent 49(Spec issue):279, 1989.
O'Sullivan DM, Tinanoff N. The association of early dental caries patterns with caries incidence in preschool children. J Public Health Dent 56(2):81, 1996.
Robb ND, Geidrys-Leeper E. The distribution of erosion in the dentitions of patients with eating disorders. Br Dent J 178:171, 1995.
Shay K. Root caries in the older patient: Significance, prevention and treatment. Dent Clin North Am 41(4):763, 1997.
Steinberg LM, et al. Remineralizing potential, antiplaque and antigingivitis effects of xylitol and sorbitol sweetened chewing gum. Clin Prev Dent 14(5):31–34, 1992.
Touger-Decker R, Sirois D. Dental care of the person with diabetes. In: Powers M (ed.). Handbook of Diabetes Nutrition Management, 2nd ed. Gaithersburg, MD: Aspen Publishers, 1995.
Touger-Decker R, et al. Effect of edentulism and dentures on diet and nutritional status. Unpublished report, 1997.
U.S. Department of Health and Human Services. CDC's Oral Health Program At-A-Glance 1996–1997. Washington, DC: U.S. DHHS Public Health Service, 1997.
U.S. Department of Health and Human Services. Food and Nutrition for Life: Malnutrition and Older Americans. Washington, DC: U.S. DHHS. December, 1994.

ADDITIONAL REFERENCES

American Dental Association ONLINE. Fluorides and Fluoridation. Available: www.ada.org/consumer/fluoride.
Anderson MH, et al. Modern management of dental caries: The cutting edge is not the dental burr. J Am Dent Assoc 124:37, 1993.
Bibby BG, et al. Oral food clearance and the pH of plaque and saliva. J Am Dent Assoc 112:333, 1986.
Boyd LD, et al. Nutrition implications of xerostomia and rampant caries caused by serotonin re-uptake inhibitors: A case study. Nutr Rev 55:362, 1997.
Faine M, et al. Dietary and salivary factors associated with root caries. Spec Care Dent 12(4):177, 1992.
Garrett NR, Perez P, Elbert C, Kapur KK. Effects of improvements of poorly fitting dentures and new dentures on masticatory performance. J Prosthet Dent 75:269, 1996.
Gedalia I, et al. Effect of hard cheese exposure, with and without fluoride prerinse, on the rehardening of softened human enamel. Caries Res 26:290, 1992.
Greska LP, et al. The dietary adequacy of edentulous older adults. J Prosthet Dent 73:142, 1995.
Gustafsson BE, et al. The Vipeholm dental caries study: The effect of different levels of carbohydrate intake on caries activity in 436 individuals observed for five years. Acta Odontol Scand 11:232, 1954.
Jensen ME, Wefel JS. Efects of processed cheese on human plaque pH and demineralization and remineralization. Am J Dent 3:217, 1990.
Kandelman D, Gagnon G. A 24-month clinical study of the incidence and progression of dental caries in relation to consumption of chewing gum containing xylitol in school preventive programs. J Dent Res 69:1771, 1990.
Kelly M, Bruerd B. The prevalence of baby bottle tooth decay among two Native American populations. J Public Health Dent 47:94, 1987.
O'Sullivan DM, Tinanoff N. Social and biological factors contributing to caries of the maxillary anterior teeth. Pediatr Dent 15:41, 1993.
Pappas AS, et al. The effects of denture status on nutrition. Spec Care Dent 18(1):17, 1998.
Rugg-Gunn AJ, et al. The effect of different meal patterns upon plaque pH in human subjects. Br Dent J 139:351, 1975.
Sebring NG, et al. Nutritional adequacy of reported intake of edentulous subjects treated with new conventional or implant-supported mandibular dentures. J Prosthet Dent 74:358, 1995.

PART 5

Medical Nutrition Therapy

Nutrition plays a primary role in growth, development, health, and fitness. As we have seen, maintaining appropriate nutrition throughout life can also prevent, or at least delay, the onset of some nutrition-related disease. This section covers the importance of nutritional care in the treatment of established disease. Today, this process is defined as Medical Nutrition Therapy (MNT).

As the knowledge base expands, the list of diseases amenable to nutrition intervention increases. Availability of sophisticated feeding and nourishment procedures places increased responsibility on those who provide nutritional care. Many nutrition professionals who are experts in their specific fields have contributed to this section.

Most of the nutrition-related diseases included here are preventable by changes in dietary practices, at least on the basis of current knowledge. Exceptions, such as some forms of neoplastic disease, are discussed in terms of both the evidence for prevention and the appropriate nutritional care in established disease.

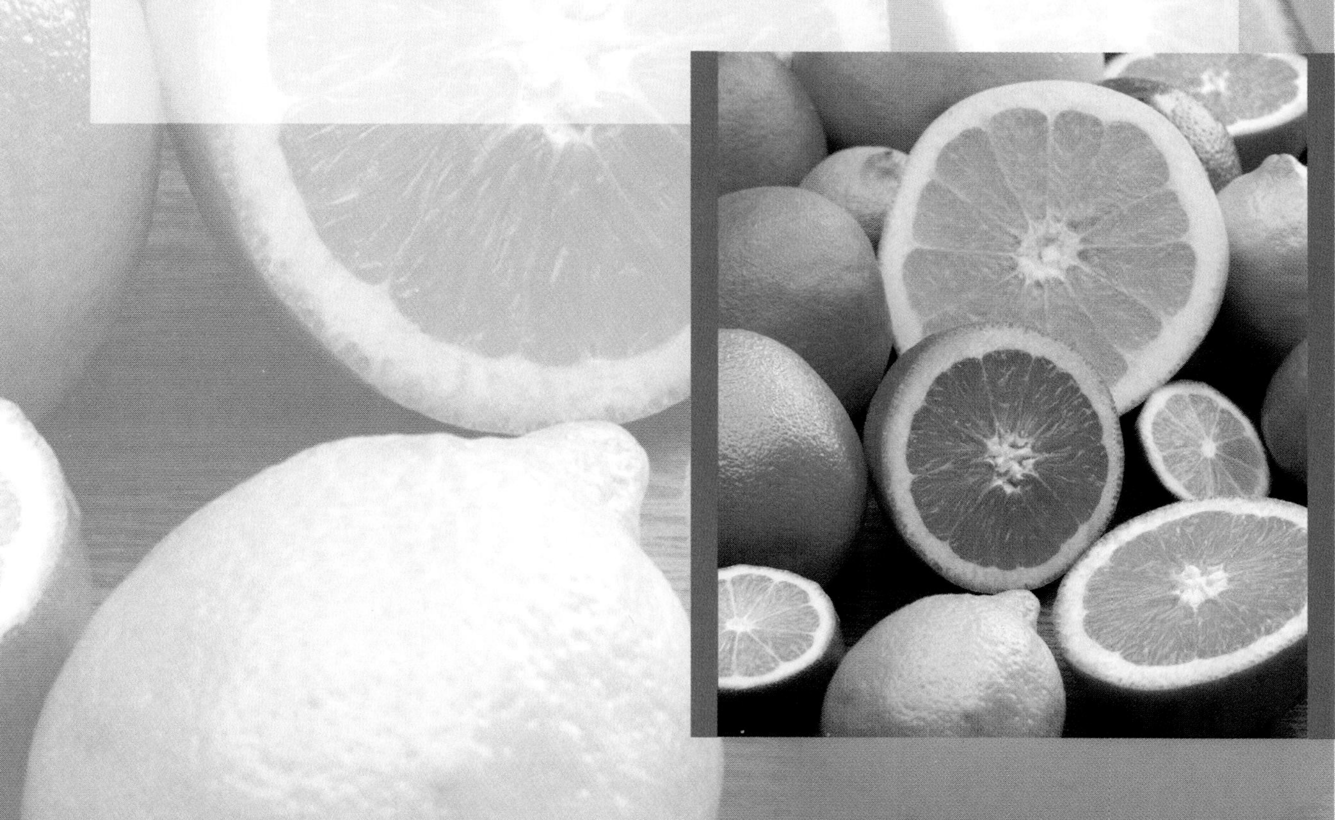

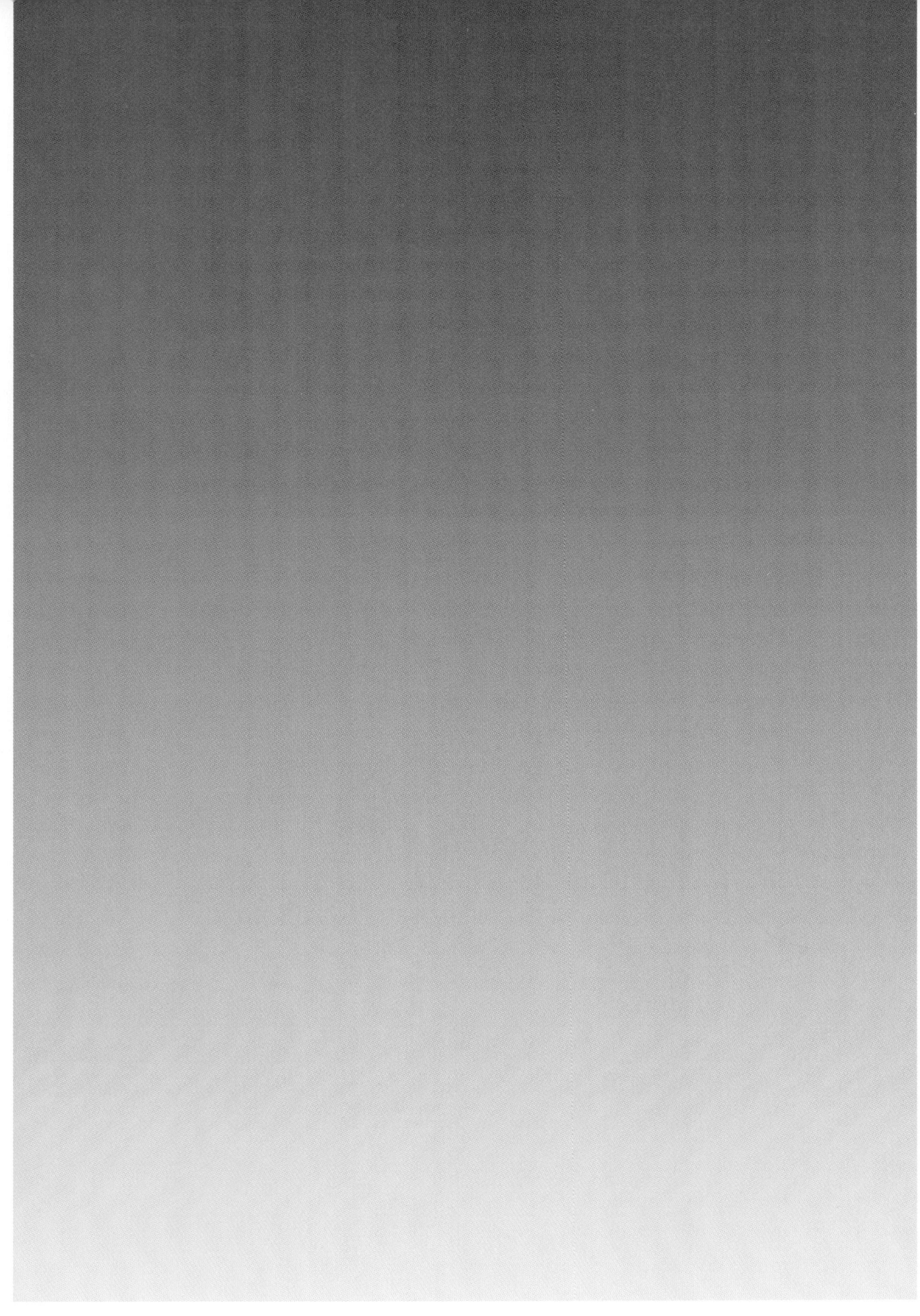

CHAPTER 30

Medical Nutrition Therapy for Upper Gastrointestinal Tract Disorders

PETER L. BEYER, MS, RD

Chapter Outline

Key Terms

ACHLORHYDRIA—absence of hydrochloric acid from maximally stimulated gastric secretions

ACHYLIA GASTRICA—absence of hydrochloric acid and pepsin in the gastric juice

ALIMENTARY HYPOGLYCEMIA—low blood glucose manifesting as weakness, perspiration, hunger, nausea, anxiety, and tremors 1 to 2 hours after a meal

ATROPHIC GASTRITIS—chronic gastritis with deterioration of the mucous membrane and glands, resulting in achlorhydria and loss of intrinsic factor

DUMPING SYNDROME—a complex physiologic response to the rapid emptying of hypertonic contents into the duodenum and jejunum

DUODENAL ULCER—a peptic ulcer situated in the duodenum

DYSPEPSIA (INDIGESTION)—a general term used to describe epigastric discomfort following meals

ENDOSCOPY—a procedure used to view the esophagus, using a flexible tube passed into the stomach

EPIGASTRIC—referring to the upper middle region of the abdomen

ESOPHAGITIS—inflammation of the esophagus

FUNDOPLICATION—a surgical procedure for the treatment of reflux esophagitis that involves mobilizing the lower end of the esophagus and wrapping the fundus of the stomach around it

GASTRIC ULCERS—lesions that are associated with disruption of the gastric mucosal barrier

GASTRITIS—inflammation of the stomach

GASTROESOPHAGEAL REFLUX—backward flow of the stomach and/or duodenal contents into the esophagus; may occur normally or as a chronic pathologic condition

HEARTBURN (PYROSIS)—a retrosternal burning related to reflux of acid fluid from the stomach into the esophagus

HELICOBACTER PYLORI—a type of bacteria that can chronically infect the stomach; thought to be a primary contributor to development of gastritis and peptic ulcers

HIATAL HERNIA—an outpouching of a portion of the stomach into the chest through the esophageal hiatus of the diaphragm

LOWER ESOPHAGEAL SPHINCTER—the last few centimeters of the esophagus which prevent reflux of gastric contents into the esophagus

MELENA—black, tarry stools indicative of gastrointestinal bleeding

MUCOSITIS—inflammation of the oral mucous membranes

PARIETAL CELLS—large cells, located on the margin of the peptic glands of the stomach, which secrete hydrochloric acid and produce intrinsic factor

PARIETAL CELL VAGOTOMY—resection or removal of the portion of the vagus nerve innervating the parietal cells for the purpose of diminishing gastric acid secretion

PEPTIC ULCER—an eroded lesion in either the esophageal, gastric, or duodenal mucosa resulting from the action of acid in gastric juice

REFLUX ESOPHAGITIS—inflammation of the esophagus related to chronic reflux of gastric contents into the esophagus

TRUNCAL VAGOTOMY—resection or removal of portions of the vagus nerve so as to decrease the cholinergic stimulation of parietal cells and reduce the cellular response to stimulants, such as gastrin

VAGUS NERVE—the 10th cranial nerve, which has many branches that supply sensory fibers to the ear, tongue, pharynx, and larynx; motor fibers to the pharynx, larynx, and esophagus; and parasympathetic and visceral afferent fibers to the thoracic and abdominal viscera

Digestive disorders are among the most common problems in health care. Approximately 30% to 40% of adults claim to have frequent indigestion, and more than 47 million visits are made annually to ambulatory care facilities for symptoms related to the digestive system. About 2.8 million endoscopies and 5 million surgical procedures involving the gastrointestinal (GI) tract are performed each year (Schappert, 1998; Kozak and Owings, 1998).

Dietary habits and specific food types can play a significant role in the onset, treatment, and prevention of many GI disorders. In many cases, diet can also play a role in improving patients' sense of well-being and quality of life and in decreasing pain, suffering, and the costs associated with gastrointestinal disease (Beyer, 1998).

TABLE 30–1 COMMON SYMPTOMS OF GASTROINTESTINAL DISEASE

SYMPTOM	POSSIBLE DISORDER
Ingestion of solid food causes distress, but liquids do not.	Esophageal stricture or tumor
Difficulty swallowing; food sticks in throat	Esophageal spasm; achalasia
Epigastric pain when eating	Gastric ulcer
Pain 2–5 hours after a meal; pain relief after eating	Duodenal ulcer
Abdominal pain several hours after ingesting a fatty meal	Pancreatic or biliary tract disease
Cramps, distention, and flatulence 18–24 hours after drinking milk	Lactose intolerance, due to lactase deficiency or rapid transit time
Heartburn after eating a large or fatty meal	Esophageal reflux

DISORDERS OF THE ESOPHAGUS

The entire esophagus functions as one tissue during swallowing. As a bolus of food is moved voluntarily from the mouth to the pharynx, the upper sphincter relaxes, the food moves into the esophagus, and the **lower esophageal sphincter** (LES) relaxes to receive the food bolus. Peristaltic waves move the bolus down the esophagus and into the stomach.

Disorders of the esophagus are caused by obstruction, inflammation, or derangement of the swallowing mechanism. Table 30–1 lists symptoms that are common in gastrointestinal disorders. Because difficulty in swallowing (*dysphagia*) is often the result of a neurologic problem, the required nutritional care for that condition is discussed in Chapter 42.

Esophagitis

Pathophysiology

Esophagitis usually occurs as a result of reflux of gastric acid and/or intestinal contents on to the lower esophageal mucosa. A common symptom associated with this mucosal inflammation is **heartburn,** which is a burning epigastric, substernal pain. Other symptoms include regurgitation and dysphagia. Figure 30–1 shows the pathophysiology of esophagitis.

Acute esophagitis is caused by ingestion of an irritating agent, viral inflammation, or intubation. Risk of chronic or **reflux esophagitis** is increased with hiatal hernia, reduced LES pressure, increased abdominal pressure (as in obstructive lung disease), delayed gastric emptying, recurrent vomiting, or other factors. When lower esophagitis is chronic, ulceration, scarring, stricture, and, eventually, dysphagia can develop.

The severity of the esophagitis resulting from **gastroesophageal reflux** is influenced by several factors. These include the composition, frequency, and volume of the gastric reflux; mucosal resistance; rate of clearance from the esophagus; and the rate of gastric emptying (Goyal, 1998).

Competency of the LES is also important. The pressure of this sphincter is influenced by many factors, including scleroderma-like disorders, smoking, and smooth muscle relaxants. LES pressures also decrease during pregnancy, in women taking progesterone-containing oral contraceptives, and even in the late stage of a normal menstrual cycle. Almost everyone experiences transient reflux episodes, but prolonged reflux can be a serious problem. Gastroesophageal reflux may further complicate matters in patients with chronic lung disease who may aspirate during sleep.

Although most cases of esophagitis are related to reflux of gastric contents, esophagitis may also be related to viral and bacterial infection, ingestion of corrosive agents, and radiation. Large doses or chronic use of aspirin and the nonsteroidal anti-inflammatory drugs (NSAIDs), and several other oral medications, may increase the risk of esophagitis in susceptible persons (Goyal, 1998).

Nutritional Care

The objectives of nutritional care are to (1) prevent pain and irritation of the inflamed esophageal mucosa during the acute phase, (2) prevent esophageal reflux, and (3) decrease the erosive capacity or acidity of gastric secretions.

In the acute inflammatory or erosive phase, the patient may prefer a liquid diet and may want to avoid foods that could obstruct the esophagus or, in rare circumstances, cause perforation (e.g., taco chips, very crisp crackers, and husks). Foods with an acid pH, such as citrus juices, tomatoes, and soft drinks, may cause pain when the esophagus is inflamed. Spices, such as chili powder and black pepper, may also result in additional irritation and dis-

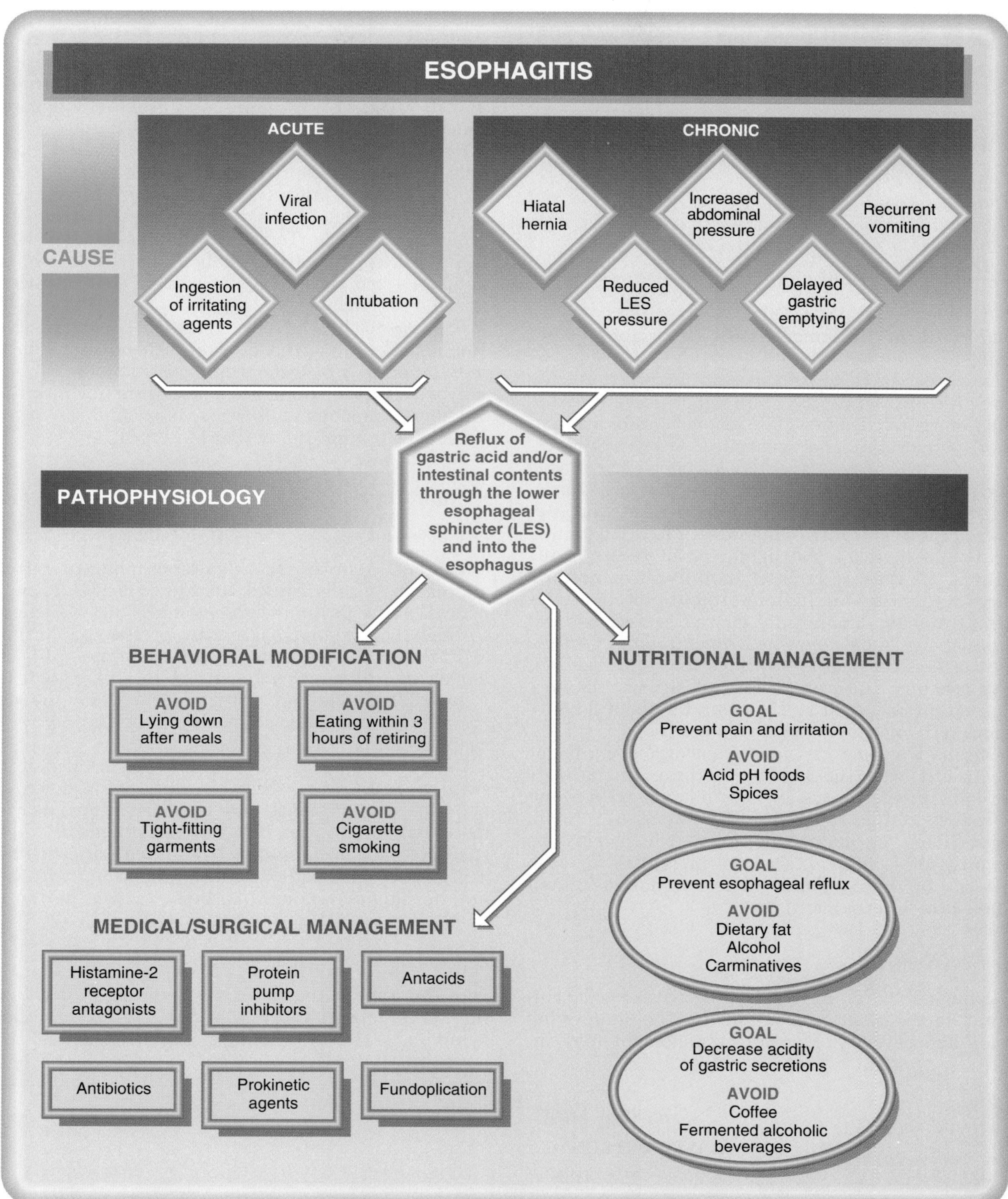

FIGURE 30–1 Pathophysiology algorithm—esophagitis. (Algorithm content developed by John Anderson, Ph.D., and Sanford C. Garner, Ph.D., 2000.)

TABLE 30–2 NUTRITIONAL CARE GUIDELINES FOR PATIENTS WITH REFLUX AND ESOPHAGITIS

1. Avoid large, high-fat meals, especially 2 to 3 hours before retiring.
2. Avoid acidic and highly spiced foods when inflammation exists.
3. Avoid chocolate, alcohol, and caffeine-containing beverages, such as coffee.
4. Avoid peppermint and spearmint oils.
5. Stay upright and avoid vigorous activity soon after eating.
6. Avoid tight-fitting clothing, especially after a meal.
7. Avoid smoking.

comfort during inflamed states (Rodriguez et al., 1998).

Avoidance of certain foods and factors that may lower LES pressure may improve or prevent symptoms of reflux. Dietary fat, alcohol, and carminatives (peppermint and spearmint) lower LES pressure. Coffee and fermented alcoholic beverages (such as beer and wine) stimulate the secretion of gastric acid. The size and timing of meals also appear to be important. Lying down after consuming meals can increase the likelihood of reflux, especially if the meal is large or high in fat or protein. Large meals that are high in fat and protein stimulate significant amounts of gastric secretions, and high-density, meals slow gastric emptying. Persons with reflux, therefore, will have fewer problems if they consume little or no food (especially meato r cheese containing fat and protein) for about 3 hours before retiring.

Obesity was once considered a contributing factor because it was thought to increase intragastric pressure. However, weight loss has not been found to reduce reflux symptoms (Kjellin et al., 1996). Tight-fitting garments, however, which may be worn by obese individuals, are thought to increase the risk of reflux. Table 30–2 summarizes nutritional care for esophagitis.

Medical/Surgical Management

Esophageal reflux may be treated with several different medications, depending on the underlying cause and severity. Medical management may include histamine-2 (H_2) receptor antagonists or proton pump inhibitors, which decrease acid secretion; antacids, which reduce gastric pH; antibiotics, which treat bacterial gastritis; various medications that increase LES pressure, and prokinetic agents, which hasten gastric emptying.

Because nicotine decreases LES pressure, cigarette smoking is contraindicated (see "*Clinical Insight:* Smoking and Gastrointestinal Function"). Medications that decrease LES pressure should be avoided if possible. To reduce the likelihood of nocturnal reflux, it is often beneficial for the patient to sleep on a bed with an upper portion that has been raised 4 to 8 inches.

The 5% to 10% of patients with severe gastroesophageal reflux who do not respond to medical therapy after 3 to 6 months may be treated surgically with **fundoplication,** a procedure in which the fundus of the stomach is wrapped around the lower esophagus to limit reflux (Perdikis et al., 1997).

Hiatal Hernia

Pathophysiology

A common contributor to gastroesophageal reflux and esophagitis is **hiatal hernia,** which is an outpouching of a portion of the stomach into the chest through the esophageal hiatus of the diaphragm (Mittal and Balaban, 1997). A major type of hiatal hernia—*paraesophageal hernia*—is illustrated in Figure 30–2. The pressure generated by the diaphragm forces acidic stomach contents up into the esophagus.

Patients with hiatal hernia may experience difficulty with deep breathing, or when lying down or bending over. Patients may experience **epigastric** discomfort after large, calorically dense meals when their stomach is distended. Not all patients with hiatal hernia have reflux, but more patients with hiatal hernia have reflux than those without hernia.

Nutritional Care

Diet therapy for hiatal hernia is aimed at decreasing symptoms in those who have reflux or other symptoms. Therapy includes the omission of the

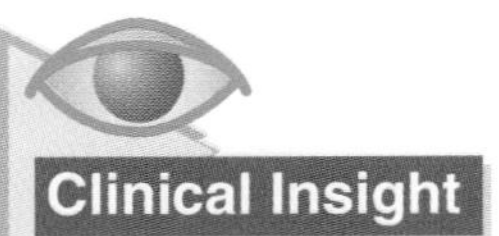

SMOKING AND GASTROINTESTINAL FUNCTION

The gastrointestinal effects of smoking include the reduction of LES and pyloric sphincter pressure, increased reflux, alteration of the nature of the gastric contents, inhibition of pancreatic bicarbonate secretion, accelerated gastric emptying of liquids, and lower duodenal pH. The acid secretory response to gastrin or acetylcholine is increased considerably. Smoking also impairs the ability of cimetidine and other drugs to lower the overnight acid secretion that is thought to play a key role in ulcerogenesis. Finally, smoking impairs spontaneous healing and increases the risk and rapidity of ulcer recurrence, as well as the likelihood that the ulcer will perforate and require surgery.

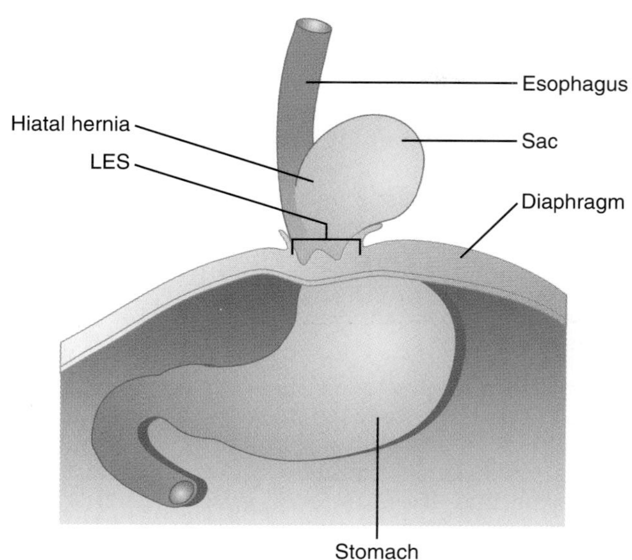

FIGURE 30–2 Diagram of a paraesophageal hiatal hernia. (*LES*, lower esophageal sphincter)

same types of foods as are contraindicated for esophagitis—that is, foods that may increase reflux or acid gastric secretions—and the consumption of smaller, low-fat meals. Surgery is not always indicated for hiatal hernia; dietary, symptom control is generally the preferred treatment.

Cancer of the Oral Cavity, Pharynx, and Esophagus

Pathophysiology

The patient who has been diagnosed with cancer of the oral cavity, pharynx, or esophagus may present with existing nutritional problems and eating difficulties caused by the tumor mass, obstruction, oral infection and ulceration, or alcoholism, a coexisting condition that is frequently associated with these tumors. Nutritional deficits may be compounded by the treatment, which commonly involves surgical resection, regional irradiation, or chemotherapy. Chewing, swallowing, salivation, and taste acuity are often affected. Extensive dental decay, osteoradionecrosis, and infections may also occur. Chemotherapy, if given, can be expected to produce nausea, vomiting, and anorexia (see Chapter 34).

Nutritional Care

Initially, nutritional support is provided via tubefeeding if the remainder of the gastrointestinal tract is functional. The extent of the resection may require long-term feeding by tube if the ability to eat cannot be regained. If oral feeding is possible after surgery, general dietary recommendations would include liquid or soft-textured, moist foods for easy mastication and swallowing, and small, frequent meals of relatively high caloric density. If steatorrhea exists, use of medium-chain triglycerides in the formula may be necessary. The use of complex carbohydrates is preferred over simple sugars.

Periodic use of an artificial saliva solution is also helpful, as is the frequent consumption of fluids to prevent dry mouth. Normal saline rinses may ameliorate **mucositis,** and topical anesthetics can be used to relieve pain. Necessary dental restorations, aggressive oral hygiene, and daily use of fluoride are recommended. Oral infections at this time are usually fungal. Unfortunately, some of the medications used in treatment may leave a metallic taste in the mouth that can further compromise the patient's desire to eat.

SURGERY OF THE MOUTH OR ESOPHAGUS

After extensive surgery of the mouth or esophagus, it may be necessary to provide oral nutrition support in liquid form. Many nutritionally complete formulas are available (see Appendices 35 through 40). To add variety to the diet, ordinary foods, such as fruits, can be puréed and mixed with water until liquefied. With more extensive oral involvement, it may be necessary to use a gastrostomy or jejunostomy tube for administering the liquid enterally. Enteral tube feedings may involve the use of ready-to-feed formulas or blenderized table foods (see Chapter 22). In rare situations, it may be necessary to provide nutritional support parenterally.

Tonsillectomy

Tonsils are lymphatic tissue and part of the immune system. Tonsillectomy is less common today than in the past, as mild inflammation of the tonsils is considered to be a natural part of the immune system's efforts to fight infection. When necessary, the doctor may remove the tonsils in an attempt to reduce the number and frequency of ear infections, tonsillitis, and sinusitis.

Because the convalescent period following a tonsillectomy is short, the nutritional adequacy of the diet is not critical. Cold, mild-flavored, soft, moist foods bring the most comfort to the patient and offer the most protection against unexpected bleeding from the surgical area. During the first 24 hours, foods that are best accepted include dairy beverages, such as milk, malted milk, and eggnogs; ice cream or frozen yogurt; fruit ice; and pear, peach, or apricot nectors. By the second day, warm fluids and soft foods may be introduced; thereafter, hot foods can be introduced cautiously as healing progresses and as these foods are tolerated. A normal diet can be instituted within 3 to 5 days.

DISORDERS OF THE STOMACH

Indigestion/Dyspepsia

Pathophysiology

Indigestion, or **dyspepsia,** is a general term that is frequently used to describe discomfort in the upper digestive tract. Symptoms of dyspepsia may include vague abdominal pain, bloating, nausea, regurgitation, and belching. Dysphagia may be relatively benign and have little consequence, or it may indicate more serious problems. Symptoms of prolonged dysphagia may be related to underlying problems, such as gastroesophageal reflux, gastritis, peptic ulcer disease, delayed gastric emptying, gallbladder disease, or cancer.

Patients who present with frequent or long-standing dyspepsia are usually evaluated for more significant problems, but many persons have symptoms that persist despite lack of specific pathology (Talley et al., 1998; McQuaid, 1998; Koch, 1997). In patients with symptoms unrelated to a specific pathologic process, diet, stress, and other life-style factors may also play a role.

Nutritional Care

Dietary indulgences—excessive volumes of food or high intake of fat, sugar, caffeine, spices, or alcohol, or both—are commonly implicated in dyspepsia (Mishkin et al., 1997; Marotta and Floch, 1991). Dietary management of uncomplicated dyspepsia is simple and has probably been passed on for generations: eat slowly, chew thoroughly, and do not eat or drink excessively. Reaction to life stresses may also contribute to abdominal distress, in which case behavioral management and emotional support may also help. If symptoms persist despite these strategies, the individual may require further evaluation.

Gastritis and Peptic Ulcer Disease

Pathophysiology

Gastritis and peptic ulceration may result when microbial, chemical, neural, or chemical abnormalities disrupt the factors that normally maintain mucosal integrity. The most common cause of gastritis and peptic ulcer is ***Helicobacter pylori*** infection (see "*Focus On: Helicobacter Pylori* Infection, Gastritis, and Peptic Ulcer Disease") but chronic use of aspirin or other NSAIDs, alcohol abuse, ingestion of erosive substances, or any combination of these factors may also be contributory (Fig. 30–3). Tobacco product use, large doses of corticosteroids, and general poor health may contribute to the onset and severity of the symptoms (Laine and Fendrick, 1997; Blum, 1996; Sontag, 1997).

The mucosa of the stomach and duodenum is normally protected from the proteolytic actions of gastric acid and pepsin by a coating of mucus secreted by glands in the epithelial walls from the lower esophagus to the upper duodenum. The mucosal

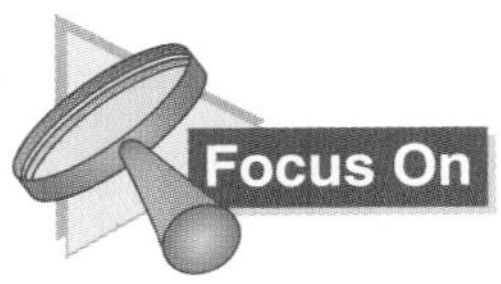

Helicobacter Pylori Infection, Gastritis, and Peptic Ulcer Disease

Helicobacter pylori infection is now known to be responsible for most of the cases of chronic inflammation of the gastric mucosa and of gastric and duodenal ulcers. *H. pylori* infection also increases the risk of some forms of atrophic gastritis and gastric cancer. The infection is typically confined to the mucosa of the stomach and is not found in the small intestine (Dunn et al., 1997). Factors that affect the occurrence and severity of symptoms include the individual's age at onset of the initial infection, the concentration of organisms, the specific strain of the organism, and often, the health of the individual (Laine and Fendrick, 1998).

H. pylori organisms are microaerophilic, gram-negative bacteria with flagella that facilitate mobility. These organisms are somewhat resistant to the acidic medium of the stomach, but additional protection is provided by their colonization beneath the protective mucous layer and by significant urease production. Urease allows the generation of ammonia to facilitate alkalinization of the immediate surroundings. The size and shape of these organisms range from spirals to coils to rods, depending on the culture media of the stomach. Prevalence of *H. pylori* infection among the adult population ranges from approximately 50% in developed countries to greater than 90% of the population in developing countries. However, only 10% to 15% of those infected by the organism develop symptomatic ulceration. The exposure and prevalence in the United States may be declining over time. Infection with *H. pylori* in young persons is now only about 10%, but the incidence in persons older than 60 years of age is about 50% (Laine and Fendrick, 1998).

Infection with the *H. pylori* organism results in a chronic inflammatory state. Infection induces inflammation from both humoral and systemic immune response, with damage resulting from cytotoxins produced by the organism during the inflammatory response by the host (Peek and Blazer, 1997; Hunt, 1997).

Treatment typically involves combination therapy of three or four medications, including bismuth, antibiotics, and antisecretory agents. The degree of microbial resistance to specific agents in different parts of the world, and the varying strains of the organism may necessitate the use of different protocols and combinations of medications. Eradication of the organism results in elimination of the inflammatory state and the symptoms (Dunn et al., 1997; Laine and Fendrick, 1998).

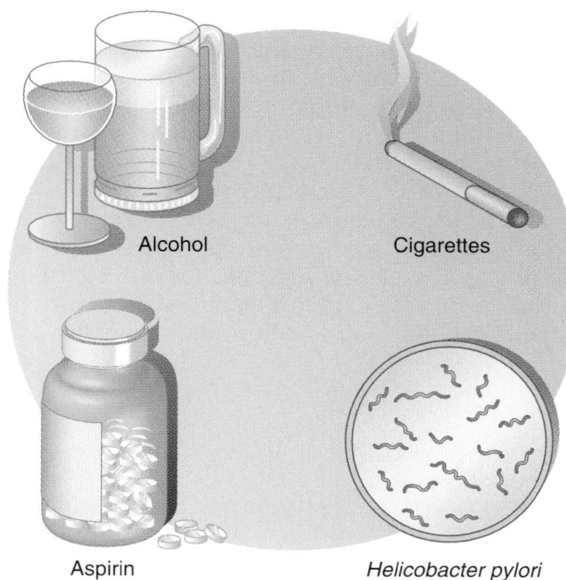

FIGURE 30–3 Common causes of gastritis.

layer is also protected from bacterial invasion by the digestive actions of pepsin and hydrochloric acid and the mucus secretions. The mucus contains acid-neutralizing bicarbonates, and additional bicarbonates are provided by the pancreatic juice secreted into the intestinal lumen.

Production of mucus is stimulated by the action of prostaglandins. Hydrochloric acid is secreted by the parietal cells in response to stimuli by acetylcholine, gastrin, and histamine (Hojgaard et al., 1996; Soll, 1998).

Gastritis

Gastritis is a general term that refers to the inflammation and tissue damage resulting from erosion of the mucosal layer and exposure of the underlying cells to gastric secretions and microbes. The most common cause of chronic gastritis is infection with *H. pylori* (see "*New Directions:* Genome of *Helicobacter pylori*"). The exposure results in general and specific inflammatory and immune responses to the gastric secretions and pathogens. Acute gastritis refers to rapid onset of inflammation and symptoms. Chronic gastritis may occur over a period of months to decades, with waxing and waning of symptoms. Gastritis may be manifested by a number of symptoms, including nausea, vomiting, malaise, anorexia, hemorrhage, and epigastric pain (Soll, 1998) (see "*Focus On:* Endoscopy").

Atrophic gastritis, which results in atrophy and loss of stomach **parietal cells**, is characterized by a loss of secretion of hydrochloric acid (**achlorhydria**) and intrinsic factor. Most cases are considered to have an autoimmune origin, although about 25% of cases may be a result of long-term *H. pylori* infection (Annibale et al., 1997).

Treatment of gastritis, which is discussed in greater detail later in this chapter, includes the eradication of pathogenic organisms (e.g., *H. pylori*) and withdrawal of any provoking agents. Antibiotics, antacids, H_2-receptor antagonists, and proton pump inhibitors may each play a role in the treatment of gastritis, depending on the precipitating cause. In individuals with atrophic gastritis, vitamin B_{12} status should be evaluated because a lack of intrinsic factor results in malabsorption of this vitamin (see the discussion on vitamin status assessment in Chapters 4, 17, and 35).

Peptic Ulcers

PATHOPHYSIOLOGY

Normal gastric and duodenal mucosa is protected from the digestive actions of acid and pepsin by the secretion of mucus, the production of bicarbonate, removal of excess acid by normal blood flow, and rapid renewal and repair of epithelial cell injury. **Peptic ulcer** refers to an ulcer that occurs as a result of the breakdown of these normal defense and repair mechanisms. Typically, more than one of the mechanisms must be malfunctioning for symptomatic peptic ulcers to develop. Unlike damage from gastritis and other forms of superficial injury, classical peptic

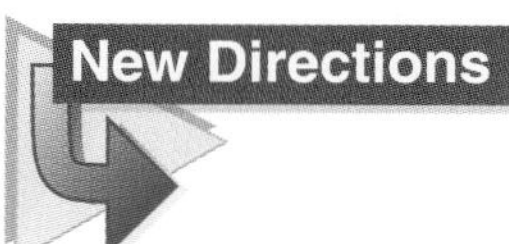

Genome of *Helicobacter Pylori*

The ability of robotic analyzers to sequence long lengths of DNA automatically and the rapidity with which computers can scan gene data banks have spawned a new discipline in the biomedical sciences: genomics. Sequencing genomes for microbial conditions offers an expeditious means of searching for novel treatments for infectious disease. *Helicobacter pylori* genome studies are important in this realm. *H. pylori* organisms live only in the human stomach, and the enzymatic pathways they need for survival in this harsh milieu are continually switched on. There are a number of antigenic variations that occur. Many genes have been found to code for iron-scavenging pathways, indicating a crucial role for iron in the survival of *H. pylori* in the stomach. The unlocking of the genome and the logical sequencing of key targets will allow the creation of novel inhibitory and bactericidal products against which no microbe has yet had the chance to become resistant (Lee, 1998).

ulcers erode through the muscularis mucosa into the submucous or muscularis propria (Fig. 30–4). Peptic ulcers typically show evidence of chronic inflammation and repair processes surrounding the lesion.

The primary causes of peptic ulcers are *H. pylori* infection, the use of aspirin and other NSAIDs (Fig. 30–5), and so-called stress ulcers. Concentrated forms of ethanol may damage gastric mucosa, worsen symptoms of peptic ulcer, and interfere with ulcer healing, but they do not appear to cause peptic ulcer. Consumption of beer and wine increases gastric secretions, whereas ethanol itself, in similar concentrations, may not. Use of tobacco products decreases bicarbonate secretion and is associated with additional complications of *H. pylori* infection. In some situations, high doses of corticosteriods have been found to increase the risk of peptic ulcer (Gutthann et al., 1997).

As a result of the early recognition of the symptoms and associated causes of peptic ulcer, the incidence and prevalence of peptic ulcer has decreased markedly in the last three decades. In particular, the eradication of *H. pylori* and the recognition of potential damage from nonsteroidal drugs have had

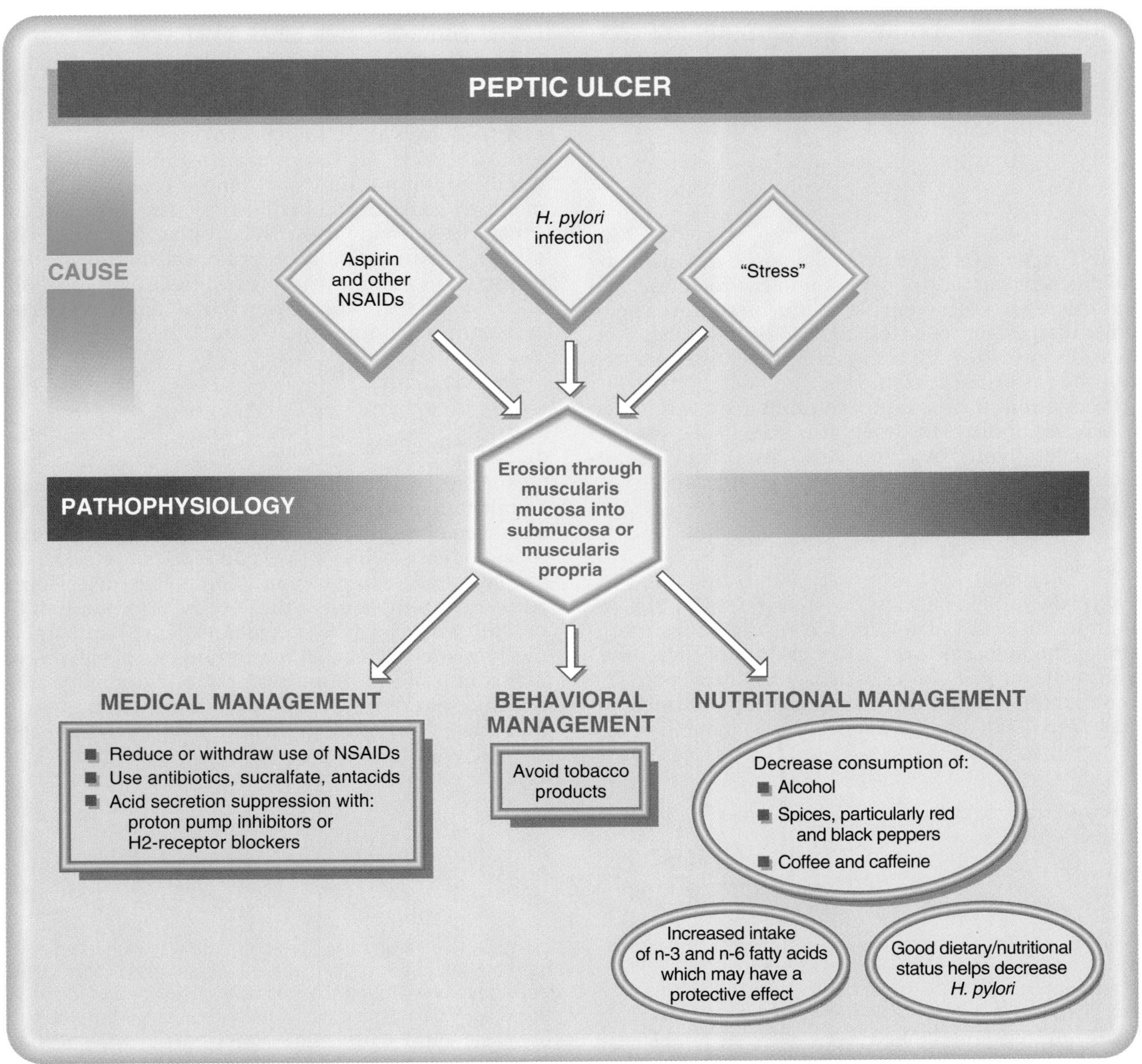

FIGURE 30–4 Pathophysiology algorithm—peptic ulcer. (Algorithm content developed by John Anderson, Ph.D., and Sanford C. Garner, Ph.D., 2000.)

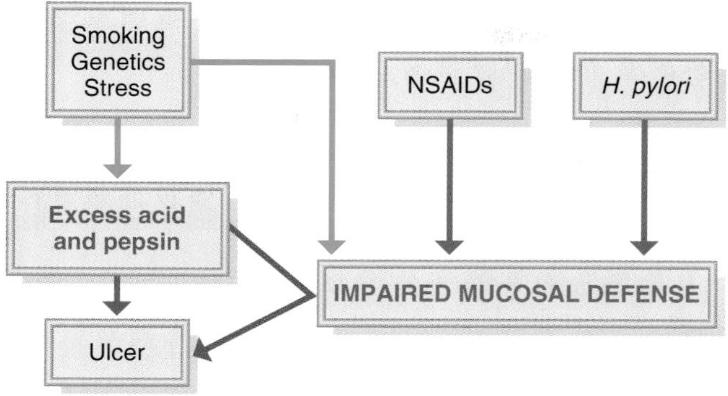

FIGURE 30–5 A model of the pathogenesis of peptic ulcer. *H. pylori* infection plus acid and peptic activity overpower mucosal defense to produce ulcers, most commonly when mucosal defense is impaired by exogenous factors. Risk factors that may increase the likelihood of peptic ulcer in those with *H. pylori* infection include smoking, alcohol consumption, genetic factors, and possibly, psychological stress. Use of nonsteroidal anti-inflammatory drugs (NSAIDs) and the hypersecretion of gastric acid that occurs in the Zollinger-Ellison syndrome are examples of causes of ulcers that occur in the absence of *H. pylori* infection.

a considerable impact in reducing the incidence of peptic ulcer.

Peptic ulcer normally involves two major regions, gastric and duodenal. Uncomplicated peptic ulcer in either region may present with signs similar to those associated with dyspepsia and gastritis. Abdominal pain or discomfort is characteristic of both gastric and duodenal ulcers, although anorexia, weight loss, nausea and vomiting, and heartburn may occur slightly more often in persons with gastric ulcer (Soll, 1998). In some patients, peptic ulcers are asymptomatic. Often, complications of hemorrhage and perforation add to the significance of the presentation.

COMPLICATIONS

Although a chronic ulcer usually follows a typical course with characteristic symptoms, occasionally, hemorrhage or perforation are the first signs of illness. Ulcers can perforate into the peritoneal cavity or penetrate into an adjacent organ (usually the pancreas), or they may erode an artery and cause massive hemorrhage. **Melena,** which refers to black, tarry stools, is a common finding associated with peptic ulcer disease in the elderly. Melena may suggest either acute or chronic gastrointestinal bleeding.

Stress Ulcers

Stress ulcers may occur as a complication of severe burns, trauma, surgery, shock, renal failure, or radiation therapy. A primary concern with stress ulceration is the potential for significant hemorrhage. Gastric ischemia is thought to be the underlying cause, but mucosal barrier changes and reflux of bile acid or pancreatic enzymes have also been implicated. The true mechanisms are not completely understood (Friedman and Peterson, 1998). Proton pump inhibitors, H_2-receptor blockers, antacids, and other medications have been used to prevent stress ulceration in high-risk patients.

Characteristics of and Comparisons Between Gastric and Duodenal Ulcers

Although gastric ulcers may occur anywhere in the stomach, most occur along the lesser curvature of the stomach (Fig. 30–6). **Gastric ulcers** typically are associated with widespread gastritis, inflammatory involvement of oxyntic (acid-producing) cells, and atrophy of acid- and pepsin-producing cells with advancing age. In some cases, gastric ulceration develops despite relatively low acid output. Antral hypomotility, gastric stasis, and increased duodenal reflux are common in gastric ulcer and, when present, may increase the severity of the gastric injury. In gastric ulcer, hemorrhage and overall mortality are higher than duodenal ulcer.

Duodenal ulcer is characterized by considerably increased acid secretion, nocturnal acid secretion, and decreased bicarbonate secretion. Most duodenal ulcers occur within the first few centimeters of the duodenal bulb, in an area immediately below the pylorus. In gastric ulcer, hemorrhage and overall mortality are higher than duodenal ulcer. Gastric outlet obstruction occurs more commonly with

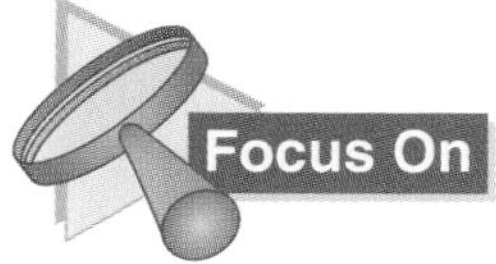

ENDOSCOPY

The stomach mucosa can be viewed, studied, and even photographed by means of **endoscopy,** a procedure that involves passing a flexible tube with a light and an eyepiece down the esophagus and into the stomach. Erosions, ulcerations, changes in the blood vessels, and destruction of surface cells can be identified. These changes can then be correlated with chemical, histologic, and clinical findings to formulate a diagnosis. This kind of study is important in the long-term monitoring of patients with chronic gastritis because of the possibility that they will develop gastric carcinoma.

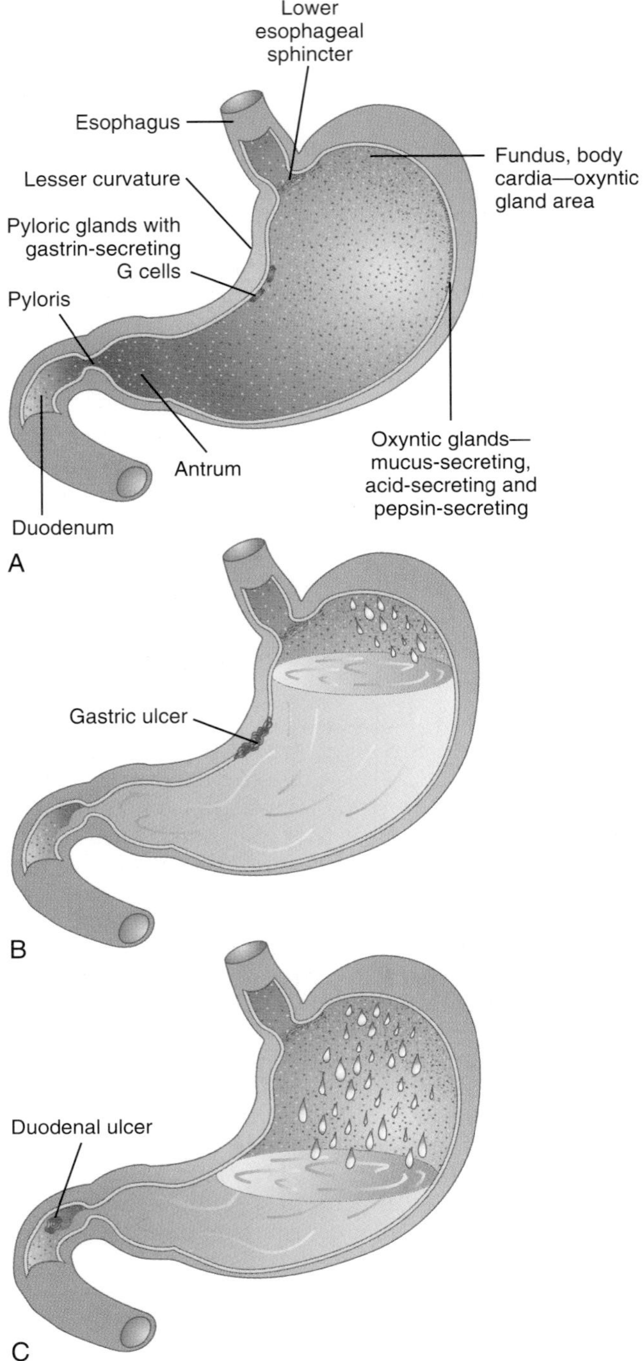

FIGURE 30–6 Diagram showing (*A*) the stomach and duodenum with eroded lesions; (*B*) a gastric ulcer; and (*C*) a duodenal ulcer.

duodenal ulcers than with gastric ulcers, and gastric metaplasia may occur in duodenal ulcer related to *H. pylori* (i.e., replacement of duodenal villous cells with gastric-type mucosal cells). Suppression of acid with H_2-receptor blockers or proton pump inhibitors may be more effective for duodenal ulcers than for gastric ulcers (Soll, 1998; Friedman and Peterson, 1998).

Management of Gastritis and Peptic Ulcer

Gastritis and Peptic Ulcers Associated with H. pylori *Infection*

Because the primary cause of gastritis and peptic ulcers is *H. pylori* infection, the primary focus of treatment in most cases is the eradication of this organism. Because of the presence of different strains of this organism and the relative resistance of the organism throughout the world, the drug protocol usually involves the use of two antibiotics. Although new antibiotic protocols will continue to be introduced and evaluated, most treatment protocols involve combination drug therapy with tetracycline and metronidazole or with metronidazole or amoxycillin plus clarithromycin (Dunn et al., 1997; Laine and Fendrick, 1998). *Bismuth,* which has been used for decades to treat various gastroduodenal disorders, is also frequently used in combination with antibiotics. Its mode of action has not been clearly established, but it appears to inhibit the growth of *H. pylori,* and it has been found to be more effective in the treatment of *H. pylori* infection and ulceration than antibiotics alone (Pounder, 1997).

In the presence of active peptic ulcer, treatment typically includes acid suppression, at least temporarily. Proton pump inhibitors, such as omeprazole or lansoprazole, and H_2-receptor blockers, such as cimetidine, famotidine, or nizatidine, are more commonly recommended than antacids. As the use of tobacco products increases the likelihood of complications and may interfere with several aspects of ulcer therapy, it should be avoided.

Ulcers Associated with the Use of NSAIDs

The first mode of treatment for ulcers associated with NSAID use is to withdraw the drug or reduce the dosage when possible. Because a significant number of persons with NSAID-induced ulcers also have concurrent *H. pylori* infection (Soll, 1998), eradication of the organism is also a focus of therapy. Proton pump inhibitors and H_2-receptor antagonists are recommended for treatment. Methods for preventing ulcers in persons at risk (the elderly, those with a past history of peptic ulcer, and those taking anticoagulants or corticosteroids) are currently being evaluated. Prostaglandins (misoprostanol) and antisecretory agents may have some value in prevention, but relatively few studies have been performed which show convincing protection in high-risk patients.

Stress Ulcers

Stress ulcers that bleed may be a significant cause of morbidity in critically ill patients, but our knowledge of effective prevention and treatment is still incomplete. Sucralfate, antacids, and acid secretion suppressors are still among the best drugs for these patients (Lasky et al., 1998; Cook et al., 1996). Efforts to prevent stress ulcers in "stressed" patients have focused on preventing or limiting conditions leading to hypotension and ischemia, respiratory disorders, and coagulopathies, in addition to avoidance of large doses of corticosteroids when possible.

Nutritional Care

For several decades, dietary factors have gained and lost favor as a significant component in the cause and treatment of dyspepsia, gastritis, and peptic ulcer disease. Since the identification of *H. pylori* as the major contributor to these disorders, the role of diet and nutritional status again must be reevaluated.

Protein foods temporarily buffer gastric secretions, but they also stimulate secretion of gastrin and pepsin. Milk or cream, which in the early days of peptic ulcer management was considered important in "coating" the stomach, is no longer considered medicinal. In animal studies, milk and cream were considered protective against peptic ulcer generation, but they were not tested against other foods (Dial et al., 1995).

The pH of a food prior to ingestion has little therapeutic importance except for patients with lesions of the mouth or the esophagus. Most foods are considerably less acidic than the normal gastric pH of 1 to 3. The pH of both orange juice and grapefruit is 3.2 to 3.6, and the pH of commonly used soft drinks ranges from approximately 2.8 to 3.5 (Flick, 1970). On the basis of their intrinsic acidity, fruit juices and soft drinks are not likely to cause peptic ulcer or appreciably interfere with healing. Some patients express discomfort with ingestion of acidic foods, but the response is not consistent among patients and, in some, symptoms may be related to heartburn.

Consumption of large amounts of alcohol from any source may cause at least superficial mucosal damage, and may worsen existing disease or interfere with treatment of the peptic ulcer. Modest consumption of alcohol does not appear to be pathogenic for peptic ulcer unless coexisting risk factors are also present. On the other hand, beers and wines significantly increase gastric secretion and should be avoided in symptomatic disease.

Both coffee and caffeine stimulate acid secretion and may also decrease LES pressure. However, neither has been strongly implicated as a cause of peptic ulcer outside of the increased acid secretion and discomfort associated with their consumption. Some spices, notably red and black pepper, can cause superficial erosions in the mucosal lining (Meyers et al., 1987). Small amounts of chili pepper may serve to increase mucosal protection by increasing production of mucus, but large amounts may cause mucosal damage, especially when consumed with alcohol or other known irritants (Abdel-Salam et al., 1995).

Because *H. pylori* infection and peptic damage result in inflammation, the use of antioxidants, ω-3 fatty acids, and various phytochemicals has been considered. Early in vitro and animal studies showed some protective effects of both ω-3 and ω-6 fatty acids, but the results have not been seen in human clinical trials (al-Shabanah, 1997; Duggan et al., 1997).

Animal and epidemiologic studies show some positive relationship between good dietary practices and nutrient status and decreased risk of complications from *H. pylori* infection (Hung et al., 1997; Aldoori et al., 1997). Malnutrition originating from either micronutrient deficiencies or generalized protein-calorie malnutrition affects rapidly dividing cells like those of the GI tract, and deficiencies could compromise wound healing. Overall, a high-quality diet and avoidance of nutrient deficiencies may offer some protection from peptic ulcer disease and may play a role in healing, but further study is warranted.

From a practical perspective, persons being treated for gastritis and peptic ulcer disease are advised to avoid the use of specific spices, alcohol, and coffee (both caffeinated and decaffeinated); to eat a good, quality diet; and to supplement for dietary inadequacies as needed. Because some patients may have significant gastric outlet obstruction, chewing thoroughly and avoiding foods with skins that are difficult to break down may be advisable, especially in those persons with dentures or missing teeth (Escamilla et al., 1994). Avoidance of specific foods and beverages known to cause discomfort or exacerbate inflammation is advised.

Meal frequency is a controversial issue in the management of peptic ulcer disease. Frequent, small meals may increase comfort, decrease the chance for acid reflux, and stimulate gastric blood flow. However, frequent meals may also increase net acid output. There is broad agreement that affected individuals should avoid consuming large meals before retiring to reduce latent increases in acid secretion. In the case of stress ulcers, continuous enteral feeding and early postoperative feeding may help maintain the mucosal barrier and gastrointestinal circulation, thus reducing the risk of stress ulceration.

Factors that increase or decrease gastric acidity are listed in Table 30–3.

Carcinoma of the Stomach

Malignant neoplasms of the stomach can lead to malnutrition as a result of excessive blood and protein losses, or more commonly, due to obstruction and mechanical interference with food intake. Most cancers of the stomach are treated by surgical resection; thus, the nutritional considerations are similar to those pertinent to partial or total gastrectomy.

The exact etiology of carcinoma of the stomach is unknown (see Chapter 39). Chronic infection with *H. pylori* is thought to increase the risk for gastric cancer, as is consumption of alcohol or smoked, cured, and pickled foods. Additionally, a diet low in fruits and vegetables is also associated with increased risk (Hwang et al., 1994; Willett and Trichopoulos, 1996).

TABLE 30–3 FACTORS THAT AFFECT GASTRIC ACIDITY

INCREASED GASTRIC ACIDITY	
Cephalic Phase of Digestion	
Thought, taste, smell of food, and chewing and swallowing initiate vagal stimulation of the parietal cells in the fundic mucosa, resulting in secretion of gastric acid.	
Gastric Phase of Digestion	
Effect of food in the stomach:	Distention of the fundus stimulates the parietal cells to produce acid.
	Increased alkalinity of antrum causes the release of gastrin, which stimulates gastric acid secretion.
	Distention of the antrum causes release of gastrin.
	Substances in certain foods and digestive products increase acidity (e.g., coffee, both with or without caffeine; alcohol; polypeptides and amino acids [products of protein digestion]).
DECREASED GASTRIC ACIDITY	
Gastric Phase of Digestion	
Acidification of the antrum reduces gastrin release and, thus, gastric acid secretion.	
Food, especially protein, has an initial buffering effect.	
Intestinal Phase of Digestion	
Fat, acid, and protein in the small intestine stimulate release of one or more gastrointestinal hormones that inhibit gastric acid secretion.	

Because symptoms are slow to manifest themselves and the growth of the tumor is rapid, carcinoma of the stomach is frequently overlooked until it is too late for an effective cure. Loss of appetite, strength, and weight frequently precede other symptoms. In some cases, **achylia gastrica** (absence of hydrochloric acid and pepsin) or achlorhydria may exist for years before the onset of gastric carcinoma.

Nutritional Care

The dietary regimen for carcinoma of the stomach is determined by the location of the cancer, the nature of the functional disturbance, and the stage of the disease. Gastrectomy is one of the possible therapies, and some patients may experience difficulties with nutrition postoperatively (see the section on dumping syndrome that appears later in this chapter). The patient with advanced, nonoperable cancer should receive a diet that is adjusted to provide comfort. Anorexia is almost always present from the early stages. Any food preferences, unless definitely harmful, are granted, and the patient should be made as comfortable as possible. In the later stages of the disease, the patient may tolerate only a liquid diet, or it may be necessary to resort to parenteral nutrition. As long as other therapeutic procedures, such as surgery, radiation therapy, or chemotherapy are being performed, the nutritional support for the patient should be equally aggressive. See Chapter 39 for further discussion of nutritional care during cancer treatment.

GASTRIC SURGERY

Peptic ulcer is primarily a medical disease, but surgery is advised when the ulcer is complicated by hemorrhage, perforation, obstruction, or intractability, or when the patient is unable to follow the medical regimen. Ulcers may recur after both medical and surgical treatment.

Vagal denervation decreases cholinergic stimulation of parietal cells and reduces cellular response to stimulants, such as gastrin. A **parietal cell vagotomy** affects only the area of gastric acid secretion. As the antrum and pylorus remain innervated by the *vagus nerve,* gastric emptying can proceed normally. However, because the surgery is difficult and time-consuming, patients who are at high risk for operative morbidity and mortality are not candidates for this procedure. A **truncal vagotomy** with *pyloroplasty* would probably be used in these circumstances. The truncal vagotomy not only interrupts innervation of the gastric parietal cells, but also results in antral and pyloric dysfunction and poor peristalsis. Incorporating pyloroplasty or gastrojejunostomy permits adequate gastric emptying; however, the postoperative side effects of dumping, diarrhea, and weight loss still occur at a rate of approximately 6%. Surgery for gastric ulcer consists of removing the ulcerated area, usually by a *partial gastric resection*.

Nutritional Care

After most types of gastric surgery (Fig. 30–7), all oral intake of foods and fluids is suspended until GI tract function returns. Once function is regained, liquids are initiated, after which the patient can progress to solids, as tolerated for volume and consistency. If the surgery requires an extended period for healing, the patient may be fed enterally through a tube, often placed as a jejunostomy. The use of total parenteral nutrition (TPN) is usually reserved for patients with postoperative complications that delay enteral feeding for an extended period (see Chapter 22).

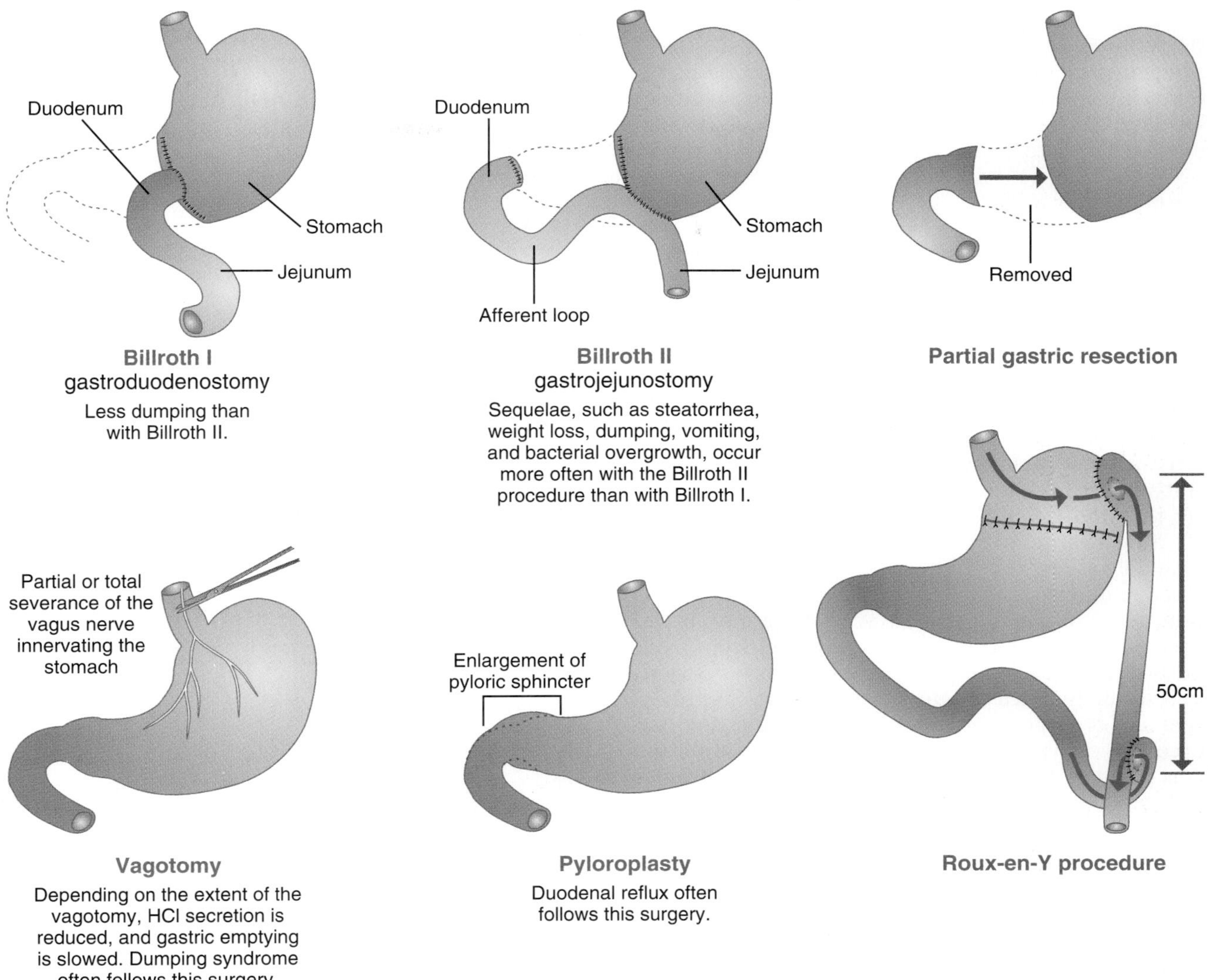
Duodenum
Stomach
Jejunum
Billroth I
gastroduodenostomy
Less dumping than with Billroth II.
Duodenum
Stomach
Jejunum
Afferent loop
Billroth II
gastrojejunostomy
Sequelae, such as steatorrhea, weight loss, dumping, vomiting, and bacterial overgrowth, occur more often with the Billroth II procedure than with Billroth I.
Removed
Partial gastric resection
Partial or total severance of the vagus nerve innervating the stomach
Vagotomy
Depending on the extent of the vagotomy, HCl secretion is reduced, and gastric emptying is slowed. Dumping syndrome often follows this surgery.
Enlargement of pyloric sphincter
Pyloroplasty
Duodenal reflux often follows this surgery.
50cm
Roux-en-Y procedure

FIGURE 30–7 Gastric surgical procedures.

The first type of fluid allowed by mouth is usually water, typically administered in the form of ice, given in small amounts and allowed to melt in the mouth, or as frequent sips of water. Some patients may tolerate water at room temperature or warm water better than iced or cold water. Later, larger amounts and varieties of fluids can be offered, followed by small amounts of soft, starchy, and low-fat protein foods. Highly spiced, fatty, or hypertonic foods may not be well tolerated by the patient. Small, frequent meals or snacks are usually better tolerated than large meals.

Nutritional impairment occurs in some patients after gastrectomy, and some have difficulty regaining normal preoperative weight because of one or both of the following: (1) inadequate food intake related to anorexia or to symptoms related to dumping syndrome, or (2) malabsorption of ingested food. Patients who have had total or almost total gastrectomy often have difficulty eating large amounts of food and so may need to make a permanent habit of eating several small meals daily.

Dumping Syndrome

The **dumping syndrome** is a complex physiologic response to the presence of larger-than-normal amounts of food and liquid in the proximal small intestine. Dumping syndrome usually occurs as a result of loss of normal regulation of gastric emptying and gastrointestinal and systemic responses to a meal. Most of the symptoms can be reproduced in normal individuals by infusing a loading dose of glucose into the jejunum (Vecht et al., 1997).

The syndrome may occur as a result of total or subtotal gastrectomy, manipulation of the pylorus, or after fundoplication (Samuk et al., 1996). The incidence of dumping ranges from approximately 5%

following minor surgical procedures to as high as 40% following total gastrectomy (Vecht et al., 1997). After surgical procedures in which portions of the stomach remain, the size of the remaining stomach can increase somewhat over a period of several months. However, many postgastrectomy patients may continue to have chronic symptoms of the dumping syndrome.

Severity of symptoms ranges from mild to relatively debilitating, depending on the nature of the surgery and the individual's dietary practices. Short-term and long-term implications are numerous, but dietary interventions, if heeded, can reduce or eliminate symptoms in most individuals. Medications that slow motility may be advised for those whose symptoms persist after changing dietary habits.

Symptoms may occur in several stages; each is related to the "dumping" of foods and beverages into the small intestine, but the mechanisms vary. Not all patients suffer all consequences or to the same degree. In the *first stage,* patients may experience abdominal fullness and nausea within 10 to 20 minutes of eating a meal. This stage may be attributed to distention of the small bowel from foods and liquids, plus a modest fluid shift from systemic circulation into the small intestine as a result of ingestion of hypertonic foods or foods that are rendered hypertonic from the action of digestive enzymes. Patients may, at the same time, experience flushing, rapid heart beat, faintness, sweating, and the need to sit or lie down. This set of systemic symptoms was originally attributed to fluid loss from the vascular space into the mesenteric bed and GI tract. Fluid does shift from systemic circulation into the gastrointestinal tract, but apparently not enough to account for the magnitude of vascular symptoms. It is now thought that patients with these early dumping symptoms are experiencing a decrease in peripheral vascular resistance and, perhaps, splanchnic (visceral) pooling of blood.

In the *intermediate stage,* which can occur from 20 minutes to more than 1 hour after eating, patients may experience abdominal bloating, increased flatulence, crampy abdominal pain, and diarrhea. The "colonic" symptoms are likely related to the increased malabsorption of carbohydrates and other foodstuffs and the subsequent fermentation of the substrates entering the colon (see Chapter 1).

The *late stage,* occurring from 1 to 3 hours after a meal, is related to reactive hypoglycemia, sometimes referred to as **alimentary hypoglycemia.** Patients may perspire; feel anxious, weak, shaky, or hungry; and may have difficulty concentrating (see Table 30–4). Rapid delivery, as well as hydrolysis and absorption of carbohydrate, produces an exaggerated rise in insulin level with a subsequent decline in blood glucose level. The rapid changes in blood glucose and the secretion of gut peptides, glucose insulinotropic polypeptide (GIP), and glucagon-like polypeptide-1 (GLP-1) appear to be at least partly responsible for the symptoms.

TABLE 30–4 NUTRITIONAL CARE GUIDELINES FOR PATIENTS WITH DUMPING SYNDROME AND ALIMENTARY HYPOGLYCEMIA

1. Small meals, spread throughout the day, are likely to result in improved net absorption and less dramatic fluid shifts.
2. High-protein, moderate-fat foods are recommended, with sufficient calories for weight maintenance or gain as needed. Complex carbohydrates included as tolerated.
3. Intake of fibrous foods slows upper GI transit and increases viscosity. However, caution should be used with large particles and fiber supplements, especially with esophageal or gastric outlet narrowing or dysmotility.
4. Lying down and avoiding activity an hour after eating may help slow gastric emptying.
5. Taking liquids with meals is thought to hasten GI transit, but adequate amounts of liquid should be consumed throughout the day, small amounts at a time.
6. Only very small quantities of hypertonic, concentrated sweets should be ingested. These include soft drinks, juices, pies, cakes, cookies, and frozen desserts (unless made with sugar substitutes).
7. Lactose, especially in milk or ice cream, may be poorly tolerated due to rapid transit, and so may need to be avoided. Cheeses and yogurt are likely to be better tolerated.
8. Medium-chain triglycerides may be helpful if steatorrhea is present.

Nutritional Complications Associated with Partial or Total Gastrectomy

Patients who are symptomatic after gastric surgery often lose weight. The weight loss may be attributable to inadequate intake resulting from the fear and anxiety that is often associated with the confusing and often distressing symptoms. Some patients may associate the symptoms with the act of eating, rather than attributing them to specific patterns, volumes, or types of foods consumed. Patients sometimes can correctly relate consumption of food types with distress, but they rarely can select appropriate foods solely on the basis of their experiences with foods or meals.

Following some forms of gastric surgery, malabsorption and steatorrhea may occur in addition to dumping and hypoglycemia. About 10% of these patients have clinically significant steatorrhea secondary to rapid transit, loss of gastric lipase, or pancreatic or biliary insufficiency. Because of disturbances in the timing of entry of food into the small intestine and the release of intestinal hormones and enzymes, efficiency of digestion may be reduced. Patients who were lactose-tolerant before gastric surgery may experience relative lactase deficiency, either because food enters the small intes-

TABLE 30–5 COMMON DRUGS USED IN THE TREATMENT OF GASTROINTESTINAL DISORDERS

TYPE OF DRUG	ACTION
Antibiotics	Eradicate *Helicobactor pylori*
Antacids	Neutralize gastric activity
Cimetidine and ranitidine	Histamine H_2-receptor antagonists that inhibit gastric acid secretion
Prostaglandins (PGs)	Methyl derivatives of PGE_2 that possess cytoprotective properties
Sucralfate	Sulfated disaccharide; coats and protects ulcer base and may increase mucosal resistance
Omeprazole	Proton pump inhibitor that decreases gastric secretions

tine further downstream, or because the rate of transit through the proximal small intestine is increased.

Anemia, osteoporosis, and select vitamin and mineral deficiencies may occur due to long-term malabsorption or limited dietary intake. Iron deficiency may be attributable to loss of acid secretion, which normally facilitates the reduction of iron compounds, allowing their absorption; rapid transit; diminished contact with sites of iron absorption; or blood loss. Vitamin B_{12} deficiency may also cause anemia. If the amount of gastric mucosa is reduced, intrinsic factor may not be produced in quantities adequate to allow for complete vitamin B_{12} absorption, and *pernicious anemia* may result. Bacterial overgrowth in the proximal small bowel or in the afferent loop can contribute to vitamin B_{12} depletion because bacteria compete with the host for utilization of the vitamin. After gastrectomy, therefore, patients generally receive prophylactic vitamin B_{12} injections.

Because of the complications associated with traditional gastrectomies, other procedures, including truncal, selective, or parietal cell vagotomy; pyloromyotomy; antrectomy; Roux-en-Y esophagojejunostomy; loop esophagojejunostomy; and gastric substitutes from ileocecal segments, have been performed as alternatives (Okuyama et al., 1997; Uras et al., 1997). *Somatostatin analogues* are used to slow gastric emptying in patients with rapid emptying and dumping syndrome. *Acarbose,* an alpha-glucoside hydrolase inhibitor that is normally used to manage type 2 diabetes mellitus, has been considered for use in some persons with dumping syndrome. Acarbose inhibits the digestion and absorption of starch, sucrose, and maltose. Acarbose may blunt the alimentary hyperglycemia/hypoglycemia related to dumping, but has the potential to worsen the colonic gas and diarrhea. Table 30–5 lists some of the other common medications used in gastrointestinal disorders.

Postgastrectomy Nutritional Care

Because of the problems that accompany eating, postgastrectomy patients frequently do not eat enough, have diarrhea from the increased intestinal activity, and become underweight, malnourished, and frustrated. The prime objective of nutritional care is to restore nutritional status and quality of life.

Proteins and fats are better tolerated than carbohydrates because they are hydrolyzed more slowly into osmotically active substances. Simple carbohydrates, such as lactose, sucrose, and dextrose, are hydrolyzed rapidly and so quantities should be limited, but complex carbohydrates (starches) can be included in the diet. Liquids enter the jejunum rapidly, so some patients may have problems tolerating liquids with meals. Patients who have severe problems with dumping may fare better if they limit the amount of liquids taken with meals, or if they take liquids only between meals, without solid food. Lying down immediately after meals may also decrease the severity of symptoms.

The use of fiber supplements can be beneficial in managing dumping syndrome, as they reduce upper GI transit time and decrease the rate of glucose absorption, thus decreasing the insulin response. *Pectin,* the dietary fiber contained in fruits and vegetables, or gums (e.g., guar) may be useful in treating dumping syndrome. These substances are thought to slow carbohydrate absorption and reduce the glycemic load and, thus, the insulin re-

CASE STUDY

Jim T. is a 45-year-old white male executive who travels extensively in his work. He is 6′0″ tall and weighs 186 lb. He recently visited his doctor complaining about upper GI distress. He reports frequent bouts of heartburn in the middle of the night, and he has lost 15 lb over the last year without intentionally dieting. Jim also occasionally experiences heartburn soon after consumption of specific meals and foods. Jim's doctor diagnosed esophageal reflux, and x-ray studies revealed a hiatal hernia.

Jim has received a good deal of advice regarding specific foods and diets from a variety of sources, but is confused about what he should eat. Jim has come to you to discuss nutritional therapies.

1. What is heartburn? Does hiatal hernia have anything to do with it?
2. Why might Jim experience heartburn in the middle of the night?
3. Why might Jim experience burning after consumption of certain foods or meals?
4. Why do you suppose Jim lost weight?
5. Do you recommend that he regain the weight?
6. What recommendations would you give for reducing or preventing Jim's symptoms?

sponse (see Appendix 54). Caution must be exercised, however, with the use of bulk fiber sources. Several cases of obstruction have been reported with the use of guar gum and other viscous substances when large amounts have been taken, especially without adequate water.

Basically, a diet that aims to avoid symptoms of dumping syndrome is moderate in fat content (30% to 40% of calories), low in simple carbohydrates, and high in protein (20% of calories). Such a diet is instituted for the purpose of achieving and maintaining the optimal weight and nutritional status of the patient. The exchange lists given in Appendix 53 can be used to calculate carbohydrate intake and teach the patient about carbohydrate control.

Milk is often not tolerated at all after gastric surgery, and small amounts are often better tolerated than large amounts. Patients who are lactose-intolerant fare better with cheeses or unsweetened yogurt than with milk (see Chapter 31). Vitamin D and calcium supplements may be needed when intake of dairy products is inadequate. Commercial lactase products are available for those with significant lactose malabsorption. When steatorrhea is a problem, those formulas whose fat content is derived primarily from medium-chain triglycerides may be better tolerated. Supplemental formulas are described in Appendices 35 to 40. Table 30–4 presents the general nutritional care guidelines for patients with dumping syndrome after gastric surgery. However, each diet must be adjusted to suit the patient, based on a careful dietary and social history.

CITED REFERENCES

Abdel-Salam OM, et al. Studies on the effect of intragastric capsaicin on gastric ulcer and on the prostacyclin-induced effect. Pharmacol Res 32:209, 1995.

Aldoori WH, et al. Prospective study of diet and the risk of duodenal ulcer in men. Am J Epidemiol 145:42, 1997.

Al-Shabanah OA. Effect of evening primrose oil on gastric ulceration and secretion induced by various ulcerogenic and necrotizing agents in rats. Food Chem Toxicol 35:769, 1997.

Beyer PL. Gastrointestinal disorders: Roles of nutrition and the dietetics practitioner. J Am Diet Assoc 98:272, 1998.

Blum AL. *Helicobacter pylori* and peptic ulcer disease. Scand J Gastroenterol 214(suppl):24, 1996.

Cook DJ, et al. Stress ulcer prophylaxis in critically ill patients. Resolving discordant meta-analyses. JAMA 275:308, 1996.

Dial EJ, et al. Gastroprotection by dairy foods against stress-induced ulcerogenesis in rats. Digest Dis Sci 40:2295, 1995.

Duggan AE, et al. Clarification of the link between polyunsaturated fatty acids and *Helicobacter pylori*–associated duodenal ulcer disease: A dietary intervention study. Br J Nutr 78:515, 1997.

Dunn BE, et al. *Helicobacter pylori.* Clin Microbiol Rev 10:720, 1997.

Escamilla C, et al. Intestinal obstruction and bezoars. J Am Coll Surg 179:285, 1994.

Flick AL. Acid content of common beverages. Am J Dig Dis 15:317, 1970.

Friedman LS, Peterson WL. Peptic ulcer and related disorders. In: Fauci AS, Braunwald E, Isselbacher KJ, et al. (eds.). Harrison's Principles of Internal Medicine, 14th ed. New York: McGraw-Hill, 1998.

Goyal RK. Diseases of the esophagus. In: Fauci AS, Braunwald E, Isselbacher KJ, et al. (eds.). Harrison's Principles of Internal Medicine, 14th ed. New York: McGraw-Hill, 1998.

Gutthann SP, et al. Individual nonsteroidal anti-inflammatory drugs and other risk factors for upper gastrointestinal bleeding and perforation. Epidemiology 8:18, 1997.

Hojgaard, et al. Peptic ulcer pathophysiology: Acid, bicarbonate, and mucosal function. Scand J Gastroenterol 216(suppl):10, 1996.

Hung CR, Neu SL. Acid-induced gastric damage in rats is aggravated by starvation and prevented by several nutrients. J Nutr 127:630, 1997.

Hunt RH. Peptic ulcer disease: Defining the treatment strategies in the era of *Helicobacter pylori*. Am J Gastroenterol 92(suppl):36S, 1997.

Hwang H, et al. Diet, *Helicobacter pylori* infection, food preservation and gastric cancer risk: Are there new roles for preventive factors? Nutr Rev 52:75, 1994.

Kjellin A, et al. Gastroesophageal reflux in obese patients is not reduced by weight reduction. Scand J Gastroenterol 31:1047, 1996.

Koch KL. Dyspepsia of unknown origin: Pathophysiology, diagnosis, and treatment. Digest Dis 15:316, 1997.

Kozak LJ, Owings MF. Ambulatory and inpatient procedures in the United States, 1995. National Center for Health Statistics. Vital Health Stat 13(135), 1998.

Laine L, Fendrick AM. *Helicobacter pylori* and peptic ulcer disease. Postgrad Med 103:231, 1998.

Lasky MR, et al. A prospective study of omeprazole suspension to prevent clinically significant gastrointestinal bleeding from stress ulcers in mechanically ventilated trauma patients. J Trauma 44:527, 1998.

Lee A. The *Helicobacter pylori* genome—New insights into pathogenesis and therapeutics. N Engl J Med 338:832, 1998.

Marotta RB, Floch MH. Diet and nutrition in ulcer disease. Med Clin North Am 75:4, 1991.

McQuaid K. Dyspepsia. In: Feldman M, Scharschmidt BF, Sleisenger MH. Gastrointestinal and Liver Disease, 6th ed. Philadelphia: WB Saunders, 1998.

Meyers BM, et al. Effect of red pepper and black pepper on the stomach. Am J Gastroenterol 82:211, 1987.

Mishkin D, et al. Fructose and sorbitol malabsorption in ambulatory patients with functional dyspepsia: Comparison with lactose maldigestion/malabsorption. Digest Dis Sci 42:2591, 1997.

Mittal RK, Balaban DH. The esophagogastric junction. N Engl J Med 336:924, 1997.

Okuyama H, et al. A comparison of the efficacy of pyloromyotomy and pyloroplasty in patients with gastroesophageal reflux and delayed gastric emptying. J Pediatr Surg 32:316, 1997.

Peek RM, Blaser MJ. Pathophysiology of *Helicobacter pylori*–induced gastritis and peptic ulcer disease. Am J Med 102:200, 1997.

Perdikis G, et al. Laparoscopic Nissen fundoplication: Where do we stand? Surg Laparosc Endosc 7(1):17, 1997.

Pounder RE. New developments in *Helicobacter pylori* eradication therapy. Scand J Gastroenterol 223 (suppl):43, 1997.

Rodriguez S, et al. Meal type affects heartburn severity. Dig Dis Sci 43:485, 1998.

Samuk I, et al. Dumping syndrome following Nissen fundoplication, diagnosis, and treatment. J Pediatr Gastroenterol Nutr 23:235, 1996.

Schappert SM. Ambulatory care visits to physician offices, hospital outpatient departments, and emergency departments: United States, 1996. National Center for Health Statistics. Vital Health Stat 13(134):1, 1998.

Soll AH. Peptic ulcer and its complications. In: Feldman M, Scharschmidt BF, Sleisenger MH. Gastrointestinal and Liver Disease, 6th ed. Philadelphia: WB Saunders, 1998.

Sontag SJ. Guilty as charged: Bugs and drugs in gastric ulcer. Am J Gastroenterol 2:1255, 1997.

Talley NJ, et al. AGA technical review: Evaluation of dyspepsia. Gastroenterology 114:582, 1998.

Uras C, et al. Restorative caecogastroplasty reconstruction after pylorus-preserving near-total gastrectomy: A preliminary study. Br J Surg 84:406, 1997.

Vecht J, et al. The dumping syndrome. Current insights into pathophysiology, diagnosis and treatment. Scand J Gastroenterol 32(suppl 223): 21, 1997.

Willet WC, Trichopoulos D. Nutrition and cancer: A summary of the evidence. Cancer Causes Control 7:178, 1996.

ADDITIONAL REFERENCES

Annibale B, et al. Atrophic body gastritis: Distinct features associated with *Helicobacter pylori* infection. Helicobacter 2:57, 1997.

Dua K, et al. Coordination of deglutitive glottal function and pharyngeal bolbus transit during normal eating. Gastroenterology 112:73, 1997.

El-Omar E, et al. *Helicobacter pylori* infection and abnormalities of acid secretion in patients with duodenal ulcer disease. Gastroenterology 109:681, 1995.

Geliebter A, et al. Reduced stomach capacity in obese subjects after dieting. Am J Clin Nutr 63:170, 1996.

Graves EJ, Owings MF. 1995 Summary: National hospital discharge summary. Advance data from vital and health statistics, number 291. National Center for Health Statistics 16(30), 1997.

Macarthur C, et al. *Helicobacter pylori*, gastroduodenal disease, and recurrent abdominal pain in children. JAMA 273:729, 1995.

Salvatore T, Giugliano D. Pharmacokinetic-pharmacodynamic relationships of acarbose. Clin Pharmacokinet 30:94, 1996.

Soll A. Medical treatment of peptic ulcer disease. JAMA 275:622, 1996.

Sung J, et al. Antibacterial treatment of gastric ulcers associated with *Helicobacter pylori.* N Engl J Med 332:139, 1995.

Sultan Khuroo M, et al. A comparison of omeprazole and placebo for bleeding peptic ulcer. 336:1054, 1997.

Tomb J, et al. The complete genome sequence of the gastric pathogen *Helicobacter pylori.* Nature 388:539, 1997.

Yip R, et al. Pervasive occult gastrointestinal bleeding in an Alaskan Native population with prevalent iron deficiency: Role of *Helicobacter pylori* gastritis. JAMA 277:1135, 1997.

CHAPTER 31

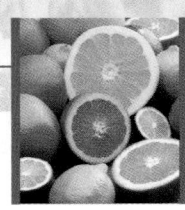

Medical Nutrition Therapy for Lower Gastrointestinal Tract Disorders

PETER L. BEYER, MS, RD

Chapter Outline

- Principles of Nutritional Care
- Common Symptoms of Intestinal Dysfunction
- Diseases of the Small Intestine
- Diseases of the Large Intestine
- Intestinal Surgery

Key Terms

BLIND LOOP SYNDROME—a disorder of bacterial overgrowth with resultant malabsorption secondary to alterations in the anatomy of the small intestine involving a loop that is disconnected from the main stream

BORBORYGMUS—intestinal rumbling

CELIAC DISEASE—common term for gluten-sensitive enteropathy

COLOSTOMY—surgical creation of an opening into the colon to permit defecation

CONSTIPATION—a condition in which the frequency or quantity of defecation is reduced

CROHN'S DISEASE—a chronic granulomatous inflammatory disease of unknown etiology involving the small or large intestine; may result in diarrhea, strictures, fistulas, malabsorption, and the need for surgical resections

DERMATITIS HERPETIFORMIS—a skin disorder that may result from a variant of celiac disease

DIARRHEA—abnormal volume and liquidity of stools

DIVERTICULITIS—inflammation of diverticula

DIVERTICULOSIS—presence of diverticula that are herniations of the mucous membrane through the muscular layers of the colonic wall

FISTULA—an abnormal passage between two internal organs, or from an internal organ to the surface of the body

FLATULENCE—the presence of excessive amounts of gas in the gastrointestinal tract

FLATUS—gas in the gastrointestinal tract that is expelled through the anus

GLUTEN-SENSITIVE ENTEROPATHY (CELIAC DISEASE)—a malabsorption syndrome precipitated by the chronic ingestion of gliadin-containing foods and characterized by a flattening of the villi of the small intestine

HIGH-FIBER DIET—a diet that contributes more than 24 g/day of dietary fiber

HYPOLACTASIA—a decrease in the amount of the intestinal enzyme lactase

ILEOSTOMY—surgical creation of an opening into the ileum through a stoma in the abdominal wall

ILEAL POUCH—surgical creation of a small reservoir, using folds of the distal ileum, which is then attached to the rectum

INFLAMMATORY BOWEL DISEASE (IBD)—a general term for inflammatory diseases of the bowel of unknown etiology, including Crohn's disease and ulcerative colitis

IRRITABLE BOWEL SYNDROME (IBS)—an abnormal stooling pattern associated with symptoms of intestinal dysfunction that persists for longer than 3 months

LACTOSE INTOLERANCE—an inability to digest lactose to galactose and glucose because of a deficiency of the enzyme lactase

MEDIUM-CHAIN TRIGLYCERIDES—triacylglycerols with fatty acids of 8 and 10 carbons in length that are short enough to be absorbed directly into the portal blood

MINIMAL-RESIDUE DIET—a diet that results in decreased fecal volume

PHYTOBEZOARS—stomach obstructions composed of partially digested plant foods

RESIDUE—the fecal contents, including bacteria and the net remains after ingestion of food and beverage, secretions into the gastrointestinal tract, and absorption

SHORT-BOWEL SYNDROME (SBS)—any of the malabsorption conditions resulting from massive resection of the small bowel; characterized by diarrhea, steatorrhea, and malnutrition

STEATORRHEA—excessive amounts of fat in the feces, as seen in malabsorption syndromes

TROPICAL SPRUE—a syndrome of unknown etiology that causes diarrhea and malabsorption, but is not responsive to gliadin-free diet therapy

ULCERATIVE COLITIS—an inflammatory disease of the colonic mucosa

The small and large intestines serve as organs of digestion, absorption, and excretion. Digestion is initiated in the mouth and stomach and continues in the duodenum and jejunum with the aid of secretions from the liver, pancreas, and small intestine. Most of the absorption of nutrients occurs in the jejunum, with only small amounts of micronutrients and macronutrients requiring absorption in the ileum. The only substances absorbed exclusively in the terminal ileum are bile salts and vitamin B_{12}. The large intestine, or colon, absorbs residual water that has not been taken up in the small intestine and excretes fecal mass (see Chapter 1).

PRINCIPLES OF NUTRITIONAL CARE

Many intestinal disorders and symptoms involve problems of motility, secretion, and absorption and occur in the absence of recognizable pathologic conditions. Although exacerbation and remission of these disorders may be due to dietary changes, the individual's diet (or specific foods in the diet) cannot always be incriminated.

Dietary modifications in disorders of the intestinal tract are designed to alleviate symptoms, correct nutritional deficiencies, and, when possible, address the primary cause of difficulty. In diseased states, treatment involves attention to the primary injury of the intestinal mucosa and the secondary conditions arising as a consequence. Increased intakes of energy, protein, vitamins, minerals, and electrolytes are frequently required to replace nutrients lost as a result of impaired digestive and absorptive capacity. Consistency of the diet may also be an important factor.

Nutritional care for all patients with diseases of the intestines must be individualized. For this reason, the principles presented in the chapter are guidelines. An internet source is found at www.niddk.nih.gov/health/digest/digest.htm.

Fiber, Roughage, and Residue

Dietary fiber is defined as that portion of food that comes largely from plant cell walls and that is not readily digested by enzymes in the human digestive tract. Although the terms fiber and roughage are sometimes used synonymously, fiber is the preferred term and includes both water-soluble and water-insoluble fractions (see Chapter 3 for a further discussion of fiber).

Dietary fiber originates in fruits, vegetables, and cereal grains. Bran, primarily from wheat, is the most effective of the insoluble fibers in absorbing water to form soft, bulky stools. Soluble fiber in fruits, vegetables, legumes, and oats forms a soft gel that slows passage of food through the intestinal tract and delays or inhibits absorption of dietary factors, such as glucose and cholesterol. Soluble fiber (hemicelluloses, pectins, and gums) makes up about 15% to 20% of the total fiber in fruits, grains, and vegetables and less than 10% of that in legumes, nuts, and seeds. Guidelines for a high-fiber diet are presented in Table 31–1.

Residue refers to the amount of net fecal mass remaining after the processes of food ingestion and gastrointestinal (GI) secretion, absorption, and fermentation. The primary components of the wet fecal residue are bacteria and water, which constitute 60% to 80% of the weight of the stool. The remaining content includes dietary fiber, sloughed mucosal cells, mucous, and varying amounts of unabsorbed starches, sugars, protein, and minerals. Increasing the consumption of fibrous foods may increase fecal residue by not only increasing the amount of unabsorbed fiber, but also by increasing bacterial mass, increasing the water content of the stool, and increasing the loss of carbohydrate, lipid, protein, and (to a lesser degree) minerals bound physically or chemically to the fibrous food (Baer et al., 1997). The fact that foods high in dietary fiber may result in slightly decreased efficiency of digestion and absorption is outweighed by the benefits of the vitamin, mineral, and phytochemical content if the sources of the fiber are fruits, vegetables, and whole grains.

Fecal residue may also be increased without increasing dietary fiber. For example, ingestion of 10 to 20 g of sorbitol, a common dietetic sweetener, or the same amount of lactose in the lactase-deficient individual may result in increased stool weight owing to the malabsorption of the sugars, increased osmolar content of the colonic lumen, and increased bacterial fecal mass (Hyams, 1983; Gudmand-Hoyer, 1994). A low- or **minimal-residue diet,** therefore, is typically used in patients with maldigestion, malabsorption, or diarrhea, and is designed to include foods that are likely to be completely digested and well absorbed and that will not unduly increase GI secretions. Foods that may affect fecal residue and may be limited in a minimal-residue diet are outlined in Table 31–2.

Because small amounts of dietary fiber may be important in maintaining normal colonic function, small amounts of particulate fiber (e.g., that found in vegetable juices, potato, plain breads, and cereals) are usually included in the diet to varying degrees.

TABLE 31–1 GUIDELINES FOR HIGH-FIBER DIETS*

1. Increase consumption of whole-grain breads, cereals, flours, and other whole-grain products (6–11 servings daily).
2. Increase consumption of vegetables, especially legumes, and fruits, especially those with edible skins, seeds, and hulls (5–8 servings daily).
3. Consume high-fiber cereals, granolas, and legumes as needed to bring fiber intake to at least 25 g daily.
4. Increase consumption of water to at least 2 L (or 2 q) daily.

*May increase stool weight, fecal water, and/or gas. The amount that causes clinical symptoms varies among individuals. The age of the individual, the presence of GI disease or malnutrition, any resection of the GI tract, and recent use of the GI tract all impact tolerance.

TABLE 31–2 FOODS TO LIMIT IN A LOW- OR MINIMAL-RESIDUE DIET

FOOD	COMMENTS	REFERENCES
Lactose (in lactose malabsorbers)	6–12 g normally tolerated in healthy, lactase-deficient individuals	Gudmand-Hoyer, 1994 Suarez et al., 1995
Fiber (excess; e.g., > 20 g)	Modest amounts (10–15 g) may help maintain normal consistency of GI contents & normal colonic mucosa in healthy states and in GI disease	Caspary, 1992; Cummings and Englyst, 1995
Resistant starch (especially raffinose and stachyose found in legumes)		Cummings and Englyst, 1995
Sorbitol, mannitol, and xylitol (excess; >10 g/day)		Rumessen and Gudmand-Hoyer, 1988
Fructose (excess; >30 g/day)		Hyams et al., 1988; Riby et al., 1993
Sucrose (excess)	Well tolerated in moderate amounts; large amounts may cause hyperosmolar diarrhea and/or decreased fecal pH with fermentation to short-chain fatty acids	Yadrick et al., 1992; Gracey, 1981
Caffeine	Increases GI secretions, colonic motility	Brown et al., 1990
Alcoholic beverages (especially wine and beer)	Increase GI secretions	Singer et al., 1987

Because the usual recommended quantities of fruits, vegetables and whole grains may be restricted with a minimum-residue diet, its use as a therapeutic diet should generally be limited to brief periods. When used any longer than for a few days, or in depleted patients, the diet should be supplemented with a multivitamin-mineral product. The optimal amount, type, and particle size of fibrous material appropriate for various disease states are still being investigated, but complete restriction of all dietary fiber is not usually recommended (Mortensen and Clausen, 1996; Eastwood and Morris, 1992). Recommendations regarding the use or type of fiber in specific GI disorders are discussed elsewhere in this chapter.

Modified-Fiber Diets

Restricted-Fiber Diet

The restricted-fiber diet is used when reduced fecal output is necessary, when the gastrointestinal tract is restricted or obstructed, or when reduced fecal residue is desired. Scarring and strictures may form after acute episodes of inflammatory bowel disease (IBD), severe cases of peptic ulcer, or GI surgeries. GI or abdominal tumors may also obstruct segments of the GI tract. Because fiber is not digested to any significant degree (except by fermentation in the colon), and because chewing is not a reliable way of reducing the size of fibrous foods, both the amount and size of fibrous material must usually be controlled. The restricted-fiber diet typically restricts fruits, vegetables, and coarse grains and usually provides less than 10 g of dietary fiber. Particularly with distal obstructions or strictures, it may be beneficial to keep the stool soft by including modest amounts of fiber, but of small particle size. In patients with GI strictures from peptic ulcer, surgical procedures, inflammatory bowel disease, radiation enteritis, or dysmotility syndromes, food bolus obstruction can occur.

These obstructions in the stomach that result from the ingestion of plant foods are called **phytobezoars** and are especially common in patients who are totally edentulous, have poor dentition, or use dentures. Foods commonly incriminated in the formation of phytobezoars include potato skins, oranges, and grapefruit, but many foods that are consumed in large segments or have skins that are difficult to chew may be problematic.

High-Fiber Diet

The **high-fiber diet** presented in Table 31–1 provides 25 g or more of dietary fiber, depending on the actual foods selected. Although the amount of dietary fiber recommended is at least 25 g daily, most Americans, on the average, consume only 10 to 15 g. A high-fiber therapeutic diet may exceed the minimum recommendation, but amounts greater than 50 g/day do not appear to improve bowel function further (Pemberton et al., 1988) and may create problems with abdominal distention and excessive flatulence. Appendix 42 provides a list of the fiber content of foods.

Ideally, fiber in the diet should be ingested in the form of foods, such as fruits, vegetables, and whole grain breads and cereals, in amounts recommended in common food guides. Realistically, fiber powders or bran concentrates may be necessary to obtain the desired fiber level in some persons. There are several available on the market that are palatable and can be added to cereals, yogurt, applesauce, juice, or soups. However, the use of foods as the fiber source results in benefits from both the fiber and the nutrients included in the foods.

Fiber is not destroyed by cooking, although the structure may be changed. Consumption of eight 8-oz glasses (2 q) of fluids daily is recommended to facilitate the effectiveness of a high fiber intake. Gastric obstruction and fecal impaction sometimes occur when boluses of fibrous gels or bran are not consumed with sufficient fluid to disperse the fiber. Appropriate cautions are also warranted for persons with GI strictures or dysmotility syndromes. In these situations, the fiber content of the diet should be increased slowly, taking almost a month to reach intakes of 25 to 30 g of fiber per day.

Upon initiation of a high-fiber diet, unpleasant side effects may occur, such as increased **flatulence, borborygmus** (intestinal rumbling), cramps, or diarrhea. A gradual increase in fiber intake helps alleviate these symptoms. If fiber supplements are used, doses should be interspersed with meals, preferably in two or more small doses per day, and fluid intake may need to be increased at the same time. Gastrointestinal disturbances associated with initial fiber ingestion usually decrease within 4 to 5 days, but some increase in flatulence is normal with high-fiber intake. The high-fiber diet is most effective after several months of compliance. The effect of high-fiber intake on mineral balance is not thought to be a problem unless cereal intakes are high and mineral intakes are low (Kelsay, 1987).

COMMON SYMPTOMS OF INTESTINAL DYSFUNCTION

Intestinal Gas and Flatulence

Pathophysiology

Intestinal gases include N_2, O_2, CO_2, H_2, and, in some individuals, CH_4 (methane). About 200 mL of gas is normally present in the GI tract, and humans excrete an average of 700 mL/day; however, there is a large range of volumes and excretion of gas in the GI tract (Strocchi and Levitt, 1998). Considerable amounts of gas may be swallowed, exchanged between the GI tract and circulating blood, and produced within the GI tract. Gases taken in or produced in the gastrointestinal tract may be absorbed into the circulation and lost in respiration, expelled through eructation (belching), or passed rectally. When individuals complain about "excessive gas," they may be referring to increased frequency of passage of gas, or they may be complaining about the abdominal distention or cramping pain associated with the accumulation of gases in the upper or lower GI tract. The association between the amount of gas in the GI tract perceived by an individual and the amount actually measured is not always accurate (Levitt et al., 1996). Inactivity, decreased GI motility, aerophagia, diet, and GI disorders can all contribute to the amount of intestinal gas and the individual's gas-related symptoms.

Gas in the upper intestinal tract results primarily from swallowing air (aerophagia) and, to a lesser extent, from chemical reactions that occur during the digestion of foods. Normally, only small amounts of swallowed air or gases dissolved in foods make their way as far as the colon. High N_2 and O_2 concentrations in rectal gas, both of which are substances that are present in the atmosphere in large quantities, result from aerophagia. Aerophagia can be avoided by eating slowly, chewing with the mouth closed, and refraining from drinking through straws.

Increased amounts of H_2 and CO_2—and sometimes, CH_4—in rectal gas indicate excessive bacterial fermentation and suggest malabsorption of a fermentable substrate. The amounts and types of gases produced may depend on the mix of microorganisms in the individual's colon. Consumption of large amounts of dietary fiber (especially soluble fiber), resistant starch, lactose in persons who are lactase deficient, or modest amounts of alcohol sugars (such as sorbitol) may result in increased gas production in the colon and increased flatulence. Consumption of unusual amounts of fructose, or even sucrose, may also result in increased amounts of fecal substrate.

When undigested carbohydrates pass into the colon, they are fermented, to varying degrees, to short-chain fatty acids and gases, primarily H_2, CO_2, and in about one-third of individuals, methane. The widely recognized propensity of legumes to produce **flatus** or gas has been traced to the presence of specific indigestible carbohydrates, namely stachyose and raffinose. The properties of other so-called "gas-forming" foods may simply be related to the nature of the fiber and carbohydrate contents of the suspected foods, to odors produced, or to individual responses to foods. Relatively little data are available to substantiate the myriad of individual responses to specific foods reported by patients. If the food or foods are important in the individual's diet, a controlled trial of adding and omitting the offending food items can be undertaken.

Constipation

Pathophysiology

Definitions of **constipation** tend to be highly subjective, but usually include hard stools, straining with defecation, and infrequent bowel movements. At least in elderly patients, hard stools, incomplete evacuation, and difficulty passing stools may be more troublesome than infrequency of bowel movements. One objective assessment defines constipation as a condition in which (1) fewer than three stools per week are passed while a person is eating a high-residue diet; (2) more than 3 days go by without the passage of a stool; or (3) the weight of stool passed in 1 day totals less than 35 g (Devroede, 1989).

Normal stool weight is approximately 100 to 200 g/per day, and normal frequency may range from one stool every 3 days to three times per day. Normal transit time through the GI tract ranges from about 18 to 48 hours. Persons consuming a diet containing the recommended amounts of dietary fiber in the form of fruits, vegetables, and whole grain breads and cereals tend to have larger, softer stools that are relatively easy to pass. Some people who believe that it is necessary to have frequent bowel movements and who ignore dietary and other health recommendations may become disturbed when this does not occur, and try to compensate with the use of medications and enemas.

The most common causes of constipation in otherwise healthy individuals include repeated lack of response to the urge to defecate, lack of fiber in the diet, insufficient fluid intake, inactivity, and chronic use of laxatives. Nervous strain or anxiety may aggravate the condition. Chronic constipation may also result from a variety of organic disorders, as outlined in Table 31–3.

Treatment

Constipation is treated by including adequate dietary fiber, fluid, and exercise in one's daily routine and heeding the urge to defecate. Patients with a laxative habit should substitute progressively milder products with an eventual goal of complete withdrawal. Treatment of more resistant cases of constipation and of constipation related to functional bowel disorders may require intensive bowel training, chronic use of stool softeners and other medications, and various forms of surgical correction (Tramonte et al., 1997).

NUTRITIONAL CARE

An essential component of treatment for patients with constipation is provision of a normal diet that is high in both soluble and insoluble fiber. Diets that are low in fiber result in prolonged transit time through the gut, permitting excessive water reabsorption and the formation of hard stools.

Normal amounts of maldigested carbohydrate and fiber may help to hydrate stools and normalize bowel function, but excesses may also cause diarrhea. The primary effects of dietary fiber on bowel function relate to its water-holding capacity, which presumably leads to larger, softer stools, and its stretching effect on the distal colon and rectum, which increases the urge to defecate. Malabsorption of large amounts of carbohydrate or fiber may result in acidification of the colonic contents, resulting from the production of short-chain fatty acids during bacterial fermentation. Production of small or normal amounts of short-chain fatty acids enhances the absorption of electrolytes and water, but larger amounts may acidify fecal contents, increase fecal osmolality and water, and stimulate bowel movement (Branski et al., 1996).

The daily diet should contain at least 25 g of dietary fiber, which can be supplied by including ample amounts of fruits, vegetables (especially legumes), and whole grains. Table 31–1 describes a high-fiber diet, and Appendix 42 lists the dietary fiber content of foods.

Brans, such as wheat bran, may be effective in promoting bulk formation and relieving constipation. However, bran should be used in moderation and increased gradually, from 1 tsp/day to 4 to 6 T/day, accompanied with adequate intake of fluids.

High-fiber diets should not be used indiscriminately. When obstructive constipation continues, even with increased or large fiber intakes, other possible causes, such as a motility disorder or a tumor, should be considered.

LAXATIVES

It is sometimes necessary to treat resistant constipation, as well as hemorrhoids, with substances that promote regular evacuation of soft stools. Bulking agents, such as cellulose, hemicellulose derivatives, psyllium seed, and ispaghula, and osmotic agents, such as lactose, magnesium hydroxide, and sorbitol, have been used. Stool softeners, such as Colace may also be used. Impactions of stool may require more stringent oral medications, rapid consumption of large volumes of fluids, enemas, or digital evacuation.

TABLE 31–3 CAUSES OF CONSTIPATION

Systemic
- Side effect of medication
- Metabolic and endocrine abnormalities, such as hypothyroidism, uremia, and hypercalcemia
- Lack of exercise
- Ignoring the urge to defecate
- Vascular disease of the large bowel
- Systemic neuromuscular disease leading to deficiency of voluntary muscles
- Poor diet, low in fiber
- Pregnancy

Gastrointestinal
- Diseases of the upper gastrointestinal tract
  - Celiac disease
  - Duodenal ulcer
  - Gastric cancer
  - Cystic fibrosis
- Diseases of the large bowel resulting in:
  - Failure of propulsion along the colon (colonic inertia)
  - Failure of passage through anorectal structures (outlet obstruction)
- Irritable bowel syndrome
- Anal fissures or hemorrhoids
- Laxative abuse

Mineral oil, particularly taken after meals, has been thought to interfere with the absorption of carotene and the fat-soluble vitamins A, D, and K. This belief may not be supported by recent studies, however.

About 3% to 5% of all pediatric outpatient visits are related to chronic constipation. In the most severe cases, there is a flaccid colon that is insensitive to distention and encopresis develops. After initial treatment with laxatives and lubricants, fiber intake is the next focus of care. Research indicates that a high-fiber diet, laxatives, and the use of mineral oil as a lubricant do not adversely affect nutritional status over a 6-month period (McClung et al., 1993).

Diarrhea

Pathophysiology

Diarrhea is characterized by the frequent evacuation of liquid stools, accompanied by an excessive loss of fluid and electrolytes, especially sodium and potassium. It occurs when there is excessively rapid transit of intestinal contents through the small intestine, decreased enzymatic digestion of foodstuffs, decreased absorption of fluids and nutrients, or increased secretion of fluids into the GI tract. Diarrhea often involves several of these mechanisms (Branski et al., 1996; Fine, 1998).

Osmotic diarrheas are caused by the presence in the intestinal tract of osmotically active solutes that are poorly absorbed. Examples include the diarrheas accompanying the dumping syndrome and following lactose ingestion in the presence of a lactase deficiency.

Secretory diarrheas are the result of active secretion of electrolytes and water by the intestinal epithelium. Acute secretory diarrheas are caused by bacterial exotoxins, viruses, and increased intestinal hormone secretion. Unlike osmotic diarrhea, secretory diarrheas are not relieved by fasting.

Exudative diarrheas are always associated with mucosal damage, which leads to an outpouring of mucus, blood, and plasma proteins, with a net accumulation of electrolytes and water in the gut. Prostaglandin release may be involved. The diarrheas associated with chronic ulcerative colitis and radiation enteritis are exudative.

Limited mucosal contact diarrheas result from conditions of inadequate mixing of chyme and inadequate exposure of chyme to intestinal epithelium, usually because of destruction or a decrease in the mucosa, as occurs in Crohn's disease or following extensive bowel resection. This type of diarrhea is usually complicated by steatorrhea resulting from bacterial overgrowth and by reduced luminal concentrations of conjugated bile acids.

Nutritional Care

Because diarrhea is a symptom of a disease state, the aim of medical treatment is to remove the cause. The next priority is to manage fluid and electrolyte replacement. Finally, attention must be given to nutrition concerns.

Losses of electrolytes, especially potassium and sodium, should be corrected early by using oral glucose electrolyte solutions with added potassium. With intractable diarrhea, especially in an infant or young child, parenteral feeding is sometimes required. Parenteral nutrition may even be necessary if exploratory surgery is anticipated, or if the patient is not expected to resume full oral intake within 5 to 7 days (see Chapter 22).

ADULTS. Nutritional care for adults with diarrhea includes the replacement of lost fluids and electrolytes by increasing the oral intake of fluids, particularly those high in sodium and potassium, such as broths and electrolyte solutions. Pectin from applesauce, or a supplement and small amounts of other hydrophilic fiber, may also help in controlling diarrhea.

When the diarrhea stops and the patient begins to tolerate food, the amounts given should be increased gradually as accepted, beginning with starches, which are likely to be well absorbed (e.g., rice, potato, plain cereals, etc.), and followed by protein foods. Fat need not be limited if the individual is otherwise healthy. Sugar alcohols, lactose, fructose, and large amounts of sucrose may worsen osmotic diarrheas and may need to be limited (see Table 31–2). Because the activity of the disaccharidases and transport mechanisms may be decreased during inflammatory and infectious intestinal disease, sugars may need to be limited.

Severe and chronic diarrhea may be accompanied by dehydration and electrolyte depletion. If accompanied by prolonged infectious, immunodeficiency, or inflammatory disease, malabsorption of vitamins, minerals, and protein and/or lipid may also occur, and the nutrients should be replaced parenterally or enterally. The loss of potassium alters bowel motility, encourages anorexia, and can introduce a cycle of bowel distress. Loss of iron from gastrointestinal bleeding may be severe enough to cause anemia. The nutritional deficiencies themselves cause mucosal changes, such as decreased villi height and reduced enzyme secretion, further contributing to malabsorption. As the diarrhea begins to resolve, the addition of more normal amounts of fiber to the diet may help to restore normal mucosal function, increase electrolyte and water absorption, and increase viscosity of the stool.

INFANTS AND CHILDREN. Acute diarrhea is most dangerous in infants and small children, who are easily dehydrated by large fluid losses. In these cases, replacement of fluid and electrolytes must be aggressive and immediate. Standard oral rehydration solutions recommended by the World Health Organization (WHO) and the American Academy of Pediatrics (AAP) contain a 2% concentration of glucose (20 g/L), 45 to 90 mEq/L of sodium, 20 mEq/L of potassium, and a citrate base (Table 31–4). Products, such as Pedialyte, Resol, Ricelyte, and Rehydralyte, are available without prescription. Pre-

TABLE 31–4 ORAL REHYDRATION SOLUTION: COMPOSITION AND RECIPE

ELEMENT	COMPOSITION
Glucose (g/100 mL)	2
Sodium (mEq/L)	90
Potassium (mEq/L)	20
Chloride (mEq/L)	80
Bicarbonate (mEq/L)	30
Osmolarity (mOsm/L)	330

Recipe

To 1 L of water add the following:

3.5 g sodium chloride
2.5 g sodium bicarbonate
1.5 g potassium chloride
20.0 g glucose

The solution should be made up fresh every 24 hours.

(Source: WHO, 1986.)

scription of a high-sugar, clear liquid diet is inappropriate for recovery from diarrhea. In children, oral rehydration therapy is less invasive than intravenous rehydration, and allows parents to assist with their children's recovery (Goepp and Katz, 1993).

A substantial proportion of children 9 to 20 months of age can maintain adequate intake when offered either a liquid or a semisolid diet during bouts of acute diarrhea (Marquis et al., 1993). Even during acute diarrhea, the intestine can absorb up to 60% of the food eaten. Physicians have been slow to adopt the practice of early refeeding after severe diarrhea in infants, despite evidence that "resting the gut" is actually more damaging (Booth, 1993). Luminal foodstuffs are needed to repair the damaged gut following infection; no controlled study has ever actually proven that fasting is beneficial in acute gastroenteritis. Early refeeding after rehydration reduces stool output and shortens the duration of illness (Meyers, 1993). Folate replacement or supplementation may be useful for acute diarrhea, possibly because it accelerates the normal regeneration of damaged mucosal epithelial cells.

Steatorrhea

Pathophysiology

Steatorrhea is a consequence of malabsorption in which unabsorbed fat remains in the stool. In contrast to the 2 to 6 g of ingested fat that is normally excreted each day, as much as 60 g may be lost with this condition. With the exception of specific carbohydrate intolerances, almost all diseases causing malabsorption cause steatorrhea. Diagnosis is usually based on a ratio of fecal fat to ingested fat or a coefficient of absorption. A 72-hour stool is collected and analyzed for fat and, at the same time, intake of dietary fat is recorded. A diet containing 75 to 100 g of fat is usually suggested.

Excessive fat excretion may result from (1) biliary insufficiency secondary to hepatic disease, biliary obstruction, blind loop syndrome, or ileal resection; (2) pancreatic insufficiency; (3) failure of normal absorption owing to mucosal damage, as in sprue and Crohn's disease, and after gastrointestinal radiation therapy; or (4) decreased fat re-esterification and decreased formation and transport of chylomicrons, as may be seen in abetalipoproteinemia and intestinal lymphangiectasia. Table 31–5 lists disorders associated with malabsorption.

Nutritional Care

Because steatorrhea is a symptom and not a disease, the underlying cause of malabsorption must be determined and treated. The presence of weight loss requires an increased energy intake. Dietary protein and carbohydrate should be high, and fats may need to be added as tolerated to meet individual needs. Multiple vitamin and mineral deficien-

TABLE 31–5 DISEASES AND CONDITIONS ASSOCIATED WITH MALABSORPTION

- Inadequate digestion
  - Pancreatic insufficiency
  - Gastric acid hypersecretion
  - Gastric resection
- Altered bile salt metabolism with impaired micelle formation
  - Hepatobiliary disease
  - Interrupted enterohepatic circulation of bile salts
  - Bacterial overgrowth
  - Drugs that precipitate bile salts
- Abnormalities of mucosal cell transport
  - Biochemical or genetic abnormalities
    - Disaccharidase deficiency
    - Monosaccharide malabsorption
    - Specific disorders of amino acid malabsorption
    - Abetalipoproteinemia
    - Vitamin B_{12} malabsorption
    - Celiac disease
  - Inflammatory or infiltrative disorders
    - Crohn's disease
    - Ulcerative colitis
    - Amyloidosis
    - Scleroderma
    - Tropical sprue
    - Gastrointestinal allergy
    - Infectious enteritis
    - Whipple's disease
    - Intestinal lymphoma
    - Radiation enteritis
    - Drug-induced enteritis
  - Endocrine and metabolic disorders
  - Short-bowel syndrome
- Abnormalities of intestinal lymphatics and vascular system
  - Intestinal lymphangiectasia
  - Mesenteric vascular insufficiency
  - Chronic congestive heart failure

cies necessitate supplemental therapy, with special emphasis on fat-soluble vitamins and minerals, such as calcium, zinc, magnesium, and iron.

MEDIUM-CHAIN TRIGLYCERIDES. Inadequate energy intake resulting from faulty digestion and absorption of fat may be alleviated by the use of **medium-chain triglycerides** (MCTs) (Craig GB, et al., 1997). These synthetic fats are made up of fatty acids that are 8 and 10 carbon atoms in length, compared with the 16- and 18-carbon chains common to most fatty acids that constitute dietary triglycerides. For this reason, MCTs are hydrolyzed more rapidly and can rely on the small amount of intestinal lipase available, rather than on pancreatic lipase for digestion. The products of hydrolysis are easily dispersed and absorbed in the absence of bile acids, which is often the cause of fat malabsorption. Short-chain fatty acids and medium-chain fatty acids are able to enter the portal venous blood for direct transport to the liver without being resynthesized into triglycerides.

MCTs are available in some enteral formulas and also as MCT oil (8.3 kcal/g; 1 T = 116 kcal). The oil is best used when it is incorporated in foods, rather than administered by spoonful. MCTs can be used to make salad dressings, sandwich spreads, or confections, and can be substituted for fats in most recipes. Normally, divided doses of less than 15 g of oil per feeding are better tolerated and absorbed than boluses.

DISEASES OF THE SMALL INTESTINE

Celiac Disease (Gluten-Sensitive Enteropathy)

Pathophysiology

Celiac disease, often called **gluten-sensitive enteropathy** or nontropical sprue, is caused by a reaction to gliadin, the alcohol-soluble component of gluten. The resulting damage to the villi of the intestinal mucosa results in potential or actual malabsorption of virtually all nutrients.

The mechanism by which gliadin damages the small bowel is unknown, but it appears that both genetic and immune components are involved. The immune response to gliadin, with the production of antigliadin antibodies, increased occurrence of products of HLA class II and other genes, and viral involvement, have been considered in the pathogenesis of celiac disease (Malnick et al., 1997; Troncone, 1996).

The disease primarily affects the mucosa of the proximal and mid-portions of the small bowel, although the more distal segments may also be involved. Atrophy and flattening of the villi severely limit the area available for nutrient absorption (Fig. 31–1). Cells of the villi become deficient in the disaccharidases and peptidases needed for digestion and also in the carriers needed to transport nutri-

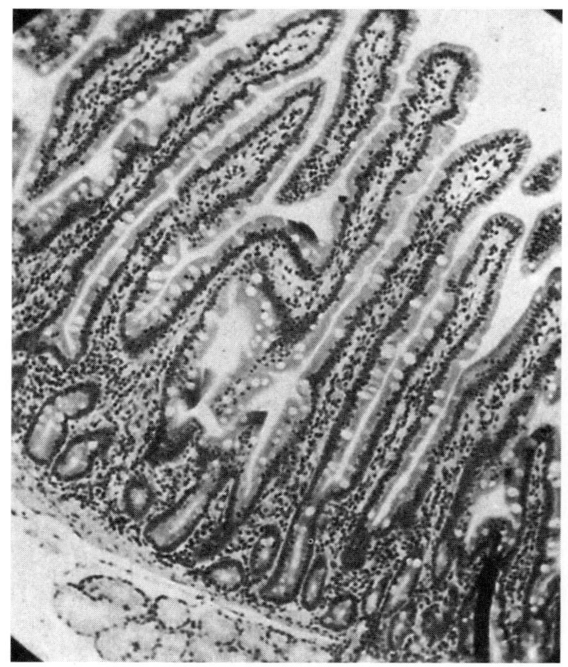

A

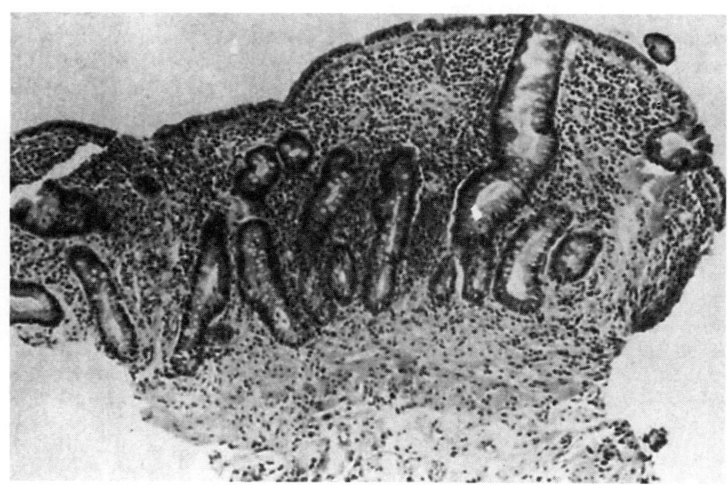

B

FIGURE 31–1 (*A*) Low-power photomicrograph (× 100) of a normal human duodenal mucosa. Note the long, thin villi. (*B*) Low-power photomicrograph (× 100) of a peroral small bowel biopsy specimen from a patient with gluten enteropathy. Note the complete loss of villi and the heavy infiltrate of white blood cells in the lamina propria. (From Floch MH. Nutrition and Diet Therapy in Gastrointestinal Disease. New York: Plenum Medical Book Co., 1981.)

ents into the bloodstream. Decreased cholecystokinin release diminishes gallbladder and pancreatic secretions, further contributing to maldigestion. Extraintestinal manifestations are listed in Table 31–6. For more information, check internet site www.csaceliacs.org/celiacdisease.html.

The classic diagnostic procedure consists of mucosal biopsy followed by a gluten-free diet, rebiopsy to document any intestinal villi improvement, and finally, a gluten challenge, followed by another biopsy 6 weeks later (Troncone, 1996). More recently, a less invasive diagnostic technique has been employed, whereby an initial biopsy is performed to demonstrate villous atrophy with hyperplasia of the crypts and abnormal surface epithelium while the patient is consuming a gluten-containing diet. Full clinical remission is then noted upon withdrawal of gliadin. Circulating antibodies to gliadin, reticulin, and endomysium, and their subsequent disappearance with consumption of a gluten-free diet, add strength to the diagnosis (Braegger and MacDonald, 1996). Use of circulating antibodies, especially endomysium, has been advocated as a noninvasive screening tool in evaluating relatives of patients with celiac disease. It is also used for further evaluation of persons who initially present with clinical symptoms similar to celiac disease, and for follow-up evaluation of patients after diagnosis and treatment (Catassi et al., 1997).

Institution of a gliadin-free diet generally reverses the process, and the intestinal mucosa reverts to normal. However, some patients may require months or even years of diet therapy for maximal recovery. Gliadin must be avoided for life (Chartrand and Seidman, 1996).

One form of celiac disease, called *refractory sprue,* does not respond to the removal of gliadin, or responds only temporarily. However, many of these patients do show a response to steroids, azothioprine, cyclosporine, or other medications classically used in inflammatory or immunologic reactions (Fig. 31–2).

Depending on the extent of involvement of the small intestine, persons with celiac disease may be relatively symptom-free, or they may present with significant GI distress, malabsorption, and malnutrition. The disease may become apparent when an infant begins eating gliadin-containing cereals, or it may not appear until middle age, when it is often unmasked by gastrointestinal surgery, stress, pregnancy, or viral infection.

The most common symptoms in children 6 months to 3 years of age are diarrhea, growth failure, vomiting, a bloated abdomen, and stools that are abnormal in appearance, odor, and quantity. Stool frequencies vary, but can be in excess of 10 stools per day. Adults may experience weight loss despite increased appetite, weakness, and fatigue, or they may present with extraintestinal symptoms, such as anemia, osteopenic bone disease, and other forms of autoimmune disease (Kemppainen et al., 1998).

Diarrhea may or may not be present. Bowel movements usually are large, putty-colored, and foul-smelling, with stools showing evidence of steatorrhea. Fifty percent to 60% of celiac patients have few or no symptoms, such as the previously identified flattening of the jejunal mucosa and regeneration following a strict dietary regimen (Marsh, 1993; Troncone et al., 1996). Subtle changes may occur over time in many individuals. The term *gluten sensitivity* is now the preferred term for patients with regular, atypical, and latent disease.

Persons with **dermatitis herpetiformis,** a papulovesicular skin disorder, show intestinal sensitivity to gliadin; 60% also have mild to severe small-bowel villous atrophy. Both the cutaneous and intestinal manifestations respond to a gluten-free diet. In some patients, it may take several years on a gliadin-free diet before the skin lesions improve.

TABLE 31–6 EXTRAINTESTINAL MANIFESTATIONS OF CELIAC DISEASE

ORGAN SYSTEM	MANIFESTATION	PROBABLE CAUSE
Hematopoietic	Anemia	Iron, folate, vitamin B_{12} or B_6 deficiency
	Hemorrhage, purpura	Hypoprothrombinemia, usually due to impaired intestinal absorption of vitamin K
Skeletal	Osteomalacia	Impaired absorption of vitamin D
	Osteoporosis, bone pain	Formation of insoluble calcium soaps by fatty acids in the intestinal lumen, leading to defective calcium transport and absorption
Muscular	Paresthesias, muscle cramps	Calcium depletion or magnesium depletion due to poor absorption
	Tetany, weakness	Hypokalemia due to potassium loss
Neurologic	Peripheral neuropathy	Deficiencies of vitamins, such as thiamin and vitamin B_{12}
Endocrine	Secondary hyperparathyroidism	Calcium and vitamin D malabsorption causing hypocalcemia
	Secondary hypopituitarism	Malnutrition due to malabsorption
	Adrenocortical insufficiency	Hypopituitarism
Integumentary	Follicular hyperkeratosis	Vitamin A deficiency
	Petechiae and ecchymoses	Hypoprothrombinemia

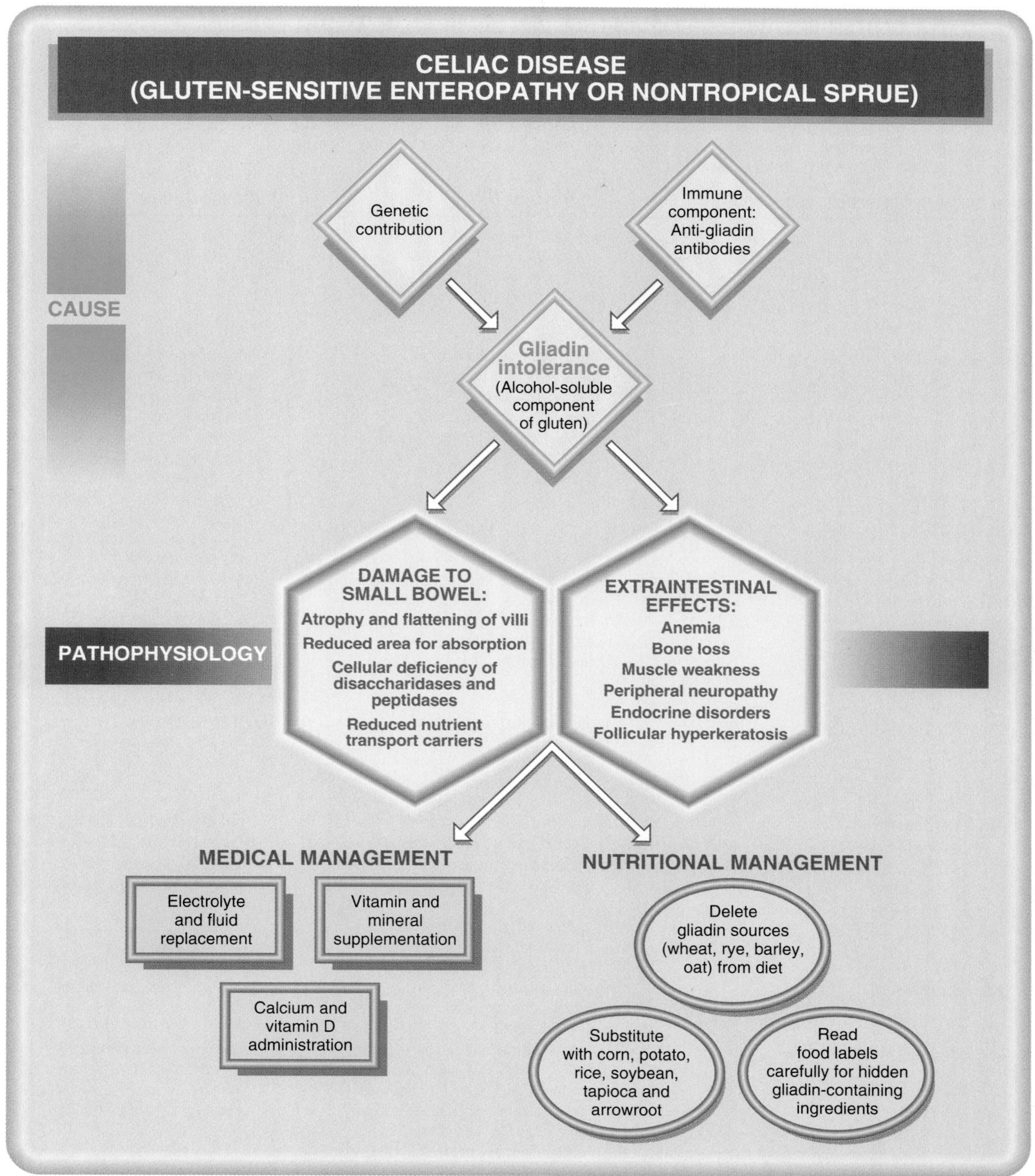

FIGURE 31–2 Pathophysiology algorithm—celiac disease (gluten-sensitive enteropathy or nontropical sprue). (Algorithm content developed by John Anderson, Ph.D., and Sanford C. Garner, Ph.D., 2000.)

TABLE 31–7 GLUTEN-RESTRICTED GLIADIN-FREE DIET* (WHEAT-, RYE-, OAT-, AND BARLEY-FREE)

General Considerations

- This diet is designed to provide adequate nutrition while eliminating wheat, rye, oats, and barley from the diet.
- Gluten may be present in foods either as a basic ingredient (i.e., listed as wheat, rye, oats, or barley) or added as a derivative when a food is processed or prepared. Thus, careful reading of labels is very important.
- Because flour and cereal products are quite often used in preparing foods, it is important to be aware of the methods of preparation used, as well as the foods themselves. This is especially true when dining out.

FOOD GROUP/RECOMMENDED DAILY INTAKE	FOODS ALLOWED	FOODS TO AVOID
Milk: ≥ 2 cups	Fresh, dry, evaporated or condensed milk; cream; sour cream,† whipping cream; yogurt;† malted milk; some commercial chocolate drinks; some nondairy creamers‡	
Meat, fish, poultry: ≥ 2 servings	All kinds of fresh meats, fish, other seafood, poultry; fish canned in oil or brine; some prepared meat products, such as hot dogs‡ and luncheon meats‡	Prepared meats that contain wheat, rye, oats, or barley, such as some sausages,‡ hot dogs,‡ bologna,‡ luncheon meats,‡ chili con carne,‡ sandwich spreads;‡ bread-containing products, such as Swiss steak, croquettes; meat loaf; tuna canned in vegetable broth;‡ and turkey with hydrolyzed vegetable protein injected as part of the basting solution
Cheeses (can be used for either meat or milk groups)	All aged cheeses, such as cheddar, Swiss, Edam, parmesan; cottage cheese,† cream cheese, pasteurized processed cheese†,#	Any cheese product containing oat gum as an ingredient
Eggs	Plain or in cooking	Eggs in sauce made from gluten-containing ingredients (e.g., a regular, wheat-based white sauce)
Potato or other starch: ≥ 1 serving	White and sweet potatoes, yams; hominy; rice; wild rice; special gluten-free noodles (Aproten, Aglutella, Ener-G);¶,# some oriental rice and bean noodles	Regular noodles; spaghetti; macaroni; most packaged rice mixes‡
Vegetables: ≥ 2 servings	All plain, fresh, frozen, or canned vegetables; dried peas and beans; lentils; some commercially prepared vegetables‡	Creamed vegetables;‡ vegetables canned in sauce;‡ some canned baked beans;‡ commercially prepared vegetables and salads‡
Fruits: ≥ 2 servings	All fresh, frozen, canned, or dried fruits; all fruit juices; some canned pie fillings	Thickened or prepared fruits; some pie fillings‡
Breads: ≥ 3 servings	Specially prepared breads using only the flours allowed; commercially available brands¶,#	All others containing wheat, rye, oat, or barley flour
Cereals: ≥ 1 serving of enriched cereal	Hot cereals made from cornmeal, cream of rice, hominy, rice, buckwheat,§ millet,§ amaranth,§ and quinoa§; cold cereals as follows: Puffed Rice, Kellogg's Sugar Pops; Post's Fruity and Chocolate Pebbles, special cereals¶,#	All others containing wheat, rye, oats or barley; bran, graham; wheat germ; malt; kaska; bulgar, spelt, kamut, and triticale
Flour and thickening agents		Wheat starch (manufacturer will state whether it contains gluten); all flours containing wheat, rye, oats, or barley
Good thickening agents	Arrowroot starch, cornstarch, tapioca starch	
Good when combined with other flours	Corn flour, cornmeal, potato flour, potato starch flour, rice bran, rice flours (plain, brown, sweet), rice polish, soy flour	
Best combined with milk and eggs in baked product	Corn flour, cornmeal, potato flour, potato starch flour, rice flours (plain, brown, sweet), rice polish, soy flour	

TABLE 31–7 **GLUTEN-RESTRICTED GLIADIN-FREE DIET* (WHEAT-, RYE-, OAT-, AND BARLEY-FREE) (continued)**

FOOD GROUP/RECOMMENDED DAILY INTAKE	FOODS ALLOWED	FOODS TO AVOID
Grainy textured products	Corn flour, cornmeal, sweet rice flour	
Drier product than with other flours	Potato flour, potato starch flour, plain and brown rice flours	
Moister product than with other flours	Sweet rice flour	
Adds distinct flavor to product (use with moderation)	Rice polish, soy flour	
Crackers and snack foods Special commercial manufacturers[¶,#]	Rice wafers;[‡] pure cornmeal tortillas; popcorn, some crackers[‡] and chips[‡]	All others containing wheat, rye, oats, or barley
Fats	Butter; margarine; vegetable oil; nuts; peanut butters; hydrogenated vegetable oils; some salad dressings;[‡] mayonnaise[‡]	Some commercial salad dressings[‡]
Soups	Homemade broth and soups made with allowed ingredients; some commercially canned soups[‡]	Most canned soups[‡] and soup mixes;[‡] bouillon
Desserts	Cakes, quickbreads, pastries, puddings prepared with allowed ingredients; cornstarch, tapioca, and rice puddings; gelatin desserts; custard; vanilla and coffee-flavored ice cream from: Arden, Carnation, Darigold, Foremost, Lucerne;[‡] some pudding mixes;[§] special commercial products[¶,#,**]	Commercial cakes, cookies, pies, etc., made with wheat, rye, oats, or barley; prepared mixes;[‡] ice cream cones; pudding[‡]
Beverages	Instant and ground coffee; instant tea; tea; carbonated beverages;[‡] pure cocoa powder; wines; rums; some root beers;[‡] vodka distilled from grapes or potatoes	Ovaltine; malted milk; ale; beer; gin; whiskies,[‖] vodka distilled from grain; herbal teas containing malted barley or other gliadin-containing grains
Sweets	Jelly; jam; honey; brown and white sugar; molasses; most syrups;[‡] some candy;[‡] chocolate; pure cocoa; coconut	Some commercial candies[‡]
Miscellaneous	Salt; pepper; herbs; extracts; food coloring; cloves; ginger; nutmeg; cinnamon; chili powder; tomato purée and paste; olives; pickles; rice, cider and wine vinegar; yeast; bicarbonate of soda; baking powder; cream of tartar; dry mustard; some other condiments;[‡] monosodium glutamate (MSG) derived from nongliadin sources	Some curry powder;[‡] some dry seasoning mixes;[‡] some gravy extracts;[‡] some meat sauces;[‡] some catsup;[‡] some mustard;[‡] horseradish;[‡] some soy sauce;[‡] chip dips;[‡] some chewing gum;[‡] distilled white vinegar[‖]

*Diet developed by Elaine I. Hartsook, PhD, RD (deceased), former Director, Gluten Intolerance Group of North America; former member, National Digestive Disease Advisory Board; Advisor, National Digestive Diseases Information Clearinghouse, National Institutes of Health, Public Health Service, U.S. Department of Health and Human Services.

†Check the type of vegetable gum used.

‡Product ingredients should be investigated.

§Although botanically different from other gluten-containing grains, it is important that these flours not be contaminated with wheat, rye, oats, or barley.

‖Distilled white vinegar uses grain as a starting material. Whiskies, including so-called corn whisky, use wheat, rye, oats, or barley in their mash. Gliadin-intolerant persons are advised to use rice, cider, or wine vinegar in preparing foods such as salad dressings or pickles, and in cooking. Avoid all whiskies.

¶Dietary Specialties, Inc., P.O. Box 227, Rochester, NY 14601.

#Ener-G Foods, Inc., P.O. Box 84487, Seattle, WA 98124-5787.

**Red Mill Farms, Inc., 290 So. 5th St., Brooklyn, NY 11211.

Commercially prepared pickles, catsup, mustard, mayonnaise, steak sauce, and other condiments are usually made with distilled grain vinegar. The maximum amount of gliadin that would be present in such products via the vinegar is probably insignificant.

Nutritional Care

Complete withdrawal of gliadin from the diet results in prompt clinical improvement. During the first few weeks of gliadin omission, the diet should be supplemented with vitamins, minerals, and extra protein to remedy deficiencies and replenish nutrient stores.

A gliadin-free diet omits the glutamine-bound fraction (glutenin and gliadin) of protein (Table 31–7). In this diet, wheat, oat, rye, and barley are excluded. Recently, the need for exclusion of oats from the diet of persons with celiac disease and dermatitis herpetiformis has been challenged (Schmitz, 1996; Hardman et al., 1997). Clinical and GI manifestations of gluten sensitivity do not appear to recur in evaluations of oat intake lasting from 6 months to 5 years. Until larger numbers of patients have been evaluated, however, some clinicians and patients may still be reluctant to add oat products to the diet.

Products made from corn, potato, rice, soybean, tapioca, arrowroot, amaranth, quinoa, millet, and buckwheat can be substituted in food products. When using the flours, it is important that they not be contaminated with a gliadin-containing flour during milling. Patients can expect differences in textures and flavors of common foods using the substitute flours, but the new recipes can also be quite acceptable once the adjustment is made. Table 31–8 provides suggestions for incorporating these substitutions into recipes.

A gluten-free diet results in a major change in the number and types of foods normally eaten. Wheat, in particular, is present in a surprising number of foods in the Western diet. A guarantee of a gliadin-free diet requires careful scrutiny of the labels of all bakery products and packaged foods. Gliadin-containing grains are used not only as a basic ingredient, but may also be added during processing or preparation of foods. Hydrolyzed vegetable protein, for example, may be made from wheat, soy, corn, or mixtures of these grains (see Table 31–9).

Freedom from symptoms after eating gliadin does not necessarily mean that the villi are undamaged. The precipitating condition usually continues to exist, and gliadin causes mucosal changes within hours. However, overt symptoms may take 8 weeks or more to reappear. It has been observed that adults who start and stop a gliadin-free diet a number of times may eventually reach a state at which they do not respond to the diet. Complications of chronic ulcerative jejunoileitis and extraintestinal manifestations may develop. Risk of malignant disease, especially lymphoma, is increased, and adherence to a gluten-free diet appears to reduce the risk (Troncone, 1996).

Lactose intolerance sometimes occurs secondary to celiac disease. A low-lactose diet, in conjunction with a gliadin-free diet, may be useful in controlling symptoms. Once the GI mucosa begins to heal after gliadin is omitted, lactase usually returns to normal levels, and the lactose intolerance disappears.

If the disease has been severe, vitamin and mineral supplementation may be required. Anemia should be treated with iron, folate, or vitamin B_{12}, depending on the type. Vitamin K may be prescribed in the presence of purpura, bleeding, or prolonged prothrombin time. Electrolyte and fluid replacement is essential in those with dehydration from severe diarrhea. Calcium and vitamin D administration may be necessary to correct osteoporosis or osteomalacia. Vitamins A and E may be necessary to replenish stores depleted by steatorrhea. A multiple vitamin-mineral supplement to at least meet recommended dietary allowances (RDAs) should be taken regularly by those who continue to have malabsorption. MCT may help provide calories and a vehicle for fat-soluble nutrients.

TABLE 31–8 SUGGESTIONS FOR SUBSTITUTIONS FOR WHEAT FLOUR IN RECIPES

Possible Substitutions for Wheat Flour in Recipes

1 cup corn flour
¾ cup coarse cornmeal
1 scant cup fine cornmeal
⅝ cup potato flour
⅞ cup rice flour

Suggestions for Improving the Eating Quality of the Final Product

1. Rice flour and cornmeal tend to have a grainy texture. A smoother texture may be obtained by mixing the rice flour or cornmeal with the liquid called for in the recipe, bringing this mixture to a boil, and then cooling the mixture before adding it to the other ingredients.
2. Soy flour must always be used in combination with another flour, not as the only flour in a recipe.
3. When using other than wheat flour in baking, longer and slower baking is required. This is particularly necessary when the product is made without milk and eggs.
4. When using coarse meals and flours in place of wheat flour, the amount of leavening must be increased. For each cup of coarse flour, use 2½ tsp of baking powder.
5. Muffins or biscuits, when made with other than wheat flour, are of better texture if baked in small sizes.
6. Dryness is a common characteristic of cakes made with flours other than wheat. Moisture may be preserved by frosting the cake or by storing it in a closed container.

(From Ohlson MA. Experimental and Therapeutic Dietetics, 2nd ed. Minneapolis: Burgess Publishing Co., 1972, p. 142.)

Tropical Sprue

Pathophysiology

Tropical sprue is a syndrome of unknown etiology that occurs in tropical areas, with the exception of Africa, south of the Sahara. It may be the sequela of an acute infectious diarrhea, with subsequent contamination of the bowel by bacteria. The intestinal organism identified may differ from one region of the tropics to the next (Farthing, 1998). Nutritional deficiency may increase susceptibility to an infectious agent. As in celiac disease, the intestinal villi are shortened, but the surface cell alterations are much less severe. The gastric mucosa may be atrophied and inflamed, with diminished secretion of hydrochloric acid and intrinsic factor.

Symptoms include diarrhea, anorexia, and abdominal distention, as well as symptoms of nutritional deficiency, such as night blindness, glossitis, stomatitis, cheilosis, pallor, and edema. Anemia may result from iron, folic acid, and vitamin B_{12} deficiencies.

Nutritional Care

Treatment involves restoration of fluids, electrolytes, and nutrients. Tropical sprue often responds promptly to antibiotics and folate therapy. Along with other nutrients as needed, folate is

TABLE 31–9 GLIADIN-CONTAINING DERIVATIVES*

INGREDIENT (AS IT APPEARS ON LABEL)[†]	ALLOWABLE	TO BE AVOIDED
"Hydrolyzed vegetable protein" (HVP)[‡]	Soy, corn	Mixtures of wheat, corn, and soya (soy)
"Flour" or "cereal products"	Rice flour, corn flour, cornmeal, potato flour, soy flour	Wheat, rye, oats, or barley
"Vegetable protein"	Soy, corn	Wheat, rye, oats, or barley
"Malt" or "malt flavoring"	Those derived from corn	Those derived from barley or barley malt syrup
"Starch"	When listed as such on an American manufacturer's ingredient list, it is cornstarch	
"Modified starch" or "modified food starch"	Arrowroot, corn, potato, tapioca, waxy maize, maize	Wheat starch
"Vegetable gum"	Carob bean, locust bean, cellulose gum, guar gum, gum arabic, gum acacia, gum tragacanth, xanthan gum	Oat gum
"Soy sauce" or "soy sauce solids"	Those that do not contain wheat (e.g., Chun King)	Those that contain wheat
"Monoglycerides and diglycerides"	Those using a gliadin-free carrier	Those that use a wheat starch carrier

*Developed by Elaine I. Hartsook, PhD, RD (deceased), former Director, Gluten Intolerance Group of North America; Advisor, National Digestive Disease Information Clearinghouse, National Institutes of Health, Public Health Service, U.S. Department of Health and Human Services.

[†]Always check the source of the following nebulous ingredients before eating any product containing them. These questionable ingredients must be cleared with the manufacturer before they are eaten. When writing the manufacturer, request information on the specific starting material(s) used in a particular ingredient. For example, when "modified food starch" appears as a labeling ingredient, ask for the specific type of starch used (i.e., potato starch, tapioca starch, etc.).

[‡]A combination of wheat, corn, and soya is primarily used as starting material for hydrolyzed vegetable protein, and thus is not allowed on a gluten-free diet. When wheat protein is "hydrolyzed," its large amino acid chains are broken down into smaller chains. Some protein researchers believe the sequence of amino acids found in these smaller chains is as toxic as the intact gliadin subfraction of the gluten protein. Thus, HVP made from wheat is not recommended for use on a gluten-free diet.

given orally, 5 mg/day, along with intramuscular vitamin B_{12} (1000 μg/month).

Intestinal Brush Border Enzyme Deficiencies

Intestinal enzyme deficiency states involve deficiencies of the brush border disaccharidases that hydrolyze disaccharides at the mucosal cell membrane. Disaccharidase deficiencies may occur as (1) rare congenital defects, such as the sucrase, isomaltase, or lactase deficiencies seen in the newborn; (2) generalized forms secondary to diseases that damage the intestinal epithelium (e.g., Crohn's disease or celiac disease); or, most commonly, (3) a genetically acquired form (e.g., lactase deficiency) that usually appears after childhood but can appear as early as 2 years of age.

Lactase Deficiency

Pathophysiology

Lactose intolerance is the most common carbohydrate intolerance and affects persons of all age groups. Intolerance to lactose is caused by a deficiency of lactase, the enzyme that digests the sugar in milk. Lactose that is not hydrolyzed into galactose and glucose remains in the gut and acts osmotically to draw water into the intestines. Colonic bacteria ferment the undigested lactose, generating short-chain fatty acids, carbon dioxide, and hydrogen gas. Consumption of quantities greater than 12 g (the amount typically found in 240 mL of milk) may result in bloating, flatulence, cramps, and diarrhea.

The condition is very prevalent in the world population, especially among blacks, Asians, and South Americans. The fact that 70% of the world's adults are unable to digest lactose has led to the proposal that lactose intolerance is the normal state and lactose tolerance is abnormal. Although it has been suggested that lactase persistence is induced by the continuation of milk in the diet after weaning, there is no evidence to support this theory. It is more likely that the maintenance of lactase through adulthood reflects the continuation of an ancient genetic mutation (see "*Focus On:* Lactose Tolerance—An Uncommon Anomaly?").

Typically, lactase activity declines exponentially at weaning to about 10% of the neonatal value. Even in adults who retain a high level of lactase levels (75% to 85% of white adults of Western European heritage), the quantity of lactase is about half that of other saccharidases, such as sucrase, α-dextrinase, or glucoamylase (Gray, 1993). The decline of lactase is commonly known as **hypolactasia.** Adult-type hypolactasia is the most common type of lactase deficiency.

Lactose intolerance can also develop secondary to an infection of the small intestine or destruction of mucosal cells from other causes. In children, it is typically secondary to other infections or conditions, such as diarrhea, acquired immunodeficiency syndrome (AIDS), or giardiasis. Lactase activity may not return after small bowel surgery or prolonged disuse of the gastrointestinal tract, such as during

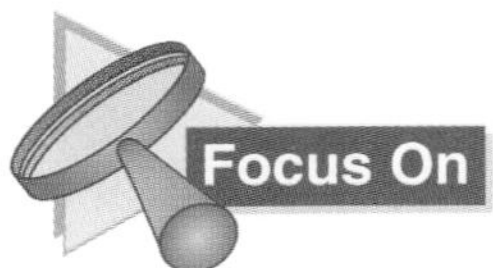

Lactose Tolerance— An Uncommon Anomaly?

When lactose intolerance was first described in 1963, it appeared to be an infrequent occurrence, arising only occasionally in the white population. However, as the capacity to digest lactose was measured in people from a wide variety of ethnic and racial backgrounds, it soon became apparent that disappearance of the lactase enzyme shortly after weaning, or at least during early childhood, was actually the predominant (normal) condition in most of the world's population. With a few exceptions, the intestinal tracts of adult mammals produce little, if any, lactase after weaning. (The milk of pinnipeds—seals, walruses, and sea lions—does not contain lactose.)

The exception of lactose tolerance has attracted the interest of geographers and others concerned with the evolution of the world's population. A genetic mutation favoring lactose tolerance appears to have arisen around 10,000 years ago when dairying was first introduced. Presumably, it would have occurred in places where milk consumption was encouraged because of some degree of dietary deprivation and in groups in which milk was not fermented prior to consumption. (Fermentation breaks down much of the lactose into monosaccharides.) The mutation would have selectively endured, because it would promote greater health, survival, and reproduction of those who carried the gene.

It is proposed that the mutation occurred in more than one location and then accompanied migrations of populations throughout the world. It continues primarily among whites from northern Europe and in ethnic groups in India, Africa, and Mongolia. The highest frequency (97%) of lactose tolerance occurs in Sweden and Denmark, suggesting an increased selective advantage in those able to tolerate lactose related to the limited exposure to ultraviolet light typical of northern latitudes. (Lactose favors calcium absorption, which is limited in the absence of vitamin D produced by skin exposure to sunlight.)

Dairying was unknown in North America until the arrival of Europeans. Thus, Native Americans and all of the non-European immigrants are among the 90% of the world's population who tolerate milk poorly, if at all. This has practical implications with respect to group feeding programs, such as school breakfasts and lunches. Fortunately, most lactose-intolerant people are able to digest milk in small to moderate amounts.

total parenteral nutrition (TPN) regimens. Usually, however, it does return, although slowly.

Lactase deficiency is typically diagnosed on the basis of (1) a history of gastrointestinal symptoms occurring after milk ingestion, (2) a test for abnormal hydrogen levels in the breath, or (3) an abnormal lactose tolerance test.

Lactose Tolerance Test. The lactose tolerance test was originally based on an oral dose of lactose equivalent to the amount in 1 q of milk (50 g). In the presence of lactose intolerance, blood glucose produced from the lactose increases less than 25 μg/100 mL of serum above the fasting level, and gastrointestinal symptoms may appear. In addition, intestinal production of hydrogen increases, as measured with the breath hydrogen test. The breath hydrogen test shows a high fasting H value and a secondary rise 60 minutes after lactose ingestion. Recently, lower doses of lactose have been used to more closely approximate the usual consumption of lactose in milk products. Many patients who demonstrate intolerance to the 50-g dose have no history of intolerance to milk and appear able to tolerate smaller amounts of milk in their diets (Suarez et al., 1995; Gudmand-Hoyer, 1994).

NUTRITIONAL CARE

The symptoms of lactose intolerance are alleviated by reduced consumption of lactose-containing foods. Most lactose-intolerant adults (lactose maldigesters) can consume some lactose (6 to 12 g) without major symptoms, especially when taken with meals or in the form of yogurt with active cultures. Some individuals attribute abdominal symptoms to lactose intolerance, but when challenged blindly with lactose, show no intolerance (Suarez et al., 1995). Many adults with intolerance to moderate amounts of milk can ultimately adapt to and tolerate 12 g or more of lactose in milk (equivalent to 8 oz of full-lactose milk) when introduced gradually, in increments, over a 6- to 12-week period (Johnson et al., 1993). Apparently, incremental or continuous exposure to a diarrheogenic quantity of fermentable sugar can lead to adaptation. This has been shown with lactulose, a nonabsorbed carbohydrate that is biochemically similar to lactose (Flourie, 1993). Regular consumption of milk by lactase-deficient persons may increase the threshold at which diarrhea occurs. Individual differences in tolerance may relate to the state of colonic adaptation.

Often, solid or semi-solid milk products, such as aged cheeses, are well tolerated because gastric emptying of these foodstuffs is slower than for liquid milk beverages, and the lactose content is low. Tolerance of yogurt may be the result of a microbial beta-galactosidase in the bacterial culture that facilitates lactose digestion in the intestine. Presence of galactosidase depends on the brand and processing method. Because this microbial enzyme is sensitive to freezing, frozen yogurt may not be as well tolerated (Montes and Perman, 1989).

Lactase enzyme and milk products treated with lactase enzyme (e.g., Lactaid) are available for lactase maldigesters who have discomfort with milk ingestion. Commercial lactase preparations may differ somewhat in their effects on both hydrogen breath excretion and symptom reduction (Ramirez et al., 1994).

Inflammatory Bowel Diseases

Pathophysiology

The two major forms of **inflammatory bowel disease (IBD)** are Crohn's disease and ulcerative colitis. The onset of IBD occurs most often in patients between the ages of 15 and 30 years, and both sexes are equally affected. In each case, the cause is unknown but genetic predisposition and immune and autoimmune phenomena are involved (Kornbluth et al., 1998; Hyams, 1996; Podolsky, 1991). Triggers for the initial onset of the diseases and subsequent exacerbations are also unknown, but they likely involve viral or bacterial interactions with immune cells lining the mucosal wall of the intestinal tract (van Dullemen et al., 1997; Miner, 1997) (see Fig. 31–3). Several specific candidate microbes have been considered but not proven.

Food intolerances of various types occur more than twice as often in persons with inflammatory bowel disease than in the population at large (Ballegaard et al., 1997). Except for a small increase in the occurrence of lactose intolerance, however, the patterns are not consistent among individuals, or even from one time to the next. Reasons for specific and nonspecific food intolerances are abundant, and may, in fact, be components of the overall symptoms of the disease. Partial GI obstructions, malabsorption, altered GI transit, increased secretions, food aversions and associations are but a few of the problems experienced by persons with IBD (Reif et al., 1997). Food allergies and other immunologic reactions to specific foods may certainly play a role in the symptoms associated with IBD, and may, to some degree, contribute to its pathology; however, the incidence of documented food allergies, compared to intolerances, is relatively small. In one objective evaluation of 375 patients with GI disease, adverse reactions to foods occurred in 32% of patients, allergies were suspected in 14.4%; allergies were confirmed in 3.2% of patients (Bischoff et al., 1996). Neither food allergies or intolerances, however, fully explain the onset or overall pathologic or clinical manifestations in all patients (see Chapter 41).

The GI tract is a major immune organ in that it is lined with large numbers of immune cells, such as macrophages and T lymphocytes, that are capable of triggering nonspecific and specific immune responses that result in the release of potent proinflammatory cytokines, eicosanoids, and destructive oxygen radicals (van Dullenmen et al., 1997; Mowat and Viney, 1997; MacDermott, 1996). Normally, when an antigenic challenge or trauma occurs, the immune response rises to the occasion; it is then turned off (and continues to be held in check) after the challenge resolves. In IBD, either the regulatory mechanisms are defective or the factors stimulating the immune and acute-phase response are enhanced, leading to tissue fibrosis and destruction. The clinical course of the disease may be mild and episodic, or severe and unremitting.

Both Crohn's disease and ulcerative colitis share some clinical features. For example, food intolerances, diarrhea, fever, weight loss, malnutrition, growth failure, and extraintestinal manifestations (arthritic, dermatologic, and hepatic) occur in both diseases. The diseases, however, also have distinctive features in terms of their genetic characteristics, clinical presentation, and treatment (Table 31–10).

Persons with IBD are at risk for several forms of malnutrition, and nutrition is a major consideration in each stage of the disease. Although malnutrition can occur in both forms of IBD, it is more likely to be a major and life-long concern in patients with Crohn's disease (Table 31–11). In both forms of IBD, the risk of malignant disease is increased with long-standing disease. The reasons for the increased risk are not firmly established, but may be associated with the increased proliferative state and nutritional factors.

CROHN'S DISEASE. **Crohn's disease** may involve any part of the GI tract, from mouth to anus. The small intestine, and especially the terminal ileum, are involved in about 75% of cases, and only about 15% to 25% of cases involve only the colon (Kornbluth et al., 1998). In the segments of bowel involved, the inflammation may be continuous; more likely, though, the inflammation will skip certain areas, so that healthy portions of bowel separate inflamed portions. Mucosal involvement in Crohn's disease is transmural in that it affects all layers of the mucosa. As inflammation, ulceration, abcesses, and fistulas resolve, fibrosis, submucosal thickening, and scarring may result, leading to narrowed segments of bowel, localized strictures, and partial or complete obstruction of the intestinal lumen.

Surgery may be necessary to repair strictures or remove portions of the bowel when medical management fails. About 50% to 70% of persons with Crohn's disease will undergo surgery related to the disease (Hyams, 1996). Surgery does not cure the disease; remission often occurs within 3 years of surgery, and the chance of reoperation sometime in the patient's life is approximately 30% to 70%, depending on the type of surgery and the age at first operation (Glotzer, 1995; Patel et al., 1997). Major resections of the intestine may result in varying degrees of malabsorption of fluid and nutrients. In extreme cases, patients may have extensive or multiple resections, resulting in dependence on parenteral nutrition to maintain adequate nutrient intake and hydration.

ULCERATIVE COLITIS. **Ulcerative colitis** involves only the colon, and the disease always extends from the rectum. Microscopic examination shows diffusely inflamed mucosa, usually with small ulcers.

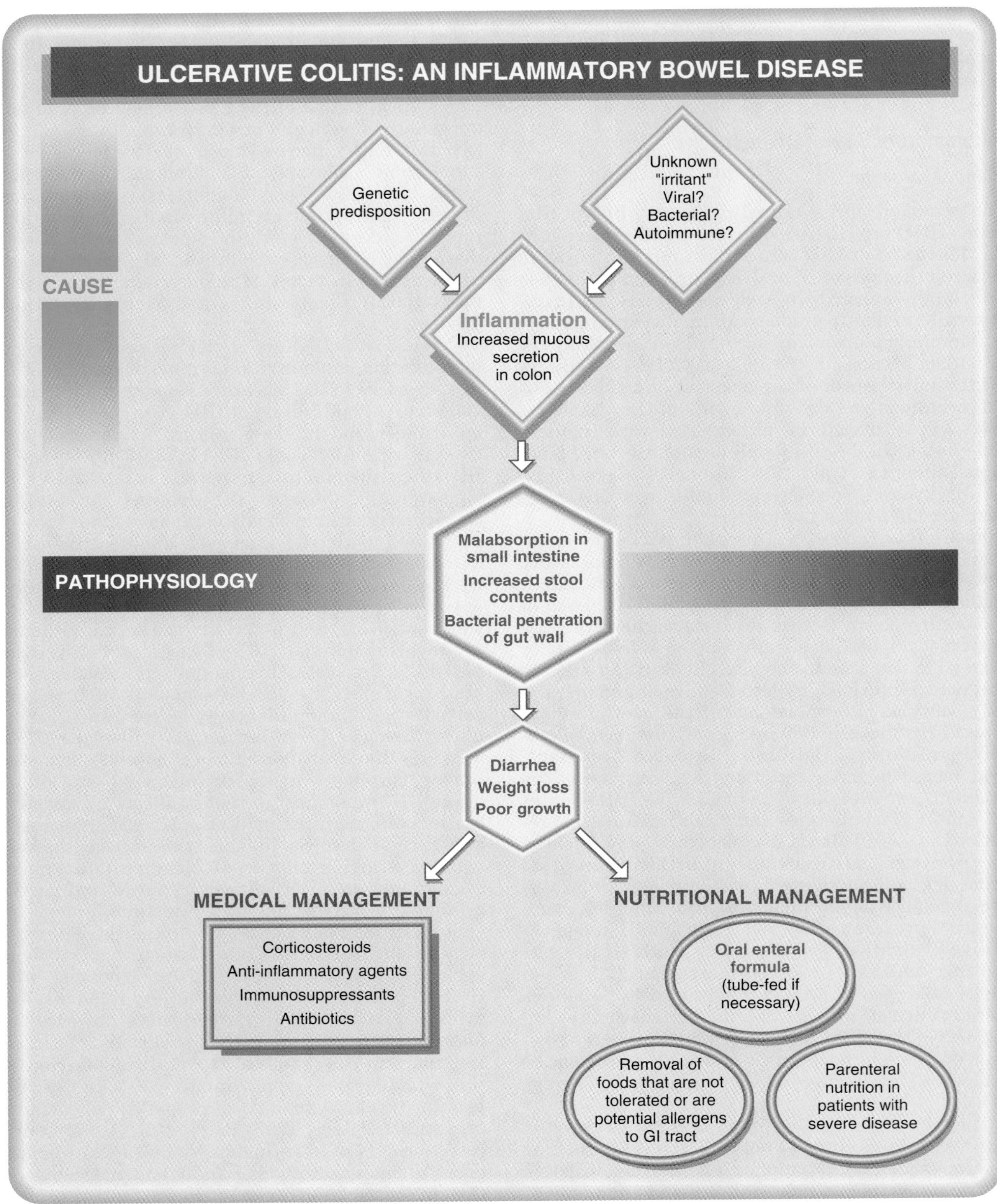

FIGURE 31–3 Pathophysiology algorithm—ulcerative colitis, an inflammatory bowel disease. (Algorithm content developed by John Anderson, Ph.D., and Sanford C. Garner, Ph.D., 2000.)

TABLE 31–10 DIFFERENTIATING BETWEEN CROHN'S DISEASE AND ULCERATIVE COLITIS

CHARACTERISTIC	REGIONAL ENTERITIS (CROHN'S DISEASE)	ULCERATIVE COLITIS
General Description		
Age at onset	Young	Young to middle-aged
Pathology and Anatomy		
Depth of involvement	Transmural (all layers of submucosa)	Mucosa and submucosa
Rectal involvement	50%	95%
Right colon involvement	Frequent	Occasional
Small bowel involvement	Involved; ileum narrowed	Usually normal
Distribution of disease	Segmental	Continuous
Inflammatory mass	Chronic and extensive	Rare (crypt abscess)
Cobblestone-like mucosa and granuloma	Common	Absent
Mesentery lymph involvement	Edema and hyperplasia	Not involved
Toxic megacolon	Occasional	Occasional
Steatorrhea	Frequent	Absent
Malignant disease	Rare	After 10 years
Fibrous stricture	Common	Absent
Clinical Manifestations		
Course of disease	Slowly progressive	Remissions and relapses
Rectal bleeding	Occasional	Common (90%–100%)
Abdominal pain	Colicky (45%)	Predefecation (60%–70%)
Hematochezia	Unusual or absent	Almost always present
Diarrhea	Present (65%–85%)	Early and frequent (80%–95%)
Vomiting	Present (35%)	Present (15%)
Nutritional deficit	Common	Common
Weight loss	Present (60%–70%)	Present (20%–50%)
Fever	Present (35%)	Present (10%)
Anal abscess	Common (75%)	Occasional (10%)
Fistula and anorectal fissure fistula	Common (80%)	Rare (10%–20%)
Systemic Manifestations		
Arthritis	Present (20%)	Uncommon (10%)
Peripheral sacroiliitis	18%	18%–20%
Hepatobiliary involvement	Uncommon	15% cholestatic dysfunction 19%–38% fatty liver 30%–50% pericholangitis
Skin: erythema nodosum, pyoderma gangrenosum	Common	Present (5%–10%)
Nephrolithiasis	Occasional	Rare

(From Black J, Matassarin-Jacobs E (eds.). Luckmann & Sorensen's Medical-Surgical Nursing, 4th ed. Philadelphia: WB Saunders, 1993, p. 1640.)

Continuous disease (rather than skipped areas) is characteristic. Serosal involvement, strictures, and significant narrowing are uncommon, but rectal bleeding or bloody diarrhea is relatively common (Jewell, 1998; Kirshner, 1996) (see Table 31–10 and Fig. 31–4). Ulcerative colitis occurs most commonly in young people aged 15 to 30 years, with a secondary peak at 50 to 60 years of age, although no age is exempt. In many cases, the colon must be removed and an ileal pouch or ileoanal anastomosis created.

Medical Management

The goals of treatment in IBD are to induce and maintain remission and to maintain nutritional status. Treatment of the primary GI manifestations appears to correct most of the extraintestinal features of the disease as well. The most effective medical agents in inducing remission during the acute stages of the disease are corticosteroids, although anti-inflammatory agents (aminosalicylates), immunosuppressive agents (cyclosporine, azathioprine, mercaptopurine), and antibiotics (metronidazole) may be used, either in combination or for maintaining remission. Each carries the potential for medical and nutritional consequences. Figure 31–5 shows an algorithm for reversing pediatric growth failure.

Investigations of various treatment modalities for the acute and chronic stages of IBD are ongoing, and include new forms of existing drugs, as well as new agents targeted to regulate cytokines, eicosanoids, or other mediators of the inflammatory/acute-phase cascade response (van Dullemen et al., 1997; Van Hogezand and Verspaget, 1996).

TABLE 31–11 POTENTIAL NUTRITION-RELATED PROBLEMS ASSOCIATED WITH INFLAMMATORY BOWEL DISEASE

- Anemias related to blood loss and poor food intake
- Gastrointestinal (GI) narrowing and strictures leading to bloating, nausea, bacterial overgrowth, and diarrhea
- Inflammation and surgical resections resulting in diarrhea and malabsorption of bile salts and micronutrients and macronutrients
- Increased GI secretions with inflammation and increased transit leading to diarrhea/malabsorption
- Abdominal pain, nausea, vomiting, bloating, diarrhea
- Food aversions, anxiety, and fear of eating related to experiences with abdominal pain, bloating, nausea, or diarrhea
- Associations of foods, or the simple ingestion of foods, with adverse symptoms of the disease (leading to anxiety and avoidance of food, which further limits intake)
- Drug-nutrient interactions
- True and perceived food allergies
- Dietary restrictions, both iatrogenic and self-imposed
- Growth failure, weight loss, micronutrient deficiencies, and protein-calorie malnutrition

Nutritional Care

Diet and nutrition play an important part in the management of exacerbations and symptoms of IBD, as well as in the remission of IBD. The ability of parenteral or enteral nutrition to induce remission of IBD has been debated for several years, and the issue is still not entirely resolved. At least in theory, use of low-residue, low-fiber liquid diets may decrease the antigenic load or reduce microbial populations in the colon. Clinical trials have been confounded by small numbers of patients, differences in study design, severity and location of the disease, differences in the nutritional formulas and whether an oral diet was continued, and differences in the definitions of acute illness, of onset, and of duration of remission. Evaluation is further confounded by the fact that the natural course of IBD is one of exacerbations and remissions.

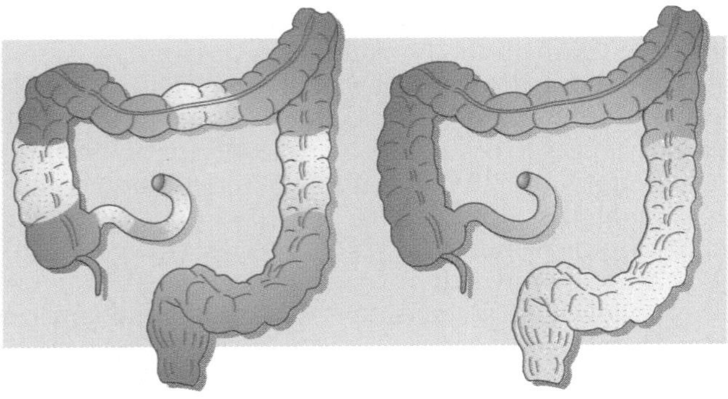

FIGURE 31–4 Crohn's disease (left) and ulcerative colitis (right). Whereas Crohn's disease typically involves the small and large intestine in a segmental manner, with intervening "skip" areas, ulcerative colitis is generally a contiguous disease process that starts in the rectum and progresses in a retrograde fashion to involve varying lengths of the colon.

Results of randomized studies and meta-analyses (Messori et al., 1996; Lindor et al., 1992; Sitrin, 1992) of several small studies with similar designs have generally concluded that "bowel rest" with parenteral nutrition is not a major requirement for achieving remission, and that enteral nutrition is the preferred means of nutritional support, and may result in greater success at inducing remission than parenteral nutrition. Commitment from the patient and caretaker to the sole use of oral enteral formulas must be high, or the formula must be fed by tube. However, enteral or parenteral intake is still not as consistently effective as corticosteroid therapy in inducing remission.

Regardless of whether or not current forms of parenteral or enteral nutrition induce remission, timely nutritional support is a vital component of therapy to restore and maintain nutritional health (Kelly and Fleming, 1995). Currently available parenteral solutions are not as well suited as complete enteral nutrition, but parenteral nutrition may be required to restore nutrition in patients with obstructions, fistulas, severe disease, and major GI resections.

Malnutrition itself compromises digestive and absorptive function and may increase the permeability of the GI tract to potential inflammatory agents (O'Keefe, 1996). Energy needs of patients with IBD are not greatly increased (unless weight gain is desired), but protein requirements may be increased by 50%, especially during active stages of the disease (Kushner and Schoeller, 1991). Supplemental vitamins and minerals may be needed because of avoidance of foods or certain food groups, malabsorption, or to correct drug-nutrient interactions.

During acute stages of the disease the diet is tailored to the individual patient. A minimal-residue diet may be effective for reducing diarrhea, whereas a diet that limits whole fibrous foods might be used when attempting to prevent obstructive symptoms. Small, frequent feedings may be tolerated better than large meals, and small amounts of isotonic, liquid, oral supplements may be valuable in restoring intake without provoking symptoms. In cases in which fat malabsorption is likely, supplements or foods made with MCTs may be valuable in adding calories and serving as a vehicle for fat-soluble nutrients.

Whether dietary factors contribute to exacerbations is not clear, but they certainly can aggravate symptoms. Although study results are inconsistent, the dietary factors commonly noted prior to exacerbations include increased sucrose intake, lack of fruits and vegetables, a low intake of dietary fiber, and altered n-6: n-3 fatty acid ratios (Reif et al., 1997; Shoda et al., 1996). In a small number of patients, specific food allergies may be identified. The significance of these factors is not clear, but they may simply reflect an overall poor-quality diet that may have increased the overall susceptibility of the

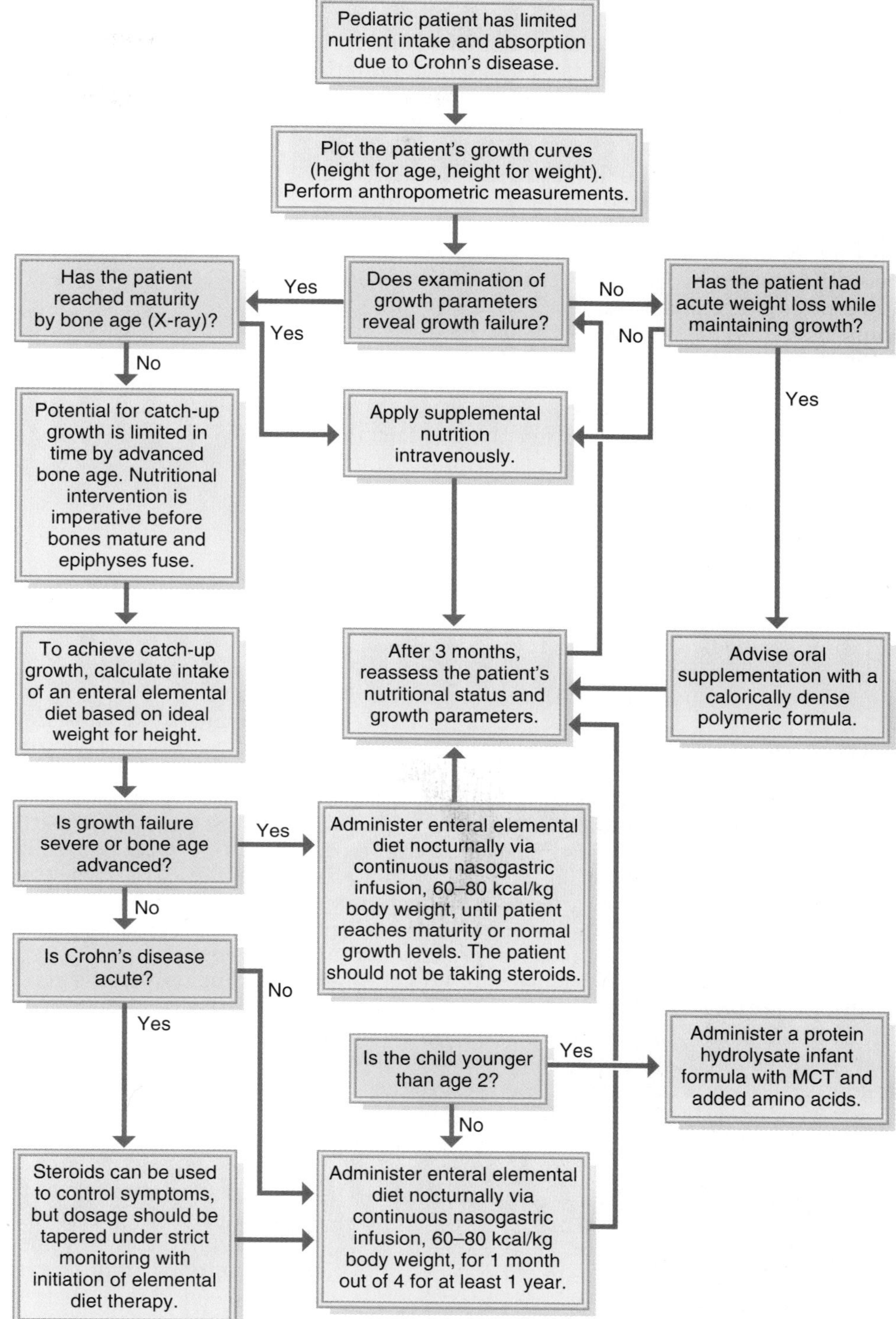

FIGURE 31–5 Algorithm for reversing growth failure in pediatric patients with Crohn's disease. (Adapted from: RD 11:5, 1991. Norwick-Eaton Pharmaceuticals: New York, NY.) *MCT,* medium-chain triglycerides.

GI tract to the disease process. Modification of oral diets and nutritional formulas with omega-3 fatty acids, specific amino acids (e.g., glutamine), and antioxidants, and the use of fermentable fibers are therapeutic strategies being considered for IBD along with medical and surgical management (Belluzi et al., 1996; O'Keefe, 1996).

In everyday life, patients may have intermittent "flares" of the disease characterized by partial obstructions, nausea, abdominal pain, bloating, or diarrhea. Patients can be taught to manage their disease by selecting appropriate foods and beverages. For example, patients might be taught to restrict foods during bouts of diarrhea (see Table 31–2) or to limit fiber (especially large particles) if partial obstruction is suspected. They can also be shown how to increase omega-3 fats so as to benefit from their anti-inflammatory effect, using supplements appropriately.

Food intolerances are very common in patients with IBD, but the foods are variable among patients, and may not be incriminated consistently from one time to the next. Patients are sometimes advised simply to eliminate the foods that they suspect are responsible for the intolerance. Often, however, the patient becomes increasingly frustrated as the diet becomes more and more limited, and symptoms may not resolve. A study by Pearson et al. (1993) revealed no significant differences in duration of remission between patients who did or did not identify food sensitivities.

Confirming true allergic GI reactions to foods is a difficult and painstaking process. The patient must be willing to consume either an amino acid diet or a very restricted diet composed of only three or four foods, with addition of each of the suspected foods one at a time. The allergen is identified on the basis of subjective and objective symptoms related to the repeated addition and elimination of the food. Circulating antibodies to food proteins have been considered to be a sign of allergy, but may in fact be a sign of increased permeability, rather than local GI allergy.

The foods that are most consistently responsible for GI symptoms (reflux, gas, bloating, and diarrhea) in a normal healthy population are likely to be the triggers for symptoms in patients with mild stages of IBD or for those in remission. Patients receive nutritional information from a variety of sources, including support groups, internet newsgroups, the audio and printed media, well-meaning friends, and food supplement salespersons. The information is sometimes inaccurate or exaggerated, or it may pertain only to one individual's situation. Education relating to the role of foods in normal GI disturbances and to the process of sorting out valid nutritional information may help to reduce the symptoms, as well as the anxiety level, of the individual.

DISEASES OF THE LARGE INTESTINE

Irritable Bowel Syndrome

Pathophysiology

Irritable bowel syndrome (IBS) is not a disease but a syndrome involving abdominal pain, bloating, and abnormal bowel movements. The most common symptoms are alternating diarrhea and constipation, abdominal pain (typically relieved by defecation), and bloating, but perception of excessive flatulence, sensation of incomplete evacuation, rectal pain, and mucus in the stool may also occur (Fig. 31–6). Painless diarrhea and chronic constipation are also variants of the syndrome, but occur less frequently. Symptoms may first present in adolescence, but most do not bring the problem to the attention of a physician until adulthood. In the United States, IBS occurs in approximately 20% of women and 10% to 15% of men. It represents about 12% of visits to family medicine clinics, 20% to 40% of visits to gastroenterologists, and is the most common reason for which patients first seek medical care (Drossman et al., 1997; Olden and Schuster, 1998).

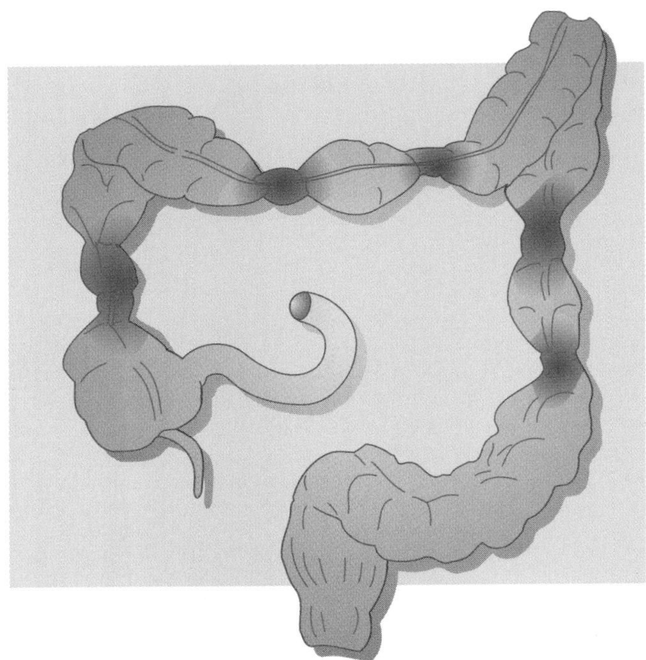

FIGURE 31–6 Irritable bowel syndrome.

The only abnormal physiologic differences appear to be altered visceral sensitivity and motility in response to GI and environmental stimuli. Persons with irritable bowel react more significantly than normal individuals to intestinal distention, dietary indiscretions, and psychosocial factors (Drossman et al., 1997). Normal individuals may experience mild GI disturbances in response to all the situations mentioned, but appear to have a milder response. Life stressors, such as divorce, employment changes, travel, relocation, or uncomfortable social situations may trigger the onset or worsen symptoms, and may override many therapeutic efforts. A history of psychosocial trauma, such as physical or sexual abuse, has been reported in 32% to 44% of cases, but the higher estimate may be somewhat exaggerated as a result of sampling technique (Drossman et al., 1997; Olden and Schuster, 1998).

Diagnosis is based on the presence of clinical symptoms of irritable bowel for three months or longer and screening for other medical or surgical conditions that may have a similar presentation. The diagnosis is further refined to categorize the syndrome to subtypes, such as alternating constipation and diarrhea, painless diarrhea, or constipation.

In addition to stress and dietary patterns, factors that may worsen symptoms and confound the diagnosis include (1) excess use of laxatives and other over-the-counter medications, (2) antibiotics, (3) caffeine, (4) previous gastrointestinal illness, and (5) lack of regularity in sleep, rest, and fluid intake. In patients with a strong family history of allergy, hypersensitivity to certain foods may be the cause of IBS (Bischoff et al., 1996). A trial of food elimination and challenge may be justified under these circumstances (see Chapter 41).

Medical Management

Management includes a combination of approaches to deal with the symptoms and the factors that may trigger them. Education, medications, counseling, and diet all play a role in the care. Depending upon the nature and severity of the symptoms, medications may include antispasmodic, anticholinergic, antidiarrheal, prokinetic, or antidepressive agents.

Nutritional Care

IBS, unlike IBD, is not life-threatening and does not result in maldigestion or malabsorption of nutrients. Dietary practices, however, may be very important in controlling symptoms.

The aim of nutritional care is to ensure adequate nutrient intake, to guide the patient toward a diet that is not likely to contribute to symptoms, and to explain the role of ordinary dietary practices in producing or avoiding GI symptoms. A normal diet is recommended, with emphasis on high-fiber foods that will add bulk to the stool, thus relieving the constricting pressure and promoting normal bowel motility. A daily fiber intake of 20 to 30 g is recommended. Additional fiber in the form of bulk laxatives (e.g., psyllium) may also be necessary. An excess of wheat bran may exacerbate mild cases; commercial fiber supplements are generally beneficial (Francis and Whorwell, 1994). It is also important that the patient drink adequate water (2 to 3 q per day) when taking fiber supplements. Excesses in dietary fat, caffeine, sugars (especially fructose and alcohol, and lactose in lactase-deficient individuals), and alcoholic beverages should be avoided. If these measures fail to control diarrhea, then the use of anticholinergic or antidiarrheal agents may be necessary. Biofeedback, relaxation, and stress reduction techniques may also be useful.

Diverticular Disease

Pathophysiology

Diverticulosis refers to sac-like herniations of the colonic wall. The outpouchings are thought to result from long-term increased colonic pressures. The cause is not known for certain, but in theory, increased intracolonic pressures and muscular thickening result from complete closure of colonic segments during contractions associated with attempts to propel small, dry, hard fecal material through the lumen of the bowel (Wess et al., 1996; Simmang and Shires, 1998) (Fig. 31–7). This theory is supported by epidemiologic studies of animals fed low-fiber diets throughout their lifetimes. In general, diverticular disease is (1) relatively rare in countries where a high-fiber diet is part of the life-long pattern, and (2) increasing where "Westernization" of the diet and increased intake of refined foods of the diet has begun. Even animals in these countries develop diverticula and suffer complications similar to those of human diverticular disease (Aldoori et al., 1994).

The incidence of diverticulosis increases with age. Thirty percent of individuals older than 50 years of age, 50% older than 70 years, and 66% older than 85 years of age develop diverticulosis (Simmang and Shires, 1998). Sigmoid involvement occurs in 99% of cases; right-sided colonic involvement occurs in Asians, but is rare in Caucasians (Deckman and Cheskin, 1993).

Complications of diverticular disease range from painless, mild bleeding and altered bowel habits to **diverticulitis,** which may include its own clinical spectrum of inflammation (abscess formation, acute perforation, acute bleeding, obstruction, and sepsis). Approximately 10% to 25% of patients with diverticulosis develop diverticulitis. One third of those admitted to hospitals for diverticular disease

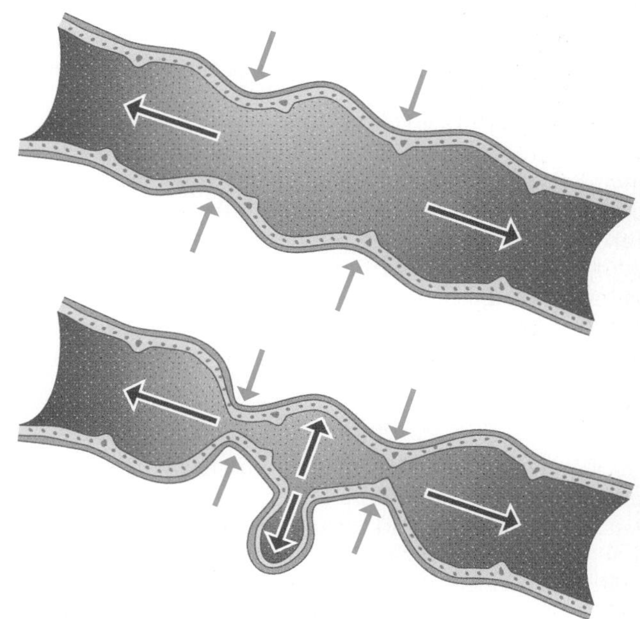

FIGURE 31–7 Mechanism by which low-fiber, low-bulk diets might generate diverticula. Where the colon contents are bulky (top), muscular contractions exert pressure longitudinally. If the lumen is small in diameter (bottom), contractions can produce occlusion and exert pressure against the colon wall, which may produce a diverticular "blow-out."

require surgery; death rates in patients requiring surgical intervention may be as high as 10% (Deckman and Cheskin, 1993).

Nutritional Care

At one time it was thought that roughage aggravated diverticular disease, so the classic diet therapy prescribed for diverticulosis consisted of a diet low in fiber or roughage. It is now recognized that a high-fiber diet promotes soft, bulky stools that pass more swiftly, require less straining with defecation, and result in lower intracolonic pressures. High-fiber intakes have been found to relieve symptoms for most patients. In one study (Deckman and Cheskin, 1993), 90% of patients using a high-fiber diet remained symptom-free after 5 years. This treatment often corrects constipation, a side benefit for many older persons.

Patients who have followed a low-fiber diet for years may require extensive encouragement to adopt the high-fiber approach. Fiber intake should be increased gradually, as it may cause bloating or gas. However, these side effects usually disappear within 2 to 3 weeks. In cases in which the patient cannot consume the necessary amount of fiber, methylcellulose and psyllium have been used with good results. Water, 2 to 3 q daily, must accompany the high-fiber intake.

For patients with an acute flare-up of diverticulitis, a low-residue diet, elemental diet or, in complicated cases, TPN may be required, followed by a gradual return to a high-fiber diet. Colonic smooth muscle contractions, which intensify after a high-fat meal, may contribute to the discomfort felt by individuals with diverticular disease (Snape, 1994). Therefore, a low-fat diet may be reasonable to suggest for these patients.

The question of whether the consumption of seeds, nuts, or skins of plant matter should be avoided—to prevent complications of diverticular disease or after bouts of diverticulitis—remains unresolved. Whether they play any role in the onset of symptoms or actually harm the diverticula needs to be evaluated, but in clear cases of perforation or obstruction, large pieces of coarse plant matter might be restricted.

Colon Cancer and Polyps

In the United States, colon cancer is the second most common cancer in adults (after lung cancer) and is also the second most common cause of death. The number of new cases of colorectal cancer in 1998 was estimated to be approximately 132,000 cases (Landis et al., 1998). Worldwide, it is the third most common malignant neoplasm and the second leading cause of cancer deaths. Colon cancer occurs more commonly in men than women (50 cases per 100,000 versus 41 cases per 100,000, respectively). The highest rates are seen in Caucasians of northern European origin in their native countries and in areas to which they have migrated. Rates in Africa and Asia are lower, but tend to rise with migration and Westernization. Colon cancer does not show a particular link to social class within any one country. Factors that increase the risk of colorectal cancer include family history, occurrence of IBD (both Crohn's disease and ulcerative colitis), familial polyposis and adenomatous polyps, and several dietary components (Steele, 1995; Eastwood, 1995; Potter et al., 1993). Polyps are considered precursors of colon cancers.

Dietary factors may include increased meat or fat intake and low intakes of vegetables, high-fiber grains, carotenoids, vitamins D, E, and folate, and the minerals calcium, zinc, and selenium (van Poppel and van-den Bergh, 1997; Singh et al., 1997). The role of dietary fat in colon carcinogenesis is not entirely clear because different dietary lipids may have different effects. Red meats, such as beef, pork, and lamb, along with their fats, may be incriminated more than other types of meats; poultry, fish, and dairy fats appear to have less of a role in carcinogenesis. Food preparation methods may also influence the carcinogenic potential of meats and fatty foods (Giovanucci and Goldin, 1997; Parodi, 1997) (see Chapter 39).

Potentially protective components of foods include omega-3 fatty acids, wheat bran, legumes, several phytochemicals, gamma-linolenic acid, and butyric acid (Craig, 1997). Butyric acid is found in dairy fats and is produced during bacterial fermentation of dietary fiber and carbohydrates in the colon. Calcium from low fat dairy products may also have a protective effect (Calcium . . . , 1999).

Depending on the point of entry of the patient into the health care system, the dietitian or nurse may be the key provider of information regarding the prevention or care of colorectal polyps or cancer. Because most Americans consume far less than the recommended amounts of fruits, vegetables (especially legumes), whole grains, and dairy products, the best advice for many patients might be to improve their diet based on the Food Pyramid Guide and to include reasonable amounts of omega-3 fatty acids (from marine sources and other sources, such as flaxseed oil). Patients who present with a diagnosis of colorectal polyps or cancer may require moderate to significant interventions, including medications, radiation therapy, chemotherapy (see Chapter 39), surgery, and/or nutritional support.

INTESTINAL SURGERY

Small Bowel Resection and Short-Bowel Syndrome

Short-bowel syndrome (SBS) refers to the consequences associated with significant resections of the small intestine. The healthy small intestine has significant reserve, but resections of 40% to 50% may lead to at least some of the consequences of SBS.

TABLE 31–12 SHORT-BOWEL SYNDROME: FACTORS AFFECTING SEVERITY OF MALABSORPTION, NUMBER OF COMPLICATIONS, AND DEPENDENCE ON PARENTERAL NUTRITION

- Length of remaining small intestine
- Loss of ileum, especially distal one third
- Loss of ileocecal valve
- Loss of colon
- Disease in remaining segment(s) of gastrointestinal tract
- Radiation enteritis
- Coexisting malnutrition
- Older age at surgery

Colonic resections alone do not produce SBS, but the risk of dehydration, electrolyte disorders, and malnutrition may increase in patients undergoing small bowel resections. The most common reasons for major resections of the intestine in adults include Crohn's disease, radiation enteritis, mesenteric infarct, malignant disease, and volvulus. In the pediatric population, most of the cases of SBS result from congenital anomalies of the GI tract, volvulus, or necrotizing enterocolitis.

Obvious complications of short-bowel syndrome include malabsorption of micronutrients and macronutrients, fluid and electrolyte imbalances, weight loss, and growth failure (in children). Gastric hypersecretion, oxalate renal stones, cholesterol gallstones, and rarely, *d*-lactic acidosis may also occur. The severity of malabsorption, the extent of complications, and the degree of dependence on parenteral nutritional support reflect the length and location of the resection, the age of the patient at operation, and the health of the remaining GI tract (Table 31–12) (Beyer, 1998; Vanderhoof, 1997).

JEJUNAL RESECTIONS

Normally, most digestion and absorption of food and nutrients occurs in the first 100 cm of small intestine. What remains to be digested or fermented and absorbed are small amounts of sugars, resistant starch, fiber, lipids, dietary fiber, and fluids. With jejunal resections, the ileum is able to perform the functions of the jejunum, especially after a period of adaptation. The motility of the ileum is comparatively slow, and hormones secreted in the ileum and colon help to slow gastric emptying and secretions. Because jejunal resections result in reduced surface area and shorter intestinal transit than normal, the functional reserve for absorption of micronutrients, excess amounts of sugars (especially lactose), and lipids is reduced.

ILEAL RESECTIONS

Significant resections of the ileum, especially the distal ileum, generally produce major nutritional and medical complications. The distal ileum is the only site for absorption of the vitamin B_{12}/intrinsic factor complex and bile salts, and the ileum normally absorbs a major portion of the several liters of fluid ingested/secreted into the GI tract (see Chapter 1). Although malabsorption of bile salts may appear to be a rather benign problem, it creates a potentially serious cascade of consequences (Beyer, 1998) (Table 31–13).

If the ileum cannot "recycle" bile salts secreted into the GI tract, hepatic production cannot maintain a sufficient bile salt pool or the secretions to emulsify lipids. The gastric and pancreatic lipases are capable of digesting some triglyceride to fatty acids and monoglycerides, but without adequate micelle formation facilitated by bile salts, lipids are poorly absorbed. This can result in significant malabsorption of fats and fat-soluble vitamins A, D, and E. In addition, malabsorption of fatty acids results in their combination with divalent cations, such as calcium, zinc, and magnesium, to form fatty acid/mineral "soaps." This results in the malabsorption of these nutrients. To compound matters, colonic absorption of oxalate, which normally is bound to the divalent cations, is increased, leading to hyperoxaluria and increased renal oxalate stones. Relative dehydration and concentrated urine, which are common with ileal resections, may further increase the risk of stone formation.

If the patient has any colon left, malabsorption of what bile salts are secreted can act as irritants to the mucosa, resulting in increased fluid and electrolyte secretion, rather than absorption, and increased colonic motility. Consumption of high-fat diets with ileal resections and retained colon may also result in the formation of hydroxy fatty acids, which also can increase fluid secretion. Cholesterol gallstones may occur more often because the ratio of bile acid, phospholipid, and cholesterol in biliary secretions is altered as a result of ileal resections. Dependence on parenteral nutrition may further increase the risk of biliary "sludge" secondary to decreased stimulus for evacuation of the biliary tract.

D-lactic acidosis is a relatively rare complication

TABLE 31–13 CONSEQUENCES OF ILEAL RESECTION

- Rapid transit of intestinal contents
- Decreased fluid absorptive area
- Malabsorption of vitamin B_{12}/intrinsic factor complex
- Malabsorption of bile salts
- Inadequate bile salts for lipid solubilization, digestion, and absorption, leading to loss of fat and fat-soluble nutrients
- Loss of secreted bile salts into colon because of decreased reabsorption
- Formation of hydroxy fatty acids by colonic bacteria from malabsorbed fat, resulting in decreased fluid and electrolyte absorption
- Malabsorption of Ca^{++}, Mg^{++}, and Zn^{++} because of formation of insoluble "soaps" with malabsorbed free fatty acids
- Increased risk of oxalate stones because of increased colonic absorption of oxalate, which normally binds to Ca^{++}, Zn^{++}, and Mg^{++}

that occurs only with severe SBS and remaining colon. The problem results from overfeeding and malabsorption of significant amounts of carbohydrate. Metabolic acidosis and production of D-lactate result from fermentation of carbohydrate, production of short-chain fatty acids, reduced colonic pH, and proliferation of acid-resistant colonic microbes that produce D-lactate (Bongaerts et al., 1997). The problem is resolved by treating the metabolic acidosis and reducing the intake of refined carbohydrates.

Medical and Surgical Management

Medications are prescribed to retard gastric emptying, decrease secretions, slow GI motility, and treat bacterial overgrowth. Recently, somatostatin and somatostatin analogues and other hormones with antisecretory, antimotility, or trophic actions have been used to retard both motility and secretions (Farthing, 1996; Ziegler et al., 1996). Surgical procedures, including reversal of segments of bowel to slow transit of GI contents, creation of reservoirs ("pouches") to serve as a form of colon, intestinal lengthening, and intestinal transplant, have been performed to help patients with major GI resections (Figueroa-Colon et al., 1996; Kurlberg et al., 1997).

Nutritional Care

Most patients who have significant bowel resections require TPN initially to restore and maintain nutritional status. The duration of TPN and subsequent nutrition therapy is based on the extent of the bowel resection, the health of the patient, and the condition of the remaining GI tract. In general, older patients with major ileal resections, patients who have lost the ileocecal valve, and patients with residual disease in the remaining GI tract fare less well. Some may require lifetime supplementation with parenteral nutrition to maintain adequate fluid and nutritional status.

The two general principles for resuming enteral nutrition after small-bowel resections are (1) to start enteral feedings early, and (2) to increase feeding concentration and volume gradually over time. The more severe the problem, the slower the progression. Small, frequent, mini-meals (6 to 10 per day) are likely to be better tolerated than larger feedings. If enteral feedings are used, continuous, dilute feedings may be better tolerated than bolus feedings with standard concentrations. Because of malnutrition and disuse of the GI tract, the digestive and absorptive function of the remaining GI tract may be compromised. The transition to more normal foods may take weeks to months, and some patients may never tolerate normal concentrations or volumes of foods (Lykins and Stockwell, 1998).

Maximal adaptation of the GI tract may take up to a year after surgery. Adaptation improves function, but does not restore normal length or capacity. Whole foods are some of the most important stimuli to the GI tract, but other nutritional measures have been considered as means of hastening the adaptive process and decreasing malabsorption. Glutamine, for example, is the preferred fuel for small intestinal enterocytes and so may be valuable in enhancing adaptation. Nucleotides may also enhance mucosal adaptation; unfortunately, they are often lacking in parenteral and enteral nutritional products. Short-chain fatty acids (e.g., butyrate, propprionate, and acetate), produced from microbial fermentation of carbohydrate and fibers, are major fuels of the colonic epithelium (Iijima et al., 1993; Reilly et al., 1995).

Patients with jejunal resections and an intact ileum and colon will likely adapt quickly to normal diets. A normal balance of protein, fat, and carbohydrate sources is satisfactory. Six small feedings, with avoidance of lactose, large amounts of concentrated sweets, and caffeine, may help to reduce the risk of bloating, abdominal pain, and diarrhea. Because the typical diet of Americans may be nutritionally lacking, and the utilization of some micronutrients may be marginal, patients should be advised that the quality of their diet is of utmost importance. A multivitamin-mineral supplement may be required to meet nutritional needs.

Patients with ileal resections require increased time and patience in the advancement from parenteral to enteral nutrition. Because of losses, fat-soluble vitamins, calcium, magnesium, and zinc may need to be supplemented. Dietary fat may need to be limited, especially in those with remaining colon. Small amounts at each feeding are more likely to be tolerated and absorbed. MCT products add to the caloric intake and serve as a vehicle for lipid-soluble nutrients. Boluses of MCT oil (e.g., taken as a medication in tablespoon amounts) may add to the patient's diarrhea, so it is best to divide the doses equally in feedings throughout the day. Fluid and electrolytes, especially sodium, should be provided frequently, again in small amounts at a time.

In patients with massive resections (e.g., when the duodenum and a few inches of jejunum are anastomosed to segments of colon), diet will only be able to provide a portion of the required nourishment. In some cases, overfeeding in an attempt to compensate for malabsorption results in further malabsorption, not only of ingested foods and liquids, but also of the increased amounts of fluids secreted in response to food ingestion. Patients with extremely short bowel are typically nutritionally dependent on large volumes of dilute parenteral solutions administered frequently. Small, frequent snacks provide some oral gratification for these patients, but only a fraction of their fluid and nutrient needs (Beyer and Frankenfield, 1987).

Blind Loop Syndrome (Bacterial Overgrowth)

Blind loop syndrome is a disorder characterized by bacterial overgrowth resulting from stasis of the intestinal tract as an outcome of obstructive disease, radiation enteritis, fistula formation, or surgical repair of the intestine. Bacteria deconjugate bile salts, which besides being cytotoxic in this form, are also less effective as micelle formers. Poor fat absorption and steatorrhea result. Carbohydrate malabsorption occurs because of injury to the brush border secondary to the toxic effects of the products of bacterial catabolism and consequent enzyme loss. The expanding numbers of bacteria use the available vitamin B_{12} for their own growth. Treatment is directed toward the removal of the blind loop or control of the bacterial growth with antibiotics. Use of a lactose-free diet, along with MCT and parenteral vitamin B_{12}, may also be useful.

Fistula Repair

A **fistula** is an abnormal passage between two internal organs, or from an internal organ to the surface of the body. Fistulas occur as a result of prenatal developmental error, trauma, or inflammatory or malignant disease processes. Fistulas of the intestinal tract can be serious threats to nutritional status because large amounts of fluid and electrolytes are lost, and malabsorption and infection can occur. Fluid and electrolyte balance must be restored; infection must be brought under control; and aggressive nutritional support is mandatory to permit spontaneous or surgical closure of the fistula and wound.

TPN or defined liquid formula diets have been used successfully in patients with fistulas (see Chapter 22). The success rate of either method depends on the location and the cause of the fistula, and the patient's overall condition.

Ileostomy or Colostomy

Patients with severe ulcerative colitis, Crohn's disease, colon cancer, or intestinal trauma frequently require the surgical creation of an opening from the body surface to the intestinal tract in order to permit defecation from the intact portion of the intestine. When the entire colon, rectum, and anus must be removed, an **ileostomy,** or opening into the ileum, is performed. If only the rectum and anus are removed, a **colostomy** can provide entrance to the colon. In some cases, a temporary opening may be made to allow surgery and healing of more distal parts of the intestinal tract.

The opening, or stoma, eventually shrinks to the size of a nickel. The output from the stoma depends on its location, as explained in Figure 31–8. The consistency of the stool from an ileostomy is liquid, whereas that from a colostomy ranges from mushy to fairly well formed. Stool from a colostomy on the left side of the colon is firmer than that from a colostomy on the right side. Odor is a major concern of the patient with an ileostomy or colostomy; however, an ileostomy stool usually has a weakly acidic odor that is not unpleasant.

Malodorous stool is usually caused by steatorrhea or bacteria acting on particular foodstuffs to produce odorous gas. Patients learn to observe their stools to determine which foods to eliminate, and this differs with individuals. Foods that tend to cause odor from a colostomy are corn, dried beans, onions, cabbage, highly spiced foods, fish, antibiotics, and some vitamin-mineral supplements. Persistent odor may be attributable to poor stoma hygiene or to an ileostomy complication that allows bacterial overgrowth in the ileum. Deodorants are available, and modern pouch appliances are odorproof. Gas production may cause the pouch to become tense and distended, and accidental dislodgment is likely. The nutritional recommendations for reducing flatulence, presented at the beginning of this chapter, may be helpful for patients with colostomies.

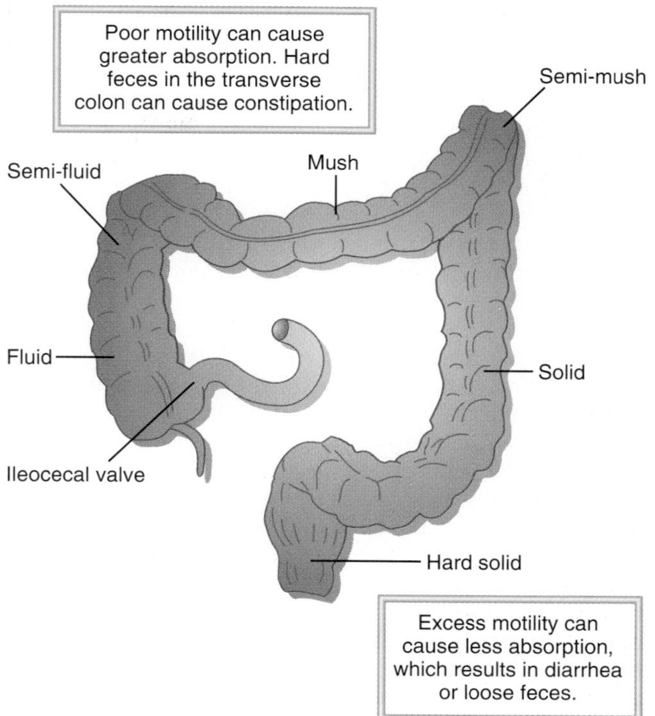

FIGURE 31–8 As the feces move from the ileocecal valve to the anus, water is absorbed and the feces become more solid. The characteristics of the output from a colostomy depend on its location in the colon.

Ileostomy adaptation does occur, in which case fecal losses will lessen and stools will become less liquid. This usually happens within 7 to 10 days. It does not happen to the same extent in patients who have had an ileal resection in addition to the ileostomy. Their ileal output will be about two to five times greater than that of the patient who has only an ileostomy. Patients with ileostomies have an above-average need for salt and water to compensate for excessive losses in stool. Inadequate water intake can result in small urine volumes and a predisposition for renal calculi. A normal diet provides adequate sodium, and the patient should be instructed to drink 2 q of water daily.

The patient with a normal, well-functioning ileostomy usually does not become nutritionally depleted. Surgical procedures, such as ileostomy, may require specific dietary changes, but no greater energy intake; caloric expenditures in these patients are similar to those of normal subjects. Vitamin E is among the antioxidant nutrients that inhibit lipoxidase enzymes and may play a role in attenuating disease activity (Coulston and Rock, 1993).

Those who also undergo resection of the terminal ileum need vitamin B_{12} supplementation. An imbalance in small bowel flora, with consequent vitamin B_{12} depletion, may occur. Patients with an ileostomy often have low vitamin C intakes because of low vegetable and fruit intakes, and so may require vitamin C supplementation. Ileostomates should be guided by their individual tolerance of foods, not by anecdotal reports.

Because it is possible for a food bolus to get caught at the point where the ileum narrows as it enters the abdominal wall, it is important to warn the patient to avoid very fibrous vegetables and to chew all food well. Other than this, patients with either an ileostomy or colostomy should be encouraged to follow their normal diet, omitting only those foods known to cause problems.

Patients with a permanent colostomy or ileostomy require considerable sympathetic understanding from the entire health care team. Acceptance of the condition and the problems involved in maintaining bowel regularity is usually difficult. Having these patients meet other people who have undergone similar surgery may help with the adjustment. Eventually, they may be encouraged by the realization that, in the future, they will not have the multiple hospitalizations or chronic disabilities that accompanied their intestinal disease.

Ileal Pouch After Colectomy

As an alternative to creation of an ileostomy for persons who have had their colons removed, surgeons can create a reservoir using a portion of the distal ileum, called an **ileal pouch.** Folds of the ileum are joined together to create a small pouch, which is then connected to the rectum and ileum. This is called an ileal pouch–anal anastomosis (IPAA). The most common pouch is the J pouch, but S and W pouches are sometimes created using additional folds of ileum (Pemberton and Phillips, 1988). Like the colon, the pouch develops a microflora capable of at least partially fermenting fiber and carbohydrate (Alles et al., 1997). Because the reservoir is smaller than the colon, bowel movements are likely to occur more frequently than normal, between 4 and 8 times daily. Vitamin B_{12} injections are usually required because, as in blind loop syndrome, the microbes may compete for and bind intraluminal vitamin B_{12}. Other problems commonly reported include obstruction, "pouchitis," increased stool output, frequency, and gas (Thompson-Fawcett et al., 1997; Pemberton and Phillips, 1998).

The incidence of obstruction may be lessened with attention to particle size of fibrous foods, chewing thoroughly, and consuming small meals frequently throughout the day. Stool frequency and volume do not return to normal, however. The normal, intact colon absorbs 80% to 90% of the liter or so of fluid entering from the ileum, leaving only 200 to 300 mL. After surgery, the remaining ileum does adapt to a small degree by increasing efficiency of fluid absorption, but even after adaption, fluid output is always in the range of 300 mL to 600 L. The same dietary measures that are used by others to reduce excessive stool output (reduced caffeine, lactose avoidance in lactose-intolerant individuals, avoidance of sorbitol, etc.) will likely reduce stool volume and frequency in persons with pouches. Adequate fluid and electrolyte intake is especially important because of the increase in intestinal losses.

Pouchitis, as implied by the name, is an inflammation of the mucosal tissue forming the pouch. The associated pathologic changes have been described as being somewhat similar to that of IBD (e.g., ulcerative colitis) (Goldstein et al., 1997). The cause of pouchitis is not entirely clear, but may be related to selected bacterial overgrowth, bile salt malabsorption, or insufficient short-chain fatty acid production. Antibiotics are the primary form of therapy, but experiments with different types of dietary fiber and other nutrient components are being investigated (Alles et al., 1997).

Rectal Surgery

Nutritional care after rectal surgery, such as hemorrhoidectomy, should be directed toward maintaining an intake that will allow wound repair and prevent infection of the wound by feces. The frequency of stools is minimized by the use of constipating drugs and a minimal-residue diet (see Table 31–2). Chemically defined diets are low in residue, and their use can reduce stool volume and frequency to as little as 50 g every 6 days, making the surgical construction of a temporary colostomy unnecessary.

CASE STUDY

Suzanne J. is a 33-year-old teacher with Crohn's disease who has been referred for evaluation because of abdominal pain, bloating, and occasional nausea and diarrhea. The physician suspects a distal small bowel stricture. The patient is seeking information on what to eat to prevent the problem from worsening during the 3-day period before her appointment at the clinic.

1. What information would be appropriate to gather about this patient before you advise her about a nutritional plan?
2. What, in terms of Mrs. J.'s symptoms, made the doctor suspect a stricture?
3. What kind of dietary advice, based solely on her presumed problem, might be warranted?

A normal diet is resumed after healing is complete, and the patient is instructed about the benefits of eating a high-fiber diet to avoid constipation in the future (see Table 31–1).

CITED REFERENCES

Aldoori WH, et al. A prospective study of diet and the risk of symptomatic diverticular disease in men. Am J Clin Nutr 60:757, 1994.

Alles MS, et al. Bacterial fermentation of fructooligosaccharides and resistant starch in patients with an ileal pouch-anal anastomosis. Am J Clin Nutr 66:1286, 1997.

Baer DJ, et al. Dietary fiber decreases the metabolizable energy content and nutrient digestibility of mixed diets fed to humans. J Nutr 127:579, 1997.

Ballegaard M, et al. Self-reported food intolerance in chronic inflammatory bowel disease. Scand J Gastroenterol 32:569, 1997.

Belluzzi A, et al. Maintaining remission in Crohn's disease: A fat chance to please. N Engl J Med 334:1557, 1996.

Beyer PL. Short bowel syndrome. In: Skipper A (ed.). Dietitian's Handbook of Enteral and Parenteral Nutrition, 2nd ed. Rockville, MD: Aspen Publishers, 1998.

Beyer PL, Frankenfield DC. Enteral nutrition in extreme short bowel. Nutr Clin Pract 2:60, 1987.

Bischoff SC, et al. Prevalence of adverse reactions to food in patients with gastrointestinal disease. Allergy 51:811, 1996.

Bongaerts GP, et al. Role of bacteria in the pathogenesis of short bowel syndrome associated d-lactic acidemia. Microb Pathog 22:285, 1997.

Booth I. Dietary management of acute diarrhea in childhood. (Commentary). Lancet 341:966, 1993.

Braegger CP, MacDonald TT. The immunologic basis for celiac disease and related disorders. Semin Gastrointest Dis 7:124, 1996.

Branski D, et al. Chronic diarrhea and malabsorption. Pediatr Clin North Am 43:307, 1996.

Brown SR, et al. Effect of coffee on distal colon function. Gut 31:450, 1990.

Calcium and the colon: Recent findings. Nutr Rev 57:124, 1999.

Caspary WF. Physiology and pathophysiology of intestinal absorption. Am J Clin Nutr 55:299S, 1992.

Catassi C, et al. Celiac disease in the general population: Should we treat asymptomatic cases? J Ped Gastroenteral Nutr 24:S10, 1997.

Chartrand LJ, Seidman G. Celiac disease is a lifelong disorder. Clin Invest Med 19:357, 1996.

Coulston A, Rock C. A Summary of the Current State of Knowledge in Clinical Nutrition and Dietetic Practice: Suggestions for Future Research in Dietetic Practice and Implications for Health Care. Chicago: The American Dietetic Association, 1993.

Craig GB, et al. Decreased fat and nitrogen losses in patients with AIDS receiving medium-chain-triglyceride-enriched formula vs those receiving long-chain-triglyceride-containing formula. J Am Diet Assoc 97:605, 1997.

Craig WJ. Phytochemicals: Guardians of our health. J Am Diet Assoc (suppl 2): S199, 1997.

Cummings JH, Englyst HN. Gastrointestinal effects of food carbohydrate. Am J Clin Nutr 61:938S, 1995.

Davenport HW. Absorption and excretion by the colon. In: Davenport HW. Physiology of the Digestive Tract, 5th ed. Chicago: Year Book Medical Publishers, 1982.

Deckman R, Cheskin L. Diverticular disease in the elderly. J Am Geriatr Soc 40:986, 1993.

Devroede G. Constipation: Mechanisms and management. In: Sleisenger MH, Fordtran JS (eds.). Gastrointestinal Disease: Pathophysiology, Diagnosis, Management, 4th ed. Philadelphia: WB Saunders, 1989.

Drossman DA, et al. Irritable bowel syndrome: A technical review for practice guideline development. Gastroenterology 112:2120, 1997.

Eastwood GL. A review of gastrointestinal epithelial renewal and its relevance to the development of adenocarcinomas of the gastrointestinal tract. J Clin Gastroenterol 21 (suppl 1):S1, 1995.

Eastwood MA, Morris ER. Physical properties of dietary fiber that influence physiological function: A model for polymers along the gastrointestinal tract. Am J Clin Nutr 55:436, 1992.

Farthing MJ. The role of somatostatin analogues in the treatment of refractory diarrhea. Digestion 57 (suppl 1):107, 1996.

Farthing MJG. Tropical malabsorption and tropical diarrhea. In: Feldman M, Sleisenger MH, Scharschmidt BF (eds.). Gastrointestinal and Liver Disease, 6th ed. Philadelphia: WB Saunders, 1998.

Figueroa-Colon R, et al. Impact of intestinal lengthening on the nutritional outcome for children with short bowel syndrome. J Pediatr Surg 31:912, 1996.

Fine KD. Diarrhea. In: Feldman M, Sleisenger MH, Scharschmidt BF. Gastrointestinal and Liver Disease, 6th ed. Philadelphia: WB Saunders, 1998.

Flourie B, et al. Can diarrhea induced by lactulose be reduced by prolonged ingestion of lactulose? Am J Clin Nutr 58:369, 1993.

Francis C, Whorwell P. Bran and irritable bowel syndrome: Time for reappraisal. Lancet 344:39, 1994.

Friedman G. Diet and the irritable bowel syndrome. Gastroenterol Clin North Am 20:313, 1991.

Giovannucci E, Goldin B. The role of fat, fatty acids, and total energy intake in the etiology of human colon cancer. Am J Clin Nutr 66:1564S, 1997.

Glotzer DJ. Surgical therapy for Crohn's disease. Gastroenterol Clin North Am 24:577, 1995.

Goepp J, Katz S. Oral rehydration therapy. Am Fam Phys 47:843, 1993.

Goldstein NS, et al. Crohn's like complications in patients with ulcerative colitis after total proctocolectomy and ileal pouch–anal anastomosis. Am J Surg Pathol 21:1343, 1997.

Gracey MS. Nutrition, bacteria and the gut. Br Med Bull 37:71, 1981.

Gray G. Intestinal lactase: What defines the decline? (Editorial). Gastroenterology 105:931, 1993.

Gudmand-Hoyer E. The clinical significance of disaccharide maldigestion. Am J Clin Nutr 59 (suppl):735, 1994.

Hardman CM, et al. Absence of toxicity of oats in patients with dermatitis herpetiformis. N Engl J Med 337:1884, 1997.

Hyams JS. Crohn's disease in children. Pediatr Clin North Am 43:255, 1996.

Hyams JS. Sorbitol intolerance: An unappreciated cause of functional gastrointestinal complaints. Gastroenterology 84:30, 1983.

Hyams JS, et al. Carbohydrate malabsorption following fruit juice ingestion in young children. Pediatrics 82:64, 1988.

Jewell DP. Ulcerative colitis. In: Feldman M, Sleisenger MH, Scharschmidt BF (eds.). Gastrointestinal and Liver Disease, 6th ed. Philadelphia: WB Saunders, 1998.

Johnson A, et al. Adaptation of lactose maldigesters to continued milk intakes. Am J Clin Nutr 58:879, 1993.

Kelly DG, Fleming CR. Nutritional considerations in inflammatory bowel diseases. Gastroenterol Clin North Am 24:597, 1995.

Kelsay J. Effects of fiber, phytic acid and oxalic acid in the diet on mineral bioavailability. Am J Gastroenterol 82:983, 1987.

Kemppainen TA, et al. Nutritional status of newly diagnosed celiac disease patients before and after the institution of a celiac disease diet—Association with the grade of mucosal villous atrophy. Am J Clin Nutr 67:482, 1998.

Kirschner BS. Ulcerative colitis in children. Pediatr Clin North Am 43:235, 1996.

Kornbluth A, et al. Crohn's disease. In: Feldman M, Sleisenger MH, Scharschmidt BF (eds.). Gastrointestinal and Liver Disease, 6th ed. Philadelphia: WB Saunders, 1998.

Kurlberg G, et al. Integrated intestinal capacity and nutritional status following small bowel transplantation. Transplant Int 10:386, 1997.

Kushner RF, Schoeller DA. Resting and total energy expenditure in patients with inflammatory bowel disease. Am J Clin Nutr 53:161, 1991.

Landis SH, et al. Cancer statistics, 1998. CA 48:6, 1998.

Levitt MD, et al. The relation of passage of gas and abdominal bloating to colonic gas production. Ann Intern Med 124:422, 1996.

Lindor KD, et al. A randomized prospective trial comparing a defined formula diet, corticosteroids, and a defined formula diet plus corticosteroids in active Crohn's disease. Mayo Clin Proc 67:328, 1992.

Lykins TC, Stockwell J. Comprehensive modified diet simplifies nutrition management of adults with short-bowel syndrome. J Am Diet Assoc 98:309, 1998.

MacDermott RP. Alterations of the mucosal immune system in inflammatory bowel disease. Gastroenterology 31:907, 1996.

Malnick SDH, et al. Celiac disease: Diagnostic clues to unmask an impostor. Postgrad Med 101:236, 1997.

Marsh M. Gluten sensitivity and latency: Can patterns of intestinal antibody secretion define the great "silent majority." Gastroenterology 104:1550, 1993.

McClung H, et al. Is combination therapy for encopresis nutritionally safe? Pediatrics 91:591, 1993.

Messori A, et al. Defined-formula diets versus steroids in the treatment of active Crohn's disease: A meta-analysis. Scand J Gastroenterol 31:267, 1996.

Meyers A. Oral rehydration therapy: What are we waiting for? (Editorial). Am Fam Phys 47:740, 1993.

Miner PB. Factors influencing the relapse of patients with inflammatory bowel disease. Am J Gastroenterol 92:1S, 1997.

Montes R, Perman J. Lactose intolerance: Pinpointing the source of nonspecific gastrointestinal symptoms. Postgrad Med 89:175, 1989.

Mortensen PB, Clausen MR. SCFA in the human colon. Scand J Gastroenterol (suppl)216:132, 1996.

Mowat AM, Viney JL. The anatomical basis of intestinal immunity. Immunol Rev 156:145, 1997.

O'Keefe SJ. Nutrition and gastrointestinal disease. Scand J Gastroenterol (suppl)220:52, 1996.

Olden KW, Schuster MM. Irritable bowel syndrome. In: Feldman M, Sleisenger MH, Scharschmidt BF (eds.). Gastrointestinal and Liver Disease, 6th ed. Philadelphia: WB Saunders, 1998.

Parodi PW. Cows' milk fat components as potential anticarcinogenic agents. J Nutr 127:1055, 1997.

Patel HI, et al. Surgery for Crohn's disease in infants and children. J Pediatr Surg 32:1063, 1997.

Pearson M, et al. Food intolerance and Crohn's disease. Gut 34:783, 1993.

Pemberton CM, et al. Mayo Clinic Diet Manual: A Handbook of Dietary Practices, 6th ed. Philadelphia: BC Decker, 1988, p. 142.

Pemberton JH, Phillips SF. Ileostomy and its alternatives. In: Feldman M, Sleisenger MH, Scharschmidt BF (eds.). Gastrointestinal and Liver Disease, 6th ed. Philadelphia: WB Saunders, 1998.

Podolsky DK. Inflammatory bowel disease (First of 2 Pts.). N Engl J Med 325:928, 1991.

Potter J, et al. Colon cancer: A review of the epidemiology. Epidemiol Rev 15:499, 1993.

Ramirez F, et al. All lactase preparations are not the same: Results of a prospective, randomized placebo-controlled trial. Am J Gastroenterol 89:566, 1994.

Reif S, et al. Pre-illness dietary factors in inflammatory bowel disease. Gut 40:754, 1997.

Riby JE, et al. Fructose absorption. Am J Clin Nutr 58:748S, 1993.

Rumessen JJ, Gudmand-Hoyer E. Functional bowel disease: Malabsorption and abdominal distress after ingestion of fructose, sorbitol, and fructose-sorbitol mixtures. Gastroenterology 95:694, 1998.

Schmitz J. Is celiac disease a lifelong disorder? Clin Invest Med 19:352, 1996.

Shoda R, et al. Epidemiologic analysis of Crohn disease in Japan: Increased dietary intake of n-6 polyunsaturated fatty acids and animal protein relates to the increased incidence of Crohn disease in Japan. Am J Clin Nutr 63:741, 1996.

Simmang CL, Shires GT. Diverticular disease of the colon. In: Feldman M, Sleisenger MH, Scharschmidt BF (eds.). Gastrointestinal and Liver Disease, 6th ed. Philadelphia: WB Saunders, 1998.

Singer MV, et al. Action of ethanol and some alcoholic beverages on gastric acid secretion and release of gastric in humans. Gastroenterology 93:1247, 1987.

Singh J, et al. Dietary fat and colon cancer: Modulating effect of types of amount of dietary fat on ras-p21 function during promotion and progression stages of colon cancer. Cancer Res 57:253, 1997.

Sitrin MD. Nutrition support in inflammatory bowel disease. Nutr Clin Pract 7:53, 1992.

Snape W. Nutrition and colonic diverticular disease. Nutrition and the MD 20:1, 1994.

Steele G. Colorectal cancer. In: Murphy GP, Lawrence W, Lenhard RE. Clinical Oncology, 2nd ed. Atlanta: The American Cancer Society, 1995.

Strocchi A, Levitt MD. Intestinal gas. In: Feldman M, Sleisenger MH, Scharschmidt BF (eds.). Gastrointestinal and Liver Disease, 6th ed. Philadelphia: WB Saunders, 1998.

Suarez FL, et al. A comparison of symptoms after the consumption of milk or lactose-hydrolyzed milk by people with self-reported severe lactose intolerance. N Engl J Med 333:1, 1995.

Thompson-Fawcett MW, et al. Ileoanal reservoir dysfunction: A problem-solving approach. Br J Surg 84:1351, 1997.

Tramonte SM, et al. The treatment of chronic constipation in adults: A systematic review. J Gen Intern Med 12:15, 1997.

Troncone R, et al. Gluten-sensitive enteropathy. Pediatr Clin North Am 43:355, 1996.

van Dulleman H, et al. Mediators of mucosal inflammation: Implications for therapy. Scand J Gastroenterol (suppl)223:92, 1997.

van Hogezand RA, Verspaget HW. Selective immunomodulation in patients with inflammatory bowel disease—Future therapy on reality? Neth J Med 48:64, 1996.

van Poppel G, van-den Berg H. Vitamins and cancer. Cancer Lett 114:195, 1997.

Vanderhoof JA, Langnas AN. Short-bowel syndrome in children and adults. Gastroenterology 113:1767, 1997.

Wess L, et al. Collagen alternation in an animal model of colonic diverticulosis. Gut 38:701, 1996.

World Health Organization. World Health Organization Guidelines for Cholera Control. WHO/COD/Ser/80.4, Rev. 1, Geneva, 1986.

Yadrick MM, et al. Comparison of the effects of diets high and low in simple sugars on bowel function in healthy, lactose-tolerant men. J Am Diet Assoc 92:1121, 1992.

Ziegler TR, et al. Gut adaptation and the insulin-like growth factor system: Regulation by glutamine and IGF-I. Am J Physiol 271:G866, 1996.

ADDITIONAL REFERENCES

American College of Physicians. Clinical guideline: Part 1. Suggested technique for fecal occult blood testing and interpretation in colorectal cancer screening. Ann Intern Med 126:808, 1997.

American Gastroenterology Association. Medical position statement: Irritable bowel syndrome. Gastroenterology 112:2118, 1997.

Beyer P. Gastrointestinal disorders: Roles of nutrition and the dietetic practitioner. J Am Diet Assoc 98:272, 1998.

Carroccio A, et al. Role of pancreatic impairment in growth recovery during gluten-free diet in childhood celiac disease. Gastroenterology 112: 1839, 1997.

Catassi C, et al. Celiac disease in the general population: Should we treat asymptomatic cases? J Pediatr Gastroenterol Nutr 24:S10, 1997.

Cheskin L, et al. Gastrointestinal symptoms following consumption of olestera or regular triglyceride potato chips. JAMA 279:150, 1998.

Emery E, et al. Banana flakes control diarrhea in enterally fed patients. Nutr Clin Pract 12:72, 1997.

Ferzoco LB, et al. Acute diverticulitis. N Engl J Med 338:1521, 1998.

Fine K, et al. The prevalence and causes of chronic diarrhea in patients with celiac sprue treated with a gluten-free diet. Gastroenterology 112:1830, 1997.

Hartsell P, et al. Early postoperative feeding after elective colorectal surgery. Arch Surg 132:518, 1997.

Janatuinen EK, et al. A comparison of diets with and without oats in adults with celiac disease. N Engl J Med 333:1033, 1995.

Juckett G. Intestinal protozoa. Am Fam Phys 53:2507, 1996.

Kaufman S, et al. Influence of bacterial overgrowth and intestinal inflammation on duration of parenteral nutrition in children with short bowel syndrome. J Pediatr 131:356, 1997.

Mora S, et al. Reversal of low bone density with a gluten-free diet in children and adolescents with celiac disease. Am J Clin Nutr 67:477, 1998.

Shaker J, et al. Hypoglycemia and skeletal disease as presenting features of celiac disease. Arch Intern Med 157:1013, 1997.

Suarez F, Saviano D. Diet, genetics, and lactose intolerance. Food Technol 51:74, 1997.

Thompson T. Do oats belong in a gluten-free diet? J Am Diet Assoc 97:1413, 1997.

Westergaard H. Short bowel syndrome. In: Feldman M, Sleisenger MH, Scharschmidt BF (eds). Gastrointestinal and Liver Disease, 6th ed. Philadelphia: WB Saunders, 1998.

Wilmore DW, et al. Factors predicting a successful outcome after pharmacological bowel compensation. Ann Surg 226:288, 1997.

Wolfsdorf J, Crigler J. Cornstarch regimens for nocturnal treatment of young adults with type I glycogen storage disease. Am J Clin Nutr 65:1507, 1997.

CHAPTER 32

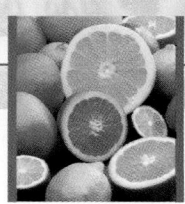

Medical Nutrition Therapy for Liver, Biliary System, and Exocrine Pancreas Disorders

JEANETTE M. HASSE, PhD, RD, FADA, CNSD AND LAURA E. MATARESE, MS, RD, FADA, CNSD

Chapter Outline

- Physiology and Functions of the Liver
- Diseases of the Liver
- Laboratory Assessment of Liver Function
- Manifestations and Complications of Cirrhosis
- Nutrition Management in Liver Disease
- Physiology and Functions of the Gallbladder
- Diseases of the Gallbladder
- Nutrition Management of Gallbladder Disorders
- Physiology and Function of the Exocrine Pancreas
- Diseases of the Exocrine Pancreas
- Nutrition Management in Pancreatic Disorders

Key Terms

ALCOHOLIC LIVER DISEASE—disease resulting from excessive alcohol ingestion characterized by fatty liver (hepatic steatosis), hepatitis, or cirrhosis

AROMATIC AMINO ACIDS—the amino acids phenylalanine, tryptophan, and tyrosine

ASCITES—accumulation of fluid, serum protein, and electrolytes within the peritoneal cavity caused by increased pressure from portal hypertension and decreased production of albumin (which maintains serum colloidal osmotic pressure)

BALLOON TAMPONADE—stoppage of blood flow by using pressure from an inflated tube or balloon

BILE—thick, viscid fluid secreted from the liver, stored in the gallbladder, and released into duodenum when fatty foods enter the duodenum; emulsifies fats in the intestine and forms compounds with fatty acids to facilitate their absorption

BRANCHED-CHAIN AMINO ACIDS—the amino acids valine, isoleucine, and leucine

CHOLANGITIS—infection in the bile ducts

CHOLECYSTECTOMY—removal of the gallbladder

CHOLECYSTITIS—inflammation of the gallbladder

CHOLEDOCHOLITHIASIS—presence of gallstones in the common bile duct

CHOLELITHIASIS—presence or formation of gallstones

CIRRHOSIS—chronic liver disease due to diffuse necrosis and regeneration leading to an increase in fibrous tissue formation disrupting the normal liver structure

ESLD—end-stage liver disease

FASTING HYPOGLYCEMIA—low blood glucose due to decreased availability of glucose from glycogen due to depressed liver function.

FATTY LIVER—a condition (hepatic steatosis) characterized by the accumulation of excess fat in the liver commonly caused by alcohol abuse, but also associated with obesity, starvation, intestinal bypass, parenteral alimentation, and diabetes mellitus

FULMINANT LIVER DISEASE—absence of preexisting liver disease with development of hepatic encephalopathy within 2 months of onset of illness

HEPATIC ENCEPHALOPATHY—a clinical syndrome developing in advanced liver disease, characterized by impaired mentation, neuromuscular disturbances, and altered consciousness; four stages of progression

HEPATIC FAILURE—condition in which liver function is diminished to 25% or less

HEPATIC STEATOSIS—fatty liver

HEPATITIS—widespread inflammation of the liver; usually viral in origin

HEPATITIS A—hepatitis caused by the hepatitis A virus that is transmitted by the fecal-oral route; recovery is usually complete, and long-term consequences are rare

HEPATITIS B—hepatitis caused by the hepatitis B virus transmitted primarily via blood and body fluids; can lead to chronic hepatitis and cirrhosis
HEPATITIS C—hepatitis caused by a blood-borne virus; transmission sources include infected needles, tainted blood products, sexual contact, or saliva; often leads to chronic hepatitis and cirrhosis
HEPATITIS D—hepatitis transmitted from intravenous or sexual sources; generally becomes chronic; dependent on hepatitis B virus for survival and propagation
HEPATITIS E—hepatitis from fecal-oral transmission, generally acute rather than chronic
HEPATOCYTE—liver cell
HEPATORENAL SYNDROME—functional renal failure without anatomic or histopathologic renal changes; associated with cirrhosis and ascites or with obstructive jaundice
JAUNDICE (ICTERUS)—a syndrome characterized by hyperbilirubinemia and deposition of bile pigment, resulting in yellowing of skin, mucous membranes, and sclera
KUPFFER CELLS—fixed phagocytes in the sinusoids of the liver
PANCREATITIS—inflammation of the pancreas caused by autodigestion of pancreatic tissue by its own enzymes
PANCREATICODUODENECTOMY (WHIPPLE PROCEDURE)—excision of the head of the pancreas along with the encircling loop of the duodenum; may include partial gastrectomy
PORTAL HYPERTENSION—abnormally increased blood pressure in the portal venous system due to the obstruction of blood flow through the liver
PORTAL SYSTEMIC ENCEPHALOPATHY—another term for hepatic encephalopathy
PRIMARY BILIARY CIRRHOSIS (PBC)—an immune-mediated chronic cirrhosis of the liver due to obstruction or infection of the small and intermediate-sized intrahepatic bile ducts while the extrahepatic biliary tree and larger intrahepatic ducts are normal; 90% of patients are women
SCLEROTHERAPY—injection of esophageal varices with a highly concentrated sclerosing agent with subsequent thrombosis, ulcer, and scar tissue formation
STEATORRHEA—presence of excess fat in the stool
VARICES—low pressure veins that become distended from increased pressure; most commonly developing in the lower esophagus and upper stomach
WERNICKE'S ENCEPHALOPATHY—condition of damage to the central nervous system from thiamin deficiency; common with alcoholism
WILSON'S DISEASE—autosomal recessive disorder of copper metabolism in which excessive accumulation of copper occurs in the liver, central nervous system, and kidney

PHYSIOLOGY AND FUNCTIONS OF THE LIVER

Structure

The liver is the largest gland in the body weighing approximately 1500 g. The liver has two main lobes—the right and left. The right lobe is further divided into the anterior and posterior segments; the right segmental fissure, which cannot be seen externally, separates the segments. The externally visible falciform ligament divides the left lobe into medial and lateral segments. The liver is supplied with blood from two sources; the hepatic artery supplies about one third of the blood from the aorta and the other two thirds enters from the portal vein, which collects blood drained from the digestive tract. Approximately 1500 mL blood per minute circulates through the liver and exits via the right and left hepatic veins into the inferior vena cava. Just as there is a system of blood vessels throughout the liver, there also exists a series of bile ducts within the liver. **Bile,** which is formed in the liver cells, exits the liver through a series of bile ducts that increase in size as they approach the common bile duct.

Functions

The liver has the ability to regenerate itself. Only 10% to 20% of functioning liver is required to sustain life, although removal of the liver will result in death within 24 hours. The liver is integral to most metabolic functions of the body and performs over 500 tasks. The main functions of the liver include metabolism of carbohydrate, protein, and fat; storage and activation of vitamins and minerals; bile formation and excretion; conversion of ammonia to urea; steroid metabolism; and action as a filter and flood chamber.

The liver plays a major role in carbohydrate metabolism. Galactose and fructose, products of carbohydrate digestion, are converted into glucose in the **hepatocyte** or liver cell. The liver stores glucose as glycogen (glycogenesis) and then returns it to the blood when glucose levels become low (glycogenolysis). The liver also produces "new" glucose (gluconeogenesis) from precursors such as lactic acid, glycogenic amino acids, and intermediates of the tricarboxylic acid cycle.

Important protein metabolic pathways occur in the liver. Transamination and oxidative deamination are two such pathways, which convert amino acids to substrates that are utilized in energy and glucose production, as well as in the synthesis of nonessential amino acids. Important serum proteins including albumin, α-globulin, β-globulin, transferrin, ceruloplasmin, and lipoproteins are formed by the liver as well as blood-clotting factors such as fibrinogen and prothrombin.

Fatty acids from the diet and adipose tissue are converted in the liver to acetyl-coenzyme A (CoA) by the process of β-oxidation to produce energy. Ketone bodies are also produced. The liver synthesizes and hydrolyzes triglycerides, phospholipids, cholesterol, and lipoproteins as well.

The liver is involved in the storage, activation, and transport of many vitamins and minerals. It stores all of the fat-soluble vitamins in addition to zinc, iron, copper, magnesium, and vitamin B_{12}. Hepatically synthesized proteins transport vitamin A, iron, zinc, and copper. Carotene is converted to vitamin A, folate to 5-methyl tetrahydrofolic acid, and vitamin D to its active form by the liver.

In addition to functions of nutrient metabolism and storage, the liver forms and excretes bile. Bile salts are metabolized and used for the digestion and absorption of fats and fat-soluble vitamins. Bilirubin is a metabolic end product from red blood cell destruction; it is conjugated and excreted in the bile.

Hepatocytes detoxify ammonia by converting it to urea, 75% of which is excreted by the kidneys. The remaining urea finds its way back to the gastrointestinal tract.

The liver also metabolizes steroids. It inactivates and excretes aldosterone, glucocorticoids, estrogen, progesterone, and testosterone. It is responsible for detoxification of substances including drugs and alcohol.

Finally, the liver acts as a filter and flood chamber by removing bacteria and debris from blood through the phagocytic action of **Kupffer cells** located in the sinusoids and by storing blood backed up from the vena cava as in right heart failure.

DISEASES OF THE LIVER

Diseases of the liver can be acute or chronic, inherited or acquired. Liver disease is classified in various ways: acute viral hepatitis, fulminant hepatitis, chronic hepatitis, alcoholic hepatitis and cirrhosis, cholestatic liver diseases, inherited disorders, and other liver diseases. Information is available at website www.liver.org.

Acute Viral Hepatitis

Acute viral **hepatitis** is a widespread inflammation of the liver and is caused by hepatitis viruses A, B, C, D, and E (Figs. 32–1B and 32–2B). Minor agents such as Epstein-Barr virus, cytomegalovirus, herpes simplex, yellow fever, and rubella can also cause an acute hepatitis syndrome.

Hepatitis A (HAV) is transmitted by the fecal-oral route and is contracted through contaminated drinking water, food, and sewage. Anorexia is the most frequent symptom and can be severe. Other common symptoms include nausea, vomiting, right upper quadrant abdominal pain, dark urine, and **jaundice.** Patients normally recover completely; however, serious complications may occur in high-risk patients. Subsequently, great attention must be given to adequate nutritional intake.

Hepatitis B (HBV) and **hepatitis C** (HCV) can lead to chronic and carrier states. HBV and HCV are transmitted via blood, blood products, semen, and saliva. For example, they can be spread from contaminated needles, blood transfusions, open cuts or wounds, splashes into the mouth or eyes, or sexual contact. Chronic active hepatitis can also develop into cirrhosis and liver failure.

The **hepatitis D** virus (HDV or Δ hepatitis) is dependent on the HBV for survival and propagation in humans. HDV may be a coinfection (occurring at the time as HBV) or a superinfection (superimposing itself on the HBV carrier state) (Seeff, 1996).

Hepatitis E virus (HEV) is rare in the United States but more frequently reported in many countries of southern, eastern, and central Asia; northern, eastern, and western Africa; and Mexico. HEV is transmitted via the oral-fecal route. Contaminated water appears to be the source of infection, which usually afflicts people living in crowded and unsanitary conditions.

The general symptoms of acute viral hepatitis are divided into four phases (Seeff, 1996). The first phase, the early *prodromal phase*, affects about 25% of patients, causing fever, arthralgia, arthritis, rash, and angioedema. This is followed by the *preicteric phase* in which malaise, fatigue, myalgia, anorexia, nausea, vomiting, dysgeusia (taste changes), and dysosmia (partial loss of speech) occur. Some patients complain of epigastric or right upper quadrant pain. The third phase is the *icteric phase* in which jaundice appears. Finally, during the *convalescent phase*, jaundice and other symptoms begin to subside. Complete recovery is expected in 95% of HAV cases, 90% of acute HBV cases, but only 15% to 30% of acute HCV cases (Seeff, 1996). Chronic hepatitis does not usually de-

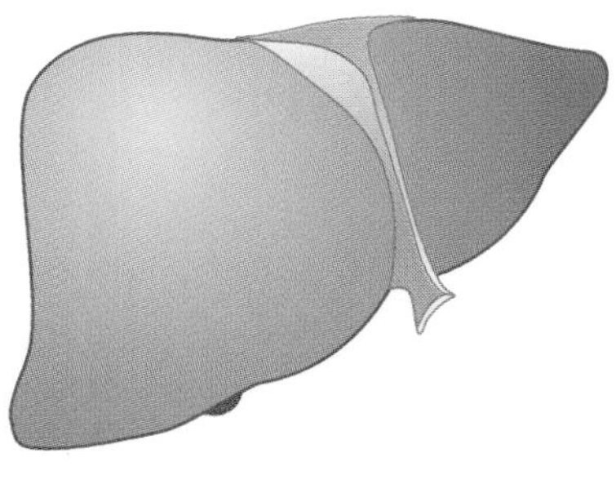

A Normal liver

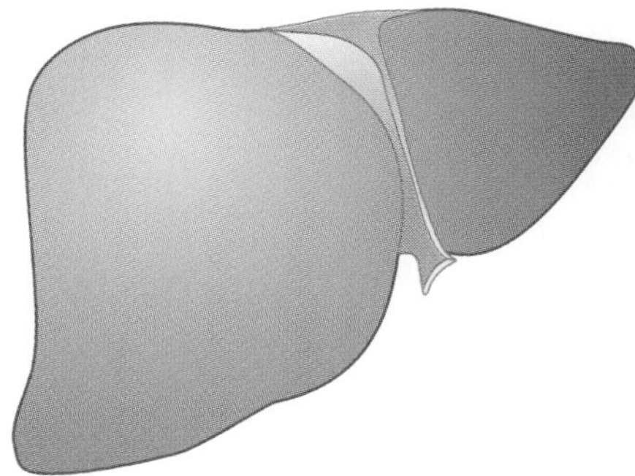

B Liver with viral hepatic damage

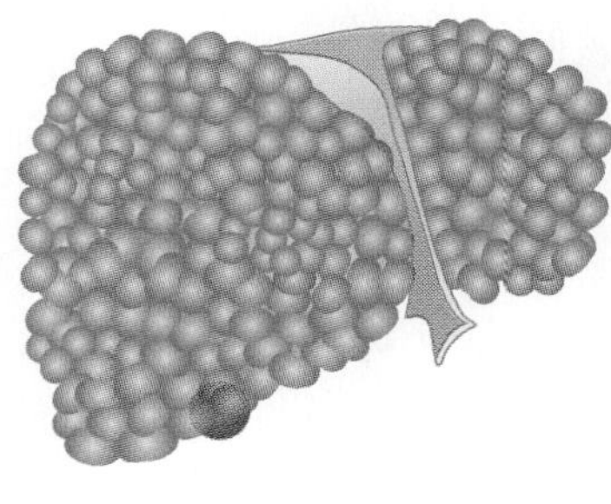

C Cirrhotic liver

FIGURE 32–1 Normal liver (*A*); liver with viral hepatic damage (*B*); and cirrhotic liver (*C*).

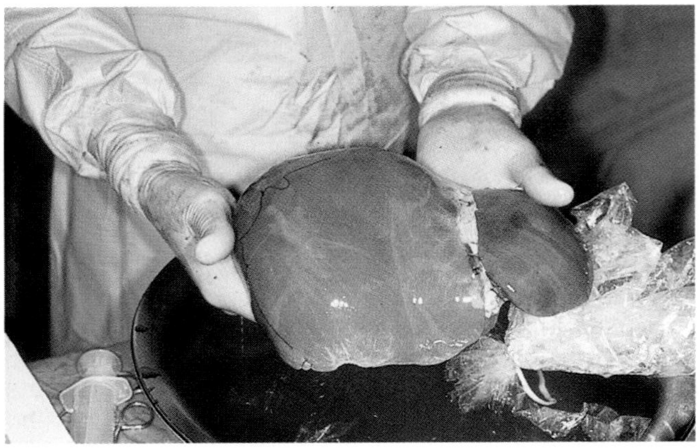

A

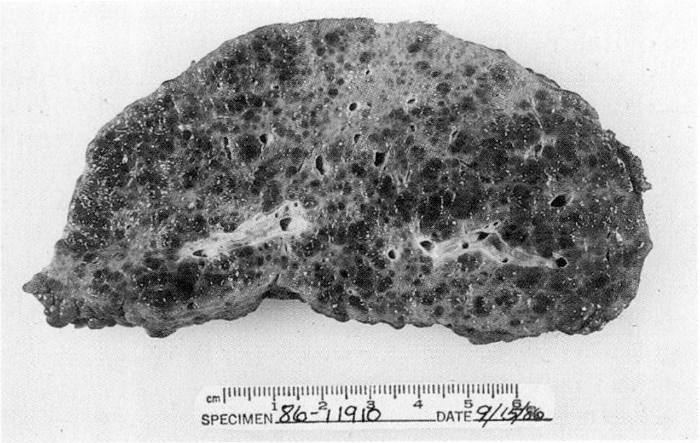

B

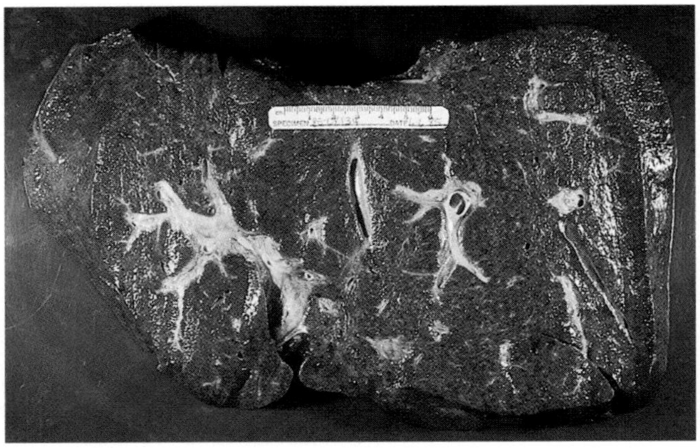

C

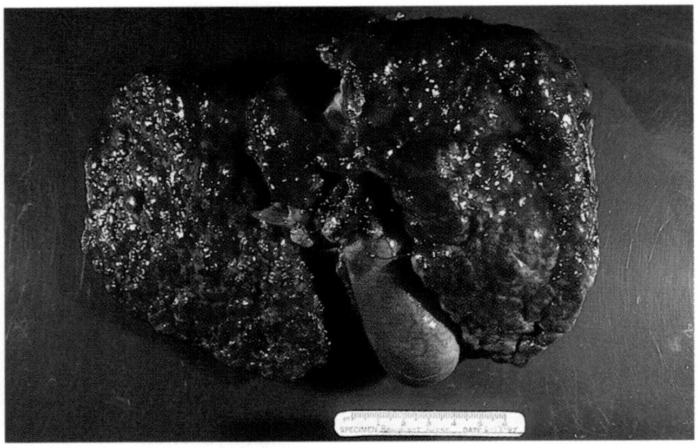

D

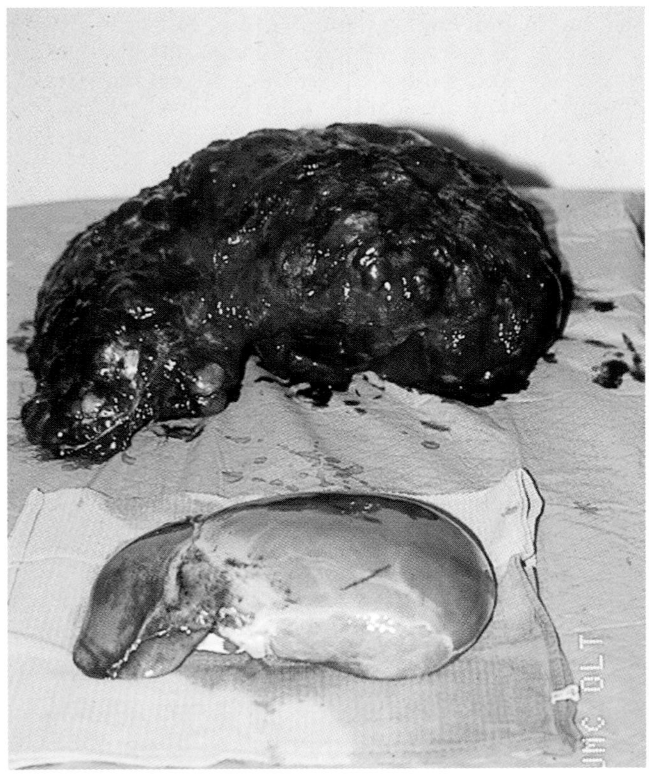

E

FIGURE 32–2 Normal liver (*A*); liver with damage from chronic active hepatitis (*B*); liver with damage from sclerosing cholangitis (*C*); liver with damage from primary biliary cirrhosis (*D*); liver with damage from polycystic liver disease (background); and normal liver (foreground) (*E*). (Reprinted with permission from Baylor Institute of Transplantation Sciences, Baylor University Medical Center, Dallas, TX.)

velop with HEV and symptoms and liver function tests usually normalize within 6 weeks (Ockner, 1996; Seeff, 1996).

Fulminant Hepatitis

Fulminant hepatitis is a syndrome in which severe liver dysfunction is accompanied by **hepatic encephalopathy. Fulminant liver disease** is defined by the absence of preexisting liver disease and the development of hepatic encephalopathy within 8 weeks of the onset of illness. The causes of fulminant hepatitis include viral hepatitis (approximately 75% of cases), chemical toxicity (e.g., acetaminophen, drug reactions, poisonous mushrooms, industrial poisons), and other causes such as Wilson's disease, fatty liver of pregnancy, Reye's syndrome, hepatic ischemia, hepatic vein obstruction, and disseminated malignancies. Extrahepatic complications of fulminant hepatitis are cerebral edema, coagulopathy and bleeding, cardiovascular abnormalities, renal failure, pulmonary complications, acid–base disturbances, electrolyte imbalances, sepsis, and pancreatitis (Douglas and Rakela, 1996).

Chronic Hepatitis

To be defined as chronic hepatitis, a patient must have at least a 6-month course of hepatitis or biochemical and clinical evidence of liver disease with confirmatory biopsy findings of unresolving hepatic inflammation (Davis, 1996).

Chronic hepatitis can have autoimmune, viral, metabolic, or toxic etiologies. Autoimmune hepatitis is diagnosed when other forms of liver disease caused by viruses, hepatotoxic agents, and metabolic diseases are excluded. The patient may exhibit serum antinuclear and smooth muscle antibodies, hypergammaglobulinemia, and other autoimmune disorders. This condition usually responds to corticosteroid administration.

Hepatic viruses, especially HCV, can also become chronic conditions. Metabolic diseases such as Wilson's disease, hemochromatosis, and α_1-antitrypsin deficiency can cause chronic hepatitis. Finally, some drugs such as α-methyldopa, nitrofurantoin, papaverine, dantrolene, clometacine, and ticrynafen can cause chronic hepatitis.

Alcoholic Hepatitis and Cirrhosis

Alcoholic liver disease is the most common liver disease in the United States and is the fourth leading cause of death among middle-aged Americans (Carithers, 1996). Acetaldehyde, a toxic by-product of alcohol metabolism, causes damage to mitochondrial membrane structure and function. Acetaldehyde is produced by multiple metabolic pathways, one of which involves alcohol dehydrogenase (see "*Focus On:* Metabolic Consequences of Alcohol Consumption"). Several variables may predispose some individuals to alcoholic liver disease. These include genetic polymorphisms of alcohol-metabolizing enzymes, gender (female more than male), coexposure to other drugs, infections with hepatotropic viruses, immunologic factors, and poor nutritional status (Diehl, 1996).

The pathogenesis of alcoholic liver disease progresses in three stages (Fig. 32–3): **hepatic steatosis, fatty liver,** (Fig. 32–4), alcoholic hepatitis, and **cirrhosis.** Fatty infiltration or hepatic steatosis is caused by a culmination of metabolic disturbances: (1) an increase in the mobilization of fatty acids from adipose tissue, (2) an increase in hepatic synthesis of fatty acids, (3) a decrease in fatty acid oxidation, (4) an increase in triglyceride production, and (5) a trapping of triglycerides in the liver. He-

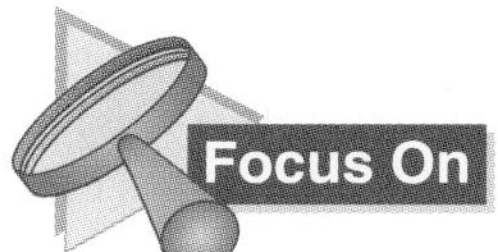

Metabolic Consequences of Alcohol Consumption

Ethanol is primarily metabolized in the liver by alcohol dehydrogenase (ADH). This results in acetaldehyde production with the transfer of hydrogen to nicotinamide adenine dinucleotide (NAD), reducing it to NADH. The acetaldehyde then loses hydrogen and is converted to acetate, most of which is released into the blood.

$$\underset{\text{ethanol}}{C_2H_2OH} + NAD \xrightarrow[\text{alcohol dehydrogenase}]{} NADH\ 1\ \underset{\text{acetaldehyde}}{CH_3\text{—}CHO}$$

$$\underset{\text{acetaldehyde}}{CH_3\text{-}CHO} + NADH + H_2O \xrightarrow[\text{alcohol dehydrogenase}]{} : NAD + H^+ + \underset{\text{acetate}}{CH_3\text{-}CHOOH}$$

Many metabolic disturbances occur because of the excess of NADH, which overrides the cell's ability to maintain a normal redox state. These include hyperlacticacidemia, acidosis, hyperuricemia, ketonemia, and hyperlipemia. The tricarboxylic acid (TCA) cycle is depressed because it requires NAD. The mitochondria, in turn, use hydrogen from ethanol, rather than from the oxidation of fatty acids, to produce energy via the TCA cycle. This leads to a decreased fatty acid oxidation and accumulation of triglycerides. In addition, NADH may actually promote fatty acid synthesis. Hypoglycemia can also occur in early alcoholic liver disease secondary to the suppression of the TCA cycle, coupled with decreased gluconeogenesis due to ethanol.

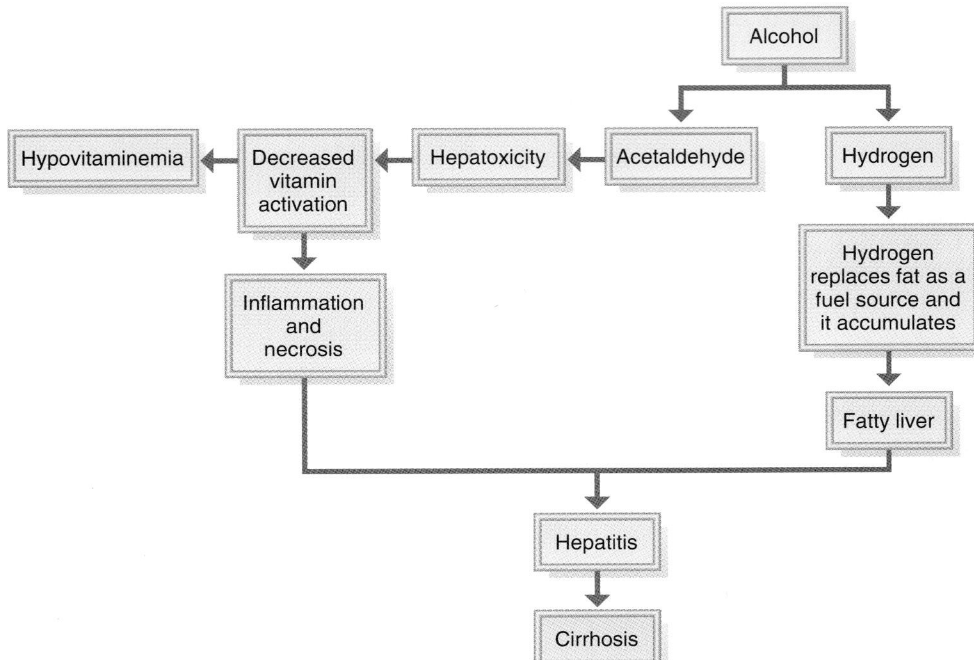

FIGURE 32–3 Complications of excessive alcohol consumption stem largely from excess hydrogen and from acetaldehyde. Hydrogen produces fatty liver and hyperlipemia, high blood lactic acid, and low blood sugar. The accumulation of fat, the effect of acetaldehyde on liver cells, and other factors as yet unknown lead to alcoholic hepatitis. The next step is cirrhosis. The consequent impairment of liver function disturbs blood chemistry, notably causing a high ammonia level that can lead to coma and death. Cirrhosis also distorts liver structure, inhibiting blood flow. High pressure in vessels supplying the liver may cause ruptured **varices** and accumulation of fluid in the abdominal cavity. There are individual differences in response to alcohol; in particular, not all heavy drinkers develop hepatitis and cirrhosis.

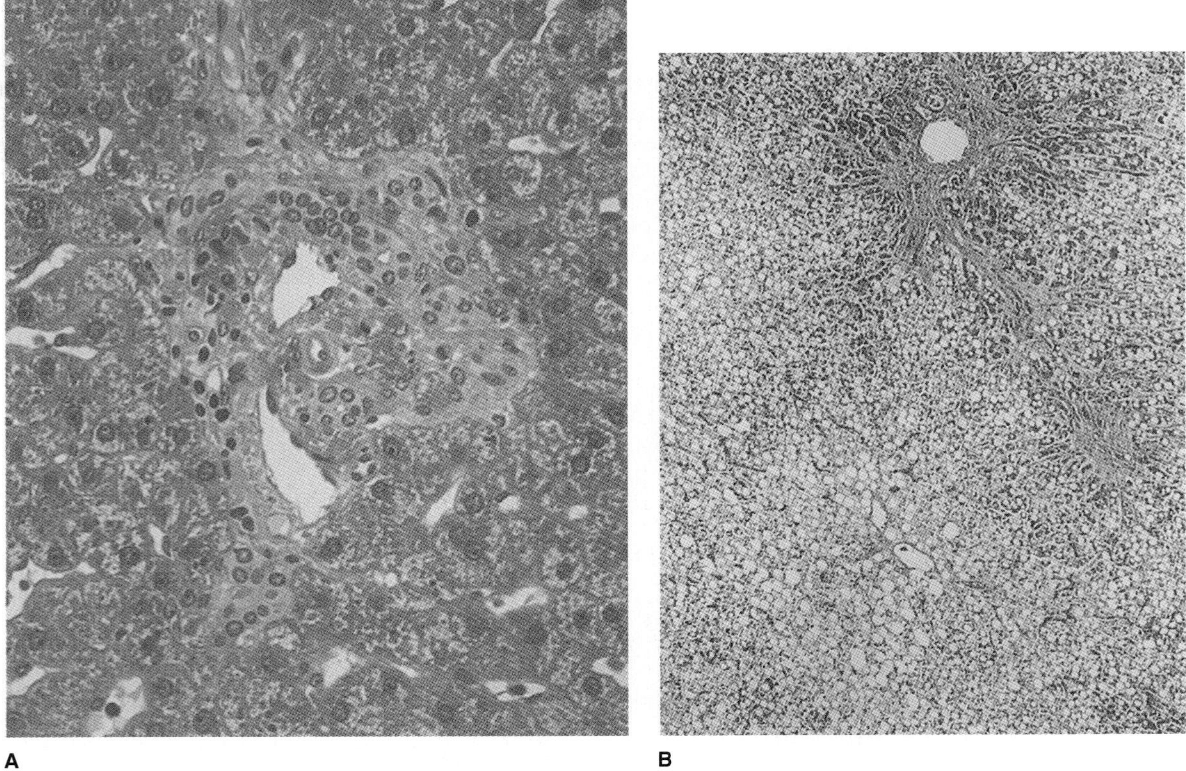

FIGURE 32–4 Microscopic appearance of (*A*) a normal liver. A normal portal tract consists of the portal vein, hepatic arteriole, one to two interlobular bile ducts, and occasional peripherally located ductules. (*B*) Acute fatty liver. This photomicrograph on low power exhibits fatty change involving virtually all the hepatocytes, with slight sparing of the liver cells immediately adjacent to the portal tract (top). (From Kanel G, Korula J. Atlas of Liver Pathology. Philadelphia: WB Saunders, 1992.)

patic steatosis is reversible with abstinence from alcohol. Conversely, if alcohol abuse continues, cirrhosis can develop.

Alcoholic hepatitis is characterized by hepatomegaly, modest elevation of transaminase levels, increased serum bilirubin concentrations, normal or depressed serum albumin concentrations, and possibly anemia and thrombocytopenia (Carithers, 1996). Patients may also have abdominal pain, anorexia, nausea, vomiting, weakness, diarrhea, weight loss, or fever. If patients discontinue alcohol intake, hepatitis may resolve. However, many individuals' condition will progress to the third stage.

Clinical features of the third stage of alcoholic cirrhosis vary. Symptoms can mimic those of alcoholic hepatitis or patients can develop **ascites,** gastrointestinal bleeding, **portal hypertension,** hepatic encephalopathy, and other symptoms of liver disease. A liver biopsy will usually reveal micronodular cirrhosis but it can be macronodular or mixed (Carithers, 1996). Prognosis depends on abstinence from alcohol and the degree of complications already developed. Ethanol ingestion creates specific and severe nutritional abnormalities (see "*Clinical Insight:* Malnutrition in the Alcoholic"). For more information, visit website www.niaaa.nih.gov.

Cholestatic Liver Diseases

Primary Biliary Cirrhosis

Primary biliary cirrhosis (PBC) is a chronic cholestatic disease caused by progressive destruction of small and intermediate-sized intrahepatic bile ducts. The extrahepatic biliary tree and larger intrahepatic ducts are normal. Ninety percent of patients with PBC are women and this disease progresses slowly eventually resulting in cirrhosis, portal hypertension, and liver transplantation or death. Primary biliary cirrhosis is an immune-mediated disease in which serum autoantibodies, elevated immunoglobulin levels, circulating immune complexes, and depressed cell-mediated immune response are present. Several nutrition complications from cholestasis can occur with PBC including osteopenia, hypercholesterolemia, and fat-soluble vitamin deficiencies (Friedman, 1996; Lindor and Dickson, 1996).

Sclerosing Cholangitis

Primary sclerosing **cholangitis** (PSC) is another chronic cholestatic liver disease. Fibrosing inflammation of segments of extrahepatic bile ducts, with or without involvement of intrahepatic ducts characterizes the disease. Progression of the disease leads to complications of portal hypertension, **hepatic failure,** and cholangiocarcinoma. Like PBC, PSC may be an immune disorder because of its strong association with human leukocyte antigen haplotypes, autoantibodies, and multiple immunologic abnormalities. Fifty to 75% of patients with PSC also have inflammatory bowel disease (especially ulcerative colitis) and 60% to 70% of individuals with PSC are men. Patients with PSC are also at increased risk of fat-soluble vitamin deficiencies and hepatic osteodystrophy due to **steatorrhea** associated with this disease (Vierling, 1996).

Inherited Disorders

Inherited disorders of the liver include hemochromatosis, Wilson's disease, α_1-antitrypsin deficiency, and others. *Hemochromatosis* is an inherited disease of iron overload. Patients with hereditary hemochromatosis may store 20 to 40 g iron compared with 0.3 to 0.8 g in normal individuals (see Chapter 35). Hepatomegaly, esophageal varices, ascites,

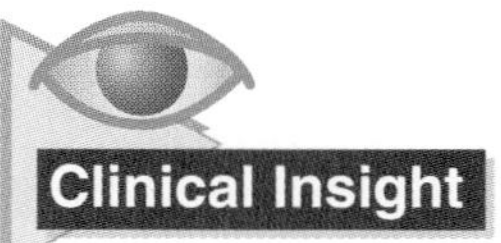

MALNUTRITION IN THE ALCOHOLIC

Several factors contribute to the malnutrition that is common in chronic alcoholics with liver disease.

1. Alcohol can replace food in the diet of moderate and heavy drinkers, displacing the intake of adequate calories and nutrients. In light drinkers it is usually an additional energy source (Lieber, 1988), also called "empty calories." Though alcohol yields 7.1 kcal/g, when it is consumed in large amounts it is not utilized efficiently as a fuel source (Mezey, 1991).

2. In the alcoholic, impaired digestion and absorption are related to pancreatic insufficiency, as well as deficiency of brush border enzymes such as lactase (Mezey, 1991). In particular, malabsorption of thiamin, vitamin B_{12}, folic acid, D-xylose, zinc, and amino acids has been found. Steatorrhea due to bile acid deficiency is also common in alcoholic liver disease. Ethanol itself has a direct effect on digestion and absorption, which is reversed by discontinuation of ethanol intake.

3. Metabolism is altered in alcoholic liver disease. Micronutrients affected include folate, thiamin, pyridoxine, vitamin A, vitamin D, zinc, and selenium (McClain et al., 1991; Mezey, 1991). For example, ethanol metabolites can cause increased degradation of the active form of pyridoxine or interfere with the formation and release of the active form of folate. Wernicke-Korsakoff syndrome from thiamin deficiency is common and is related to deranged metabolism. Magnesium and phosphorus can also be added to the list of micronutrients found to be deficient in alcoholics (Shronts and Fish, 1993).

TABLE 32–1 COMMON LIVER FUNCTION TESTS

LABORATORY TEST	COMMENT
Hepatic Excretion	
• Total serum bilirubin	• When increased, may indicate bilirubin overproduction or defect in hepatic uptake or conjugation
• Indirect serum bilirubin	• Unconjugated bilirubin; increased with excessive bilirubin production (hemolysis), immaturity of enzyme systems, inherited defects, and drug effects
• Direct serum bilirubin	• Conjugated bilirubin; increased with depressed bilirubin excretion, hepatobiliary disease, intrahepatic or extrahepatic cholestasis, benign postoperative jaundice and sepsis, and congenital conjugated hyperbilirubinemia
• Urine bilirubin	• More sensitive than total serum bilirubin; confirms if liver disease is the cause of jaundice
• Urine urobilinogen	• Used when obstructive jaundice is expected; rarely used
• Serum bile acids	• Reflects efficacy of ileal reabsorption and hepatic extraction of bile acids from portal circulation; levels increase with liver disease; little clinical utility
Cholestasis Tests	
• Serum alkaline phosphatase	• Enzyme widely distributed in liver, bone, placenta, intestine, kidney and leukocytes; mainly bound to canalicular membranes in liver; increased levels suggest cholestasis, but can be increased with bone disorders, pregnancy, normal growth, and some malignancies
• 5′-nucleotidase (5′ NT)	• Enzyme present in canalicular and plasma membranes of hepatocytes; also in heart and pancreas; increased with liver disease
• Leucine aminopeptidase (LAP)	• Cellular peptidase; usually increased in cholestasis and suggests hepatobiliary origin of elevation of alkaline phosphatase; may also increase with pregnancy
• γ-Glutamyl transpeptidase (GGT)	• Enzyme associated with microsomes and plasma membranes in hepatocytes; also present in kidney, pancreas, heart, and brain; increased with liver disease but also after myocardial infarction, in neuromuscular disease, pancreatic disease, pulmonary disease, diabetes mellitus, and during alcohol ingestion
Hepatic Enzymes	
• Alanine aminotransferase (ALT, formerly SGPT)	• Located in cytosol of hepatocyte; found in several other body tissues but highest in the liver; increased with liver cell damage
• Aspartate aminotransferase (AST, formerly SGOT)	• Located in cytosol and mitochondria of hepatocyte; also in cardiac and skeletal muscle, brain, pancreas, kidney, and leukocytes; increased with liver cell damage
• Serum lactic dehydrogenase (LDH)	• Located in liver, red blood cells, cardiac muscle, kidney; increased with liver disease but lacks sensitivity and specificity because it is found in most other body tissues
Serum Proteins	
• Prothrombin time (PT)	• Most blood coagulation factors are synthesized in the liver; vitamin K deficiency and decreased synthesis of clotting factors increase prothrombin time and risk of bleeding
• Partial thromboplastin time (PTT)	• Assesses the "intrinsic" clotting mechanism; reflects activity of all clotting factors except platelet factor e, factors VII and XII; complementary to PT
• Serum albumin	• Main export protein synthesized in the liver and most important factor in maintaining plasma oncotic pressure; decreased synthesis occurs with liver dysfunction; synthesis is influenced by thyroid and glucocorticoid hormones, plasma colloid osmotic pressure, and toxins; increased losses occur with protein-losing enteropathy, nephrotic syndrome, burns, gastrointestinal bleeding, exfoliative dermatitis
• Serum globulin	• α_1- and α_2-globulins are synthesized in the liver; increased with chronic liver disease; limited diagnostic use in hepatobiliary disease
• Mitochondrial antibody	• 90% of patients with PBC have antibodies in their serum against a lipoprotein component of the inner mitochondrial membrane; also present in 25% of patients with chronic active hepatitis and postnecrotic cirrhosis
• Antinuclear and smooth muscle antibodies	• May be present in patients with chronic active hepatitis (usually not associated with HBV or HCV) and in a minority of patients with PBC; not organ or species specific
Markers of Specific Liver Diseases	
• Serum ferritin	• Major iron storage protein; increased level is a sensitive indicator of genetic hemochromatosis
• Ceruloplasmin	• Major copper-binding protein synthesized by the liver; decreased in Wilson's disease
• α-Fetoprotein	• Major circulating plasma protein; increased with hepatocellular carcinoma
• α_1-Antitrypsin	• Main function is to inhibit serum trypsin activity; decreased in α_1-antitrypsin deficiency, which can cause liver and lung damage
Specific Tests for Viral Hepatitis	
• IgM anti-HAV	• Marker for hepatitis A; indicates current or recent infection or convalescence
• IgG anti-HAV	• Marker for hepatitis A; indicates current or previous infection and immunity
• HBsAg	• Marker for hepatitis B; positive in most cases of acute or chronic infection
• HBeAg	• Marker for hepatitis B; transiently positive during active virus replication; reflects concentration and infectivity of virus
• IgM or IgG Anti-HBc	• Marker for hepatitis B; positive in all acute and chronic cases; positive in carriers; not protective
• Anti-HBe	• Marker for hepatitis B; transiently positive during convalescence and in some chronic cases and carriers; not protective; reflects low infectivity
• Anti-HBs	• Marker for hepatitis B; positive late in convalescence; protective
• Anti-HCV	• Marker for hepatitis C; positive 5–6 weeks after onset of HCV; not protective; reflects infectious state
• HCV-RNA	• Marker for hepatitis C

TABLE 32–1 COMMON LIVER FUNCTION TESTS (continued)

• IgM or IgG Anti-HDV	• Markers for hepatitis D; indicates infection; not protective
• IgM Anti-HEV	• Marker for hepatitis E; indicates current or recent infection; not protective
• IgG Anti-HEV	• Marker for hepatitis E; indicates current or previous infection and immunity
Miscellaneous Tests	
• Ammonia	• Liver converts ammonia to urea; may increase with hepatic failure and portal-systemic shunts

(Data from Baker AL. Liver chemistry tests. In: Kaplowitz N (ed.). Liver and biliary diseases, 2nd ed. Baltimore: Williams & Wilkins, 1996, p. 207; Kamath PS. Clinical approach to the patient with abnormal liver test results. Mayo Clin Proc 71:1089, 1996; Lindsay KL, Hoofnagle JH. Serologic tests for viral hepatitis. In: Kaplowitz N (ed.). Liver and biliary diseases, 2nd ed. Baltimore: Williams & Wilkins, 1996, p. 221; Ockner RK: Acute viral hepatitis. In: Bennett JC, Plum F (eds.). Cecil textbook of medicine, 20th ed. Philadelphia: WB Saunders, 1996, p. 762; Weisiger RA. Laboratory tests in liver disease. In: Bennett JC, Plum F (eds.). Cecil textbook of medicine, 29th ed. Philadelphia: WB Saunders, 1996, p. 759.)

impaired hepatic synthetic function, abnormal skin pigmentation, glucose intolerance, cardiac involvement, hypogonadism, arthropathy, and hepatocellular carcinoma may develop. If diagnosed early, phlebotomy will improve a patient's condition (Bacon and Brown, 1996).

Wilson's disease is an autosomal recessive disorder associated with impaired biliary copper excretion. Copper accumulates in various tissues including the liver, brain, cornea, and kidneys. Low serum ceruloplasmin levels and the presence of Kayser-Fleischer rings confirm the diagnosis, although patients with this disease may present before the development of these confirming symptoms (Maher, 1996). Patients can present with acute, fulminant, or chronic active hepatitis secondary to Wilson's disease. Often neurologic signs may be the first indication of illness (Sokol, 1996). Copper-chelating agents and possibly zinc supplementation (to inhibit intestinal copper absorption and binding in the liver) are used to treat Wilson's disease once diagnosed. A low-copper diet is implemented if other therapies are unsuccessful. If not diagnosed until onset of fulminant failure, survival is not possible without transplantation (Sokol, 1996).

α_1*-Antitrypsin deficiency* is another inherited disorder and can cause both liver and lung disease (Maher, 1996). α_1-Antitrypsin is a glycoprotein found in serum and body fluids and inhibits several proteolytic enzymes. Cholestasis or cirrhosis is caused by this deficiency (Whitington, 1996) and there is no treatment except liver transplantation.

Other Liver Diseases

There are several other causes of liver disease. Liver tumors can be primary or metastatic, benign or malignant (LaBreque, 1996). The liver can be affected in the presence of systemic diseases such as rheumatoid arthritis, systemic lupus erythematosus, polymyalgia, rheumatic/temporal arteritis, polyarteritis nodosa, systemic sclerosis, and Sjögren's syndrome (Bonaciní, 1996). Liver disease can also occur due to nonalcoholic steatohepatitis caused by obesity, diabetes mellitus, parenteral nutrition, and jejunoileal bypass. When hepatic blood flow is altered as in acute ischemic and chronic congestive hepatopathy, Budd-Chiari syndrome, and hepatic veno-occlusive disease, hepatic dysfunction occurs (Bacon et al., 1996). Parasitic, bacterial, fungal, and granulomatous liver diseases also occur. There are even liver diseases of pregnancy (Riely, 1996). Finally, *cryptogenic cirrhosis* is any cirrhosis for which the etiology is unknown.

LABORATORY ASSESSMENT OF LIVER FUNCTION

Biochemical laboratory markers are used to evaluate and monitor patients having or suspected of having liver disease. Enzyme assays measure the release of liver enzymes and other tests measure liver function. Table 32–1 summarizes common laboratory tests.

MANIFESTATIONS AND COMPLICATIONS OF CIRRHOSIS

Cirrhosis has many clinical manifestations as illustrated in Figure 32–5. Several major complications of **end-stage liver disease (ESLD)** have nutritional implications.

Portal Hypertension

Portal hypertension increases collateral blood flow and can result in varices in the gastrointestinal tract. These varices often bleed causing a medical emergency. Treatment includes administration of β-adrenergic blockers to decrease heart rate, endoscopic **sclerotherapy** or variceal ligation, and radiologic or surgical placement of shunts. During an acute bleeding episode, somatostatin analogue may be administered to decrease bleeding, or a nasogastric tube equipped with an inflatable **balloon** will be placed to **tamponade** bleeding vessels (Crippin, 1996).

During acute bleeding episodes, nutrition cannot be administered enterally. Repeated endoscopic therapies may cause esophageal strictures or impair a patient's swallowing. Finally, surgically or radiologically placed shunts may increase the incidence of encephalopathy and reduce nutrient metabolism because blood is shunted past the liver cells.

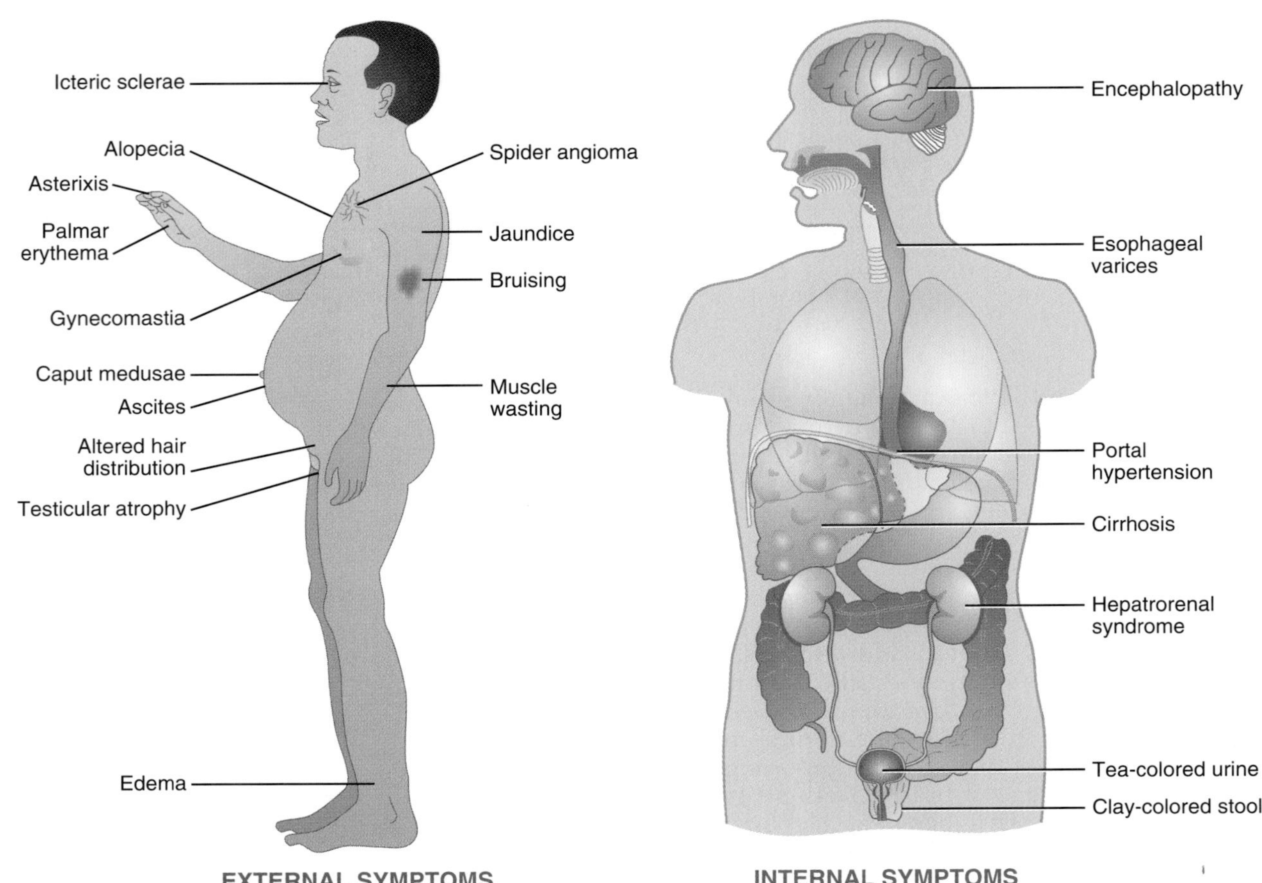

FIGURE 32–5 Clinical manifestations of cirrhosis.

Ascites

Ascites is the accumulation of fluid in the abdominal cavity due in part to portal hypertension. Sodium restriction is the primary therapy for ascites, but diuretic therapy is also used. Diuretics frequently alter electrolyte balance, which must be considered when providing nutrition. Large-volume paracentesis to relieve ascites impairs nutritional status by removing protein.

Hepatic Encephalopathy

Hepatic or **portal systemic encephalopathy** results in neuromuscular and behavior alterations. Table 32–2 describes the four stages of hepatic encephalopathy.

There are multiple precipitating causes of hepatic encephalopathy including gastrointestinal bleeding, fluid and electrolyte abnormalities, uremia, infection, use of sedatives, constipation, and alkalosis. Hepatic encephalopathy is precipitated by excessive dietary protein intake in approximately 7% to 9% of patients with liver failure (Leevy and Davison, 1967).

Just as there are multiple causes of hepatic encephalopathy, there are multiple theories as to the mechanism by which hepatic encephalopathy occurs. Ammonia is considered to be an important etiologic factor in the development of encephalopathy (Latifi et al., 1991). When the liver fails, it is unable to detoxify ammonia to urea, and ammonia is a direct cerebral toxin. Although serum and cerebrospinal fluid levels do not correlate well with the degree of hepatic encephalopathy, treatment is based on lowering these levels. Ammonia metabolites such as glutamine and α-ketoglutarate in cerebrospinal fluid have, however, correlated more closely with severity of encephalopathy. The main source of ammonia is the endogenous production by the gastrointestinal tract (i.e., from the degradation

TABLE 32–2 FOUR STAGES OF HEPATIC ENCEPHALOPATHY

STAGE	SYMPTOMS
I	Mild confusion, agitation, irritability, sleep disturbance, decreased attention
II	Lethargy, disorientation, inappropriate behavior, drowsiness
III	Somnolence but arousable, incomprehensible speech, confusion, aggression when awake
IV	Coma

of bacteria and blood from gastrointestinal bleeding). Therefore, drugs such as lactulose and neomycin are given. Lactulose is a nonabsorbable disaccharide. It acidifies colonic contents, retaining ammonia as the ammonium ion. It also acts as an osmotic laxative to remove the ammonia. Neomycin is a nonabsorbable antibiotic that helps decrease colonic ammonia production.

Exogenous protein is also a source of ammonia. Some clinicians suggest that dietary protein causes an increase in ammonia levels and subsequently hepatic encephalopathy, but this has not been proven in studies. One study even showed that patients with worsening hepatic encephalopathy often have decreased protein intakes and increased blood urea nitrogen and creatinine levels. Patients with improved encephalopathy had higher protein intakes and lower blood urea nitrogen and creatinine levels (Morgan et al., 1995).

Another major hypothesis for the pathogenesis of portal systemic encephalopathy has been termed the *altered neurotransmitter theory*. A plasma amino acid imbalance exists in **ESLD** in which **branched-chain amino acids** (BCAAs) are decreased and **aromatic amino acids** (AAAs) plus methionine, glutamine, asparagine, and histidine are increased (Table 32–3). The BCAAs furnish as much as 30% of energy requirements for skeletal muscle, heart, and brain when gluconeogenesis and ketogenesis are depressed (Latifi et al., 1991). This causes serum BCAA levels to fall. At the same time, plasma AAAs and methionine are released into circulation by muscle proteolysis but the synthesis into protein and liver clearance of AAAs is depressed (Hiyama and Fischer, 1988). This changes the plasma molar ratio of BCAA to AAA and may contribute to the development of hepatic encephalopathy; AAAs may limit the cerebral uptake of BCAAs because they compete for carrier-mediated transport at the blood–brain barrier (Latifi et al., 1991).

Studies evaluating the benefit of supplements enriched with BCAAs and restricted in AAAs have varied in study design, sample size, composition of BCAA-enriched formulas, level of encephalopathy, type of liver disease, duration of therapy, and control groups (Hasse et al., 1997). Even though it is difficult to compare the studies, most experts agree that BCAA-enriched formulas are indicated for patients with encephalopathy who do not tolerate standard proteins, and who have not responded to lactulose and neomycin therapy (Ichida et al., 1996; Mendenhall et al., 1993; Nompleggi and Bonkovsy, 1994; Plauth et al., 1997).

Other theories postulate that vegetable and casein protein-based diets may improve mental status compared with meat protein (Bianchi et al., 1993; Mullen and Weber, 1991). Casein-based diets are lower in AAAs and higher in BCAAs than meat-based diets. The potential advantage of vegetable protein is that it is low in methionine and ammonigenic amino acids as well as BCAA enriched. The high-fiber content of a vegetable–protein diet may also play a role in the excretion of nitrogenous compounds.

Several other substances have been implicated in the development of hepatic encephalopathy such as short-chain fatty acids, mercaptans, phenols, and γ-aminobutyric acid (Latifi et al., 1991). Another final dietary theory implicates zinc deficiency, types of fatty acids, or the amino acid tryptophan in the development of hepatic encephalopathy (Mullen and Weber, 1991).

TABLE 32–3 AMINO ACIDS COMMONLY ALTERED IN LIVER DISEASE

Aromatic amino acids—serum levels increased
Tyrosine
Phenylalanine*
Free tryptophan*
Branched-chain amino acids—serum levels decreased
Valine*
Leucine*
Isoleucine*
Other amino acids—serum levels increase
Methionine*
Glutamine
Asparagine
Histidine*

*Denotes essential amino acids.

Renal Insufficiency and Hepatorenal Syndrome

Acute renal failure can occur in patients with ESLD. If conservative therapies, including discontinuation of nephrotoxic drugs, optimization of intravascular volume status, and monitoring of fluid intake and output fail, dialysis may be required. In any case, renal insufficiency and failure necessitates alteration in fluid, sodium, potassium, and phosphorus intake.

Osteopenia

Osteopenia has been identified as a problem particularly in patients with primary biliary cirrhosis, sclerosing cholangitis, and alcoholic liver disease. Depressed osteoblastic function and osteoporosis also can occur in patients with hemochromatosis, and osteoporosis is prevalent in patients who have had long-term treatment with corticosteroids. Corticosteroids increase bone resorption and suppress osteoblastic function, and affect sex hormone secretion, intestinal absorption of dietary calcium, renal excretion of calcium and phosphorus, and the vitamin D system (Epstein et al., 1995; Katz and Epstein, 1992).

Prevention or treatment options for osteopenia include weight maintenance, ingestion of a well-balanced diet, adequate protein to maintain muscle mass, 1500 mg calcium per day, and adequate vitamin D from the diet or supplements, avoidance of alcohol, and monitoring for steatorrhea with diet adjustments as needed to minimize nutrient losses (Hasse et al., 1997).

NUTRITION MANAGEMENT IN LIVER DISEASE

The objectives of nutrition therapy are to (1) maintain or improve nutritional status or correct malnutrition; (2) prevent further liver cell injury and enhance regeneration; (3) prevent or alleviate hepatic encephalopathy and other metabolic disturbances amenable to nutrition therapy.

Malnutrition in Liver Disease

Moderate to severe malnutrition is a common finding in patients with advanced liver disease (Akerman et al., 1993 Caregaro et al., 1996; Pikul et al., 1993) (Fig. 32–6). This is extremely significant considering that malnutrition plays a major role in the pathogenesis of liver injury and has a profound negative impact on prognosis.

Numerous coexisting factors are involved in the development of malnutrition in liver disease (Fig. 32–7). Inadequate oral intake, a major contributor, is caused by anorexia, dysgeusia, early satiety, nausea, and vomiting associated with liver disease and the drugs used to treat it including diuretics, bile acid sequestrants, neomycin, and lactulose (Francisco-Ziller and DiCecco, 1997; Hasse et al., 1997). Other causes of inadequate intake are related to dietary restrictions and unpalatable hospital diets.

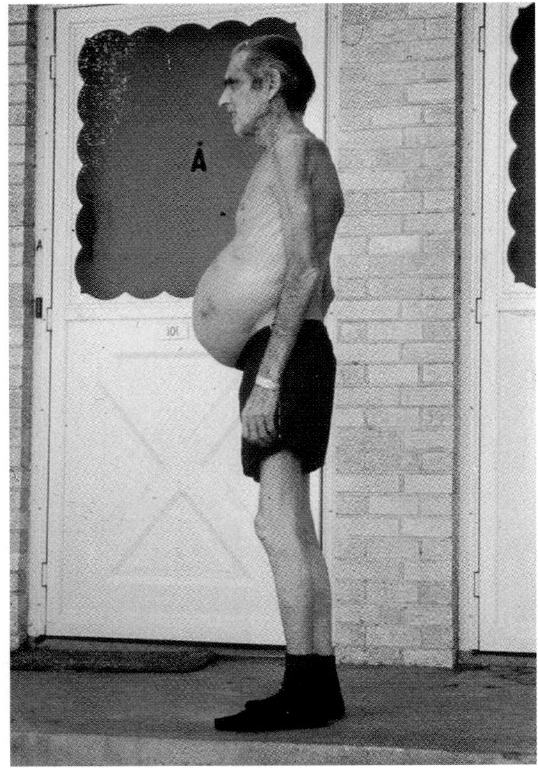

FIGURE 32–6 Severe malnutrition and ascites in a man with end-stage liver disease.

Maldigestion and malabsorption also play a role in the malnutrition of liver disease. Steatorrhea is common in cirrhosis, especially relating to diseases involving bile duct injury and obstruction. The medications previously mentioned may also cause specific malabsorptive losses. In addition, altered metabolism secondary to liver dysfunction causes malnutrition in various ways. Micronutrient function is affected by altered storage in the liver, decreased transport by liver-synthesized proteins, and renal losses associated with alcoholic and advanced liver disease. Abnormal macronutrient metabolism and increased energy expenditure can also contribute to malnutrition. Finally, protein losses can occur from large-volume paracentesis (Hasse et al., 1997).

Assessment of Nutritional Status

Objective Parameters

Many traditional markers of nutritional status are affected by liver disease and its consequences, making assessment very difficult. Table 32–4 summarizes factors that affect interpretation of nutritional assessment parameters in patients with liver dysfunction. Objective parameters that may be helpful when monitored serially include anthropometric measurements and dietary intake (Francisco-Ziller and DiCecco, 1997; Harrison et al., 1997; Plauth et al., 1997). The best way to perform a nutritional assessment may be to combine these parameters with the subjective global assessment approach.

Subjective Global Assessment

Subjective global assessment (SGA) has been used in liver disease and transplantation and has demonstrated an acceptable level of reliability and validity (Detsky et al., 1987; Hasse, 1993). This method uses a few readily available parameters obtained by an experienced clinician (see Chapter 16). The SGA gives a broad perspective but is not sensitive to changes in nutritional status. Other available parameters should also be reviewed for their impact on the patient's overall health status. The elements of SGA in evaluating nutritional status are summarized in Table 32–5.

Nutrition Therapy in Liver Disease

At least one study suggests that malnutrition in patients with cirrhosis is associated with liver function deterioration, but is not an independent risk factor for death (Merli et al., 1996). Other studies

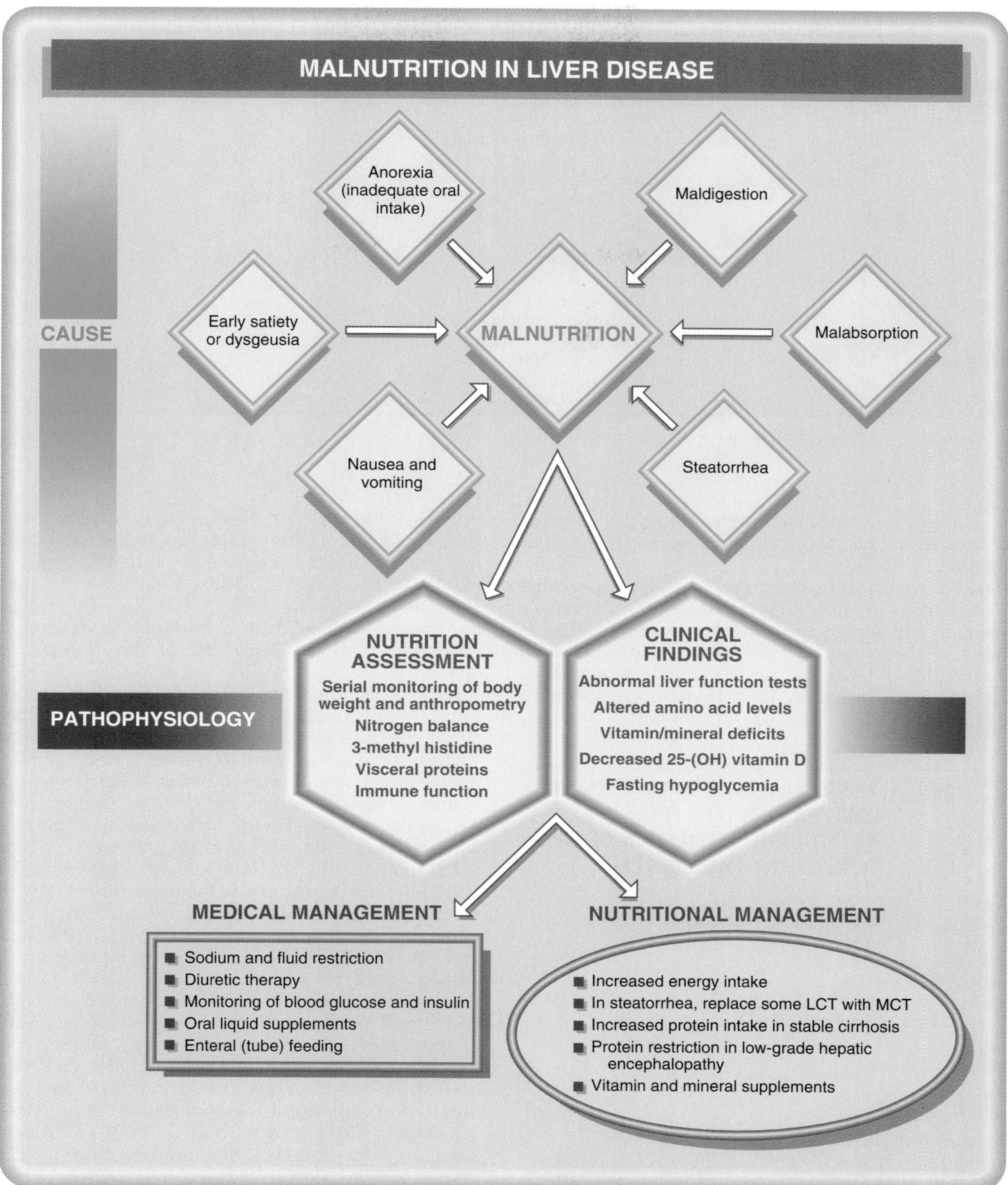

FIGURE 32–7 Pathophysiology algorithm—malnutrition in liver disease. (Algorithm content developed by John Anderson, Ph.D., and Sanford C. Garner, Ph.D., 2000.)

TABLE 32–4 FACTORS THAT AFFECT INTERPRETATION OF NUTRITION ASSESSMENT TESTS IN PATIENTS WITH END-STAGE LIVER DISEASE

PARAMETER	FACTORS AFFECTING INTERPRETATION
Body weight	• Affected by edema, ascites, and diuretic use.
Anthropometric measurements	• Questionable sensitivity, specificity, and reliability. • Multiple sources of error. • Question if skinfold measurements reflect total body fat. • References do not account for variation in hydration status and skin compressibility.
Creatinine–height index	• Affected by malnutrition, aging, decreased body mass, and protein intake. • Affected by renal function. • Creatinine is a metabolic end product of creatine, which is synthesized in the liver; therefore, severe liver disease alters creatinine synthesis rates.
Nitrogen balance studies	• Nitrogen is retained in the body in the form of ammonia. • Hepatorenal syndrome can affect the excretion of nitrogen.
3-Methyl histidine excretion	• Affected by dietary intake, trauma, infection, and kidney function.
Visceral protein levels	• Synthesis of visceral proteins is decreased. • Affected by hydration status, malabsorption, and kidney insufficiency.
Immune function tests	• Affected by liver failure, electrolyte imbalances, infection, and kidney insufficiency.

(Reprinted with permission from Hasse J. Nutritional aspects of adult liver transplantation. In: Busuttil RW, Klintmalm GB (eds.). Transplantation of the liver. Philadelphia: WB Saunders, 1996, p. 359.)

have associated increased mortality with moderate malnutrition and inadequate intake (Mendenhall et al., 1993).

When appropriate nutrition therapy is provided to patients with liver disease, malnutrition can be reversed and clinical outcomes improved. Studies to date have been able to show positive outcomes with parenteral and enteral nutrition in malnourished patients with cirrhosis, including improvement in nutritional status and clinical complications of cirrhosis such as ascites, encephalopathy, and infection, in addition to decreased mortality (Campillo et al., 1995; Hirsch et al., 1993; Kearns et al., 1992; Nompleggi and Bonkovsky, 1994). Specific nutrient requirements depend on a patient's disease state, symptoms, and the acuteness of the disease condition.

TABLE 32–5 SUBJECTIVE GLOBAL ASSESSMENT (SGA) PARAMETERS FOR NUTRITIONAL EVALUATION OF LIVER TRANSPLANT CANDIDATES

History
Weight change (consider fluctuations resulting from ascites and edema)
Appetite
Taste changes and early satiety
Dietary recall (calories, protein, sodium)
Persistent gastrointestinal problems (nausea, vomiting, diarrhea, constipation, difficulty chewing or swallowing)

Physical
Muscle wasting
Fat stores
Ascites or edema

Existing Conditions
Disease state and other problems that could influence nutritional status such as hepatic encephalopathy, gastrointestinal bleed, renal insufficiency, infection

Nutritional Rating (Based on Results of Above Parameters)
Well nourished
Moderately (or suspected of being) malnourished
Severely malnourished

(Reprinted with permission from Hasse J. Nutritional aspects of adult liver transplantation. In: Busuttil RW, Klintmalm GB (eds.). Transplantation of the liver. Philadelphia: WB Saunders, 1996, p. 367.)

ENERGY. Energy requirements vary among patients with cirrhosis. Several studies have measured resting energy expenditure (REE) in patients with liver disease to determine energy requirements. Some found patients with ESLD to be normometabolic and others hypo- or hypermetabolic. Although several studies concluded that patients with cirrhosis did not require any more calories than did healthy controls, Dolz and colleagues (1991) determined that ascites increases energy expenditure slightly. Other studies have found inverse relationships between severity of liver disease and energy expenditure without a significant increase in REE (Kondrup and Müller, 1997).

In general, energy requirements for patients with ESLD and without ascites are approximately 120% of the basal energy expenditure (BEE). However, requirements increase to 150% to 175% of BEE if ascites, infection, or malabsorption is present or if nutritional repletion is desired (Hasse et al., 1997). This equates to approximately 25 to 35 calories/kg. Estimated dry body weight should be used in calculations to prevent overfeeding.

CARBOHYDRATE. Determining carbohydrate needs is often challenging in liver failure because of the liver's primary role in carbohydrate metabolism. Metabolically stable cirrhotic patients behave similarly to normal individuals experiencing prolonged starvation. Liver failure reduces glucose production and peripheral glucose utilization. The rate of gluconeogenesis is increased with preference for lipids and amino acids for energy (Hasse, 1996; Hasse et al., 1997; Plauth et al., 1997). Alterations in the hormones insulin, glucagon, cortisol, and epinephrine are responsible in part for the preference for alternative fuels.

Glucose intolerance occurs in almost two thirds of patients with cirrhosis and 10% to 37% of patients will develop overt diabetes. Glucose intolerance in patients with liver disease occurs due to insulin resistance in peripheral tissues. Hyperinsulinism also occurs in patients with cirrhosis possibly because insulin production is increased, hepatic clearance is decreased, portasystemic shunting occurs, there is a defect in the insulin-binding action at the receptor site, or there is a postreceptor defect.

Fasting hypoglycemia can occur because of the decreased availability of glucose from glycogen in addition to the failing gluconeogenic capacity in ESLD. Hypoglycemia occurs more often in acute or fulminant liver failure rather than in chronic liver disease. Hypoglycemia may also occur after alcohol consumption in patients whose glycogen stores are depleted by starvation due to the block of hepatic gluconeogenesis by ethanol. Patients with hypoglycemia should eat frequently to prevent this condition (see "*Clinical Insight:* Fasting Hypoglycemia").

LIPID. In cirrhosis, plasma free fatty acids, glycerol, and ketone bodies are increased in the fasting state. The body prefers lipids as an energy substrate and lipolysis is increased with active mobilization of lipid deposits, but the net capacity to store exogenous lipid is not impaired. A range of 25% to 40% of calories as fat is generally recommended (Plauth et al., 1997).

Fat absorption may be impaired in liver disease. Possible causes include decreased bile salt secretion (as in PBC, sclerosing cholangitis, and biliary strictures), administration of neomycin or cholestyramine, and pancreatic enzyme insufficiency. Stools may be greasy, floating, or light or clay colored, signifying malabsorption, which can be verified by a 72-hour fecal fat study (see Chapter 31). If significant steatorrhea is present, replacement of some of the long-chain triglycerides (LCT) or dietary fat with medium-chain triglycerides (MCT) may be useful. MCTs do not require bile salts and micelle formation for absorption so they are readily taken up via the portal route. Some nutrition supplements (see Appendices 35 through 40) contain MCT, which can be used in addition to liquid MCT oil. Fifteen milliliters, three to four times per day is recommended (15 mL provides 115 kcal, or about 7.7 kcal/g).

Significant stool fat losses may warrant a trial of a low-fat diet. If diarrhea does not resolve, the fat restriction should be discontinued because it decreases the palatability of the diet and severely hampers adequate calorie intake (Corish, 1997).

PROTEIN. Protein is by far the most controversial nutrient in liver failure, and also the most complex. Cirrhosis has long been thought of as a catabolic disease with increased protein breakdown and inadequate resynthesis, resulting in depletion of visceral protein stores and muscle wasting. Protein kinetic studies have only been able to demonstrate increased nitrogen losses in patients with fulminant hepatic failure or decompensated disease, but not in patients with stable cirrhosis (McCullough and Tavill, 1991). Patients with cirrhosis also have increased protein utilization (Nielsen et al., 1995).

At least one study (Nielsen et al., 1995) suggests that 0.8 g protein/kg per day is the mean protein requirement to achieve nitrogen balance in patients with stable cirrhosis. This is higher than the requirement for normal individuals (0.6 g/kg) and malnourished patients without disease (0.4 to 0.5 g/kg) (Kondrup and Müller, 1997). Therefore, in uncomplicated hepatitis or cirrhosis without encephalopathy, protein requirements range from 0.8 to 1.0 g/kg dry weight per day to achieve nitrogen balance. To promote nitrogen accumulation or positive balance, at least 1.2 to 1.3 g/kg per day is needed (Nielsen et al., 1995).

The practice of protein restriction in patients with low-grade hepatic encephalopathy is based on empirical evidence assuming that protein intolerance causes hepatic encephalopathy, but has never

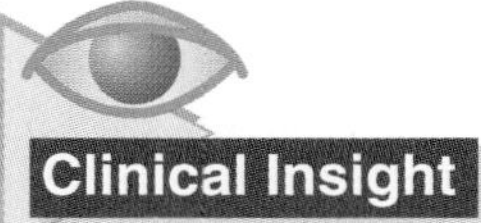

FASTING HYPOGLYCEMIA

Two thirds of the glucose requirement in an adult is used by the central nervous system. During fasting, plasma glucose concentrations are maintained for use by the nervous system and the brain because liver glycogen is broken down, or new glucose is made from nonglucose precursors such as alanine (Polonsky, 1992). Fasting hypoglycemia occurs with reduced synthesis of new glucose or reduced liver glycogen breakdown.

Causes of fasting hypoglycemia include cirrhosis, consumption of alcohol, extensive intrahepatic cancer, deficiency of the hormones cortisol and growth hormone, or non-beta cell tumors of the pancreas. The method for detecting it involves measuring plasma insulin when plasma glucose is low. The diagnostic hallmark of an insulinoma is altered insulin secretion in the presence of hypoglycemia. Fasting hypoglycemia may also be caused by spontaneously produced antibodies. All individuals with liver or pancreatic disease should be monitored for fasting hypoglycemia. Nutritional therapy involves balanced meals with small frequent snacks to avoid periods of fasting. Monitoring of blood glucose and insulin levels will be required.

been proven in a study that it will improve mental state (Kondrup and Müller, 1997). Unnecessary protein restriction may only worsen body protein losses, and therefore must be avoided. In situations of stress such as alcoholic hepatitis or decompensated disease (sepsis, infection, gastrointestinal bleeding, severe ascites), at least 1.5 g protein/kg per day should be provided. Patients with encephalopathy often do not receive adequate protein.

VITAMINS AND MINERALS. Vitamin and mineral supplementation is needed in all patients with ESLD because of the liver's intimate role in nutrient transport, storage, and metabolism, in addition to the side effects of drugs (Table 32–6).

Deficiencies of fat-soluble vitamins have been found in all types of liver failure, especially in cholestatic diseases where malabsorption and steatorrhea occur. Therefore, supplementation is necessary, using water-soluble forms. Intravenous or intramuscular vitamin K is often given for 3 days to rule out vitamin K deficiency as the cause of hypoprothrombinemia. Water-soluble vitamin deficiencies associated with alcoholic liver disease include thiamin (which can lead to **Wernicke's encephalopathy**), pyridoxine (B_6), cyanocobalamin (B_{12}), folate, and niacin (B_3). Large doses (100 mg) of thiamin are given daily for a limited time if deficiency is suspected.

Mineral nutriture is also altered in liver disease. Elevated serum copper levels are found in cholestatic liver diseases (PBC and PSC). Because copper and manganese are excreted primarily via bile, supplementation should not be provided.

Wilson's disease is a disorder of abnormal copper metabolism in which urinary excretion is high, serum levels are low, and excess copper in various organs causes severe damage. Chelating agents such as zinc acetate or D-penicillamine are the primary treatment. A vegetarian diet may be useful adjunctive therapy because copper is less available (Brewer et al., 1993). Dietary copper restriction (Table 32–7) is not routinely prescribed unless other therapies are unsuccessful.

Zinc and magnesium levels are low in liver disease related to alcoholism, due in part to diuretic therapy. Calcium as well as magnesium and zinc may be malabsorbed with steatorrhea. Therefore, at least standard doses to meet RDAs for these minerals should be provided.

FLUIDS AND ELECTROLYTES. Fluid retention is common, and ascites is a serious consequence of liver disease. Portal hypertension, hypoalbuminemia, lymphatic obstruction, and renal retention of sodium and fluid contribute to fluid retention. Increased release of catecholamines, renin, angiotensin, aldosterone, and antidiuretic hormone secondary to peripheral arterial vasodilation causes renal retention of sodium and water.

Though dilutional hyponatremia may exist, it usually represents water overload in excess of sodium retention. Therefore, treatment includes sodium and fluid restriction, in addition to diuretic therapy. Sodium is commonly restricted to 2 g/day (see Chapter 36 for discussion of low-sodium diets). More severe limitations may be imposed; however, caution is warranted because of the limited palatability of these diets.

Hyponatremia occurs because of decreased ability to excrete water due to persistent release of antidiuretic hormone, sodium losses via paracentesis, excessive diuretic use, or overly aggressive sodium restriction. Fluid intake is usually restricted to 1 to 1.5 L/day, depending on the severity of the edema and ascites. Daily fluid intake may be restricted to as little as 500 to 750 mL/day plus urinary losses if hyponatremia is severe and persistent (Hasse et al., 1997).

Diuretic therapy often includes spironolactone

TABLE 32–6 VITAMIN/MINERAL DEFICITS IN SEVERE HEPATIC FAILURE

VITAMIN OR MINERAL	PREDISPOSING FACTORS	SIGNS OF DEFICIENCY
Vitamin A	Steatorrhea, neomycin, cholestyramine, alcoholism	Dermatitis, night blindness
Vitamin D	Steatorrhea, glucocorticoids, cholestyramine	Osteomalacia
Vitamin E	Steatorrhea, cholestyramine	Edema, peripheral neuropathy
Vitamin K	Steatorrhea, antibiotics, cholestyramine	Bleeding
Vitamin B_6	Alcoholism	Mucous membrane lesions, dermatitis
Vitamin B_{12}	Alcoholism, cholestyramine	Megaloblastic anemia, glossitis, CNS dysfunction
Folate	Alcoholism	Megaloblastic anemia, glossitis, irritability
Niacin	Alcoholism	Dermatitis, dementia, diarrhea, inflammation of mucous membranes
Thiamin	Alcoholism, high-carbohydrate diet	Neuropathy, ascites, edema, CNS dysfunction
Zinc	Diarrhea, diuretics, alcoholism	Immunodeficiency, impaired taste acuity, poor wound healing, decreased protein synthesis
Magnesium	Alcoholism, diuretics	Neuromuscular irritability, hypokalemia, hypocalcemia
Iron	Chronic bleeding	Stomatitis, microcytic anemia, malaise
Potassium	Diuretics, anabolism, insulin use	Muscular weakness, malaise, respiratory or cardiac arrest
Phosphorus	Alcoholism, anabolism	Anorexia, weakness, cardiac failure, glucose intolerance

(Adapted from Shronts EP: Nutritional assessment of adults with end-stage hepatic failure. Nutr Clin Pract 3:113, 1988.)
CNS, central nervous system.

TABLE 32–7 COPPER CONTENT OF COMMONLY USED FOODS*

FOOD GROUPS	HIGH (>0.2 mg/PORTION COMMONLY USED†) (AVOID)	MODERATE (0.1–0.2 mg/PORTION) (NO MORE THAN 6 SERVINGS/DAY)	LOW (0.1 mg/PORTION COMMONLY USED†) (MAY BE EATEN AS DESIRED)
Meat and meat substitutes	Lamb; pork; pheasant; quail; duck; goose; squid; salmon; all organ meats including liver, heart, kidney, brain; all shellfish, including oysters, scallops, shrimp, lobster, clams, and crab; meat gelatin; soy protein meat substitutes; tofu; all nuts and seeds	All other fish (3 oz); dark meat turkey (3 oz); peanut butter (2 Tbsp)	Beef; cheese; cottage cheese; eggs; light meat turkey; cold cuts and frankfurters that do not contain pork, dark turkey, or organ meats; all others not listed on high or moderate list
Fats and oils	Avocado	Olives (2 med); cream (½ cup)	Butter; cream; margarine; mayonnaise; nondairy cream substitutes; oils; sour cream; salad dressings (made from allowed ingredients); all others not listed on high or moderate list
Milk	Chocolate; cocoa; soy milk		All other dairy products; milk flavored with carob
Starch	Dried beans including soybeans, lima beans, baked beans, garbanzo beans, pinto beans; dried peas; lentils; millet; barley; wheat germ; bran breads and cereals; cereals with >0.2 mg copper per serving (check label); soy flour; soy grits; sweet potatoes (fresh)	Whole-wheat bread (1 slice); potatoes in any form (½ cup or 1 small); pumpkin (¾ cup); melba toast (4); whole-wheat crackers (6); parsnips (⅔ cup); winter squash (½ cup); green peas (½ cup); instant oatmeal (½ cup); instant Ralston™ (½ cup); cereals with 0.1–0.2 mg of copper per serving (check labels); dehydrated and canned soups (1 cup)	Breads and pasta from refined flour; canned sweet potatoes; rice; regular oatmeal; cereals with <0.1 mg of copper per serving (check label); all others not listed on high or moderate list
Vegetables	Mushrooms; vegetable juice cocktail	Bean sprouts (1 cup); beets (½ cup); spinach (½ cup cooked, 1 cup raw); tomato juice and other tomato products (½ cup); broccoli (½ cup); asparagus (½ cup)	All others, including fresh tomatoes
Fruits	Nectarines; dried fruits including raisins, dates, and prunes (dried fruits are permitted if dried at home)	Mango (½ cup); pears (1 medium); pineapple (½ cup); papaya (¼ average)	All others
Desserts	Desserts that contain significant amounts of any foods high in copper		All others
Sugar and sweets	Chocolate; cocoa	Licorice (1 oz); syrups (1 oz)	All others including jams, jellies, and candies made with allowed fruits; carob; flavoring extracts
Miscellaneous	Brewer's yeast	Ketchup	
Beverages‡	Instant breakfast beverages; mineral water; alcohol§	Postum™ and other cereal beverages	All others including fruit-flavored beverages; lemonade

(From Pemberton CM et al. Mayo Clinic diet manual: A handbook of nutrition practices, 7th ed. St. Louis: Mosby-Yearbook, 1994.)

*Data that are available on the average copper content of foods vary greatly. There is disagreement on the copper content of the usual American diet, with estimates that range from 1 mg of copper a day to 5 mg/day. The concentration of copper in foods is affected by many factors, including soil conditions, geographic location, species, diet, processing method, and contamination in processing. The exact copper content of foods is difficult to verify. It is estimated that avoidance of high-copper foods and restriction of moderate-copper foods results in a diet of approximately 1 mg/day. For practical purposes, diets are designed to limit foods with a higher copper content than other foods, and not to achieve a specific level of copper in the diet.

†Portions commonly used are those generally accepted as typical portion sizes in various nutrient data source manuals.

‡A water sample from the patient's home water supply should be analyzed for copper content. Demineralized water should be used if the water contains more than 100 μg/L.

§Although not necessarily high in copper, alcoholic beverages are discouraged because of their action as a hepatotoxin.

and furosemide. These drugs are often used in combination for best effect. Furosemide, a loop diuretic, has a stronger natriuretic effect, but spironolactone is more effective in increasing sodium excretion in patients with ESLD (Gurk-Turner, 1997). Major side effects of loop diuretics include hyponatremia, hypokalemia, hypomagnesemia, hypocalcemia, and hypochloremic acidosis. Conversely, spironolactone is potassium-sparing. Serum potassium levels must therefore be monitored carefully and supplemented or restricted if necessary because deficiency or excess may contribute to metabolic abnormalities.

Weight, abdominal girth, urinary sodium concentration, and serum levels of urea nitrogen, creatinine, albumin, uric acid, and electrolytes should be monitored during diuretic therapy.

Problems in Feeding. Great care should be taken to serve food that is attractive and appetizing. Because anorexia, nausea, dysgeusia, and other gastrointestinal symptoms are common, adequate nutrition intake is difficult to achieve. With ascites, early satiety is also a frequent complaint. Smaller, more frequent meals are better tolerated than three traditional meals. In addition, evidence suggests that frequent feedings also improve nitrogen balance and prevent hypoglycemia. Oral liquid supplements should be encouraged and, when necessary, enteral tube feedings used. Adjunctive nutrition support should be given to malnourished patients with liver disease if their intake is less than 0.8 g protein/kg and less than 30 calories/kg per day and if they are at risk for fatal complications of disease (Kondrup and Müller, 1997). Esophageal varices are usually not a contraindication for tube feeding.

Nutrition Therapy in Liver Resection and Transplantation

Liver resection is fairly common now that problem areas can be located by means of tomography and arteriography. As with any major surgery, protein and energy needs increase after liver resection. Needs are also increased to promote liver cell regeneration. Enteral nutrition is vital because of the role of portal hepatotrophic factors necessary for liver cell proliferation. Optimal nutrition is most important for patients with poor nutritional status prior to hepatectomy (e.g., patients with hepatocellular carcinoma or cholangiocarcinoma). Nutrition support may be occasionally required.

Liver transplantation has become an established treatment for ESLD. If malnutrition is present, nutrition support is required prior to transplant. In the acute post-transplant phase, nutrient needs are increased to promote healing, deter infection, provide energy for recovery, and replenish depleted body stores (Hasse, 1998). Nitrogen requirements are elevated in the acute post-transplant phase and can be met with early postoperative tube feeding (Hasse et al., 1995). Multiple medications used after transplant have nutritional side effects such as anorexia, gastrointestinal upset, hypercatabolism, diarrhea, hyperglycemia, hyperlipidemia, sodium retention, hypertension, hyperkalemia, and hypercalciuria. Therefore, dietary modification is based on the specific side effects of drug therapy (Table 32–8). During the chronic post-transplant phase, nutrient requirements are adjusted to prevent or treat problems of obesity, hyperlipidemia, hypertension, diabetes mellitus, and osteopenia (Hasse, 1997; Weseman and McCashland, 1998). Table 32–9 summarizes nutrient needs following liver transplantation.

PHYSIOLOGY AND FUNCTIONS OF THE GALLBLADDER

The gallbladder lies on the undersurface of the right lobe of the liver, as shown in Figure 32–8. The main function of the gallbladder is to concentrate,

TABLE 32–8 MEDICATIONS COMMONLY USED AFTER LIVER TRANSPLANTATION

IMMUNOSUPPRESSANT DRUG	POSSIBLE NUTRITION SIDE EFFECTS	PROPOSED NUTRITION THERAPY
• Azathioprine	• Macrocytic anemia	• Folate supplements
	• Mouth sores	• Soft foods if needed
	• Nausea, vomiting, diarrhea, anorexia, sore throat, stomach pain, decreased taste acuity	• Adjust food/meals as needed, monitor intake
• Antithymocyte globulin	• Nausea, vomiting	• Adjust food/meals as needed, monitor intake
• Cyclosporine	• Sodium retention	• Decrease sodium intake
	• Hyperkalemia	• Decrease potassium intake
	• Hyperlipidemia	• Limit fat and simple carbohydrate intake
	• Hyperglycemia	• Decrease simple carbohydrate intake
	• Decreased serum magnesium level	• Increase magnesium intake; give magnesium supplements
	• Nausea, vomiting	• Adjust food/meals as needed; monitor intake
• Glucocorticoids	• Sodium retention	• Decrease sodium intake
	• Hyperglycemia	• Decrease simple carbohydrate intake
	• Hyperlipidemia	• Limit fat and simple carbohydrate intake
	• False hunger	• Avoid overeating
	• Protein wasting with high doses	• Increase protein intake
	• Decreased absorption of calcium and phosphorus	• Increase calcium and phosphorus intake; give supplements as needed
• Muromonab-CD3	• Nausea, vomiting, anorexia	• Adjust food/meals as needed, monitor intake
• Mycophenolate mofetil	• GI symptoms: nausea, vomiting, diarrhea	• Adjust food/meals as needed, monitor intake
• Sirolimus	• Possible hyperglycemia	• Decrease simple carbohydrate intake
	• Possible GI symptoms	• Adjust food/meals as needed, monitor intake
	• Hyperlipidemia	• Limit fat and simple carbohydrate intake
• Tacrolimus	• Hypertension	• Adjust food/meals as needed; monitor intake
	• Hyperglycemia	• Decrease simple carbohydrate intake
	• Hyperkalemia	• Decrease potassium intake
	• Nausea, vomiting	• Adjust food/meals as needed; monitor intake
	• GI symptoms (diarrhea)	• Adjust food/meals as needed; monitor intake
• 15-Deoxysperagualin	• GI symptoms	• Adjust food/meals as needed; monitor intake

(Adapted with permission from Hasse J. Role of the dietitian in the nutrition management of adults after liver transplantation. J Am Diet Assoc 91:473, 1991.)
GI, gastrointestinal.

TABLE 32–9 NUTRITION CARE GUIDELINES FOR LIVER TRANSPLANTATION

	PRETRANSPLANTATION	IMMEDIATE POST-TRANSPLANTATION (FIRST 2 POST-TRANSPLANT MONTHS)	LONG-TERM POST-TRANSPLANTATION
Calories	High calorie (basal + 20% or more)	Moderate calorie (basal + 15–30%)	Weight maintenance (basal + 10–20%)
Protein*	Moderate protein (1–1.5 g/kg/day—minimize need for restriction)	High protein (1.2–1.75 g/kg/day)	Moderate protein (1 g/kg/day)
Fat	As needed	20–30% of nonprotein calories	Low fat (≤ 30% of calories)
Carbohydrate	High carbohydrate (complex and simple)	70% of nonprotein calories	Reduced simple carbohydrate
Sodium	2–4 g/day (as indicated)	2–4 g/day (as indicated)	2–4 g/day (as indicated)
Fluid	Restrict to 1000–1500 mL/day (as indicated)	As needed	As needed
Calcium	800–1200 mg/day	800–1200 mg/day	1200–1500 mg/day
Vitamins	Daily multivitamin/mineral supplement to RDA levels; additional water- and fat-soluble vitamins as indicated	Daily multivitamin/mineral supplement to RDA levels; additional water- and fat-soluble vitamins as indicated	Daily multivitamin/mineral supplement to RDA levels for first post-transplant year

(Adapted with permission from Porayko MK et al. Impact of malnutrition and its therapy on liver transplantation. Semin Liver Dis 11(4):305, 1991.)
* Use estimated dry or ideal weight.
RDA, recommended dietary allowance.

store, and excrete bile, which is produced by the liver. During the concentration process, water and electrolytes are reabsorbed by the gallbladder mucosa. The chief constituents of bile are cholesterol, bilirubin, and bile salts. *Bilirubin,* the main bile pigment, is derived from the release of hemoglobin from red blood cell destruction. It is transported to the liver, where it is conjugated and excreted via bile. *Bile salts,* made by liver cells from cholesterol, are essential for the digestion and absorption of fats, fat soluble vitamins, and some minerals (see Chapter 1). Excreted into the small intestine via bile, bile salts are then reabsorbed into the portal system (enterohepatic circulation). Bile also contains immunoglobulins that support the integrity of the intestinal mucosa. In addition, it is the primary excretory pathway for the minerals copper and manganese.

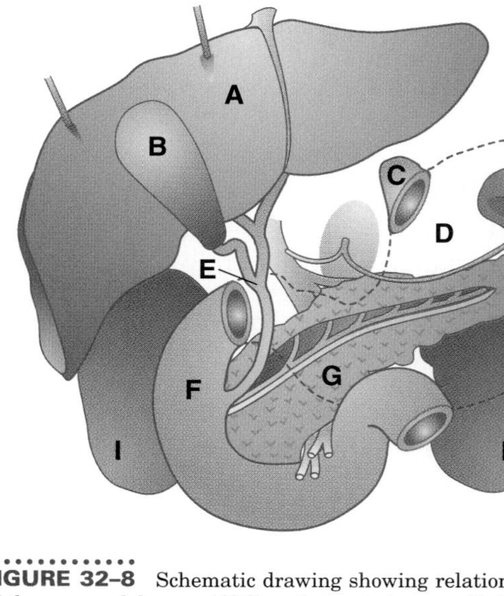

Bile is removed by the liver via bile canaliculi that drain into intrahepatic bile ducts. The ducts lead to the left and right hepatic ducts, which leave the liver and join to become the common hepatic duct. The bile is directed to the gallbladder via the cystic duct for concentration and storage. The cystic duct joins the common hepatic duct to form the common bile duct. The bile duct then joins the pancreatic duct, which carries digestive enzymes. During the course of digestion, food reaches the duodenum, causing the release of intestinal hormones, such as cholecystokinin and secretin. This stimulates the gallbladder and pancreas and causes the sphincter of Oddi to relax, allowing pancreatic juice and bile to flow into the duodenum at the ampulla of Vater to assist in fat digestion. For this reason diseases of the gallbladder, liver, and pancreas are often interrelated.

FIGURE 32–8 Schematic drawing showing relationship of organs of the upper abdomen. (**A**) liver (retracted upward); (**B**) gallbladder; (**C**) esophageal opening of stomach; (**D**) stomach (shown in dotted outline); (**E**) common bile duct; (**F**) duodenum; (**G**) pancreas and pancreatic duct; (**H**) spleen; (**I**) kidneys.

DISEASES OF THE GALLBLADDER

Disorders of the biliary tract affect millions of people each year, causing significant suffering and even death by precipitating pancreatitis and sepsis. The common diseases of the biliary tract are cholelithiasis, choledocholithiasis, and cholecystitis. Other diseases include PSC, PBC, and bile duct cancer. Treatment may involve diet, medication, and/or surgery.

Cholelithiasis

The formation of gallstones (calculi) in the absence of infection of the gallbladder is called **cholelithiasis.** Virtually all gallstones form within the gallbladder. With rare exceptions, stones form behind biliary duct strictures due to stasis in bile ducts after cholecystectomy. Gallstone disease affects millions of Americans each year and causes significant morbidity. In most cases, gallstones are asymptomatic. However, symptomatic gallstone disease can have serious complications.

Gallstones that pass from the gallbladder into the common bile duct may remain there indefinitely without causing symptoms, or they may pass into the duodenum with or without symptoms. **Choledocholithiasis** develops when stones slip into the bile ducts, producing obstruction, pain, and cramps. If passage of bile into the duodenum is interrupted, cholecystitis can develop. In the absence of bile in the intestine, lipid absorption is impaired, and without bile pigments, stools become light in color (acholic). If uncorrected, bile backup can result in jaundice and liver damage (*secondary biliary cirrhosis*). Obstruction of the distal common bile duct can lead to pancreatitis if the pancreatic duct is blocked (see next section).

Most gallstones in the United States are unpigmented cholesterol stones, composed primarily of cholesterol, bilirubin, and calcium salts (Johnston and Kaplan, 1993). Risk factors for cholesterol stone formation include female gender, pregnancies, age, family history, obesity and truncal body fat distribution, diabetes mellitus, inflammatory bowel disease, and drugs (lipid-lowering medications, oral contraceptives, and estrogens) (Everhart, 1993; Hoy et al., 1994). Certain ethnic groups are at greater risk of stone formation (i.e., Pima Indians, Scandinavians, Mexican Americans). Rapid weight loss (as with jejunoileal and gastric bypass and fasting or severe calorie restriction) is associated with a high incidence of biliary sludge and gallstone formation (Liddle et al., 1989; Marks et al., 1992).

Low-grade chronic infections produce changes in the gallbladder mucosa, which affect its absorptive capabilities. Excess water or excess bile acid may be absorbed as a result. Cholesterol may then precipitate out and cause gallstone formation (Johnston and Kaplan, 1993). High dietary fat intake over a prolonged period of time may predispose a person to gallstone formation because of the constant stimulus to produce more cholesterol for bile synthesis required in fat digestion.

Pigmented stones typically consist of bilirubin polymers or calcium salts. They are associated with chronic hemolysis. Risk factors associated with these stones are age, sickle cell anemia and thalassemia, biliary tract infection, cirrhosis, alcoholism, and long-term total parenteral nutrition (TPN) (Diehl, 1991).

Treatment of gallstone disease includes surgical removal of the gallbladder (**cholecystectomy**), especially if the stones are numerous, large, or calcified. The cholecystectomy may be done as a traditional open laparotomy or as a less invasive, laparoscopic procedure. Chemical dissolution with the administration of bile salts, chenodeoxycholic acid, and ursodeoxycholic acid (litholytic therapy) or dissolution by extracorporeal shock wave lithotripsy (ESWL) may also be used, but these are much less common than surgical techniques. Patients with gallstones that have migrated into the bile ducts may be candidates for *endoscopic retrograde cholangiopancreatography (ERCP)* techniques (Johnston and Kaplan, 1993).

Cholecystitis

Inflammation of the gallbladder is known as **cholecystitis** and may be chronic or acute. It is usually caused by gallstones obstructing the bile ducts (*calculous cholecystitis*), leading to the backup of bile. Bilirubin, the main bile pigment, gives bile its greenish color. When biliary tract obstruction prevents bile from reaching the intestine, it backs up and returns to the circulation. Bilirubin has an affinity for elastic tissues; therefore, when it overflows into the general circulation it causes the yellow skin pigmentation and eye discoloration typical of jaundice. Acute cholecystitis without stones (*acalculous cholecystitis*) may occur in critically ill patients such as those with sepsis, shock, multiple trauma, or burns (Adam and Roddi, 1991). Acalculous cholecystitis seems to arise when the gallbladder and its bile are stagnant. The walls of the gallbladder become inflamed and distended, and infection can occur. During such episodes, the patient experiences upper quadrant pain accompanied by nausea, vomiting, and flatulence. Acute cholecystitis requires surgical intervention unless medically contraindicated. Without surgery, the condition may either subside or progress to gangrene.

Acute Cholangitis

Inflammation of the bile ducts is known a cholangitis. Patients with *acute cholangitis* need resuscitation with fluids and broad-spectrum antibiotics. If the patient does not improve with conservative treatment, placement of a percutaneous biliary stent, endoscopic papillotomy with stone extraction or positioning of an internal or nasobiliary stent, or open surgery may be necessary (te Boekhorst, 1988).

Sclerosing Cholangitis

Sclerosing cholangitis can result in sepsis and liver failure. Most patients have multiple intrahepatic strictures, which make surgical intervention difficult if not impossible. Patients are generally on broad-spectrum antibiotics. Percutaneous ductal dilatation may provide short-term bile duct patency in some patients. When sepsis is recurrent, patients may require chronic antibiotic therapy.

Cholestasis

Cholestasis is a condition of sludge-like buildup in the gallbladder due to the lack of stimulation or release of bile. This can occur in patients without oral or enteral feeding for a prolonged period, such as those requiring TPN. This can predispose to acalculous cholestasis. Prevention includes stimulation of intestinal and biliary motility and secretions by at least minimal enteral feedings (Hager, 1994). If this is not possible, then drug therapy is used.

NUTRITION MANAGEMENT OF GALLBLADDER DISORDERS

There is no specific dietary treatment to prevent cholelithiasis in susceptible individuals. Nutritionally related factors include obesity and severe fasting and these should be corrected where possible. In cholecystitis, dietary treatment includes a low-fat diet to prevent gallbladder contractions. There is conflicting data as to whether or not intravenous lipids stimulate gallbladder contraction (De Boer et al., 1992; Kalfarentzos et al., 1991; Priori et al., 1997).

Acute Cholecystitis

In an acute attack, oral feedings are discontinued. Parenteral nutrition may be indicated if the patient is malnourished and it is anticipated that he or she will be NPO for a prolonged period of time. When feedings are resumed, a low-fat diet is recommended to decrease gallbladder stimulation. A hydrolyzed low-fat formula (see Appendices 35 through 40), or an oral diet consisting of 30 to 45 g fat per day can be given. Studies have failed to show a relationship between dietary cholesterol and gallstone formation. Table 32–10 shows a combination of foods that provides this amount of fat.

Chronic Cholecystitis

Patients with chronic conditions may require a long-term low-fat diet that contains 25% to 30% of total kilocalories as fat. Stricter limitation is undesirable because fat in the intestine is important for some stimulation and drainage of the biliary tract.

The degree of food intolerance varies widely among individuals with gallbladder disorders, but many complain of foods that cause flatulence and bloating. It is best to determine with the patient any foods that should be eliminated for this reason. See Chapter 31 for a discussion of potential gas-forming foods.

Administration of water-soluble forms of fat-soluble vitamins may be of benefit in individuals with chronic gallbladder conditions or in those in whom fat malabsorption is suspected.

Gallbladder Surgery

Following surgical removal of the gallbladder, oral feedings are usually resumed with the return of bowel sounds and after the patient can tolerate nasogastric drainage tube removal. The diet can be advanced as tolerated to a regular diet. In the absence of the gallbladder, bile is secreted directly by the liver into the intestine. The biliary tract dilates forming a "simulated pouch" over time, to allow bile to be held in a manner similar to the original gallbladder.

PHYSIOLOGY AND FUNCTION OF THE EXOCRINE PANCREAS

The pancreas is an elongated, flattened gland that lies in the upper abdomen behind the stomach. The head of the pancreas is in the right upper quadrant below the liver within the curvature of the duodenum and the tapering tail slants upward to the hilum of the spleen. This glandular organ has both an endocrine and exocrine function. Pancreatic cells manufacture glucagon, insulin, and somatostatin for absorption into the bloodstream (endocrine function) for regulation of glucose homeostasis. Other cells secrete enzymes and other substances directly into the intestinal lumen, where they aid in digesting proteins, fats, and carbohydrates (exocrine function). In the vast majority of cases, the pancreatic duct, which carries the exocrine pancreatic secretions, merges with the common bile duct into a unified opening through which bile and pancreatic juices drain into the duodenum at the ampulla of Vater. Many factors regulate exocrine secretion from the pancreas. Neural and hormonal responses play a role, with the presence and composition of ingested foods being a large contributor. The two primary hormonal stimuli for pancreatic secretion are secretin and cholecystokinin (see Chapter 1).

DISEASES OF THE EXOCRINE PANCREAS

Pancreatitis

Pancreatitis is an inflammation of the pancreas characterized by edema, cellular exudate, and fat necrosis. The disease can range from mild and self-limiting to severe, with autodigestion, necrosis, and hemorrhage of pancreatic tissue. Ranson and colleagues (1974) identified 11 signs that could be measured during the first 48 hours of admission, which have prognostic significance (Table 32–11). By using these observations one can determine the likely outcome of hospitalization. Surgical intervention may be necessary. Pancreatitis is classified as acute or chronic, the latter with pancreatic destruction so extensive that exocrine and endocrine function are severely diminished, and maldigestion and diabetes may result.

The symptoms of pancreatitis can range from continuous or intermittent pain of varying intensity to severe upper abdominal pain, which may radiate to the back. Symptoms may worsen with the ingestion of food. Clinical presentation may also include nausea, vomiting, abdominal distention, and steatorrhea. Severe cases are complicated by hypoten-

TABLE 32–10 FAT-RESTRICTED DIET*

FOODS ALLOWED	FOODS EXCLUDED
Beverages Skim milk or buttermilk made with skim milk; coffee, tea, Postum, fruit juice, soft drinks, cocoa made with cocoa powder and skim milk	**Beverages** Whole milk, buttermilk made with whole milk, chocolate milk, cream in excess of amounts allowed under fats
Bread and Cereal Products Plain, nonfat cereals, spaghetti, noodles, rice, macaroni; plain whole grain or enriched bread, air-popped popcorn, bagels, English muffins	**Bread and Cereal Products** Biscuits, breads, egg or cheese bread, sweet rolls made with fat, pancakes, doughnuts, waffles, fritters, popcorn prepared with fat, muffins, natural cereals and breads to which extra fat is added
Cheese Cottage, ¼ cup to be used as substitute for 1 oz of cheese, or low-fat cheeses containing less than 5% butterfat	**Cheese** Whole-milk cheeses
Desserts Sherbet made with skim milk; nonfat frozen yogurt; nonfat frozen nondairy desserts; fruit ice; sorbet; gelatin; rice, bread, cornstarch, tapioca, or pudding made with skim milk; fruit whips with gelatin, sugar, and egg white; fruit; angel food cake; graham crackers; vanilla wafers; meringues	**Desserts** Cake, pie, pastry, ice cream, or any dessert containing shortening, chocolate, or fats of any kind, unless especially prepared using part of fat allowance
Eggs 3 per week prepared only with fat from fat allowance; egg whites as desired; low-fat egg substitutes	**Eggs** More than 1/day unless substituted for part of the meat allowed
Fats Choose up to the limit allowed among the following (1 serving in the amount listed equals 1 fat choice): 1 tsp butter or margarine 1 T reduced-fat margarine 1 tsp shortening or oil 1 tsp mayonnaise 2 tsp Italian or French dressing 1 T reduced-fat salad dressing 1 strip crisp bacon ⅛ avocado (4 in. diameter) 2 T light cream 1 T heavy cream 6 small nuts 5 small olives	**Fats** Any in excess of amount prescribed on diet; all others
Fruits As desired	**Fruits** Avocado in excess of amount allowed on fat list
Lean Meat, Fish, Poultry, and Meat Substitutes Choose up to the limit allowed among the following: poultry without skin, fish, veal (all cuts), liver, lean beef, pork, and lamb, all with visible fat removed—1 oz cooked weight equals 1 equivalent; ¼ cup water-packed tuna or salmon equals 1 equivalent; tofu or tempeh—3 oz equals 1 equivalent	**Meat, Fish, Poultry, and Meat Substitutes** Fried or fatty meats, sausage, scrapple, frankfurters, poultry skins, stewing hens, spareribs, salt pork, beef unless lean, duck, goose, ham hocks, pig's feet, luncheon meats (unless reduced fat), gravies unless fat-free, tuna and salmon packed in oil, peanut butter
Milk Skim, buttermilk, or yogurt made from skim milk	**Milk** Whole, 2%, 1%, chocolate, buttermilk made with whole milk
Seasonings As desired	**Seasonings** None
Soups Bouillon, clear broth, fat-free vegetable soup, cream soup made with skimmed milk, packaged dehydrated soups	**Soups** All others
Sweets Jelly, jam, marmalade, honey, syrup, molasses, sugar, hard sugar candies, fondant, gumdrops, jelly beans, marshmallows, cocoa powder, fat-free chocolate sauce, red and black licorice	**Sweets** Any candy made with chocolate, nuts, butter, cream, or fat of any kind
Vegetables All plainly prepared vegetables	**Vegetables** Potato chips; buttered, au gratin, creamed, or fried potatoes and other vegetables unless made with allowed fat; casseroles, or frozen vegetables in butter sauce

TABLE 32–10 FAT-RESTRICTED DIET* (continued)

DAILY FOOD ALLOWANCES FOR A 40-g FAT DIET		
Food	Amount	Approximate Fat Content (g)
Skim milk	2 cups or more	0
Lean meat, fish, poultry	6 oz or 6 equivalents	18
Whole egg or egg yolks	3 per week	2
Vegetables	3 servings or more, at least 1 or more dark green or deep yellow	0
Fruits	3 or more servings, at least 1 citrus	0
Breads, cereals	As desired, fat-free	0
Fat exchanges*	4–5 exchanges daily	20–25
Desserts and sweets	As desired from permitted list	0
	Total fat	38–43

*Fat content can be reduced further by reducing the fat exchanges. 1 fat exchange = 5 g fat.

sion, oliguria, and dyspnea. Laboratory evaluation will usually reveal elevations of serum amylase or lipase levels. However, the serum amylase test is nonspecific for pancreatitis and may be falsely negative or falsely positive. Serum lipase has the same degree of sensitivity as amylase but greater specificity. Severe cases of pancreatitis may lead to hemorrhage, shock, or death.

There are numerous causes of pancreatitis, including chronic alcoholism, biliary tract disease, gallstones, certain drugs, trauma, hypertriglyceridemia, hypercalcemia, and some infections such as viruses (Banks, 1998; Calleja and Barkin, 1993). Whereas alcohol is the leading cause of chronic pancreatitis in most Western societies (Holt, 1993), gallstones are the most common cause of acute pancreatitis (Steinberg and Tenner, 1994). Pancreatitis is associated with serious complications and significant mortality. For alcoholic pancreatitis, the overall mortality rate is about 5%; for gallstone-associated and idiopathic pancreatitis, it is 10% to 25% (de Beaux et al., 1995; Mann et al., 1994).

The exact mechanisms that lead to pancreatic injury have not been fully defined. One theory involves blockage or reflux of the ductal contents into the pancreatic duct (Calleja and Barkin, 1993). It appears that a common characteristic is premature activation of the enzymes within the pancreas, resulting in autodigestion within the pancreatic cells (Pisters and Ranson, 1992). The enzymes released by destroyed pancreatic cells eventually reach the bloodstream, causing elevated serum amylase and lipase levels. Usually a hallmark finding in acute pancreatitis, these markers alone are not always diagnostic nor do they indicate the extent of pancreatic injury. Further evaluation of the extent or severity of pancreatic injury is best done with radiographic imaging (computed tomography, ultrasound) studies.

It should be noted that in cases of chronic pancreatitis involving extensive destruction of pancreatic tissue with subsequent fibrosis, enzyme production is diminished and serum amylase and lipase may appear normal. However, absence of enzymes to aid in the digestion of food leads to steatorrhea and malabsorption. Table 32–12 describes several tests used to determine the extent of pancreatic destruction.

TABLE 32–11 RANSON'S CRITERIA FOR CLASSIFYING THE SEVERITY OF PANCREATITIS*

At admission or diagnosis:
- Age over 55 y
- White blood cell count >16,000/m^3
- Blood glucose level >200 mg/100 mL
- Lactic dehydrogenase >350 IU/L
- Aspartate transaminase >250 U/L

During the initial 48 hours:
- Hematocrit decrease of >10 mg/dL
- Blood urea nitrogen increase of >5 mg/dL
- Arterial PO_2 <60 mm Hg
- Base deficit >4 mEq/L
- Fluid sequestration >6000 mL
- Serum calcium level <8 mg/mL

(Modified with permission from Ranson JH et al. Prognostic signs and the role of operative management in acute pancreatitis. Surg Gynecol Obstet 139:69, 1974.)

*Five observations are made on admission; six observations are made 48 hours later. If three or more of these parameters are present, more than 60% of patients subsequently expire of the disease during that hospitalization. Six other clinical parameters have a significant impact on outcome if they develop over the first 48 hours after admission.

TABLE 32–12 SOME TESTS OF PANCREATIC FUNCTION

TEST	SIGNIFICANCE
Secretin stimulation test	Measures pancreatic secretion, particularly bicarbonate, in response to secretin stimulation
Glucose tolerance test	Assesses endocrine function of the pancreas by measuring insulin response to a glucose load
72-hr stool fat test	Assesses exocrine function of the pancreas by measuring fat absorption that reflects pancreatic lipase secretion

NUTRITION MANAGEMENT IN PANCREATIC DISORDERS

Acute Pancreatitis

Pain associated with pancreatitis is partially related to the secretory mechanisms of pancreatic enzymes and bile. The nutrition care is therefore adjusted to provide minimal stimulation of these systems (Fig. 32–9). The pancreas is put "at rest." During acute attacks, all oral feeding is withheld and hydration is maintained intravenously. In less severe attacks, a clear liquid diet with negligible fat may be given in a few days. The patient should be monitored for any symptoms of pain, nausea, or vomiting. The diet should be progressed as tolerated to easily digested foods with a low fat content, and then advanced as tolerated. Foods may be better tolerated if they are divided into six small meals. The low-fat diet described in Table 32–10 can be used.

Severe acute pancreatitis results in a hypermetabolic and catabolic state. Metabolic demands have been compared to that of a patient with sepsis (Pisters and Ranson, 1992). Amino acids are released from muscle and used for gluconeogenesis. These patients often exhibit signs of malnutrition such as decreased serum levels of albumin, transferrin, and lymphocytes. Attention should also be given to a nutrition regimen with adequate protein, in an effort to achieve positive nitrogen balance. Energy expenditure has been shown to be up to 49% greater than predicted in these patients (Bouffard et al., 1989).

In severe, prolonged pancreatitis, TPN may be necessary. Whether the infusion of lipid emulsion leads to significant pancreatic stimulation remains controversial; however, it appears that patients with mild to moderate stress can tolerate dextrose-based solutions, whereas patients with more severe stress require a mixed fuel system of dextrose and lipid to avoid complications of glucose intolerance. Lipid emulsion should not be included in a TPN regimen if hypertriglyceridemia is the cause of the pancreatitis (Pisters and Ranson, 1992). A serum triglyceride level should be obtained before TPN with lipids is initiated. Lipids may be given to patients with triglyceride values less than 300 mg/dL. Due to the possibility of pancreatic endocrine abnormalities as well as a relative insulin resistance, close glucose monitoring is also warranted. H_2-receptor antagonists may be prescribed to decrease hydrochloric acid production, which will reduce stimulation of the pancreas. Somatostatin is considered to be the best inhibitor of pancreatic secretion and may be added to the TPN solution (Latifi and Dudrick, 1996).

Depressed serum calcium levels are often identified in patients with acute pancreatitis. Possible causes include hypoalbuminemia with subsequent third-spacing of fluid. The calcium, which is bound to the albumin, is thus affected. Another possible explanation is a "soap" formation by the calcium and fatty acids created by the fat necrosis. Checking an ionized calcium level is a method of determining available calcium.

Aggressive nutrition support may also include attempts to use the gastrointestinal tract. Placing a feeding tube into the jejunum beyond the ligament of Treitz and using a hydrolyzed, low-fat formula should be considered in a stable patient as the acute pancreatitis resolves (Kalfarentzos et al., 1997; Ragins et al., 1973). Close observation for patient tolerance is important. Chapter 22 discusses jejunal feedings in detail. When the patient is allowed to eat, supplemental pancreatic enzymes may be needed to treat steatorrhea. See Chapter 37 for a discussion of enzyme use.

Chronic Pancreatitis

In contrast to acute pancreatitis, chronic pancreatitis usually evolves insidiously over many years. Nutrition care for people with chronic pancreatitis involves several other considerations. Chronic pancreatitis is characterized by recurrent attacks of abdominal pain. The pain can be precipitated by meals. Associated nausea, vomiting, or diarrhea make it difficult to maintain adequate nutritional status. In addition, there is an increase in REE; weight loss may result (Hebuterne, 1996). Large meals with high-fat foods and alcohol should be avoided. Supplemental pancreatic enzymes may provide pain relief by decreasing exocrine secretions. When pancreatic function is diminished by approximately 90%, enzyme production and secretion are insufficient. Maldigestion and malabsorption of protein and fat thus become a problem (Holt, 1993). Pancreatic enzyme replacement is mandatory at this time.

Malabsorption of the fat-soluble vitamins may occur in patients with significant steatorrhea. Also, deficiency of pancreatic protease, necessary to cleave vitamin B_{12} from its carrier protein, could potentially lead to vitamin B_{12} deficiency. With appropriate supplemental enzyme therapy, vitamin absorption should be improved; however, the patient should still be monitored periodically for vitamin deficiencies. Water-soluble forms of the fat-soluble vitamins or parenteral administration of vitamin B_{12} may be necessary. (See Chapter 35 for a discussion of B_{12} administration.)

Pancreatic enzyme replacements are given orally with meals; the dosage should be at least 30,000 IU lipase with each meal. To promote weight gain, the level of fat in the diet should be the maximum a patient can tolerate without increased steatorrhea or pain. Additional therapies that may be tried to maintain nutritional status and minimize symptoms in patients with maximal enzyme supplementation include a lower fat diet (40 to 60 g/day) or substitution of some dietary fat with MCT oil to further improve fat absorption and weight gain.

Because pancreatic bicarbonate secretion is frequently defective, medical management may also

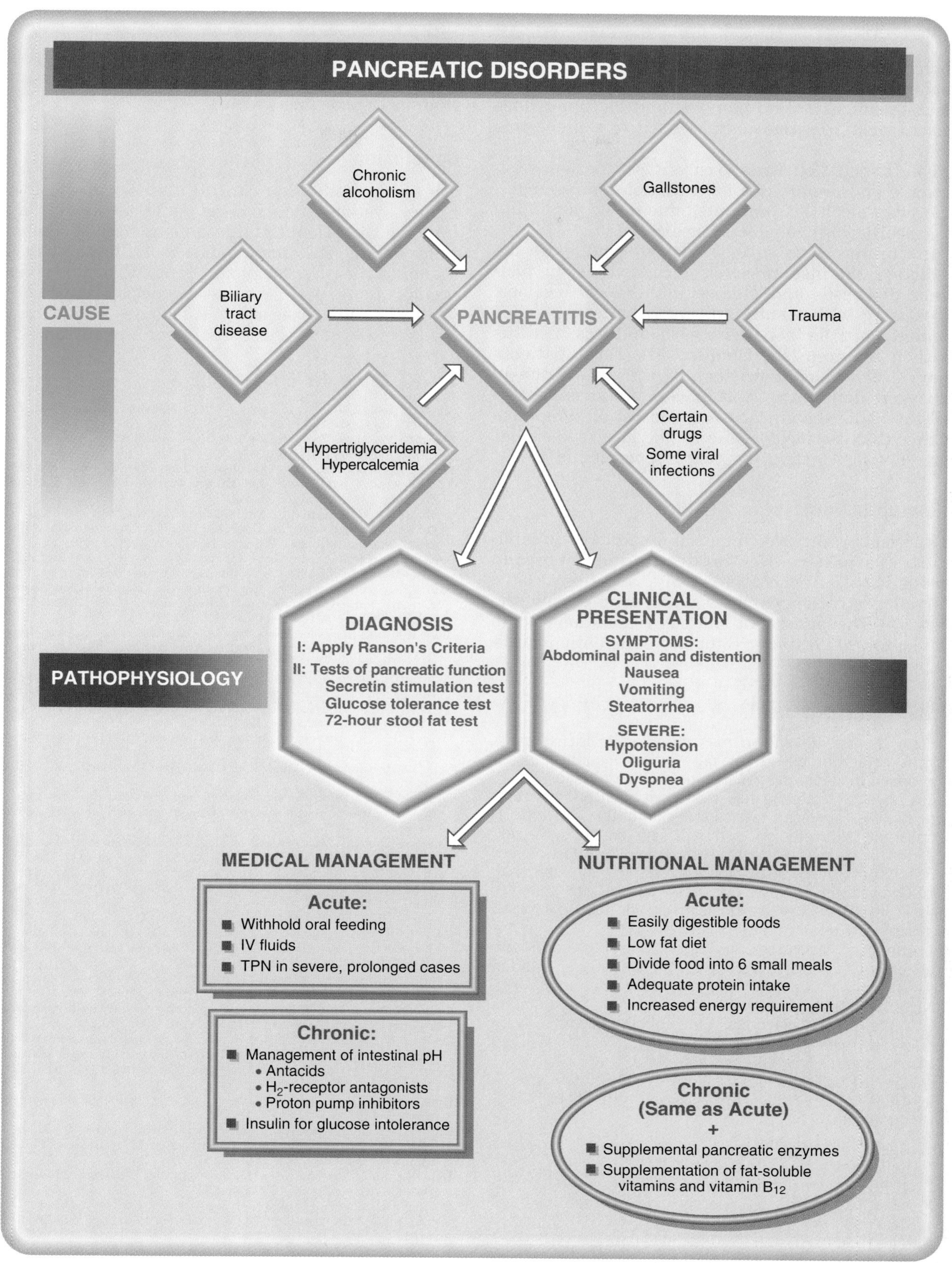

FIGURE 32–9 Pathophysiology algorithm—pancreatic disorders. (Algorithm content developed by John Anderson, Ph.D., and Sanford C. Garner, Ph.D., 2000.)

include maintenance of an optimal intestinal pH to facilitate enzyme activation. Antacids, H_2-receptor antagonists, or proton pump inhibitors that reduce gastric acid secretion may be used to achieve this effect.

Effort should be made to cater to the patient's tolerances and preferences for nutrition management. However, alcohol is prohibited due to the possibility of exacerbating the pancreatic disease.

In chronic cases with extensive pancreatic destruction, the insulin-secreting capacity of the pancreas decreases and glucose intolerance develops. Treatment with insulin and nutrition care similar to that used for a patient with diabetes mellitus is then required (see Chapter 34). These patients may also develop refractory hypoglycemia due to glucagon deficiency (Holt, 1993). Management is delicate and should focus on control of symptoms rather than normoglycemia as the goal (see earlier box, "*Clinical Insight:* Fasting Hypoglycemia").

Pancreatic Surgery

A surgical procedure often used for pancreatic carcinoma is a **pancreaticoduodenectomy (Whipple procedure).** A cholecystectomy, vagotomy, or a partial gastrectomy may also be done during the surgery. The pancreatic duct is reanastamosed to the jejunum. Partial or complete pancreatic insufficiency can result, depending on the extent of the pancreatic resection. Nutrition care is similar to that for chronic pancreatitis.

CASE STUDY

Frank T. is a 40-year-old man admitted to the hospital with chief complaints of right upper quadrant pain, anorexia, nausea, dysgeusia, and frequent loose stools. On physical exam he has mild peripheral edema with a slightly jaundiced appearance. Muscle wasting is apparent. No asterixis is noted. The patient's mental status is clear, but he appears lethargic. There is no history of portal hypertension, ascites, or gastrointestinal bleeding. Muscle wasting is noted along with stomatitis. The patient has a significant alcohol abuse history spanning 15 years.

Abnormal laboratory values include elevated liver enzymes and total bilirubin; serum albumin, 2.5 g/dL; transferrin, 150 mg/dL; megaloblastic anemia profile; NH_3, 55 mmol/L.

A preliminary diagnosis of alcoholic hepatitis with possible mild pancreatic insufficiency is made. On biopsy, steatosis and fibrosis are found.

Nutritional data includes: height, 177.8 cm; weight, 67 kg; IBW, 75 kg ± 10%; UBW, 82 kg (5 years ago), 73 kg (6 months ago).

1. Based on available data, what vitamin or mineral deficiencies may exist?
2. What nutritional therapy would you prescribe?
3. What nutritional parameters are affected by the patient's liver dysfunction?
4. What is Frank's overall nutritional status?
5. What conditions may be leading to his frequent loose stools?
6. What further information would you require or obtain to complete your assessment?

Conclusion

The goal of nutrition care in diseases of the liver, biliary system, and exocrine pancreas should be to improve nutritional status and to support the patient during the acute phases of illness. Understanding the physiology and function of these vital organs along with the pathogenesis that results when they are diseased will decrease patient morbidity and lead to better treatment and outcomes.

CITED REFERENCES

Adam A, Roddi ME. Acute cholecystitis: Radiologic management. Baillieres Clin Gastroenterol 5(4):787,1991.

Akerman PA, et al. Preoperative nutrition assessment in liver transplantation. Nutrition 9(4):350, 1993.

Bacon BR, Brown KE. Iron metabolism and disorders of iron overload. In: Kaplowitz N (ed.). Liver and Biliary Diseases, 2nd ed. Baltimore: Williams & Wilkins, 1996, p. 349.

Bacon BR, et al. Ischemia, congestive failure, Budd-Chiari syndrome, and veno-occlusive disease. In: Kaplowitz N (ed.). Liver and Biliary Diseases, 2nd ed. Baltimore: Williams & Wilkins, 1996, p. 469.

Baker AL. Liver chemistry tests. In: Kaplowitz N (ed.). Liver and Biliary Diseases, 2nd ed. Baltimore: Williams & Wilkins, 1996, p. 207.

Banks PA. Acute and chronic pancreatitis. In: Feldman M, et al. (eds.). Sleisenger and Fordtran's Gastrointestinal and Liver Disease. Philadelphia: WB Saunders, 1998, p. 809.

Bianchi GP, et al. Vegetable versus animal protein diet in cirrhotic patients with chronic encephalopathy: A randomized crossover comparison. J Intern Med 233:385, 1993.

Bonacini M. Liver in systemic diseases. In: Kaplowitz N (ed.). Liver and Biliary Diseases, 2nd ed. Baltimore: Williams & Wilkins, 1996, p. 439.

Bouffard YH, et al. Energy expenditure during severe acute pancreatitis. J Parent Enter Nutr 13:26, 1989.

Brewer G, et al. Does a vegetarian diet control Wilson's disease? J Am Coll Nutr 12:527, 1993.

Calleja GA, Barkin JS. Acute pancreatitis. Med Clin North Am 77:1037, 1993.

Campillo B, et al. Short-term changes in energy metabolism after 1 month of a regular oral diet in severely malnourished cirrhotic patients. Metabolism 44(6):765, 1995.

Caregaro L, et al. Malnutrition in alcoholic and virus-related cirrhosis. Am J Clin Nutr 63:602, 1996.

Carithers RL Jr. Alcoholic hepatitis and cirrhosis. In: Kaplowitz N (ed.). Liver and Biliary Diseases, 2nd ed. Baltimore: Williams & Wilkins, 1996, p. 377.

Corish C. Nutrition and liver disease. Nutr Rev 55(1):17, 1997.

Crippin JS. Monitoring and care of the patient before transplantation. In: Busuttil RW, Klintmalm GB (eds.). Transplantation of the Liver. Philadelphia: WB Saunders, 1996, p. 348.

Davis GL. Chronic hepatitis. In: Kaplowitz N (ed.). Liver and Biliary Diseases, 2nd ed. Baltimore: Williams & Wilkins, 1996, p. 327.

de Beaux AC, et al. Factors influencing morbidity and mortality in acute pancreatitis: An analysis of 279 cases. Gut 37:121, 1995.

De Boer SY, et al. Effect of intravenous fat on cholecystokinin secretion and gallbladder motility in man. J Parent Enter Nutr 16:16, 1992.

Detsky AS, et al. What is subjective global assessment? J Parent Enter Nutr 11:8, 1987.

Diehl AK. Epidemiology and natural history of gallstone disease. Gastroenterol Clin North Am 20:1, 1991.

Diehl AM. Liver disease in the alcoholic: Clinical aspects. In: Zakim D, Boyer TD (eds.). Hepatology: A Textbook of Liver Disease. Philadelphia: WB Saunders, 1996, p. 1050.

Dolz C, et al. Ascites increases the resting energy expenditure in liver cirrhosis. Gastroenterology 100:738, 1991.

Douglas DD, Rakela J. Fulminant hepatitis. In: Kaplowitz N (ed.). Liver and Biliary Diseases, 2nd ed. Baltimore: Williams & Wilkins, 1996, p. 317.

Epstein S, et al. Organ transplantation and osteoporosis. Curr Opin Rheumatol 7:255, 1995.

Everhart J. Contributions of obesity and weight loss to gallstone disease. Ann Intern Med 119:1029, 1993.

Francisco-Ziller N, DiCecco S. Nutritional care of the pretransplant patient. Top Clin Nutr 13(2):1, 1998.

Friedman SL. Cirrhosis of the liver and its major sequelae. In: Bennett JC, Plum F (eds.). Cecil Textbook of Medicine, 20th ed. Philadelphia: WB Saunders, 1996, p. 788.
Gurk-Turner C. Management of the metabolic complications of liver disease: An overview of commonly used pharmacologic agents. Support Line 19(4):17, 1997.
Hager LA. Hepatic complications associated with total parenteral nutrition. Support Line 16(3):1, 1994.
Harrison J, et al. A prospective study on the effect of recipient nutritional status on outcome in liver transplantation. Transplant Int 10:369, 1997.
Hasse J. Role of the dietitian in the nutrition management of adults after liver transplantation. J Am Diet Assoc 91:473, 1991.
Hasse J. Nutritional aspects of adult liver transplantation. In: Busuttil RW, Klintmalm GB (eds.). Transplantation of the Liver. Philadelphia: WB Saunders, 1996, p. 359.
Hasse JM. Diet therapy for organ transplantation. Nurs Clin North Am 32(4):863, 1997.
Hasse JM. Recovery after organ transplantation in adults: The role of postoperative nutrition therapy. Top Clin Nutr 13(2):15, 1998.
Hasse J, et al. Subjective global assessment—Alternative nutritional assessment technique for adult liver transplant candidates. Nutrition 9:330, 1993.
Hasse JM, et al. Early enteral nutrition support in patients undergoing liver transplantation. J Parent Enter Nutr 19:437, 1995.
Hasse J, et al. Nutrition therapy for end-stage liver disease: A practical approach. Support Line 19(4):8, 1997.
Hebuterne X, et al. Resting energy expenditure in patients with alcoholic chronic pancreatitis. Dig Dis Sci 41:533, 1996.
Hirsch S, et al. Controlled trial on nutrition supplementation in outpatients with symptomatic alcoholic cirrhosis. J Parent Enter Nutr 17:119, 1993.
Hiyama DT, Fischer JE. Nutritional support in hepatic failure. Nutr Clin Pract 3:96, 1988.
Holt S. Chronic pancreatitis. South Med J 86:201, 1993.
Hoy M, et al. Reduced risk of liver-function-test abnormalities and new gallstone formation with weight loss on 3350-kj (800-kcal) formula diets. Am J Clin Nutr 60:249, 1994.
Ichida T, et al. Clinical study of an enteral branched-chain amino acid solution in decompensated liver cirrhosis with hepatic encephalopathy. Nutrition 11(suppl 2):238, 1996.
Johnston D, Kaplan M. Pathogenesis and treatment of gallstones. N Engl J Med 328:412, 1993.
Kalfarentzos F, et al. Gallbladder contraction after administration of intravenous amino acids and long-chain triacyglycerols in humans. Nutrition 7:347, 1991.
Kalfarentzos F, et al. Enteral nutrition is superior to parenteral nutrition in severe acute pancreatitis: Results of a randomized prospective trial. Br J Surg 84:1665, 1997.
Kamath PS. Clinical approach to the patient with abnormal liver test results. Mayo Clin Proc 71:1089, 1996.
Katz IA, Epstein S. Posttransplant bone disease. J Bone Miner Res 7:12, 1992.
Kearns PJ, et al. Accelerated improvement of alcoholic liver disease with enteral nutrition. Gastroenterology 102:200, 1992.
Kondrup J, Müller MJ. Energy and protein requirements of patients with chronic liver disease. J Hepatol 27:239, 1997.
LaBrecque DR. Neoplasia of the liver. In: Kaplowitz N (ed.). Liver and Biliary Diseases, 2nd ed. Baltimore: Williams & Wilkins, 1996, p. 391.
Latifi R, Dudrick S. Nutrition support of acute pancreatitis. In: Latifi R, Dudrick S (eds.). Current Surgical Nutrition. New York: Chapman & Hall, 1996, p. 226.
Latifi R, et al. Nutritional support in liver failure. Surg Clin North Am 71:567, 1991.
Leevy CM, Davison E. Portal hypertension and hepatic coma. Postgrad Med J 41:84, 1967.
Liddle RA, et al. Gallstone formation during weight reduction dieting. Arch Intern Med 149:1750, 1989.
Lieber CS. The influence of alcohol on nutritional status. Nutr Rev 46:241, 1988.
Lindor KD, Dickson ER. Primary biliary cirrhosis. In: Kaplowitz N (ed.). Liver and Biliary Diseases, 2nd ed. Baltimore: Williams & Wilkins, 1996, p. 339.
Lindsay KL, Hoofnagle JH. Serologic tests for viral hepatitis. In: Kaplowitz N (ed.). Liver and Biliary Diseases, 2nd ed. Baltimore: Williams & Wilkins, 1996, p. 221.
Maher JJ. Inherited, infiltrative, and metabolic disorders involving the liver. In: Bennett JC, Plum F (eds.). Cecil Textbook of Medicine, 20th ed. Philadelphia: WB Saunders, 1996, p. 785.
Mann DV, et al. Multicentre audit of death from acute pancreatitis. Br J Surg 81:890, 1994.
Marks JW, et al. The sequence of biliary events preceding the formation of gallstones in humans. Gastroenterology 103:566, 1992.
McClain CJ, et al. Trace metals in liver disease. Semin Liver Dis 11:321, 1991.
McCullough AJ, Tavill AS. Disordered energy and protein metabolism in liver disease. Semin Liver Dis 11:265, 1991.
Mendenhall CL, et al. A study of oral nutritional support with oxandrolone in malnourished patients with alcoholic hepatitis: Results of a Department of Veterans Affairs cooperative study. Hepatology 17:564, 1993.
Merli M, et al. Does malnutrition affect survival in cirrhosis? Hepatology 23:1041, 1996.
Mezey E. Interaction between alcohol and nutrition in the pathogenesis of alcoholic liver disease. Semin Liver Dis 11:340, 1991.
Morgan TR, et al. Protein consumption and hepatic encephalopathy in alcoholic hepatitis. J Am Coll Nutr 14:152, 1995.
Mullen KD, Weber FL. Role of nutrition in hepatic encephalopathy. Semin Liver Dis 11(4):292, 1991.
Nielsen K, et al. Long-term oral refeeding of patients with cirrhosis of the liver. Br J Nutr 74:557, 1995.
Nompleggi DJ, Bonkovsky HL. Nutritional supplementation in chronic liver disease: An analytical review. Hepatology 19:518, 1994.
Ockner RK. Acute viral hepatitis. In: Bennett JC, Plum F (eds.). Cecil Textbook of Medicine, 20th ed. Philadelphia: WB Saunders, 1996, p. 762.
Pikul J, et al. Degree of preoperative malnutrition is predictive of postoperative morbidity and mortality in liver transplant recipients. Transplantation 57:469, 1994.
Pisters PWT, Ranson JHC. Nutritional support for acute pancreatitis. Surg Gynecol Obstet 175:275, 1992.
Plauth M, et al. ESPEN guidelines for nutrition in liver disease and transplantation. Clin Nutr 16:43, 1997.
Polonsky K. A practical approach to fasting hypoglycemia. N Engl J Med 326:1020, 1992.
Porayko MK, et al. Impact of malnutrition and its therapy on liver transplantation. Semin Liver Dis 11:305, 1991.
Priori P, et al. Stimulation of gallbladder emptying by intravenous lipids. J Parent Enter Nutr 21(6):350, 1997.
Ragins H, et al. Intrajejunal administration of an elemental diet at neutral pH avoids pancreatic stimulation: Studies in dog and man. Am J Surg 126:606, 1973.
Ranson JH, et al. Prognostic signs and the role of operative management in acute pancreatitis. Surg Gynecol Obstet 139:69, 1974.
Riely CA. Liver diseases of pregnancy. In: Kaplowitz N (ed.). Liver and Biliary Diseases, 2nd ed. Baltimore: Williams & Wilkins, 1996, p. 483.
Seeff LB. Acute viral hepatitis. In: Kaplowitz N (ed.). Liver and Biliary Diseases, 2nd ed. Baltimore: Williams & Wilkins, 1996, p. 289.
Shronts EP, Fish J. Hepatic failure. In: Gottschlich MM, et al. (eds.). Nutrition Support Dietetics—Core Curriculum. Silver Spring, MD: A.S.P.E.N., 1993, p. 311.
Sokol RJ. Copper storage diseases. In: Kaplowitz N (ed.). Liver and Biliary Diseases, 2nd ed. Baltimore: Williams & Wilkins, 1996, p. 363.
Steinberg W, Tenner S. Acute pancreatitis. N Engl J Med 330:1198, 1994.
te Boekhorst T, et al. Etiological factors of jaundice in severely ill patients. J Hepatol 7:111, 1988.
Vierling JM. Hepatobiliary complications of ulcerative colitis and Crohn's disease. In: Zakim D, Boyer TD (eds.). Hepatology: A Textbook of Liver Disease. Philadelphia: WB Saunders, 1996, p. 1366.
Weisiger RA. Laboratory tests in liver disease. In: Bennett JC, Plum F (eds.). Cecil Textbook of Medicine, 20th ed. Philadelphia: WB Saunders, 1996, p. 759.
Weseman RA, McCashland TM. Nutritional care of the chronic posttransplant patient. Top Clin Nutr 13(2):27, 1998.
Whitington PF. Metabolic liver diseases of childhood. In: Kaplowitz N (ed.). Liver and Biliary Diseases, 2nd ed. Baltimore: Williams & Wilkins, 1996, p. 511.

ADDITIONAL REFERENCES

Banks PA. Modern concepts in pancreatitis. Mount Sinai J Med 60:170, 1993.
Hasse JM, et al. Solid organ transplantation. In: Gottschlich MM, et al. (eds.). Nutritional support in acute pancreatitis. Gastroenterol Clin North Am 18:525, 1989.
Kondrup J, et al. Nutritional therapy in patients with liver cirrhosis. Am J Clin Nutr 46:239, 1992.
Kalfarentzos FE, et al. Total parenteral nutrition in severe acute pancreatitis. J Am Coll Nutr 10:156, 1991.
Kern F. Effects of dietary cholesterol on cholesterol and bile acid homeostasis in patients with cholesterol gallstones. J Clin Invest 93:1186, 1994.
Lebenthal E, et al. Enzyme therapy for pancreatic insufficiency: Present status and future needs. Pancreas 9:1, 1994.
Lieber CS. Herman Award lecture, 1993: A personal perspective on alcohol, nutrition, and the liver. Am J Clin Nutr 58:430, 1993.
Matarese LE, Shronts EP (eds.). Nutrition Support Dietetics—Core Curriculum. Silver Springs, MD: A.S.P.E.N., 1993.
Runyon B. Care of patients with ascites. N Engl J Med 330:337, 1994.
Schneeweiss B, et al. Energy metabolism in patients with acute and chronic liver disease. Hepatology 11:387, 1990.

CHAPTER 33

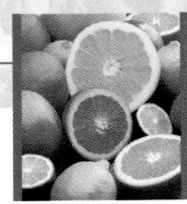

Medical Nutrition Therapy for Metabolic Stress: Sepsis, Trauma, Burns, and Surgery

MARION F. WINKLER, MS, RD, CNSD
AND SUSAN MANCHESTER, RD, CNSD

CHAPTER OUTLINE

Key Terms

ACUTE-PHASE PROTEINS—secretory proteins in the liver, concentrations of which are altered in response to injury or infection; positive acute-phase proteins, C-reactive protein, α_1-antitrypsin, and fibronectin are increased; negative acute-phase proteins, immunoglobulin G and M, complement, prealbumin, transferrin, ceruloplasmin, and albumin are decreased

ADRENOCORTICOTROPHIC HORMONE (ACTH) OR CORTICOTROPIN—a hormone secreted by the anterior pituitary gland that acts primarily on the adrenal cortex, stimulating its growth and secretion of corticosteroids

BACTERIAL TRANSLOCATION—morphologic changes resulting from acute insult to the gastrointestinal tract that allows entry of bacteria from the gut lumen to the body and initiates a systemic inflammatory response that may contribute to multiple organ dysfunction syndrome

CATECHOLAMINES—hormones released by the adrenal medulla in response to shock and a higher glucagon/insulin ratio; stimulate hepatic glycogenolysis, fat mobilization, and gluconeogenesis; include epinephrine and norepinephrine

CYTOKINES—proinflammatory proteins released by macrophages that acts as a mediator of shock, multiple organ dysfunction syndrome, and sepsis; examples include tumor necrosis factor, interleukin-1, interleukin-6

EBB PHASE—initial response to bodily insult characterized by lower blood pressure, cardiac output, body temperature, and oxygen consumption associated with hypovolemia, hypoperfusion, and lactic acidosis

FLOW OR ADAPTIVE PHASE—a neuroendocrine response to physiologic stress that follows the ebb phase and is characterized by hypermetabolism and hypercatabolism

GLASCOW COMA SCALE (GCS)—system for determining the degree of neurologic insult and a patient's level of consciousness by assessing responses to eye opening and motor and verbal response

GLUTAMINE—an amino acid that is the preferential fuel for enterocytes in the gut mucosa, especially during stress; it enhances cell mass and height of the mucosal villi

GROWTH HORMONE—an anabolic agent mediated by insulin-like growth factor 1 (IGF-1); thought to accelerate growth in children and improve protein synthesis in injured patients

GUT-ASSOCIATED LYMPHOID TISSUE (GALT)—a component of the gut intestinal mucosal barrier that may provide protection against multiple organ dysfunction syndrome; contains 40% of the immune effector cells in the body

INTERLEUKIN-1—a cytokine mediator induced by tumor necrosis factor (TNF) and produced by endothelial cells and monocytes; induces fever by stimulating prostaglandin production

MULTIPLE ORGAN DYSFUNCTION SYNDROME (MODS)—organ dysfunction resulting from direct injury or trauma, disease, or in response to inflammation; the response usually is in an organ remote from the original site of infection or injury

SEPSIS—the systemic response to an identifiable infectious agent

SEPTIC SHOCK—a severe form of sepsis with hypotension, hypoperfusion, lactic acidosis, oliguria, and an acute change in mental status

SHORT-CHAIN FATTY ACIDS (SCFA)—by-products of dietary fiber fermentation in the colon that have beneficial effects on the gastrointestinal tract; include proprionate, acetate and butyrate

STRUCTURED LIPID—fat composed of a rearranged triglycerides containing both medium- and long-chain fatty acids; may improve hepatic protein synthesis and reduce protein catabolism and energy expenditure

SYSTEMIC INFLAMMATORY RESPONSE SYNDROME (SIRS)—the sepsis syndrome that occurs without evidence of invasive bacterial or fungal infection; can result in multiple organ dysfunction syndrome

TUMOR NECROSIS FACTOR—a cytokine produced by activated cells, Kupffer cells in the liver, and macrophages that is stimulated by endotoxin, bacteria, virus, and fungal infection; initiates an inflammatory response; stimulates skeletal muscle catabolism

---

Trauma from motor vehicle accidents, gunshots, stab wounds, falls, and burns is a major cause of death and disability. It is the leading cause of death for persons from 1 to 44 years of age and the third leading cause of death for persons of all ages, following cardiovascular disease and cancer. Injury results in profound metabolic alterations beginning at the time of injury and persisting until wound healing and recovery are complete. Whether the event is sepsis (infection), trauma (including burns), or surgery, once the systemic response is activated, the physiologic and metabolic changes that follow are similar (Fig. 33–1). Variability in the response is related in part to the patient's age, previous state

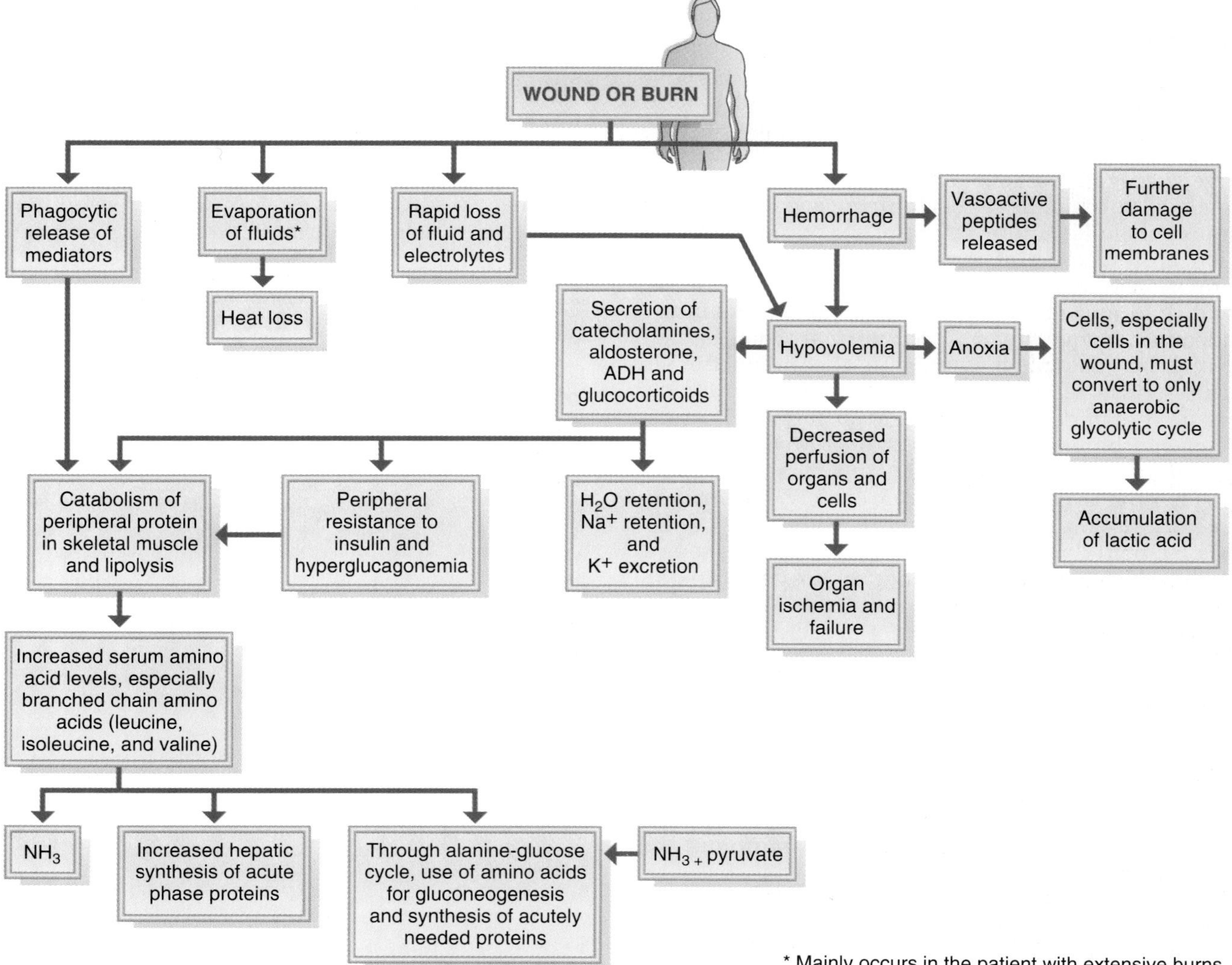

FIGURE 33–1 Physiologic and metabolic changes immediately after an injury or burn. The extent of these changes depends on the severity of the trauma. ADH, antidiuretic hormone; NH_3, ammonia.

TABLE 33–1 CHARACTERISTICS OF METABOLIC PHASES OCCURRING AFTER SEVERE INJURY

EBB PHASE RESPONSE	FLOW PHASE	
	Acute Response	Adaptive Response
Hypovolemic shock	*Catabolism predominates*	*Anabolism predominates*
↓ tissue perfusion ↓ metabolic rate ↓ oxygen consumption ↓ blood pressure ↓ body temperature	↑ glucocorticoids ↑ glucagon ↑ catecholamines Release of cytokines, lipid mediators Production of acute phase proteins ↑ excretion of nitrogen ↑ metabolic rate ↑ oxygen consumption Impaired utilization of fuels	Hormonal response gradually diminishes ↓ hypermetabolic rate Associated with recovery Potential for restoration of body protein Wound healing depends in part on nutrient intake

(Source: Enteral Nutrition Support in Critical Care. Ross Products Division, Abbott Laboratories, 1994. Permission obtained.)

of health, preexisting disease, type of infection, and presence of multiple organ dysfunction syndrome.

METABOLIC RESPONSE TO STRESS

The metabolic response to critical illness, traumatic injury, sepsis, burns, or major surgery is complex and involves most metabolic pathways. This state is characterized by an accelerated catabolism of lean body or skeletal mass that clinically results in negative nitrogen balance and muscle wasting. The goals of nutritional support during sepsis and after injury include minimization of starvation, prevention or correction of specific nutrient deficiencies, provision of adequate calories to meet energy needs, and fluid and electrolyte management to maintain adequate urine output and normal homeostasis. Nutrition also plays a role in the production of acute-phase reactants and other secretory proteins, wound healing, and the support of cellular host defense mechanisms. It is important to recognize that the provision of nutritional support alone cannot abolish the hypermetabolic response and the subsequent muscle breakdown seen in acute injury or illness. Critically ill patients who are injured, septic, or bedridden cannot be expected to gain weight, lean body mass, or strength until the source of hypermetabolism is treated or corrected and physical therapy or exercise is begun.

The response to critical illness, injury, and sepsis characteristically involves both the ebb and flow phases (Cuthbertson, 1979) (Table 33–1). The **ebb phase,** occurring immediately following injury, is associated with hypovolemia, shock, and tissue hypoxia. Typically, this phase is manifested by decreased cardiac output, oxygen consumption, and body temperature. Insulin levels fall in direct response to the increase in glucagon, most likely as a signal to increase hepatic glucose production (Souba and Wilmore, 1994). The **flow phase,** which follows fluid resuscitation and restoration of oxygen transport, is characterized by increased cardiac output, oxygen consumption, body temperature, energy expenditure, and total body protein catabolism. Physiologically, a marked increase occurs in glucose production, free fatty acid release, circulating levels of insulin, **catecholamines,** glucagon, and cortisol. The magnitude of hormonal response appears to be associated with the severity of the injury.

Hormonal and Cell-Mediated Response

Metabolic stress is associated with an altered hormonal state that results in increased flow of substrate but poor utilization of carbohydrate, protein, fat, and oxygen (Table 33–2). Counter-regulatory hormones, which are elevated after injury and sep-

TABLE 33–2 METABOLIC RESPONSES DURING SEPSIS

ORGAN	RESPONSE
Liver	↑ glucose production ↑ amino acid uptake ↑ acute-phase protein synthesis ↑ trace metal sequestration
Central Nervous System	Anorexia Fever
Circulation	↑ glucose ↑ triglycerides ↓ amino Acids ↑ urea ↓ iron ↓ zinc
Skeletal muscle	↑ amino acid efflux (especially glutamine), leading to loss of muscle mass
Intestine	↓ amino acid uptake from both luminal and circulating sources, leading to gut mucosal atrophy
Endocrine	↑ ACTH ↑ cortisol ↑ growth hormone ↑ epinephrine ↑ norepinephrine ↑ glucagon ↑ insulin (usually)

(From Michie HR. Metabolism of sepsis and multiple organ failure. World J Surg 20:461, 1996.)

sis, play a role in the accelerated proteolysis that is characteristically seen. Glucagon promotes gluconeogenesis, amino acid uptake, ureagenesis, and protein catabolism. Cortisol, which is released from the adrenal cortex in response to stimulation of **adrenocorticotropic hormone,** enhances skeletal muscle catabolism and promotes hepatic utilization of amino acids for gluconeogenesis, glycogenolysis and acute-phase protein synthesis. After injury or sepsis, energy production becomes increasingly protein dependent. Branched-chain amino acids (BCAA; leucine, isoleucine, and valine) are oxidized from skeletal muscle as a source of nitrogen, energy for the muscle, and carbon skeletons for the glucose alanine cycle and muscle **glutamine** synthesis. The fate of amino acid generation from muscle catabolism is shown in Figure 33–2.

The mobilization of **acute-phase proteins** results in rapid loss of lean body mass and an increased negative nitrogen balance, which continues until the cause of the stress is relieved. Breakdown of protein tissue also causes increased urinary losses of potassium, phosphorus, and magnesium.

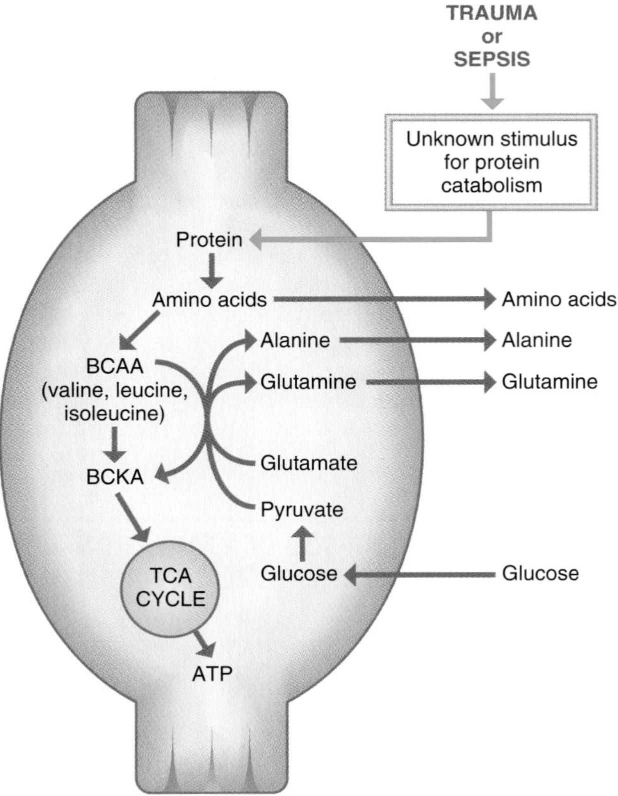

FIGURE 33–2 Skeletal muscle proteolysis. Breakdown of skeletal muscle protein leads to increases in amino acid levels. Amino acids are transaminated with glutamate or pyruvate to form alanine and glutamine. The muscle preferentially uses branched-chain amino acids (BCAA) for energy through transamination with the formation of branched-chain ketoacids (BCKA), which can enter the tricyclic acid (TCA) cycle for energy production. (From Simmons RL, Steed DL. Basic Science Review for Surgeons. Philadelphia: WB Saunders, p. 120, 1992.)

Lipid metabolism is also altered in stress and sepsis. There is an increased circulation of free fatty acids thought to result from increased lipolysis due to elevated catecholamines and cortisol as well as a marked elevation in the ratio of glucagon to insulin. The free fatty acids can be oxidized and used to form ketones, which provide energy to non–glucose-dependent tissues, or to resynthesize triglyceride.

Most notable is the hyperglycemia observed during stress. This initially results from a marked increase in glucose production and uptake secondary to gluconeogenesis, and elevated levels of hormones including epinephrine that diminish insulin release. Stress also initiates the release of aldosterone, a corticosteroid that causes renal sodium retention, and antidiuretic hormone (ADH), which stimulates renal tubular water resorption. The action of these hormones results in conservation of water and salt and support of the circulating blood volume.

The response to injury is also regulated by metabolically active **cytokines** such as **interleukin-1** (IL-1), interleukin-6 (IL-6), and **tumor necrosis factor** (TNF), which are released by phagocytic cells in response to tissue damage, infection, inflammation, and some drugs and chemicals. The involvement of cytokines in response to injury is illustrated in Figure 33–3. Cytokines are thought to stimulate hepatic amino acid uptake and protein synthesis, accelerate muscle breakdown, and induce gluconeogenesis. IL-1 appears to have a major role in stimulating the acute-phase response. This includes fever, leukocytosis, skeletal muscle proteolysis, and acute-phase protein synthesis (Bessey, 1993). As part of the acute-phase response, serum iron and zinc levels also decrease and levels of ceruloplasmin increase primarily due to sequestration and in the case of zinc, increased urinary zinc excretion. The net effect of the hormonally and cell-mediated response is an increase in oxygen supply and a greater availability of substrates for metabolically active tissues.

STARVATION VERSUS STRESS

The metabolic response to stress differs from starvation as depicted in Figure 33–4, as do the changes that occur in energy and nutrient utilization (Table 33–3). Starvation is characterized by decreased energy expenditure, utilization of alternative fuel sources, and decreased protein wasting. The response to chronic inadequate food intake is adaptive, aimed at preserving lean body mass. Stored glycogen, the primary fuel source in early starvation, is depleted in about 24 hours. After the depletion of glycogen, glucose is available from the breakdown of protein to amino acids. The depressed glucose levels lead to decreased insulin secretion and an increase in glucagon. Unlike the stressed state, counter-regulatory hormones such as catecholamines, cortisol, and growth hormone are not

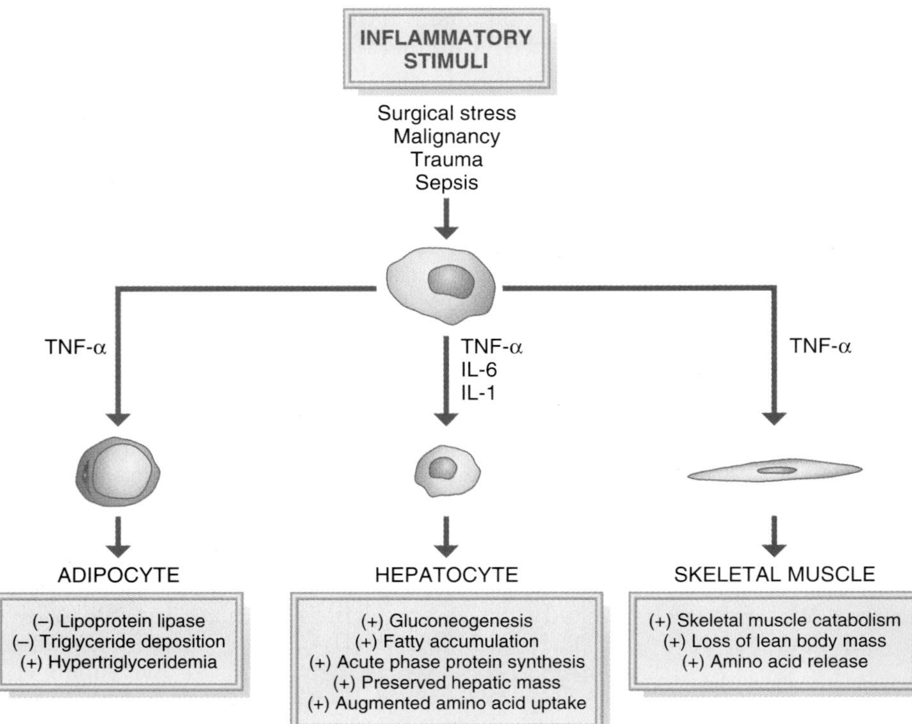

FIGURE 33–3 The involvement of cytokines in response to injury response. (From Espat NJ, et al. Cytokines, inflammation, and nutrition. Support Line XVI(1):2, 1994.)

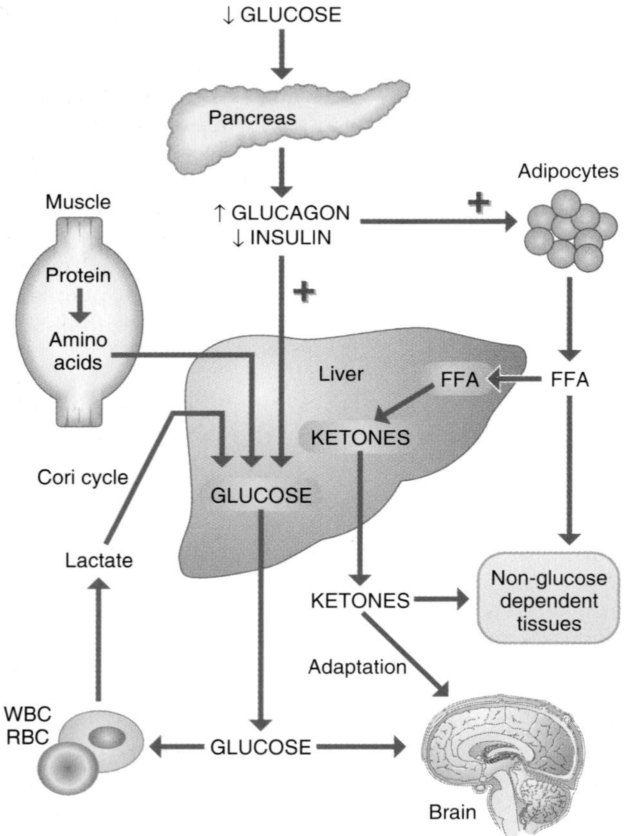

FIGURE 33–4 Metabolic changes in starvation. FFA, free fatty acids; RBC, red blood cells; WBC, white blood cells. (From Simmons RL, Steed DL. Basic Science Review for Surgeons. Philadelphia: WB Saunders, p. 118, 1992.)

elevated. In late starvation, fatty acids, ketones, and glycerol provide the energy source for all tissues except the glucose-obligated brain, nervous system, and red blood cells. During the adaptive state of starvation, protein catabolism is reduced and hepatic gluconeogenesis decreases. Lipolytic activity is also different in starvation and in stress. After 1 week of fasting or food deprivation, a state of ketosis develops in which ketones constitute an effective substitute for glucose, thus reducing the need for gluconeogenesis and conserving body protein to the greatest possible extent. In late starvation as in

TABLE 33–3 COMPARISON OF STARVATION AND STRESS HYPERMETABOLISM*

	STARVATION	STRESS HYPERMETABOLISM
Resting energy expenditure	Decreased	Increased
Respiratory quotient	(0.6–0.7)	(0.8–0.9)
Mediator activation	—	+++
Primary fuels	Fat	Mixed
Proteolysis	+	+++
Branched-chain oxidation	+	+++
Hepatic protein synthesis	+	+++
Ureagenesis	+	+++
Urinary nitrogen loss	+	+++
Gluconeogenesis	+	+++
Ketone body production	++++	+

(Source: Barton RG. Nutrition support in critical illness. Nutr Clin Pract 9:127, 1994. With permission.)

*Patients fall in a continuum between the extremes of starvation and stress hypermetabolism.

stress, ketone body production is increased and fatty acids serve as a major energy source.

SYSTEMIC INFLAMMATORY RESPONSE SYNDROME (SIRS)/MULTIPLE ORGAN DYSFUNCTION SYNDROME (MODS)

The term **systemic inflammatory response syndrome (SIRS)** is the preferred terminology to describe the widespread inflammation that can occur in infection, pancreatitis, ischemia, burns, multiple trauma, hemorrhagic shock, and immunologically mediated organ injury (Bone, 1992). The inflammation is usually present in areas remote from the primary site of injury and affects otherwise healthy tissue. Each condition leads to release of cytokines, proteolytic enzymes, or toxic oxygen species and activation of the complement cascade. The term **sepsis** is used when a patient has a documented infection and an identifiable organism. Bacteria and their toxins lead to a stronger inflammatory response. Other microorganisms that lead to an inflammatory response include viruses, fungi, and parasites. The diagnosis for SIRS is made according to the following criteria: body temperature above 38° C or less than 36° C; heart rate more than 90 beats/min; respiratory rate greater than 20 breaths/min (tachypnea) or $PaCO_2$ of less than 32 mm Hg (hyperventilation); white blood cell count above 12,000/mm^3 or less than 4,000/mm^3 or the presence of more than 10% bands (immature neutrophils) in the absence of chemotherapy induced neutropenia and leukopenia (Bone et al., 1992). The diagnosis of sepsis is made when SIRS is present and there is documentation of infection.

A frequent complication of SIRS is the development of **multiple organ dysfunction syndrome (MODS).** The syndrome generally begins with lung failure followed by failure of the liver, intestine, and kidney. Hematologic and myocardial failure usually manifest later; however, central nervous system changes can occur at any time in the syndrome (Deitch, 1992). MODS can be primary, the direct result of injury to an organ from trauma. Examples of primary MODS include pulmonary contusion, renal failure due to rhabdomyolysis, or coagulopathy from multiple blood transfusions (Bone, 1992). Secondary MODS occurs in the presence of inflammation or infection in organs remote from the initial injury (Fig. 33–5). Clinically, patients with SIRS/MODS are hypermetabolic and exhibit high cardiac output, low oxygen consumption, high venous oxygen saturation, and lactic acidemia. Patients generally have a strong positive fluid balance associated with massive edema and a decrease in plasma protein concentrations.

Multiple hypotheses have been proposed to explain the development of SIRS/MODS. In some animal models and clinical studies, SIRS leading to MODS appears to be mediated by excessive production of proinflammatory cytokines and other mediators of inflammation. Much of the research has focused on trying to understand what triggers this mediator production. The gut hypothesis suggests that the trigger is injury or disruption of the gut barrier function with corresponding translocation of enteric bacteria into the mesentary lymph nodes, liver, and other organs (Fig. 33–6).

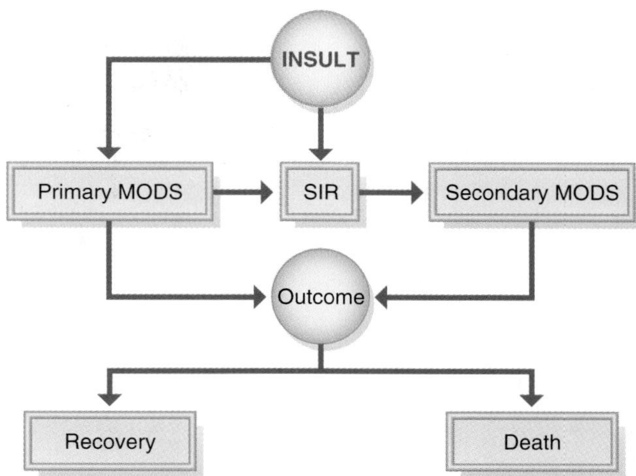

FIGURE 33–5 The different causes and results of primary and secondary multiple organ dysfunction syndrome (MODS). SIR, systemic inflammatory response. (From Bone RC, et al. ACCP/SCCM Consensus Conference: Definitions for sepsis and organ failure and guidelines for the use of innovative therapies in sepsis. Chest 101:1644, 1992.)

A major component of the gut barrier is the **gut-associated lymphoid tissue (GALT)** which contains 40% of the immune effector cells in the body. (Langkamp-Henken, 1992). However, circulating endotoxins, which are easily detectable early after injury, and increased cytokine activity did not correlate with the development of SIRS, sepsis, or death in burn and trauma patients (Kelly et al., 1997). Studies of gut decontamination using oral antibiotics have failed to consistently eliminate endotoxin or affect clinical outcome (Reynolds, 1996). Enteral feeding, on the other hand, restores gut function and influences the clinical course. Although the mechanism is not entirely known, enteral nutrition may act at several levels by altering antigen exposure, modulating splanchnic immune responses, enhancing mucosal protection, or influencing oxygenation and blood supply to the mucosa (Reynolds, 1996).

It is thought that poor gut function associated with parenteral nutrition or the lack of enteral stimulation might be due to an exaggerated cytokine response due to loss of intestinal barrier function (Swank, Deitch, 1996). Alterations in intestinal gut barrier function associated with malnutrition are thought to occur through intestinal weight loss and villous atrophy, yet at least one study found normal gastrointestinal morphology by biopsy in both malnourished and well-nourished patients (Reynolds, 1996). The presence of one or more antibodies (IgG and β-lactoglobulin) more strongly correlated with the degree of malnutrition.

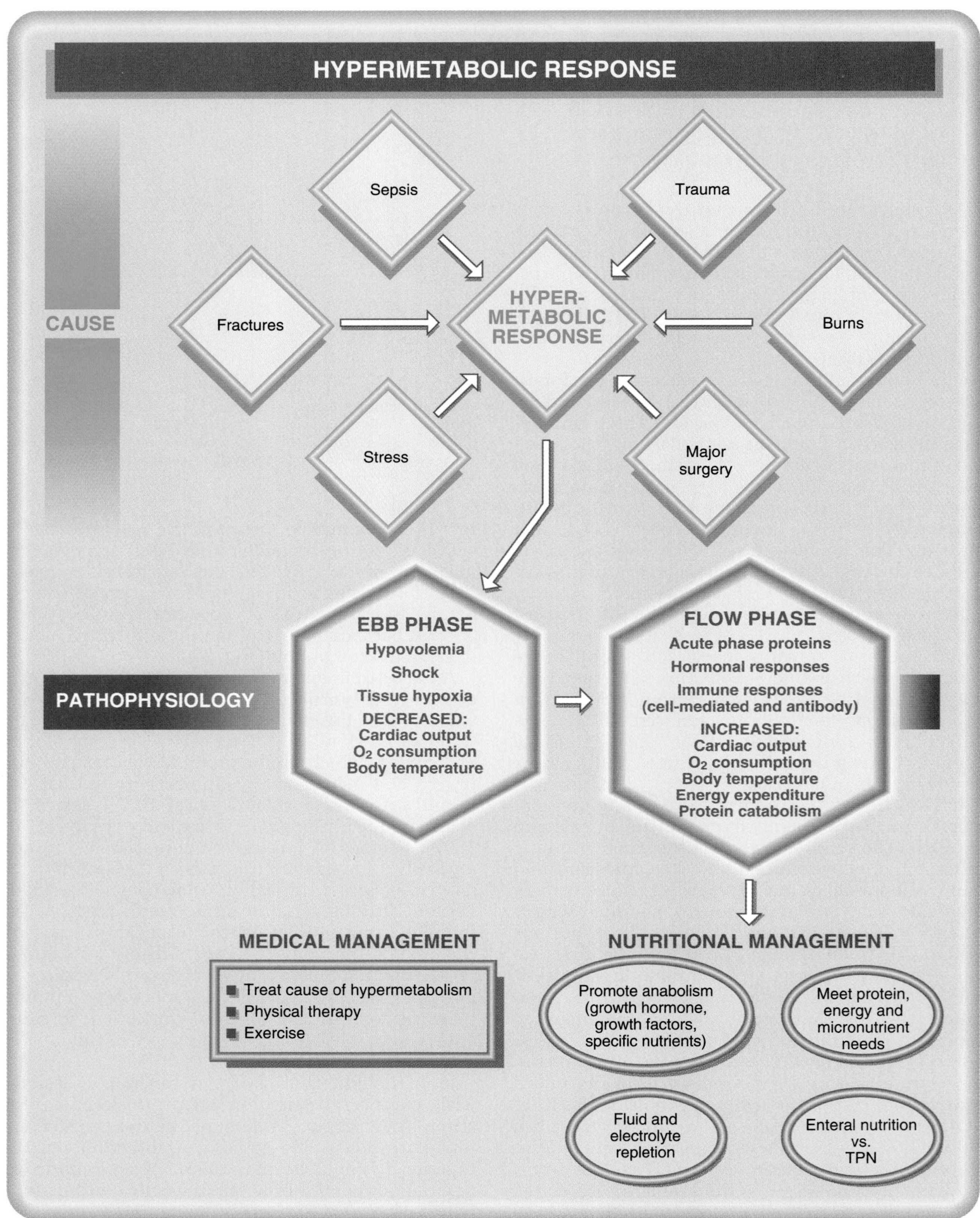

FIGURE 33–6 Pathophysiology algorithm—hypermetabolic response to stress. (Algorithm content developed by John Anderson, Ph.D., and Sanford C. Garner, Ph.D., 2000.)

Much of the current research does suggest that the route of nutrient delivery is important in the prevention and treatment of **bacterial translocation** (Fig. 33–7), the movement of bacteria from the gut lumen to the body. Because enteral feeding maintains the villous height and brush border enzymes, feedings may be better tolerated when initiated promptly while this absorptive area remains intact. It has been stated that the greatest impact of the current focus on the gut hypothesis is a better understanding of normal gastrointestinal flora in host defense and an evolving awareness of the role of enteral nutrients in the maintenance of optimal metabolic homeostasis (Marshall and Girotti, 1995). Future research will likely focus on questions that try to answer: does enteral nutrition truly modulate gut barrier function in humans or is tube feeding tolerance simply a marker of a healthy intestine? (Reynolds, 1996); and are specialized formulas that are believed to enhance immune status helpful in preventing septic complications in trauma patients? (Richardson, 1998).

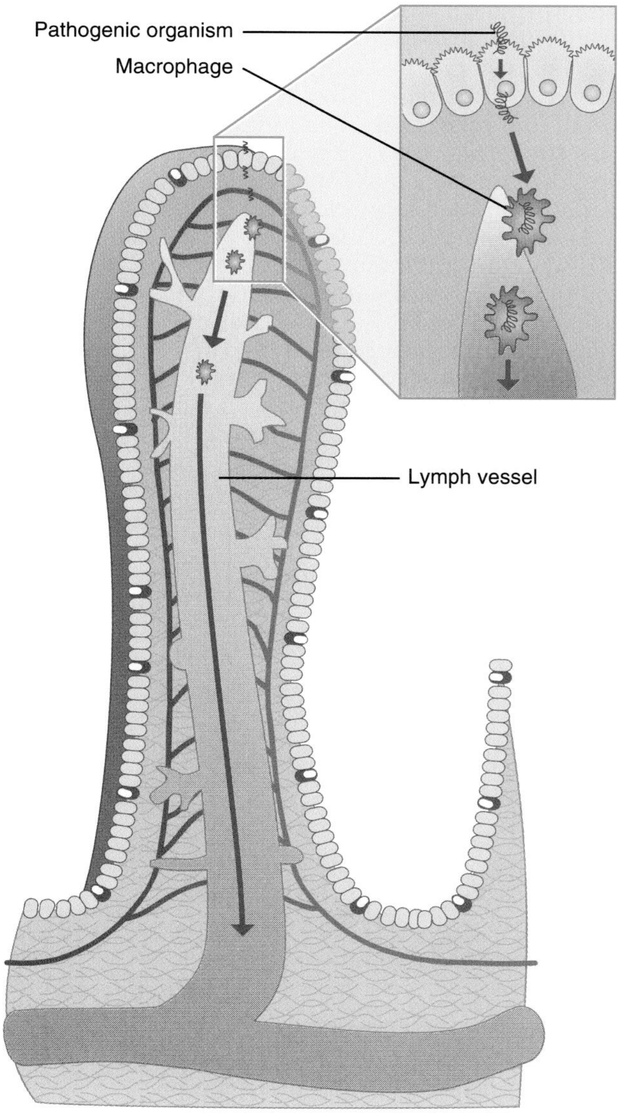

FIGURE 33–7 Bacterial translocation across microvilli and how it spreads into the bloodstream.

Nutritional Assessment

Traditional methods of assessing nutritional status are often of limited value in the critical care setting. The severely injured patient is typically unable to provide a dietary history, values for weight may be erroneous following fluid resuscitation, anthropometic measurements are not sensitive to acute changes, and plasma protein concentrations are affected by the stress response, independent of nutritional status. Urine urea nitrogen (UUN) excretion in grams per day has been used to evaluate the degree of hypermetabolism, with a UUN value of 0 to 5 corresponding with normometabolism, 5 to 10 with mild hypermetabolism or level 1 stress, 10 to 15 with moderate hypermetabolism or level 2 stress, and greater than 15 with a severe hypermetabolic state or level 3 stress (Blackburn et al., 1977; Cerra et al., 1984). Because of the difficulties in conducting a nutritional assessment in a critically ill patient, clinical judgment must play a major role in deciding when to offer nutritional support. The ability to predict the clinical course and when the patient will resume adequate oral food intake are key components of this process (Pomp et al., 1988).

The objectives of optimal metabolic and nutritional support in injury, trauma, burns, or sepsis are to (1) detect and correct preexisting malnutrition; (2) prevent progressive protein calorie malnutrition; and (3) optimize the patient's metabolic state by managing fluid and electrolytes (ASPEN Board of Directors, 1993). The first emphasis of care is fluid resuscitation and the removal of the inflicting stress through wound repair, abscess drainage, burn wound debridement and grafting, or treatment of infection. Nutritional support should begin as soon as the patient is hemodynamically stable (vital functions are stable, fluid and electrolyte and acid–base balance are achieved, and tissue perfusion is adequate to allow transport of oxygen and fuel). Nutritional support during the catabolic phase will probably not result in positive nitrogen balance, but it may slow the loss of body protein. However, undernutrition can lead to inadequate protein synthesis, weakness, and eventually MODS or death.

DETERMINATION OF NUTRIENT REQUIREMENTS

Energy

It is now generally recognized that injured hypermetabolic patients do not require the massive caloric loads that were once thought appropriate

(Barton and Cerra, 1991; Elwyn, 1980). Although it is essential to provide adequate energy to metabolically stressed patients, excess calories could result in complications such as hyperglycemia, hepatic steatosis, and excess carbon dioxide production, which can exacerbate respiratory insufficiency or potentially prolong weaning from mechanical ventilation. Persistent hyperglycemia can also lead to a glucose-obligated diuresis, which may make fluid and electrolyte management more complicated.

Energy requirements can be estimated using the Harris-Benedict equation (see Chapter 2) and an appropriate stress factor applied. Because it is important to avoid overfeeding the critically ill stressed patient, it may be prudent to add a factor for stress of 1.3. Once the patient is hemodynamically stable and is ambulating or undergoing rehabilitation, caloric delivery can be in a higher anabolic range. Energy requirements can also be estimated at 25 to 30 nonprotein calories per kilogram per day (ASPEN Board of Directors, 1993). (See "*Clinical Insight:* Estimating Energy and Protein Requirements.") Either method may overestimate the caloric requirements of mechanically ventilated and sedated patients in whom neuromuscular paralysis may decrease energy requirements in even septic patients by as much as 30%.

The use of indirect calorimetry provides a better evaluation of the energy expenditure of the critically ill hypermetabolic patient. Trauma patients have significantly greater elevations in measured energy expenditure than nontrauma patients; however, the magnitude of increase does not often exceed 30% above the predicted value (Winkler et al., 1988). It is also possible to derive energy expenditure from oxygen consumption data when a pulmonary artery catheter is in place for hemodynamic monitoring. Samples of arterial and mixed venous blood gases, cardiac output measurements, and hemoglobin concentration are needed.

When designing a parenteral nutrition formulation, glucose is the primary caloric substrate. The maximum rate of glucose oxidation is approximately 5 to 7 mg/kg/min or 7.2 g/kg/day (Wolfe et al., 1979). Part of this glucose load is provided endogenously via gluconeogenesis. Carbohydrate should constitute approximately 60% to 70% of the nonprotein calories. Insulin should be administered to maintain blood glucose levels at less than 220 mg/dL (ASPEN Board of Directors, 1993). Fat provides the remainder of the nonprotein calories, at about 15% to 40% of the calories. Fat is used not only to prevent essential fatty acid deficiency, but to meet the elevated energy requirements, particularly in the presence of glucose intolerance. Recent reports have cautioned against the use of intravenous fat emulsion in stressed and trauma patients. Fatty acids have been shown to modulate the immune response both in experimental and clinical settings (Grimm et al., 1994).

The proposed mechanisms for fat emulsion induced immunosuppression include: blocking of the reticuloendothelial system by particles in the emulsion (Seidner et al., 1989), altered production of metabolites due to changes in the availability of fatty acid precursors, altered cell membrane composition, and increased oxygen-free radical production (Grimm et al., 1994). Lipid-induced alterations in immune function may further compromise the immunosuppressed state associated with major injury by leading to MODS. A recent study compared T-cell function in trauma patients who were randomized to receive total parenteral nutrition (TPN) with and without lipids (Battistella et al., 1997). In this study carbohydrate content was kept the same so TPN differed in the calorie content and one group received a hypocaloric regimen. Results demonstrated that the lipid group had a significantly longer period of mechanical ventilation, intensive care unit stay, and hospitalization. Patients in the lipid group had an average of 2.4 infections per patient, primarily pneumonia, compared to 1.4 infections per patient in the group receiving no lipids. Although the increased incidence in infection may be due to the prolonged course of mechanical venti-

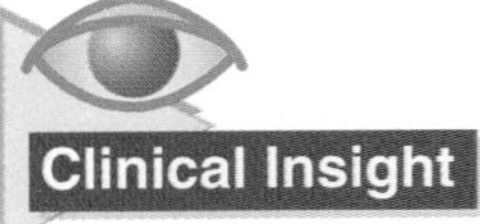

Estimating Energy and Protein Requirements

A 64-year-old man underwent surgery for a ruptured colonic diverticulum. He developed an intra-abdominal abcess that drained through the wound, and he had repeated temperature spikes. On x-ray, an ileus was noticed. Physical examination revealed an edematous, toxic-appearing patient with a poorly healing abdominal wound. His preoperative weight was 147 lb (67 kg), and his height 5′9″ (180 cm).

1. Using the Harris-Benedict Equation:

   BEE (male) = 66.47 + 13.75 (W) + 5 (H) − 6.76 (age) = 1455 kcal

2. Using an injury factor of 1.3 to account for surgical stress and sepsis:

   1455 kcal × (1.3) = 1892 kcal
   Nonprotein calorie:nitrogen ratio 100:1
   (1892/100 = 18.92 g N × 6.25 g = 118 g protein)

3. Using the ASPEN guidelines:

   25–30 nonprotein kcal/kg = 1675–2010 kcals
   1.5–2.0 g protein/kg = 100–134 g

lation, the authors do conclude that the intravenous fat emulsion was associated with a prolonged depression in T-cell function and therefore prolonged the postinjury immune dysfunction and increased the patient's susceptibility to infection.

Protein

Amino acids are supplied to critically ill patients as part of the total nutritional regimen, to support the synthesis of proteins required for defense and recovery, to spare lean body mass, and to reduce the amount of endogenous protein catabolism for gluconeogenesis. The optimal protein requirement for critically ill patients is 1.5 to 2.0 g/kg/day (ASPEN Board of Directors, 1993). The suggested nonprotein calorie/gram of nitrogen ratio for critically ill patients is 100:1 (Bessey, 1990). There appears to be no advantage in providing excessive protein in terms of protein-sparing activity or in promoting nitrogen balance in septic patients. Providing exogenous amino acids does not alter the catabolic state, but it does decrease the characteristic negative nitrogen balance by supplying the liver with substrates for protein synthesis and subsequently reducing the need for endogenous proteins from peripheral tissue (Gilder, 1986). BCAA have been shown to be reduced in the plasma of humans following injury or sepsis. Clinically, BCAA-enriched nutrition solutions have been associated with improved nitrogen retention, improved hepatic protein synthesis, decreased protein degradation, and achievement of nitrogen equilibrium in less time (Cerra et al., 1987).

Vitamins, Minerals, and Trace Elements

No specific guidelines exist for the provision of vitamins, minerals, and trace elements in metabolically stressed individuals. Some evidence indicates that vitamin requirements of critically ill, stressed patients may be higher than in nonstressed individuals (Winkler and Albina, 1990). With increased caloric intake there may be an increased need for B vitamins, particularly thiamine and niacin. Catabolism and loss of lean body tissue increase the loss of potassium, magnesium, phosphorus, and zinc. Gastrointestinal and urinary losses, organ dysfunction, and acid–base imbalance necessitate that mineral and electrolyte requirements be determined and adjusted individually. Fluid and electrolytes should be provided to maintain adequate urine output and normal serum electrolytes. One recent study demonstrated increased urinary excretion of copper, zinc, and selenium in injured patients (Berger et al., 1996). Copper levels normalized quickly and this was explained by ceruloplasmin being an acute phase protein, but zinc excretion remained high resulting in prolonged depressed serum zinc levels. Because of zinc losses via the gastrointestinal tract and its role in wound healing, it may be prudent to supplement zinc in acutely injured patients. The hypozincemia is thought to be due to the acute-phase response, hemodilution (zinc is bound to albumin), and incompletely replaced blood and enteric losses.

NUTRITIONAL CARE PLAN

The preferred route for nutrient delivery is an oral diet. However, critically ill patients are often unable to eat because of endotracheal intubation and ventilator dependence. Furthermore, oral feeding may be delayed by impairment of chewing, swallowing, or anorexia induced by pain-relieving medications or post-traumatic shock and depression. Patients who are able to eat may not be able to meet the increased energy and nutrient requirements associated with metabolic stress and recovery, and often require oral nutritional supplements or enteral tube nutrition. When enteral nutrition fails to meet nutritional requirements, or when gastrointestinal feeding is contraindicated, parenteral nutritional support should be initiated (Fig. 33–8).

Timing and Route of Feeding

Successful enteral nutrition for surgical or stressed patients may require access to the small bowel. Although critically ill patients are presumed to be at a higher risk of aspiration due to conditions such as respiratory insufficiency, gastric dysmotility, or neuromuscular paralysis, recent studies in surgical patients have demonstrated that the rate of aspiration in patients fed into the stomach or small bowel is not significantly different (Fox et al., 1995). Gastric motility is usually impaired for 12 to 24 hours after laparotomy, whereas a colonic ileus may last up to 5 days. Generally, small bowel motility returns within 4 to 6 hours postoperatively.

Consideration should be given to placing an enteric feeding tube if the patient is expected to be unable to consume food by mouth for an extended period. Tubes can be placed under x-ray guidance, endoscopically, or intraoperatively into the stomach or small bowel (see Chapter 22). Initially, patients with multiple intestinal injuries, small bowel ileus, high-output intestinal fistulas, severe pancreatitis, or other severe intestinal insults may require TPN. However, because of the demonstrated benefits of early enteral nutrition, tube feedings can often be administered simultaneously at low rates to maintain gut integrity (Zaloga et al., 1992). This allows adequate nutrient delivery while helping to preserve the intestinal mucosa.

Although early enteral feeding has proven benefits, it is still important to wait until the patient is hemodynamically stable before beginning. There are differences in anaerobic metabolism during shock and following resuscitation, and the aggressive delivery of enteral nutrients in a state of intestinal hypoperfusion may result in increased intestinal ischemia and necrosis (Tappenden et al., 1998).

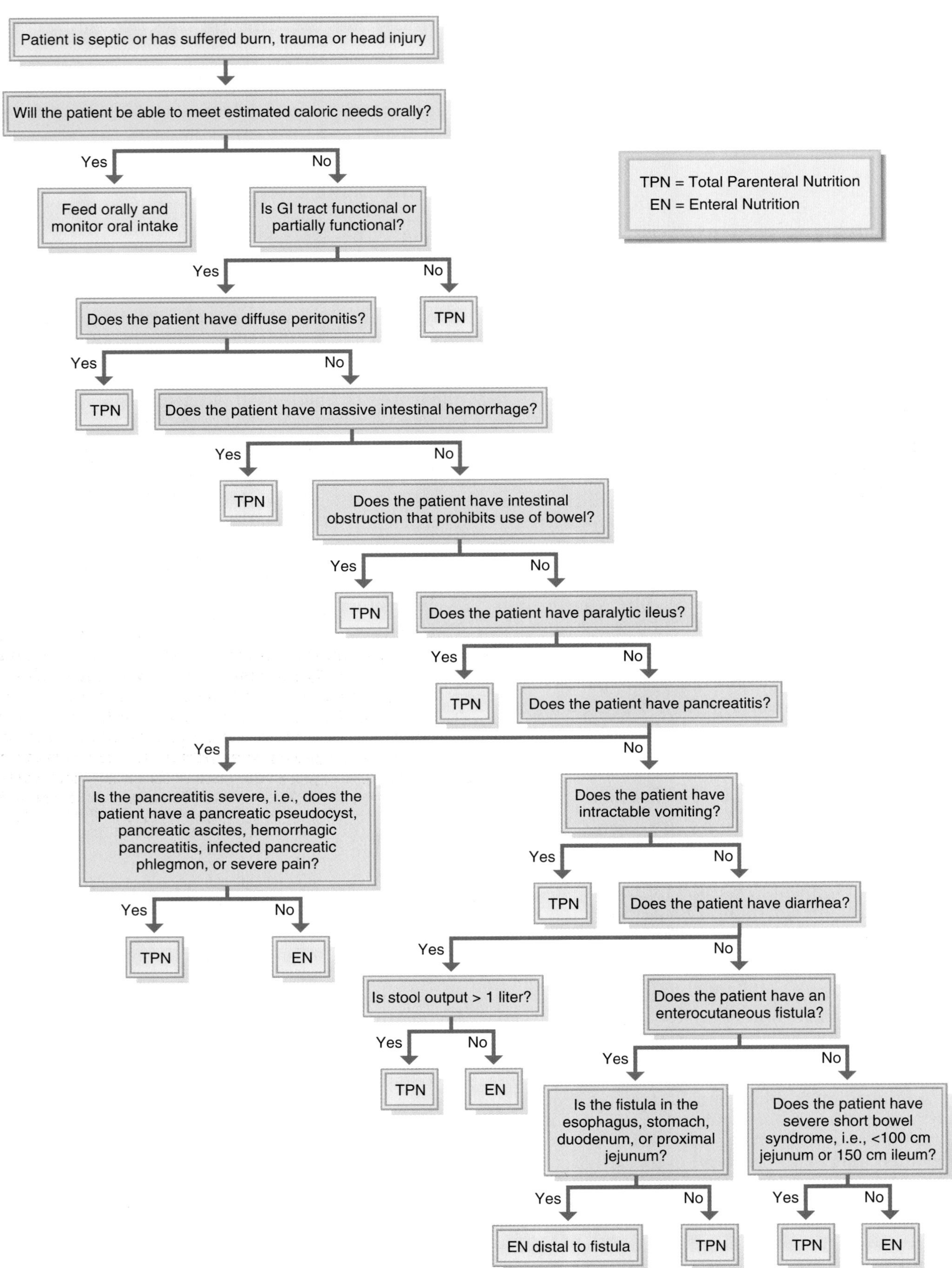

FIGURE 33–8 Determining route of nutrition support in the critically ill. (From The ASPEN Nutrition Support Practice Manual. Silver Spring, MD: ASPEN, p. 18-6, 1998.)

Product Selection

Choosing an enteral product should be based on fluid, energy, and nutrient requirements as well as gastrointestinal function. Most standard polymeric enteral formulas can be used to feed the critically ill patient. The ratio of nonprotein calories to nitrogen in these products ranges from approximately 100:1 to 150:1. Some critically ill patients demonstrate intolerance to standard diets, because of the fat content of the formula, and temporarily require a lower fat diet or a product containing a higher ratio of medium-chain triglycerides. Several commercially available products are marketed specifically for trauma and metabolic stress. These products typically have a nonprotein calorie/nitrogen ratio of 100:1 and a higher ratio of BCAA or additional glutamine or arginine (see Appendices 35–40).

In addition to the simple presence of food in the gut, specific substances such as glutamine, short-chain fatty acids, and fiber have been investigated for their role in maintaining the intestinal mucosa. Figure 33–9 depicts glutamine metabolism and demonstrates its uptake by the kidney and the intestine as a preferential fuel for enterocytes. It has been suggested that a glutamine deficiency develops during critical illness and negatively affects gut health. Parenteral nutrition formulations have not traditionally contained glutamine because of instability in the solution and, as a result, TPN has been thought to contribute to this deficiency. Glutamine supplementation of TPN solutions has been shown to partially reverse mucosal atrophy, attenuate the reduction of intestinal immunoglobulin A, and improve upper respiratory immunity to influenza virus in mice (Li, 1997). Other animal studies comparing glutamine-rich versus glutamine-free diets do not demonstrate structural changes in the gastrointestinal mucosa (Wusteman et al., 1995). When glutamine is supplemented in the diets of patients who have short bowel syndrome or who have undergone bone marrow transplantation, improved clinical outcomes have been documented (Byrne et al., 1995).

Dietary fiber is known to maintain colonic integrity. The colonic fermentation of fiber and other nondigestible carbohydrates produces **short-chain fatty acids (SCFA)** (proprionate, acetate and butyrate). These substances are readily absorbed and trophic to the colonocyte, stimulate water and sodium absorption, and may provide a significant source of calories. Much of the experimental work has focused on whether SCFA could improve im-

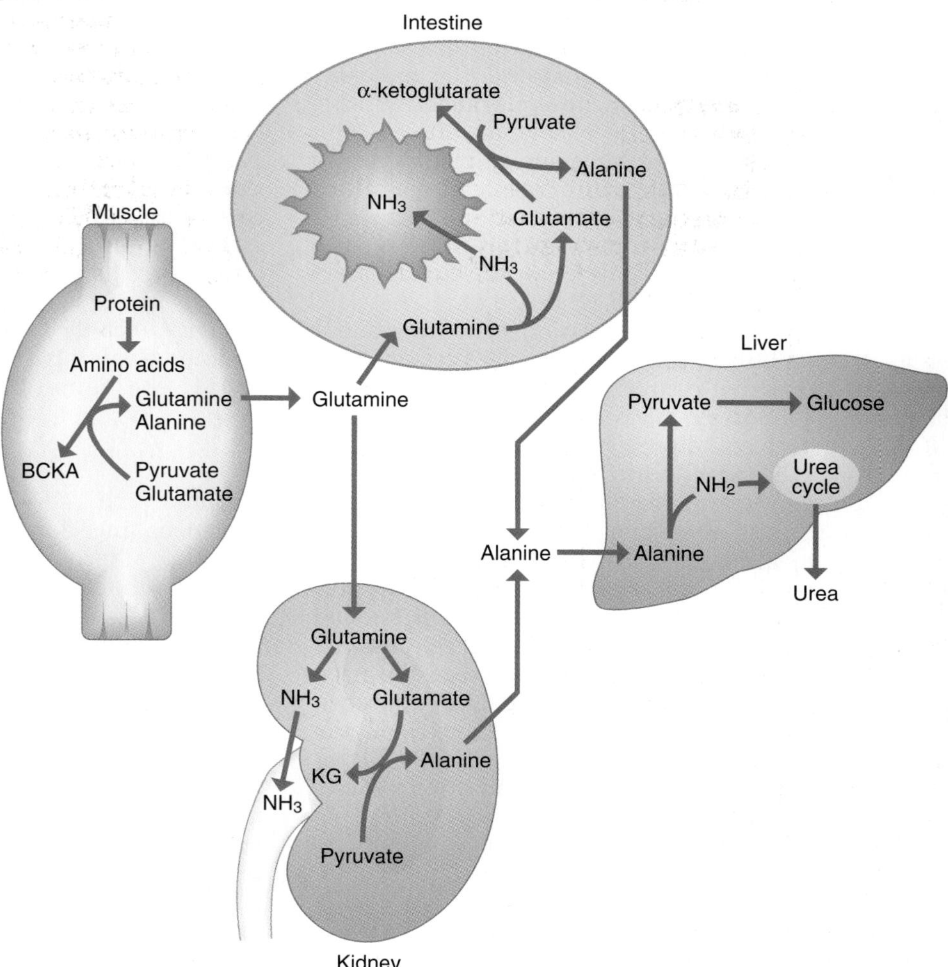

FIGURE 33–9 Glutamine metabolism. Glutamine is generated by skeletal muscle from glutamate by transamination. Glutamine is taken up by the intestine and kidney, where deamination and ammonia elimination occur. The glutamate formed is transaminated with pyruvate to form alanine, which goes to the liver for gluconeogenesis, and α-ketoglutarate (KD), which can be used for energy production by the muscle or kidney. NH_2, amine; NH_3, ammonia. (From Simmons RL, Steed DL. Basic Science Review for Surgeons. Philadelphia: WB Saunders, p. 122, 1992.)

munocompetence by maintaining the gastrointestinal mucosal barrier in patients with intestinal atrophy and immunosuppression (Koruda et al., 1986). SCFA resulting from dietary fiber fermentation in the colon or added as a supplement to TPN have been shown in rats to prevent the TPN-associated mucosal atrophy (Tappenden et al., 1997) and improve nonspecific immunity after small bowel resection (Pratt et al., 1996). It is not known whether the effects of SCFA are through stimulation of gastrointestinal growth factors or direct action on the enterocyte (Tappenden et al., 1996).

Promoting Anabolism

Combinations of anabolic hormones, growth factors and specific nutrients have been used to enhance nutritional support and modify the metabolic response to trauma and critical illness. **Growth hormone** stimulates growth, antagonizes the action of insulin, and has lipolytic activity. In trauma patients with low growth hormone levels, the administration of human growth hormone has been shown to improve protein and fat metabolism (Jeevanandam et al., 1992). The use of human growth hormone was also associated with improved nitrogen balance and normalization of plasma free amino acid levels in hypermetabolic and acute trauma patients (Jeevanandam et al., 1995). Patients with severe short bowel syndrome receiving growth hormone, glutamine, and a modified oral diet have enhanced nutrient absorption and marked improvement in bowel function (Byrne et al., 1995). The administration of growth hormone to mechanically ventilated patients with acute respiratory failure promotes marked nitrogen retention and increased fat-free mass and total body water, yet these results are not accompanied by improved muscle strength or shortened ventilator days (Pichard et al., 1996).

Growth hormone administration with nutritional support could have a role in improving protein economy and enhancing recuperation in the face of catabolic illness related to *insulin-like growth factor-1 (IGF-1)* (Young and Persinger, 1994). Clinical findings associated with growth hormone therapy include hyperglycemia, insulin resistance, and mild sodium and fluid retention. There is also at least one reported announcement by a manufacturer of growth hormone, that therapy in a large multicenter European trial may be associated with a twofold higher mortality in intensive care unit patients (Ziegler, 1998). These findings underscore the need to carefully evaluate clinical trials and appropriately apply the results to practice. Caution in the use of growth hormone therapy in critically ill patients in intensive care units is currently warranted.

HEAD INJURY

Patients with *traumatic brain injury (TBI)* are severely hypermetabolic and catabolic. The more severe the head injury, the greater is the release of catecholamines (norepinephrine and epinephrine) and cortisol and the hypermetabolic response. Although most brain-injured patients are well nourished before injury, without aggressive nutritional support, rapid loss in lean body mass and immunosuppression can occur. With evidence that neurons are capable of regenerating, it becomes even more crucial to provide an environment conducive for repair (Ott and Young, 1991). The **Glascow Coma Scale (GCS)** is a frequently used tool for quantifying a patient's state of consciousness. A score of 14 to 15 indicates minor head injury, 9 to 13 corresponds to moderate injury, and a score of less than 8 reflects severe injury (Hester, 1993).

Energy Requirements

Most studies show that the measured energy expenditure in patients with TBI is about 40% greater than predicted by the Harris-Benedict equation (Hadley et al., 1986; Ott and Young, 1991). Patients with GCS of 4 to 5 often have the highest energy expenditure. Brain-dead patients, or those receiving sedatives, barbiturates, or musculoskeletal blocking agents, often have lower than predicted energy expenditures, averaging about 14% less (Hester, 1993; Ott and Young, 1991). Although the hypermetabolism of head-injured patients was thought to be related to steroid administration, recent evidence shows this is not true (Konvolinka, Morell, 1991). The use of indirect calorimetry is helpful in determining the caloric requirements of these patients, because over- or underfeeding can be harmful. A study comparing predictive formulas like the Harris-Benedict equation to measured energy expenditure determined by indirect calorimetry demonstrated significant discrepancies (Sunderland and Heilbrun, 1992). In the absence of indirect calorimetry, energy requirements should be estimated for patients with TBI using the Harris-Benedict equation and applying a stress factor of 1.4 (Annis et al., 1991) (see Chapter 2).

Protein Requirements

Patients with TBI will probably be in a negative nitrogen balance for 2 to 3 weeks, regardless of the quantity of protein provided (Annis et al., 1991). Steroid administration can further increase urinary nitrogen losses during the first 6 days after the injury (Greenblatt et al., 1989), but then nitrogen losses remain similar regardless of steroid administration (Annis et al, 1991; Robertson et al., 1985). The administration of BCAA may aid in restoring plasma amino acid profiles and improving nitrogen balance (Ott and Young, 1991). Protein requirements are generally estimated at 1.5 to 2.2 g/kg of body weight (Hester, 1993). Provision of more protein results in a heightened nitrogen excretion (Hadley et al., 1986). An adequate amount of nonprotein calories is essential for protein sparing. Because achieving early nitrogen equilibrium is very difficult, minimizing catabolism is paramount.

Vitamins, Minerals, and Fluid

Although the requirements for vitamins and minerals are not well established for brain-injured individuals, studies have shown decreases in plasma levels of many B vitamins and vitamin C. Urinary zinc excretion increases significantly during stress and serum zinc levels are often low. Because salt-wasting occasionally occurs in the brain-injured patient, treatment may consist of restricting fluids, providing additional sodium, or both. Additionally, osmotic dehydration may be performed to control cerebral swelling.

Methods of Nutritional Support

Brain injured individuals are often unable to take oral nutrition. However, patients with a GCS greater than 12 are usually able to consume food (Ott and Young, 1991). Thirty percent or more of brain-injured patients experience dysphagia. The impairment can be physiologic or cognitive. These individuals may have a delayed or absent swallowing reflex, reduced lingual control, prolonged oral transit time, reduced pharyngeal peristalsis, or laryngeal incompetence. Patients may be easily distracted, which greatly prolongs mealtime and results in inadequate intake. Conversely, some brain injured patients eat rapidly, consuming excessive amounts of food, and even nonfood items (Wood, 1990). Early nutritional support is essential. In addition to providing adequate nutrition, early enteral feeding may help blunt the stress response by decreasing the intestinal permeability to toxins, which could otherwise stimulate the release of toxic inflammatory mediators (Annis et al., 1991). Furthermore, prompt use of the gut should maintain the intestinal absorptive area. Patients frequently experience impaired gastric emptying, which hinders the ability to feed via a nasogastric or gastrostomy tube. Access to the small bowel has allowed for successful enteral feeding in many instances, and parenteral and enteral nutritional support are frequently combined.

MAJOR BURNS

Major burns result in severe trauma. Energy requirements can increase as much as 100% above resting energy expenditure (REE), depending on the extent and depth of the injury (Fig. 33–10). This hypermetabolism is accompanied by exaggerated protein catabolism and increased urinary nitrogen excretion. Protein is also lost through the burn wound exudate. Burn patients are particularly susceptible to infection, and this markedly increases requirements for both energy and protein. Because patients with major burns may develop an ileus (loss of intestinal peristalsis or lack of effective coordinated peristalsis) and are anorectic, nutritional support can be a real challenge.

Fluid and Electrolyte Repletion

The first 24 to 48 hours of treatment for thermally injured patients are devoted to fluid and electrolyte replacement. A variety of formulas have been developed to calculate the volume of resuscitation fluid needed. Most agree that half of the calculated vol-

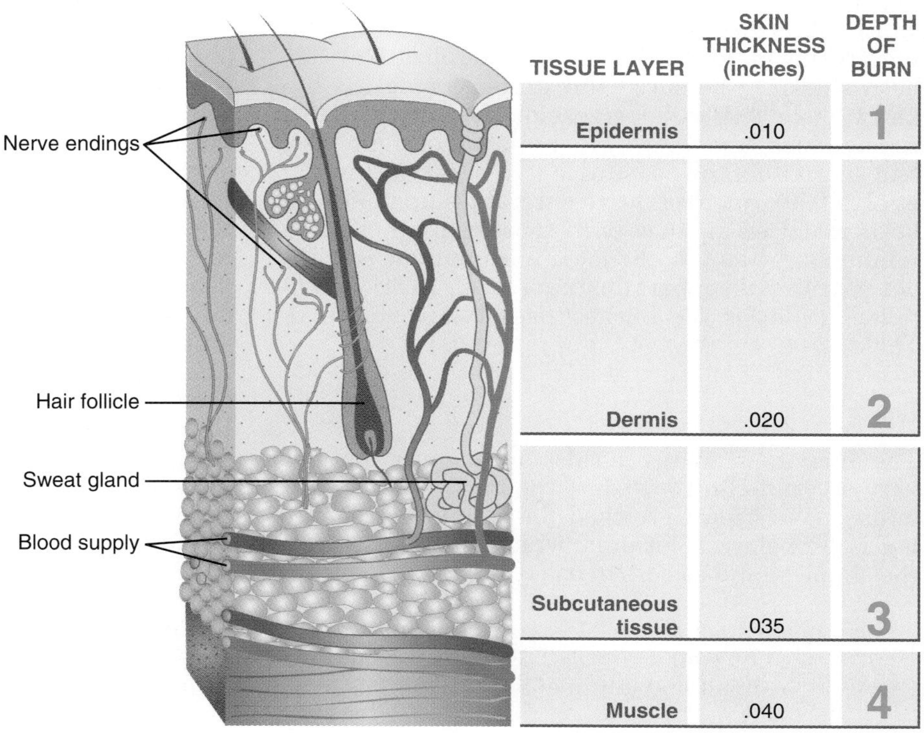

FIGURE 33–10 Interpretation of burn classification based on damage to the integument.

ume for the first 24 hours be given during the first 8 hours, because this is the period of greatest intravascular loss.

The volume of fluid needed is based on the age and weight of the patient and the extent of the burn. Variations of a standard known as the Lund and Browder chart (Herndon et al., 1985; Lund and Browder, 1944) can be used to determine the percentage of total body surface area (TBSA) burned. Once resuscitation is complete, ample fluids must be given to cover both maintenance requirements and evaporative losses that continue through open wounds. Evaporative water loss can be estimated at 2.0 to 3.1 mL/kg of body weight per 24 hours per % TBSA burn. Serum sodium, osmolar concentrations, and body weight are used to monitor fluid status. Providing adequate fluids and electrolytes as early as possible after injury is paramount for maintaining circulatory volume and preventing ischemia (Warden, 1992).

Wound Management

Wound management depends on the depth and extent of the burn. Current surgical management promotes early debridement, excision, and grafting. Energy expenditure may be reduced slightly by the practice of covering wounds as early as possible to reduce evaporative heat and nitrogen losses and to prevent infection.

Nutritional Care

Along with early wound coverage and infection control, nutritional support is recognized as one of the most significant aspects of care for the burned patient. Wound healing can occur only in an anabolic state. Feeding should be initiated soon after resuscitation is complete. In fact, very early enteral feeding (within 4 to 12 hours of hospitalization) has been shown to be successful in decreasing the hypercatabolic response, decreasing the release of catecholamines and glucagon, reducing weight loss, and shortening the hospital length of stay (Chiarelli et al., 1990). Intraoperative enteral feeding has also been practiced at some burn centers in an effort to minimize the length of time a burn patient is without nutritional support (Jenkins et al., 1994). Nutritional goals for the burned patient are shown in Table 33–4.

Energy

The increased energy needs of the burn patient vary according to the size of the burn. Various formulas have been developed for estimating energy needs. The Curreri formula, which follows, is one of the simplest and easiest to use (Curreri, 1979):

kcal needed per day = 24 kcal × kg usual body weight + 40 kcal × % TBSA burned
(using a maximum of 50% burn)

TABLE 33–4 NUTRITIONAL CARE GOALS FOR BURNED PATIENTS

1. Minimizing metabolic response by:
   - controlling environmental temperature
   - maintaining fluid and electrolyte balance
   - controlling pain and anxiety
   - covering wounds early
2. Meeting nutritional needs by:
   - providing adequate calories to prevent weight loss of greater than 10% of usual body weight
   - providing adequate protein for positive nitrogen balance and maintenance or repletion of circulating proteins
   - providing vitamin and mineral supplementation as indicated
3. Preventing Curling's ulcer by:
   - providing antacids or continuous enteral feedings

Once burns exceed 50% to 60% TBSA, minimal increases in energy expenditure occur (Waymack and Herndon, 1992). Some formulas do not establish an upper limit to the number of kilocalories required. When these formulas are used, it should be noted that the maximum caloric load that the body can handle is approximately 100% above resting metabolic expenditure (2 × REE) (Cunningham et al., 1989). The measurement of metabolic rate by indirect calorimetry has confirmed that the Curreri formula exceeds actual energy expenditure (Saffle et al., 1990).

Additional calories may be required to meet the needs of fever, sepsis, multiple trauma, or the stress of surgery. Although weight gain may be desirable for the severely underweight patient, this is generally not feasible until after the acute illness. Weight maintenance should be the goal for overweight patients until the healing process is complete. Obese individuals may be at higher risk of wound infection and graft disruption. The energy requirement for the obese burned person is probably more than that calculated when ideal body weight is used, but less than that calculated when actual body weight is used. Indirect calorimetry is the most accurate method of determining the energy needs of the obese patient (Gottschlich, 1993).

An accurate formula for calculating the nutritional needs of the pediatric burn patient remains to be developed. Because basic requirements depend on the stage of growth and development, it is difficult to provide a formula to cover all age groups. Commonly used, the Galveston formula estimates the caloric requirements equal to 1800 kcal/m^2 + 2200 kcal/m^2 of burn (Waymack and Herndon, 1992). For children less than 3 years old, the Polk formula estimates calorie needs at (60 kcal × kg weight) + (35 kcal × % burn) (Gottschlich, 1993).

Energy Sources

Carbohydrates are excellent for protein-sparing. However, even though carbohydrate is recommended as the chief energy source in burn patients, there appears to be a maximum glucose load of 7 mg/kg/min above which glucose is not oxidized, but rather is converted to fat (Wolfe et al., 1979). This state of lipogenesis causes increased oxygen consumption and carbon dioxide production. Excessive carbohydrate can aggravate hyperglycemia, causing osmotic diuresis, dehydration, and respiratory difficulty.

Although lipids are a concentrated source of calories, high levels of lipids may cause deleterious immunologic responses and increased susceptibility to infections (Gottschlich et al., 1990). The composition of the lipid is important because diets high in ω-3 fatty acids may result in improved immune response and in tube feeding tolerance (Alexander and Gottschlich, 1990). The ω-3 fatty acids inhibit the production of prostaglandin E_2 and leucotrienes, which have immunosuppressive properties. The administration of a low-fat nutrition solution, both enterally and parenterally, results in less pneumonia, improved respiratory function, faster recovery of nutritional status, and a 21-day shorter length of care (Garrel et al., 1995). A reasonable approach is to begin by limiting lipid to 15% to 20% of the nonprotein calories, giving attention to indicators of immune function, feeding tolerance, and serum triglycerides before higher amounts are used (Gottschlich, 1993).

Both medium-chain triglycerides and **structured lipids** are currently under investigation. Medium-chain triglycerides are theoretically preferentially oxidized, leaving little tendency for deposition in adipose tissue, or clogging of the reticuloendothelial system of the mitochondria (Tredget and Yu, 1992). See box, "*Focus On:* Advantages of Medium-Chain Triglycerides" in Chapter 22. Structured lipids may improve hepatic protein synthesis and reduce protein catabolism and energy expenditure.

Protein

The protein needs of burned patients are elevated because of losses through urine and wounds, increased use in gluconeogenesis, and wound healing. Recent evidence promotes the use of high-protein feeding. Provision of 20% to 25% of total calories as protein of high biologic value is suggested (Gottschlich, 1993). It is generally agreed that the protein need for thermally injured children is higher than the recommended dietary allowance. Feeding 2.5 to 3.0 g protein per kilogram of body weight has been suggested (Cunningham et al., 1990). The ability of pediatric burn patients to tolerate protein depends on their renal function and fluid balance.

The BCAAs seem to have no beneficial effect in burn patients (Alexander, Gottschlich, 1990). The conditionally essential amino acid, arginine, may improve cell-mediated immunity and wound healing (Gottschlich, 1993; Tredget and Yu, 1992). Arginine may also affect anabolic hormone production (Gottschlich et al., 1990). A recent study showed that glutamine enhances the ability of neutrophils to kill certain bacteria (Ogle et al., 1994). For all patients receiving high-protein diets, blood urea nitrogen, serum creatinine, and hydration must be monitored.

Assessment of Energy and Protein Adequacy

The adequacy of protein and energy intake is best evaluated by following wound healing, graft take, and basic nutritional assessment parameters. Wound healing or graft take may be delayed if weight loss exceeds 10% of the usual weight. An exact evaluation of weight loss may be difficult to obtain because of fluid shifts or edema, or because of differences in the weights of dressings or splints. The coordination of weight measurement with dressing changes or hydrotherapy may allow recording of a weight without dressings and splints (Gottschlich, 1993). Generally, the fluid gained during the resuscitation period is lost within 2 weeks. Weight change trends can then be identified.

Nitrogen balance is frequently used to evaluate the efficacy of a nutritional regimen, but it cannot be considered accurate without accounting for wound losses. The following formulas have been used to estimate wound nitrogen losses (Gottschlich, 1993).

< 10% open wound = 0.02 g nitrogen/kg/day
11 to 30% open wound = 0.05 g nitrogen/kg/day
> 31% open wound = 0.12 g nitrogen/kg/day

During the first 4 weeks, nitrogen balance studies may be the most reflective measure in nutritional monitoring (Carlson et al., 1991). Nitrogen excretion should begin to decrease as wounds heal or are grafted or covered; however, serum albumin levels usually remain depressed until major burns are healed. Proteins with shorter half-lives, such as serum prealbumin, retinol-binding protein, and transferrin, show promise for helping to assess the protein status of burn patients (see Chapter 17).

Vitamins and Minerals

It is generally agreed that vitamin needs are increased for burn patients, but exact requirements have not been established. Supplements may be needed for patients eating food; however, most patients receiving tube feeding or TPN receive amounts of vitamins in excess of the RDAs because of the high calorie intake. Vitamin C is involved in collagen synthesis and immune function, and may be required in increased amounts for wound healing. Doses of 500 mg twice daily is the routine protocol at some burn centers (Gottschlich, 1993). Vitamin A is also an important nutrient for immune function and epithelialization. Provision of 5000 IU of vitamin A per 1000 calories of enteral nutrition is often recommended (Gottschlich, 1993).

Electrolyte imbalances involving serum sodium or potassium are usually corrected by adjusting fluid therapy. Hyponatremia may be seen in patients whose evaporative losses are reduced drastically by the application of dressings or grafts, with changes in maintenance fluids, or in those treated with silver nitrate soaks, which tend to draw sodium from the wound. Restricting the oral consumption of free water and sodium-free fluids may help correct hyponatremia. Hypokalemia often occurs after the initial fluid resuscitation and during protein synthesis. A slightly elevated serum potassium may indicate inadequate hydration.

Depression of serum calcium levels may be seen in patients with burns involving more than 30% TBSA. Hypocalcemia often accompanies hypoalbuminemia. Calcium losses may be exaggerated if the patient is immobile or being treated with silver nitrate soaks. Early ambulation and exercise should help minimize these losses. Administration of calcium supplements may be necessary to treat symptomatic hypocalcemia.

Hypophosphatemia has also been identified in patients with major burns. This occurs most commonly in patients receiving large volumes of resuscitation fluid along with parenteral infusion of glucose solutions and large amounts of antacids for stress ulcer prophylaxis. Serum levels need to be monitored, and appropriate phosphate supplementation provided. Magnesium levels may also require attention because a significant amount of magnesium can be lost from the burn wound. Supplemental phosphorus and magnesium are often given parenterally to avoid gastrointestinal irritation.

A depressed serum zinc level has been reported in burn patients, but it is unclear whether this is representative of total body zinc nutriture or an artifact of hypoalbuminemia, because zinc is bound to serum albumin. Zinc is a cofactor in energy metabolism and protein synthesis. Supplementation with 220 mg zinc sulfate is appropriate (Gottschlich, 1993). The anemia initially seen following a burn is usually unrelated to iron deficiency and is treated with packed red blood cells.

Methods of Nutritional Support

Methods of nutritional support need to be implemented on an individual basis. Most patients with burns of less than 20% TBSA are able to meet their needs with a regular, high calorie and protein diet. Often the use of concealed nutrients such as adding protein to puddings, milks, and gelatins is helpful because consuming large volumes of foods can be overwhelming to the patient and can lead to overeating after the burns are healed. Patients with major burns, extraordinarily high energy expenditure, or poor appetites usually require tube feeding or TPN.

Enteral feeding is the preferred method of nutritional support for burn patients, but parenteral nutrition may be necessary with early excision and grafting, to avoid the frequent interruptions in enteral nutritional support required for anesthesia. TPN may be the method of choice for patients with persistent ileus who do not tolerate tube feedings or who have a high risk of aspiration. Because ileus is often present only in the stomach, severely burned patients can be successfully fed into the small bowel. With careful monitoring, central lines for TPN can be maintained through burn wounds. The use of IGF-1 and human growth hormone in conjunction with nutritional support has been shown to blunt the stress response and improve nitrogen balance in burn patients (Goodwin, 1993; Waymack and Herndon, 1992). Anabolic steroids such as *oxandrolone*, when combined with a high-protein diet (2 g/kg/day) have also been shown to significantly increase the rate that patients restore lost weight after burn injury (Demling and Desanti, 1997).

Ancillary Measures

Physical therapy helps prevent muscle wasting and atrophy (Goodwin, 1993). A warm environment minimizes heat loss and the expenditure of energy to maintain body temperature. Thermal blankets, heat lamps, and individual heat shields are often used to maintain environmental temperature near 30°C. Minimizing fear and pain with reassurance from the staff and adequate pain medication can also reduce catecholamine stimulation, helping to avoid increases in energy expenditure.

Antacids should be given to patients with major burns to prevent formation of stress-related Curling's ulcers in the gastric or duodenal mucosa.

SURGERY

Although surgical morbidity correlates best with the extent of the primary disease and the nature of the operation performed, malnutrition may compound the severity of complications (Mullen et al., 1979). A well-nourished patient usually tolerates major surgery better than a severely malnourished patient because malnutrition is associated with a high incidence of operative complications and death (Campos and Mequid, 1992). Of interest are the recent findings of the National Veterans Affairs Surgical Risk Study, which evaluated 87,000 noncardiac surgeries in 44 Veterans Administration medical centers, that preoperative serum albumin was the strongest predictor of postoperative mortality (Khuri et al., 1997). An internet site for more information from the American College of Surgeons is www.facs.org.

Preoperative Nutritional Care

In the perioperative period, nutritional support has been used for patients with inadequate intake who require a major operation but cannot undergo immediate surgery, and for candidates for immediate surgery who have significant nutritional deficits (ASPEN Board of Directors, 1993). Except for patients who are unable to take food enterally or who are malnourished, there is no conclusive evidence that perioperative nutritional support (other than in the form of oral intake) is effective in reducing operative complications and death. A chemically defined or elemental liquid diet with minimal residue can be used preoperatively for patients at nutritional risk. A large multicenter study of surgical patients in Veterans Administration hospitals concluded that the use of preoperative TPN should be limited to patients who exhibit signs of severe malnutrition unless other specific indications exist (Veterans Affairs TPN Cooperative Study Group, 1991). Severely malnourished patients may benefit from initiation of nutritional support within 1 to 3 days of hospital admission and provision of adequate amounts of nutrition for 7 to 10 days before surgery (ASPEN Board of Directors, 1993).

It is important that the stomach be empty of food at the time of the operation to avoid the danger of vomitus aspiration during the induction of anesthesia or on awakening. In elective cases, no food is allowed by mouth for at least 6 hours before surgery. In emergency cases, gastric lavage is advisable to remove stomach contents before anesthesia is started.

Before abdominal surgery, the colon should be free of residue to prevent postoperative infection. Colonic bacteria are reduced when less food residue is present. Low-fiber foods or a liquid diet are commonly given for 2 to 3 days preceding surgery, and the patient receives an enema a few hours before going to the operating room. Enteral products that are low in residue can be used as a colon prep prior to surgery.

Postoperative Nutritional Care

In the postoperative period, nutritional support is used to reduce nutritional deficits that ordinarily develop in untreated patients during the period of NPO (nothing by mouth) following surgery. The length of time a patient can tolerate remaining NPO after surgery without complications is unknown, but it is probably influenced by the patient's preexisting nutritional status, the severity of the operative stress, and the nature and severity of the illness. If the period of postoperative starvation is expected to be longer than 1 week, nutritional support may be beneficial even for a mildly malnourished individual; however, institution of nutritional support within 1 to 3 days postoperatively is judicious in severely malnourished patients (ASPEN Board of Directors, 1993).

The introduction of solid food depends on the condition of the gastrointestinal tract. Oral feeding is often delayed for the first 24 to 48 hours following surgery to await the return of bowel sounds or passage of flatus. A general practice has been to progress over a period of several meals from clear

CASE STUDY

Michael P., a 22-year-old man, was involved in a motor vehicle accident as an unbelted rear seat passenger and sustained a skull fracture, left subdural hematoma, and a right pneumothorax requiring a chest tube. Glasgow Coma Scale was 10. His weight on admission to the surgical intensive care unit was 162 lb; height, 6′4″. He has no previous significant medical or nutritional history.

MP was stabilized, given slightly less than his maintenance fluid requirements and a diuretic to prevent brain swelling. He was maintained on a respirator. A nasogastric tube was placed for drainage.

On hospital day 4, TPN was initiated because of continued high nasogastric drainage. The patient began running high fevers. The diuretic was discontinued and the fluid restriction was liberalized because MP was becoming too dehydrated. Using the Harris-Benedict equation with an injury factor of 1.4, energy requirements were calculated at 2681 kcal. Indirect calorimetry indicated that MP's measured energy expenditure (MEE) was 2990 kcal/day. The nutritional goal was to feed the patient his actual measured energy needs. Protein requirements were calculated to provide approximately 1.5 g/kg, or 110 g of protein per day. The serum albumin level of 4.3 g/dL on admission dropped to 2.9 g/dL after rehydration.

A concentrated intact nutrient formula was started at 20 cc/h via the nasogastric tube on hospital day 6. Feedings were successfully advanced to the goal rate of 85 cc/h by day 9. This provided 3060 kcal and 124 g protein per day. TPN was discontinued as MP continued to tolerate enteral nutrition. Rapid turnover proteins were low; retinol-binding protein was 1.3 mg/dL (normal 3.0 to 6.0 mg/dL) and prealbumin was 4.8 mg/dL (normal 10 to 40 mg/dL). Zinc was normal at 83 (63 to 147 μg/dL). Total urinary nitrogen excretion was 27 g/day.

On hospital day 11, a nasojejunal tube replaced the nasogastric tube to lessen the risk of aspiration for this unresponsive patient. MP continued to run a fever and was often treated with a cooling blanket. Because of anticipated continued ventilator dependence and neurologic impairment, gastrostomy (G-tube) and jejunostomy (J-tube) tubes were surgically placed. Since the initiation of nutritional support, MP had received 90% or more of his measured nutritional requirements. His weight is now 132 lb. Diarrhea and copious airway secretions began during hospital week 3. An infectious cause of diarrhea was ruled out. A less concentrated tube feeding formula was provided for hydration and to perhaps lessen stooling.

1. What indications of hypermetabolism are evident in this patient's history?
2. Compare Michael's measured energy expenditure to that calculated by the Harris-Benedict equation. What are the differences? Also compare it in kilocalories per kilogram.
3. What nutritional recommendations would you make for the remainder of his hospital stay?

liquids to full liquids, and finally to solid foods. There is, however, no physiologic reason why solid foods should not be introduced once the gastrointestinal tract is functioning and a few liquids are being tolerated. Multiple studies have now demonstrated that after surgery, patients can be fed a regular solid food diet rather than a clear liquid diet (Bickel et al., 1992; Jeffery et al., 1996; Martindale, 1998). If oral feeding is not possible, or an extended NPO period is anticipated, access for enteral feeding should be obtained at the time of surgery. Combined gastrostomy-jejunostomy tubes offer significant advantages over standard gastrostomies because they allow for simultaneous gastric drainage from the gastrostomy tube and enteral feeding via the jejunal limb.

CITED REFERENCES

Alexander JW, Gottschlich MM. Nutritional immunomodulation in burn patients. Crit Care Med 18:S149, 1990.

Annis K, et al. Nutritional support of the severe head-injured patient. Nutr Clin Pract 6:245, 1991.

ASPEN Board of Directors: Guidelines for the use of parenteral and enteral nutrition in adult and pediatric patients. J Parenter Enteral Nutr 17 (suppl): 1993.

Barton RG, Cerra FB. Metabolic and nutritional support. In: Moore EE, et al. (eds.). Trauma. Norwalk, CT: Appleton & Lange, 1991.

Battistella FD, et al. A prospective, randomized trial of intravenous fat emulsion administration in trauma victims requiring total parenteral nutrition. J Trauma 43:52, 1997.

Berger MM, et al. Copper, selenium, and zinc status and balances after major trauma. J Trauma 40:103, 1996.

Bessey PQ. Nutritional support in critical illness. In: Dietch EA (ed.). Multiple Organ Failure: Pathophysiology and Basic Concepts in Therapy. New York: Thieme, 1990.

Bessey PQ. Parenteral nutrition and trauma. In: Rombeau J, Caldwell MD (eds.). Parenteral Nutrition, 2nd ed. Philadelphia: WB Saunders, 1993.

Bickel A, et al. Early oral feeding following removal of nasogastric tube in gastrointestinal operations. Arch Surg 127:287, 1992.

Blackburn GL, et al. Nutritional and metabolic assessment of the hospitalized patient. J Parenter Enteral Nutr 1:11, 1977.

Bone RC. Toward an epidemiology and natural history of SIRS (systemic inflammatory response syndrome). JAMA 268:3452, 1992.

Bone RC, et al. ACCP/SCCM Consensus Conference: Definitions for sepsis and organ failure and guidelines for the use of innovative therapies in sepsis. Chest 101:1644, 1992.

Byrne TA, et al. Growth hormone, glutamine, and a modified diet enhance nutrient absorption in patients with severe short bowel syndrome. J Parenter Enteral Nutr 19:296, 1995.

Campos A, Meguid M. A critical appraisal of the usefulness of perioperative nutritional support. Am J Clin Nutr 55:117, 1992.

Carlson DW, et al. Evaluation of serum visceral protein levels as indicators of nitrogen balance in thermally injured patients. J Parenter Enteral Nutr 15:440, 1991.

Cerra FB, et al. The effect of stress level, amino acid formula, and nitrogen dose on nitrogen retention in traumatic and septic stress. Ann Surg 205:282, 1987.

Chiarelli A, et al. Very early nutrition supplementation in burned patients. Am J Clin Nutr 51:1035, 1990.

Cunningham J, et al. Measured and predicted calorie requirements of adults during recovery from severe burn trauma. Am J Clin Nutr 49:404, 1989.

Cunningham J, et al. Calorie and protein provision for recovery from severe burns in infants and young children. Am J Clin Nutr 51:553, 1990.

Curreri PW. Nutritional replacement modalities. J Trauma 19:904, 1979.

Cuthbertson DP. The metabolic response to injury and its nutritional implications: Retrospect and prospect. J Parenter Enteral Nutr 3:108, 1979.

Deitch EA. Multiple organ failure. Ann Surg 216:117, 1992.

Demling RH, Desanti L. Oxandrolone, an anabolic steroid, significantly increases the rate of weight gain in the recovery phase after major burns. J Trauma 43:47, 1997.

Elwyn DH. Nutritional requirements of adult surgical patients. Crit Care Med 8:9, 1980.

Fox KA, et al. Aspiration pneumonia following surgically placed feeding tubes. Am J Surg 170:560, 1995.

Garrel DR, et al. Improved clinical status and length of care with low-fat nutrition support in burn patients. J Parenter Enteral Nutr 19:482, 1995.

Gilder H. Parenteral nourishment of patients undergoing surgical or traumatic stress. J Parenter Enteral Nutr 10:88, 1986.

Goodwin CW. Parenteral nutrition in thermal injuries. In: Rombeau J, Caldwell MD (eds.). Clinical Nutrition–Parenteral Nutrition. 2nd ed. Philadelphia: WB Saunders, 1993.

Gottschlich MM. Burns. In: Gottschlich MM, et al. (eds.). Nutrition Support Dietetics Core Curriculum, 2nd ed. Silver Spring, MD: American Society for Parenteral and Enteral Nutrition, 1993.

Gottschlich MM, et al. Differential effects of three enteral dietary regimens on selected outcome variables in burn patients. J Parenter Enteral Nutr 14:225, 1990.

Gottschlich MM, et al. Significance of obesity on nutritional, immunologic, hormonal, and clinical outcome parameters in burns. J Am Diet Assoc 93:1261, 1993.

Greenblatt SH, et al. Catabolic effect of dexamethasone in patients with major head injuries. J Parenter Enteral Nutr 13:372, 1989.

Grimm H, et al. Immuno-regulation by parenteral lipids: Impact of the ω-3 to ω-6 fatty acid ratio. J Parenter Enteral Nutr 18:417, 1994.

Hadley MN, et al. Nutritional support and neurotrauma: A critical review of early nutrition in forty-five acute head injury patients. Neurosurgery 19:367, 1986.

Herndon DN, et al. Treatment of burns in children. Pediatr Clin N Am 32:1311, 1985.

Hester DD. Neurologic impairment. In: Gottschlich MM, et al. (eds.). Nutrition Support Dietetics Core Curriculum, 2nd ed. Silver Spring, MD: American Society for Parenteral and Enteral Nutrition, 1993.

Jeevanandam M, et al. Decreased growth hormone levels in the catabolic phase of severe injury. Surgery 111:495, 1992.

Jeevanandam M, et al. Adjuvant recombinant human growth hormone normalizes plasma amino acids in parenterally fed trauma patients. J Parenter Enteral Nutr 19:137, 1995.

Jeffery KM, et al. The clear liquid diet is no longer a necessity in the routine postoperative management of surgical patients. Am Surg 62:167, 1996.

Jenkins ME, et al. Enteral feeding during operative procedures in thermal injuries. J Burn Care Rehabil 15:199, 1994.

Kelly JL, et al. Is circulating endotoxin the trigger for the systemic inflammatory response syndrome seen after injury? Ann Surg 225:530, 1997.

Khuri SF, et al. Risk adjustment of the postoperative mortality rate for the comparative assessment of the quality of surgical care: Results of the National Veterans Affairs Surgical Risk Study. J Am Coll Surg 185:315, 1997.

Konvolinka CW, Morell VO. Nutrition in head trauma. Nutr Clin Pract 6:251, 1991.

Koruda MJ, et al. Effect of parenteral nutrition supplemented with short-chain fatty acids on adaptation to massive small bowel resection. Gastroenterology 95:715, 1986.

Langkamp-Henken B, et al. Immunologic structure and function of the gastrointestinal tract. Nutr Clin Pract 7:100, 1992.

Li J, et al. Effect of glutamine-enriched total parenteral nutrition on small intestinal gut-associated lymphoid tissue and upper respiratory tract immunity. Surgery 121:542, 1997.

Lund CL, Browder NC. The estimation of areas of burns. Surg Gynecol Obstet 79:352, 1944.

Marshall JC, Girotti MJ. From premise to principle: The impact of the gut hypothesis on the practice of critical care surgery. Can J Surg 38:132, 1995.

Martindale R. Clear liquid diets: Tradition or intuition? Nutr Clin Pract 13:186, 1998.

Mullen JL, et al. Implication of malnutrition in the surgical patient. Arch Surg 114:121, 1979.

Ogle CK, et al. Effect of glutamine on phagocytosis and bacterial killing by normal and pediatric burn patient neutrophils. J Parenter Enteral Nutr 18:128, 1994.

Ott L, Young B. Nutrition in the neurologically injured patient. Nutr Clin Pract 6:223, 1991.

Pichard C, et al. Lack of effects of recombinant growth hormone on muscle function in patients requiring prolonged mechanical ventilation: A prospective, randomized, controlled study. Crit Care Med 24:403, 1996.

Pomp A, et al. Specialized nutritional support in surgical patients. Prob Gen Surg 5:271, 1988.

Pratt VC, et al. Short-chain fatty acid-supplemented TPN improves nonspecific immunity after intestinal resection in rats. J Parenter Enteral Nutr 20:264, 1996.

Reynolds JV. Gut barrier function in the surgical patient. Br J Surg 83:1668, 1996.

Reynolds JV, et al. Impaired gut barrier function in malnourished patients. Br J Surg 83:1288, 1996.

Richardson JD. What's new in trauma and burns. J Am Coll Surg 184:210, 1997.
Robertson CS, et al. Steroid administration and nitrogen excretion in the head-injured patient. J Neurosurg 63:714, 1985.
Saffle JR, et al. A randomized trial of indirect calorimetry-based feedings in thermal injury. J Trauma 30:776, 1990.
Seidner DL, et al. Effects of long chain triglyceride emulsions on reticuloendothelial system function in humans. J Parenter Enteral Nutr 13:614, 1989.
Souba W, Wilmore D. Diet and nutrition in the case of the patient with surgery, trauma and sepsis. In: Shils ME, et al. (eds.). Modern Nutrition in Health and Disease, vol. 2, 8th ed., Philadelphia: Lea & Febiger, 1994.
Sunderland PM, Heilbrun MP. Estimating energy expenditure in traumatic brain injury: Comparison of indirect calorimetry with predictive formulas. Neurosurgery 31:246, 1992.
Swank GM, Deitch EA. Role of the gut in multiple organ failure: Bacterial translocation and permeability changes. World J Surg 20:411, 1996.
Tappenden KA, et al. Short-chain fatty acids increase proglucagon and ornithine decarboxylase messenger RNAs after intestinal resection in rats. J Parenter Enteral Nutr 20:357, 1996.
Tappenden KA, et al. Short-chain fatty acid-supplemented total parenteral nutrition enhances functional adaptation to intestinal resection in rats. Gastroenterology 112:792, 1997.
Tappenden KA, et al. Early enteral nutrition may have detrimental effects in patients with gastrointestinal hypoperfusion. Abstract. Presented at the 22nd Clinical Congress, American Society for Parenteral and Enteral Nutrition, January 1998.
Tredget EE, Yu YM. The metabolic effects of thermal injury. World J Surg 16:68, 1992.
Veterans Affairs Total Parenteral Nutrition Cooperative Study Group. Perioperative total parenteral nutrition in surgical patients. N Engl J Med 325:525, 1991.
Warden GD. Burn shock resuscitation. World J Surg 16:16, 1992.
Waymack JP, Herndon DN. Nutritional support of the burned patient. World J Surg 16:80, 1992.
Winkler MF, Albina JE. Vitamin status of TPN patients. J Parenter Enteral Nutr 14:16S, 1990.
Winkler MF, et al. Energy expenditure in TPN patients. Presented at the American Dietetic Association, San Francisco, CA, September 1988.
Wolfe R, et al. Glucose metabolism in man: Responses to intravenous glucose infusion. Metabolism 28:210, 1979.
Wood P. Managing dysphagia in patients with traumatic brain injury. News & Views. Mead Johnson Nutritionals Newsletter (2) 1, 1990.
Wusteman M, et al. The effect of enteral glutamine deprivation and supplementation on the structure of rat small-intestine mucosa during a systemic injury response. J Parenter Enteral Nutr 19:22, 1995.
Young LS, Persinger RL. The utility of growth hormone in nutrition support. Support Line XVI:6, 1994.
Zaloga GP, et al. Effect of rate of enteral nutrient supply on gut mass. J Parenter Enteral Nutr 16:39, 1992.
Ziegler TR. Anabolic agents in nutritional support. Presented at the 22nd Clinical Congress, American Society for Parenteral and Enteral Nutrition, January 1998.

ADDITIONAL REFERENCES

Starvation

Cahill GF. Starvation in man. N Engl J Med 282:668, 1980.

Critical Illness and Stress

Barton RG. Nutrition support in critical illness. Nutr Clin Pract 9:127, 1994.
Kemper M, et al. Caloric requirements and supply in critically ill surgical patients. Crit Care Med 20:344, 1992.
Mueller C. Inflammatory response and sepsis. In: Matarese LE, Gottschlich MM (eds.). Contemporary Nutrition Support Practice. Philadelphia: WB Saunders, 1998.
Winkler MF. Nutritional assessment in critical care. In: Simko MD, et al. (eds.). Nutrition Assessment: A Comprehensive Guide for Planning Intervention. Rockville, MD: Aspen Publishers, 1995.

Early Enteral Feeding

Moore FA, et al. Early enteral feeding, compared with parenteral reduces postoperative septic complications: The results of a meta-analysis. Ann Surg 216:172, 1992.

Burns

Ireton-Jones CS, Baxter CR. Nutrition for adult burn patients: A review. Nutr Clin Pract 6:3, 1991.
Mayes T, Gottschlich MM. Burns. In: Matarese LE, Gottschlich MM (eds.). Contemporary Nutrition Support Practice. Philadelphia: WB Saunders, 1998.

Head Trauma

Magnuson B, et al. Pentobarbital coma in neurosurgical patients: Nutritional considerations. Nutr Clin Pract 9:146, 1994.
Ott L, et al. Altered gastric emptying in the head injured patient: Relationship to feeding intolerance. J Neurosurg 74:738, 1991.

Surgery

Albina JE. Nutrition and wound healing. J Parenter Enteral Nutr 18:367, 1994.
Winkler M. Surgery and wound healing. In: Skipper A (ed.). Dietitian's Handbook of Enteral and Parenteral Nutrition. Gaithersburg, MD: Aspen Publishers, 1998.

Trauma

Kudsk KA, et al. A randomized trial of isonitrogenous enteral diets after severe trauma: An immune enhancing diet reduces septic complications. Ann Surg 224:531, 1996.

CHAPTER 34

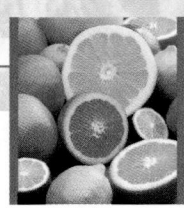

Medical Nutrition Therapy for Diabetes Mellitus and Hypoglycemia of Nondiabetic Origin

MARION J. FRANZ, MS, RD, LD, CDE

Chapter Outline

- Glucose Intolerance Classifications and Pathophysiology
- Diagnostic and Screening Criteria for Diabetes Mellitus
- Insulin and the Counterregulatory Hormones
- Management of Diabetes Mellitus
- Acute Complications
- Long-Term Complications
- Surgery and Diabetes
- Diabetes and Age-Related Issues
- Implementing Nutritional Self-Management
- Pathophysiology of Hypoglycemia of Nondiabetic Origin
- Types of Hypoglycemia
- Diagnosis of Hypoglycemia
- Treatment of Hypoglycemia
- Avoiding the Symptoms of Hypoglycemia

Key Terms

ADRENERGIC SYMPTOMS—symptoms of hypoglycemia that arise from the action of the autonomic nervous system

COMBINATION THERAPY—a form of therapy for diabetes using combinations of oral medications or a combination of oral medication(s) and insulin injection(s)

COUNTERREGULATORY (STRESS) HORMONES—hormones, including glucagon, epinephrine (adrenaline), norepinephrine, cortisol, and growth hormone, released during stressful situations, which have the opposite effect of insulin and cause the liver to release glucose from stored glycogen and the adipose cells to release fatty acids for extra energy; these hormones counterbalance declining glucose levels

DAWN PHENOMENON—an increase in blood glucose levels between 4 AM and 8 AM, when natural adrenaline begins to function; possibly caused by a diurnal variation in growth hormone

DIABETES CONTROL AND COMPLICATIONS TRIAL (DCCT)—a 10-year study, sponsored by the National Institutes of Health, in which more than 1400 people with type 1 diabetes were treated with either conventional therapy (usually, two insulin injections per day) or intensive therapy (multiple insulin injections or an insulin pump); follow-up evaluations proved that tight blood glucose control reduces the risk of diabetic complications

DIABETIC KETOACIDOSIS (DKA)—severe, uncontrolled diabetes, resulting from insufficient insulin, in which ketone bodies (acids) build up in the blood; if left untreated (with immediate administration of insulin and fluids), can lead to coma and even death

FASTING HYPOGLYCEMIA—low blood glucose that occurs in the food-deprived state

GESTATIONAL DIABETES MELLITUS (GDM)—glucose intolerance, the onset or first recognition of which occurs during pregnancy

GLUCAGON—a hormone, produced by the alpha cells of the pancreas, which causes an increase in blood glucose levels by stimulating the release of glucose from liver glycogen stores

GLYCATED HEMOGLOBIN—a blood test that measures an individual's average blood glucose levels, expressed as a percentage of total hemoglobin with glucose attached, over the preceding 2 or 3 months; may also be called glycosylated hemoglobin or glycohemoglobin

HONEYMOON PHASE—the period after initial diagnosis of diabetes when there may be some recovery of beta-cell function and a temporary decrease in exogenous insulin requirement

HYPERGLYCEMIA—an excessive amount of glucose in the blood (generally ≥180 mg/dL) caused by too little insulin, insulin resistance, or increased food intake; symptoms include frequent urination, increased thirst, and weight loss

HYPEROSMOLAR HYPERGLYCEMIC NONKETOTIC (HHNK) SYNDROME—extremely high blood glucose levels with absence of or only slight ketosis and profound dehydration

HYPOGLYCEMIA (OR INSULIN REACTION)—low blood glucose level (usually ≤70 mg/dL), which can be caused by the administration of excessive insulin or oral medications, too little food, delayed or missed meals or snacks, increased amounts of exercise or other physical activity, or alcohol intake without food

HYPOGLYCEMIA OF NONDIABETIC ORIGIN—low levels of blood glucose that lead to neuroglycopenia symptoms which are ameliorated by the ingestion of carbohydrate

IMMUNE-MEDIATED DIABETES MELLITUS—a form of type 1 diabetes resulting from cell-mediated autoimmune destruction of the beta cells of the pancreas

IMPAIRED GLUCOSE HOMEOSTASIS—metabolic stages of impaired glucose use, intermediate between normal glucose homeostasis and diabetes, which are considered to be risk factors for future diabetes and cardiovascular disease

INSULIN—a hormone released from the beta cells of the pancreas that enables cells to metabolize and store glucose and other fuels

INSULIN RESISTANCE—an impaired biologic response to either exogenous or endogenous insulin; insulin resistance and insulin deficiencies are usual causes of type 2 diabetes

INTENSIVE DIABETES MANAGEMENT—a method of treatment for diabetes that attempts to maintain near-normal glycemia by using all available resources

MACROVASCULAR DISEASES—diseases of the large blood vessels, including coronary artery disease, cardiovascular disease, and peripheral vascular disease

MEAL-PLANNING APPROACHES—educational tools used to teach meal planning and to implement the nutrition prescription

MICROVASCULAR DISEASES—diseases of the small blood vessels, including retinopathy and nephropathy

NEUROGLYCOPENIA—neurological symptoms of hypoglycemia that are related to an insufficent supply of glucose to the brain

NUTRITION PRESCRIPTION—a treatment plan that identifies the number of calories, macronutrient composition, number of meals and snacks, and timing of meals for an individual with diabetes

ORAL GLUCOSE-LOWERING MEDICATIONS—drugs, administered orally, that are used to control or lower blood glucose levels, including first- and second-generation sulfonylureas, biguanides, alpha-glucosidase inhibitors, thiazolidinediones, and meglitinide

POLYDIPSIA—excessive thirst

POLYURIA—excessive urination

POSTPRANDIAL BLOOD GLUCOSE—a blood glucose test performed 1 to 2 hours after eating

POSTPRANDIAL (REACTIVE) HYPOGLYCEMIA—low blood glucose within 2 to 5 hours after eating

PREPRANDIAL BLOOD GLUCOSE—a blood glucose test performed before eating

SELF-MANAGEMENT TRAINING SKILLS—comprehensive skills in both diabetes management (decision making to enable appropriate self-care) and life-style improvement (problem-solving that allows a more flexible lifestyle)

SELF-MONITORING OF BLOOD GLUCOSE (SMBG)—a method whereby individuals can test their own blood glucose levels; using a chemically treated strip and visually comparing the strip to a color chart, or by inserting the strip into a meter that measures the glucose level

SOMOGYI (REBOUND) EFFECT—hypoglycemia followed by "rebound" hyperglycemia caused by an overproduction of counterregulatory hormones; insulin doses should not be increased at this time

"SURVIVAL" SKILLS—basic information needed at the time of diagnosis of diabetes or when changes are made in the treatment regimen

TARGET BLOOD GLUCOSE GOALS—levels for capillary blood glucose tests that are reasonable for an individual and that can be achieved without risk of serious hypoglycemia

TYPE 1 DIABETES—a type of diabetes that usually occurs in persons younger than 30 years of age; previously known as insulin-dependent diabetes mellitus (IDDM) or juvenile-onset diabetes; can be either immune-mediated or idiopathic

TYPE 2 DIABETES—a type of diabetes usually occurring in persons older than 30 years of age; previously known as non–insulin-dependent diabetes mellitus (NIDDM) or maturity-onset diabetes

WHIPPLE'S TRIAD—a triad of clinical features that includes (1) low blood glucose levels, (2) accompanied by symptoms, which are (3) relieved by administration of glucose

---

Diabetes mellitus is a group of diseases characterized by high blood glucose levels resulting from defects in insulin secretion, insulin action, or both. Abnormalities in the metabolism of carbohydrate, protein, and fat are also present. Persons with diabetes have bodies that do not produce or respond to **insulin,** a hormone produced by the beta cells of the pancreas that is necessary for the use or storage of body fuels. Without effective insulin, hyperglycemia occurs, which can lead to both the short-term and long-term complications of diabetes mellitus.

Diabetes mellitus affects approximately 16 million Americans, roughly 5.9% of the total population. About 10.3 million people in the United States have been diagnosed as having diabetes, and another 5.4 million have diabetes but remain undiagnosed. The incidence of diabetes varies according to age group: for those 65 years of age or older, it is 18.4%; for those 20 years of age or older, it is 8.2%; and for those younger than 20 years of age, it is 0.16% (Centers for Disease Control and Prevention, 1997).

Prevalence of diabetes increases with increasing age, with about 50% of the cases occurring in people older than 55 years of age. Diabetes is particularly prevalent in minorities; indeed, the prevalence of type 2 diabetes is highest in ethnic minorities in the United States, such as the Hispanic populations (Latinos and Mexican Americans), Native Americans and Alaska Natives, African Americans, Asian Americans, and Pacific Islanders. Overall, the

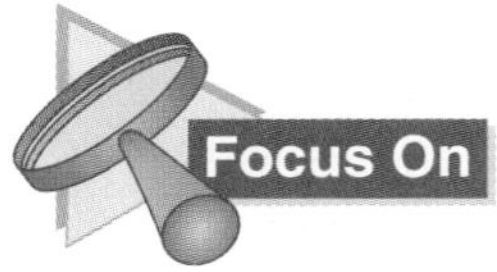

Diabetes Does Discriminate!

Diabetes strikes particularly hard at minorities. The prevalence of diabetes in the United States is highest in ethnic minorities, such as Hispanic populations (Mexican and Latino Americans), African Americans, and Native Americans. Mexican Americans and Latino Americans (Puerto Ricans and Cubans) are twice as likely to have diabetes as non-Hispanic whites of similar age. Non-Hispanic blacks are 1.7 times as likely to have diabetes as non-Hispanic whites (Centers for Disease Control and Prevention, 1997).

Certain environmental or life-style factors may increase the risk of developing type 2 diabetes in susceptible populations. For example, the increased incidence rate in Mexican Americans is probably attributable both to genetic factors and to an increased prevalence of risk factors, such as obesity. An increase in prevalence is also observed in populations that have migrated to more urbanized locations, compared with people of the same group who remained in their traditional home. Urbanization is usually related to major changes in diet, physical activity, and socioeconomic status, as well as increased obesity.

Adoption of a "Western" life-style (which may include a diet high in fat and a sedentary way of life) is associated with a dramatically increased rate of type 2 diabetes in the Pima Indians of Arizona. The rapidly increasing incidence of type 2 diabetes is one of the most serious health problems facing Native Americans today. Among the Pima Indians of Arizona, about 55% of adults older than 35 years of age have type 2 diabetes. This disease is increasingly being diagnosed in Native Americans younger than 30 years of age, and has been diagnosed in some as young as 7 years of age.

Ravussin et al. (1994) surveyed a closely related population of Pima Indians living in Maycoba, a small village in a remote, mountainous region of northwestern Mexico. They found that individuals in this community ate a diet lower in fat than is typically consumed in Arizona, and both men and women were very physically active. The men and women of Maycoba weighed, on the average, 50 lb less than a comparable group of Pimas from the Phoenix area. More importantly, diabetes was diagnosed in about 10% of the Maycoba Pimas, compared to almost 50% of the Arizona Pimas. These results suggest that a more traditional life-style may help protect against the development of diabetes (Ravussin, 1994).

The main staples of the Maycoba Pimas' diet are beans, corn (as tortillas), and potatoes. Several essential nutrients are lacking because of the relative absence of fruits and vegetables. Diet analysis reveals a diet composed of 13% protein, 23% fat, 63% carbohydrate, and <1% alcohol and containing more than 50 g of fiber. This is in sharp contrast to the present high-fat diet of the Arizona Pimas. Even more striking than the low-fat diet of the Maycoba population, however, was the high level of physical activity in this population; more than 40 hours a week were spent engaged in hard physical work (Ravussin, 1994).

The results imply that intervention approaches involving diet and exercise may be effective in reducing the incidence of obesity and type 2 diabetes in high-risk populations. This approach may help to reduce the diabetes epidemic that affects many developing countries, as well as the underprivileged in industrialized nations (King and Rewers, 1993).

prevalence in adults is slightly higher in women than in men, especially in African-American women. (See "*Focus On:* Diabetes Does Discriminate!")

Diabetes mellitus contributes to a considerable increase in morbidity and mortality, which can be reduced by early diagnosis and treatment. In 1997, diabetes costs in the United States were $98 billion. Direct medical expenditures, such as inpatient care, outpatient services, and nursing home care, totaled $44.1 billion. Indirect costs, totaling $54.1 billion, were associated with lost productivity, including premature death and disability. Total medical expenditures incurred by people with diabetes totaled $77.7 billion or $10,071 per person, as compared with $2,669 per person without diabetes (American Diabetes Association, 1997). See website www.diabetes.org.

GLUCOSE INTOLERANCE CLASSIFICATIONS AND PATHOPHYSIOLOGY

In 1997, new recommendations for the classification and diagnosis of diabetes mellitus, put forth by an expert committee, were accepted and supported by the American Diabetes Association, the National Institute of Diabetes and Digestive and Kidney Diseases (NIDDKD), and the Centers for Disease Control and Prevention, Division of Diabetes Translation. Along with the new classifications, a recommendation was made to eliminate the terms "insulin-dependent diabetes mellitus (IDDM)" and "non–insulin-dependent diabetes mellitus (NIDDM)," and to keep the terms "type 1" and "type 2" diabetes, but to use Arabic rather than Roman numerals (Expert Committee on the Diagnosis and Classification of Diabetes Mellitus, 1997) (Table 34–1).

Type 1 Diabetes

Type 1 diabetes is characterized by beta-cell destruction, usually leading to absolute insulin deficiency, and may account for 5% to 10% of all diagnosed cases of diabetes. Persons with type 1 diabetes are dependent on exogenous insulin to prevent ketoacidosis and death. Although it may occur at any age, even in the eighth and ninth decades of life, most cases are diagnosed in people younger than 30 years of age, with a peak incidence at around ages 10 to 12 years in girls and ages 12 to 14 years in boys. In the United States, about 123,000 individuals younger than 20 years of age have diabetes, and about 300,000 to 500,000 individuals of all ages have type 1 diabetes (National Diabetes Data Group, 1995). It is difficult to estimate the true prevalence of type 1 diabetes because the distinction between type 1 diabetes and insulin-treated type 2 diabetes is often unclear.

Type 1 diabetes has two forms: immune-mediated diabetes mellitus and idiopathic diabetes mellitus. **Immune-mediated diabetes mellitus** results from a cell-mediated autoimmune destruction of the beta cells of the pancreas. *Idiopathic type 1 diabetes mellitus* refers to forms of the disease that have no known etiology. Although only a minority of persons with type 1 diabetes falls into this category, of those who do, most are of African or Asian origin (Expert Committee on the Diagnosis and Classification of Diabetes Mellitus, 1997).

At diagnosis, people with type 1 diabetes are usually lean and are experiencing excessive thirst, frequent urination, and significant weight loss. The primary defect of type 1 diabetes is pancreatic beta-cell destruction, usually leading to absolute insulin deficiency and resulting in **hyperglycemia, polyuria, polydipsia,** weight loss, dehydration, electrolyte disturbance, and ketoacidosis. The rate of beta-cell destruction is quite variable, proceeding rapidly in some individuals (mainly infants and children) and slowly in others (mainly adults). The capacity of a healthy pancreas to secrete insulin is far in excess of what is needed normally; therefore, the clinical onset of diabetes may be preceded by an extensive asymptomatic period of months to years, during which beta cells are undergoing gradual destruction (see Fig. 34–1).

The etiology of immune-mediated diabetes involves a genetic predisposition and an autoimmune destruction of the islet beta cells that produce insulin. Genetic factors involve the association between type 1 diabetes and certain histocompatibility locus antigens (HLA), with linkage to the DQA and B genes, and influenced by the DRB genes. These HLA-DR/DQ alleles can be either predisposing or protective (Expert Committee on the Diagnosis and Classification of Diabetes Mellitus, 1997).

At diagnosis, the 85% to 90% of patients with type 1 diabetes have one or more circulating autoantibodies to islet cells, endogenous insulin, or other antigens that are constituents of islet cells. Antibodies identified as contributing to the destruction of beta cells are (1) islet cell autoantibodies (ICAs); (2) insulin autoantibodies (IAAs), which may occur in persons who have never received insulin therapy; and (3) autoantibodies to glutamic acid decarboxylase (GAD), a protein on the surface of beta cells. GAD autoantibodies appear to provoke an attack by the T cells (killer T lymphocytes), which may be what destroys the beta cells in diabetes. If persons genetically at risk for type 1 diabetes are screened with a combination of ICA and IAA assays, in about 90%, an abnormality can be detected before diabetes is diagnosed. The combination of high-titer ICA and IAA tests and decreased first-phase insulin secretion is predictive of the onset of type 1 diabetes within 5 years. One attractive hypothesis is that a viral infection, toxic chemical agents, or other diseases may trigger an autoimmune reaction through molecular mimicry in genetically susceptible individuals (Skyler, 1998).

Frequently, after diagnosis and the correction of hyperglycemia, metabolic acidosis, and ketoacidosis, endogenous insulin secretion recovers. During this **"honeymoon phase,"** exogenous insulin requirements decrease dramatically for up to 1 year. However, the need for increasing exogenous insulin replacement is inevitable, and within 8 to 10 years after clinical onset, beta-cell loss is complete and insulin deficiency is absolute.

TABLE 34–1 TYPES OF DIABETES AND IMPAIRED GLUCOSE HOMEOSTASIS

CLASSIFICATION	DISTINGUISHING CHARACTERISTICS
Type 1 diabetes	Affected persons usually are lean, have abrupt onset of symptoms before the age of 30 years (although it may occur at any age), and are dependent on exogenous insulin to prevent ketoacidosis and death. This condition was previously called insulin-dependent diabetes mellitus (IDDM) or juvenile-onset diabetes.
Type 2 diabetes	Affected persons usually are obese and are older than 30 years of age at diagnosis. Although not dependent on exogenous insulin for survival, individuals may require it for adequate glycemic control. This condition was previously known as non–insulin-dependent diabetes mellitus (NIDDM), or adult-onset diabetes.
Gestational diabetes mellitus (GDM)	A condition of glucose intolerance affecting pregnant women, the onset or discovery of which, occurs during pregnancy.
Other specific types	Diabetes that results from specific genetic syndromes, surgery, drugs, malnutrition, infections, and other illnesses.
Impaired glucose homeostasis	Metabolic stages of impaired glucose homeostasis (impaired fasting glucose [IFG] or impaired glucose tolerance [IGT]) that are intermediate between normal glucose values and diabetes.

(From Expert Committee on the Diagnosis and Classification of Diabetes Mellitus. Report of the Expert Committee on the Diagnosis and Classification of Diabetes Mellitus. Diabetes Care 20:1183, 1997.)

Type 2 Diabetes

Type 2 diabetes may account for 90% to 95% of all diagnosed cases of diabetes. Risk factors for type 2 diabetes include older age, obesity, a family history of diabetes, a prior history of gestational diabetes, impaired glucose homeostasis, physical inactivity, and race or ethnicity (see the box, p. 740). Although approximately 80% of these people are obese or have a history of obesity at the time of diagnosis, type 2 diabetes can occur in nonobese individuals as well, especially in the elderly (see Fig. 34–2).

Type 2 diabetes is characterized by insulin resistance and relative (rather than absolute) insulin de-

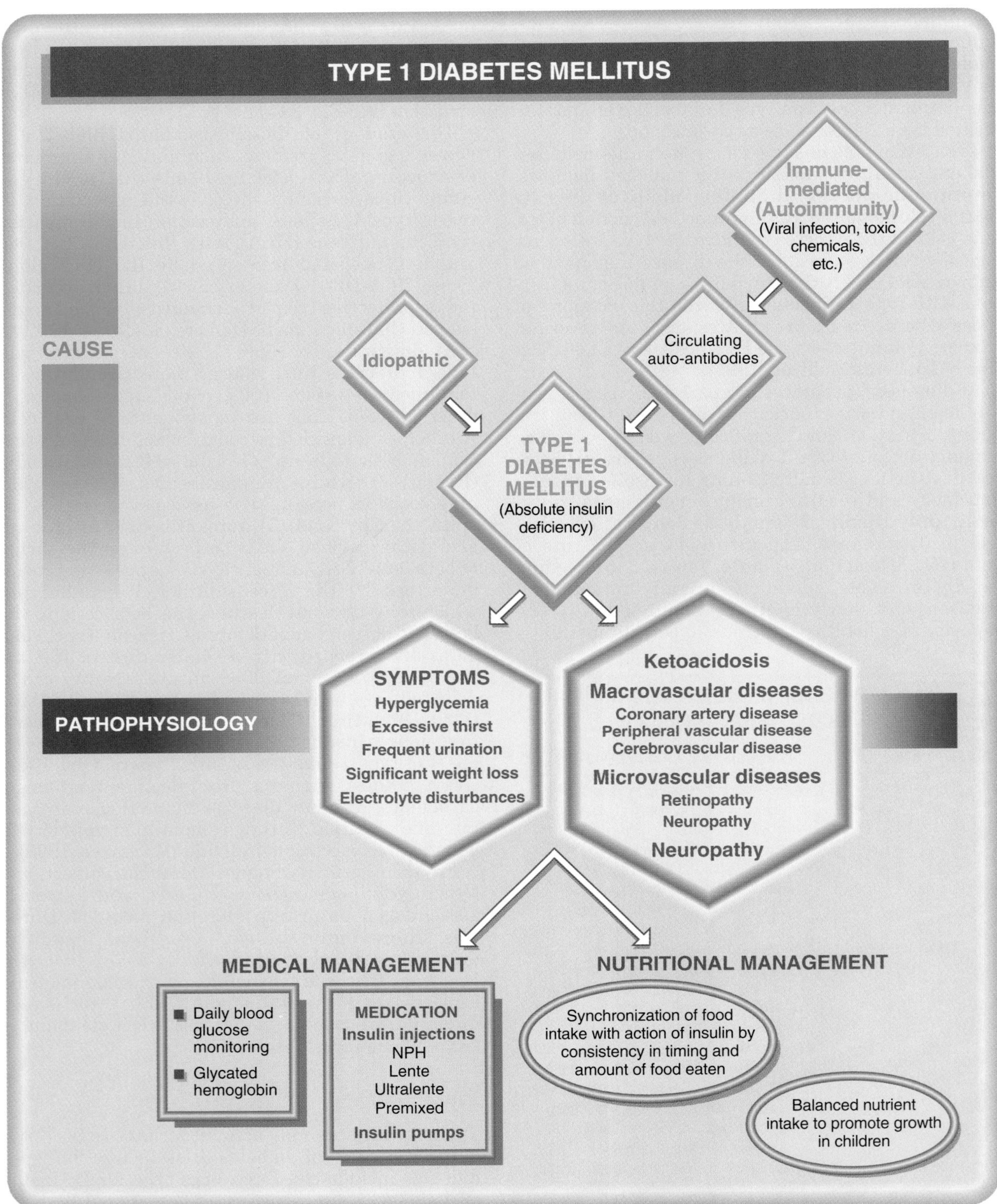

FIGURE 34–1 Pathophysiology algorithm—diabetes mellitus, type 1. (Algorithm content developed by John Anderson, Ph.D., and Sanford C. Garner, Ph.D., 2000.)

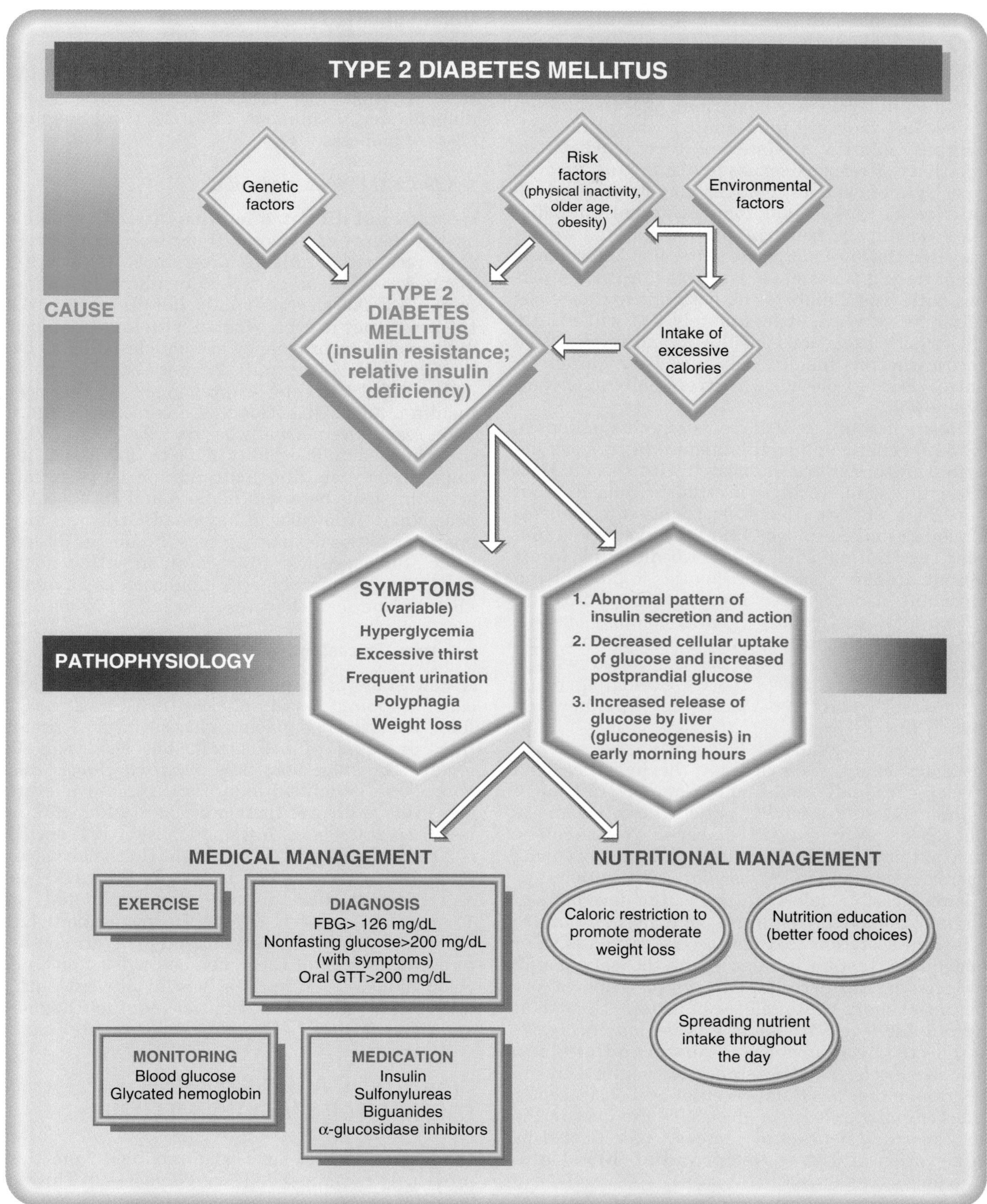

FIGURE 34–2 Pathophysiology algorithm—diabetes mellitus, type 2. (Algorithm content developed by John Anderson, Ph.D., and Sanford C. Garner, Ph.D., 2000.)

ficiency. People with type 2 diabetes can range from being predominantly insulin-resistant (with relative insulin deficiency) to predominantly deficient in insulin secretion with insulin resistance. Endogenous insulin levels may be normal, depressed, or elevated, but they are inadequate to overcome concomitant **insulin resistance** (decreased tissue sensitivity or responsiveness to insulin); as a result, hyperglycemia ensues. Persons may or may not experience the classic symptoms of uncontrolled diabetes (polydipsia, polyuria, polyphagia, and weight loss), and they are not prone to develop ketoacidosis except during times of severe stress. Although persons with type 2 diabetes do not require exogenous insulin for survival, approximately 40% will eventually require exogenous insulin for adequate blood glucose control. Insulin may also be required for control during periods of stress-induced hyperglycemia.

The etiology of type 2 diabetes remains unknown, but both genetic and environmental factors are important. Although not associated with specific HLA tissue types, identical twin studies indicate that there is a 58% to 75% concordance for diabetes (Maclaren and Atkinson, 1992). Unlike type 1 diabetes, circulating islet cell antibodies are rarely present. Intake of excessive calories is probably an important factor. Older age, physical inactivity, and obesity, particularly intra-abdominal obesity, are probably the most powerful risk factors, and even small weight losses are associated with a change in glucose levels toward normal in many persons with this type of diabetes (Zimmerman, 1998).

This form of diabetes frequently goes undiagnosed for many years because the hyperglycemia develops gradually and is often not severe enough in the early stages for the patient to notice any of the classic symptoms of diabetes. Nevertheless, such patients are at increased risk of developing macrovascular and microvascular complications.

Three possible defects influence the development of type 2 diabetes. The first is an abnormal pattern of insulin secretion that can be either excessive or inadequate. Insulin is released by the pancreas in two phases, and persons with type 2 diabetes lose the initial sharp acute release of insulin. Second, at the cellular level, uptake of glucose may decrease, as reflected by an increase in **postprandial blood glucose** levels. This resistance to insulin may result from either a cellular receptor or a postreceptor defect. Finally, release of glucose by the liver in the early morning hours may increase, as reflected by an elevation in fasting **(preprandial) blood glucose** levels.

Hyperglycemia plays a central role in initiating and sustaining hyperglycemia. The syndrome that develops—glucose toxicity—compounds the initial problems of defective insulin secretion and insulin resistance, leading to continued hyperglycemia, hence, the importance of achieving near-euglycemia in persons with type 2 diabetes.

Other Specific Types of Diabetes

This category includes diabetes associated with specific genetic syndromes, surgery, drugs, malnutrition, infections, and other illnesses. Such types of diabetes may account for 1% to 2% of all diagnosed cases of diabetes.

Gestational Diabetes Mellitus

Gestational diabetes mellitus (GDM) is defined as any degree of glucose intolerance with onset or first recognition during pregnancy. It occurs in about 4% of all pregnancies, resulting in approximately 135,000 cases annually, but disappears when the pregnancy is over. Women with known diabetes mellitus before pregnancy are not classified as having GDM. GDM is usually diagnosed during the second or third trimester of pregnancy. At this point, insulin-antagonist hormone levels increase, and insulin resistance normally occurs (see Chapter 7).

Because fetal morbidity may be increased, it is important to identify this condition by performing screening tests between the 24th and 28th weeks of pregnancy. Women who have had GDM are at increased risk for developing type 2 diabetes later. In some studies, nearly 40% of women with a history of GDM subsequently were diagnosed as having diabetes (American Diabetes Association, 1999a).

Impaired Glucose Homeostasis

A new stage of **impaired glucose homeostasis,** called *impaired fasting glucose* (IFG), has been defined as a fasting plasma glucose level of greater than or equal to 110 mg/dL but less than 126 mg/dL. The stage known as *impaired glucose tolerance* (IGT) is defined as an oral glucose tolerance test value of greater than or equal to 140 mg/dL but less than 200 mg/dL. Although neither IFG nor IGT is a clinical entity in its own right (in the absence of pregnancy), both are risk factors for future diabetes and cardiovascular disease. It is estimated that 13.4 million persons (7% of the population) have IFG. Research is being conducted to determine how to predict which of these persons will go on to develop diabetes, as well as how to prevent such a progression (Expert Committee on the Diagnosis and Classification of Diabetes Mellitus, 1997).

DIAGNOSTIC AND SCREENING CRITERIA FOR DIABETES MELLITUS

Diagnostic criteria have been modified from those previously recommended (see Table 34–2). Three diagnostic methods may be used to diagnose diabetes; however, the fasting plasma glucose (FPG) test is preferred. At this time, *hemoglobin A1c (HbA1c),* a measure of average blood glucose levels during the past 6 to 8 weeks, is not recommended for diagnosis. Furthermore, in pregnant women, different criteria are applied in establishing the diagnosis of

TABLE 34–2 DIAGNOSIS OF DIABETES MELLITUS AND IMPAIRED GLUCOSE HOMEOSTASIS

DIAGNOSIS	CRITERIA
Diabetes	FPG ≥126 mg/dL (≥7.0 mmol/L) CPG ≥200 mg/dL (≥11.1 mmol/L) plus symptoms 2hPG ≥200 mg/dL (≥11.1 mmol/L)
Impaired Glucose Homeostasis	
Impaired Fasting Glucose	FPG ≥110 and <126 mg/dL (≥6.1 and <7.0 mmol/L)
Impaired Glucose Tolerance	2hPG ≥140 and <200 mg/dL (≥7.8 and <11.1 mmol/L)
Normal	FPG <110 mg/dL (<6.1 mmol/L) 2hPG <140 mg/dL (<7.8 mmol/L)

(From Expert Committee on the Diagnosis and Classification of Diabetes Mellitus. Report of the Expert Committee on the Diagnosis and Classification of Diabetes Mellitus. Diabetes Care 20:1183, 1997.)

FPG, fasting plasma glucose (preferred testing method); *CPG*, casual plasma glucose; *2hPG*, 2-hour plasma glucose level (measured 2 hours after an oral glucose tolerance test with administration of 75 g of glucose).

gestational diabetes. The following revised criteria are applicable to diagnosis; they are not treatment criteria or goals of therapy. One of the following three tests should be used at a second test date to confirm the diagnosis:

- A confirmed FPG value of greater than or equal to 126 mg/dL indicates a diagnosis of diabetes. Previously, a value greater than or equal to 140 mg/dL had been required for diagnosis.
- In the presence of symptoms of diabetes, a confirmed nonfasting plasma glucose (casual) value of greater than or equal to 200 mg/dL is indicative of diabetes. "Casual" refers to any time of the day, without regard to the elapsed time since one's last meal. Symptoms of diabetes include the classic ones of polyuria, polydipsia, and unexplained weight loss.
- An oral glucose tolerance test, involving administration of 75 g of glucose and measurement of the plasma glucose level 2 hours later, can be used for diagnosis, with confirmed glucose values of greater than or equal to 200 mg/dL indicating a diagnosis of diabetes.

In asymptomatic, undiagnosed individuals, testing or screening for diabetes should be considered in all individuals aged 45 years and older. If test results are normal, screening should be repeated at 3-year intervals. According to the Expert Committee on the Diagnosis and Classification of Diabetes Mellitus (1997) testing should be considered at a younger age, or be carried out more frequently, in individuals who:

- Are obese
- Have a first-degree relative with diabetes
- Are members of a high-risk ethnic population
- Are women with a history of having babies weighing more than 9 lb at birth or having GDM
- Are hypertensive (blood pressure >140/90 mm Hg)
- Have a high-density lipoprotein (HDL) cholesterol level less than 35 mg/dL and/or a triglyceride level exceeding 250 mg/dL
- Had IGT or IFG on previous testing

Some time during the 24th to 28th weeks of pregnancy, an oral glucose challenge (which does not have to be preceded by fasting) with a 50-g glucose load is recommended. Low-risk women who do not need to be screened must meet all of the following criteria: younger than 25 years of age; normal body weight; no family history of diabetes; and not a member of an ethnic or racial group with a high prevalence of diabetes. An elevated plasma glucose level (≥140 mg/dL [≥7.8 mmol/L]) 1 hour later is considered to be an indication of the need for diagnostic testing. The criterion for the diagnosis of GDM is based on a 100-g oral glucose tolerance test (OGTT) (Table 34–3). During normal pregnancy, fasting plasma glucose levels are decreased (normal of 60 to 90 mg/dL), and a normal 1- to 2-hour postprandial glucose level is less than 120 mg/dL (Expert Commission on the Diagnosis and Classification of Diabetes Mellitus, 1997).

INSULIN AND THE COUNTERREGULATORY HORMONES

Optimal control of diabetes requires the restoration of normal carbohydrate, protein, and fat metabolism. Insulin is both anticatabolic and anabolic and facilitates cellular transport (Table 34–4). In general, the **counterregulatory hormones** (glucagon, growth hormone, cortisol, epinephrine, and norepinephrine) have the opposite effect of insulin.

MANAGEMENT OF DIABETES MELLITUS

Diabetes is a chronic disease that requires changes for a lifetime. The management of diabetes includes medical nutrition therapy (MNT), medications, exer-

TABLE 34–3 DIAGNOSIS OF GESTATIONAL DIABETES MELLITUS (GDM)

TYPE OF TEST	RESULTS
Screening during pregnancy—a 50-g oral glucose challenge (does not have to be fasting) at 24 to 28 weeks gestation	A plasma glucose level ≥140 mg/dL (≥7.8 mmol/L) 1 hour later indicates the need for further diagnostic testing.
Oral glucose tolerance test with an abnormal screen	After a 100-g oral glucose load, GDM may be diagnosed if two plasma glucose values equal or exceed: **Fasting:** 105 mg/dL (5.8 mmol/L) **1 hr:** 190 mg/dL (10.5 mmol/L) **2 hr:** 165 mg/dL (9.2 mmol/L) **3 hr:** 145 mg/dL (8.1 mmol/L)

(From Expert Committee on the Diagnosis and Classification of Diabetes Mellitus. Diabetes Care 20:1183, 1997.)

TABLE 34–4 THE ACTION OF INSULIN ON CARBOHYDRATE, PROTEIN, AND FAT METABOLISM

EFFECT	CARBOHYDRATE	PROTEIN	FAT
Anticatabolic (prevents breakdown)	Decreases breakdown and release of glucose from glycogen in the liver	Inhibits protein degradation; diminishes gluconeogenesis	Inhibits lipolysis; prevents excessive production of ketones and ketoacidosis
Anabolic (promotes storage)	Facilitates conversion of glucose to glycogen for storage in liver and muscle	Stimulates protein synthesis	Facilitates conversion of pyruvate to free fatty acids, stimulating lipogenesis
Transport	Activates the transport system of glucose into muscle and adipose cells	Lowers blood amino acids in parallel with blood glucose levels	Activates lipoprotein lipase, facilitating transport of triglycerides into adipose tissue

cise, blood glucose monitoring, and self-management education. An important goal of treatment is to provide the individual with the necessary tools to achieve the best possible glycemic control to prevent, delay, or arrest the microvascular and macrovascular complications of diabetes while minimizing hypoglycemia and excess weight gain (Table 34–5) (American Diabetes Association, 1999b).

Evidence relating hyperglycemia and other metabolic consequences of insulin deficiency to the development of complications comes from a series of studies in Europe and North America. However, the **Diabetes Control and Complications Trial (DCCT)** demonstrated beyond a doubt the clear link between glycemic control and development of complications. The DCCT, sponsored by the National Institutes of Health, was a long-term, prospective, randomized, controlled, multicenter trial that studied approximately 1400 young adults (aged 13 to 39 years) with type 1 diabetes who were treated with either intensive therapeutic regimens (multiple injections of insulin or use of insulin infusion pumps guided by blood glucose monitoring results) or conventional regimens (one or two insulin injections per day) (Diabetes Control and Complications Trial Research Group, 1995). Patients who achieved control similar to that of the intensively treated patients in the study could expect a 50% to 75% reduction in the risk of progression to retinopathy, nephropathy, and neuropathy after 8 to 9 years (Diabetes Control and Complications Trial Research Group, 1993).

Previously, small studies had demonstrated the relationship of blood glucose control to complications in type 2 diabetes (Ohkubbo et al., 1995; Kuusisto et al., 1994). However, the reports of the United Kingdom Prospective Diabetes Study (UKPDS) in 1998 demonstrated conclusively that elevated blood glucose levels cause long-term complications in type 2 diabetes just as in type 1 diabetes (U.K. Prospective Diabetes Study Group, 1998a). The UKPDS recruited and followed 5102 newly diagnosed individuals with type 2 diabetes for an average of 10–11 years. Subjects randomized into a group treated conventionally, primarily with diet therapy, had an average HbA1c of 7.9% compared to subjects randomized into an intensively treated group, initially treated with sulfonylureas, who had an average HbA1c of 7.0%. In the intensive therapy group, the microvascular complications rate decreased significantly by 25% and the risk of macrovascular disease decreased by 16%. For every point decrease in HbA1c, there was a 35% reduction in risk of complications. Combination therapy (mixing insulin or metformin with sulfonylureas) was needed in both groups to meet glycemic goals. Aggressive treatment of even mild-to-moderate hypertension was also beneficial in both groups (U.K. Prospective Diabetes Study, 1998b). This study clearly illustrates the progressive nature of type 2 diabetes. In both groups loss of glycemic control was noted over the 10-year trial. The ability to prevent or at least slow this rise in glycemia may be facilitated by newer glucose-lowering drugs that were not available to the UKPDS and by providing follow-up and aggressive treatment of type 2 diabetes.

Persons with diabetes, their families, and health care teams must set treatment goals together. To do this requires open communication and appropriate patient self-management education. Treatment goals should be individualized, realistic, and achievable. Diabetes control is assessed by individuals at home by self-monitoring of blood glucose (SMBG) and measurement of urine ketones.

Longer-term glycemic control is assessed by results of **glycated hemoglobin** tests. When hemoglobin and other proteins are exposed to glucose, the glucose becomes attached to the protein in a

TABLE 34–5 INDICES OF GLYCEMIC CONTROL IN NONPREGNANT ADULTS

BIOCHEMICAL INDEX	NONDIABETIC	GOAL	ACTION SUGGESTED
Fasting/preprandial glucose level	<110 mg/dL (<6.1 mmol/L)	80–120 mg/dL (4.4–6.7 mmol/L)	<80 or >140 mg/dL (<4.4 or >7.8 mmol/L)
Bedtime glucose level	<120 mg/dL (<6.7 mmol/L)	100–140 mg/dL (5.6–7.8 mmol/L)	<100 or >160 mg/dL (<5.6 or >8.9 mmol/L)
Hemoglobin A_{1c}*	<6%	<7%	>8%

(Reprinted with permission from American Diabetes Association. Standards of care (Position Statement). Diabetes Care 22(suppl 1):S33, 1999.)

* Referenced to hemoglobin A_{1c} nondiabetic range (4%–6%).

slow, nonenzymatic, and concentration-dependent fashion. Measurements of glycated proteins—primarily hemoglobin and serum proteins—best reflect the average plasma glucose concentration over the preceding weeks and months, thereby complementing day-to-day testing (Goldstein et al., 1995).

Glycated hemoglobin can be assayed by several methods that measure different components of the glycated product. In nondiabetic persons, total glycated hemoglobin (GHb) values are 5.0% to 8.0%, whereas HbA1c values are 4.0% to 6.0%. These values correspond to mean blood glucose levels of about 90 mg/dL (or approximately 5 mmol/L). Depending on the method used, actual test results, including normal ranges, will vary, and results from different laboratories cannot be compared directly (Goldstein et al., 1995).

Nutrition Therapy

MNT is integral to total diabetes care and management. However, health care professionals and persons with diabetes report that adherence to nutrition and meal planning principles is one of the most challenging aspects of diabetes care. Adherence to meal planning principles often requires some difficult life-style changes.

To integrate nutrition effectively into the overall management of diabetes requires a coordinated team effort, including a dietitian who is knowledgeable and skilled in implementing current principles and recommendations for diabetes. MNT requires an individualized approach and effective nutrition self-management education. Dietitians must also take responsibility for evaluating outcomes. Monitoring glucose and glycated hemoglobin levels, lipid values, blood pressure, weight, and quality-of-life issues is essential in evaluating the success of nutrition-related recommendations. If desired outcomes from MNT are not met, changes for overall diabetes care and management should be recommended (Kulkarni et al., 1998).

The American Diabetes Association's nutrition recommendations underscore the importance of individualized nutrition care. They depart from previous guidelines in not setting optimal levels for macronutrient intake (Table 34–6), but instead recommend that macronutrient intake be based on a nutrition assessment, modification of usual eating habits, treatment goals, and monitoring of desired metabolic outcomes (American Diabetes Association, 1999c).

Just as no one insulin regimen works for everyone, no one diet can be recommended for everyone with diabetes. Nutrition interventions, including the nutrition prescription and educational tools, should be based on a thorough assessment of each person's usual and customary intake and nutritional status. Interventions are ongoing throughout the lifespan and should be outcome-driven. Of major concern is what the individual with diabetes is able and willing to do. To facilitate adherence, cultural, ethnic, and financial considerations are of prime importance. Educators must also use creative teaching tools that match the varying educational levels and diabetes management goals of persons with diabetes (American Diabetes Association, 1999c). Preventive care, including nutrition, saves millions of dollars in hospital costs and makes good sense (Santiago, 1993).

Goals

The overall goal is to assist individuals with diabetes to make necessary life-style changes that lead to desired metabolic outcomes, not just to increased knowledge. However, there are also more specific goals for nutrition therapy (Table 34–7). The primary goal of nutrition self-management is to assist persons with diabetes to maintain a blood glucose level that is as near-normal as possible by balancing food, insulin (exogenous or endogenous), and physical activity. Furthermore, each person with diabetes needs to have reasonable, individualized goals for ranges of blood glucose levels.

The prevalence of macrovascular diseases in persons with diabetes is increased twofold to fourfold. Therefore, it is important for persons with diabetes to achieve optimal lipid levels. Nutrition plays a primary role in achieving desirable lipid outcomes (Table 34–8) (American Diabetes Association, 1999d) (see Chapter 26).

Adequate calories to maintain or attain reasonable weight for an adult should be provided. Reasonable body weight for the individual is defined as the level of weight that both the patient and health care professionals acknowledge as achievable and

TABLE 34–6 HISTORICAL PERSPECTIVE ON NUTRITION RECOMMENDATIONS FOR DIABETES MELLITUS

YEAR	DISTRIBUTION OF CALORIES FROM CHO (%)	DISTRIBUTION OF CALORIES FROM PROTEIN (%)	DISTRIBUTION OF CALORIES FROM FAT (%)
Before 1921	Starvation Diets		
1921	20	10	70
1950	40	20	40
1971	45	20	35
1986	up to 60	12–20	<30
1994	A	10–20	A, B

(Reprinted with permission from American Diabetes Association: Nutrition recommendations and principles for people with diabetes mellitus (Position Statement). Diabetes Care 22(suppl 1):S45, 1999.)

CHO, carbohydrate; *A*, based on nutrition assessment and treatment goals; *B*, <10% saturated fat.

TABLE 34–7 GOALS OF MEDICAL NUTRITION THERAPY FOR DIABETES MELLITUS

- Maintenance of as near-normal blood glucose levels as possible
- Achievement of optimal lipid levels
- Provision of adequate calories
  - For maintaining or attaining reasonable weight for adults
  - For normal growth and development in children and adolescents
  - For meeting pregnancy and lactation needs
  - For recovery from catabolic illness
- Prevention and treatment of the acute complications of insulin-treated diabetes
  - Hypoglycemia
  - Short-term illnesses
  - Exercise-related problems
- Prevention and treatment of the long-term complications of diabetes
  - Renal disease
  - Autonomic neuropathy (gastrointestinal)
  - Hypertension
  - Cardiovascular disease
- Improvement of overall health through optimal nutrition

(Adapted with permission from American Diabetes Association. Nutrition recommendations and principles for people with diabetes mellitus (Position Statement). Diabetes Care 22(suppl 1):S42, 1999.)

maintainable, both short- and long-term. This usually is not the same as traditionally defined desirable or ideal body weight. For persons using exogenous insulin, preventing weight gain is an important issue. For persons with type 2 diabetes, moderate weight loss, regardless of the initial weight, has been shown to reduce hyperglycemia, insulin resistance, dyslipidemia, and hypertension.

A caloric level should be prescribed that provides for normal growth and development in children and adolescents. The meal plan is not a restriction of calories; it is intended to ensure a reasonably consistent food intake and a nutritionally balanced diet. Parents of young children and adolescents need to learn to adjust insulin rather than to restrict food to control blood glucose levels.

Adequate calories are also needed to meet the increased metabolic requirements of pregnancy and lactation. Monitoring blood glucose levels, urine ketone levels, appetite, and weight gain allows for the appropriate caloric adjustments.

Nutrition also plays a role in preventing and treating acute complications of insulin-treated diabetes, such as hypoglycemia, short-term illnesses, and exercise-related blood glucose problems. It is also critical in treating the long-term complications of diabetes, such as renal disease, gastrointestinal neuropathy, hypertension, and lipid abnormalities.

Dietary Guidelines for Americans and the Food Guide Pyramid (see Chapter 15), which outline and illustrate nutrition guidelines and nutrient needs for all healthy Americans, can be useful aids for persons with diabetes and their family members. Family members and significant others are encouraged to follow the same life-style recommendations as the person with diabetes.

TABLE 34–8 CARDIOVASCULAR RISK BASED ON LIPID LEVELS FOR ADULTS

	LOW	BORDERLINE	HIGH
Cholesterol	<200 mg/dL (<5.2 mmol/L)	200–239 mg/dL (5.2–6.2 mmol/L)	>240 mg/dL (>6.2 mmol/L)
LDL cholesterol	<100 mg/dL (<2.6 mmol/L)	100–129 mg/dL (2.6–3.3 mmol/L)	≥130 mg/dL (≥3.35 mmol/L)
HDL cholesterol	>45 mg/dL (>1.2 mmol/L)	35–45 mg/dL (0.9–1.2 mmol/L)	<35 mg/dL (<0.9 mmol/L)
Triglycerides	<200 mg/dL (<2.3 mmol/L)	200–399 mg/dL (2.3–4.5 mmol/L)	≥400 mg/dL (≥4.5 mmol/L)

(Adapted with permission from American Diabetes Association: Management of dyslipidemia in adults with diabetes (Position Statement). Diabetes Care 22(suppl. 1):S56, 1999.)
LDL, low-density lipoprotein; HDL, high-density lipoprotein.

Strategies for Nutrition Therapy and Type 1 Diabetes

Day-to-day consistency in the timing and amount of food eaten is important for persons receiving conventional insulin therapy (i.e., two injections of insulin per day). The ideal management plan integrates insulin therapy with the individual's usual eating and exercise habits. It is not necessary to create unnatural or artificial divisions of meals and snacks. Rather, it is recommended that individuals (1) eat at consistent times synchronized with the action of insulin; (2) monitor blood glucose levels; and (3) adjust insulin doses for the amount of food usually eaten and required (American Diabetes Association, 1999c; Franz et al., 1994).

Intensive diabetes management, involving multiple injections (three or more insulin injections per day) or use of an insulin infusion pump, gives the individual increased flexibility in choosing when and what to eat. Persons can be taught to adjust their premeal insulin doses to compensate for departures from their meal plan, to delay premeal insulin for late meals, and to administer insulin for snacks that are not part of their plan (Farkas-Hirsch, 1998). However, even with intensive insulin therapy, consistency in food intake and an individualized meal plan facilitate improved glycemic control (Delahanty and Halford, 1993). Implementing nutrition practice guidelines for type 1 diabetes has also been shown to improve patient outcomes (Kulkarni, 1998).

Strategies for Nutrition Therapy and Type 2 Diabetes

The primary nutrition goals for persons with type 2 diabetes are to achieve and maintain normal blood glucose and lipid levels. A number of strategies can be implemented to achieve these goals. Learning new life-style behaviors and attitudes are essential (American Diabetes Association, 1999c; Franz et al., 1994).

Caloric restriction and moderate weight loss (10 to 20 lb [4.5 to 9.0 kg]) have been shown to improve diabetes control, even if a desirable body weight is not achieved (Watts et al., 1990). Weight loss appears to improve glucose uptake, increase insulin sensitivity, and normalize hepatic glucose production. Weight loss may be most beneficial soon after type 2 diabetes is diagnosed, when insulin secretion is still adequate.

A hypocaloric diet, however, has been shown to have an important regulatory effect on glucose control in persons with type 2 diabetes, independent of any effects from weight loss (Kelley et al., 1993; Wing et al., 1994). When calories are restricted, hyperglycemia improves more rapidly than with weight loss. Furthermore, when calories are increased after weight reduction, glucose levels increase despite no regain of weight. This suggests that caloric intake is more important than weight.

A genetic predisposition to obesity and possible impaired metabolic and appetite regulation make it difficult to lose and, more importantly, to maintain weight loss. Because of the psychological and physiologic impact of dieting, individuals should be encouraged to attain and maintain a reasonable body weight. Emphasis should be on blood glucose control, a nutritionally adequate intake, and moderate caloric restriction (250 to 500 kcal less than the average daily intake as calculated from nutrition assessment), rather than weight loss. Exercise, behavior modification of eating habits, and psychological support are also important. Other nutrition related strategies that may be useful include making better food choices, especially reducing fat intake (Boden and Chen, 1995); adequately spacing meals; and spreading nutrient intake throughout the day instead of consuming only two to three meals (Jenkins et al., 1992; Bertelsen et al., 1993).

Patterns of therapy vary according to type of diabetes, age, age at diagnosis, duration of diabetes, and race. It has been reported that 64% of adults with diabetes follow a prescribed diet all or most of the time. This varies slightly by type of diabetes: diets are followed by 73% of adults with type 1 diabetes and 63% of adults with type 2 diabetes. By necessity, people with type 1 diabetes require insulin injections; thus, they rarely use oral glucose-lowering medications. Among adults with type 2 diabetes, insulin use increases from 22% to at least 58% with increasing duration of diabetes, whereas use of oral medications follows the opposite pattern. Nearly 64% of adults with type 2 diabetes use oral therapy during the first 5 years after diagnosis, but this is reduced to 37% after 20 years of diabetes duration (American Diabetes Association, 1996).

Blood glucose monitoring provides the necessary feedback to adjust nutrition and medications. Frequent follow-up with a dietitian as outlined in nutrition practice guidelines for type 2 diabetes can provide the problem-solving techniques, encouragement, and support that life-style changes require (Franz et al., 1995).

Carbohydrate

An adequate intake of carbohydrate is recommended for all healthy Americans, including those with diabetes. Grains, vegetables, and fruits are good sources of vitamins, minerals, and dietary fiber. The belief that sucrose must be restricted was based on the assumption that sugars, such as sucrose, are more rapidly digested and absorbed than starches, and thus aggravate hyperglycemia. However, scientific evidence does not justify restricting sugars or sucrose based on this belief. In at least 12 to 15 studies in which sucrose was substituted for other carbohydrates, no adverse effects of sucrose on glycemia were found (Bantle et al., 1993; Rickard et al., 1998; Wheeler et al., 1996). The glycemic effect of carbohydrate foods varies, but cannot be predicted by their structure (i.e., starch versus sugar) owing to the efficiency of the human digestive tract in reducing starch polymers to glucose. Research conducted over the past decade has shown that starches have a higher glycemic index than fruits, milk, or sucrose (Wolever et al., 1994) (see Appendix 54). Starches are rapidly metabolized into 100% glucose during digestion, in contrast to sucrose, which is metabolized into glucose and fructose. Fructose has a lower glycemic index, which has been attributed to its slow rate of absorption and its storage in the liver as glycogen (Nuttall et al., 1992).

Although various starches do have different glycemic responses, from a clinical perspective, first priority is given to the total amount of carbohydrate consumed, rather than to the source of the carbohydrate (American Diabetes Association, 1999c). This is the basis of carbohydrate counting, whereby food portions contributing 15 g of carbohydrate (regardless of the source) are considered to be one carbohydrate choice.

Fiber

Although soluble fiber (from legumes, oats, fruits, and some vegetables) is capable of inhibiting glucose absorption from the small intestine, the clinical significance of this effect is probably insignificant (American Diabetes Association, 1999c). However, dietary fiber may be beneficial in treating or preventing several benign gastrointestinal disorders and colon cancer. Diets containing 20 g/day of soluble fibers may be capable of modestly reducing fasting circulating total and low-density lipoprotein (LDL) cholesterol when administered in conjunction with a diet containing at least 50% carbohydrate (Nuttall, 1993). However, it is difficult to consume that level of soluble fiber in foods alone. The recommendations for fiber intake for persons with diabetes are, therefore, similar to those for the general public: that is, approximately 20 to 35 g/day of dietary fiber. Daily inclusion of a fiber-containing breakfast cereal, whole-grain products, fruits, vegetables, and legumes are useful.

Sweeteners

Even though sucrose restriction cannot be justified on the basis of its glycemic effect, it is still good advice to suggest that persons with diabetes be careful in their consumption of foods containing significant amounts of sucrose. Besides being high in total carbohydrate content, they may also contain significant amounts of fat. It is important that individuals learn how to substitute sucrose-containing foods for other carbohydrate-containing foods in their meal plan.

There appears to be no significant advantage of alternative nutritive sweeteners over sucrose (American Diabetes Association, 1999c). *Fructose* provides 4 kcal/g, as do other carbohydrates, and even though it does have a lower glycemic response than sucrose and other starches, large amounts (double the usual intakes) of fructose have reportedly had an adverse effect on blood cholesterol levels, especially LDL cholesterol levels (Bantle et al., 1992). However, there is no reason to recommend that people with diabetes avoid fructose, which occurs naturally in fruits and vegetables, as well as in foods sweetened with fructose. Fruit juice concentrate, honey, molasses, and corn syrup are other natural sweeteners with no significant advantages over sucrose (American Diabetes Association, 1999c).

Sorbitol, mannitol, and *xylitol* are common sugar alcohols that also have a lower glycemic response and lower caloric content than sucrose and other carbohydrates. Because they are not soluble in water, they are often combined with fat; therefore, foods sweetened with sugar alcohols may have a caloric content that is similar to that of the foods they are replacing. Some individuals report gastric discomfort after eating foods sweetened with these products, and consuming large quantities may cause diarrhea. *Starch hydrolysates* are formed by the partial hydrolysis of edible starches. The reducing activity of starch hydrolysates can then be eliminated by hydrogenation, whereupon the product becomes a polyol (American Diabetes Association, 1999c).

Saccharin, aspartame, acesulfame K, and *sucralose* are noncaloric sweeteners currently approved for use in the United States. Food and Drug Administration (FDA) approval is being sought for *alitame* and *cyclamates.* All such products must undergo rigorous testing by the manufacturer and scrutiny from the FDA before they are approved and marketed to the public (Powers, 1999).

The FDA determines an acceptable daily intake (ADI) for food additives, including nonnutritive sweeteners, which is defined as a safe amount for daily consumption over a lifetime. The ADI includes a 100-fold safety factor and greatly exceeds average consumption levels. For example, aspartame consumption (14-day average) in persons with diabetes is 2 to 4 mg/kg/day, well below the U.S. ADI of 50 mg/kg/day (Butchko and Kotsonis, 1991). All FDA-approved nonnutritive sweeteners can be used by individuals with diabetes, including pregnant women; however, because saccharin can cross the placenta, other sweeteners are better choices (American Diabetes Association, 1999c).

Protein

The rate of protein degradation and conversion of protein to glucose in type 1 diabetes may depend on the state of insulinization and the degree of glycemic control. With less than optimal insulinization, conversion of protein to glucose can occur rapidly, adversely influencing glycemic control. In poorly controlled type 2 diabetes, gluconeogenesis is also accelerated and may account for the majority of increased glucose production in the postabsorptive state (Henry, 1994). However, the independent influence of dietary protein on glycemia and insulin sensitivity in well-controlled type 1 diabetes (Peters and Davidson, 1993) and type 2 diabetes (Nuttall et al., 1984) is minimal. The reason why ingested protein does not increase blood glucose levels remains unclear. However, even though amino acids provide substrate for new hepatic glucose synthesis, they do not increase the rate of hepatic glucose release (Franz, 1997).

At present, there is no evidence that protein requirements increase or decrease in persons with uncomplicated diabetes, so the Recommended Dietary Allowance (RDA) for protein intake—0.8 g/kg/day—for nondiabetic adults is also appropriate for adults with diabetes. Typically, protein accounts for roughly 12% to 20% or more of the total calories consumed. At present, scientific evidence does not support either an increased or decreased protein intake for the person with diabetes, and protein intake in the range of 10% to 20% of daily calories is recommended (American Diabetes Association, 1999c).

With the onset of nephropathy, restricted-protein diets may modify the underlying glomerular injury and, along with control of hypertension and hyperglycemia, delay the progression of renal failure. Generally, the response to low-protein diets in studies with diabetic subjects has been beneficial in terms of slowing progression of renal disease (Zeller et al., 1991; Pedrini et al., 1996) (see Chapter 38). A protein intake of 0.8 g/kg/day, or approximately 10% of total calories consumed, is recommended (American Diabetes Association 1999c). With a lower protein intake of 0.6 g/kg/day, evidence of protein malnutrition is noted. Decreased muscle strength and increased body fat with no change in total body weight were reported after just 12 weeks of severe protein restriction (Brodsky et al., 1992).

Several studies suggest that animal rather than vegetable protein may be an important determinant in the progression of renal disease. Studies, although preliminary, are based on evidence that vegetable proteins have significantly different renal effects than animal proteins (Nakamura et al., 1993; Wheeler, 1999).

Fat

If dietary protein contributes 10% to 20% of the total daily calories, 80% to 90% of total remains to be distributed between dietary carbohydrate and fat. It is generally agreed that reducing saturated fat (to less than 10% of total calories) and cholesterol (to less than 300 mg) is an important nutritional goal, but how dietary carbohydrate and fat (monounsaturates and polyunsaturates) should be distributed is controversial.

Persons with type 1 diabetes do not have lipid levels that differ from those of matched nondiabetic persons, but they are still at increased risk for cardiovascular disease. Therefore, the National Cholesterol Education Program (NCEP) recommendations are appropriate for most individuals with type 1 diabetes who are at a healthy weight and have normal lipid values (American Diabetes Association, 1999c) (see Chapter 26).

Type 2 diabetes is associated with a twofold to fourfold increase in the prevalence of dyslipidemia, including increased triglyceride levels, decreased HDL cholesterol levels, and total cholesterol and LDL cholesterol levels that are similar to age-matched nondiabetics. The percentage of calories from fat in the diet depends on desired glucose, lipid, and weight outcomes. If obesity and weight loss are the primary concerns, a reduced dietary fat intake should be considered. If LDL cholesterol is the primary concern, the NCEP Step II Diet guidelines should be implemented (see Chapter 26). If triglyceride and very low-density lipoprotein (VLDL) cholesterol levels are the primary concerns, one approach that may be tried is a moderate increase in monounsaturated fat intake, consumption of less than 10% of calories from saturated fats, and a moderate carbohydrate intake (American Diabetes Association, 1999c).

Several studies have suggested that a moderate-fat diet (up to 40% of total calories) can improve serum lipid levels as well as or better than fat-restricted diets, provided the additional fat is predominantly monounsaturated fatty acids (MUFAs) (Garg et al., 1994). Because major sources of MUFAs are olive, canola, and peanut oils, increasing fat intake beyond that achieved by substituting these oils in cooking can be difficult. However, the incorporation of olives, avocados, and nuts into meals and snacks may be beneficial in this regard.

Another option is a low-fat, low-calorie diet. Pascale et al. (1995) found no adverse effects on lipid levels or glycemic control from a low-calorie or low-fat diet in individuals with type 2 diabetes. Adding dietary fat restriction to the calorie-counting diet improved weight loss and maintenance. It appears that high-carbohydrate diets that are also low in calories do not cause an elevation in serum triglycerides.

Alcohol

The effect of alcohol on blood glucose levels depends not only on the amount of alcohol ingested but also on its relationship to food intake. The same precautions that apply to alcohol consumption for the general population apply to persons with diabetes. However, in the fasting state, alcohol may cause hypoglycemia in persons taking exogenous insulin. Alcohol cannot be converted to glucose (although it can be used as a source of calories and is metabolized in a manner similar to fat), and it blocks gluconeogenesis. It also augments or increases the effects of insulin by interfering with the counterregulation response to insulin-induced hypoglycemia. All of these factors contribute to the development of hypoglycemia when alcohol is consumed without food (Franz, 1999a).

For most individuals, blood glucose levels are not affected by moderate use of alcohol when diabetes is well controlled (Koivisto et al., 1993). For persons using insulin, up to two drinks for men and one drink for women (1 drink = 12 oz beer, 5 oz of wine, or 1½ oz of distilled spirits) of an alcoholic beverage can be consumed with, and in addition to, the regular meal plan. No food should be omitted given the possibility of alcohol-induced hypoglycemia and the fact that alcohol does not require insulin to be metabolized. Persons whose blood glucose levels are out of control, those with elevated triglyceride levels, and pregnant women should avoid alcohol. For persons concerned with total energy intake, alcohol is best substituted for fat exchanges or calories. Alcohol is high in calories (7 kcal/g) and is metabolized in a manner similar to fat (Franz, 1999a).

Sodium

People differ in their sensitivity to sodium and its effect on blood pressure. However, there does appear to be a relationship between diabetes and hypertension. In type 2 diabetes, hypertension is associated with obesity, but the association of hypertension with diabetes can exist even in the absence of obesity in both type 1 and type 2 diabetes. There is also evidence that persons with type 2 diabetes are more sodium-sensitive than the general public (Wylie-Rosett, 1999).

Because sodium-sensitive individuals are not easily identified, intake recommendations for people with diabetes are the same as for the general population: approximately 2400 to 3000 mg/day of sodium. For persons with mild to moderate hypertension, an intake of 2400 mg/day or less of sodium is recommended. For people with hypertension and nephropathy, a sodium intake of 2000 mg/day or less is recommended (American Diabetes Association, 1999c) (see Chapter 27).

Vitamins and Minerals

There appears to be no justification for routinely prescribing vitamin and mineral supplements for most persons with diabetes (Mooradian et al., 1994). Antioxidant therapies, such as probucol, vitamin E, and vitamin C, are currently being studied (Reaven et al., 1995).

Because the response to supplements is largely determined by an individual's nutritional status, only persons with micronutrient deficiencies are likely to respond favorably. Those at greatest risk of deficiency who may benefit from prescription of vitamin and mineral supplements, include patients consuming extreme calorie-restricted diets, strict vegetarians, the elderly, pregnant or lactating women, those taking medication known to alter micronutrient metabolism, patients in poor metabolic control (glycosuria), and patients in critical care environments (Franz, 1999b).

Chromium deficiency in animal models is associated with elevated blood glucose, cholesterol, and triglyceride levels. However, it is unlikely that most individuals with diabetes are chromium-deficient. In three double-blind crossover studies of chromium supplementation in individuals with diabetes, no improvement in blood glucose control was noted. In individuals with IGT who consumed a diet deficient in chromium for 4 weeks, chromium supplementation improved glucose tolerance (Mooradian et al., 1994). The response to chromium supplementation is related to the degree of chromium deficiency, the degree of glucose intolerance, and the duration of the study (Anderson, 1998). However, before chromium supplementation can be recommended, double-blind crossover studies in people with diabetes with known dietary intake of chromium using chromium supplements that may be better absorbed than older supplements need to be undertaken (Franz, 1999b).

Magnesium replacement may be required for patients with poor glycemic control or those receiving diuretics. Magnesium depletion has been associated with insulin insensitivity, which may improve with oral supplementation, especially in type 2 diabetes (American Diabetes Association, 1992).

Medications

Insulin

Persons with type 1 diabetes depend on insulin to survive. In persons with type 2 diabetes, insulin may be needed to restore glycemia to near normal. Circumstances that require the use of insulin in type 2 diabetes include failure to achieve adequate control with administration of oral glucose-lowering medications; periods of acute injury, infection, or surgery; pregnancy; and allergy or serious reactions to sulfonylurea agents.

Insulin has four properties: action, concentration, purity, and source. These properties determine its onset, peak, and duration (Table 34–9). Regular and Lispro insulins are *short-acting* and provide a burst of insulin to cover the meal that is just about to be eaten. Regular insulin needs to be taken 30 to 45 minutes before eating. Lispro insulin, an analogue with two amino acids reversed in position starts to work very quickly, so it should be taken immediately before eating. Both insulins may be used in combination with a background or intermediate-acting insulin, and may also be used independently during acute illness, in insulin pumps, and in multiple daily injection regimens.

Background or *intermediate-acting* insulins include NPH and Lente. Their appearance is cloudy, and their onset, peak, and duration are similar. Ultralente is a slightly *longer-acting* insulin than the intermediate-acting insulins. Premixed insulins are also available: 70/30, which is 70% NPH and 30% regular; and 50/50, which is 50% NPH and 50% regular.

TABLE 34–9 COMPARATIVE ACTIONS OF INSULIN

INSULIN	ONSET	PEAK EFFECT	DURATION
Short-acting Insulins (clear)			
Lispro (Humalog)	5–15 minutes	30–75 minutes	2–3 hours
Regular (R)	30–45 minutes	2–3 hours	4–6 hours
Background Insulins (cloudy)			
NPH (N)	2–4 hours	4–10 hours	10–18 hours
Lente (L)	2–4 hours	4–10 hours	10–18 hours
Ultralente (U)	3–5 hours	8–14 hours	18 hours
Premixed Insulins (short-acting and background together)			
70/30 or 50/50	30–60 minutes	2–12 hours	Up to 18 hours

(Reprinted with permission from My Insulin Plan. Minneapolis: International Diabetes Center, 1998.)

U-100 is the concentration of insulin available in the United States. This refers to insulin activity per milliliter of insulin; therefore, U-100 means 100 units/mL.

Human or highly purified animal insulins are now standard and contain less than 1 ppm of impurities. They are associated with fewer insulin antibodies, less insulin allergy, and less lipoatrophy at the injection site than previous preparations. The source of insulin is important because it affects the speed of absorption, peak, and duration of action. Animal insulins come from the pancreas of cows and pigs. However, since 1984, human insulin has been produced synthetically. Human insulins are generally absorbed more rapidly, peak earlier, and have a shorter duration time than animal insulins. A major advantage of human insulin is that it produces fewer antibodies and, as a result, can also be used for intermittent periods of insulin treatment, such as during surgery and pregnancy. Most newly diagnosed patients are started on human insulin.

The type and timing of insulin regimens should be individualized, based on eating and exercise habits and blood glucose levels. A single dose of insulin is seldom effective for optimal blood glucose control in either type of diabetes. A commonly used regimen combines a short-acting and background (NPH or Lente) insulin, given twice a day. The prebreakfast dose consists of about one third regular and two thirds NPH. The presupper dose is usually divided into equal amounts of NPH and regular insulin (Fig. 34–3).

Another common regimen combines a short-acting and background insulin prebreakfast, a short-acting insulin presupper, and background insulin, such as NPH, at bedtime. The background insulin is administered at bedtime to control the early morning surge in blood glucose levels (dawn phenomenon). Other intensive insulin regimens consist

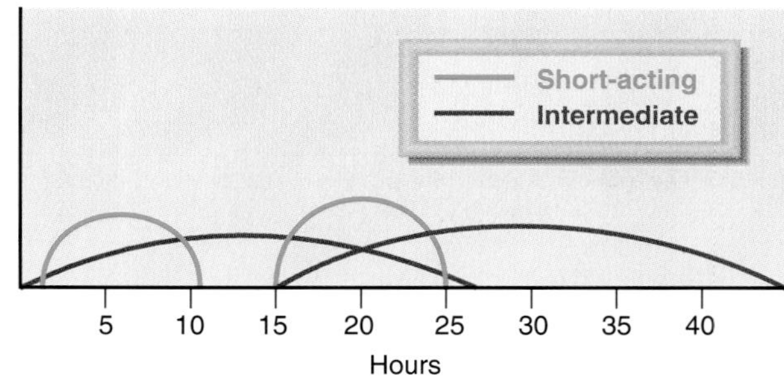

FIGURE 34–3 Time actions of two-injection insulin regimens.

of multiple daily injections or insulin infusion pump therapy. A short-acting insulin is given before meals to provide bolus insulin replacement, and a background insulin is given once or twice a day (Fig. 34–4). These types of regimens allow increased flexibility in the type and timing of meals. The amount of short-acting insulin can be adjusted based on the composition of the meal.

Insulin infusion pump therapy provides basal short-acting insulin pumped continuously by a mechanical device in micro amounts through a subcutaneous catheter that is monitored 24 hours a day. Boluses of the short-acting insulin are then given before meals. Pump therapy requires a committed and motivated person who is willing to do a minimum of four blood glucose tests per day, keep blood glucose and food records, and learn the technical features of pump usage. Pump therapy is also more expensive than other insulin regimens.

Oral Glucose-Lowering Medications

The use of the newer **oral glucose-lowering medications,** alone or in combination, provides numerous options for achieving euglycemia in persons with type 2 diabetes. Persons with mild to moderate hyperglycemia that is not adequately controlled by MNT alone can be treated with metformin, alpha-glucosidase inhibitors, or thiazolidinediones. With modest insulin deficiencies, sulfonylurea agents, alone or in combination with other oral medications, can be given to restore glycemic control. As

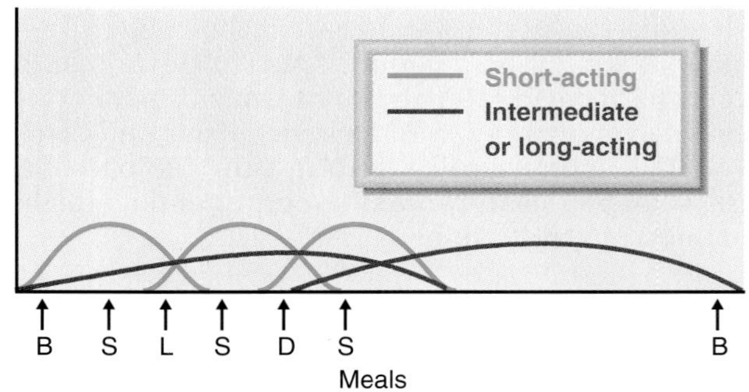

FIGURE 34–4 Time actions of multiple-injection insulin regimens. *B*, breakfast; *S*, snack; *L*, lunch; *D*, dinner.

endogenous insulin effectiveness deteriorates, insulin can be used with oral medications; eventually, multiple injections of insulin alone may be necessary (Lebovitz, 1994). Although new diabetes medications have entered the marketplace recently, additional diabetes-related medications are being developed and are being ushered from research and clinical testing toward FDA approval.

Sulfonylureas work by stimulating the beta cells in the pancreas to release more insulin. They have been on the market for the longest period of time and are generally the most economical to use. Over extensive periods, however, these drugs may exhaust beta-cell activity. Disadvantages of their use include weight gain, and they can cause hypoglycemia. First- and second-generation sulfonylurea drugs differ from one another in their potency, pharmacokinetics, and metabolism. The new sulfonylurea drugs may be taken alone or with other diabetes drugs. Their reduced frequency of dosage can promote adherence to the drug regimen (Table 34–10).

Meglitinide is a new class of nonsulfonylurea hypoglycemic agents for type 2 diabetes. Repaglinide (prandin) is quick in onset and short-acting and, therefore, is taken before each meal. Administering this short-acting agent just before meals affords immediate hypoglycemic activity and decreases the risk of hypoglycemia between meals and at night. It works by improving insulin secretion in response to glucose levels by binding to a different site than the sulfonylureas (Malaisse, 1995).

Another drug class—the *biguanides*—offers clinicians yet another treatment alternative. In the liver, biguanides suppress glucose production and lower insulin resistance, but do not stimulate insulin secretion. Glucophage (metformin) was approved for use in the United States in 1994, but it has been used in other countries for many years. It is not associated with hypoglycemic reactions, it may cause small weight losses when therapy begins, and it improves lipid levels. A rare side effect is severe lactic acidosis, which can be fatal. The acidosis usually occurs in patients who use alcohol, have renal dysfunction, or have liver impairments. Biguanides can be used alone or in combination with other diabetes medications (Hermann et al., 1994).

Thiazolidinediones are another new class of antidiabetic drugs. Rezulin (troglitazone) acts by lowering insulin resistance to injected or endogenous insulin and enhances insulin action in muscle, adipose tissue, and liver cells. It is approved for use as monotherapy, or in combination with sulfonylureas or insulin. Patients with liver disease or severe heart failure should not be given troglitazone. Avandia (rosiglitazone) and Actos (pioglitazone) are two new thiazolidinediones reported to be less likely to cause liver toxicity. The ability to reduce insulin resistance may make these drugs useful in preventing type 2 diabetes (Nolan et al., 1994).

Alpha-glucosidase inhibitors work in the small intestine to inhibit enzymes that digest carbohydrates, thereby delaying carbohydrate absorption

TABLE 34–10 COMPARATIVE ACTIONS OF GLUCOSE-LOWERING MEDICATIONS

CLASS	MEDICATION	MODE OF ACTION	USUAL STARTING DOSE	MAXIMUM DOSE
Second-generation sulfonylureas	Glipizide (Glucotrol)	Stimulate insulin secretion in the pancreas	5 mg before breakfast	40 mg/day
	Glipizide (Glucotrol XL)		5 mg with first meal of the day	20 mg
	Glyburide (Glynase)		1.5–3 mg/day with first meal of the day	12 mg
	Glimepiride (Amaryl)		1–2 mg with breakfast or with first main meal	8 mg
Meglitinide	Repaglinide (Prandin)	Stimulates insulin secretion in presence of glucose	0.5 mg before each meal for HbA1c <8% 1–2 mg before each meal for HbA1c ≥8%	4 mg before each meal (16 mg/day)
Biguanide	Metformin (Glucophage)	Decreases hepatic glucose production	500 mg or 850 mg once daily with meal	2550 mg
Alpha-glucosidase inhibitors	Acarbose (Precose)	Delay absorption of glucose from the GI tract	25 mg before dinner, increasing to 25 mg TID before each meal	300 mg/day
	Miglitol (Glyset)		25 mg before dinner, increasing to 25 mg TID before each meal	300 mg/day
Thiazolidinediones	Troglitazone (Rezulin)	Decrease insulin resistance in peripheral tissues	200 mg with food, once daily	600 mg/day
	Rosiglitazone (Avandia)		2 mg	6 mg
	Pioglitazone (Actos)		30 mg	50 mg

and lowering postprandial glycemia. For example, Precose (acarbose) and Glyset (miglitol) are competitive inhibitors of intestinal brush-border alpha-glucosidases required for the breakdown of starches, dextrins, maltose, and sucrose to absorbable monosaccharides. They do not cause hypoglycemia or weight gain when used alone, but frequently may cause flatulence, diarrhea, cramping, or abdominal pain. Symptoms may be alleviated by initiating therapy at a low dose and gradually increasing the dose to therapeutic levels (Coniff, 1995).

Some persons may benefit from **combination therapy** with oral medications and newer antidiabetic drugs, or with oral medications and insulin. Candidates for insulin and combination therapy are those whose blood glucose level is poorly controlled by oral medications. Frequently, intermediate-acting insulin is given at bedtime to control fasting glucose levels, and the oral medication is used to control glucose levels during the day (Yki-Jarvinen et al., 1992).

Exercise

Exercise should be an integral part of the treatment plan for persons with diabetes. Exercise helps all persons with diabetes improve insulin sensitivity, reduce cardiovascular risk factors, control weight, and bring about a healthier mental outlook. Given appropriate guidelines, people with diabetes can exercise safely. The exercise plan will vary depending on interest, age, general health, and level of physical fitness.

When the nondiabetic person exercises, insulin levels decline while counterregulatory hormones (primarily glucagon) rise. In this way, increased glucose utilization by the exercising muscle is matched precisely with increased glucose production by the liver.

In persons with type 1 diabetes, the glycemic response to exercise varies depending on overall diabetes control, plasma glucose and insulin levels at the start of exercise, intensity and duration of the exercise, previous food intake, and previous conditioning. An important variable is the level of plasma insulin during and after exercise. Excessive insulin levels can potentiate hypoglycemia because of insulin-enhanced muscle glucose uptake by the exercising muscle. In contrast, because insulin levels are too low in a poorly controlled (underinsulinized) exerciser, production of glucose and free fatty acids (FFAs) continues with minimal uptake. This results in large increases in plasma glucose and ketone levels (Wasserman and Zinman, 1994).

In persons with type 2 diabetes, blood glucose control can improve with exercise, largely because of decreased insulin resistance and increased insulin sensitivity, which results in increased peripheral use of glucose not only during but also after the activity. Because enhanced insulin sensitivity is lost within 48 hours after exercise, repeated periods of exercise at regular intervals are needed to reduce the glucose intolerance associated with type 2 diabetes. This exercise-induced enhanced insulin sensitivity occurs without changes in body weight. Exercise also decreases the effects of counterregulatory hormones; this, in turn, reduces the hepatic glucose output, contributing to improved glucose control.

Timing the exercise session for persons with type 2 diabetes may be advantageous. For example, exercise performed later in the day has been shown to reduce overnight hepatic glucose output and fasting glycemia. Exercise after eating can also be beneficial, reducing postprandial hyperglycemia, which is common in type 2 diabetes.

Potential Problems with Exercise

Hypoglycemia is a potential problem associated with exercise in persons taking insulin or oral medications. Hypoglycemia is more common after exercise than during exercise because of the need to replete liver and muscle glycogen, which can take up to 24 to 30 hours.

Hyperglycemia and worsening ketosis can result from insulin deficiency if exercise is started when blood glucose levels are higher than 250 to 300 mg/dL. With elevated fasting blood glucose and urine ketones, exercise should be postponed until control improves (American Diabetes Association, 1999e). Exercise of high intensity can also result in hyperglycemia owing to the effects of counterregulatory hormones (Mitchell et al., 1988; Purdon et al., 1993).

In persons with preexisting cardiovascular disease, exercise may precipitate arrhythmias, myocardial ischemia, or infarction. For some time, it has been thought that patients with proliferative retinopathy are at increased risk for retinal or vitreous hemorrhage, or retinal detachment, during exercise. However, few or no data support this contention. Some ophthalmologists in certain situations may still caution patients not to exercise during specific times, or to avoid certain types of exercise (Wasserman and Zinman, 1994). The presence of peripheral neuropathy increases the risk of foot, soft tissue, and joint injury. High-quality footwear should be used.

Exercise Guidelines

Before starting an exercise program, the person with diabetes should seek medical clearance from a physician. In designing an exercise regimen, a physical activity assessment should be performed, and the medical history, diabetes management plan, and clinical status of the individual should all be taken into consideration (American Diabetes Association, 1999e).

SMBG, both preexercise and postexercise, is the key to safety and understanding how exercise affects diabetes control. Frequent postexercise testing may be especially important. Blood glucose monitoring provides feedback that can be used to guide insulin and carbohydrate adjustments. The choice between increasing carbohydrate or decreasing medication depends on the individual and his or her diabetes management goals.

In general, 1 hour of increased exercise requires an additional 15 g of carbohydrate, either before or after exercise. For more strenuous exercise, 30 g of carbohydrate per hour may be needed. Moderate exercise for less than 30 minutes rarely requires any additional carbohydrate or insulin adjustment; however, a small snack may be needed if the blood glucose level is less than 100 mg/dL (<5.5 mmol/L) (Table 34–11) (Franz and Barry, 1993).

It is often necessary to adjust the insulin dosage to prevent hypoglycemia. This occurs most often with strenuous activity lasting more than 45 to 60 minutes. For most persons, a modest decrease (of approximately 10% to 20%) in the insulin component corresponding to the period of exercise is sufficient to prevent hypoglycemia. For prolonged vigorous exercise, a larger decrease in the total daily insulin dosage (by as much as one third to half) may be necessary to prevent repeated hypoglycemic episodes. In addition to these acute reductions in insulin dosages, individuals participating in a regular, long-term fitness program often find their usual total dosage of insulin decreasing by as much as 15% to 20% (Wasserman and Zinman, 1994).

Exercise Prescription

The type of exercise individuals choose to perform should be tailored to their physical capacity and interests. A complete exercise program includes warm-up and cool-down periods. These not only prepare muscles for an aerobic workout, but also improve range of motion. Cardiovascular conditioning is also helpful. Most people can at least undertake a walking program safely. Ideally, the aerobic portion of an exercise session should last a minimum of 20 minutes, with a goal of 30 to 40 minutes. However, even three sessions of 10 minutes of activity during the day can improve physical fitness. Muscle-strengthening exercises, such as lifting light weights, are also an important component of an exercise session. Muscles dispose of glucose, so this type of exercise can also improve glucose control.

TABLE 34–11 CARBOHYDRATE ADJUSTMENTS FOR EXERCISE

TYPE OF ACTIVITY	BLOOD GLUCOSE LEVEL	CARBOHYDRATE ADJUSTMENT
Short duration and low intensity (30 minutes or less; e.g., walking ½ mile, leisurely biking)	<100 mg/dL	10–15 g of carbohydrate (CHO) (1 CHO choice)
	>100 mg/dL	No extra CHO needed
Moderate duration and moderate intensity	<100 mg/dL	30–45 g CHO (2–3 CHO choices)
(30–60 minutes; e.g., tennis, swimming, jogging, bicycling, etc.)	100–180 mg/dL	15 g CHO (1 CHO choice)
	180–300 mg/dL*	No extra CHO needed
Long duration, moderate intensity (≥1 hour; e.g., football, hockey, basketball, strenuous bicycling)	<100 mg/dL	45 g CHO (3 CHO choices)
	100–180 mg/dL	30–45 g CHO (2–3 CHO choices)
	180–300 mg/dL*	15 g CHO/hour

(Adapted with permission from Franz MJ, Barry B. Diabetes and Exercise. Guidelines for Safe and Enjoyable Activity. Minneapolis: International Diabetes Center, 1993, p. 16.)

* If fasting blood glucose level exceeds 250 mg/dL before exercise, check urine for ketones. If ketones are moderate to large, delay exercising until the blood glucose level is better controlled.

Blood Glucose Monitoring

Self-monitoring of blood glucose (SMBG) can be used to manage diabetes effectively and safely. However, laboratory measurement of glycated hemoglobin provides the best available index of overall diabetes control.

Self-Monitoring of Blood Glucose Levels

The health care team should work together to implement blood glucose monitoring and establish individual **target blood glucose goals.** The frequency of monitoring depends on the type of diabetes and overall therapy.

SMBG can be performed up to seven times per day—before breakfast, lunch, and dinner; at bedtime; 1 to 2 hours after meals; during the night (once a week); or to determine causes of hypoglycemia or hyperglycemia. It is frequently recommended that persons with type 1 diabetes test glucose levels four times a day, before each meal and at bedtime. Those with type 2 diabetes may perform glucose monitoring one to four times a day, but only 3 or 4 days per week (American Diabetes Association, 1994b).

It is important that the results of SMBG be written in a record book, and that individuals be taught how to adjust their management program based on the results. The first step in using such records is to learn how to identify patterns in blood glucose levels and how to adjust basic insulin doses. After this is mastered, algorithms for insulin dose changes can be added.

In using blood glucose monitoring records, it should be remembered that factors other than food affect blood glucose levels. An increase in blood glucose levels can be the result of insufficient insulin or oral medications, too much food, or increases in glucagon and other counterregulatory hormones as a result of stress, illness, or infection. Factors contributing to hypoglycemia include too much insulin or oral medications, not enough food, unusual amounts of exercise, and skipped or delayed meals. Urine glucose testing, frequently used in the past, has so many limitations that it should not used.

Urine testing, however, remains the only practical way to detect ketones. Testing for ketonuria should be performed regularly during periods of illness and when blood glucose levels consistently exceed 240 mg/dL (13.3 mmol/L). The presence of persistent, moderate, or large amounts of ketones, along with elevated blood glucose levels, requires insulin adjustments. Persons with type 2 diabetes rarely have ketosis. However, ketone testing should be done in the presence of a serious illness.

Self-Management Education

Diabetes management is a team effort. Persons with diabetes must be at the center of the team because they have the responsibility for day-to-day management. Dietitians, nurses, physicians, and other health care providers contribute their expertise to developing therapeutic regimens that help the person with diabetes achieve the best metabolic control possible. The goal is to provide individuals with the knowledge, skills, and motivation to incorporate self-management into their daily life-styles. Individualized education is a planned process that requires time, materials, space, and professional expertise.

For newly diagnosed patients, a staged approach to education should be used. Initial education focuses on the skills needed for survival (Table 34–12). In-depth information and additional topics are added after the patient has time to adjust to the diagnosis. The numerous topics vary according to the type of diabetes and the characteristics and needs of the individual. The knowledge and skills needed to implement nutritional recommendations cannot be acquired in one session; therefore, nutrition education must be an ongoing component of diabetes care. Because food is an important component of diabetes treatment and health, continued nutrition education is essential (Table 34–13).

Optimal self-management of diabetes requires changes in existing behaviors in addition to the adoption of new ones. Successful behavioral change requires comprehensive education, skill development, and motivation. This is best accomplished through a coordinated team effort in which the dietitian must be an active participant.

ACUTE COMPLICATIONS

Hyperosmolar Hyperglycemic Nonketotic (HHNK) Syndrome

Hypoglycemia, diabetic ketoacidosis, and **hyperosmolar hyperglycemic nonketotic (HHNK) syndrome** are acute complications related to diabetes. Hypoglycemia and diabetic ketoacidosis are discussed in greater detail later in this section. HHNK syndrome is defined as an extremely high blood glucose level, absence of or only small amounts of ketones, and profound dehydration. Glucose levels

TABLE 34–12 INITIAL SELF-MANAGEMENT EDUCATION (SURVIVAL SKILLS)

Basic Survival Skills for Medical Nutrition Therapy for All Persons with Diabetes

- Basic food/meal plan guidelines
- Exercise guidelines
- Signs, symptoms, treatment, and prevention of hypoglycemia
- Nutritional management during short-term illness
- Self-monitoring of blood glucose levels
- Plan for continuing care

(Reprinted with permission from Monk A, et al. Practice guidelines for medical nutrition therapy by dietitians for persons with non–insulin-dependent diabetes mellitus. J Am Diet Assoc 95:999, 1995.)

TABLE 34–13 ESSENTIAL NUTRITION EDUCATION TOPICS FOR SELF-MANAGEMENT

Topics Emphasized Based on Patient's Life-Style, Level of Nutrition Knowledge, and Experience in Planning, Purchasing, and Preparing Food and Meals

- Sources of carbohydrate, protein, fat
- Nutrition labels
- Grocery shopping guidelines
- Guidelines for eating out: restaurant, cafeteria, and fast-food choices
- Modification of fat intake
- Use of sugar-containing foods
- Alcohol consumption guidelines
- Snack choices
- Use of blood glucose monitoring for problem solving and identification of blood glucose patterns
- Meal time adjustments
- Flexible meal planning
- Dietetic foods and sweeteners
- Exchanges
- Recipes, menu ideas, cookbooks
- Adjustment of food intake for exercise
- Behavior modification techniques
- Problem-solving tips
- Birthdays, special occasions, holidays
- Brown-bag lunches
- Travel, schedule changes
- Vitamin, mineral, and other nutritional supplements
- Work shift rotation, if needed

(Reprinted with permission from Monk A, et al. Practice guidelines for medical nutrition therapy by dietitians for persons with non–insulin-dependent diabetes mellitus. J Am Diet Assoc 95:999, 1995.)

generally range from greater than 600 to 2000 mg/dL (>33.3 to 111.1 mmol/L), with an average of approximately 1000 mg/dL (55.5 mmol/L). Patients who have HHNK syndrome have sufficient insulin to prevent lipolysis and ketosis. This condition occurs rarely, usually in older patients with type 2 diabetes. Treatment consists of hydration and small doses of insulin to correct the hyperglycemia.

Hyperglycemia/Diabetic Ketoacidosis

Hyperglycemia can lead to **diabetic ketoacidosis (DKA),** a life-threatening but reversible complication characterized by severe disturbances in carbohydrate, protein, and fat metabolism. DKA is always the result of inadequate insulin for glucose utilization. As a result, the body depends on fat for energy, and ketones are formed. Acidosis results from increased production and decreased utilization of acetoacetic acid and 3-beta-hydroxybutyric acid from fatty acids. These ketones spill into the urine, hence the reliance on urine testing for ketones.

DKA is characterized by elevated blood glucose levels (≥250 mg/dL [≥13.9 mmol/L]) and the presence of ketones in the blood and urine. Symptoms include polyuria, polydipsia, hyperventilation, dehydration, the fruity odor of ketones, and fatigue. SMBG, testing for urine ketones, and medical intervention can all help prevent DKA. If left untreated, DKA can lead to coma and death. Treatment includes supplemental insulin, fluid and electrolyte replacement, and medical monitoring. Acute illnesses, such as flu, colds, vomiting, and diarrhea, if not managed appropriately, can lead to the development of DKA. Patients need to know the steps to take during acute illness to prevent DKA (Table 34–14).

TABLE 34–14 SICK-DAY GUIDELINES FOR PERSONS WITH DIABETES

1. During acute illnesses, take usual doses of insulin. The need for insulin continues, or may even increase, during periods of illness. Fever, dehydration, infection, or the stress of illness can trigger the release of counterregulatory or "stress" hormones, causing blood glucose levels to become elevated.
2. Monitoring of blood glucose levels and urine testing for ketones should be done at least four times daily (before each meal and at bedtime). Blood glucose readings exceeding 240 mg/dL and moderate to large urine ketones are danger signals indicating that additional insulin is needed.
3. If regular foods are not tolerated, liquid or soft carbohydrate-containing foods (such as regular soft drinks, soup, juices, and ice cream) should be eaten. At least 50 g of carbohydrate (3 to 4 carbohydrate choices) should be consumed every 3 to 4 hours in small, frequent feedings.
4. Ample amounts of liquid should be consumed every hour. If nausea or vomiting occurs, small sips—1 or 2 T every 15 to 30 minutes—should be consumed. If vomiting continues, the health care team should be notified.
5. The health care team should be called if illness continues for more than 1 day.

(Adapted with permission from Franz MJ, Joynes JO. Diabetes and Brief Illness. Minneapolis: International Diabetes Center, 1993, p. 4.)

Hypoglycemia

Hypoglycemia is a common side effect of insulin therapy. Autonomic symptoms are generally the first signs of mild hypoglycemia, and include shakiness, sweating, palpitations, and hunger. Moderate and advanced hypoglycemic symptoms are related to neuroglycopenia and include headaches, confusion, lack of coordination, blurred vision, anger, seizures, and coma. There are several common causes of hypoglycemia (see Table 34–15). In gen-

TABLE 34–15 COMMON CAUSES OF HYPOGLYCEMIA

Medication errors
Excess insulin or oral medications
Inadvertent or deliberate errors in insulin doses
Improper timing of insulin in relation to food intake
Intensive insulin therapy
Inadequate food intake
Omitted or inadequate meals or snacks
Delayed meals or snacks
Increased exercise or activity
Unplanned activities
Prolonged duration or increased intensity of exercise
Alcohol intake without food

(Adapted with permission from Skyler JS (ed.). Medical Management of Type 1 Diabetes, 3rd ed. Alexandria, VA: American Diabetes Association, 1998, p. 137.)

eral, treatment begins with 15 g of carbohydrate. Commercially available glucose tablets have the advantage of being premeasured to help prevent overtreatment (Table 34–16). If patients are unable to swallow, administration of subcutaneous or intramuscular glucagon may be needed. Parents, roommates, and spouses should be taught how to mix, draw up, and administer glucagon so that they are properly prepared for emergency situations. Kits that include a syringe prefilled with diluting fluid are available.

Some individuals experience hypoglycemia unawareness, which means that they do not experience the usual symptoms. Patients need to be reminded of the need to treat hypoglycemia, even in the absence of symptoms. SMBG is essential for prevention and treatment. Changes in insulin injections, eating, exercise schedules, and travel routines warrant increased frequency of monitoring (Cryer et al., 1994). Patients with recurrent hypoglycemia may not be good candidates for intensive insulin therapy.

Hyperglycemia after Hypoglycemia

Hypoglycemia followed by "rebound" hyperglycemia is also called the **Somogyi effect.** This phenomenon originates during hypoglycemia with the secretion of counterregulatory hormones (glucagon, epinephrine, growth hormone, and cortisol). Hepatic glucose production is stimulated, thus raising blood glucose levels. If rebound hyperglycemia goes unrecognized and insulin doses are increased, a cycle of overinsulinization may result.

Dawn Phenomenon

The amount of insulin required to normalize blood glucose levels during the night is less in the predawn period (from 1 to 3 AM) than at dawn (4 to 8 AM). This rise in blood glucose levels may be increased if insulin levels decline between predawn and dawn, or if hypoglycemia occurs during the predawn period. Blood glucose level is monitored at bedtime and at 2 to 3 AM to identify the **dawn phenomenon.** Consuming extra food at bedtime or administering an insulin form that does not peak at 1 to 3 AM should be considered to prevent morning hyperglycemia. Taking intermediate-acting insulin at bedtime or substituting it with a longer-acting insulin may also be effective.

TABLE 34–16 TREATMENT OF HYPOGLYCEMIA

- Immediate treatment with carbohydrate is essential.
  - If the blood glucose level falls below 70 mg/dL (3.9 mmol/L), treat with 15 g of carbohydrate, which is equivalent to:
    3 glucose tablets
    Fruit juice or regular soft drinks, ½ cup
    Saltine crackers, 6
    Sugar or honey, 1 T
- Wait 15 minutes and retest. If the blood glucose level remains ≤70 mg/dL (≤3.9 mmol/L), treat with another 15 g of carbohydrate.
- Repeat testing and treatment until the blood glucose level returns to within normal range.
- Evaluate the time to the next meal or snack to determine the need for additional food. If it is more than an hour to next meal add an additional 15 g of carbohydrate.

(Adapted with permission from Skyler JS (ed.). Medical Management of Type 1 Diabetes, 3rd ed. Alexandria, VA: American Diabetes Association, 1998, p. 139.)

LONG-TERM COMPLICATIONS

MNT is important in managing several long-term complications of diabetes. Nutrition is also a major component in reducing risk factors for chronic complications, especially those related to macrovascular disease. Obesity, especially intra-abdominal obesity or the android distribution of adipose tissue (a waist-to-hip ratio >1.0 in men and >0.8 in women), is associated with dyslipidemia, hypertension, glucose intolerance, and increased prevalence of cardiovascular disease (see Chapter 23). Other risk factors include smoking, lack of exercise, renal failure, and microalbuminuria.

Macrovascular Diseases

Macrovascular diseases—including coronary heart disease (CHD), peripheral vascular disease (PVD), and cerebrovascular disease (CVD)—are more common, tend to occur at an earlier age, and are more extensive and severe in people with diabetes. Lipid abnormalities are one of the risk factors contributing to accelerated atherosclerotic vascular disease (see Chapter 26). Generally, total cholesterol and LDL cholesterol are comparable between persons with diabetes and the general population. However, patients with type 2 diabetes typically have smaller, more dense LDL particles, which increases atherogenicity even if the total LDL cholesterol level is not significantly increased. Elevated plasma triglyceride and very low-density lipoprotein (VLDL) cholesterol levels and lower HDL cholesterol levels are more common with type 2 diabetes. Cardiovascular risk based on lipid levels for adults is outlined in Table 34–8. Treatment decisions for adults are based on LDL cholesterol levels. With CHD, PVD, or CVD, MNT and drug therapy are initiated when LDL cholesterol levels exceed 100 mg/dL, with a goal of reducing this value to 100 mg/dL or less. Without CHD, PVD, or CVD, MNT is initiated when LDL cholesterol levels exceed 100 mg/dL; drug therapy is appropriate at LDL cholesterol levels of 130 mg/dL or higher (American Diabetes Association, 1999d).

Dyslipidemia

In general, treatment for dyslipidemia involves improved glucose control, an individualized meal plan designed to result in gradual, moderate weight loss, food choices low in saturated fats and cholesterol, and increased physical activity. Nutrition recommendations for reducing elevated serum triglyceride levels may include a moderate increase in monounsaturated fat intake and a more moderate intake of carbohydrate; however, saturated fats should still be less than 10% of total calories.

Patients should be treated aggressively with diet, exercise, and glucose control. If these measures fail to achieve LDL cholesterol goals, the addition of cholesterol- and triglyceride-lowering drugs, such as HMG-CoA reductase inhibitors (pravastatin or simvastatin), or fibric acid derivatives (gemfibrozil) is warranted (American Diabetes Association, 1999d).

Hypertension

Treatment of hypertension in persons with diabetes should also be vigorous to reduce the risk of macrovascular and microvascular disease. The goal for blood pressure control is less than 130/85 mm Hg (American Diabetes Association, 1993). Besides sodium restriction (<2400 mg/day), other clearly beneficial nutrition interventions include weight reduction and restricted alcohol intake (see Chapter 27).

Microvascular Diseases

Microvascular diseases associated with diabetes involve the small blood vessels and may include retinopathy and nephropathy.

Retinopathy

Diabetic retinopathy is a leading cause of new blindness among adults; ~5000 new cases of blindness related to diabetes are estimated to occur each year in the United States (Zimmerman, 1998). More than 80% of all patients with diabetes have some form of retinopathy 15 years after diagnosis. However, laser photocoagulation can reduce the loss of vision associated with proliferative retinopathy and macular edema by 50% if the conditions are identified in time (Zimmerman, 1998). In both types of diabetes, the development and progression of retinopathy is duration-dependent and associated with increased glycemic levels. In patients with type 1 diabetes, retinopathy rarely occurs before the fifth year of the disease and rarely before the onset of puberty, even in patients with diabetes of 5 years' duration or longer. The hormonal changes of puberty seem to exert an accelerating influence on the development of retinopathy.

There are three stages of diabetic retinopathy. The early stages of *nonproliferative diabetic retinopathy (NPDR)* are characterized by microaneurysms, a pouch-like dilation of a terminal capillary; lesions that include cotton-wool spots (also referred to as soft exudates); and the formation of new blood vessels as a result of the retina's great metabolic need for oxygen and other nutrients supplied by the bloodstream.

As the disease progresses to the middle stages of moderate, severe, and very severe NPDR, gradual loss of the retinal microvasculature occurs, resulting in retinal ischemia. Extensive intraretinal hemorrhages and microaneurysms are common reflections of increasing retinal nonperfusion.

The most advanced stage—termed *proliferative diabetic retinopathy (PDR)*—is the final and most vision-threatening stage of diabetic retinopathy. It is characterized by the onset of ischemia-induced new vessel proliferation at the optic disk or elsewhere in the retina. The new vessels are fragile and prone to bleeding, resulting in vitreous hemorrhage. With time, the neovascularization tends to undergo fibrosis and contraction, resulting in retinal traction, retinal tears, vitreous hemorrhage, and retinal detachment. *Diabetic macular edema*, which involves thickening of the central (macular) portion of the retina, and glaucoma, in which fibrous scar tissue increases intraocular pressure, are other clinical findings in retinopathy (Aiello et al., 1998).

The DCCT and the UKPDS have demonstrated that, in patients with diabetes, intensive treatment that lowers average glucose levels to near normal, prevents or ameliorates retinopathy. No other treatment to reduce the occurrence of retinopathy has been identified. In addition, because photocoagulation decreases the loss of vision by about 50% in patients with PDR and macular edema, identification of patients at risk is of major importance. All patients with type 2 diabetes should have annual eye examinations, including a complete visual history, visual acuity examination, and careful ophthalmoscopic examination with a dilated pupil, starting at the time of diagnosis. Patients with type 1 diabetes should have an annual detailed ocular examination 5 years after diagnosis; the examination need not be done before puberty unless the patient has eye symptoms or evidence of other diabetic complications (American Diabetes Association, 1999b).

Nephropathy

Although *nephropathy* develops in a higher percentage of persons with type 1 diabetes, nephropathy is more commonly attributable to type 2 diabetes because of the greater prevalence of type 2 diabetes. More than 20% of persons with both types of diabetes have overt nephropathy after 15 to 20 years of diabetes, and this may progress to end-stage renal disease (ESRD) requiring dialysis or renal transplantation (National Diabetes Data Group, 1995).

The earliest clinical evidence of nephropathy is the appearance of low but abnormal urine albumin levels (>30 mg/day or 20 μg/min), referred to as microalbuminuria or incipient nephropathy. Without specific interventions, approximately 80% of persons with type 1 diabetes over a period of 10 to 15 years will progress to overt nephropathy or clinical albuminuria (≥300 mg/day or 200 μg/min) with hypertension. Without interventions, the glomerular filtration rate (GFR) will gradually decline over a period of years, with ESRD developing in 50% of persons with type 1 diabetes within 10 years and more than 75% of these patients by 20 years. Without specific interventions, 20% to 40% of patients with type 2 diabetes and with microalbuminuria progress to overt nephropathy, but by 20 years after onset of overt nephropathy, only about 20% will have progressed to ESRD (American Diabetes Association, 1999f).

Although diabetic nephropathy cannot be cured, there are persuasive data that indicate that the clinical course of the disease can be modified. The most important factor that can influence progression of nephropathy is the optimization of metabolic control. Evidence also suggests that the frequency of nephropathy may decrease with the use of more effective antihypertensive therapy. Angiotensin converting enzyme (ACE) inhibitors can reduce the amount of proteinuria and slow the progression of nephropathy (Lewis et al., 1993, Ravid et al., 1993). ACE inhibitors are recommended as the primary treatment for all hypertensive patients with diabetes and microalbuminuria or overt nephropathy. In patients with type 1 diabetes and microalbuminuria, ACE inhibitors are recommended, even with normal blood pressure (American Diabetes Association, 1999f).

As discussed earlier, with evidence of macroalbuminuria, a daily protein intake of about 0.8 g/kg of body weight (roughly 10% of daily calories) is recommended. However, once the GFR begins to decline, further restriction to 0.6 g/kg/day may prove useful in slowing the decline of GFR in selected patients. In hypertensive or edematous patients with nephropathy, dietary sodium intake restriction is required; intake should not exceed 2000 mg of sodium per day (see Chapter 36). Smoking should be strongly discouraged and regular physical activity encouraged (American Diabetes Association, 1999f).

Neuropathy

Chronic high blood glucose levels are also associated with nerve damage. *Neuropathy* can be present in both type 1 and type 2 diabetes. Peripheral neuropathy usually affects the nerves controlling sensation in the feet and hands. Autonomic neuropathy affects nerve function controlling various organ systems. Cardiovascular effects include postural hypotension and decreased responsiveness to cardiac nerve impulses, leading to painless or silent ischemic heart disease. Sexual function may be affected, with impotence the most common manifestation. Damage to nerves innervating the gastrointestinal (GI) tract can cause a variety of problems. Neuropathy can be manifested in the esophagus as nausea and esophagitis, in the stomach as unpredictable emptying, in the small bowel as loss of nutrients, and in the large bowel as diarrhea or constipation.

Gastroparesis (impaired gastric motility) affects about 25% of this population and is perhaps the most frustrating condition that patients and dietitians experience. It results in delayed or irregular contractions of the stomach, leading to various GI symptoms, such as feelings of fullness, bloating, nausea, vomiting, diarrhea, or constipation. It can cause detrimental effects on blood glucose control.

Treatment first involves minimizing abdominal stress. Small, frequent meals may be better tolerated than three full meals a day. These meals should be low in fiber and fat. If solid foods are not well tolerated, liquid meals may need to be recommended. As much as possible, the timing of insulin administration should be adjusted to match the usually delayed nutrient absorption. This may even require insulin injections after eating. Frequent blood glucose monitoring is important to determine appropriate insulin therapy.

Brittle Diabetes

Less than 5% of persons with diabetes are unable to participate in normal activities of daily living because of recurrent episodes of severe metabolic decompensation, termed *brittle diabetes*. The term should be reserved for those individuals in whom diabetic instability is manifested by recurrent episodes of ketosis or ketoacidosis, severe hypoglycemia, or both, and is significant enough to result in an inability to maintain a normal life-style or to endanger life. It is not appropriate to use the term to describe persons with diabetes who maintain a relatively normal life-style despite less-than-optimal glycemic control (persistently elevated or fluctuating blood glucose levels).

The causes of brittle diabetes are often difficult to determine. Noncompliance is common, including missed insulin doses, surreptitious insulin administration, failure to monitor glucose levels, or fabrication of monitoring results. Eating disorders, such as anorexia nervosa and bulimia, as well as induced glycosuria (caused by omission of insulin), severe family problems, and drug or alcohol abuse, may also be associated with brittle diabetes. Nearly all cases of brittle diabetes are believed to be the result of emotional, family, or psychiatric disturbance; cases that have an entirely physiologic basis occur infrequently. Therefore, aggressive psychosocial or psychiatric evaluation is essential.

SURGERY AND DIABETES

A person with diabetes who undergoes surgery may present special challenges. After surgery, blood glucose levels may be difficult to regulate because of a variety of factors: dextrose-containing intravenous solutions, unpredictable eating patterns, and the influence of counterregulatory hormones or metabolic stress leading to elevated glucose levels (see Chapter 33). This greater risk of hyperglycemia contributes to an increased incidence of ketoacidosis, infection, and poor wound healing. Blood glucose monitoring is essential to ensure that adequate insulin is given.

Fluid management in the postsurgical period is aimed at achieving adequate vascular volume. Intravenous dextrose is often continued until adequate oral or enteral food and fluid intakes are established. Patients requiring clear- or full-liquid diets should receive approximately 200 g of carbohydrate spread evenly throughout the day at meal and snack times to prevent "starvation ketosis." Liquids should not be sugar-free. Patients require carbohydrate and calories, and sugar-free liquids do not meet these nutritional needs. Diabetes medications need to be adjusted to achieve and maintain metabolic control (American Diabetes Association, 1999g).

Enteral nutrition (EN) may be administered intermittently or continually. Although bolus feedings increase the risk of aspiration, they may be most similar to usual patterns of food intake. GI tolerance may, however, increase when formula is administered at a constant infusion rate. Standard high-carbohydrate EN formulas can interfere with glycemic control, so EN products modified for diabetes may be beneficial (see Appendix 37). Insulin administration and blood glucose monitoring must be tailored to all feeding regimens (McMahon, 1999).

PREVENTING DIABETES

Several trials are underway to determine if diabetes can be prevented. Evidence from previous life-style interventions suggests the possibility for the prevention of type 2 diabetes. As a result, the National Institutes of Health, National Institute of Diabetes and Digestive and Kidney Diseases has begun a 27-center randomized controlled trial (Diabetes Prevention Program, or DPP) to investigate the effects of life-style intervention and pharmacologic intervention (metformin) on prevention of diabetes in those at high risk because of having impaired glucose tolerance. The life-style intervention goals are to lose ≥7% of body weight, to increase exercise to ~700 kcal/week, and to sustain these changes throughout the 6-year trial (Wing, 1999).

Two prevention trials for type 1 diabetes are also underway. In the United States, the Diabetes Prevention Trial–Type 1 (DPT–1) is studying the possibility of delaying or even preventing the autoimmune destruction of the beta cells by giving insulin. In Part 1, individuals with a 25% to 50% risk of developing type 1 diabetes are randomized into a group taking capsules of crystallized insulin or a control group. In Part 2, individuals with a greater than 50% risk are randomized into a group taking insulin by injections or a control group. Another prevention trial, European-Canadian Nicotinamide Diabetes Intervention Trial (ENDIT), is also underway. The hypothesis is that the rate of type 1 diabetes can be substantially reduced with the use of pharmacologic doses of nicotinamide. In pilot studies, nicotinamide has been reported to protect or strengthen the pancreatic beta cells by making them more resistant to autoimmune destruction (Gale, 1996).

DIABETES AND AGE-RELATED ISSUES

Pregnancy

Normalization of blood glucose levels during pregnancy is extremely important for women who have preexisting diabetes or who develop gestational diabetes. MNT is important not only to meet the increased nutrient needs of the mother and the developing fetus, but also to assist in optimizing blood glucose levels.

Preexisting Diabetes and Pregnancy

Preconception counseling and the ability to achieve near-normal blood glucose levels before pregnancy have been shown to effectively reduce the incidence of anomalies in infants born to women with preexisting diabetes to nearly that of the general population (Kitzmiller et al., 1996). Normal blood glucose levels are 7 to 14 mg/dL (0.39 to 78 mmol/L) lower during pregnancy. Table 34–17 outlines blood glucose goals during pregnancy for preexisting diabetes and for GDM (Jovanovic-Peterson, 1995).

As a result of hormonal changes during the first trimester, blood glucose levels are often erratic. Although caloric needs do not differ from those preceding pregnancy, the meal plan may need to be adjusted to accommodate the metabolic changes. Women should be educated about the increased risk

TABLE 34–17 BLOOD GLUCOSE GOALS DURING PREGNANCY

TEST	PRE-EXISTING DIABETES	GESTATIONAL DIABETES
Fasting	60–90 mg/dL (3.3–5 mmol/L)	90 mg/dL (5.0 mmol/L)
Premeal	60–105 mg/dL (3.3–5.8 mmol/L)	
1 hr postprandial	100–120 mg/dL (5.5–6.7 mmol/L)	140 mg/dL (7.8 mmol/L)
2 hr postprandial	90–120 mg/dL (5–6.67 mmol/L)	120 mg/dL (6.7 mmol/L)
2 to 6 hr postprandial	60–120 mg/dL (3.3–6.67 mmol/L)	
Normal values during pregnancy		
Fasting: 60–90 mg/dL (3.3–5 mmol/L)		
1–2 hr postprandial: 120 mg/dL (6.67 mmol/L)		

(Adapted with permission from Jovanovic-Peterson L (ed.). Medical Management of Pregnancy Complicated by Diabetes, 2nd ed. Alexandria, VA: American Diabetes Association, 1995, pp. 34 and 82.)

of hypoglycemia during pregnancy and cautioned against overtreatment. The importance of between-meal snacks should be stressed.

There is an increased need for insulin during the second and third trimesters of pregnancy. This is the reason for screening for GDM between the 24th and 28th week of pregnancy. Insulin needs and levels peak 38 to 40 weeks' postconception at two to three times prepregnancy levels. Pregnancy-associated hormones that are antagonistic to the action of insulin lead to an elevation of blood glucose levels. For women with preexisting diabetes, this increased insulin need must be met by increased exogenous insulin.

Meal plan adjustments are necessary to provide the additional calories required to support fetal growth, and regular follow-up visits are needed to monitor weight gain, caloric and nutrient intake, blood glucose control, and starvation ketosis. Urine ketones during pregnancy signal starvation ketosis. This can be caused by inadequate caloric or carbohydrate intake, omission of meals or snacks, or prolonged intervals between meals (e.g., more than 10 hours between the bedtime snack and breakfast). Women should be instructed to test their urine periodically before breakfast. Ketonemia during pregnancy has been associated with reduced IQ scores in children (Rizzo et al., 1991).

Nutrition therapy is individualized according to the nutrition history, prepregnancy weight, and physical activity levels. Generally, an additional 100 to 300 kcal/day is added to the meal plan at the beginning of the second trimester (Durnin, 1991). The increased calorie requirement can easily be met by one or two additional cups of reduced-fat or skim milk and 1 to 2 oz of meat or meat substitute. This also provides adequately for the increased protein need of 10 g/day. Small meals and more frequent snacks are recommended. A late-evening snack is especially important to decrease the likelihood of starvation ketosis.

The appropriateness of the caloric intake can be evaluated by monitoring weight gain. Records of food intake and blood glucose values are essential for determining whether glycemic goals are being met and for preventing and correcting ketosis.

Gestational Diabetes Mellitus

The overall nutrition recommendations for preexisting diabetes also apply to GDM, although the diagnosis is generally not made before the second or third trimester. Limited research has been done to determine the ideal diet for GDM. The goal of nutrition therapy is to provide adequate calories and optimal nutrition during pregnancy without hyperglycemia or ketonemia. Individualization of the meal plan is recommended, as the ideal percentage and type of carbohydrate is controversial. Monitoring blood glucose levels, urine ketones, appetite, and weight gain can aid in developing an appropriate, individualized meal plan and in adjusting the meal plan throughout pregnancy (American Diabetes Association, 1999c; Franz et al., 1994).

Although MNT guidelines for GDM vary across the country, one consistent recommendation involves limiting carbohydrate intake at breakfast. Some women can tolerate only 30 g or less of carbohydrate at breakfast; larger amounts are generally tolerated later in the day. Foods high in total amounts of carbohydrate are also limited. Frequent small feedings throughout the day may also facilitate blood glucose control without the need for exogenous insulin.

For obese women with GDM, a 30% to 33% caloric restriction (an intake of about 1800 kcal/day) has been shown to reduce hyperglycemia with no increase in ketonuria (Knopp et al., 1991). Therefore, obese women with a body mass index (BMI) exceeding 30 may do well with moderate caloric restriction.

Exercise can also assist in overcoming peripheral resistance to insulin and in controlling postprandial hyperglycemia. The safest form of exercise is one that does not cause fetal distress, uterine contractions, or maternal hypertension. Appropriate exercises use the upper body muscles or place little mechanical stress on the leg and trunk regions (Durak et al., 1990).

Self-monitoring of blood glucose is essential for all women with GDM. It is the only means of determining whether normal blood glucose levels are being achieved. If blood glucose levels remain above normal values for pregnancy, exogenous insulin is required. Only human insulin should be used, though, to reduce the likelihood of insulin-antibody formation in both mother and fetus.

After delivery, approximately 90% of all women with GDM become normoglycemic. However, women with GDM have up to a 60% chance of developing type 2 diabetes later. This prevalence rate can be decreased with maintenance of a desirable body weight after pregnancy. With an appropriate weight loss and exercise program, these women can improve their health and lower their risk of developing diabetes in the future (Metzger, 1992).

Children and Adolescents

Involvement of a multidisciplinary team, including a physician, dietitian, nurse, and behavioral specialist, all trained in pediatric diabetes, is the best means of achieving optimal diabetes management in youth. The most important team members, however, are the child and his or her family.

A complete nutrition assessment, which is the basis for the meal plan for youth with diabetes, includes anthropometric measurements, nutrition assessment and food history, biochemical indices, assessment of feelings and family concerns related to nutrition and diabetes, and typical activity patterns.

A major nutrition goal for children and adolescents with type 1 diabetes is maintenance of normal growth and development (Drash, 1993). Possible causes of poor weight gain and linear growth include poor glycemic control, inadequate insulin, and over-restriction of calories. The last may be a consequence of the common erroneous belief that restricting food, rather than adjusting insulin, is the way to control blood glucose. Other reasons unrelated to diabetes management include thyroid abnormalities and malabsorption syndromes. Excessive weight gain can be due to excessive caloric intake, overtreatment of hypoglycemia, or overinsulinization. Other causes include low physical activity levels and hypothyroidism (accompanied by poor linear growth).

The nutrition prescription is based on the nutrition assessment. Newly diagnosed children often present with weight loss and hunger; as a result, the initial meal plan must be based on adequate calories to restore and maintain appropriate body weight. In approximately 4 to 6 weeks, the initial caloric level may need to be modified to meet more usual caloric requirements. Children have a natural ability to know how much to eat for normal growth and development. Several formulas can be used to confirm that a child or adolescent is receiving the minimum number of calories necessary for growth and development (Table 34–18). Height and weight should be recorded on growth charts every 3 to 6 months to make sure children are growing normally. If not, the overall diabetes management plan needs to be assessed. Caloric needs in children change continuously, so food intake should be evaluated every 3 to 6 months.

Daily eating patterns in children generally require three meals and two or three snacks, depending upon the length of time between meals and the child's physical activity level. The purpose of the snacks is to prevent hypoglycemia between meals and to provide adequate calories.

TABLE 34–18 ESTIMATING CALORIC REQUIREMENTS FOR YOUTH

- Base calories on nutrition assessment.
- Validate caloric needs.

Method 1

1000 kcal for 1st year
Add 100 kcal/yr up to age 11.
Girls 11–15 years of age: Add 100 kcal/yr.
Girls >15 years of age: Calculate as an adult.
Boys 11–15 years of age: Add 200 kcal/yr.
Boys >15 yr of age: 23 kcal/lb (50 kcal/kg) if very active
18 kcal/lb (40 kcal/kg) if usual activity level
15–16 kcal/lb (30–35 kcal/kg) if sedentary

Method 2

1000 kcal for 1st year
Boys: Add 125 kcal × age.
Girls: 100 kcal × age.
Up to 20% additional kcal for activity

- Toddlers (between 1 and 3 years of age): 40 kcal/inch of length

(Reprinted with permission from American Diabetes Association. Maximizing the Role of Nutrition in Diabetes Management. Alexandria, VA: American Diabetes Association, 1994a, p. 48.)

Realistic blood glucose goals should be determined and discussed with the youth and family. Youth with diabetes are also more likely than their age- and sex-matched nondiabetic peers to be at risk for cardiovascular disease. It is therefore essential to reduce risk factors in youth with type 1 diabetes. Lipid levels should be monitored regularly, and NCEP treatment guidelines for children and adolescents should be followed (Expert Panel, 1992) (see Chapter 26). After the appropriate nutrition prescription has been determined, the meal planning approach can be selected. Most pediatric educators agree that it is better to start with a more precise meal plan and then teach flexibility than to start with flexibility and try to teach precise planning later. A number of meal planning approaches can be used. Carbohydrate counting for food planning provides youth and their families with guidelines that facilitate glycemic control while still allowing the choice of many common foods that children and adolescents enjoy. However, whatever approach to food planning is used, the youth and family must find it understandable and applicable to their life-style.

The nutrition education process begins with an assessment following the diagnosis of diabetes, and continues over a lifetime. Continuous reassessment and self-management education allow for changes in growth and development, changes in school routines, and the change accompanying seasonal sports, vacation, and camping excursions—just some of the factors that may necessitate a change in caloric intake and meal plans. Blood glucose records help the dietitian and other team members integrate insulin regimens into usual nutrition and exercise patterns.

Elderly

The prevalence of diabetes and IGT increases dramatically as people age. Many factors predispose the elderly to diabetes: age-related decreases in insulin, age-related insulin resistance, adiposity, decreased physical activity, multiple prescription medications, genetics, and coexisting illnesses. A major factor appears to be insulin resistance. Controversy persists as to whether the insulin resistance is itself a primary change or is attributable to reduced physical activity, decreased lean body mass, and increased adipose tissue, which are all frequently seen in the elderly. Abdominal obesity also correlates with insulin resistance in the elderly (Kohrt et al., 1993). Furthermore, medications used to treat coexisting diseases may complicate diabetes therapy in older persons.

Despite the increase of glucose intolerance with age, aging per se should not be a reason for suboptimal control of blood glucose. Even if it is incorrectly assumed that preventing long-term diabetic complications is not relevant to the care of the elderly, persistent hyperglycemia has deleterious effects on the body's defense mechanisms against infection. It also increases the pain threshold by exacerbating neuropathic pain, and it has a detrimental effect on the outcome of cerebrovascular accidents.

Malnutrition, not obesity, is often the more prevalent nutrition-related problem of the elderly. It often remains subclinical or unrecognized because the result of malnutrition—excessive loss of lean body mass—resembles the signs and symptoms of the aging process. Until a primary disease develops or chronic problems are exacerbated by illness or some other stress, malnutrition may remain unrecognized. Both malnutrition and diabetes adversely affect wound healing and defense against infection, and malnutrition is associated with depression and cognitive deficits (see Chapter 13).

Because of concern over malnutrition, it is essential that the elderly, especially those in long-term care settings, be provided a diet that meets their nutritional needs, enables them to attain or maintain a reasonable body weight, helps control blood glucose, and is palatable. Weight loss in the elderly is common and often signifies a decline in health status. Long-term care residents with diabetes may do well with the regular diet served to all residents (American Diabetes Association, 1999g). In long-term care facilities, meals and snacks are served at regular times and are planned so that similar types and amounts of foods are served. This contrasts with many elderly patients' often erratic pattern of eating, especially if they live alone.

In the elderly, acute hyperglycemia and dehydration can lead to a serious complication of diabetes: HHNK syndrome. As discussed previously, patients with HHNK syndrome have a very high blood glucose level (ranging from 400 to 2800 mg/dL [22.2 to 155.5 mmol/L], with an average of 1000 mg/dL [55.5 mmol/L]) without ketones. Patients are markedly dehydrated, and mental status often ranges from mild confusion to hallucinations or coma. Treatment includes provision of adequate fluids, as well as blood glucose control.

IMPLEMENTING NUTRITIONAL SELF-MANAGEMENT

The components of nutritional self-management include assessment, establishment of behavioral and medical goals, implementation and education, evaluation and documentation, and follow-up and ongoing care. Throughout the process, there must be rapport between the person with diabetes and the dietitian if the nutrition care plan is to be successful (Tinker et al., 1994).

Step One: Assessment and the Nutrition Prescription

When a nutritional care plan and prescription is developed, many parameters are assessed, including anthropometric measures, biochemical indices and laboratory data, clinical signs, nutrition history, learning style, cultural heritage, and socioeconomic status. Table 34–19 provides a summary of such assessment data. A complete nutrition assessment should be done at the onset of nutrition therapy to familiarize the health care team with the individual's life-style and eating habits. The **nutrition prescription** is based on the assessment and begins with a food and eating history. Food histories can be done several ways (see Chapter 16). The objective for the dietitian is to determine a schedule and pattern of eating that will be the least disruptive to the life-style of the individual with diabetes and, at the same time, will facilitate improved glycemic control. With this objective in mind, asking the individual to either record or report what, how much, and when he or she typically eats during a 24-hour period may be the most useful. Another approach is to ask the individual to keep and bring with them a 3-day or 1-week food intake record. This request can be made when an appointment with the dietitian is scheduled. Assessment of the most typical daily pattern can then be made.

It is essential first to learn about the individual's daily routine and schedule. The following information is needed about the individual: (1) time of waking; (2) usual meal and eating times; (3) work schedule or school hours; (4) type, amount, and timing of exercise; and (5) usual sleep habits.

The history can also reveal other useful information, including (1) usual caloric intake; (2) quality of the usual diet; (3) times, size, and content of meals and snacks; (4) food idiosyncrasies; (5) frequency with which meals are eaten in restaurants; (6) who usually prepares food; (7) eating problems (e.g., as related to dental, GI, or other problems); (8) alcoholic beverage intake; and (9) supplements used.

Using the nutrition assessment and food history information, the dietitian can then design a preliminary meal plan and sample menus. Calculations for the nutrition prescription can be done using a form, such as the one shown in Figure 34–5. It is not necessary to begin with a set calorie or macronutrient prescription. The nutrition prescription is determined by modifying the usual food intake as necessary.

The nutrient information from the exchange lists can be a useful tool for evaluating the food history and determining the nutrition prescription. Table 34–20 lists the macronutrient and caloric values for the exchange lists.

TABLE 34–19 NUTRITION ASSESSMENT

- *Minimal referral data:* treatment regimen; medical history; medications; laboratory data (glycated hemoglobin, cholesterol level and fractionations, blood pressure, renal function if applicable); team goals; clearance for exercise
- *Clinical data:* exercise history; psychosocial and economic issues; blood glucose monitoring; knowledge; skill level; attitudes; motivation
- *Nutrition history:* current eating habits with beginning modifications

	Meal/Snack/Time										
Food Group	Breakfast	Snack	Lunch	Snack	Dinner	Snack	Total servings/ day	CHO (g)	Protein (g)	Fat (g)	Calories
Starches								15	3	1	80
Fruit								15			60
Milk								12	8	1	90
Vegetables								5	2		25
Meats/ Substitutes									7	5(3)	75(55)
Fats										5	45
							Total				
							Calories	X4=	X4=	X9=	Total=
							Percent calories				

Calculations are based on medium-fat meats and skim/very low-fat milk. If diet consists predominantly of low-fat meats, use the factor 3 g instead of 5 g fat; if predominantly high-fat meats, use 8 g fat. If low-fat (2%) milk is used, use 5 g fat; if whole milk is used, use 8 g fat.

FIGURE 34–5 Worksheet for assessment and design of a meal or food plan. *CHO,* carbohydrate.

Using the form in Figure 34–5, the dietitian begins by totaling the number of exchanges from each list and multiplying this number by the grams of carbohydrate, protein, and fat contributed by the total exchanges. Next, the grams of carbohydrate, protein, and fat are totaled from each column; the grams of carbohydrate and protein are then multiplied by 4 (4 kcal/g of carbohydrate and protein) and the grams of fat are multiplied by 9 (9 kcal/g of fat). Total calories and percentage of calories from

TABLE 34–20 MACRONUTRIENT AND CALORIC VALUES FOR EXCHANGE LISTS

GROUPS/LISTS	CARBOHYDRATE (g)	PROTEIN (g)	FAT (g)	CALORIES
Carbohydrates				
Starch	15	3	≤1	80
Fruit	15	—	—	60
Milk				
Skim	12	8	0–3	90
Reduced-fat	12	8	5	120
Whole	12	8	8	150
Other carbohydrates	15	Variable	Variable	Variable
Vegetables	5	2	—	25
Meat and Meat Substitutes				
Very lean	—	7	0–1	35
Lean	—	7	3	55
Medium-fat	—	7	5	75
High-fat	—	7	8	100
Fat	—	—	5	45

(Reprinted with permission from American Diabetes Association and American Dietetic Association. Exchange Lists for Meal Planning. Alexandria, VA: American Diabetes Association, 1995b, p. 3.)

	Meal/Snack/Time										
	Breakfast	Snack	Lunch	Snack	Dinner	Snack	Total servings/ day	CHO (g)	Protein (g)	Fat (g)	Calories
Food Group	*7:30 AM*	*10:00*	*12:00*	*3:00*	*6:30*	*10:00*					
Starches	*2*	*1*	*2—3*	*1*	*2—3*	*1—2*	*10*	15 *150*	3 *30*	1 *10*	80
Fruit	*1*		*1*		*1*	*0—1*	*3*	15 *45*			60
Milk	*1*				*1*		*2*	12 *24*	8 *16*	1 *2*	90
Vegetables			✓		✓			5 *10*	2 *4*		25
Meats/ Substitutes			*2—3*		*3—4*		*6*		7 *42*	5(3) *30*	75(55)
Fats	*1*	*0—1*	*1—2*	*0—1*	*1—2*	*0—1*	*5*			5 *25*	45
	3—4 CHO	*1 CHO*	*3—4 CHO*	*1 CHO*	*4—5 CHO*	*1—2 CHO*	Total	*229*	*92*	*67*	
							Calories	X4= *916*	X4= *368*	X9= *603*	Total=
							Percent calories	*50*	*19*	*30*	*1900—2000*

1900—2000 calories
230 gm CHO-50%
90 gm protein-20%
65 gm fat-30%

Calculations are based on medium-fat meats and skim/very low-fat milk. If diet consists predominantly of low-fat meats, use the factor 3 g, instead of 5 g fat; if predominantly high-fat meats, use 8 g fat. If low-fat (2%) milk is used, use 5 g fat; if whole milk is used, use 8 g fat.

FIGURE 34–6 An example of a completed worksheet from the assessment, the nutrition prescription, and a sample 1900- to 2000-calorie meal plan. *CHO,* carbohydrate.

each macronutrient can then be determined. Numbers derived from these calculations are then rounded off. Figure 34–6 provides an example of a nutrition prescription and preliminary meal plan. In this example, the nutrition prescription would be the following:

1900–2000 calories
230 g carbohydrate (50%)
90 g protein (20%)
65 g fat (30%)

The number of carbohydrate choices for each meal and snack is the total of the starch, fruit, and milk servings. The carbohydrate choices are circled under each meal and snack column.

The next step is to evaluate the preliminary meal plan from Figure 34–6. First, and foremost, does the individual with diabetes think it is feasible to implement the meal plan into his or her life-style? Second, are the calories appropriate? Third, is it appropriate for diabetes management? Fourth, does it encourage healthful eating?

To answer the first question concerning the feasibility of the meal plan, begin by reviewing with the individual the meal plan and sample menu in terms of general food intake. Go over the timing of meals and snacks and approximate portion sizes and types of foods. Later, a meal-planning approach will be selected that will assist the individual in making his or her own food choices. At this point, it needs to be determined if this meal plan is reasonable for the individual with diabetes. Table 34–21 illustrates a sample menu for the nutrition prescription of 1900 to 2000 calories.

Next, determine whether the number of calories is appropriate for the individual. Caloric requirements are dependent on several factors, such as age, gender, height, weight, and activity level. Table 34–22 outlines two methods for determining approximate caloric requirements. The simpler approach multiplies weight by approximate calories needed per lb (or kg) of body weight. Many dietitians use handheld calculators to determine caloric requirements. The Harris-Benedict equation, with modifications, generally is used in the calculations (see Chapter 2).

It should be emphasized that both methods for determining caloric requirements are only approximate. On a practical basis, they do provide a starting point for evaluating the caloric adequacy of the meal plan. Adjustments in calories can be made during follow-up visits.

The determination of a caloric level and nutrition prescription for a child or adolescent also is based

TABLE 34–21 SAMPLE MENU FOR 1900 TO 2000 KILOCALORIE MEAL PLAN

MEAL/TIMING	FOOD SELECTIONS
Breakfast—7:30 AM	
3–4 Carbohydrate choices (i.e., 2 starch, 1 fruit, 1 milk)	Raisin bran cereal, ½ cup Bagel, ½ Cantaloupe (5-inch), ⅓ Skim milk, 1 cup
1 fat	Reduced-fat cream cheese, 1 T
Snack—10:00 AM	
1 Carbohydrate choice (i.e., 1 starch or fruit)	Bagel, ½
0–1 fat	Reduced-fat cream cheese, 1 T
Lunch—12:00 Noon	
3–4 Carbohydrate choices (i.e., 2–3 starch, 1 fruit)	Whole wheat bread, 2 slices Vegetable-beef soup, 1 cup Apple, 1 small
Vegetable	Lettuce and tomato slices
2–3 Meats	Turkey, 2 oz
1–2 fat	Reduced-fat mayonnaise, 1 T
Snack—3:00	
1 Carbohydrate choice (i.e., 1 starch or fruit)	Pretzels, ¾ oz
0–1 fat	
Dinner—6:30	
4–5 Carbohydrate choices (i.e., 2–3 starch, 1 fruit, 1 milk)	Baked potato, 1 medium Dinner roll, 1 Mandarin oranges, ¾ cup Skim milk, 1 cup
Vegetables	Broccoli spears, ½ cup Dinner salad, 1 small
3–4 meats	Chicken breast, baked, 3 oz
1–2 fats	Sour cream, regular, 2 T Reduced-fat salad dressing, 2 T
Snack—10:00 PM	
1–2 Carbohydrate choices (i.e., 1–2 starch, 0–1 fruit)	Ice cream, light, ½ cup Strawberries, 1-¼ cup
0–1 fat	

on the nutrition assessment. Two formulas, as shown in Table 34–18, can be used to confirm that the child is receiving the minimum necessary calories.

To determine the appropriateness of the meal plan for diabetes management, distribution of the meals and snacks and the macronutrient percentages are assessed. Appropriateness is based on the treatment goals and on the types of medications prescribed.

For individuals requiring insulin, the timing of meals and snacks is extremely important. Once insulin is injected, the rate of absorption from the injection site is mainly dependent on the kind and amount of insulin administered. Food must be eaten in synchronization with the time of actions of insulin. To prevent overnight hypoglycemia, many patients require a bedtime snack. Many individuals who use intermediate-acting insulins (NPH or Lente) also require an afternoon snack. Children and adolescents generally require a morning snack, and often do better with two afternoon snacks, especially if their school lunch period is early and the family dinner relatively late.

Individuals using rapid-acting insulin (Humalog) do not need a snack. This insulin is taken immediately before eating. Besides peaking very quickly, it has about a 2- to 3-hour duration of action.

Persons with type 2 diabetes often do better with smaller meals and snacks. However, snacks cannot be in addition to the usual meals. A portion of the meal should be saved to be eaten as a snack between meals.

The best way to ensure that the meal plan encourages healthful eating is to encourage patients to eat a variety of foods from all of the food groups. The Food Guide Pyramid, with its suggested number of servings from each food group, can be used to compare the patient's meal plan with the nutrition recommendations for all Americans.

Step Two: Behavioral and Medical Goals

Both short- and long-term behavioral and medical goals should be mutually identified by the individual with diabetes and medical professionals. *Short-term goals* (days/weeks) are often behavioral goals and relate to life-style changes. The primary behavioral goals are consistent and appropriate food intake, regular physical activity, correct medication dosage (if needed), and frequent blood glucose monitoring. *Long-term goals* (months/years) generally focus on diabetes management goals for desired outcomes—blood glucose and lipid levels, and body weight—that lead to improved or maintained metabolic control. Primary medical goals are normal (or as near normal as possible) blood glucose, glycated

TABLE 34–22 METHODS FOR DETERMINING CALORIC REQUIREMENTS OF ADULTS

1. Caloric requirements of adults
   - Obese or very inactive adults, chronic dieters: 10 to 12 kcal/lb (20 kcal/kg)
   - Adults older than 55 years of age, active women, sedentary men: 13 kcal/lb (28 kcal/kg)
   - Active men or very active women: 15 kcal/lb (30 kcal/kg)
   - Thin or very active men: 20 kcal/lb (40 kcal/kg)
2. Harris-Benedict equation for determining caloric requirements of adults

   (Measure of Resting Energy Expenditure [REE])

   Women: REE = 655 + 9.63W(kg) + (1.83H(cm) – 4.73A(yr)

   Men: REE = 66 + 13.73W(kg) + 5.3H(cm) – 6.83A(yr)

   Obese adults: W = ([actual wt. – DBW] × 0.25) + DBW

   Activity factors: restricted, 1.1; sedentary, 1.2; aerobic activity = 3×/wk, 1.3; 5×/wk, 1.5; 7×/wk, 1.6; true athlete, 1.7

   (REE × activity factor = total caloric requirements).

W, weight; *H*, height; *A*, age; DBW, desired body weight hemoglobin, lipid, and blood pressure values. In addition, even a modest weight loss for persons with type 2 diabetes may make a significant difference in blood glucose and lipids, and weight loss should be viewed as a means to an end rather than an end in itself.

Step Three: Implementation and Education

This step involves selecting an appropriate meal-planning approach and identifying strategies for behavioral change that enhance motivation and adherence to necessary life-style changes. As mentioned earlier, a number of **meal-planning approaches** are available, ranging from simple guidelines or menus to more complex counting methods (Table 34–23). Use of *Exchange Lists for Meal Planning* has been a common approach (American Diabetes Association and The American Dietetic Association, 1995b) (see Appendix 53). The exchange list's macronutrient values are a useful tool for dietitians to evaluate food intake. However, they may not be the appropriate educational tool for many persons with diabetes. No single meal-planning approach has been shown to be more effective than any other, and the tool selected depends on the patient's stage of learning and needs. A meal-planning approach should be selected that interprets the nutrition prescription so the individual with diabetes can select appropriate foods for meals and snacks.

Educational Resources

The First Step in Diabetes Meal Planning (American Diabetes Association and The American Dietetic Association, 1995c) provides general guidelines for meal planning based on the Food Guide Pyramid and is designed to be used for meal planning until an individualized meal plan can be implemented. However, for some individuals, there may be no need to advance to more complex meal planning approaches if metabolic outcomes are being achieved.

EXCHANGE LISTS. The word *exchange* refers to the fact that each item on a particular list, in the portion listed, may be interchanged with any other item on the list. An exchange can be explained to patients as a substitution, choice, or serving. Foods are divided into three groups: carbohydrates, meat and meat substitutes, and fat. The carbohydrate group includes the starch, fruit, milk, and other carbohydrates lists. Vegetables are also carbohydrates, but, unless three or more servings are eaten in a meal, can be considered "free." Meats are divided into very lean, lean, medium-fat, and high-fat choices, based on their fat content, and the fat list is divided into saturated, monounsaturated, and polyunsaturated fat choices. A free food list is based on servings of food that contribute 20 kcal or less per serving. The final lists are combination and fast foods that are commonly used by individuals. A meal plan outlines the daily number of choices the patient can select from each list at meal and snack times.

CARBOHYDRATE COUNTING. A very popular approach to meal planning is carbohydrate counting. It can be used as a basic meal planning approach or for more intensive management. Several carbohydrate counting educational tools are available. All are based on the concept that, after eating, it is the carbohydrate in foods that is the major predictor of postprandial blood glucose levels. One carbohydrate choice contributes 15 g of carbohydrate.

The American Diabetes Association and The American Dietetic Association have developed three carbohydrate counting booklets (1995a). *Carbohydrate Counting: Getting Started* is an introduction to carbohydrate counting and encourages individuals to eat consistent amounts of carbohydrates at meals and snacks. *Carbohydrate Counting: Moving On* focuses on identifying patterns in blood glucose levels as related to food intake, diabetes medication (if used), and physical activity. The individual is taught to interpret records and take action based on blood glucose patterns. *Carbohydrate Counting: Using Carbohydrate/Insulin Ratios* is designed for people using multiple daily insulin injections or an insulin pump. The relationship between food eaten and insulin injected can be shown as a carbohydrate-to-insulin ratio. This ratio is used by the individual to determine how to adjust premeal insulin when eating more or less than usual.

My Food Plan (International Diabetes Center, 1996) combines both carbohydrate counting and caloric control in a simplified approach. It groups carbohydrate choices, meat and meat substitutes, and fats by approximate portion sizes. General guidelines for food planning are given, and a form for an individualized meal plan is included.

Facilitating Behavioral Changes

The transtheoretical model, discussed in "*Focus On:* Stages of Change" in Chapter 21 (p. 453), has been proposed by Prochaska as a general model of intentional behavior change (Prochaska, 1994). It includes a sequence of stages along a continuum of behavioral change. Different intervention strategies may be needed for individuals at different stages of the change process. Motivational interventions may work best with individuals in the earlier contemplative stages, whereas specific skill-training interventions may be most appropriate for persons who have decided to change. Relapse and recycling through the stages occur quite frequently, as individuals attempt to modify behaviors.

Staging Education

Information must be provided to persons over a period of time; nutrition self-management education is a continual process. Education begins with initial, basic, or **"survival" skills** education. In-depth education provides more detailed information. It

TABLE 34–23 MEAL-PLANNING APPROACHES FOR DIABETES AND RELATED RESOURCES

MEAL-PLANNING APPROACH	RESOURCES	DESCRIPTION
Diabetes nutrition guidelines	***The First Step in Diabetes Meal Planning*** (American Diabetes Association, The American Dietetic Association)	Emphasizes diabetes principles that apply to current eating habits—consistent meal times coordinated with endogenous or exogenous insulin.
	Healthy Food Choices (American Diabetes Association, The American Dietetic Association)	A pamphlet that promotes healthy eating. It is divided into two sections: (1) guidelines for making healthy food choices and (2) simplified exchange lists.
	Healthy Eating for People with Diabetes (International Diabetes Center, Minneapolis, MN)	A low-literacy booklet based on the "plate method" of selecting foods; includes general information on the role of meal planning in diabetes.
	Eating Healthy Foods (American Diabetes Association, The American Dietetic Association)	A booklet designed specifically for persons with minimal reading skills. The amount of text is limited; symbols and color codes are used, and concepts and foods are presented visually.
Menu approaches	***Month of Meals 1, Month of Meals 2, Month of Meals 3, Month of Meals 4, Month of Meals 5*** (American Diabetes Association)	Separate booklets, each of which contains 28 days of complete menus for breakfast, lunch, dinner, and snacks. Menus are written for a basic meal plan of 1500 kcal/day with instructions on how to adjust the calorie level upward or downward. Although certain elements are consistent in each volume, each volume has unique features: *book 1* includes a special occasion section; *book 2* adds more ethnic foods; *book 3* emphasizes time-saving meals; *book 4* features family favorites; and *book 5* is vegetarian.
Counting approaches	***Exchange Lists for Meal Planning*** (American Diabetes Association, The American Dietetic Association)	Groups foods into lists called exchanges. Each list is a group of measured foods that contribute approximately the same number of calories and the same amount of carbohydrate, protein, and fat; therefore foods on each list can be substituted or "exchanged" with other foods on the same list. Persons with diabetes need an individualized meal plan that outlines the number of choices from each list that should be included for each meal and for snacks.
	Carbohydrate Counting: Getting Started, Moving On, Using Carbohydrate/Insulin Ratios (American Diabetes Association, The American Dietetic Association)	Booklets, in three levels of complexity, emphasize the close relationship of total carbohydrate intake to glycemic control. Each booklet stresses the need for appropriate modifications in activity or medications if carbohydrate intake deviates from the usual meal plan.
	My Food Plan (International Diabetes Center, Minneapolis, MN)	Groups foods into simplified categories containing approximate portions of common foods. Carbohydrate choices are grouped together. A personalized food plan panel allows individualization. General guidelines are included for making healthful food choices.
	Carbohydrate Counting (International Diabetes Center, Minneapolis, MN)	A booklet that explains carbohydrate counting and how it can be added to the exchange system of meal planning to give persons with diabetes greater flexibility in food choices. One choice from either the starch, fruit, or milk list supplies approximately 15 g of carbohydrate, and each is one carbohydrate choice. A meal plan outlines the number of carbohydrate choices each person can select for meals and for snacks.
	High Carbohydrate–High Fiber (HCF) and High-Fiber Maintenance (HCF Nutrition Research Foundation, Lexington, KY)	Follows a format similar to that of *Exchange Lists for Meal Planning,* but adds a beans and cereals exchange list. Emphasizes intake of fiber, particularly water-soluble fiber, from food sources.
	Calorie Point System (Nutrition Education Center, Overland Park, KS)	A simplified method of counting daily intake of calories, with each calorie point equaling 75 kcal. Each food portion size is assigned a specific number of calorie points.
	Total Available Glucose (TAG) (Medical University of South Carolina, Charleston, SC)	The TAG value of any portion of food is calculated by adding 100% of the grams of carbohydrate, 58% of the grams of protein, and 10% of the grams of fat. The TAG values are used to individualize insulin requirements.

(Adapted with permission from Holler HJ, Pastors JG (eds.). Diabetes Medical Nutrition Therapy: A Guide to Management and Nutrition Education Resources. Chicago: The American Dietetic Association, 1997.)

TABLE 34–24 ADULT LEARNING PRINCIPLES

The learner must feel the need to learn.
The environment should be conducive to change.
Goals should be developed mutually.
The learner needs to participate actively.
Learning should be based on past experiences.

(Reprinted with permission from American Diabetes Association: Maximizing the Role of Nutrition in Diabetes Management. Alexandria, VA: American Diabetes Association, 1994a, p. 55.)

presents the rationale for the meal plan, expands on selection of healthy foods, and provides additional practical tips for meal planning. Principles of adult learning are outlined on Table 34–24.

Continued in-depth and ongoing education allows the individual to integrate and use nutrition information to better manage her or his diabetes. It provides skills that allow for flexibility, optimal control of diabetes, and improved quality of life. Flow sheets can be useful in documenting what and when information is covered and in reviewing this information on a regular basis.

Step Four: Evaluation and Documentation

Outcomes must be identified and the effectiveness of nutrition interventions documented. Throughout the entire education process, the activities of both the educator and the individual with diabetes should be evaluated to determine the effectiveness of the nutritional care plan. Monitoring of medical and clinical outcomes should be done after the second or third visit, to determine whether the individual is making progress toward established goals. If no progress is evident, the individual and educator need to reassess and perhaps revise the nutritional care plan. If altering food intake alone isn't achieving metabolic target ranges, the dietitian should recommend that medications be added or adjusted.

Finally, documentation is essential for communication and reimbursement. Table 34–25 lists the areas of the nutrition intervention that require documentation.

TABLE 34–25 NUTRITION CARE DOCUMENTATION AREAS

Short- and long-term goals
Nutrition prescription
Food/meal plan
Educational topics covered
Patient acceptance and understanding
Anticipated compliance
Successful behavioral changes
Additional needed skills or information
Additional recommendations
Plans for ongoing care

(Reprinted with permission from Monk A, et al. Practice guidelines for medical nutrition therapy by dietitians for persons with non–insulin-dependent diabetes mellitus. J Am Diet Assoc 95:999, 1995.)

Step Five: Follow-Up and Ongoing Nutritional Therapy

Diabetes is a chronic disease that requires ongoing nutritional care at least every 6 to 12 months. Asking the patient to keep 3-day or weekly food diaries between visits provides valuable information. Food diaries can be compared to the meal plan, which will help determine whether the initial meal plan needs changing. Food diaries can be integrated with the blood glucose monitoring records to determine changes that can lead to improved glycemic control. For patients receiving insulin, it can then be determined whether blood glucose values that are outside target ranges can be corrected with adjustments in the meal plan or adjustments in the insulin regimen.

After the basic food and nutrition strategies have been mastered, other aspects of nutrition education should be presented to increase flexibility in food choices and life-style while still maintaining glucose control. Of particular importance is information on eating out and the use of information from food labels. Persons using insulin also need information on how to make adjustments in food intake when schedules are disrupted.

Nutritional follow-up visits should provide encouragement and ensure realistic expectations for the patient. A change in eating habits is not easy for most people, and they become discouraged without appropriate recognition of their efforts. Patients should be encouraged to speak freely about problems they are having with food and eating patterns. Furthermore, there may be major life changes that require changes in the meal plan. Job and schedule changes, travel, illness, and other factors all have an impact on the meal plan.

PATHOPHYSIOLOGY OF HYPOGLYCEMIA OF NONDIABETIC ORIGIN

Hypoglycemia has been defined as a clinical syndrome with diverse causes in which low levels of plasma glucose eventually lead to neuroglycopenia (Service, 1995). Hypoglycemia literally means low (*hypo*) blood glucose (*glycemia*). Normally, the body is remarkably adept at maintaining fairly steady blood glucose levels—usually between 60 to 100 mg/dL (3.3 to 5.6 mmol/L)—despite the intermittent ingestion of food. Maintaining normal levels of glucose is important because body cells, especially the brain, must have a steady and consistent supply of glucose to function properly. Under physiologic conditions, the brain depends almost exclusively on glucose for its energy needs.

In a small number of people, however, blood glucose levels become too low. If the brain and nervous system are deprived of the glucose they need to function, symptoms, such as sweating, shaking, weakness, hunger, headaches, and irritability, can develop. Hypoglycemia can be difficult to diagnose because these typical symptoms can be caused by many different health problems besides hypoglycemia. For example, adrenaline (epinephrine), released as a result of anxiety and stress, can trigger the symptoms of hypoglycemia. The only way to determine whether hypoglycemia is causing these symptoms is to measure blood glucose levels while an individual is experiencing the symptoms. If blood glucose levels are low while the symptoms are present, and if the symptoms disappear within 10 to 15 minutes of eating, hypoglycemia is probably responsible for the symptoms.

Hypoglycemia, therefore, can best be defined by the presence of three features known as **Whipple's triad:** (1) a low plasma or blood glucose level; (2) symptoms of hypoglycemia at the same time as the low blood glucose values; and (3) amelioration of the symptoms by correction of the hypoglycemia (Prince, 1997). Hypoglycemic syndromes are classically divided into fasting hypoglycemia (food-deprived) or postprandial (reactive) hypoglycemia, which occurs in response to food. Alternative classifications have been proposed based on the clinical appearance of the patient (i.e., healthy-appearing patient, ill-appearing patient, hospitalized patient) (Service, 1995). The discussion in this chapter is based on the more traditional classification.

A fairly steady blood glucose level is maintained by the interaction of several mechanisms. After eating, food is broken down into glucose and enters the bloodstream. As blood glucose levels rise, the pancreas responds by releasing the hormone insulin, which allows glucose to leave the bloodstream and enter various body cells where it fuels the body's activities. Some glucose is also taken up by the liver and stored there for later use. When the glucose levels from the last meal decline, the body goes from a "fed" to a "fasting" state. Insulin levels also decrease, which keeps the blood glucose levels from falling too low. In addition, stored glucose is released from the liver back into the bloodstream with the help of **glucagon,** a hormone which is also released from the pancreas. Normally, the body's ability to balance glucose, insulin, and glucagon (and other counterregulatory hormones) keeps glucose levels within the normal range. Glucagon provides the primary defense against hypoglycemia; without it, full recovery does not occur. Epinephrine is not necessary for counterregulation when glucagon is present. In the absence of glucagon, however, epinephrine has an important role (Cryer, 1993).

It is important to keep blood glucose levels within normal limits; the various body cells, particularly those of the brain and central nervous system, must receive a steady and consistent supply of glucose to function properly. Even with hunger, either because it is many hours since food was eaten, or because the last meal was small, blood glucose levels remain fairly consistent.

Symptoms of hypoglycemia have been recognized at plasma glucose levels of about 60 mg/dL, and impaired brain function has occurred at levels of approximately 50 mg/dL (Mitrakou et al., 1991). Symptoms have been classified into two major groups: those that arise from the action of the autonomic nervous system and those related to an insufficient supply of glucose to the brain. **Adrenergic symptoms** include sweating, trembling, feelings of warmth, anxiety, or nausea. Symptoms of neuroglycopenia include dizziness, confusion, tiredness, difficulty speaking, headaches, and inability to concentrate. Hunger, blurred vision, drowsiness, and weakness are other symptoms some people experience. Symptoms differ for different people, but are consistent from episode to episode for any one person. Furthermore, there is not a consistent chronological order to the evolution of symptoms; autonomic symptoms do not always precede neuroglycopenic ones. In many persons, neuroglycopenic symptoms are the only ones observed (Hepburn et al., 1991). Hypoglycemia is the cause for any of these symptoms only if blood glucose levels are determined to be below normal at the time the symptoms occur.

TYPES OF HYPOGLYCEMIA

If blood glucose levels fall below normal limits within 2 to 5 hours after eating, this is often referred to as reactive hypoglycemia (named because the body is reacting to food), or postprandial hypoglycemia. **Postprandial hypoglycemia** can be caused by alimentary hyperinsulinism, idiopathic reactive hypoglycemia, or rare syndromes, such as hereditary fructose intolerance, galactosemia, or leucine sensitivity. *Alimentary hyperinsulinism* is the most common type of documented postprandial hypoglycemia and is seen in patients who have undergone gastrectomy or some other type of gastric surgery. These procedures are associated with rapid delivery of food to the small intestine, rapid absorption of glucose, and exaggerated insulin response. These patients respond best to multiple, frequent feedings (Prince, 1997) (see Chapter 30).

The ingestion of alcohol after a prolonged fast, or the ingestion of large amounts of alcohol and carbohydrate on an empty stomach ("gin-and-tonic" syndrome), may also cause hypoglycemia within 3 to 4 hours in some healthy persons.

Idiopathic reactive hypoglycemia is characterized by normal insulin secretion but increased insulin sensitivity and, to some extent, reduced response of glucagon to acute hypoglycemia. The increase in insulin sensitivity associated with a deficiency of glucagon secretion leads to hypoglycemia late postprandially (Leonetti et al., 1996). Idiopathic reactive hypoglycemia has been inappropriately overdiagnosed by both physicians and patients, to the point that some physicians doubt its existence. Although rare, it does exist, but can only be documented in individuals with hypoglycemia that occurs spontaneously and who meet the criteria of Whipple's triad.

Fasting hypoglycemia may occur in response to having gone without food for 8 hours or more. However, generally, fasting hypoglycemia is the result of a serious underlying medical condition. Causes of fasting hypoglycemia include hormone deficiency states (e.g., hypopituitarism, adrenal insufficiency, catecholamine or glucagon deficiency), acquired liver disease, renal disease, certain drugs (e.g., alcohol, propranolol, salicylate), insulinoma (of which most are benign, but 6% to 10% can be malignant), and other nonpancreatic tumors. *Factitious hypoglycemia,* or self-administration of insulin or sulfonylurea in persons who do not have diabetes, is a common cause as well (Prince, 1997). Symptoms related to fasting hypoglycemia tend to be particularly severe, and can include a loss of mental acuity, seizures, and unconsciousness. If the underlying problem can be resolved, hypoglycemia is no longer a problem.

DIAGNOSIS OF HYPOGLYCEMIA

One of the criteria used to confirm the presence of hypoglycemia is a blood glucose level of less than 50 mg/dL (<2.8 mmol/L). Previously, the oral glucose tolerance test was the standard test for this condition. However, this test is not helpful because it involves a nonphysiologic stimulus and because results show little correlation with individuals who later are documented to have hypoglycemia (Palardy et al., 1989). Recording fingerstick blood glucose measurements during spontaneously occurring symptomatic episodes at home is a method that is often used to establish the diagnosis. An alternative method is to perform a glucose test in a medical office setting, in which case the patient is given a typical meal that has been documented in the past to lead to symptomatic episodes; Whipple's triad can be confirmed if symptoms occur (Prince, 1997). If blood glucose levels are low during the symptomatic period, and if the symptoms disappear upon eating, hypoglycemia is probably responsible.

Disorders resulting in hypoglycemia are heterogeneous in their etiology and clinical manifestations. Many patients with postprandial symptoms have been shown to have a hypoglycemic disorder. It is essential to make a correct diagnosis in patients with fasting hypoglycemia, because the implications for therapy are serious.

TREATMENT OF HYPOGLYCEMIA

The treatment of hypoglycemic disorders involves two distinct components: the relief of neuroglycopenic symptoms by the restoration of blood glucose levels to the normal range, and the correction of the underlying cause. The immediate treatment is to eat foods or beverages containing carbohydrate. As the glucose from the breakdown of carbohydrate is absorbed into the bloodstream, it will increase the level of glucose in the blood and relieve the symptoms. If an underlying problem is causing hypoglycemia, appropriate treatment of this disease or disorder is essential.

Almost no research has been done to determine what type of food-related treatment is best for the prevention of hypoglycemia. Traditional advice has been to avoid foods containing sugars and to eat protein- and fat-containing foods. However, recent research on the glycemic index and sugars (Wolever et al., 1994) has raised questions about the appropriateness of restricting only sugars, as these foods have been reported to have a lower glycemic index than many of the starches which were encouraged in the past (see Appendix 54). Restriction of sugars may contribute to a decreased intake in total carbohydrate, which may be more important than the source of the carbohydrate.

Previous nutrition-related recommendations for hypoglycemia have tended to be based on the experiences of the clinician as to what works. Bell et al. (1985) reported on survey returns (n = 76) identifying 35 diet manuals that contained dietary modifications for reactive hypoglycemia. A severely or moderately restricted carbohydrate diet was recommended by 83% of the hospitals. Most institutions (74%) recommended that caloric intake be adjusted to attain or maintain ideal body weight. There was wide agreement regarding limitation of simple sugar in the diet (97%), and all recommended more than three meals per day. Most institutions made no recommendations concerning fiber, alcohol, or caffeine.

It may be helpful to review what is known about the metabolism of carbohydrates, protein, and fat; their effects on blood glucose levels; and their relationship to insulin secretion. It should be remembered that this research has been conducted using normal subjects, not subjects who have been diagnosed with hypoglycemia.

After digestion, the major macronutrients absorbed are glucose, fructose, galactose, amino acids, and fatty acids that are reconstituted into triglycerides in chylomicrons. Glucose, fructose, and galactose are the major absorbed products of carbohydrate-containing foods, with approximately 75% from glucose, 22% from fructose, and 3% from galactose. The effect of these absorbed sugars on plasma glucose levels and insulin response is different for each (Nuttall and Gannon, 1991b) (see Chapters 1 and 3).

Most studies indicate little difference in the maximal glucose concentration reached, but rather a prolongation in the time interval over which the glucose level remains elevated. Blood glucose levels generally return to premeal levels after approximately 4 hours, but with smaller amounts of carbohydrate, this time span is shortened. This has been attributed to a regulated metering of glucose from the stomach (Gannon and Nuttall, 1987).

Insulin secretory rate is primarily determined by the absolute ambient glucose concentration to which the beta cells in the pancreatic islets are exposed. Superimposed on this regulation is a transient and large increase of insulin in response to a rapid rise in glucose, referred to as first-phase insulin secretion. After ingestion of glucose (or a mixed meal), these two phases become indistinguishable (Nuttall and Gannon, 1991b).

The amount of insulin secreted after glucose ingestion depends more on the amount of glucose ingested than on the magnitude of the glucose increase (Castro et al., 1970). Quantitatively, the increase in insulin concentration greatly exceeds the increase in glucose concentration. For example, the maximal glucose concentration typically does not exceed 50% of the premeal value, whereas the increase in insulin concentration is commonly 800% to 900%.

Overall, the system is designed to maintain the circulating glucose concentration in the nonfed state within narrowly defined limits. It is also designed to allow only a modest rise in glucose after carbohydrate-containing meals, and to return glucose concentrations rapidly to the nonfed state. Most of the insulin secreted during a 24-hour period is secreted during times of the day when ingested food is not being assimilated, the basal insulin secretion (Nuttall and Gannon, 1991b).

Fructose ingestion in normal subjects results in little or no change in insulin concentrations, and little increase in glucose concentrations (Crapo et al., 1980). Ingestion of galactose results in only a modest increase in peripheral glucose concentrations and a modest rise in insulin, which is attributable to the rise in glucose. Galactose is ingested, however, in the form of lactose (milk sugar), which is equimolar amounts of glucose and galactose. Galactose is primarily used for glycogen synthesis in the liver, and insulin has little effect on galactose metabolism (Niewoehner et al., 1990).

Ingested protein does not raise the plasma glucose concentrations in normal subjects, even when ingested in large amounts. This lack of change in glucose concentration occurs, although 50% to 70% of the ingested protein can be accounted for by deaminated amino acids and urea synthesis in the liver. Presumably, most deaminated amino acids are converted to glucose (Nuttall and Gannon, 1991a).

Although fat does not independently stimulate insulin secretion, it also does not affect the circulating glucose concentration. However, when ingested with carbohydrate, the plasma glucose and insulin responses are modified. This is an area that requires additional research (Nuttall and Gannon, 1991b). Preliminary evidence also suggests that a high fat intake may contribute to insulin resistance (Boden and Chen, 1995).

Using the information just presented, guidelines for the prevention of hypoglycemia have been published (International Diabetes Center, 1998).

AVOIDING SYMPTOMS OF HYPOGLYCEMIA

The goal of treatment is to adopt eating habits that will keep blood glucose levels as static as possible. Recommended guidelines are listed in Table 34–26.

Table 34–21 presents a sample menu. Patients with hypoglycemia may also benefit from learning carbohydrate counting and limiting carbohydrate servings (15 g of carbohydrate per serving) to two to four at a meal and one to two for snacks. Foods containing protein that are also low in fat can be eaten at meals or with snacks. These foods would be expected to have a limited effect on blood glucose levels and can add extra food for satiety and for calories without having a detrimental effect on blood glucose levels. However, because protein, as well as carbohydrate, stimulates insulin release, a moderate intake may be advisable.

In summary, nutrition is a challenging aspect of the management of diabetes and hypoglycemia of nondiabetic origin. Attention to nutrition and meal-planning principles is essential for glycemic control and overall good health. A registered dietitian who is knowledgeable and skilled in implementing current nutrition principles and making recommenda-

TABLE 34–26 GUIDELINES FOR AVOIDING HYPOGLYCEMIC SYMPTOMS

1. Eat small meals, with snacks interspersed between meals and at bedtime. This means eating five to six small meals rather than two to three large meals to steady the release of glucose into the bloodstream.
2. Spread the intake of carbohydrate foods throughout the day. Eating large amounts of carbohydrate at one time produces increased amounts of glucose and stimulates the release of increased amounts of insulin, which can cause blood glucose levels to drop. Most individuals can eat two to four servings of carbohydrate foods at each meal and one to two servings at each snack. Furthermore, if carbohydrate is removed from the diet, the body loses its ability to handle carbohydrate properly. Carbohydrate foods include starches, fruits and fruit juices, milk and yogurt, and foods containing sugar.
3. Avoid foods that contain large amounts of carbohydrate. Examples of these foods are regular soft drinks, syrups, candy, regular fruited yogurts, pies, and cakes.
4. Avoid beverages and foods containing caffeine. Caffeine can cause the same symptoms as hypoglycemia and make the individual feel worse (Kerr et al., 1993).
5. Limit or avoid alcoholic beverages. Drinking alcohol on an empty stomach and without food can lower blood glucose levels by interfering with the liver's ability to release stored glucose (gluconeogenesis) (Franz, 1999a). If an individual chooses to drink alcohol, it should be done in moderation (one or two drinks no more than twice a week), and food should always be eaten along with the alcoholic beverage.
6. Decrease fat intake. A high-fat diet, especially saturated fat, has been shown to affect the body's ability to use insulin (insulin resistance). Decreasing fat intake can also help with weight loss, if weight is a problem. Excess weight also interferes with the body's ability to use insulin.

CASE STUDY 1

Type 1 Diabetes

Ellen D. is a 15-year-old with newly diagnosed type 1 diabetes. She is 5'2", 115 lb, and active in cheerleading and basketball in high school. She is receiving insulin therapy; her physicians are regulating the dosage and timing while she is hospitalized.

Her grandmother has diabetes and is supportive of Ellen's need for education. Ellen's parents are divorced, and she now lives with her grandmother. What steps should you, as her nutrition counselor, take?

1. What food and meal-planning information needs to be shared with the health care team as insulin therapy is integrated into Ellen's normal eating and exercise habits?
2. What guidance should you offer regarding Ellen's sports activities?
3. Ellen is worried about keeping up with her peers. How will you help her adapt to the need for frequent snacks during a busy school day and during activities with her friends?
4. When Ellen travels on field trips or vacations, what types of snacks can she pack to take along?
5. What signs and symptoms of lack of diabetes control must Ellen understand in order to manage her disease? Which problem is she more likely to experience—hyperglycemia or hypoglycemia?

tions for people with diabetes or hypoglycemia of nondiabetic origins is the medical team member who should plan, implement, and evaluate MNT. Outcomes must be identified and the effectiveness of nutrition interventions continually documented.

CASE STUDY 2

Type 2 Diabetes

Debra J. is a 45-year-old woman with a known diagnosis of type 2 diabetes for 5 years. She has not had a medical check-up for 3 years. She returns at this time with a primary complaint of chronic fatigue. Her laboratory test results show the following: HbA_{1c}, 8.3%; serum cholesterol, 214 mg/dL; triglycerides, 275 mg/dL. Her current weight is 175 lb and her height is 64 in. She states she hasn't returned for any follow-up visits because the only advice she gets is to lose weight and not to eat sugar, neither of which she is able to do.

1. What advice will you offer to improve Debra's metabolic parameters and, in particular, to improve her blood glucose control?
2. What suggestions will you have about fat intake?
3. What information will you share about exercise?
4. What meal-planning method do you suggest for her?
5. What will you recommend regarding her sugar intake?

CITED REFERENCES

Aiello LP, et al. Diabetic retinopathy (Technical Review). Diabetes Care 21:143, 1998.

American Diabetes Association. Magnesium supplementation in the treatment of diabetes (Consensus Statement). Diabetes Care 15:1065, 1992.

American Diabetes Association. Treatment of hypertension in diabetes (Consensus Statement). Diabetes Care 16:1394, 1993.

American Diabetes Association. Maximizing the Role of Nutrition in Diabetes Management. Alexandria, VA: American Diabetes Association, 1994a.

American Diabetes Association. Self-monitoring of blood glucose (Consensus Statement). Diabetes Care 17:81, 1994b.

American Diabetes Association. Diabetes—1996 Vital Statistics. Alexandria, VA: American Diabetes Association, 1996.

American Diabetes Association. Economic consequences of diabetes mellitus in the U.S. in 1997. Diabetes Care 21:296, 1997.

American Diabetes Association. Gestational diabetes mellitus (Position Statement). Diabetes Care 22(suppl 1):S74, 1999a.

American Diabetes Association. Standards of medical care for patients with diabetes mellitus (Position Statement). Diabetes Care 22(suppl 1):S32, 1999b.

American Diabetes Association. Nutrition recommendations and principles for people with diabetes mellitus (Position Statement). Diabetes Care 22(suppl 1):S42, 1999c.

American Diabetes Association. Management of dyslipidemia in adults with diabetes (Position Statement). Diabetes Care 22(suppl 1):S56, 1999d.

American Diabetes Association. Diabetes mellitus and exercise (Position Statement). Diabetes Care 22(suppl 1):S49, 1999e.

American Diabetes Association. Diabetes nephropathy (Position Statement). Diabetes Care 22(suppl 1):S66, 1999f.

American Diabetes Association. Translation of the diabetes nutrition recommendations for health care institutions. Diabetes Care 22(suppl 1):S46, 1999g.

American Diabetes Association and The American Dietetic Association. Carbohydrate Counting: Getting Started, Moving On, Using Carbohydrate/Insulin Ratios. Alexandria, VA: American Diabetes Association, 1995a.

American Diabetes Association and The American Dietetic Association. Exchange Lists for Meal Planning. Alexandria, VA: American Diabetes Association, 1995b.

American Diabetes Association and The American Dietetic Association. The First Step in Diabetes Meal Planning. Alexandria, VA: American Diabetes Association, 1995c.

Anderson RA. Chromium, glucose intolerance and diabetes. J Am College of Nutrition 17:548, 1998.

Bantle JP, et al. Metabolic effects of dietary fructose in diabetic subjects. Diabetes Care 15:1468, 1992.

Bantle JP, et al. Metabolic effects of dietary sucrose in type II diabetic subjects. Diabetes Care 16:1301, 1993.

Bell LS, et al. Dietary strategies in the treatment of reactive hypoglycemia. J Am Diet Assoc 85:1141, 1985.

Bertelsen JC, et al. Effect of meal frequency on blood glucose, insulin, and free fatty acids in NIDDM subjects. Diabetes Care 16:3, 1993.

Boden G, Chen X. Effects of fat on glucose uptake and utilization in patients with non–insulin-dependent diabetes. J Clin Invest 96:1261, 1995.

Brodsky IG, et al. Effects of low-protein diets on protein metabolism in insulin-dependent diabetes mellitus patients with early nephropathy. J Clin Endocrinol Metab 75:351, 1992.

Butchko HH, Kotsonis FN. Acceptable intake vs actual intake: The aspartame example. Am J Clin Nutr 56:258, 1991.

Castro A, et al. Plasma insulin and glucose responses of healthy subjects to varying glucose loads during three-hour oral glucose tolerance tests. Diabetes 19:842, 1970.

Centers for Disease Control and Prevention. National Diabetes Fact Sheet: National Estimates and General Information on Diabetes in the United States. Atlanta, GA: U.S. Department of Health and Human Services, Centers for Disease Control and Prevention, 1997.

Coniff RF, et al. Reduction of glycosylated hemoglobin and postprandial hyperglycemia by acarbose in patients with NIDDM. Diabetes Care 18:817, 1995.

Crapo P, et al. Effects of oral fructose in normal, diabetic, and impaired glucose tolerance subjects. Diabetes Care 3:375, 1980.

Cryer PE, et al. Hypoglycemia (Technical review). Diabetes Care 17:734, 1994.

Cryer RE. Glucose counterregulation: The physiological mechanisms that prevent or correct hypoglycemia. In: Frier BM, Fisher BM (eds.). Hypoglycemia and Diabetes: Clinical and Physiological Aspects. London: Edward Arnold, 1993, p. 34.

Delahanty LM, Halford BN. The role of diet behaviors in achieving improved glycemic control in intensively treated patients in the Diabetes Control and Complications Trial. Diabetes Care 16:1453, 1993.

Diabetes Control and Complications Trial Research Group. The effect of intensive treatment of diabetes on the development and progression of long-term complications in insulin-dependent diabetes mellitus. N Engl J Med 329:977, 1993.

Diabetes Control and Complications Trial Research Group. Implementation of treatment protocols in the Diabetes Control and Complications Trial. Diabetes Care 18:36, 1995.

Drash A. The child, the adolescent and the Diabetes Control and Complications Trial. Diabetes Care 16:1515, 1993.

Durak EP, et al. Comparative evaluation of uterine response to exercise on five aerobic machines. Am J Obstet Gynecol 162:754, 1990.

Durnin J. Energy requirements of pregnancy. Diabetes 40(suppl 2):152, 1991.

Expert Committee on the Diagnosis and Classification of Diabetes Mellitus. Report of the Expert Committee on the Diagnosis and Classification of Diabetes Mellitus. Diabetes Care 20:1183, 1997.

Expert Panel on Blood Cholesterol Levels in Children and Adolescents: Report of the expert panel on blood cholesterol levels in children and adolescents. Pediatrics 90(suppl):525, 1992.

Farkas-Hirsch R (ed.). Intensive Diabetes Management, 2nd ed. Alexandria, VA: American Diabetes Association, 1998.

Franz MJ. Protein: Metabolism and effect on blood glucose levels. Diabetes Educator 23:643, 1997.

Franz MJ. Alcohol and diabetes. In: Franz MJ, Bantle JP (eds.). American Diabetes Association Guide to Medical Nutrition Therapy for Diabetes. Alexandria, VA: American Diabetes Association, 1999a, p. 192.

Franz MJ. Micronutrients and diabetes. In: Franz MJ, Bantle JP (eds.). American Diabetes Association Guide to Medical Nutrition Therapy for Diabetes. Alexandria, VA: American Diabetes Association, 1999b, p. 165.

Franz MJ, Barry B. Diabetes and Exercise. Guidelines for Safe and Enjoyable Activity. Minneapolis: International Diabetes Center, 1993.

Franz MJ, et al. Nutrition principles for the management of diabetes and related complications (Technical review). Diabetes Care 17:490, 1994.

Franz MJ, et al. Nutrition practice guidelines and basic care by dietitians for persons with non-insulin-dependent diabetes mellitus: Medical and clinical outcomes. J Am Diet Assoc 95:1009, 1995.

Franz MJ, Joynes JO. Diabetes and Brief Illness. Minneapolis: International Diabetes Center, 1993.

Gale EAM. Theory and practice of nicotinamide trials in pre-type 1 diabetes. J Pediatr Endocrinol Metab 9:375, 1996.

Gannon MC, Nuttall FQ. Factors affecting interpretation of postprandial glucose and insulin area. Diabetes Care 10:759, 1987.

Garg A, et al. Effects of varying carbohydrate content of diet in patients with non–insulin-dependent diabetes mellitus. JAMA 271:1421, 1994.

Goldstein DE, et al. Tests of glycemia in diabetes (Technical review). Diabetes Care 18:896, 1995.

Henry RR. Protein content of the diabetic diet (Technical review). Diabetes Care 17:1502, 1994.

Hepburn DA, et al. Symptoms of acute insulin-induced hypoglycemia in humans with and without IDDM: Factor-analysis approach. Diabetes Care 14:949, 1991.

Hermann LS, et al. Therapeutic comparison of metformin and sulfonylurea alone and in various combinations: A double-blind controlled study. Diabetes Care 17:1100, 1994.

Holler HJ, Pastors JG (eds.). Diabetes Medical Nutrition Therapy: A Guide to Management and Nutrition Education Resources. Chicago: The American Dietetic Association, 1997.

International Diabetes Center. My Food Plan. Minneapolis: International Diabetes Center, 1996.

International Diabetes Center. Reactive and Fasting Hypoglycemia. Minneapolis: International Diabetes Center, 1998.

Jenkins DJA, et al. Metabolic advantages of spreading nutrient load: Effects of increased meal frequency in non–insulin-dependent diabetes. Am J Clin Nutr 55:461, 1992.

Jovanovic-Peterson L (ed.). Medical Management of Pregnancy Complicated by Diabetes, 2nd ed. Alexandria, VA: American Diabetes Association, 1995.

Kelley DE, et al. Relative effects of caloric restriction and weight loss in non–insulin-dependent diabetes mellitus. J Clin Endocrinol Metab 77:1287, 1993.

Kerr D, et al. Effect of caffeine on the recognition of and responses to hypoglycemia in humans. Ann Intern Med 119:799, 1993.

King H, Rewers M. Diabetes in adults is now a third world population problem. Diabetes Care 16:157, 1993.

Kitzmiller JL, et al. Preconception care of diabetes, congenital malformations, and spontaneous abortions (Technical review). Diabetes Care 19:514, 1996.

Knopp RH, et al. Metabolic effects of hypocaloric diets in management of gestational diabetes. Diabetes 40(suppl 2):165, 1991.

Kohrt WM, et al. Insulin resistance in aging is related to abdominal obesity. Diabetes 42:273, 1993.

Koivisto VA, et al. Alcohol with a meal has no adverse effects on postprandial glucose homeostasis in diabetic patients. Diabetes Care 16:1612, 1993.

Kulkarni K, et al. Nutrition practice guidelines for type 1 diabetes mellitus positively affect dietitian practices and patient outcomes. J Am Diet Assoc 98:62, 1998.

Kuusisto JL, et al. NIDDM and its metabolic control predict coronary heart disease in elderly subjects. Diabetes 43:960, 1994.

Lebovitz HE. Stepwise and combination drug therapy for the treatment of NIDDM. Diabetes Care 17:1542, 1994.

Leonetti F, et al. Increased nonoxidative glucose metabolism in idiopathic reactive hypoglycemia. Metabolism 45:606, 1996.

Lewis JL, et al. The effect of angiotensin-converting-enzyme inhibition on diabetic nephropathy. N Engl J Med 329:1456, 1993.

Maclaren N, Atkinson M. Is insulin-dependent diabetes environmentally induced? Editorial. N Engl J Med 327:348, 1992.

Malaisse WJ. Stimulation of insulin release by non-sulfonylurea hypoglycemic agents: The meglitinide family. Hormone Metab Res 27:263, 1995.

McMahon MM. Nutrition support and diabetes. In: Franz MJ, Bantle JP (eds.). American Diabetes Association Guide to Medical Nutrition Therapy for Diabetes Alexandria, VA: American Diabetes Association, 1999, p. 335.

Metzger BE. Summary and recommendations of the Third International Workshop—Conference on Gestational Diabetes Mellitus. Diabetes 40(suppl 2):197, 1992.

Mitchell TH, et al. Hyperglycemia after intense exercise in IDDM subjects during continuous subcutaneous insulin infusion. Diabetes Care 11:311, 1988.

Mitrakou A, et al. Hierarchy of glycemic thresholds for counterregulatory hormone secretions, symptoms, and cerebral dysfunction. Am J Physiol 260:E67, 1991.

Monk A, et al. Practice guidelines for medical nutrition therapy by dietitians for persons with non–insulin-dependent diabetes mellitus. J Am Diet Assoc, 95:999, 1995.

Mooradian AD, et al. Selected vitamins and minerals in diabetes mellitus (Technical review). Diabetes Care 17:464, 1994.

Nakamura H, et al. Renal effects of different types of protein in healthy volunteer subjects and diabetic patients. Diabetes Care 16:1071, 1993.

National Diabetes Data Group. Diabetes in America, 2nd ed. Bethesda, MD: National Institutes of Health, National Institute of Diabetes and Digestive and Kidney Diseases, NIH Publication No. 95-1468, 1995.

Niewoehner CB, et al. Hepatic uptake and metabolism of oral galactose in adult fasted rats. Am J Physiol 259:E804, 1990.

Nolan JJ, et al. Improvement in glucose tolerance and insulin resistance in obese subjects treated with troglitazone. N Engl J Med 331:1188, 1994.

Nuttall FQ. Dietary fiber in the management of diabetes. Diabetes 42:503, 1993.

Nuttall FQ, et al. Effect of protein ingestion on the glucose and insulin response to a standardized oral glucose load. Diabetes Care 7:465, 1984.

Nuttall FQ, et al. The metabolic responses to various doses of fructose in type II diabetic subjects. Metabolism 41:510, 1992.

Nuttall FQ, Gannon MC. Metabolic responses to dietary protein in persons with and without diabetes mellitus. Diabetes Nutr Metab Clin Exp 4:71, 1991a.

Nuttall FQ, Gannon MC. Plasma glucose and insulin response to macronutrients in nondiabetic and NIDDM subjects. Diabetes Care 14:824, 1991b.

Ohkubbo Y, et al. Intensive therapy prevents the progression of diabetic complications in Japanese patients with non–insulin-dependent diabetes mellitus: A randomized prospective 6-year study. Diabetes Res Clin Pract 28:103, 1995.

Palardy J, et al. Blood glucose measurements during symptomatic episodes in patients with suspected postprandial hypoglycemia. N Eng J Med 321:1421, 1989.

Pascale RW, et al. Effects of a behavioral weight loss program stressing calorie restriction versus calorie plus fat restriction in obese individuals with NIDDM or a family history of diabetes. Diabetes Care 18:1241, 1995.

Pedrini MT, et al. The effect of protein restriction on the progression of diabetic and nondiabetic renal diseases: A meta-analysis. Ann Intern Med 124:627, 1996.

Peters AL, Davidson MB. Protein and fat effects on glucose response and insulin requirements in subjects with insulin-dependent diabetes mellitus. Am J Clin Nutr 58:555, 1993.

Powers M. Sugar alternatives and fat replacers. In: Franz MJ, Bantle JP (eds.). American Diabetes Association Guide to Medical Nutrition Therapy for Diabetes. Alexandria, VA: American Diabetes Association, 1999, p. 148.

Prince MJ. Hypoglycemia of nondiabetic origin. Curr Ther Endocrinol Metab 6:454, 1997.

Prochaska JO, et al. Changing for Good. New York: Morrow Press, 1994.

Purdon C, et al. The roles of insulin and catecholamines in the glucoregulatory response during intense exercise and early recovery in insulin-dependent diabetic and control subjects. J Clin Endocrinol Metab 76:566, 1993.

Ravid M, et al. Long-term stabilizing effect of angiotensin-converting enzyme inhibitor on plasma creatinine and on proteinuria in normotensive type 2 diabetic patients. Ann Intern Med 118:577, 1993.

Ravussin E, et al. Effects of a traditional lifestyle on obesity in Pima Indians. Diabetes Care 17:1067, 1994.
Reaven PD, et al. Effects of vitamin E on susceptibility of low-density lipoprotein and low-density lipoprotein subfractions to oxidation and on protein glycation in NIDDM. Diabetes Care 18:807, 1995.
Rickard KA, et al. Lower glycemic response to sucrose in the diets of children with type 1 diabetes. J Pediatr 133:429, 1998.
Rizzo T, et al. Correlations between antepartum maternal metabolism and intelligence of offspring. N Engl J Med 325:911, 1991.
Santiago J. Lessons from the diabetes control and complications trial. Diabetes 42:1549, 1993.
Service FJ. Hypoglycemic disorders. N Engl J Med 17:1144, 1995.
Skyler JS (ed.). Medical Management of Type 1 Diabetes, 3rd ed. Alexandria, VA: American Diabetes Association, 1998.
Suter SL, et al. Metabolic effects of new oral hypoglycemic agent CS-045 in NIDDM subjects. Diabetes Care 15:193, 1992.
Tinker LF, et al. Commentary and translation: 1994 Nutrition recommendations for diabetes. J Am Diet Assoc 94:507, 1994.
U.K. Prospective Diabetes Study Group. Intensive blood-glucose control with sulphonylureas or insulin compared with conventional treatment and risk of complications in patients with type 2 diabetes (UKPDS 34). Lancet 352:854, 1998a.
U.K. Prospective Diabetes Study Group. Tight blood pressure control and risk of macrovascular and microvascular complications in type 2 diabetes (UKPDS 38). BMJ 317:703, 1998b.
Wasserman DH, Zinman B. Exercise in individuals with IDDM (Technical review). Diabetes Care 17:924, 1994.
Watts NB, et al. Prediction of glucose response to weight loss in patients with non–insulin-dependent diabetes mellitus. Arch Intern Med 150:803, 1990.
Wheeler ML. Nephropathy and medical nutrition therapy. In: Franz MJ, Bantle JP (eds.). American Diabetes Association Guide to Medical Nutrition Therapy for Diabetes. Alexandria, VA: American Diabetes Association, 1999 p. 312..
Wheeler ML, et al. Controlled portions of presweetened cereals present no glycemic penalty in persons with insulin-dependent diabetes mellitus. J Am Diet Assoc 96:458, 1996.
Wing RR. Lifestyle and the prevention of diabetes. In: Franz MJ, Bantle JP (eds.). American Diabetes Association Guide to Medical Nutrition Therapy for Diabetes. Alexandria, VA: American Diabetes Association, 1999, p. 351.
Wing RR, et al. Caloric restriction per se is a significant factor in improvements in glycemic control and insulin sensitivity during weight loss in obese NIDDM patients. Diabetes Care 17:30, 1994.
Wolever TMS, et al. Determinants of diet glycemic index calculated retrospectively from diet records of 342 individuals with non–insulin-dependent diabetes. Am J Clin Nutr 59:1265, 1994.
Wylie-Rosett J. Hypertension and medical nutrition therapy. In: Franz MJ, Bantle JP (eds.). American Diabetes Association Guide to Medical Nutrition Therapy for Diabetes. Alexandria, VA: American Diabetes Association, 1999, p. 295.
Yki-Jarvinen H, et al. Comparison of insulin regimens in patients with non-insulin-dependent diabetes mellitus. N Engl J Med 327:1426, 1992.
Zeller KR, et al. Effect of restricting dietary protein on the progression of renal disease in patients with insulin-dependent diabetes mellitus. N Engl J Med 324:78, 1991.
Zimmerman BR (ed.). Medical Management of Type 2 Diabetes, 4th ed. Alexandria, VA: American Diabetes Association, 1998.

ADDITIONAL REFERENCES

American Diabetes Association. Consensus development conference on insulin resistance (Consensus Report). Diabetes Care 21:310, 1998.
American Diabetes Association. Implications of the Diabetes Control and Complications Trial (Position Statement). Diabetes Care 21(suppl 1):S88, 1998.
American Diabetes Association and The American Dietetic Association. Single-Topic Diabetes Resources. Alexandria, VA: American Diabetes Association, 1996.
American Dietetic Association. Nutrition Practice Guidelines for Type 1 and Type 2 Diabetes. Chicago: The American Dietetic Association, 1996.
Anderson BJ, Rubin RR (eds.). Practical Psychology for Diabetes Clinicians. Alexandria, VA: American Diabetes Association, 1996.
Clement S. Diabetes self-management education (Technical review). Diabetes Care 18:1204, 1995.
Franz MJ, Bantle JP (eds.). American Diabetes Association Guide to Medical Nutrition Therapy for Diabetes. Alexandria, VA: American Diabetes Association, 1999.
Funnell M, et al. (eds.). A Core Curriculum for Diabetes Educators, 3rd ed. Chicago: American Association of Diabetes Educators, 1999.
Funnell MM, Haas LB. National standards for diabetes self-management education programs (Technical review). Diabetes Care 18:100, 1995.
Hollenbeck CB, et al. The effects of variations in percent of naturally occurring complex and simple carbohydrates on plasma glucose and insulin response in individuals with non–insulin-dependent diabetes mellitus. Diabetes 34:151, 1985.
International Diabetes Center. Healthy Eating for People with Diabetes. Minneapolis: International Diabetes Center, 1997.
Is chromium supplementation effective in managing type II diabetes? Nutr Rev, 56:302, 1998.
Jones TW, et al. Decreased epinephrine response to hypoglycemia during sleeps. N Engl J Med 338:1657, 1998.
Powers M (ed.). Handbook of Diabetes Medical Nutrition Therapy, 2nd ed. Rockville, MD: Aspen Publishers, 1996.
Prochaska JO, et al. In search of how people change: Application to addictive behaviors. Am Psychol 47:1102, 1992.
Schafer RG, et al. Translation of the diabetes nutrition recommendations for health care institutions (Technical Review). Diabetes Care 20:96, 1997.
Warshaw H, et al. Fat replacers: Their use in foods and role in diabetes medical nutrition therapy (Technical Review). Diabetes Care 19:1294, 1996.
Wheeler ML, et al. Macronutrient and energy database for the 1995 Exchange Lists for Meal Planning: A rationale for clinical practice decisions. J Am Diet Assoc 96:1165, 1996.
Wheeler ML, Kulkarni KD (eds.). The art of nutrition: Multiple aspects of diabetes medical nutrition therapy. Diabetes Spectrum 9:97, 1996.

CHAPTER 35

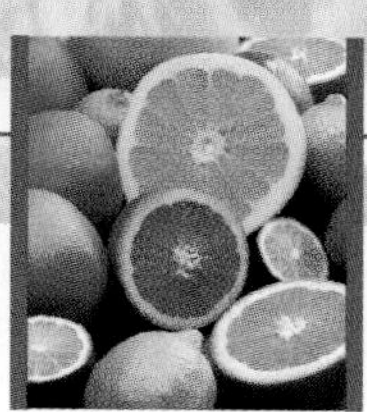

Medical Nutrition Therapy for Anemia

TRACY STOPLER KASDAN, MS, RD

CHAPTER OUTLINE

- Iron-Related Blood Disorders
- Megaloblastic Anemias
- Other Nutritional Anemias
- Nonnutritional Anemias

Key Terms

ANEMIA—a deficiency in the size or number of red blood cells or the amount of hemoglobin they contain, which limits the exchange of oxygen and carbon dioxide between the blood and the tissue cells

APLASTIC ANEMIA—a normochromic-normocytic anemia accompanied by a deficiency of all of the formed elements in the blood; can be caused by exposure to toxic chemicals, ionizing radiation, or medications, although the cause is often unknown

FERRITIN—an iron apoferritin complex; one of the chief storage forms of iron

HEMATOCRIT—the volume percentage of erythrocytes in the blood

HEME—the nonprotein, iron protoporphyrin constituent of hemoglobin

HEME IRON—the organic form in which iron occurs in meat, fish, and poultry

HEMOCHROMATOSIS—a genetically determined form of iron overload that results in progressive hepatic, pancreatic, cardiac, and other organ damage

HEMOGLOBIN—a conjugated protein containing four heme groups and globin; the oxygen-carrying pigment of the erythrocytes

HEMOLYTIC ANEMIA—anemia caused by shortened survival of mature red blood cells

HOLOTRANSCOBALAMIN II (HOLO TC II)—vitamin B_{12} attached to the B-globulin, which is the major circulating vitamin B_{12} delivery protein

HOMOCYSTEINE—a sulfur-containing amino acid which, in normal metabolism, is converted to methionine; an elevated serum homocysteine level is thought to be a risk factor for cardiovascular disease

HYPOCHROMIC—characterized by deficient hemoglobin content of red blood cells

INTRINSIC FACTOR (IF)—a glycoprotein, secreted by the gastric glands, that is necessary for the absorption of exogenous vitamin B_{12} by ileal cell surface receptors for IF-B_{12} complexes

MACROCYTIC ANEMIA—a form of anemia characterized by larger-than-normal red blood cells and increased mean corpuscular volume and mean corpuscular hemoglobin

MEGALOBLASTIC ANEMIA—a form of anemia characterized by the presence of large, immature, abnormal, red blood cell progenitors in the bone marrow; 95% of cases are attributable to folic acid or vitamin B_{12} deficiency

MICROCYTIC—characterized by smaller-than-normal erythrocytes and less circulating hemoglobin; characteristic of iron deficiency and thalassemia

NEGATIVE B_{12} BALANCE—a vitamin B_{12} predeficiency stage

NONHEME IRON—iron that is not a part of the heme complex and that is present in foods, such as eggs, grains, vegetables, and fruits; also present in small amounts in meat, fish, and poultry

PERNICIOUS ANEMIA—a macrocytic, megaloblastic anemia caused by a deficiency of vitamin B_{12}, secondary to lack of intrinsic factor

PROTOPORPHYRIN—an iron-containing portion of the respiratory pigments which, when combined with protein, forms hemoglobin or myoglobin

SICKLE CELL ANEMIA—a chronic hemolytic anemia, occuring most commonly in blacks, that is due to homozygous inheritance of HbS, resulting in a defective hemoglobin synthesis that causes the red blood cells to become sickle-shaped

SIDEROBLASTIC ANEMIA—a microcytic, hypochromic anemia characterized by a derangement in the final pathway of heme synthesis leading to a buildup of iron-containing immature red blood cells; responsive to pharmacologic doses of vitamin B_6

THALASSEMIA—anemia secondary to defective synthesis of the globin part of the hemoglobin

TOTAL IRON BINDING CAPACITY—the capacity of transferrin to take on or become saturated with iron

This chapter was reviewed by Victor Herbert, MD, JD.

TRANSFERRIN—globulin that binds and transports iron from the gut wall to the tissue cells

TRANSFERRIN SATURATION—a measure of the amount of iron bound to transferrin; a gauge of iron supply to the tissues

Anemia is a condition in which a deficiency in the size or number of erythrocytes, or the amount of hemoglobin they contain, limits the exchange of oxygen and carbon dioxide between the blood and the tissue cells. Classification is based on cell size—*macrocytic* (large), *normocytic* (normal), and *microcytic* (small)—and on hemoglobin content—*hypochromic* (pale color) and *normochromic* (normal color) (Table 35–1). Most anemias are caused by a lack of nutrients required for normal erythrocyte synthesis, principally iron, vitamin B_{12}, and folic acid. Others result from a variety of conditions, such as hemorrhage, genetic abnormalities, chronic disease states, or drug toxicity.

The anemias that result from an inadequate intake of iron, protein, certain vitamins (B_{12}, folic acid, pyridoxine, and ascorbic acid), copper, and other heavy metals are frequently called nutritional anemias. The most common nutritional anemias in the United States result from iron or folic acid deficiency.

IRON-RELATED BLOOD DISORDERS

Iron Deficiency Anemia

Iron deficiency anemia is characterized by the production of small (microcytic) erythrocytes and a diminished level of circulating hemoglobin. This is actually the last stage of iron deficiency, and it represents the end point of a long period of iron deprivation.

Pathophysiology

There are many possible causes of iron deficiency anemia (Fig. 35–1). The condition can arise from (1) inadequate iron intake secondary to a poor diet (such as a vegetarian life-style with insufficient heme iron); (2) inadequate absorption resulting from diarrhea, achlorhydria, intestinal disease, atrophic gastritis, partial or total gastrectomy, or

TABLE 35–1 MORPHOLOGIC CLASSIFICATION OF ANEMIA

MORPHOLOGIC TYPE OF ANEMIA	UNDERLYING ABNORMALITY	CLINICAL SYNDROMES/CAUSES	TREATMENT
Macrocytic (MCV > 94; MCHC > 31)			
Megaloblastic	Vitamin B_{12} deficiency	Pernicious anemia	Vitamin B_{12}
	Folic acid deficiency	Nutritional megaloblastic anemias, sprue, and other malabsorption syndromes	Folic acid
	Inherited disorders of DNA synthesis	Orotic aciduria	Treatment based on the nature of the disorder
	Drug-induced disorders of DNA synthesis	Chemotherapeutic agents, anticonvulsants, oral contraceptives	Discontinue offending drug and administer folic acid
Nonmegaloblastic	Accelerated erythropoiesis	Hemolytic anemia	Treatment of underlying disease
	Increased membrane surface area		
Hypochromic Microcytic (MCV < 80; MCHC < 31)			
	Iron deficiency	Chronic loss of blood, inadequate diet, impaired absorption, increased demands	Ferrous sulfate and correction of underlying cause
	Disorders of globin synthesis	Thalassemia	Nonspecific
	Disorders of porphyrin and heme synthesis	Pyridoxine-responsive anemia	Pyridoxine
	Other disorders of iron metabolism		
Normochromic Normocytic (MCV 82–92; MCHC > 30)			
	Recent blood loss	Various	Transfusion, iron
			Correction of underlying condition
	Overexpansion of plasma volume	Pregnancy	Restore homeostasis
	Hemolytic diseases	Overhydration	Treatment based on the nature of the disorder
	Hypoplastic bone marrow	Aplastic anemia	Transfusions
		Pure red blood cell aplasia	Androgens
	Infiltrated bone marrow	Leukemia, multiple myeloma, myelofibrosis	Chemotherapy
	Endocrine abnormality	Hypothyroidism, adrenal insufficiency	Treatment of underlying disease
	Chronic disorders		Treatment of underlying disease
	Renal disease	Renal disease	Treatment of underlying disease
	Liver disease	Cirrhosis	Treatment of underlying disease

(Adapted from Wintrobe MM, et al. Clinical Hematology, 8th ed. Philadelphia: Lea & Febiger, 1981.)

MCV, mean corpuscular volume: 5 volume of one red blood cell expressed in femtoliters (fL); *MCHC*, mean corpuscular hemoglobin concentration: 5 concentration of hemoglobin expressed in g/dL.

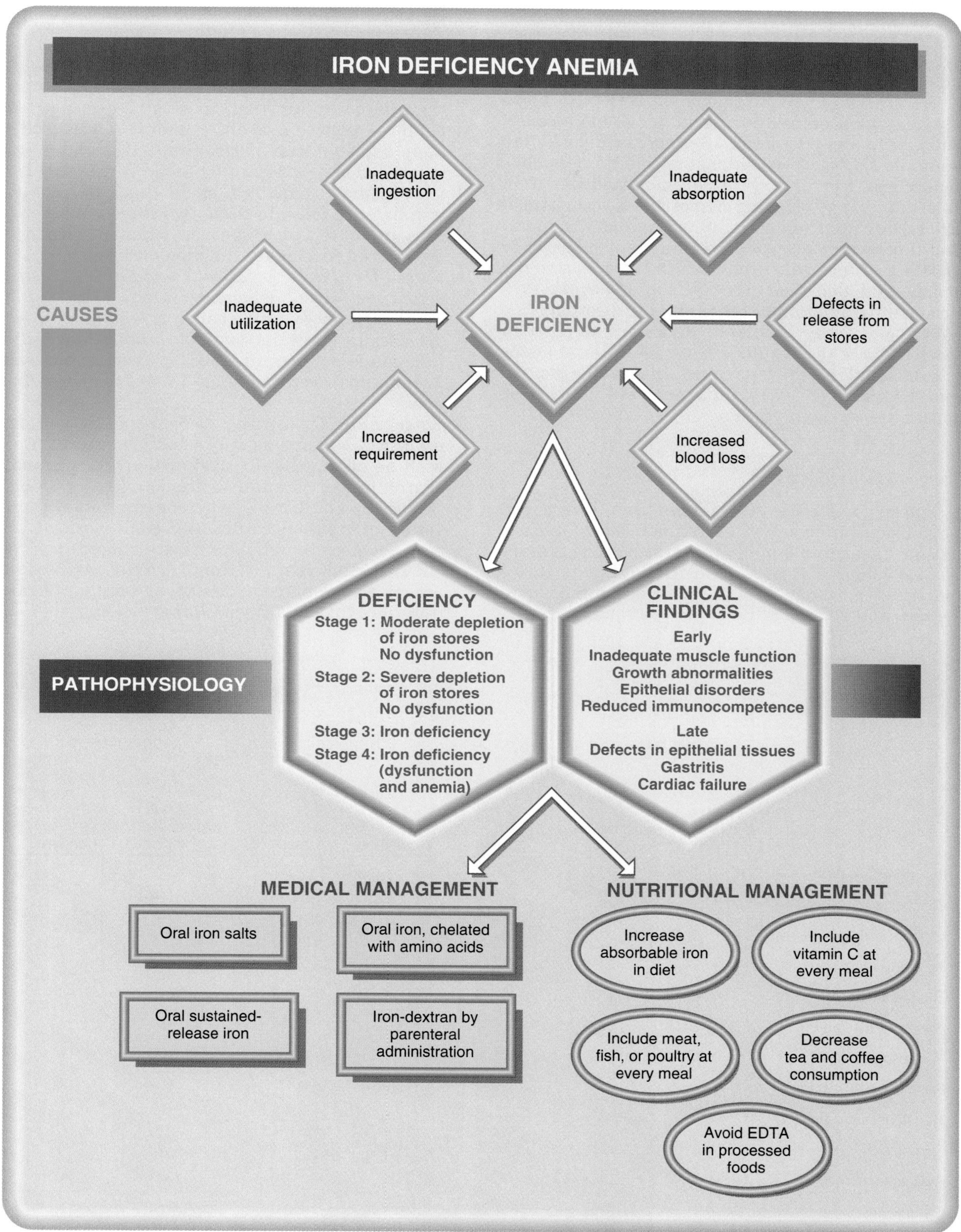

FIGURE 35–1 Pathophysiology algorithm—iron deficiency anemia. *EDTA,* ethylenediaminetetra-acetic acid. (Algorithm content developed by John Anderson, Ph.D., and Sanford C. Garner, Ph.D., 2000.)

drug interference (antacids, cholestyramine, cimetidine [Tagamet], pancreatin, ranitidine [Zantac], and tetracycline); (3) inadequate utilization secondary to chronic gastrointestinal disturbances; (4) increased iron requirement for growth of blood volume, which occurs during infancy, adolescence, pregnancy, and lactation; (5) increased excretion owing to excessive menstrual blood (in females); hemorrhage from injury; or chronic blood loss from a bleeding ulcer, bleeding hemorrhoids, esophageal varices, regional enteritis, ulcerative colitis, parasites (hookworm disease), or malignant disease; or (6) defective release of iron from iron stores into the plasma and defective iron utilization owing to a chronic inflammation or other chronic disorder.

With few exceptions, iron deficiency anemia in male adults is the result of blood loss. Large losses of menstrual blood can cause iron deficiency in women, many of whom are unaware that their menses are unusually heavy.

Stages of Deficiency

As shown in Figure 35–2, one's iron status can range from iron overload to iron deficiency anemia. Routine measurement of iron status is necessary because about 6% of Americans have a negative iron balance, about 10% have a gene for positive balance, and about 1% have iron overload.

Deviations from normal iron status have been summarized by Herbert (1992) as follows:

- *Stages I and II negative iron balance (i.e., iron depletion)*—In these stages, iron stores are low and there is no dysfunction. In stage I negative iron balance, reduced iron absorption produces moderately depleted iron stores. Stage II negative iron balance is characterized by severely depleted iron stores. More than 50% of all cases of negative iron balance fall into these two stages. When persons in these two stages are treated with iron, they never develop dysfunction or disease.
- *Stages III and IV negative iron balance (i.e., iron deficiency)*—Iron deficiency is characterized by inadequate body iron, causing dysfunction and disease. In stage III negative iron balance, dysfunction is not accompanied by anemia; however, anemia does occur in stage IV negative iron balance.
- *Stages I and II positive iron balance*—Stage I positive iron balance usually lasts for several years with no accompanying dysfunction. Supplements of iron and/or vitamin C promote progression to dysfunction or disease, whereas iron removal prevents progression to disease. Iron overload disease develops in individuals with stage II positive balance after years of iron overload have caused progressive damage to tissues and organs. Again, iron removal stops disease progression.

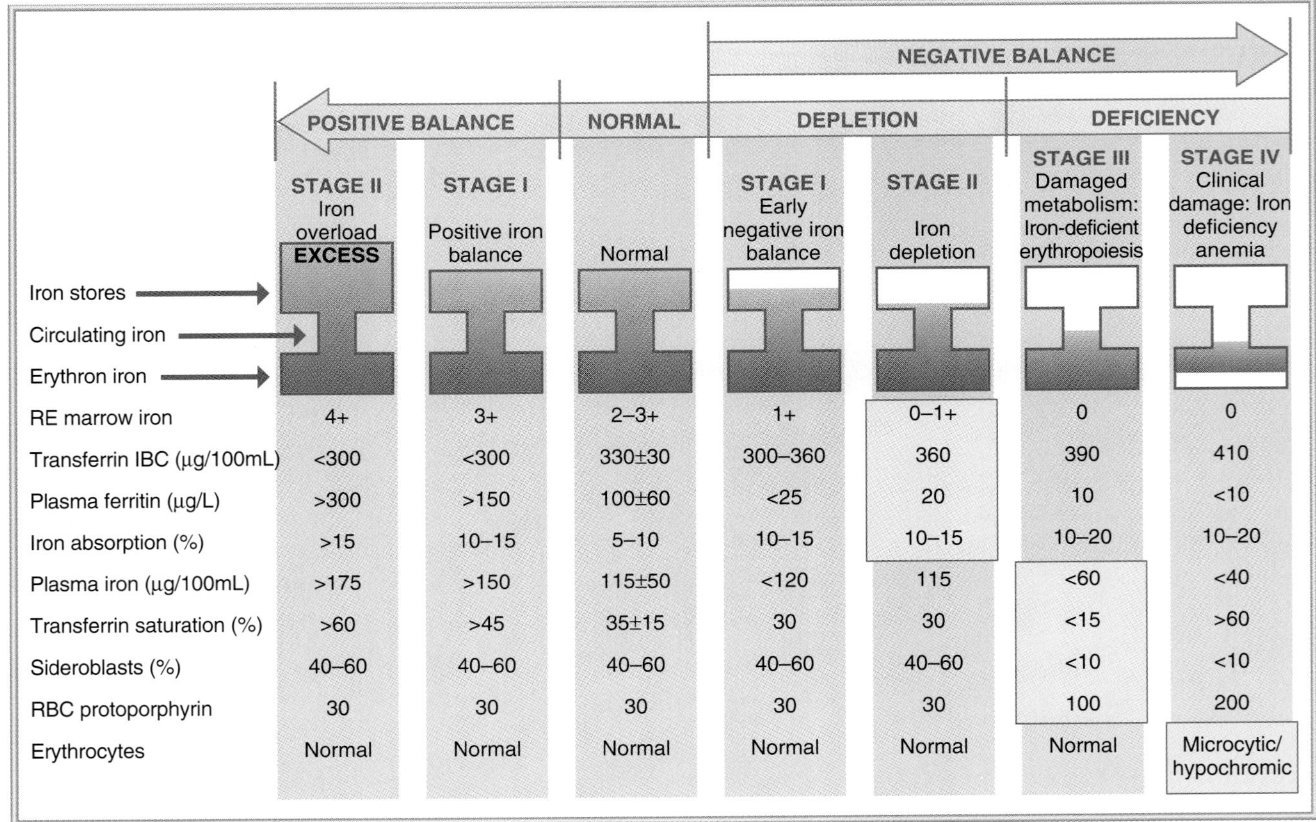

NEGATIVE BALANCE
POSITIVE BALANCE
NORMAL
DEPLETION
DEFICIENCY
STAGE II Iron overload
EXCESS
STAGE I Positive iron balance
Normal
STAGE I Early negative iron balance
STAGE II Iron depletion
STAGE III Damaged metabolism: Iron-deficient erythropoiesis
STAGE IV Clinical damage: Iron deficiency anemia
Iron stores
Circulating iron
Erythron iron
RE marrow iron 4+ 3+ 2–3+ 1+ 0–1+ 0 0
Transferrin IBC (μg/100mL) <300 <300 330±30 300–360 360 390 410
Plasma ferritin (μg/L) >300 >150 100±60 <25 20 10 <10
Iron absorption (%) >15 10–15 5–10 10–15 10–15 10–20 10–20
Plasma iron (μg/100mL) >175 >150 115±50 <120 115 <60 <40
Transferrin saturation (%) >60 >45 35±15 30 30 <15 >60
Sideroblasts (%) 40–60 40–60 40–60 40–60 40–60 <10 <10
RBC protoporphyrin 30 30 30 30 30 100 200
Erythrocytes Normal Normal Normal Normal Normal Normal Microcytic/hypochromic

FIGURE 35–2 Sequential stages of iron status. (From Herbert V, et al. Vitamin C–driven free radical generation from iron. J Nutr 126: 1214S, 1996. © 1990, 1995 by Victor Herbert.) *RE*, reticuloendothelial cells; *TIBC*, total iron-binding capacity; *RBC*, red blood cell.

There are a variety of indicators of iron status. Serum ferritin levels are in equilibrium with body iron stores. Very early (stage I) positive iron balance may best be recognized by measuring **total iron-binding capacity (TIBC).** Conversely, measurement of serum ferritin levels may best reveal early (stages I and II) negative iron balance, although serum total iron-binding capacity may be as good an indicator.

Clinical Findings

Because anemia is the last manifestation of chronic, long-term iron deficiency, the symptoms reflect a malfunction of a variety of body systems. Inadequate muscle function is reflected in decreased work performance and exercise tolerance. Neurologic involvement is manifested by behavioral changes, such as fatigue, anorexia, and pica, especially pagophagia (ice eating) (see Chapter 7). Abnormal cognitive development in children suggests the presence of iron deficiency before it has developed into overt anemia (Pollitt et al., 1986). Growth abnormalities, epithelial disorders, and a reduction in gastric acidity are common. A possible sign of early iron deficiency is reduced immunocompetence, particularly defects in cell-mediated immunity and the phagocytic activity of neutrophils, which may lead to an increased propensity for infection.

As iron deficiency anemia becomes more severe, defects arise in the structure and function of the epithelial tissues, especially of the tongue, nails, mouth, and stomach. The skin may appear pale, and the inside of the lower eyelid may be light pink instead of red. Fingernails can become thin and flat, and eventually, *koilonychia* (spoon-shaped nails) may be noted (Fig. 35–3). Mouth changes include atrophy of the lingual papillae, burning, redness, and, in severe cases, a completely smooth, waxy, and glistening appearance to the tongue (*glossitis*). *Angular stomatitis* may also occur, as may a form of *dysphagia* (difficulty in swallowing). Gastritis occurs frequently and may result in achlorhydria. Progressive, untreated anemia results in cardiovascular and respiratory changes that can eventually lead to cardiac failure.

Some behavioral symptoms of iron deficiency seem to respond to iron therapy before the anemia is cured, suggesting they may be the result of tissue depletion of iron-containing enzymes rather than of a decreased level of hemoglobin (see Chapter 5).

Diagnosis

Progressive stages of iron deficiency can be evaluated by four different measurements.

1. The plasma **ferritin** level provides a measure of iron stores.
2. **Transferrin saturation** can be used as a gauge of iron supply to the tissues. It is calculated by dividing serum iron by TIBC; levels less than 16% are considered to be inadequate for erythropoiesis.

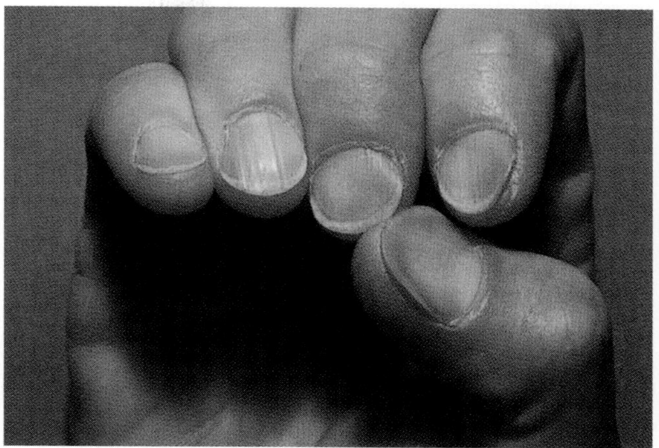

FIGURE 35–3 Fingernails with cup-like depressions (koilonchia) are a sign of iron deficiency in adults. (From Callen JP, Greer KE, Hood AF, Paller AS, Swinyer LJ. Color Atlas of Dermatology. Philadelphia: WB Saunders, 1993.)

3. Both **hemoglobin** and **hematocrit** measurements can indicate anemia. Most patients develop symptoms of anemia when the hemoglobin level is approximately 8 to 11 g/dL (see Fig. 35–2).
4. The ratio of zinc **protoporphyrin** (ZnPP; erythrocyte protoporphyrin) to heme is a sensitive indicator of the iron supply to the developing red blood cells. When insufficient substrate iron is available to incorporate into porphyrin, zinc is then substituted. Although it can combine with globin and circulate, this zinc-containing molecule cannot bind oxygen.

A definitive diagnosis of iron deficiency anemia requires more than one method of iron evaluation and preferably includes the first three of the measurements just listed. The evaluation should also include an assessment of cell morphology. The serum or plasma ferritin level is the most sensitive parameter of negative iron balance, as it decreases only in the presence of true iron deficiency, as with transferrin saturation. By contrast, the ZnPP:heme ratio and hemoglobin levels are affected by chronic infection and other factors that can produce a condition that mimics iron deficiency anemia when, in fact, iron is adequate. The TIBC declines and serum ferritin levels rise in chronic disease unrelated to iron metabolism (see Table 35–1). By itself, hemoglobin concentration is unsuitable as a diagnostic tool in cases of suspected iron deficiency anemia for three reasons: (1) it is affected only late in the disease; (2) it cannot distinguish iron deficiency from other anemias; (3) hemoglobin values in normal individuals vary widely.

Treatment

Treatment should focus primarily on the underlying disease or situation leading to the anemia, although this is often very difficult to determine. Repletion of iron stores, not merely alleviation of the anemia, should be the goal.

SUPPLEMENTATION

The chief treatment for iron deficiency anemia involves oral administration of inorganic iron in the ferrous form. At a dose of 30 mg, absorption of ferrous iron is three times greater than if the same amount were given in the ferric form. At larger doses, the difference is even more marked. The most widely used preparation is ferrous sulfate, and the dose is calculated in terms of the amount of elemental iron provided. Other salts absorbed to about the same degree are the ferrous forms of lactate, fumarate, glycine sulfate, glutamate, and gluconate.

Iron is best absorbed when the stomach is empty; however, under these conditions, it tends to cause gastric irritation. Gastrointestinal side effects of nausea, epigastric discomfort and distention, heartburn, diarrhea, or constipation can be minimized by increasing the dose slowly over a few days until the required dosage is reached, and by giving the iron in divided doses at least three times per day. Use of a chelated form of iron (bound to amino acids) can result in improved absorption and can reduce the likelihood of gastrointestinal distress. Sustained-release iron preparations reduce gastrointestinal side effects by preventing rapid dissolution of iron, but they may also allow the iron to bypass the jejunum, which is the most active site of iron absorption. Side effects are dose-related, so smaller dosages and a longer therapeutic program may be advisable.

Depending on the severity of the anemia and the individual's tolerance of iron supplementation, the daily dose of elemental iron should be 50 to 200 mg for adults and 6 mg/kg for children. Ascorbic acid greatly increases iron absorption through its capacity to maintain iron in the reduced state.

Absorption of 10 to 20 mg of iron per day permits red blood cell production to rise to about three times the normal rate and, in the absence of blood loss, hemoglobin concentration to rise at a rate of 0.2 g/dL/day. Increased reticulocytosis is seen within 2 to 3 days after iron administration, but affected individuals may report subjective improvements in mood and appetite even sooner. The hemoglobin level will begin to increase by day 4 of treatment. Iron therapy should be continued for several months, even after restoration of normal hemoglobin levels, to allow for repletion of body iron reserves.

If iron supplementation fails to correct the anemia, one should consider the following possibilities: (1) the patient may not be taking the medication as prescribed, most likely because of unpleasant side effects; (2) bleeding may be continuing at a rate faster than the erythroid marrow can replace blood cells; or (3) the supplemental iron is not being absorbed, possibly as a result of malabsorption secondary to steatorrhea, celiac sprue, or hemodialysis. In these circumstances, parenteral administration of iron, in the form of iron-dextran, may be necessary. Although replenishment of iron stores by this route is faster, it is more expensive and not as safe as oral administration.

NUTRITIONAL INTERVENTION

In addition to iron supplementation, attention should be given to the amount of absorbable dietary iron consumed. Liver, kidney, beef, egg yolk, dried fruits, dried peas and beans, nuts, green leafy vegetables, molasses, whole-grain breads and cereals, and fortified cereals are among the foods that rank highest in terms of their iron content (see Table 35–2 and Appendix 41 for a more complete list).

It is estimated that 1.8 mg of iron must be absorbed daily to meet the needs of 80% to 90% of adult women and adolescent males and females. Because typical Western diets generally contain 6 mg/1000 kcal of iron, the bioavailability of iron in the diet is clearly more important in correcting or preventing iron deficiency than the total amount of dietary iron consumed.

Bioavailability of Dietary Iron. Several factors influence the bioavailability of dietary iron. The rate of absorption depends on the iron status of the individual, as reflected in the level of iron stores. The lower the iron stores, the greater will be the rate of iron absorption. Individuals with iron deficiency anemia absorb about 20% to 30% of dietary iron, compared to the 5% to 10% absorbed by those without iron deficiency.

Absorption is also influenced by the form of iron in the diet. **Heme iron,** present in meat, fish, and poultry (MFP), is much better absorbed than **nonheme iron,** which can also be found in MFP, as well as in eggs, grains, vegetables, and fruits. The absorption rate of nonheme iron varies between 3% and 8%, depending on the presence of dietary enhancing factors, specifically, ascorbic acid and MFP. Ascorbic acid is not only a powerful reducing agent, it also binds iron to form a readily absorbed complex. The mechanism by which MFP potentiates the absorption of nonheme iron in other foodstuffs is unknown. MFP digestion may lead to the release of amino acids (particularly cysteine) and polypeptides in the upper small bowel, which then chelate with nonheme iron to form soluble, absorbable complexes (Mulvihill et al., 1998).

Iron absorption can be inhibited to varying degrees by a number of factors that chelate iron, including carbonates, oxalates, phosphates, and phytates (unleavened bread, unrefined cereals, and soybeans). Factors in vegetable fiber may inhibit nonheme iron. Taken with meals, tea can reduce iron absorption by 50% through the formation of insoluble iron compounds with tannin. Ethylenediaminetetra-acetic acid (EDTA), a food preservative, causes a 50% reduction in nonheme iron absorption. Iron in egg yolk is poorly absorbed because of the presence of phosvitin.

In summary, then, to maximize iron absorption and prevent iron deficiency anemia, one should (1) improve food choices to increase total dietary iron intake; (2) include a source of vitamin C at every meal; (3) include MFP at every meal, if possible; (4) avoid drinking large amounts of tea or coffee

TABLE 35–2 IRON CONTENT OF SOME COMMON FOODS

FOOD	PORTION SIZE	IRON (mg)*
Protein Group		
Chicken, light meat	3 oz	0.9
Chicken, dark meat	3 oz	1.2
Turkey, dark meat	3 oz	2.0
Pork chop	3 oz	0.7
Tenderloin steak	3 oz	1.3
Venison, roasted	3 oz	3.0
Liver, beef	3 oz	5.8
Liver, chicken	3 oz	7.2
Liver, pork	3 oz	15.2
Tuna fish	3 oz	0.6
Swordfish	3 oz	1.1
Oysters, raw	3 oz	5.5
Tofu, raw	½ cup	4.0
Black beans	½ cup	1.8
Chickpeas	½ cup	2.4
Kidney beans	½ cup	2.6
Lentil beans	½ cup	3.3
Egg	1 whole	0.6
Cashew nuts	1 oz	1.7
Pistachio nuts	1 oz	1.9
Sunflower seeds	1 TBS	1.9
Dairy Group		
Milk	1 cup	0.1
Ricotta, part-skim	½ cup	0.6
Fruit Group		
Apricots	3 raw	0.6
Apple, dried	10 rings	0.9
Figs, dried	1	0.4
Peaches, dried	5 halves	2.6
Raisins	½ cup	1.5
Strawberries	1 cup, frozen	1.2
Vegetable Group		
Artichoke, cooked	1 cup	5.1
Baked potato	1 medium	2.7
Broccoli	1 medium stalk	2.1
Green pepper	1 medium	0.9
Lima beans	½ cup	2.1
Spinach	1 cup	1.5
Grain Group		
Pasta (enriched)	1 cup	2.0
Rice (enriched)	1 cup	1.8
Whole wheat bread	1 slice	1.0
Bagel	1	1.8
Cereals		
Grapenuts	½ cup	18.0
Product 19	¾ cup	18.0
Total	1 cup	18.0
Wheat germ	1 oz (¼ cup)	2.6
Cream of wheat, instant	¾ cup	8.2
Oatmeal, plain, instant	1 packet	6.7
Other		
Brown sugar	1 cup	4.8
Molasses, blackstrap	1 TBS	5.0

*Absorbability of iron from animal foods averages 15%; from plant foods, it averages only 3%.

with meals, as both contain tannin; (5) avoid high quantities of EDTA by checking food labels for its presence in foods; and (6) reduce milk consumption to no more than 3 cups per day and replace it with iron-containing foods.

Hemochromatosis

Hemochromatosis is a genetically determined form of iron overload that is present, in heterozygous form, in about 12% of non-blacks and about 30% of blacks (see website www.niddk.nih.gov/health/hematol). About 1 in 200 nonblacks and about 1 in 100 blacks are homozygous. Homozygotes will die of iron overload unless they donate blood frequently. In women, monthly menses slow the associated organ damage until after menopause.

Pathophysiology

Men are particularly susceptible to hemochomatosis because they have no physiologic mechanisms, such as menstruation, pregnancy, or lactation, for losing iron. The excessive iron intake usually stems from accidental incorporation of iron into the diet from environmental sources. In developing countries, the iron overload can result from eating foods cooked in cast-iron cooking vessels or contaminated by iron-containing soils.

After absorption, iron is transported by plasma **transferrin,** a β_1-globulin that binds iron derived from either the gastrointestinal tract, iron storage sites, or hemoglobin breakdown and transports it to the bone marrow (hemoglobin synthesis), endothelial cells (storage), or placenta (fetal needs). The protein HFE is the product of the gene responsible for hemochromatosis. It is this protein that interacts with the transferrin receptors on the surface of cells, thus regulating the cells' ability to take up the transferrin-bound iron from the circulation (Cohen, 1998).

Excess iron is stored as ferritin and hemosiderin in the macrophages of the liver, spleen, and bone marrow. The body has a limited capacity to excrete iron. Approximately 1 mg of iron is excreted daily through the gastrointestinal tract, urinary tract, and skin. To maintain a normal iron balance, the daily obligatory loss must be replaced by the absorption of heme and nonheme food iron. Individuals with iron overload excrete increased amounts of iron, especially in the feces, to partially compensate for the increased absorption and higher stores (Fairbanks, 1994).

Clinical Findings

In hemochromatosis, iron absorption is enhanced, resulting in a gradual, progressive accumulation of iron. This disease, associated in whites with an abnormal HLA-A gene located on the short arm of chromosome 6, is often underdiagnosed. Most affected people do not know they have the disease. In its early stages, iron overload may result in symptoms similar to iron deficiency, such as fatigue and weakness; later, it can cause chronic abdominal pain, aching joints, impotence, and menstrual irregularities. A progressive positive iron balance may result in a variety of serious problems, including hepatomegaly, skin pigmentation, diabetes mellitus, arthritis, cancer, heart disease, and hypogonadism. Mortality from hemochromatosis is preventable if excess body iron is removed by phlebotomy therapy before hepatic cirrhosis develops.

Diagnosis

If an iron overload is suspected, the following screening tests should be performed: serum ferritin level (storage iron), serum iron concentration, total iron binding capacity (TIBC), and percent transferrin saturation ([serum iron/TIBC] × 100). Iron overload may be present if the percent transferrin saturation is greater than 50 in women and 60 in men, and if the serum iron level is greater than 180 mg/dL. DNA testing, using blood or cheek cell samples, is also available for early detection of hemochromatosis.

The individual with iron overload may simultaneously be anemic as a result of damage to the bone marrow or an inflammatory disorder (i.e., arthritis), cancer, internal bleeding, or chronic infection. Iron supplements should not be taken until the cause of the anemia is known.

Treatment

For patients with significant iron overload, weekly phlebotomy for 2 to 3 years may be required to eliminate all excess iron. Treatment for iron overload may also involve iron depletion with intravenous desferrioxamine-B, a chelating agent that is excreted by the kidneys. Calcium disodium EDTA can also be used. Individuals who are diagnosed as having hemochromatosis should inform all blood relatives so that they, too, can be evaluated.

NUTRITIONAL INTERVENTION

Individuals with iron overload should ingest less heme iron (i.e., from MFP) compared to nonheme iron (plant groups). Persons with iron overload should also avoid alcohol and vitamin C supplements because both enhance iron absorption. In addition, vitamin C supplements may cause release of harmful free-radical–generating excess iron from body stores.

Iron Toxicity

Other disorders associated with iron overload include thalassemia minor, sideroblastic anemia, chronic hemolytic anemia, aplastic anemia, ineffective erythropoiesis, transfusional iron overload (secondary to multiple blood transfusions), porphyria cutanea tarda, and alcoholic cirrhosis. Excess dietary iron intake (as occurs in South African [Bantu] blacks who absorb excess dietary iron from alcoholic beverages fermented in iron stills and food cooked in iron pots) or an overdose of iron medication (as may occasionally occur in children who mistake iron tablets for candy) can be fatal in doses of 3 to 10 g. Iron can cause irritation of the mucosa with ulceration and bleeding, hypoxia, metabolic acidosis, alveolar and hepatic damage, and renal failure. Death can occur in 12 to 48 hours.

Hyperhomocysteinemia

Deficiency of either vitamin B_{12} or folic acid causes the circulating level of the sulfur-containing amino acid **homocysteine** to rise. Elevated serum levels of homocysteine are toxic to blood vessels, producing coronary artery clots (with heart attacks), thrombotic (clotting) strokes, and peripheral vein (particularly in the leg) thrombosis. Approximately 20% of all heart attacks, 40% of clotting strokes, and 60% of all peripheral vein occlusions (including those in pregnant women) are attributable to abnormally high serum homocysteine levels (Flynn et al., 1997). (See Chapters 4 and 26 for a further discussion of homocysteine and cardiovascular disease.)

High homocysteine levels are usually treated with vitamin B_6 in infants and small children (see Chapter 44), with folic acid in fertile females, and with oral vitamin B_{12} in the elderly (food vitamin B_{12} gradually becomes nonabsorbable in the elderly due to gastric atrophy).

MEGALOBLASTIC ANEMIAS

Megaloblastic anemia reflects a disturbed synthesis of DNA, which results in morphologic and functional changes in erythrocytes, leukocytes, platelets, and their precursors in the blood and bone marrow. Megaloblastic anemia is usually caused by a deficiency of vitamin B_{12} or folic acid, both of which are essential to the synthesis of nucleoproteins. Hematologic changes are the same for both; however, the folic acid deficiency is the first to appear. Normal body folate stores are depleted within 2 to 4 months in individuals consuming folate-deficient diets; by contrast, vitamin B_{12} stores are depleted only after several years of a vitamin B_{12}–deficient diet. In individuals with vitamin B_{12} deficiency, folic acid supplementation can mask B_{12} deficiency (Markle, 1997). In correcting the anemia, the vitamin B_{12} deficiency may remain undetected, leading to the irreversible neuropsychiatric damage that is only prevented with B_{12} supplementation.

Pernicious and Other Vitamin B_{12} Deficiency Anemias

Pathophysiology

Pernicious anemia is a megaloblastic macrocytic anemia caused by a deficiency of vitamin B_{12}. Most commonly, the vitamin deficiency is secondary to a lack of **intrinsic factor (IF),** a glycoprotein in the gastric juice that is necessary for the absorption of dietary vitamin B_{12}. Very rarely, vitamin B_{12} deficiency anemia occurs in strict vegetarians whose diet contains no vitamin B_{12} except for traces found in plants contaminated by microorganisms capable of synthesizing vitamin B_{12}. Other causes are shown in Table 35–3.

Ingested vitamin B_{12} is freed from protein by gastric acid and gastric and intestinal enzymes. The free vitamin B_{12} attaches to salivary R binder which, at an acid pH (2.3), such as that found in the stomach, has a higher affinity for the vitamin than does IF. IF, secreted by parietal cells of the gastric mucosa, is necessary for the absorption of exogenous vitamin B_{12}.

The release of pancreatic trypsin into the proximal small intestine destroys R binder and releases vitamin B_{12} from its complex with R protein. At an alkaline pH (6.8), as may be found in the intestine, IF then binds the vitamin B_{12}.

The vitamin B_{12}–IF complex is then carried to the ileum where, in the presence of ionic calcium (Ca^{++}) and a pH of greater than 6, it attaches to the surface vitamin B_{12}–IF receptors on the ileal cell brush border.

At the brush border, the vitamin B_{12}–IF complex enters the ileal cell, where the vitamin B_{12} is released, attaching to **holotranscobalamin II (holo TC II).** Like IF, holo TC II plays an active role in binding and transporting vitamin B_{12}. The TC II–vitamin B_{12} complex then enters the portal venous

TABLE 35–3 CAUSES OF VITAMIN B_{12} DEFICIENCY

- I. Inadequate ingestion
  - A. Poor diet (lacking microorganisms and animal foods, which are the sole sources of vitamin B_{12})
    - 1. Strict vegetarianism (eating no meat, fowl, seafood, eggs, milk, or any products thereof)
    - 2. Chronic alcoholism (no vitamin B_{12} or folate in hard liquor; folate deficiency occurs first and is more common, partly because body stores of vitamin B_{12} last much longer than those of folate)
    - 3. Poverty, religious tenets (Hinduism, Seventh Day Adventism, certain Catholic orders), dietary faddism
- II. Inadequate absorption
  - A. Gastric disorder producing inadequate or absent secretion by gastric parietal cells of intrinsic factor
    - 1. Addisonian pernicious anemia (PA): that form of vitamin B_{12} deficiency disease that is attributable to inadequate intrinsic factor secretion of uncertain cause
      - a) Hereditary absence of normal intrinsic factor secretion: Absent secretion at birth (circulating antibody to intrinsic factor never present) supports the theory that antibody occurs only when antigenic stimulus is produced by intrinsic factor, which enters blood from damaged parietal cells and is recognized as foreign by the immunologic surveillance system; rare
      - b) Congenital production of defective intrinsic factor molecule (three published cases)
      - c) Autoimmunity-associated gastric atrophy: Affected patients usually are nondiagnostic-for-pernicious-anemia circulating parietal cell antibody, which is an index only of past or present gastric damage and not of the amount of intrinsic factor secretion (circulating diagnostic-for-PA antibody to intrinsic factor is always present in individuals younger than 21 years of age; there is a gradual decrease in measurable antibody, however, so that, by the age of 65 years, only two thirds of patients present with measurable circulating antibody to intrinsic factor)
        - (1) Juvenile pernicious anemia (usually presents between the ages of 3 and 14 years)
        - (2) Hereditarily determined degenerative gastric atrophy (gradually progresses with increasing age; almost 50% of all adult PA cases fall into this category)
        - (3) Acquired gastric atrophy as the end result of superficial inflammatory gastritis; superficial gastritis with atrophy (almost 50% of all adult PA cases fall into this category, which includes acquired gastric damage related to iron deficiency or alcohol)
        - (4) Endocrine disorders (hypothyroidism, polyendocrinopathy) associated with gastric damage
    - 2. Gastrectomy
      - a) Total
      - b) Subtotal (approximately 20% develop PA within 10 years after surgery; associated with atrophy of remaining parietal cells)
        - (1) Proximal
        - (2) Distal
        - (3) Lesions that destroy the gastric mucosa (ingested corrosives, linitis plastica)
        - (4) Intrinsic factor inhibitor in gastric section
      - c) Antibody to intrinsic factor (in saliva or gastric juice)
        - (1) "Blocking" antibody (attaches to intrinsic factor to block ability of intrinsic factor to take up vitamin B_{12})
        - (2) "Binding" antibody (attaches to intrinsic factor at a site distal to the site of vitamin B_{12} attachment)
      - d) Small intestinal disorder (affecting ileum, which is the main site of vitamin B_{12} absorption)
        - (1) Gluten-induced enteropathy (childhood and adult celiac disease); idiopathic steatorrhea; nontropical sprue
        - (2) Tropical sprue (Vitamin B_{12} is often the first nutrient to be subnormally absorbed and the last to return to normal absorption.)
        - (3) Regional enteritis
        - (4) Strictures or anastomoses of the small bowel; other "stagnant bowel" syndromes
        - (5) Intestinal resection
        - (6) Cancers and granulomatous lesions involving the small intestine
        - (7) Other conditions characterized by chronically disturbed intestinal function
        - (8) Drugs inhibiting or preventing vitamin B_{12} absorption
          - (a) Para-aminosalicylic (PAS) acid
          - (b) Colchicine
          - (c) Neomycin

TABLE 35–3 CAUSES OF VITAMIN B_{12} DEFICIENCY (continued)

(d) Ethanol
(e) Metformin (and possibly other biguanide agents)
(9) Specific malabsorption for vitamin B_{12}
(a) Long-term ingestion of calcium chelating agents
(10) Inadequately alkaline pH in ileum (Zollinger-Ellison syndrome, pancreatic disease)
(11) Unknown causes (lack of intestinal receptors for vitamin B_{12} intrinsic factor complex? Absence of "releasing factor"?)
(a) Congenital disorder (Imerslund-Graesbeck syndrome; receptors probably functional)
(b) Acquired disorder (forme fruste of sprue; receptors possibly absent or nonfunctional)
e) Competition for vitamin B_{12} by intestinal parasites or bacteria
(1) Fish tapeworm (*Diphyllobothrium latum*)
(2) Bacteria: the blind loop syndrome
f) Pancreatic disease (normal pancreatic exocrine secretion of trypsin and bicarbonate required for normal vitamin B_{12} absorption)
g) Human immunodeficiency virus (HIV) infection (acquired immunodeficiency syndrome [AIDS]) leading to gastrointestinal dysfunction and malabsorption

III. Inadequate utilization
A. Vitamin B_{12} antagonists
1. Substituted vitamin B_{12} amides and anilides (experimental agents)
2. Cobaloximes (experimental agents)
3. Anti–vitamin B_{12} analogues?
B. Congenital or acquired enzyme deficiency or deletion
1. Methylmalonyl-CoA mutase
2. Methyltetrahydrofolate-homocysteine methyltransferase
3. Vitamin B_{12a} reductase
4. Vitamin B_{12r} reductase
5. Deoxyadenoxyltransferase
6. Other enzyme reduction or deletion
C. Abnormal vitamin B_{12}–binding protein in serum that irreversibly binds vitamin B_{12}, making it unavailable to tissues
1. Increased TC I or TC III glycoprotein (myeloproliferative disorders; "granulocyte-related" vitamin B_{12} binders)
2. Increased TC II protein (liver disease; "liver-related" vitamin B_{12} binders)
3. Other abnormal vitamin B_{12} binding (a glycoprotein in some cases of hepatoma)
D. Inadequate serum vitamin B_{12}–binding protein (congenital or acquired)
1. TC II protein (the lack of which produces megaloblastic anemia; it delivers vitamin B_{12} to blood cells as transferrin delivers iron)
2. TC I glycoprotein (the lack of which is not known to produce megaloblastic anemia; it is mainly a storage protein for vitamin B_{12}, somewhat akin to ceruloplasmin for copper)
3. TC III (increasing amounts produced in vitro by granulocytes)

IV. Increased requirement (normal adult daily requirement for exogenous sources is 0.1 μg (0.073 nmol)
A. Hyperthyroidism
B. Increased hematopoiesis?
C. Infancy
D. Parasitization
1. By fetus
2. By malignant tissue?

V. Increased excretion
A. Inadequate vitamin B_{12}–binding protein in serum
B. Liver disease (inadequate storage capacity for vitamin B_{12})
C. Renal disease?

VI. Increased destruction by antioxidants
A. Pharmacologic doses of ascorbic acid

(From Herbert V, Das KC. Folic acid and vitamin B_{12}. In: Shils ME, Olson JA, Shike M (eds.). Modern Nutrition in Health and Disease, 8th ed, vol. 1. Philadelphia: Lea & Febiger, 1994, p. 414.)

blood. Other binding proteins in the blood include haptocorrin, also known as *transcobalamin* I, and transcobalamin III (TC I and TC III). These are alpha-globulins—larger, macromolecular-weight glycoproteins—that make up the R binder component of the blood. Unlike IF, the R proteins are capable of binding not only vitamin B_{12} itself, but also many of its biologically inactive analogues.

Although approximately 75% of the vitamin B_{12} in human serum is bound to haptocorrin and roughly 25% is bound to TC II, *only TC II is important in delivering vitamin B_{12} to all the cells that need it*. After transport through the bloodstream, TC II is recognized by receptors on cell surfaces. Patients with haptocorrin abnormalities have no symptoms of vitamin B_{12} deficiency. Those lacking TC II rapidly develop megaloblastic anemia (Herbert, 1998).

As a result of normal enterohepatic circulation—that is, excretion of vitamin B_{12} and analogues in bile and reabsorption of mainly vitamin B_{12} in the ileum—it generally takes decades for strict vegetarians who are not receiving vitamin B_{12} supplementation, to develop a vitamin B_{12} deficiency. Vitamin B_{12} is also excreted in urine.

STAGES OF DEFICIENCY

Figure 35–4 shows the sequential biochemical and hematologic stages of vitamin B_{12} deficiency. The sequence of events involves four stages of depletion.

*Stage 1—**negative vitamin B_{12} balance***—begins when vitamin B_{12} intake is low or absorption is poor, depleting TC II, the primary delivery protein, resulting in a low TC II level (Herzlich and Herbert, 1988). A low TC II (<40 pg/mL) may be the earliest

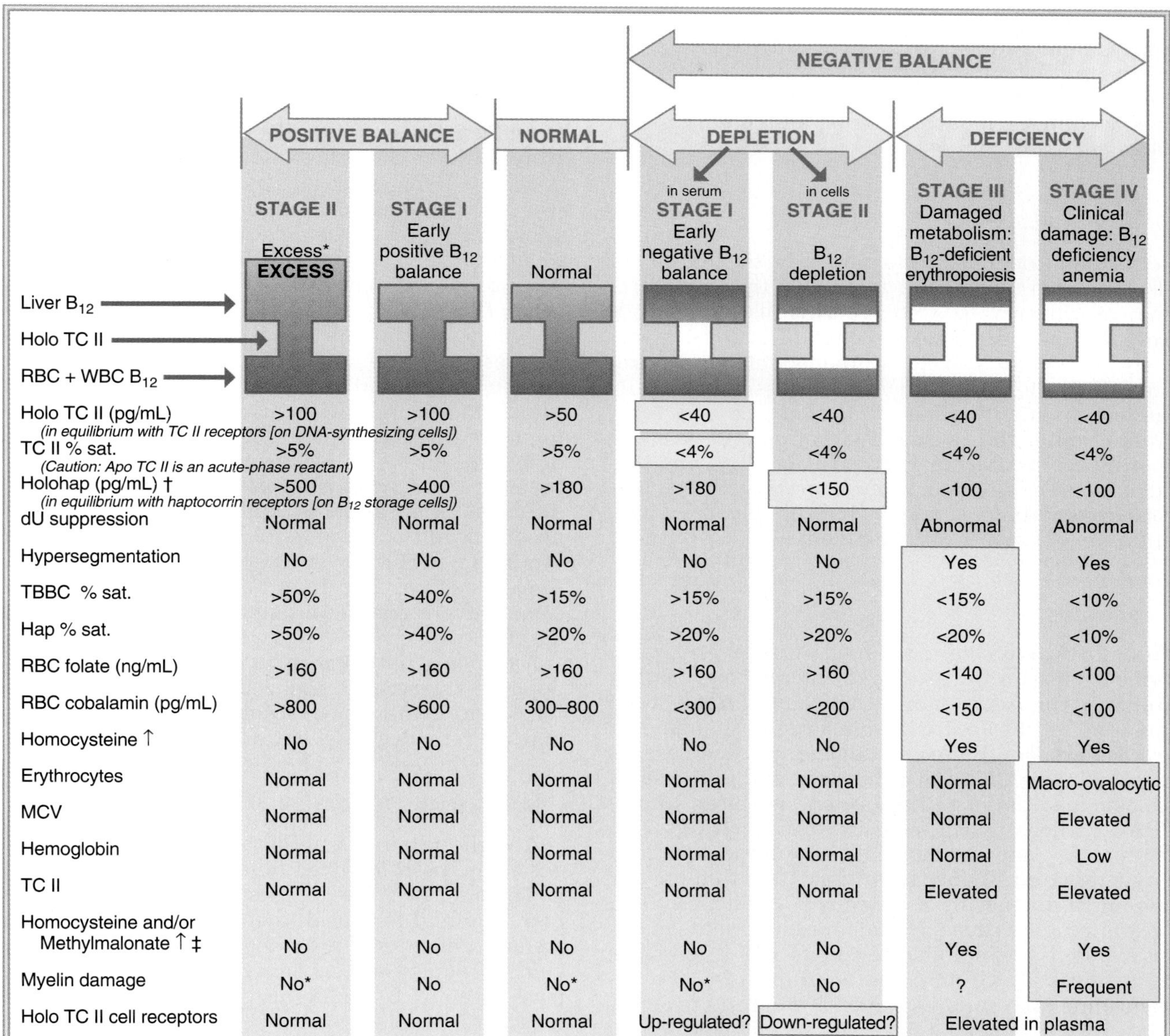

	POSITIVE BALANCE		NORMAL	NEGATIVE BALANCE: DEPLETION		NEGATIVE BALANCE: DEFICIENCY	
	STAGE II Excess* EXCESS	STAGE I Early positive B_{12} balance	Normal	in serum STAGE I Early negative B_{12} balance	in cells STAGE II B_{12} depletion	STAGE III Damaged metabolism: B_{12}-deficient erythropoiesis	STAGE IV Clinical damage: B_{12} deficiency anemia
Holo TC II (pg/mL) (in equilibrium with TC II receptors [on DNA-synthesizing cells])	>100	>100	>50	<40	<40	<40	<40
TC II % sat. (Caution: Apo TC II is an acute-phase reactant)	>5%	>5%	>5%	<4%	<4%	<4%	<4%
Holohap (pg/mL) † (in equilibrium with haptocorrin receptors [on B_{12} storage cells])	>500	>400	>180	>180	<150	<100	<100
dU suppression	Normal	Normal	Normal	Normal	Normal	Abnormal	Abnormal
Hypersegmentation	No	No	No	No	No	Yes	Yes
TBBC % sat.	>50%	>40%	>15%	>15%	>15%	<15%	<10%
Hap % sat.	>50%	>40%	>20%	>20%	>20%	<20%	<10%
RBC folate (ng/mL)	>160	>160	>160	>160	>160	<140	<100
RBC cobalamin (pg/mL)	>800	>600	300–800	<300	<200	<150	<100
Homocysteine ↑	No	No	No	No	No	Yes	Yes
Erythrocytes	Normal	Normal	Normal	Normal	Normal	Normal	Macro-ovalocytic
MCV	Normal	Normal	Normal	Normal	Normal	Normal	Elevated
Hemoglobin	Normal	Normal	Normal	Normal	Normal	Normal	Low
TC II	Normal	Normal	Normal	Normal	Normal	Elevated	Elevated
Homocysteine and/or Methylmalonate ↑ ‡	No	No	No	No	No	Yes	Yes
Myelin damage	No*	No	No*	No*	No	?	Frequent
Holo TC II cell receptors	Normal	Normal	Normal	Up-regulated?	Down-regulated?	Elevated in plasma	

Holo TC II, holotranscobalamin II; *TBBC,* total B_{12} binding capacity; *% sat.,* percent saturation; *RBC,* red blood cell; *MCV,* mean corpuscular volume.

* Cyanocobalamin excesses (injected or intranasal) produce transient increases in B_{12} delivery protein (TC II); the significance of such increases is unknown. Cyanocobalamin acts as an anti-B_{12} agent in a rare congenital defect in B_{12} metabolism.

† In serum and urine.

‡ Low holohaptocorrin correlates with **liver cell** B_{12} depletion, except in liver disease and myeloproliferative disorders, in which serum B_{12} and binding proteins are artificially elevated.

There may be hematopoietic cell and glial cell B_{12} depletion **prior to** liver cell depletion, and those cells may be in stage III or IV negative B_{12} balance, whereas liver cells are still in stage II.

FIGURE 35–4 Sequential stages of vitamin B_{12} status. (From Herbert V. Staging vitamin B_{12}. In: Ziegler EE, Filer LJ (eds.). Present Knowledge in Nutrition, 7th ed. Washington, DC: International Life Sciences Institute (ILSI) Press, 1996, p. 195. © 1990, 1995 by Victor Herbert.)

detectable sign of a vitamin B_{12} deficiency (Herbert, 1990).

In *stage 2 (vitamin B_{12} depletion)*, besides the low B_{12} on TC II, there is also a low B_{12} on haptocorrin (holohap <150 pg/mL), the storage protein.

Stage 3—damaged metabolism or *vitamin B_{12}–deficient erythropoiesis*—includes an abnormal deoxyuridine (dU) suppression, hypersegmentation, a decreased TIBC and holohap percent saturation, and a low red blood cell folate level (<140 ng/mL).

Stage 4—clinical damage or vitamin B_{12} deficiency anemia—includes all preceding stages, in addition to macro-ovalocytic erythrocytes, elevated mean corpuscular volume, elevated TC II levels, an increased methylmalonate level, and, often, myelin damage.

Clinical Findings

Pernicious anemia affects not only the blood but also the gastrointestinal tract and the peripheral and central nervous systems. This distinguishes it from folic acid deficiency anemia. The overt symptoms, which are caused by inadequate myelinization of the nerves, include paresthesia (especially numbness and tingling in the hands and feet), diminution of the senses of vibration and position, poor muscular coordination, poor memory, and hallucinations. If the deficiency is prolonged, the nervous system damage may be irreversible, even with initiation of vitamin B_{12} treatment.

Diagnosis

Vitamin B_{12} stores are depleted after several years without vitamin B_{12} intake. As microbiologic assays are very time-consuming, they have largely been replaced by the less time-consuming, though still precise, are simultaneous radioassays. Radioassays measure more than one component within the same biologic medium (e.g., the Becton-Dickinson SimulTRAC Radioassay Kit measures the levels of serum vitamin B_{12} and serum folate simultaneously in a single test tube). Other laboratory tests that may be helpful in diagnosing a vitamin B_{12} deficiency and determining its cause, include measurements of unsaturated B_{12} binding capacity (UBBC), intrinsic factor antibody (IFAB), the Schilling test, the deoxyuridine (dU) suppression test, and tests to determine serum homocysteine and serum methionine levels.

The IFAB and Schilling urinary excretion tests can determine whether the deficiency is caused by a lack of IF. The IFAB assay is performed on a patient's serum, whereas the Schilling test requires that the patient first swallow radioactive B_{12} alone, and then a second time with IF.

The vitamin B_{12} assay is performed on the patient's urine after both steps of the Schilling test are completed. Patients with pernicious anemia excrete very little vitamin B_{12} during the first step because little or no vitamin B_{12} is absorbed; during the second step, however, the urinary excretion becomes almost normal because more vitamin B_{12} is absorbed with the addition of the IF. Vitamin B_{12} deficiency secondary to malabsorption syndrome is manifested by a decrease in urinary excretion of B_{12} that remains unchanged with IF administration. A low holo TC II value is a sign of early B_{12} deficiency.

Treatment

Prior to 1926, pernicious anemia was incurable, and the diagnosis invariably meant death in a relatively short time. In 1926, Minot and Murphy reported on the effectiveness of liver therapy, and active concentrates of liver suitable for oral use were soon developed. By 1936, relatively purified extracts of liver were available for intramuscular injection. In 1948, vitamin B_{12} was determined to be the active agent in liver, and it is now available for either oral or parenteral administration. Treatment usually consists of an intramuscular or subcutaneous injection of 100 μg of vitamin B_{12} once per week. After an initial response is elicited, the frequency of administration is reduced until remission can be maintained indefinitely with monthly injections of 100 μg. Very large oral doses of vitamin B_{12} (1000 μg daily) are also effective, even in the absence of IF, because about 1% of vitamin B_{12} will be absorbed by diffusion. A nasal gel is available that is also well absorbed. Initial doses should be increased when vitamin B_{12} deficiency is complicated by debilitating illness, such as infection, hepatic disease, uremia, coma, severe disorientation, or marked neurologic damage.

A response to treatment is evidenced by improved appetite, alertness, and cooperation, followed by improved hematologic results, as manifested by marked reticulocytosis within hours of an injection.

NUTRITIONAL INTERVENTION

A high-protein diet (1.5 g/kg of body weight) is desirable, both for liver function and for blood regeneration. Because green leafy vegetables contain both iron and folic acid, the diet should contain increased amounts of these foods. Liver should be included frequently because it carries a good supply of iron, vitamin B_{12}, folic acid, and other important nutrients. Meats (especially beef and pork), eggs, milk, and milk products are particularly rich in vitamin B_{12}, although the cholesterol content must also be considered (Table 35–4).

Folic Acid Deficiency Anemia

Pathophysiology

Folic acid deficiency anemia is associated with tropical sprue, can affect pregnant women, and occurs in infants born to mothers with folic acid defi-

TABLE 35–4 VITAMIN B_{12} CONTENT OF SOME COMMON FOODS*

FOOD	PORTION SIZE	VITAMIN B_{12} (µg)
Protein Group		
Chicken/turkey	3 oz	0.3
Hamburger	3 oz	8.0
Pork chop	3 oz	0.9
Tenderloin steak	3 oz	0.5
Liver, chicken	3 oz	16.5
Liver, pork	3 oz	15.8
Kidney, pork	3 oz	6.6
Swordfish	3 oz	1.7
Sardines (tomato sauce)	3 oz	7.7
Salmon	3 oz	5.8
Egg	1 whole	0.5
Dairy Group		
Milk (all varieties)	1 cup	0.9
Yogurt	1 cup	1.4
Cottage cheese	½ cup	0.6
Cheese	1 oz	
Mozzarella/American		0.2
Ricotta/provolone		0.4
Swiss		0.5

*Essentially, vitamin B_{12} is in everything that walks, swims, and flies, and is not in anything that grows in the ground.

ciency. Prolonged inadequate diets; faulty absorption and utilization of folic acid, and increased requirements due to growth are believed to be the most frequent causes (Table 35–5). Because alcohol interferes with the folate enterohepatic cycle, most alcoholics have a negative folate balance, and the majority are folate-deficient. Alcoholics comprise the only group that generally has all six causes of folic acid deficiency simultaneously—inadequate ingestion, absorption, and utilization and increased excretion, requirement, and destruction of folic acid.

Folate absorption takes place in the small intestine. Enzyme conjugases (pteroylpolyglutamate hydrolase, commonly called folate conjugase), found in the brush border of the small intestine, reduce polyglutamates to dihydrofolate and tetrahydrofolate (THFA) in the small intestine epithelial cells (enterocytes). From the enterocytes, these forms are transported to the circulation, where they are bound to protein and transported as methyltetrahydrofolate into the cells of the body.

In the absence of vitamin B_{12}, *5-methyltetrahydrofolate* (5-methyl THFA), the major circulating and storage form of folic acid, is metabolically inactive. To be activated, the 5-methyl group is removed and THFA is cycled back into the folate pool, where it functions as the main 1-carbon-unit acceptor in mammalian biochemical reactions. THFA may then be converted to the coenzyme form of folate required to convert deoxyuridylate to thymidylate, which is necessary for DNA synthesis.

METHYLFOLATE TRAP

Vitamin B_{12} deficiency can result in a folic acid deficiency by causing folate entrapment in the metabolically useless form of 5-methyl THFA (Fig. 35–5). The lack of vitamin B_{12} to remove the 5-methyl unit means that metabolically dead methyl THFA is trapped. It cannot release its 1-carbon methyl group to become THFA, the basic 1-carbon carrier that picks up 1-carbon units from one molecule and delivers them to another. Hence, a functional folic acid deficiency results.

Stages of Deficiency

Folate deficiency develops in four stages: two that involve depletion, followed by two marked by deficiency (Fig. 35–6) (Herbert et al., 1999).

- *Stage 1: Early negative nutrient balance (negative serum balance; serum depletion)*—This stage is characterized by a reduction in serum folate levels to less than 3 ng/mL.
- *Stage 2: Negative cell balance (cell depletion)*—Folate depletion is indicated by a decrease in erythrocyte folate levels to less than 160 ng/mL.

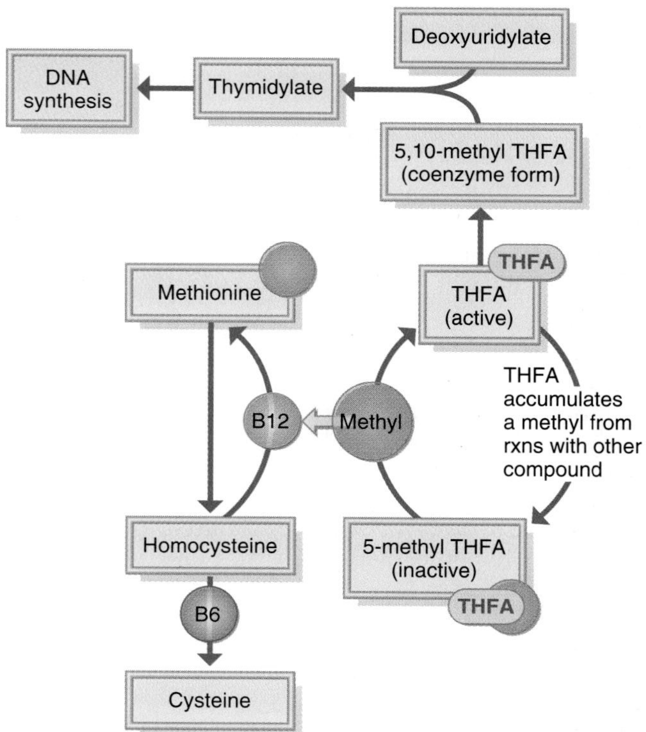

FIGURE 35–5 Methylfolate trap. A deficiency of vitamin B_{12} can result in a deficiency of folic acid because folate is trapped in the form of 5-methyltetrahydrofolate (5-methyl THFA), which cannot be converted to tetrahydrofolate (THFA) by the vitamin B_{12}-dependent pathway.

TABLE 35–5 CAUSES OF FOLATE DEFICIENCY

I. Inadequate ingestion
    A. Poor diet (lack of unprocessed, fresh, uncooked, or slightly cooked food or fruit juices [folates are heat labile])
        1. Nutritional megaloblastic anemia
            a) Tropical
            b) Nontropical
            c) Scurvy (diets low in vitamin C are also low in folate)
        2. Chronic alcoholism, with or without cirrhosis

II. Inadequate absorption (affecting the upper third of the small intestine, which is the main site of folate absorption. Because most food folates are in polyglutamate forms, biliary and intestinal g-glutamyl conjugases are necessary to split off excess glutamates to make folates absorbable.)
    A. Malabsorption syndromes
        1. Gluten-induced enteropathy (childhood and adult celiac disease; idiopathic steatorrhea; nontropical sprue; coincident vitamin B_{12} malabsorption only in rare cases)
        2. Any other chronic functional or structural disorder involving the upper small intestine
            a) Tropical sprue (coincident vitamin B_{12} malabsorption almost invariably present)
            b) Associated with herpetic and other skin disorders
        3. Drugs
            a) Anticonvulsants (e.g., phenytoin, primidone)
            b) Barbiturates
            c) Cycloserine
            d) Ethanol
            e) Metformin
            f) Amino acid excess (glycine or methionine)
            g) Nitrofurantoin? (antimicrobial)
            h) Glutethimide? (sedative)
            i) Cholestyramine
            j) Sulfasalazine (Azulfidine)
    B. Specific malabsorption for folate
        1. Congenital nonconjugase defects (four cases published)
        2. Acquired nonconjugase defects
        3. Inadequate biliary or intestinal conjugases
        4. Conjugase inhibitors (such as those contained in some beans)
    C. Blind loop syndrome (more commonly, bacteria make folate and actually raise the serum folate level of host.)

III. Inadequate utilization (metabolic block)
    A. Folic acid antagonists (dihydrofolate reductase inhibitors)
        1. 4-amino-4-deoxyfolates, i.e., methotrexate (chemotherapy, immunosuppression, psoriasis)
        2. 2-4-diaminopyrimidine, e.g., pyrimethiamine, trimethoprim (malaria, toxoplasmosis, antibacterial)
        3. Triamterene (diuretic)
        4. Diamidine compounds, i.e., pentamidine, isothionate (*Pneumocystis carinii*, protozocidal)
    B. Diphenylhydantoin and possibly other anticonvulsants (which may block cell uptake or use folate)
    C. Enzyme deficiency
        1. Congenital
            a) Formiminotransferase
            b) Dihydrofolate reductase
            c) Methyltetrahydrofolate transmethylase
            d) Other enzymes (some of which affect folate secondarily)
        2. Acquired
            a) Liver disease
                (1) Formiminotransferase
                (2) Other enzymes
    D. Vitamin B_{12} deficiency (reduced folate uptake and retention)
    E. Alcohol (both specific and nonspecific damage)
    F. Ascorbic acid deficiency
    G. Dietary amino acid excess (glycine, methionine)

IV. Increased requirement
    A. Extra tissue demand
        1. By fetus
        2. By malignant tissue (especially in lymphoproliferative disorders)
        3. By breast-fed infant
    B. Infancy
    C. Increased hematopoiesis
    D. Increased metabolic activity
    E. Lesch-Nyhan syndrome
    F. Drugs (l-dopa?)

V. Increased excretion
    A. Vitamin B_{12} deficiency (possible obligatory excretion of folate in urine and bile)
    B. Liver disease?
    C. Kidney dialysis
    D. Chronic exfoliative dermatitis

VI. Increased destruction
    A. Oxidant in diet?

(From Herbert V, Das KC. Folic acid and vitamin B_{12}. In: Shills ME, Olson JA, Shike M (eds.). Modern Nutrition in Health and Disease, 8th ed, vol. 1. Philadelphia: Lea & Febiger, 1994, p. 420.)

- *Stage 3: Biochemical deficiency, with folate-deficient erythropoiesis*—This stage is characterized by slowed DNA synthesis, manifested by an abnormal diagnostic deoxyuridine (dU) suppression test correctable in vitro by folates, granulocyte nuclear hypersegmentation, and macro-ovalocytic red cells.
- *Stage 4: Clinical folate deficiency*—This stage is manifested by an elevated mean corpuscular volume (MCV) and anemia.

Clinical Findings

Because of their interrelated roles in protein synthesis, a deficiency of either vitamin B_{12} or folic acid will result in the same clinical sign—that is, a megaloblastic anemia. Erythrocyte protein cannot be synthesized properly in the deficient state, and large (macrocytic), immature (megaloblastic) blood cells are the result.

The common clinical signs of folic acid deficiency include fatigue, dyspnea, sore tongue, diarrhea, irritability, forgetfulness, anorexia, glossitis, and weight loss.

Diagnosis

Normal body folate stores are depleted within 2 to 4 months on a folate-deficient diet, resulting in a macrocytic megaloblastic anemia. This state is also characterized by a decreased number of erythrocytes, leukocytes, and platelets. Folate deficiency

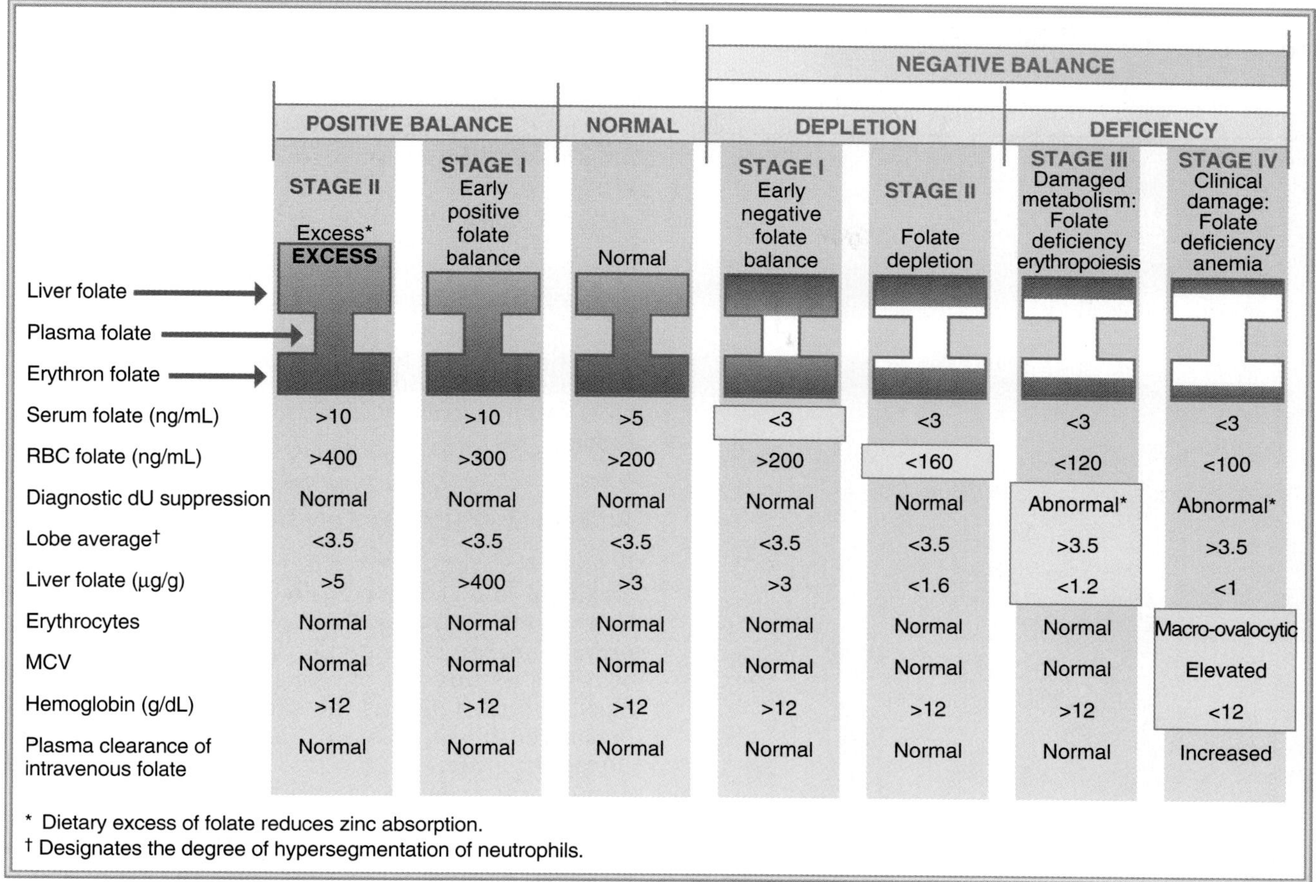

	POSITIVE BALANCE		NORMAL	NEGATIVE BALANCE: DEPLETION		NEGATIVE BALANCE: DEFICIENCY	
	STAGE II Excess* EXCESS	STAGE I Early positive folate balance	Normal	STAGE I Early negative folate balance	STAGE II Folate depletion	STAGE III Damaged metabolism: Folate deficiency erythropoiesis	STAGE IV Clinical damage: Folate deficiency anemia
Serum folate (ng/mL)	>10	>10	>5	<3	<3	<3	<3
RBC folate (ng/mL)	>400	>300	>200	>200	<160	<120	<100
Diagnostic dU suppression	Normal	Normal	Normal	Normal	Normal	Abnormal*	Abnormal*
Lobe average†	<3.5	<3.5	<3.5	<3.5	<3.5	>3.5	>3.5
Liver folate (µg/g)	>5	>400	>3	>3	<1.6	<1.2	<1
Erythrocytes	Normal	Normal	Normal	Normal	Normal	Normal	Macro-ovalocytic
MCV	Normal	Normal	Normal	Normal	Normal	Normal	Elevated
Hemoglobin (g/dL)	>12	>12	>12	>12	>12	>12	<12
Plasma clearance of intravenous folate	Normal	Normal	Normal	Normal	Normal	Normal	Increased

* Dietary excess of folate reduces zinc absorption.
† Designates the degree of hypersegmentation of neutrophils.

FIGURE 35–6 Sequential stages of folate status. *RBC,* red blood cell; *dU,* deoxyuridine; *MCV,* mean corpuscular volume. (From Herbert V. Folic acid. In: Shils ME, Olson JA, Shike M (eds.). Modern Nutrition in Health and Disease, 9th ed. Philadelphia: Lea & Febiger, 1998. © 1990, 1995 Victor Herbert.)

anemia is manifested by very low serum folate levels (less than 3 ng/mL) and red cell folate (RCF) levels (less than 140 ng/mL). Whereas a low serum folate level merely diagnoses a negative balance at the time the blood is drawn, an RCF level measures actual body folate stores and so is the superior measurement for determining folate nutriture. To differentiate folate deficiency from vitamin B_{12} deficiency, levels of serum folate, RCF, serum vitamin B_{12}, and vitamin B_{12} bound to TC II can be measured simultaneously using a radioassay kit. Also diagnostic for folate deficiency is an elevated level of *formiminoglutamic acid* (FIGLU) in the urine, as well as the dU suppression test in bone marrow cells or peripheral blood lymphocytes.

Treatment

Before treatment is initiated, it is important to diagnose the cause of the megaloblastosis correctly. Administration of folate will correct megaloblastosis due to either folate or vitamin B_{12} deficiency, but it can mask the neurologic damage of vitamin B_{12} deficiency, allowing the nerve damage to progress to the point of irreversibility.

A dosage of 1 mg of folate, taken orally every day for 2 to 3 weeks, will replenish folate stores. Maintaining repleted stores requires an absolute minimum oral intake of 50 to 100 µg of folic acid daily. When folate deficiency is complicated by alcoholism or other conditions that suppress hematopoiesis, increase folate requirements, or reduce folate absorption, therapy should begin at a dosage of 500 to 1000 mg/day.

Symptomatic improvement, as evidenced by increased alertness, cooperation, and appetite, may be apparent within 24 to 48 hours, long before hematologic values revert to normal, a gradual process that takes about a month. After the anemia is corrected, the patient should be instructed to eat at least one fresh, uncooked fruit or vegetable or to drink a glass of fruit juice daily. One cup of orange juice supplies about 135 µg of folic acid (see Table 35–6 for a list of common foods containing folate).

TABLE 35–6 FOLIC ACID CONTENT OF SOME COMMON FOODS

FOOD	PORTION SIZE	FOLATE (μg)
Protein Group		
Chicken, light meat	3 oz	3.0
Chicken, dark meat	3 oz	7.2
Turkey, dark meat	3 oz	7.9
Pork chop	3 oz	5.2
Tenderloin steak	3 oz	5.0
Liver, chicken	3 oz	654.0
Liver, pork	3 oz	139.0
Tuna fish	3 oz	3.5
Sardines (tomato sauce)	3 oz	21.0
Salmon	3 oz	13.0
Tofu, raw	½ cup	37.0
Egg	1	23.0
Black beans	½ cup	128.0
Kidney beans	½ cup	18.0
Lentil beans	½ cup	36.0
Soybean nuts	½ cup	122.0
Cashew nuts	1 oz	19.6
Dairy Group		
Milk (all varieties)	1 cup	13.0
Yogurt	1 cup	28.0
Cottage cheese	½ cup	10.5
Fruit Group		
Apricots	3 raw	9.1
Orange	1	40.0
Orange juice	1 cup	136.0
Strawberries, frozen	1 cup	9.7
Banana	1	22.0
Vegetable Group		
Baked potato	1 medium	22.0
Sweet potato	1 medium	26.0
Broccoli	1 cup	62.0
Brussel sprouts	½ cup	47.0
Endive	½ cup	36.0
Spinach	½ cup	108.0
Grain Group		
Barley	½ cup	13.0
Whole wheat bread	1 slice	14.0
Wheat germ	¼ cup	99.0
Grapenuts cereal	¼ cup	101.0

Fresh, uncooked fruits and vegetables are good sources of folate because folate can easily be destroyed by heat.

OTHER NUTRITIONAL ANEMIAS

Copper Deficiency Anemia

Copper and other heavy metals are essential for the proper formation of hemoglobin. *Ceruloplasmin*, a copper-containing protein, is required for normal mobilization of iron from its storage sites to the plasma. In a copper-deficient state, iron cannot be released, leading to low serum iron and hemoglobin levels, even in the presence of normal iron stores. Other consequences of copper deficiency suggest that copper proteins are needed for utilization of iron by the developing erythrocyte and for optimal functions of the erythrocyte membrane (see Chapter 5).

The amounts of copper needed for normal hemoglobin synthesis are so minute that they are usually amply supplied by an adequate diet. However, copper deficiency may occur in infants who are fed cow's milk or a copper-deficient infant formula. It may also be seen in children or adults who have a malabsorption syndrome or who are receiving long-term total parenteral nutrition that does not supply copper.

Anemia of Protein-Energy Malnutrition

Protein is essential for the proper production of hemoglobin and red blood cells. Because of the reduction in cell mass and, thus, oxygen requirements in protein-energy malnutrition (PEM), fewer red blood cells are required to oxygenate the tissue. Because blood volume remains the same, this reduced number of red blood cells with a low hemoglobin level (**hypochromic,** normocytic anemia) which can mimic an iron deficiency anemia, is actually a physiologic (nonharmful) rather than pharmacologic (harmful) anemia. In acute PEM, the loss of active tissue mass may be greater than the reduction in the number of red blood cells, leading to polycythemia. The body responds to this red blood cell production, which is not a reflection of protein and amino acid deficiency, but of an oversupply of red blood cells. Iron released from normal red blood cell destruction is not reused in red blood cell production but is stored, so that iron stores are often adequate. Iron deficiency anemia can reappear with rehabilitation when red blood cell mass expands rapidly.

The anemia of PEM may be complicated by deficiencies of iron and other nutrients, and by associated infections, parasitic infestation, and malabsorption. A diet lacking in protein is usually deficient in iron, folic acid, and, less frequently, vitamin B_{12}. The nutrition counselor plays an important role in assessing recent and typical dietary intake of these nutrients.

Sideroblastic (Pyridoxine-Responsive) Anemia

Sideroblastic anemia has four primary characteristics: (1) microcytic and hypochromic red blood cells; (2) high serum and tissue iron levels (causing increased transferrin saturation); (3) the presence of an inherited defect in the formation of D-aminolevulinic acid synthetase, an enzyme involved in heme synthesis (pyridoxal-5-phosphate is necessary in this reaction), and (4) a build-up of iron-containing immature red blood cells (sideroblasts, for which the anemia is named). The iron that cannot be used for heme synthesis is stored in the mitochondria of immature red blood cells. These iron-laden mitochrondia do not function normally, and the development and production of red blood cells become ineffective. The symptoms are those of both anemia and iron overload. The neurologic and cutaneous manifestations of vitamin B_6 deficiency are not observed. The anemia responds to the administration of pharmacologic doses of pyridoxine, and thus is referred to as vitamin B_6 (pyridoxine)–responsive anemia, to distinguish it from anemia *caused* by a dietary vitamin B_6 deficiency.

Treatment consists of a therapeutic trial dose of 50 to 200 mg/day of pyridoxine or pyridoxal phosphate, which is 25 to 100 times the recommended dietary allowance (RDA). If the anemia responds to one or the other, pyridoxine therapy is continued for life. However, the anemia is only partially corrected; a normal hematocrit value is never regained. Patients respond to this treatment to varying degrees, and some may achieve near-normal hemoglobin levels.

Unlike the familial sideroblastic anemia just mentioned, acquired sideroblastic anemias, such as those attributable to drug therapy (isoniazid, chloramphenicol), copper deficiency, hypothermia, and alcoholism, are not vitamin B_6 (pyridoxine)–responsive.

Vitamin E–Responsive Anemia

Hemolytic anemia occurs when defects in red blood cell membranes lead to oxidative damage and, eventually, to cell lysis. Vitamin E, an antioxidant, is involved in protecting the membrane against oxidative damage, and one of the few signs noted in vitamin E deficiency is early hemolysis of red blood cells. Vitamin E–responsive hemolytic anemia in neonates is discussed in Chapters 8 and 9.

NONNUTRITIONAL ANEMIAS

Sickle Cell Anemia

Sickle cell anemia, a chronic hemolytic anemia also known as hemoglobin S disease, affects 1 out of 600 blacks in the U.S. as a result of homozygous inheritance of hemoglobin S. This results in defective hemoglobin synthesis, which produces sickle-shaped red blood cells with oxygen deprivation. The disease is usually diagnosed toward the end of the first year of life.

Clinical Findings

In addition to the usual symptoms of anemia, sickle cell anemia is characterized by episodes of pain resulting from the occlusion of small blood vessels by the abnormally shaped erythrocytes. The occlusions frequently occur in the abdomen, causing acute, severe, abdominal pain. The hemolytic anemia and vasoocclusive disease result in impaired liver function, jaundice, gallstones, and deteriorating renal function. The constant hemolysis of erythrocytes increases iron stores in the liver. Iron deficiency anemia and sickle cell anemia can coexist. Iron overload is less common, and is usually a problem only in those who have received multiple blood transfusions.

Treatment

No specific treatment exists for sickle cell anemia other than relieving pain during a crisis and, possibly, administering an exchange transfusion. It is important that sickle cell anemia not be mistaken for iron deficiency anemia that can be treated with iron supplements, as iron stores in the patient with sickle cell anemia secondary to transfusions are frequently excessive.

To be low in absorbable iron, the diet should emphasize vegetable proteins. Iron-rich foods, such as liver, iron-fortified formula, and iron-fortified cereals, are excluded. Substances, such as alcohol and ascorbic acid supplements, both of which enhance iron absorption and free-radical release from iron, should be avoided. It is important to remember, however, that iron deficiency may be present in some patients with sickle cell anemia owing to repeated phlebotomies, excessive transfusions, hematuria secondary to renal papillary necrosis, or other factors (see the accompanying box, "*Clinical Insight:* Nutritional Care for Sickle Cell Anemia").

Zinc can increase the oxygen affinity of both normal and sickle-shaped erythrocytes. Thus, zinc supplements may be beneficial in managing sickle cell disease, especially since decreased plasma zinc is common in children with the SS genotype sickle cell disease, and is associated with decreased linear growth and skeletal growth, muscle mass, and sexual maturation (Leonard et al., 1998). Curiously this growth and development retardation is more aparent in males than females (Modebe and Ifenu, 1993). Because zinc competes with copper for binding sites on proteins, the use of high doses of zinc may precipitate copper deficiency.

The diet should be high in folate (400 to 600 μg daily) because the increased production of erythrocytes needed to replace the cells being continuously destroyed also increases folic acid requirements (see Table 35–6 for a list of common foods containing folate).

Thalassemia Minor

Thalassemia minor is a hemolytic anemia characterized by microcytic, hypochromic, and short-lived red blood cells due to defective hemoglobin synthesis, which affects mostly persons of Mediterranean

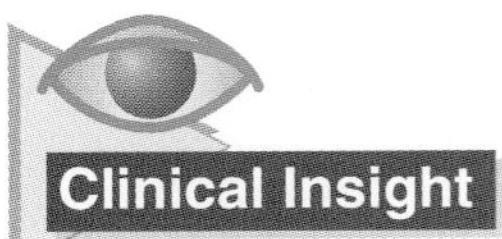

Nutritional Care for Sickle Cell Anemia

Individuals with sickle cell anemia should receive instruction as to how they can develop a well-balanced food plan providing enough calories and protein for growth and development. Their intake can be low due to the abdominal pain characteristic of the disease. There may also be an increased metabolic rate leading to a need for a higher caloric intake (Singhal et al., 1993).

Their diets must promote foods high in the vitamin folate (see Table 35–6), and the trace minerals zinc and copper. (See Chapter 5 for sources of these minerals.) In addition, they may have intakes low in vitamins A, C, and E, and this needs to be addressed in food choices (Williams et al., 1997).

When assessing the nutritional status of individuals with sickle cell anemia, the following questions must be given special attention in addition to the usual questions:

1. Do you take any vitamin and/or mineral supplements?
2. Do you consume any alcohol?
3. What are the sources of protein in your diet?

The following 1-day vegetarian menu plan, which is presented along with its nutritional analysis, is an example of how one can meet the dietary requirements of an individual with sickle cell anemia, although a vegetarian diet is not necessary. Obtaining adequate calories, protein, and zinc for growth and development is more important than eliminating animal proteins because of their heme source of well-absorbed iron. The same animal proteins are also good sources of copper and zinc (Henderson et al., 1994).

A multivitamin/mineral supplement containing 50% to 150% of the recommended dietary allowance (RDA) for folate, zinc, and copper (not iron) is also recommended; 2 to 3 quarts of water daily is also important. Lastly, it is important to remember that individuals with sickle cell disease may require higher than RDA amounts of protein.

MEAL PLAN

BREAKFAST	LUNCH	DINNER	SNACKS
1 cup shredded wheat	1 cup cottage cheese	2 cups pasta	1 cup frozen yogurt
1 banana	1 cup melon	½ cup marinara sauce	¼ cup nuts (unsalted)
1 cup low-fat milk	1 roll	1 cup beans	
	1 T peanut butter	1 cup broccoli	

NUTRITIONAL ANALYSIS*

NUTRITIONAL COMPONENT	AMOUNT	RDA, AI†, OR ESADDI‡ FOR ADULTS OLDER THAN 25 YEARS OF AGE
Calories	2204	
Protein	108.3 (19%)	
Carbohydrate	328 (58%)	
Fat	57 (23%)	
Cholesterol	48 mg	300 mg
Dietary fiber	35 g	15–35 g
Calcium	1100 mg	1000–1300 mg
Iron	17 mg	10 mg (males); 15 mg (females)
Folate	507 μg	400 μg
Zinc	12.4 mg	15 mg (males); 12 mg (females)
Copper	2.4 mg	1.5–3.0 mg*
Vitamin C	212 mg	60 mg

*Not including a vitamin/mineral supplement.
†*AI*, Adequate intake.
‡*ESADDI*, Estimated safe and adequate daily dietary intake.

origin. In thalassemia minor, one should expect to find a very low MCV, a normal to high red blood cell count and red cell distribution width (RDW), and normal levels of serum iron, serum ferritin, and TIBC. When thalassemia minor is combined with iron deficiency anemia, the MCV remains very low, but the RDW increases, the red cell count becomes normal or low, the level of serum iron and serum ferritin becomes low, and TIBC becomes high.

Sports Anemia (Hypochromic Microcytic Transient Anemia)

Increased red blood cell destruction, along with decreased hemoglobin, serum iron, and ferritin concentrations, may occur at the initiation and early stages of a vigorous training program. Once called "march hemoglobinuria," this anemia was believed to arise in soldiers as a result of mechanical trauma incurred by erythrocytes (red blood cells) during long marches. The red blood cells in the capillaries are compressed every time the foot lands, until they burst, releasing hemoglobin. A similar situation can exist in runners, especially long distance runners (see Chapter 25).

Athletes having hemoglobin concentrations below that needed for optimal oxygen delivery may benefit from consuming nutrient- and iron-rich foods, ensuring that their diets contain adequate protein, and avoiding certain foods (tea, coffee) and drugs (antacids, H_2-blockers, and tetracycline) that inhibit iron absorption. No athlete should take iron supplements unless iron deficiency is diagnosed. The diagnosis can be established after the following laboratory tests are run: complete blood cell count with differential; serum ferritin level, serum iron level, TIBC, and percent saturation of iron-binding capacity. Athletes who are female, vegetarian, involved in endurance sports, or entering a growth spurt are also at risk for iron deficiency anemia, and should, therefore, undergo periodic monitoring.

The dietitian, nurse, or health instructor is often the first person who assesses for sports anemias (see Chapter 25).

CASE STUDY

Mary Jo B. is a 20-year-old black woman who was recently diagnosed as having sickle cell disease. She is a runner and complains about frequent periods of dizziness and weakness. Her hemoglobin level is normal, but recent laboratory studies indicate a low serum folate and vitamin B_{12} level. Her mother has suggested that she take an over-the-counter multiple vitamin/mineral supplement. Mary Jo has called you for guidance. What steps would you recommend that she take?

1. What are the risks of taking a multiple vitamin/mineral supplement when one has sickle cell anemia?
2. What other laboratory data should you obtain before discussing her case with her doctor?
3. What foods could be included in her diet that would be beneficial yet that would not contain too much of any single vitamin or mineral?
4. Are there any problems with her usual daily intake of 1 or 2 citrus fruits and a quart of juice?
5. What other suggestions would you offer Mary Jo?

CITED REFERENCES

Cohen L. Iron overload gene. Proc Natl Acad Sci 95:1472, 1998.

Fairbanks VF. Iron in medicine and nutrition. In: Shils ME, Olson JA, Shike M (eds.). Modern Nutrition in Health and Disease, 8th ed., vol. 1. Philadelphia: Lea & Febiger, 1994, p. 185.

Flynn MA, et al. Atherogenesis and the homocysteine-folate-cobalamin triad: Do we need standardized analyses? J Am Coll Nutr 16:258, 1997.

Green R. Disorders of inadequate iron in diagnosis and treatment of iron disorders. Hosp Pract Symposium Suppl 26(suppl. 3): 25, 1991.

Henderson RA, et al. Prevalence of impaired growth in children with homozygous sickle cell anemia. Am J Med Sci 307:405, 1994.

Herbert V. Everyone should be tested for iron disorders. J Am Diet Assoc 92:1502, 1992.

Herbert V. Staging vitamin B_{12} status in vegetarians. Am J Clin Nutr 59(suppl): 1213s, 1993.

Herbert V. Vitamin B_{12}. In: Ziegler EE, Filer LJ (eds.). Present Knowledge in Nutrition, 7th ed. Washington, DC: International Life Sciences Institute Press, 1996, p. 191.

Herbert V. Folic acid. In: Shils M, et al. (eds.). Modern Nutrition in Health and Disease, 9th ed., vol. 1. Philadelphia: Lea & Febiger, 1999, p. 433.

Herbert V, et al. Low holotranscobalamin is the earliest serum marker for subnormal vitamin B_{12} (cobalamin) absorption in patient with AIDS. Am J Hematol 34:132, 1990.

Herzlich B, Herbert V. Depletion of serum holotrans cobalamin II: An early sign of negative B_{12} balance. Lab Invest 58:3,332, 1988.

Kanazawa S, et al. Enhancement by human bile of the binding of free and intrinsic factor-bound cobalamin (vitamin B_{12}) to small bowel epithelial cell receptors. Am J Gastroenterol 80:964, 1985.

Leonard MB, et al. Plasma zinc status, growth, and maturation in children with sickle cell disease. J Pediatr 132:467, 1998.

Markle HV. Unmetabolized folic acid and masking of cobalamin deficiency. Am J Clin Nutr 66:1480, 1997.

Modebe O, Ifenu SA. Growth retardation in homozygous sickle cell disease: role of calorie intake and possible gender-related differences. Am J Hematol 44:149, 1993.

Mulvihill B, et al. Effect of myofibrillar proteins in vitro on bioavailability of non-haem iron. Int J Food Sci Nutr 49:187, 1998.

Pollitt E, et al. Iron deficiency and behavioral development in infants and preschool children. Am J Clin Nutr 43:555, 1986.

Singhal A et al. Resting metabolic rate in homozygous sickle cell disease. Am J. Clin Nutr 57:32, 1993.

Williams R, et al. Nutrition assessment in children with sickle cell disease. J Assoc Minn Phys 8:44, 1997.

ADDITIONAL REFERENCES

Cuthbert JA. Iron, HFE, and hemochromatosis: Update. J Invest Med 45:518, 1997.

Dallman PR. Iron deficiency and the immune response. Am J Clin Nutr 46:329, 1987.

Das KC, Herbert V. In vitro DNA synthesis by megaloblastic bone marrow: Effect of folates and cobalamins on thymidine incorporation and de novo thymidine synthesis. J Hematol 31:11, 1989.

Hallberg L, et al. Iron absorption in man: Ascorbic acid and dose-dependent inhibition by phytate. Am J Clin Nutr 49:140, 1989.

Herbert V. Vitamin B_{12} and folic acid supplementation. Am J Clin Nutr 66:1479, 1997.

Herbert V, Bigaoutte J. Call for endorsement of a petition to the Food and Drug Administration to always add vitamin B_{12} to any folate fortification or supplement. Am J Clin Nutr 65:572, 1997.

Herbert V, et al. Total Nutrition: The Only Nutrition Guide You'll Ever Need. (By the staff of Mount Sinai School of Medicine). New York: St Martin's Press, 1995.

Herbert V, et al. Vitamin C–driven free radical generation from iron. J Nutr 126(suppl 4):121, 1996.

Hine RJ. Folic acid: Contemporary clinical perspective. In: Chernoff R (ed.). Perspectives in Applied Nutrition, vol. 1. St. Louis: CV Mosby, 1993, p. 3.

Monsen ER. Iron nutrition and absorption: Dietary factors [that] impact iron bioavailability. J Am Diet Assoc 88:786, 1988.
Monsen ER, Balintfy JL. Calculating dietary iron bioavailability: Refinement and computerization. J Am Diet Assoc 80:307, 1982.
Oski F. Iron deficiency in infancy and childhood. N Engl J Med 329:190, 1993.
Pan W, Habicht J. The non-iron deficiency-related differences in hemoglobin concentration between men and women. Am J Epidemiol 134:1410, 1991.
Pellegrini B, et al. Zinc, copper and iron and their interrelations in the growth of sickle cell patients. Arch Latinoam Nutr 45:198, 1995.
Reed JD, et al. Nutrition and sickle cell disease. Am J Hematol 24:441, 1987.
Wintrobe MM, et al. Clinical Hematology, 8th ed. Philadelphia: Lea & Febiger, 1981.
Yip R, Dallman P. The roles of inflammation and iron deficiency as causes of anemia. Am J Clin Nutr 48:1295, 1988.

CHAPTER 36

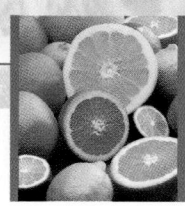

Medical Nutrition Therapy for Heart Failure and Transplant

DEBRA KRUMMEL, PhD, RD

Chapter Outline

- Congestive Heart Failure
- Cardiac Transplantation

Key Terms

CACHECTIC HEART—a soft, flabby heart characterized by loss of myocardial mass as the result of extreme malnutrition

CARDIAC CACHEXIA—a profound state of malnutrition characterized by a predominant loss of lean muscle mass

CONGESTIVE HEART FAILURE (CHF)—a clinical syndrome characterized by progressive deterioration of left ventricular function, inadequate tissue perfusion, fatigue, shortness of breath, and congestion

LEFT VENTRICULAR HYPERTROPHY—enlargement of the left ventricle of the heart, a major risk factor for congestive heart failure

LOW SALT SYNDROME—a syndrome characterized by hyponatremia, hypochloremia, and eventually, azotemia, that occurs when glomerular filtration rate decreases as the result of salt depletion

MILD SODIUM RESTRICTION—restriction of dietary sodium to 2 g (87 mEq) per day

MODERATE SODIUM RESTRICTION—restriction of dietary sodium to 1 g (43 mEq) per day

NO ADDED SALT DIET—a diet containing 4 g (174 mEq) of sodium per day

ORTHOPNEA—respiratory distress while in a recumbent position

SEVERE SODIUM RESTRICTION—restriction of dietary sodium to 250 mg (11 mEq) per day

STRICT SODIUM RESTRICTION—restriction of dietary sodium to 500 mg (22 mEq) per day

Some categories of heart disease, such as congestive heart failure and cardiac cachexia, are characterized by gradual failure of the heart to act as a pump. Nutritional care in these conditions is concerned primarily with the consequences of poor circulation throughout the body. In end-stage heart disease, cardiac transplantation becomes necessary.

CONGESTIVE HEART FAILURE

Pathophysiology

Normally, the heart pumps adequate blood to perfuse tissues and meet metabolic needs (Fig 36–1). **Congestive heart failure (CHF)** is a complex of symptoms (fatigue, shortness of breath, and congestion) that occurs when an impaired left ventricle cannot provide adequate blood flow to the rest of the body (Cohn, 1996). Most people with CHF have left ventricular systolic dysfunction. Table 36–1). Many cardiovascular diseases end up in this common pathway to CHF. Specifically, diseases of the heart (valves, muscle, vessels, arteries) and vasculature (hypertension) can lead to CHF (Fig 36–2).

Over the last 15 years, at least 60% to 65% of CHF cases were attributable to coronary heart disease (Massie and Shah, 1997). Once the disease is established, other conditions, such as myocardial infarction, dietary sodium excess, medication noncompliance, arrhythmias, pulmonary embolism, infection, and anemia, can precipitate CHF (Rich, 1997). The prognosis for CHF depends on the causative factors and the individual's response to treatment. Overall, the prognosis is poor, with the 5-year mortality rates for advanced CHF approaching 50% and the risk of sudden death being six- to nine-fold higher than that for the general population (Deedwania, 1997).

Prevalence and Incidence

CHF has become a major public health problem in the United States over the last 15 years (Starling, 1998). Unlike other cardiovascular diseases, the

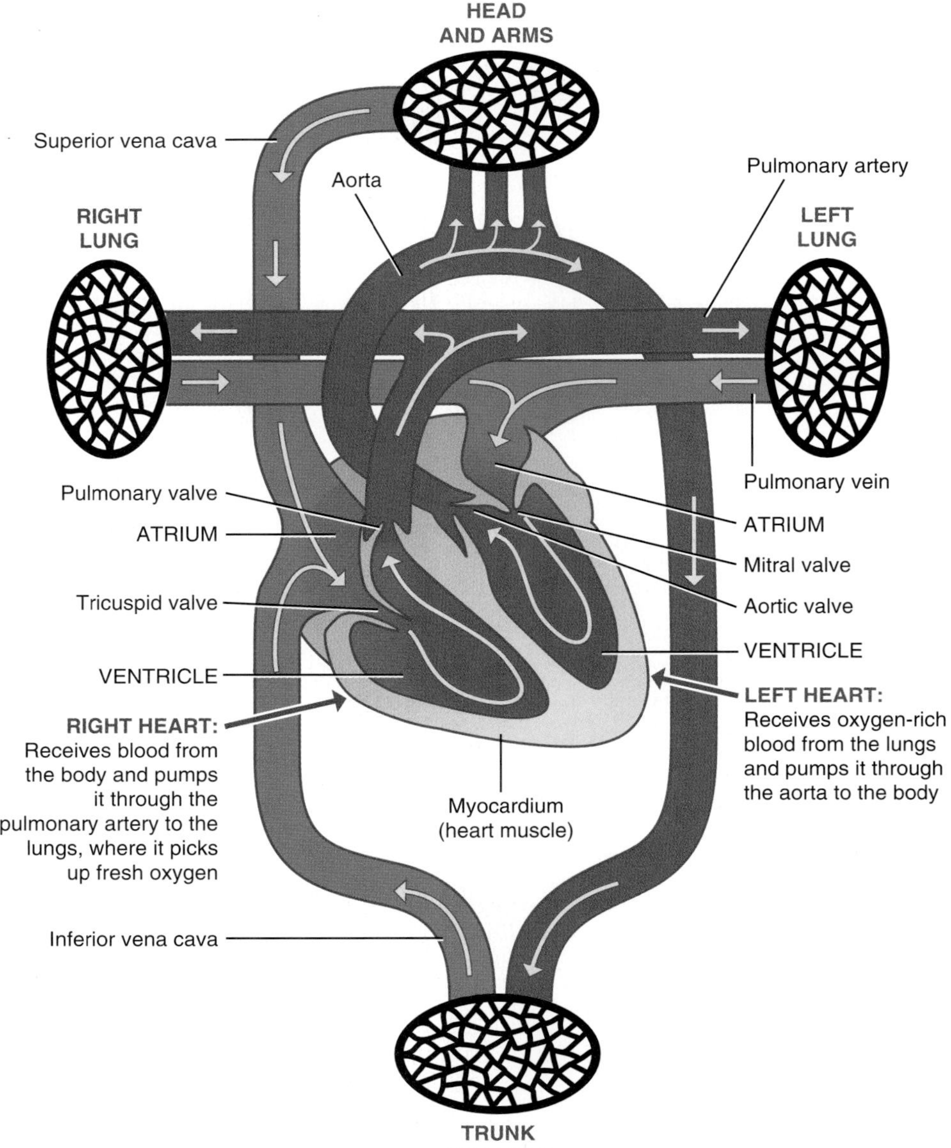

FIGURE 36–1 The structure of the heart pump.

prevalence and incidence of CHF are increasing. Approximately 5 million Americans have CHF, and between 1979 and 1995, the death rate associated with this disease increased 115% (American Heart Association, 1997). Most deaths from CHF occur in people older than 65 years (Mortality from Congestive Heart Failure, 1994). For the Medicare population, CHF is the most common diagnosis, second only to hypertension as the precipitating cause for physician office visits (Rich, 1997). CHF has a profound effect on the quality of life. Estimated costs to manage CHF are in the range of $10 to $15 billion per year (Massie and Shah, 1997).

The incidence of heart failure has risen in the last decade due to an aging population and the increased number of people being saved from premature death secondary to myocardial infarction. Approximately 465,000 new cases are diagnosed each year, affecting men more often than women and blacks more often than whites (Massie and Shah, 1997). In persons older than 65 years of age, the incidence of CHF approaches 10 per 1000 people (American Heart Association, 1997). Long-term survival after diagnosis of CHF is poorer in men than in women, but only 15% of affected women live longer than 8 to 12 years after diagnosis (American Heart Association, 1997).

Risk Factors

The Framingham Study is a 50-year epidemiologic study of the incidence, prevalence, and risk factors for cardiovascular diseases (see the box, "*Focus On:* Framingham Heart Study," Chapter 26). In the Framingham population, the risk factors for CHF are hypertension, **left ventricular hypertrophy,** coronary heart disease, and diabetes. The mean age of onset is 70 years, and 91% of the Framingham cohort had hypertension before CHF (Ho et al., 1993; Levy et al., 1996).

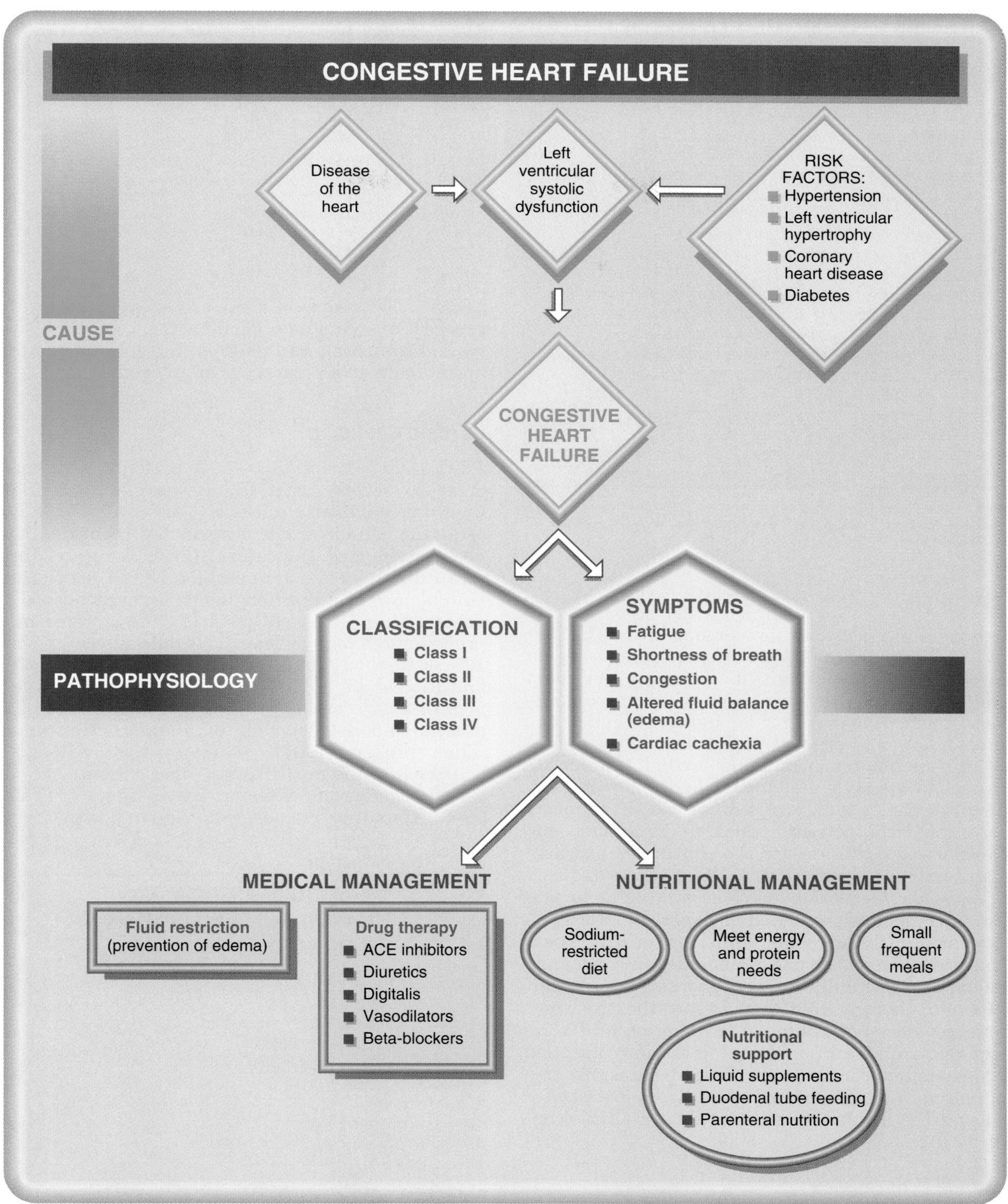

FIGURE 36–2 Pathophysiology algorithm—congestive heart failure. (Algorithm content developed by John Anderson, Ph.D., and Sanford C. Garner, Ph.D., 2000.)

TABLE 36–1 LESS COMMON CAUSES OF LEFT VENTRICULAR SYSTOLIC DYSFUNCTION

Infectious agents: viral, bacterial, fungal
Acute rheumatic fever
Infiltrative disorders: amyloid, hemochromatosis, sarcoid
Toxic: heroin, cocaine, alcohol, amphetamines, adriamycin, cyclophosphamide, sulfonamides, lead, arsenic, cobalt, phosphorus, ethylene glycol
Nutritional deficiencies: protein, thiamine, selenium
Electrolyte disorders: hypocalcemia, hypophosphatemia, hyponatremia, hypokalemia
Collagen vascular disorders: lupus erythematosus, rheumatoid arthritis, systemic sclerosis, polyarteritis nodosa, hypersensitivity vasculitis, Takayasu's syndrome, polymyositis, Reiter's syndrome
Endocrine and metabolic diseases: diabetes, thyroid disease (both hypo- and hyper-), hypoparathyroidism with hypocalcemia, pheochromocytoma, acromegaly
Tachycardia-induced: incessant supraventricular tachyarrhythmias or atrial fibrillation with rapid ventricular rates
Miscellaneous: hypereosinophilic syndrome, peripartum cardiomyopathy, sleep apnea syndrome, Whipple's disease, L-carnitine deficiency

(From American College of Cardiology/American Heart Association Task Force on Practice Guidelines. Guidelines for evaluation and management of heart failure. J Am Coll Cardiol 26:1384, 1995.)

Prevention

Because survival rates for persons with CHF are low (24% of men and 31% of women after a 5-year period), prevention is critical. *Primary prevention* strategies include the treatment of underlying diseases, such as hypertension, hyperlipidemia, and diabetes, so as to prevent CHF before left ventricular dysfunction or symptoms occur. Appropriate changes in life-style may include a diet low in saturated fat, cholesterol, and sodium; weight management; physical activity; smoking cessation; and pharmacologic therapy for those who are not compliant with or unresponsive to life-style strategies.

Secondary prevention involves strategies to prevent CHF once left ventricular dysfunction or coronary artery disease has been diagnosed. These strategies include the use of angiotensin-converting enzyme (ACE) inhibitors, beta-blockers, antihyperlipidemia therapy, anticoagulation therapy, hormone replacement therapy (in women), and coronary revascularization. Early detection, correction of presymptomatic left ventricular dysfunction, and aggressive management of risk factors are needed to lower the incidence and mortality of CHF (Kannel, 1996).

Disease Progression

In CHF, the heart can compensate for poor cardiac output by (1) increasing the force of contraction, (2) increasing in size, (3) pumping more often, and (4) stimulating the kidneys to conserve sodium and water. For a time, this compensation maintains near-normal circulation, but eventually the heart can no longer maintain a normal output *(decompensation).* The stages of CHF are categorized by the severity of symptoms (Table 36–2). In CHF, advanced symptoms can develop in weeks or months, and sudden death can occur at any time.

TABLE 36–2 CLASSIFICATIONS OF HEART FAILURE

Class I	No undue symptoms associated with ordinary activity and no limitation of physical activity
Class II	Slight limitation of physical activity; patient comfortable at rest
Class III	Marked limitation of physical activity; patient comfortable at rest
Class IV	Inability to carry on physical activity without discomfort; symptoms of cardiac insufficiency or chest pain at rest

(Reprinted with permission from Bender JR: Heart valve disease. In Zaret BL, Moser M, and Cohen LS (eds): Yale University School of Medicine Heart Book. New York, Hearst Books, 1992.)

Cardiac Cachexia

Thirty-five percent to 53% of patients with moderate to severe heart failure have malnutrition, known as **cardiac cachexia** (Carr et al., 1989). Because no standardized criteria for cachexia have been established, indicators of body fat stores, protein nutriture, and immunity have all been used. Unlike normal starvation, which is characterized by adipose tissue loss, cachexia is characterized by a predominant loss of lean body mass greater than 10% of the body total (Anker et al., 1997; Freeman and Roubenoff, 1994). This loss of lean body mass further exacerbates CHF due to the loss of cardiac muscle and development of a **cachectic heart.** (Zhao and Zeng, 1997).

Although it is unclear why some patients become cachectic, a variety of factors may play a role (Table 36–3). Impaired fat absorption occurs with severe

TABLE 36–3 FACTORS ASSOCIATED WITH THE DEVELOPMENT OF CARDIAC CACHEXIA

Generalized cellular hypoxia
Decreased energy intake
Anorexia secondary to ascites or drug therapy
Unpalatable diet and fluid restriction
Breathlessness and exhaustion from eating
Altered taste and smell
Depression
Nausea and vomiting
Elevated blood tumor necrosis factor level
Decreased energy assimilation
Increased myocardial oxygen consumption
Increased work of breathing
Elevated basal metabolic rate
Fat malabsorption
Fever
Nutrient losses
Certain diuretics (Zn, Mg, K losses)
Renal protein loss
Poor absorption due to congestion of intestinal veins

CHF and contributes to cachexia (King et al., 1996). Other metabolic changes include decreased plasma sodium values and increased catabolic catecholamine (norepinephrine, epinephrine, cortisol) and tumor necrosis factor levels. *Tumor necrosis factor* is a cytokine that causes weight loss in animals and is elevated moderately in CHF patients and markedly in cachectic patients and in patients with other wasting disorders (Zhao and Zeng, 1997). Increased levels of tumor necrosis factor are associated with lowered BMI and plasma total protein levels and decreased skinfolds, which indicate a catabolic state. It appears that CHF progresses to cardiac cachexia when the balance between catabolism and anabolism is impaired (Anker et al., 1997). Cardiac cachexia can also occur in any case of extreme malnutrition (see Chapter 24).

The cachectic patient who must undergo cardiac surgery is at increased risk for delayed wound healing, increased time for weaning from ventilator support, susceptibility to postoperative acute renal failure, and death. In general, cachectic patients have poorer outcomes and incur higher hospitalization costs than other cardiac patients (Freeman and Roubenoff, 1994). Therefore nutritional support and rehabilitation should begin before surgery.

Symptoms

Three symptoms—fatigue, shortness of breath, and congestion—are the hallmarks of CHF. *Shortness of breath (dyspnea)* upon exertion is the earliest symptom. The shortness of breath gets worse and occurs at rest (**orthopnea**) or at night *(paroxysmal nocturnal dyspnea)*. Other symptoms that reflect inadequate blood supply to the abdominal organs include anorexia, nausea, a feeling of fullness, constipation, abdominal pain, malabsorption, an enlarged liver, and liver tenderness. Decreased cranial blood supply can lead to mental confusion, memory loss, anxiety, insomnia, and headache. The latter symptoms are more common in older patients and often are the only symptoms; this can lead to a delay in diagnosing (Tresch, 1997). Often, the first symptom in the elderly is a dry cough with generalized weakness and anorexia.

Treatment

The short-term goals for treatment of CHF are to relieve symptoms and to improve the quality of life (Cohn, 1996). The degree to which these goals are met by treatment can be assessed by conducting a patient interview. The long-term goal of treatment is to prolong life by lessening, stopping, or reversing left ventricular dysfunction (Cohn, 1996). Unfortunately, there is no sensitive indicator for the effectiveness of long-term therapy.

Initial management of CHF includes a mild sodium restricted diet (2 g/day) and regular activity (as symptoms permit). Bed rest is no longer recommended except for those with acute failure. The heart becomes deconditioned as with less exercise, whereas with exercise, peak exercise capacity can be increased (Cohn, 1996). Fluids are restricted if hyponatremia develops (serum sodium level < 130 mEq/L) (Aronow, 1997).

The goals for medical nutritional therapy are to provide optimal nourishment with the least amount of stress to the heart and to reduce and prevent edema. Commonly used medications include diuretics (e.g., furosemide), vasodilators (e.g., hydralazine), and glycosides (e.g., digoxin). Basically, these drugs reduce excess fluid, dilate blood vessels, and increase the strength of the heart's contraction, respectively. ACE inhibitors (e.g., captopril, enalapril) improve symptoms, quality of life, exercise tolerance, and survival, and are considered a primary component of CHF treatment. Most of these drugs can affect nutritional status as shown in Table 36–4. For a discussion of the interrelationships between these drugs and other risk factors for heart disease, refer to Chapters 18 and 27, and to the American Heart Association website at www.amhrt.org.

TABLE 36–4 DRUGS USED TO TREAT CONGESTIVE HEART FAILURE THAT AFFECT NUTRITIONAL STATUS

DRUG CLASS/ GENERIC NAME*	NUTRITIONAL CONSIDERATIONS†
ACE Inhibitor	
Enalapril	Avoid taking with salt substitutes, potassium substitutes, or natural licorice. GI side effects: anorexia, taste loss, dry mouth, glossitis, stomatitis, nausea/vomiting, abdominal pain, diarrhea, constipation
Diuretics	
Furosemide	Avoid taking with natural licorice. GI side effects: anorexia, increased thirst
Hydrochlorothiazide	Avoid taking with a natural licorice. Use with caution if taken with calcium supplements. GI side effects: anorexia, increased thirst, dry mouth, nausea/vomiting, GI irritation, diarrhea, constipation
Digitalis	
Digoxin	Avoid taking with foods containing high bran fiber, foods with high pectin content, and natural licorice. Use caution if taken with calcium or magnesium supplements. GI side effects: anorexia, nausea/vomiting, diarrhea
Vasodilator	
Hydralazine HCl	Avoid taking with natural licorice. GI side effects: anorexia, increased thirst, dry mouth, unpleasant taste, nausea/vomiting, GI distress, diarrhea, constipation
Beta-blocker	
Metoprolol	Avoid taking with natural licorice. GI side effects: dry mouth, nausea, dyspepsia, GI upset, flatulence, diarrhea, constipation

(†Data from Pronsky ZM. Powers and Moore's Food Medication Interactions, 8th ed. Pottstown, PA, Food Medication Interactions, 1993.)
GI, gastrointestinal.
*Drugs are those recommended in Armstrong and Moe, 1994.

Nutritional Care

Assessment

Altered fluid balance complicates assessment of the patient with CHF. Weight can be either normal or increased in malnourished patients with CHF, because of fluid retention. However, the patient with cardiac cachexia may lose 10% to 15% of body weight. Because of the dilutional effect of excess extracellular fluid, the usual biochemical nutrition markers (serum albumin, transferrin) may be disproportionately low. To assess lean body mass, therefore, anthropometrics and diet history must be used. Measurement of calf and thigh circumferences, along with measurement of the mid–upper arm circumference, are the most sensitive indicators of lean body mass in cardiac patients retaining fluid (Poindexter et al., 1989). All patients with CHF should be assessed for cardiac cachexia, especially if they are awaiting surgery.

Dietary Components

ENERGY

Along with the usual factors, the energy needs of patients with CHF depend on their current weight, activity restrictions, and the severity of the heart failure. Overweight patients with limited activity must achieve and maintain an appropriate weight that will not stress the myocardium. For the obese patient, hypocaloric diets (1000 to 1200 kcal/day) will reduce the stress on the heart and facilitate weight reduction. In the undernourished patient with severe congestive heart failure, energy needs are increased by 30% to 50% above basal level as a result of the increased energy expenditure of the heart and lungs. Patients with cardiac cachexia may require further increases in energy [1.6 to 1.8 × resting energy expenditure (REE)] for nutritional repletion.

PROTEIN

Protein requirements are 0.8 to 1.0 g of protein per kilogram of body weight if the intake is oral, or 1.5 g/kg if given parenterally (Porter, 1989). The arterial pCO_2 value (see Chapter 37) and the presence of hyperglycemia determine the amount of carbohydrate in the diet. Hypoperfusion of the pancreas, as well as certain medications used to treat CHF, can lead to acute hyperinsulinemia and insulin resistance.

NUTRITIONAL SUPPORT

Because of anorexia, early satiety, ascites, altered taste, and labored efforts to eat, patients with CHF may need nutritional support. Nutrient-dense liquid supplements are the first choice for supplementing intake. If the patient is unable to meet nutritional goals with oral feedings, duodenal tube feeding can be initiated. Feedings begin slowly (30 mL/hour) and are increased gradually. Fluid and electrolyte status must be carefully monitored (see Chapter 22). Overly aggressive nutritional support can worsen CHF, resulting in pulmonary edema. The nutritional formula should have a high calorie: volume ratio (2 kcal/mL) and a moderate to low sodium content (see Appendix 36–C). Continuous nasoenteric feeding can produce a gain in lean body mass and a loss in body weight (as extracellular fluid is lost) in patients with CHF without compromising cardiac status.

When both oral and tube feedings fail, parenteral nutrition is started. As with enteral feeding, parenteral therapy begins slowly. Because of the increased blood volume, 1500 mL/day is often the initial volume for infusion. In the cachectic patient, infusion rates as low as 600 mL/day have been used to avoid metabolic stress for the patient. Central venous pressure, pulse rate, arterial blood pressure, and urine output are monitored as fluid volume is increased.

At the first sign of inadequate intake, enteral or parenteral therapy should begin as progression is slow and nutritional goals take longer to attain. Complete nutritional rehabilitation takes a minimum of 3 weeks.

SODIUM

Edema in patients with decompensated CHF results from impaired cardiac function. Inadequate blood flow to the kidneys leads to aldosterone and antidiuretic hormone secretion. Both of these hormones act to conserve fluid. Aldosterone promotes sodium resorption, and antidiuretic hormone promotes water conservation in the distal tubules of the nephron. Sodium and fluid thus accumulate in the tissues. Even asymptomatic patients with mild heart failure (Class I to II) and no congestion can retain sodium and water if consuming a high-salt diet (6 g or 250 mEq/day of sodium) (Volpe et al., 1993).

The degree to which sodium and, possibly, fluids are restricted depends on the individual, but most clinicians recommend a 2-g sodium restriction diet (American College of Cardiology, 1995; Aronow, 1997). Patients with moderate or severe cardiac failure may require sodium to be restricted to 1 g/day. This can be liberalized to 3 g/day if the patient improves. It is unknown whether a 3-g sodium restriction diet is best for most patients, or if 2-g sodium restriction is required (Dracup et al., 1994). In the rare patient whose sodium intake must be restricted to only 500 mg/day, the period of restriction should be limited; as such a diet is unpalatable and nutritionally inadequate. Indeed, it would be more appropriate to maintain a higher intake of sodium and to increase the use of diuretics. Low-sodium diets enhance the sodium-depleting effects of diuretics. Thus, the use of these diets in conjunction with diuretics often yields the best results.

Sodium-Restricted Diets. The five most common forms of sodium-restricted diets are described as follows (see also the accompanying box, "*Clinical Insight:* Sodium and Salt Measurement Equivalents"):

4 g (174mEq) of Sodium per day / ***No-Added-Salt Diet.*** High-sodium foods are limited. An intake of no more than ½ teaspoon of table salt is allowed daily.

2 g (87 mEq) of Sodium per day / ***Mild Sodium Restriction.*** High-sodium foods are eliminated; moderate-sodium foods are limited. An intake of no more than ¼ teaspoon of table salt is allowed daily.

1 g (43 mEq) of Sodium per day / ***Moderate Sodium Restriction.*** High-sodium and moderate-sodium foods are eliminated. Table salt is not allowed. Canned or processed foods containing salt are omitted. Frozen peas, lima beans, mixed vegetables, and corn are omitted because brine is used during processing. Regular bread and baked goods are limited. This diet may be difficult to maintain at home.

500 mg (22 mEq) of Sodium per day / ***Strict Sodium Restriction.*** High-sodium and moderate-sodium foods are eliminated. Table salt is not allowed. Canned or processed foods containing salt are omitted. The frozen vegetables mentioned in the 1-g sodium diet are omitted, as are the following vegetables, which are naturally high in sodium: beets, beet greens, carrots, kale, spinach, celery, white turnips, rutabagas, mustard greens, chard, and dandelion greens. Low-sodium bread replaces regular bread. Meat is restricted to 6 oz daily. This diet is unpalatable and should be used only for short periods of time. It can be nutritionally deficient if not planned carefully.

250 mg (11 mEq) of Sodium per day / ***Severe Sodium Restriction.*** High-sodium foods and moderate-sodium foods are eliminated. Table salt is not allowed. Canned or processed foods containing salt are omitted. Low-sodium bread is used, and low-sodium milk replaces regular milk. Foods high in natural sodium (protein foods) are eliminated or limited, as are the high-sodium vegetables already mentioned. This is an extreme diet that is rarely used.

Designing a Sodium-Restricted Diet. The type of sodium restriction prescribed should be the least restrictive diet that will still achieve the desired results. The first step is to minimize or eliminate the use of table salt and high-sodium foods. Table 36–5 lists serving sizes for some common high-sodium foods that should only be used sparingly in the sodium-restricted diet. Other foods that should be limited are shown in Table 36–6. As the restriction becomes more severe, attention is directed toward foods prepared with salt or sodium-containing compounds (see Table 36–7). Finally, the intake of foods that naturally contain sodium—milk, meat, and vegetables—must be considered. Table 36–8 lists the sodium content of food groups and the number of servings from each group that can be included at each level of sodium restriction. Table 36–9 presents a plan for a 2-g sodium diet.

It is important to keep in mind the variety of ways in which dietary goals can be attained. For example, a patient may prefer to follow a 1-g sodium plan, in which regular bread is limited and canned vegetables are omitted, in order to be allowed to use ½ teaspoon of salt (1150 mg of sodium) on food throughout the day. This would bring the total sodium intake to 2 g/day.

Experience has shown that patients eating a diet of low-sodium foods do not make up the sodium difference when allowed use of a salt shaker ad libitum. This supports the hypothesis that a substantial reduction in dietary sodium is possible if low-sodium foods are consumed in conjunction with ad libitum use of table salt, and that acceptable dietary saltiness can be achieved with less salt (Beauchamp et al., 1987).

Dietary Sources of Sodium. Dietary sources of sodium include (1) salt used at the table, (2) salt or sodium compounds added during preparation or processing of foods (see Table 36–7), (3) inherent sodium in foods, and (4) chemically softened water. The average American consumes approximately 4 to 6 g of sodium daily, much more than the minimum 250 mg (9 mEq) required by the human to maintain life. Up to 20% comes from salt added to food during preparation or at the table. Between

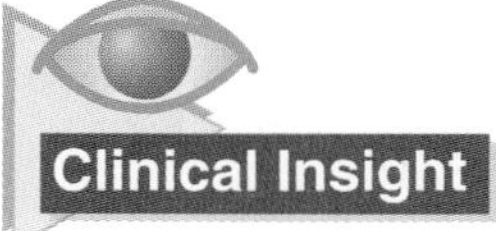

Clinical Insight

Sodium and Salt Measurement Equivalents

Sodium chloride is approximately 40% (39.3%) sodium and 60% chloride. To convert a specified weight of sodium chloride to its sodium equivalent, multiply the weight by 0.393.

Sodium is also measured in milliequivalents (mEq). To convert milligrams of sodium to mEq, divide by the atomic weight of 23.

To convert sodium to sodium chloride (salt), multiply by 2.54.

Millimoles (mmol) and milliequivalents (mEq) of sodium are the same. For example:

1 tsp of salt = approximately 6 g NaCl
= 6096 mg NaCl
6096 mg NaCl × 0.393 = 2396 mg Na (about 2400 mg)
2396 mg Na/23 = 104 mEq Na
1 g Na = 1000 mg/23 = 43 mEq or mmol

TABLE 36–5 EQUIVALENT HIGH-SODIUM FOODS, EACH OF WHICH CONTAINS 400 MG OF SODIUM

Meats
1 small hot dog or 1 slice of lunchmeat
4 slices bacon
1½ oz cooked pork sausage
1½ oz ham or corned beef
1½ oz regular canned tuna
1½ oz regular canned crab
3 oz regular canned salmon
¾ cup cottage cheese
2 oz cheese

Grains
20 small pretzels
¼ of 12 in. thin-crust cheese pizza

Vegetables
2 servings (½ cup each) regular canned vegetables
⅓ cup canned regular sauerkraut
½ large dill pickle
1 oz (approximately 20) potato chips

Soups
(All soups listed are canned soups diluted with equal amounts of water.)
⅔ cup beef broth or vegetarian vegetable
½ cup tomato, chicken gumbo, cream of celery
⅓ cup cream of mushroom

Miscellaneous
¼ tsp salt, scant
1 tsp soy sauce
4 tsp Worcestershire sauce
2⅓ T catsup
2 T mustard, chili sauce, or barbecue sauce
4⅔ T tartar sauce
2 T French dressing
4 medium olives
4 T sweet pickle relish

(Adapted from American Dietetic Association: Manual of Clinical Dietetics, 5th ed., 1996.)

35% and 80% of dietary sodium comes from processed foods (Mattes and Donnelly, 1991).

Animal protein foods, such as milk, cheese, eggs, meat, poultry, and fish, have a relatively high sodium content. This is because, like human muscle cells, animal tissue cells are surrounded by sodium chloride. Thus, these foods must be limited in strict to severe sodium restriction diets. These foods are also restricted because of their saturated fat content in order to prevent further heart disease. Because Kosher meats and poultry are soaked in salt water for 1 hour after slaughter to remove the blood, even though the meat is washed thoroughly before cooking, the sodium content of such foods may still be increased as much as four times, to a level of 90 to 115 mg/oz. Acceptable alternatives are to boil the meat and discard the broth before eating, or to use low-sodium kosher meats that are available.

TABLE 36–6 HIGH-SODIUM FOODS

1. Smoked, processed, or cured meats and fish (e.g., ham, bacon, corned beef, cold cuts, frankfurters, sausage, tongue, salt pork, chipped beef, pickled herring, anchovies, tuna, sardines)
2. Meat extracts, bouillon cubes, meat sauces
3. Salted snacks (potato chips, tortilla chips, corn chips, pretzels, salted nuts, popcorn, and crackers)
4. Prepared salad dressings, condiments, relishes, Worcestershire sauce, barbecue sauce, soy sauce, commercial salad dressings, salsa, catsup, pickles, mustard, olives, sauerkraut
5. Prepackaged frozen foods (although plain vegetables not soaked in brine are excluded): packaged mixes for sauces, gravies, casseroles, and noodle, rice, or potato dishes; oriental foods; spaghetti; pot pies
6. Canned soup, unless made without salt
7. Cheeses (processed and cheese spreads)

TABLE 36–7 SODIUM-CONTAINING ADDITIVES

NAME	FOODS LIKELY TO CONTAIN
Disodium phosphate	Cereals, cheeses, ice cream, bottled drinks
Monosodium glutamate	Accent (a flavor enhancer), meats, condiments, pickles, soups, candy, baked goods
Sodium alginate	Ice cream, chocolate milk
Sodium benzoate	Fruit juices
Sodium hydroxide	Pretzels, sour cream, cocoa products, canned peas
Sodium propionate	Breads
Sodium sulfite	Dried fruits, cut salad greens
Sodium pectinate	Syrups and toppings, ice cream, sherbet, salad dressings, jams and jellies
Sodium caseinate	Ice cream and other frozen products
Sodium bicarbonate	Baking powder, tomato soup, self-rising flour, sherbets, confections

Between 4% and 27% of dietary sodium comes from ingested water. The amount of sodium in drinking water is an issue for the person restricted to a 500-mg sodium diet if the sodium concentration in the water is greater than 40 ppm (40 mg or 2 mEq/L). Typical water softeners exchange sodium ions for calcium and other ions that cause water hardness. Use of distilled water may be necessary; alternatively, only the hot water can be chemically softened.

SODIUM LABELING. With enactment of the Nutrition Labeling and Education Act (NLEA) of 1990, the Food and Drug Administration (FDA) revised regulations to require labeling of sodium content on foods and provided legal definitions for the terms "low sodium," "moderately low sodium," and "reduced sodium" (Table 36–10). The Daily Value for sodium was set at 2400 mg/day. Patients can use the Percent Daily Value to determine whether a certain food would fit into a diet that contains 2400 mg sodium. The expression of sodium content in milligrams can also help patients determine whether the food is appropriate for their restriction level (see Table 36–11).

NON-NUTRIENT SOURCES OF SODIUM. "Low-sodium" *salt substitutes,* which contain one-third to one-half as much sodium as regular table salt, can be calculated into a mildly restricted diet. Vegetized salts, which use powdered dehydrated vegetables, may

TABLE 36–8 FOOD SERVINGS FOR SODIUM-CONTROLLED DIETS

FOOD GROUP	SERVING SIZE	SODIUM CONTENT		SUGGESTED NUMBER OF SERVINGS FOR VARIOUS RESTRICTED DIETS				
		mg Na⁺	mEq Na⁺	4g	2g	1g	500 mg	250 mg
Milk, low sodium	8 oz	7	—				1	2
Milk, regular	8 oz	120	5	2	2	2	1	—
Buttermilk, salted	8 oz	280	13	—	—	—	—	—
Cottage cheese, regular	¼ cup	130	6	1	1	1	—	—
Cheese, regular	1 oz	200	9	1	—	—	—	—
Meat, fish, poultry, unsalted cheese, tofu (½ cup)	1 oz	25	1	6	6	6	5	4
Fresh shellfish	1 oz	50	2	1	1	—	—	—
Peanut butter, regular	1 T	80	3	1	1	—	—	—
Egg	1	70	3	Not restricted		1	1	—
Vegetables, cooked, fresh, frozen	½ cup	10	—			Not restricted		
Vegetables, naturally higher in sodium	½ cup	40	2		Not restricted		1	—
Vegetables, canned, regular	½ cup	230	10	—	—	—	—	—
Vegetable juices, canned	½ cup	200	9	—	—	—	—	—
Fruits	½ cup	2	—			Not restricted		
Bread, regular	1 slice	150	7	4	4	1	—	—
Bread, low sodium	1 slice	5	—			Not restricted		
Quick bread, muffin	1 serving	300	14	1	—	—	—	—
Cereal, ready-to-eat, salted	1 cup	300	14	1	—	—	—	—
Cereal, unsalted	½ cup	5	—			Not restricted		
Butter or margarine, salted	1 tsp	50	2	3	3	2	—	—
Butter or margarine, unsalted	1 tsp	1	—			Not restricted		
Mayonnaise, regular	1½ tsp	50	2	1	1	1	1	1
Salad dressing, regular	1 T	350	16	1	—	—	—	—
Soup, regular	1 cup	900	42	—	—	—	—	—
Soup, low sodium	1 cup	25	1			Not restricted		
Desserts, regular	1 serving	300	14	1	—	—	—	—
Desserts, low sodium	1 serving	15	—			Not restricted		
Salt	1 tsp	2300	10	½ tsp	¼ tsp	—	—	—

contain considerable quantities of sodium and should, therefore, be used only when their sodium content is counted as part of the total intake. Most commercial salt substitutes are mineral bases consisting of potassium chloride, calcium chloride, or ammonium chloride and thus do not contain sodium chloride.

Spices, herbs, and other seasonings (horseradish, tabasco, lemon juice, and vinegar) can be used to improve the flavor of low-sodium foods. Most spices contain less than 0.05% sodium, and almost all contain less than 0.1%. Any of the herb or spice salts, such as garlic salt, should be avoided.

NONDIETARY SOURCES OF ADDED SODIUM. In addition to the sodium in food and water, incidental amounts may be ingested in the form of medicines and toothpastes. Barbiturates, sulfonamides, antibiotics, and other drugs, as well as cough medications, stomach alkalizers, laxatives, toothpastes, and mouthwashes, may contain large amounts of sodium. For example, some over-the-counter chewable antacid tablets can add 1200 to 7000 mg of sodium daily when used as therapy for ulcer or gastric distress. Aspirin supplies about 50 mg of sodium per tablet. Most medicine contain less than 5 mg of sodium per dose; only those containing 80 to 120 mg per dose contribute substantially to sodium intake.

LOW-SODIUM OR LOW-SALT SYNDROME. Severe sodium restriction is generally reserved for the hospitalized patient whose sodium tolerance is unusually low. Care should be taken to avoid hyponatremia, hypochloremia, and, eventually, azotemia as the glomerular filtration rate decreases. **Low-salt syndrome** can also result from adrenal insufficiency, severe and prolonged vomiting, diarrhea, and burns. Symptoms of potential low-sodium syndrome or salt depletion are weakness, lassitude, anorexia, vomiting, abdominal cramps, aching skeletal muscles, and mental confusion.

POTASSIUM

Some diuretics (e.g., *hydrochlorothiazide*) increase potassium excretion. Potassium depletion may lead to *digitalis toxicity,* which is characterized by anorexia, nausea and vomiting, abdominal discomfort, hallucinations, depression, drowsiness, and cardiac arrhythmias. For some patients, the inclusion of high-potassium foods in the diet is enough. Other patients require the use of potas-

TABLE 36–9 2-GRAM SODIUM DIET

FOOD CATEGORY	FOOD RECOMMENDED	FOOD EXCLUDED
Beverages	Milk (limit to 16 oz daily), buttermilk (limit to 1 cup/wk); eggnog; all fruit juices; low-sodium, salt-free vegetable juices; low-sodium, carbonated beverages	Malted milk, milkshake, chocolate milk; regular vegetable or tomato juices; commercially softened water used for drinking or cooking
Breads and cereals	Enriched white, wheat, rye, and pumpernickel bread, hard rolls, and dinner rolls; muffins, cornbread, and waffles; most dry cereals, cooked cereal without added salt; unsalted crackers and breadsticks; low-sodium or homemade bread crumbs	Breads, rolls, and crackers with salted tops; quick breads; instant hot cereals; pancakes; commercial bread stuffing; self-rising flour and biscuit mixes; regular bread crumbs or cracker crumbs
Desserts and sweets	All; desserts and sweets made with milk should be within allowance	Instant pudding mixes and cake mixes
Fats	Butter or margarine; vegetable oils; unsalted salad dressings, regular salad dressings limited to 1 tbsp; light, sour, and heavy cream	Regular salad dressings containing bacon fat, bacon bits, and salt pork; snack dips made with instant soup mixes or processed cheese
Fruits	Most fresh, frozen, and canned fruits	Fruits processed with salt or sodium-containing compounds (ie, some dried fruits)
Meats and meat substitutes	Any fresh or frozen beef, lamb, pork, poultry, fish, and shrimp; canned tuna or salmon, rinsed; eggs and egg substitutes; low-sodium cheese including low-sodium ricotta and cream cheese; low-sodium cottage cheese; regular yogurt; low-sodium peanut butter; dried peas and beans; frozen dinners (<500 mg sodium)	Any smoked, cured, salted, koshered, or canned meat, fish, or poultry including bacon, chipped beef, cold cuts, ham, hot dogs, sausage, sardines, anchovies, crab, lobster, imitation seafood, marinated herring, and pickled meats; frozen breaded meats; pickled eggs; regular hard and processed cheese, cheese spreads and sauces; salted nuts
Potatoes and potato substitutes	White or sweet potatoes; squash; enriched rice, barley, noodles, spaghetti, macaroni and other pastas cooked without salt; homemade bread stuffing	Commercially prepared potato, rice, or pasta mixes; commercial bread stuffing
Soups	Low-sodium commercially canned and dehydrated soups, broths, and bouillons; homemade broth and soups without added salt and made with allowed vegetables; cream soups within milk allowance	Regular canned or dehydrated soups, broths, or bouillon
Vegetables	Fresh, frozen vegetables and low-sodium canned vegetables	Regular canned vegetables, sauerkraut, pickled vegetables, and others prepared in brine; frozen vegetables in sauces; vegetables seasoned with ham, bacon, or salt pork
Miscellaneous	Salt substitute with physician's approval; pepper, herbs, spices; vinegar, lemon or lime juice; hot pepper sauce; low-sodium soy sauce (1 tbsp); hot pepper sauce; low-sodium condiments (ketchup, chili sauce, mustard) in limited amount (1 tsp); fresh ground horseradish; unsalted tortilla chips, pretzels, potato chips, popcorn, salsa (1/4 cup)	Any seasoning made with salt including garlic salt, celery salt, onion salt, and, seasoned salt; sea salt, rock salt, kosher salt; meat tenderizers; monosodium glutamate; regular soy sauce, barbecue sauce, teriyaki sauce, steak sauce, Worcestershire sauce, and most flavored vinegars; canned gravy and mixes; regular condiments; salted snack foods, olives

TABLE 36–10 FOOD LABELING GUIDE FOR SODIUM

Sodium-free:	Less than 5 mg per standard serving; cannot contain any sodium chloride
Very low sodium:	35 mg or less per standard serving
Low sodium:	140 mg or less per standard serving
Reduced sodium:	At least 25% less sodium per standard serving than in the regular food
Light in sodium:	50% less sodium per standard serving than in the regular food
Unsalted, without added salt, or no salt added:	No salt added during processing; the product it resembles is normally processed with salt
Lightly salted:	50% less added sodium than is normally added; product must state "not a low sodium food" if that criterion is not met

TABLE 36–11 SODIUM AND SALT IN GRAM AND MILLIEQUIVALENT MEASURES

mEq Na^+ (APPROXIMATE)	Mg Na^+	g NaCl (APPROXIMATE)
11	250	0.6
22	500	1.3
43	1000	2.5
65	1500	3.8
87	2000	5.0
130	3000	7.6
174	4000	10.2
217	5000	12.7

TABLE 36–12 NUTRIENT CARE FOR CARDIAC TRANSPLANT PATIENTS

PHASE	MAJOR NUTRITIONAL CONCERNS	ACTIONS
Pre-transplant	Cardiac cachexia Sodium and fluid restriction	Evaluate diet, weight history, and functional status. Apply strategies to boost intake. Consider maximally concentrated nutrition support.
Immediate post-transplant	Sufficient calories and protein to promote healing and to help withstand rejection episodes Metabolic and nutritional effects of immunosuppressive regimen	Monitor pertinent assessment data.* Apply strategies to encourage adequate intake. Ensure appropriate calcium intake.
Long-term post-transplant	Hypercholesterolemia and accelerated graft atherosclerosis Long-term metabolic and nutritional effects of immunosuppressive regimen (weight gain, glucose intolerance)	Monitor pertinent assessment data.* Encourage lipid-lowering diet. Apply strategies for weight control. Promote diabetes management.

(Data from Rock CL, Leonard LB. Nutrition care of cardiac transplant patients. Top Clin Nutr 5(1):1, 1990.)

*Body weight, height (in children), dietary intake; serum albumin, prealbumin, glucose, potassium, sodium, magnesium, calcium, and phosphorus levels; hemoglobin, hematocrit values; total blood cholesterol, total fasting triglyceride values; high-density, low-density, and very-low-density lipoprotein cholesterol levels.

sium supplements. Another source of potassium is salt substitutes, which can provide between 500 and 2000 mg (13 to 72 mEq) of potassium per teaspoon. However, salt substitutes are contraindicated in patients with renal failure and in those receiving certain medications used to treat CHF (see Table 36–4). Consequently, the approval of a physician should always be sought prior to their use.

FLUIDS

During hospitalization, fluids are commonly restricted for CHF patients. Intake may be limited to 500 to 2000 mL/day. Occasionally, foods having a high fluid content also must be limited. Fluid status should be monitored by measuring urine specific gravity and serum electrolyte values, and by observing for clinical signs of edema. Restrictions are often discontinued upon the patient's discharge from the hospital.

OTHER NUTRIENTS

A normal intake of other nutrients is recommended. Caution must be used with vitamin/mineral supplements, especially calcium and magnesium, as these nutrients may aggravate cardiac arrhythmias.

MEAL PLAN

Patients with CHF often tolerate small, frequent feedings better than larger, infrequent meals, as the latter are more tiring to consume, can contribute to abdominal distention, and markedly increase oxygen consumption. All of these factors tax the already stressed heart.

CARDIAC TRANSPLANTATION

Nutritional care of the heart transplant patient can be divided into three phases: pre-transplant, immediate post-transplant, and long-term post-transplant (Table 36–12). *Pre-transplant nutritional goals* for transplant candidates with adequate nutriture are (1) a body weight that is within 90% to 110% of ideal body weight, (2) a positive nitrogen balance of 3 to 4 g/day, (3) a sodium intake of 2 g/day, (4) a protein intake of 1.0 to 1.2 g/kg of body weight, and (5) a caloric intake of 30 kcal/kg of body weight (Poindexter et al., 1992). Patients with poor nutritional status would require additional protein (1.5 to 2.0 g/kg) and calories (35 to 40 kcal/kg) for anabolism.

Patients awaiting cardiac transplant also need to be evaluated for osteopenic bone disease secondary to prolonged periods of inactivity, malnutrition, and use of loop diuretics (Francisco-Ziller and DiCecco, 1998). Nutritional treatment for osteopenia includes calcium supplementation (1 to 1.5 g/day) and water-miscible vitamin D supplements (see Chapter 28). If oral intake is inadequate, slow infusions (30 mL/hour) of isotonic, low-fat enteral feedings are the first alternative. Patients with comorbid condi-

TABLE 36–13 TUBE-FEEDING FORMULAS FOR POST-TRANSPLANT PATIENTS

CONDITION	SUGGESTED TUBE-FEEDING FORMULA
Normal digestion, immediately post-transplant	Polymeric, high-nitrogen formula
Fluid overload	Concentrated polymeric formula
Hyperglycemia	Diabetic formula
Hypercarbia	High-fat formula
Fat malabsorption	Low-fat formula or formula containing medium-chain triglycerides
Diarrhea or constipation	High-fiber formula (provide adequate fluid)
Renal failure	Renal formula (concentrated formula with limited potassium, sodium, and phosphorus)
Impaired digestion or immediate postintestinal transplant	Semi-elemental or glutamine-enhanced formula

(From Hasse J. Recovery after organ transplantation in adults: The role of postoperative nutrition therapy. Top Clin Nutr 13(2):15, 1998.)

TABLE 36–14 ELECTROLYTE DISTURBANCES IN POST-TRANSPLANT PATIENTS

ELECTROLYTE ABNORMALITY	POSSIBLE CAUSE(S)	SUGGESTED TREATMENT
Hypernatremia	Dehydration; excess sodium intake	Increase fluid intake; decrease sodium intake.
Hyponatremia	Overhydration; total body sodium deficit	Restrict fluid intake; increase sodium intake if there is a total body sodium deficit.
Hyperkalemia	Drugs such as tacrolimus, cyclosporine, potassium-sparing diuretics; renal insufficiency; metabolic acidosis	Restrict potassium intake; administer potassium binder.
Hypokalemia	Potassium-wasting diuretics; refeeding syndrome; diarrhea; fistula; inadequate potassium intake	Increase dietary potassium intake; administer supplements.
Hyperphosphatemia	Renal insufficiency	Restrict phosphorus intake; administer phosphate binders.
Hypophosphatemia	Refeeding syndrome; glucocorticoids	Increase intake of high-phosphorus foods; administer phosphorus supplements.
Hypermagnesemia	Renal insufficiency	Limit magnesium intake.
Hypomagnesemia	Cyclosporine; refeeding syndrome; diabetic ketoacidosis; diuretics; diarrhea	Increase intake of high-magnesium foods; administer magnesium supplements.
Decreased bicarbonate	Increased exocrine drainage (pancreas transplant); intestinal drainage (intestinal transplant)	Administer bicarbonate supplements; if patient is receiving total parenteral nutrition; provide acetate.

(From Hasse J. Recovery after organ transplantation in adults: The role of postoperative nutrition therapy. Top Clin Nutr 13(2):15, 1998.)

tions require other tube-feeding formulas (Table 36–13).

There are four goals of medical nutritional therapy for post-transplant patients: (1) to promote healing, (2) to fight infection, (3) to provide nutrients for ambulation and physical therapy, and (4) to replenish nutrient stores (Hasse, 1998). In the *immediate post-transplant* period, nutrient needs are increased, as is the case after any major surgery. High caloric and protein intakes (1.3 to 1.5 × basal energy expenditure and 1.2 to 2.0 g/kg of body weight, respectively), are initial goals. Protein intakes are increased because of steroid-induced catabolism, surgical stress, anabolism, and wound healing. Particular attention should be paid to protein intakes when corticosteroid doses are high, as the rate of protein catabolism is proportional to the dose. Patients progress from clear liquids to a soft diet given in small, frequent feedings. Electrolyte disorders secondary to drug therapy and other post-transplant consequences often require nutritional treatment (Table 36–14). Nutritional monitoring in the immediate post-transplant phase is extensive (Table 36–15). Nutrient intake is often maintained by using liquid supplements and foods of high caloric content. In patients with poor appetites, persistence usually is the key to achievement of nutritional goals.

Because of longer survival time, many transplant patients experience complications, such as hyper-

TABLE 36–15 NUTRITIONAL MONITORING FOLLOWING TRANSPLANTATION

MONITORING TOOL	INDICATIONS
Indirect calorimetry	When it is difficult to estimate caloric needs and when a patient is receiving adequate nutrition, according to estimates, but is not thriving
Body weight	Daily
Fluid intake and output	Every 8 to 12 hours daily
Nutrient intake	Daily until adequate
Serum glucose concentration	Every 6 hours initially; less frequently when level normalizes
Serum potassium concentration	Daily
Serum phosphorus level	At least twice per week
Serum bicarbonate level	Daily for small-intestine and pancreas transplant recipients
Serum magnesium level	Once or twice per week

(Reprinted from Hasse JM, DiCecco SR. Solid organ transplantation. In: Skipper A (ed.). The Dietitian's Handbook of Enteral and Parenteral Nutrition, 2nd ed, Aspen Publishers, Inc., Gaithersburg, MD, 1998.)

CASE STUDY

Evelyn S. is a 76-year-old white woman with a 25-year history of mild hypertension, controlled by diet and a diuretic. Recently, she has been complaining of a dry cough, headache, dizziness, and shortness or breath while doing yard work. She was admitted to your hospital with the diagnosis of congestive heart failure. During her 3-week stay, she has been given oxygen because her PO_2 level was 48 on admission and is now only 60. Laxis, Inderal, and Zaroxolyn have been prescribed. She lives alone and her two grown daughters live out of state. What types of discharge planning and instructions should you consider?

1. What are the effects of her medications on Evelyn's nutritional status?
2. She is currently following a 2-g sodium diet but will be following a no-added-salt diet at home. Her favorite foods are ethnic German foods, including sauerkraut, cabbage dishes, pork, and sausage. What dietary adaptations do you suggest?
3. Because shopping is difficult for Mrs. S., what types of agency referrals should you seek? What advice will you offer to her daughters who have called to talk about dietary changes?
4. If Mrs. S. is discharged to a nursing home, write a draft discharge nutrition summary to send to the dietitian there. What key pieces of information are relevant?

TABLE 36–16 COMMON NUTRITIONAL SIDE EFFECTS OF IMMUNOSUPPRESSIVE MEDICATIONS

DRUG	MECHANISM OF ACTION	SIDE EFFECTS
Cyclosporine A (Sandimmune, Neoral)	Inhibits the response of cytotoxic T cells to interleukin-2 (IL-2) and prevents helper T lymphocytes from producing IL-2	Nephrotoxocity, neurotoxicity (e.g., headache, tremor, seizure); hypertension; hyperglycemia; hyperlipidemia; hyperkalemia; hypomagnesemia; gingival hyperplasia)
Tacrolimus (Prograf, FK506)	Inhibits the proliferation of cytotoxic T cells and the synthesis of IL-2	Nephrotoxicity; neurotoxicity; hypertension; hyperglycemia (diabetogenic effects); hyperkalemia; nausea and vomiting; gastrointestinal symptoms (diarrhea)
Corticosteroids (Prednisone, Prednisolone, Solumedrol, Solucortef)	Anti-inflammatory response at the arterial site; inhibits IL-1 and decreases IL-2, which suppresses lymphocyte proliferation and decreases circulating lymphocytes	Altered fluid/electrolyte balance; hypertension; adrenal-axis suppression; mood swings (depression, euphoria); peptic ulcer disease; hyperphagia; hyperlipidemia; poor wound healing; cataracts
Azathioprine (Imuran)	Inhibits RNA and DNA synthesis to prevent cytotoxic T-cell and B-cell proliferation and antibody production	Bone marrow suppression (leukopenia, thrombocytopenia, pancytopenia, macrocytic anemia); nausea and vomiting; diarrhea; hepatotoxicity
Mycophenolate mofetil (Cellcept, RS-61443)	Decreases lymphocyte activation and replication by suppressing enzymes in the purine salvage pathway, thereby creating a purine deficiency and inhibiting T- and B-cell proliferation; also suppresses antibody formation	Gastrointestinal symptoms (nausea, vomiting, diarrhea); leukopenia
Antithymocyte globulin (ATGam)	Decreases circulating lymphocytes	Anaphylactic reaction; fever and chills; nausea and vomiting; leukopenia
Muromonab CD3 (OKT3)	Binds to mature T cells to decrease their effector function	Anaphylactic reaction; pulmonary edema (usually first dose only); severe flu-like symptoms; headache; increased incidence of lymphoproliferative disorders
Sirolimus (Rapamycin)	Inhibits T- and B-cell proliferation while not affecting IL-2 production	Possible hyperglycemia; possible gastrointestinal symptoms; hyperlipidemia
15-Deoxysperagualin	Inhibits T and B lymphocytes	Leukopenia; thrombocytopenia; gastrointestinal symptoms

(Reprinted from Hasse JM, DiCecco SR. Solid organ transplantation. In: Skipper A. (ed.). The Dietitian's Handbook of Enteral and Parenteral Nutrition, 2nd ed, Aspen Publishers, Inc., Gaithersburg, MD, 1998.)

lipidemia, hypertension, obesity, diabetes, and osteopenia (Weseman and McCashland, 1998). Immunosuppressive drugs have a marked impact on nutritional status and thus influence *long-term post-transplant nutrition goals* (Table 36–16). Weight gain and hyperlipidemia are two main sequelae of immunosuppressive drug therapy. Factors found to pose a significant risk for the development of hypercholesterolemia after transplantation are prednisone dose, baseline cholesterol level, blood glucose levels, and weight gain (Kubo et al., 1992). Because graft atherosclerosis is the leading cause of death in long-term survivors, a Step Two diet (30% of calories derived from fat, less than 7% from saturated fatty acids, and an intake of less than 200 mg of cholesterol/day), along with restriction of sodium to 2 to 4 g per day, is recommended (see Chapter 26). Stricter diets and the use of pharmacologic agents may be necessary to normalize blood lipid levels. Ideal body weight should be achieved and maintained; increasing activity level is important for weight maintenance and the attainment of lipid goals.

CITED REFERENCES

American College of Cardiology/American Heart Association Task Force on Practice Guidelines. Guidelines for evaluation and management of heart failure. J Am Coll Cardiol 26:1376, 1995.

American Heart Association. 1998 Heart and Stroke Statistical Update. Dallas, TX: American Heart Association, 1997.

Anker SD, et al. Hormonal changes and catabolic/anabolic imbalance in chronic heart failure and their importance for cardiac cachexia. Circulation 96:526, 1997.

Armstrong PW, Moe GW. Medical advances in the treatment of congestive heart failure. Circulation 88:2941, 1994.

Aronow WS. Treatment of congestive heart failure in older patients. J Am Geriatr Soc 45:1252, 1997.

Beauchamp GK, et al. Modification of salt taste. Ann Intern Med 98:763, 1987.

Cohn JN. The management of chronic heart failure. N Engl J Med 335:490, 1996.

Deedwania PC. Underutilization of evidence-based therapy in heart failure. Arch Intern Med 157:2409, 1997.

Dracup K, et al. Management of heart failure. II. Counseling, education, and lifestyle modifications. JAMA 272:1442, 1994.

Francisco-Ziller N, DiCecco S. Nutritional care of the pretransplant patient. Top Clin Nutr 13(2):1, 1998.

Freeman LM, Roubenoff R. The nutrition implications of cardiac cachexia. Nutr Rev. 52:340, 1994.

Hasse JM. Recovery after organ transplantation in adults: The role of postoperative nutrition therapy. Top Clin Nutr 13(2):15, 1998.

Ho KL, et al. The epidemiology of heart failure: The Framingham Study. J Am Coll Cardiol 22 (suppl A): 6A, 1993.

Kannel WB. Need and prospects for prevention of cardiac failure. Eur J Clin Pharmacol 49:S3, 1996.

King D, et al. Fat malabsorption in elderly patients with cardiac cachexia. Age Ageing 25(2):144, 1996.

Kubo SH, et al. Factors influencing the development of hypercholesterolemia after cardiac transplantation. Am J Cardiol 70:520, 1992.

Levy D, et al. The progression from hypertension to congestive heart failure. JAMA 275:1557, 1996.

Massie BM, Shah NB. Evolving trends in the epidemiologic factors of heart failure: Rationale for preventive strategies and comprehensive disease management. Am Heart J 133:703, 1997.

Mattes RD, Donnelly D. Relative contributions of dietary sodium sources. J Am Coll Nutr 10:383, 1991.

Mortality from Congestive Heart Failure: United States, 1980–1990. MMWR 43:77, 1994.

Poindexter SM, et al. Potential parameters of nutritional assessment in the congestive heart failure and cardiac transplant patient: Circumference measures of waist, lower thigh, and calf. J Am Diet Assoc 89:A65, 1989.

Poindexter SM, et al. Nutrition support in cardiac transplantation. Top Clin Nutr 7(3):12, 1992.

Porter, K. Cardiac cachexia. In: Blackburn GL, Bell SJ, Mullen JL (eds.). Nutritional Medicine: A Case Management Approach. Philadelphia: WB Saunders, 1989.

Rich MW. Epidemiology, pathophysiology, and etiology of congestive heart failure in older adults. J Am Geriatr Soc 45:968, 1997.
Starling RC. The heart failure pandemic: Changing patterns, costs, treatment strategies. Cleve Clin J Med 65:351, 1998.
Tresch DD. The clinical diagnosis of heart failure in older patients. J Am Geriatr Soc 45:1128, 1997.
Volpe M, et al. Abnormalities of sodium handling and cardiovascular adaptations during high salt diet in patients with mild heart failure. Circulation 88:1620, 1993.
Weseman RA, McCashland TM. Nutritional care of the chronic posttransplant patient. Top Clin Nutr 13(2):27, 1998.
Zhao S-P, Zeng L-H. Elevated plasma levels of tumor necrosis factor in chronic heart failure with cachexia. Int J Cardiol 58:257, 1997.

ADDITIONAL REFERENCES

American Dietetic Association: Handbook of Clinical Dietetics, 2nd ed. New Haven, CT: Yale University Press, 1992.
Bagatell CJ, Heymsfield SB. Effect of meal size on myocardial oxygen requirements: Implications for postmyocardial infarction diet. Am J Clin Nutr 39:421, 1989.
Carr JG, et al. Prevalence and hemodynamic correlates of malnutrition in severe congestive heart failure secondary to ischemic or idiopathic dilated cardiomyopathy. Am J Cardiol 63:709, 1989.
Funk M, Krumholz HM. Epidemiologic and economic impact of advanced heart failure. J Cardiovasc Nurs 10:1, 1996.
Garg R, et al. Heart failure in the 1990s: Evolution of a major public health problem in cardiovascular medicine. J Am Coll Cardiol 22 (suppl A): 3A, 1993.
Heart Failure Guideline Panel. Heart Failure: Management of patients with left ventricular systolic dysfunction. Am Fam Phys 50:603, 1994.
Levine B, et al. Elevated circulating levels of tumor necrosis factor in severe chronic heart failure. N Engl J Med 323:236, 1990.
Moore CE, et al. Heart transplant nutritional programs: A national survey. J Heart Lung Transplant 10:50, 1991.
Poole-Wilson PA. Relation of pathophysiologic mechanisms to outcome in heart failure. J Am Coll Cardiol 22 (suppl A): 22A, 1993.
Rock CL, Leonard LB. Nutrition care of cardiac transplant patients. Top Clin Nutr 5(1):1, 1990.
Warnold I, Lundholm K. Clinical significance of preoperative nutritional status in 215 noncancer patients. Ann Surg 199:299, 1984.

CHAPTER 37

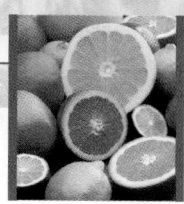

Medical Nutrition Therapy for Pulmonary Disease

DONNA H. MUELLER, PHD, RD, FADA

Chapter Outline

- Relationships between Nutrition and the Pulmonary System
- Overview of Medical Nutrition Therapy in Pulmonary Disease
- Bronchopulmonary Dysplasia
- Cystic Fibrosis
- Chronic Obstructive Pulmonary Disease
- Asthma
- Aspiration
- Lung Cancer
- Pneumonia and Tuberculosis
- Respiratory Failure
- Future Directions

Key Terms

ADULT RESPIRATORY DISTRESS SYNDROME—a life-threatening condition characterized by severe hypoxia, bilateral pulmonary fluid infiltration, and decreased lung compliance, usually occurring without prior lung disease but secondary to catastrophic illness

ASTHMA—a condition of hypersensitive airways from allergic and nonallergic causes, generated by immunologic responses

BRONCHOPULMONARY DYSPLASIA (BPD)—a chronic lung disease of infancy that commonly arises following respiratory distress syndrome (RDS) and treatment with oxygen; characterized by broncheolar metaplasia and interstitial fibrosis

CHRONIC BRONCHITIS—a chronic, productive cough with inflammation of one or more of the bronchi and secondary changes in lung tissue

CHRONIC OBSTRUCTIVE PULMONARY DISEASE (COPD)—a process characterized by the presence of chronic bronchitis, emphysema, or both, leading to the development of airway obstruction

COEFFICIENT OF FAT ABSORPTION (CFA)—the amount of fat absorbed, based on a 72-hour record of fat intake and a fecal fat collection; calculated by the following equation: CFA = fat intake − fecal fat/fat intake

COR PULMONALE—a heart condition characterized by right ventricular enlargement and failure that arises due to increased pressure within the pulmonary arteries

CYSTIC FIBROSIS (CF)—an autosomal recessive disorder characterized by dysfunction of the exocrine glands and production of abnormally thick secretions that obstruct airway, pancreatic, and other ducts

DISTAL INTESTINAL OBSTRUCTION SYNDROME (DIOS)—recurrent distal intestinal impaction; formerly termed meconium ileus equivalent

DYSPNEA—shortness of breath

EMPHYSEMA—a condition of the lung characterized by abnormal, permanent enlargement of alveoli, accompanied by destruction of their walls without obvious fibrosis

PANCREATIC ENZYME REPLACEMENT THERAPY—Use of exogenous pancreatic enzymes to produce more normal digestion in people with pancreatic insufficiency

PULMONARY ASPIRATION—the drawing of foreign bodies, such as food or liquid, into the lungs during inspiration

PULMONARY FUNCTION TESTS—a group of procedures designed to measure the ability of the respiratory system to exchange oxygen and carbon dioxide

RESPIRATORY DISTRESS SYNDROME (RDS)—a condition affecting newborn infants, particularly premature neonates, that is marked by dyspnea with cyanosis

RESPIRATORY QUOTIENT—the ratio of the volume of carbon dioxide expired to the volume of oxygen inspired (CO_2/O_2)

SURFACTANT—a substance composed of phospholipids (especially dipalmitophosphatidylcholine) and proteins that is produced by type II cells of the alveolar epithelium; it lowers surface tension so as to permit gas exchange at the gas-liquid interface

SWEAT TEST—a test performed using pilocarpine iontophoreses to determine levels of sodium and chloride in sweat; elevated levels are diagnostic of cystic fibrosis

TACHYPNEA—Abnormal rapidity of respiration which, if prolonged, can lead to excess loss of CO_2 and respiratory alkalosis

RELATIONSHIPS BETWEEN NUTRITION AND THE PULMONARY SYSTEM

Optimal nutrition throughout life promotes anatomic development and physiologic function of the pulmonary system. The respiratory structures include the nose, pharynx, larynx, trachea, bronchi, bronchioles, alveolar ducts, and alveoli. Supporting structures include the skeleton and the muscles (e.g., the intercostal, abdominal, and diaphragm muscles). Nerves, blood, and lymph supply all tissues (Fig. 37–1). Within a month after conception, pulmonary system structures are recognizable. The pulmonary system grows and matures during gestation and childhood. Aging results in diminished lung integrity (Rossi et al., 1996).

Gas exchange is the major function of the pulmonary system. The lungs enable the body to obtain the oxygen needed to meet its cellular metabolic demands and to remove the carbon dioxide produced by these processes. The lungs also function to filter, warm, and humidify inspired air; synthesize surfactant; regulate body acid-base balance; synthesize arachidonic acid; and convert angiotensin I to angiotensin II. See website www.lungusa.org or www.nih.gov.

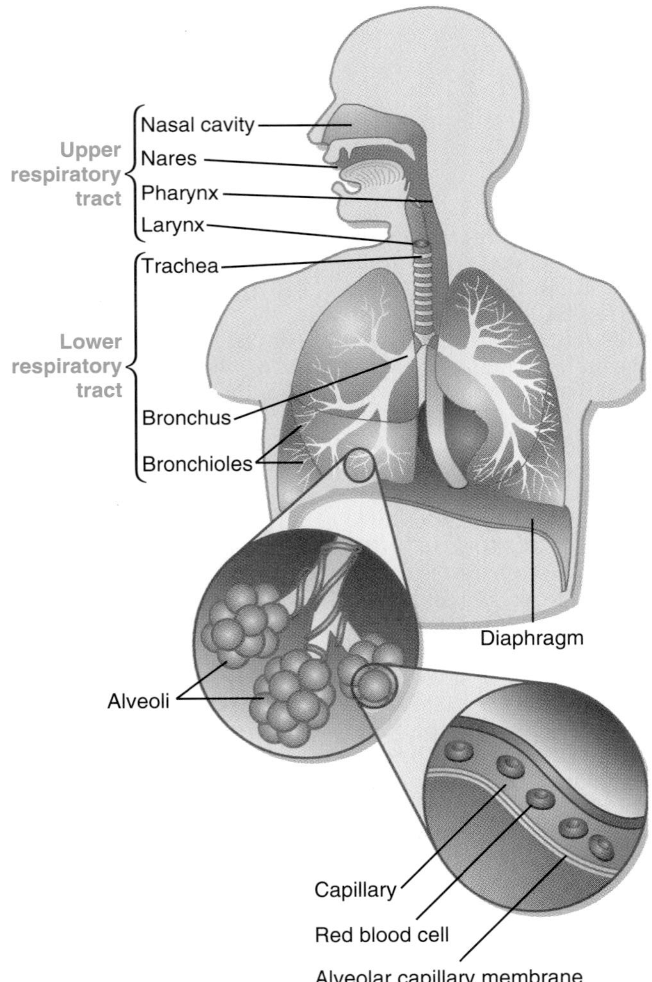

FIGURE 37–1 Anatomy of the pulmonary system.

Impact of Malnutrition on the Pulmonary System

The relationship between malnutrition and respiratory disease has long been recognized (Pingleton, 1998). Malnutrition adversely affects lung structure, elasticity, and function; respiratory muscle mass, strength, and endurance; lung immune defense mechanisms; and control of breathing. For example, protein and iron deficiency result in low hemoglobin levels, resulting in diminished oxygen-carrying capacity of the blood. Low levels of other minerals, such as calcium, magnesium, phosphorus, and potassium, compromise respiratory muscle function at the cellular level. Hypoproteinemia contributes to the development of pulmonary edema by decreasing colloid osmotic pressure, which allows body fluids to move into the interstitial space. Decreased levels of **surfactant,** a compound synthesized from proteins and phospholipids, contribute to the collapse of alveoli and thus increase the work of breathing. The supporting connective tissue of the lungs is composed of collagen, which requires vitamin C for its synthesis. Normal airway mucus is a substance consisting of water, glycoproteins, and electrolytes. Weight loss from inadequate energy intake is significantly correlated with a poor prognosis in people with pulmonary diseases.

The association of malnutrition with impaired immunity places any malnourished patient at high risk for developing respiratory infections. Malnourished pulmonary patients requiring hospitalization are likely to have lengthy hospital stays and are prone to increased morbidity and mortality.

Impact of Pulmonary System Disease on Nutritional Status

Pulmonary disease substantially increases energy requirements. This factor explains the rationale for including body composition and weight parameters in nearly all medical, surgical, pharmacologic, and nutritional research studies of people with respiratory diseases.

The complications of pulmonary diseases or their treatments can make adequate intake, digestion, absorption, circulation, cellular utilization, storage, and excretion of many foods and most nutrients difficult. Some adverse effects of lung disease on nutritional status are listed in Table 37–1. Drug-nutrient interactions of medications commonly used in pulmonary disease, such as bronchodilators, antibiotics, steroids, and diuretics, are described in Chapter 18.

TABLE 37–1 ADVERSE EFFECTS OF LUNG DISEASE ON NUTRITIONAL STATUS

Increased energy expenditure
- Increased work of breathing
- Chronic infection
- Medical treatments (e.g., bronchodilators, chest physical therapy)

Reduced intake
- Fluid restriction
- Shortness of breath
- Decreased oxygen saturation when eating
- Anorexia due to chronic disease
- Gastrointestinal distress and vomiting

Additional limitations
- Difficulty preparing food due to fatigue
- Lack of financial resources
- Impaired feeding skills (for infants and children)
- Altered metabolism

OVERVIEW OF MEDICAL NUTRITION THERAPY IN PULMONARY DISEASE

Individualized nutritional assessment, intervention, and counseling are integral components of care for each patient with pulmonary system disease. Respiratory alterations can occur at any time throughout the life cycle—from the premature infant with insufficient surfactant production, to the emaciated teenager with anorexia nervosa, to the young adult with street-drug overdose, to the older adult with severe osteoporosis. Pulmonary system disorders may be categorized as primary, such as tuberculosis (TB), bronchial asthma, and cancer of the lung, or secondary, such as those associated with cardiovascular disease, obesity, acquired immunodeficiency disease (AIDS), sickle cell disease, and scoliosis. Examples of acute conditions include aspiration of enteral feeding liquids, airway obstruction from foods like peanuts, and anaphylaxis from consumption of shellfish. Examples of chronic conditions include cystic fibrosis (CF) and emphysema. Table 37–2 presents a summary of some pulmonary diseases with nutritional implications.

To determine pulmonary status, the clinician uses the results of numerous diagnostic and monitoring tests, such as imaging procedures, **pulmonary function tests,** arterial blood gas determinations, sputum cultures, and biopsies. Assessment of the cardiovascular, renal, neurologic, and hematologic systems is also important, as diseases involving these systems often produce complications affecting pulmonary anatomy, physiology, and biochemistry.

Nutritionally relevant, common, presenting signs and symptoms of pulmonary diseases include cough, early satiety, anorexia, weight loss, dyspnea during preparing food and eating, and fatigue. As pulmonary disease progresses, other related conditions may interfere with food intake or overall nutritional status, especially abnormal production of sputum, vomiting, **tachypnea** (rapid breathing), hemoptysis, thoracic pain, nasal polyps, anemia, depression, and altered taste secondary to medications.

BRONCHOPULMONARY DYSPLASIA

Bronchopulmonary dysplasia (BPD) is a chronic lung condition of infancy that occurs most frequently in premature infants following **respiratory distress syndrome (RDS)** in the neonatal period. Infants with severe disease often require prolonged intensive medical care. Therapies, such as mechanical ventilation, supplemental oxygen, medications, or tube feedings, may be required long after the infant's discharge from the hospital. Because the pathophysiology of BPD is incompletely understood, medical treatment and nutritional intervention are empirically based, and often have limited scientific rationale (Hazinski, 1998).

Nutritional Status and Assessment

Because of the fragile nature of affected infants, careful and consistent nutritional assessment is imperative (Mueller, 1998). Growth of infants with BPD is followed closely because it is a major outcome indicator of medical and nutritional status (Farrell and Fiascone, 1997). Because lung size is stature-dependent, linear growth is important for the growth of healthy lung tissue and for the resolution of the condition. Observations of growth patterns of infants with BPD suggest that these infants grow more slowly, thereby requiring careful assessment of both respiratory and nutritional

TABLE 37–2 SELECTED PULMONARY CONDITIONS HAVING NUTRITIONAL IMPLICATIONS

CATEGORY	EXAMPLES
Neonate	Bronchopulmonary dysplasia (BPD)
Obstruction	Cystic fibrosis (CF)
	Chronic obstructive pulmonary disease (COPD)
	• Emphysema
	• Chronic bronchitis
	Asthma
	Aspiration (foreign body, food, fluid)
Tumor	Lung cancer
Infection	Pneumonia
	Tuberculosis (TB)
Respiratory failure	Acute respiratory failure (ARF)
	Lung transplantation
Other system abnormalities	
Neuromuscular	Muscular dystrophy
Skeletal	Paralysis
	Osteoporosis
	Scoliosis
Cardiovascular	Pulmonary edema
Endocrine	Severe obesity
	Prader-Willi syndrome

status (de Meer et al., 1997; Giacoia et al., 1997; Gregoire et al., 1998).

Reasons for growth failure among infants with BPD include increased energy needs combined with inadequate dietary intake, gastroesophageal reflux, emotional deprivation, and chronic hypoxia (Johnson et al., 1998). Brief episodes of decreased oxygen saturation are thought to occur frequently in infants with BPD, especially during feeding. Thus, whenever growth languishes, low oxygen saturation should be evaluated as a contributing factor. Growth should be evaluated and compared to that of other infants of the same postconceptional age (see Chapter 9). Factors to include in a nutritional assessment are listed in Table 37–3.

Nutritional Requirements and Care

Infants with BPD have special short- and long-term nutritional requirements and care considerations related both to their prematurity (see Chapter 9) and their pulmonary status. The general goal of nutritional care is to supply adequate nutrient intakes, promote linear growth, maintain fluid balance, and develop age-appropriate feeding skills. Meeting energy and nutrient needs is a major challenge in the care of infants and toddlers with BPD (Brunton et al., 1998).

Energy

Increased energy needs are well recognized in infants with BPD. Resting energy expenditure for infants with BPD has been documented to be 25% to 50% greater than that in age-matched controls. Infants with BPD who have growth failure may have energy needs that are 50% higher than those who are growing well (Kurzner et al., 1988). Energy needs also vary over the course of the disease. In the acute phase, when infants are kept in controlled temperature environments, fed parenterally, remain relatively inactive, and are not growing or are growing slowly, energy requirements may be 50 to 85 kcal/kg/day. In contrast, during the convalescent phase, when infants are growing rapidly, being fed orally, and using additional energy for temperature regulation, activity, and the work of breathing, they may require 120 to 130 kcal/kg/day or more (Oh, 1986).

Macronutrients

Protein intake should be within the advised range for infants of comparable postconceptional age. As the caloric density of the diet is increased by the addition of fat and carbohydrate, protein should continue to provide 7% or more of total calories. Lesser amounts may be inadequate for growth.

Additions of fat or carbohydrate should be made to formula only after it has been concentrated to 24 kcal/oz to keep protein at an acceptable level. Fat provides essential fatty acids (EFAs) and helps meet energy demands when tolerance for fluid and carbon dioxide load is limited. Excess sources of carbohydrate may abnormally increase the respiratory quotient (RQ) and the output of CO_2. Continuous calculations of the proportions of the macronutrients related to respiratory status are major considerations in any nutritional evaluation.

To maintain fluid balance, infants with BPD may require fluid restriction, sodium restriction, and long-term treatment with diuretics, all of which have nutritional implications. When fluid intake is restricted, the use of parenteral lipids or calorically dense enteral feedings may help the infant meet energy needs.

Vitamins and Minerals

Adequate supplies of all vitamins and minerals are essential. Special attention is focused on those related to prematurity, infections, oxygen therapy, and drug-nutrient interactions.

Because of their role in cell membrane integrity and as antioxidants, adequate supplies of vitamins A, C, E, and, perhaps, inositol (see Chapter 4) are crucial. Of special interest is vitamin A because of its role in the proper development and maintenance

TABLE 37–3 COMPONENTS OF NUTRITIONAL ASSESSMENT FOR INFANTS WITH BRONCHOPULMONARY DYSPLASIA

HISTORICAL	MEDICAL	NUTRITIONAL	FEEDING HISTORY	ENVIRONMENTAL
Birth weight	Respiratory status	Weight	Volume of intake	Parent–child interaction
Gestational age	Oxygen saturation	Length	Frequency of feedings	Home facilities
Medical history	Use of medications	Head circumference	Behavior during feedings	Community resources
Nutritional history	Emesis	Hemoglobin and hematocrit values	Formula composition	Economic resources
Previous growth pattern	Stool pattern	Serum electrolytes	Use of solids	
	Urine output	Other biochemical tests as needed (e.g., serum albumin, alkaline phosphatase, phosphorus levels)	Feeding milestones	
	Urine specific gravity			

(Adapted from Sirois LW. Nutritional assessment and management of the infant with bronchopulmonary dysplasia. Nutr Support Serv 4:62, 1984.)

of the epithelial cells of the respiratory tract (Verma et al., 1996). Indeed, vitamin A supplements have been reported to decrease the length of stay in neonatal intensive care units (Robbins and Fletcher, 1993).

Mineral intake and retention should be monitored regularly and supplemented as needed to maintain normal levels. Determination of mineral requirements is complicated by growth delay and the multiple medications prescribed for infants and toddlers with BPD. Medications include diuretics, bronchodilators, antibiotics, cardiac antiarrhythmics, and corticosteroids. Collectively, these medications are associated with increased urinary loss of minerals, especially chloride, potassium, and calcium (see Chapter 18).

Additional chloride losses may occur in infants with chronic CO_2 retention and respiratory acidosis because of metabolic correction for the acidosis. Deficiencies of chloride or potassium are associated with muscle weakness and impaired growth.

Infants with BPD are at risk for inadequate bone mineralization. Besides limited nutrient intake, other risk factors include inadequate stores of calcium and phosphorus related to prematurity, intermittent respiratory acidosis, chronic use of medications, and insufficient physical activity.

For infants sensitive to sodium loads, formulas with lower sodium content can be selected (see Appendix 39 and Table 8–5). Also, the sodium content of medications, water, and foods must be considered.

Diet Modification

The nutritional care of infants with BPD is a major challenge. Barriers to adequate intake include anorexia, fatigue, poor coordination of breathing and swallowing, and weakness of suck. To meet energy needs, calorically dense formulas; small, frequent feedings; use of a soft nipple; and nasogastric or gastrostomy tube feedings may be needed. When calorically dense formulas are used (>24 kcal/oz), the adequacy of fluid intake and urinary output must be monitored closely.

If gastroesophageal reflux is evident, lung disease may worsen owing to aspiration. Associated vomiting with expulsion of feedings leads to inadequate nutritional intake. Treatment includes thickened feedings; prone positioning; medications, like antacids or histamine H_2-receptor antagonists; and, in severe cases, surgical fundoplication. To thicken formula, ½ to 1 T of infant cereal is added per ounce of formula, with adjustments made as necessary.

Feeding difficulties frequently occur among infants with BPD. Risk factors include a history of unpleasant oral experiences (e.g., intubation, frequent suctioning, or recurrent vomiting), a history of non-oral feedings, delayed introduction of solids, or discomfort or choking associated with eating solids. Infants may tire easily while breast-feeding or bottle-feeding. Useful approaches that may facilitate feeding acceptance include providing a pleasant and calm mealtime environment, providing oral stimulation during tube feedings, using consistent and appropriate feeding techniques, and gradually introducing progressive texture and flavor changes. An interdisciplinary approach involving the primary caregiver is recommended.

CYSTIC FIBROSIS

Cystic fibrosis (CF) is a complex, multisystem disorder that is inherited in an autosomal recessive fashion. The first comprehensive description of CF in the United States was published in 1938 (Andersen, 1938); in 1989, the disease's underlying genetic basis was presented (Riordan et al., 1989; Kerem et al., 1989). The CF gene, named the cystic fibrosis transmembrane regulator (CFTR), is located on the long arm of chromosome 7. It encodes a protein product involved in regulating chloride ion transport. Multiple mutations have been identified (Sharer et al., 1998).

Although CF remains the most common lethal genetic disorder prevalent in whites, it is expressed in other population groups as well. About 2% to 5% of white populations are heterozygotes, with an incidence of CF of 1:2500 live births. Survival has dramatically improved owing to scientific advancements and improvements in diagnostic and treatment procedures, including nutrition. Of the approximately 30,000 people treated at CF centers in the United States, the median age of patients is approximately 30 years (Cystic Fibrosis Foundation, 1999) (see website www.cff.org). Women with CF have delivered healthy babies, and some have chosen to breast-feed their unaffected infants (Michel and Mueller, 1994).

Pathophysiology and Diagnostic Criteria

The expression of the CF gene is largely restricted to epithelial cells. Almost all exocrine glands are affected by secretion of abnormally thick, tenacious mucus that obstructs glands and ducts in various organs. The clinical features are dominated by involvement of the respiratory tract, sweat and salivary glands, intestine, pancreas, liver, and reproductive tract. Pulmonary complications include acute and chronic bronchitis, bronchiectasis, pneumonia, atelectasis, and peribronchial and parenchymal scarring. Pneumothorax and hemoptysis are common. In advanced stages, cor pulmonale or infection with *Burkholdteria cepacia* may be present, signifying a poor prognosis (Aitken and Fiel, 1993) (see Fig. 37–2).

Several methods are available for diagnosing CF. For families with previously identified CF, prenatal analysis may be possible. Several countries and some states in the United States conduct routine

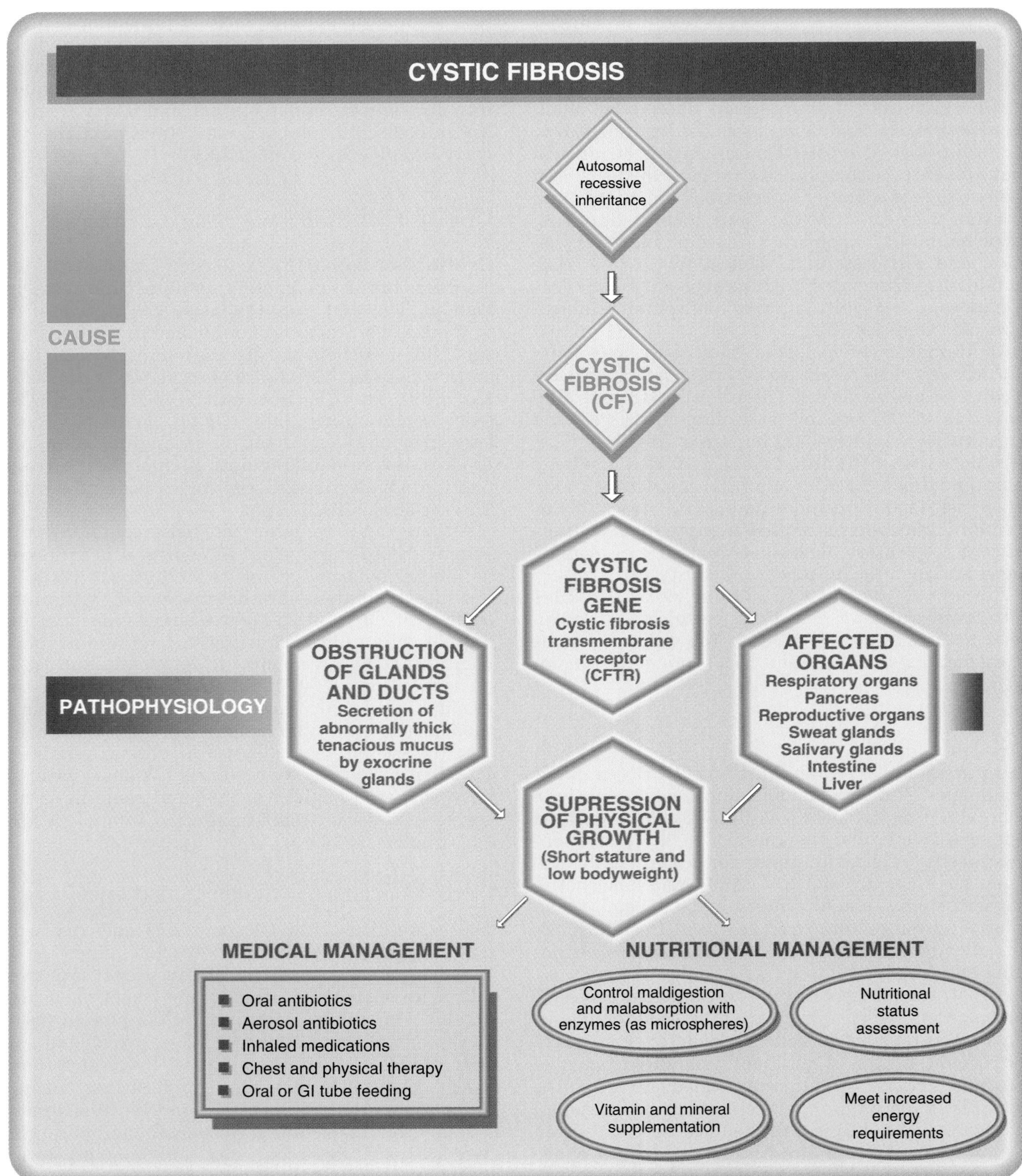

FIGURE 37–2 Pathophysiology algorithm—cystic fibrosis. (Algorithm content developed by John Anderson, Ph.D., and Sanford C. Garner, Ph.D., 2000.)

neonatal screening for the disease (Farrell et al., 1997). The most reliable clinical diagnostic test, known as the **sweat test,** is performed by pilocarpine iontophoresis. Elevated levels of sodium and chloride (>60 mEq/L) in collected sweat samples are indicative of CF. Criteria for the diagnosis of CF include a positive result on a sweat test and the presence of chronic lung disease, failure to thrive and malabsorption, or a family history of CF.

CF can have a profound impact on the digestive system. Approximately 85% of individuals with CF have pancreatic insufficiency. Plugs of thick mucus reduce the quantity of digestive enzymes released from the pancreas into the small intestine. The resultant enzyme insufficiency causes maldigestion of food and malabsorption of nutrients. Decreased bicarbonate secretion can further reduce digestive enzyme activity. Decreased bile acid reabsorption contributes further to fat malabsorption. The presence of excessive mucus lining the small intestinal tract may interfere with nutrient absorption by the microvilli. Gastrointestinal complications include bulky, foul-smelling stools; cramping and intestinal obstruction; rectal prolapse; and liver involvement. As the disease progresses, damage to the endocrine portion of the pancreas can cause impaired glucose tolerance and development of CF-related diabetes mellitus (Zipf et al., 1990). The prevalence of insulin-requiring diabetes is estimated to be 7% in the entire population with CF, and up to 15% in the adult CF population. As many as 50% of adults with CF may demonstrate glucose intolerance.

Nutritional Status and Assessment

Individuals with CF are at high risk for malnutriton (Gaskin, 1993). Maldigestion and malabsorption, as well as the progressive complications of the disease, make it difficult to meet increased nutrient needs. Factors interfering with adequate intake and retention of nutrients include dyspnea, coughing and cough-induced vomiting, gastrointestinal discomfort, anorexia during episodes of infection, possible impaired sense of smell and taste, and glucosuria. Growth retardation and difficulty maintaining desired weight for height are common problems. Before diagnosis, infants with CF often demonstrate growth failure. With treatment, growth generally improves, and when energy intake is adequate, growth appropriate for age can usually be achieved (see Fig. 37–3).

As lung disease progresses, growth velocity in children, and weight for height in adults, may decline. The long-term relationship between nutritional support, growth, and survival is not known; however, improved nutritional status on a long-term basis continues to be suggested as a contributing factor to increased survival. Comprehensive nutritional assessment in individuals with CF was codified by the Cystic Fibrosis Foundation (Ramsey et al., 1992) and is summarized in Table 37–4.

Nutritional Requirements and Care

Because of all the intricate manifestations and complications of CF, nutritional requirements and care must be individually determined for each affected person. Moreover, nutritional requirements and intervention need to be integrated with other therapies, including oral and aerosol antibiotics, other inhaled medications, and chest physical therapy (Creveling et al., 1997).

Based upon clinical research and experience, the goals of nutritional care in CF are to control maldigestion and malabsorption; provide adequate nutrients to promote optimal growth or maintain

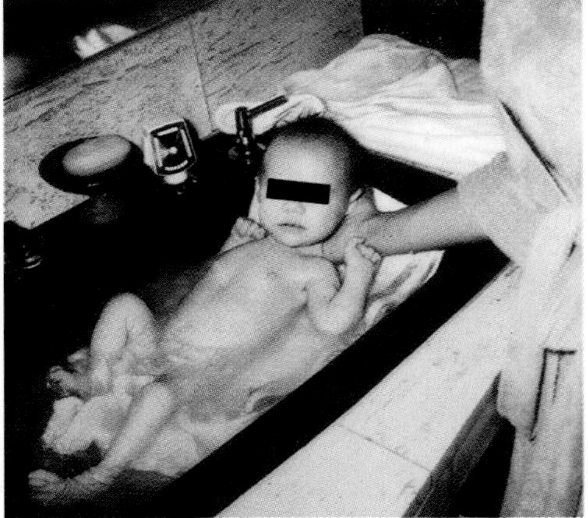

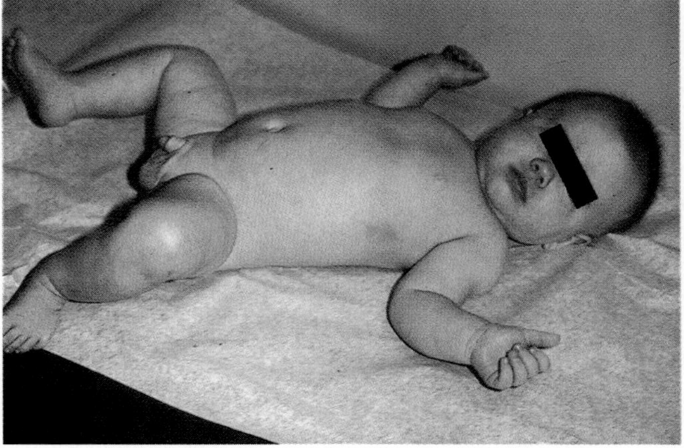

FIGURE 37–3 (*A,B*) Response to therapy in a child with cystic fibrosis. BF was admitted to the hospital in respiratory failure, with a history of cough, tachypnea, and failure to thrive since 4 weeks of age. Diagnosis of cystic fibrosis was made on finding sweat chloride of 105 mEq/L and undetectable enzyme levels in duodenal secretions. (Courtesy of Daniel V. Schidlaw, M.D., St. Christopher's Hospital for Children, Philadelphia, PA.)

TABLE 37–4 NUTRITIONAL ASSESSMENT IN CYSTIC FIBROSIS

INDEX	MINIMUM FREQUENCY	INDICATION
Anthropometry		
Weight	Every 3 months	Routine care
Height (children ≥ 2 years old); length (children < 2 years old)	Every 3 months	Routine care
Head circumference	Every 3 months until age 2 years	Routine care
Mid-arm circumference	Every 3 months	Routine care
Triceps skinfold thickness	Every 3 months	Routine care
Nutritional assessment		
Dietary intake*	Yearly	Routine care, diagnosis
3-d fat balance†	As indicated	Weight loss, growth failure, clinical deterioration, diagnosis
Anticipatory dietary guidance	Yearly	Routine care, diagnosis
Laboratory studies		
Complete blood count‡	Yearly	Routine care, diagnosis
Serum or plasma retinol value	Yearly	Routine care, diagnosis
Serum or plasma α-tocopherol value	Yearly	Routine care, diagnosis
Albumin level	As indicated	Weight loss, growth failure, clinical deterioration, diagnosis
Electrolytes and acid-base status	As indicated	Prolonged fever, summer heat, infancy, breast-feeding, diagnosis

(From Ramsey BW, et al. Nutritional assessment and management in cystic fibrosis: A consensus report. Am J Clin Nutr 55:108, 1992.)

*Usually consists of a 24-hr recall with assessment of dietary pattern; should be obtained by a dietitian.

†Includes both a diet record to determine energy and fat intake as well as a determination of stool fat excretion. This permits calculation of the coefficient of fat absorption (CFA) and assessment of the degree of malabsorption in malnourished patients.

‡If there is any evidence of iron deficiency, iron status must be measured (i.e., serum iron, iron-binding capacity, and serum ferritin levels).

weight for height and pulmonary function; and prevent nutritional deficiencies (Bruno et al., 1995; Salamoni et al., 1996; Williams, 1998). Those individuals at especially high risk include infants, children, adolescents, and pregnant and lactating women. Table 37–5 summarizes a graded approach to nutritional management.

Pancreatic enzyme replacement therapy is the first step taken to correct maldigestion and malabsorption. The introduction of enteric-coated enzyme microspheres in the early 1980s was a major advance in nutritional management. The microspheres, designed to withstand the acidic environment of the stomach, release enzymes in the duodenum, where they digest protein, fat, and carbohydrate.

The quantity of enzymes to be taken with food depends on the degree of pancreatic insufficiency, the quantity of food eaten, the fat and protein content of food consumed, and the type of enzymes used (Borowitz et al., 1995). Enzyme dosage—limited to 2500 lipase units per kilogram of body weight per

TABLE 37–5 CATEGORIES FOR NUTRITIONAL MANAGEMENT OF PATIENTS WITH CYSTIC FIBROSIS (CF)

CATEGORY	TARGET GROUP	GOALS
Routine management	All patients with CF	Nutritional education, dietary counseling, pancreatic enzyme replacement (for patients with pulmonary insufficiency), vitamin supplementation (for patients with pulmonary insufficiency)
Anticipatory guidance	Patients with CF who are at risk of developing energy imbalance (i.e., severe pulmonary insufficiency, frequent pulmonary infections, periods of rapid growth), but who are maintaining a weight–height index ≥ 90% of ideal weight	Further education to prepare patients for increased energy needs; increased monitoring of dietary intake; increased caloric density in diet as needed; behavioral assessment and counseling
Supportive intervention	Patients with decreased weight gain velocity and/or a weight–height index 85%–90% of ideal weight	All of the above, plus oral supplements as needed
Rehabilitative care	Patients with a weight–height index consistently < 85% of ideal weight	All of the above, plus enteral supplementation via nasogastric tube or enterostomy, as indicated
Resuscitative and palliative care	Patients with a weight–height index < 75% of ideal weight, or progressive nutritional failure	All of the above, plus continuous enteral feeds or total parenteral nutrition.

(From Ramsey BW, et al. Nutritional assessment and management in cystic fibrosis: A consensus report. Am J Clin Nutr 55:108, 1992.)

meal—is adjusted empirically to control gastrointestinal symptoms, including steatorrhea, and to promote growth appropriate for age. If gastrointestinal symptoms cannot be controlled, enzyme dosage, patient adherence, and enzyme type should be reevaluated. Fecal fat or nitrogen balance studies may help to evaluate the adequacy of enzyme supplementation.

For infants or children unable to swallow capsules, the capsules can be opened and the microspheres mixed with a soft food, such as applesauce. Microspheres should not be mixed with foods that have a pH greater than 6.0, such as dairy products (e.g., milk, custard, and ice cream), because the enteric coating will dissolve and the enzymes exposed to the gastric acidity will be inactivated. For the same reason, to retain benefits of the enteric coating, microspheres should not be chewed or crushed.

Distal intestinal obstruction syndrome (DIOS), also known as recurrent intestinal impaction or (formerly) *meconium ileus equivalent,* sometimes occurs in children and adults. Prevention or treatment of DIOS involves adequate enzymes and fluids, an increased-fiber diet, exercise, laxatives, and stool softeners (Gavin et al., 1997).

Energy

The energy needs of those with CF vary widely from individual to individual, and even in the same individual throughout the course of life (Duggan and Gilbert, 1996; Murphy et al., 1995). Factors to consider are gender, age, basal metabolic rate, physical activity, respiratory infection, severity of lung disease, and severity of malabsorption. When indirect calorimetry measurement of energy requirements is unavailable, initial equations for calculating caloric recommendations are available (see "*Clinical Insight:* Estimation of Daily Energy Requirements in Cystic Fibrosis"). Patients with CF should not be encouraged to decrease their activity levels, but to increase their energy intake instead (Boas, 1997; Michel and Mueller, 1995). Relatively healthy children with CF may be able to maintain normal growth and energy stores when fed a high-energy, moderate-fat diet complemented with sufficient pancreatic enzyme supplementation (Kawchak et al., 1996).

Macronutrients

Dietary protein levels are increased in CF as a result of malabsorption. However, when energy needs are adequately met, individuals with CF generally can meet their protein needs by following a typical North American diet, with at least 15% to 20% of the total calories consumed as proteins or the appropriate RDA for protein for the individual's gender, age, and height being met.

Fat intake should provide 35% to 40% or more of total kilocalories as tolerated. Dietary fat helps to provide the required energy, EFAs, and fat-soluble vitamins. Moreover, fat limits the volume of food required to meet energy demands and improves the palatability of the diet.

Indications of fat intolerance include an increase in the number of stools, greasy stools, or abdominal cramping. Among patients with CF who have pancreatic insufficiency and who are treated with enzymes to control malabsorption, clinical signs of EFA deficiency are rare, although blood and tissue lipid levels may be abnormal (Levy et al., 1993). Essential fatty acid deficiencies may be present, even among patients who are treated adequately with pancreatic enzymes to control malabsorption. Although such visible signs of EFA deficiency as the typical skin lesions may not be noticeable, the clinician should consider routinely testing for abnormal blood lipid profiles. Additionally, patients need to be encouraged to include sources of EFAs (e.g., canola, flaxseed, soybean, or corn oil) as part of their daily fat intake (Benabdeslam et al., 1998; Levy et al., 1993; Winklhofer-Roob, 1998).

As the disease progresses, changes in carbohydrate intake may be necessary. Lactose intolerance may become evident and pancreatic endocrine involvement may require carbohydrate adjustments (see Chapter 34).

Vitamins and Minerals

With pancreatic enzyme supplementation, the water-soluble vitamins appear to be adequately absorbed in patients with CF, and requirements under normal conditions can usually be met by diet. However, individual variations are important to monitor.

Even with pancreatic enzyme supplementation, fat-soluble vitamins usually remain inadequately absorbed (Sokol, 1991). Low serum concentrations of vitamin A despite increased hepatic stores have been documented in CF, suggesting impaired mobilization/transport of the vitamin from the liver (Farrell and Hubbard, 1983). Decreased levels of vitamin D metabolites have been observed. This is one of several factors that may be related to the decreased bone mineral content that has been described in populations with CF (Mischler et al., 1979; Reiter et al., 1985). Low vitamin E levels have been associated with hemolytic anemia and abnormal neurologic findings (Cynamon et al., 1988; Peters and Kelly, 1996). Individuals with CF may be at risk for vitamin K deficiency secondary to long-term use of antibiotics or liver disease, as well as malabsorption. Although most patients maintain normal prothrombin times without supplementation, decreased biologic activity of vitamin K has been reported (Beker et al., 1997). For all of these reasons, vitamin K supplementation is recommended.

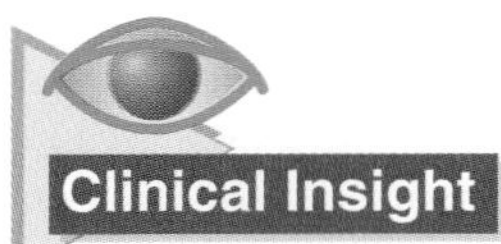

Estimation of Daily Energy Requirement in Cystic Fibrosis

To estimate a caloric prescription, you need the following data:

1. Gender
2. Age
3. Weight
4. Basal metabolic rate
5. Physical activity coefficient
6. Lung disease coefficient
7. Coefficient of fat absorption

If the child is growing adequately or the adult is maintaining weight, and if the pulmonary status and steatorrhea are under good control, the total daily energy requirement (DER) is reflective of the person's typical energy use and intake. Compare the typical intake to the recommended dietary allowance (RDA) for gender and age. To enable the child/adult to achieve and maintain healthy growth and body composition, the caloric prescription may approximate the RDA.

If the child is not growing adequately or the adult is not maintaining weight or body composition, use the following steps to estimate the DER.

STEP 1

Calculate the basal metabolic rate (BMR) using the World Health Organization (WHO) equations for predicting BMR from body weight (wt).

EQUATIONS FOR PREDICTING BMR (Kcal) FROM BODY WEIGHT (Kg)

AGE RANGE (YRS)	FEMALES	MALES
0–3	61.0wt – 51	60.9wt – 54
3–10	22.5wt + 499	22.7wt + 495
10–18	12.2wt + 746	17.5wt + 651
18–30	14.7wt + 496	15.3wt + 679
30–60	8.7wt +829	11.6wt + 879

STEP 2

Calculate daily energy expenditure (DEE) by multiplying the BMR by the activity coefficient (AC) and adding the disease coefficient (DC).

$$DEE = BMR \times (AC + DC)$$

Activity Coefficient (AC)

- Confined to bed = 1.3
- Sedentary = 1.5
- Active = 1.7

Disease Coefficient (DC)

- Normal lung function = 0.0
  (forced expiratory volume in 1 second (FEV_1) ≥ 80% of that predicted)
- Moderate lung disease = 0.2
  (FEV_1 40%–79% of that predicted)
- Severe lung disease = 0.3
  (FEV_1 < 40% of that predicted)
- Very severe lung disease = 0.4–0.5
  (FEV_1<< 40% of that predicted)
- If pulmonary function tests (PFTs) are unavailable, severity of lung disease is assessed clinically.

Sample Calculation

Data: Male patient; 22 years old; weight = 54 kg; FEV_1 60% of that predicted; attends college; relatively sedentary

Calculation: DEE = BMR × (1.5 + 0.2)
= [15.3 (54) + 679] × 1.7
= [826.2 + 679] × 1.7 = 1505.2 × 1.7

DEE = 2559 Kcal

STEP 3

Calculate the total daily energy requirement (DER)* from the daily energy expenditure (DEE), taking into account the degree of steatorrhea.

- Pancreatic sufficiency = DER = DEE
  (coefficient of fat absorption [CFA] ≥ 93% of intake, including patients on enzymes)
- Pancreatic insufficiency = DER = DEE (0.93/CFA)
  (CFA must be determined as a fraction of fat intake)
- Stool fat collection unavailable = DER = DEE (0.93/0.85)
  (approximate value of 0.85 may be used in the calculation; if possible, obtain fecal fat collection)

Sample Calculation

Assuming the patient had pancreatic insufficiency and was taking enzymes, the daily energy requirement would be computed as follows:

Data: Laboratory analysis of 72-hour fecal fat collection reveals that CFA = 78% of intake.

Calculation: DER = DEE × (0.93/CFA)
= 2559 × (0.93/0.78) = 2559 × 1.19

DER = 3045 Kcal/day

***NOTE:** The DER may be further modified due to infection, fever, or other systemic conditions, such as body composition, cystic fibrosis–related diabetes mellitus, or pregnancy. Careful and frequent reassessment must be accomplished on an anticipatory basis.

(Adapted from Ramsey BW, et al. Nutritional assessment and management in cystic fibrosis: A consensus report. Am J Clin Nutr 55:108, 1992, pp 115–116.)

Sodium requirements are increased in CF owing to increased losses in sweat. When sodium intake is inadequate, lethargy, vomiting, and dehydration may occur. Adequate salt is consumed by most children and adults following a typical North American diet with processed foods. However, supplemental salt is required under some conditions. Infants require extra salt owing to the low-sodium content of breast milk, formula, and infant foods; ⅛ to ¼ tsp/day is usually adequate in this situation. Children and adults need additional salt during periods of fever, hot weather, or physical exertion. Table

TABLE 37–6 VITAMIN AND MINERAL SUPPLEMENTATION IN CYSTIC FIBROSIS

NUTRIENT	QUANTITY
Vitamin A	1–2 times the RDA/day*
Vitamin D	1–2 times the RDA/day*
Vitamin E	
Infants	25–50 IU/day†
Children ≤ 10 years old	100 IU/day
Children > 10 years old	200–400 IU/day
Vitamin K	
Infants (< 1 year old)	2.5–5.0 mg weekly
Children and adults receiving long-term antibiotic therapy or with liver disease	2.5–5.0 mg twice weekly
Sodium	
Infants	¼ tsp. salt daily
Children and adults at times of vigorous exercise, heat stress, or profuse diarrhea	250 mg–2 g, 2–3 times per day

(Adapted from Ramsey BW, et al. Nutritional assessment and management in cystic fibrosis: A consensus report. Am J Clin Nutr 55:108, 1992.)
*Vitamins A and D can be provided by 1 to 2 multivitamins daily.
†Vitamin E is provided in a water-soluble form.

salt or proprietary electrolyte replacement solutions are used.

Other minerals are not routinely supplemented, although mineral status should be evaluated on an individual basis. Decreased bone mineralization, low iron stores, and low magnesium levels have all been described in CF (Green et al., 1985; Pond et al., 1996). Plasma zinc levels may be low in cases of moderate to severe malnutrition (Durie and Pencharz, 1989). Table 37–6 summarizes recommendations for initial vitamin and mineral supplementation in CF. This regimen can be adjusted on an individual basis over time.

TABLE 37–7 SUGGESTIONS FOR INCREASING ENERGY INTAKE

Include foods of high-energy density.
Include snacks regularly, especially before bedtime. Serve snacks at least 2 hours before the next meal.
Keep foods readily accessible for snacking.
Soft foods and beverages may be easier to eat when there is shortness of breath.
To enhance appetite, pay attention to appearance, texture, and aroma of the foods offered.
Simplify food preparation by using convenience foods or preprepared foods.
Identify financial and food resources in the community to help meet needs.
Encourage companionship at meals.

(Adapted from Adams EJ. Nutrition care in cystic fibrosis. Nutr News 51:1, 1988. Courtesy of National Dairy Council®.)

Diet Modification

Diet modification is the first approach for meeting the increased nutritional requirements of CF (Bentur et al., 1996; Collins et al., 1997; Michel and Mueller, 1989). Along with adequate dietary modification, positive eating behaviors must be established (Stark et al., 1997). Intake can be enhanced by regular and enjoyable mealtimes, larger food portions at meals, extra snacks, and foods selected for high-nutrient density (Table 37–7). Table 37–8 shows how energy intake can be boosted throughout the day. Homemade or proprietary nutritional supplements, such as fortified beverages and puddings, can also help the individual with CF attain nutritional goals.

Supplementation by feeding tube is an alternative for those unable to meet nutritional needs by the oral route. Formulas are provided by continuous infusion through a nasogastric, gastrostomy, or je-

TABLE 37–8 SAMPLE MENU: TYPICAL LUNCH WITH INCREASED NOURISHMENT

TYPICAL LUNCH	CALORIES	BOOSTED LUNCH	CALORIES
Soup		**Soup**	
Tomato (½ cup) made with water	50	Tomato, made with ½ cup fortified milk*	162
		and 1 tsp margarine	36
Sandwich		**Sandwich**	
Bologna (1 oz)	88	Bologna (2 oz)	176
Cheese (1 oz)	107	Cheese (2 oz)	214
Mustard (1 tsp)	4	Mayonnaise (1 tsp)	34
Bread (2 slices)	124	Bread (2 slices)	124
Salad		**Salad**	
Lettuce & tomato with French dressing	70	Carrot-raisin with mayonnaise	153
Dessert		**Dessert**	
Applesauce (⅓ cup)	91	Baked apple (with sugar and margarine)	188
Beverage		**Beverage**	
Whole milk (½ cup)	80	Fortified milk* (½ cup)	112
TOTAL KILOCALORIES	**614**	TOTAL KILOCALORIES	**1199**

(Adapted from Michel SH, Mueller DH. Practical approaches to nutrition care of patients with cystic fibrosis. Top Clin Nutr 4:46, 1989, p. 53.)
*Fortified milk = 1 cup whole milk plus 4 T powdered nonfat milk.

junostomy tube, often while the person sleeps (see Chapter 22). Elemental and nonelemental formulas with enzymes have both been used effectively. Enzyme powder can be added directly to the formula. If the nocturnal method is chosen, capsules can be taken by mouth when the feeding is started and again once or twice during the night. Factors to consider in the decision to proceed with night-time supplementation include nutritional status, medical status (e.g., factors such as the presence of nasal polyps and the degree of oxygenation during sleep), risks associated with tube feeding (e.g., aspiration), and the psychosocial and financial impact (Bowser, 1990). Intensive supplementation has been associated with improved weight gain, slowed decline in pulmonary function, decreased incidence of respiratory infection, and improved sense of well-being (Dalzell et al., 1992).

Although the short-term benefits of supplementation have been well documented, nutritional status is likely to regress when supplementation is discontinued. The long-term impact of intensive supplementation on disease course has not been determined. Parenteral nutrition is best used for short-term support in patients with clearly evident needs, such as in those recuperating from gastrointestinal surgery.

For infants with CF and their families, the immunologic and psychosocial benefits of breast-feeding are well established, and breast-feeding should not be discouraged (Marcus et al., 1991; Cannella et al., 1993). For the infant with pancreatic insufficiency, enzyme microspheres can be added to a small amount of baby food or placed directly in the infant's mouth. Supplementation with high-calorie formula may be necessary to meet growth goals. For formula-fed infants, standard formulas (20 to 27 kcal/oz), given with supplemental enzymes, are usually adequate. Protein hydrolysate formulas with medium-chain triglycerides may also be used (see Appendix 39).

CHRONIC OBSTRUCTIVE PULMONARY DISEASE

Chronic obstructive pulmonary disease (COPD) is characterized by slowly progressive obstruction of the airways. COPD may be subdivided into two categories: **emphysema** (type I) and **chronic bronchitis** (type II). Tobacco smoking is the most important causative factor (Fig. 37-4).

Nutritionally, patients with emphysema are thin, often cachectic. They are generally older and have mild hypoxemia and normal hematocrit values. **Cor pulmonale** develops late in the course of the disease. Conversely, patients with chronic bronchitis are of normal weight and, indeed, are often overweight. Hypoxemia is prominent in these patients, hematocrit values are increased, and cor pulmonale develops early.

Nutritional Status and Assessment

Nutritional depletion is evidenced clinically by low body weight for height and reduced triceps fatfold measurements. Besides decreased food intake, depletion appears related to pulmonary complications, such as the degree of airflow obstruction, gas diffusing capacity, CO_2 retention, respiratory and limb muscle strength, and altered muscle function. Mal-

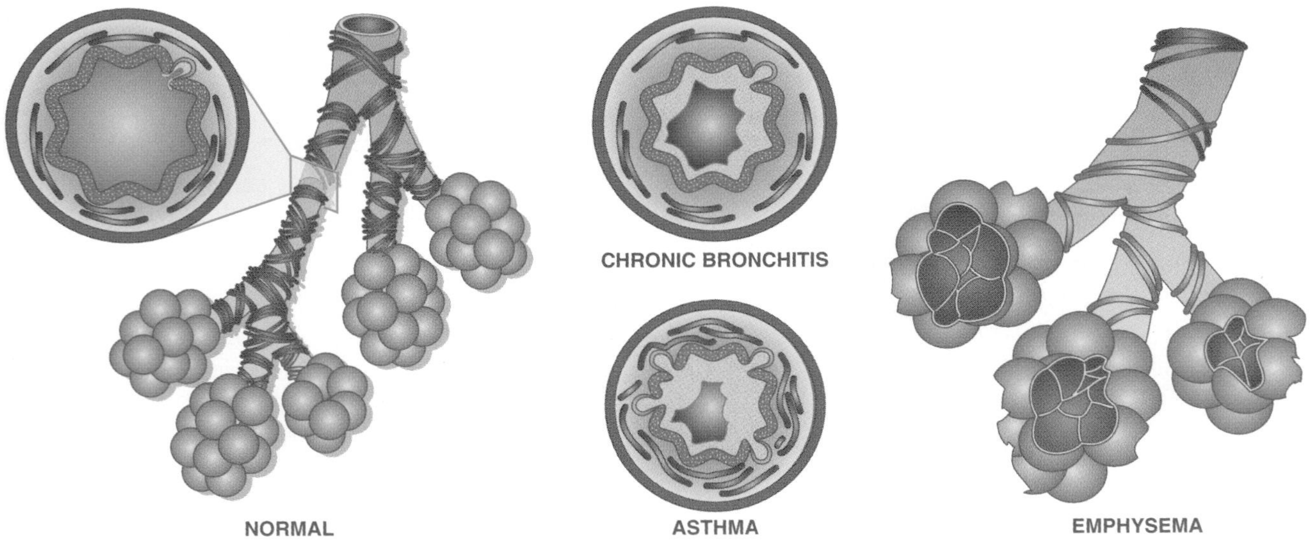

FIGURE 37–4 Selected airway disorders. *A,* Normal lung anatomy showing open bronchioles and normal-sized alveoli and adequate bronchi elastic recoil. *B,* Chronic bronchitis characterized by inflammation and narrowing of the lumen of the bronchi. *C,* Asthma characterized by extreme spasmatic narrowing of the bronchi lumen. *D,* Emphysema characterized by enlargement of air spaces distal to the terminal bronchioles, destruction of alveolar membranes, and loss of bronchi elastic recoil.

nourished patients with COPD have a worse prognosis than those who are well nourished.

Components of the nutritional assessment in COPD are listed in Table 37–9. Determination of body composition helps to differentiate lean muscle mass from adipose tissue, and overhydration from dehydration. Indirect calorimetry is a useful assessment tool. In patients with cor pulmonale resulting in fluid retention, weight maintenance or gain may camouflage actual wasting of lean body mass. Thus, for patients retaining fluids, careful interpretation of both anthropometric measurements and biochemical indicators of nutritional status is necessary, especially since the latter are depressed by hemodilution. Morning headache and confusion from *hypercapnia* (excessive carbon dioxide in the blood) must be identified, as these symptoms may interfere with food preparation or intake.

The medication profile should be assessed for food and nutrient interactions. Examples of drugs with potential nutritional implications are bronchodilators, expectorants, and corticosteroids (see Chapter 18). Other pertinent assessments focus on blood oxygen saturation, fatigue, anorexia, difficulty chewing and swallowing from **dyspnea,** constipation from low-fiber food selections, or diarrhea from impaired peristalsis secondary to lack of oxygen to the gastrointestinal tract.

Nutritional Requirements and Care

The primary goals of nutritional care for patients with COPD are to facilitate nutritional well-being, maintain an appropriate lean body mass:adipose tissue ratio, correct fluid imbalance, and manage drug-nutrient interactions (Celli, 1997; Chapman and Winter, 1996; Cordova and Criner, 1997; Saudny-Unterberger et al., 1997).

Energy

Energy requirements are elevated in COPD, and they vary for each individual. The factors listed in Table 37–1 can make meeting energy needs difficult. For patients participating in pulmonary rehabilitation programs, adjusted energy requirements will depend on the intensity of daily therapy (Dore et al., 1997) (see Chapter 2).

Macronutrients

In the individual with stable COPD, requirements for protein, fat, and carbohydrate are determined by the underlying lung disease, oxygen therapy, medications, weight status, and any acute fluid fluctuations. Sufficient protein, 1.0–1.5 gram/kg dry body weight, is necessary to maintain or restore lung and muscle strength, as well as promote immune function. A balanced ratio of protein (15 to 20% of calories) with fat (30 to 45% of calories) and carbohydrate (40 to 55% of calories) is important to preserve a satisfactory respiratory quotient (RQ) from substrate utilization (see Chapter 2). Repletion, but not overfeeding, is the hallmark of nutritional care (Ryan et al., 1993). Often, other concurrent disease processes exist, such as cardiovascular or renal disease, cancer, or diabetes mellitus. These underlying conditions affect the total amount and kind of protein, fat, and carbohydrate prescribed.

Vitamins and Minerals

As with macronutrients, vitamin and mineral requirements for individuals with stable COPD depend on the underlying lung pathology, other concurrent diseases, medical treatments, and weight status. For people continuing to smoke tobacco, additional vitamin C may be necessary. Research indicates that people who smoke about one pack of cigarettes per day appear to require about 16 mg more ascorbate per day, whereas those who smoke two packs need about 32 mg as replacement (Cross and Halliwell, 1993).

The role of minerals, such as magnesium and calcium, in muscle contraction and relaxation may be important for people with COPD. Intakes at least equivalent to the recommended dietary allowance (RDA) or adequate intake (AI) level should be pro-

TABLE 37–9 COMPONENTS OF NUTRITIONAL ASSESSMENT FOR ADULTS WITH CHRONIC OBSTRUCTIVE PULMONARY DISEASE

HISTORICAL	MEDICAL	NUTRITIONAL	DIET HISTORY	ENVIRONMENTAL
Medical history Nutritional history Usual weight	Respiratory status Oxygen saturation Dental status Senses of smell and taste Gastrointestinal function	Weight Height Skinfold measurements Hemoglobin and hematocrit values Serum electrolytes Serum proteins Additional biochemical tests as needed (e.g., immunologic testing, creatinine height index, nitrogen balance)	Usual home diet Use of supplements Where meals are eaten Social companionship with meals	Home facilities Physical abilities Financial resources

vided. Patients who are receiving aggressive nutritional support should undergo routine monitoring of magnesium and phosphorus levels because of their cofactor roles in adenosine triphosphate (ATP) generation. Reduced bone mass, measured by dual-energy x-ray absorptiometry (DXA), has been demonstrated in patients with COPD, thus providing evidence for the nutritional and exercise concerns related to osteoporosis in this population (Nishimura et al., 1997).

Some patients with cor pulmonale and fluid retention require sodium and fluid restriction. Depending upon the diuretics prescribed, increased dietary intake of potassium may be required (see Chapter 18).

Diet Modification

A modified oral diet usually is preferred. When abdominal bloating is a problem, limitation of foods associated with gas formation may be helpful (see Chapters 30 and 31). Adequate exercise, fluids, and easily chewed dietary fiber enhance gastrointestinal motility. Patients and their families benefit from specific suggestions for enhancing appetite, promoting oral intake, and lessening fatigue when eating. Some suggestions are resting before meals, eating small portions of nutrient-dense foods, and planning expectorant medication usage apart from mealtimes. Patients with disease-related physical limitations may be helped by assistance with food shopping and meal preparation. Linkage with community resources, such as congregate meal programs or the Meals on Wheels program, may also be helpful (see Chapter 14).

Enteral nutritional supplementation by mouth or by feeding tube can increase total caloric and nutrient intake for some patients with COPD. Decisions to implement this method of nutritional support must take into consideration patient anxiety, labor to perform, and cost. It must be understood that the patient's nutritional status may be improved as long as enteral nutrition is continued, but will revert if and when supplementation is discontinued. Besides the potential for aspiration, other negative consequences of nocturnal tube feedings must be considered. Even in healthy adults, oxygen consumption decreases by 15% to 25% during sleep (Schwab, 1995).

ASTHMA

Unlike CF and COPD, **asthma,** also known as "hyperactive airways," is classified as a reversible obstructive respiratory disorder. However, continued inadequate management can lead to a life-threatening situation known as status asthmaticus. Asthmatic symptoms may be related to allergen exposure, including foods (see Chapter 41). The underlying pathophysiology of primary pulmonary asthma is unclear.

A common sign of asthma is persistent mouth breathing. In young children, this can result in permanent oral structure malformation lasting into adulthood. The resulting open bite can make biting into nourishing foods, such as sandwiches or fresh fruits and vegetables, difficult.

Nutritional Requirements and Care

Research results remain controversial but encouraging, and food and nutrients are being studied for possible roles in asthma's etiology or treatment (Monteleone and Sherman, 1997; Weiss, 1997; Ziment, 1997). Examples include omega-3 and omega-6 fatty acids, antioxidants, the cations sodium and magnesium, and methylxanthines (Broughton et al., 1997; Hill et al., 1997a; Leichsenring et al., 1995; Schwartz and Weiss, 1992; Soutar et al., 1997). In addition, because of magnesium's function as a cation with smooth muscle relaxant and anti-inflammatory effects, treatment of the acute asthmatic attack with either inhaled or intravenous magnesium sulfate as a pharmacologic agent is being investigated (Ciarallo et al., 1996; Hill et al., 1996b; Nannini and Hofer, 1997). The availability of DXA as a nutrition assessment test is allowing the study of the effect of the chronic use of prescribed corticosteroids on bone mineral density (Gagnon et al., 1997) (see Chapter 28).

To treat asthma, medications are routinely prescribed, including bronchodilators to relax the airway smooth muscle and anti-inflammatory agents to suppress airway inflammation. Patients may experience numerous, nutritionally relevant, side effects. These include dry mouth and throat, nausea, vomiting, diarrhea, increased serum glucose levels, sodium retention, and hypokalemia, as well as hand tremors, headache, and dizziness (see Chapter 18). Another possible nutritionally related side effect of medications or chronic coughing is gastroesophageal reflux (Paterson, 1997) (see Chapter 30).

ASPIRATION

Pulmonary aspiration, or the movement of food or fluid into the lungs, can result in pneumonia or even death. Proper body positioning when eating is essential for everyone. At increased risk are infants, toddlers, elderly people, and individuals with oral, upper gastrointestinal, neurologic, or muscular abnormalities. Besides liquids, foods that are most easily aspirated include those that are round in shape, such as nuts, popcorn, hot dog pieces, or chunks of inadequately chewed foods, like meat or raw vegetables. Close attention must be given to people receiving enteral tube feedings (see Chapter 22).

LUNG CANCER

Lung cancer almost always is the result of persistent tobacco smoking for many years. However, since the pulmonary system is exposed to the environment, other inhaled pollutants may initiate the malignant condition. The primary sites are usually the bronchi, with subsequent metastasis to other organs, such as the bone, brain, liver, or skin.

In cigarette smokers, food components and specific nutrients have been investigated as either preventive or therapeutic modalities for lung cancer. Findings indicate that high-dose beta-carotene supplements may have a negative impact, but that increased consumption of fruits and vegetables may be beneficial (Handelman, 1997; Ziegler et al., 1996). Because neither successful prevention nor successful management of lung cancer has been elucidated, the possible role of whole foods or its various components in lung cancer's initiation or promotion is receiving worldwide attention (Berwick and Schantz, 1997; El-Bayoumy et al., 1997; Potter, 1997; Menon et al., 1998).

Currently, the medical treatment of lung cancer involves radiation therapy, chemotherapy, and surgery, which are accompanied by various nutritional side effects (see Chapters 33 and 39). Patients with lung cancer experience the added stress of respiratory fatigue and diminished residual capacity. Weight loss, along with an associated decline in other anthropometric and laboratory indicators of cancer-related malnutrition, portends a changing prognosis (Chlebowski et al., 1996.)

Because of the pulmonary constraints in people with lung cancer, purchasing and preparing foods may be overwhelming tasks. Eating may become an unenjoyable activity owing to severe pain, dyspnea, and dyspepsia. Thus, providing foods, beverages, and nutritional supplements in the forms and at the times best tolerated by the patient is essential. Administering oral medications with calorically dense nutritional supplements is another means of supplying needed nutrients (see Chapter 34).

PNEUMONIA AND TUBERCULOSIS

Among the pulmonary infections with nutritional implications are pneumonia and tuberculosis (TB) (Nardell and Kent, 1998). Pneumonia usually occurs as a nosocomial infection or as a consequence of food, fluid, or secretion aspiration. Optimal nutritional status and proper feeding techniques aid in preventing this pulmonary infection (Riquelme et al., 1997). Aspiration is common in babies, children, and adults who are frail, have frequent coughing spasms, are unable effectively to chew or swallow their foods and beverages, or have inadequate head and neck control during eating. Suggestions for preventing aspiration of secretions or food and fluids are located in Chapter 42 and in Table 42–6.

TB has traditionally been diagnosed among economically disadvantaged population groups (e.g., immigrants, homeless persons, and children) or those living in close quarters (e.g., prisoners, refugees), but recently, it is increasingly being recognized as a complication of human immunodeficiency virus (HIV)/AIDS (Madebo et al., 1997) (see Chapter 40). Nutritionally related symptoms of TB include night sweats, fatigue, and hemoptysis.

In both of these pulmonary infections, multiple medications, especially antibiotics, are prescribed. A common medication prescribed in TB is isoniazid (INH). This drug depletes pyridoxine (vitamin B_6) and interferes with vitamin D metabolism. This, in turn, can decrease absorption of calcium and phosphorus (see Chapter 18). Patients thus require increased vitamin and mineral intake, along with increased kilocalories and fluids, and consistent monitoring of laboratory values.

RESPIRATORY FAILURE

Respiratory failure (RF) occurs when the pulmonary system is unable to perform its functions. The causes may be traumatic, surgical, or medical. *Multiple organ dysfunction syndrome (MODS)* is the term used to denote abnormal interaction among the organ systems, culminating in relentless dysfunction of all organ systems. The **adult respiratory distress syndrome (ARDS)** is a common complication of critical illness. Ultimately, in respiratory failure from any cause, the patient requires oxygen, provided through nasal cannula or by mechanical ventilator support, for varying lengths of time and at various levels of oxygen. Central factors in failure to wean from oxygen support or mechanical ventilation are respiratory muscle weakness and retention of carbon dioxide. The prognosis is precarious for patients with underlying chronic pulmonary disease, such as CF or emphysema, or for those who are otherwise medically compromised, malnourished, or elderly. Lung transplantation may be a viable option for some patients, especially for those with cystic fibrosis (Beck et al., 1997; Holcombe and Resler, 1994; Pingleton, 1998.)

Nutritional Status and Assessment

Nutritional needs vary widely within this group of patients, depending on the underlying disease process, prior nutritional status, and the patient's age. Hypercatabolism or hypermetabolism may be present.

As with most pulmonary diseases, body composition fluctuations are the hallmark nutritional assessment indicators for individuals with RF. Most patients become severely underweight. Thus, a battery of accurate anthropometric measurements is crucial over the entire course of treatment, sometimes spanning the patient's lifetime. Accurate interpretation of laboratory results may be confounded by fluid imbalances, medications, and ventilator support. Other nutritionally relevant factors to assess include immunocompetence, chronic mouth breathing, aerophagia, dyspnea, exercise tolerance, and depression.

Nutritional Requirements and Care

The goals of nutritional care in patients with RF are to meet basic nutritional requirements, preserve lean body mass, restore respiratory muscle mass and strength, maintain fluid balance, improve resistance to infection, and facilitate weaning from oxygen support and mechanical ventilation by providing energy substrates without exceeding the respiratory system's capacity to clear carbon dioxide. Methods to provide nutritional support depend on the underlying disease, whether the patient is critically or chronically ill, and whether ventilator support is necessary (Donahoe, 1997; Thomsen, 1997) (see Chapter 22).

Energy

Because of hypercatabolism and hypermetabolism, energy needs are elevated in RF, and sufficient energy must be supplied to prevent the use of the body's own reserves of protein and fat. Energy requirements fluctuate, and so are best determined by continuous individual assessment. To estimate initial caloric requirements, the Harris-Benedict equation, modified for stress as well as the underlying disease, can be used (see Chapter 2). Thereafter, indirect calorimetry is most useful, except for some patients who are mechanically ventilated, as their ventilation procedures may negate the results. Overfeeding should be avoided (Barton et al., 1997).

Macronutrients

Because the patient with RF may be in negative nitrogen balance, protein should be supplied to restore balance. However, enterally supplied protein or parenterally supplied amino acids do affect the respiratory quotient. The basic requirements for carbohydrate and fat as actual nutrients for nourishment are influenced by the underlying organ system decompensation, the patient's respiratory status, and the ventilation methods used. Controversy persists concerning the optimal ratio of protein, fat, and carbohydrate supplied to patients with RF. By general consensus, the most important factor is to provide adequate, but not excessive, kilocalories (Pingleton, 1996.) For example, for the energy prescription, some clinicians start with 1.2–1.4 × REE. Protein is calculated as 1.5–2.0 grams/kg dry body weight. Nonprotein calories are evenly divided between fat and carbohydrate. Daily monitoring of each patient's intake is crucial.

Water requirements must be individualized based upon the method of oxygen delivery and environmental factors, coupled with underlying progressive disease processes and prescribed medications.

Vitamins and Minerals

Exact requirements for specific vitamins and minerals in RF are unknown. It is assumed that vitamins and minerals need to be supplied at least at the level of the RDA, plus repletion, based on the gender and age of the patient. The intake of vitamins and minerals necessary for anabolism, wound healing, and immunity, as well as of those with antioxidant functions, may need to be increased. For example, during anabolism, mineral balance must be monitored in an anticipatory manner to prevent the refeeding syndrome (see Chapter 22). Minerals that function as electrolytes need to be monitored closely, especially because of fluid imbalances and the occurrence of respiratory acidosis or alkalosis. As a side effect of medications, potassium, calcium, and magnesium may be lost in the urine.

Diet Modification

Diet composition and food selections should be planned to accommodate the nutritional requirements, individual preferences, and living arrangements of the patient. Some people participate in outpatient pulmonary rehabilitation programs. Most patients who are not intubated or who have tracheostomies will be able to meet all or most of their nutritional needs by mouth. Small portions and favorite foods enhance oral food intake. Consumption must be monitored to maintain appropriate caloric levels and a suitable ratio of protein, fat, and carbohydrate. Provision of adequate oxygen is crucial for proper digestion and absorption of food. Patients receiving inadequate oxygen may complain of anorexia, early satiety, malaise, bloating, and constipation or diarrhea. Intubated patients usually require enteral tube feedings or parenteral feedings. The gastrointestinal route is preferred, although aspiration and bacterial overgrowth are concerns. Feeding procedures that minimize aspiration include the use of a continuous method of feeding rather than large bolus feedings, tube placement in the duodenum rather than the stomach, chest elevation to at least 45 degrees, frequent evaluation for gastric residuals, and endotracheal tube cuff inflation (Laaban et al., 1993; Schols, 1997).

FUTURE DIRECTIONS

Tremendous advancements have been made in the understanding of pulmonary system physiology, biochemistry, molecular biology, and pharmacology, as well as in medical, surgical, and nutritional technology. A balanced approach to nutritional care, coupled with close individualized assessment and monitoring of each patient's pulmonary condition, is vital. Research studies discovering the mechanisms

CASE STUDY

Sam I. is a 2-year-old with recent weight loss, chronic sinus and ear infections, and wheezing, which caused the pediatrician to investigate for cystic fibrosis. Sweat test results were positive. The family has scheduled an appointment to see you. You have a 3-day food record and dietary pattern on which to base your recommendations. Sam is now using pancreatic enzymes with his meals.

1. What nutritional screening and assessment information would you want before the family arrives for the visit?
2. What foods or nutrients will you highlight in Sam's diet?
3. What is the goal for weight gain? How long should it take, provided Sam's medicines are effective?
4. The family has recently heard about gene therapy and asks you about it. How would you respond?
5. Sam goes to a day care center during the week. What types of lunches could his mother pack for him? What types of instructions should be shared with the day care staff?

for generating energy at the cellular level in respiratory diseases, the methods to promote and maintain body composition of patients, and the specific roles of nutrients and phytonutrients in the etiology or treatment of pulmonary conditions offer promise (Cook et al., 1997; Loft and Poulsen, 1996; Schunemann et al., 1997; Yan et al., 1997).

CITED REFERENCES

Aitken ML, Fiel SB. Cystic fibrosis. Dis Mon 39:1, 1993.

Andersen DH. Cystic fibrosis of the pancreas and its relation to celiac disease: A clinical and pathologic study. Am J Dis Child 56:344, 1938.

Barton RG, et al. Chemical paralysis reduces energy expenditure in patients with burns and severe respiratory failure treated with mechanical ventilation. J Burn Care Rehabil 18:461, 1997.

Beck CE, et al. Improvement in the nutritional and pulmonary profiles of cystic fibrosis patients undergoing bilateral sequential lung and heart-lung transplantation. Nutr Clin Pract 12:216, 1997.

Beker LT, et al. Effect of vitamin K1 supplementation on vitamin K status in cystic fibrosis patients. J Pediatr Gastroenterol Nutr 24:512, 1997.

Benabdeslam H, et al. Biochemical assessment of the nutritional status of cystic fibrosis patients treated with pancreatic enzyme extracts. Am J Clin Nutr 67:912, 1998.

Bentur L, et al. Dietary intakes of young children with cystic fibrosis: Is there a difference? J Pediatr Gastroenterol Nutr 22:254, 1996.

Berwick M, Schantz S. Chemoprevention of aerodigestive cancer. Cancer Metastasis Rev 16:329, 1997.

Boas SR. Exercise recommendations for individuals with cystic fibrosis. Sports Med 24:17, 1997.

Borowitz DS, et al. Use of pancreatic enzyme supplements for patients with cystic fibrosis in the context of fibrosing colonopathy. Consensus Committee. J Pediatr 127:681, 1995.

Bowser EK. Evaluating enteral nutrition support in cystic fibrosis. Top Clin Nutr 5:55, 1990.

Broughton KS, et al. Reduced asthma symptoms with n-3 fatty acid ingestion are related to 5-series leukotriene production. Am J Clin Nutr 65:1011, 1997.

Bruno MJ, et al. Maldigestion associated with exocrine pancreatic insufficiency: Implications of gastrointestinal physiology and properties of enzyme preparations for a cause-related and patient-tailored treatment. Am J Gastroenterol 90:1383, 1995.

Brunton JA, et al. Growth and body composition in infants with bronchopulmonary dysplasia up to 3 months corrected age: A randomized trial of a high energy nutrient enriched formula fed after hospital discharge. J Pediatr 133:340, 1998.

Cannella PC, et al. Feeding practices and nutrition recommendations for infants with cystic fibrosis. J Am Diet Assoc 93:297, 1993.

Celli BR. ATS standards for the optimal management of chronic obstructive pulmonary disease. Respirology 2(suppl 1):S1, 1997.

Chapman KM, Winter L. COPD: Using nutrition to prevent respiratory function decline. Geriatrics 51:37, 1996.

Chlebowski RT, et al. Recent implications of weight loss in lung cancer management. Nutrition 12(suppl):S43, 1996.

Ciarallo L, et al. Intravenous magnesium therapy for moderate to severe pediatric asthma: Results of a randomized, placebo-controlled trial. J Pediatr 129:809, 1996.

Collins CE, et al. Fat gram target to achieve high energy intake in cystic fibrosis. J Paediatr Child Health 33:142, 1997.

Cook DG, et al. Effect of fresh fruit consumption on lung function and wheeze in children. Thorax 52:628, 1997.

Cordova FC, Criner GJ. Management of advanced chronic obstructive pulmonary disease. Compr Ther 23:413, 1997.

Creveling S, et al. Cystic fibrosis, nutrition, and the health care team. J Am Diet Assoc 97(suppl 2):S186, 1997.

Cross C, Halliwell B. Nutrition and human disease: How much extra vitamin C might smokers need? Lancet 341:1091, 1993.

Cynamon HA, et al. Effect of vitamin E deficiency on neurologic function in patients with cystic fibrosis. J Pediatr 113:637, 1988.

Cystic Fibrosis Foundation: Facts about cystic fibrosis. Available at: http://www.cff.org/facts.htm. Accessed May 12, 1999.

Dalzell AM, et al. Nutritional rehabilitation in cystic fibrosis: A 5-year follow-up study. J Pediatr Gastroenterol Nutr 15:141, 1992.

de Meer K, et al. Total energy expenditure in infants with bronchopulmonary dysplasia is associated with respiratory status. Eur J Pediatr 156:299, 1997.

Donahoe M. Nutritional support in advanced lung disease. The pulmonary cachexia syndrome. Clin Chest Med 18:547, 1997.

Dore MF, et al. Role of the thermic effect of food in malnutrition of patients with chronic obstructive pulmonary disease. Am J Respir Crit Care Med 155:1535, 1997.

Duggan MB, Gilbert K. An experimental estimate of the maintenance energy requirement in children with cystic fibrosis. Eur J Clin Nutr 50:251, 1996.

Durie PR, Pencharz PB. A rational approach to the nutritional care of patients with cystic fibrosis. J R Soc Med 82:11, 1989.

El-Bayoumy K, et al. Dietary control of cancer. Proc Soc Exp Biol Med 216:221, 1997.

Farrell PA, Fiascone JM. Bronchopulmonary dysplasia in the 1990s: A review for the pediatrician. Curr Probl Pediatr 27:129, 1997.

Farrell PM, Hubbard VS. Nutrition in cystic fibrosis: Vitamins, fatty acids and minerals. In: Lloyd-Still JD (ed.). Textbook of Cystic Fibrosis. Boston: John Wright-PSG, 1983.

Farrell PM, et al. Nutritional benefits of neonatal screening for cystic fibrosis. N Engl J Med 337:963, 1997.

Gagnon L, et al. Influence of inhaled corticosteroids and dietary intake on bone density and metabolism in patients with moderate to severe asthma. J Am Diet Assoc 97:1401, 1997.

Gaskin KJ. Cystic fibrosis: Nutritional problems and their management. Semin Pediatr Gastrol Nutr 4:9, 1993.

Gavin J, et al. Dietary fibre and the occurrence of gut symptoms in cystic fibrosis. Arch Dis Child 76:35, 1997.

Giacoia GP, et al. Follow-up of school-age children with bronchopulmonary dysplasia. J Pediatr 130:400, 1997.

Green CG, et al. Symptomatic hypomagnesemia in cystic fibrosis. J Pediatr 107:425, 1985.

Gregoire MC, et al. Health and developmental outcomes at 18 months in very preterm infants with bronchopulmonary dysplasia. Pediatrics 101:856, 1998.

Handelman GJ. High-dose vitamin supplements for cigarette smokers: Caution is indicated. Nutr Rev 55:369, 1997.

Hazinski TA. Bronchopulmonary dysplasia. In: Chernick V, Boat TF (eds.). Kendig's Disorders of the Respiratory Tract in Children, 6th ed. Philadelphia: WB Saunders, 1998.

Hill J, et al. Investigation of the effect of short-term change in dietary magnesium intake in asthma. Eur Respir J 10:2225, 1997a.

Hill J, et al. Studies of the effects of inhaled magnesium on airway reactivity to histamine and adenosine monophosphate in asthmatic subjects. Clin Exp Allergy 27:546, 1997b.

Holcombe BJ, Resler R. Nutrition support for lung transplant patients. Nutr Clin Pract 9:235, 1994.

Johnson DB, et al. Nutrition and feeding in infants with bronchopulmonary dysplasia after initial hospital discharge: Risk factors for growth failure. J Am Diet Assoc 98:649, 1998.

Kawchak DA, et al. Longitudinal, prospective analysis of dietary intake in children with cystic fibrosis. J Pediatr 129:119, 1996.

Kerem BS, et al. Identification of the cystic fibrosis gene: Genetic analysis. Science 245:1073, 1989.

Kurzner SI, et al. Growth failure in infants with bronchopulmonary dysplasia: Nutrition and elevated resting metabolic expenditure. Pediatrics 81:379, 1988.

Leichsenring M, et al. (n-6)-Fatty acids in plasma lipids of children with atopic bronchial asthma. Pediatr Allergy Immunol 6:209, 1995.

Levy E, et al. Lipoprotein abnormalities associated with cholesteryl ester transfer activity in cystic fibrosis patients: The role of essential fatty acid deficiency. Am J Clin Nutr 57:573, 1993.
Loft S, Poulsen HE. Cancer risk and oxidative DNA damage in man. J Mol Med 74:297, 1996.
Madebo T, et al. HIV infection and malnutrition change the clinical and radiological features of pulmonary tuberculosis. Scand J Infect Dis 29:355, 1997.
Marcus MS, et al. Nutritional status of infants with cystic fibrosis associated with early diagnosis and intervention. Am J Clin Nutr 54:578, 1991.
Menon LG, et al. Effect of isoflavones genistein and diadzein in the inhibition of lung metastasis in mice induced by B16F-10 melanoma cells. Nutr Cancer 30:74, 1998.
Michel SH, Mueller DH. Practical approaches to nutrition care of patients with cystic fibrosis. Top Clin Nutr 4:46, 1989.
Michel SH, Mueller DH. Impact of lactation on women with cystic fibrosis and their infants: A review of five cases. J Am Diet Assoc 94:159, 1994.
Michel SH, Mueller DH. Nutrition and cystic fibrosis. J Respir Care Pract/RT April/May:27, 1995.
Mischler EH, et al. Demineralization in cystic fibrosis. Am J Dis Child 133:632, 1979.
Monteleone CA, Sherman AR. Nutrition and asthma. Arch Intern Med 157:23, 1997.
Mueller DH. Timeliness of codifying nutrition ABCDEs for BPD. J Pediatr 133:315, 1998.
Murphy MD, et al. Resting energy expenditures measured by indirect calorimetry are higher in preadolescent children with cystic fibrosis than expenditures calculated from prediction equations. J Am Diet Assoc 95:30, 1995.
Nannini LJ Jr, Hofer D. Effect of inhaled magnesium sulfate on sodium metabisulfite-induced bronchoconstriction in asthma. Chest 111:858, 1997.
Nardell EA, Kent D. Respiratory infections in the economically disadvantaged. In: Fishman AP, et al. (eds.). Fishman's Pulmonary Diseases and Disorders, 3rd ed., vol. 2. New York: McGraw-Hill, 1998.
Nishimura Y, et al. Relationship between changes of bone mineral content and twelve-minute walking distance in men with chronic obstructive pulmonary disease: A longitudinal study. Intern Med 36:450, 1997.
Oh W. Nutritional management of infants with bronchopulmonary dysplasia. Bronchopulmonary dysplasia and related chronic respiratory disorders. In: Report of the 90th Ross Conference on Pediatric Research, Ross Laboratories, Columbus, OH, 1986.
Paterson WG. Extraesophageal complications of gastroesophageal reflux disease. Can J Gastroenterol 11 (suppl B):45B, 1997.
Peters SA, Kelly FJ. Vitamin E supplementation in cystic fibrosis. J Pediatr Gastroenterol Nutr 22:341, 1996.
Pingleton SK. Enteral nutrition in patients with respiratory disease. Eur Respir J 9:364, 1996.
Pingleton SK. Nutrition in acute respiratory failure. In: Fishman AP, et al. (eds.). Fishman's Pulmonary Diseases and Disorders, 3rd ed., vol. 2. New York: McGraw-Hill, 1998.
Pond MN, et al. Functional iron deficiency in adults with cystic fibrosis. Respir Med 90:409, 1996.
Potter JD. Beta-carotene and the role of intervention studies. Cancer Lett 114:329, 1997.
Ramsey BW, et al. Nutritional assessment and management in cystic fibrosis: A consensus report. Am J Clin Nutr 55:108, 1992.
Reiter EO, et al. Vitamin D metabolites in adolescents and young adults with cystic fibrosis: Effects of sun and season. J Pediatr 106:21, 1985.
Riordan J, et al. Identification of the cystic fibrosis gene: Cloning and characterization of the complementary DNA. Science 245:1066, 1989.
Riquelme R, et al. Community-acquired pneumonia in the elderly. Clinical and nutritional aspects. Am J Respir Crit Care Med 156:1908, 1997.
Robbins ST, Fletcher AB. Early vs delayed vitamin A supplementation in very-low-birth weight infants. J Parenter Enteral Nutr 17:220, 1993.
Rossi A, et al. Aging and the respiratory system. Aging 8:143, 1996.
Salamoni F, et al. Bone mineral content in cystic fibrosis patients: Correlation with fat-free mass. Arch Dis Child 74:314, 1996.
Saudny-Unterberger H, et al. Impact of nutritional support on functional status during an acute exacerbation of chronic obstructive pulmonary disease. Am J Respir Crit Care Med 156(3 Pt. 1):794, 1997.
Schols AM. Nutrition and outcome in chronic respiratory disease. Nutrition 13:161, 1997.
Schunemann HJ, et al. Oxidative stress and lung function. Am J Epidemiol 146:939, 1997.
Schwab RJ. Control of respiration during sleep. In: Grippi MA. (ed.). Pulmonary Pathophysiology. Philadelphia: JB Lippincott, 1995.
Schwartz J, Weiss ST. Caffeine intake and asthma symptoms. Ann Epidemiol 2:627, 1992.
Sharer N, et al. Mutations of the cystic fibrosis gene in patients with chronic pancreatitis. N Engl J Med 339:645, 1998.
Sokol RJ, et al. Fat-soluble vitamins in infants identified by cystic fibrosis newborn screening. Pediatr Pulmonol [Suppl] 7:52, 1991.
Soutar A, et al. Bronchial reactivity and dietary antioxidants. Thorax 52:166, 1997.
Stark LJ, et al. Descriptive analysis of eating behavior in school-age children with cystic fibrosis and healthy control children. Pediatrics 99:665, 1997.
Thomsen C. Nutritional support in advanced pulmonary disease. Respir Med 91:249, 1997.
Tomezsko JL, et al. Dietary intake of healthy children with cystic fibrosis compared with normal control children. Pediatrics 90:547, 1992.
Verma RP, et al. Vitamin A deficiency and severe bronchopulmonary dysplasia in very low birthweight infants. Am J Perinatol 13:389, 1996.
Weiss ST. Diet as a risk factor for asthma. Ciba Found Symp 206:244, 1997.
Williams CP. Pediatric Manual of Clinical Dietetics. Chicago: American Dietetic Association, 1998.
Winklhofer-Roob, B. Nutritional status in cystic fibrosis: Where to go from here? Am J Clin Nutr 67:817, 1998.
Yan L, et al. Effect of dietary supplementation of selenite on pulmonary metastasis of melanoma cells in mice. Nutr Cancer 28:165, 1997.
Ziegler RG, et al. Nutrition and lung cancer. Cancer Causes Control 7:157, 1996.
Ziment I. Alternative therapies for asthma. Curr Opin Pulmon Med 3:61, 1997.
Zipf W, et al. Consensus conference on CF-related diabetes mellitus. In: Concepts in Care, vol. 1, sect. IV, pt. 7. Bethesda, MD: Cystic Fibrosis Foundation, 1990, p. 1.

ADDITIONAL REFERENCES

Andreoli TE, et al. Cecil Essentials of Medicine, 4th ed. Philadelphia: WB Saunders, 1997.
Collins FS. Cystic fibrosis: Molecular biology and therapeutic implications. Science 256:774, 1992.
Dodge JA. Nutrition in cystic fibrosis: A historical overview. Proc Nutr Soc 51:225, 1992.
Dumas C, et al. Body composition of children with chronic lung disease. Pediatr Pulmonol [Suppl] 16:174, 1997.
Durie PR. Cystic fibrosis: Gastrointestinal and hepatic complications and their management. Semin Pediatr Gastroenterol Nutr 4:3, 1993.
Durie PR. Pancreatitis and mutations of the cystic fibrosis gene (Editorial). N Engl J Med 339:687, 1998.
Escott-Stump S. Nutrition and Diagnosis-Related Care, 4th ed. Baltimore: Williams & Wilkins, 1998.
Matarese LE. Contemporary Nutrition Support Practice: A Clinical Guide. Philadelphia: WB Saunders, 1997.
Ryan CF, et al. Energy balance in stable malnourished patients with chronic obstructive pulmonary disease. Chest 103:1038, 1993.
Vrlenich LA, et al. The effect of bronchopulmonary dysplasia on growth at school age. Pediatrics 95:855, 1995.
West JB. Pulmonary Pathophysiology: The Essentials. Baltimore: Williams & Wilkins, 1998.

CHAPTER 38

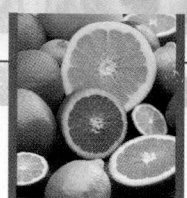

Medical Nutrition Therapy for Renal Disorders

KATY G. WILKENS, MS, RD

Chapter Outline

- Physiology and Function of the Kidneys
- Diseases of the Kidney
- Progressive Nature of Renal Disease
- End-Stage Renal Disease
- Human Immunodeficiency Virus and Renal Disease

Key Terms

ACUTE GLOMERULONEPHRITIDES—a group of diseases characterized by inflammation of the capillary loops of the glomerulus

AZOTEMIA—the accumulation in the blood of abnormal quantities of urea, uric acid, creatinine, and other nitrogenous wastes

L-CARNITINE—an amino acid synthesized in the kidney; required for mitochondrial oxidation of long-chain fatty acids; usually low in dialysis patients; supplementation associated with improved muscle function and less leg cramping

CONTINUOUS ARTERIOVENOUS HEMOFILTRATION (CAVH)—a method of acute renal failure management in which an ultrafiltration membrane, powered by the patient's own blood, produces an ultrafiltrate that can then be replaced by parenteral nutrition fluids

DIALYSATE—the solution used in dialysis to remove waste products and excess fluids from the blood; similar to plasma but without waste products

END-STAGE RENAL DISEASE—a disease characterized by the kidney's inability to excrete waste products, maintain fluid and electrolyte balance, and produce hormones

ERYTHROPOIETIN—a hormone secreted chiefly by the kidney in the adult and by the liver in the fetus, which acts on stem cells of the bone marrow to stimulate red blood cell production

GLOMERULAR FILTRATION RATE (GFR)—the quantity of glomerular filtrate formed per unit in all nephrons of both kidneys

HEMODIALYSIS—a method of clearing waste products from the blood in which blood passes by the semipermeable membrane of the artificial kidney and waste products are removed by diffusion

ISCHEMIC ACUTE TUBULAR NECROSIS—extensive kidney tissue destruction resulting from a prolonged episode of blood deprivation

METASTATIC CALCIFICATION—the deposition of calcium in tissues as a result of abnormalities in calcium and phosphate levels in the blood and fluids

NEPHRITIC SYNDROME—the syndrome of hematuria, hypertension, and mild loss of renal function that results from acute inflammation of the capillary loops of the glomerulus

NEPHROLITHIASIS—a condition marked by the presence of renal calculi (stones)

NEPHROTIC SYNDROME—a condition resulting from loss of the glomerular barrier to protein; characterized by massive edema, proteinuria, hypoalbuminemia, hypercholesterolemia, hypercoagulability, and abnormal bone metabolism

OLIGURIA—the condition of having urinary volumes of less than 500 mL/day

OSTEITIS FIBROSA CYSTICA—inflammation of the bone with fibrous degeneration and formation of cysts secondary to parathyroid gland hyperfunction

PERITONEAL DIALYSIS—a method of removing waste products from the blood in which diffusion carries them from the blood through the semipermeable peritoneal membrane and into the dialysate

PYELONEPHRITIS—urinary tract infection

RENAL FAILURE—the inability of a kidney to excrete the daily load of wastes

RENAL OSTEODYSTROPHY—metabolic bone disease as a complication of end-stage renal disease

RENAL TUBULAR ACIDOSIS—a defect in tubular handling of bicarbonate, treated by different methods that are cause specific

RENIN–ANGIOTENSIN MECHANISM—a major control of blood pressure involving kidney-secreted renin that acts in the plasma to form angiotensin I, which is converted to angiotensin II, a powerful vasoconstrictor and potent stimulus of aldosterone secretion by the adrenal gland

This chapter was generously reviewed by Kerri Wiggins, MS, RD, Renal Dietitian, Skagit Valley Kidney Center, Mt. Vernon, WA.

SOLUTE LOAD—the end waste products of metabolism

UREMIA—a clinical syndrome of malaise, weakness, nausea and vomiting, muscle cramps, itching, metallic mouth taste, and often neurologic impairment, which is brought about by an unacceptable level of nitrogenous wastes in the blood

PHYSIOLOGY AND FUNCTION OF THE KIDNEYS

The main function of the kidney is to maintain homeostatic balance with respect to fluids, electrolytes, and organic solutes. The normal kidney has the ability to perform this function over a wide range of dietary fluctuations in sodium, water, and various solutes. This task is accomplished by the continuous filtration of blood and by alterations (secretion and reabsorption) in this filtered fluid. The kidney receives 20% of cardiac output, which allows the filtering of approximately 1600 L/day of blood. Approximately 180 liters of fluid (ultrafiltrate) is produced in filtering this blood, and through active processes of reabsorbing certain components and secreting others, the composition of this fluid is changed into the 1.5 liters of urine excreted in an average day.

Each kidney consists of approximately 1 million functioning units called nephrons (Fig. 38–1). The *nephron* consists of a *glomerulus* connected to a series of *tubules*, which can be broken into functionally different segments: the proximal convoluted tubule, loop of Henle, distal tubule, and collecting duct. Each nephron functions independently in producing a contribution to the final urine, although all are under similar control and are thus coordinated. Nevertheless, when one segment of a nephron is destroyed, that complete nephron is no longer functional.

The glomerulus is a spherical mass of capillaries surrounded by a membrane, *Bowman's capsule.* The function of the glomerulus is to produce the large amount of ultrafiltrate, which the ensuing segments of the nephron then modify. The ultrafiltrate produced in the glomerulus is very similar in composition to blood. Due to its barrier function,

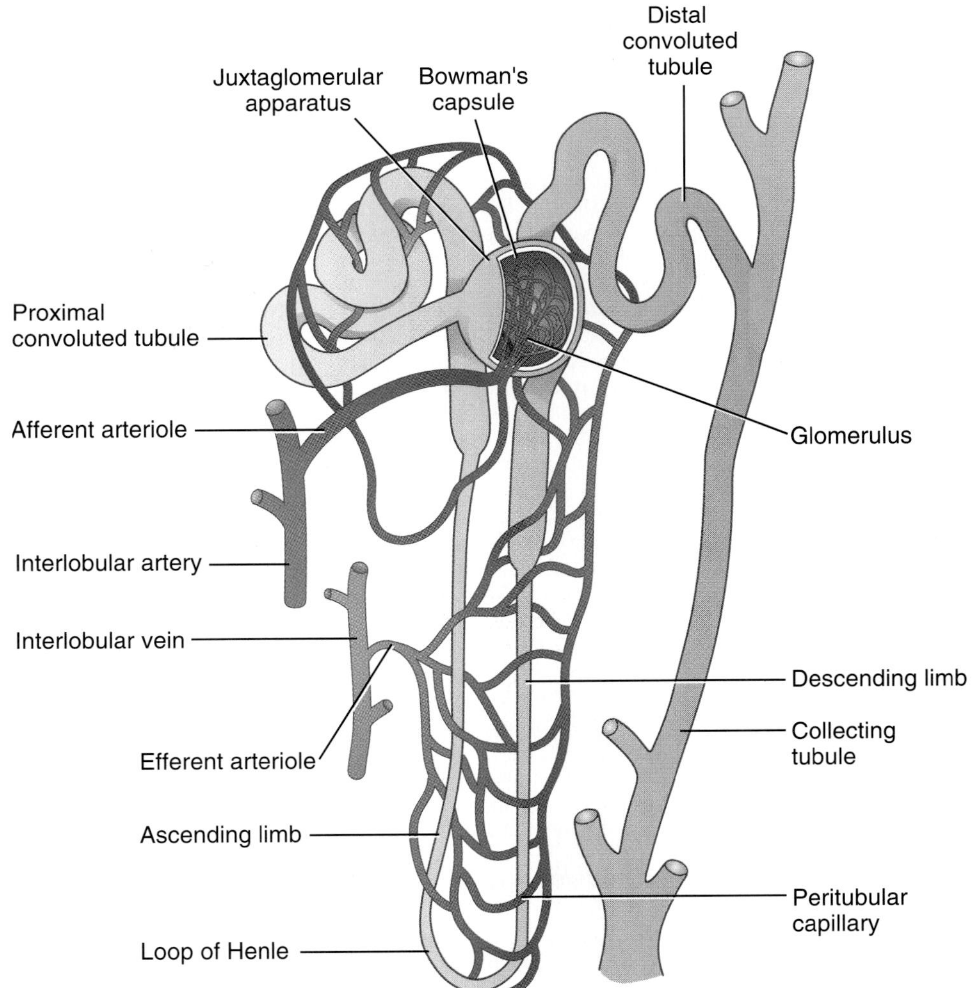

FIGURE 38–1 The nephron.

the glomerulus blocks blood cells as well as molecules of molecular weight greater than 6500, most notably protein. The production of ultrafiltrate is mainly passive, relying on the perfusion pressure generated by the heart and supplied by the renal artery.

The tubules reabsorb the vast majority of components that compose the ultrafiltrate. Much of this process is active and requires a large expenditure of energy in the form of adenosine triphosphate. Due to a unique structure, differences in permeabilities between the various segments, and the response to hormonal control, the tubule is able to produce a final urine, which can vary widely in concentration of sodium, potassium, other electrolytes, osmolality, pH, and volume.

Ultimately, the final urine produced is funneled into common *collecting tubules* and into the *renal pelvis*. The renal pelvis narrows into a single *ureter* per kidney, and each ureter carries urine into the bladder, where it accumulates before elimination.

Although the homeostatic mechanisms are interrelated to a large extent, occasional demands are placed on the kidney to regulate one substance while sacrificing tight control of others. In this regard, the control of circulating blood volume predominates over the control of all other parameters. Thus sodium, the most important molecule in determining the body's circulating volume, is regulated at the expense of all other substances. A gain or loss of 1% of circulating volume is reflected in marked changes in urine as well as in serum composition of potassium, bicarbonate, and water.

The kidney has almost unlimited ability to regulate water homeostasis. Owing to its ability to form a large concentration gradient between its inner medulla and outer cortex, the kidney can excrete urine as dilute as 50 mOsm or as concentrated as 1200 mOsm. Given a daily fixed **solute load** of about 600 mOsm (the solute load representing the end waste products of normal metabolism), the kidney can get rid of as little as 500 mL of concentrated urine or as much as 12 liters. Control of water excretion is regulated by *antidiuretic hormone* (ADH), a small peptide hormone secreted by the posterior pituitary. An excess of relative body water, indicated by a fall in osmolality, leads to prompt shutoff of all ADH secretion. Likewise, a small rise in osmolality brings about marked ADH secretion and retention of water. However, the need to conserve sodium sometimes leads to a sacrifice of the homeostatic control of water for the sake of volume.

The minimum urinary volume capable of eliminating a relatively fixed 600 mOsm of solute is 500 mL, assuming that the kidney is capable of maximum concentration. Urinary volume of less than 500 mL/day is called **oliguria;** it is impossible for such a small urine volume to eliminate all of the daily waste.

The majority of the solute load consists of nitrogenous wastes, largely the end products of protein metabolism. Urea predominates in amounts depending on the protein content of the diet; uric acid, creatinine, and ammonia are present in small amounts. If these normal waste products are not eliminated appropriately, they collect in abnormal quantities in the blood, a condition known as **azotemia.** The ability of the kidney to adequately eliminate nitrogenous waste products is known as *renal function*; **renal failure** is the consequence of inability to excrete the daily load of these wastes.

The kidney also performs functions unrelated to excretion. One of these involves the **renin–angiotensin mechanism,** a major control of blood pressure. Decreased blood volume causes cells of the glomerulus (the *juxtaglomerular apparatus*) to react by secreting renin, a proteolytic enzyme. Renin acts in the plasma to form *angiotensin I,* which is converted to *angiotensin II*, a powerful vasoconstrictor and a potent stimulus of aldosterone secretion by the adrenal gland. As a consequence, sodium is reabsorbed, and blood pressure is returned to normal.

The kidney also produces the hormone **erythropoietin,** a critical determinant of erythroid activity in the bone marrow. Deficiency of erythropoietin is a factor in the severe anemia present in chronic renal disease.

Maintenance of *calcium–phosphorus homeostasis* involves the complex interactions of parathyroid hormone (PTH), calcitonin, vitamin D, and three effector organs, the gut, kidney, and bone. The role of the kidney includes production of the active form of vitamin D—$1,25(OH)_2D_3$—as well as elimination of both calcium and phosphorus. Active vitamin D promotes efficient absorption of calcium by the gut and is one of the substances necessary for bone remodeling and maintenance (see Chapter 28).

DISEASES OF THE KIDNEY

The manifestations of renal disease are a direct consequence of the portion of the nephron most affected. These manifestations include (1) nephrotic syndrome, (2) nephritic syndrome, (3) acute renal failure (ARF), (4) tubular defects, (5) renal stones, and finally (6) end-stage renal disease (ESRD). Objectives of nutritional care depend on the abnormality being treated.

Glomerular Diseases

The functions of the glomerulus that are important with respect to disease are production of an adequate ultrafiltrate and prevention of certain substances from entering this ultrafiltrate.

Nephrotic Syndrome

Nephrotic syndrome consists of a heterogeneous group of diseases whose common manifestations derive from a loss of the glomerular barrier to protein. Large protein losses in the urine lead to hypoalbuminemia with consequent edema, hypercholesterolemia, hypercoagulability, and abnormal bone metabolism.

More than 95% of the cases of nephrotic syndrome stem from three systemic diseases (diabetes mellitus, systemic lupus erythematosus [SLE], and amyloidosis) and four diseases primarily of the kidney (minimal change disease [disease seen only with electron microscopy], membranous nephropathy, focal glomerulosclerosis, and membranoproliferative glomerulonephritis). Although renal function can deteriorate during the course of these diseases, it is not a consistent feature (Hricik et al., 1998).

NUTRITIONAL CARE

The primary objective is to manage the symptoms associated with the syndrome (edema, hypoalbuminemia, and hyperlipidemia), decrease the risk of progression to renal failure, and maintain nutritional stores. Patients with an established severe protein deficiency who continue to lose protein may require an extended time of carefully supervised nutritional care.

The diet should attempt to provide sufficient protein and energy to maintain a positive nitrogen balance and to produce an increase in plasma albumin concentration and disappearance of edema. An increase in albumin and positive nitrogen balance are not always acheiveable, as a high protein diet often leads to increased urinary losses (Mitch, 1996). The dietary protein level for patients with nephrotic syndrome remains controversial. Historically, these patients received diets high in protein (up to 1.5 g/kg/day) in an attempt to increase serum albumin and prevent protein malnutrition. However, studies have shown that a reduction of protein intake to as low as 0.8 mg/kg/day can decrease proteinuria without adversely affecting serum albumin. To allow for optimal protein use, three fourths of the protein should be from sources of high biologic value (HBV), and energy intake should be about 35 kcal/kg/day for adults and 100 to 150 kcal/kg/day for children (Kaysen, 1997).

Edema, the most clinically apparent manifestation of this group of diseases, indicates a state of total body sodium overload. Yet, due to the low oncotic pressure in the circulating blood volume that results from hypoalbuminemia, the volume of circulating blood may be reduced. Attempts to limit sodium intake more than modestly, and attempts to eliminate large amounts of extra sodium with diuretics, can result in marked hypotension, exacerbation of the coagulopathy, and deterioration of renal function. Control of edema in this group of diseases should therefore not be complete, should rely to some extent on elastic full-length support hose, and should entail only modest sodium restriction, approximately 3 g of sodium daily (see Chapter 36).

The important consequence of hypercholesterolemia lies in the potential for inducing cardiovascular disease. Although a satisfactory answer is not apparent, it is believed that patients with longstanding nephrotic syndrome are at increased risk (Toto, 1996). Many pediatric patients with frequently relapsing or resistant nephrotic syndrome are at particular risk for premature atherosclerosis. Certain lipid-lowering agents, when combined with a cholesterol-lowering diet, can reduce total cholesterol, low-density lipoprotein (LDL) cholesterol, and triglycerides in patients with nephrotic syndrome (see Chapter 26).

Nephritic Syndrome

Nephritic syndrome incorporates the clinical manifestations of a group of diseases characterized by inflammation of the capillary loops of the glomerulus. These diseases, also referred to as **acute glomerulonephritides,** are sudden in onset, last a short time, and proceed to either complete recovery, development of chronic nephrotic syndrome (as already discussed), or ESRD.

The primary manifestation of these diseases is *hematuria* (blood in the urine), a consequence of the capillary inflammation that damages the glomerular barrier to blood cells. The syndrome is also characterized by hypertension and by mild loss of renal function. The most common presentation follows a streptococcal infection and is usually, although not always, self-limiting. Other causes include primary kidney diseases, such as IgA nephropathy and hereditary nephritis, as well as secondary diseases, such as SLE, vasculitides, and glomerulonephritis associated with endocarditis, abscesses, or infected ventriculoperitoneal shunts.

NUTRITIONAL CARE

The treatment of acute glomerulonephritis attempts to maintain good nutritional status while allowing time for the disease to resolve spontaneously. In patients in whom an underlying disease is responsible, treatment of that disease predominates and largely determines outcome. There is no reason to restrict protein or potassium intake unless significant uremia or hyperkalemia develops. When hypertension is present, it is related mainly to extracellular volume excess and should be treated with sodium restriction.

Diseases of the Tubules and Interstitium

To a great extent, the functions of the kidney tubules make them susceptible to injury. The enormous energy requirements and expenditures of the tubules in performing the work of active secretion and reabsorption leave this part of the kidney particularly vulnerable to ischemic injuries. High local concentrations of many toxic drugs can destroy or damage various segments of the tubules. Finally, the high-solute concentration generated in the medullary interstitium exposes it to the damage from oxidants and precipitation of calcium–phosphate product (extraosseous calcification) and favors the sickling of red blood cells in sickle cell anemia.

Acute Renal Failure

Acute renal failure (ARF) is characterized by a sudden reduction in **glomerular filtration rate (GFR)** and an alteration in the ability of the kidney to excrete the daily production of metabolic waste (Fig. 38–2). It can occur in association with either a reduction in urine output (*oliguria,* strictly defined as production of less than 500 mL in 24 hours) or normal urine flow. ARF typically occurs in previously healthy kidneys. Its duration varies from a few days to several weeks. The causes of ARF are numerous and often several occur simultaneously (Table 38–1). These causes are generally classified into three categories: (1) inadequate renal perfusion (*prerenal*), (2) diseases within the renal parenchyma *(intrinsic),* and (3) obstruction (*postrenal*). Generally, if careful attention is directed at diagnosing and correcting the prerenal and obstructive causes, ARF is short-lived and requires no particular nutritional intervention.

Intrinsic ARF can result from toxic drug exposure, a local allergic reaction to drugs, rapidly progressive glomerulonephritis, or a prolonged episode of ischemia leading to **ischemic acute tubular necrosis.** Of these, the latter is the most devastating. Typically, patients develop this illness as a complication of sustained shock due to an overwhelming infection, severe trauma, surgical accident, or cardiogenic shock.

The clinical course and outcome depend mainly on the underlying cause. Patients with ARF caused by drug toxicity generally recover fully after they stop taking the drug. On the other hand, the mortality rate associated with ischemic acute tubular necrosis due to shock is approximately 70%. Typically, these patients are highly catabolic, and extensive tissue destruction occurs in the early stages. Hemodialysis is used to reduce the acidosis, correct the uremia, and control hyperkalemia.

If recovery is to occur, it generally takes place within 2 to 3 weeks of the time when the underlying insults have been corrected. The recovery (diuretic) phase is characterized first by an increase in urine output and later by a return of waste elimination. During this period, dialysis may still be required, and careful attention must be paid to fluid and electrolyte balance and appropriate replacement.

NUTRITIONAL CARE

Nutritional care in ARF is particularly important because the patient not only has uremia, metabolic acidosis and fluid and electrolyte imbalance, but usually also suffers from physiologic stress (e.g., infection or tissue destruction) that increases protein needs. The problem of balancing protein and energy needs with treatment of acidosis and excessive nitrogenous waste is complicated and delicate (see Chapter 33).

In the early stages of ARF, the patient is often moribund and is unable to eat. It has been clearly shown that early attention to nutritional status, often in the form of total parenteral nutrition (TPN) and early dialysis, have a positive impact on patient survival (Molina, 1995).

Replacement of renal function during ARF can be carried out as standard hemodialysis, peritoneal dialysis, or **continuous arteriovenous hemofiltration (CAVH).** CAVH uses a small ultrafiltration membrane powered by the patient's own blood to produce an ultrafiltrate that can be replaced by parenteral nutrition fluids. This allows parenteral feeding without fluid overload.

TABLE 38–1 SOME CAUSES OF ACUTE RENAL FAILURE

PRERENAL
Severe dehydration
Circulatory collapse
INTRINSIC
Acute tubular necrosis
Trauma, surgery
Septicemia
Nephrotoxicity
Antibiotics, contrast agents and other drugs
Vascular disorders
Bilateral renal infarction
Acute glomerulonephritis of any cause
Poststreptococcal infection
Systemic lupus erythematosus
POSTRENAL OBSTRUCTION
Benign prostatic hypertrophy
Carcinoma of the bladder or prostate
Ureterovesical stricture

PROTEIN

At the onset of ARF, when few patients can tolerate oral feedings because of vomiting and diarrhea, intravenous (IV) preparations can be used to reduce protein catabolism. Giving carbohydrate alone (e.g., 100 g over a 24-hour period) only reduces protein breakdown by 50%. The preferred treatment is parenteral administration of glucose, lipids, and a mixture of essential and nonessential amino acids. This reduces the protein catabolism and urea production to a minimum until the patient can tolerate oral feeding.

Considerations regarding the amount of protein that should be given to the patient with ARF must balance the extraordinary catabolic needs of a patient in intensive care with the inability to excrete

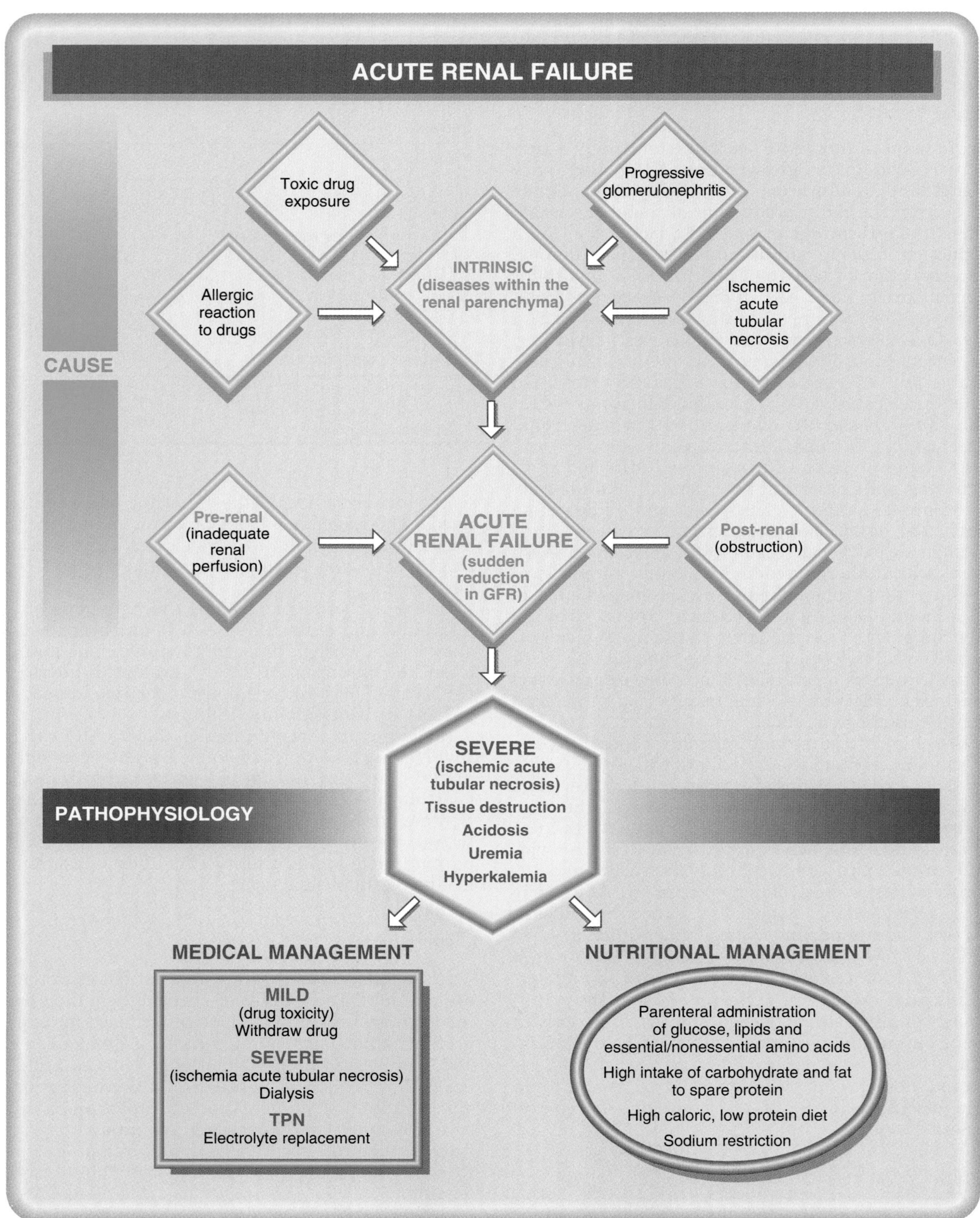

FIGURE 38–2 Pathophysiology algorithm—acute renal failure. (Algorithm content developed by John Anderson, Ph.D., and Sanford C. Garner, Ph.D., 2000.)

the fluid, electrolytes, and solute that this treatment requires. Often these patients can receive continuous renal replacement therapies, such as CAVH, or *continuous venovenous hemofiltration (CVVH),* which are ongoing treatments, rather than periodic dialysis. A large protein load may otherwise necessitate more frequent dialysis, often in a patient who is not hemodynamically stable, and the patient is at high risk for dialysis complications. This issue is therefore quite controversial. The amount of protein recommended is influenced by the underlying cause of ARF and the presence of other conditions. A range of recommended levels can be found in the literature, from 0.5 to 0.8 g/kg for nondialysis patients, to 1.0 to 2.0 g/kg for dialyzed patients. As the patient's overall medical status stabilizes and improves, metabolic requirements decrease, and dialysis becomes less hazardous. During this stable period before renal function returns, it is generally agreed that a daily protein intake of 0.8 to 1.0 g/kg of ideal body weight (IBW) should be given.

ENERGY

Energy requirements are determined by the underlying cause of ARF and comorbidity. Energy needs can be measured at the bedside by indirect calorimetry in most intensive care settings. If this equipment is not available, calorie needs should be estimated at 30 to 40 kcal/kg dry weight/day. Excessive calorie intake can lead to excess CO_2 production. If peritoneal dialysis or *continuous renal replacement therapy (CRRT)* is used, the amount of glucose absorbed can add significantly to the daily energy intake and should be calculated. Large intakes of carbohydrate and fat will prevent the use of protein for energy production. For patients receiving TPN, high concentrations of both carbohydrate and lipid can be administered to fulfill these needs, as long as respiratory concerns are monitored.

A high-calorie, low-protein diet may be used in cases where dialysis or hemofiltration are unavailable. In addition to the usual dietary sources of refined sweets and fats, special high-calorie, low-protein, and low-electrolyte formulas have been developed to augment the diet. Care must be taken with these products, however, because hyperglycemia is not uncommon secondary to glucose intolerance. Insulin is often needed (see Appendix 37).

FLUID AND SODIUM BALANCE

During the early (often oliguric) phase of ARF, meticulous attention to fluid status is essential. Ideally, fluid and electrolyte intake should balance the net output. With negligible urine output, significant contributions to total body water output include emesis and diarrhea, body cavity drains, and skin and respiratory losses. If fever is present, skin losses can be excessive, whereas if the patient is on humidified air, almost no respiratory losses occur. Table 38–2 provides an example of a water requirements calculation. Due to the numerous IV drugs as well as blood and blood products necessitated by the underlying disease, the challenge in managing patients at this point becomes how to cut fluid intake as much as possible while providing adequate protein and energy.

Sodium is restricted depending on the level of urinary excretion. In the oliguric phase when the sodium output is very low, an attempt is made to keep intake low as well, perhaps as low as 20 to 40 mEq/day. However, it is often impossible to limit sodium, due to the requirement for many IV solutions (including IV antibiotics, medications for blood pressure, and TPN). The administration of these solutions in electrolyte-free water, in the face of oliguria, quickly leads to water intoxication (hyponatremia). For this reason, all fluid above the daily calculated water loss should be presented in a balanced salt solution.

POTASSIUM BALANCE

Most of the excretion of potassium and the control of potassium balance are normal functions of the kidney. When renal function is impaired, potassium balance should be scrutinized carefully. In addition to dietary sources, all body tissues contain large amounts of potassium; thus tissue destruction can lead to tremendous overload. Potassium levels can shift abruptly and need to be monitored fre-

TABLE 38–2 SAMPLE CALCULATION OF FLUID REQUIREMENTS IN ACUTE RENAL FAILURE

LOSSES	
Measured urine output of previous 24 h	–200 mL
Insensible water loss in 24 h (varies with room temperature, room humidity, and body temperature)	–500 mL
Total water loss in 24 h	–700 mL
INPUT	
Water produced by metabolism in 24 h (provided catabolism and weight loss are not occurring)	500 mL
Water to allow for fluid gain	1000 mL
Water in usual diet in 24 h	500 mL
Additional fluid intake needed in 24 h to replace losses in urine	200 mL
Total fluid gain in 24 h	1700 mL
Total fluid gain minus total fluid loss = fluid gain for 24 h	1700 mL – 700 mL = 1000mL
24-h fluid gain times 2 days between dialyses	1000 × 2 = 2 L fluid gain between dialysis treatments

quently. Potassium intake needs to be individualized according to serum levels.

The primary mechanism of potassium removal during ARF is dialysis. Control of serum potassium levels between dialysis administrations relies mainly on IV infusions of glucose, insulin, and bicarbonate, all of which serve to drive potassium into cells.

Exchange resins such as Kayexalate, which exchange K^+ for Na^+ in the gastrointestinal tract, can be used to treat high K^+ concentrations, but for many reasons these resins are less than ideal. The treatment is unpleasant, regardless of whether it is given orally or by retention enema. In addition, because it can gel in the gastrointestinal tract causing obstruction, it must be given with sorbitol, a nonabsorbable sugar that induces diarrhea. Administration requires a functioning gastrointestinal tract with respect to both absorption and motility, which the critically ill patient often does not have. Finally, the exchanged sodium leads to volume overload, which must also be controlled mainly by dialysis during renal failure. Table 38–3 summarizes medical nutrition therapy for ARF.

Other Tubular or Interstitial Diseases

There is a wide variety of diseases or disorders of the tubules and interstitium. They share common manifestations and can be considered together with respect to dietary management.

Chronic interstitial nephritis can occur as a result of analgesic abuse, sickle cell disease, diabetes mellitus, or vesicoureteral reflux and manifests primarily as an inability to concentrate the urine and as mild renal insufficiency. A hereditary disorder of the interstitium, *medullary cystic disease,* also presents this picture. Dietary management consists of adequate fluid intake, which can require several liters of extra fluid. This is generally quite well tolerated by the patient, except when intercurrent illness occurs.

Fanconi syndrome is characterized by an inability to reabsorb the proper amount of glucose, amino acids, phosphate, and bicarbonate in the proximal tubule, leading to excretion of these substances in the urine. Adults with this syndrome present with acidosis, hypokalemia, polyuria, or osteomalacia, whereas children present with polyuria, growth retardation, rickets, or vomiting. No specific medical treatment is usually available; therefore, dietary treatment is the main form of management. Replacement therapy usually consists of large volumes of water, as well as dietary supplements of bicarbonate, potassium, phosphate, calcium, and vitamin D.

Other tubular defects, generally affecting reabsorption of only a single solute, are treated with replacement of that particular solute. **Renal tubular acidosis (RTA),** a defect in tubular handling of bicarbonate, can be caused by either a *proximal tubular defect (type 2)* or a *defect in the distal tubule (type 1).* The proximal lesion can be associated with other proximal defects, such as in the Fanconi syndrome, and has very little clinical significance by itself, whereas distal RTA leads to severe osteomalacia, kidney stones, and often nephrocalcinosis (calcification of the kidney). Distal RTA is treated with small amounts of bicarbonate, 70 to 100 mEq/day, with complete resolution of disease manifestations. *Isolate proximal RTA* in the adult is a benign disease, which is often made worse with bicarbonate treatment and should therefore not be treated.

Pyelonephritis

Pyelonephritis, also commonly known as urinary tract infection, does not require extensive dietary management. In chronic cases, however, the use of cranberry juice to reduce bacteriuria has been verified in a double-blind study (Avorn et al., 1994). Concentrated tannins or proanthocyanidins in cranberry juice and apparently blueberry juice seem to inhibit the adherence of *Escherichia coli* bacteria to the epithelial cells of the urinary tract (Howell et al., 1998). The factor does *not* appear to be hippuric acid, acting to make the urine more acidic.

Nephrolithiasis (Kidney Stones)

About 10% of men and 3% of women have a kidney stone during adulthood (Coe et al., 1992a). Kidney stones are formed when the concentration of components in the urine reaches a level in which crystallization is possible. They generally are composed of calcium salts, uric acid, cystine, or struvite (triple salt of ammonium, magnesium, and phosphate). Although the clinical manifestations of these stones is similar, their pathogenesis and treatment differ. Several long-term follow-up studies suggest that

TABLE 38–3 SUMMARY OF MEDICAL NUTRITION THERAPY FOR ACUTE RENAL FAILURE

NUTRIENT	AMOUNT
Protein	0.8–1.0 g/kg IBW increasing as GFR returns to normal. 60% should be HBV protein.
Energy	30–40 kcal/kg body weight.
Potassium	30–50 mEq/day in oliguric phase (depending on urinary output, dialysis, and serum K^+ level); replace losses in diuretic phase.
Sodium	20–40 mEq/day in oliguric phase (depending on urinary output, edema, dialysis, and serum Na^+ level); replace losses in diuretic phase.
Fluid	Replace output from the previous day (vomitus, diarrhea, urine) plus 500 mL.
Phosphorus	Limit as needed.

GFR, glomerular filtration rate; *HBV,* high biologic value; *IBW*, ideal body weight.

stones will recur in most patients who pass a single stone. For this reason, most authors suggest it is important that there be a stone analysis as well as metabolic evaluation after the first or second stone (Coe et al., 1992a). Analysis of stone type is not as important as identifying and treating the underlying metabolic abnormality.

Regardless of the type of stone or its cause, the encouragement of large volumes of fluid intake (1.5 to 3 L/day) to produce at least 2 liters of urine daily, is an essential component of effective prophylactic treatment. A recent study of 199 stone formers found that those who increased fluid intake to maintain daily urine volume over 2 liters had significantly lower recurrence rate (27%) of stones than those who only maintained urine volumes at 1 liter per day (Borghi et al., 1996). The goal of rigorous hydration is to keep the urine dilute, preventing the crystallization of stone-forming minerals.

Recently, the Nurse's Health Study found that during 8 years of follow-up the relative risk for stone development among 81,003 women was 38% lower in women drinking over 2.5 liters of fluid daily compared with those drinking less than 1.4 liters of fluid daily. Each additional 8 oz of fluid either as tea, decaffeinated coffee, regular coffee, or wine was associated with an 8%, 9%, 10%, or 59% reduction of risk, respectively. Interestingly each additional 8 oz of fluid as milk, soda, and juice did not affect the risk except for grapefruit juice. Each additional 8 oz of grapefruit juice increased the risk of stone development by 44% (Curhan et al., 1998).

Calcium Oxalate and Calcium Phosphate Stones

About 80% of stones are composed of *calcium oxalate* (alone or with a nucleus of calcium phosphate [hydroxyapatite]) and are most common in middle-aged men. Their causes are multiple, including hyperparathyroidism, hyperuricosuria, idiopathic hypercalciuria, low urine citrate level, distal RTA, hyperoxaluria and possibly infection with nanobacteria (Kajander and Ciftcioglu, 1998).

The primary treatment involves correction of the specific defect. This includes the removal of parathyroid adenoma for hyperparathyroidism, dietary protein reduction, and medication with allopurinol for hyperuricosuria, protein restriction or diurectic use for hypercalciuria, and medication with bicarbonate and potassium for RTA.

Overproduction of oxalate, or *primary hyperoxaluria*, is a rare inherited metabolic disorder that leads to recurrent calcium oxalate stones and eventually deposition of calcium oxalate in the renal parenchyma, progressive renal insufficiency, and usually death before the third decade of life. A recent long-term study (average length of follow-up was 10 years) found optimal treatment seems to include early diagnosis and treatment with large doses of pyridoxine, a cofactor in the defective enzymatic pathway leading to oxalate overproduction, and oral orthophosphate. Orthophosphate therapy reduces the urinary calcium oxalate and thus renal deposition of calcium oxalate (Milliner et al., 1994).

Another form of hyperoxaluria, *enteric hyperoxaluria*, results from gut overabsorption of oxalate, commonly seen in small intestinal diseases such as Crohn's disease, celiac sprue, and intestinal bypass surgery, or pancreatic insufficiency. It is also possible that excessive intakes of vitamin C over 1000 mg per day may increase urinary oxalate. It is not clear whether the vitamin C conversion to oxalate occurs in vivo or after the urine has left the body (Liebman et al., 1997).

Treatment of this disorder requires 800 to 1200 mg/day of oral calcium (which binds oxalate) as well as a low-oxalate intake (see Appendix 45). Even though foods can have high levels of oxalate, to date only eight foods have been shown to actually raise urinary oxalate excretion (Table 38–4). If these foods are eliminated from the diet, a low-oxalate intake results (Brinkley et al., 1990; Finch et al., 1981). Changes in urinary oxalate excretion exert more influence on the formation of calcium oxalate crystals in the urine than do changes in urinary calcium concentration (Massey and Sutton, 1993).

Also to consider are the wide variations in individuals' abilities to degrade dietary oxalate in the gut. Oxalate is degraded by *oxalobacter formigenes*, anaerobic microflora in the human intestine. The presence of these microbes and the amount of degradation of dietary oxalate in the gut could influence the amount of oxalate absorbed, and thus the level in the urine. This may be the reason for the enteric hyperoxaluria—an alteration in the presence of the oxalate-degrading microbes (Allison et al., 1986).

Hypercalciuria (more than 200 mg of calcium in a 24-hour urine collection) may be the single most important condition underlying calcium stone formation. This condition can be either *absorptive* (increased intestinal absorption of calcium), *renal* (impaired renal tubular absorption of calcium; a renal "leaker"), or *resorptive* (excessive resorption of calcium from bone due to primary hyperparathyroidism, which is treated with surgery). The ab-

TABLE 38–4 FOODS THAT RAISE URINARY OXALATE EXCRETION

Rhubarb
Spinach
Strawberries
Chocolate
Wheat bran
Nuts
Beets
Tea

(Data from Brinkley LJ, et al. A further study of oxalate bioavailability in foods. J Urol 144:94, 1990; French AM, et al. Urine compositions in normal subjects after oral ingestion of oxalate-rich foods. Clin Sci 60:411, 1981; Massey LK, et al. Effect of dietary oxalate and calcium on urinary oxalate and risk of formulation of calcium oxalate kidney stones. J Am Diet Assoc 93:901, 1993.)

sorptive and renal forms are referred to as *idiopathic hypercalciuria,* which is by far the most common type of hypercalciuria (Coe et al., 1992a).

The only situation in which a low-calcium diet (400 to 600 mg daily) would be appropriate is the patient who is a "renal leaker," and even then it poses a threat of bone loss. Also, no studies show that reduced calcium intake, which can reduce urinary calcium, makes a difference in stone recurrence (Coe et al., 1992a).

In most other cases, it may be appropriate to increase calcium intake, as suggested by a study of about 45,000 men aged 40 to 75 years. Those with the highest dietary calcium intake were one third less likely to develop a stone than those who consumed the smaller amount. The authors speculated that increased calcium intake reduces the body's supply of urinary oxalate, another component of most kidney stones. Increased binding of oxalate by calcium may occur in the gastrointestinal tract (Curhan et al., 1993).

The general policy of calcium restriction for patients with kidney stones containing calcium is not appropriate. Findings provide no support for the belief that a diet low in calcium reduces the risk of kidney stones. A recent study of about 1300 women showed that those with a history of renal stones had significantly lower dietary calcium intakes (Sowers et al., 1998). A low-calcium intake may increase the risk for stones by increasing the degree of calcium oxalate saturation of the urine if hyperoxaluria also exists (Bataille et al., 1983). In fact, higher dietary calcium intake may decrease the incidence of kidney stones by making more calcium available in the gut to form insoluble calcium oxalate that will not be absorbed (Massey et al., 1993). Supplementation with calcium citrate does not appear to increase the calcium oxalate saturation of the urine even though urinary calcium does increase. Concomitant increases in urinary citrate also seem to leave the calcium oxalate stone-forming potential of the urine unchanged (Coe et al., 1992b; Levine et al., 1994).

Patients with idiopathic hypercalciuria have been treated effectively with ample fluid intake and thiazide diuretics, which decrease urinary calcium. Maximal effectiveness of thiazides is accomplished by mildly restricting sodium intake to 4 to 5 g/day. Dramatic drops in urine calcium have been reported with more severe dietary sodium restriction (Goldfarb, 1988).

Hyperuricosuria usually leads to the formation of calcium oxalate rather than uric acid stones. Uric acid crystals may form a nidus on which calcium oxalate precipitates. Uric acid also encourages calcium oxalate growth by binding calcium oxalate inhibitors.

Dietary intake of animal protein is directly related to risk of stone formation. Animal protein intake increases the excretion of uric acid and calcium and lowers urinary citrate excretion, all of which are risk factors for stone formation. Hyperuricosuria is treated by limiting protein intake to the level of the recommended dietary allowance (RDA).

Potassium supplementation leads to a reduction in calcium excretion in healthy adults and reduces the risk of stone formation (Lemann et al., 1991).

Some salt-loading studies have shown that urinary calcium excretion increases about 1 mmole (40 mg) for each 100 mmole (2300 mg) increase in dietary sodium in normal adults. Thus, decreased intake of sodium may help decrease the risk of calcium stone formation (Massey and Whiting, 1995).

Uric Acid Stones

Uric acid stones are associated with gout and malignant disease as well as some gastrointestinal diseases characterized by diarrhea. Drugs such as aspirin or probenecid can increase uric acid excretion, and thus can lead to stone formation. The most important factor involved in forming uric acid stones appears to be the production of an acid urine (Coe and Favus, 1986). For this reason, the cornerstone of management of uric acid stones, in addition to fluid ingestion, is to raise the normally slightly acidic urine pH to within the range of 6.0 to 6.5. This can be accomplished with a high-alkaline ash diet, supplemented with citrate or bicarbonate (see *Clinical Insight:* "Acid Ash" and "Alkaline Ash" Diets). Protein may be decreased to the RDA if hyperuricosuria is extreme.

More recent studies have identified calculations for the potential renal acid load and renal net acid excretion of foods to modify urine pH and to decrease recurrent urolithiasis (Remer and Manz, 1995). Implications of these studies suggest future uses that include altering diets for sports activities or for reducing osteoporosis.

Cystinine Stones

Cystinine stones, caused by a hereditary disorder of amino acid transport, represent a rare and exceedingly difficult management problem. Treatment consists of extremely high oral intakes of fluid (>4 L/day), often necessitating getting up during the night to drink and urinate. In addition, an alkaline ash diet and alkaline therapy are needed to raise the urinary pH to 7.5. If these measures alone do not control stone formation, the addition of penicillamine has been beneficial but can have serious systemic side effects. Cystinine stones usually cause relentless, progressive renal destruction.

Struvite Stones

Struvite stones, which constitute 5% to 15% of stones, contain ammonium, magnesium, and phosphate and are usually seen in women. They are formed when the urinary tract is infected with urease-splitting organisms. These organisms, most commonly *Proteus* or *Klebsiella*, produce high concentrations of ammonium on cleavage of urea. Large stones typically lodge in the renal pelvis,

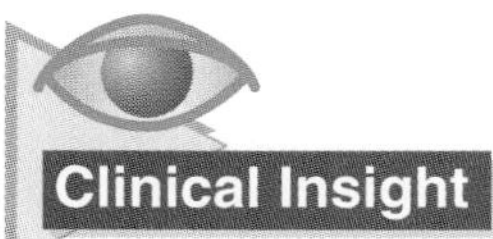

Clinical Insight

"Acid Ash" and "Alkaline Ash" Diets

Dietary intake influences the acidity or alkalinity of the urine (Sherman and Gettler, 1912). The *acid-forming potential* is contributed by chloride, phosphorus, and sulfur (anions) and the *base-forming potential* by sodium, potassium, calcium, and magnesium (cations). In general, fruits and vegetables contribute alkaline "ash" to the urine, except in the case of prunes, plums, and cranberries. These fruits contain benzoic and quinic acids that are excreted in the urine as hippuric acid. However, the effectiveness of these foods, particularly cranberry juice, as urine acidifiers is poorly established (Soloway and Smith, 1988).

High-protein foods (meat, fish, poultry, eggs, and cheese), and breads and cereals are the primary contributors of acid "ash." Milk contributes to both categories. However, because factors of digestion, absorption, use of salt or medications, hormonal status, and homeostatic mechanisms all affect renal excretion and urine production, urine pH cannot be predicted by calculation of intake. Such information can be obtained only by direct measurement of the urine (Dwyer et al., 1985).

The following food lists serve as a guide to influencing urine pH. They are usually used to supplement the effect of medication in altering urine pH; therefore, it may be sufficient to avoid excessive use of particular foods rather than to avoid them completely.

Potentially Acid or Acid-Ash Foods*

Meat:	Meat, fish, fowl, shellfish, eggs, all types of cheese, peanut butter, peanuts
Fat:	Bacon, nuts (Brazil nuts, filberts, walnuts)
Starch:	All types of bread (especially whole-wheat), cereal, crackers, macaroni, spaghetti, noodles, rice
Vegetables:	Corn, lentils
Fruits:	Cranberries, plums, prunes
Desserts:	Plain cakes, cookies

Potentially Basic or Alkaline-Ash Foods

Milk:	Milk and milk products, cream, buttermilk
Fat:	Nuts (almonds, chestnuts, coconut)
Vegetables:	All types (except corn, lentils), especially beets, beet greens, Swiss chard, dandelion greens, kale, mustard greens, spinach, turnip greens
Fruit:	All types (except cranberries, prunes, plums)
Sweets:	Molasses

Neutral Foods

Fats:	Butter, margarine, cooking fats, oils
Sweets:	Plain candies, sugar, syrup, honey
Starches:	Arrowroot, corn, tapioca
Beverages:	Coffee, tea

* Adapted from Pemberton CM, et al. Mayo Clinic Diet Manual, 6th ed. Toronto: BC Decker, p. 256, 1988.

forming staghorn calculi. Recurrent pyelonephritis and progressive renal failure usually develop with eventual obstruction. Treatment consists of long-term effective antibiotics as well as surgical or ultrasonic removal of stones. Dietary management has no significant role in this form of stone disease.

PROGRESSIVE NATURE OF RENAL DISEASE

A wide range of kidney lesions are characterized by a slow, steady decline in renal function. A number of the diseases discussed earlier lead to renal failure in some patients, whereas other patients have a benign course without loss of renal function. The factors involved in producing a benign disease in one patient and renal failure in another patient are not clear. However, it has been recognized in all kidney diseases that once approximately three quarters of kidney function has been lost, regardless of the underlying disease, progressive further loss of kidney function ensues. This is true even in diseases in which the underlying cause has been eliminated completely, such as in vesicoureteral reflux, cortical necrosis of pregnancy, or analgesic abuse. The nature of this progressive loss of function has been the subject of an enormous amount of basic and clinical research during the past several decades and the subject of several excellent reviews (Hricik et al., 1998; Remuzzi and Bertani, 1998).

It is currently believed that in response to a decreasing GFR, the kidney undergoes a series of adaptations to prevent this decrease. Although in the short term this leads to improvement in filtration rate, in the long term it leads to an accelerated loss of nephrons and progressive renal insufficiency. The nature of these adaptations involves a change in the hemodynamic characteristics of the remaining glomeruli, specifically leading to increased glomerular pressure. Factors that increase glomerular pressure tend to accelerate this process, whereas factors that decrease glomerular pressure tend to alleviate it.

The role of dietary protein has been championed as a factor that increases glomerular pressure and thus leads to accelerated loss of renal function (Brenner and Lazarus, 1988). Numerous studies in experimental models of moderate renal insufficiency demonstrate a significant decline in this process with protein restriction. Clinical studies appear to corroborate the experimental models, demonstrating a role for protein restriction in the management of patients with mild to moderate renal insufficiency, for the purpose of preserving renal function (Giordano, 1981; Ihle et al., 1989; Remuzzi and Bertani, 1998). Though it must be pointed out that these clinical studies are small, often retrospective, and uncontrolled, the bulk of scientific evidence favors such a role.

A large multicenter trial, Modification of Diet in Renal Disease, attempted to determine the role of protein, phosphorus restriction, and blood pressure control in the progression of renal disease. In patients with early renal insufficiency, the projected mean decline in the glomerular filtration rate at 3 years did not differ significantly between the diet groups. In patients with more progressed renal deterioration, those on a very low-protein diet using ketoanalogues had a somewhat lower rate of decline than those on a low-protein diet only. "In both groups there was no delay in the time to the occurrence of ESRD or death" (Klahr, 1994).

As a result of this and other related studies, the National Institute of Diabetes and Digestive and Kidney Diseases of the National Institutes of Health convened a conference to develop recommendations for the management of patients with progressive renal disease (www.niddk.nih.gov/health/kidney). Recommendations for dietary protein intake in progressive renal failure are 0.8 g/kg/day 60% HBV, for patients whose GFR is greater than 55 mL/min, and 0.6 g/kg/day 60% HBV, for patients whose GFR is 25 to 55 mL/min (Beto, 1994).

These studies pointed out that systemic hypertension, another factor that mitigates the progressive loss of renal function, must be well controlled to produce benefits from protein restriction. Also important, in the control of the progression of renal failure in diabetics, is good blood sugar control. In a national multicenter trial, the Diabetes Control and Complications Trial, blood sugar control was more important than protein restriction in delaying the onset of renal failure in diabetics (see Chapter 34).

The potential benefits of protein restriction in the patient with moderate renal insufficiency must be weighed against the potential hazards of such treatment, namely, protein malnutrition. Much controversy still remains, based mainly on this consideration. If protein restriction is elected, careful monitoring, and anthropomorphic studies should be carried out periodically (see Chapters 16 and 17).

END-STAGE RENAL DISEASE

End-stage renal disease (ESRD) can result from a wide variety of different kidney diseases. Currently, 90% of patients reaching ESRD have chronic (1) diabetes mellitus, (2) glomerulonephritis, or (3) hypertension. With ESRD comes a myriad of problems related to the kidney's inability to excrete waste products, maintain fluid and electrolyte balance, and produce hormones. As renal failure slowly progresses, a point is reached at which the level of circulating waste products leads to symptoms of uremia (Fig. 38–3).

Uremia is defined as the clinical syndrome of malaise, weakness, nausea and vomiting, muscle cramps and itching, metallic taste in the mouth, and often neurologic impairment that is brought about by an unacceptable level of nitrogenous wastes in the body. The manifestations are somewhat nonspecific and vary from one patient to another. No reliable laboratory parameter corresponds directly with the beginning of symptoms. However, as a rule of thumb, a blood urea nitrogen (BUN) above 100 mg/dL and a creatinine of 10 to 12 mg/dL are usually quite close to this threshold.

Medical Treatment

Treatment of ESRD requires either transplantation or dialysis. If transplantation is anticipated, it is important to maintain optimal nutritional status so that the patient will be a good candidate for the transplant.

Transplantation

Transplantation involves the surgical implantation of a kidney from a living related donor, a living nonrelated donor, or a cadaver (Fig. 38–4). Rejection of the foreign tissue is a major complication. Currently, patients awaiting transplantation far outnumber the donated kidneys available.*

*Registration as an organ donor can be done easily at a local driver's licensing bureau.

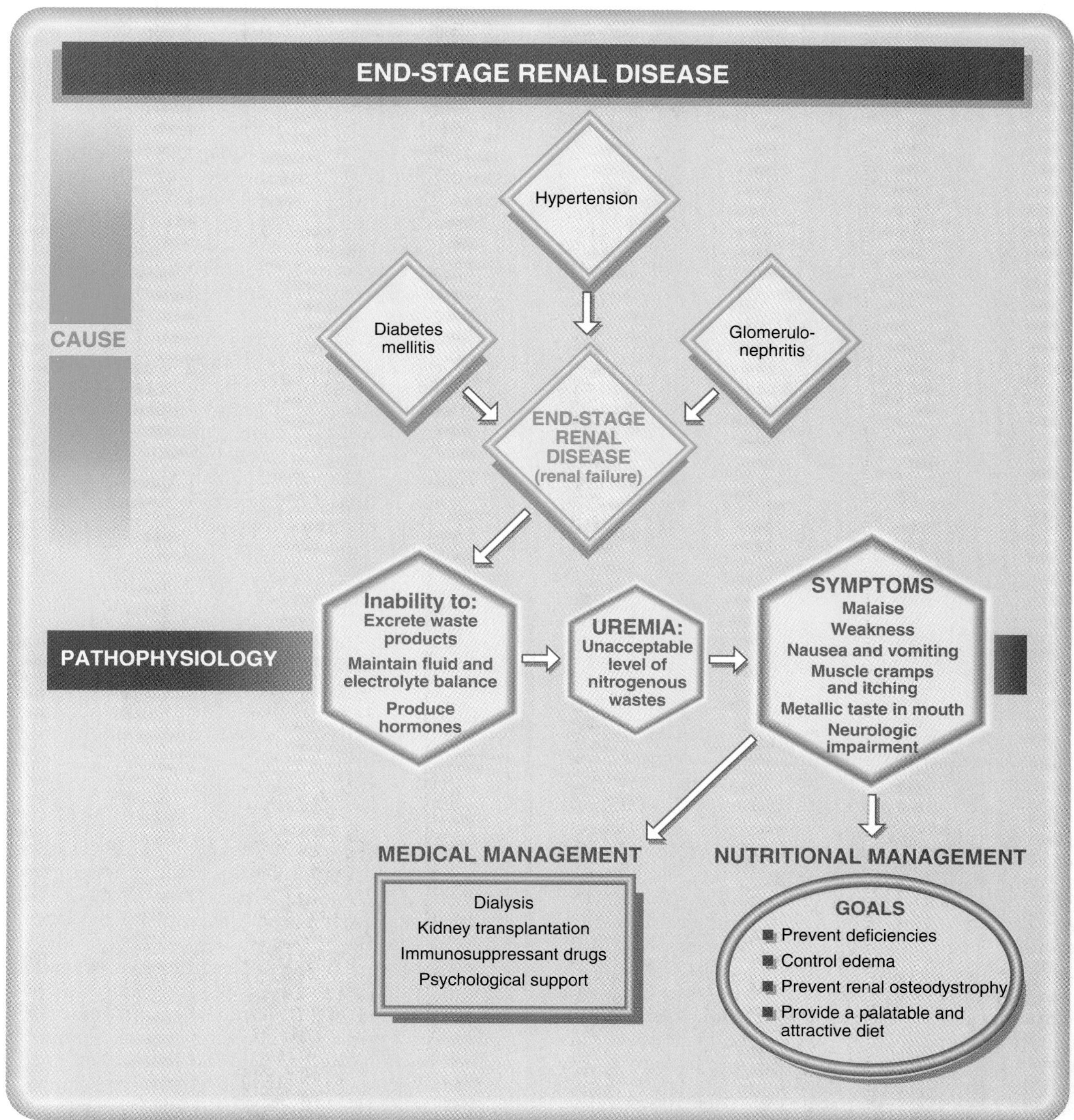

FIGURE 38–3 Pathophysiology algorithm—end-stage renal disease. (Algorithm content developed by John Anderson, Ph.D., and Sanford C. Garner, Ph.D., 2000.)

NUTRITIONAL CARE

The nutritional care of the adult patient who has received a transplanted kidney is based mainly on the metabolic effects of the required immunosuppressive therapy. Medications typically used long term include steroids, cyclosporine, azathioprine, and mycophenolate mofetil. FK506 and OKT3 are typically used short term (initially or with acute rejection).

Corticosteroids are associated with accelerated protein catabolism, hyperlipidemia, sodium retention, weight gain, glucose intolerance, and inhibition of normal calcium, phosphorus, and vitamin D metabolism. Cyclosporine therapy is associated with hyperkalemia, hypertension, and hyperlipi-

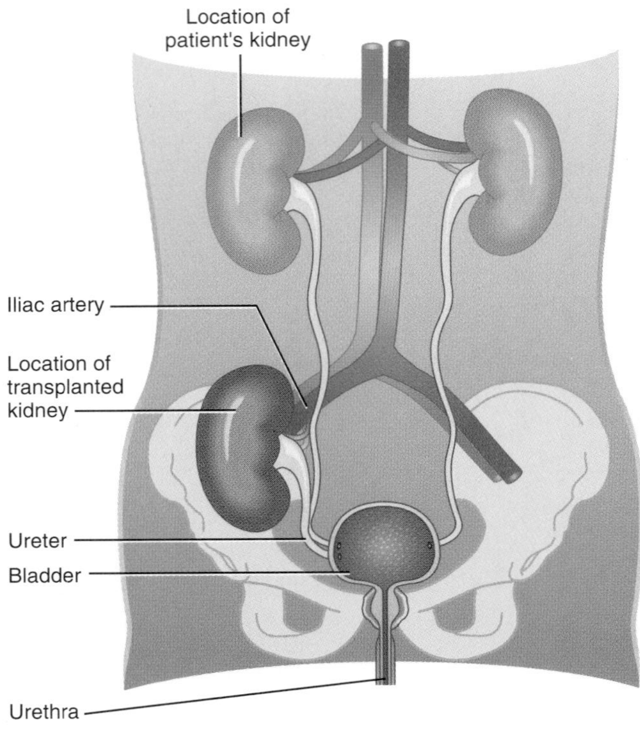

FIGURE 38–4 Location of a transplanted kidney.

demia (see Chapter 18). The doses of these medications used after transplantation are decreased over time until a "maintenance level" is reached.

During the first month after transplantation, and during high-dose steroid therapy used for acute rejection episodes, a high-protein diet (1.3 to 1.5 g/kg body weight) with an energy intake of 30 to 35 kcal/kg is recommended to prevent negative nitrogen balance (Gray, 1993, 1994). Higher amounts of protein, 1.6 to 2.0 g/kg, are required in cases of increased needs, such as fever, infection, and increased surgical or traumatic stresses. A moderate sodium restriction (80 to 100 mEq/day) during this period minimizes fluid retention and helps to control blood pressure. After this time, protein intake can be decreased to 1 g/kg, and calorie intake should be at a level sufficient to achieve and maintain an appropriate weight for height. Sodium intakes are individualized, based on fluid retention and blood pressure.

Hyperkalemia, commonly associated with cyclosporine therapy, warrants dietary potassium restriction, although this is usually only temporary. Following transplantation, many patients exhibit hypophosphatemia and mild hypercalcemia (due to bone resorption) associated with persistent hyperparathyroidism and the effects of steroids on calcium, phosphorus, and vitamin D metabolism. The diet should contain adequate amounts of calcium and phosphorus (1200 mg of each daily), and serum levels should be monitored periodically. Supplemental phosphorus may be necessary to correct hypophosphatemia.

The majority of transplant recipients have elevated serum triglycerides or cholesterol, or both. The etiology of this hyperlipidemia is multifactorial, and it is unclear whether treatment should be given, and if so, what treatment. Intervention consists of calorie restriction for those who are overweight, limiting cholesterol intake to less than 300 mg/day, and limiting total fat (see Chapter 26). In patients exhibiting glucose intolerance, limiting simple carbohydrates and maintaining a regular moderate exercise regimen are appropriate (Perez, 1993).

In one study of patients who were receiving cyclosporine, during their first year posttransplant the use of 6 g of fish oil, providing ω-3 fatty acids, had a beneficial effect on renal hemodynamics and blood pressure. The 1-year graft survival was also better for those taking the fish oils. The authors speculate that the effect of fish oils on eicosanoid production is probably important and this may enhance the immunosuppressive effects of cyclosporine (van der Heide et al., 1993).

Dialysis

Dialysis can be accomplished either by hemodialysis or by peritoneal dialysis (Pastan and Bailey, 1998). The most common method is **hemodialysis,** in which blood passes by the semipermeable membrane of the artificial kidney and waste products are removed by diffusion.

HEMODIALYSIS

Hemodialysis requires permanent access to the bloodstream through a fistula created by surgery to connect an artery and a vein (Fig. 38–5). Fistulas are often made near the wrist, causing the forearm veins to become greatly enlarged. If the patient's blood vessels are fragile, an artificial vessel called a graft may be surgically implanted. Large needles are inserted into the fistula or graft before each dialysis and removed when dialysis is complete.

The dialysis fluid is similar to that of normal plasma. Waste products and electrolytes move by osmosis from the blood into the **dialysate** and are removed (Fig. 38–6). Hemodialysis usually requires treatment of 3 to 5 hours three times per week (Fig. 38–7). Dietary protein needs are about 1 to 1.2 g/kg to make up for some losses through the dialysate (Table 38–5).

PERITONEAL DIALYSIS

Peritoneal dialysis makes use of the semipermeable membrane of the peritoneum. A catheter is surgically implanted in the abdomen and into the peritoneal cavity (Fig. 38–8). Dialysate containing a high-dextrose concentration is instilled into the peritoneum, where diffusion carries waste products

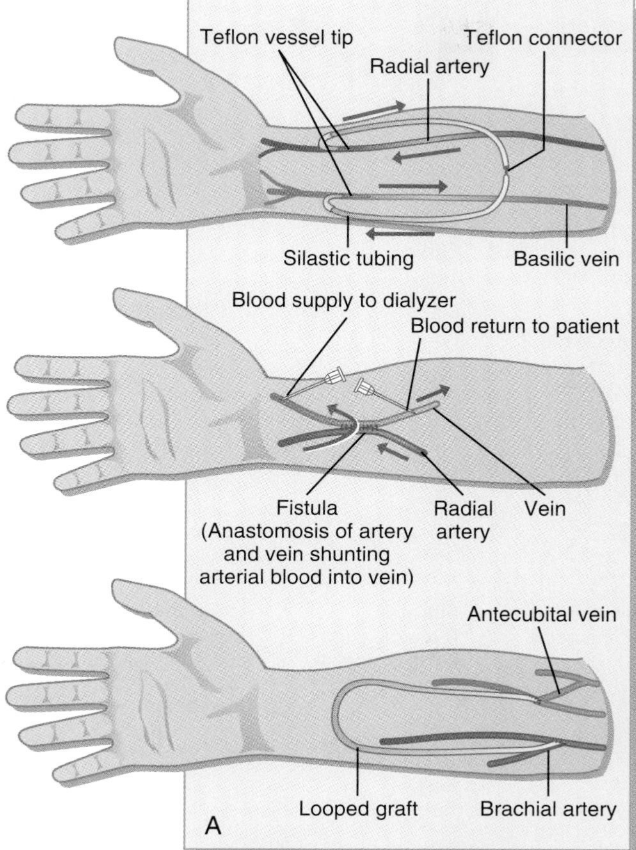

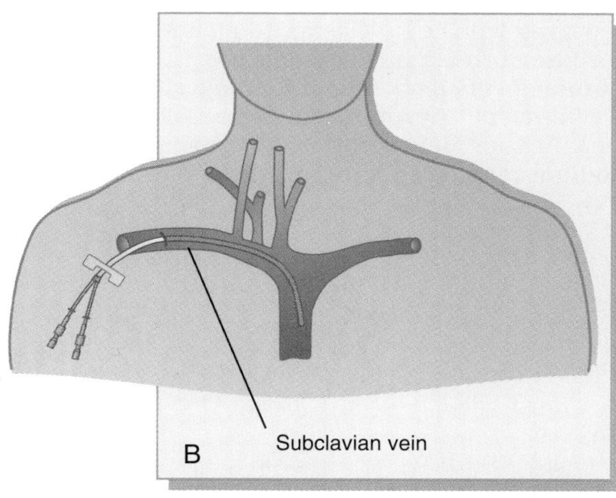

FIGURE 38–5 Types of access for hemodialysis. *A,* Cannula (rarely used now). *B,* AV (arteriovenous fistula). *C,* artificial loop graft. *D,* subclavian catheter (usually temporary).

from the blood through the peritoneal membrane and into the dialysate. This fluid is then withdrawn and discarded, and new solution is added.

Peritoneal dialysis is a less efficient method of removing waste products from the blood. Treatments usually last longer than hemodialysis, about 10 to 12 h/day, three times per week. Patients with peritoneal dialysis have higher protein needs (about 1.2 to 1.5 g protein/kg) because of greater protein losses.

Continuous ambulatory peritoneal dialysis (CAPD) is similar to peritoneal dialysis, except that the dialysate is left in the peritoneum and exchanged manually so that no machine is required. Exchanges of dialysis fluid are done four to five times daily, making it a 24-hour treatment. Protein losses are somewhat higher than those from regular peritoneal dialysis. Advantages of this form of treatment are avoidance of large fluctuations in blood chemistry and the ability of the patient to achieve a more normal life-style.

Patients with CAPD have more liberal fluid, sodium, and potassium allowances because the therapy is continuous and more of these products are removed. The loss of sodium can be as much as 6 g/day; thus, these patients may need higher sodium intakes, as shown in Table 38–5. Complications associated with CAPD include peritonitis, hypotension requiring additional fluid and sodium replacement, and weight gain. The weight gain is experienced by most patients with CAPD as a result of absorbing 600 to 800 calories/day from the glucose in the dialysate. This may be desirable in patients who are underweight, but eventually dietary intake will have to be modified to account for the energy absorbed from dialysate.

Psychological Support

Patients with renal failure must deal not only with conflicting feelings about being dependent on artificial means of elimination, but also with changes in the quality of their lives and the necessity for adapting to a chronic, progressive illness. Control becomes a central issue because they must devote large quantities of time to dialysis, follow fairly strict dietary regimens, and often take several medications. Those who work with renal dialysis patients must be especially empathic to their feelings of thirst, anorexia when faced with eating, and taste changes due to uremia. See website www.kidney.org.

Nutritional Care

Goals of nutritional care in the management of ESRD are:

1. To prevent deficiency and maintain good nutritional status (and growth, in the case of children) through adequate protein, energy, vitamin, and mineral intake
2. To control edema and electrolyte imbalance by controlling sodium, potassium, and fluid intake
3. To prevent or retard the development of renal osteodystrophy by controlling calcium, phosphorus, and vitamin D intake
4. To enable the patient to eat a palatable, attractive diet that fits his or her life-style as much as possible

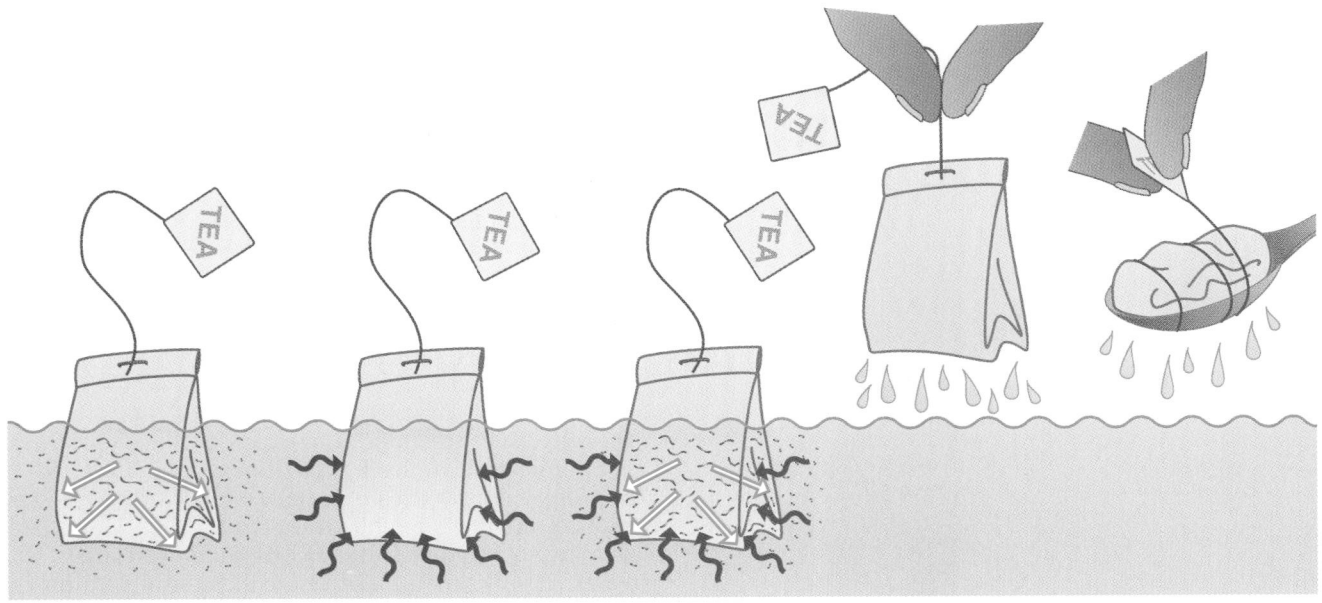

Diffusion is the passage of particles through a semipermeable membrane. Tea, for example, diffuses from a tea bag into the surrounding water.

Osmosis is the movement of fluid across a semipermeable membrane from a lower concentration of solutes to a higher concentration of solutes.

Diffusion and **Osmosis** can occur at the same time.

Filtration is the passage of fluids through a membrane.

Ultrafiltration provides additional pressure to squeeze extra fluid through the membrane.

FIGURE 38–6 Dialysis: How it works. (Adapted from Core Curriculum for the dialysis Technician: A Comprehensive Review of Hemodialysis, AMGEN INC).

Even with the development of dialysis methods and transplantation techniques, nutritional care remains essential to enhance dialysis, maintain optimal nutritional status, and prevent complications.

Because treatment is on an outpatient basis, or dialysis is done at home, patients with ESRD assume responsibility for their diet. Most long-term patients know their diets very well (Fig. 38–9), having been instructed by a dietitian many times at their dialysis unit. Patients who are relatively new to dialysis may require much more intensive education. Regardless of length of time on dialysis, all patients facing long-term compliance with a difficult diet regimen are helped by periodic professional counseling. Monitoring the patient's long-term nutritional status is an important role of the dietitian. Table 38–6 presents a guide for teaching patients about their blood values and control of their disease.

Fluid and Sodium Balance

The ability of the kidney to handle sodium and water in ESRD must be assessed frequently through measurement of blood pressure, presence of edema, serum sodium level, and dietary intake. The diet and fluid intake are then modified accordingly.

Although sodium is retained by most patients with ESRD, it may be lost by others. Examples of diseases with a salt-losing tendency are polycystic disease of the kidney, chronic obstructive uropathy, chronic pyelonephritis, and analgesic nephropathy. To prevent hypotension, hypovolemia, cramps, and further deterioration of renal function, extra sodium may be required in these patients. Usually

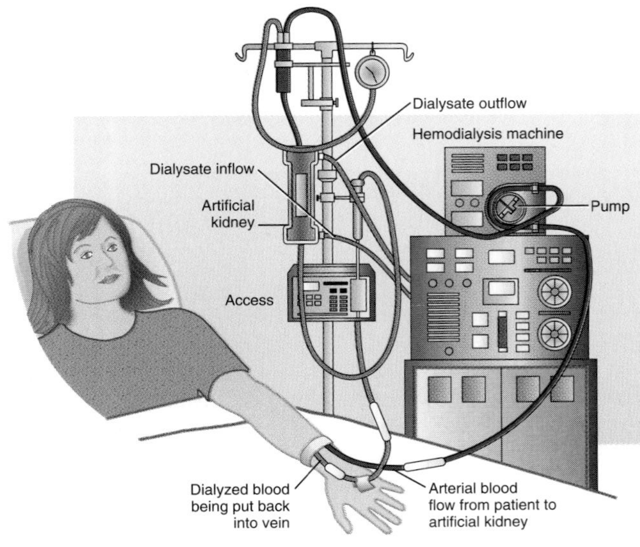

FIGURE 38–7 Hemodialysis. Treatment is usually for 3 to 6 hours, three times per week.

TABLE 38–5 NUTRIENT REQUIREMENTS FOR ADULTS WITH RENAL DISEASE BASED ON TYPE OF THERAPY

THERAPY	ENERGY	PROTEIN	FLUID	SODIUM	POTASSIUM	PHOSPHORUS
Impaired renal function (predialysis)	30–40 kcal/kg IBW	0.6 –0.8 g/kg BW	Ad libitum	Variable, 2–3 g/day	Variable, usually ad libitum or increased to cover losses with diuretics	1–1.2 g/day
Hemodialysis	35 kcal/kg IBW	1–1.2 g/kg BW (1.2–1.5 g/kg for repletion)	1000 mL/day + urine output	2–3 g/day	2–3 g/day	1–1.2 g/day
Intermittent peritoneal dialysis (IPD)	30 kcal/kg IBW (40–50 kcal/kg for repletion)	1.2 g/kg BW (1.5 g/kg for repletion)	1000 mL/day + urine output	2–3 g/day	2–3 g/day	1–1.2 g/day
Continuous ambulatory peritoneal dialysis (CAPD)	25 kcal/kg IBW (40–50 kcal/kg for repletion)	1.2 g/kg BW (1.5 g/kg for repletion)	Ad libitum (minimum of 2000 mL/day + urine output)	6–8 g/day	3–4 g/day	1.5–2 g/day
Diabetic on hemodialysis IPD or CAPD	35 kcal/kg IBW (40–50 kcal/kg for repletion)	1.5 g/kg BW	Same as for hemodialysis, IPD, or CAPD. Monitor thirst, blood sugar, and weight changes.		Same as for hemodialysis, IPD, or CAPD. (Increased blood sugar may cause increased potassium.)	1–1.2 g/day (often liberalized due to other restrictions)
Transplant, 4–6 weeks after transplant	30–35 kcal/kg IBW	1.5–2 g/kg BW	Ad libitum	Variable	Variable; may require restriction with cyclosporine-induced hyperkalemia	1.2 g/day Calcium 1.2 g/day
6 weeks or longer after transplant Carbohydrate—limit simple carbohydrate Fat < 35% of calories Cholesterol no more than 400 mg/day Polyunsaturated/saturated fat ratio of > 1.0	To achieve/maintain IBW	1 g/kg BW	Ad libitum	Variable	Variable	Calcium 1.2 g/day

IBW, ideal body weight.

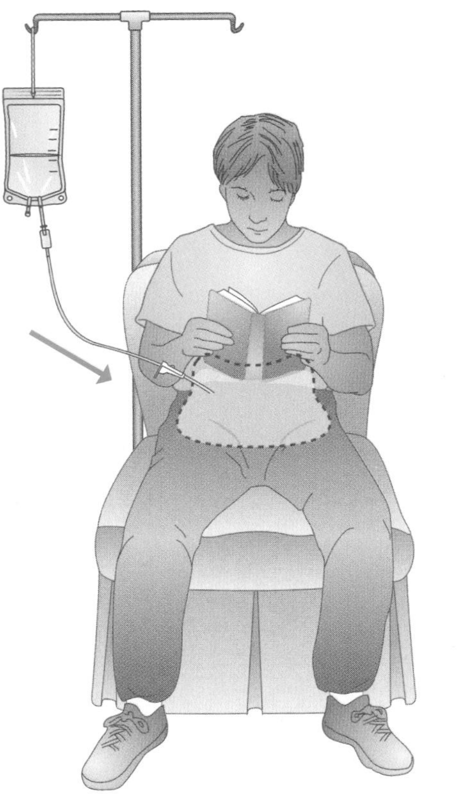

The peritoneal cavity is filled with dialysate, using gravity.

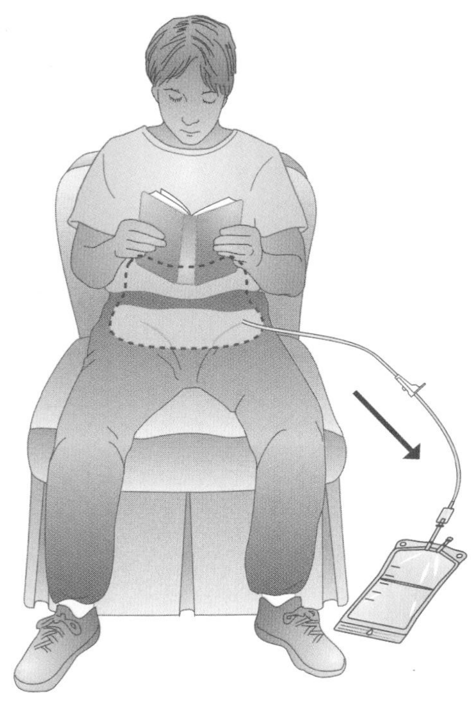

At the end of the exchange, the dialysate is drained into the bag, again using gravity.

FIGURE 38–8 Continuous ambulatory peritoneal dialysis; 20 minute exchanges usually are given four to five times daily, every day.

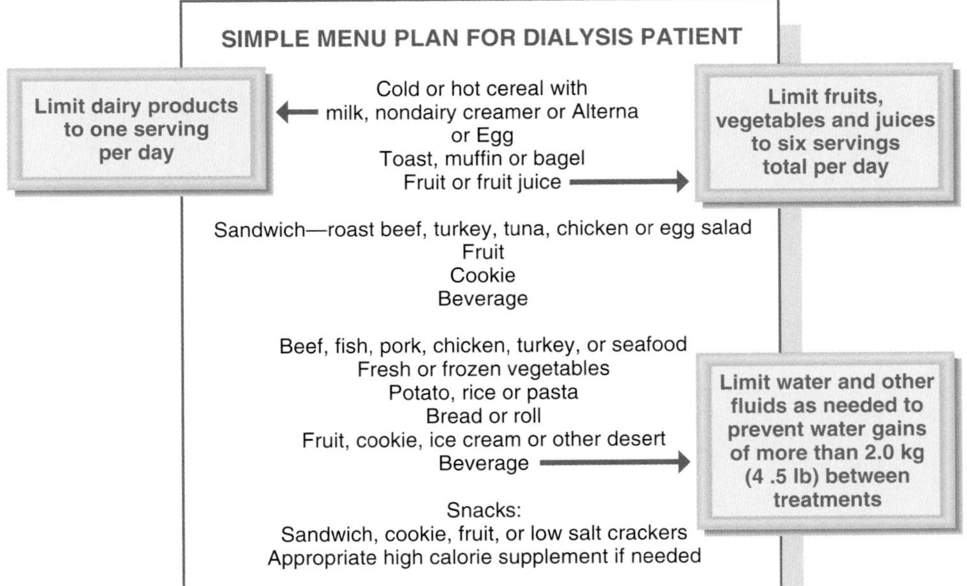

SIMPLE MENU PLAN FOR DIALYSIS PATIENT
Limit dairy products to one serving per day
Cold or hot cereal with
milk, nondairy creamer or Alterna
or Egg
Toast, muffin or bagel
Fruit or fruit juice
Limit fruits, vegetables and juices to six servings total per day
Sandwich—roast beef, turkey, tuna, chicken or egg salad
Fruit
Cookie
Beverage
Beef, fish, pork, chicken, turkey, or seafood
Fresh or frozen vegetables
Potato, rice or pasta
Bread or roll
Fruit, cookie, ice cream or other desert
Beverage
Limit water and other fluids as needed to prevent water gains of more than 2.0 kg (4 .5 lb) between treatments
Snacks:
Sandwich, cookie, fruit, or low salt crackers
Appropriate high calorie supplement if needed

FIGURE 38–9 A simple menu plan for a patient on dialysis. The diet should allow for no more than a 5% weight gain between dialyses.

TABLE 38–6 DIALYSIS PATIENT'S GUIDE TO BLOOD VALUES*

This guide is to help in the understanding of lab reports. The normal values are for people with good kidney function. Acceptable values for dialysis patients are given in the next column. Blood values should fall within the range for dialysis patients. Many things affect blood values, and diet is one of these. Understanding blood chemistry will help diet control.

BLOOD TEST†	NORMAL VALUES	VALUES FOR DIALYSIS PATIENTS	FUNCTION	DIET CHANGES
Sodium	136–145 mEq/L	Same	Found in salt and many preserved foods. A diet high in sodium will make you thirsty. When you drink too much fluid, it may dilute the sodium and it will look low. If you eat too much sodium and do not drink water, it may be high. Always check your weight gains against your sodium value.	High: Eat less salt and salty foods. Make sure you are gaining about 4% of your body weight between dialyses and are not dehydrated. Low: Probably drinking too much fluid. Limit weight gains to 4% of your body weight between dialyses. Eat less salt and fewer salty foods if weight gains exceed 4% of your body weight.
Potassium	3.5–5.5 mEq/L	Same	Found in most high-protein foods, fruits, and vegetables. It affects muscle action, especially the heart. High levels can cause your heart to stop. Low levels can also cause symptoms, such as weakness.	High: Avoid foods with over 250 mg potassium per serving and limit daily intake to 2000 mg. Consult a dietitian. Low: Add one 250-mg potassium food per day and recheck blood level.
Chloride	97–108 mEq/L	Same	Usually associated with amount of sodium in the blood.	No dietary changes.
Total CO_2	23–30 mEq/L	Lower than normal	Total CO_2 is a measure of how acidic your blood is. Your kidneys usually keep this normal. When they fail, your blood becomes more acidic, and your CO_2 is lower.	No dietary changes. If low, may need more dialysis.
Creatinine	0.7–1.5 mg/dL	10–15 mg/dL	A normal waste product of muscle breakdown. This value is controlled by dialysis. You have a higher amount because the artificial kidney is not working all the time like the normal kidney does.	No dietary changes; dialysis controls creatinine.
Glucose	60–125 mg/dL	Same (higher for diabetic)	This sugar in the blood is made from the food that you eat, especially the starches and sugars. The body uses glucose for energy. For diabetics: a high blood sugar can make you thirsty.	You need a minimum of 4 servings of breads/starches or cereals and 2–3 servings of fruit to provide energy. For diabetics: Avoid concentrated sweets unless your blood sugar is low.
Calcium	8.5–10.5 mg/dL	8.5–11 mg/dL	Found in dairy products, meats, and green vegetables. It is used by the body to make bone and help muscle movement. It is closely related to phosphorus; vitamin D is needed for its absorption.	High: Eat fewer milk products. Check with a doctor if you are taking a calcium supplement or active vitamin D.

(continued)

TABLE 38–6 DIALYSIS PATIENT'S GUIDE TO BLOOD VALUES* (continued)

BLOOD TEST†	NORMAL VALUES	VALUES FOR DIALYSIS PATIENTS	FUNCTION	DIET CHANGES
			Calcium and phosphorus are needed for strong bones. They have a "see-saw" relationship, thus when phosphorus is up, calcium is don. The ratio should be kept within normal for strong bones.	Low: Increase calcium in diet (if phosphorus is normal) by adding more milk products. You may need a calcium supplement or active vitamin D. Check with your doctor.
Phosphorus	2.3–6.0 mg/dL	Same	Found in milk products, dried beans, peas, nuts, and meat. It is also used to build bones.	High: Limit milk and milk products to 1 serving per day. Take phosphate binders as prescribed. Low: Add 1 serving milk product or other high-phosphorus food per day and recheck blood level.
BUN	4–22 mg/dL	< 100 mg/dL	Waste product of protein breakdown. Unlike creatinine, this is affected by the amount of protein in your diet. Dialysis removes urea nitrogen.	High: Limit intake of meat, fish, chicken, and dairy products to about 3 servings per day and contact the dietitian. Low: May be low if you are not eating and are losing weight. May also increase with loss of muscle. Contact the dietitian.
Uric acid	4.0–8.5 mg/dL	Same	A waste product of purine. A high level may be related to symptoms of gout. Purines are found in a variety of foods. (See Chapter 43.)	No dietary changes. Because purines are found in most foods, you would have to stop eating! If you have gout, your doctor can prescribe a medicine to lower the uric acid level.
Alkaline phosphatase	30–115 IU/L	Same	Found in normal bone. Released from bone when calcium is being removed.	Keep calcium and phosphorus within normal range.
LDH	80–220 IU/L	Same	Enzymes released when tissue is damaged. Increased in infection, heart problems, liver damage, and damage of any tissue.	No dietary changes.
SGOT	0–41 IU/L	Same		No dietary changes.
Cholesterol	150–240 mg/dL	Often lower	Found in high-fat foods from animal sources (e.g., meat, milk, eggs). Your body can also make its own if there is not enough in your diet. Within normal levels, cholesterol is not harmful. Low cholesterol is a sign of not eating well.	High: May need to limit cholesterol intake. Low: Increase intake of eggs, fats, and protein rich foods. Check with dietitian.

TABLE 38–6 DIALYSIS PATIENT'S GUIDE TO BLOOD VALUES* (continued)

BLOOD TEST†	NORMAL VALUES	VALUES FOR DIALYSIS PATIENTS	FUNCTION	DIET CHANGES
Total protein	6.0–8.2 g/dL	Same	Proteins make up all body cells. Albumin is a type of protein. Globulins are used to fight infection. Both are needed by the body. Protein is lost with dialysis. In peritoneal dialysis protein loss is much more than hemodialysis, so you need even more protein.	Low: Increase intake of protein-rich foods: meat, fish, chicken, eggs. Ask your dieti--tian for high-protein recipes.
Albumin‡	3.5–5.0 g/dL (BCG test) 3.0–4.5 (BCP test)	Same Same	If albumin is low, fluid will "leak" from blood vessels into tissue, causing edema. When fluid is in the tissue, it is more difficult to remove with dialysis.	
HCT	35–45%	Usually lower 30–36%	This is the percentage of red blood cells in the blood. Red blood cells carry oxygen to the cells. Everyone's value is different; learn what is normal for you.	If hematocrit is dropping, check with your doctor.
Serum ferritin	100–200 μg/L (men) 100–150 mg/L (women)	100–300 μg/L 100–300 μg/L	Ferritin is the form of iron stored in the liver. If iron stores are low, you cannot make new red blood cells.	Iron in food is not well enough absorbed. Ask your doctor about an iron supplement. Do not take iron at the same time as your phosphate binders.
Hepatitis B surface antigen (hepatitis)	Negative		A protein in your body if you have serum hepatitis, a liver disease.	No dietary changes.

*Developed by Linda Peterson, RN, and Katy Wilkens, RD, Northwest Kidney Center, Seattle, Washington.
†*Alk phos,* alkaline phosphatase; *BUN,* blood urea nitrogen; *HCT,* hematocrit; *LDH,* lactic dehydrogenase; *SGOT,* serum glutamic oxaloacetic transaminase.
‡Normal range depends on type of laboratory testing done (Blagg et al., 1993).
§*BCG,* bromocresol green
||*BCP,* bromocresol purple

the diet contains 130 mEq (3 g) or higher of sodium per day, which is the amount in a normal diet without added salt. Needs for extra sodium can be met by adding salt or salty foods. The number of patients requiring this higher sodium intake is few, but serves as an example of why each patient must be looked at individually when determining a diet prescription.

Dialysis patients with hypertension and edema may need to restrict intakes of sodium and fluids (see Chapter 36). Even those who do not experience these symptoms, but who put out minimal urine, will benefit from a reduced sodium intake, to limit their thirst and prevent large intradialytic fluid gains. The recommended intake of sodium for the vast majority of patients is 2 to 3 g/day. Because solid foods in the average diet contribute approximately 500 to 800 mL of fluid, these foods will replace the 500 mL of net insensible water loss as shown in Table 38–2. Additional fluid is given to replace urinary and vomitus losses.

Fluid and sodium requirements can increase in the presence of perspiration, vomiting, or fever. Hypotension and the possibility of clotting at the shunt site must be avoided from overrestriction of fluid and sodium intake.

In the patient who is maintained with dialysis, sodium intake and fluid intake are regulated to allow for a weight gain from increased fluid in the vasculature of 4 to 5 lb (2 to 3 kg) between dialyses (Oldenburg, 1988). Other studies support a fluid gain of 2% to 5% of body weight (Sherman et al., 1995). This means a sodium intake of 130 mEq (3 g) daily and a more liberal fluid intake, usually about 1000 mL/day plus the amount equal to the urine output. Care must be taken to avoid overrestriction of the patient's intake and malnutrition, while meeting the clinical needs for a stable fluid balance. In these situations, interaction between the dietitian and nursing staff is invaluable.

A 130-mEq sodium diet allows for light salting of foods during cooking but no additional salt at the table and no salted, smoked, or cured meat or fish, salted snack foods, canned soups, or high-sodium convenience foods. In relation to sodium intake, it is important to remember that the easiest way to reduce the patient's thirst and fluid intake, is to decrease the sodium intake. Chapter 36 gives the details of a low-sodium meal plan.

When educating about fluid balance, the health care provider must teach the patient how to deal with thirst without drinking. Sucking on a few ice chips, cold sliced fruit, or sour candies; using a spray mouthwash; or chewing "sports gum" containing citric acid may help to alleviate the dryness.

Patients must be taught to measure their fluid intake and urine output, examine their ankles for edema, weigh themselves regularly each morning, and record their weight. Occasionally (in about 15% to 20% of patients), hypertension is not alleviated even after meticulous attention to fluid and water balance. In these patients, hypertension is usually perpetuated by a high level of renin secretion and requires medication for control.

Potassium

Potassium (K^+) usually requires restriction, depending on the individual's body size, the serum K^+ level, and the frequency of dialysis. High intakes are not tolerated with less frequent dialysis. The daily intake of potassium for most Americans is 75 to 100 mEq (3 to 4 g). This is usually reduced in ESRD to 40 to 65 mEq (1.5 to 2.5 g) per day and is reduced for the anuric patient on dialysis to 51 mEq (2 g) per day. Some patients, those on high-flux dialysis, or with increased dialysis times, may be able to tolerate higher intakes. Again, a close monitoring of the patient's laboratory values, K^+ content of the dialysate bath, and dietary intake is invaluable.

The potassium content of foods is listed in Appendix 41. Care should be taken when counseling patients on a low-potassium diet, to point out to them the many low-sodium foods that contain KCl, as a salt substitute, rather than NaCl. Salt substitues, "Lite Salt," and low-sodium herb mixtures must all be carefully checked to be sure they do not contain a dangerous level of potassium. Low-sodium soy sauces, sauerkraut, and other special dietary products may need particular review by a trained professional. It is also good to check this not only with the patient but with other people who may be cooking for the patient, such as a church group or neighbors, who may be using salt substitutes in the mistaken belief they are helping the patient avoid salt.

Protein

Dialysis is a drain on body protein, and the daily intake should be increased to compensate for this. Protein losses of 20 to 30 g can occur during a 24-hour peritoneal dialysis, with an average of 1 g/h. Hourly losses in hemodialysis are similar. Patients receiving peritoneal dialysis three times per week or continuous ambulatory dialysis require a daily protein intake of at least 1.2 to 1.5 g/kg body weight. Those receiving hemodialysis three times per week should have 1 to 1.2 g/kg body weight. Recent studies of patients on dialysis indicate that those with low albumin levels have a much higher mortality rate; consequently, more emphasis is placed on adequate protein intake. Protein requirements for patients on different types of dialysis are summarized in Table 38–5. Serum BUN and serum creatinine levels, uremic symptoms, and weight should be monitored, and the diet should be adjusted accordingly.

Although serum albumin is an excellent indicator of protein status, it is important to know the laboratory's methodology for measuring serum albumin. The bromocresol purple (BCP) test yields lower results than the bromocresol green (BCG) test (see Table 38–6). (Blagg et al., 1993).

Kinetic Modeling

A recent trend in evaluating the efficacy of dialysis relies on measuring the removal of urea from the patient's blood over a given period of time. This method, often referred to as *KT/V* (where K is the urea clearance of the dialyzer, T is the time between drawings of the blood, and V is the patient's total body water volume), should ideally produce a result higher than 1.2. The method for calculating the efficacy of peritoneal dialysis is somewhat different, but a weekly KT/V of 2.0 is the goal. The KT/V can be altered by several patient- and dialysis-associated variables. The calculations for KT/V can also be used to determine the patient's *protein catabolic rate (PCR),* which is a simplified nitrogen balance test in the dialysis patient. The PCR values should be above 1.0 g/kg.

A similar method looks at the reduction in urea before and after dialysis. The patient is well dialyzed when there is a 65% or greater reduction in the serum urea. Patients who are poorly dialyzed tend to have lower albumin levels and a higher risk of death (Owen et al., 1993).

Most patients find it difficult, if not impossible, to consume adequate protein and still have a palatable diet. In addition, the uremia itself causes some taste aberrations, notably to red meats, sometimes making it difficult to achieve the high HBV/low biologic value (LBV) protein ratio (Klahr, 1994).

Table 38–7 contains the exchange lists quantified for controlled intakes of protein, sodium, phosphorus, and kilocalories. Although the exchange lists may simplify calculation of the diet, some patients may prefer to learn the actual protein, phosphorus, and sodium content of foods and adjust their intake accordingly. Sodium, potassium, and protein values of foods are given in Appendix 41.

TUBE FEEDING

Patients with ESRD who require enteral tube feeding often do quite well on standard formulas used for most tube-fed patients. Before changing to a "specialty" formula a trial with these feedings is recommended because they are usually less expensive and typically have lower osmolality than the specific renal products. If eletrolyte or fluid concerns arise, patients can be changed to one of the formulas now available specifically designed for

TABLE 38–7 EXCHANGE LISTS FOR PROTEIN, KILOCALORIES, SODIUM, AND PHOSPHORUS*

FOOD	PROTEIN (g)	Kcal	SODIUM (mg)	PHOSPHORUS (mg)
Milk choices	4	120	80	110
Nondairy milk substitutes	0.5	140	40	30
Meat choices	7.0	65	25	65
Starch choices	2.0	90	80	35
Vegetable choices	1.0	25	15	20
Fruit choices	0.5	70	0	15
Fat choices	Trace	45	55	5
High-calorie choices	Trace	100	15	5
Salt choices	—	—	250	—

MILK CHOICES

Average per choice: 4 g protein, 120 Kcal, 80 mg sodium, 110 mg phosphorus

Milk (nonfat, low-fat, whole)	½ cup
Lo Pro	1 cup
Buttermilk, cultured	½ cup
Chocolate milk	½ cup
Light cream or half and half	½ cup
Ice milk or ice cream	½ cup
Yogurt, plain or fruit-flavored	½ cup
Evaporated milk	¼ cup
Sweetened condensed milk	¼ cup
Cream cheese	3 T
Sour cream	4 T
Sherbet	1 cup

NONDAIRY MILK SUBSTITUTES

Average per choice: 0.5 g protein, 140 Kcal, 40 mg sodium, 30 mg phosphorus

Dessert, nondairy frozen	½ cup
Dessert topping, nondairy frozen	½ cup
Liquid nondairy creamer, polyunsaturated	½ cup

MEAT CHOICES

Average per choice: 7 g protein, 65 Kcal, 25 mg sodium, 65 mg phosphorus

Prepared without added salt

Beef	1 oz
Round, sirloin, flank, cubed, T-bone, and porterhouse steak; tenderloin rib, chuck, and rump roast; ground beef or ground chuck	
Pork	1 oz
Fresh ham, tenderloin chops, loin roast, cutlets	
Lamb	1 oz
Chops, leg, roasts	
Veal	1 oz
Chops, roasts, cutlets	
Poultry	1 oz
Chicken, turkey, Cornish hen, domestic duck, goose	
Fish	1 oz
Fresh and frozen fish	1 oz
Lobster, scallops, shrimp, clams	1 oz
Crab, oysters	1½ oz
Canned tuna, canned salmon (canned without salt)	1 oz
Sardines (canned without salt)	1 oz
Wild game	1 oz
Venison, rabbit, squirrel, pheasant, duck, goose	
Egg	
Whole	1 large
Egg white or yolk	2 large
Low-cholesterol egg product	¼ cup
Chitterlings	2 oz
Organ meats	1 oz

Prepared with added salt

Beef	1 oz
Deli-style roast beef	
Pork	1 oz
Boiled or deli-style ham	
Poultry	1 oz
Deli-style chicken or turkey	
Fish	
Canned tuna, canned salmon	1 oz
Sardines	1 oz
Cheese	
Cottage	¼ cup

The following are high in sodium phosphorus and/or saturated fat. They should be used in your diet only as advised by your dietitian.

- Bacon
- Black beans, black-eyed peas, great northern beans, lentils, lima beans, navy beans, pinto beans, red kidney beans, soybeans, split peas, turtle beans
- Frankfurters, bratwurst, Polish sausage
- Luncheon meats including bologna, braunschweiger, liverwurst, picnic loaf, summer sausage salami
- Nuts and nut butters
- All cheeses except cottage cheese

STARCH CHOICES

Average per choice: 7 g protein, 90 Kcal, 80 mg sodium, 35 mg phosphorus

Breads and rolls

Bread (French, Italian, raisin, light rye, sourdough, white)	1 slice
Bagel	½ small
Bun, hamburger or hot dog type	½
Danish pastry or sweet roll, no nuts	½ small
Dinner roll or hard roll	1 small
Doughnut	1 small
English muffin	½
Muffin, no nuts, bran, or whole-wheat	1 small (1 oz)
Pancake	1 small (1 oz)
Pita or "pocket" bread	½ 6-in diameter
Tortilla, corn	2 6-in diameter
Tortilla, flour	1 6-in diameter
Waffle	1 small (1 oz)

TABLE 38–7 EXCHANGE LISTS FOR PROTEIN, KILOCALORIES, SODIUM, AND PHOSPHORUS*

Food	Amount
Cereals and grains	
Prepared without added salt	
Cereals, ready-to-eat, most brands	¾ cup
Puffed rice	2 cups
Puffed wheat	1 cup
Cereals, cooked	
Cream of Rice or Wheat, Farina, Malt-O-Meal	½ cup
Oat bran or oatmeal, Ralston	⅓ cup
Cornmeal, cooked	¾ cup
Grits, cooked	½ cup
Flour, all-purpose	2½ T
Pasta (noodles, macaroni, spaghetti), cooked	½ cup
Pasta made with egg (egg noodles), cooked	⅓ cup
Rice, white or brown, cooked	½ cup
Starchy vegetables	
Prepared or canned without added salt	
Corn	⅓ cup or ½ ear
Green peas	¼ cup
Potatoes, boiled or mashed	½ cup
Potatoes, baked, white or sweet	1 small (3 oz)
Potatoes, French fried	½ cup or 10 small
Potatoes, hashed brown	½ cup
Squash, butternut, mashed	½ cup
Squash, winter, baked (all other varieties), cubed	1 cup
Crackers and snacks	
Crackers: saltines, round butter	4 crackers
Graham crackers	3 squares
Melba toast	3 oblong
RyKrisp	3 crackers
Popcorn, plain	1½ cups, popped
Potato chips	1 oz, 14 chips
Tortilla chips	¾ oz, 9 chips
Pretzels, sticks or rings	¾ oz, 10 sticks
Pretzels, sticks or rings, unsalted	¾ oz, 10 sticks
Desserts	
Cake, angel food	1/20 cake or 1 oz
Cake	2 × 2-in square or 1½ oz
Sandwich cookie	4 cookies
Shortbread cookie	4 cookies
Sugar cookie	4 cookies
Sugar wafer	4 cookies
Vanilla wafer	10 cookies
Fruit pie	⅛ pie
Sweetened gelatin	½ cup

The following foods are high in poor-quality protein and/or phosphorus. They should be used only when advised by your dietitian.

- Bran cereal or muffins, Grape Nuts cereal, granola cereal or bars
- Boxed frozen or canned meals, entrees or side dishes
- Black beans, black-eyed peas, great northern beans, lentils, lima beans, navy beans, pinto beans, red kidney beans, soybeans, split peas
- Pumpernickel, dark rye, whole wheat, or oatmeal bread
- Whole wheat cereals
- Whole wheat crackers

High sodium—each serving counts as 1 Starch choice and 1 Salt choice.
High phosphorus.

TABLE 38–7 EXCHANGE LISTS FOR PROTEIN, KILOCALORIES, SODIUM, AND PHOSPHORUS*

VEGETABLE CHOICES

See Starch choices for other vegetables. Average per choice: 1 g protein, 25 Kcal, 15 mg sodium, 20 mg phosphorus

Prepared or canned without added salt unless otherwise indicated

1 cup serving	
Alfalfa sprouts	Escarole
Cabbage	Lettuce, all varieties
Celery	Pepper, green, sweet
Cucumber (or ½ whole)	Radishes, sliced (or 15 small)
Eggplant	Turnips
Endive	Watercress
1/2 cup serving	
Artichoke	Onions
Bamboo shoots	Parsnips
Bean sprouts	Pumpkin
Beans, green or wax	Rutabagas
Beets	Sauerkraut
Carrots (or 1 small)	Squash, summer
Cauliflower	Tomato (or 1 medium)
Chard	Tomato juice, unsalted
Chinese cabbage	Tomato juice, canned with salt
Collards	
Kale	Tomato puree
	Turnip greens
Kohlrabi	Vegetable juice cocktail, unsalted
Mushrooms, fresh raw (or 4 medium)	Vegetable juice cocktail, canned with salt
1/4 cup serving	
Asparagus (or 2 spears)	Mushrooms, fresh cooked
Avocado (¼ whole)	Mustard greens
Beet greens	Okra
Broccoli	Snow peas
Brussels sprouts	Spinach
Chili pepper	Tomato sauce

Prepared or canned with salt

Vegetables canned with salt (use serving size listed above)

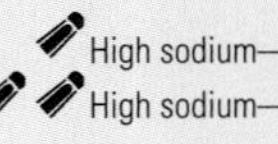

High sodium—each serving counts as *1 Vegetable choice* and *1 Salt choice.*
High sodium—each serving counts as *1 Vegetable choice* and *2 Salt choices.*
High sodium—each serving counts as *1 Vegetable choice* and *3 Salt choices.*
High phosphorus.

FRUIT CHOICES

Average per choice: 0.5 g protein, 70 Kcal, 15 mg phosphorus

1 cup serving	
Apple (1 medium)	Papaya nectar
Apple juice	Peach nectar
Applesauce	Pear nectar
Cranberries	Pear, canned or fresh (1 medium)
Cranberry juice cocktail	Tangerine (1 medium)
½ cup serving	
Apricot nectar	Lemon (½ medium)

TABLE 38–7 **EXCHANGE LISTS FOR PROTEIN, KILOCALORIES, SODIUM, AND PHOSPHORUS***

Banana (½ small)	Lemon juice
Blueberries	Mango (½ medium)
Figs, canned	Nectarine (½ medium)
Fruit cocktail	Orange (½ medium)
Grapes (15 small)	Peach, canned or fresh (½ medium)
Grape juice	
Grapefruit (½ medium)	Pineapple
Grapefruit juice	Plums, canned or fresh (1 medium)
Gooseberries	
Kiwifruit (½ medium)	Rhubarb
	Strawberries
	Watermelon
¼ cup serving	
Apricots (2 halves)	Honeydew melon (⅛ small)
Apricots, dried (2)	Orange juice
Blackberries	Papaya (¼ medium)
Cantaloupe (⅛ small)	Prune juice
Cherries	Prunes, cooked (5)
Dates (2 T)	Raisins (2 T)
Figs, dried (1 whole)	Raspberries

FAT CHOICES

Average per choice: trace protein, 45 Kcal, 55 mg sodium, 5 mg phosphorus	
Unsaturated fats	
Margarine	1 tsp
Reduced-calorie margarine	1 T
Mayonnaise	1 tsp
Low-calorie mayonnaise	1 T
Oil (safflower, sunflower, corn, soybean, olive, peanut, canola)	1 tsp
Salad dressing (mayonnaise-type)	2 tsp
Salad dressing (oil-type)	1 T
Low-calorie salad dressing (mayonnaise-type)	2 T
Low-calorie salad dressing (oil-type)	2 T
Tartar sauce (high sodium)	1½ tsp
Saturated fats	
Butter	1 tsp
Coconut	2 T
Powdered coffee whitener	1 T
Solid shortening	1 tsp

(High sodium symbol) High sodium—each serving counts as *1 Fat choice* and *1 Salt choice.*

HIGH-CALORIE CHOICES

Average per choice: trace protein, 100 Kcal, 15 mg sodium, 5 mg phosphorus	
Beverages	
Carbonated beverages (fruit flavors, root beer; colas or pepper-type) (high phosphorus)	1 cup
Kool-Aid	1 cup
Limeade	1 cup
Lemonade	1 cup
Cranberry juice cocktail	1 cup
Tang	1 cup
Fruit-flavored drink	1 cup
Wine[†]	½ cup
Frozen desserts	
Fruit ice	½ cup
Popsicle (3 ounces)	1 bar
Juice bar (3 ounces)	1 bar
Sorbet	½ cup
Candy and sweets	
Butter mints	14
Candy corn	20 or 1 oz
Chewy fruit snacks	1 pouch
Cranberry sauce or relish	¼ cup
Fruit chews	4
Fruit Roll Ups	2
Gumdrops	15 small
Honey	2 T
Hard candy	4 pieces
Jam or jelly	2 T
Jelly beans	10
LifeSavers or cough drops	12
Marmalade	2 T
Marshmallows	5 large
Sugar, brown or white	2 T
Sugar, powdered	3 T
Syrup	2 T
Special low-protein products	
Ask your dietitian for information on how to obtain these products.	
Low-protein gelled dessert	½ cup
Low-protein bread	1 slice
Low-protein cookies	2
Low-protein pasta	½ cup
Low-protein rusk	2 slices

The following foods are high in poor-quality protein and/or phosphorus. They should be used only when advised by your dietition.

- Beer[†]
- Chocolate
- Nuts and nut butters

(High phosphorus symbol) High phosphorus.

[†]Check with a physician before using alcohol.

SALT CHOICES

Average per choice: 250 mg sodium	
Salt	⅛ tsp
Seasoned salts (onion, garlic, etc.)	⅛ tsp
Accent	¼ tsp
Barbecue sauce	2 T
Bouillon	⅓ cup
Catsup	1½ T
Chili sauce	1½ T
Dill pickle	⅙ large or ½ oz
Mustard	4 tsp
Olives, green	2 medium or ⅓ oz
Olives, black	3 large or 1 oz
Soy sauce	¾ tsp
Light soy sauce	1 tsp
Steak sauce	2½ tsp
Sweet pickle relish	2½ tsp
Taco sauce	2 T
Tamari sauce	¾ tsp
Teriyaki sauce	1¼ tsp
Worcestershire sauce	1 T

(Reprinted with permission from the American Dietetic Association. A Healthy Food Guide: Kidney Disease, The National Renal Diet. Chicago: The American Dietetic Asscoiation, 1993.)

renal patients, Nepro (Ross Labs), Magnacal Renal (Mead Johnson), Travasorb Renal (Travenol), and Novasource Renal (Novartis), to name a few (Emery, 1997). If patients are receiving these "renal" products only, they may develop problems with a low phosphorus level, if they are experiencing "re-feeding syndrome," or if they are on phosphate binders. The dosage of the phosphate binders may need to be adjusted or eliminated. In some cases patients may need a phosphorus supplement or the addition of milk to their feeding to maintain an acceptable serum phosphorus level.

Some enteral feeding products contain only essential amino acids. These products are designed to be used just as the low-protein diet is used in predialysis patients, as a way to lower exogenous protein waste products. One such product is Amin-Aid (McGaw), which contains only the essential amino acids plus histidine in the amount required and which, when mixed with water, provides amino acids, carbohydrate, and a few electrolytes (see Appendix 38). A side effect of this formulation may be diarrhea due to the high osmolality.

Electrodialyzed whey (lactalbumin treated to remove the electrolytes) combined with glucose and water provides HBV protein with adequate calories and few electrolytes. However, unless the patient is experiencing severe shifts in electrolytes or requires a very large volume, most standard house tube feedings can be tailored to meet the requirements.

Energy

Energy intake must be adequate to spare protein for tissue protein synthesis and to prevent its metabolism for energy. Depending on the patient's nutritional status and degree of stress, between 25 and 40 kcal/kg body weight should be provided, with the lower amount for transplant and peritoneal dialysis patients. The higher level would be appropriate for the nutritionally depleted patient.

Calcium, Phosphorus, and Vitamin D

A major complication of ESRD is metabolic bone disease or **renal osteodystrophy.** The disease is essentially of three types: *osteomalacia,* or bone demineralization; osteitis fibrosa cystica, caused by hyperparathyroidism; and metastatic calcification of joints and soft tissues.

As the GFR decreases, phosphorus, whose level is controlled by renal excretion, is retained in the plasma. Serum calcium level declines for several reasons. Decreased 1,25-$(OH)_2D_3$, brought about by decreased ability of the kidney to convert the inactive form, appears to be most important. In addition, the calcium–phosphate product, which increases as phosphate increases, leads to extraosseus calcifications throughout the body and brings about a decreased calcium level. The low calcium level triggers several mechanisms by which the healthy body increases calcium to normal. These include the release of PTH from the parathyroid glands as well as increased synthesis of the active form of vitamin D by the kidney. This in turn acts on the gut to increase absorption of both calcium and phosphate and, in concert with PTH, acts to increase bone resorption, thus liberating both calcium and phosphate.

Parathormone also acts on the kidney to increase secretion of phosphate while retaining extra calcium. With decreased ability to produce 1,25-$(OH)_2D_3$, the patient with failing kidneys cannot increase gut absorption of calcium and must therefore rely on the effects of PTH to keep calcium levels up and phosphate down through bone resorption, and to increase renal elimination of phosphate. The dependence of calcium–phosphate control on increasing levels of PTH thus leads to a characteristic hyperplastic demineralized bone disease, **osteitis fibrosa cystica.** The disease is characterized by dull aching bone pain.

Even though the serum calcium level is elevated in response to PTH, the serum phosphate concentration remains high as the GFR falls lower. If the product of the serum calcium level (mg/100 mL) multiplied by the serum phosphate level (mg/100 mL) is greater than 70, **metastatic calcification** is imminent. Clinical management aims to keep the product below 70 by preventing transient elevations in serum phosphate concentration.

In essence, calcium and phosphorus intake must be controlled to as great a degree as possible to avoid aggravation of the delicate situation posed by hyperparathyroidism, phosphate retention, and hypocalcemia in renal failure. *In practical terms, calcium intake is kept high and phosphorus intake is kept low.* This is a problem as far as food is concerned because most of the high-calcium foods (milk and milk products) are also high in phosphorus. Consequently, methods in addition to dietary manipulation must be relied on.

Calcium intake is increased with calcium supplements in the form of calcium carbonate (e.g., Tums), acetate, (Phos-lo) lactate, malate, or gluconate along with the 300 to 500 mg calcium provided in the diet. These supplements are given between meals to increase calcium absorption. Starting calcium supplementation early is more likely to prevent hyperparathyroidism.

Calcium is present in the dialysate bath, and the amount can be somewhat adjusted to help stabilize low calcium values, or to decrease serum calcium in patients who have developed hypercalcemia due to active vitamin D administration.

Phosphate intake is lowered by restricting dietary sources to 1200 mg or less (see Table 38–7). A better way to estimate phosphorus restriction is to allow about 17 mg/kg body weight/day. A regression equation exists for estimating phosphorus intake based on protein intake.

128 + 14 (grams of protein in diet) = milligrams phosphorus per day in the diet.

Dietary restrictions alone are not adequate to control serum phosphorus, and nearly all patients undergoing dialysis will require phosphate-binding medication. In the past, aluminum hydroxide products such as Basaljel and Amphojel were used, but the resulting aluminum toxicity in many ESRD patients caused this treatment to be largely abandoned (Andress, 1986; Coburn and Norris, 1986). Current treatment relies on the use of calcium agents to bind phosphorus in the gut. Calcium carbonate, acetate, lactate, or gluconate are routinely used with each meal or snack (Schiller et al., 1989). Calcium citrate is avoided because of its ability to increase aluminum absorption. A complication of use of these calcium-based binders with committant use of active vitamin D is hypercalcemia. Because of this, some clinicians have returned to limited use of aluminum binders, in combination with calcium-based binders, and sometimes, even of magnesium-based binders. Obviously, serum levels of aluminum and magnesium need to be watched closely in these patients. A new phosphate-binding resin, Renagel (sevelamer hydrochloride), because of its composition, is able to reduce serum phosphorus without raising serum calcium.

Severe constipation leading to intestinal impaction is a potential risk of excessive consumption of phosphate binders. Occasionally, this may lead to perforation of the intestine, resulting in peritonitis and death. Constipation is often the reason why patients will not take the prescribed phosphate binders. Suggestions for using bran or other high-fiber foods and regular light exercise may contribute to patient compliance. Bulking agents such as Citrucel and Metamucil are low in phosphorus and potassium and are often used; however, they require the use of extra fluid to be mixed with them, which needs to be considered when using these products.

As with calcium supplementation, the early initiation of phosphate reduction therapies is advantageous for delaying hyperparathyroidism and bone disease. Unfortunately, most patients are asymptomatic during the early phase of hyperparathyroidism and are not attentive about following a modified diet and taking the calcium supplements and phosphate binders with meals. However, they should be encouraged to do so.

Because of potential *hypermagnesemia*, which can exacerbate the already existent bone disease, magnesium-containing antacids such as Maalox, Gelusil, Milk of Magnesia,or Mylanta should not be used.

Many patients on dialysis suffer from hypocalcemia, despite calcium supplementation. Because of this, the routine drug of choice is 1,25-$(OH)_2D_3$, which is available as calcitriol (Rocaltrol, Roche Labs; and Calcijex, Abbot Labs). Analogues such as 1-α,$(OH)D_3$ and 1-α,25-$(OH)_2D_3$ DHT (Roxane Labs), which have similar configurations, have been produced and are also available. Both the oral and IV types are effective.

Hemodialysis or peritoneal dialysis does not alleviate osteodystrophy. However, it can reduce the progression of the disease because the infused calcium results in decreased PTH secretion. Patients must still be responsible for following a low-phosphorus diet and for taking calcium to bind the phosphate.

Fluoride

High levels of fluoride in the serum of the uremic patient appear to aggravate the existing bone disease, possibly by enhancing bone demineralization. Increased serum fluoride levels in dialyzed uremic patients have been reported and may possibly be attributed to the fluoride content of the dialysate bath. It is recommended that water from fluoridated supplies be deionized before it is used in dialysis (Rao and Friedman, 1975).

Iron

The hypoproliferative, normochromic, normocytic anemia of chronic renal failure usually stabilizes with dialysis; however, it manifests itself in complaints of fatigue. It is caused by both an inability of the kidney to produce **erythropoietin (EPO),** a hormone that stimulates the bone marrow to produce red blood cells, and an increased destruction of red blood cells secondary to the circulating uremic waste products.

A synthetic form of EPO, *recombinant human erythropoietin (rHuEPO),* is used to treat the anemia of ESRD. Clinical trials have demonstrated a dramatic effect in the correction of anemia, as well as in the restoration of a general sense of well-being (Eschbach et al., 1987). EPO occasionally causes a rise in serum K^+. Whether this is due to increased blood viscosity impairing dialysis, increased breakdown of erythrocytes causing increased K^+, or an increase in the patient's appetite due to the increased sense of well-being is not clear.

Patients should be monitored closely while EPO dose is adjusted, and they may need increased dialysis or a lower level of K^+ in the dialysate bath. Accompanying the rise in hematocrit is almost always an increased need for iron, requiring supplementation both orally and intravenously. Oral iron itself is not effective in maintaining adequate iron stores in patients taking EPO. Unless there is a documented allergic reaction, allmost all patients on EPO will require periodic IV or intramuscular iron. For patients who are allergic to IV iron, oral iron is the only alternative and is usually given in three divided doses. Because of its ability to bind with phosphate binders, oral iron should be taken between meals and not with calcium phosphate binders.

Blood transfusion is not recommended for most patients with ESRD because of (1) its depression of erythropoiesis in the bone marrow, (2) the possibility of overexpansion of the blood volume, (3) the risk of hepatitis, and (4) hemochromatosis and hemosiderosis due to increased iron stores and the administration of parenteral iron.

Serum ferritin is an accurate indicator of iron overload. Patients who have received several transfusions and who are storing extra iron may have serum ferritin levels of 800 to 5000 ng/mL. (A normal level is 68 ng/mL for women and 150 ng/mL for men; see Chapter 35.) In patients who are receiving EPO, ferritin is kept above 100 ng/dL, although some recommendations are for levels up to 300 ng/dL. When ferritin values fall below 100 ng/mL, IV iron is usually given. The percent of iron saturation is another useful indicator of iron status in these patients. The percent saturation should be greater than 20%.

Vitamins

One of the several causes of vitamin deficiency in uremia is the decreased dietary intake due to the restriction of dietary phosphorus and potassium. Water-soluble vitamins are usually abundant in high-potassium foods such as citrus fruits and vegetables and high-phosphorus foods, such as milk. Diets for patients on dialysis tend to be low in folacin, niacin, riboflavin, and vitamin B_6. Ascorbic acid is marginal. With frequent episodes of anorexia or illness, the vitamin intake is decreased even further.

Altered metabolism and excretory function as well as drug administration also may alter vitamin levels. Little is known about gastrointestinal absorption in uremia, but it may be significantly decreased. It is possible that uremic toxins interfere with the activity of some vitamins; for example, the phosphorylation of pyridoxine (vitamin B_6) and its analogues may be inhibited.

Water-soluble vitamins are also lost during dialysis. In general, ascorbic acid and most of the B-complex vitamins are dialyzable. Because vitamin B_{12} is protein bound, losses of this B vitamin during dialysis are minimal.

Levels of fat-soluble vitamins do not usually change as much as levels of the water-soluble vitamins in renal disease. Circulating levels of retinol-binding protein are high in patients with renal failure, normally indicating vitamin A toxicity. Whether this indicates toxicity in these patients is unclear. They may have an increased capacity to tolerate vitamin A, due to the extra carrying capacity. Because little is known about this, supplementation of vitamin A is not usually recommended. Vitamin D, of course, should only be given in the active D_3 form by prescription, because ESRD patients do not activate this vitamin, in the form that it is normally in the diet or given in usual supplements. Little is known about vitamin E supplementation in chronic renal failure, although there is some evidence that it does help protect against red blood cell fragility in the uremic patient. However, supplementation is not routinely recommended. Vitamin K supplements are usually avoided due to the large number of patients taking anticoagulants such as coumadin.

Several vitamin supplements are now available that fit the needs of the uremic patient or the patient receiving dialysis (Nephrocaps, Fleming and Co.; Tabron, Parke-Davis; Neph-ron FA, Nephro-Tech Inc.; and Nephrovits, R & D Labs). A supplement of vitamin B complex and vitamin C is often used. Additional supplements of folic acid and pyridoxine may also be given. Folic acid supplementation is recommended at 1 mg/day. This level is above that allowed in over-the-counter vitamin preparations and requires a prescription.

It is worth noting that many dialysis patients routinely use some form of oral nutritional supplement, the majority of which contain complete vitamin supplementation to the level of the RDAs in 3 to 4 cans. Patients may be getting a significant amount of their vitamin nutriture from these supplements and may not require oral vitamin preparations in addition to their diets. A thorough analysis of the patient's intake is needed.

Carbohydrate

Glucose intolerance with both hyperglycemia and hypoglycemia is frequently observed in patients with ESRD. It seems to reflect a delayed and erratic action of insulin due to tissue resistance to insulin action or to an insulin antagonism by the products of uremia. In any case, this glucose intolerance rarely requires administration of insulin but might require control of the carbohydrate in the diet. If there are problems with hypoglycemia, the addition of dextrose to the dialysate usually alleviates the problem.

Lipid

Atherosclerotic cardiovascular disease is the most frequent cause of death among patients maintained on long-term hemodialysis. This appears to be a function of both underlying disease (e.g., diabetes mellitus, hypertension, nephrotic syndrome) and a lipid abnormality common among patients with ESRD. Typically, the patient with ESRD has an elevated triglyceride level with or without an increase in cholesterol. The lipid abnormality likely represents both increased synthesis of very-low-density lipoprotein and decreased clearance.

Treatment of hyperlipidemia with diet or pharmacologic agents remains controversial. Epidemiologic evidence demonstrating increased incidence of atherosclerotic coronary disease is balanced by studies demonstrating that patients with clearly defined clinical evidence of atherosclerosis at the initiation of dialysis are at no increased risk for a cardiovascular event over age-matched cohorts (Ma et al., 1992).

Although routine treatment appears unwarranted, a good case can be made for dietary and pharmacologic treatment of patients with ESRD with underlying lipid disorders and evidence of accelerated atherosclerosis. The new generation of lipid-lowering drugs, including lovastatin, may have a significant impact on future management (see Chapter 26).

Improvement of the plasma lipid profile in ESRD may also result from supplementation with the amino acid **L-carnitine.** Because the kidney is a major site of carnitine synthesis, dialysis patients typically have abnormal carnitine metabolism and low plasma-free carnitine levels. Research has shown the effectiveness of carnitine supplementation in increasing free and acyl carnitine levels in these patients. Carnitine supplementation has been associated with improved muscle function and less cramping, fewer hypotensive episodes and less protein catabolism (American Association for Kidney Patients, 1994; Wolk, 1993).

Parenteral Nutrition

When a patient with ESRD becomes too ill to maintain an adequate oral intake, and when tube feeding is not advisable due to gastrointestinal complications, parenteral nutrition should be considered (see Chapter 22).

Parenteral nutrition in ESRD is similar to parenteral nutrition used for other malnourished patients. The use of essential amino acid solutions, such as Nephramine, used to be recommended in cases of ARF or when a patient was not receiving dialysis treatment, but this practice has been discontinued because these patients seem to tolerate regular amino acid infusions well. Patients receiving dialysis therapy tolerate routine amino acid solutions, such as Freeamine (McGaw), Travasol 8.5 (Clintec), and Aminosyn (Abbot Labs).

Vitamins and Minerals

Most researchers agree that vitamin needs for ESRD are different from normal requirements during parenteral nutrition, but do not agree on their recommendations for individual nutrients. It is generally accepted that folate, pyridoxine, and biotin should be supplemented, and that vitamin A should not be provided parenterally unless retinol-binding protein is monitored, because it is elevated in patients with renal failure. Table 38–8 presents vitamin supplementation guidelines.

Little information is available relating to trace mineral supplementation in renal failure. Because most trace minerals, including zinc, chromium, and magnesium, are excreted in the urine, a close monitoring of these minerals in the serum seems to be appropriate.

Hypophosphatemia is a potential complication of parenteral nutrition in ESRD. When the patient is consuming some food, and receiving phosphate binders, this may be of even greater concern. If adequate protein and calories are provided and the patient becomes anabolic, the phosphate-binder regime may need to be altered to prevent hypophosphatemia and potential respiratory arrest.

TABLE 38–8 GUIDELINES FOR DAILY PARENTERAL VITAMIN SUPPLEMENTATION IN TOTAL PARENTERAL NUTRITION FOR PATIENTS WITH RENAL FAILURE*

VITAMIN	SILBERMAN	KOPPLE
A, as retinol (IU)	3300	0
E, tocopherol (IU)	10	10
K (mg)		7.5
Niacin (mg)	40	20
Thiamin HCl (mg)	3	2
Riboflavin (mg)	3.6	2
Pantothenic acid (mg)	15	10
Pyridoxine (mg)	5	10
Ascorbic acid (mg)	100	100
Biotin (mg)	60	200
Folic acid (mg)	1	2
B_{12} (mg)	5	3

(From Kouba J. Vitamin and electrolytes in patients with renal failure requiring total parenteral nutrition. Dietitians in Critical Care. Chicago: American Dietetic Association, p. 5, December 1985.)

*These are general guidelines and may need more specific evaluation and adjustment in patients in severe stress or with gastrointestinal losses from diarrhea, ostomies, fistula drainage, etc.

Intradialytic Parenteral Nutrition

Malnourished patients with chronic renal failure who are on hemodialysis have easy access to potential parenteral nutrition due to the requirements of the dialysis therapy itself. Because direct access to the blood must be made at every treatment, parenteral nutrition can be administered if necessary without additional invasive procedures or surgery.

Typically, *intradialytic parenteral nutrition (IDPN)* is administered through a connection to the venous side of the extracorporeal circuit during dialysis (Olsham and Schwartz, 1987). Due to the high blood flow rate achieved through use of the surgically created fistula and the high blood pump speeds attained, hypertonic glucose and protein can be administered without danger of phlebitis. Lipids may also be administered (Tables 38–9, 38–10, and 38–11). Reimbursement issues surrounding this therapy are complex and should be investigated related to the particular patient's geographic area before initiating this treatment.

COMPLICATIONS

Complications are similar to those encountered in TPN with the exception of *postdialysis hypoglycemia* due to the abrupt ending of the glucose supply. To avoid this problem, glucose administration is typically tapered up and down during the first and last half hour of the 3- to 4-hour treatment. Insulin is often given, usually in the bag of dextrose–amino acid solution, so that the patient

TABLE 38–9 REGIMEN FOR PARENTERAL NUTRITION BY PERIPHERAL VEIN FOR DIALYSIS PATIENTS*

INFUSION	QUANTITY	CALORIES (kcal)	VOLUME (mL)
10% Glucose	50 g glucose	170	500
10% Amino acids	40–50 g protein	160	500
10% Lipid emulsion	50 g fat	550	500
Total		880	1500†
Monitor serum glucose, sodium, potassium, bicarbonate, phosphate, triglycerides			

*Developed by Katy Wilkens, RD, Northwest Kidney Center, Seattle, Washington.
†Additional volume may include insulin and vitamins.

does not become hypoglycemic if the infusion must be stopped. Blood sugar levels are typically monitored during the therapy. Additionally, some patients may benefit from a snack of complex carbohydrate toward the end of the treatment.

Amino acid losses through the dialysate average about 10%. Vitamins and trace minerals are typically not administered with these solutions because patients are able to tolerate oral vitamin preparations and also have some oral dietary intake.

Other potential methods of nutritional support are the use of a hemodialysis dialysate solution containing amino acids and the use of a peritoneal dialysate solution containing amino acids as well as dextrose. These methods are currently in limited usage.

ESRD in Patients with Diabetes

Because renal failure is a complication of diabetes, approximately 35% of all new patients starting dialysis have diabetes. Because of the need to control blood sugar, these patients require even more specialized diet therapy. The diet for diabetes management (as discussed in Chapter 34) can be modified for the patient on dialysis.

In the presence of hyperglycemia, most patients with diabetes experience thirst, and fluid overload may become a serious problem. Increased osmolarity due to high serum levels of glucose may cause water and potassium to be pulled out of cells, with resultant hyperkalemia.

In addition, the diabetic patient on dialysis often has other complications, such as retinopathy, neuropathy, gastroparesis, and amputation, all of which can place this patient at high nutritional risk.

ESRD in Children

Renal failure may occur in children at any age, from the newborn infant through the adolescent. As with all children, the major concern is to promote normal growth and development. Without aggressive monitoring and encouragement, the child rarely meets his or her nutritional requirements. If the renal disease is present from birth, nutritional support needs to begin immediately, to avoid losing the growth potential of the first few months of life.

Growth in children with ESRD is usually retarded. Although no specific therapy ensures normal growth, factors capable of responding to therapy include metabolic acidosis, electrolyte depletion, osteodystrophy, chronic infection, and protein-calorie malnutrition. Energy and protein needs for children with chronic renal disease are at least equivalent to the RDA for normal children of the same height and age. If nutritional status is poor, energy needs may be even higher to promote weight gain and linear growth. Parenteral nutrition or feeding by tube may be necessary in the presence of poor intake, particularly in the critical growth period of the first 2 years of life. Gastrostomy tubes are often placed in these children to enhance nutritional intake and faciltate growth. Table 38–12 presents the nutritional requirements of children with renal failure.

Control of calcium and phosphorus balance is especially important for maintaining good growth. The goal is to restrict phosphorus intake while promoting calcium absorption with the aid of 1,25-

TABLE 38–10 REGIMEN FOR INTERMITTENT PARENTERAL NUTRITION ADMINISTERED DURING HEMODIALYSIS THERAPY*

INFUSION	QUANTITY	CALORIES (kcal)	VOLUME (mL)
70% Glucose	350 g glucose	1160	500
15% Amino acids	25 g protein	Protein should not be counted on to provide calories.	250
20% Lipid emulsion	50 g fat	550	250
Totals		1810	1000†
Monitor serum glucose, sodium, potassium, bicarbonate, phosphate, triglycerides			

*Developed by Katy Wilkens, RD, Northwest Kidney Center, Seattle, Washington.
†Additional volume may include insulin and vitamins.

TABLE 38–11 REGIMEN FOR TOTAL PARENTERAL NUTRITION BY SUBCLAVIAN VEIN FOR DIALYSIS PATIENTS*

INFUSION	QUANTITY	CALORIES (kcal)	VOLUME (mL)
70% Glucose	700 g glucose	2380	1000
15% Amino acids	50 g protein	Protein should not be counted on to provide calories.	500
20% Lipid emulsion	100 g fat	1100	500
Total		3480	2000[†]
Monitor serum glucose, sodium, potassium, bicarbonate, phosphate, triglycerides			

*Developed by Katy Wilkens, RD, Northwest Kidney Center, Seattle, Washington.
[†]Additional volume may include insulin and vitamins.

$(OH)_2D_3$. This helps prevent renal osteodystrophy, which can cause severe growth retardation during childhood. Use of calcium carbonate formulations to supplement the dietary intake enhances calcium intake while binding excess phosphorus. Aluminum-containing preparations are used only in patients with extreme hyperphosphatemia and only on a short-term basis. Aluminum binders should never be used routinely in children under the age of 10 years.

Persistent metabolic acidosis is often associated with growth failure in infancy. In chronic acidosis, the titration of acid by the bone causes calcium loss and contributes to bone demineralization. Bicarbonate may be added to the formula to counteract this effect.

Restriction of protein in pediatric diets is controversial. The so called "protective" effect on kidney function must be weighed against the clearly negative effect of possible protein malnutrition on growth. The RDA for protein for age is usually the minimum amount to be given (see Table 10–1).

Each child's diet should be adjusted to his or her food preferences, family eating patterns, and biochemical needs. This is often not an easy task. In addition, care must be taken not to place too much emphasis on the diet to avoid its becoming a manipulative tool and an attention-getting device.

Special encouragement, creativity, and attention are required to help the child with ESRD consume the necessary energy. When possible, *continuous cyclic peritoneal dialysis (CCPD),* dialysis which is intermittent during the day and continuous at night, appears to be a viable therapy of choice for children because it allows liberalization of the diet. The child is more likely to meet nutritional requirements with fewer dietary restrictions, and therefore experience better growth.

New developments that may help with treatment of renal disease in children include the use of rHuEPO and *rDNA-produced growth hormone (rHGH).* Correction of anemia with the use of rHuEPO may increase appetite, intake, and feeling of well-being, but it has not been found to affect growth, even with seemingly adequate nutritional support. Daily rHGH has been shown to increase growth in children with chronic renal failure and ESRD, even when these children have normal endogenous production of growth hormone (Fine et al., 1994).

HUMAN IMMUNODEFICIENCY VIRUS AND RENAL DISEASE

Exposure to human immunodeficiency virus (HIV) may occur in patients with renal disease. HIV infection with eventual development of acquired immunodeficiency syndrome (AIDS) may then occur (see Chapter 40).

Drugs often used in the treatment of patients with HIV may be nephrotoxic and cause reversible kidney disease. Sepsis, common in the patient with HIV, may also lead to renal failure. The prognosis of patients with HIV who develop ARF appears to be somewhat improved if they receive repetitive dialysis therapy.

The patient with ESRD with previously diagnosed renal disease who develops *positive HIV antibodies* has a somewhat better prognosis. Survival on dialysis treatment may range from 3 months to several years, with death resulting from other complications of renal failure or the development of AIDS.

Several cases of patients becoming infected with HIV as a result of *organ transplantation* from an HIV-positive donor, either living related or cadaveric, have been reported. The Centers for Disease Control and Prevention recommend that no person from a high-risk category should be considered as a donor for organ transplantation and that HIV testing should be performed on all donors.

Conversely, transplantation of a kidney to an HIV-positive patient may be contraindicated because the immunosuppressive drugs may shorten the time required to develop AIDS. The 2-year survival rate for asymptomatic HIV-positive patients who have had transplants has been reported to be significantly lower than for non–HIV-positive transplant recipients.

Nutritional Care

Weight loss and malnutrition are common findings in patients with AIDS, apparently due to malabsorption, altered metabolism, and altered organ

TABLE 38–12 NUTRIENT REQUIREMENTS BASED ON TYPE OF THERAPY FOR CHILDREN WITH RENAL DISEASE*

THERAPY	ENERGY	PROTEIN		FLUID	SODIUM	POTASSIUM	PHOSPHORUS
		Creatinine Clearance	Protein Requirement				
Impaired renal function (predialysis)	Infant (under 1 y): 120–150 kcal/kg	10–50	1.5 g/kg	35 mL/100 kcal + urine output	23–69 mg/kg/day (1–3 mEq/kg/day)	29–87 mg/kg/day (1–3 mEq/kg/day)	0.5–1 g/day
	Child: First 10 kg = 100 kcal/kg	<10	1 g/kg				
	Second 10 kg = 50 kcal/kg Every kg thereafter: 20 kcal/kg	<5	0.3–0.5 g/kg				
		Weight of Child					
Hemodialysis	Same as above	10–20 kg	2 g/kg	Same as above, plus losses from dialysis. Child's fluid gains should be about 5% of body weight	57 mg/kg/day (2.5 mEq/kg/day)	Same as above	0.5–1 g/day
		20–30 kg	1.5 g/kg				
		30–40 kg	1.0–1.5 g/kg				
		40+ kg	1.0 g/kg				
Intermittent peritoneal dialysis (IPD)	Same as above	10–20 kg	2 g/kg	Same as above	Same as above		
		20–40 kg	1.5 g/kg				
		40+ kg	1.0–1.5 g/kg				
Continuous ambulatory peritoneal dialysis (CAPD)	100–120 kcal/kg	10–20 kg	2–3 g/kg	100–160 mL/kg/day + urine output	Same as above	Same as above	0.5–1 g/day
		20–40 kg	1.5–2 g/kg				
		40+ kg	1.0–1.5 g/				
Transplant	Normal energy requirement for age. Tendency toward obesity due to steroids. Not more than 35% of total calories from fat. Low saturated fat.		2–3 g/kg	Ad libitum	Variable	Variable, usually ad libitum	Ad libitum Supplement if necessary. Calcium ad libitum, supplement if necessary. Vitamin D as necessary.

*Developed by Anne Hetrick, RD, Shands Teaching Hospital, University of Florida, Gainesville.

CASE STUDY 1

Hemodialysis

Mark M. is a 36-year-old man with a history of drug abuse and cocaine addiction. Recently, he was admitted to the local hospital with acute renal failure and has been started on hemodialysis. He has no prior medical problems or hypertension. His labs include BUN, 90; creatinine, 7; potassium, 6.1; all other labs are currently normal. He is 6′ 2″ and weighs 190 lb.

1 What suggestions do you have for the dialysis nutrition prescription?
2. His doctor suggests daily use of a multivitamin supplement containing B-complex vitamins but not the fat-soluble vitamins. Why?
3. What level of protein would you suggest during dialysis? With this factor, how much should Mark be receiving in the way of protein foods?
4. If he goes home without dialysis but has chronic renal failure, what might his doctor suggest for a protein level?
5. What foods will be monitored, using the National Renal Diet?

function (see Chapter 40). Problems with nutritional treatment in such patients are compounded by restrictions on sodium, potassium, and fluid. As in any renal disease patient with malnutrition, all restrictions not absolutely necessary for the patient's immediate well-being are usually omitted.

CASE STUDY 2

Peritoneal Dialysis

Kelsey W. is a 33-year-old woman with glomerulonephritis who has been on dialysis 8 years. Current laboratory values:

Na: 135	K: 5.9	CO_2: 16
Creat: 9	Ca: 8.7	PO_4: 6.9
Alb: 3.4	Ferritin: 82	Wt: 57.2 kg
Ht: 172	Fluid gains: 2.9–3.7 kg	BUN: 70
AMA: <50%	AFA: >8%	

1. Explain why you would expect to see each of the laboratory value discrepancies and what could be done nutritionally to affect each value. Also assess the patient's weight and anthropometric values to determine appropriate nutritional therapy.
2. Kelsey takes the following medications: erythropoietin, Benadryl, folic acid, prednisone, Nephrocaps, Basagel, and Tums. The patient dialyzes against the following dialysate fluid: 3 mEq K, 3.5 mg calcium, bicarbonate, 200 g dextrose. Comment on the appropriateness of each. What are they used for? Would you suggest any changes? Any additional medications?
3. The patient is currently awaiting a cadaveric transplant. She asks you how her diet will change with the transplant. If the transplant does not happen soon, she is considering peritoneal dialysis to give her more freedom from the machine. What would be the nutritional concerns if this were to happen?

The emphasis is on providing adequate oral intake tolerated by the patient.

Parenteral nutrition, either total or intermittent, may be used as an adjunctive treatment in these patients. Open communication with these terminally ill patients is required among the patient, family, and health care team to provide the patient with adequate but not heroic treatment.

CITED REFERENCES

American Association for Kidney Patients Carnitine Renal Dialysis Consensus Group. Role of L-carnitine in treating renal dialysis patients. Dialysis and Transplantation 23:177, 1994.

Allison MJ, et al. Oxalate degradation by gastrointestinal bacteria from humans. J Nutr 116:455, 1986.

Andress DL. Aluminum-associated bone disease in chronic renal failure: High prevalance in the long-term dialysis population. J Bone Miner Res 1:391, 1986.

Avorn J, et al. Reduction of bacteriuria and pyuria after ingestion of cranberry juice. JAMA 271:751, 1994.

Bataille P, et al. Effect of calcium restriction on renal excretion of oxalate and the probability of stones in various pathophysiological groups with calcium stones. J Urol 130:218, 1983.

Beto J. Highlights of the consensus conference on prevention of progression in chronic renal disease: Implications for dietetic practice. J Renal Nutr 4:122, 1994.

Blagg C, et al. Serum albumin concentration: HCFA quality assurance criterion is method dependent. Am J Kidney Dis 21:138, 1993.

Borghi L, et al. Urinary volume, water and recurrence in idiopathic calcium nephrolithiasis: A 5 year randomized prospective study. J Urol 155:839, 1996.

Brenner BM, Lazarus JM (eds.). Acute Renal Failure, 2nd ed. New York: Churchill-Livingstone, 1988.

Brinkley LJ, et al. A further study of oxalate bioavailability in foods. J Urol 144:94, 1990.

Coburn JW, Norris KC: Diagnosis of aluminum-related bone disease and treatment of aluminum toxicity with desferoxamine. Semin Nephrol 4:12, 1986.

Coe FL, Favus MJ. Disorders of stone formation. In: Brenner BM, Rector FC (eds.). The Kidney, 3rd ed. Philadelphia: WB Saunders, 1986.

Coe FL, et al. The pathogenesis and treatment of kidney stones. N Engl J Med 327:1141, 1992a.

Coe FL, et al. Stone forming potential of milk or calcium fortified orange juice in idiopathic hypercalciuric adults. Kidney Int 41:139, 1992b.

Curhan GC, et al. A prospective study of dietary calcium and other nutrients and the risk of symptomatic kidney stones. N Engl J Med 328:833, 1993.

Curhan GC, et al. Beverage use and risk for kidney stones in women. Ann Int Med 128: 534, 1998.

Dwyer J, et al. Acid/alkaline ash diets: Time for assessment and change. J Am Diet Assoc 85:841, 1985.

Emery E. Enteral feedings for renal patients: A primer. Renal Nutritional Forum16 (Spring):1, 1997.

Eschbach J, et al. Correction of the anemia of end-stage renal disease with recombinant human erythropoietin. N Engl J Med 316:73, 1987.

Finch AM, et al. Urine composition in normal subjects after oral ingestion of oxalate-rich foods. Clin Sci 60:411, 1981.

Fine RN, et al. Growth after recombinant human growth hormone treatment in children with chronic renal failure: Report of a multicenter randomized double-blind placebo-controlled study. J Pediatr 124:324, 1994.

Giordano C. Early diet to slow the course of chronic renal failure. In: Zurukzoglu W, Papadimetrious M (eds.). Eighth International Congress of Nephrology, June 1981. Basel: S Karger, 1981.

Goldfarb S. Dietary factors in the pathogenesis and prophylaxis of calcium nephrolithiasis. Kidney Int 34:544, 1988.

Gray LB. Nutritional implications of renal transplantation, Pt. I. Renal Nutrition Forum 12(4):1, 1993; Pt. II, Renal Nutrition Forum 13(1):1, 1994.

Hricik DE, et al. Glomerulonephritis. N Engl J Med 339:888, 1998.

Howell A, et al. Inhibition of the adherence of P-fimbriated *Escherichia coli* to uroepithelial-cell surface by proanthocyanidin extracts from cranberries (Letter), N Engl J Med 339:1085, 1998

Ihle BU, et al. The effect of protein restriction on the progression of renal inefficiency. N Engl J Med 321:1773, 1989.

Kajander EO, Ciftcioglu N. Nanobacteria: An alternative mechanism for pathogenic intra and extracellular calcification and stone formation. Proc Natl Acad Sci U S A 95:8274, 1998.

Kaysen G. Nutritional management of nephrotic syndrome. In: Kopple

JD, Massery SG (eds.). Nutritional Management of Renal Disease. Baltimore: Williams & Wilkens, 1997, p. 533.
Klahr S. The effects of dietary protein restriction and blood pressure control on the progression of chronic renal disease. N Engl J Med 330:877, 1994.
Lemann J, et al. Potassium administration reduces and potassium deprivation increases urinary calcium excretion in healthy adults. Kidney Int 39:973, 1991.
Levine BS, et al. Effect of calcium citrate supplementation on urinary calcium oxalate saturation in female stone formers: Implications for prevention of osteoporosis. Am J Clin Nutr 60:592, 1994.
Liebman M, et al. Effects of supplemental ascorbate and orange juice on urinary oxalate. Nutr Res 17:415, 1997.
Ma KW, et al. Cardiovascular risk factors in chronic renal failure and hemodialysis populations. Am J Kid Dis 19:505, 1992.
Massey LK, Sutton RAL. Modification of dietary oxalate and calcium reduces urinary oxalate in hyperoxaluric patients with kidney stones. J Am Diet Assoc 93:1305, 1993.
Massey LK, Whiting SJ. Dietary salt, urinary calcium, and kidney stone disease. Nutr Rev 53:131, 1995.
Massey LK, et al. Effect of dietary oxalate and calcium on urinary oxalate and risk of formation of calcium oxalate kidney stones. J Am Diet Assoc 93:901, 1993.
Molina M. Nutrition support in the patient with renal failure. Crit Care Clin 11:685, 1995.
Milliner DS, et al. Results of long-term treatment with orthophosphate and pyridoxine in patients with primary hyperoxaluria. N Engl J Med 331:1553, 1994.
Mitch WE. Nutritional therapy for the nephrotic syndrome. In: Brenner BM (ed.). The Kidney, 5th ed., vol. 2. Philadelphia: WB Saunders, 1996.
Oldenburg B. Factors influencing excessive thirst and fluid intakes in dialysis patients. Dialys Transplant 17:21, 1988.
Olsham AR, et al. Intradialytic parenteral nutrition administration during outpatient hemodialysis. Dialysis Transplantation 16:495, 1987.
Owen W, et al. The urea reduction ratio and serum albumin concentration as predictors of mortality in patients undergoing hemodialysis. N Engl J Med 329:1001, 1993.
Pastan S, Bailey J. Dialysis therapy. N Engl J Med 338:1428, 1998.
Perez N. Managing nutrition problems in transplant patients. Nutr Clin Pract 8(1):28, 1993.
Rao TKS, Friedman EA. Fluoride and bone disease in uremia. Kidney Int 7:125: 1975.
Rao T, Friedman E. The types of renal disease in the acquired immunodeficiency syndrome. N Engl J Med 316:1062, 1987.
Remer T, Manz F. Potential renal acid load of foods and its influence on urine pH. J Am Diet Assoc 95:791, 1995.
Remuzzi G, Bertani T. Pathophysiology of progressive nephropathies. N Engl J Med 339:1448, 1998.
Schiller LR, et al. Effect of the time of administration of calcium acetate on phosphorous binding. N Engl J Med 320:1110, 1989.
Sherman HC, Gettler AO. The balance of acid forming and base forming elements in food and its relation to ammonia metabolism. J Biol Chem 11:323, 1912.
Sherman RA, et al. Interdialytic weight gain and nutrition parameters in chronic hemodialysis patients. Am J Kidney Dis 25:579, 1995.
Toto RD. Treatment of dyslipidemia in chronic renal failure, lipid abnormalies in patients with renal failure. Blood Purif 14:75, 1996.
Soloway MS, Smith RA. Cranberry juice as a urine acidifier. JAMA 260:1465, 1988.
Sowers MRF, et al. Prevalence of renal stones in a population-based study with dietary calcium, oxalates, and mediaction exposures. Am J Epidemiol 147:914, 1998.
van der Heide JJH, et al. Effect of dietary fish oil on renal function and rejection in cyclosporine-treated recipients of renal transplants. N Engl J Med 329:769, 1993.
Wolk R. Micronutrition in dialysis. Nutr Clin Pract 8:267, 1993.

ADDITIONAL REFERENCES

Baron P, Waymack JP. A review of nutrition support for transplant patients. Nutr Clin Pract 8:12, 1993.
Brinkley L, et al. Bioavailability of oxalate in foods. J Urol 17:534, 1981.
Council on Renal Nutrition. Pocket Guide to Nutritional Assessment of the Adult Renal Patient. New York: National Kidney Foundation, 1993.
Evanoff GV, et al. Effect of dietary protein restriction on the progression of diabetic nephropathy. Arch Intern Med 147:492, 1987.
Furst P. Principles of essential amino acid therapy in uremia. Am J Clin Nutr 31:1744, 1978.
Georgalas A, Goffi J. Nutritional strategies for the treatment of chronic renal failure in children. Nutrition Today 28(4):24, 1993.
Hruska KA, Teitelbaum SL. Renal osteodystrophy. N Engl J Med 333:166, 1995.
Koch VH, et al. Accelerated growth after recombinant human growth hormone treatment of children with chronic renal failure. J Pediatr 113:365, 1989.
Kopple JD. The nutrition management of the patient with acute renal failure. J Parenter Enteral Nutr 20:3, 1996.
Larsson L, Tiselius H-G. Hyperoxaluria. Miner Electrolyte Metab 13:242, 1987.
Levine SL. Enteral nutrition in ESRD. In: Stover J (ed.). A Clinical Guide to Nutrition Care in ESRD, 2nd ed. Chicago: American Dietetic Association, 1994.
Maschio G, et al. Effects of dietary protein and phosphorus restriction in the progression of early renal failure. Kidney Int 22:371, 1982.
Mitch WE, Klahr S. Nutrition and the Kidney, 2nd ed. Boston: Little, Brown, 1993.
Pachter L. Culture and clinical care: Folk illness beliefs and behaviors and their implications for health care delivery. JAMA 271:690, 1994.
Seidner D. Nutritional care of the critically ill patient with renal failure. Semin Nephrol 14(1):53, 1994.
Stover J (ed.). A Clinical Guide to Nutrition Care in End-Stage Renal Disease, 2nd ed. Chicago: American Dietetic Association, 1994.
Stover J, Nelson P. Nutritional recommendations for infants, children and adolescents with ESRD. In: Stover J (ed.). A Clinical Guide to Nutrition Care in End-Stage Renal Disease, 2nd ed. Chicago: American Dietetic Association, 1994.
Walser M. 1988 Herman Award Lecture: Effect of ketoanalogues in chronic renal failure and other disorders. Am J Clin Nutr 49:17, 1989.
Wiggins K, Wilkens K (eds.). Suggested Guidelines for Nutrition Care of Renal Patients, 3rd ed. Chicago: American Dietetic Association, 1999.
Zerwekh JE. Pathogenesis of hypercalciuria. In: Pak CYC (ed.). Renal Stone Disease. Pathogenesis, Prevention and Treatment. Boston: Martinus Nijhoff, 1987.
Ziegler VS, et al. Southeast Asian renal exchange list. J Am Diet Assoc 89:85, 1989.

CHAPTER 39

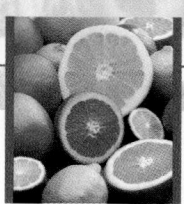

Medical Nutrition Therapy for Neoplastic Disease

CAROL B. FRANKMANN, MS, RD, LD, CNSD

CHAPTER OUTLINE

- Nutrition in the Etiology of Cancer
- Nutritional Effects of Cancer
- Nutritional Effects of Cancer Therapy
- Nutritional Care of the Patient with Cancer

Key Terms

AGEUSIA—inability to taste

ALLOGENEIC MARROW TRANSPLANTATION—transfer of marrow from a donor to another person (often a relative, such as a sibling) who is not genetically identical; a *syngeneic* marrow transplantation occurs from a twin

ANTINEOPLASTIC AGENTS—chemical agents (cytotoxics, immunologic preparations, hormones) or medications used to treat cancer

AUTOLOGOUS MARROW TRANSPLANTATION—transfer of marrow using the patient's own tissue (from hematopoietic stem cells)

CANCER CACHEXIA—the weak, malnourished, and emaciated condition that often results from cancer

CARCINOGENS—substances that induce cancer in humans and animals

CARCINOGENESIS—a multistage, biologic process that proceeds on a continuum, but is often described as initiation, promotion, and progression phases

CASE CONTROL STUDIES—studies in which the diets of individuals with cancer are compared with those of cancer-free controls matched for age, sex, and other key factors

COHORT STUDIES—studies in which diets of different groups of subjects are determined prior to cancer onset, and the incidences of developing cancers in each group are compared

CYTOKINES—protein mediators produced by inflammatory cells in response to exogenous stimuli

DYSGEUSIA—impaired taste

GRAFT-VERSUS-HOST DISEASE (GVHD)—a disease caused by the immune response of histoincompatible, immunocompetent donor cells against the tissues of an immunoincompetent host; an immunologic reaction of allogeneic donor cells (graft) reacting against the patient (host) tissues

HYPOGEUSIA—decreased taste acuity

INITIATION—the initial stage of tumorigenesis involving transformation of cellular DNA

METASTASIS—growth of malignant tissue that spreads to surrounding tissues

NEOPLASM—a new and abnormal formation of tissue that serves no useful function

NEUTROPENIA—a reduction in white blood cell count (neutrophils) that can be caused by chemotherapy or radiation therapy, and that, in turn, results in increased susceptibility to infections which can be life-threatening

PANCYTOPENIA—a reduction in all cellular elements of the blood

PHYTOCHEMICALS—nonnutritive compounds in plants thought to influence the process of tumorigenesis

PROGRESSION—the phase in which tumor cells aggregate, grow autonomously, and form benign tumors that eventually lead to a malignant phenotype with the capacity for tissue invasion and metastasis

PROMOTION—the stage of tumorigenesis in which initiated cells are activated by a promoting agent to multiply and form a discrete tumor

RADIATION-INDUCED ENTERITIS—a condition of inflammation that can occur after radiation to the intestinal tract and that leads to diarrhea and malabsorption

TUMOR NECROSIS FACTOR (CACHECTIN)—a hormone-like protein that releases fat from fat stores, reduces the concentration of enzymes required for the production and storage of fat, and induces a state of anorexia

VENO-OCCLUSIVE DISEASE (VOD)—a symptomatic occlusion of the small hepatic venules caused by hepatotoxins and radiation; may resolve after removal of the offending agent, or may progress to portal hypertension and liver failure

XEROSTOMIA—mouth dryness

Cancer can be regarded as a disease of the body's cells. Its development involves damage to the DNA of cells; this damage accumulates over time. When these damaged cells escape the mechanisms that are in place to protect the organism from the growth and spread of such cells, a **neoplasm** is established. Classification of tumors is based on their tissue of origin, their growth properties, and their invasion of other tissues. The growth of a malignant neoplasm usually destroys surrounding tissue and may eventually spread to distant tissues, a process termed **metastasis.** As cancer occurs in cells that are replicating, the patterns of cancer are quite different in children and adults. In early life, the brain, nervous system, bones, muscles, and connective tissue are still growing. Thus, in children, these tissues are more commonly involved with cancerous lesions than in adults. Conversely, the common adult tumors involve epithelial linings and are rare in children. Leukemias and lymphomas, tumors of the immune system, occur in both children and adults, although the natural history of the disease differs depending on whether they occur early or late (Food, Nutrition, and the Prevention of Cancer, 1997).

The study of diet and nutrition as it relates to cancer addresses both the causes and consequences of cancer. **Carcinogenesis** is thought to be a multistage process that proceeds on a continuum but is often described in three progressive phases: initiation, promotion, and tumor progression (Fig. 39–1). **Initiation** involves a transformation of the cell produced by the interaction of chemicals, radiation, or viruses with cellular DNA. The transformation occurs rapidly, but the resultant cell remains dormant for a variable period until activated by a promoting agent. During **promotion,** initiated cells multiply to form a discrete tumor. From there, **progression** proceeds, leading eventually to a fully malignant neoplasm with the capacity for tissue invasion and metastasis.

Diagnosis of cancer includes tissue evaluation (biopsy), serum markers (AFP, CEA, PSA, B-HCG, etc.), and staging (radiographic, surgical, or T-N-M staging for tumor size, nodes, metastasis). Goals of treatment may include cure, palliation, or adjuvant therapy. Response is documented as complete, partial, no change, or progression.

Although the exact mechanisms are unknown, nutrition may modify the carcinogenic process at any stage, including carcinogen metabolism, cellular and host defenses, cell differentiation, and tumor growth. Nutrition itself is also adversely affected, both by the tumor and by the medical treatment given, posing special problems for nutritional care. An effective internet site for more information is www.cancer.org.

NUTRITION IN THE ETIOLOGY OF CANCER

If the estimate that 80% to 90% of cancer is related to environmental factors is correct, including an estimated 35% related to diet, then most human cancers are potentially preventable. The strong influence of environmental factors is readily seen in studies of migration between cultures. These studies have revealed that the pattern of occurrence of many types of cancer changes to resemble that of the new country. For example, in Japan, mortality from breast and colon cancer is low and mortality from stomach cancer is high, whereas the reverse is true in the United States. After two or three generations, the cancer pattern of Japanese immigrants to the United States becomes similar to that of their new country. The change coincides with differences in environmental exposure, lifestyle, and diet.

Studies evaluating the role of diet in the etiology of cancer seek to identify relationships between the diet of the population groups or categories of individuals and the incidence of specific cancers. Sets of individuals are compared in **case control, cohort,** or cross-sectional studies. Information from these forms of epidemiologic research is statistically more powerful than that gathered from population studies. The strongest evidence comes from consistent findings using different types of epidemiologic studies in diverse populations.

The sheer complexity of diet presents a difficult challenge when contemplating a study of its relationship to cancer. There are literally thousands of chemicals, some well known, others little known and unmeasured. Diets contain both inhibitors and enhancers of carcinogenesis. In addition, when one major component of the diet is altered, other changes take place simultaneously. For example, decreasing animal protein also decreases animal fat. This makes the interpretation of research findings difficult because the effects cannot be clearly associated with a single factor. Many tumors have a long latency period, in which case the diet at the time of initiation or promotion, not at the time of diagnosis, may be important. Some prospective epidemiologic studies attempt to circumvent this difficulty by measuring diet at one point in time and following the same subjects for several years.

Studies done with laboratory animals are used to test the effect of food and nutrition on cancer. Since the early part of this century, laboratory scientists have shown that various nutritional manipulations influence the occurrence of tumors in animals. In concert with epidemiologic work, animal studies can be used to provide hypotheses to guide epidemiologic research and reveal modifiable pathways to cancer in humans.

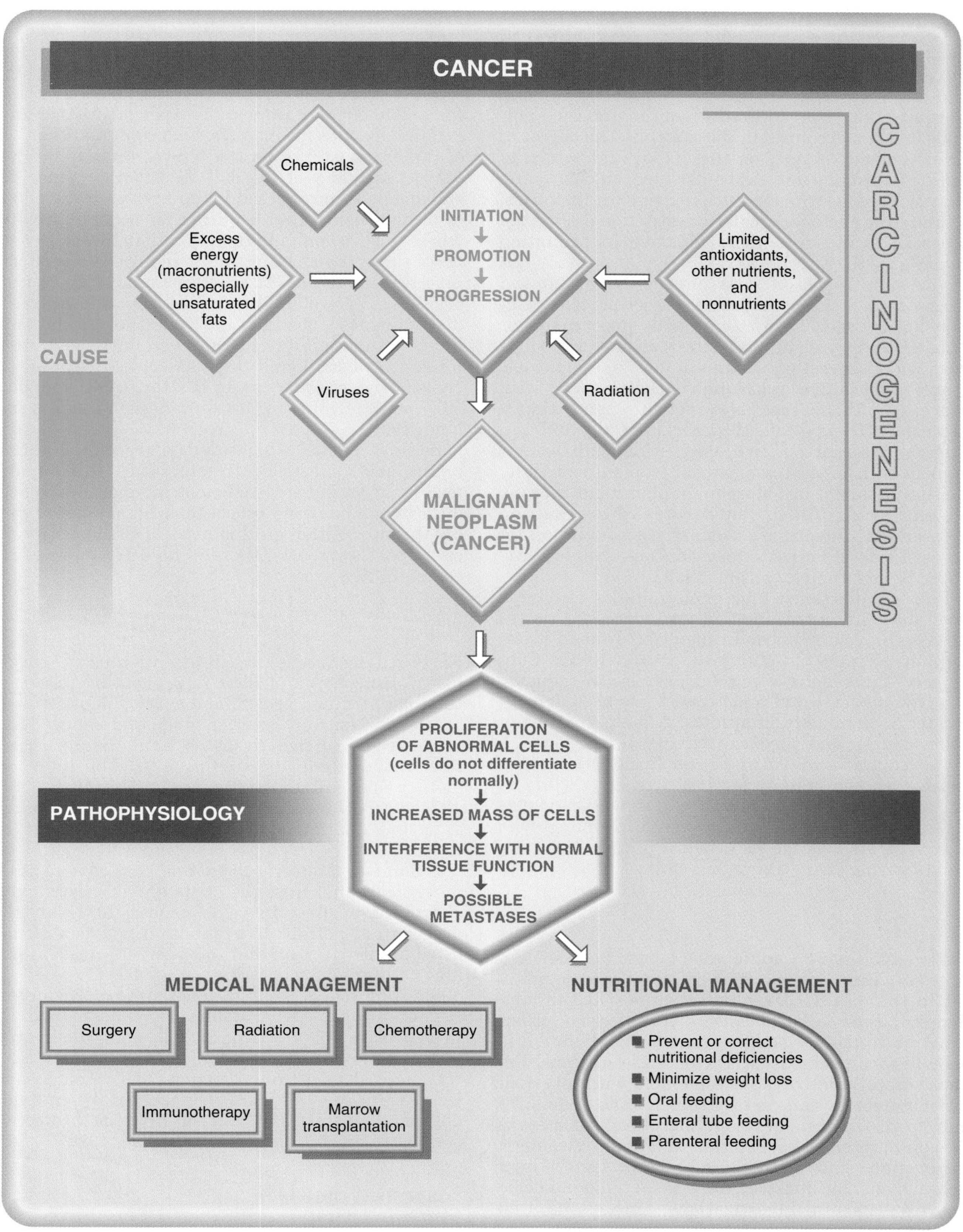

FIGURE 39–1 Pathophysiology algorithm—carcinogenesis. (Algorithm content developed by John Anderson, Ph.D., and Sanford C Garner, Ph.D., 2000.)

Energy Balance and Exercise

In animal studies, chronic restriction of food inhibits the growth of most experimentally induced tumors and the occurrence of many spontaneous tumors. This effect is observed even when the underfed animals ingest more fat than the controls. The degree of effect depends mainly on the extent and timing of caloric restriction and the tumor type. Underfeeding is most effective when maintained during all phases; if limited to one phase, caloric restriction during the progression phase is more effective in inhibiting tumor growth (Kritchevsky, 1997).

The significance of data on energy intake and cancer risk in humans remains unclear. The relationship between body weight, body mass index, or relative body weight and site-specific cancer has been widely investigated, and in most epidemiologic studies, a positive association has been seen with cancers of the breast, endometrium, and kidney (Trentham-Dietz et al., 1997; Olson et al., 1995). In breast cancer, a positive association with weight gain is seen in postmenopausal women, especially those who do not use hormone replacement therapy (Huang et al., 1997). Rapid rates of growth and greater adult height are also associated with an increased risk of breast cancer (Barnes-Josiah et al., 1995; Brinton and Swanson, 1992).

Physical inactivity, high energy intake, and large body mass are associated with an increased risk of developing colon cancer in men and women (Slattery et al., 1997a; Martinez et al., 1997). Conversely, the benefit of regular exercise in reducing the risk of breast and colon cancer has been demonstrated in a number of studies. A meta-analysis of colon cancer and physical activity levels found a 50% reduction in colon cancer incidence among those with the highest level of activity (Colditz et al., 1997). An equally significant reduction in the risk for breast cancer was observed in women who exercised an average of 4 hours per week during child-bearing years (Bernstein et al., 1994).

Fat

Some experimental and epidemiologic data show a link between some neoplasms and the amount of fat in the diet. Geographic variations in the incidence and mortality of cancers of the breast, colon, lung, and prostate suggest that high fat intake is related to an increased risk of these cancers. Because dietary fat intake is correlated with intake of other nutrients and dietary components, it is difficult to distinguish between the effects of dietary fats and protein, total calories, and fiber. A complex interaction of fat with these or other factors may account for inconsistent results of epidemiologic and experimental investigations. Perhaps no area is more controversial than the proposed link between dietary fat and the development of breast cancer (see "*New Directions:* The Role of Fat in Breast Cancer").

Protein

Understanding the role of protein in tumor development is complicated by the fact that most diets high in protein are also high in meat and fat and low in fiber. The effect of protein on experimental carcinogenesis depends on the tissue of origin and the type of tumor, as well as on the type of protein and the caloric adequacy of the diet. In general, tumor development is suppressed by diets containing levels of protein below that required for optimal growth, whereas it is enhanced by protein levels two to three times the amount that is required. The effects may be attributable to specific amino acids, a general effect of protein, or, in the case of low-protein diets, depressed food intake. Epidemiologic data are limited and conflicting. However, increased meat intake has been found to be associated with an increased risk of colon cancer (Potter, 1996) and, possibly, with advanced prostate cancer (Giles and Ireland, 1997).

Because animal studies demonstrate that certain amino acid deficiencies inhibit some tumors, the feeding of amino acid–deficient diets or amino acid antagonists has been proposed as an adjunct to cancer therapy. Although this hypothesis has theoretical appeal, currently, there is no active clinical research in this area.

Fiber

Early studies focused much attention on the possible protective role of fiber in preventing cancer of the colon, rectum, breast, and ovaries. Most studies of the relationship between fiber and cancer have measured fiber-rich foods or total dietary crude fiber rather than fiber components. The intake of dietary fiber influences the intake of meat, fat, and refined carbohydrates, as well as a number of nutrients and nonnutrients with identified impact on cancer risk.

A number of observational and case control studies indicate that fiber-rich diets are associated with a protective effect in colon cancer; however, the data do not permit discrimination between effects attributable to fiber and nonfiber effects attributable to vegetables (Trock et al., 1990; Howe et al., 1992). The role of genetics must also be considered. Higher intakes of vegetables were associated inversely with colon cancer risk in one case control study; however, the association with dietary fiber was limited to proximal tumors and to older subjects (Slattery et al., 1997b). The most recent study does not support the role of fiber as protective against colorectal cancer (Fuchs et al., 1999).

Fruits and Vegetables

Generally, fruits and vegetables are low in energy and are good sources of fiber, vitamins, minerals, and other bioactive substances. Numerous epidemiologic studies have examined the relationship be-

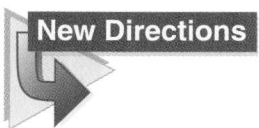

Role of Fat in Breast Cancer

Pro: Fat Amount and Type Do Affect Breast Cancer

It has been hypothesized that a high-fat diet promotes the development of postmenopausal breast cancer. This contention is supported by data showing international correlations between fat intake and breast cancer rates, modest positive associations with a high-fat diet in case control studies, and animal model studies that have consistently demonstrated that dietary fat influences mammary cancer development at several stages in the carcinogenic process. A number of plausible biologic mechanisms have been suggested that may explain the promotional effects of fat. The only conflicting findings are from *cohort studies,* which have shown that fat is unrelated to the risk of breast cancer.

In the absence of data from *dietary intervention trials,* the weight of available evidence suggests that the type and amount of fat in the diet are related to postmenopausal breast cancer, and that the inability to detect associations within populations (cohort studies) is attributable to measurement error and the relative homogeneity of diets measured. It is expected that the results from intervention trials will clarify this issue (Wynder et al., 1997).

Some epidemiologic evidence suggests that monosaturated fat, and olive oil in particular, may reduce the risk of breast cancer when substituted for other types of fat (Willett, 1997). However, the largest individual prospective study to date found no evidence that lower intake of total fat or particular types of fat over 14 years of follow-up was associated with a decreased risk of breast cancer (Holmes et al., 1999). Most types of epidemiologic studies provide indirect support for a protective effect of energy restriction and reduced growth rates against breast cancer, which is consistently observed in animal studies of mammary carcinogenesis (Willett, 1997).

Con: Fat Amount and Type Do Not Affect Breast Cancer

Results from large, prospective studies do not support the concept, derived from animal and ecologic evidence, that dietary fat intake in mid-life is associated with breast cancer risk. Thus, if fat is relevant to breast cancer, it is probably only at extremely low fat intakes or during early life. An emerging hypothesis that increased energy intake and growth rate in childhood and adolescence increase risk deserves further study (Hunter and Willett, 1996).

Rates of breast cancer vary approximately 5-fold among countries and are strongly correlated with national per capita availability of dietary fat. However, this relation may be substantially confounded by many other factors associated with affluent life-styles, such as reduced parity and physical inactivity.

The observation that women in provinces in China who consume approximately 25% of their energy from fat have much lower rates of breast cancer than U.S. women with similar fat intakes provides additional evidence that factors other than dietary fat account for these large international differences.

Conclusion

Epidemiologic studies have not provided conclusive evidence of an association between dietary fat and breast cancer, partly because studies that focus on a single nutrient cannot always readily evaluate the interactive effects of other life-style factors or the limitations of measurement tools. Research is needed that focuses on a comprehensive approach to diet, lifestyle choices, and breast cancer risk while emphasizing a fat-caloric intake-obesity linkage.

The best hope for a definitive answer may rest with randomized, controlled, clinical trials. Two such trials—the Women's Health Initiative and the Women's Intervention Nutrition Study—are currently being conducted (Greenwald et al., 1997). The role of fat in weight gain is an important aspect to consider in women diagnosed with breast cancer (Demark-Wahnefried et al., 1997). Changes in metabolic rate, physical activity, and overall intake also warrant further study.

tween fruit and vegetable intake and the incidence of cancer. As Table 39–1 shows, a statistically significant protective effect of fruit and vegetable consumption was found in 128 of 156 dietary studies (Block et al., 1992).

For most cancer sites, except the prostate, persons with low fruit and vegetable intake experience about twice the risk of cancer as those with high intake, even after controlling for potentially confounding factors. Fruits in particular are significantly protective against cancers of the esophagus, oral cavity, and larynx. Strong evidence of a protective effect of fruit and vegetable consumption is seen with cancers of the pancreas and stomach, as well as in colorectal and bladder cancers, and cancers of the cervix, ovary, and endometrium (Block et al., 1992).

Other investigators report that consumption of the following groups and types of vegetables and fruits is comparatively low in those who subsequently develop cancer: raw and fresh vegetables, leafy green vegetables, cruciferae (i.e., broccoli and cabbage), lettuce, carrots, and raw and fresh fruit. Other data suggest that foods high in phytoestrogens, particularly soy, or high in precursor compounds that can be metabolized by gut bacteria into active agents, such as grains and vegetables with woody stems that contain lignans, may be associated with a lower risk of sex-hormone-related cancers (Potter and Steinmetz, 1996; Steinmetz and Potter, 1991a). Consumption of soybeans is thought to contribute to the low incidence of breast and prostate cancer in Japan (Messina et al., 1994).

Possible mechanisms by which vegetable and fruit intake may alter cancer risks have been proposed. A large number of potentially anticarcino-

TABLE 39–1 SUMMARY OF EPIDEMIOLOGIC STUDIES OF FRUIT AND VEGETABLE INTAKE AND CANCER PREVENTION BY SITE

SITE	NO. OF STUDIES	PROTECTIVE ($p < 0.05$)	HARMFUL ($p < 0.05$)
All sites	170	132	6
All sites except prostate	156	128	4
Lung	25	24	0
Larynx	4	4	0
Oral cavity, pharynx	9	9	0
Esophagus	16	15	0
Stomach	19	17	1
Colorectal	27	20	3
Bladder	5	3	0
Pancreas	11	9	0
Cervix	8	7	0
Ovary	4	3	0
Breast	14	8	0
Prostate	14	4	2
Miscellaneous	8	6	0

(Adapted from Block G, Patterson B, Subar A. Fruit, vegetables, and cancer prevention: A review of the epidemiological evidence. Nutr Cancer 18:3, 1992.)

genic agents are found in these foods, including carotenoids, vitamins C and E, selenium, and dietary fiber, as well as **phytochemicals,** such as dithiolthiones, glucosinolate and indoles, lycopene, isothiocyanates, flavonoids, phenols, phytates, protease inhibitors, plant sterols, allium compounds, lignans, ellagic acid, and limonene (see Chapter 12). Most of the data for observations of the anticarcinogenic potential of all of these compounds have been derived from animal and in vitro studies (Potter and Steinmetz, 1996; Craig, 1997).

These agents have both complementary and overlapping mechanisms of action, including the induction of detoxification enzymes, inhibition of nitrosamine formation, provision of substrate for formation of antineoplastic agents, dilution and binding of carcinogens in the digestive tract, alteration of hormone metabolism, and antioxidant effects. It appears extremely unlikely that any one substance is responsible for all of the associations seen.

Possible adverse effects of a high vegetable and fruit consumption include the presence of aflatoxin, pesticides, nitrates, alar, goitrogens, and plant-produced pesticides (Steinmetz and Potter, 1991b).

Chemoprevention

Cancer chemoprevention seeks to reverse carcinogenesis in the premalignant phase. Studies have been directed at reversing precancerous lesions, preventing disease in populations at high risk for recurrent or new disease, and reducing the incidence of specific tumors in the general population. Several large-scale, randomized, intervention trials have examined the effects of vitamin/mineral supplementation, with mixed results.

A study in Finland with male smokers who received either alpha-tocopherol, betacarotene, or both, or placebo revealed a 16% higher incidence of lung cancer associated with betacarotene supplementation (ATBC Cancer Prevention Study Group, 1994). A second large study (CARET) of betacarotene and lung cancer also revealed negative effects; that is, a 28% greater incidence of lung cancer and a 17% greater death rate in the group receiving the supplement (Omenn et al., 1996). In both of these studies, heavy alcohol intake appeared to increase the negative effects. Trials with higher doses and longer duration are warranted. The Physician's Health Study found neither increased risk nor benefit from betacarotene supplementation after 12 years of follow-up studies in patients with lung cancer; however, only 11% of the group studied were current smokers (Hennekens et al., 1996).

Two large studies were conducted in Linxian, China, to test the effects of vitamin/mineral supplements on cancer incidence in an area that has one of the highest esophageal/gastric cancer mortality rates in the world and a diet low in micronutrients. After 5 years, the group receiving two to three times the RDA for betacarotene, vitamin E, and selenium showed significant reduction in mortality due to cancer, especially stomach cancer. No significant effect on mortality was observed for other supplement regimens (Blot et al., 1993; Blot, 1994). A recent investigation found that calcium supplementation is associated with a moderate reduction in the risk of recurrent colorectal adenomas (Baron et al., 1999).

Chemoprevention is also an active area of clinical research that holds promise for patients with cancers commonly associated with recurrence, such as head and neck cancers, as well as for identified high-risk populations, such as former smokers with bronchial metaplasia. The development of second primary tumors is a major cause of treatment failure in patients with head and neck cancers treated in an early stage. Early clinical trials with isotretinoin, a retinoid, decreased the incidence of recurrence; however, there were significant side effects that prevented one third of the patients from completing the treatment (Hong et al., 1990). Subsequent studies have identified doses that reduce toxicity and show mixed results in reducing recurrence of disease. Trials with precursor lesions are more promising. Antioxidant compounds have been shown to be effective in reversing oral leukoplakia, precursor lesions with a high rate of transformation to malignant disease. To date, chemoprevention studies are in a developmental stage, with no agent showing clear efficacy in reducing incidence or improving survival. However, new agents are under development, including peigallacatchin gallate (green tea) and curcumin, and there is renewed interest in folic acid (Berwick and Schantz,

1997), as well as genistein (soy) and lycopene (tomatoes).

Alcohol

Epidemiologic studies indicate that alcohol has a causal role in carcinogenesis, especially for cancers of the mouth, pharynx, larynx, and esophagus. Alcohol appears to have an increased effect on those tissues directly exposed to it during its consumption and tends to act synergistically with tobacco (Marshall and Boyle, 1996). The malnutrition associated with alcoholism is also likely to be important in the increased risk for certain cancers in the alcoholic individual.

Alcohol, especially beer consumption, has been associated with an increased risk for colorectal cancer in a number of studies (Kune and Vitetta, 1992). The positive relationship between alcohol intake and breast cancer risk has been documented repeatedly, and this correlation has been supported by studies showing that moderate alcohol intake increases endogenous estrogen levels (Hunter and Willett, 1996).

Coffee and Tea

Coffee intake has been investigated as a possible risk factor for a variety of cancers. Regular consumption of coffee or tea has no significant relationship with the risk of cancer at any site. In fact, some studies indicate that regular drinking of green tea possibly reduces the risk of stomach cancer (Yu et al., 1995). Consumption of very hot drinks has been associated with an increased risk of esophageal cancer (Cheng and Day, 1996).

Artificial Sweeteners

Artificial sweeteners have been investigated, primarily in relation to bladder cancer. In 1970, cyclamate was banned from use as a food additive in the United States based on the results of a study demonstrating a significant increase in bladder tumors in rats fed a mixture of cyclamate and saccharin at doses up to 2500 mg/kg/day (Renwick, 1990). During the next 15 years, several intensive reviews were completed. To date, the manufacturer's petition to resume use remains pending.

The weight of evidence from metabolic studies, short-term tests, animal bioassays, and epidemiologic studies indicates that cyclamate itself is not carcinogenic; however, evidence from in vitro and in vivo studies in animals implies that it may have cancer-promoting or cocarcinogenic activities. Epidemiologic studies indicate that no measurable overall increase in the risk of bladder cancer has been noted in individuals who have used these non-nutritive sweeteners (cyclamate and saccharin).

Aspartame has not been found to be carcinogenic in experimental studies, and clinical studies have shown no ill effect in humans consuming large doses (Newberne and Conner, 1986). Epidemiologic data are not available because its approval for use is relatively recent.

Nitrates, Nitrites, and Nitrosamines

Nitrates and nitrites have received attention because of their relationship with nitrosamines, which are potent **carcinogens** in various species. Nitrate can be readily reduced to nitrite, which in turn can interact with dietary substrates, such as amines and amides, to produce *N*-nitroso compounds, or nitrosamines and nitrosamides. This conversion, known as *N*-nitrosation, has been demonstrated to occur in saliva as well as in the stomach, colon, and bladder.

Nitrates are present in a variety of foods, but the main dietary sources are vegetables and drinking water. Sodium and potassium nitrates are used in the processes of salting, pickling, and curing foods; they also give hot dogs and luncheon meat their pink color. Nitrosamines are present in tobacco and tobacco smoke.

Epidemiologic studies do not provide evidence of an etiologic role for nitrate intake in stomach cancer risk.

Method of Food Preparation

Cooking methods can cause contamination of food by carcinogens, especially polycyclic aromatic hydrocarbons (e.g., benzo[*a*]pyrene) and heterocyclic aromatic amines (Miller and Miller, 1986). These toxic substances are formed during combustion of carbon fuel and pyrolysis of protein, which commonly occurs during charcoal broiling, frying, and smoking of meats. Several investigators have found mutagenic activity in foods after frying and charcoal broiling. Epidemiologic studies have indicated an increased risk of stomach and esophageal cancers associated with the frequent intake of smoked and fried foods (Wu-Williams et al., 1990; Yu et al., 1988).

Case control and limited cohort studies have revealed that a high salt intake is associated with an increased risk for stomach cancer (Kono and Hirohata, 1996). The potential interaction between salty foods and *Helicobacter pylori* infection in the development of stomach cancer needs further investigation. Consumption of fruits and vegetables appears to provide a protective effect (Hirohata and Kono, 1997).

Dietary Recommendations

The National Cancer Institute and the Committee on Diet and Health, the Food and Nutrition Board of the National Research Council, as well as several privately funded organizations, have made recommendations for diet and life-style practices that may contribute to cancer prevention. These recommendations of the American Cancer Society include

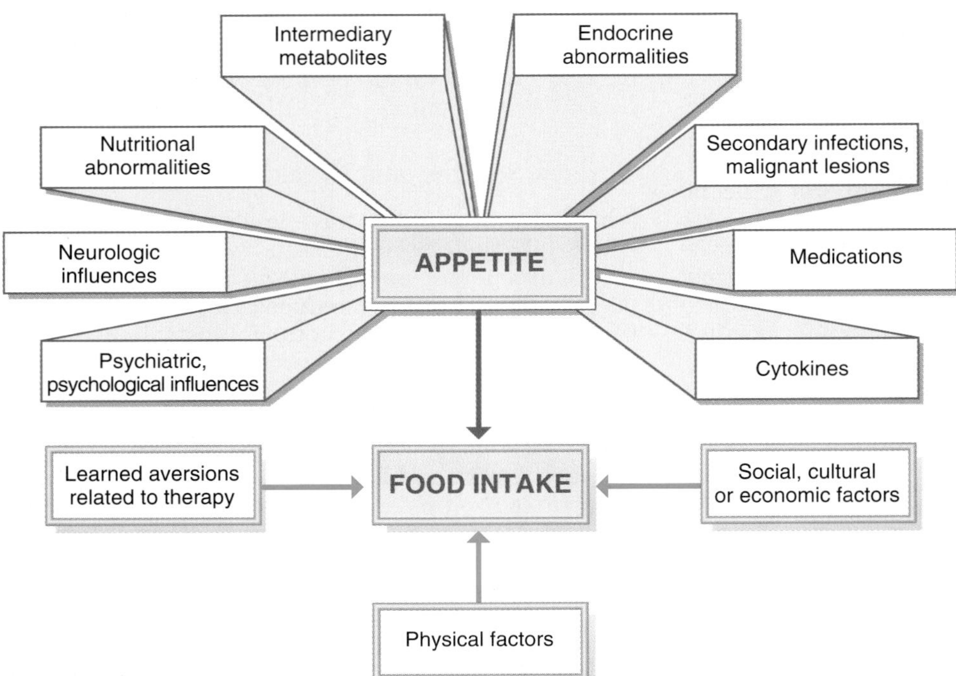

FIGURE 39–2 Factors that affect appetite, an especially important consideration in cancer patients. (AICR. Food, nutrition, and prevention of cancer: A global perspective.)

choosing most foods from plant sources (especially cruciferous vegetables); limiting intake of high-fat foods, especially from animal sources; becoming physically active; achieving and maintaining a healthy body weight; and limiting consumption of alcoholic beverages (Lenhard, 1996.)

Studies indicate that adults who strongly believe in a diet–cancer connection decreased the percentage of energy derived from fat and increased their fiber intake. Food composition knowledge and perceived pressure to eat a healthful diet were not significantly related to changes in fiber intake, fat intake, or weight (Patterson et al., 1996). Perceived ease of eating a healthful diet was a strong predictor of intake (Harnack et al., 1997). These findings challenge dietitians to design diet and health promotion programs that address the barriers to dietary change, as well as educate people about the relationship of diet to health. The importance of lifestyle changes are evident in recommendations from the American Institute for Cancer Research.

NUTRITIONAL EFFECTS OF CANCER

The adverse nutritional effects of cancer can be severe and may be compounded by effects of the treatment regimens and the psychological impact of cancer. The result is often a profound depletion of nutrient stores. Data suggest an association between weight loss and shortened survival (Langstein and Norton, 1991) and imply a relationship between nutritional status and the outcome of malignant disease (Fig. 39–2).

Cachexia

Cancer cachexia is a syndrome of progressive weight loss, anorexia, asthenia, anemia, and abnormalities in protein, fat, and carbohydrate metabolism. The etiology of this complex metabolic derangement remains unknown. Recent work has focused on the role of **cytokines,** which through broad physiologic actions, produce metabolic changes and wasting in the tumor-bearing host that are similar, but not identical, to those seen in sepsis and inflammation.

Cytokines that are thought to play a role include **tumor necrosis factor (cachectin),** interleukin-1, interleukin-6, and interferon-g. These cytokines have overlapping physiologic activities, which makes it likely that no single substance is the sole cause of cancer cachexia (Tisdale, 1997; Matthys and Billiau, 1997). A pool of anticytokine antibodies or other cytokine inhibitors might be considered as a potential intervention for the treatment of cachectic patients. Trials with single agents and metabolic inhibitors (pentoxyfylline and hydrazine sulfate) have failed to show benefit (Ottery et al., 1998). However, administration of thalidomide, an inhibitor of tumor necrosis factor–alpha, has resulted in weight gain in patients with human immunodeficiency virus (HIV) (Haslett, 1998). Thalidomide, when administered at therapeutic doses, may cause significant and incapacitating drowsiness.

A number of other pharmacologic agents are also being investigated in the management of the anorexia-cachexia syndrome, including corticosteroids, progestational agents, and recombinant human growth hormone. Trials indicate that corticosteroids require escalating doses to maintain increased appetite and are associated with negative side effects. Recombinant growth hormone has been studied in patients with wasting associated with HIV. An acute anabolic effect was achieved, but this was transient. A number of well-designed trials have shown an increase in appetite, food intake, and weight in cancer patients treated with megestrol acetate (Megace), a progestational appetite stimulant that is very well tolerated (Ottery et al., 1998).

Energy Metabolism

In chronic starvation, the metabolic rate is reduced as the body adapts to conserve energy and preserve body tissue. However, when compared to control groups, cancer patients have been reported to have reduced, normal, or increased energy expenditure. Studies using indirect calorimetry have shown increased resting energy expenditure (REE) in individuals with some tumor types, but not in others (Fredrix et al., 1991; Dickerson et al., 1995). In a study of patients with lung cancer, hypermetabolism and weight loss were associated with enhanced levels of inflammatory mediators and acute-phase proteins (Staal van den Brekel et al., 1995). When REE in malnourished patients with esophageal cancer was expressed as a function of fat-free mass or body weight, energy expenditure was similar to the REE of age- and height-matched controls (Thomson et al., 1990). One study of the impact of malignant disease on REE revealed that REE returned to normal levels in patients with lung cancer after curative surgery (Fredrix et al., 1991).

Substrate Metabolism

Energy metabolism is intimately related to carbohydrate, protein, and lipid metabolism, all of which are altered by tumor growth. Tumors exert a consistent demand for glucose. Neoplastic cells exhibit a characteristically high rate of anaerobic metabolism, yielding lactate as the end product. This expanded lactic acid pool requires an increased rate of host gluconeogenesis via Cori cycle activity, which is increased in some patients with cancer but not in others. Both protein breakdown and lipolysis take place at increasing rates to maintain high rates of glucose synthesis. A relative state of insulin resistance may develop, characterized by excess fatty oxidation and decreased uptake and use of glucose, especially in muscle (Puccio and Nathanson, 1997).

Alterations in protein metabolism appear to be directed toward providing adequate amino acids for tumor growth. Most notable is the loss of skeletal muscle protein; however, visceral organ atrophy and hypoalbuminemia also occur. Abnormalities of protein metabolism include inappropriate elevations in whole-body protein turnover and increases in skeletal muscle protein synthesis, catabolism, and liver protein synthesis. These changes occur in the presence of reduced nitrogen intake, suggesting an inability to adapt to diminished protein intake by reducing protein turnover. Albumin synthesis rates appear to be similar to those in healthy individuals (Fearon et al., 1998); hypoalbuminemia occurs because of increased total body water associated with cancer cachexia, which is more pronounced than the increase in albumin synthesis (Langstein and Norton, 1991).

Lipid metabolism is altered, as evidenced by inappropriate mobilization of free fatty acids from adipose tissues and subsequent depletion of total body fat. Disorders may also be seen in the form of decreased lipid clearance from serum and elevated plasma free fatty acid levels. Supporting evidence suggests that tumors produce lipolytic substances that are directly responsible for increased fat mobilization (Langstein and Norton, 1991).

Other Metabolic Abnormalities

Fluid and electrolyte imbalances are seen in patients with advanced cancer. Hypercalcemia may be seen in bone-metastasizing tumors of the breast, lung, and pancreas, as well as in nonmetastatic tumors that induce parathyroid hormone–like peptides. Dietary calcium should not be restricted.

Severe imbalances in fluid and electrolyte status may be present in patients with cancers that promote excessive diarrhea or vomiting. Severe diarrhea can result from tumors secreting serotonin (carcinoid syndrome), calcitonin, or gastrin (Zollinger-Ellison syndrome). Persistent vomiting is associated with intestinal obstruction or intracranial tumors.

The activities of several enzyme systems are affected, as are certain endocrine functions, and the nature of the alterations varies by tumor type. Host immunologic function is impaired, apparently as the result of both the neoplasm and progressive malnutrition.

In addition to the cancer-induced metabolic effects, the mass of the tumor may anatomically alter the normal physiology of specific organ systems.

Sensory Changes

Alterations in taste and smell sensations are common, and they contribute to the anorexia frequently seen in patients with cancer. Studies of taste sensitivity in malignant disease have shown variable results. Reports include an elevated recognition threshold for sweet, a lowered threshold for bitter, and some increase in thresholds for sour and salt (Kamath et al., 1983). However, another study found no threshold differences between matched controls and untreated patients with esophageal cancer (Boock and Reddick, 1991). Taste alterations are associated with the disease, certain antineoplastic agents, and irradiation or surgery involving the head and neck. Chemotherapy-induced, learned taste aversions have been reported in both adults and children (Charuhas, 1993).

Patients may also experience a heightened sense of smell that results in a sensitivity to food preparation odors, as well as aversions to nonfood items, such as soaps or perfumes. Interventions that decrease the aroma of foods, such as serving foods cold instead of hot may be helpful (Ottery, 1996; Paserot et al., 1997).

These sensation abnormalities do not consistently correlate with the tumor site, extent of tumor involvement, tumor response to therapy, or food preferences and intake.

NUTRITIONAL EFFECTS OF CANCER THERAPY

Antitumor therapy may involve chemotherapy, radiation, surgery, immunotherapy, or a combination of these. Certain hematologic malignant diseases (leukemias, lymphomas, multiple myelomas), as well as solid tumors, can be treated by bone marrow transplantation. Autologous marrow transplantation also may be used to ameliorate the dose-limiting hematologic toxicity of chemotherapy, allowing higher levels of antineoplastic agents to be given. Each of these therapeutic programs contributes to nutritional alterations in patients by interfering with their ability to ingest, digest, and absorb adequately (Table 39–2).

TABLE 39–2 SIDE EFFECTS OF CANCER THERAPY WITH NUTRITIONAL IMPLICATIONS

Radiation
Myelosuppression
Nausea, vomiting, and general loss of appetite
Taste and smell changes
Dental problems
Mucositis and xerostomia
Esophageal stricture from irradiation of the thorax
Diarrhea and malabsorption from bowel damage
Depressed immune function
Chemotherapy
Myelosuppression
Taste abnormalities
Mucositis, cheilosis, glossitis, stomatitis, and esophagitis
Diarrhea and malabsorption from gastrointestinal toxicity
Nausea, vomiting, and anorexia
Anemias
Depressed immune function
Immunotherapy
Fatigue
Flu-like symptoms
Fever
Nausea and vomiting
Immune stimulation, including reversal of neutropenia
Weight loss
Marrow Transplantation
Nausea, vomiting, and anorexia
Mucositis, stomatitis, and esophagitis
Taste and salivary changes
Diarrhea and malabsorption from bowel damage
Acute and chronic graft-versus-host disease
Veno-occlusive disease
Pulmonary disease
Renal disease

Chemotherapy

Chemotherapy is the use of chemical agents or medications to treat cancer. Whereas surgery and radiation therapy are used to treat localized tumors, chemotherapy is a systemic therapy that affects the whole body. The action of chemotherapeutic agents is not limited to malignant tissue; it affects normal cells as well. As a result, major organ toxicities are seen, and dietary intake and nutritional status are adversely affected. Food intake is inhibited by mucositis (Fig. 39–3), cheilosis, glossitis, stomatitis, and esophagitis caused by many drugs. Table 39–3 summarizes the side effects of common oncologic medications. Side effects are dependent on the specific agent, dosage, duration of treatment, accompanying drugs, and individual response (see Chapter 18).

Nausea and vomiting may occur with **antineoplastic agents.** However, the concomitant administration of antiemetics (e.g., serotonin receptor antagonists, Zofran, Kytril, Anzemet) when given in combination with corticosteroids, eliminate or greatly reduce nausea and vomiting in up to 80% of patients. Aggressive use of antiemetics, antidiarrheals, and antibiotics allow most patients to incur only minimal side effects or to recover more quickly from more serious side effects. The reality is that in spite of the supportive care, many patients still suffer significant side effects, especially in "dose-intense" chemotherapy regimens. These days, neutropenia and myelosuppression are the primary limiting factors for administration of chemotherapeutic agents.

Taste abnormalities lead to anorexia and *oligophagy* (eating few foods). Diarrhea may be induced, or constipation or *adynamic ileus* (inhibition of bowel motility) may occur. Symptoms of gastrointestinal toxicity are usually not long lasting; however, some combination chemotherapeutic programs have severe and prolonged gastrointestinal effects. Some agents, especially corticosteroids, cause tissue breakdown and promote excessive urinary loss of protein, potassium, and calcium. The intestinal mucosa and digestive processes are affected, altering digestion and absorption to some degree. Protein, energy, and vitamin metabolism may be impaired, although the consequences of this are not known. Total lymphocyte count is depressed and does not accurately reflect nutritional status following antineoplastic agent administration.

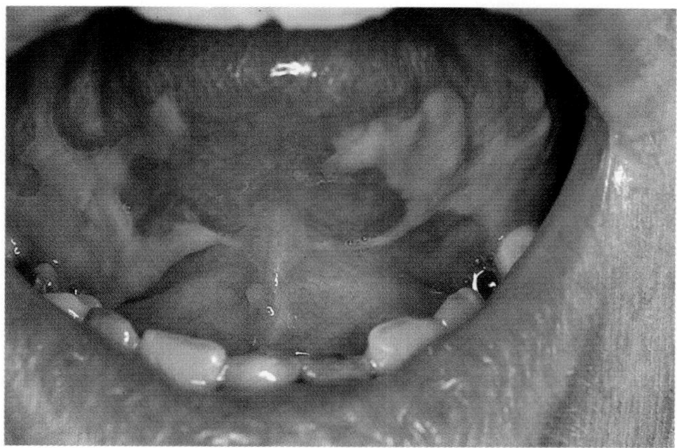

FIGURE 39–3 Severe oral mucositis following marrow transplantation. The patient also received a course of high-dose cyclophosphamide and whole-body radiation.

Radiation Therapy

The effects of radiation therapy vary according to the region irradiated. Radiation to the head and neck causes a variety of food ingestion problems, including sore throat, mucositis, permanent **xerostomia** (mouth dryness), severe dental and gum destruction, and altered taste and smell.

These symptoms appear within 10 to 17 days of the initiation of therapy. Anorexia, fatigue, and weight loss are common in these patients (Hunter, 1996). Radiation treatment to the thorax induces esophagitis with accompanying dysphagia. Esophageal stricture, leading to obstruction, can occur. Radiation to the abdomen may produce acute gastritis or enteritis with nausea, vomiting, diarrhea, and anorexia; severe gastrointestinal damage is accompanied by malabsorption of disaccharides, fats, and electrolytes. Total body radiation may cause all of the aforementioned acute symptoms to some extent. As with chemotherapy, radiation therapy depresses immune function, thus limiting the usefulness of this parameter in assessing nutritional status. Most of the side effects experienced are temporary, generally resolving within 2 to 4 weeks after completion of radiation treatments.

Radiation-induced enteritis can develop into a chronic form of the condition, with symptoms of ulceration or obstruction intensifying the risk of malnutrition. Chronic radiation enteritis combined with massive bowel resection, which results in extensive bowel dysfunction, is referred to as *short bowel syndrome*. The severity of this condition depends on the length and location of the nonfunctional or resected bowel; it is generally diagnosed when the individual has less than 150 cm of small intestine remaining. The sequelae include maldigestion, malabsorption, malnutrition, dehydration, and potentially lethal metabolic aberrations. Initially, total parenteral nutrition (TPN) is required, and frequent monitoring of fluids and electrolytes may be required for weeks or months. The diet may need to be restricted to defined formula tube feedings or frequent small meals that are high-complex carbohydrate, low-fat, low-oxalate, lactose-free, and high-protein. Medications can be given to decrease intestinal motility. Multivitamin supplements that include vitamin B_{12}, folic acid, and vitamins A, E, and K should be given to prevent deficiencies. Serum concentrations of various minerals should be monitored and adjusted as needed (see Chapter 31).

In the absence of continued underlying intrinsic disease, some degree of adaptation occurs; however, this frequently requires more than a year. Enteral feedings are paramount in the adaptive response. As enteral intake increases, TPN is reduced (Grant et al., 1996; see also Chapter 22). Radiation enteritis can be prevented in patients with gynecologic malignant disease by use of an “intestinal mesh sling,” which is surgically placed prior to therapy to elevate the small bowel above the pelvic external beam radiation field (Rodier et al., 1995). In patients with head and neck cancer, careful mouth care and dental management are necessary in order to reduce the risk of debilitating tooth and gum damage or osteoradionecrosis.

Surgery

Surgery is a primary mode of treatment for patients with gastrointestinal malignant lesions, and it may be combined with preoperative or postoperative adjuvant chemotherapy or radiation therapy. When the tumor involves the gastrointestinal tract, significant nutritional problems may be associated with both surgical resection and the disease process.

Patients with head and neck cancer have im-

TABLE 39–3 COMMON PROBLEMS ASSOCIATED WITH ONCOLOGIC MEDICATIONS

POTENTIAL PROBLEMS	MEDICATIONS
Anorexia, nausea, and vomiting	Carmustine, cisplatin, cyclophosphamide, dacarbazine, mechlorethamine, streptozocin, carboplatin, cytarabine, doxorubicin, methotrexate, procarbazine, altretamine, gemcitabine, idarubicin, ifosfamide, mitoxantrone, topotecan, anastrozole, docetaxel, etoposide, 5-fluorouracil, irinotecan, mitomycin, and paclitaxel
Mucositis	5-fluorouracil, methotrexate, vinblastine, bleomycin, dactinomycin, doxorubicin, and hydroxyurea
Constipation	Vincristine and vinblastine
Fluid retention	Hormonal therapy
Liver toxicity	Fluorouracil, mercaptopurine, and methotrexate
Reaction to monoamine oxidase inhibitors	Procarbazine

(Adapted from Kouba J. Nutritional care of the individual with cancer. Nutr Clin Pract 3:176, 1988.)

paired ingestion due to the tumor mass, and they often have a history of chronic, heavy alcohol intake. Surgery results in temporary or permanent dependence on tube feeding. Patients who resume oral intake often have dysphagia and require modifications of food consistency and extensive training in chewing and swallowing (Kyle, 1990). Referrals to a speech therapist can yield dramatic positive results.

Surgical treatment of esophageal tumors may require partial or total ablation of the esophagus. The stomach is usually used for esophageal replacement. A feeding nasojejunostomy or jejunostomy tube can be placed at the time of surgery, permitting early postoperative tube feedings. Usually, the patient is able to progress to a regular diet. If weight loss and malabsorption occur, a low-fat diet with small, frequent feedings of nutrient-dense foods is prescribed (Grant et al., 1996). New research studies support the use of glutamine-enriched tube-feeding formulas or glutamine supplementation to aid in healing after gastrointestinal surgery (see Chapters 22 and 31).

Chylous fistula is a well-known complication of radical neck dissection that results from injury to the thoracic duct as it enters the left subclavian vein. Until the fistula closes, fat intake should be restricted to medium-chain triglycerides.

Pancreatic cancer, with its attendant surgical resection, has several nutritional consequences. When more than 70% of the pancreas is removed, insulin is required to regulate glucose metabolism, and a carbohydrate-controlled diet may be warranted. Up to 90% of the pancreas must be removed before clinical symptoms of malabsorption result. Pancreatic enzyme replacement is used to aid digestion, and a fat-restricted diet may be required (Grant et al., 1996).

Total gastrectomy commonly leads to malnutrition secondary to reduced dietary intake and malabsorption. Placement of a jejunostomy feeding tube at surgery is advisable, and enteral nutrition support is generally feasible within 4 to 5 days after surgery. Fat intolerance may be seen, especially if the vagus nerves are severed. Administration of pancreatic enzymes with meals may be beneficial for patients in whom the mixing of food and pancreatic juices is inadequate.

When partial gastrectomy is in the lower remnant of the stomach, *dumping syndrome* is possible as a result of the rapid transit of foods or liquids (especially those high in simple carbohydrate content) and the dilutional response of the small remnant to highly osmotic bolus feedings. The most common nutritional problem is anemia secondary to malabsorption of iron, folate, and, less commonly vitamin B_{12} (Grant et al., 1996). Patients may benefit from consumption of 6 to 8 small meals per day, with fluids taken between meals.

Partial or total colectomies may induce profound losses of fluid and electrolytes, the severity of which is related to the length and site of the resection. Ileal resections of as little as 15 cm of the terminal ileum can result in bile salt losses that exceed the liver's capacity for resynthesis, and vitamin B_{12} absorption is affected. With depletion of the bile salt pool, steatorrhea develpos. Calcium carbonate should be administered orally to minimize oxalate absorption (Grant et al., 1996). Nutritional support consists of a diet low in fat, osmolality, lactose, and oxalate. See Chapter 31 for more information.

Immunotherapy

Biologic response modifiers are natural products that are made in quantities through cloning and genetic engineering. Used directly as cytotoxic agents or indirectly as stimulators of the patient's own natural defenses, biological agents can kill tumor cells. Alpha-interferon is used to treat hairy-cell leukemia. Interleukin-2 is utilized in the treatment of patients with melanoma and renal cell carcinoma. Colony-stimulating factors—cytokines that stimulate the marrow to develop faster—are being used to shorten periods of neutropenia for patients and to enrich the graft for myeloid precursors prior to harvest of marrow from donors (Isola et al., 1997). Patients in whom these agents are used may experience fatigue, chills, fever,and flu-like symptoms, which can result in decreased food intake.

Marrow Transplantation

Marrow transplantation is performed for the treatment of certain hematologic malignant diseases, such as leukemia and lymphoma, and for solid tumors. The preparative regimen includes cytotoxic chemotherapy, with or without total body irradiation, to suppress immunologic reactivity and eradicate malignant cells. This treatment regimen is followed by intravenous infusion of bone marrow or peripheral stem cells from a suitable donor.

With improved tissue typing using DNA techniques and several million donors worldwide, **allogeneic marrow transplantation** from an unrelated donor has become a clinical option for many patients who would not previously have been candidates for marrow transplantation (Ringden, 1997) (Fig. 39–4). Diseases with marrow failure or leukemic infiltration of the bone marrow generally require allogeneic transplantation. Autologous transplantation is often preferable for malignant lesions without marrow infiltration. Acute toxic reactions, such as nausea, vomiting, and diarrhea, usually diminish 24 to 48 hours after the administration of preconditioning therapy. Delayed effects during the first month after transplantation include mucositis, stomatitis, esophagitis, salivary and taste alterations, fatigue, and gut damage. Patients typically have little or no oral intake during the first few weeks post-transplant, and so require enteral or parenteral nutrition support.

Graft-versus-host disease (GVHD) is a major complication after allogeneic transplantation. Donor marrow cells react against the tissues of the

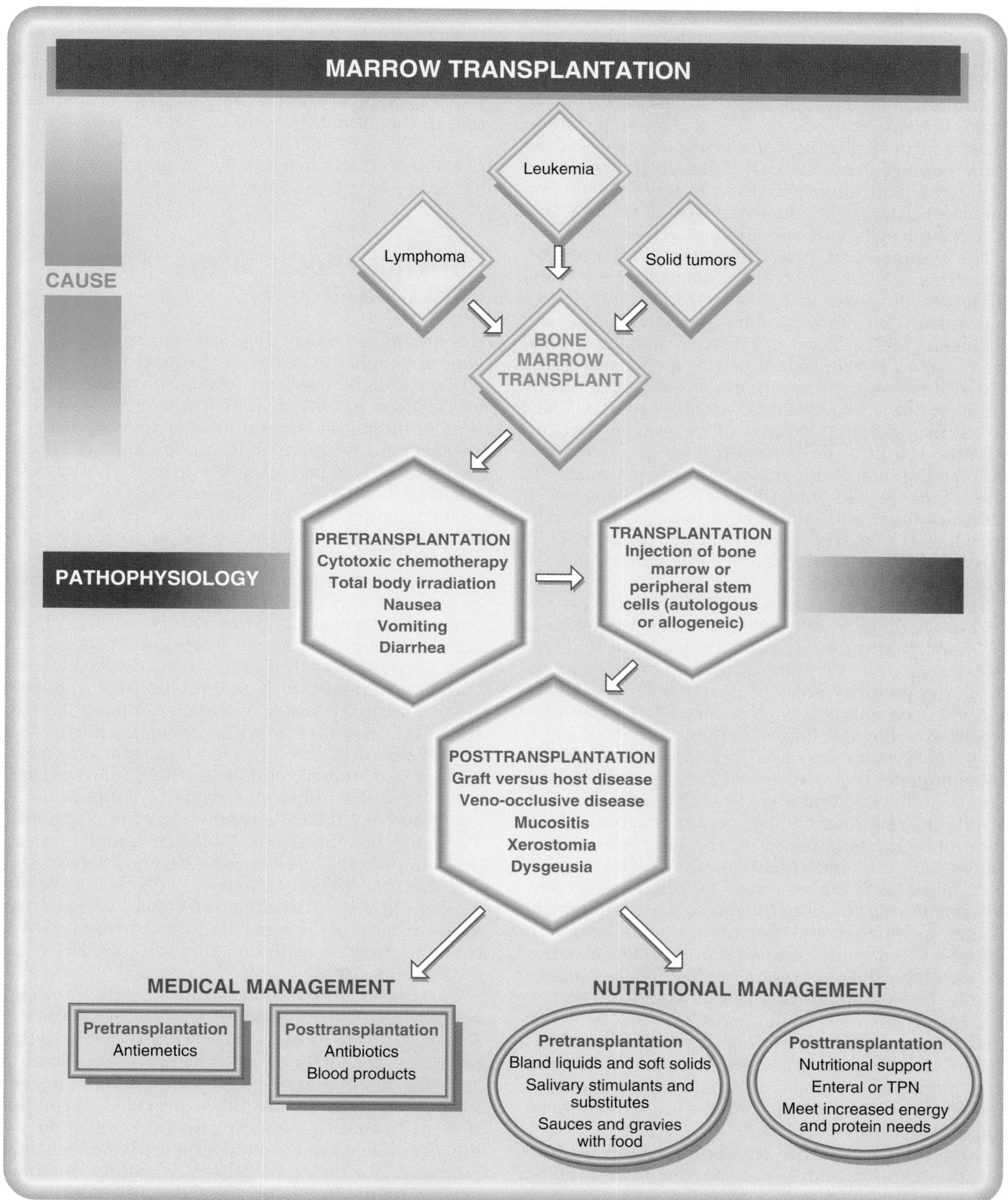

FIGURE 39–4 Pathophysiology algorithm—marrow transplantation. (Algorithm content developed by John Anderson, Ph.D., and Sanford C. Garner, Ph.D., 2000.)

"foreign" host. The functions of several target organs (skin, liver, gut, lymphoid cells) are disrupted, and susceptibility to infection is increased. Acute GVHD is usually manifested within 3 months post-transplant, and may be seen as early as 7 to 10 days. It may resolve, or it may develop into a chronic form requiring long-term treatment and dietary management. GVHD of the liver, evidenced by icterus and abnormal liver function tests, frequently accompanies gastrointestinal GVHD, further complicating nutritional management.

The symptoms of gastrointestinal GVHD are severe. The volume of secretory diarrhea may reach 10 L per day and is an indicator of the degree and extent of mucosal damage (Herrmann and Petruska, 1993). Total gut rest is indicated until the diarrhea is reduced. Nitrogen losses associated with diarrhea can be severe and are compounded by the high-dose corticosteroids used to treat GVHD. Initial oral feedings consist of beverages that are isotonic, low-fat, and lactose-free so as to compensate for the loss of intestinal enzymes secondary to alterations in the intestinal villi and mucosa. If these are tolerated, solids of the same nature can be introduced. Dietary restrictions are progressively reduced as foods are gradually introduced and tolerance is established.

Veno-occlusive disease (VOD) of the liver is characterized by chemotherapy-induced damage to the hepatic venules. It can develop 1 to 3 weeks post-transplant. Symptoms of hepatomegaly, ascites, and jaundice occur in nearly 50% of patients. A fraction of patients with severe VOD experience progressive hepatic failure leading to encephalopathy, multisystem organ failure, and death. Nutritional support requires concentrated parenteral nutrients, judicious fluid and electrolyte management, close monitoring, and adjustment of macronutrients and micronutrients based on the tolerance and response of the individual patient. The use of branched-chain amino acid formulas is recommended for encephalopathic patients, although the benefit is controversial. Serum ammonia level may not be a reliable indicator of protein tolerance or of the development of encephalopathy. These patients usually have minimal oral intake and are receiving multiple antibiotics, so ammonia may not be generated in their gastrointestinal tract (Miller, 1997). Other acute or chronic complications of marrow transplantation include pulmonary disease, rejection of the graft, growth abnormalities in children, and infection.

Autologous marrow transplantation involves the use of the patient's own marrow to reestablish hematopoietic cell function after the administration of high-dose chemotherapy. It can be performed in older patients with comparative safety, and there is only a small risk of GVHD. The use of mobilized stem cell progenitors has, in some cases, replaced autologous bone marrow as the source of hematopoietic progenitors for transplantation. Their use has shortened the period of **pancytopenia** when patients are at risk for bleeding and serious infections that may lead to sepsis. These advances, along with improved prophylactic antibiotic regimens that are relatively easy to administer, have allowed patients to receive autologous marrow transplantation in the outpatient setting. This change has substantially reduced the cost of the procedure and, hence, has made it available to an increased number of patients (Meisenberg et al., 1997).

NUTRITIONAL CARE OF THE PATIENT WITH CANCER

A common secondary diagnosis in patients with advanced neoplastic disease is protein-energy malnutrition. Weight loss and altered nutritional status are evident in 50% of patients with cancer at the time of diagnosis (Langstein and Norton, 1991). In an early study, even small amounts of weight loss (less than 5% of body weight) prior to therapy were associated with a poor prognosis (DeWys et al., 1980), reinforcing the importance of early nutritional assessment and intervention as a preventive measure.

Although the detrimental effect of malnutrition on survival is evident, the favorable influence of nutritional intervention is not always as clear. Nutritional support improves nutritional indices and may improve overall patient performance status in oncology patients with malnutrition secondary to gastrointestinal obstruction or treatment toxicity. However, in patients with cancer cachexia, little improvement is noted in lean body mass or overall patient performance status (ASPEN Board of Directors, 1993). Except in one study of patients undergoing marrow transplant who were supported with TPN, the beneficial effect of nutritional intervention on survival has not been demonstrated (Klein and Koretz, 1994). Moreover, TPN is unlikely to benefit patients with advanced cancer whose malignant disease is documented as unresponsive to chemotherapy or radiation therapy (ASPEN Board of Directors, 1993).

Parenteral nutritional support may, however, benefit some severely malnourished patients with cancer as well as those in whom gastrointestinal toxicities are likely to prevent oral nutritional intake for more than 1 week. Nutritional intervention, when possible, should be provided in conjunction with oncologic therapy to improve quality of life. Specialized nutritional support is not routinely indicated for well-nourished or mildly malnourished patients in whom adequate oral intake is anticipated. TPN administration may be restricted in patients undergoing aggressive anticancer therapy due to use of the TPN access (double- or triple-lumen) for chemotherapy, blood products, and other medication administration. The risk of infection in the immunocompromised patient is also a concern in the decision to utilize TPN.

The controversy persists regarding the merits of nutritional support for patients with cancer. Nevertheless, the adverse effects of malnutrition are clear. Nutritional support is a means of both preventing and treating malnutrition, and as such, plays an important role in the care of the patient with cancer (Bloch, 1994).

Goals of Nutritional Care

The goals of nutritional care of patients with cancer are to prevent or correct nutritional deficiencies and to minimize weight loss. Early intervention is essential. Screening for the risk of nutritional problems should be done at the time of diagnosis and nutritional monitoring should continue throughout treatment. With the recent shift of care from the hospital setting to outpatient settings, it is essential that screening be conducted at all clinical sites. Tools for patient-generated nutritional screening or assessment have been published (McMahon et al., 1998; American Dietetic Association, 1997). Nutritional assessment and intervention must be timely and must anticipate nutritional needs (see Chapters 16 and 17).

Oral Nutritional Management Strategies

Strategies for modifying nutrient intake depend on the specific feeding problem and the extent of depletion. The oral route is the preferred mode of feeding, but it may be resisted by the patient who experiences nausea, altered taste sensations, and dysphagia. Oral intake may be encouraged with modifications of food and its presentation (Charuhas, 1993). Patients with altered taste acuity (**dysgeusia, hypogeusia, ageusia**) may benefit from increased use of flavorings and seasonings during food preparation. Meat aversions may require the elimination of red meats, which tend to be strong in flavor, or the substitution of alternative protein sources. Dysphagia secondary to lesions involving the oral and esophageal tissues can be lessened with the intake of foods that are soft or liquefied and served at moderate or room temperature (see Chapter 42).

Artificial saliva preparations and saliva stimulants are useful in cases of diminished salivation, as are foods with high moisture content and plenty of fluids throughout the day and with meals. Patients with intestinal damage may require dietary modifications involving lactose, fat, and fiber content, as well as alterations in texture. Commercial nutritional supplements can be included in many dietary plans. Guidelines for oral feedings are presented in Table 39–4. Management of diarrhea and steatorrhea is discussed in Chapter 31.

Chemotherapy-induced nausea and vomiting are commonly classified as anticipatory, acute, or delayed emesis, each of which is manifested by distinct pathophysiologic events and requires different therapeutic interventions. Currently, the most effective agents for treating acute emesis are the 5-hydroxytryptamine receptor antagonists. Although costly, they are used in conjunction with highly and moderately emetogenic chemotherapeutic regimens. Delayed emesis is not sufficiently controlled by these agents, and there are few treatment options available (Ettinger, 1995). The anticipatory form of nausea and vomiting is a conditioned response that develops by the third or fourth cycle of treatment in about one third of patients. It is primarily a psychological issue and so responds best to behavioral interventions, such as relaxation training or systematic desensitization (Fessele, 1996).

The timing of food presentation also deserves consideration. Patients with cancer often complain of a decreased ability to eat as the day progresses, which means that the morning is often the best time for eating. This phenomenon may be attributable to sluggish digestion and gastric emptying as a result of decreased production of digestive secretions, gastrointestinal mucosal atrophy, and gastric muscle atrophy. Frequent, small feedings, with particular emphasis on morning feedings, are suggested in such cases.

The timing of meals or snacks relative to gastrointestinal toxic therapy may have a bearing on subsequent learned food aversions. These aversions develop when specific foods are associated with unpleasant symptoms, such as nausea and vomiting, and psychological stimuli, such as anxiety. The effect may not be limited to new food items, but may also involve foods that were included in the patient's usual diet before treatment. Exposure of patients to a "scapegoat" food or beverage just before chemotherapy and (probably) radiotherapy can markedly reduce the incidence of treatment-related aversions to foods in the patient's usual diet (Mattes, 1994; Puccio and Nathanson, 1997).

Enteral Tube Feeding

Efforts to encourage oral intake sometimes fail or are inappropriate, necessitating more aggressive feeding methods. If the gut is functional, enteral tube feeding may be utilized. Nasogastric or nasoenteric tubes are used for short-term support; patients requiring enteral feeding for more than 6 weeks may be better served with a more permanent tube. Using laparotomy, laparoscopy, fluoroscopy, or endoscopy, tubes can be placed in the stomach, duodenum, or jejunum (Minard, 1994). This allows feeding distal to metastatic or obstructive tumors or areas of surgical resection (Ellis et al., 1992; see also Chapter 22).

The selection of the enteral solution is determined by several factors, including the functional capacity of the gut, the intubation site, the patient's metabolic status, and considerations of cost and convenience, especially in home use. Appendices 35 through 40 describe available enteral preparations.

Commercial milk-based or soy-based formulas serve most needs. Patients with radiation enteritis, cancer of the gastrointestinal tract, or existing mal-

TABLE 39–4 GUIDELINES FOR ORAL FEEDING DURING ANTITUMOR THERAPY

PROBLEM	DIET	SUPPLEMENTS AND AIDS	FOODS TO AVOID
Acute gastrointestinal toxicity; nausea and emesis	Clear, cold nonacidic liquids Light, low-fat foods	None	Milk products, cream soups, fried foods, sandwiches, sweet desserts
Stomatitis, esophagitis	Liquid and soft diet (broth-based soups, fruit ades, carbonated beverages, melons) Alterations in texture and temperature	Mild-flavored supplements, frequent oral hygiene, frequent saline rinses	Juices, especially citrus; bananas; crisp or raw foods; meats; spicy entrees; textured or granular foods; coarse bread products; extremely hot or cold foods
Production of viscous mucus, xerostomia (mouth dryness)	Soft, nonirritating diet; tea with lemon; fruit ades; juices; popsicles; carbonated beverages, broth-based soups; thinned hot cereal	Artificial saliva, frequent saline rinses and oral hygiene	Thick nectars and liquids, thick cream soups, thick hot cereals, bread products, gelatin, oily foods
Decreased salivation	Regular diet with high-moisture foods (gravies, sauces, casseroles, chicken, fish, beverages with foods, citric acid–containing foods, sherbet, melons, vegetables with sauces)	Artificial saliva; saliva stimulants, such as sugarless lemon drops and gum; frequent saline rinses	Dry foods, bread products, meats, crackers, bananas, excessively hot foods, alcohol
Mouth blindness (hypogeusia)	Regular diet with strongly flavored (spicy) foods Emphasis on aroma and texture	Flavored supplements, frequent saline rinses	Bland foods, plain meats, unsalted foods
Taste alterations (dysgeusia)	Regular diet with many cold foods; milk products Emphasis on experimentation with foods	Fruit-flavored supplements	Red meats, chocolate, coffee, tea
Early satiety	High-calorie diet with calorically dense foods Meat, fish, poultry, eggs, whole milk, cheese, cream soups, ice cream, whole-milk yogurt, creamed vegetables, rich desserts Small, frequent feedings	Calorically dense supplements	Low-fat or nonfat milk products; broth-based soups; green salads; steamed, plain vegetables; low-calorie beverages
Constipation	Regular diet with fiber added; extra fluids	Fiber-enriched supplements, bulking agents	Gas-forming foods and beverages
Myelosuppression (neutropenia)	Safe food diet; well-cooked foods; eliminate foods that could potentially be contaminated with pathogenic organisms	Hand-washing; safe food-handling practices	Raw fish, meats; mold-containing, unpasteurized cheeses, tempe, all miso products, raw fruit and vegetables, dried fruit and raw or fresh roasted nuts, Brewers yeast, unpasteurized honey, commercial cream-filled pastries requiring refrigeration, dry/fresh spices added after cooking, herbal supplements

nutrition may have multiple malabsorption problems, and so may benefit from elemental or peptide-based formulas. Beneficial effects have been reported with the use of specialized nutritional formulas supplemented with glutamine (Ziegler et al., 1992, 1998) or arginine, ribonucleic acids, and omega-3 fatty acids (Daly et al., 1995).

Parenteral Nutrition

If the gastrointestinal tract is not functioning or enteral support is not adequate, parenteral nutrition must be considered. This mode of feeding involves the administration of concentrated nutrient solutions via infusion into a large-diameter vein, usually the subclavian vein (see Chapter 22).

The ideal parenteral formula for patients with cancer has not yet been determined. Energy and protein are usually administered as glucose and a mixture of amino acids. Required energy intake is generally estimated to be 25 to 35 kcal/kg; protein intake is 1.2 to 2 g/kg (Herrmann and Petruska, 1993; Barton, 1994). Indirect calorimetry should be used to assess the energy needs of hypermetabolic and septic patients. The complications of excess calories include hyperglycemia, excess CO_2 production, lipogenesis, and hepatic steatosis. Intravenous fat may provide 25% to 30% of the total kilocalories, with a maximum recommended infusion rate of 1 to 1.4 g/kg/day. Maximum glucose oxidation rate in the septic patient is 5 mg/kg/min (Barton, 1994). Electrolytes are added to the solution, as are trace minerals and vitamins. Details regarding the nutrient composition and administration of parenteral formulas are given in Chapter 22.

Parenteral nutrition is associated with an increased rate of infection in patients treated with chemotherapy. This has led to the hypothesis that the absence of glutamine in most commercially available parenteral formulations promotes disruption of the mucosal barrier, facilitating bacterial translocation and bacteremia. Two studies have compared the clinical efficacy of glutamine enriched TPN with standard TPN in patients who received marrow transplantation; one study demonstrated benefit derived from the enriched formula (Klein and Koretz, 1994).

Lipids have also been considered to be potential contributors to the increased infection rate in patients receiving parenteral nutrition. Lenssen et al. have determined that providing 25% to 30% of calories from intravenous lipid is not associated with an increased incidence of bacterial or fungal infection in patients undergoing marrow transplantation (Lenssen et al., 1998).

Intense monitoring and specialized care are required for patients receiving TPN. Successful outpatient use of TPN can be achieved when the patient and family are cooperative and are instructed properly.

Home Enteral and Total Parenteral Nutrition

Cancer is the largest single diagnosis for patients starting home enteral nutrition (HEN) or TPN. The mean survival time of patients with cancer is 6 months after starting nutritional support, but 25% live beyond a year and 20% resume full oral intake. The outcome is better for children and for patients with leukemia, lymphoma, or small bowel or liver neoplasms. Patients with cured cancer but severe radiation enteritis requiring home TPN, can expect to survive 8 to 10 years and seem to benefit from home parenteral nutrition therapy (Howard, 1993). Clinical pathways have been developed to provide a clear, concise, standardized method for monitoring home nutritional support. The average variance from the pathway may be more frequent for oncology patients because of complications and unexpected events (Ireton-Jones et al., 1997).

Pediatric Patients

Like the adult patient with cancer, the child with cancer can suffer adverse nutritional consequences as a result of both the malignant disease and the treatment. The incidence of malnutrition ranges from 6% to 50% in the pediatric population, depending on the type, stage, and location of the tumor. It is usually more severe in the presence of aggressive tumors in the later stages of the disease (Andrassy and Chwals, 1998).

Creative efforts are required to minimize the psychological effects of fear, unpleasant hospital routines, unfamiliar foods, learned food aversions, and pain. Oral feeding programs should stress the maximal use of favorite, nutrient dense foods during times when intake is likely to be best and food aversions are least likely to occur. Oral nutritional supplements can be useful, but their acceptance is often a problem, so the child should be offered a selection from which to choose.

Families may express their fears of dying through an extreme preoccupation with eating and maintaining weight. Psychogenic food refusal in children requires interventions that address underlying psychological issues (Mauer et al., 1990).

Enteral nutrition by nasogastric tube is indicated for selected children who are able to cooperate and who have a functional gastrointestinal tract. Some children have even been taught to pass their own nasogastric tube for intermittent or night-time feedings (Mauer et al., 1990). It should be remembered, though, that aspiration is always a potential risk. One study confirmed that enteral nutrition support via gastrostomy tubes is safe and effective in reversing malnutrition in some children who are undergoing intensive chemotherapy (Aquino et al., 1995).

TPN is indicated for children receiving intense treatment associated with severe gastrointestinal toxicity, and for children who are malnourished or have a high risk of developing malnutrition. TPN is seldom indicated for children with advanced cancer associated with significant deterioration or with diseases that are unresponsive to antineoplastic therapy (ASPEN Board of Directors, 1993).

The nutritional requirements of pediatric patients with cancer are similar, with an adjustment for activity level, to those of normal growing children. Often, pediatric patients with cancer are not bedridden, but are as active as their healthy peers. Factors that may alter nutrient requirements in cancer include the impact of the malignant disease on host metabolism, the catabolic effects of antineoplastic therapy, and physiologic stress, such as surgery, fever, malabsorption, and infection. Fluid requirements are increased during anticancer (cytoreductive) therapy or in the presence of fever, diarrhea, or renal failure. Micronutrients may require supplementation during periods of poor intake, stress, or malabsorption. The best long-term indicator of adequate nutrient intake is growth.

The long-term nutritional effects of cancer and its treatment in children are not well documented. Deficiencies in energy and protein can be expected to affect growth adversely, although the impact may be temporary, and catch-up growth may occur after successful tumor therapy is discontinued. However, some treatment regimens may have an effect on growth that is independent of nutritional deprivation. With the increasing survival rates for several childhood cancers, further studies of the long-term effects should be feasible.

Children receiving radiation therapy to the head and neck are at risk for maxillofacial abnormalities. The current practice of including the whole vertebral body in the radiation field has reduced the incidence of scoliosis, which was a late effect of prior treatment procedures (DeLatt and Lampkin, 1992).

Children also have increased nutritional requirements for growth and development that must be met despite extended periods of cancer treatment (ASPEN Board of Directors, 1993). There is a special vulnerability during the adolescent growth spurt. Ewing's sarcoma is frequently associated with malnutrition, probably because it is most common in the second decade of life (Mauer et al., 1990). Another reason children with advanced cancer are at a greater risk of severe nutritional depletion than adults is the frequent use of more aggressive, multimodal treatment. Marrow transplantation is now an accepted and increasingly successful intensive therapy for a wide range of disorders in children. Many supportive therapies may be safely managed in the outpatient arena, reducing the period of hospitalization (Fidler and Hibbs, 1997).

Marrow Transplant Patients

The marrow transplantation procedure is associated with severe nutritional consequences and requires prompt, aggressive, nutritional intervention. Nausea, vomiting, and diarrhea are caused by the cytotoxic conditioning regimen, and may later accompany antibiotic administration. Antiemetics may be helpful.

Following marrow transplantation, complications of delayed onset include varying degrees of mucositis, xerostomia, and dysgeusia. Mucositis, which is often severe and extremely painful, develops in more than 75% of patients in whom a marrow transplant is performed (see Fig. 39-3). Herpes simplex virus and *Candida albicans* account for most oral infections (Eisen et al., 1997). Bland liquids and soft solids are best tolerated by patients with mucositis. Salivary stimulants and substitutes are beneficial for temporary relief of dry mouth; in addition, liquids and foods with sauces and gravies are suggested. Changes in taste acuity persist for weeks post-transplant. Strong-flavored or spicy foods are better accepted without mucositis.

Patients may be able to tolerate little or no oral intake during the first few weeks, and so will require nutritional support via enteral or parenteral routes. Because the function of the gastrointestinal tract is compromised, TPN is often used. Some investigators who have compared TPN with enteral nutrition support in marrow transplantation cases have established the feasibility of enteral feeding in some, but not all, patients (Papdopoulou et al., 1997; Miller, 1997; Szeluga, 1987). Roberts and Miller (1998) report the successful use of gastrostomy tubes for long-term nutritional support in marrow transplant recipients. TPN should be reserved for patients who cannot tolerate enteral feeding.

Most studies estimate energy requirements to be 1.3 to 1.5 times the basal energy expenditure (BEE) and protein needs to be 1.5 g/kg/day. Increased needs may be observed in children and patients with severe stress, GVHD, fever, or intestinal losses (Herrmann and Petruska, 1993). Some investigators report that the use of supplemental glutamine in patients receiving TPN improves clinical outcome, as evidenced by fewer infections and shortened hospital stays (Ziegler et al., 1992), and it may promote lymphocyte recovery (Ziegler et al., 1998).

The nutritional management of patients receiving outpatient marrow transplantation requires frequent assessment and intervention by the dietitian. There is a clinical pathway for providing medical nutritional therapy to outpatients receiving peripheral blood stem cell rescue during high-dose chemotherapy (Dickson, 1997).

A significant improvement in long-term, disease-free survival has been demonstrated in marrow transplant patients who receive TPN compared with those who do not (Klein and Koretz, 1994). The administration of optimal levels of TPN is complicated, however, by the frequent need to interrupt it for the infusion of antibiotics, blood products, and drugs. This, in turn, necessitates the use of more concentrated nutrient solutions, increased flow rates, and occasionally, double- and triple-lumen catheters.

Nutrition-related problems associated with marrow transplantation may persist. A study of patients 1 year post-transplant revealed weight loss, oral sensitivity, and xerostomia in 20% to 25%; in 5% to 10%, anorexia, reflux symptoms, stomatitis, diarrhea, steatorrhea, and dysgeusia persisted. Problems were observed more frequently in the 44% of patients with extensive, chronic GVHD. These findings support the need for ongoing, community-based monitoring after discharge from a transplant center (Lenssen et al., 1990).

Patients with Terminal Cancer

The use of aggressive nutritional support techniques may prolong life. However, TPN is unlikely to benefit patients with advanced cancer whose malignant disease has been documented as unresponsive to chemotherapy or radiation therapy (ASPEN Board of Directors, 1993).

Hydration in the terminally ill patient has been another subject of controversy. Large volumes of fluid may be detrimental (Smith, 1997). Consideration should be given to the pathophysiology of dehydration, which is not painful. "Comfort measures" that use intravenous solutions may not prolong life. In fact, decreased pain, increased mental acuity, and decreased apnea have been demonstrated in hospice patients who are not hydrated artificially (Smith, 1997).

A more appropriate priority is that oral feedings be provided "as tolerated," along with emotional support. The pleasurable aspects of eating should be emphasized, without concern for quantity or nutrient content.

Complementary and Alternative Nutrition Therapies

Complementary and alternative therapies have gained in popularity in recent years, paralleled by significant changes in the U.S. health care system. In 1992, the Office of Alternative Medicine (OAM) was established at the National Institutes of Health to provide a structure for the study of alternative and complementary therapies. To facilitate the grant review process, the OAM classified alternative therapies into seven major categories: alternative systems of practice, bioelectromagnetic applications, manual healing methods, mind/body control, pharmacologic and biologic treatments, herbal medicine, and diet/nutrition/life-style changes (Barrocas, 1997).

Eisenberg (1997) reports that patients explore alternative therapies when (1) health promotion and disease prevention are sought, (2) conventional therapies have been exhausted, (3) conventional therapies are of indeterminate effectiveness or are commonly associated with side effects or significant risks, (4) no conventional therapy is known to relieve the patient's condition, or (5) the conventional approach is perceived to be emotionally or spiritually without benefit. Studies indicate that those who use alternative or complementary therapies tend to be white, more affluent, better educated (Lerner and Kennedy, 1992), and older than nonusers (Newman et al., 1998). In a study of patients at risk for recurrence of breast cancer, 80% reported the use of dietary supplements. The use of herbal and vitamin compounds was inversely related to the months since diagnosis; use of miscellaneous supplements, such as shark cartilage, was directly associated with more advanced disease (Newman et al., 1998). When it is a child who has the malignant disease, the use of alternative medicines may be increased by all members of the family (Mottonen and Uhari, 1997).

In general, alternative or complementary therapies commonly reported by cancer patients include metabolic therapy, dietary treatments, vitamin/mineral supplementation, and herbal therapies. The latter is discussed extensively in Chapter 19.

Metabolic therapy is a term used for a variety of cancer management methods, including unproven and disproved diagnostic methods and treatments. Metabolic practitioners generally claim that diseases, including cancer, are caused by an accumulation of toxic substances in the body. They allege that if these toxins are removed, the body can heal itself naturally. Three basic steps are common to metabolic therapy: detoxification, strengthening of the immune system, and the use of special modalities to attack cancer.

Therapy regimens generally include colonic cleansing, special diets, and vitamin and mineral supplements. The major medical complications of these regimens result from colonic irrigation, which generally involves the use of coffee, wheatgrass, or other substances. Electrolyte imbalance, toxic colitis, bowel perforation, and sepsis have been reported with colonic irrigation. Except for the Gerson diet, the dietary component of metabolic therapy appears to be less restrictive than other regimens and thus causes fewer problems. Most regimens promote "natural" and "organic" foods and recommend restriction of animal products, refined flours and sugars, and foods that are processed or contain artificial ingredients.

Another form of metabolic therapy is *oxymedicine*, the use of compounds, such as ozone and hydrogen peroxide, that contain reactive forms of oxygen to help destroy tumors. These hyperoxygenerators have no demonstrated benefits, and both hydrogen peroxide (administered enterally and parenterally) and ozone (administered rectally) can be harmful because of excess free radical production and oxidation of tissue (American Cancer Society, 1991).

Dietary treatments for cancer generally are based on the "you are what you eat" principle. A number of diet therapies exist, consisting of specific foods prepared and consumed in a specified manner.

The *macrobiotic diet* is a quasi-religious/philosophical system popularized in the United States by Michio Kushi. Currently, the diet derives 50% to 60% of its calories from whole grains, 25% to 30% from vegetables, and the remainder from beans, seaweed, and soups. Meat and certain vegetables are avoided, and soybean consumption is promoted. Past research determined that the diet was deficient in calcium and vitamin B_{12}. Recently, the OAM funded a pilot study of the macrobiotic diet, the principal investigator of which is Lawrence Kushi, ScD, a member of the faculty of the University of Minnesota School of Public Health and the son of Michio Kushi (Cassileth and Chapman, 1996).

Megavitamin therapy, another frequently practiced therapy, is characterized by the use of large doses of one or more vitamins. The treatment is based on the belief that the body's ability to destroy the tumor is enhanced by large doses of vitamins, antioxidants, and other substances, including coenzyme Q10 and pangamic acid (Roberts, 1998).

Miscellaneous substances that may be used by patients with cancer include enzymes, which are purported to treat cancer by dissolving the coating of cancer cells so as to allow the immune system to destroy the cancer; melatonin, a hormone that promotes sleep and has strong antioxidant properties; and dehydroepiandrosterone (DHEA), a hormone with unknown safety and effectiveness (Roberts, 1998).

A nutritional history and assessment should always address the patient's use of alternative therapies. Patients frequently do not inform their health providers about their use of alternative therapies either because they are not asked, or they are afraid of the reaction (Roberts, 1998). Communication that utilizes open-ended questions, listening with empathy, and an unbiased approach is essential to successful intervention. In that context, the dietitian can then provide reliable, scientific information about alternative therapies so that the patient can make informed choices and avoid undesired risks.

Patient Rehabilitation

Rehabilitation is an important concept that pervades cancer care in all settings. The effect of cancer and cancer treatment on the patient's quality of life is addressed throughout the treatment period and continues until the patient is able to successfully resume activities of daily living (Body et al., 1997; Blesch, 1996).

Regardless of which mode of feeding is utilized, nutritional goals should be specific, achievable, and limited in scope to encourage patient cooperation. The goals need to be directed toward a visible means of feedback, such as body weight or some other meaningful index. Instruction of the patient and family members regarding expected problems and their possible solutions should be initiated early in the cancer therapy course, and should continue in conjunction with follow-up nutritional assessment.

CASE STUDY

Janice K. is a 48-year-old mother of four. Recently she was diagnosed with breast cancer (estrogen-receptor positive) and has been prescribed tamoxifen. In the next 3 weeks, she will undergo a modified radical mastectomy followed by radiation therapy. She is 5 feet, 8 inches tall, weighs 185 lbs, and has a history of mild hypertension controlled with dietary measures. She also is attracted to the use of multiple vitamins and supplements as well as alternative therapies for reducing her cancer recurrence risk.

1. What recommendations do you have to prepare Janice for surgery?
2. After radiation therapy, what side effects might Janice experience? List some dietary strategies Janice may follow if she experiences the following: weight gain, persistent queasiness, a slight difficulty in swallowing (esophagus is in the radiation field). She is also likely to be inactive from fatigue and the radiation treatments.
3. Is Janice at her ideal body weight? If not, what suggestions would you recommend? Consider her hypertension, planned surgery, and radiation therapy.
4. What dietary recommendations, if any, are appropriate for a regimen of tamoxifen?
5. What guidance should be provided in regard to the appropriate use of vitamin-mineral supplements and ways to evaluate alternative therapies? How does soy affect estrogen-receptor positive forms of breast cancer?

Fatigue and impairment of physical performance are common and severe problems of cancer patients. Psychological, as well as physical factors, play a role. Poor nutrition contributes to fatigue; conversely, fatigue may hinder eating and nutritional support regimens. The goal is to minimize the side effects of treatment and to maximize the patient's nutritional parameters (Kalman and Villani, 1997). Appropriate exercise may be helpful in treating primary fatigue (Dimeo et al., 1998).

Patients need to be encouraged to care for themselves and to maintain their nutritional intake. Patient support groups can be formed for mutual encouragement. Recent studies indicate that an increasing number of patients with cancer are able to return to full function and regain their quality of life, in addition to maintaining their earning potential and employment status (Harrison et al., 1997).

CITED REFERENCES

American Cancer Society. Unproven methods of cancer management: Laetrile. Cancer 41:187, 1991.

American Dietetic Association. Medical Nutrition Therapy Across the Continuum of Care. Chicago: American Dietetic Association, 1997.

American Society for Parenteral and Enteral Nutrition (ASPEN) Board of Directors. Guidelines for the use of parenteral and enteral nutrition in adult and pediatric patients. J Parenter Enteral Nutr 17(suppl):15, 1993.

Andrassy RJ, Chwals WJ. Nutritional support of the pediatric oncology patient. Nutrition 14:124, 1998.

Aquino VM, et al. Enteral nutrition support by gastrostomy tube in children with cancer. J Pediatr 127:58, 1995.

The ATBC Cancer Prevention Study Group. The effect of vitamin E and beta-carotene on the incidence of lung cancer and other cancers in male smokers. N Engl J Med 330:1029, 1994.

Barnes-Josiah D, et al. Early body size and subsequent weight gain as predictors of breast cancer incidence. Cancer Causes Control 6:112, 1995.

Baron JA, et al. Calcium supplements for the prevention of colorectal adenomas. N Engl J Med 340:101, 1999.

Barrocas A. Complementary and alternative medicine: Friend, foe or OWA? J Am Diet Assoc 97:1373, 1997.

Barton RG. Nutrition support in critical illness. Nutr Clin Pract 9:127, 1994.

Bernstein L, et al. Physical exercise and reduced risk of breast cancer in young women. J Natl Cancer Inst 86:1403, 1994.

Berwick M, Schantz S. Chemoprevention for aerodigestive cancer. Cancer Metast Rev 16:329, 1997.

Blesch KS. Rehabilitation of the cancer patient at home. Semin Oncol Nurs 12:219, 1996.

Bloch AS. Feeding the cancer patient: Where have we come from, where are we going? Nutr Clin Pract 9:87, 1994.

Block G, et al. Fruit, vegetables, and cancer prevention: A review of the epidemiologic evidence. Nutr Cancer 18:1, 1992.

Blot WJ. Prevention of esophageal cancer: The nutrition intervention trials in Linxian, China. Linxian Nutrition Intervention Trials Study Group. Cancer Res 54(suppl):2029S, 1994.

Blot WJ, et al. Nutrition intervention trials in Linxian, China: Supplementation with specific vitamin/mineral combinations, cancer incidence, and disease-specific mortality in the general population. J Natl Cancer Inst 85:1483, 1993.

Body JJ, et al. The concept of rehabilitation of cancer patients. Curr Opin Oncol 9:332, 1997.

Boock CA, Reddick JE. Taste alterations in bone marrow transplantation patients. J Am Diet Assoc 91:1121, 1991.

Brinton LA, Swanson CA. Height and weight at various ages and risk of breast cancer. Ann Epidemiol 2:597, 1992.

Cassileth BR, Chapman CC. Alternative cancer medicine: A ten-year update. Cancer Invest 14:396, 1996.

Charuhas PM. Dietary management during antitumor therapy of cancer patients. Top Clin Nutr 9:42, 1993.

Cheng KK, Day NE. Nutrition and esophageal cancer. Cancer Causes Control 7:33, 1996.

Colditz GA, et al. Physical activity and reduced risk of colon cancer: Implications for prevention. Cancer Causes Control 8:649, 1997.

Craig WJ. Phytochemicals: Guardians of our health. J Am Diet Assoc 97(suppl 2):S199, 1997.

Daly JM, et al. Enteral nutrition during multimodal therapy in upper gastrointestinal cancer patients. Ann Surg 221:327, 1995.

DeLatt CA, Lampkin BC. Long-term survivors of childhood cancer: Evaluation and identification of sequelae of treatment. Cancer 42:263, 1992.

Demark-Wahnefried W, et al. Weight gain in women diagnosed with breast cancer. J Am Diet Assoc 97:519, 1997.

DeWys WD, et al. Prognostic effect of weight loss prior to chemotherapy in patients. Am J Med 60:491, 1980.

Dickerson RN, et al. Resting energy expenditure of patients with gynecologic malignancies. J Am Coll Nutr 14:409, 1995.

Dickson TC. Clinical pathway nutrition management for outpatient bone marrow transplantation. J Am Diet Assoc 97:61, 1997.

Dimeo F, et al. Aerobic exercise as therapy for cancer fatigue. Med Sci Sports Exerc 30:475, 1998.

Eisen D, et al. Oral cavity complications of bone marrow transplantation. Semin Cutan Med Surg 16:265, 1997.

Eisenberg DM. Advising patients who seek alternative medical therapies. Ann Intern Med 127:61, 1997.

Ellis LM, et al. Laparoscopic feeding jejunostomy tube in oncology patients. Surg Oncol 1:245, 1992.

Ettinger DS. Preventing chemotherapy-induced nausea and vomiting: An update and a review of emesis. Semin Oncol 22(4 suppl 10):6, 1995.

Fearon KC, et al. Albumin synthesis rates are not decreased in hypoalbuminemic cachectic cancer patients with an ongoing acute-phase protein response. Ann Surg 227:249, 1998.

Fessele KS. Managing the multiple causes of nausea and vomiting in the patient with cancer. Oncol Nurs Forum 23:1409, 1996.

Fidler PA, Hibbs CJ. Bone marrow transplant today—Home tomorrow. Ambulatory care issues in pediatric marrow transplantation. J Pediatr Oncol Nurs 14:228, 1997.

Food, Nutrition, and the Prevention of Cancer: A global perspective. Washington, DC: World Cancer Fund/American Institute for Cancer Research, 1997.

Fredrix EWHM, et al. Effects of different tumor types on resting energy expenditure. Cancer Res 51:6138, 1991.

Fuchs CS, et al. Dietary fiber and the risk of colorectal cancer and adenoma in women. N Engl J Med 340:169, 1999.

Giles G, Ireland P. Diet, nutrition, and prostate cancer. Int J Cancer 10(suppl):13, 1997.

Grant JP, et al. Malabsorption associated with surgical procedures and its treatment. Nutr Clin Pract 11:43, 1996.

Harnack L, et al. Association of cancer prevention–related nutrition knowledge, beliefs, and attitudes to cancer prevention dietary behavior. J Am Diet Assoc 97:957, 1997.

Harrison LB, et al. Detailed quality of life assessment in patients treated with primary radiotherapy for squamous cell cancer of the base of the tongue. Head Neck 19:169, 1997.

Haslett PA. Anticytokine approaches to the treatment of anorexia and cachexia. Semin Oncol 25(2 suppl 6):53, 1998.

Hennekens CH, et al. Lack of effect of long-term supplementation with beta-carotene on the incidence of malignant neoplasms and cardiovascular disease. N Engl J Med 334:1145, 1996.

Herrmann VM, Petruska PJ. Nutrition support in bone marrow transplant recipients. J Parenter Enteral Nutr 8:19, 1993.

Hirohata T, Kono S. Diet/nutrition and stomach cancer in Japan. Int J Cancer [Suppl] 10:34, 1997.

Holmes MD, et al. Association of dietary intake of fat and fatty acids with risk of breast cancer. JAMA 281:914, 1999.

Hong WK, et al. Prevention of second primary tumors with isotretinoin in squamous-cell carcinoma of the head and neck. N Engl J Med 323:795, 1990.

Howard L. Home parenteral and enteral nutrition in cancer patients. Cancer 72(suppl):3531, 1993.

Howe GR, et al. Dietary intake of fiber and decreased risk of cancer of the colon and rectum: Evidence from the combined analysis of 13 case-control studies. J Natl Cancer Inst 24:1887, 1992.

Huang Z, et al. Dual effects of weight and weight gain on breast cancer risk. JAMA 278:1407, 1997.

Hunter AMB. Nutrition management of patients with neoplastic disease of the head and neck treated with radiation therapy. Nutr Clin Pract 11:157, 1996.

Hunter DJ, Willett WC. Nutrition and breast cancer. Cancer Causes Control 7:56, 1996.

Hunter DJ, et al. A prospective study of vitamins C, E, A and risk of breast cancer. N Engl J Med 329:234, 1993.

Ireton-Jones C, et al. Clinical pathways in home nutrition support. J Am Diet Assoc 97:1003, 1997.

Isola LM, et al. A pilot study of allogeneic bone marrow transplantation using related donors stimulated with G-CSF. Bone Marrow Transpl 20:1033, 1997.

Kalman D, Villani LJ. Nutritional aspects of cancer-related fatigue. J Am Diet Assoc 97:650, 1997.

Kamath S, et al. Taste thresholds of patients with cancer of esophagus. Cancer 52:386, 1983.

Klein S, Koretz RL. Nutrition support in patients with cancer: What do the data really show? Nutr Clin Pract 9:91, 1994.

Kono S, Hirohata T. Nutrition and stomach cancer. Cancer Causes Control 7:41, 1996.

Kritchevsky D. Caloric restriction and experimental mammary carcinogenesis. Breast Cancer Res Treat 46:161, 1997.

Kune GA, Vitetta L. Alcohol consumption and the etiology of colorectal cancer: A review of the scientific evidence from 1957 to 1991. Nutr Cancer 18:97, 1992.

Kyle UG. The patient with head and neck cancer. In: Bloch AS (ed.). Nutrition Management of the Cancer Patient. Rockville, MD: Aspen Publishers, 1990.

Langstein HN, Norton JA. Mechanisms of cancer cachexia. Hematol/Oncol Clin North Am 5:103, 1991.

Lenhard R. American Cancer Society nutrition guidelines. CA 46:323, 1996.

Lenssen P, et al. Intravenous lipid dose and incidence of bacteremia and fungemia in patients undergoing bone marrow transplantation. Am J Clin Nutr 67:927, 1998.

Lenssen P, et al. Prevalence of nutrition-related problems among long-term survivors of allogeneic marrow transplantation. J Am Diet Assoc 90:835, 1990.

Lerner IJ, Kennedy BJ. The prevalence of questionable methods of cancer treatment in the United States. Cancer 42:181, 1992.

Marshall JR, Boyle P. Nutrition and oral cancer. Cancer Causes Control 7:101, 1996.

Martinez ME, et al. Leisure-time physical activity, body size, and colon cancer in women. Nurses' Health Study Res Group. J Natl Cancer Inst 89:948, 1997.

Mattes RD. Prevention of food aversions in cancer patients during treatment. Nutr Cancer 21:13, 1994.

Matthys P, Billiau A. Cytokines and cachexia. Nutrition 13:763, 1997.

Mauer AM, et al. Special nutritional needs of children with malignancies: A review. J Parenter Enteral Nutr 14:315, 1990.

McMahon K, et al. Integrating proactive nutritional assessment in clinical practices to prevent complications and cost. Semin Oncol 25(2 suppl 6):20, 1998.

Meisenberg BR, et al. Outpatient high-dose chemotherapy with autologous stem-cell rescue for hematologic and nonhematologic malignancies. J Clin Oncol 15:11, 1997.

Messina MJ, et al. Soy intake and cancer risk: A review of the in vitro and in vivo data. Nutr Cancer 21:13, 1994.

Miller EC, Miller JA. Carcinogens and mutagens that may occur in foods. Cancer 58:1795, 1986.

Miller JE. Hepatic veno-occlusive disease: A challenging complication of bone marrow transplantation. Support Line 19:10, 1997.

Minard G. Enteral access. Nutr Clin Prac 9:172, 1994.

Mottonen M, Uhari M. Use of micronutrients and alternative drugs by children with acute lymphoblastic leukemia. Med Pediatr Oncol 28:5, 1997.

Newberne PM, Conner MW. Food additives and contaminants: An update. Cancer 58:1851, 1986.

Newman V, et al. Dietary supplement use by women at risk for breast cancer recurrence. J Am Diet Assoc 98:285, 1998.

Olson SH, et al. Body mass index, weight gain, and risk of endometrial cancer. Nutr Cancer 23:141, 1995.

Omenn GS, et al. Effects of a combination of beta-carotene and vitamin A on lung cancer and cardiovascular disease. N Engl J Med 334:1150, 1996.

Ottery F. Supportive nutritional management of the patient with pancreatic cancer. Oncology 10:26, 1996.

Ottery FD, et al. Pharmacologic management of anorexia/cachexia. Semin Oncol 25(2 suppl 6):35, 1998.

Papdopoulou A, et al. Enteral nutrition after bone marrow transplantation. Arch Dis Child 77:131, 1997.

Paserot D, et al. Evaluation of sensitive alterations in cancer patients treated by chemotherapy: First report. Proc Annu Meeting Am Soc Clin Oncol 16:A274, 1997.

Patterson RE, et al. Do beliefs, knowledge, and perceived norms about diet and cancer predict dietary change? Am J Publ Health 86:1394, 1996.

Potter JD. Nutrition and colorectal cancer. Cancer Causes Control 7:127, 1996.

Potter JD, Steinmetz K. Vegetables, fruit and phytoestrogens as preventive agents. IARC Sci Publ 139:61, 1996.

Puccio M, Nathanson L. The cancer cachexia syndrome. Semin Oncol 24:277, 1997.

Renwick AG. Acceptable daily intake and the regulation of intense sweeteners. Food Add Contamin 7:463, 1990.

Ringden O. Bone marrow transplantation using unrelated donors for hematological malignancies. Med Oncol 14:11, 1997.

Roberts S. Alternative nutrition therapies used by oncology patients. Support Line 20:10, 1998.

Roberts SR, Miller JE. Success using PEG tubes in marrow transplant recipients. Nutr Clin Pract 13:74, 1998.

Rodier JF, et al. Prevention of radiation enteritis and pelvic floor reconstruction by a polyglactin 910 (Vicryl) mesh in gynecologic malignancies. Int J Oncol 7(suppl):963, 1995.

Slattery ML, et al. Energy balance and colon cancer—beyond physical activity. Cancer Res 57:75, 1997a.

Slattery ML, et al. Plant foods and colon cancer: An assessment of specific foods and their related nutrients (United States). Cancer Causes Control 8:575, 1997b.

Smith S. Controversies in hydrating the terminally ill patient. J Intravenous Nurs 20:193, 1997.

Staal van den Brekel AJ, et al. Increased resting energy expenditure and weight loss are related to a systemic inflammatory response in lung cancer patients. J Clin Oncol 13:600, 1995.

Steinmetz KA, Potter JD. Vegetables, fruit, and cancer. I. Epidemiology. Cancer Causes Control 2:325, 1991a.

Steinmetz KA, Potter JD. Vegetables, fruit, and cancer. II. Mechanisms. Cancer Causes Control 2:427, 1991b.

Szeluga PJ, et al. Nutritional support of bone marrow transplant recipients: A prospective randomized clinical trial comparing total parenteral nutrition to an enteral feeding program. Cancer Res 47:3309, 1987.

Thomson SR, et al. Resting metabolic rate of esophageal carcinoma patients: A model for energy expenditure measurement in a homogeneous cancer population. J Parenter Enteral Nutr 14:119, 1990.

Tisdale MJ. Biology of cachexia. J Natl Cancer Inst 89:1763, 1997.

Trentham-Dietz A, et al. Body size and risk of breast cancer. Am J Epidemiol 145:1011, 1997.

Trock B, et al. Dietary fiber, vegetables, and colon cancer: Critical review and meta-analyses of the epidemiologic evidence. J Natl Cancer Inst 82:650, 1990.

Willett WC. Fat, energy, and breast cancer. J Nutr 127(5 suppl):9215, 1997.

Wynder EL, et al. Breast cancer: Weighing the evidence for a promoting role of dietary fat. J Natl Cancer Inst 89:766, 1997.

Yu G-P, et al. Green-tea consumption and risk of stomach cancer: A population-based case-control study in Shanghai, China. Cancer Causes Control 6:532, 1995.

Ziegler TR, et al. Clinical and metabolic efficacy of glutamine-supplemented parenteral nutrition after bone marrow transplantation. Ann Int Med 116:821, 1992.

Ziegler TR, et al. Effects of glutamine supplementation on circulating lymphocytes after bone marrow transplantation: A pilot study. Am J Med Sci 315:4, 1998.

ADDITIONAL REFERENCES

Etiology

Ballard-Barbash R, et al. Dietary fat, serum estrogen levels, and breast cancer risk: A multifaceted story. J Natl Cancer Inst 91:492, 1999.

Boyd N, et al. Effects at two years of a low-fat, high carbohydrate diet on radiologic features of the breast: Results from a randomized trial. J Natl Cancer Inst 89:488, 1997.

Day R. Future need for more cancer research. J Am Diet Assoc 98:523, 1998.

Djuric Z, et al. Oxidative DNA damage levels in blood from women at high risk for breast cancer are associated with dietary intakes of meats, vegetables and fruits. J Am Diet Assoc 98:524, 1998.

Doerr T, et al. Zinc deficiency in head and neck cancer patients. J Am Coll Nutr 16:418, 1997.

Doyle T, et al. The association of drinking water source and chlorination by-products with cancer incidence among postmenopausal women in Iowa: A prospective cohort study. Am J Publ Health 87:1168, 1997.

Greenwald P, et al. Fat, caloric intake, and obesity: Lifestyle risk factors for breast cancer. J Am Diet Assoc 97(7 suppl):S24, 1997.

Holt P, et al. Modulation of abnormal colonic epithelial cell proliferation and differentiation by low-fat dairy foods. J Am Med Assoc 280:1074, 1998.

Horn-Ross P. Diet and the risk of salivary gland cancer. Am J Epidemiol 146:171, 1997.

Kaplan S, et al. Nutritional factors in the etiology of brain tumors: Potential role of nitrosamines, fat, and cholesterol. Am J Epidemiol 146:832, 1997.

Nutritional Care

Alberts D, et al. Randomized, double-blinded, placebo-controlled study of effect of wheat bran fiber and calcium on fecal bile acids in patients with resected adenomatous colon polyps. J Natl Cancer Inst 88:81, 1996.

Bartels CL, Miller SJ. Herbal and related remedies. Nutr Clin Pract 12:5, 1998.

Cohen L. Colorectal cancer: A primary care approach to screening. Geriatrics 51:45, 1996.

Imai K, et al. Cancer-preventive effects of drinking green tea among a Japanese population. Prev Med 26:769, 1997.

Spaulding-Albright N. A review of some herbal and related products commonly used in cancer patients. J Am Diet Assoc 97(suppl 2):S208, 1997.

Walker MS, et al. Oncology Nutrition Patient Education Materials. Chicago: American Dietetic Association, 1998

CHAPTER 40

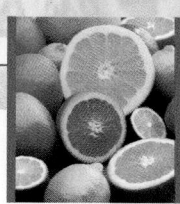

Medical Nutrition Therapy for Human Immunodeficiency Virus (HIV) Infection and Acquired Immunodeficiency Syndrome (AIDS)*

MARCY FENTON, MS, RD
AND ELLYN SILVERMAN, MPH, RD, CHES

Chapter Outline

- Pathophysiology, Etiology, and Classification
- Perinatal Considerations
- Manifestations and Treatment of HIV Infection
- Relationship Between Malnutrition and AIDS
- Medical Nutrition Therapy
- Food and Water Safety and Infection Control
- Complementary and Alternative Nutrition Therapies

Key Terms

ACQUIRED IMMUNE DEFICIENCY SYNDROME (AIDS)—HIV infection along with a CD4 cell count of 200 or less (or less than 14%); or dementia, wasting syndrome, or malignant diseases, such as Kaposi's sarcoma or non-Hodgkin's lymphoma; or one of 26 opportunistic infections

ACUTE HUMAN IMMUNODEFICIENCY VIRUS (HIV) INFECTION—an acute syndrome characterized by fever, malaise, lymphadenopathy, pharyngitis, headache, myalgia, and sometimes, rash

AIDS ENTEROPATHY—changes in the small and large bowel thought to be attributable to direct HIV infection and with no other identifiable pathogen; manifested as chronic diarrhea and possibly, malabsorption

AIDS WASTING SYNDROME (AWS)—involuntary weight loss of 10% of baseline body weight plus either chronic diarrhea (two loose stools per day for more than 30 days) or chronic weakness and documented fever (for 30 days or more, intermittent or constant) in the absence of a concurrent illness or other condition that would explain the findings

CONSTITUTIONAL DISEASE—another name for AIDS wasting syndrome

DRUG RESISTANCE—a situation in which treatment does not completely suppress HIV replication; virus mutations are produced that outnumber the original "wild type" virus, and the virus loses its sensitivity to a drug

HIGHLY ACTIVE ANTIRETROVIRAL THERAPY (HAART)—a new drug therapy which acts to reduce viral concentrations in the blood; contains at least three antiviral agents

HIV-ASSOCIATED NEPHROPATHY (HIVAN)—a syndrome of progressive renal failure with HIV infection

HIV ENCEPHALOPATHY (AIDS DEMENTIA)—degenerative disease of the brain due to infection with HIV

KAPOSI'S SARCOMA—a malignant neoplastic vascular proliferation characterized by the development of bluish-red cutaneous nodules, usually on the surface of the skin or oral cavities

LIPODYSTROPHY—a disturbance of fat metabolism that involves the loss of the thin layer of fat, making veins seem to protrude; characterized by wasting of the face and limbs with the accumulation of fat on the abdomen (both under the skin and within the body cavity) or between the shoulder blades

LYMPHADENOPATHY SYNDROME (LAS)—swollen, firm, and sometimes tender lymph nodes secondary to any of a number of causes ranging from infection, such as HIV, influenza, or mononucleosis, to lymphoma (cancer of the lymph nodes)

*This chapter is a revision of a chapter, contributed by Barbara Eldridge, RD, CD, that appeared in the previous edition.

MYALGIA—diffuse muscle pain, usually accompanied by malaise (vague feeling of discomfort or weakness)

OPPORTUNISTIC INFECTION—infection by an organism that does not ordinarily cause disease but which becomes pathogenic under certain circumstances, such as impaired immune response

PERINATAL HIV TRANSMISSION (PHT)—transmission of HIV infection from mother to infant in utero, during birth, or during breast-feeding

RETROVIRUS—a virus, such as HIV, which replicates using an enzyme (reverse transcriptase) to copy RNA into DNA when RNA is its natural genetic state; most cells have DNA in their natural state and transcribe to RNA during replication

The **acquired immunodeficiency syndrome (AIDS)** was first described by the Centers for Disease Control (CDC) in 1981. Several young adults were reported to have unusual opportunistic infections—*Pneumocystis carinii* pneumonia, cytomegalovirus, or candidiasis—or a rare skin cancer, Kaposi's sarcoma, associated with severe depression of cellular immunity. These cases represented a previously unknown disorder. In 1983, researchers isolated the etiologic agent, a **retrovirus** which was named *human immunodeficiency virus* (HIV) (Barre-Sinoussi, 1983). In 1998, the oldest case of human infection by the virus was confirmed using a 1959 blood sample of a man from the Belgian Congo (Brown, 1998a).

Two recent major developments have greatly changed the way HIV disease is managed and its subsequent outcomes. The first is the use and application of viral load testing. Viral load tests measure the quantity of free virus circulating in the bloodstream (HIV-RNA copies per milliliter of blood plasma); the optimal test result is "undetectable" using the most sensitive test available. Viral load tests with CD4+ cell counts help predict the likelihood of AIDS-related illness and death (Tables 40–1 and 40–2), (Mellors et al., 1997) and represent the "essential parameter in decisions to initiate or change antiretroviral therapies" (Panel on Clinical Practices, 1997).

The second major development is the explosion of new antiretroviral drugs that are available and used in combination with each other. Antiretroviral drugs act to destroy HIV or suppress its replication, and were credited in 1997 for reducing death rates up to 60% in some areas of the United States (Russell, 1998). The use of only one antiretroviral drug has been recognized as leading to drug-resistant mutants of the virus, and its use has been discontinued. In addition to the remarkable decrease in deaths with the advent of new therapies, rates of opportunistic infections have declined significantly since 1996. The largest decreases have been seen in the incidences of *Pneumocystis carinii* pneumonia, wasting syndrome, Kaposi's sarcoma, *Mycobacterium avium* complex, and cytomegalovirus retinitis and, to a lesser extent, toxoplasmosis, dementia, esophageal candidiasis, cryptococcal meningitis, and cryptosporidiosis (Michaels et al., 1998).

More than 612,000 cases of AIDS have been reported in the United States. Of the affected individuals, 61% have died (CDC,1997a). In June of 1997, the CDC reported AIDS cases by exposure category: 49% of the cases occurred among men who had sex with men, 26% among intravenous drug users, 9% among those having heterosexual contact, and 6% among men who had sex with men and injected drugs. Others affected included hemophiliacs and other recipients of blood transfusions, and infants born to mothers with HIV infection.

HIV disease is the second leading cause of death for Americans between the ages of 25 and 44 years, with as many as 50% of new HIV infections occurring among individuals younger than 25 years of age. Whites account for 45.6% of cases, African Americans for 35.4%, Latinos for 17.8%, and Asian Americans for 0.71%. At the end of 1996, the percentages of persons living with AIDS in the United States were as follows: adult men, 80%; adult women, 18.6%; and pediatric population (<13 years old), 1.4% (CDC, 1997a). State and federal correctional facilities have an occurrence of AIDS that is 14-fold greater than that of the general U.S. population (Pérez, 1997). The 1995 death rate from AIDS for blacks was more than three times higher than the death rate for all other people (Day, 1998).

TABLE 40–1 INDICATIONS FOR THE INITIATION OF ANTIRETROVIRAL THERAPY IN THE CHRONICALLY HIV-INFECTED PATIENT

CLINICAL CATEGORY	CD4+ T CELL COUNT AND HIV RNA	RECOMMENDATION
Symptomatic (AIDS, thrush, unexplained fever)	Any value	Treat
Asymptomatic	CD4+ T Cells < 500/mm^3 or HIV RNA > 10,000 (bDNA) or > 20,000 (RT-PCR)	Treatment should be offered. Strength or recommendation is based on prognosis for disease-free survival and willingness of the patient to accept therapy.[1]
Asymptomatic	CD4+ T Cells > 500/mm^3 and HIV RNA < 10,000 (bDNA) or < 20,000 (RT-PCR)	Many experts would delay therapy and observe; however, some experts would treat.

[1]Some experts would observe patients with CD4+ T cell counts between 350-500/mm^3 and HIV RNA levels < 10,000 (bDNA) or < 20,000 (RT-PCR)

Centers for Disease Control and Prevention. Guidelines for the use of antiretroviral agents in HIV-infected adults and adolescents. MMWR. June 17, 1998; updated The Living Document, May 5, 1999, www.hivatis.org.

TABLE 40–2 CLASSIFICATION SYSTEM FOR HIV INFECTION AND EXPANDED AIDS SURVEILLANCE CASE DEFINITION FOR ADOLESCENTS AND ADULTS

Clinical Categories

The clinical categories are defined as follows:

Category A—one or more of the conditions listed here occurring in an adolescent or adult with documented HIV infection. Conditions listed in categories B and C must not have occurred.

- Asymptomatic HIV infection
- Persistent generalized lymphadenopathy (PGL)
- Acute (primary) HIV infection with accompanying illness or a history of acute HIV infection

Category B—symptomatic conditions occurring in an HIV-infected adolescent or adult that are not included among conditions listed in clinical category C, and that meet at least one of the following criteria:

1. the conditions are attributed to HIV infection and/or are indicative of a defect in cell-mediated immunity
2. the conditions are considered by physicians to have a clinical course or management that is complicated by HIV infection.

Examples of conditions in clinical category B include, but are not limited to, the following:

- Bacterial endocarditis, meningitis, pneumonia, or sepsis
- Candidiasis (vulvovaginal) that is persistent (1 month duration) or poorly responsive to therapy
- Candidiasis, oropharyngeal (thrush)
- Cervical dysplasia, severe; or carcinoma
- Constitutional symptoms, such as fever (≥38.5°C) or diarrhea lasting >1 month
- Hairy leukoplakia, oral
- Herpes zoster (shingles), involving at least two distinct episodes or more than one dermatome
- Idiopathic thrombocytopenic purpura
- Listeriosis
- *Mycobacterium tuberculosis* infection, pulmonary
- Nocardiosis
- Pelvic inflammatory disease
- Peripheral neuropathy

Category C—any condition listed in the 1987 surveillance case definition for AIDS and affecting an adolescent or adult. The conditions in clinical category C are strongly associated with severe immunodeficiency, occur frequently in HIV-infected individuals, and cause serious morbidity or mortality. Among the conditions listed in the 1993 AIDS surveillance case definition (assuming HIV positivity) are the following:

- Candidiasis of bronchi, trachea, or lungs
- Candidiasis, esophageal
- CD4 lymphocyte counts < 200, or a CD4 percent of total lymphocytes < 14 if the absolute count is not available
- Cervical cancer, invasive
- Coccidioidomycosis, disseminated or extrapulmonary (Valley fever)
- Cryptococcosis, extrapulmonary
- Cryptosporidiosis, chronic intestinal (>1 month duration)
- Cytomegalovirus disease (other than liver, spleen, or nodes)
- Cytomegalovirus retinitis (with loss of vision)
- HIV encephalopathy
- Herpes simplex: chronic ulcer(s) (>1 month duration); or bronchitis, pneumonitis, or esophagitis
- Histoplasmosis, disseminated or extrapulmonary
- Isosporiasis, chronic intestinal (>1 month duration)
- Kaposi's sarcoma (KS)
- Lymphoma, Burkitt's (or equivalent term)
- Lymphoma, immunoblastic (or equivalent term)
- Lymphoma, primary in brain
- *Mycobacterium avium* complex or *M. kansasii*, disseminated or extrapulmonary
- *Mycobacterium tuberculosis*, any site, pulmonary or extrapulmonary
- Mycobacterium, other species or unidentified species, disseminated or extrapulmonary
- *Pneumocystis carinii* pneumonia (PCP)
- Pneumonia, recurrent
- Progressive multifocal leukoencephalopathy (PML)
- Salmonella septicemia, recurrent
- Toxoplasmosis of brain
- Wasting syndrome secondary to HIV

CD4+ CELL COUNT CATEGORIES (AIDS-INDICATOR CELL COUNT)	CLINICAL CATEGORIES		
	A (Asymptomatic or PGL)	B (Symptomatic, not A or C Conditions)	C (AIDS-Indicator Condition)
> 500/mm^3	A1	B1	C1
200–499/mm^3	A2	B2	C2
< 200/mm^3	A3	B3	C3

(From Centers for Disease Control. 1993 Revised classification system for HIV infection and expanded surveillance case definition for AIDS among adolescents and adults. MMWR 41[No. RR-17], 1992.)

PGL, persistent generalized lymphadenopathy.

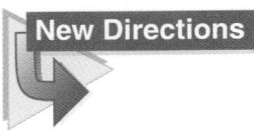

The Changing Face of AIDS

When AIDS was first identified in 1983, it was seen almost exclusively in the homosexual male population. However, the incidence of the disease is changing. People of color (African Americans, Latinos, Asian/Pacific Islanders, American Indians, and Alaska Natives) now constitute 54% of the total number of people with AIDS, and African Americans and Latinos have been disproportionately affected (CDC, 1997a).

Heterosexual HIV transmission accounts for an increasing number of U.S. AIDS cases. The number of heterosexual-contact cases reported in 1993 had increased 130% over those reported in 1992, compared to a 109% increase for all other transmission categories combined. Adolescents and young adults, women, blacks, and Hispanics are at highest risk for heterosexually acquired HIV infection. Persons at highest risk for heterosexual HIV transmission are those who have multiple sex partners, sex with a high-risk partner, or sexually transmitted diseases.

Although representing a small percentage of the total number, older HIV-infected adults are often misdiagnosed. Moreover, this age group was found to use condoms at 1/6th the rate of 20-year-olds, and were 1/5th as likely to get tested for HIV. Postmenopausal women, who are often uninformed of the dangers of HIV transmission, may become increasingly sexually active with more partners who use condoms less. The physiology of these women may increase the risk of transmission, as the vaginal walls are thin, vaginal lubrication decreases, and there is an increased risk of tearing vaginal membranes, providing easy access for the virus (Engle, 1998).

The CDC suggests that HIV prevention programs should focus on promoting behavior change in populations at risk. Therefore, the CDC has expanded efforts to assist health departments in planning HIV prevention programs at the community level (CDC, 1994).

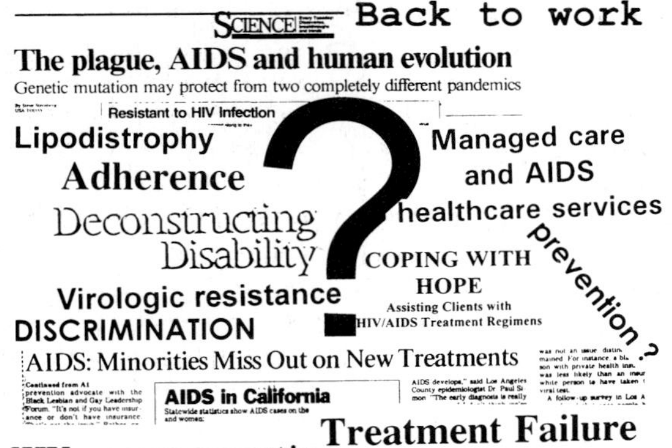

The decline in AIDS severity and deaths is welcomed good news. However, there is still a pressing need for:

1. better HIV prevention programs directed at populations at risk, including education on all sexually transmitted diseases, and federal- and state-funded needle exchange and drug prevention programs to slow the spread of HIV-infection among IV drug users
2. better HIV treatment programs for all populations in all economic strata.

The reporting of cases of AIDS has been mandated federally. Mandatory names-reporting upon HIV diagnosis has been a sensitive social issue with health care implications. Some contend that, without HIV names-reporting, significant problems arise, including those related to the tracking of trends in HIV infection, contact and partner notification, and monitoring of individuals to ensure that they receive needed services (Steinbrook, 1997). Others maintain that the reporting of names of people testing positive for HIV, without a confidential and protective coding system, will ultimately hinder efforts to stop the spread of the virus, deter individuals from being tested for the virus, and jeopardize security of one's home, job, health insurance, and family. Further, the current system already is discriminatory and does not allocate adequate resources to provide needed services and medications to people who are currently HIV-infected (Adams et al., 1998; Horberg and Schatz, 1998; Krieger, 1998).

Global Trends

Childbearing age women are the fastest growing subset of HIV infected population; vertical transmission from mother to child is also increasing (Li et al., 1998). In Botswana, Zimbabwe, and soon, South Africa, 25% of all adults are infected (Daley, 1998). All must contend with the social, economic, and political realities facing developing nations. For example, many developing countries spend less than $10 per person per year on health care (Clarke et al., 1998). The short course of AZT therapy used in the Thailand study costs approximately $50 per woman, compared to $1000 for the cost of the 076 regimen in developed countries (Brown, 1998b).

In the United States, where one of every two new infections is derived from a dirty needle, needle exchange and drug use reduction programs are a top priority. The rising number of infections stemming from the use of methamphetamines, both oral and injectable, must be addressed in HIV prevention programs, especially in certain urban U.S. communities.

The number of incarcerated HIV-infected individuals continues to rise, as does the number of infected heterosexual adults older than 50 years of age (see "*New Directions:* The Changing Face of AIDS").

In the United States, it is estimated that 60,000 new infections occur annually, with between 650,000 and 950,000 people living with HIV infection (CDC, 1997a). According to the Third National Health and Nutrition Examination Survey (NHANES III), the HIV prevalence rate in the United States is 0.32% of the general population, with men four times more likely to be infected than women, depending upon race and ethnicity. African-American and Mexican-American men are three times more likely to be HIV-positive than women in these groups, and white men are six times more likely to be HIV-infected than white women.

The number of women diagnosed as having AIDS, regardless of race or route of exposure, increased by 63% between 1991 and 1995, more than any other group. Compared to the rate in white women, the AIDS rate for black women is 17 times higher, and the rate for Latinos is six times higher (CDC, 1997a). The CDC and the American College Health Association estimate that 1 in 500 college students are HIV-infected (CDC, 1995). Among Americans older than 50 years of age, the number testing positive for HIV has risen to greater than 10% (CDC, 1997); older women are becoming infected at a higher rate than men (Engle, 1998).

The costs and numbers of individuals covered by Medicare and Medicaid have continued to grow. Compared to the number of people with AIDS covered in 1990, it was projected that, in the year 2000, those numbers will be six times greater with Medicare, and almost three times greater with Medicaid (Office of the Actuary, 1995).

One of the most profound, recent developments has been that, for 2 years in a row, the number of deaths and severe illnesses attributable to complications of AIDS has sharply declined. In the United States, the number of AIDS deaths dropped 44% in the first half of 1997, compared to the same period in 1996 when the number of AIDS cases dropped only 12%. This recent decline is attributed to the use of **highly active antiretroviral therapy (HAART),** which reduces concentrations of virus in the blood (Maugh, 1998), and, to some extent, safer sex practices (Wasowica, 1998). HAART usually consists of a combination of at least three antiretroviral agents, one of which may be, but is not necessarily, a protease inhibitor. However, the following major concerns about HAART have surfaced:

1. As many as 25% to 45% of all patients receiving triple combination therapies may develop **drug resistance** (Berger, 1998), and resistant mutants have been reported (Mayers, 1999).
2. Complicated drug schedules and meal and food requirements demand daily adherence, or the patient risks suboptimal dosing and viral breakthrough, which will contribute to the development of drug-resistant strains. In one study, the frequency of missing at least one dose was 12% for the previous day, 11% for the day before that, 13% for the day before that, and 30% for the last 3 days. For 36% of the participants, the primary reason for missed doses was lack of understanding of the drug regimen's special instructions; women and mothers with infected children were less likely than men to understand (Hect et al., 1998).
3. Antiretroviral drugs are not tolerated by all patients. Side effects often occur at the start of treatment and may include anorexia, nausea, vomiting, pain, diarrhea, rash, and headache.
4. A number of disturbing physical and biochemical alterations have been recognized as affecting a yet unknown percentage of persons taking potent antiretroviral therapies, in particular, the protease inhibitors. Loosely termed "lipodystrophy syndrome," these alterations include increased abnormal fat deposition on the back of the neck ("buffalo hump") (Fig. 40–1) and on the abdomen ("protease paunch"), enlarged breasts in women, thinning of the arms and legs, increased wrinkling of the face (especially in the nasolabial folds) with loss of buccal fat. Metabolic alterations include low serum testosterone concentrations in both women and men, elevations in serum triglyceride and sometimes, cholesterol values, and hypertension (Kotler and Muurahainen, 1998; Engelson et al., 1996). A derangement in glucose metabolism has also been reported (Dubé and Sattler, 1998). Some patients experiencing these physical changes opt to discontinue medications, undergo liposuction, begin anabolic therapy, switch antiretroviral medications, or do a combination of these.
5. Medication costs can be about $15,000 annually per person, and medications are not available to all patients. Although there are exceptions, many state-based AIDS Drug Assistance Programs (ADAP) and private health insurance policies do not cover all these medications.

Another recent medical development is the use of immune-based therapies. These treatments either affect the activity of the immune system in general or some specific activity of one of its components. They may help restore immune responsiveness,

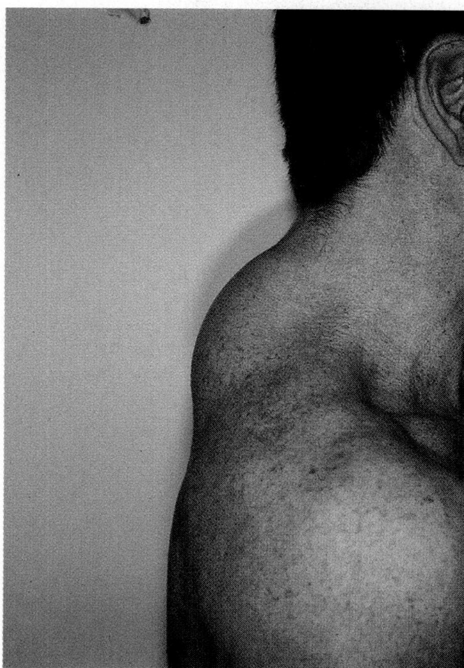

FIGURE 40–1 Buffalo hump, abnormal fat deposition in neck area. (Courtesy Derek H. Jones, M.D.)

suppress viral infections, or even counteract the bone marrow toxicity of some anti-HIV drugs (Bitton et al., 1999).

The problems with drug therapy contribute to the growing disparity in AIDS care between various ethnic and economic groups with HIV infection in the United States.

PATHOPHYSIOLOGY, ETIOLOGY, AND CLASSIFICATION

Primary infection with HIV is the underlying cause of AIDS. HIV invades the genetic core of the CD4+ or T-helper lymphocyte cells (Bowen et al., 1985). Although HIV needs CD4+ cells to be activated before it can replicate, CD4+ cells are the principal agents involved in protection against infection. Distinct viral compartments that have been identified are blood, semen, vaginal secretions, the lymph system, and the central nervous system. HIV infection causes a progressive depletion of CD4+ cells, which eventually leads to immunodeficiency, constitutional disease, neurologic complications, opportunistic infections, and neoplasms (see Table 40–2).

The virus can be transmitted via any one of five body fluids: blood, semen, preseminal fluid, vaginal fluid, and breast milk. Saliva, tears, and urine do not contain enough virus to transmit the virus. The most common way HIV is transmitted is via blood and semen during unprotected anal, vaginal, or oral sex (Clum, 1996). Transmission can also occur by sharing of contaminated needles and injection of contaminated blood products, as well as by transfer across the placenta from an infected mother to her baby (Health and Public Policy Committee, 1986). The virus is not transmitted by casual contact—touching, hugging, or kissing—or through using the same plates, silverware, or drinking glasses. All persons should use universal precautions to protect both themselves and others when working with body fluids.

PERINATAL CONSIDERATIONS

Perinatal HIV transmission (PHT) can happen three ways: (1) in utero, (2) during birth while moving through the birth canal, or (3) during breastfeeding. The risk to babies born to mothers with confirmed HIV infection may be as high as 26% (Landers, 1995). In the United States, 500 infants are infected with HIV each year, compared to 2000 before 1994–1995. Use of AZT and HIV testing are credited for the 43% drop in PHT from 1992 to 1996 (Vasquez, 1998). Highly active antiretroviral therapies essentially eliminate HIV in vaginal secretions and in the blood, both of which are believed to be routes of exposure to HIV for neonates during birth.

The pediatric AIDS Clinical Trial Group (ACTG) 076 study showed that, with the use of oral AZT, initiated at 14 to 34 weeks of gestation, administered intravenously during labor, and then administered to the infant for 6 weeks after birth, PHT transmission could be reduced by about two thirds, to about 8% (Connor et al., 1997). In 1998, a shorter and less costly course of AZT therapy was shown to reduce PHT by about 50%, raising the possibility that cases of PHT worldwide may be avoidable (Brown, 1998b). However, AZT monotherapy is considered to be substandard therapy (Carpenter et al., 1997), and several clinical trials in the United States are now underway to evaluate the efficacy of combination antiretroviral treatments in preventing PHT.

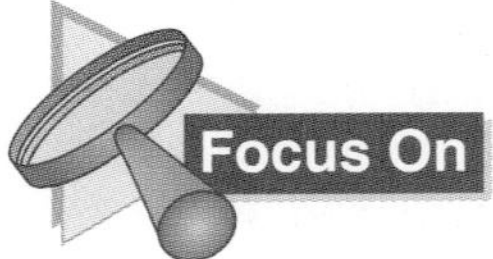

PEDIATRIC HIV/AIDS

Not long ago, 80% of patients with HIV/AIDS died of malnutrition. Today, the important role of nutrition support is well recognized. Although children born to mothers with HIV are often born with weight and height below the 50th percentile, uninfected children catch up, whereas HIV-infected children do not. An earlier and more pronounced deficit in height for age is noted, especially by 15 months of age (Saavedra et al., 1995). Every child with the infection should be assessed at baseline, and every 1–3 months thereafter, to determine risk of nutritional compromise (Heller, 1997).

Protein needs in these children are considered to be 1.5 to 2 times the RDA for age and gender. Energy needs may vary from 100% to 200% of the RDA; those children with severe encephalopathy may be bed-fast and require fewer total calories. Weight loss may be attributable to poor energy intake, malabsorption, and opportunistic infections.

A multivitamin supplement is needed to provide at least 100% of the RDAs. In adults, supplements up to 55% RDA for riboflavin and thiamine have improved survival rates (Heller, 1997). Stunting and failure to thrive (FTT) have been identified in up to 94% of HIV-infected children. Skinfold measurements should be taken for comparison. The goal is simply to preserve lean body mass.

Poor absorption may be a problem for vitamins A, C, B_6, B_{12}, folate, iron, selenium, and zinc (Heller, 1997). Abnormal serum or plasma protein or micronutrient levels were less common in one cohort study of HIV-infected children, and growth retardation was the more common concern (Henderson et al., 1997). Routine monitoring is unnecessary in the absence of specific clinical indicators of deficiency.

Tube-feeding via gastrostomy tube may improve the weight and fat mass of children with HIV. Higher age-adjusted CD4 cell counts and lower weight-for-height scores at baseline have been significant predictors of a positive response to gastrostomy tube feedings (Miller et al., 1995).

TABLE 40–3 IMMUNOLOGIC CATEGORIES FOR HIV-INFECTED CHILDREN BASED ON AGE-SPECIFIC CD4+ T-LYMPHOCYTE COUNTS AND PERCENTAGE OF TOTAL LYMPHOCYTES

IMMUNOLOGIC CATEGORY	CELL COUNTS (Cells/μL [%]*) ACCORDING TO AGE		
	<12 Months	1–5 Years	6–12 Years
No evidence of suppression	≥1500 (≥25)	≥1000 (≥25)	≥500 (≥25)
Evidence of moderate suppression	750–1499 (15–24)	500–999 (15–24)	200–499 (15–24)
Severe suppression	<750 (<15)	<500 (<15)	<200 (<15)

(Adapted from Centers for Disease Control and Prevention. 1997 USPHS/IDSA guidelines for the prevention of opportunistic infection in persons infected with human immunodeficiency virus. MMWR 46 (No. RR-12):27, 1997.)
*Percentage of total lymphocytes.

Short of definitive studies, 1997 guidelines called for antiretroviral therapy in pregnant women to be the same as in nonpregnant adults (Panel on Clinical Practices, 1997). A consideration of lesser importance, although still significant, is that poor nutritional status in infected mothers increases the risk of PHT, with the related risk factors identified as (1) poor prenatal nutrition (specifically, vitamin A deficiency), and (2) low hemoglobin levels (Semba et al., 1994; Grant and DeCock, 1998).

Nutrition status during both fetal and neonatal periods is a factor affecting PHT (Stiehm, 1995). Poor prenatal nutrition, apart from HIV status, can result in delayed growth of the fetus and inadequate growth for gestational age, contributing to decreased cellular immunity and low T-cell levels, small thymus size, and increased rate of infection (Stiehm, 1995). Nutrient deficiencies can result from the increased nutritional demands for fetal growth and development. These demands are further increased by HIV, especially in developing countries, where deficiencies of vitamin A, folate, iron, and zinc are common. Indeed, it is likely that nutritional deficiencies contribute to an increased rate of PHT (Landers, 1995). (See "*Focus On:* Pediatric HIV/AIDS".)

In developed countries, it is recommended that HIV-positive mothers be discouraged from breastfeeding (Life Sciences Research Office, FASEB, 1990). The risk of breast milk transmission is estimated to range from 14% to 22% in some developing countries. Banked milk may be an option for some mothers. Table 40–3 describes the categories of HIV infection in children.

MANIFESTATIONS AND TREATMENT OF HIV INFECTION

Four stages of HIV disease have been characterized: acute HIV infection, asymptomatic HIV infection, symptomatic HIV infection, and AIDS.

ACUTE HIV INFECTION. **Acute HIV infection** is the 4 to 7 week period immediately after primary infection when there is rapid viral replication and when 30% to 60% of newly infected persons develop an acute syndrome characterized by fever, malaise, **lymphadenopathy syndrome,** pharyngitis, headache, **myalgia,** and sometimes, rash, which may last for a week to a month. The time period between the initial HIV infection and seroconversion, that is, the development of HIV antibodies, varies from 1 week to several months or more (HIV/AIDS Treatment Information Center, 1997). Once antibodies to HIV appear in the blood, individuals with and without symptoms will test positive for HIV at this time (Carey, 1988).

ASYMPTOMATIC HIV. *Asymptomatic HIV* is the stage where few, if any, noticeable symptoms occur. Prior to the era of HAART, this stage could last an average of 10 years (Clum, 1996). Subclinical and underrecognized changes have been reported, including a decrease in lean body mass without apparent total body weight change, vitamin B_{12} deficiency, and increased susceptibility to food- and water-borne pathogens.

SYMPTOMATIC HIV. *Symptomatic HIV* occurs when symptoms appear (see Table 40–4). These symptoms may include fevers, sweats, skin problems, fatigue, or other symptoms that are not usually considered AIDS-defining conditions. A decline in nutrient status or body composition may also occur.

AIDS. The diagnostic term AIDS is reserved for those persons with at least one well-defined, life-threatening clinical condition that is clearly linked to HIV-induced immunosuppression (Goedert and Blattner, 1988) (see also AIDS-defining conditions, Category C, in Table 40–2).

Whether all HIV-infected persons eventually develop AIDS is uncertain at this time. A small proportion of persons infected with the virus develop AIDS and die within months following primary infection, whereas approximately 5% of HIV-infected individuals exhibit no signs of disease progression even after 12 or more years (Pantaleo et al., 1995; Cao et al., 1995). This latter group of long-term nonprogressors comprises individuals who have been infected for more than 7 years, who received no antiretroviral therapy, who showed no decline in CD4 cells, and who had a comparatively lower viral burden in the peripheral blood and in lymph nodes than those with active AIDS (Pantaleo et al., 1995). A lowered viral load set point, lesser virulence of the virus, and protective genetic mutations appear to contribute to this state.

TABLE 40–4 CONDITIONS ASSOCIATED WITH CD4 CELL COUNT IN HIV INFECTION

CD4+ CELL COUNT	CONDITION	COMMON PHYSICAL PROBLEMS AND SYMPTOMS
200–500 mm^3	Oral thrush	Loss of appetite, white plaques, mouth discomfort, change in taste
	Kaposi's sarcoma	Slightly raised, purplish lesions on the skin, mucous membranes, or lymph nodes; usually painless
	Tuberculosis reactivation	Cough, blood-stained sputum (hemoptysis), fever, night sweats, weight loss, chest pain, prolonged fatigue, anorexia
	Herpes zoster (shingles) virus	Vesicular skin lesions along dermatomes, pain
	Bacterial sinusitis/pneumonia	Inflammation of the nasal cavity and sinuses, congestion, fever, pain, tearing of the eyes, and sensitivity to light
	Herpes simplex (virus)	Weeping skin lesions (oral, perirectal), bleeding, rectal discharge, pain
100–200/mm^3	*Pneumocystis carinii* pneumonia (PCP) (fungi)	Fever, chills, night sweats, cough with or without sputum production, shortness of breath, antibiotic side effects, weight loss, weakness
50–100/mm^3	Systemic fungal infections	
	Cryptococcal meningitis (or others)	Headache and fevers, malaise, nausea, fatigue, loss of appetite
	Histoplasmosis	Fever, weight loss, skin lesions, difficulty breathing, anemia, lymphodenopathy, possibly pneumonia
	Primary tuberculosis	Cough, blood-stained sputum (hemoptysis), fever, night sweats, weight loss, chest pain, prolonged fatigue, anorexia
	Cryptosporidiosis (protozoal) infection of large and small bowels	Severe chronic, watery diarrhea (up to 15–20 times a day), severe weight loss, weakness, electrolyte imbalance, abdominal cramping, fever, nausea, vomiting, enlarged lymph nodes
	Cerebral toxoplasmosis (protozoa)	Fevers, swollen glands, headaches
	Progressive multifocal leukoencephalopathy (PML)	Progressive weakness and dementia, speech problems, forgetfulness, perceptual problems, visual problems, incontinence
	Peripheral neuropathy	Painful, burning feet, or numbness in the feet and/or hands
	Cervical carcinoma	Watery, blood-tinged vaginal discharge, seen most often after sexual intercourse
0–50/mm^3	Cytomegalovirus disease (CMV) (virus)	Blindness or visual loss (retinitis), fever, fatigue/severe malaise, weight loss, facial edema (secondary to adrenalitis), enteritis or colitis
	Disseminated *Mycobacterium avium* complex (MAC) (bacteria)	Fever, severe weight loss/cachexia, abdominal pain, diarrhea, malabsorption, antibiotic side effects
	Non-Hodgkin's lymphoma	Depends on location; lumps, fatigue, and/or pain
	AIDS dementia complex	Loss of coordination, mood swings, loss of inhibitions, widespread cognitive dysfunctions

(Adapted from Martin J, Hughes A, Franks P. AIDS Home Care and Hospice Manual, 2nd ed. San Francisco: Visiting Nurses and Hospice of San Francisco, 1990; and Phair JP, Murphy R. Contemporary Diagnosis and Management of HIV/AIDS Infections. Health Care Co., 1997.)

HIV Medical Management

The goals of medical management of HIV are to:

1. Prolong life and improve the quality of life for the long term
2. Suppress the virus to as low a level as possible for as long as possible
3. Optimize and extend the usefulness of currently available therapies
4. Minimize drug toxicity and manage side effects. Table 40–5 lists the side effects of steroid medications used in the management of HIV.

Disease progression differs among individuals; therefore treatment decisions must be individualized. The CDC classification system for HIV infection outlines clinical and CD4+ categories (see Table 40–2). With the advent of viral load testing and HAART, clinical and therapeutic management of HIV-infected individuals is based upon the following (NIH Panel, 1997):

1. Viral load levels (HIV-RNA) which predict the risk of HIV disease progression, as well as when to initiate or change therapy
2. Current and lowest CD4+ counts, which indicate the extent of HIV-induced immune damage and the risk of development of opportunistic infections
3. Current and past clinical conditions and symptoms of HIV disease, including history of treatment outcomes

AIDS wasting syndrome (AWS), also known as **constitutional disease,** is diagnostic of AIDS in the HIV-positive individual for whom no other cause of the symptoms has been identified (CDC, 1987a). Common constitutional signs of HIV infection include persistent fever, often with night sweats; chronic or intermittent fatigue and malaise; and diarrhea of unknown etiology. Involuntary weight loss of 10% to 15% is common. Leading researchers and physicians suggest redefining AWS to include those in whom there is at least a 5% involuntary weight loss (Gorbach, 1997). As little as a 5% weight loss has been associated with a significantly increased risk of opportunistic complications and death (Wheeler et al., 1998).

TABLE 40–5 HIV MEDICATIONS AND NUTRITIONAL COMPLICATIONS—STEROIDS

MEDICATION	RX	D	C	N	V	FT	H	F WITH	F WITHOUT	CONTRA	OTHERS
STEROIDS (INCLUDING ANABOLIC) + OTHER MEDS USED FOR WASTING	X			X			X	Take with food	Take on empty stomach		Anabolics in general: Skin problems, e.g. acne Hair growth (hirsutism) Menstrual irregularities Change in libido and potency (altered desire for sex, ability to have erection and ejaculation) Fluid retention Abnormal liver enzymes/hepatitis (jaundice) Altered blood glucose, even diabetes
Dexamethasone (Decadron)	X						X	Take with food			Stomach upset/ulcers, indigestion, weight gain, increased urination, depression
Testosterone *Injections:* testosterone cypionate, testosterone enathanate; (Depo-testosterone); *Patches:* Testosterm, Androderm	X			X							Mood changes: increase in hemoglobin/hematocrit (red blood cell count = RBC)
Nandrolone (Deca-Durabolin)	X	X		X	X					Not with severe hepatic dysfunction	Sore tongue, chills
Oxandrolone (Oxandrin)	X	X		X	X						Sore tongue
Oxymetholone (Anadrol)	X	X		X	X					Not with severe hepatic dysfunction	Masculinization, alterations in cholesterol
Pentoxifylline (Trental)				Y	Y			Take with food			GI(NVD); headache
Recombinant human growth hormone (Serostim)	X	X		X			X			Caution with diabetes; do not take if active tumor present	Musculoskeletal discomfort of hands and feet; increased blood sugar, triglycerides
Thalidomide (Thalomid)	X		X			X	X		Take on empty stomach	Can cause birth defects if taken when pregnant	Drowsiness, rash, dry mouth, edema, acne, insomnia, sedation

X or Y, possible; Rx, prescription; D, diarrhea; C, constipation; N, nausea; V, vomiting; Ft, fatigue; H, headache; F with, with food; F without, without food; Contra, contraindication; Others, more concerns.

Reprinted by permission of Nutrition & HIV Program, AIDS Project Los Angeles, mfenton@apla.org (323-993-1612).

Opportunistic Infections

Opportunistic infections with bacteria, fungi, protozoa, or viruses are common. They are often the cause of diarrhea, malabsorption, fever, and weight loss, as well as many other symptoms. Common infections, their relationships to CD4+ counts, and their manifestations are summarized in Table 40–6.

Malignant Disease

Kaposi's sarcoma (KS) is a malignant disease of the peripheral blood mononuclear cells which manifests as purple nodules on the skin, mucous membranes, lymph nodes, or throughout the gastrointestinal tract. KS lesions in the oral cavity or esophagus may cause pain and difficulty with chewing and swallowing. KS lesions in the intestinal tract have been implicated in diarrhea and intestinal obstruction. Localized KS lesions can be treated with surgery or radiation therapy, and chemotherapy is often used to treat persons with disseminated disease. Usually, disseminated disease is difficult to control because chemotherapy can further suppress immune function in persons with already existing HIV-related complications. Cases of KS have declined recently with use of new HAART therapy.

Lymphomas, including non-Hodgkin's lymphoma and Burkitt's lymphoma, that involve the small bowel can cause malabsorption, diarrhea, or intestinal obstruction. Primary lymphoma in the brain can cause alterations in personality and in motor

TABLE 40–6 SIDE EFFECTS, DRUG AND FOOD INTERACTIONS OF COMMONLY USED HIV THERAPIES

MEDICATIONS	INDICATIONS	POSSIBLE GASTROINTESTINAL INTERACTION(S)	COMMENT(S)
Trimethoprim-sulfamethoxazole (Bactrim)	*Pneumocystis carinii* pneumonia (PCP)	Nausea, vomiting	Ensure adequate hydration.
	Drug-resistant tuberculosis	Glossitis/stomatitis, hyponatremia	
Pentamidine (Nebupent)	PCP treatment and prophylaxis	Alterations in taste, hypoglycemia and hyperglycemia, nausea, vomiting	IV administration may cause changes in blood glucose levels and may lower blood pressure. Maintain adequate hydration.
Pyrimethamine (Daraprim)	Administered with sulfadiazine for toxoplasmosis	Megaloblastic anemia, vomiting, anorexia, tongue tenderness	Take with food.
Acyclovir (Zovirax)	Herpes simplex, Herpes zoster infection	Nausea, headache	Ensure adequate hydration.
AZT (Retravir)	Inhibition of HIV replication	Nausea, vomiting, bone marrow suppression	Monitor the patient for anemia, headache.
Ganciclovir (Cytovene)	Cytomegalovirus (CMV)	Diarrhea (rarely), anorexia, vomiting (rarely), lowering of white blood cell count	Monitor patient's status with a complete blood cell count (CBC), especially if this agent is combined with AZT.
Ketoconazole (Nizoral)	Candidiasis, histoplasmosis	Nausea, vomiting, bowel changes	This agent requires an acidic gastric environment for absorption. Avoid alcohol; take with food.
ddI-didanosine (Videx)	Inhibition of HIV replication	Peripheral neuropathy, diarrhea, vomiting, nausea	Avoid antacids containing magnesium or aluminum.
Megestrol (Megace)	Treatment of anorexia	Sexual dysfunction, shortness of breath	
Clarithromycin (Biaxin)	*Mycobacterium avium* complex (MAC)	Diarrhea, taste alterations, nausea	
Isoniazid (INH)	Tuberculosis	Potential liver problems if alcohol is used.	Avoid alcohol; take with food. B_6 vitamin supplementation may be required.
ddc (Zalcitabine)	Inhibition of HIV replication	GI distress, diarrhea	Peripheral neuropathy; pancreatitis can result.
Saquinavir mesylate (Invirase)	Protease inhibitor	Diarrhea, nausea	High fat diet increases absorption; lipodystrophy; abnormal LFT.
Hydroxyurea (Hydrea)	Immune system enhancer	Anorexia, diarrhea	Caution with renal impairment.
Nevirapine (Viramune)	Reverse transcriptase inhibitor	Nausea, headache	Rash may occur.

and cognitive abilities. Lymphomas of these types often respond poorly to the multi-agent chemotherapies indicated, because preexisting immune suppression often limits the amount and frequency of treatment. Other malignant diseases seen in some homosexual men include *squamous cell carcinoma* of the tongue and *cloacogenic carcinoma* of the colon. However, it is yet unknown if these are related to HIV (Carey, 1988; CDC, 1997b).

Neurologic Diseases

Immediately following infection, HIV enters the brain and may result in **AIDS dementia** (also known as **HIV encephalopathy**), myelopathy, peripheral neuropathy, and myopathy. Secondary neurologic complications may result from toxoplasma encephalitis, progressive multifocal leukoencephalopathy, cytomegalovirus (CMV) encephalitis, radiculomyelitis, cryptococcal meningitis, primary central nervous system (CNS) lymphoma, and neurosyphilis.

In one study, AIDS dementia was reported to occur at a rate of 7% per year of survival after AIDS diagnosis, and to occur in about 20% of those with HIV disease. Symptoms of AIDS dementia may include deterioration in cognition (concentration, recall, new memory development, and language), motor function (coordination, gait, bladder control) and behavior (psychosis, depression, withdrawal). Viral load in the brain and the level of neurologic decline are not strongly correlated. The presence of one or more secondary factors may be necessary for AIDS dementia: cytokines, calcium-mediated toxicity, excitatory amino acids (glutamate, quinolinic acid), arachidonic acid, oxidative mechanisms, platelet-activating factor, or apoptosis (programmed cell death).

Myelopathy (disease of the spinal cord) may occur in as many as 25% of those with advanced HIV disease, and can result in partial paralysis of the lower extremities (paraparesis). Myelopathy affects motor and sensory functions and is manifested by spasticity and, in some, weakness in the legs and bladder. Approximately 20% of patients with AIDS experience *peripheral neuropathy,* characterized by sensory loss, pain, and weakness, as well as wasting of muscle in the hands or legs and feet. The first signs are tingling, burning, or numbness in the toes and fingers. Peripheral neuropathy may be caused by the virus or by drugs (zacitabine, didanosine, stavudine).

Myopathy—progressive muscle weakness—is usually a result of HIV infection or toxicity from AZT. If AZT is the underlying cause, creatine kinase levels are usually elevated (Clifford, 1997).

Other Affected Organ Systems

Nutritionally pertinent organs affected by HIV infection or its treatment include the liver, the kidney, the gastrointestinal tract, and the pancreas. *Mycobacterium avium complex* (MAC) can be seen in the lymph nodes, liver, bone marrow, blood, and urine of patients with AIDS. Liver function may also be compromised by infection with cytomegalovirus (CMV), cryptosporidia, and hepatitis B, or by hepatic malignant diseases, such as KS or lymphoma. CMV can affect the eye, causing retinitis, and if left untreated, it may progress to blindness. It is estimated that up to 25% of persons with AIDS may have CMV retinitis.

Millions of people in the United States are infected with hepatitis C (HVC), including many HIV-infected persons. Those with both HIV and HVC have a faster progression to AIDS and death (Piroth et al., 1998), and current HVC treatments do not seem to alter outcome in HIV-infected persons (Kotler and Engelson, 1998).

Although most cases of tuberculosis (TB) affect the lungs, the disease may also occur, especially in HIV-infected persons, in extrapulmonary sites, such as in the larynx, lymph nodes, brain, kidneys, or bones. TB is caused by *Mycobacterium tuberculosis.* Medical conditions that increase the risk of TB infection include HIV infection, a body weight that is 10% or more below ideal weight, immunosuppressive therapy, and hematologic disorders, such as leukemia and lymphomas. Other risk factors include being underfed, alcoholism, intravenous (IV) drug use, and homelessness.

It is estimated that 10% of all HIV-infected persons may be tuberculin-positive (Jacobson, 1992) and that, although only 10% of all people with inactive TB develop the active form, those with TB and HIV are 40 times more likely to develop active TB (Clum, 1996), chiefly as a result of reactivation of latent TB infection. It is common for those with TB infection to have HIV infection also. *M. tuberculosis* coinfection causes immune activation and a rapid increase in the rate of HIV replication (Goletti et al., 1996; Blanchard et al., 1997).

Early and aggressive treatment of TB and HIV is critical to controlling the progression of both diseases. Dietary recommendations include liberal amounts of protein and calories; sufficient, but not excessive, calcium and vitamin D, as well as iron; supplemental vitamin B_6 and vitamin A (as carotene is poorly converted); adequate fluids (unless contraindicated); and adjustments of TB medications because of nutrient-drug interactions (Table 40–6).

A syndrome of progressive renal failure, identified as **HIV-associated nephropathy (HIVAN),** has been reported (Sreepada Rao, 1988). Proteinuria may also result from repeated infections, volume depletion, or nephrotoxic drugs. Twenty percent of hospitalized HIV-infected patients are reported to have acute renal failure (creatine >2.0 mg/dL) (Valeri and Neusy, 1991), and 30% to 60% have hyponatremia, associated with increased morbidity and mortality (Tang et al., 1993). The number of dialysis centers serving HIV-infected patients has increased (see Chapter 38).

Chronic diarrhea may persist in the absence of identifiable enteric pathogens as a result of what is known as **AIDS enteropathy.** It has been suggested that the intestinal injury that appears is related to specific complications, rather than to the immunodeficiency caused by HIV (Kotler, 1999). Persons with HIV enteropathy may have subtotal villous atrophy and abnormal results on tests of small bowel function, including 72-hour fecal fat, d-xylose, and para-aminobenzoic acid (PABA) absorption (Cello, 1997).

RELATIONSHIP BETWEEN MALNUTRITION AND AIDS

Wasting and Metabolic Disorders

Malnutrition is an important and complicated consequence of HIV infection. *Protein-energy malnutrition* (PEM) is a frequent complication of AIDS. Weight loss, body cell mass depletion, decreased skinfold thickness and midarm circumference, decreased iron-binding capacity, and hypoalbuminemia are frequently reported (Collins, 1988; Kotler, 1995).

AIDS wasting syndrome is the second most commonly reported AIDS-defining condition for adults, and the fourth for children younger than 13 years of age (CDC, 1996). Weight loss and wasting are considered multi-factorial, with major contributing factors being: lack of adequate intake, malabsorption, metabolic irregularities, uncontrolled opportunistic infection, and lack of physical activity. Decreased oral intake, identified as the most common cause of weight loss (Macallan et al., 1995), can be the result of anorexia secondary to medications; depression; infection; symptoms, such as nausea, vomiting, diarrhea, dyspnea, or fatigue; or neurologic disease.

Low oral intake can also be attributable to disorders of the mouth and esophagus, such as candidiasis, herpes simplex, aphthous ulcers, or CMV. Malabsorption, often suspected when there are loose stools, diarrhea, or vomiting, can be caused by medications; HIV infection; opportunistic infections, such as CMV, MAC, or cryptosporidiosis; or developed intolerances to lactose, fat, and possibly, gluten. At the same time, energy and protein needs may be increased by fevers and infection. HIV-induced metabolic changes and host responses are poorly understood. Resting energy expenditure is elevated in asymptomatic HIV-infected persons and relates to viral load (Mulligan et al., 1997). Lipid metabolism and transport may also be affected by infection, causing lean body wasting.

Women have been found to lose more body fat than lean body mass during both the early and advanced stages of wasting, whereas men lose greater amounts of lean body mass while sparing body fat. Further, women have less growth hormone resistance as a function of weight loss as compared to men (Office of AIDS Research, 1998).

Immune changes associated with PEM are similar to those seen in AIDS (Gray, 1983; Jain and Chandra, 1984). Both conditions are marked by multiple opportunistic infections of viral, bacterial, parasitic, and fungal origin. KS and B-cell lymphomas have been reported in individuals in Central and East Africa, where PEM is common.

Malnutrition may contribute to the frequency and severity of infection seen in AIDS by compromising immune function (Chlebowski, 1985). Deficiencies of protein, calories, copper, zinc, selenium, iron, essential fatty acids, pyridoxine, folate, and vitamins A, C, and E all interfere with immune function (Fabris et al., 1988; Falutz et al., 1988). Severe weight loss can also result in organ damage, which may increase the risk for a fatal outcome from infections.

The malnutrition associated with HIV infection and AIDS is both similar to other infectious processes and unique to HIV. Nutritional status is a major factor in survival. In the absence of disease, starvation leads to death at 66% of ideal body weight. Body cell mass—the amount of functional protoplasm in nonadipose tissue (muscle and viscera)—may be the best predictor of death (Flier and Underhill, 1992). It has been reported that, as the wasting of lean body mass nears 55% of normal for age, sex, and height in persons with AIDS, death is imminent, regardless of the causes of malnutrition (Kotler, 1992; Keusch and Thea, 1993). Body fat is not a predictable marker of wasting; persons with AIDS, especially men, tend to lose body cell mass with little loss of fat, in contrast to uncomplicated starvation, in which fat stores are depleted. As with AIDS wasting syndrome, host resistance to infection causes changes in metabolism, as mediated by cytokines. The search for host mediators of metabolic disturbances initially resulted in the cachectin hypothesis, related to tumor necrosis factor (TNF) (see Chapter 39). Other theories have since been evaluated.

Direct and indirect mechanisms are responsible for the impact of nutrition on HIV. Directly, nutritional factors are required for specific immune-cell triggering, interactions, and expression. Clinical trials with supplementation of specific nutrients at different stages of HIV disease have been recommended (Timbo and Tollefson, 1994). Indirectly, nutritional factors are essential for DNA and protein synthesis, as well as the physiologic integrity of cell tissues and organ systems, including lymphoid tissues.

Prescriptive drug treatments used to prevent weight and body cell mass loss have become available. Megestrol acetate (Megace), dronabinol (Marinol), and experimentally, medical marijuana, are appetite stimulants commonly used to combat HIV anorexia. Megace, the more powerful appetite stimulant, reduces testosterone levels and increases body fat, and Marinol, a derivative of marijuana, produces undesired central nervous side effects. Adequate exercise is necessary to assure gain in lean body mass. Hormonal therapies, anabolic steroids and human growth hormone are options in the treatment of underlying hormonal irregularities and documented losses in body cell mass and wasting. HIV-infected men and women should be monitored and corrected for testosterone deficiency. Testosterone is obtainable in injected, patches, and oral synthetic forms. Anabolic steroids require adequate intake to maintain and build, and progressive resistance exercise to maximize increases in body cell mass. Recombinant human growth hormone, a lipolytic agent, promotes body cell mass at the expense of fat stores and adequate intake is necessary. Side effects vary depending upon the individual drug and include mood changes, skin problems, hair growth, menstrual irregularities, changes in libido and potency, fluid retention, abnormal liver enzymes and altered blood glucose, even diabetes. (See Table 40–5.)

Because nutrient deficiencies may play an important role in the pathogenesis of HIV disease, medical nutrition therapy and counseling are critical aspects of treatment. The general goals of nutrition intervention are to (1) preserve optimal somatic and visceral protein status; (2) prevent nutrient deficiencies or excesses known to compromise immune function; (3) minimize nutrition-related complications that interfere with either intake or absorption of nutrients; (4) support optimal therapeutic drug levels; and (5) enhance the quality of life. Figure 40–2 is a decision tree for assessing HIV patients.

MEDICAL NUTRITION THERAPY

Achieving nutritional health and preventing malnutrition are essential in maintaining positive health outcomes for persons with HIV, and medical nutrition therapy in HIV care must be included as a primary component of total health care (Fenton and Fitz, 1997). Medical nutrition therapy requires six distinct components: screening, referral, assessment, intervention, outcomes evaluation and communication (American Dietetic Association, 1996). The first steps are described here.

Nutritional Screening

Ideally, all persons with HIV infection should be screened for nutritional problems and concerns at the time of their first contact with a health care professional, and routine monitoring should be performed on an ongoing basis. Time and the occur-

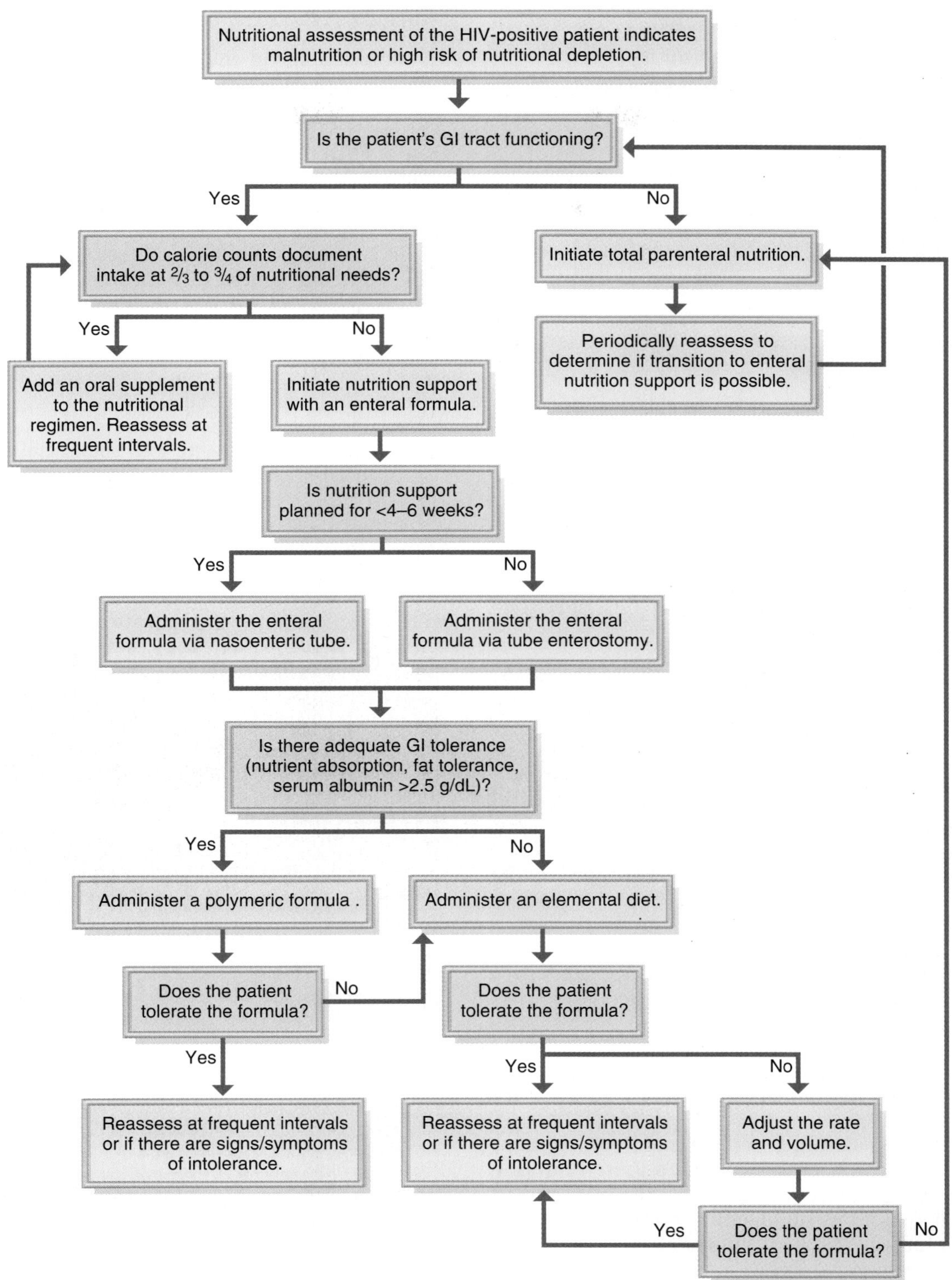

FIGURE 40–2 Algorithm of nutritional support for persons with HIV infection.

rence of nutrition-related symptoms should trigger automatic referrals for nutrition intervention as identified by any member of the health care team. Table 40–7 presents nutrition screening information, whereas Table 40–8 provides screening information specific to pediatric patients.

Nutrition Referral

Referral information should include the following:

- Consent to release medical information (usually necessary when clients are seen outside of their primary medical setting)

TABLE 40–7 SCREENING FOR MEDICAL NUTRITION THERAPY IN HIV-INFECTED ADULTS AND ADOLESCENTS OLDER THAN 18 YEARS OF AGE

Referral is automatic when any one of the following conditions exist:

1. Newly diagnosed HIV infection or never been seen by a registered dietitian
2. If asymptomatic: not seen by a registered dietitian in the past 6 months to 1 year
3. Newly diagnosed HIV with symptoms or AIDS
4. If HIV with symptoms or AIDS: not seen by a dietitian in the past 6 months or more
5. >5% unintentional weight loss from usual body weight within the last 6 months, or since the last visit (% *weight loss formula:* usual body weight − current body weight/usual body weight × 100)
6. Poor oral intake of food or fluid
7. Change in stools (color, consistency, frequency, smell)
8. Persistent gas, bloating, heartburn
9. Persistent diarrhea or constipation
10. Persistent nausea or vomiting
11. Difficulty chewing, swallowing, mouth sores, thrush or herpes simplex type 1
12. Severe dental caries
13. Changes in perception of taste or smell
14. Food allergies/food intolerance (fat, lactose, wheat, etc.)
15. Economically unable to meet caloric and nutrient needs
16. Concomitant diabetes mellitus, hypertension, hepatic or renal insufficiency, heart disease, cancer, pregnancy, or other nutrition-related condition
17. Visible wasting or < 90% ideal body weight
18. Albumin < 3.2 mg/dL
19. Cholesterol < 120 mg/dL or > 200 mg/dL
20. Triglycerides > 450 mg/dL
21. Scheduled chemotherapy or radiation therapy
22. Medication regimen that involves food or meal modification
23. Need for enteral or parenteral nutrition
24. Patient- or MD-initiated weight management, obesity, vitamin-mineral supplementation, vegetarianism or complementary/alternative diet therapies

(Adapted from Fenton M. Nutrition referral screening for adults (18+ years) with HIV/AIDS. AIDS Project Los Angeles, 1997. In: Guidelines and Protocol of Care for Providing Medical Nutrition Therapy to HIV-Infected Persons, Standards of Care Committee, Los Angeles County Commission on HIV Health Services, 1997.)

- Current diagnosis and medical history
- Referring health care provider's nutrition prescription or desired outcome
- Clinical symptoms and feeding route
- Weight history and body composition
- Recent biochemical data
- Current medications, including prescription and nonprescription drugs, vitamins, minerals, and other dietary supplements
- Use of complementary and alternative therapies
- Functional status
- Life-style, psychosocial status, and activity/exercise routine, including substance use patterns

See Chapter 16 for a further discussion of nutritional screening.

Nutritional Assessment

A comprehensive nutritional assessment should then be performed. Factors to be considered include not only HIV infection–associated symptoms, but dietary patterns, the use of nontraditional therapies, and the impact of these treatments on the person (see Chapter 16).

The diet should be evaluated for nutrient adequacy, especially of nutrients involved with immune function. When working with persons with HIV infection contracted through IV drug use or with a history of using drugs, one should take into consideration their typically erratic, and usually inadequate intakes. Individuals following nontraditional diet therapies should be made aware of any potentially harmful effects.

Psychosocial conditions should also be assessed. Fear, anxiety, depression, and social isolation all affect appetite and nutrient intake. Illness or ostracism often leads to a lack of employment and subsequent loss of social contacts, as well as income and medical insurance.

Evaluating weight in terms of the *percentage of usual weight,* rather than published height and weight tables, is more accurate for this population, although percent ideal body weight is an important marker. Monitoring changes in anthropometric measurements over time is feasible because many patients will have multiple clinic visits and hospitalizations. Useful measurements include height, weight, hip-to-waist ratio, neck circumference, and

TABLE 40–8 SCREENING FOR PEDIATRIC PATIENTS (<18 YEARS OF AGE) WITH HIV/AIDS FOR MEDICAL NUTRITION THERAPY

In addition to the conditions listed in Table 40–7, referral to a registered dietitian is automatic when any one of the following conditions exist:

1. Weight for age <10 percentile (National Center for Health Statistics [NCHS])
2. Height for age <10th percentile if weight for age is also <10th percentile for age (NCHS)
3. Downward crossing of one major weight-for-age percentile
4. Poor appetite; food or fluid refusals
5. Prolonged bottle-feeding and/or severe dental caries
6. Change in stools (color, consistency, frequency, smell)
7. Children 0–12 months old: low birth weight
8. Children 0–12 months old: no weight gain for 1 month
9. Children 0–12 months old: diarrhea or vomiting for ≥2 days
10. Children 0–12 months old: poor suck
11. Children 1–3 years old: no weight gain for 2 consecutive months
12. Children 1–3 years old: diarrhea or vomiting for ≥ 3 days
13. Children 4–16 years old: no weight gain for 3 consecutive months
14. Children 4–16 years old: diarrhea or vomiting for ≥ 4 days
15. Albumin < 3.5 mg/dL
16. Cholesterol < 65 mg/dL or > 175 mg/dL
17. Triglycerides < 40 mg/dL or > 160 mg/dL

(Adapted from Fenton M, Heller L. Nutrition referral screening for pediatrics (<18 years) with HIV/AIDS. AIDS Project Los Angeles, 1997. In: Guidelines and Protocol of Care for Providing Medical Nutrition Therapy to HIV-Infected Persons, Standards of Care Committee, Los Angeles County Commission on HIV Health Services, 1997.)

measurements of either lean body mass (using triceps skinfold and midarm muscle circumference) or body cell mass (using bioelectric impedance analysis or other techniques). These calculations should be compared to each other, rather than to published reference data (Collins, 1988) (see Chapter 16).

Laboratory values, such as serum albumin, prealbumin, retinol-binding protein, transferrin, and total iron-binding capacity, can be used to monitor changes in visceral protein status (see Chapter 17). These parameters are especially useful when compared over time. Total lymphocyte count and delayed hypersensitivity skin testing should not be used, as these immune functions are impaired in this population and are, therefore, not indicative of nutritional status (Collins, 1988). Evaluation of drug therapy is essential, as many side effects complicate nutritional status (see Fig. 40–3 and "*Clinical Insight:* HIV Medications").

Nutrition Intervention

It is recommended that all persons with HIV infection and AIDS receive early and on-going medical nutrition therapy. The goals for nutrition therapy should be to educate these individuals about the importance of consuming a well-balanced diet, to provide adequate nutrition for maintenance or improvement in nutritional status, and to prevent PEM and vitamin and mineral deficiencies. Counseling should be individualized and supported with practical written guidelines (Table 40–9). Mapping out one's meal and medication schedule is part of medical nutrition therapy, and is an important component for supporting adherence to a drug regimen.

Energy and Activity

Energy and protein needs vary depending on the health status of the individual at the time of HIV infection, the progression of the disease, and the development of complications that impair nutrient intake and utilization. The Harris–Benedict equation (see Chapter 2) can be used to determine basal energy expenditure (BEE), which can be multiplied by a stress factor to allow for maintenance and anabolism. An adjustment must also be made in the presence of fever. Energy requirements increase by 13% and protein requirements by 10% for every degree Celsius of temperature elevation above normal (Hyman and Kaufman, 1989). Several studies (Keusch and Thea, 1993) suggest the following guidelines for determining energy requirements:

$$\text{BEE} \times 1.3 \text{ for maintenance}$$

$$\text{BEE} \times 1.5 \text{ for weight gain}$$

Activity can also affect energy requirements. Chronic exercise and high-fat diets have often been associated with immune suppression. One study of HIV-infected individuals found that exercise has mixed effects, and that a high-fat diet has no adverse effect on runners' immune systems (Venkatraman et al., 1997). CD8 suppressor T-cell levels were higher in men than in women; numbers of killer cells were 2.5 times higher after exercise than at rest, and were positively related to dietary fat levels. In men, but not in women, levels of proinflammatory cytokines were lower after exercise than at rest. Activity can be successfully planned for this population.

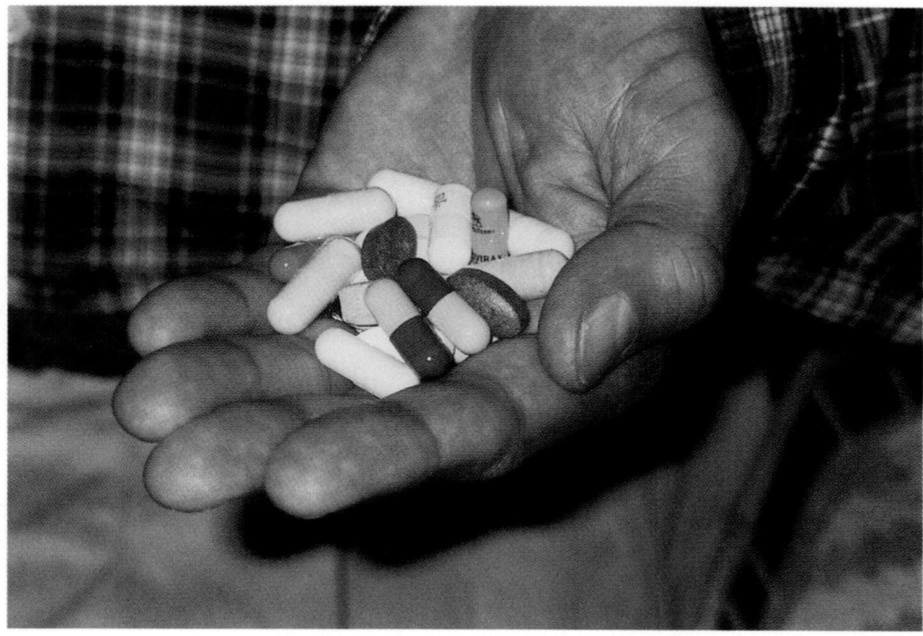

FIGURE 40–3 A patient with AIDS holding his typical amount and mix of meds taken at one time during the day.

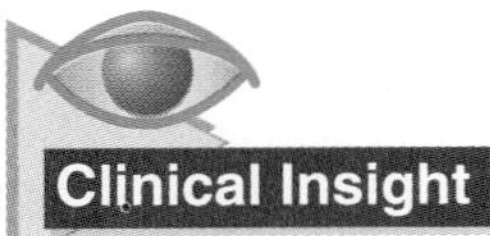

HIV Medications

Medications may be categorized as reverse transcriptase inhibitors (AZT, ddI, ddC, d4T, 3TC) and protease inhibitors (saquinavir, indinavir, ritonavir, nelfinavir). Only nelfinavir has been approved for use in pediatrics. Disguising the taste of these medications is important. This is best done by adding a small amount to cold foods, such as ice cream, milk shakes, fruit ices; thick, sweet foods, such as honey, jellies, or frozen juice; or small amounts of peanut butter, pudding, applesauce, or yogurt. Using small quantities of food ensures that all of the medicine is consumed.

Saquinavir is best absorbed after a high-energy, high-fat meal. However, because it contains some lactose, it may cause diarrhea or nausea. *Indinavir* is best absorbed on an empty stomach or with a light, nonfat snack. Fluids need to be increased and juice works well since the calories in juice are usually also needed. Nausea, vomiting, change in taste, or diarrhea can occur. *Ritonavir* should be taken with a high-energy, high-fat meal. Its side effects include weakness, diarrhea, nausea and vomiting, loss of appetite, abdominal pain, abnormal mouth sensations of burning or prickling, and elevated plasma cholesterol or triglyceride levels. *Nelfinavir* should be taken with food; loose stools or diarrhea can occur. *Nevirapine* can be taken with food or on an empty stomach; mouth sores and rash can occur, as can general fatigue.

Protein

Studies to clarify the ability of a high-protein diet to reverse HIV-associated malnutrition and body composition changes are still needed. High-protein diets might safely promote positive nitrogen balance and lean body mass repletion. HIV-infected persons, like the uninfected, have an unimpaired metabolic response to a high-protein diet; protein supplementation stimulates protein metabolism (Engelson et al., 1998). Protein requirements may be estimated at 1.0 to 1.4 g/kg for maintenance and 1.5 to 2.0 g/kg for repletion (Shronts, 1989). Because of the increased protein requirements, protein restriction is indicated only in persons with severe hepatic or renal disease. Dietary intervention for these further compromised patients is the same as for noninfected persons.

Fat

Tolerance to fat varies from person to person. In individuals with malabsorption or diarrhea, use of a low-fat diet may aid in management. Studies suggest that the use of medium-chain triglyceride (MCT) oil is better than long-chain triglyceride–based supplements for decreasing stool fat and stool nitrogen content and in reducing the number of bowel movements and abdominal symptoms. MCT is more readily absorbed than long-chain triglycerides (Craig et al., 1997).

Fish oil (omega-3 fatty acids), when given with MCT oil, may improve immune function because this combination is less inflammation-promoting than the usual omega-6 fatty acids (Balog, 1998; Bell et al., 1991). However, if triglyceride and cholesterol levels are increased, leading clinicians have speculated that following the guidelines established in the National Cholesterol Education Program could be beneficial (see Chapter 26).

Fluids and Electrolytes

Fluid needs in HIV-infected individuals are similar to those of well individuals, and are calculated to be 30 to 35 mL/kg (8 to 12 cups for adults), with additional amounts to compensate for losses from diarrhea, nausea and vomiting, night sweats, and prolonged fever (Fields-Gardner et al., 1997). Replacement of electrolyte losses (sodium, potassium, and chloride) in the presence of vomiting and diarrhea is also recommended.

Vitamins and Minerals

Recent studies have begun to identify the vitamin and mineral needs of HIV-positive persons and those with AIDS. These studies suggest the need for increased intake of the following micronutrients: beta-carotene, vitamin E, ascorbic acid, vitamin B_{12}, vitamin B_6, and folic acid (Raiten, 1990; Coodly et al., 1993; Prabhala et al., 1990). Although the exact requirements for vitamins and minerals are still unknown at this time, it is suggested that persons consuming an inadequate diet use a vitamin-mineral supplement providing 100% of the RDAs (ADA, 1994). Use of doxorubin hydrochloride, for example, requires adequate riboflavin to reduce drug toxicity. Excellent nutritional status enhances the ability to fight subsequent infections (McKinley et al., 1994).

Special Concerns in Pediatric Patients

In addition to supporting optimal function of the immune system, nutrition is especially critical in children, as it provides the best opportunity for normal growth and development (Heller, 1997). Children should be growing consistently, and weight gain and linear growth must be monitored carefully from baseline and at least every 3 months (see Table 40–8). In some studies, the incidence of failure to thrive and growth stunting has been identified in up to 94% of HIV-infected children (McKinney, 1993); further, changes in adipose and muscle stores may occur as a result of metabolic changes. The goal is to preserve lean body mass, and serum prealbumin, a sensitive predictor of visceral protein stores, is used to measure the effectiveness of nutrition intervention (Heller, 1997).

Each infected child should undergo a baseline nu-

TABLE 40–9 PRACTICAL EATING SUGGESTIONS FOR SYMPTOM MANAGEMENT

SYMPTOM/PROBLEM	MANAGEMENT
Nausea	Small, frequent meals Avoidance of high-fat, greasy foods Cool or room-temperature foods Avoidance of lying down flat after eating
Sore mouth/throat	Soft, moist foods Avoidance of spicy or acidic foods Experimentation with temperature of foods (avoidance of very hot or very cold foods; cool or room-temperature foods are best) Use of nutrient- and energy-dense foods to maximize oral intake
Xerostomia (dry mouth)	Use of foods that are moist or served with a sauce or gravy Consumption of liquids at mealtimes and extra fluids between meals Emphasis on good oral hygiene: flossing, brushing, and rinsing; regular dental care Use of fluoride gels or mouthwashes Consideration of prophylactic antifungal therapy Chewing of sugarless gum or sucking of mints
Difficulty with breathing	Use of easy to eat foods Use of nutrient- and energy-dense foods
Diarrhea	Fluid and electrolyte replacement Low-insoluble, high-soluble fiber diet Possible benefits from low-lactose diet Low-fat diet (may be indicated) Avoidance of gas-causing foods and beverages Avoidance of caffeine
Constipation	Increased fluid intake Increased dietary fiber intake
Inadequate oral intake	Use of nutrient- and energy-dense foods, including nutritional supplements Use of small, frequent meals and snacks Consideration of alternative nutrition support or appetite stimulant such as Megace, Marinol
Fatigue	Adequate sleep, relaxation, exercise Adequate diet, especially foods rich in vitamins B_{12}, A, C, folate, and carotene or zinc, as inadequate levels may cause fatigue (Coodley, 1993; Tang, 1996) Avoidance of caffeine, alcohol, cigarette smoking, and recreational drug use Avoidance of stress and treatment of anxiety or depression Identification and management of possible causes for anemia: • Medications: AZT, bactrim, dapsone, gancyclovir, interferon, pyrimethamine • Other causes: alcohol abuse, bleeding, *Mycobacterium avium* complex, tuberculosis, fungal infections, cytomegalovirus
Body cell mass loss	Adequate diet Resistance exercise Correct for testosterone deficiency Consider anabolic agents (Rx from MD)

tritional assessment, with follow-up every 4 to 6 months, depending on the child's age, nutritional status, and nutritional symptoms (see Tables 40–8 and 40–9). As in adults, nutrition changes in children with HIV/AIDS are not always apparent, and poor intake is usually the major reason for weight loss. General nutrition recommendations for children include high-energy, high-protein, nutrient-dense foods, as protein needs may vary from 150% to 200% of the RDA, and energy needs may vary from 100% to 200% of the RDA (Bentler, 1993). Nutrient and caloric intake must be assessed. A multivitamin supplement that provides 100% of the RDA should be given, regardless of intake.

Treatment for children with HIV includes the use of potent antiretroviral medications. The protease inhibitor nelfinivir is most commonly prescribed in children. As in adults, these medications, used in children, are associated with adverse side effects, as well as difficulties with maintaining a rigid dosage schedule. Children and their caregivers need assistance from a dietetics professional in identifying creative ways of adhering to medication schedules and reducing the flavor and smells of medications. Medications can be mixed into foods or beverages, such as shakes, ice cream, or applesauce, so that they are consumed in sufficient quantities to be effective. Table 40–6 presents HIV medications, along with their dietary considerations and side effects. Although reducing fat intake may decrease difficulty with diarrhea and malabsorption, decreasing fat in a child's diet, especially before the age of 2 years, may directly and negatively impact the growth and development of the child (Leung, 1989).

Mild to severe developmental delays are estimated to occur in up to 80% of HIV-infected children, and as a result, feeding skills may also be impaired (Heller, 1997). A child's oral/motor and self-feeding skills, especially during the first 3 years of life, should be monitored closely. Oral and esophageal manifestations, such as Candida or herpes simplex infections, can make it painful for the child to eat. In such cases, the family may benefit from guidelines and suggestions as to soft, cold, and nonacidic foods and beverages that can help support the child's nutrition status.

When working with the HIV-infected child, the total family unit and environment must be considered, including social/financial issues, cultural issues, and caregiver support in dealing with a chronically ill child. The health care professional's role in these areas may be direct, or may involve referral to an appropriate agency or individual. Resolving barriers to adequate nutrition intake, such as assuring regular access to food, eliminating stress in the environment, and increasing financial resources, can help to improve the child's nutrition status.

Nutritional Complications

If the disease progresses, signs and symptoms of HIV infection and AIDS will be manifested, along with an increase in nutritional complications. Pre-HAART studies have shown that wasting and diarrhea will occur sooner or later during the course of AIDS. In many persons, death appears to be determined more by nutritional status than by any particular opportunistic infection (Keusch and Thea, 1993). Other common nutrition-related complications are anorexia, fatigue, fever, dehydration, nausea, and fat and metabolic abnormalities. Successful lowering of viral load, especially through the use of potent protease inhibitors, helps to maintain nutritional status.

Diarrhea and Malabsorption

Persons with the greatest risk of developing diarrhea are those with a $CD4^+$ cell count of less than 200 to 250 cells/mm^3. Fifty percent of all persons with HIV/AIDS will develop diarrhea at sometime during the clinical course of their disease (Cello, 1997). Diarrhea and malabsorption are the major nutritional problems for this population, and they are often the most difficult problems to resolve. Abnormal d-xylose absorption and steatorrhea are common. Malabsorption of fat, monosaccharides, disaccharides, nitrogen, vitamin B_{12}, folate, minerals, and trace elements occurs in patients with intestinal infections of the small bowel. When the large bowel is infected, malabsorption of fluids and electrolytes is seen. Diarrhea and malabsorption can lead to subtherapeutic blood levels of HIV and other medications, thereby negatively influencing treatment outcomes (Patel et al., 1995).

The causes of diarrhea can be multifactorial, and its etiology, although sometimes difficult to identify, must be pursued. In one study, 80% to 85% of persons with AIDS-associated diarrhea were found to have one or more identifiable enteric pathogens (Cello et al., 1991). These pathogens and other factors causing diarrhea are listed in Table 40–10.

Whether or not the cause of diarrhea is identified, intervention and treatment must be pursued. Treatment is often empiric and uses a combination of antidiarrheal agents, including luminal agents, such as cholestyramine, and fiber supplements; antimotility agents, such as codeine phosphate, Lomotil, Imodium, morphine, and paragoric; and hormones, such as octreotide (Sandostatin) (Dieterich, 1997). Table 40–11 provides information on the nutritional management of diarrhea.

TABLE 40–10 POSSIBLE CAUSES OF HIV-RELATED DIARRHEA

CATEGORY	SPECIFIC AGENTS/CONDITIONS
Bacteria	Campylobacter species
	Clostridium difficile
	Enteroadherent *Escherichia coli*
	Mycobacterium avium complex/ *M. tuberculosis*
	Salmonella species
	Shigella
	Vibrio
Parasites	Cryptosporidium
	Cyclospora
	Giardia
	Isospora
	Microsporidia
	Entamoeba histolytica
Fungi	*Histoplasma capsulatum*
Viruses	Adenovirus
	Cytomegalovirus
	Herpes simplex
	HIV (possibly)
Nutritional causes	Fat malabsorption
	High-fiber diet
	Hypoalbuminemia
	Lactose intolerance
	Kaposi's sarcoma
	Malnutrition
	Caffeine
	Sorbitol
Drugs	
Antacids	Mg^{++}-containing
Antiretrovirals	Didanosine (Videx, ddI)
	Nelfinavir (Viracept)
	Ritonavir (Norvir)
	Saquinavir (Fortovase)
Antimicrobials	Amphotericin
	Macrolide antibiotics
	Azithromycin
	Clorithromycin
	Pentamidine
Gastrointestinal agents	Propulsid
Vitamins (high dose)	Vitamin C
	Vitamin E

(Adapted from Dieterich DT. Diarrhea in the HIV/AIDS Patient. Medical Education Collaborative and Oestreicher Medical Communications, Inc., 1997.)

Disorders of the Oral Cavity and Esophagus

Oral candidiasis is common in persons with AIDS. Symptoms include soreness of the mouth and tongue, often described as a "burnt" feeling, and pain or difficulty with swallowing. *Dysgeusia* may also be present secondary to medication, zinc and other nutrient deficiencies, candidiasis, xerostomia, or excessive mucus production.

KS or herpes in the oropharyngeal or esophageal area can also inhibit normal chewing and swallowing, limiting nutritional intake. Patients with extensive or chronic lesions may require alternative nutritional support, such as enteral or parenteral nutrition. Use of specially designed formulas may slow the progressive decline toward malnutrition. Table 40–9 lists suggestions for improving the dietary intake of the patient with AIDS who has a painful mouth.

Neurologic Disorders

CNS manifestations of AIDS, ranging from psychomotor impairment to severe dementia, can significantly affect the ability of an infected individual to maintain adequate nutrition. Moreover, decreased sensory perception when chewing and swallowing can increase the risk of aspiration. In helping the patient to maintain adequate nutritional intake, it is important to work closely with occupational and physical therapists, speech pathologists,

TABLE 40–11 NUTRITION INTERVENTION FOR DIARRHEA

TYPE OF DIARRHEA	INTERVENTION
Treatable diarrhea	Maintain adequate nutritional intake for bowel regeneration. Enhance absorption by using elemental diets. Control infection and symptoms with antibiotics and antidiarrheals.
Diarrhea resistant to treatment	Promote patient comfort. Maintain adequate hydration; intravenous hydration may be indicated. Provide fiber-containing nutritional supplements. Control symptoms by using antidiarrheals or antispasmodics. TPN may be indicated.
Diarrhea resulting from AIDS enteropathy	Avoid lactose. Reduce high-fructose–containing foods (apple and pear juices, grapes, honey, dates, nuts, figs, soft drinks). Limit sorbitol, hexitols, and mannitol (apple and pear juices, "sugar-free" gums and mints). Limit fat if steatorrhea is present; try using medium-chain triglyceride (MCT) oil. Increase fluid intake. Try bulking agents, like psyllium-containing products. Consider prescriptive pancreatic enzymes Consider L-gutamine (.4 g/kg up to 30 g/d for 5–14 days, followed by 5-10 g/day) Avoid caffeinated beverages. Incorporate small, frequent meals into meal plans. Use an elemental diet to enhance absorption. Consider a lactobacillus replacement if the patient is receiving long-term antibiotic therapy. Recommend a multivitamin-mineral supplement. Gradually reintroduce suspect foods, one at a time, and check for tolerance.
General guidelines for diarrhea	Consume foods at room temperatures. Limit sources of bran-type fibers. Avoid foods that cause gas.

the nursing staff, and others involved in overall patient care.

Alterations in Metabolism and Body Shape

The use of potent anti-HIV therapies, especially protease inhibitors, has increased the incidence of insulin resistance, type 2 diabetes, hypercholesterolemia, pancreatitis, and hypertriglyceridemia in the HIV/AIDS population. Principles developed for diabetes or the Step 2 diet of the National Cholesterol Education Program are used in an effort to control these conditions (see Chapters 26 and 34). Oral hypoglycemics and insulin are being used, as are lipid-lowering drugs, such as Lipitor. Supplements often promoted for these conditions include omega-3 fatty acids, alpha-lipoic acid, and L-carnitine.

The body shape changes seen include increased abdominal fat, decreased peripheral subcutaneous fat stores (arms, legs, and face), buffalo hump and enlarged breasts, prominent veins, and ingrown toenails, among others. Treatment in such cases is both difficult and confusing. Discontinuing antiretroviral therapy is not viewed as a favorable option, although switching therapies to less offending regimens is being considered. One report of successful treatment with growth hormone has been published (Torres, 1998), and this approach awaits further study. Monitoring body composition and measuring waist-hip ratio, midarm, breast, and neck circumferences, in addition to weight and bioelectrical impedance analysis (BIA), will provide a clearer picture of body shape changes over time. BIA does not seem to be effective in identifying fat redistribution, as it reflects trends, more than truncal adiposity. Expensive studies, such as computed tomography (CT) scans and magnetic resonance imaging (MRI), are used exclusively for research, but provide the most accurate assessment of these body composition changes.

FOOD AND WATER SAFETY AND INFECTION CONTROL

Because of the vulnerability of persons with immune suppression to food- and water-borne pathogens, food and water safety is a concern. Persons with HIV and their caregivers should be instructed in food and water safety practices at home, as well as when eating out or traveling abroad. In 1995, the CDC&P published *Cryptosporidiosis: A Guide for Persons with HIV/AIDS,* which listed strategies for reducing the risk of contracting this disease (CDC&P, 1995) (Table 40–12).

The CDC has emphasized the need to consider blood and other body fluids from all persons to be potentially infective (CDC, 1987a). In the hospital setting, nursing and nutrition service employees should follow their institution's appropriate univer-

TABLE 40–12 STRATEGIES FOR REDUCING THE RISK OF CRYPTOSPORIDIOSIS

1. Wash your hands.
2. Avoid sex that involves contact with stool.
3. Avoid touching farm animals.
4. Avoid touching the stool of pets.
5. Wash and/or cook your food.
6. Exercise caution when swimming in lakes, rivers, or pools, or using Jacuzzi tubs.
7. Drink safe water.
   - Boil water for 1 minute at a rapid boil. Store boiled water in a clean, closed container.
   - Filter tap water (using a filter tested and certified by NSF standard 53 for cyst removal or reduction).
   - Use bottled water (reverse osmosis–treated, distilled, or filtered through an absolute 1-μm [or smaller] filter).
8. Exercise caution consuming foods or beverages when traveling.

(From Centers for Disease Control and Prevention. Cryptosporidiosis: A Guide for Persons with HIV/AIDS. Atlanta: CDC, 1995.)

sal precaution policies and procedures to prevent the transmission of HIV. Hospital personnel need not wear gowns, masks, or gloves while performing general patient care, unless respiratory or strict isolation is indicated.

COMPLEMENTARY AND ALTERNATIVE NUTRITION THERAPIES

People with HIV disease often become frustrated with the lack of definitive medical therapies. In their search for answers, some turn to unconventional nutritional therapies. The term "alternative medicine" has been used to describe treatments and practices that (1) lack sufficient documentation of safety and effectiveness against specific diseases and conditions, (2) are not generally taught in U.S. medical schools, and (3) are not generally reimbursable by health insurance providers (Stehlin, 1995).

The National AIDS Health Fraud Task Force uses the definition of AIDS fraud as "the sale, advertising, or promotion (usually for profit) of products, therapies or services to diagnose, prevent, cure or treat HIV disease or AIDS which are unproven, unscientific or harmful" (California AIDS Fraud Task Force, 1996).

Among the major questions to consider in assessing therapies are the following:

- Is the product or treatment harmful?
- Are there harmful drug–drug interactions with prescription or over-the-counter medications or nutrients?
- Are unproven treatments being used, while delaying effective conventional treatment(s) and possibly missing important windows of opportunity?
- Does the therapy work?
- Is the financial expense worth the benefit?

TABLE 40–13 NUTRITION RELATED COMPLEMENTARY AND ALTERNATIVE THERAPIES

REGIMEN/THERAPY	DESCRIPTION/PURPORTED ACTION	COMMENT(S)
Herbs/botanicals		
Astragalus (Huang ch'i)	Used in China to stimulate the immune system	Overdose may cause suppression of the immune system.
Cat's claw (*Uncaria tomentosa* or una de gato)		
Echinacea (*Echinacea angustifolia*)	Used to treat ailments ranging from the common cold to chronic infections; immune stimulation effects derived from (1) stimulating phagocytosis, (2) increasing respiratory activity, and (3) increasing mobility of leukocytes	Not recommended for use in patients with tuberculosis, HIV, or other autoimmune diseases. Prolonged use may result in immune system depression secondary to overstimulation. No information on potential drug interaction is available.
Garlic (*Allium sativum*)	Used to fight infection and as an antioxidant, antibacterial, and immune stimulant; may decrease low-density lipoprotein and increase high-density lipoprotein cholesterol levels; may reduce blood pressure; inhibits aggregation of blood platelets	Avoid large doses of garlic when taking aspirin and other anticoagulants. Other adverse effects may include gastrointestinal disturbances (e.g., heartburn and gas).
Ginseng (Korean or Asian-Panax ginseng)	Used to enhance cellular immune function, as well as mental and physical capacity	Reported adverse effects include initial nervousness and excitation, estrogenic effects in women, hypoglycemic effects, involvement in the cytochrome P-450 system, and interaction with warfarin
St. John's Wort (*Hypericum performatum*)	Used as an antidepressant; currently being studied as a treatment for viral infections, such as herpes and HIV	Side effects may include photosensitivity, bloating, gas, allergic reactions.
Homeostatic macrobiotic diet	Based on the Zen Buddhist philosophy that advocates maintaining the proper balance between yin and yang foods. The standard form of this diet usually includes 50%–60% whole grains and cereals; 20%–25% vegetables; 5%–10% sea vegetables and beans; 5% miso or tamari broth soup. Emphasis placed on fluid restriction	Diet may be deficient in calories, protein, iron, calcium, vitamin D, vitamin B_{12}, folic acid, riboflavin, and ascorbic acid.
Yeast-free diet (also known as anti-Candida diet)	Used to prevent opportunistic yeast infections that can further weaken the immune system; involves the elimination of foods containing yeast and foods with high concentrations of simple sugars	Diet claims are unsubstantiated by research and questioned by the American College of Allergy and Immunology Practice Standards Committee, although some doctors support its use.
Megadoses of vitamins and minerals	High doses of vitamins A, C, E, B_{12}, and selenium and zinc that are used to strengthen and "revitalize" the immune system	Effects are unproven, and toxicities can result from chronic and excessive intake.
Antiviral AL-721 and homemade formulas	"AL" or "active lipid," in the ratio of 7:2:1, is made from soy or egg yolk lecithin, can be given orally or by injection, and has been reported to reduce or inhibit HIV replication.	AL-721 is approved for use in clinical trials by the FDA. Homemade formulas or generic substitutions are not approved, and may be impure.
Dr. Berger's Immune Power Diet and Maximum Immunity Diet	Designed to boost and "revitalize" the immune system	Diet claims are unsubstantiated.
Medical marijuana	Reduce nausea; increase appetite	Undergoing limited clinical trials.

CASE STUDY

Jon M. is a 24-year-old, HIV-positive patient who was recently admitted to your facility. His serum albumin level is 3.2 g/dL; his BUN and creatinine levels are slightly elevated; his blood glucose is 90 mg/dL. He has not eaten for 48 hours because of diarrhea and vomiting. He is currently receiving IV fluids, antibiotics, and acyclovir, AZT, and amphotericin-B. He is 6 foot, 4 inches tall and weighs 195 lb.

1. Calculate Jon's reported daily intake of protein and calories. How does this compare with the recommended amount for his age, sex, and size?
2. What recommendations would you make at this point about the use of an oral diet?
3. What dietary suggestions would you offer to Jon relative to his drug regimen? What side effects is Jon likely to experience with this therapy?
4. Would you recommend parenteral nutrition? Why or why not?

One must be wary of products or services when their promotion uses sensationalism, testimonials, or claims that it is based on a secret formula, or when promotional literature accuses the government or Western doctors of neglect.

Complementary and alternative therapies for HIV/AIDS often include alternative systems of medical practice (Chinese traditional medicine, Ayurvedic, Tibetan), homeopathy, naturopathy, dietary systems (macrobiotics, yeast-free diets, special foods and nutrients, herbs, and other supplements), integrative mind-body approaches (yoga, biofeedback, visualization), and manual healing techniques (massage, acupuncture, acupressure). Use of complementary and alternative therapies should be acknowledged as a part of the MNT assessment and intervention (Fenton et al., 1998). Table 40–13 summarizes some complementary and alternative therapies that have attracted patients with HIV infection or AIDS. (See Chapter 19.)

CITED REFERENCES

Adams M, et al. Battling HIV on many fronts. N Engl J Med 338:198, 1998.

The American Dietetic Association. Position of the American Dietetic Association and The Canadian Dietetic Association: Nutrition intervention in the care of persons with human immunodeficiency virus infection. J Am Diet Assoc 94:1042, 1994.

The American Dietetic Association (ADA), HIV/AIDS Medical Nutrition Therapy Protocol. Medical Nutrition Therapy Across the Continuum of Care, 2nd ed. Chicago: ADA, 1998.

Balog DL, et al. HIV wasting syndrome: treatment update. Ann Pharmacother 32:446, 1998.

Bell SJ, et al. Alternative lipid sources for enteral and parenteral nutrition: Long- and medium-chain triglycerides, structured triglycerides, and fish oils. J Am Diet Assoc 91:74, 1991.

Berger DS. Understanding and managing resistance. Positively Aware Jan/Feb 1998, p. 21.

Bitton N, et al. Gene therapy approaches to HIV-infection: immunological strategies—Use of T bodies and universal receptors to redirect cytolytic T cells. Front Biosci 4:386, 1999.

Blanchard A, et al. Influence of microbial infections on the progress of HIV disease. Trends Microbiol 5:326, 1997.

Bowen DL, et al. Immunopathogenesis of the acquired immune deficiency syndrome. Ann Intern Med 103:704, 1985.

Brown D. AIDS virus identified in blood sample taken from African man in 1959. Washington Post, February 4, 1998a, p. a5.

Brown D. AZT's success in pregnancy may help expand AIDS treatment for the poor. Washington Post, February 19, 1998b, p. a10.

California AIDS Fraud Task Force. Stop AIDS Health Fraud (pamphlet). Los Angeles: California AIDS Fraud Task Force, 1996.

Cao Y, et al. Virologic and immunologic characterization of long-term survivors of human immunodeficiency virus type 1 infection. N Engl J Med 332:201, 1995.

Carey JT. The clinical spectrum. In: Blanchet KD (ed.). AIDS: A Health Care Management Response. Rockville, MD: Aspen Publishers, 1988.

Carpenter CC, et al. Antiretroviral therapy for HIV infection in 1997. JAMA 277:1962, 1997.

Cello JP. Gastrointestinal tract manifestations of AIDS. In: Sande MA, Voberding PA (eds.). The Medical Management of AIDS. Philadelphia: WB Saunders, 1997.

Cello JP, et al. Effect of octreotide on refractory AIDS-associated diarrhea. Ann Intern Med 115:705, 1991.

Centers for Disease Control. HIV/AIDS Surveillance Report. MMWR 36 (suppl 2S): 3S, 1987a. Available at www2.cdc.gov/mmwr.

Centers for Disease Control. Recommendations for prevention of HIV transmission in health care settings. MMWR 36:1, 1987b.

Centers for Disease Control. HIV/AIDS Surveillance Report, 2nd quarter, 1993. MMWR 5(2), 1994. Available at www2.cdc.gov/mmwr.

Centers for Disease Control and Prevention. Cryptosporidiosis: A Guide for Persons with HIV/AIDS. Atlanta: CDC, 1995. Available at www2.cdc.gov/mmwr.

Centers for Disease Control and Prevention. HIV/AIDS Surveillance Report. 8(2):1, 1996. Available at www2.cdc.gov/mmwr.

Centers for Disease Control and Prevention. HIV/AIDS Surveillance Report, Midyear Edition, vol. 9(1). Atlanta: CDC, 1997a. Available at www2.cdc.gov/mmwr.

Centers for Disease Control and Prevention. 1997 USPHS/IDSA guidelines for the prevention of opportunistic infection in persons infected with human immunodeficiency virus. MMWR 46(No. RR-12):27, 1997b. Available at www2.cdc.gov/mmwr.

Chlebowski RT. Significance of altered nutritional status in acquired immunodeficiency syndrome (AIDS). Nutr Cancer 7:85, 1985.

Clarke M, et al. Ethical issues facing medical research in developing countries. Lancet 351:286, 1998.

Clifford DB, et al. HAART improves prognosis in HIV-associated progressive multifocal leukoencephalopathy. Neurology 52:623, 1999.

Clum N. Take Control: Living with HIV and AIDS. Los Angeles: AIDS Project, 1996, p. 46.

Collins CL. Nutrition care in AIDS. Diet Curr 15:1, 1988.

Connor EM, et al. Reduction of maternal-infant transmission of human immunodeficiency virus type 1 with Zidovudine treatment. N Engl J Med 331:1173, 1997.

Coodley GO, et al. β-carotene in HIV infection. J AIDS 6:272, 1993.

Craig GB, et al. Decreased fat and nitrogen losses in patients with AIDS receiving medium-chain-triglyceride–enriched formula vs. those receiving long-chain-triglyceride–containing formula. J Am Diet Assoc 97:605, 1997.

Daley S. A post-apartheid agony: AIDS on the March 1998. The New York Times International, July 23, 1998, p. A1.

Day D. Better AIDS prevention can close health gap. New York Times, January 29, 1998.

Dubé MP, Sattler FR. Metabolic complications of antiretroviral therapies. AIDS Clin Care 10:1, 1998.

Engelson ES, et al. Nutrition and testosterone status of HIV+ women, (Abstract no. Tu. B 2382). International Conference on AIDS, Jul 7–12, 1996, vol. 11, p. 1, 332.

Engelson ES, et al. Effect of a high protein diet upon protein metabolism in HIV-infected men and women. [Abstract No. 32166]. 12th World AIDS Conference, Geneva, Switzerland, 1998.

Engle L. Old AIDS. Body Positive, XI:11, 1998.

Fabris N, et al. AIDS, zinc deficiency and thymic hormone failure. JAMA 259:839, 1988.

Falutz J, et al. Zinc as a cofactor in human immunodeficiency virus—induced immunosuppression. JAMA 259:2850, 1988.

Fenton M. Nutrition referral screening for adults (18+ years) with HIV/AIDS. AIDS Project Los Angeles, 1997. In: Guidelines and Protocol of Care for Providing Medical Nutrition Therapy to HIV-Infected Persons, Standards of Care Committee, Los Angeles County Commission on HIV Health Services, 1997.

Fenton M, Fitz P. Principles and Guidelines: Comments. Letter on the Report of the NIH Panel to Define Principles of Therapy of HIV Infection, and Guidelines for the Use of Antiretroviral Agents in HIV-Infected Adults and Adolescents, July 21, 1997.

Fenton M, Heller L. Nutrition referral screening for pediatrics (<18 years) with HIV/AIDS. AIDS Project Los Angeles, 1997. In: Guidelines and Protocol of Care for Providing Medical Nutrition Therapy to HIV-Infected Persons, Standards of Care Committee, Los Angeles County Commission on HIV Health Services, 1997.

Fenton M, et al. HIV/AIDS Adults: Medical Nutrition Therapy Across the Continuum of Care, 2nd ed. Chicago: The American Dietetic Association, 1998.

Fields-Gardner C, et al. A Clinician's Guide to Nutrition in HIV and AIDS. Chicago: The American Dietetic Association, 1997.
Flier J, Underhill L. Metabolic disturbances and wasting in the acquired immunodeficiency syndrome. N Engl J Med 327:329, 1992.
Goedert JJ, Blattner WA. The epidemiology and natural history of human immunodeficiency virus. In: DeVita VT, Hellman S, Rosenberg SA (eds.). AIDS Etiology, Diagnosis, Treatment and Prevention, 2nd ed. Philadelphia: JB Lippincott, 1988, p. 33.
Goletti D, et al. Effect of *Mycobacterium tuberculosis* on HIV activation: Role of immune activation. J Immunol 157:1271, 1996.
Gorbach S. Report to the International AIDS Wasting Conference, Ft. Lauderdale, FL, November 16–19, 1997.
Grant AD, DeCock KM. The growing challenge of HIV/AIDS in developing countries. Br Med Bull 54:369, 1998.
Gray RH. Similarities between AIDS and PCM. Am J Public Health 73:1332, 1983.
Hect FM, et al. Adherence and effectiveness of protease inhibitors in clinical practice. Presented at the 5th Conference on Retroviruses and Opportunistic Infections, Chicago, IL, February 1–5, 1998.
Heller L. Nutrition support for children with HIV/AIDS. J Am Diet Assoc, 97:473, 1997.
Henderson R, et al. Serum and plasma markers of nutritional status in children infected with the human immunodeficiency virus. J Am Diet Assoc 97:1377, 1997.
HIV/AIDS Treatment Information Service. Glossary Of HIV/AIDS–Related Terms, 2nd ed. Washington, DC: U.S. Department Of Health and Human Services, March, 1997.
Horberg M, Schatz B. To The Editor. N Engl J Med 338:198, 1998.
Hyman C, Kaufman S. Nutritional impact of acquired immune deficiency syndrome: A unique counseling opportunity. J Am Diet Assoc 89:520, 1989.
Jacobson MA. Sande MA, Volberding PA (eds.). Medical Management of AIDS, 3rd ed. Philadelphia: WB Saunders, 1992.
Jain VK, Chandra RD. Does nutritional deficiency predispose to acquired immune deficiency syndrome? Nutr Res 4:537, 1984.
Joint United Nations Programme On HIV/AIDS. Report On The Global HIV/AIDS Epidemic, World AIDS Day, New York, December 1, 1997.
Keush GT, Thea DM. Malnutrition in AIDS. Med Clin North Am 77:795, 1993.
Kotler DP. Characterization of intestinal disease associated with human immunodeficiency virus infection and response to antiretroviral therapy. J Infect Dis 179:4545, 1999.
Kotler DP. Nutritional effects and support in the patient with acquired immunodeficiency syndrome. J Nutr 122:723, 1992.
Kotler DP, Muurahainen N. Nutritional and gastrointestinal syndromes: Complications of HIV infection and treatment. Clinical Care Options for HIV, Conference Summaries, 5th Conference on Retroviruses and Opportunistic Infections. Available: www.healthcg.com. (2/3/98).
Kreiger L. City urged to require doctors to report HIV. San Francisco Examiner Online (1/26/98), CDC, NCHSTP Daily News Update.
Landers DV. 1995 Nutrition and Immune Function II: Maternal Factors Influencing Transmission. Nutrition in Pediatric HIV Infection: Setting the Research Agenda, Bethesda, MD, September, 1995.
Li Q, et al. Vertical transmission of human immunodeficiency virus type 1: Frequency and correlation of transmission. Int J Mol Med 1:589, 1998.
Life Sciences Research Office, FASEB. Nutritional Therapy and Nutrition Education in the Care and Management of AIDS Patients. Tentative Report, Task Order 7. Washington, DC: Center for Food Safety and Nutrition, FDA, DHHS, 1990.
Macallan D, et al. Energy expenditure and wasting in human immunodeficiency virus infection. N Engl J Med 333:83, 1995.
Maugh TH II. AIDS deaths down 44% in US: New cases drop. Los Angeles Times, February 3, 1998.
Mayers D. Maintenance antiretroviral treatment in HIV infection. JAMA 281:497, 1999.
McKinley M, et al. Improved body weight status as a result of nutrition intervention in adult, HIV-positive outpatients. J Am Diet Assoc 94:1014, 1994.
Michaels S, et al. Differences in the incidence rates of opportunistic processes before and after the availability of protease inhibitors. 5th Conference on Retrovirus and Opportunistic Infections, Chicago, IL, February 1–5, 1998.
Miller G, et al. Gastrostomy tube supplementation for HIV-infected children. Pediatrics 96:696, 1995.
Mulligan K, et al. Energy expenditure in human immunodeficiency virus. N Engl J Med 336:70, 1997.
National Institutes of Health (NIH) Panel To Define Principles Of Therapy Of HIV Infection. Draft Report of the NIH Panel To Define Principles of Therapy of HIV Infection. Bethesda, MD: Office of AIDS Research of The National Institutes of Health, 1997, p. 7.
Office of the Actuary. Estimated Medicaid and Medicare costs of AIDS and numbers of individuals covered. Washington, DC: Health Care Financing Administration, February 27,1995.
Office of AIDS Research in Collaboration with the NIH Institutes, Centers, and Divisions. Report on Current NIH-Supported Research Activities on Women and HIV/AIDS. Bethesda, MD, May, 1998.
Panel On Clinical Practices For Treatment Of HIV Infection. The Guidelines for the Use of Antiretroviral Agents in HIV-Infected Adults And Adolescents. Bethesda, MD: Department Of Health and Human Services and Henry J. Kaiser Family Foundation. November, 1997.
Pantaleo G, et al. Studies in subjects with long-term non-progressive human immunodeficiency virus infection. N Engl J Med 332:209, 1995.
Patel KB, et al. Drug malabsorption and resistant tuberculosis in HIV-infected patients. N Engl J Med 332:336, 1995.
Pérez JH. AIDS behind bars: We should all care. Body Positive 10:1, 1997.
Piroth L, et al. Does hepatitis C virus coinfection accelerate clinical and immunological evolution of HIV-infected patients? AIDS 12:381, 1998.
Prabhala RH, et al. Immunomodulation in humans caused by beta-carotene and vitamin A. Nutr Res 10:1473, 1990.
Raiten DJ. Nutrition and HIV Infection: A Review and Evaluation of the Extant Knowledge of the Relationship Between Nutrition and HIV Infection (FDA Contract No. 223-88-2124). 1990.
Russell S. AIDS deaths drop 60% in CA. San Francisco Chronicle, January 9, 1998.
Saavedra J, et al. Longitudinal assessment of growth in children born to mothers with human immunodeficiency virus infection. Arch Pediatr Adolesc Med 149:497, 1995.
Semba RD, et al. Maternal vitamin A deficiency and mother-to-child transmission of HIV-1. Lancet 343:1593, 1994.
Semba RD, et al. Infant mortality and maternal vitamin A deficiency during human immunodeficiency virus infection. Clin Infect Dis 21:966, 1995.
Shronts EP. Nutrition Support Dietetics Core Curriculum 1989. Rockville, MD: Aspen Publishers, 1989, p. 221.
Sreepada Rao TK. Renal complications in patients with AIDS. J Crit Illness 3:55, 1988.
Stehlin, IB. An FDA guide to choosing medical treatments. FDA Consumer, June, 1995.
Steinbrook R. Battling HIV on many fronts. N Engl J Med 337:779, 1997.
Stiehm RE. Newborn factors in maternal-infant transmission of pediatric HIV infection. In: Nutrition in Pediatric HIV Infection: Setting The Research Agenda. Bethesda, MD: NIH, September, 1995.
Tang W, et al. Hyponatremia in hospitalized patients with acquired immunodeficiency syndrome. Am J Med 94:164, 1993.
Tang A, et al. Characterizations of the acute clinical illness associated with HIV infection. Arch Intern Med 148:945, 1996.
Timbo B, Tollefson L. Nutrition: A cofactor in HIV disease. J Am Diet Assoc 94:1018, 1994.
Valeri A, Neusy A. Acute and chronic renal disease in hospitalized patients. Clin Nephrol 33:110, 1991.
Vasquez E. News briefs. Positively Aware, vol. 11, January/February, 1998, p. 15.
Venkatraman J, et al. Influence of the level of dietary lipid intake and maximal exercise on the immune status in runners. Med Sci Sports Exercise 29:333, 1997.
Wasowica L. California AIDS Deaths Plummet 60 Percent. UPI, January 9, 1998.
Wheeler D, et al. Weight loss as a predictor of survival and disease progression in HIV infection. J AIDS Hum and Retroviral 18:80, 1998.

ADDITIONAL REFERENCES

American Gastroenterological Association Patient Care Committee. American Gastroenterological Association medical position statement: Guidelines for the management of malnutrition and cachexia, chronic diarrhea, and hepatobiliary disease in patients with human immunodeficiency virus infection. Gastroenterology 111:1722, 1996.
Chesney M, Ickovics J. For the Recruitment Adherence and Retention Committee of the AIDS Clinical Trials Group (ACTG). Adherence to combination therapy in AIDS clinical trials (1997). Presented at the Annual Meeting of the AIDS Clinical Trials Group, Washington, DC, July, 1997.
Dieterich D. Hepatitis and HIV. 8th Clinical Care Options for HIV Symposium. Clinical Care Options for HIV Online Journal 4:2, 1998.
Grunfeld C, Feingold K. Body weight as essential data in the management of patients with human immunodeficiency virus infection and acquired immunodeficiency syndrome. Am J Clin Nutr 58:317, 1993.
Mellors JW, et al. Plasma viral load and CD4+ lymphocytes as prognostic markers of HIV-1 infection. Ann Intern Med 126:946, 1997.
Rabeneck L, et al. A randomized controlled trial evaluation of nutrition counseling with or without oral supplementation in malnourished HIV-infected patients. J Am Diet Assoc 98:433, 1998.
Salomon S, et al. An elemental diet containing medium-chain triglycerides and enzymatically hydrolyzed protein can improve gastrointestinal tolerance in people infected with HIV. J Am Diet Assoc 98:460, 1998.
Salomon S, et al. Living Well With HIV and AIDS. Chicago: The American Dietetic Association, 1993.

San Francisco AIDS Foundation. Viral load and CD4 T-Cell testing, Drug Resistance, and Adherence to HAART. San Francisco: Treatment Education And Advocacy Department, The San Francisco AIDS Foundation, December, 1997.

Stack J, et al. High-energy, high-protein, oral, liquid nutrition supplementation in patients with HIV infection: Effect on weight status in relation to incidence of secondary infection. J Am Diet Assoc 96:337, 1996.

Tang A, et al. Low serum vitamin B-12 concentrations are associated with faster human immunodeficiency virus type 1 (HIV-1) disease progression. J Nutr 127:345, 1997.

Young J. HIV and medical nutrition therapy. J Am Diet Assoc 97:S161, 1997.

Wu K, et al. Effects of dietary n-3 fatty acid supplementation in men with weight loss associated with the acquired immune deficiency syndrome: Relation to indices of cytokine production. J AIDS Hum Retroviral 11:258, 1998.

CHAPTER 41

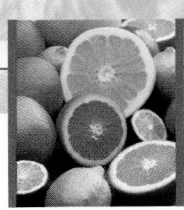

Medical Nutrition Therapy for Food Allergy and Food Intolerance

SHERRY HUBBARD WILSON RD, LD

Chapter Outline

- Immunologic Basis
- Symptoms
- Common Food Allergens
- Risk Factors for the Development of Food Allergy
- Food Intolerances
- Diagnosis
- Treatment
- Natural History
- Food Allergy in Infancy
- Diet and Prevention of Allergic Disease

Key Terms

ADVERSE FOOD REACTION—any undesired response to a food that is not documented to be allergy-based

ALLERGEN—substance foreign to the body which, upon interaction with the immune system, causes an allergic reaction

ANAPHYLAXIS—an acute, often severe, and sometimes fatal immune response that may affect one or more organ systems

ANTIBODIES—immunoglobulins produced in response to an antigen or allergen

ATOPY—tendency toward allergies, determined genetically

CAP-RAST FEIA (FLUROSCEIN-ENZYME IMMUNOASSAY)—a test, more sensitive than the radioallergosorbent test (RAST), that provides quantitative assessment of food-specific IgE antibodies

CELL-MEDIATED IMMUNITY—immunity that is mediated by T lymphocytes, either through the release of lymphokines or by direct cytotoxicity

CROSS-REACTIVITY—an allergic response to a food or substance either within a given group (i.e., crustacea, legumes) or with unrelated substances (e.g., banana, kiwi, or chestnuts with latex)

DOUBLE-BLIND, PLACEBO-CONTROLLED FOOD CHALLENGE (DBPCFC)—a test of reaction to a food where the food is disguised such that neither the patient nor researcher knows it is being given; the "gold standard" for establishing food allergy

ECZEMA—a skin rash characterized by small red and white bumps that itch; often a symptom of allergy; also called atopic dermatitis

ELIMINATION DIET—an eating plan that omits one or more foods suspected to cause an adverse food reaction

FOOD ALLERGY—an adverse food reaction that is mediated by an immunoglobulin E (IgE) immunologic mechanism; the reaction occurs consistently after consumption of a particular food and causes functional changes in target organs; IgE-mediated food hypersensitivity

FOOD HYPERSENSITIVITY DISORDERS—IgE-mediated disease (food allergy) or sensitivity induced by cell-mediated or immune-complex disease

FOOD INTOLERANCE—an adverse reaction to a food caused by toxic, pharmacologic, metabolic, or idiosyncratic reactions to the food or chemical substances in the food

FOOD AND SYMPTOM DIARY—a subjective tool for recording food and drink consumed and onset, intensity, and duration of symptoms

HUMORAL IMMUNITY—immunity mediated by antibodies produced by B lymphocytes

IMMUNOGLOBULIN E (IgE)–MEDIATED REACTION—rapid onset of symptoms occurring after ingestion of a specific allergen that cross-links the antigen-specific IgE molecule to mast cells and basophils

MAST CELLS—tissue cells that release histamine or other substances causing allergic symptoms

RADIOALLERGOSORBENT TEST (RAST)—a test that measures specific IgE antibodies in serum; used as an alternative to skin tests

SENSITIZATION—exposure to an antigen or allergen that results in the development of hypersensitivity

SKIN TEST—a test in which an antigen is applied directly to the skin and then pricked or scratched through with a needle or a specifically designed prick/scratch implement, in order to observe the histamine response

THYMUS AND TONSILS—tissues of lymphoid material that contribute to immunity

Food allergy continues to be a term that is misused and misunderstood by the general public. Indeed, surveys completed for the Food Allergy Center in 1989, 1992, and 1993 indicate that 16.2%, 16.6%, and 13.9% of the respondents respectively, believed that a member of their household had a food allergy. These figures are much different than the estimated 0.1% to 8% who actually have a food allergy confirmed by double-blind, placebo-controlled food challenge (DBPCFC) (Sampson and Ho, 1997; Altman and Chiaramonte, 1996). A frequent misconception is that all reactions to food are allergy-based. Until actual food allergy is properly diagnosed, the term **adverse food reaction,** an umbrella term used for any undesired food reaction, should be used (website addresses for updates on food allergy and adverse reactions is: www.foodallergy.org and www.aaaai.org).

IMMUNOLOGIC BASIS

Definition

The term adverse food reaction encompasses two categories: food hypersensitivity and food intolerance. **Food intolerance** is an adverse reaction to a food caused by toxic, pharmacologic, metabolic, or idiosyncratic reactions to food or chemical substances in the food. **Food hypersensitivity** occurs when the immune system reacts to a substance (food) that is usually harmless because the immune system erroneously assumes it is harmful. Food hypersensitivity includes Immunoglobulin E (IgE) and non-IgE type reactions. Most food allergies are type I or **IgE-mediated reactions** with an immunopathologic process that is reproducible through a "cause-and-effect relationship" (Taylor et al., 1999; Hide, 1994; Grote et al., 1998). IgE reactions usually occur immediately or within 2 hours of exposure, and their severity ranges from mild to life-threatening.

Persons who have a genetic predisposition to allergic disease, also called **atopy,** have an increased probability of developing food allergies. These same individuals may never develop food allergy symptoms, but could experience other atopic disease, such as asthma, allergic rhinitis, or atopic dermatitis. The incidence of food allergy appears to decrease with age. Infants younger than 2 years of age are more likely to develop food allergies than are older children or adults. Estimates of the incidence of food allergy in the population range from 5% to 8% in children to 1.5% in adults (Sampson and Ho, 1997; Plaut, 1997).

Antigen Exclusion

When an allergic food reaction occurs, proteins from the food, called antigens or **allergens,** must be absorbed from the gastrointestinal tract, interact with the immune system, and produce a response. Under normal conditions, the gastrointestinal tract and the immune system provide a barrier that prevents the absorption of most intact proteins. When this barrier fails, allergic **sensitization** may occur, in which case re-exposure produces an allergic reaction.

Immune System

The immune system functions to clear the body of foreign substances (or antigens), such as viruses, bacteria, blood cells, and tissue cells. Normally, when antigens interact with cells of the immune system, they are cleared from the body without an adverse reaction. Three types of cells respond to antigens presented: B lymphocytes, T lymphocytes, and macrophages. The lymphocytes arise from stem cells in the bone marrow and, along with T cells originating from stem cells in the thymus, are the basis for the function of the two branches of the immune system: the humoral pathway and the cell-mediated pathway.

Humoral immunity involves **antibodies** (immunoglobulins) and has an important role in food allergy. Antigen-specific antibodies are produced by the B lymphocytes (B cells) in response to the antigen presented. The union of an antigen and its antibody results in the production of chemical mediators or direct cellular damage, which, in turn, causes symptoms. Five classes of antibodies have been identified. IgG, IgM, and IgD antibodies protect the body against bacteria and viruses. Secretory IgA antibodies in breast milk provide breast-feeding infants with local intestinal protection against viruses and bacteria. IgA antibodies, present in saliva and intestinal secretions, block the absorption of antigens. IgE antibodies help to eliminate parasites from the body, and are also responsible for classic allergic reactions.

Cellular or **cell-mediated immunity** involves the action of T lymphocytes (T cells). T cells do not produce antibodies, but do recognize antigens. When antigens stimulate T-cell growth, the T cells produce lymphokines and cytokines, substances that help regulate the activities of other cells or that cause direct cellular damage to target cells, resulting in the destruction of antigens. Cellular immunity has an important role in resistance to viruses, fungi, tumor cells, and other foreign cells. Certain reactions, such as contact dermatitis and the tuberculin reaction, are also mediated by T cells. The role of cellular immunity in food allergy is unclear.

Tissue macrophages, derived from monocytes present in the blood, also have important roles in the recognition and clearance of antigens. Through the process of phagocytosis, the macrophage engulfs and destroys antigens. B cells, T cells, and macrophages are all thought to interact (Fig. 41–1).

The **thymus and tonsils** also play a role in immunity. The thymus is a ductless, gland-like organ which, because of its T-cell production, is essential to the development of peripheral lymphoid tissue. Although the thymus is largest and most active prior to puberty, the mature T cells it exports exert their effect into adulthood. Removal of the thymus during adulthood has little effect on a person's resistance to disease.

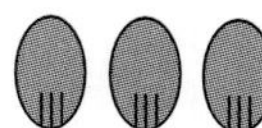

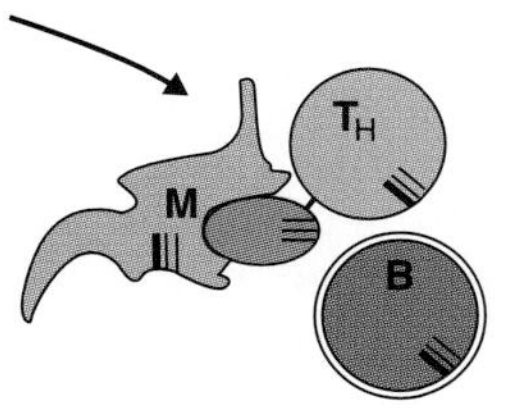

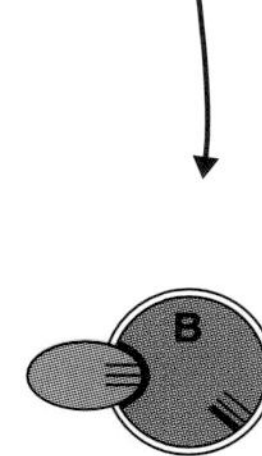

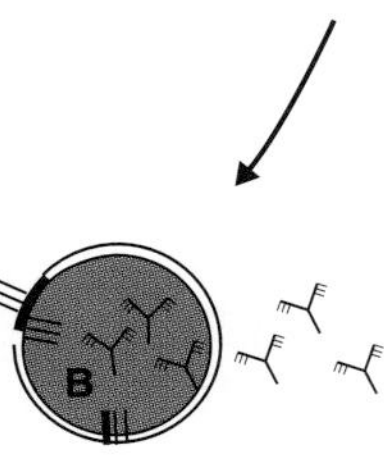

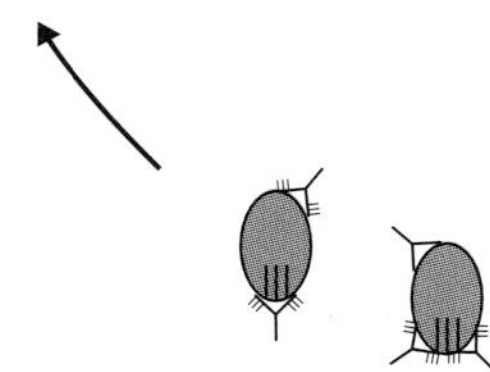

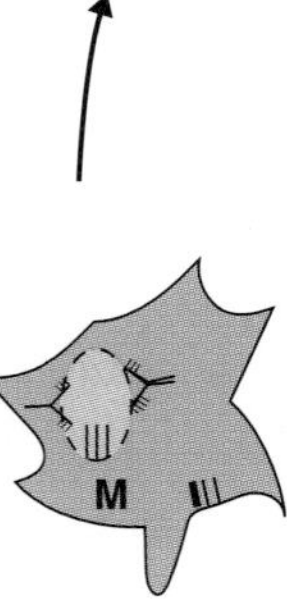
M
6. Antibody binding causes cellular events and attracts other leukocytes to the complex. The interaction of other leukocytes along with the cellular events results in the neutralization, destruction, or elimination of the antigen.

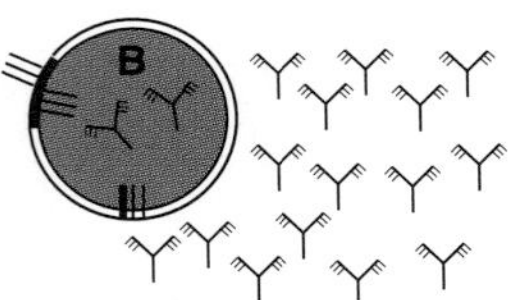

FIGURE 41–1 Sequence of events stimulating antibody-mediated immunity. (Reprinted with permission from Ignatavicius DD, Workman ML, Mishler MA. Medical-Surgical Nursing (3rd ed.). Philadelphia: WB Saunders, 1999.

The tonsils consist of two small, rounded masses of lymphoid tissue that lie in the path of inspired air and all ingested food and liquids. Foreign material that is inspired into the airways and that becomes trapped in the tonsillar crypts comes in contact with antigen-processing cells. Their surgical removal, especially during childhood, may impair or delay the development of an individual's immunity to disease.

Allergic Reactions

Allergic reactions are unusual responses of the immune system and represent altered reactivity to an antigen. The antigens involved in allergic reactions are called allergens. Allergic reactions are classified into four types: types I, II, and III, which are antibody-dependent, and type IV, which is T-cell–dependent (Table 41–1).

Immediate hypersensitivity (type I), which involves IgE, is the most common allergic reaction and has the most clearly understood mechanism. The combination of an allergen with allergen-specific IgE fixed to tissue **mast cells** or circulating basophils causes the release of chemical mediators, including histamine, serotonin, kinins, and others. When released, these inflammatory mediators can cause itching, contraction of smooth muscle, vasodilation, and secretion of mucus. IgE-mediated allergic reactions have an important role in food allergy. Manifestations, which are most often systemic, in-

TABLE 41–1 TYPES OF ALLERGIC REACTIONS

REACTION/CLASSIFICATION	MECHANISM	COMMENTS
Type I Immediate hypersensitivity, anaphylactic IgE-mediated, or reaginic reaction	The allergen binds with sensitized IgE antibody on mast cells (specialized granular cells in the intestines, skin, and respiratory tract) or basophils (similar cells in blood). This results in release of mediators (histamine, eosinophilic chemotactic factor, bradykinin, etc.). IgG has also been identified as being involved in this type of reaction.	Applies to hay fever, anaphylaxis, most food allergies. Symptoms occur within seconds or up to 2 hours. Symptoms of food reactions may include laryngeal edema, nausea, vomiting, severe abdominal pain, bloating, diarrhea, angioedema, eczema, erythema, itching, hoarseness, wheezing, cough, chest tightness, hypotension, bronchospasm, and shock.
Type II Cytotoxic	IgG antibody reacts with the cell membrane or an antigen associated with the cell membrane.	Results from transfusion of incompatible blood types. No food reactions have been demonstrated.
Type III Antigen-antibody complex Arthus reaction	Antigen and antibodies (IgG and IgM) form a complex called a "precipitating antibody." The antigen-antibody complex is known as an Arthus reaction when it occurs in soft tissues, like blood vessels, lungs, or kidneys; and as serum sickness when the complex circulates. Complement is also activated in some cases.	Occurs in some food reactions. Milk precipitins have been found in the lungs of some children with chronic respiratory infection, and in the gastrointestinal tract of those with gastroenteropathy. Reactions usually take 6 hours or more to appear and may take several days to become clinically apparent.
Type IV Delayed or cell-mediated hypersensitivity	T cells interact directly with antigen.	Usual mechanism of graft rejection. Possibly involved in some food allergies, such as protein-losing enteropathies.

(Adapted from Butkus SN, Mahan LK. Food allergies: Immunological reactions to foods. © The American Dietetic Association. Reprinted by permission from Journal of the American Dietetic Association, 86:601, 1986.)

volve the skin, gastrointestinal tract, or respiratory system (Table 41–2).

The contribution of non-IgE–mediated immunologic reactions to food hypersensitivity is not as clear. Circulating food-specific antibodies (IgG, IgA, and IgM) occur commonly. It has also been postulated that antigen-antibody complexes (type III reaction) may have a role in several food-related inflammatory diseases. These include celiac disease, various forms of colitis, enteritis with bleeding, malabsorptive disorders, ulceration, and chronic pneumonitis (Heiner's syndrome). Cell-mediated hypersensitivity (type IV reaction) may have a role in celiac disease, protein-losing enteropathies, eosinophilic gastroenteritis, and inflammatory bowel disorders, such as ulcerative colitis.

SYMPTOMS

A wide range of symptoms has been attributed to food allergy (see Table 41–2). Gastrointestinal symptoms occur most frequently, followed by symptoms involving the skin and respiratory system (Fig. 41–2). Gastrointestinal symptoms have been reported in 70% of the children studied, whereas cutaneous symptoms have been reported in 24%, and respiratory symptoms have been found in 6%. Although the distribution of symptoms reported varies with the population evaluated, respiratory symptoms are thought to be the least common and occur most often in association with other symptoms (Bock, 1986; Novembre et al., 1988).

Food-induced **anaphylaxis** is an acute, often severe, and sometimes fatal immune response that usually occurs within a limited time following exposure to an antigen. Anaphylaxis may affect any body system. The most dangerous allergic reaction is systemic anaphylaxis, which can include abdominal pain, nausea, vomiting, cyanosis, a drop in blood pressure, angioedema, chest pain, urticaria, diarrhea, shock, and death. Peanuts are the most common cause of death from anaphylaxis in the United States. People with known anaphylactic reactions to any food allergen should carry an Epi-Pen at all times.

Food-related, exercise-induced anaphylaxis (FREIA) is a distinct form of physical allergy. FREIA may occur within 2 hours after rigorous activity followed by a meal containing one or more specific foods that are normally well tolerated (Anderson, 1994; Caffarelli et al., 1996). Investigators have reported an increase in histamine release and mast cell degeneration in this disorder (Perkins, 1994).

TABLE 41–2 SYMPTOMS OF FOOD ALLERGY

Gastrointestinal Manifestations
Abdominal pain
Nausea
Vomiting
Diarrhea
Gastrointestinal bleeding
Protein-losing enteropathy
Oral and pharyngeal pruritus
Cutaneous Manifestations
Urticaria (hives)
Angioedema
Eczema
Erythema (skin inflammation)
Itching
Respiratory Manifestations
Rhinitis
Asthma
Cough
Laryngeal edema
Milk-induced syndrome with respiratory disease (Heiner's syndrome)
Systemic Manifestations
Anaphylaxis
Hypotension
Controversial or Unproven Manifestations
Behavioral conditions
Tension-fatigue syndrome
Attention-deficit and hyperactivity disorder (ADHD)
Otitis media
Psychiatric disorders
Neurologic disorders
Musculoskeletal disorders
Migraine headache

Unclear or Unproven Relationships

The role of food allergy in behavioral, psychological, neurologic, and musculoskeletal disorders remains largely unproven. Behavioral symptoms, such as hyperactivity and the tension fatigue syndrome, often anecdotally described, have not been reproduced in controlled challenge studies (Bock, 1986). Symptoms, such as irritability and fussiness, have been observed only in conjunction with gastrointestinal, skin, or respiratory symptoms (Bock, 1986 and 1987). A relationship between food allergy and migraine headaches has been suggested by some studies (Egger et al., 1983; Mansfield et al., 1985). However, these studies were conducted without double-blind, placebo-controlled tests, which makes their results controversial. In children with migraine headaches and epilepsy, avoidance of specific foods has been purported to decrease migraine headaches and seizure activity (Egger et al., 1989). However, the available data are too limited to establish food allergy as an important cause for migraine headaches or seizures. Some studies have demonstrated that patients may benefit from the elimination of specific foods if those foods are shown to be precipitating factors in food allergy (Weber et al., 1991). However, without DBPCFC tests to verify the food as a precipitating factor, foods may be restricted or eliminated inappropriately. When otitis media, migraine headaches, and headaches associated with intractable epilepsy do not respond to other treatments, evaluation of food allergy may be warranted (see Chapter 42).

Most documented allergic reactions to foods occur within 2 hours of ingestion. Symptoms vary with the amount of antigen (allergen) ingested and absorbed, the types of reactions that occur, and the sensitivity of the target organ.

COMMON FOOD ALLERGENS

Although many foods have been implicated in food allergy, relatively few foods have been documented as causing an allergic reaction. The most common food allergens are foods with high-protein content, especially those of plant or marine origin (see Table 41–3). However, food allergy may develop in response to any food included in the diet. As food allergens are highly specific, avoidance of entire botanical families or food groups usually is not necessary (Sampson, 1988).

Peanuts, tree nuts, shellfish and fish, cow's milk, chicken egg, soy, and wheat are the most frequently identified food allergens (American Academy of Allergy, Asthma, and Immunology, 1998). Although frequently described, allergic reactions to chocolate and strawberry have not been documented (Bock, 1986).

The antigens in food are often large, water-soluble glycoproteins (M.W. of 10,000 to 70,000 daltons). Individual foods contain many different proteins, of which only a few may be highly allergenic. For example, cow's milk contains more than 20 different proteins, of which beta-lactoglobulin, casein, and alpha-lactalbumin are among the most allergenic. **Cross-reactivity** between antigens may occur, especially between foods within the same bio-

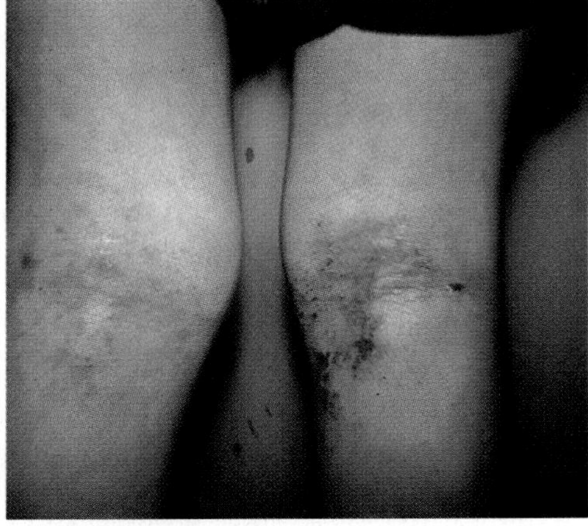

FIGURE 41–2 Atopic eczema. IgE-mediated skin reaction to a food allergen. Commonly seen on the back of knees and the inside of elbows.

TABLE 41–3 MOST COMMON ALLERGENS ACCORDING TO AGE GROUP

INFANTS/CHILDREN	ADULTS
Egg	Fish
Fish	Nuts
Milk	Peanuts
Peanuts	Shellfish
Soy	Wheat

logic family. For example, an infant who is allergic to cow's milk may be allergic to goat's milk. A child who is allergic to ragweed pollen may not tolerate melons, banana, or avocado. However, allergy to one food or pollen does not necessarily mean that there will be allergy to all related foods. In children, clinically significant cross-reactivity between legumes, such as peanuts and soybeans, is rare (Bernhisel-Broadbent and Sampson, 1989). Adverse idiosyncratic reactions to each food must be documented.

Although many allergens are unaffected by denaturation from heat and acid, the allergenicity of some proteins can be altered by heating. Antigens of some foods are removed by processing. For example, individuals sensitive to soybeans, cottonseed, peanuts, or corn usually tolerate the respective oils of these plants (Bush et al., 1984; Taylor et al., 1981). However, caution is advised for those with a history of severe anaphylactic reactions. Peanuts, other legumes, shellfish, fish, tree nuts, eggs, and milk are the foods most frequently associated with anaphylactic reactions (Joint Task Force on Practice Parameters [JTFPP], 1998).

RISK FACTORS FOR THE DEVELOPMENT OF FOOD ALLERGY

The risk of developing food allergy depends on heredity, exposure to a food (antigen), gastrointestinal permeability, and environmental factors. Heredity is thought to play a major role in the development of allergy. Atopy, the tendency to develop IgE-mediated reactions, appears to be familial. A child's risk of being atopic is estimated to be 47% to 100% when both parents are atopic and only 13% when neither parent is atopic (Ziegler et al., 1989).

Exposure to an antigen is a prerequisite for the development of food allergy. After the initial exposure to an antigen and sensitization of the immune cells, allergic reactions may occur. Infants may become sensitized to an antigen in breast milk, in which case allergic reactions may occur the first time an infant eats the antigen in food (Anderson, 1994). Susceptibility to food allergy also depends on gastrointestinal permeability, which allows antigen penetration. Gastrointestinal permeability is thought to be greatest in early infancy and to decline with intestinal maturation. Other conditions, such as gastrointestinal disease, malnutrition, prematurity, and immunodeficiency states, may also be associated with increased permeability and the risk of developing food allergy (Fig. 41–3).

The amount of antigen presented and environmental factors can also influence the development of food allergy. The effects of foods and other antigens may be additive. Clinical symptoms of food allergy may increase when inhalant allergies are exacerbated by seasonal or environmental changes. Common inhalant allergens include house dust, mites, feathers, animal dander, pollens, molds, and grain dust. Similarly, the effects of environmental factors, such as tobacco smoke, stress, exercise, and cold, may enhance the clinical symptoms of food allergy. For example, in Japan, rice is a more common allergen than it is in the United States.

FOOD INTOLERANCES

Food intolerances are adverse reactions to foods caused by nonimmunologic mechanisms, including toxic, pharmacologic, metabolic, or idiosyncratic reactions (Table 41–4). Symptoms caused by food intolerances include gastrointestinal, cutaneous, and respiratory disorders and are often the same as those related to food allergy. Therefore, food intolerances must be considered in the differential diagnosis of food allergy. Although symptoms of food intolerance may be similar to those of food allergy, different treatment may be required depending on the mechanism involved. Allergy skin testing is not useful in the diagnosis and treatment of these conditions.

Food Additives

Historically, food additives, such as preservatives, flavor enhancers, and coloring agents, have been linked to adverse reactions. Additives implicated include tartrazine (FD&C No. 5), azo dyes and other coloring agents, benzoic acid, sodium nitrate, butylated hydroxyanisole (BHA), butylated hydroxytoluene (BHT), and sulfites (Ortolani et al., 1988) (see Table 41–4).

Overall, adverse reactions to coloring agents and preservatives benzoic acid, sodium nitrate, BHA, and BHT appear to be rare, even in the groups thought to be at greatest risk. Early reports suggest that intrinsic asthmatics and aspirin-sensitive asthmatics are the most likely to react to food additives. However, more recent controlled studies reveal that challenge with tartrazine, azo dyes, and benzoic acid elicit symptoms of asthma in up to 21% of the intrinsic asthmatics studied, whereas BHA and BHT challenges elicit no response (Stevenson et al., 1986; Weber et al., 1979). Similarly, in populations with chronic urticaria, challenge with tartrazine, sodium nitrate, and benzoate is linked to

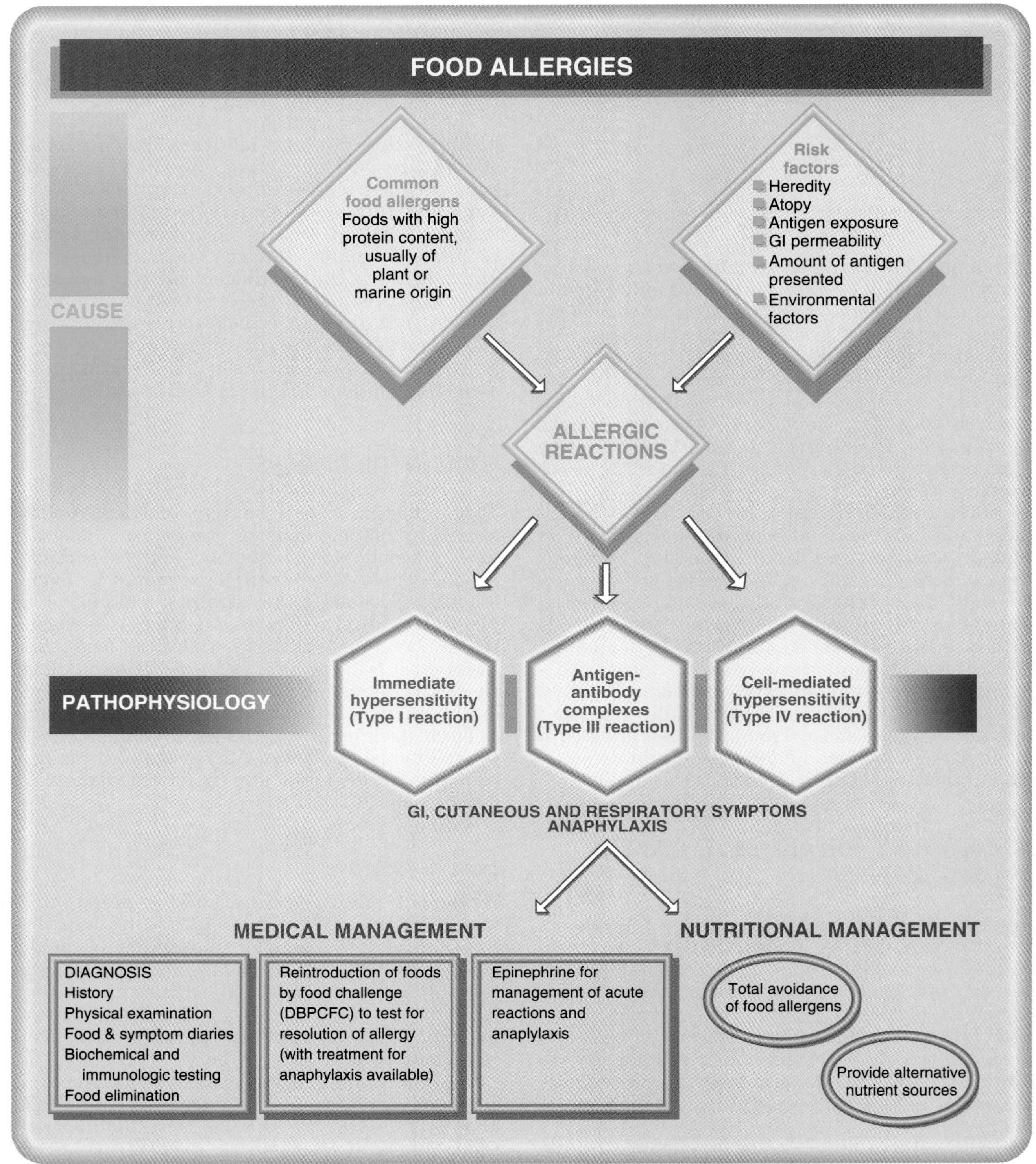

FIGURE 41–3 Pathophysiology algorithm—food allergies. (Algorithm content developed by John Anderson, Ph.D., and Sanford C. Garner, Ph.D., 2000.)

TABLE 41–4 REPRESENTATIVE NONIMMUNOLOGIC REACTIONS TO FOOD

CAUSE	ASSOCIATED FOODS	SYMPTOMS
Gastrointestinal Disorders		
Enzyme deficiency		
Lactase	Foods containing lactose and milk	Bloating, flatulence, diarrhea, abdominal pain
Glucose-6-phosphate dehydrogenase	Fava or broad beans	Hemolytic anemia
Disease		
Cystic fibrosis Gallbladder disease Enteropathies	Symptoms may be precipitated by many foods, especially high-fat foods or certain proteins	Bloating, loose stools, abdominal pain
Inborn Errors of Metabolism		
Phenylketonuria	Foods containing phenylalanine	Elevated serum phenylalanine levels, mental retardation
Galactosemia	Foods containing lactose or galactose	Vomiting, lethargy, failure to thrive
Psychological Reactions	Symptoms may be precipitated by any food.	Wide variety of symptoms involving any system
Reactions to Pharmacologic Agents in Foods		
Vasoactive amines		
Phenylethylamine	Chocolate, aged cheese, red wine	Migraine headaches
Tyramine	Cheddar cheese, French cheeses, brewers' yeast, Chianti wine, canned fish	Migraine headaches, cutaneous erythema, urticaria and hypertensive crisis in patients taking monoamine oxidase (MAO) inhibitors
Histamine	Fermented cheeses, fermented foods (e.g., sauerkraut, pork sausages, canned tuna, anchovies, sardines)	Erythema, headaches, decreased blood pressure
Histamine-releasing agents	Shellfish, chocolate, strawberries, tomatoes, peanuts, pork, wine, pineapple	Urticaria, eczema, pruritus
Reactions to Food Additives		
Tartrazine or FD&C Yellow No. 5	Yellow or yellow-orange colored foods, soft drinks, medicine	Hives, rash, asthma
Benzoic acid or sodium benzoate	Soft drinks and some cheeses, salt-free margarines, and processed potato products	Hives, rash, asthma
Sulfites		
Sodium sulfite, potassium sulfite, sodium metabisulfite, potassium metabisulfite, sodium bisulfite, potassium bisulfite, sulfur dioxide	Shrimp, many processed foods, avocado, instant potatoes, dried fruits, vegetables, acidic juices, wine, beer	Acute asthma and anaphylaxis, loss of consciousness
Reactions to Microorganism Contamination of Foods		
Proteus causes histidine to break down to a histamine-like substance (anaphylactic type reaction)	Unrefrigerated scombroid fish (tuna, bonita, mackerel); heat-stable toxin produced	Scombroid fish poisoning (itching, rash, vomiting, diarrhea)
Gonyaulax catenella (red tide)	Mussels and clams that ingest the organism that produces saxitoxin, a heat-stable neurotoxin	Paralytic shellfish poisoning (progressive numbness from head to arms); frequently fatal

(Adapted from Butkus SN, Mahan LK. Food allergies: Immunological reactions to foods. © The American Dietetic Association. Reprinted by permission from Journal of the American Dietetic Association, 86:601, 1986.)

urticaria in only 1% to 4% of those evaluated (Ortolani et al., 1988; Stevenson et al., 1986).

Adverse reactions to monosodium glutamate (MSG) are reported to include headache, nausea, flushing, abdominal pain, and asthma, and they generally occurr 1 to 14 hours after ingestion (Raiten et al., 1995). Whether or not MSG actually causes this response is still controversial. MSG is thought to be safe for most people. It is found naturally in tomatoes, parmesan cheese, and mushrooms. Restaurant meals prepared without MSG are usually available.

Although reports of an association between the use of food additives, dyes, and sugars and the occurrence of behavioral symptoms, such as hyperactivity, have been published in the popular literature, these relationships have not been supported by most controlled challenge studies (Mahan et al., 1985) (see Chapter 10). Improved behavior has been reported in preschool boys with attention-deficit and hyperactivity disorder (ADHD) who consume an additive-free and caffeine-free diet that is low in sugar; however, these effects may be related to a reduction of caloric intake in the treatment diet (Kaplan et al., 1989). Alternatively, it is possible that some food additives are related to behavioral changes in a subset of this population. However, elimination diets cannot be recommended for the routine management of hyperactivity. When families choose to pursue an additive-free diet in conjunction with recommended therapy, advice on implementing an adequate and safe diet should be provided.

Sulfites

Adverse reactions to sulfites in foods have been well documented (Steinman, 1996; Taylor, 1992). Sulfiting agents are added to many foods and beverages to prevent browning, control microbial growth and spoilage, modify texture, and bleach certain foods. Sulfites are also used as antioxidants in pharmaceuticals. Although the prevalence of sulfite sensitivity in the general population is unknown, adverse reactions among nonasthmatics have been reported (Simon, 1989). Sulfite sensitivity is most likely to occur in the asthmatic population, in whom the prevalence ranges from 2% to 8%; steroid-dependent asthmatics are at increased risk.

The diagnosis of sulfite sensitivity requires controlled, provocative challenge with sulfites. Guidelines for challenge have been outlined; most adverse reactions occur with doses of 20 to 50 mg of sulfite administered in solution (Simon, 1989). Reactions to sulfites present in foods may differ, however. Sulfite-sensitive asthmatics may not always react after ingestion of sulfite-containing foods. The occurrence of reactions depends on the nature of the food, the level of residual sulfite, the sensitivity of the individual, and, perhaps, the form of residual sulfite and the mechanism of the sulfite-induced reaction (Taylor et al., 1988).

Management of sulfite sensitivity requires avoidance of sulfite-containing foods. Foods containing high levels of sulfites are listed in Table 41–4. Since 1986, Food and Drug Administration (FDA) regulations have banned the use of sulfites on fresh fruits and vegetables other than potatoes that are served raw (see "*Focus On:* Sulfites"). Current regulations of the FDA and the Bureau of Alcohol, Tobacco, and Firearms also require labeling of packaged foods that contain sulfites added as a preservative and alcoholic beverages containing 10 ppm or more sulfite (Food and Drug Administration, 1988).

Carbohydrate Intolerance

Lactase deficiency is the most common enzyme deficiency worldwide. Individuals with a deficiency of the intestinal enzyme lactase have a decreased ability to digest lactose, which is the sugar in milk. Related symptoms following ingestion of lactose include abdominal cramping, flatulence, and diarrhea. Because the symptoms are similar, lactose intolerance is often confused with allergy to cow's milk. Deficiencies of lactase and other carbohydrate-digesting enzymes are discussed further in Chapter 31.

Gastrointestinal symptoms following the ingestion of fruit juice are commonly reported in infants and children. These symptoms may be related to carbohydrate intolerance rather than to food allergy. Carbohydrate malabsorption has been documented following ingestion of pear, apple, and grape juices. A brief restriction of fruit juices may be useful in the evaluation of infants and children with chronic, nonspecific diarrhea (see Chapter 10).

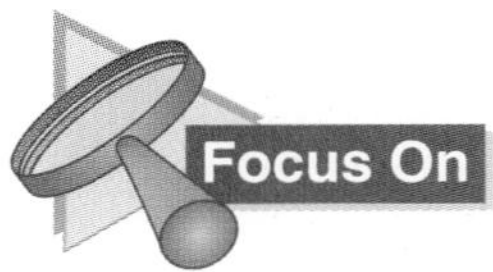

SULFITES

Approximately 5% of the estimated 9 million asthmatics in the United States are sensitive to sulfur-containing compounds that are frequently encountered in foods. In extreme cases, manifestations may include bronchospasms. Since 1985, four deaths (occuring in restaurants) attributable to this cause have been confirmed. Nonasthmatics may also be affected, but these individuals react with less severe symptoms.

Sulfur-containing compounds have, for many years, been added to a number of foods to prevent oxidation, microbial infestation, and bleaching of colors. When sulfites in the final product exceed more than 10 ppm, the label must carry the chemical name (e.g., "potassium bisulfate"). Because sulfites destroy thiamin, they are not permitted in foods that are considered to be significant sources of this vitamin (e.g., meats, some fish, and crab). (Information about foods in which added sulfites are "generally recognized as safe" can be found in the Code of Federal Regulations, 21 Food and Drugs, Parts 182 and 184.)

Sulfite-sensitive individuals can avoid offending foods by reading the labels on packaged foods. However, such labeling protection has not historically been available for sulfite-treated foods that are served fresh, such as salad-bar ingredients and menu items that are delivered to restaurants in pre-prepared forms. (Sulfites are used to prevent browning of salad greens and preserve the whiteness of peeled, raw potatoes.) Although the original packaging or containers for items, such as raw French fries and hash browns, may be properly labeled, restaurant patrons have generally not been afforded this information.

This potential hazard to asthmatics was addressed by the Food and Drug Administration (FDA) in 1986 with the prohibition of sulfite use on fresh fruits and vegetables intended to be sold or served raw or presented to the consumer as fresh. In February of 1990, a similar ban was applied to potatoes. However, the latter ban was appealed on the basis of a legal technicality related to the FDA hearings, and in May of that year, the regulation was overturned by a federal court. Alternatives are being explored by the FDA. At present, however, the safest way for the sensitive consumer to order potatoes at a restaurant is to order potatoes baked or otherwise cooked in their skins (Information, 1990).

DIAGNOSIS

No simple test can be used to diagnose food allergy. Diagnosis requires identification of the suspected food, proof that the food causes an adverse response, and verification of immunologic involvement. Nonallergic mechanisms must be ruled out. The omission of foods from the diet on the basis of improper diagnosis can and has threatened nutritional status (Altman and Chiaramonte, 1996).

A clinical history is the first tool used in diagnosis. The information gathered should include a description of symptoms, the time of food ingestion relative to the onset of symptoms, a description of the most recent reactions, a list of suspected foods, and an estimate of the quantity of food required to produce a reaction. Because food allergy may be linked to the introduction of new foods, early feeding history should be explored. Early introduction of highly allergenic foods (e.g., peanuts or other nuts) into the diet can increase the likelihood of an allergy (Sampson and Ho, 1997). Any family history of allergy should also be reviewed.

Physical examination includes measurements of weight and height (and head circumference for an infant), which are plotted on a growth chart and are evaluated in relationship to earlier measurements. Decreased weight for height measurements may be related to malabsorption and food allergy. Therefore, patterns of growth and their relationship to the onset of symptoms should be explored. Clinical signs of malnutrition should be assessed, including the evaluation of fat and muscle stores (see Chapter 16). Evidence of chronic conditions, such as **eczema** (itchy rash with red and white bumps) rhinitis, and asthma, are also evaluated.

A 7- to 14-day **food and symptom diary** may be useful if there is a perceived general food reaction with chronic symptoms but no specific suspect food, if symptoms are not well defined by the history, or when atopic dermatitis has been diagnosed. A 24-hour recall is helpful when reactions occur less frequently. Both the food diary and the 24-hour recall should include the time food is eaten, as well as the quantity, and type of food; the time symptoms appear relative to the time of food ingestion; and any medications taken before or after the onset of symptoms, as medications may alter the symptoms observed. Sometimes, the information obtained indicates something other than a food reaction. The more information obtained when a reaction occurs, the more useful the diary or recall. The 1- to 2-week diary record can also serve as a baseline for future intervention. It is especially useful when reactions to food preservatives or additives are suspected.

Biochemical testing can rule out nonallergenic causes of symptoms. A complete blood count and differential; tests of stool for reducing substances, ova, parasites, or occult blood; and a sweat chloride test for the exclusion of cystic fibrosis are examples of tests that may be useful.

Immunologic testing is useful for screening patients, but it cannot be used to diagnose food allergy. Immunologic tests may help to identify suspected allergenic foods or to confirm an immunologic mechanism (IgE-mediated food allergies). Positive immunologic test results must be confirmed by a DBPCFC, the "gold standard" for identifying food-induced symptoms (Bock et al., 1988; Plaut, 1997; Beyer et al., 1997). Reliable immunologic tests include the skin-prick test, the **radioallergosorbent test (RAST),** and the enzyme-linked immunosorbent assay (ELISA) (Table 41–5). The **CAP-RAST FEIA (fluroscein-enzyme immunoassay)** also appears promising in diagnosing food allergy because it provides a quantitative assessment of allergen-specific IgE antibody, and higher levels of antibodies are predictors of clinical symptoms (Sampson and Ho, 1997). Unfortunately, thus far, only six foods have been approved for this test—egg, milk, peanut, fish, soy, and wheat.

Skin-prick tests are the most economical and provide results within 15 to 30 minutes. Control comparisons using histamine skin-prick test results provide both positive and negative wheal diameters necessary for accurate readings (Fig. 41–4). All skin-prick tests are compared to the control wheal. Test wheals that are 3 mm greater than the negative control indicate a positive result. Negative skin-prick skin tests have excellent *negative* predictive accuracy and suggest the absence of an IgE-mediated reaction. For children younger than 2 years of age, the **skin test** is reserved to confirm im-

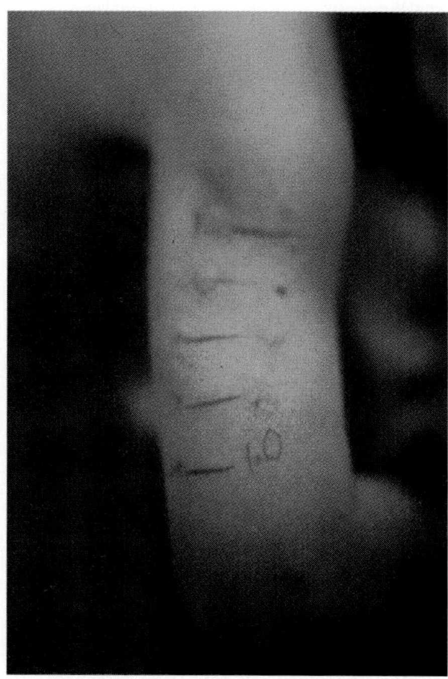

FIGURE 41–4 A skin-prick test showing the wheal and flare of the reaction to the allergen as compared to the reaction to the histamine control.

TABLE 41–5 **DIAGNOSTIC TESTS**

TYPE OF TEST	DESCRIPTION	COMMENTS
Skin testing (scratch, prick, or puncture)	A drop of antigen is placed on the skin, and the skin is then scratched or punctured to allow penetration.	Screening test; cannot be relied upon as sole diagnostic tool; a history of food-symptom relationship also important; must be followed by a DBPCFC
Radioallergosorbent test (RAST)	Serum is mixed with food on a paper disk and then washed with radioactively labeled IgE.	No more accurate than the skin test, but more costly; may be useful in people who have skin disease
Enzyme-linked immunosorbent assay (ELISA)	This test is much like RAST, except no radioactive material is used.	Same as for RAST
CAP-RAST fluroscein-enzyme immunoassay (FEIA)	Compared to RAST, this test binds more allergen.	New test for food allergy; available for only six foods as of October 1998; shows promise as a component in diagnostic process for food allergy
Cytotoxic testing	Allergen is mixed with whole blood or serum leukocyte suspension; lysed leukocytes are then counted.	Unreliable
Sublingual testing	Drops of allergen extract are placed under the tongue and symptoms are recorded.	Unreliable
Provocation testing and neutralization	Subcutaneous injection of allergen extract elicits symptoms; this is then followed by injection of a weaker or stronger preparation to neutralize symptoms.	Unreliable
Kinesiologic testing	The subject's arm is extended and foods to be tested are placed in the hand. The test is considered to yield positive results if the arm moves more easily after the food has been placed in the hand.	Unreliable

munologic mechanisms after symptoms have been confirmed by a positive test result from a food challenge, or when the history of the reaction is impressive.

RAST and ELISA are as reliable as the skin-prick test, but are more costly. Both tests may be useful for people who have had anaphylaxis or who have skin diseases, such as widespread atopic dermatitis. Many children wih atopic dermatitis have a food allergy that can be diagnosed using a skin-prick test for seven foods (milk, egg, peanut, soy, wheat, cod or catfish, and cashew); these foods account for 89% of positive food challenge tests (Burks et al., 1998).

Unreliable tests include cytotoxic testing, sublingual testing, provocative and neutralization testing, and kinesiologic testing (American Academy of Allergy, Asthma and Immunology, 1981; David, 1987) (see Table 41–5).

Food elimination is the next step in diagnosis. A food record is kept during the elimination phase. This record is used to ensure that all forms of suspected foods have been eliminated from the diet (see Fig. 41–5). It is also used to evaluate the diet's nutritional adequacy. If a limited diet continues for several weeks, vitamin or mineral supplementation may be necessary. An **elimination diet** should be personalized, when possible, for more accurate results, eliminating only one or two suspect foods at a time for each 2-week period. If multiple foods in general are indicated, a variation of the "strict" elimination diet shown in Table 41–6 should be used. Any food on the list that is suspect or that is eaten more often than once every 4 months should be substituted with a food that is rarely or almost never eaten. If the individual or the health care provider continues to suspect foods, then an elemental diet should be considered. This is the most severe form of elimination diet. It prevents malnutrition, but because it is expensive and is not always accepted, it should be reserved for the most severe cases.

Products such as Neocate or Neocate One Plus for infants and young children, and Tolerex or L-Emental formulas for teenagers and adults, can be used. Foods are added back into the diet one at a time while the individual is receiving the elemental formula. The elimination process will determine whether symptoms resolve with avoidance. If symptoms persist with careful avoidance of suspect foods, other causes for the allergy should be considered. If a positive result has been obtained on a skin test and symptoms improve unequivocally with the elimination of one or two foods, those foods can be eliminated from the diet empirically until it is appropriate to rechallenge. However, if symptoms improve only with the elimination of multiple foods, multiple food challenges are needed. If symptoms improve or resolve, a DBPCFC is indicated for confirmation (Bock et al., 1988).

Food Challenge

A food challenge is conducted once symptoms have resolved. Foods are reintroduced (challenged) one at a time on different days while the person is carefully observed in a medical setting for the recurrence of symptoms. Only one food should be challenged at a time to eliminate confusion. An initial dose of 1/10 the amount thought to cause a reaction has been recommended (Bock, 1985). The

TABLE 41–6 THREE STAGES OF ELIMINATION DIETS

	FOODS ALLOWED	FOODS TO AVOID
Elimination Diet 1: Milk-, Egg-, and Wheat-Free		
Animal protein sources	Lamb, chicken, turkey, beef, pork	Cow's milk, chicken eggs
Vegetable protein sources	Soy milk, soybeans, other beans, lentils	
Grains or alternative starches	White potato, sweet potato, yams, rice, tapioca, arrowroot, buckwheat, corn, barley, rye, millet, oats	Wheat
Vegetables	All vegetables	
Fruits	All fruits and juices	
Sweeteners	Cane or beet sugar, maple syrup, corn syrup	
Oils	Soy oil, corn oil, safflower oil, coconut oil, vegetable oil, olive oil, peanut oil, milk-free margarines	Butter and margarines that include milk
Other	Salt, all spices	
Elimination Diet 2: Stricter Elimination Diet		
Animal protein sources	Lamb	All other animal protein, including meat, fish, poultry, eggs, and milk
Vegetable protein sources	None	Soy milk, soybeans, peas, other beans, lentils, peanuts, bean sprouts, all nuts
Grains or alternative starches	White potato, sweet potato, yams, rice, tapioca, buckwheat, arrowroot, corn	Wheat, oats, barley, millet, rye
Vegetables	Most vegetables	Peas, tomatoes
Fruits	Most fruits and juices	Citrus fruits, strawberries
Sweeteners	Cane or beet sugar, maple syrup, corn syrup	
Oils	Safflower oil, coconut oil, olive oil, sesame oil	Butter, margarine, vegetable oils, soy oil, corn oil, peanut oil, nonspecific shortening, or fats of animal origin
Other	Salt, pepper, all spices,* vanilla or lemon extract, baking soda, cream of tartar	Chocolate, coffee, tea, colas and other soft drinks, alcoholic beverages
Elimination Diet 3: Severe Restriction†		
Rice in any form (rice cakes and rice cereal being especially helpful) Pineapple Apricots Cranberries Peaches Pears Apples including canned fruit and juices of these Lamb Chicken Asparagus Beets Carrots Lettuce Sweet potatoes White Vinegar Olive oil Honey Cane or beet sugar Salt Safflower oil		All other foods

*Suggest limiting number to five to minimize dietary variables.
†This is not a nutritionally complete diet and must only be used with the advice of a physician or nutritionist for short periods (2 weeks or less).
(Adapted from Bock SA. Food Allergy. A Primer for People. New York: Vantage Press, Inc., 1988, p. 39.)

dose is gradually increased until a reaction occurs or a usual serving has been consumed under observation in a controlled setting. The amount tolerated under observation can then be offered at home.

The most accurate challenge is the **double-blind, placebo-controlled food chalenge (DBPCFC),** which provides objective results, eliminating outside influences. DBPCFC is considered to be the "gold standard" when attempting to establish a food and symptom relationship, and is used to confirm food allergy. In a double-blind food challenge, neither the person administering the challenge nor the person being challenged knows which food is being offered. Each DBPCFC must be personalized. Recipes for double-blind food challenge studies must be carefully developed to avoid any hint of the flavor, color, or texture of the allergen, so that the patient does not detect the differences between the active food and the placebo food (Huijbers, 1994).

Because severe reactions can occur during a challenge, a physician must be in attendance and emergency supplies must be at hand. The first presentation may contain either the suspect food or placebo. The suspect food is concealed in a food or beverage known to be tolerated, such as applesauce, juice, or a specially prepared cookie. When the suspect food is first presented, the amount should be less than the amount believed to be necessary to trigger a reaction, which can be determined from the history reported. The quantity of food offered is then doubled with each presentation until 8 to 10 g of dried food or 60 to 100 g of fresh food has been consumed. One to three placebos should be placed randomly throughout the challenge presentations (Bock et al., 1988). Reactions have been observed in children after consumption of 20 mg to 8 g of dried food (Bock, 1986) and in adults after consumption of 5 to 100 g of fresh food (Atkins et al., 1985).

The last presentation is an open challenge of the suspect food. Reactions have occurred during the open challenge that did not occur in the blinded challenges. The risk of reaction may be reduced by mixing fresh suspect food with foods that are tolerated rather than offering dried suspect food in capsules. Occasionally, symptoms may accompany the last presentation if the threshold is greater than indicated by the history. Rechallenge is then necessary, using a greater amount than at the first challenge. Most allergic reactions occur within 2 hours of the challenge. Non–IgE-mediated reactions may occur more than 24 hours after challenge. The individual should continue to be monitored during this time (Bock et al., 1988).

Although most food allergies are not fatal, approximately 1000 Americans experience anaphylactic shock each year after eating foods to which they are extremely allergic (Schardt, 1994). The most likely triggers are peanuts, fish, nuts, shellfish, milk, eggs, and soybeans. To minimize risks to patients, all challenges that may cause an anaphylactic reaction should be carried out in a physician's office or hospital. The patient should be observed for an additional 2 hours before discharge. If there is a clear history of a life-threatening anaphylactic reaction after eating a specific food, that food should not be challenged unless there is sufficient evidence that the person is no longer reacting to the allergen and skin test results are negative.

A single-blind food challenge, in which the person receiving the challenge does not know what has been offered, may be useful in similar situations and is easier to implement. However, challenges carried out for research purposes should be DBPCFC as specifically explained (Bock, 1986 and 1988).

TREATMENT

Total avoidance of a food allergen is the only proven treatment for food allergy (Sampson, 1989; Plaut, 1997; Joint Task Force, 1998). Although many food intolerances may allow some ingestion of the offending food, food hypersensitivities do not. Families and individuals need guidelines and suggestions for avoiding allergenic foods, substituting permissible foods for restricted foods in meal planning and preparation, and selecting nutritional replacement foods. Nutritional counseling is essential and should be given the same consideration as other medical therapies (Tiainen, 1995; Carroll, 1994).

Foods to be avoided may be hidden in the diet in unfamiliar forms. To help identify and avoid offending foods, allergy-specific lists that describe foods to avoid, list key words for ingredient identification, and present acceptable substitutes may be useful (Tables 41–7 through 41–11). Caretakers should be cautioned to read labels carefully before purchasing food.

When a food-sensitive individual ingests a hidden allergen, the most common reason is that the "safe" food was contaminated. This may happen as a result of using common serving utensils, such as at an ice cream parlor, at a salad bar, or in a deli (where the meat slicer may be used to slice both meat and cheese). Another situation that may lead to the unknowing ingestion of an allergenic food occurs when

TABLE 41–7 EGG ALLERGY

Foods to Avoid*

Albumin	egg yolk	meringue
apovitellin	flavoprotein	ovalbumin
avidin	frozen eggs	ovogycoprotein
bernaise sauce	globulin	ovomucin
dried eggs	hollandaise sauce	ovomucoid
eggnog	imitation egg product	ovomuxoid
egg solids	livetin	powdered egg
egg substitutes	lysozyme	Simplesse
egg white	mayonnaise	

Egg Substitutes (Equivalent to 1 Egg)

egg replacer, such as Ener G (ENERG-G Foods Inc.), 1½ tsp + 1 T of water	1 packet plain gelatin + 2 T warm water (Do not mix until ready to use.)
½ tsp baking powder + 1 T liquid + 1 T vinegar	3 T puréed apple
1 tsp yeast dissolved in ¼ cup warm water	1 medium banana
1 T apricot purée	
1½ T water + 1½ T oil + 1 tsp baking powder	

(From Burns-Ogle G, Doerr J, Martin B [eds.]. Manual of Medical Nutrition Therapy, 3rd ed. Oklahoma City: Oklahoma Dietetic Association, 1996.)

*Eliminate the following foods, as well as any foods containing any of these ingredients, from your diet.

TABLE 41–8 COW'S MILK ALLERGY

Foods to Avoid*,†		
acidophilus milk	creamed candies	milk (whole, 2%, 1½%, 1%, ½%, skim, non-fat condensed milk)
artificial butter flavor	cultured buttermilk	semi-sweet chocolate
butter	dry milk (whole, lowfat, nonfat)	sherbet
butter fat	eggnog	sour cream
butter oil	evaporated milk	sour cream dressings
caramel candy	goat's milk ‡	sour cream solids
carob candies	half & half cream	sour milk solids
cheese (e.g., cheddar, Colby, cream, Edam, Gouda, Monterey Jack, mozzarella, Muenster, Neufchâtel, parmesan, provolone, ricotta, Romano, Swiss, cottage)	ice cream	sweetened condensed milk
chocolate milk	imitation milk, low-sodium	whipping cream
	light cream	yogurt, frozen
	low-fat ice cream	yogurt, regular
	malted milk	
	milk chocolate	
ammonium caseinate	magnesium caseinate	sodium caseinate
calcium caseinate	potassium caseinate	
casein	lactoglobulin	pudding
casein hydrolysate	lactose	rennet casein
curds	lactulose	sweet whey
custard	milk protein	whey
delactosed whey	milk protein hydrolysates	whey protein hydrolysate
lactalbumin	nougat	whey protein concentrate
lactalbumin phosphate	protein hydolysate	
Ingredients Potentially Made with Cow's Milk Products		
caramel flavoring	brown sugar flavoring	Simplesse
Bavarian cream flavoring	butter flavoring	
coconut cream flavoring	natural flavoring	
Milk Substitutes to Use in Recipes (Use to replace 1 cup of cow's milk)		
1 cup soy-based infant formula		
1 cup water		
1 cup light-colored fruit juice (e.g., apple, orange, white grape)		
1 cup soy milk (e.g., Edensoy, Westsoy, Vitasoy)		
Infant Formulas		
Elemental		
Neocate (Scientific Hospital Supplies International, Ltd.; 1-800-365-7354)		
Neocate One+ (Scientific Hospital Supplies International, Ltd.)		
Protein Hydrolysates§		
Nutramigen (Mead Johnson; 415-474-2169)		
Alimentum (Ross Laboratories; 614-624-7578)		
Ultracare for Kids (Metagenics 800-338-3948)		

(From Burns-Ogle G, Doerr J, Martin B [eds.]. Manual of Medical Nutrition Therapy, 3rd ed. Oklahoma City: Oklahoma Dietetic Association, 1996.)

†Individuals who must avoid all cow's milk sources frequently need a calcium supplement. The most readily absorbed nonmilk calcium sources are calcium citrate and calcium carbonate.

‡Goats milk protein is similar to cow's milk protein. Those with cow's milk allergy may experience similar symptoms with goat's milk ingestion. Goats milk is not recommended as a cow's milk substitute.

§Protein hydrolysate–containing formulas may cause symptoms in some infants.

*Eliminate the following foods, as well as any foods containing any of these ingredients, from your diet.

one product is used to make a second product, and only ingredients of the second product are listed on the food label. An example would be the listing of mayonnaise as an ingredient in a salad dressing without specifically listing egg as an ingredient of the mayonnaise. Lastly, manufacturing plants or restaurants may use the same equipment to produce two different products (e.g., peanut butter and almond butter) and despite cleaning, traces of an allergen may remain on the equipment between uses. Alternatively, a restaurant may use the same oil to fry both potatoes and fish (Table 41–12). (See "*Clinical Insight:* Does "Pareve" Really Mean Milk-Free?")

When foods are removed from the diet, alternative nutrient sources must be provided. Table 41–13 defines levels of nutritional risk based on the types of food removed from the diet. For example, when dairy products are omitted, other foods must provide calcium, vitamin D, protein, riboflavin, and energy. The nutritional adequacy of the diet should be monitored by conducting an ongoing evaluation of the patient's growth and nutritional status and by

TABLE 41–9 PEANUT ALLERGY

Foods to Avoid*

beer nuts
chopped peanuts
cold-pressed peanut oil
defattened peanuts
egg rolls
expelled or expressed peanut oil
fresh peanuts
granulated peanuts
ground nuts
high-protein food
hydrolyzed plant protein
hydrolyzed vegetable protein
marzipan
mixed nuts
nougat
peanut flour
peanut soup
peanuts, roasted
peanut butter
peanut oil
peanut flakes
peanuts, shelled
peanuts, whole, roasted in-shell

Additional Products That May Contain Peanuts

pie crusts
cheese cake crusts
chocolate candy
ice cream
baked goods
sauces
chili
candy
hamster feed
peanut meal
live stock feed

(From Burns-Ogle G, Doerr J, Martin [eds.]. Manual of Medical Nutrition Therapy, 3rd ed. Oklahoma City: Oklahoma Dietetic Association, 1996.)

*Eliminate all sources of peanuts from your diet. DO NOT eat any food that has touched peanuts or use any utensils used in preparing peanut-containing dishes.

Remember that peanut powder, peanut butter, and peanuts may be used in casseroles, sprinkled on top of dishes, or used as an ingredient (e.g., in vegetable dishes, fruit dishes, cookies, cakes, pastries, desserts, chili, soups, stews, egg rolls, etc.). BE CAREFUL WHEN EATING AT SOCIAL FUNCTIONS OR WHEN DINING OUT! TAKE EXTRA PRECAUTIONS WHEN DINING AT ASIAN, CHINESE, THAI, MEDITERRANEAN, AND INDIAN RESTAURANTS, AS THESE RESTAURANTS USE MANY DIFFERENT PEANUT FORMS IN MULTIPLE WAYS. YOU ARE ENCOURAGED TO AVOID RESTAURANTS THAT SERVE FOODS THAT WOULD PUT YOU AT RISK.

When possible call the manager of a restaurant 2 or 3 days before dining out. Explain why you must avoid peanuts. Find out if any form of peanuts is used as a recipe ingredient or as garnish, or if the food is cooked in peanut oil.* Explain that you have severe reactions to peanuts. NEVER, NEVER assume a dish is peanut-free just because the menu description does not mention peanut. Many restaurant dishes are purchased prepared to heat and serve. This includes more expensive restaurants. Be sure to emphasize why you are requesting this information.

Some sauces served in Mexican restaurants may contain peanuts. When dining at any restaurant, always ask your waitperson or the restaurant manager which dishes may contain peanuts. If you are not satisfied with the answer, choose a different dish or restaurant.

TABLE 41–10 SOY ALLERGY

Foods to Avoid*

chee-fan
deep-fried mature soy seed
fermented soybean paste
fermented soybeans
hamanatto
immature green soy seed
ketjap
metiauza
miso
natto
soy flour
soy grits
soy protein concentrates
soy protein isolates
soy protein shake
soy sauce
soybean curd
soybean hydrolysates
soybean lecithin[†]
soybean milk
soybean oil
soybean sprouts
sufu
tao-cho
tao-si
taotjo
tempeh
textured soy protein
textured vegetable protein (TVP)
tofu
whey-soy drink

Ingredients Potentially Made from Soybean Products

hydrolyzed plant protein
hydrolyzed soy protein
hydrolyzed vegetable protein
natural flavoring
vegetable broth
vegetable gum
vegetable starch

Soy and Milk Substitutes

rice milk
fruit juices

Infant Formulas

Elemental

Neocate (Scientific Hospital Supplies International, Ltd.; 1-800-365-7354)
Neocate One+ (Scientific Hospital Supplies International, Ltd.)

Protein Hydrolysates[‡]

Nutramigen (Mead Johnson; 415-474-2169)
Alimentum (Ross Laboratories; 614-624-7578)

(From Burns-Ogle G, Doerr J, Martin B [eds.]. Manual of Medical Nutrition Therapy, 3rd ed. Oklahoma City: Oklahoma Dietetic Association, 1996.)

*Eliminate the following foods, as well as any foods containing any of these ingredients, from your diet.

‡Note: Protein hydrolysate–containing formulas may cause symptoms in some infants. Ask your allergist, physician, or dietitian to recommend the best formula for your infant.

†Several studies indicate that soybean lecithin and soy oil are frequently tolerated by individuals who are soy-allergic.

TABLE 41–11 WHEAT ALLERGY

Foods to Avoid*

atta	laubina	wheat protein powder
bal ahar	leche alim	wheat bran
bread flour	malted cereals	wheat bread
bulgar	minchin	wheat bread crumbs
cake flour	multigrain breads	wheat flakes
cereal extract	multigrain flours	wheat germ
couscous	puffed wheat	wheat gluten
cracked wheat	red wheat flakes	wheat meal
durum flour	rolled wheat	wheat pasta
durum	semolina	wheat protein beverage
enriched flour	shredded wheat	wheat starch
farina	soft wheat flour	wheat tempeh
gluten	spelt	white flour
graham flour	superamine	whole wheat berries
high-gluten flour	triticale	whole wheat flour
high-protein flour	vital gluten	winter wheat flour
kamut flour	vitalia macaroni	

Ingredients Potentially Made from Wheat Products

hydrolyzed vegetable protein
vegetable starch
starch
gelatinized starch
modified starch
modified food starch
vegetable gum

Substitutions

When substituting any flour—either nongluten– or low-gluten–containing flour—use a recipe developed specifically for that flour. No nonwheat flour will produce an acceptable end product when substituted for wheat flour in a wheat flour–based recipe. A variety of recipes have been developed specifically for these particular grains as a replacement for wheat-containing products. See list of cookbooks on page 929.

Leavening Agents

More leavening is required in nongluten and low-gluten–containing flours.
Try adding 2 to 2½ T. baking powder per cup of nongluten or low-gluten flours.

(From Burns-Ogle G, Doerr J, Martin B [eds.]. Manual of Medical Nutrition Therapy, 3rd ed. Oklahoma City: Oklahoma Dietetic Association, 1996.)
* Eliminate the following foods, as well as any foods containing any of these ingredients, from your diet.

periodic evaluation of food records. Malnutrition and poor growth have been documented in children consuming inadequate elimination diets (David et al., 1984; Isolauri et al., 1998). Vitamin and mineral supplementation may be needed, especially when multiple foods are omitted (Tiainen, 1995).

Unless a clear diagnosis of food allergy is established, the physician may be well advised to allow the patient to return to a normal diet. The efficacy of the restricted diet and the patient's acceptance of it must be monitored by long-term follow-up studies. If symptoms persist or reappear, a review of intake will determine if all forms of suspected foods have been omitted from the diet. If symptoms persist even with adherence to the diet, other causes for the allergy should be investigated. Because food is an important part of an individual's culture, the social aspects of eating can make adherence difficult. Continued support from health care providers is needed to minimize the impact of dietary changes on family and social life. The strategies listed in Table 41–14 may help families and individuals cope with food allergies.

Desensitization treatments or medications are not viable alternatives for managing food allergy. The efficacy of desensitization shots and oral desen-

TABLE 41–12 REASONS WHY ALLERGENS MAY CONTAMINATE A FOOD

- Common serving utensils used to serve different foods
- Manufacture of two different food products using the same equipment, but without proper cleansing in between
- Misleading labels (e.g., nondairy creamers that contain sodium caseinate)
- Ingredients, added for a specific purpose, are listed on the label only in general terms of their purpose, rather than as a specific ingredient (e.g., egg white that is simply listed as an "emulsifier")
- Addition of an allergenic product to a second product that bears a label listing only the ingredients of the second product (e.g., mayonnaise)
- Switching of ingredients by food manufacturers (e.g., a shortage of one vegetable oil prompting substitution with another)
- An ingredient that is present in a food, but in such a low percentage that it does not *have* to be listed on a label

(Adapted from Steinman HA. Hidden allergens in foods. J Allergy Clin Immunol 98:241, 1996.)

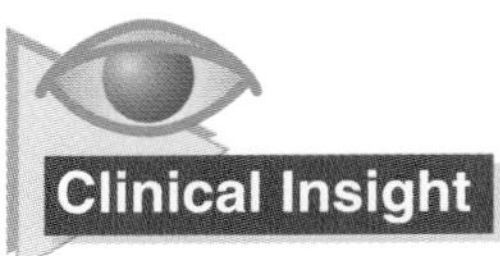

Clinical Insight

DOES "PAREVE" REALLY MEAN MILK-FREE?

by Leila Beker, M.D.

For many years, milk allergic individuals have used the kosher designation "pareve" foods to mean that the food is milk-free and therefore "safe."

Pareve products are considered milk-free from a religious standpoint and meet Jewish Dietary Law requirements. However, from a food allergy standpoint, Pareve (parev, Parve) may NOT be 100% milk-free. Equipment that has been cleaned to the Kosher Dietary Law specifications may contain trace amounts of milk or trace contamination from airborne dust in a food plant. These trace amounts of milk in products labeled Pareve do not violate religious law and these products are still considered Pareve. However, these products could present a problem to a milk allergic individual. Kosher labeling does help identify products that do have milk: kosher dairy (D), dairy equipment (DE), but relying on Parve-labeled products as 100% milk-free is NOT recommended.

The Food Allergy Network no longer recommends relying on Pareve-labeled products for milk-free diets. (Regenstein, 1998)

sitization for food allergy is unproven, and the treatments may place the patient at risk for anaphylaxis (Cohen et al., 1979).

NATURAL HISTORY

Food allergy is initiated by either IgE or non-IgE mechanisms. Hypersensitivity is most common in the first 1 to 2 years of life, and most infants outgrow their sensitivities by the age of 3 years. One third of children and adults lose their reactivity after 1 to 2 years of allergen avoidance, but those who are reactive to peanuts, nuts, fish, and shellfish rarely lose their sensitivity (Sampson and Metcalfe, 1992).

In a prospective study of 480 children who underwent follow-up evaluation until 36 months of age, 80% of the initial complaints of adverse reactions to foods occurred during the first year of life (Bock, 1987). Most restricted foods were returned to the diet within 9 months of the initial complaint, and all but 4 of the 37 confirmed or probable reactions resolved by 3 years of age. Allergies to cow's milk, soy, and egg were judged to be most likely to resolve with age (Bock, 1982). It should be noted that RAST or skin testing results for IgE sensitization may remain positive even after the food can be eaten without symptoms (Eggleson, 1987).

Because symptoms of food allergy tend to resolve with age, nutrient-dense allergenic foods should be reintroduced by food challenge every 6 to 12 months to ensure that they are not being restricted unnecessarily. After two to three positive open challenges, blinded challenges may be useful in overcoming any bias that has developed.

TABLE 41–13 NUTRITIONAL RISK IN FOOD ALLERGY MANAGEMENT

LEVEL OF RISK	FOOD CHARACTERISTICS/EXAMPLES
Low risk	Any food that can easily be eliminated with minimal or no nutritional risk to the patient **Example:** Avoidance of a specific fruit or vegetable
Moderate risk	Any food that may be encountered frequently through the food supply, yet whose elimination does not significantly limit food choices or vital nutrient sources **Example:** Avoidance of fish, crustaceans, and tree nuts
Complex risk	Any food that permeates the food supply, providing a significant source of specific nutrients that are not readily available through other foods that are a part of the normal diet, whose elimination results in a significant life-style and dietary change owing to the difficulty of avoiding that food and products containing that food **Example:** Avoidance of wheat, soy, egg, milk, peanuts, or multiple foods

(From Burns-Ogle G, Doerr J, Martin B [eds.]. Manual of Medical Nutrition Therapy, 3rd ed. Oklahoma City: Oklahoma Dietetic Association, 1996.)

FOOD ALLERGY IN INFANCY

Cow's milk or protein-containing dairy products are the most common single allergen for infants. Prevalence is approximately 2.5% in the first 3 years of life (Hoffman et al., 1997) (Fig. 41–5). In a study involving three groups of infants classified according to their reactions to cow's milk, symptoms in 53% were characterized by pallor, vomiting, and diarrhea 45 minutes to 20 hours after milk ingestion. Twenty-seven percent had predominantly urticarial and angioedematous symptoms within 5 minutes of drinking milk and displayed positive skin test reactions to milk and elevated total and milk-specific IgE antibody levels. Twenty percent of the infants displayed eczematous, bronchitic, or diarrheal symptoms, most of which developed more than 1 day after milk ingestion. These infants were the most difficult to identify clinically and had a history of chronic ill health and poor growth (Hill et al., 1986; Hill et al., 1995).

Recent studies suggest that some cases of constipation among infants and children may be related

TABLE 41–14 STRATEGIES FOR COPING WITH FOOD ALLERGY

Food Substitutions

Try to substitute item-for-item at meals. For example, if the family is eating ice cream for dessert, substitution of another type of frozen dessert may be better accepted than a dissimilar dessert, such as cookies.

Dining Out and Eating Away from Home

Eating meals away from home can be risky for individuals with food allergies. Whether at a fancy restaurant or a fast-food establishment, inadvertent exposure to an allergen can occur, even among the most knowledgeable individuals. Here are some precautions to take:

- Bring "safe" foods along to make eating out easier. For breakfast, bring along soy milk if others will be having cereal with milk.
- Alert the waitstaff to the potential severity of your food allergy/allergies.
- Question the waitstaff carefully about ingredients.
- Always carry medications.

Special Occasions

Call the host family in advance to determine what foods will be served. Offer to provide an acceptable dish that all can enjoy.

Grocery Shopping

Be informed about what foods are acceptable, and read labels carefully. Product ingredients change over time; continue to read the labels on foods, even if they were previously determined to be "safe" foods. Allow for the fact that shopping will take extra time.

Label Reading

New labeling legislation makes it easier for individuals with food allergies to identify certain potential allergens from the ingredient list on food labels. For example, when food manufacturers use protein hydrolysates or hydrolyzed vegetable protein, they must now specify the source of protein used (e.g., hydrolyzed soy or hydrolyzed corn). Although reactions to food colors or food dyes are rare, individuals who suspect an intolerance will find them listed separately on the food label, rather than categorized simply as "food color."

Substitutions in Cooking

- *Milk:* Use soy or rice milk, or fruit juice in recipes calling for milk. Use soy or rice milk for milk replacement. Use a 1:1 replacement ratio. Infant formulas, such as Neocate, Neocate One Plus, Nutramigen, or Alimentum, can also be used.
- *Egg:* In baking, achieve the emulsifying effect of one egg by combining 2 T whole wheat flour, ½ tsp oil, ½ tsp baking powder, and 2 T milk, water, or fruit juice. Egg-free substitutes are also available.
- *Chocolate:* Use carob powder, measure for measure, when substituting for cocoa. As a substitute for one square of chocolate, use 3 T carob powder plus 2 T milk, water, butter, or margarine.
- *Wheat:* Wheat flour replacements and tips for cooking without wheat are available from many sources. (See "Cookbooks for People with Food Allergies" on page 929.)

to cow's milk allergy. When symptom-free, 21 of 27 infants and 44 of 65 children were consuming a diet free of cow's milk protein (CMP). Hypersensitivity and constipation may have an allergenic pathogenesis in this population (Iacono et al., 1998). Gastroesophageal reflux as an allergic symptom has also been noted in infants allergic to cow's milk (Iacono et al., 1996).

Recommendations for Infant Feeding

Human milk is the preferred food for all infants. When use of human milk is not possible, soy protein or cow's milk protein hydrolysate formulas are alternatives to standard cow's milk formulas. If symptoms continue, Neocate, an amino-based formula, may be offered (Hill et al., 1995, Vanderhoof, 1997). Of infants allergic to cow's milk, 15% to 50% may also develop an allergy to soy (Sampson et al., 1991). Use of a protein hydrolysate formula instead of a soy formula in infants who are showing clinical symptoms of an allergic reaction to cow's milk is recommended to reduce the likelihood of sensitization to soy protein also. The American Academy of Pediatrics recommends the use of human milk or casein or whey protein hydrolysates with peptides having a molecular weight of less than 1200 daltons for infants with clinical symptoms of cow's milk or soy allergy. Commercially available casein protein hydrolysate formulas (Nutramigen, Pregestimil, and Alimentum) that meet this criterion have routinely been used to feed infants allergic to cow's milk protein, and adverse reactions have only rarely been reported. However, some whey protein hydrolysate formulas (Good Start) contain larger peptides and are not an acceptable alternative for these infants (American Academy of Pediatrics, 1989).

The use of goat's milk as an alternative to cow's milk is not recommended because of the potential cross-reactivity with beta-lactoglobulin in cow's milk. In addition, goat's milk is deficient in several nutrients and has a high renal solute load. It is especially low in folic acid, containing about 1/10 the level present in whole cow's milk or human milk. Infants receiving goat's milk instead of infant formula require supplements of iron, folacin, and vitamins A, C, and D. Goat's milk must be diluted to three-quarters strength, and carbohydrates must be added to decrease the renal solute load.

Name ______

	DAY 1 DATE ___	DAY 2 DATE ___	DAY 3 DATE ___	DAY 4 DATE ___	DAY 5 DATE ___	DAY 6 DATE ___	DAY 7 DATE ___
SYMPTOMS							
B R E A K F A S T							
SNACK SUPPLEMENTS							
SYMPTOMS							
L U N C H							
SNACK SUPPLEMENTS							
SYMPTOMS							
D I N N E R							
SNACK							
SYMPTOMS							
MEDICATION							

FIGURE 41–5 Food and symptom diary.

Sensitivity to breast milk has been reported. Allergens in the mother's diet, such as cow's milk or eggs, can pass into the breast milk and cause an allergic reaction in the infant. Sometimes, the reaction does not occur until the allergenic food is actually eaten by the infant (Cantani and Gagliesi, 1996). Infants with atopic dermatitis should be evaluated for possible food allergies. If the infant is still nursing, the mother should be placed on a 2-week diet free of milk, eggs, peanut, and soy. Food challenges are then accomplished by having the mother eat the suspect food prior to breast-feeding. If a food is judged to yield a positive test result through challenge, that food is eliminated from the mother's diet until the infant is weaned.

Foods in the mother's diet may also be associated with nonallergic reactions, usually gastrointestinal upset. Implicated foods include caffeinated beverages, chocolate, some herbal teas, cabbage, onions, turnips, garlic, radishes, rhubarb, spinach, and spices. Avoidance of the problem food by the mother may alleviate her infant's symptoms. This is preferable to discontinuing breast-feeding.

Colic

The association between colic and food allergy remains controversial. Symptoms of colic, sleeplessness, and irritability are rarely the result of an immune-mediated reaction to cow's milk protein (American Academy of Pediatrics, 1989). However, persistent colic may warrant trial of an elimination diet for the breast-feeding mother or trial of a fiber-enriched, casein hydrolysate formula for the infant receiving cow's milk or soy formula, or an amino acid–based formula, such as Pregestimil. The nutritional adequacy of the mother's diet should be monitored when foods, especially cow's milk, are omitted from her diet. A calcium supplement with vitamin D can help meet the adequate intake (AI) for calcium and vitamin D during lactation. (See Chapter 7.)

DIET AND PREVENTION OF ALLERGIC DISEASE

The role of early feeding in the development of food allergy and allergic disease remains an area of controversy. Breast-feeding, together with maternal avoidance of allergens, may delay the development of allergic disease in high-risk infants (Kendall and Gloeckner, 1994; Cantani and Gagliesi, 1996). Reduced exposure to allergenic foods during infancy has been associated with a decreased prevalence of food allergy during the first year and a delay in the onset of atopic dermatitis (Steinman, 1994). Breast-feeding the infant is strongly encouraged, even if only for the first few days of life. Breast milk is always best, but a casein hydrolysate formula or amino acid–based formula can be used for infants at risk for atopic disease. When possible, the infant should be exclusively breast-fed for the first 6 months of life. A protein hydrolysate or amino acid–based formula can be used to supplement as necessary. Withholding highly allergenic foods, such as milk, eggs, peanuts, tree nuts, and fish, from children at high risk for allergy for the first 2 to 3 years of life has been recommended (Sampson and Scanlon, 1989; Cantani and Gagliesi, 1996).

TABLE 41–15 FOODS KNOWN TO CROSS-REACT IN LATEX ALLERGY

Banana	Potato
Avocado	Cherry
Kiwi	Grape
Chestnut	Celery
Papaya	Tomato
Passion fruit	Carrot
Pineapple	Wheat
Peach	Hazelnut
Nectarine	Rye
Fig	Apple
Melon	Pear

Latex Allergy

The diagnosis of latex allergy has increased remarkably since 1989. Symptoms include contact dermatitis (type IV) and immediate allergic reactions (type I), as manifested by rhinitis, asthma, conjunctivitis, angioedema, urticaria, anaphylaxis, and death (Sussman and Gold, 1996). Cross-reactivity between latex and multiple foods has been reported as well, and certain foods must be avoided (Beezhold et al., 1999; Slater, 1994; Brehler et al., 1997) (Table 41–15). In addition, latex gloves should

CASE STUDY

Sally J. is 4 years old. As an infant, she was unable to tolerate a standard cow's milk–based formula. The pediatrician recommended that Mrs. J. switch to a casein hydrolysate formula, which Sally tolerated well. As she became older, Sally was able to tolerate cow's milk, but when she ate peanuts or eggs, she experienced a variety of symptoms, including wheezing, runny eyes, and hives.

Until now, Mrs. J. was able to monitor carefully what Sally ate. Preparing meals without the offending foods has not posed a problem. In the fall, however, Sally will be entering kindergarten. Mrs. J is worried because she heard that the snack most frequently served in school is peanut butter on crackers.

1. What is the best dietary intervention for Sally?
2. What are some measures Mrs. J will have to take regarding Sally's food allergies in school?
3. What other circumstances may arise that may warrant special instructions to caregivers?
4. As Sally gets older, what can Mrs. J. begin to teach her that will help Sally manage her food allergies independently?

not be worn while preparing foods for these individuals. Individuals who work in the latex industry, health care workers, and children with spina bifida who tend to be atopic are considered to be at increased risk for allergic reactions (Committee Report, 1993; Slater, 1994). It should also be noted that individuals with food allergies may also have latex allergy. Thus, careful history taking is critical when working with those belonging to a high-risk group (e.g., patients with spina bifida). Research continues to try to define this cross-reactivity and the foods that need to be avoided. More information can be found at www.execpc.com/~alert.

Genetic Engineering

Genetic engineering can transfer an allergen from one food into another, usually from expression of one or more proteins (Fuchs and Astwood, 1996; Metcalfe et al., 1996; Nordlee et al., 1996). Further engineering may someday be available to reduce levels of specific antigens in the food supply.

CITED REFERENCES

Altman D, Chiaramonte L. Clinical aspects of allergic disease. J Allergy Clin Immunol 97:1247, 1996.

American Academy of Allergy, Asthma, and Immunology. Position statement: Controversial techniques. J Allergy Clin Immunol 67:333, 1981.

American Academy of Allergy, Asthma, and Immunology. Position Statement on anaphylaxis in school and other childcare settings. J Allergy Clin Immunol 102:173, 1998.

American Academy of Pediatrics, Committee on Nutrition: Hypoallergenic infant formulas. Pediatrics 83:1068, 1989.

Anderson JA. Tips when considering the diagnosis of food allergy. Top Clin Nutr 9:11, 1994.

Atkins FM, et al. Evaluation of immediate adverse reactions to foods in adult patients. Part II: A detailed analysis of reaction patterns during oral food challenge. J Allergy Clin Immunol 75:356, 1985.

Beezhold DH, et al. Latex allergy can induce clinical reactions to specific foods. Clin Exp Allergy 26:416, 1996.

Bernhisel-Broadbent J, Sampson H. Cross-allergenicity in the legume botanical family in children with food hypersensitivity. J Allergy Clin Immunol 83:435, 1989.

Beyer K, et al. Severe allergic reactions to foods are predicted by increases of CD4+CE45RO+ T cells and loss of L-selectin expression. J Allergy Clin Immunol 99:522, 1997.

Bock SA. A critical evaluation of clinical trials in adverse reactions to foods in children. J Allergy Clin Immunol 78:165, 1986.

Bock SA. The natural history of food sensitivity. J Allergy Clin Immunol 69:173, 1982.

Bock SA. Natural history of severe reactions to foods in young children. J Pediatr 107:676, 1985.

Bock SA. Prospective appraisal of complaints of adverse reactions to foods in children during the first 3 years of life. Pediatrics 79:683, 1987.

Bock SA, et al. Double-blind, placebo-controlled food challenge (DBPCFC) as an office procedure: A manual. J Allergy Clin Immunol 82:986, 1988.

Burks A, et al. Atopic dermatitis and food hypersensitivity reactions. J Pediatr 132:132, 1998.

Bush RK, et al. Soybean oil is not allergenic to soybean-sensitive individuals. J Allergy Clin Immunol 73:176, 1984.

Butkus SN, Mahan LK. Food allergies: Immunological reactions to foods. J Am Diet Assoc 86:601, 1986.

Caffarelli C, et al. Respiratory pathophysiologic responses: Reduced pulmonary function in multiple food-induced, exercise-related episodes of anaphylaxis. J Allergy Clin Immunol 98:4, 1996.

Cantani A, Gagliesi D. Severe reactions to cow's milk in very young infants at risk of atopy. Allergy Asthma Proc 17:205, 1996.

Carroll P. Guidelines for counseling patients with food sensitivities. Top Clin Nutr 9(3):33, 1994.

Cohen SH, et al. Acute allergic reaction after composite pollen ingestion. J Allergy Clin Immunol 64:270, 1979.

David TJ. Unorthodox allergy procedures. Arch Dis Child 62:1060, 1987.

David TJ, et al. Nutritional hazards of elimination diets in children with atopic eczema. Arch Dis Child 59:323, 1984.

Egger J, et al. Is migraine food allergy? Lancet 2:805, 1983.

Egger J, et al. Oligoantigenic diet treatment of children with epilepsy and migraine. J Pediatr 114:51, 1989.

Eggleson PA. Prospective studies in the natural history of food allergy. Ann Allergy 59:179, 1987.

Fuchs R, Astwood J. Allergenicity assessment of foods derived from genetically modified plants. Food Technol 50:83, 1996.

Grote M, et al. In situ localization of a high molecular weight cross-reactive allergen in pollen and plant-derived food by immunogold electron microscopy. J Allergy Clin Immunol 101:250, 1998.

Hide D. Food Allergy Child. Clinical Experimental Allergy 24:1, 1994.

Hill DJ, et al. Allergens, IgE, mediators, inflammatory mechanisms. J Allergy Clin Immunol 96:386, 1995.

Hill DJ, et al. Manifestations of milk allergy in infancy: Clinical and immunologic findings. J Pediatr 109:270, 1986.

Hoffman KM, et al. Evaluation of the usefulness of lymphocyte proliferation assays in the diagnosis of allergy to cow's milk. J Allergy Clin Immunol 99:3, 360, 1997.

Huijbers G, et al. Masking foods for food challenge: Practical aspects of masking foods for a double-blind, placebo-controlled food challenge. J Am Diet Assoc 94:645, 1994.

Iacono G, et al. Gastroesophageal reflux and cow's milk allergy in infants: A prospective study. J Allergy Clin Immunol 97:822, 1996.

Iacono G, et al. Intolerance of cow's milk and chronic constipation in children. N Engl J Med, 339:1100, 1998.

Information on foods containing sulfiting agents. Seattle District, WA: Food and Drug Administration, March 1990.

Joint Task Force on Practice Parameters (JTFPP) representing the American Academy of Allergy, Asthma and Immunology; American College of Allergy, Asthma and Immunology; and the Joint Council of Allergy, Asthma and Immunology: The Diagnosis and Management of Anaphylaxis. J Allergy Clin Immunol 101 (pt. 2): S488, 1998.

Kaplan BJ, et al. Dietary replacement in preschool-aged hyperactive boys. Pediatrics 83:7, 1989.

Kendall P, Gloeckner J. Managing food allergies and sensitivities. Top Clin Nutr 9(3):1, 1994.

Latex allergy can induce clinical reactions to specific foods. In: Clinical and Experimental Allergy, vol. 26, 1996, p. 416.

Mahan LK, et al. Sugar allergy and children's behavior. J Allergy Clin Immunol 75:177, 1985.

Mansfield LE, et al. Food allergy and adult migraine: Double-blind and mediator confirmation of allergic etiology. Ann Allergy 55:126, 1985.

Metcalfe D, et al. Assessment of the allergenic potential of food derived from genetically engineered crop plants. Crit Rev Food Sci Nutr 36(suppl):S165, 1996.

Nordlee J, et al. Identification of a brazil-nut allergen in transgenic soybeans. N Engl J Med 334:688, 1996.

Novembre E, et al. Foods and respiratory allergy. J Allergy Clin Immunol 81:1059, 1988.

Ortolani C, et al. Chemicals and drugs as triggers of food-associated disorder. Ann Allergy 60:358, 1988.

Perkins J. Update on food allergy research. Top Clin Nutr 9:22, 1994.

Plaut MD. Workshop synopses: New directions in food allergy research. J Allergy Clin Immunol 100:7, 1997.

Raiten D, et al. Executive summary from the report: Analysis of adverse reactions to monosodium gutamate (MSG). J Nutr 125:2892S, 1995.

Regenstein JM. Are "Pareve" products really milk-free? Food Allergy News, 17(6):1, 1998.

Sampson H, Ho D. Relationship between food-specific IgE concentrations and the risk of positive food challenges in children and adolescents. J Allergy Clin Immunol 100:444, 1997.

Sampson H, Metcalfe D. Primer on allergic and immunologic diseases. JAMA 268:2840, 1992.

Sampson HA. Food allergy. J Allergy Clin Immunol 84(pt. 2):1062, 1989.

Sampson HA. The role of food allergy and mediator release in atopic dermatitis. J Allergy Clin Immunol 81:635, 1988.

Sampson HA, Scanlon S. Natural history of food hypersensitivity in children with atopic dermatitis. J Pediatr 115:23, 1989.

Sampson HA, et al. Safety of casein hydrolysate formula in children with cow's milk allergy. J Pediatr 118:520, 1991.

Simon RA. Sulfite challenge for the diagnosis of sensitivity. Allergy Proc 10:357, 1989.

Slater J. Latex allergy. J Allergy Clin Immunol. 94:2, part 2, 1994.

Steinman HA. Hidden allergens in foods. J Allergy Clin Immunol 98:241, 1996.

Stevenson DD, et al. Adverse reactions to tartrazine. J Allergy Clin Immunol 78:182, 1986.

Sulfite ban deemed null and void. Tufts University Diet Nutr Lett 8(8):1, October, 1990.

Sussman G, Gold M. Guidelines for the Management of Latex Allergies and Safe Latex Use in Health Care Facilities. Arlington Heights, IL: American College of Allergy, Asthma, and Immunology, March, 1996, http://allergy.meg.edu.

Taylor S. The 48th Annual Meeting of the American Academy of Allergy and Immunology. Food Safety Note 3:13, 1992.

Taylor SL, et al. Peanut oil is not allergenic for peanut-sensitive individuals. J Allergy Clin Immunol 68:372, 1981.
Taylor SL, et al. Sensitivity to sulfited foods among sulfite-sensitive subjects with asthma. J Allergy Clin Immunol 81:1159, 1988.
Taylor SL, et al. Food allergies and avoidance diets. Nutr Today, 34(1):15, 1999.
Tiainen J, et al. Diet and nutritional status in children with cow's milk allergy. Euro Clin Nutr 49:605, 1995.
Vanderhoof JA. Intolerance to protein hydrolysate infant formulas: An underrecognized cause of gastrointestinal symptoms in infants. J Pediatr 131:741, 1997.
Weber RW, et al. Incidence of bronchoconstriction due to aspirin, azo dyes, non-azo dyes, and preservatives in a population of perennial asthmatics. J Allergy Clin Immunol 64:32, 1979.
Weber RW, Vaughn TR. Food and migraine headache. Immunol Allergy Clin N Am, 11:831, 1991.
Ziegler RS, et al. Effect of combined maternal and infant food-allergen avoidance on development of atopy in early infancy: A randomized study. J Allergy Clin Immunol 84:72, 1989.

ADDITIONAL REFERENCES

Bock SA. Food sensitivity: A critical review and practical approach. Am J Dis Child 134:973, 1980.
Chandra R, et al. Food allergy and atopic disease: Pathogenesis, diagnosis, prediction of high risk, and prevention. Ann Allergy 71:495, 1993.
Clinical management of latex allergy. Nutr in Clin Prac 12:68, 1997.
Ferguson A. Food sensitivity or self-deception? N Engl J Med 323:476, 1990.
Food allergy. Peanut anaphylaxis. Allergy Proc 10:249, 1989.
Hattevig G, et al. Clinical symptoms and IgE responses to common food proteins and inhalants in the first 7 years of life. Clin Allergy 17:571, 1987.
Katsunama T, et al. Wheat-dependent exercise-induced anaphylaxis: Inhibition by sodium bicarbonate. Am Allergy 68:184, 1992.
Lessof M. Food Intolerance. New York: Routledge, Chapman and Hall, 1992.
Munoz-Furlong A. The food allergy network. Top Clin Nutr 9(3):38, 1994.
Panaush RS. Delayed reactions to foods, food allergy and rheumatic disease. Ann Allergy 56:500, 1986.
Parker S, et al. Foods perceived by adults as causing adverse reactions. J Am Diet Assoc 93:40, 1993.
Perkin J. Food Allergies and Adverse Reactions. Gaithersburg, MD: Aspen Publishers, 1990.
Poysa L, et al. Atopy in children with and without a family history of atopy. Part 1: Clinical manifestations with special reference to diet in infancy. Acta Paediatr Scand 78:896, 1989.
Roesler TA, et al. Factitious food allergy and failure to thrive. Arch Pediatr Adolesc Med 148:1150, 1994.
Van Bever HP, et al. Food and food additives in severe atopic dermatitis. Allergy 44:588, 1989.
Van Hooser B, Crawford LV. Allergy diets for infants and children. Comp Therapy 15:38, 1989.

ORGANIZATIONS THAT PROVIDE INFORMATION ON FOOD ALLERGY

Allergy and Asthma Network/Mothers of Asthmatics, Inc.
3554 Chain Bridge Road
Suite 200
Fairfax, VA 22030-2709
http://www.podi.com/health/aanma

American Academy of Allergy, Asthma and Immunology
611 East Wells Street
Milwaukee, WI 53202
http://www.aaaai.org

American College of Allergy, Asthma and Immunology
85 West Algonquin Road
Suite 550
Arlington Heights, IL 60005
http://allergy.mcg.edu

The American Dietetic Association
216 West Jackson Boulevard
Suite 800
Chicago, IL 60606
http://www.eatright.org

The Asthma and Allergy Foundation of America
1125 15th Street, N.W.
Suite 502
Washington, DC 20005

The Food Allergy Network
10400 Eaton Place
Suite 107
Fairfax, VA 22030-2208
http://www.foodallergy.org

Allergy to Latex Education and Resource Team, Inc.
P.O. Box 13930
Milwaukee, WI 53212-0930
Phone: 1-888-97ALERT
http://www.execpc.com/~alert

International Food Information Council (IFIC) Foundation
1100 Connecticut Avenue, NW, Suite 430
Washington, DC 20036
Phone: 202-296-6540
FAX: 202-296-6547
http://ificinfo.health.org

COOKBOOKS FOR PEOPLE WITH FOOD ALLERGIES

- *The Allergy Cookbook: Diets Unlimited for the Limited Diet*
  by Jerry Dolovich, M.D.
  Allergy Information Association
  Room 7, 25 Poynter Avenue
  Weston, Ontario, Canada M9R 1K8
  Phone: 416/244-9312
- *The Allergy Cookbook and Food Buying Guide*
  by Pamela Nonken and S. Roger Hirsch, M.D.
  Warner Publishers
  307 5th Avenue
  New York, NY 10016
  Phone: 212/725-4500
- *Allergy Recipes*
  American Dietetic Association
  208 South LaSalle Street
  Suite 1100
  Chicago, IL 60604-1003
- *Baking for People with Food Allergies*
  by U.S. Department of Agriculture
  Superintendent of Documents
  U.S. Government Printing Office
  Washington, DC 20402
  Home and Garden Bulletin #137
- *The Complete Food Allergy Cookbook: "The Foods You've Always Loved with the Ingredients You Can't Have!"*
  Prima Publishing
  P.O. Box 1260BK

Rocklin, CA 95677
Phone: 916/632-4400
$22.95; quantity discounts available

- *Cooking for the Allergic Child*
  by Judy Moyer
  Collegiate Pride, Inc.
  Publishing Division
  3019 Enterprise Drive
  State College, PA 16801
  Phone: 814/237-4377
- *Cooking Without—Recipes for the Allergic Child and Family*
  by Margaret Williams
  Tricor, Inc.
  P.O. Box 3
  Milford, PA 18337
  Phone: 201/293-3466
- *Cooking for People with Food Allergies*
  by USDA Human Nutrition Information Service
  Superintendent of Documents
  U.S. Government Printing Office
  Washington, DC 20402
  Stock #: 001-000-04512-1; $1.50
- Ener-G Foods, Inc.
  P.O. Box 24723
  Seattle, WA 98124
  This company sells specialty foods for wheat-, milk, soy-, gluten, and egg-free diets. Mail order is available.
- *Going Against the Grain: Wheat-Free Cookery*
  by Phyllis Potts
  Central Point Publishing
  21861 S. Central Point Road
  Oregon City, OR 97045
  $14.95
- *Special Recipes and Allergy Aids Booklet*
  General Foods Consumer Center
  Nutrition Series
  250 North Street
  White Plains, NY 10625
- *Wheat-, Milk- and Egg-Free Recipes Allergy Booklet*
  Consumer Services Department
  Quaker Oats Company
  Chicago, IL 60654

CHAPTER 42

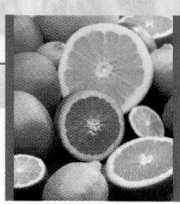

Medical Nutrition Therapy for Neurologic Disorders

LEEANN R. SHIVELEY, MPH, RD
AND PATRICK J. CONNOLLY, MD

Chapter Outline

- Neurologic Disease Classification
- Nervous System Wiring and Lesions
- Localizing Signs of Mass Lesions
- Medical Nutrition Therapy
- Neurologic Diseases Arising from Nutritional Deficiencies or Excesses: Primary Prevention Strategies
- Neurologic Diseases with Non-Nutritional Etiologies: Secondary Intervention Strategies

Key Terms

AGNOSIA—loss of comprehension that occurs as a manifestation of Alzheimer's disease
ANOMIA—inability to remember names of objects; a common manifestation of Alzheimer's disease
APRAXIA—inability to perform purposeful movements although there is no sensory or motor impairment
ASPIRATION—inhalation of foreign object(s) into the lungs
ASPIRATION PNEUMONIA—pulmonary bacterial infection induced by reflux of gastrointestinal contents, thus introducing the bacterial load of the oral cavity to the lungs
ATAXIA—impaired muscular movement, especially voluntary movement
COMMINUTION—splintering of bone into many fragments
CORPUS CALLOSUM—the bridge between the two hemispheres of the brain, consisting of white matter
CORTICAL BLINDNESS—blindness resulting from a lesion of visual area of cerebral cortex
DEGLUTITORY DYSFUNCTION—swallowing irregularity
DIFFUSE AXONAL INJURY—injury of axons throughout the brain, usually in the brain stem
DYSARTHRIA—impairment of the tongue or other muscles essential to speech, which makes speaking difficult
DYSGEUSIA—impaired taste
DYSPHAGIA—difficulty swallowing
ECHOLALIA—repeating spoken words by others, manifestation of Alzheimer's disease and psychotic disorders
EMBOLIC STROKE—occlusion of an artery by cholesterol plaque, depriving part of the brain's oxygen supply
EPIDURAL HEMATOMA—usually from trauma, bleeding between the skull and the dura mater
FAUCES—the constricted opening leading from the mouth and the oral pharynx
HEMIPARESIS—weakness affecting only one side of the body
HEMIANOPSIA—blindness for half of the visual field or vision in one eye
HEMOTYMPANUM—fluid or blood behind the eardrum or leaking from the ear, suggesting a skull base fracture
HYDROCEPHALUS—accumulation of cerebrospinal fluid within ventricles of the brain
MYCOPLASMA—a bacterial organism associated with Guillain-Barré syndrome
MYELOPATHY—any pathologic condition of the spinal cord
NYSTAGMUS—constant, involuntary movement of the eyeball
OTORRHEA—clear fluid running from the ear, suggesting a skull base fracture
PARESTHESIA—numbness sensation, heightened sensitivity, experienced in central and peripheral nerve lesions and in locomotor ataxia
PERIPHERAL NEUROPATHY—functional disturbance or pathologic changes in the peripheral nervous system; noninflammatory lesions in the peripheral nervous system
PETIT MAL SEIZURE—one of three former classifications of epilepsy; "absence" seizure
SUBARACHNOID HEMORRHAGE (SAH)—bleeding into subarachnoid space, often caused by a ruptured aneurysm in the arteries at the base of the brain
SUBDURAL HEMATOMA—blood collection between dura mater and arachnoid membrane
THROMBOEMBOLIC EVENT—obstruction of a blood vessel by a thrombus that has become detached from its site of formation
THROMBOTIC STROKE—the rupturing of a cholesterol plaque in an artery with subsequent platelet aggregation to clot an already narrowed artery
TRANSIENT ISCHEMIC ATTACK (TIA)—a brief attack lasting from a few minutes to hours of cerebral dysfunction of vascular origin with no persistent neurologic defect
TONIC-CLONIC SEIZURE—"grand mal" seizure

Despite knowledge and understanding of the nutrients required to prevent neurologic diseases, diseases of the nervous system continue to pose serious health problems of worldwide magnitude and are still seen in epidemic proportions. Between 1991 and 1994, when sudden economic and political changes occurred in Cuba, the Cuban Ministry of Public Health reported over 50,000 cases of optic and peripheral neuropathy among its population of 10.8 million. The pathogenesis was associated with an acute nutritional deficiency combined with the toxic effects of tobacco. A significant number of patients improved after treatment with parenteral administration of vitamin B-complex vitamins (high doses of thiamine, riboflavin, B_6, and B_{12}); oral supplements of vitamins A, E, and folic acid; and consumption of a high-protein diet for 10 days. Prophylactic vitamin supplements were subsequently distributed to the entire population and after only 2 months, the incidence of disease had plummeted (Ordunez-Garcia et al., 1996).

NEUROLOGIC DISEASE CLASSIFICATION

Nutritional issues associated with neurologic disease can be classified into two types. The first type is neurologic disease arising from nutritional deficiencies or excesses as described above. Primary prevention is the cornerstone of management for this first group and can usually be translated to correction of a deficiency.

Because overnutrition is so prevalent in developed countries, one would not expect the prevalence of nutritional deficiencies to be as high as it is. Most often, diseases of the nervous system having a nutritional etiology are attributed to alcoholism, malnutrition, and malabsorption (Table 42–1). For malabsorptive states refer to Chapter 30. Although many neurologic dysfunctions occur secondarily to a deficiency of a single or several vitamins, other diseases of the nervous system may be attributed to dietary excess. For a comprehensive list of neurologic diseases having nutritional, prevention, and treatment strategies, refer to Table 42–2.

The second category of neurologic disease has an etiology that is not nutritional, but has nutritional considerations that are integral to medical management. Specific nutritional therapies are adjuncts to disease management. Many elements of nutrition in neurologic disease are similar, regardless of the origin of the disease process.

NERVOUS SYSTEM WIRING AND LESIONS

The central nervous system (CNS) in mammals is functionally differentiated in three dimensions. This implies that lesions of the nervous system can leave a unique "calling card" of localized dysfunction. A primer of localizing lesions is given, with particular emphasis afforded to nutritionally significant dysfunction.

TABLE 42–1 SOME CAUSES OF NEUROLOGIC DISORDER DUE TO MALABSORPTION

Defective intraluminal hydrolysis	Gastric resection Pancreatic insufficiency Exclusion or deficiency of bile salts
Primary mucosal cell abnormality	Celiac disease Abetalipoproteinemia
Inadequate absorption surface	Massive small gut resection Ileal resection or bypass Jejunal bypass Jejunocolic fistula Gastroileostomy
Abnormalities of intestinal wall	Ileojejunitis Amyloidosis Radiation injury
Lymphatic obstruction and stasis	Lymphoma Tuberculosis
Bacterial overgrowth and parasitic infections	Blind loops Jejunal diverticula Scleroderma Whipple's disease Tropical sprue D-lactic acidosis
Miscellaneous	Diabetic neuropathy Hypoparathyroidism Hypothyroidism

(From Glickman R. Pathophysiology and diagnosis. In: Wyngaarden JB, Smith LH Jr. (eds.). Cecil's Textbook of Medicine, 16th ed. Philadelphia: WB Saunders, p. 678, 1982.)

Nerve tracts coming to and from the brain cross to opposite sides in the CNS (Fig. 42–1). Therefore, a lesion in the brain that affects the right arm would be found on the left side of the brain. Signs of weakness are the most quantifiable clinical signs of nervous system disease.

The neurons in the motor strip (upper motor neurons) receive input from all parts of the brain and project their axons all the way to their destinations in the spinal cord. Here they connect to the spinal cord motor neurons (lower motor neurons). These neurons extend from the spinal cord to muscles without interruption. The location of a lesion in the nervous system can often be deduced clinically by observing stereotypical abnormalities of either upper or lower motor neurons (Table 42–3).

LOCALIZING SIGNS OF MASS LESIONS

The frontal lobes are the source of our most complex activities, and therefore commonly offer the most complex presentations. Psychiatric manifestations such as depression, mania, or personality change may herald a tumor or other frontal lobe mass, either right or left. If the tumor is near the base of the skull, one may lose the sense of smell or have visual changes because the olfactory and optic nerves track along the bottom of the frontal lobes.

TABLE 42–2 NEUROLOGIC SYNDROMES ATTRIBUTED TO NUTRITIONAL DEFICIENCY OR EXCESS

NUTRITIONAL DEFICIENCY

Site of Major Syndrome	Name
Encephalon	Hypocalcemia (lack of vitamin D), tetany, seizures
	Mental retardation (protein-calorie deprivation)
	Cretinism (lack of iodine)
	Wernicke-Korsakoff syndrome (thiamine)
Corpus callosum	Marchiafava-Bignami disease
Optic nerve	Nutritional deficiency optic neuropathy ("tobacco-alcohol amblyopia")
Brain stem	Central pontine myelinolysis
Cerebellum	Alcoholic cerebellar degeneration
	Vitamin E deficiency in bowel disease
Spinal cord	Combined system disease (B_{12} deficiency)
	Tropical spastic paraparesis (some forms?)
Peripheral nerves	Beriberi (thiamine), pellagra (nicotinic acid)
	Hypophosphatemia (?)
	Tetany (vitamin D deficiency)
Muscle	Myopathy of osteomalacia

NUTRITIONAL EXCESS

Syndrome	Condition	Agent
Increased intracranial pressure	Self-medication	Vitamin A
Encephalopathy	Phenylketonuria	Phenylalanine
	Water intoxication	Water
	Hepatic encephalopathy	Protein (and NH_3)
	Ketotic or nonketotic coma in diabetes	Glucose
Strokes	Hyperlipidemia	Lipid
Peripheral neuropathy	Hypochondriasis	Pyridoxine
	Insomnia, anxiety	Tryptophan, contaminated
Myopathy	Anorexia nervosa, bulimia	Emetine, ipecac
Myoglobinuria	Constipation	Licorice

Lesions in the central portion of the frontal lobes may present as a motor **apraxia.** Here, the patient cannot properly execute a complex activity, although he or she is strong and understands a request to perform the activity. The frontal lobes are larger than normally appreciated, and the posterior portions of the frontal lobes are where the motor strips are located. Lesions here will exhibit upper motor neuron signs in the part of the body governed by this cortex. Temporal lobes offer memory and speech functions, so lesions here may affect these. Although any lesion of cerebral gray matter may produce seizures, the temporal lobes are particularly prone to seizures. In the right parietal lobe, masses may cause a chronic inability to focus attention in which the patient completely ignores the left side of the body. The speech centers are located near the junction of the left temporal, parietal, and frontal lobes. Pathology in this region may cause speech problems.

TABLE 42–3 CLINICAL DIFFERENCES BETWEEN UPPER AND LOWER MOTOR NEURON LESIONS

UPPER MOTOR NEURON FINDINGS	LOWER MOTOR NEURON FINDINGS
Weakness	Weakness
Stiff limbs	Floppy limbs
Sensory loss less common	Sensory loss more common
Increased reflexes	Decreased reflexes

The occipital lobes are reserved for vision, and dysfunction here may bring about **cortical blindness** of varying degrees. In this condition, the patient is unaware that he or she cannot see. Lesions at other points along the visual pathway can cause several different types of visual field deficits.

Lesions of the cerebellum and brain stem may obstruct the ventricular system where it is most narrow. This obstruction may precipitate life-threatening **hydrocephalus,** a condition of increased intracranial pressure (ICP) that may quickly result in death. Other signs of hydrocephalus include trouble with balance, walking and coordination abnormalities, and marked sleepiness. The patient may complain of a headache that is worse on awakening. Lesions in the brain stem may infiltrate any of the cranial nerves (Table 42–4), which enervate structures of the face and head, including the eyes, ears, jaw, tongue, pharynx, and the facial muscles. These may often have consequences for nutrition because the patient is often unable to eat without risking aspiration of food or liquids into the lung. Other means of nutrition are often necessary. Tumors or other lesions in the medulla may infiltrate

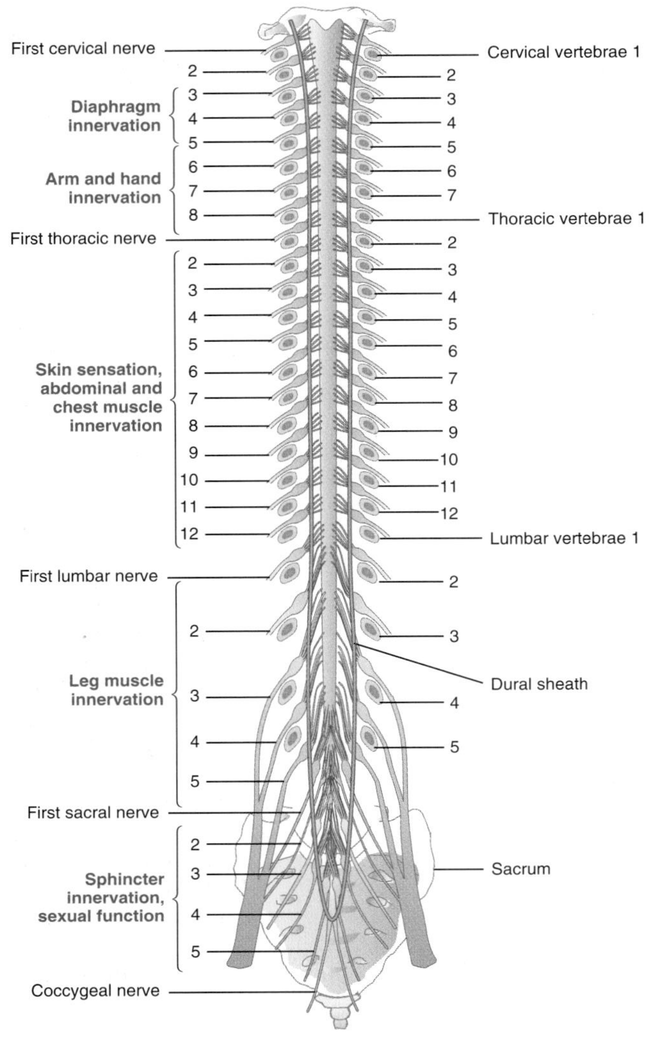

FIGURE 42–1 Spinal cord lying within the vertebral canal. Spinal nerves are numbered on the left side; vertebrae are numbered on the right side; body areas supplied by various levels are in blue.

respiratory and cardiac centers, and dysregulation of these centers has grim consequences.

Lesions in the spinal cord ordinarily cause lower motor neuron signs at the level(s) of the mass and upper motor signs in segments below the level of the mass. Spinal cord injury is the most common cause of pathology in this region. Other examples of spinal cord abnormalities are multiple sclerosis, tumor, syrinx (fluid collection), chronic meningitis, vascular insufficiency, and mass lesions of the epidural space.

Lesions of the pituitary gland and hypothalamus are often heralded by systemic manifestations that may include electrolyte and metabolic abnormalities secondary to adrenocortical, thyroid, and antidiuretic hormone dysregulation. Because of the proximity to the visual pathways, visual field, acuity, and binocular deficits are also often present. The syndrome of inappropriate secretion of antidiuretic hormone is often a complication, and consideration of volume status is important here; hyponatremia is essential to the diagnosis. Because the hypothalamus is the regulatory center for hunger and satiety, lesions here may present as anorexia or overeating.

Finally, disorders of peripheral nerves and the neuromuscular junction can certainly affect one's ability to maintain proper nutrition. Disorders such as Guillain-Barré syndrome or myasthenia gravis may aggravate the patient's natural efforts to maintain metabolic balance. Note that many parts of the nervous system are required to eat and drink, so a problem at any step along the way can result in an inability to meet the body's metabolic demands independently.

MEDICAL NUTRITION THERAPY

The nutritional management of patients with neurologic disease is complex. Often severe neurologic impairments compromise the mechanisms and cognitive abilities needed for adequate nourishment. Not only do many of these patients have dysphagia, but the ability to obtain, prepare, and present food to the mouth are compromised (Kelly and Buchholz,

TABLE 42–4 BASIC FUNCTIONS OF CRANIAL NERVES

(NUMBER)	CRANIAL NERVE MOTOR FUNCTION	SENSORY FUNCTION
Olfactory (I)	None	Smell
Optic (II)	None	Vision
Oculomotor (III)	1. Eye movement 2. Pupil constriction	None
Trochlear (IV)	Eye movement	None
Trigeminal (V)	Mastication	1. Facial heat, cold and touch 2. Noxious odors 3. Input for corneal reflex
Abducens (VI)	Eye movement	None
Facial (VII)	1. All muscles of facial expression 2. Corneal reflex	1. Facial pain 2. Taste on anterior two thirds of tongue
Vestibulocochlear (VIII)	None	Hearing and head acceleration and input for oculocephalic reflex
Glossopharyngeal (IX)	1. Swallowing 2. Gag reflex	Palatal, glossal and oral sensation
Vagus (X)	1. Heart rate, GI activity, sexual function 2. Cough reflex	Taste on posterior third of tongue
Spinal accessory (XI)	1. Trapezius 2. Sternocleido-mastoid	None
Hypoglossal (XII)	Tongue movement	None

1996). As a result, all neurologic patients are at risk for malnutrition. Early recognition of signs and symptoms, implementation of an appropriate care plan to meet the nutritional requirements of the individual, and counseling for the patient and family members on dietary choices are first steps. Regular evaluation of the patient's nutritional status in relation to the disease management, with the ultimate goal of improving outcomes and the patient's quality of life, is also essential.

Nutritional assessment is the first step in managing the patient. It should include a detailed diet history as well as a history of weight loss or gain. The diet history is helpful to assess patterns of normal chewing, swallowing, and rate of ingestion. Weight loss history establishes a baseline weight. A weight loss of 10% or more is indicative of nutritional risk. Anemias should be noted because the synthesis of the neurotransmitters dopamine and serotonin require adequate iron nutriture (Connor and Beard, 1997). For explicit information on nutrition assessment, refer to Chapters 16 and 17.

Procurement of Food

In chronic neurologic disease, there is a decline in function and in the ability to care for oneself. Fulfillment of basic needs including the procurement of food may depend on the involvement of family, friends, or professionals. In acute insults, such as trauma, stroke, or Guillain-Barré syndrome, the entire process of eating can be interrupted abruptly and the patient may require enteral nutrition support for a period of time until overall function improves and eating can be resumed.

Meal Preparation

Problems of impaired vision and ambulation may occur and make eating less enjoyable by turning meal preparation into a difficult task. In this situation, reliance on convenience foods is repeated. Comfort foods, prepackaged single servings of food, or convenience foods often permits independent preparation of meals.

Feeding Issues: Presentation of Food to the Mouth

The patient with neurologic disease may be unable to feed himself or herself due to limb weakness, poor body positioning, hemianopsia, apraxia, confusion, or neglect. The region of the CNS that is damaged determines the resulting disability (Table 42–5).

If limb weakness or paralysis occurs on the dominant side of the body, uncoordination resulting from a new reliance on the nondominant side may make eating difficult and unpleasant. Small frequent feedings can help if fatigue or early satiety is a problem. The patient may not only have to adjust to eating with one hand, but also to using the nondominant hand. An occupational therapist may be helpful with recommendations for specific adaptive eating utensils. **Hemiparesis,** or weakness that causes the body to slump toward the affected side, may increase the patient's risk of aspiration. It is important to make the patient sit as upright (at a 90° angle) as possible. If the patient must be in bed during mealtime, pillows can be used to bank and support the paretic side.

Hemianopsia is blindness for one half of the

TABLE 42–5 COMMON DISORDERS OF NEUROLOGIC DISEASES

SITE IN THE BRAIN	IMPAIRMENT	RESULTS
Cortical lesions of the parietal lobe (perception of sensory stimuli)	Sensory deficits	Fine regulation of muscle activities impossible if the patient is unable to perceive joint position, and motion and tension of contracting muscles
Lesions of the nondominant hemisphere	Hemi-inattention syndrome (neglect)	Patient neglects that side of the body
Optic tract lesions (usually of the middle cerebral artery or the artery near the internal capsule)	Visual field cuts	Patient reads one half of a page, eats from only half of the plate, and so forth.
Loss of subcortically stored pattern of motor skills	Apraxia	Inability to perform a previously learned task (e.g., walking, rising from a chair), but paralysis, sensory loss, spasticity, and incoordination are not present
No identification with a particular brain disorder or a specifically located lesion	Language apraxia	Inability to produce meaningful speech, even though oral muscle function is intact and language production has not been affected
Lesion of Broca's area	Nonfluent aphasia	Thought and language formulation are intact, but the patient is unable to connect them into fluent speech production
Lesion of Wernicke's area	Fluent aphasia	Flow of speech and articulation seem normal, but language output makes little or no sense
Extensive brain damage	Global aphasia	Both expression and speech perception are severely impaired
Brain stem lesions Bilateral hemispheric lesions Cerebellar disorders	Dysarthria	Inability to produce intelligible words with proper articulation

(From Steinberg FU. Rehabilitating the older stroke patient: What's Possible? Geriatrics 41:85, 1986.)

field of vision. The patient must learn to recognize that he or she no longer has a normal field of vision and to compensate by turning the head. *Neglect* is inattention to a weakened or paralyzed side of the body and occurs when the nondominant (right) parietal side of the brain is affected. The patient ignores the affected body part, and his or her perception of the body's midline is shifted. Hemianopsia and neglect can occur together, impairing the patient's function severely. For example, a patient may eat only half of the contents of a meal because he or she recognizes only half of it (Fig. 42–2).

Another potential interference with self-feeding is apraxia, in which the patient has difficulty with perceptual motor planning. Even though the patient knows what needs to be done and has the physical ability to do it, he or she is unable to carry out an action and cannot follow directions. It may be possible to do the action after a demonstration; however, this may affect judgment and result in the performance of dangerous tasks, making it unsafe to leave the patient alone. Confusion or dementia may prevent a patient from safely preparing meals or even remembering to eat regularly. Supervision, or even assistance with feeding, may be required.

Eating: The Oral Process

This is the stage where patients begin to report difficulties with eating. Reports of coughing and unusually long mealtimes are associated with tongue, facial, and masticator muscle weakness. Observation during meals allows the nurse or dietitian to screen informally for signs of dysphagia problems and bring them to the attention of the health care team.

Proper position for swallowing should be to sit bolt upright with the head in a chin-down position. Concentrating on the swallowing process can also help reduce choking. Environmental distractions and conversation during mealtime increase the risk for **aspiration** or inhalation of food into the lungs. However, families should be encouraged to maintain as normal mealtime behavior as possible.

Dysphagia, or difficulty in swallowing, is a common problem in those with neurologic disease. Symptoms associated with dysphagia may include drooling, choking, or coughing during or after meals, inability to suck from a straw, holding pockets of food in the buccal recesses (of which the patient may be unaware), absent gag reflex, chronic upper respiratory infections, weight loss, and anorexia. Other signs are a gurgly voice quality or a moist cough after eating or drinking. A swallowing evaluation by a speech pathologist is in order. Dysphagia often leads to malnutrition because of inadequate intake.

Swallowing

Initiation of the swallow begins voluntarily, but is completed reflexively. Normal swallowing allows for safe and easy passage of food from the oral cavity through the pharynx and esophagus into the stomach. This occurs by means of propulsive muscular force with some benefit from gravity. The process of swallowing can be organized into three phases as shown in Figure 42–3.

ORAL PHASE. During the preparatory and oral phases of swallowing, food is placed in the mouth where it is combined with saliva, chewed if necessary, and formed into a bolus by the tongue. The tongue pushes the food to the rear of the oral cavity by gradually squeezing it backward against the

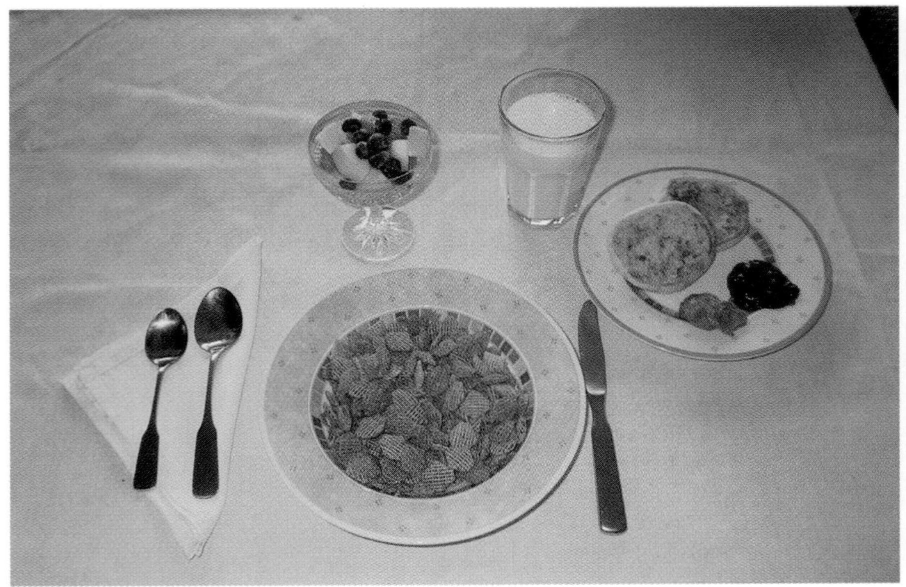

A

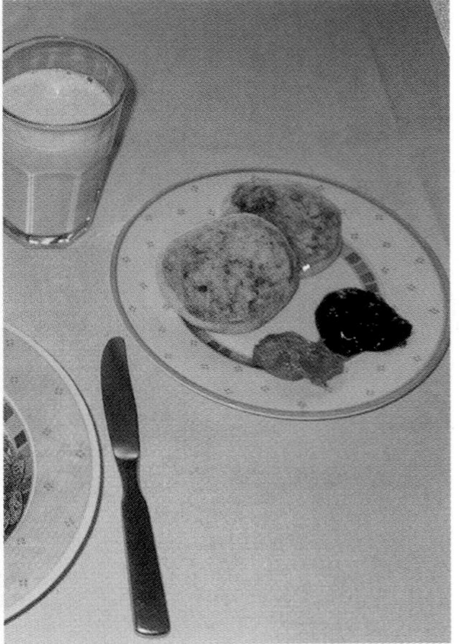

B

FIGURE 42–2 (A) Normal vision; (B) hemianopsia.

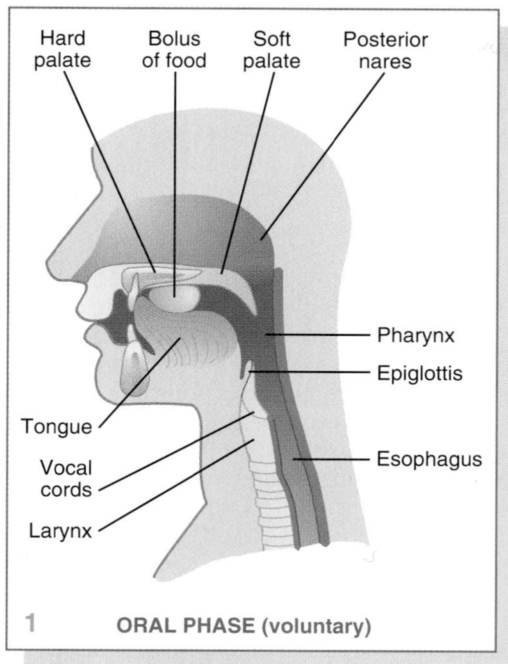

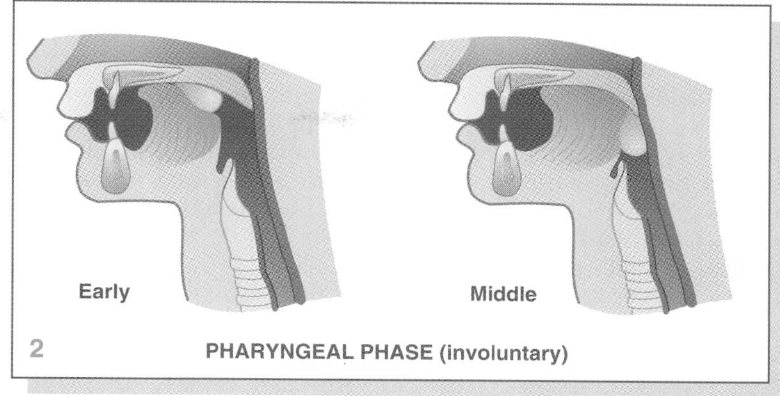

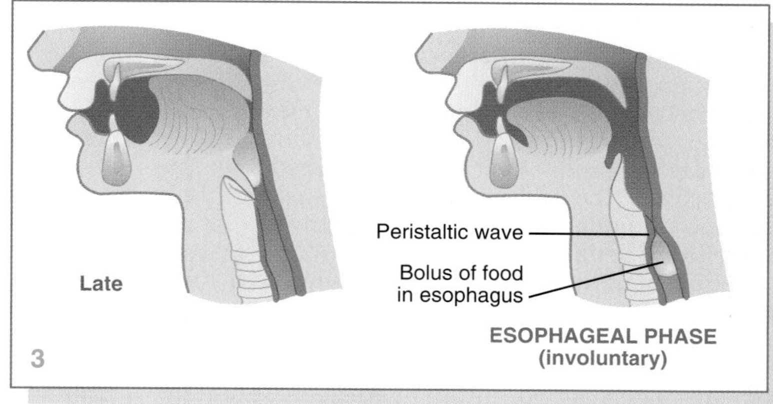

FIGURE 42–3 Swallowing occurs in three phases: (1) Voluntary or oral phase. The tongue presses food against the hard palate, forcing it toward the pharynx. (2) Involuntary, pharyngeal phase. Early: wave of peristalsis forces a bolus between the tonsillar pillars. Middle: soft palate draws upward to close posterior nares and respirations cease momentarily. Late: vocal cords approximate and the larynx pulls upward, covering the airway and stretching the esophagus open. (3) Involuntary, esophageal phase. Relaxation of the upper esophageal (hypopharyngeal) sphincter allows the peristaltic wave to move the bolus down the esophagus.

hard and soft palate (see Fig. 42–3). Increased ICP or cranial nerve damage may result in weakened or poorly coordinated tongue movements, leading to problems in completing the oral phase of swallowing. Weakened lip muscles result in the inability to completely seal the lips, form a seal around a cup, or suck through a straw. Patients are embarrassed by drooling and may not want to eat in front of others. The patient may have difficulty forming a cohesive bolus and moving it through the oral cavity. Food can become pocketed in the buccal recesses, especially if sensation in the cheek is lost or facial weakness exists.

PHARYNGEAL PHASE. The pharyngeal phase is initiated when the bolus is propelled past the **faucial** arches. Four events must occur in rapid succession during this phase. The soft palate elevates to close off the nasopharynx and prevent oropharyngeal regurgitation. The hyoid and larynx elevate, and the vocal cords adduct to protect the airway. The pharynx sequentially contracts while the cricopharyngeal sphincter relaxes, allowing the food to pass into the esophagus. Breathing resumes at the end of the pharyngeal phase. Symptoms of uncoordination during this phase include gagging, choking, and nasopharyngeal regurgitation.

ESOPHAGEAL PHASE. The final or esophageal phase, during which the bolus continues through the esophagus into the stomach, is completely involuntary. Any difficulties that occur during this phase are generally the result of a mechanical obstruction, but neurologic disease cannot be ruled out. For example, impaired peristalsis can arise from brain stem infarct.

Liquids

Swallowing liquids of thin consistency (water) requires the most coordination and control. Liquids are easily aspirated into the lungs and may pose a life-threatening event because **aspiration pneumonia** may ensue, even from sterile water in the lungs. Sterile water is no longer sterile once it is introduced to the bacterial load of the oral cavity. If a patient has difficulty consuming thin liquids, fluid requirements may be met by thickening liquids. Liquids of all types can be thickened with nonfat dry milk powder, cornstarch, modular carbohydrate supplements, or commercial thickeners that contain a modified cornstarch thickener, such as Thick-It or Thick n Easy. Thick liquids containing a high percentage of water need to be emphasized to maintain fluid balance. Popsicles, ice, and fresh fruit are additional sources of free water. Encourage noncaffeinated sources because caffeine has a diuretic effect contributing to dehydration, fatigue, and thickened saliva. Often the patient presents with fatigue and malaise, which may be associated with a "mild chronic dehydration" due to decreased fluid intake.

Milk is considered a liquid with unique properties. Often, intake of milk is associated with symptoms of excess mucus production. However, no statistically significant data have proven a link between milk or dairy products and symptoms of mucus production (Pinnock et al., 1990). However, the dysphagic patient often reports increased phlegm after milk consumption, which may actually be a consequence of poor swallowing ability rather than mucous production. It is suggested that patients "chase" the milk products with appropriately thickened liquids, to help flush the throat, rather than eliminate dairy products.

Neurogenic bladder is a common sign and management issue in patients with a **myelopathy,** or spinal cord injury. Its main feature is urinary retention. This predisposes to urinary tract infection and miscalculation of fluid balance. Alternately, myelopathy and spinal cord injury may result in urinary urgency, frequency, and incontinence. To minimize these problems, it is helpful to distribute fluids evenly throughout the waking hours and to limit them before bedtime. Some patients limit fluid intake severely to decrease frequency of urination. This increases the risk of urinary tract infection (UTI). One nontraumatic source of myelopathy and neurogenic bladder is multiple sclerosis (MS). Individuals with MS have a higher incidence of UTIs. Increased intake of cranberry juice can reduce the frequency of this uncomfortable condition (see Chapter 38).

Textures

As chronic disease progresses, cranial nerves become damaged leading to neurologic deficits manifested by dysphagia and the elimination of entire food groups. Vitamin and mineral supplementation may be necessary. If chewable supplements are not handled safely, liquid forms may be added to acceptable foods. Nutritional intervention should be individualized according to the type and extent of dysfunction. The dietitian can ensure that the diet remains palatable and nutritionally adequate by recommending changes in food consistency to mechanical soft or pureed consistency to reduce the need for oral manipulation and to conserve energy while eating (Table 42–6). Small, frequent meals may also encourage increased intake. Swallowing can also be improved by emphasizing the taste, texture, and temperature of foods. Juices can be substituted for water and will provide taste, nutrients, and calories. A cool temperature facilitates the swallowing mechanism and therefore cold food items may be better tolerated. Carbonation may also be better tolerated because there is the beneficial effect of texture. Sauces and gravies lubricate foods for ease in swallowing and can help prevent fragmentation of foods in the oral cavity. Moist pastas, casseroles, and egg dishes are well tolerated.

Nutrition Support

Acute and chronic neurologic diseases often have periods in their clinical courses when nutrition support is required. For acute disease, nutrition support may be required in the early term until a degree of function is regained, whereas chronic neurologic disease may require nutrition support in the late stages of the disease to meet metabolic demands. Nutrition support helps to avert complications of aspiration, pneumonia, and sepsis, which can compound the deteriorating effects of these diseases. Enteral tube feedings may be necessary if the risk of aspiration from eating is high, or if the patient cannot eat enough to meet his or her needs. In the latter case, nocturnal tube feedings can bridge the gap between oral intake and actual nutritional requirements. This should allow the normal sensation of hunger to be generated and provide freedom from tube feeding during the day.

In most instances the gastrointestinal tract function remains intact and enteral rather than parenteral nutrition is the preferred method of administering nutrition support. (A noted exception occurs after spinal cord injury. In this instance, ileus is a common sequela for 7 to 10 days after the insult. See Chapter 33.) Although a nasogastric tube can be a short-term option, a percutaneous endoscopic gastrostomy or (PEG) tube or PEG/J (gastrostomy-jejunostomy tube) placed under local anesthesia is preferred for long-term management. These should be considered for patients whose swallowing function is inadequate to ensure nutritional health (see Chapter 22).

In the acute setting, when a previously well-nourished individual is unable to resume oral alimentation within 7 days, nutrition support may be required to prevent decline in nutritional health and to aid recovery. For the majority of patients, this intervention is commonly used to tide the patient over until he or she can resume oral nourishment. Conversely, in the chronic setting, nutrition support is an issue that each patient must eventually face, because it may result in prolonged therapy. However, adequate nutriture can maintain health of the individual longer, and may be a welcome relief to the patient who has become overburdened with the difficulties of sustenance. One study of patients with amyotrophic lateral sclerosis demonstrated improved survival after 6 months of nutritional support via PEG (Mazzini et al., 1995).

On the other hand, some patients may decline

TABLE 42–6 GUIDELINES FOR FEEDING THE DYSPHAGIC PATIENT

The following considerations are intended only as a starting point from which an individual's diet can be planned. Coordinated efforts between the dietitian and the swallowing therapist will determine the dietary prescription.

NEUROLOGIC DISORDERS

Condition	Dietary Consideration	Rationale
Slow/weak/uncoordinated swallow	Include highly seasoned, flavorful, aromatic foods; add sugar, spices	Maximize stimulus for swallow
	Serve food at very cold temperatures	Maximize stimulus for swallow
	Include highly textured foods, such as diced cooked vegetables, diced canned fruit	Maximize stimulus for swallow
	Maintain semisolid consistencies that form a cohesive bolus	Need to avoid consistencies that will tend to fall apart in the pharynx
	Avoid sticky or bulky foods	Reduce risk of airway obstruction
	Caution with thin liquids (water, juices, milk, carbonated beverages) Try: Carbonated beverages (carbonation may stimulate reflex) Iced tart juices or crushed popsicles—banana and vanilla melt slowest (flavor and temperature may stimulate reflex) Medium or spoon-thick liquids may be substituted Thickening thin liquids with nonfat dry milk powder, fruit flakes, or commercial thickeners (Thick-It)	They are difficult to control, unpredictable, and may spill into pharynx prior to swallow reflex
	Small, frequent meals	Minimize fatigue; optimize food temperature and total nutrient intake
Weakened or poor oral-muscular control	Maintain semisolid consistencies that form a cohesive bolus	Requires less oral manipulation; purees are difficult to control
	Avoid slippery, sticky foods	
	Avoid thin liquids (see earlier description of thin liquids and recommendation)	See earlier rationale
	Small, frequent meals	Minimize fatigue, optimize total nutrient intake
Reduced oral sensation	Position food in most sensitive area	Maximize sensation
	Do not mix textures (e.g., vegetable soup)	Simplify swallow; minimize risk of aspirating thinner liquids
	Use colder temperatures	Maximize sensation; avoid potentially burning oral mucosa with liquids at too hot a temperature
	Use highly seasoned, flavorful foods	Maximize sensation
Cricopharyngeal dysfunction	Maintain liquid-puréed diet if no other contraindications are present	Liquids and purees pass into the esophagus more easily
Decreased laryngeal elevation	Limit diet to medium- and spoon-thick liquids, soft solids	Thin liquids easily penetrate the larynx
	Avoid sticky or bulky foods or food that will fall apart	Reduce the risk of airway obstruction
Decreased vocal cord closure	Avoid thin liquids	Easy, quick laryngeal penetration
	Avoid foods that will fall apart	Reduce risk of small pieces entering the larynx after the swallow

EXAMPLES OF FOOD CONSISTENCIES

Solids		Liquids	
Foods that form a cohesive bolus	***Foods that fall apart***	***Thin liquids***	***Medium-thick liquids***
Egg dishes: soufflés, quiches	Dry, crumbly breads	Apple juice	Vegetable juice
Poached or scrambled eggs	Crackers	Cranberry juice	Blenderized or cream soups
Egg, tuna, or meat salad	Thin, pureed foods: applesauce	Orange juice	Ensure Plus or Sustacal HC
Macaroni salad	Plain, chopped raw vegetables and fruits	Grape juice	Nectars
Soft cheeses	Plain rice	Broth	Milkshakes, malts
Canned fruit	Cooked peas, corn	Milk	Eggnog
Macaroni or rice casseroles	Plain ground meats	Chocolate milk	
Ground meats with gravy	Thin hot cereals	Coffee	***Spoon-thick liquids***
Moist, soft meat, or fish loaf		Tea	Yogurt
Custard	***Sticky or bulky foods***	Water	Pureed fruit
Cheesecake with sauce	Fresh white bread	Soda	Ice cream
Pudding	Peanut butter	Alcohol	Sherbet or sorbet
Aspic	Plain mashed potatoes	Ensure or Isocal	Pudding
Mousse	Bananas	Hot chocolate	Frozen shakes
Finger gelatin	Refried beans		Popsicles
Whipped gelatin	Bran cereals		Frozen juices
Hot cereals	Chunks of plain meats		Frozen sodas
Vegetables in sauces	Raw vegetables or fruits		

(Adapted from The American Dietetic Association. Manual of Clinical Dietetics. Chicago: The American Dietetic Association, 1992. Courtesy of Megan S. Veldee, MS, RD, and Robert M. Miller, PhD, Seattle Veterans Administration Medical Center, Seattle WA.)

early placement of a feeding tube because of the emotional and physical impact of this choice. In advanced stages of disease one may refuse tube feedings, choosing not to prolong life. Nutrition support should enhance the quality of life and the health care team has an important role in alleviating patient concerns and fostering informed decisions. The patient needs to be fully informed about the impact of tube feeding on daily life. Discussion of both the advantages and the disadvantages of nutritional support with the patient and family should be initiated well ahead of need. Discussion of tube feeding options should include a description of feeding schedules, tube placement procedures and appropriate training.

NEUROLOGIC DISEASES ARISING FROM NUTRITIONAL DEFICIENCIES OR EXCESSES: PRIMARY PREVENTION STRATEGIES

For information on beriberi and pellagra, see Chapter 4.

Pernicious Anemia

Historically, pernicious anemia, or vitamin B_{12} (cobalamin) deficiency has been one of the most common neurologic syndromes caused by a single nutrient. The classic triad of anemia, neurologic deficits, and epithelial atrophy of the tongue was well recognized at the turn of the century. Until 1926 when replacement therapy was introduced, the term "pernicious" appropriately described the outcome of events for those afflicted with this disease—"destructive, harmful, and fatal." Consumption of liver was prescribed empirically, and only in 1948 was vitamin B_{12} recognized as the healing agent (Rowland, 1995).

Given the technology for measuring vitamin B_{12} levels in the blood, early detection during the preclinical phase of disease is the rule. As a result, pernicious anemia is rarely seen in medical centers in developed countries. For those who develop pernicious anemia only 20% are younger than age 50; most are over 60. The effectiveness of diagnosis and treatment has been remarkable. Over 90% of symptomatic patients regain independence in conducting activities of daily living (ADL). See Chapter 35 on anemias.

Etiology and Pathophysiology

In the nervous system, lesions occur initially in the myelin sheaths of optic nerves, cerebral white matter, and peripheral nerves. The biochemical abnormality responsible for the neurologic dysfunction is part of lipid metabolism and appears to involve vitamin B_{12} and its role as a coenzyme that normally transforms methylmalonyl coenzyme A (CoA) to succinyl CoA, a step in propionate metabolism. Failure of the cobalamin-dependent enzyme, methylmalonyl CoA mutase leads to the accumulation of methylmalonyl CoA and its precursor, propionyl CoA. Propionyl CoA displaces succinyl CoA inserting irregular fatty acids into membrane lipids similar to the myelin lesions that characterize this disease. Conceivably, the presence of abnormal fatty acids may explain the structural changes observed in central and peripheral myelin of these patients (Adams et al., 1997).

Clinical Findings and Treatment

Most neurologic manifestations of vitamin B_{12} deficiency are associated with the typical macrocytic anemia of pernicious anemia. General weakness and especially **paresthesias** constitute the earliest and most common symptoms. Patients may report tingling or the feeling of "pins and needles" in either hands or feet. This tends to be constant and steadily progressive. If left untreated, the following signs may ensue as the disease progresses: impaired taste **(dysgeusia);** impaired gait, spasticity and contracture; mental signs of irritability, apathy, somnolence, emotional instability, marked confusion, and depression; and visual impairment. Fortunately, for the majority of patients today, the disease can be detected before neurologic symptoms or signs develop.

Early diagnosis of pernicious anemia can be somewhat complicated, however, because hematologic and neurologic signs do not always correlate. A significant component of primary prevention is the determination of serum vitamin B_{12} because it is the best, most readily available test for evaluating vitamin B_{12} status. Levels less than 150 mg/mL are considered to represent deficiency (Jacob and Milne, 1993). A more definitive test, the Schilling test, is used to confirm B_{12} malabsorption from a lack of *intrinsic factor* (see Chapter 17).

The duration of symptoms before treatment is the factor most likely to influence treatment response; neurologic manifestations that occur less than 3 months are rapidly and completely reversible. Amelioration of symptoms occurring between 6 to 12 months is variable and in extreme cases, arrest of disease progression is the most that can be accomplished. Prompt initiation of therapy is imperative. Initially, daily intramuscular injections of 1000 mg cyanocobalamin are administered for several weeks. Subsequently, weekly doses of 100 mg cyanocobalamin are administered for several months followed by monthly maintenance doses of 100 mg cyanocobalamin administered for life if lack of intrinsic factor is apparent.

Nutritional Considerations

For the majority of individuals with pernicious anemia, inadequate dietary intake of vitamin B_{12} is unrelated to this disease. However, for individuals who consume vegetables exclusively (vegans), inadequate dietary intake of vitamin B_{12} may correlate to vitamin B_{12} deficiency. In this situation, oral therapy may be appropriate or the individual may consider consuming certain foods that contain sources of this nutrient, such as eggs, milk, and cereals with high amounts of vitamin B_{12}. For a complete description of foods containing vitamin B_{12}, refer to Chapters 4 and 35.

Wernicke-Korsakoff Syndrome

Wernicke-Korsakoff syndrome (WKS) is a disease of the cerebellum and brain stem resulting from chronic B_1 deficiency. It most commonly occurs in alcoholics and WKS is one of the gravest consequences of alcoholism (Zubaran et al., 1996). WK syndrome is actually two separate diseases, Wernicke disease and Korsakoff psychosis, but their frequent association has led to their inclusion into one syndrome.

The incidence of WKS may be underreported because it is often undiagnosed. Alcoholism is more prevalent in the homeless populations who have limited access to medical care. Due to the fact that clinical findings are subtle, diagnosis of WKS is often made at autopsy. One pilot study revealed 17 undiagnosed cases of Wernicke's encephalopathy of 31 (55%) at autopsy, whereas only 2 of the 17 had been suspected of having Wernicke's based on clinical findings (Naidoo, 1991).

Although the epidemiology of WKS cannot be precisely quantified, the risk factors can be accurately described. In North America and Europe, this nutritional disorder is the most frequently encountered manifestation acquired from thiamin deficiency, usually occurring in the presence of alcoholism. It has also been seen in patients who are nutritionally depleted from either gastrointestinal disease or acquired immunodeficiency syndrome (AIDS).

Etiology and Pathophysiology

Thiamin deficiency is the accepted primary cause of WKS. Depletion of body stores of thiamin can happen rapidly, within 7 to 8 weeks, especially in alcoholics. The pathology in this acute and severe nutritional deficiency is restricted to the CNS, but not all regions of the nervous system are affected equally (Langlais, 1996).

The exact relationship between the lesions induced by thiamin deficiency and their effect on the brain remain unclear. A synergistic effect of alcohol and thiamin deficiency on the severity of disease has been proposed (Kril, 1993). However, one thing that is certain is the effect that treatment has on outcome. Wernicke's encephalopathy is responsive to thiamin, whereas Korsakoff's psychosis is not and unfortunately, the mental derangements precipitated by Korsakoff's psychosis are irreversible.

Clinical Findings and Treatment

Wernicke's disease is characterized by the "classic triad" of disturbances in mentation (encephalopathy), vision **(nystagmus),** and gait **ataxia,** but they are present simultaneously in only 10% to 33% of cases (Greenberg, 1997). This is one reason why clinical diagnosis is deferred until it is confirmed at autopsy. Korsakoff's psychosis and an amnestic-confabulatory state present as a mental disorder in which retentive memory is significantly impaired as compared to other cognitive functions. Memory is diminished, there is an inability to learn new things, conceptual or perceptual functions decline, and as the disease progresses, confabulation lying vanishes.

Treatment should be started immediately with thiamin if WKS is suspected, or administered prophylactically to alcoholics because thiamin can prevent disease progression and even reverse the brain abnormalities that are not yet permanent changes (Zubaran et al., 1996). From 50 to 100 mg thiamin should be administered parenterally for several days because the possibility of gastrointestinal malabsorption exists. It is also important that glucose never be given before thiamin because sudden increases in brain glucose levels may precipitate symptoms of WKS in patients with marginal thiamin reserves. Glucose and metabolic stress also increase requirements for thiamin (Adams et al., 1997).

The response to therapy depends on the conversion of thiamin to its active form in the liver. With concomitant liver disease response may be delayed. However, ophthalmologic symptoms generally respond rapidly to thiamin, whereas ataxia and encephalopathy respond more slowly. Mental deficits of Korsakoff's psychosis do not improve. A decrease in erythrocyte transketolase activity also correlates well with improvement in the clinical picture, as a normal value is a sensitive measure of adequate thiamin nutriture.

Nutritional Considerations

First and foremost, the nutritional deficiency should be corrected if possible. In the situation of thiamin deficiency, not only should therapeutic thiamin supplementation be administered, but nutrient-dense foods containing thiamin, such as whole-grain or enriched breads and cereals, should be incorporated into the patient's diet as well. Alcohol must be eliminated. Because no singular food item contains large amounts of thiamin, one serving of a nutrient-dense food item contributes about 10% of an individual's daily need. A diet consisting of a variety of food items is required to ensure that the recommended dietary allowance (RDA) for thiamin is met (see Chapter 4).

In the presence of concomitant encephalopathy, repletion of dietary protein may be limited or restricted. For a complete discussion of nutritional therapy in liver disease refer to Chapter 32.

Stroke

Stroke is the most rampant clinical entity of cerebrovascular disease in developed countries. It is defined as an acute onset of focal or global neurologic deficit lasting more than 24 hours, and attributable to diseases of the intra- or extracranial neurovasculature. Often, severe strokes may be preceded by **transient ischemic attacks (TIA).**

Stroke is the third most common cause of death in the United States, accounting for 150,000 deaths annually or 7.1% of all annual deaths (Balaban, 1992). Old age is the most significant risk factor. Among modifiable risk factors, hypertension and smoking contribute the most to the risk of stroke. Other factors include coronary heart disease, atrial fibrillation, diabetes, and oral contraceptive use, particularly by female smokers. Stroke is a disease of the 20th century, resulting in large part from tobacco use and overnutrition. Although the incidence of stroke has declined over the past 30 years, the cost of the disease is approximately $5 billion annually (Balaban, 1992). This high cost may be attributed in part to the high degree of disability imparted by cerebrovascular events. More information is available on the internet at http://www-medstanford.edu/school/stroke.

Etiology and Pathology

Eighty-five percent of strokes are incited by a **thromboembolic event.** Atherosclerosis is a key risk factor for thromboembolic events and risk is heightened by the presence of other common diseases such as hypertension, diabetes, and gout (Fig. 42–4). **Embolic stroke** occurs when a cholesterol plaque is dislodged from a proximal vessel and travels to the brain and blocks an artery, most commonly the *middle cerebral artery (MCA).* In patients with dysfunctional cardiac atria, clots may be dislodged from here and embolize. **Thrombotic stroke** is common in the coronary vessels, extracranial vessels, and the basilar artery, but less so in the cerebral vessels (De Girolami et al., 1994). Here a cholesterol plaque in an artery ruptures and, subsequently, platelets aggregate to clog an already narrowed artery.

Intracranial hemorrhage is less common (15% of strokes), but more often fatal immediately. There are two varieties, and both occur more commonly in individuals with hypertension. The first is *intraparenchymal hemorrhage*. Among patients with intraparenchymal hemorrhage, the prevalence of hypertension is 80%. This event occurs when a vessel inside the brain ruptures. A variation of intraparenchymal hemorrhage is a lacunar (Latin: lake) infarct. These smaller infarcts occur in the deep structures of the brain such as the internal capsule, basal ganglia, pons, thalamus and cerebellum. Even a small lacunar infarct can produce significant disability because the brain tissue in the deep structures is so densely functional. The second type of intracranial hemorrhage is **subarachnoid hemorrhage (SAH).** This occurs most commonly as a result of head trauma, but almost as often as a result of a ruptured aneurysm of a vessel in the subarachnoid space. Ruptured aneurysms more commonly result in clinically significant SAH than does trauma.

Clinical Findings and Treatment

The history can give some evidence about the mechanism of a new infarct. Hemorrhage is suspected when the patient presents with headache, decreased level of consciousness, and vomiting, all of which evolve over minutes to hours. A thromboembolic stroke is more likely when the patient is fully conscious, but there is a sudden onset of motor or sensory findings (Greenberg, 1997). As with all neurologic disease, the clinical presentation depends on the location of the abnormality. An infarction of a particular cerebrovascular territory can be suspected by seeking out various constellations of neurologic deficits. An MCA occlusion will betray itself by producing paresis and sensory deficits of limbs on the opposite side of the body because this artery supplies the motor and sensory strips. If the left MCA is occluded, aphasias may also be present.

In the past, treatment for embolic stroke was supportive, focusing on prevention of further brain infarction and rehabilitation. Recently, use of thrombolytic or "clot-busting" drugs has allowed reversal of brain ischemia by lysing thromboembolic clots in selected patients. Evaluation and initiation of therapy needs intervention to occur within 6 hours of the onset of symptoms. Use of aspirin may be of some value in preventing further cerebrovascular events, but its effectiveness has not yet been demonstrated definitively.

Treatment of intracranial hemorrhage revolves around controlling ICP while maintaining sufficient perfusion of the brain. This may include surgical evacuation of large volumes of intracranial blood, ventricular drainage, or other neurosurgical interventions. Rehabilitation is a key component of therapy. Hemorrhage, particularly SAH, commonly has more severe functional consequences, and therefore has a longer period of convalescence than ischemic stroke.

Nutritional Management

Primary prevention is the cornerstone for managing stroke. This can be accomplished in part by dietary means as well as by other life-style behaviors. These nutrition-related factors have shown a salutary effect on reducing the incidence of stroke and have been compiled from various large population-based prospective studies in Table 42–7.

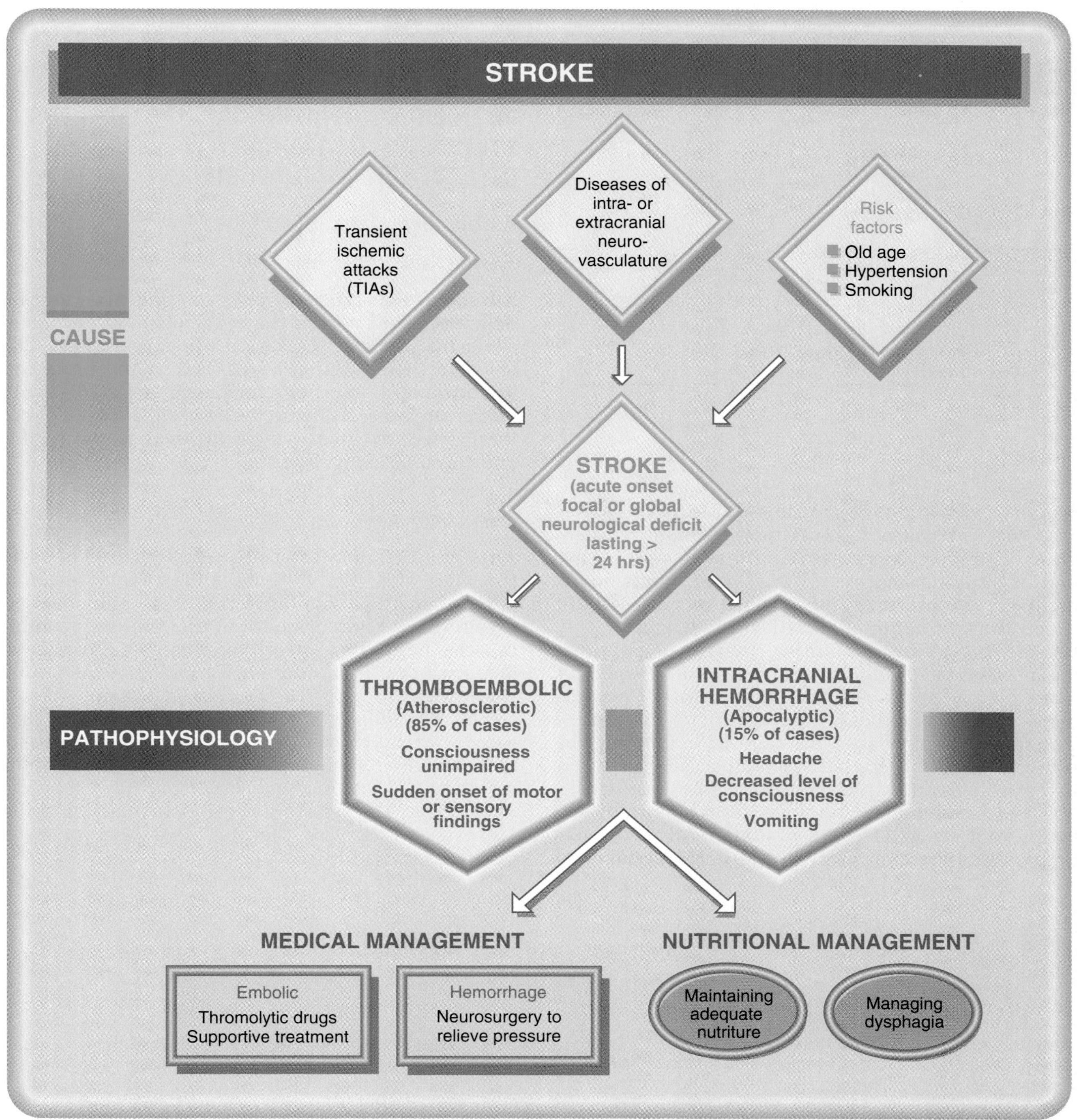

FIGURE 42–4 Pathophysiology algorithm—stroke. (Algorithm content developed by John Anderson, Ph.D., and Sanford C. Garner, Ph.D., 2000.)

Given the large prevalence of stroke and its associated burden of disease, treatment for those afflicted with this disease cannot be ignored. Malnutrition predicts a poor outcome. Once stroke does occur, dietary reduction of cholesterol, fat, and salt are of questionable benefit. Efforts should be directed toward maintaining the overall health of the patient. Under ideal circumstances, nutritional status is maintained. However, even in the presence of adequate intake, nutriture of the patient is not always guaranteed (Davalos et al., 1996).

The feeding difficulties experienced by stroke victims are determined by the extent of the stroke and the area of the brain affected. Dysphagia frequently occurs with stroke and it contributes to

TABLE 42–7 NUTRITION-RELATED FACTORS AND STROKE RISK

RISK FACTORS FOR STROKE
BMI > 27 kg/m^2 in women
Weight gain > 11 kg over 16 years in women
Waist-to-hip ratio > .92 in men
Diabetes
Hypertension
Cholesterol in hemorrhagic stroke
PROTECTIVE FACTORS FOR STROKE
High intake of total dietary fat
Daily consumption of fresh fruit
Flavonoid consumption > 4.7 cup green tea/day
Fish consumption in white and black women and black men
Cholesterol in ischemic stroke

BMI, body mass index.

complications and poor outcome. It has been associated with increased malnutrition, pulmonary infections, disability, increased length of hospital stay, and institutional care, and is also an independent predictor of mortality (Smithard et al., 1996). Given that, patients admitted to the hospital after stroke who exhibit difficulties chewing or swallowing should be promptly evaluated for dysphagia and dietary interventions implemented accordingly. For specific dietary interventions in dysphagia, refer to Table 42–6 on page 939. In some instances, nutrition support is temporarily required to maintain nutritional health until oral alimentation can be resumed. As motor functions improve, eating and other ADL are fundamental to the patient's rehabilitation process and necessary for resuming independence. (See "*Focus On:* Cholesterol and Stroke.")

NEUROLOGIC DISEASES WITH NON-NUTRITIONAL ETIOLOGIES: SECONDARY INTERVENTION STRATEGIES

Adrenomyeloleukodystrophy

Etiology and Pathophysiology

Adrenomyeloleukodystrophy is a congenital enzyme deficiency that affects the metabolism of very-long-chain fatty acids (VLCFA) in the paroxisomes. This leads to accumulation of VLCFA in the brain and the adrenal glands. The incidence is 1/20,000 male births. It is an X-linked recessive disorder characterized by myelopathy, **peripheral neuropathy,** and cerebral demyelination.

Clinical Findings and Treatment

First clinical manifestations usually occur between the ages of 4 and 8 years and may manifest as adrenal insufficiency or cerebral decompensation. **Dysarthria** (impairment of the tongue or other muscles needed for speech) or dysphagia may interfere with oral alimentation. Bronzing of the skin is a late clinical sign. In the face of adrenal insufficiency, physiologic replacement of steroids is indicated, which may improve neurologic symptoms and prolong life. Numerous therapies have been directed at the root of the disorder but have been disappointing. The selective use of bone marrow transplant is one current therapy; gene therapy holds promise for the future.

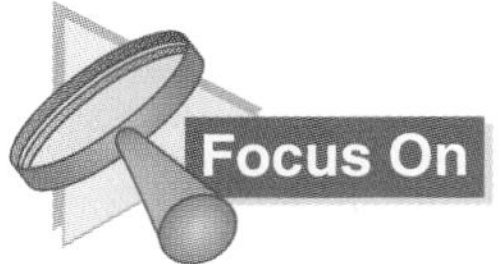

CHOLESTEROL AND STROKE

Although the role of cholesterol in heart disease is well known, cholesterol's role in predisposing an individual to stroke is less well established. This may come as a surprise given the ostensibly similar origin of coronary artery disease and cerebrovascular disease.

One prospective study demonstrated no association between cholesterol levels and first stroke, but the authors here pointed out that this finding may, if segregated, reveal a positive association between cholesterol levels and ischemic stroke while revealing a negative association between cholesterol and hemorrhagic stroke. The authors did, however, find an association between increased diastolic blood pressure and stroke risk (Prospective Studies Collaboration, 1995). A 1994 meta-analysis concluded that there was no decreased risk of stroke from cholesterol-lowering diets or medications in middle-aged men (Atkins et al., 1993).

However, data from the Diabetes Control and Complications Trial (DCCT) showed that those individuals under intensive treatment for diabetes had nearly one half the number of cerebrovascular events as conventionally treated patients (DCCT, 1995). They also found in the study that low-density lipoproteins, so-called bad cholesterol, total cholesterol, and triglycerides were significantly lower in the group receiving intensive treatment. This suggests a beneficial effect of intensive diabetes treatment on macrovascular disease in insulin-dependent diabetes.

Despite cholesterol's role in coronary artery disease, its role in ischemic stroke, outside of insulin-dependent diabetes, is still unclear. Current research will continue to delineate cholesterol's role in stroke and will guide future recommendations on cholesterol reduction. It should be remembered though that reducing serum cholesterol does have a proven role in prevention of coronary artery disease.

Nutritional Considerations

Nutritional therapy by dietary avoidance of VLCFA has not been proven. It does not lead to biochemical change because of endogenous synthesis. A specialty product, Lorenzo's oil, does lower the VLCFA level; however, the clinical course is not altered (Rowland, 1995).

Alzheimer's Disease

Alzheimer's disease (AD) is the most common form of dementia. It is named after Alois Alzheimer who first described the clinical features and pathologic changes. Originally, diagnosis was confirmed if onset was at less than age 65. Today, senile dementia with onset later than at age 65 is also considered to be AD. Senile dementia is both clinically and pathologically similar to AD except for age of onset (Rowland, 1995).

The incidence rate (new cases) of AD is similar for both sexes and throughout the world, increasing exponentially after age 40. The incidence rate approximates three new cases per year per 100,000 persons below age 60 and 125 new cases per 100,000 people over age 60 (Adams et al., 1997). Given the growth rate of the elderly population in the United States, it is estimated that by the year 2000, there will be 2 million persons with AD. The prevalence rate is three times higher among women than men; the higher prevalence rate seen in women is a result of a lower overall mortality than that of men. Given its prevalence, the personal, familial, financial, and clinical impact of AD is staggering (Adams et al., 1997). More information about Alzheimer's disease is available at http://www.Alzheimers.org.

Etiology and Pathophysiology

No one single factor has been established as a risk factor for AD, as debate surrounds the issue of causality. The risk factors commonly associated with AD are birth order, mother's age at birth, head injury, level of education, and presence of Down syndrome (Fig. 42–5). There is general agreement that a genetic factor is common. β-Amyloid protein and endoplasmic reticulum-associated binding protein are central to the pathophysiology and are targeted for therapy (Geula et al., 1998; Yan et al., 1997).

A familial occurrence accounts for less than 1% of all cases of AD, which is believed to be inherited by an autosomal dominant pattern. Some report greater concordance in monozygotic twins than dizygotic twins, which if true, would discount the single autosomal dominant gene theory of inheritance. Several genes have been identified as increasing the susceptibility for developing AD, but only one, the allele apolipoprotein-E4 (Apo-E4), has possible nutritional implications. Apo-E4, a protein located on chromosome 19, binds β-amyloid, which is involved in the transport of cholesterol. This association has been identified not only in familial cases of AD, but in sporadic cases as well (Rowland, 1995).

Clinical Findings and Treatment

Alzheimer's disease is diagnosed by histopathology. Clinically, the diagnosis is presumptive and one of exclusion. As a result, studies may be subjected to criticism due to the absence of a confirmatory diagnosis and until recently, there was speculation that AD may have actually represented unrecognized cases of thiamin deficiency (Folstein, 1996; Rowland, 1995).

Manifestations of AD result in a progressive dementia with increasing loss of memory, intellectual function, and disturbances in speech. Initially, day-to-day events are forgotten—possessions are misplaced and appointments are forgotten—while memories are retained. Cerebral function declines, but only becomes evident after the loss in memory is pronounced. Speech becomes impaired—names of objects are not remembered **(anomia),** words spoken by others are repeated **(echolalia),** and there is a loss of comprehension **(agnosia).** Over time, motor skills deteriorate as evidenced by changes in reflexes and a shuffling gate. Clinical findings are consistent when disease progression reaches the terminal stage; bowel and bladder control is lost, there is limb weakness and or contractures, and intellectual activity ceases. The patient becomes completely incapacitated in a vegetative state as death approaches.

There is no effective treatment; cerebral vasodilators, stimulants, L-dopa, and mega doses of vitamins B, C, and E remain unproven therapies. Certain drugs may be effective in suppressing aberrant behavior or aiding disturbed sleep. Estrogen administration seems to be beneficial for some postmenopausal women (Wickelgren, 1997). Tacrine use has resulted in a modest improvement in both noncognitive function and cognition as well (Raskind et al., 1997). Primary care management is the effective treatment. Assessment of the following four domains is fundamental to maximizing health, function, and quality of life of patients and family members (Cohen, 1994):

- Patient
- Individual family caregivers
- Family function
- Availability of community services

Determination of the nutritional status of the patient goes hand in hand with this approach because this population is often malnourished, and "unless detected and corrected, poor nutrition has untoward consequences on health and well-being" (Cohen, 1994).

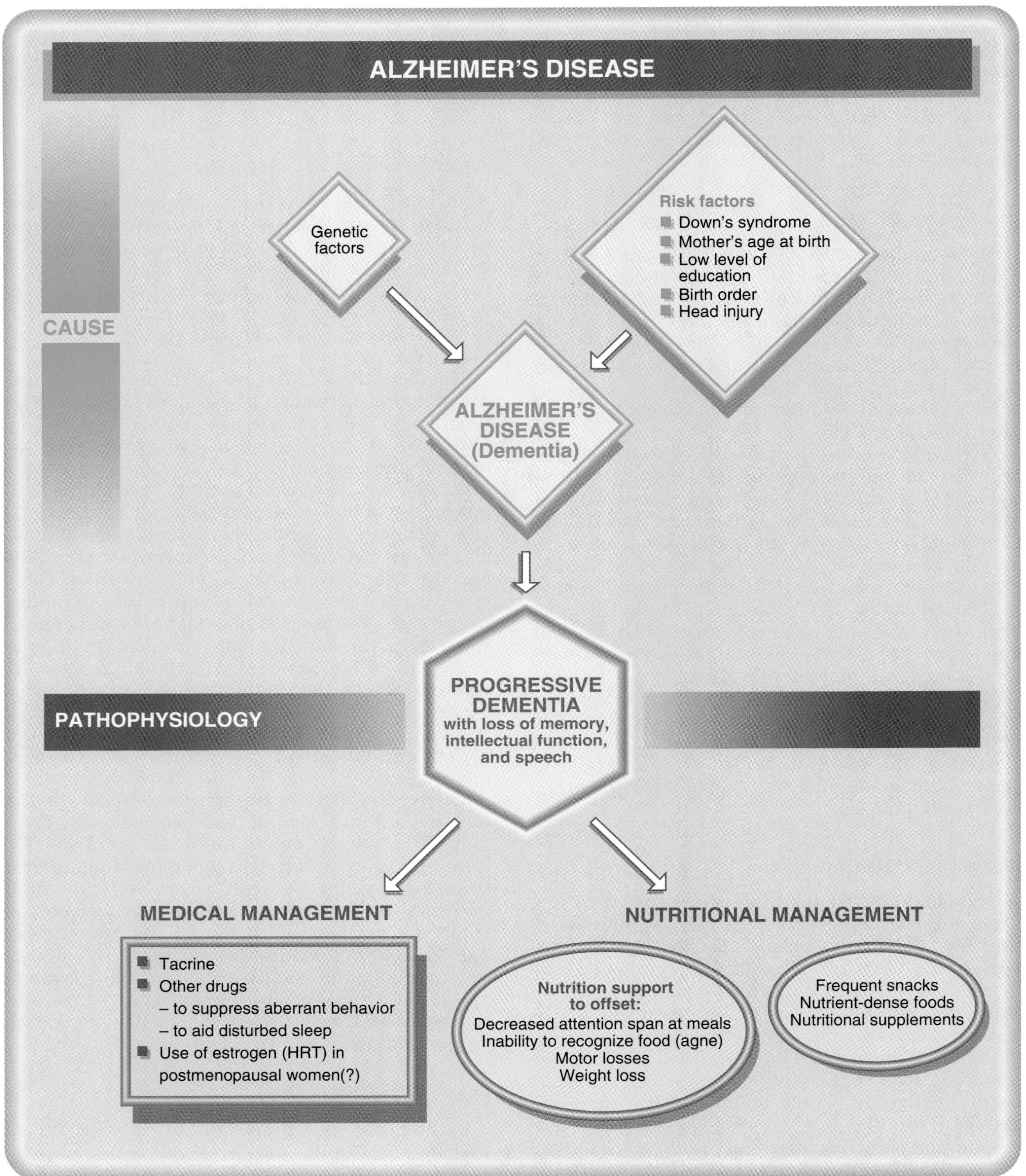

FIGURE 42–5 Pathophysiology algorithm—Alzheimer's disease. (Algorithm content developed by John Anderson, Ph.D., and Sanford C. Garner, Ph.D., 2000.)

Nutritional Management

Although a gluttonous appetite may develop in some individuals with AD, generally the global nutritional finding is weight loss (Barrett-Connor et al., 1996). It is not clear if there is an increase in the resting metabolic rate or if weight loss is a result of increased energy expenditure. The latter is probably true because energy output associated with constant pacing may be increased. For others, eating is neglected and weight loss is due to an inadequate food intake resulting from decreased independence and impaired self-feeding. In still other cases, weight loss may be secondary to a higher basal energy expenditure as a result of higher rates of infection. (See "*Focus On:* Herbs, Nutrients, and Ginkgo in Alzheimer's Disease and Other Neurologic Disorders.")

Alzheimer's disease is a disease of cortical neurons. The frontal lobe controls behavior, reasoning, emotion, and cognition; the temporal lobe controls hearing, memory, smell, and language; and the parietal lobe controls sensory perception, hearing, and body image. As a result, a wide range of neurologic functions are impaired that interfere with numerous activities involved with eating.

Cognitive losses impair attention span, reasoning, and judgment. This includes the ability to recognize feelings of hunger, thirst, and satiety. As the disease progresses, the attention span decreases and meals may be forgotten as soon as they are eaten or meals may not be eaten at all. Dehydration is also a problem; recognizing thirst and then seeking water is often neglected. These individuals are easily distracted so attempts should be made to minimize distractions at mealtimes. Noise can be distracting and therefore the radio or television should be turned off during mealtime. Food may need to be placed on small plates or bowls and given one at a time so as not to stress the individual by offering a choice of foods. As social inhibitions decrease, the patient may take another person's food. The patient consuming inedible items, spoiled foods, or hazardous fluids reflects impaired reasoning. These patients should be served first and be closely supervised during meals.

With sensory losses, perception of the surrounding world and related auditory, visual, or tactile recognition are distorted; this is called *agne*. Visual agne, the inability to recognize food, is manifested by not eating. The touch or smell of food is needed to initiate eating responses. Another example of a sensory loss is the inability to recognize food when it is served in a bowl the same color as the food item. Use of colored bowls and plates that are in contrast to the color of the food may be necessary so that food can be distinguished from the place setting. Patients may also have difficulties using eating utensils, but they can model behaviors if demonstrated by staff or caregivers.

Motor losses occur over the course of the illness. Some clients may need hand guidance to initiate eating. Usually, after the activity has been initiated, the patient can continue the activity as long as verbal cues continue. As motor skills decline, use of eating utensils will become limited; over time the patient may be able to use only a spoon. Eating

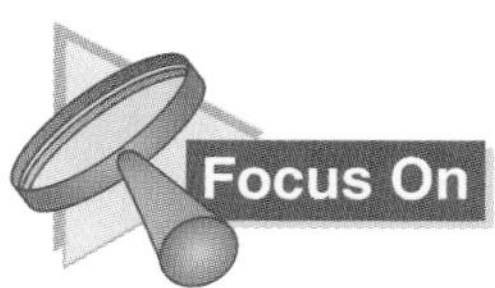

Herbs, Nutrients, and Ginko in Alzheimer's Disease and Other Neurologic Conditions

The tight microglial cellular junctions that form the blood–brain barrier (BBB) protect the CNS from large molecules. Diseases such as Alzheimer's disease (AD) and stress can make the BBB more permeable (Friedman et al., 1996). Proper inclusion of specific nutrients, such as antioxidants, may play a role in maintaining this barrier.

Antioxidants, especially vitamin E, have been studied for their role in AD. α-tocopherol and the drug, selegiline, have been found to be useful in slowing the progression of moderately severe AD (Sano et al., 1997). Antioxidants in foods have been shown to be effective in maintaining memory; folate, vitamin C, and β-carotene seem to be the best protective agents in fruits and vegetables (Warsama Jama et al., 1996; Tufts University Newsletter, 1998). Cognitive ability is also supported by adequate intakes of vitamins B_6 and B_{12} in addition to folate.

Ginkgo biloba extract (GBE) has been promoted in Asian countries and was recently approved for use in Germany to treat dementia (LeBars et al., 1997). Studies in the United States have tested the effectiveness of ginko in a 1-year double-blind, randomized trial. Results found no improvement in memory or functioning in the treatment group, but significant worsening among the placebo group. Although the mechanism is not yet clear, there may be a role for this extract in the dementia population.

St. John's Wort is currently under study for use in counteracting depression. This plant appears to have the same ingredients as some types of antidepressants. Interestingly, nondemented elderly persons with depression symptoms are at risk for subsequent dementia (Devanand et al., 1996). Products on the market do not always provide predictable levels of the effective ingredient, and home remedies may not be safe to use because they may have other contaminants. Further study is warranted (see Chapter 19).

Echinacea is a product that should be avoided with autoimmune disorders such as multiple sclerosis and lupus because of its stimulating impact on the immune system. As with all prescribed and over-the-counter products, controlled studies are needed to verify efficacy and effectiveness of all of these substances.

utensils should not be removed prematurely because this may contribute to agitation, excessive disability, lack of eating, and eventually weight loss.

Assessment of motor skills should be done routinely. Finger foods may be useful when use of utensils becomes difficult, but only if the patient has no difficulty with chewing or swallowing and is not inclined to swallow large boluses of food. In the latter case, finger foods are not appropriate.

Although adaptive equipment is useful in certain situations, it may be unfamiliar to the patient with AD and not as helpful. As end-stage disease approaches, swallowing often becomes impossible; dysphagia should be assessed to prevent the risk of aspiration (Finley, 1997). Table 42–8 lists additional interventions for eating-related behavioral problems in individuals with dementia. To combat weight loss, frequent snacks, nutrient-dense foods, and nutritional supplements need to be provided. Behavior modification along with altered food items will improve the quality of life of the individual for as long as possible. Evaluation of nutritional status is needed throughout the stages of AD to ensure that objectives of nutritional therapy continue to be met.

TABLE 42–8 EXAMPLES OF PRACTICAL INTERVENTION FOR EATING-RELATED BEHAVIORAL PROBLEMS COMMON IN INDIVIDUALS WITH DEMENTIA

BEHAVIORAL PROBLEM	INTERVENTION
Attention/ concentration deficit	Verbally direct client through each step of eating process
	Place utensils in hand
	Make food/fluids available and visible
Combative, throws food	Identify provocative agent, remove
	Feeder stands/sits on nondominant side
	Provide nonbreakable dishes with suction holder
	Give one food at a time
	Reward appropriate mealtime behavior
Chews constantly	Tell client to stop chewing after each bite
	Serve soft foods to reduce the need to chew
	Offer small bites
Eats nonedible things	Remove nonedibles from reach
	Provide finger foods
	Provide edible centerpiece or table decorations
Eats too fast	Set utensils down between bites
	Offer food items separately
	Offer bulky foods that require chewing
	Use a smaller spoon/cup
Eats too slowly	Monitor eating place/provide verbal cues "chew," "take a bite"
	Serve first to allow more time
	Use insulated dishes to maintain proper temperatures
Forgetful/ disoriented	Simple routines
	Constant environment
	Assigned seating
	Minimize distractions
	Limit choices
Forgets to swallow	Tell client to swallow
	Feel for swallow before offering next bite
	Stroke upward on larynx
Inappropriate emotional expression	Engage in conversation
	Ignore emotional display
	Provide quiet environment
Paces	Sit beside client at table
	Change dining location
	Aerobic exercise before meals
	Finger foods
	Cups with covers/spout
Plays in food	Serve one food at a time
	Fill glass/plate half full at refill
	Finger food
	Cups with covers/spout
Shows paranoia	Provide structured routine
	Present food in a consistent manner
	Serve foods in closed containers
	Do not put medicine in food
Spits	Evaluate chewing/swallowing ability
	Tell client not to spit
	Place away from others who would be offended
	Provide mealtime supervision
Will not go into dining room	Ask why
	Change dining location
	Provide a single dining partner versus a group
	Serve meals in room

(Adapted with permission from the Nutrition Screening Initiative, a project of the American Academy of Family Physicians, The American Dietetic Association, and the National Council on the Aging, Inc., and funded in part by a grant from Ross Products Division, a division of Abbott Laboratories.)

Amyotrophic Lateral Sclerosis

Amyotrophic lateral sclerosis (ALS), also referred to as Lou Gehrig's disease after the famous baseball player afflicted with the disease, is the most common type of motor system disease. It involves progressive denervation atrophy and weakness of muscles, hence the term amyotrophy, and is the hallmark sign and symptom of ALS. Both upper and lower motor neurons are lost in the spinal cord, brain stem, and motor cortex thus contributing to the clinical manifestations characterized by generalized skeletal muscular weakness, atrophy, and hyperreflexia. The natural history of disease for ALS is unpleasant; the course is relentless and without remissions, relapses, or plateaus; it finally progresses to death in 2 to 6 years (Adams et al., 1997).

Epidemiology and Pathophysiology

There are not consistent risk factors of occupation, trauma, diet, or socioeconomic status. The prevalence is constant throughout the world, and men are affected more than women. The average age of onset is the mid-fifties, but varies considerably, ranging from the late teens to the eighties (Mitsumoto, 1994). ALS is known as the neurodegenerative disease of the aging nervous system. The etiology of ALS is unknown. The pathologic basis of weakness in ALS is the selective death of motor neurons in the ventral gray matter of the spinal cord and in the motor cortex (Kasarskis and Neville, 1996).

The disease is not inherited except for 5% of cases. Genetic analysis of patients with familial, chromosome 21-linked ALS suggests that mutations in the copper-zinc superoxide dismutase (SOD1) gene may be involved in the etiology (Rosen et al., 1993). The possible role of antioxidant status in prevention and therapeutic intervention needs to be investigated. Studies involving the use of vitamin C and vitamin E are recommended to further define the role of antioxidant therapy in ALS.

The disease is also associated with a defect in high-affinity glutamate transport with region and chemical specificity (Rothstein et al., 1992). Defects in extracellular glutamate clearance could lead to neurotoxic levels, and thus be pathogenic in ALS.

Clinical Findings and Treatment

Given the classic signs of this disease, ALS can be accurately diagnosed by clinical examination 95% of the time. The typical presentation is evidenced with both lower motor neuron (weakness, wasting, fasciculation) and upper motor neuron deficits (hyperactive tendon reflexes, Hoffman signs, Babinski signs, or clonus). Muscle weakness commences in the legs and hands and progresses to the proximal arms and oropharynx. As these motor nerves deteriorate, almost all of the voluntary skeletal muscles are at risk for atrophy and complete loss of function. This loss of spinal motor neurons causes the denervation of voluntary skeletal muscle of the neck, trunk, and limbs resulting in muscle wasting, flaccid weakness, and fasciculations leading to loss of mobility. The progressive loss of function in cortical motor neurons can lead to spasticity of jaw muscles resulting in dysarthria (slurred speech) and dysphagia (Kasarskis and Neville, 1996).

The onset of dysphagia is usually insidious and the functional deficits affect dysphagia and speech similarly; swallowing difficulties usually follow speech difficulties. Despite the presence of impaired speech, patients often do not report difficulties swallowing. Although some weight loss is inevitable given the muscle atrophy, consistent or dramatic loss may be an indicator of probable chewing difficulties or dysphagia (Strand et al., 1996).

The relationship of dysphagia and respiratory status in disease progression is worth noting. As ALS progresses, there is a progressive loss of function in bulbar and respiratory muscles contributing to oral and pharyngeal dysphagia. In a longitudinal study, Strand and others noted that when respiratory status was compromised (vital capacity <1 liter), the functional status of swallowing was significantly impaired such that nutrition support was required. At this point, the respiratory status is impaired such that the patient is not a good candidate for PEG placement. Although the PEG is placed under local anesthesia, the patient may not be able to lie prone for tube placement without respiratory decompensation. This reinforces the need for early versus late education about dysphagia management and initiation of discussion about whether or not to place a feeding tube. This decision is predicated on respiration not swallowing status.

Eye movement and eye blink are spared, as are the sphincter muscles of the bowel and bladder. Incontinence is rare. Sensation remains intact and, except in rare cases, mental acuity is maintained. Although mechanical ventilation can extend the life of patients, the majority decline this option because the quality of life with advanced ALS is poor. There is no effective therapy for curing or even slowing the disease progression. Research has shown no benefit from immunosuppression, immunoenhancement, plasmapheresis, lymph node irradiation, glutamate antagonists, nerve growth factors, or antiviral agents. These treatments remain uncorroborated. Therefore, only supportive measures can be used to maintain the optimal quality of life.

The Amyotrophic Lateral Sclerosis Severity Scale (ALSSS) developed by Hillel and colleagues is one guideline used to assess the functional level of swallowing, speech, and upper and lower extremities (Hillel et al., 1989). Once the severity of deficits have been identified the appropriate interventions can be implemented (Table 42–9).

Nutritional Management

The changes in nutriture during the different stages of ALS have not been well documented. However, Kasarskis et al. (1996) studied the effects ALS has on nutritional status with relation to the proximity of death, to characterize the natural history of ALS with regard to nutritional status (Table 42–10). Their results demonstrate decreases in body fat, lean body mass, muscle power, and nitrogen balance, and an increase in resting energy expenditure as death approaches.

The clinician should become familiar with common clinical findings throughout the natural history of disease progression to prevent secondary complications of malnutrition and dehydration. The functional status of each patient should be monitored closely so that timely intervention with the appropriate management techniques can be started. In particular, dysphagia should be monitored closely. Oropharyngeal weakness affects survival in ALS by placing the patient at continuous risk of aspiration, pneumonia, and sepsis and by curtailing the adequate intake of energy and protein (Kasarskis and Neville, 1996). These problems can compound the deteriorating effects of the disease. Therefore, Strand and colleagues (1996) have outlined the timing of dysphagia intervention on a continuum of five stages that correlate to the severity scale.

1. Normal Eating Habits (ALS Severity Scale Rating 10–9). Early assessment and intervention are critical for maintaining nutritional health in ALS. This is the appropriate time to begin educating the patient, before the development of speech or swallowing symptoms. Hydration and maintenance of nutritional health are critical at this stage. Fluid

TABLE 42–9 AMYOTROPHIC LATERAL SCLEROSIS SEVERITY SCALE

SWALLOWING SCALE

Rating	
	NORMAL EATING HABITS
10	Normal Swallowing: Person denies any difficulty chewing or swallowing. Examination demonstrates no abnormality.
9	Nominal Abnormality: Only the individual with ALS notices slight indicators such as food lodging in the recesses of the mouth or sticking in the throat.
	EARLY EATING PROBLEMS
8	Minor Swallowing Problems: Complains of some swallowing difficulties. Maintains essentially a regular diet. Isolated choking episodes.
7	Prolonged Time or Small Bite Size: Mealtime has significantly increased and smaller bite sizes are necessary. Must concentrate on swallowing liquids.
	DIETARY CONSISTENCY CHANGES
6	Soft Diet: Diet is limited primarily to soft foods. Requires some special meal preparation.
5	Liquified Diet: Oral intake adequate. Nutrition limited primarily to liquified diet. Thin liquid intake usually a problem. May force self to eat.
	NEEDS TUBE FEEDING
4	Supplemental Tube Feedings: Oral intake alone is no longer adequate. Person uses or needs a tube to supplement intake. Person continues to take significant nutrition (greater than 50%) by mouth.
3	Tube Feeding with Occasional Oral Nutrition: Primary nutrition and hydration accomplished by tube. Receives less than 59% of nutrition by mouth.
	NOTHING BY MOUTH
2	Secretions Managed with Aspirator/Medication: Cannot safely manage any oral intake. Secretions managed by aspirator and/or medications. Swallows reflexively.
1	Aspiration of Secretions: Secretions cannot be managed noninvasively. Rarely swallows.

SPEECH SCALE

Rating	
	NORMAL SPEECH PROCESSES
10	Normal Speech: Individual denies any difficulty speaking. Examination demonstrates no abnormality.
9	Nominal Speech Abnormality: Only the individual with ALS or spouse notices that speech has changed. Maintains normal rate and volume.
	DETECTABLE SPEECH DISTURBANCE
8	Perceived Speech Changes: Speech changes are noted by others, especially during fatigue or stress. Rate of speech remains essentially normal.
7	Obvious Speech Abnormalities: Speech is consistently impaired. Affected are rate, articulation, and resonance. Remains easily understood.
	BEHAVIORAL MODIFICATIONS
6	Repeats Messages on Occasion: Rate is much slower. Repeats specific words in adverse listening situations. Does not limit complexity or length of message.
5	Frequent Repeating Required: Speech is slow and labored. Extensive repetition or a "translator" is commonly needed. Person probably limits the complexity or length of message.
	USE OF AUGMENTATIVE COMMUNICATION
4	Speech Plus Augmentative Communication: Speech is used in response to questions. Intelligibility problems need to be resolved by writing or a spokesperson.
3	Limits Speech to One-Word Response: Vocalizes one-word response beyond yes/no; otherwise writes or uses a spokesperson. Initiates communication nonvocally.
	LOSS OF USEFUL SPEECH
2	Vocalizes for Emotional Expression: Uses vocal inflection to express emotion, affirmation, and negation.
1	Nonvocal: Vocalization is difficult, limited in duration, and rarely attempted. May vocalize for crying or pain.
X	Tracheostomy

UPPER EXTREMITIES SCALE RATING

Rating	
	NORMAL FUNCTION
10	Normal Function: Person denies any weakness of unusual fatigue of upper extremities. Examination demonstrates no abnormality.
9	Suspected Fatigue: Person suspects fatigue in upper extremities during exertion. Cannot sustain work for as long as normal. Atrophy not evident on examination.
	INDEPENDENT AND COMPLETE SELF-CARE
8	Slow Self-Care Performance: Dressing and hygiene performed more slowly than usual.
7	Laborious Self-Care Performance: Requires significantly more time (usually double or more) and effort to accomplish self-care. Weakness is apparent on examination.
	INTERMITTENT ASSISTANCE
6	Mostly Independent: Handles most aspects of dressing and hygiene alone. Adapts by resting, modifying (electric razor), or by avoiding some tasks (e.g., buttons, tie).
5	Partial Independence: Handles some aspects of dressing and hygiene alone. However, routinely requires assistance for many tasks such as makeup, combing, shaving, etc.
	NEEDS ATTENDANT FOR SELF-CARE
4	Attendant Assists Person: Attendant must be present for dressing and hygiene. Person performs the majority of each task with the assistance of the attendant.
3	Person Assists Attendant: The attendant assists the person with ALS for most all tasks. The person moves in a purposeful manner to assist the attendant. Does not initiate self-care tasks.
	TOTAL DEPENDENCE
2	Minimal Movement: Minimal movement of one or both arms. Cannot reposition arms.
1	Paralysis: Flaccid paralysis. Unable to move upper extremities.

LOWER EXTREMITIES SCALE

Rating	
	NORMAL
10	Normal Ambulation: Person denies any weakness or fatigue. Examination detects no abnormality.
9	Fatigue Suspected: Person suspects weakness or fatigue in lower extremities during exertion.
	EARLY AMBULATION PROBLEM
8	Difficulty with Uneven Terrain: Difficulty and fatigue when walking long distances, climbing stairs, and walking over uneven ground (even thick carpet).
7	Observed Changes in Gait: Noticeable change in gait. Pulls on railing when climbing stairs. May use leg brace.
	WALKS WITH ASSISTANCE
6	Walks with Mechanical Device: Needs or uses canes, walker, or assistant to walk. Probably uses wheelchair away from home.

5	Walks with Mechanical Device and Attendant: Does not attempt to walk without an attendant. Ambulation limited to less than 50 feet. Avoids stairs.
	FUNCTIONAL MOVEMENT ONLY
4	Able to Support Weight: At best can shuffle a few steps with the help of an attendant for transfers.
3	Purposeful Leg Movements: Unable to take steps but can position legs to assist an attendant in transfers. Moves legs purposefully to maintain mobility in bed.
	NO PURPOSEFUL LEG MOVEMENT
2	Minimal Movement: Minimal movement of one or both legs. Cannot reposition legs independently.
1	Paralysis: Flaccid paralysis. Cannot move lower extremities.

(From Hillel AD, et al. ALS Severity Scale. J Neuroepidemiol 8:142, 1989. Reproduced with permission of J. Karger AG, Basel.)

intake of at least 2 q/day from noncaffeinated sources is important because caffeine has a diuretic effect contributing to dehydration. Dehydration contributes to fatigue and thickens saliva. For patients with spinal ALS, emphasis on fluids is important because they may intentionally limit fluid intake because of difficulties with toileting. The diet history is helpful to assess patterns of normal chewing, swallowing, and the rate of ingestion; weight loss history establishes a baseline weight. A weight loss of 10% or more is indicative of nutritional risk.

2. and 3. Early Eating Problems (Severity Scale Rating 8–7) and Dietary Consistency Changes Severity Scale Rating 6–5). At this point, patients begin to report difficulties eating; reports of coughing and unusually long mealtimes are associated with tongue, facial, and masticator muscle weakness. Dietary intervention is focused on modification of consistency, avoidance of thin liquids, and use of foods that are easier to chew and swallow. As these symptoms progress, the oral transport of food becomes difficult as dry crumbly foods will tend to break apart and cause choking. Foods that require more chewing, raw vegetables or steak, are typically avoided. As dysphagia progresses, ingestion of thin liquids, especially water, may become more problematic. Often the patient has fatigue and malaise, which may be associated with a mild chronic dehydration due to a decreased fluid intake. Dietary intervention should be geared toward changes in food consistency to mechanical soft or pureed to reduce the need for oral manipulation and to conserve energy (Table 42–11). Small, frequent meals may also increase intake (Asbeck and Burns, 1988). Thick liquids containing a high percentage of water to maintain fluid balance as well as attempts to increase fluid intake need to be emphasized. Popsicles, Jello, ice, and fresh fruit are additional sources of free water. Liquids can be thickened with a modified cornstarch thickener.

Swallowing can be improved by emphasizing taste, texture, and temperature. Juices can be substituted for water to provide taste, nutrients, and calories. A cool temperature facilitates the swallowing mechanism and therefore cold food items may be better tolerated (see Table 42–6). Heat does not provide the same advantage. Carbonation may also be better tolerated as there is a beneficial effect of texture.

Instructions for preventing aspiration should be addressed. Proper position for safe swallowing should be to sit bolt upright with the head in a chin-down position. Concentrating on the swallowing process can also help reduce choking. Environmental distractions and conversation during mealtime increase the risk for aspiration; however, families should be encouraged to maintain as normal mealtime behavior as possible. As dysphagia progresses, the limitation of food consistencies may result in the exclusion of entire food groups. Vitamin and mineral supplementation may be necessary. If chewable supplements are not handled safely, liquid forms may be added to acceptable foods. Fiber may also need to be added along with fluids for constipation problems.

4. Tube Feeding (Severity Scale Rating 5–4). Dehydration will occur acutely before malnutrition, a more chronic state, is exhibited. This may be an early indication of the need for nutrition support. Weight loss resulting from muscle wasting and

TABLE 42–10 NUTRITIONAL AND METABOLIC CHANGES DURING THE PROGRESSION OF AMYOTROPHIC LATERAL SCLEROSIS

	EARLY PHASE	LATE PHASE
Pathophysiology	Cycles of muscle denervation, muscle catabolism and atrophy, reinnervation, and protein synthesis	Net muscle catabolism and atrophy
Functional status	Mild functional restriction of physical activity Mild impairment of respiration	Progressive limitation of physical activity Increased work of ventilation
Nutritional and metabolic changes	Positive nitrogen balance Normal resting energy expenditure Probable neutral energy balance	Negative nitrogen balance Increased resting energy expenditure Decrease in body fat

(Source: Kasarskis EJ, et al. Nutritional status of patients with amyotrophic lateral sclerosis: Relation to the proximity of death. Am J Clin Nutr 63:130, 1996. Printed in USA. © 1996 Am. J. Clin. Nutr. American Society for Clinical Nutrition.)

TABLE 42–11 DIET FOR EASY CHEWING AND SWALLOWING

TYPE OF FOOD	FOODS GENERALLY INCLUDED	FOODS COMMONLY EXCLUDED
Fluids	Thick juices,* sherbet,* sherbet shakes,* popsicles,* gelatin,* thin liquids thickened with Thick-It[†]	Water, thin juices, milk, coffee, tea
Bread and cereals	Bread, toast, cooked cereal, quick breads without nuts and raisins, pancakes, moist pastas, and casseroles	Crackers, dry rice, dry cereal flakes, crumbly bread, soft white bread
Dairy products	Butter, margarine, creamy or blenderized cottage cheese, soft cheeses, yogurt, thickened milk or dairy substitutes, and ice cream if tolerated	Dry cottage cheese, melted hot cheese
Eggs	Medium-cooked, poached, scrambled, soft omelet, custard	Runny eggs, thin eggnogs
Meat, fish, and poultry	Moist ground meat in casseroles, meatloaf, meatballs, ground meat with sauces and gravies, moist, tender fish without bones	Dry ground meat, chunky meats, dry fish, or fish with bones
Fruits	Soft canned fruits with seeds, pits, and skin removed; ripe bananas, chilled, thick pureed fruits, soft fruits in gelatin	Raw fruits except bananas, thin pureed fruits, stringy pineapple
Vegetables	Soft canned vegetables, baked, mashed, or boiled potatoes with margarine or gravy, whipped squash with margarine, scalloped potatoes, thick pureed vegetables, minced vegetables in gelatin	Raw vegetables, chunky vegetables such as diced beets, stringy vegetables such as spinach, corn, firm peas
Soups	Thick soups (blenderized)	Thin soups or chunky style soups
Desserts	Fruit whip, gelatin,* apple or peach crisp, moist cookies without nuts or raisins, custard, pudding, sherbet, ice cream if tolerated	Dry cakes and cookies, dessert with raisins, nuts, seeds, or coconut, hard candies and chocolate

*Safety with these foods may depend on oral retention times because they melt in the mouth and become difficult to manage.
[†]Thick-It is a modified cornstarch used to thicken both hot and cold liquids. Made by Milani and available nationwide.

dysphagia will eventually lead to placement of a PEG tube for nutrition and protection against aspiration due to dysphagia. Enteral nutrition support is preferred over parenteral nutrition support because the gastrointestinal tract should be functioning properly. Given the progressive nature of ALS, placing feeding tubes when dysphagia and dehydration are evident is probably better than initiating this therapy later in the course after the patient has become overtly malnourished or after respiratory status is marginal. The decision of whether to place a feeding tube for nutrition support is part of the decision-making process each patient must face. However, it might be added that adequate nutriture can maintain health of the individual longer. One study demonstrated improved survival after 6 months by administering nutritional support via a PEG (Mazzini et al., 1995). The initiation of nutrition support may be a welcome relief for the patient who has become overburdened with all of the difficulties of sustaining himself. The purpose of nutrition support should be to enhance the quality of life.

Although a nasogastric tube can be a short-term option, a PEG tube, placed under local anesthesia, is preferred for long-term management (Mathus-Vliegen et al., 1994). Long-term access should be considered via a PEG or percutaneous endoscopic jejunostomy (PEJ) tube (see Chapter 22).

5. NPO (Severity Scale Rating 2–1). The final level of dysphagia is reached when the patient cannot eat orally. Nor can the patient manage his or her own oral secretions. Although saliva production is not increased, it tends to pool in the front of the mouth due to a declining swallow response. Once the swallowing mechanism is absent, mechanical ventilation is required to manage saliva flow. Tube feeding is permanent at this stage.

Epilepsy

Epilepsy is an intermittent derangement of the nervous system due presumably to a sudden, excessive, disorderly discharge of cerebral neurons. It is estimated that 1.65 million individuals in the United States have epilepsy. Most seizures begin in early life, but there is a resurgence of epileptic events after age 60. Internet information is available at www.efa.org at the Epilepsy Foundation.

Etiology and Pathophysiology

The first occurrence of a seizure in adults should prompt investigation into a cause. Usually, a clinical workup reveals no anatomic abnormalities, and the cause of the seizure remains unknown or idiopathic. In other instances cerebrovascular disease, trauma, or a named syndrome is identified (Rowland, 1995). The medical history is the key component for suggesting further avenues of diagnostic investigation, especially in children. An electroencephalogram can help to delineate seizure activity. It is most helpful in localizing partial complex seizures.

Clinical Findings and Treatment

There are two peaks of seizure incidence. The first occurs in the infants less than 2 years of age. The second occurs after the age of 60. Often, the patient will have normal cognition and development, and a physical examination will reveal nothing suspect.

The dramatic **tonic-clonic seizure** is the most common image of a seizure, yet there are numerous classifications of seizures, each with a different and often less dramatic clinical presentation. A generalized seizure is one that involves or appears to involve the entire brain cortex from its beginning phases. The tonic-clonic seizure comes under this heading. After such a seizure the patient will wake up slowly after a time; he or she will be groggy and disoriented for minutes to hours after the event. This is termed the postictal phase. The **petit mal seizure** or absence seizure is also generalized in nature. A patient with absence seizures may appear to be daydreaming during an episode, but he or she recovers consciousness within a few seconds and has no postictal fatigue or disorientation.

Partial seizures occur when there is a discrete focus of epileptogenic brain tissue. A simple partial seizure involves no loss of consciousness, whereas a complex partial seizure is characterized by a change in consciousness. This implies a spread to the brain stem areas that govern consciousness. Partial seizures may also secondarily generalize. This means that the electrical activity in the seizure focus spreads across the entire brain.

Determining the seizure type is key to implementing effective therapy. Generalized seizures are ordinarily managed with valproate or phenytoin. These drugs are difficult to use because they interact with other drugs metabolized in the liver and have a proclivity to cause liver damage. Liver enzymes and serum drug levels must be monitored periodically. Phenytoin's metabolism has unusual kinetics; thus, toxic levels may be attained with very small dosage adjustments. Gabapentin has been introduced recently, and it is rapidly gaining popularity because of its safety and ease of use.

Carbamazepine or phenytoin can usually control partial seizures. Failure of partial seizure control may prompt consideration of seizure surgery. A localized focus resected from nonessential brain will render a patient seizure free in 75% of cases. A discussion of phenobarbital is avoided here because its use is controversial. It has been associated with decreased intelligence quotient (IQ) when used in children. It is occasionally considered for use after failure of other antiepileptic drugs.

Medications used in anticonvulsant therapy may alter the nutritional status of the patient. Phenobarbital, phenytoin, and primidone interfere with intestinal absorption of calcium by increasing vitamin D metabolism in the liver. Long-term therapy with these drugs may lead to osteomalacia in adults or rickets in children. Vitamin D supplementation is recommended. Folic acid supplementation interferes with phenytoin metabolism so it contributes to difficulties in achieving therapeutic levels. For this reason, sporadic folic acid supplementation should be avoided (see Chapter 18). Phenytoin and phenobarbital are bound primarily to albumin in the bloodstream. Decreased serum albumin levels in malnutrition or with reduced albumin synthesis secondary to advanced cirrhosis limit the amount of drug that can be bound. This results in an increased free drug concentration and possible drug toxicity with a standard dose.

Continuous enteral feeding inhibits the absorption of phenytoin, necessitating an increase in the dose to achieve a therapeutic level. Holding the tube feeding before and after drug administration has not been shown to be effective in achieving therapeutic drug levels (Ozuna and Friel, 1984). In the event that tube feedings are stopped, the dose of phenytoin needs to be adjusted to avoid toxicity.

Alcohol consumption results in the loss of the intended effect of phenytoin, possibly causing seizures. Absorption of phenobarbital is delayed by the consumption of food; therefore, administration of the drug must be staggered around mealtimes.

Nutritional Management

The ketogenic diet is often reserved as a last resort for treatment of all types of seizures in children in whom all drug therapies have failed. This treatment is considered to be unconventional despite having minimal side effects and being inexpensive. Not only is this unconventional therapy an effective form of secondary treatment for epilepsy, it also has the potential to be curative. The diet will completely control epilepsy in one third of the children whose seizures are otherwise uncontrollable. For another one third of children, the diet will either markedly decrease the frequency of seizures or allow medications to be reduced (Freeman et al., 1996). More information can be found on the Web page of the Epilepsy Foundation at www.efa.org.

The diet is designed to create and maintain a state of ketosis. Its mechanism of action is not clearly understood, but the beneficial effect in epilepsy may be due to a change in neuronal metabolism, whereby a ketone body behaves as an inhibitory neurotransmitter, producing an anticonvulsant effect on the body (American Dietetic Association, 1992). Mild dehydration is important with this diet to prevent dilution of the level of ketones circulating at any time (Berryman, 1997).

Two forms of the ketogenic diet are in use: the "traditional" approach, developed in the 1920s and the medium-chain triglyceride (MCT)-based approach. With either approach the child fasts in the hospital for 24 to 72 hours until a 4+ ketonuria is produced. For the majority of patients, if the diet is going to work, it will usually work during the initial fasting period. It should also be noted that antiepileptic drugs need to be stopped when administering the ketogenic diet.

In the traditional approach, once ketosis is established, caloric intake is resumed in a 4:1 ratio of fat/protein and carbohydrate kilocalories. Kilocalories are calculated to provide 75% of the recommended dietary allowance (RDA) for a child's ideal weight and height. Protein is calculated to provide appropriate intake for growth (about 1 g/kg/day). Carbohydrates are added to make up the remaining portion of protein and carbohydrate calories, which is usually a minimal to negligible amount. The Exchange Lists (see Appendices) can be used to adjust the carbohydrate amount. Fluids are also carefully controlled—about 65 mL/kg/day but not to exceed 2 L/day is recommended (Kinsman et al., 1992). A multiple vitamin and calcium supplement is recommended to ensure that the diet is nutritionally complete and this should be provided in a sugar-free form.

The MCT-based ketogenic diet replaces the long-chain fats of the traditional diet with MCT. MCT oil is available as an odorless, colorless, tasteless oil and was originally used as a means of improving the palatability of the diet. A greater amount of nonketogenic foods such as fruits and vegetables and small amounts of bread and other starches can be allowed because ketosis from MCT can be more readily achieved (Table 42–12). Fluids are not limited in this diet.

The ketogenic diet may be unpalatable and complex, making compliance difficult to maintain. Long-term, children may benefit from behavioral techniques while parents often require substantial psychosocial support. For the child whose epilepsy is controlled on the diet, complying with the diet is much easier than dealing with devastating seizures. Fortunately, the duration of the diet is limited; it can usually be discontinued after 2 to 3 years.

Guillain-Barré Syndrome

Guillain-Barré syndrome (GBS) is an acute onset, inflammatory, demyelinating polyneuropathy that has a predilection for proximal motor nerves, including the cranial nerves and the diaphragm. The incidence is approximately 2/100,000. Like myasthenia gravis, this disorder is most likely mediated by the immune system. In 60% of cases, the disorder follows an infection. Some of the more common organisms are *Campylobacter jejuni*, *Mycoplasma*, and some herpes viruses (Griffin, 1996). There are several pathologic varieties, and the nature of the distinction is related to the segment of the immune system inflicting nerve damage. The clinical course of GBS is similar regardless of subtype, although GBS following from *Campylobacter* infection tends to be more severe.

The loss of function in affected nerves occurs because of demyelination. Myelin is the specialized fatty insulation that envelops the conducting part of the nerve, the axon. In GBS the immune system recognizes myelin and mounts an attack against it. Presumably, myelin shares a common characteristic with the pathogen from the antecedent infection, so the immune system cannot differentiate what is foreign (the pathogen) from what is native (myelin). When myelin is removed from a nerve, its ability to conduct signals is severely impaired, and this results in neuropathy.

Clinical Features and Treatment

The most common sequence of symptoms is areflexia, followed by proximal limb weakness, followed finally by cranial nerve weakness and respi-

TABLE 42–12 TYPICAL KETOGENIC DIET MENU USING MCT OIL

FOOD ITEM	AMOUNT (g)	CARBOHYDRATE (g)	PROTEIN (g)	FAT (g)	ENERGY (kcal)
Breakfast					
White bread	5	2.8	0.4	0.2	13
Egg, scrambled	48		6.1	5.5	74
Cream, heavy whipping	10	0.3	0.3	3.8	36
Margarine	5			5	45
MCT oil	12			12	108
Fat	11			11	99
Koolaid, with non-nutritive sweetner	240				
Total		2.8	6.8	37.5	375
Lunch					
American cheese	12	2.2	2.8	3.6	52
Ham	23	0.7	3.7	3.9	53
MCT oil mayonnaise	11			11	99
Fat	19			19	171
Koolaid, with non-nutritive sweetner	240				
Total		2.9	6.5	37.5	375
Dinner					
Turkey	19		6.3	0.7	32
Tomato	10	0.5	0.1	0.0	3
Green beans	10	0.6	0.2	0.0	3
Potatoes	12	1.7	0.2	0.0	8
Margarine	15			15	135
MCT oil mayonnaise	11			11	99
Fat	10			10	90
Koolaid, with non-nutritive sweetner	240				
Total		2.8	6.8	36.7	370
Daily Total:		8.5	20.1	111.7	1120

ratory insufficiency. These symptoms may progress for up to 1 month, but normally peak by 2 weeks. Diagnosis is ordinarily made on clinical grounds, but nerve conduction studies are revealing. Before the clinical course is apparent, myelopathic disorders need to be considered. GBS will reveal itself in a matter of days.

Because of the potentially precipitous progression of GBS, hospitalization is in order, if only for observation. Vital capacity and swallowing function may rapidly deteriorate such that intensive care is sometimes necessary. Intubation and respiratory support should be instituted early in the face of respiratory decline, to avoid resusitation. Plasmapheresis, the exchange of the patient's plasma for albumin, is often helpful. This reduces the load of circulating antibodies. Also, intravenous immunoglobulin has been shown to be of benefit. Steroids may be used in conjunction with the above measures (Cecil and Underlie, 1997).

Nutritional Management

Guillain-Barré syndrome evolves quickly, and during this acute stage, the metabolic response of GBS is similar to the stress response that occurs in neurotrauma. Researchers studied 21 patients with GBS admitted to an intensive care unit. Energy needs assessed by indirect calorimetry were 40 to 45 nonprotein kcal/kg and protein needs assessed by 24-hour urine urea nitrogen were 2.0 to 2.5 g/kg. Supportive care by immediate attainment of positive energy balance provided by high-energy and protein tube feedings, may help to reestablish a positive nitrogen balance and attenuate muscle wasting (Roubenoff et al., 1992).

For a small percentage of patients, oropharyngeal muscles may be affected, leading to dysphagia and dysarthria. In this situation, a visit by the dietitian at mealtime can be an invaluable way to observe any difficulties the patient may have with chewing or swallowing. Such difficulties warrant evaluation by a swallowing specialist. The swallow therapist can evaluate the degree of dysphagia and make appropriate dietary recommendations pertaining to texture. The nutritionist can then ensure that patients are adequately nourished (Curran, 1997).

Migraine Headache

The syndrome is defined clinically as an episodic intense, throbbing head pain, usually on one side of the head. Classically, it is associated with a prodrome of visual disturbances or unusual olfactory and gustatory perception.

Etiology and Pathophysiology

The migraine headache is thought to be vascular in origin. The leading theory proposes that dural blood vessels become dilated, and the pulsatile blood flow through these vessels distends and irritates the highly pain-sensitive dura mater. This would explain the throbbing quality of the headache. An inflammatory component to migraine headache has also been proposed.

Clinical Findings and Treatment

A thorough history is the key to diagnosis here. To qualify for a diagnosis of migraine headache, the headache must be throbbing, episodic, and supremely intense. The excruciating headache must not be prematurely considered migraine. A history of intercurrent nausea, vomiting, photophobia, and visual or olfactory auras should be sought. Less commonly, the examiner can elicit a neurologic deficit.

Numerous medicines are used to prevent or abort migraine, indicating a less than crystal clear understanding of its pathophysiology. Nonsteroidal anti-inflammatories are often the first line, followed by sympathomimetics and serotonin agonists such as sumitriptan. Prophylaxis can include calcium channel antagonists, β-adrenergic blockers, and serotonin antagonists.

Nutritional Management

The proposed mechanisms that predicate migraine headache on nutritional factors are poorly understood. One recent study suggests that riboflavin may be beneficial because its derivatives participate in mitochondrial dysfunction that plays a part in migraine pathogenesis (Schoenen et al., 1998). Migraine attacks are triggered by a variety of factors, including food, and respond to a variety of treatments. Foods implicated in one individual may not trigger attacks in another, and food intolerance thresholds vary over time. Therefore, it is ill-advised to make general recommendations about food avoidance.

Another obstacle to dietary management occurs when dietary restriction of the offending foods contributes to inadequate nutritional intake. Because suspect food items can only be correctly identified if eliminated and then reintroduced into the diet, the dietitian should offer alternative food suggestions so eliminated dietary items are replaced with foods having similar nutritional value to ensure adequate food intake and nutritional status.

Foods responsible for contributing to migraine attacks include citrus fruits, tea (flavonoids), coffee, pork, chocolate, milk, nuts, vegetables, and cola drinks. Substances causing modification in vascular tone are tyramine, phenylalanine, phenolic flavonoids, alcohol, food additives (sodium nitrate, monosodium glutamate, aspartame), and caffeine. Foods thought to trigger migraines subsequent to hypoglycemia are chocolate, cheese, citrus fruits, bananas, nuts, cured meats, dairy products, cereals, beans, hot dogs, pizza, food additives, coffee, tea, cola drinks, alcoholic drinks such as red wine, beer or whiskey distilled in copper stills (Leira and

Rodriguez, 1996; American Dietetic Association, 1993). Initiation of therapy will require trial and error and extensive record-keeping of symptoms and food intake on the part of the patient.

Myasthenia Gravis

Myasthenia gravis (MG) is not only the most well known disorder of the neuromuscular junction, but it is also one of the most well-characterized autoimmune diseases, a class of disorders in which the body's immune system raises a response to acetylcholine receptors (AChR). The incidence of MG is 3/100,000 people.

Etiology and Pathophysiology

The neuromuscular junction is the site on the striated muscle membrane where a spinal motor neuron connects. Here, the signal from the nerve is carried to the muscle via a submicron-sized gap, a synapse. The molecule that carries the signal from the nerve ending to the muscle membrane is acetylcholine (ACh), and AChR populate the muscle membrane. These receptors translate the chemical signal of ACh into an electrical signal that is required for contraction of muscle fibers.

In MG, the body unwittingly makes antibodies to AChR. These antibodies are the same that fight off colds and give immunity. The AChR antibodies bind to AChR and make them unresponsive to ACh. There is no disorder of nerve conduction, and no intrinsic disorder of muscle. The characteristic weakness in MG occurs because the nervous system's signal to muscle is garbled at the neuromuscular junction. Patients with MG commonly have an overactive thymus gland. This gland resides in the anterior thorax, and plays a role in the maturation of B lymphocytes, the cells that are charged with synthesizing antibodies (see Chapter 41).

Clinical Features and Treatment

Relapsing and remitting weakness and fatigability, the period of which varies from minutes to days, characterize MG. The most common presentation is diplopia (double vision) due to extraocular muscle weakness, followed by dysarthria, facial muscle weakness, and dysphagia. It is estimated that 33% of patients with MG have significant swallowing disorders due to fatigue following mastication (Miller, 1997). In 10% of this population, muscular wasting has been encountered, primarily in patients with malnutrition due to dysphagia (Rowland, 1995). Less commonly, proximal limb weakness (i.e. in hips and shoulders) may be present. In 10% of patients, severe diaphragmatic weakness can result in respiratory difficulty. There is no involvement of sensory nerves.

Anticholinesterases are medicines that inhibit acetylcholinesterase. They serve to increase the amount of ACh in the neuromuscular junction. Removal of the thymus results in symptomatic improvement in most patients. Corticosteroids are considered as a means of immunosuppression. In the event that respiratory failure occurs, intubation and temporary cessation of anticholinesterases are the proper course of action until the crisis resolves (Greenberg, 1997).

Nutritional Management

Chewing and swallowing are often compromised in MG. Because this occurs with fatigue, it is important to provide nutritionally dense foods at the beginning of meals before the patient tires. Small frequent meals that are easy to chew and swallow are helpful. Difficulties holding a bolus on the tongue have also been observed, suggesting that foods that do not fall apart easily may be better tolerated. For patients treated with anticholinesterase drugs, it is crucial to time medication with feeding to facilitate optimal swallowing.

Physical activity should be limited before mealtime to ensure maximal strength to eat a meal. In certain patients, even nonstrenuous activities such as talking can mean the difference between consuming an oral diet versus requiring enteral nutrition support (Miller, 1997). It is also a good idea not to encourage food consumption once the patient begins to tire because this may contribute to aspiration. It is more likely that respiratory exacerbations requiring intubation and artificial ventilation occur from aspiration of oral secretions (Rowland, 1995). If and when respiratory crisis occurs, it is usually temporary. Nutrition support via nasogastrointestinal tube may be implemented in the interim to assist in maintaining the vital function of the patient until the crisis subsides. Once extubated, a swallow evaluation using cinefluoroscopy is appropriate to assess degree of **deglutitory dysfunction** or swallowing irregularity, and risk of aspiration associated with resuming an oral diet.

Multiple Sclerosis

Multiple sclerosis (MS) is a chronic disease affecting the CNS characterized by destruction of the myelin sheath whose function is to transmit electrical nerve impulses. MS is called "multiple" because multiple areas of optic nerves, spinal cord, and brain undergo "sclerosis" whereby myelin is replaced with sclera or scar tissue. The signs and symptoms of MS are easily distinguished features, despite remitting to a varying extent, and they recur over the natural history of this disease. The prevalence is less than 1/100,000 in equatorial areas; 6 to 14/100,000 in the southern United States and southern Europe; and 30 to 80/100,000 in Canada, northern Europe, and the northern United States. An internet site is www.nmss.org.

Etiology and Pathophysiology

The precise cause of MS remains undetermined and the epidemiology is difficult to establish in view of the uncertainty of the diagnosis and relative rarity of the disease. A number of well-established findings have been incorporated into a hypothesis to explain the etiology of MS. Although a familial predisposition to MS has been noted in a minority of cases, familial tendency is not well established; no consistent pattern of Mendelian inheritance has emerged (Adams et al., 1997). The tendency exists to consider diseases having an increased familial incidence as inherited; however, instances of the same condition in several family members may reflect exposure to a common agent. Hence, environmental factors compete for this distinction and two of these are latitude and diet.

Epidemiologic studies have linked the incidence of MS to geographic location rather than to a particular ethnic group. This increased incidence from the equator northward has been explained by the sun. Recently, exogenous 1,25-dihydroxyvitamin D_3 (hormonal form of vitamin D_3) has been associated with preventing experimental autoimmune encephalomyelitis (EAE) in mice. This association has focused attention on the possible relationship of MS to vitamin D. Researchers hypothesize that the degree of sunlight exposure catalyzing the production of vitamin D_3 in skin is an environmental factor and that the hormonal form of vitamin D_3 is a selective immune system regulator inhibiting this autoimmune disease (Hayes et al., 1997). Low sunlight exposure yields insufficient vitamin D_3, which limits 1,25-dihydroxyvitamin D_3 and increases the risk for MS.

Diet is another environmental risk factor associated with the development of MS. One ecologic study compared sex-specific mortality rates of MS from the World Health Statistics to the consumption of various saturated fats obtained from the food balance sheets of the United Nations Food and Agriculture Organization (FAO). A higher prevalence of disease was noted in populations consuming diets rich in animal fats containing saturated fatty acids. Ecologic studies are a good starting point in determining whether or not an association exists. However, the exposure (dietary fat) and outcome (incidence of disease) data for each individual are unknown and therefore a causal relationship of dietary fat to the incidence of MS cannot be concluded (Gordis, 1996). It appears that both environmental factors are compelling, but circumstantial evidence warrants further studies.

Clinical Findings and Treatment

Currently there is no proven treatment for changing the course of MS, preventing future attacks, or preventing deterioration. Initially, recovery from relapses is nearly complete, but over time, neurologic deficits remain (Fig. 42–6). Therefore, it is imperative that measures to maximize recovery from initial attacks or exacerbations prevent fatigue and infection, and use all of the available rehabilitative measures to postpone the bedridden stage of disease. Physical and occupational therapies are standard for weakness, spasticity, tremor, uncoordination, and other symptoms.

Steroid therapy is used in treating exacerbations; adrenocorticotrophic hormone (ACTH) and prednisolone are the drugs of choice. However, treatment is not consistently effective and tends to be more useful in cases of less than 5 years' duration. Side effects of short-term steroid treatment include increased appetite, weight gain, fluid retention, nervousness, and insomnia. Methotrexate may also be used with ACTH, causing anorexia and nausea. Drug therapies may, therefore, be a challenge (see Chapter 18). Reduced cerebrospinal fluid and serum levels of vitamin B_{12} and folate have been noted in MS patients receiving high-dose steroids. Because a deficiency of these two nutrients has been associated with cerebral demyelination and subacute combined degeneration of the spinal cord, it might be desirable to administer B_{12} and folate or at least monitor the levels of these nutrients (Frequin et al., 1993). A more recent therapy involves use of β-interferon (Avonex, Betaseron, Copaxone) because it interferes with viruses and inhibits secretion of γ-interferon. Treatment with β-interferon seems to delay neurological deterioration. The drawback is expense.

Nutritional Management

With respect to nutritional research, verifying the role of environmental factors such as nutrition, has dominated over therapeutic trials aimed at treating the disease once it has occurred. However, several dietary regimens for managing MS have been studied, including low-fat, gluten-free diets, and fatty acid supplements, all yielding equivocal results.

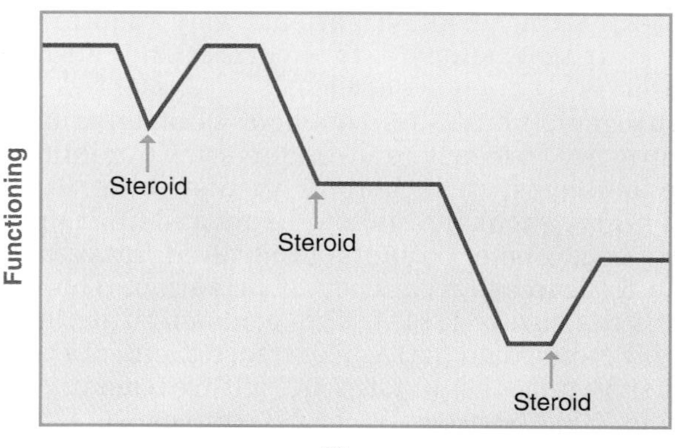

FIGURE 42–6 The progression of multiple sclerosis.

Swank and Dugan reported findings from a 35-year study that showed an improvement in disease progression with a low-fat diet. However, the theory has not been accepted because of a lack of controls (Swank and Dugan, 1991). Other data suggest that dietary supplementation with linoleic acid (safflower oil, soybean oil) may have some beneficial effects not only on the severity and duration of relapses, but also on the progression of disability when patients are treated early in the course of the disease, although this therapy remains investigational (Wozniak-Wowk, 1993). Other trials have used 1.7 g/day of eicosapentanoic acid (EPA) and 1.1 g/day of docosahexaenoic acid (DHA), with the controls receiving 10 g/day of oleic acid (olive oil) for a period of 2 years. Evidence favoring treatment with EPA and DHA is inconclusive (Wozniak-Wowk, 1993).

Past trials of various diets such as allergen-free, gluten-free, pectin-free, and fructose-restricted diets, the raw food Evers diet, the MacDougal diet (no gluten, low sugar and no refined sugar, low-fat diet high in polyunsaturated fatty acids, and megadoses of vitamins/minerals), the Cambridge liquid diet (330 kcal/day with 22 g protein), and vitamin/mineral therapies (zinc phosphates, calcium, other combinations) have generally been ruled ineffective (Wozniak-Wowk, 1993).

Although there have not been any valid clinical trials supporting the efficacy of nutrition in delaying the progression of MS, it is imperative that the clinical dietitian evaluate the nutritional health status of the patient, maximizing nutrition status as an adjunct to the medical care plan. As the disease progresses, neurologic deficits, in particular dysphasia, may occur as the result of damaged cranial nerves. Hence, diet consistency may need to be modified from solids to mechanical soft or pureed items and even progressing to thick liquids to prevent aspiration. Additional problems include impaired vision, dysarthria, and poor ambulation making eating less enjoyable by turning meal preparation into a difficult task. In this situation, reliance on comfort foods, prepackaged, single-serving, or convenience foods often permits independent preparation of meals. Given the chronic nature of this debilitating disease, patients may require enteral nutrition support to hydrate and sustain themselves.

Neurogenic bladder is common, causing urinary incontinence, urgency, and frequency. To minimize these problems, it is helpful to distribute fluids evenly throughout the waking hours and limit them before bed. Some patients limit fluid intake severely to decrease frequency of urination. This increases the risk of UTI. UTI is common in patients with MS, and some patients increase their intake of cranberry juice as a form of self-treatment (see Chapter 38). Neurogenic bowel can cause either constipation or diarrhea and incidence of fecal impaction is increased in MS. A diet that is high in fiber with additional prunes and adequate fluid can moderate both problems.

Parkinson's Disease

Parkinson's disease (PD) is a progressive and disabling disease due to decreased dopamine (a neurotransmitter) transmission to the basal ganglia. Although the natural history of this disease can be remarkably benign in some cases, approximately 66% of patients are disabled within 5 years and 80% after 10 years (Adams et al., 1997). PD is one of the most common neurologic diseases in North America, affecting approximately 1% of the population over 65 years of age. The incidence is similar across socioeconomic groups, though PD is less common in African Americans and Asians as compared to whites. It most commonly occurs between the ages of 40 and 70 (Adams et al., 1997), with a mean age of onset of 55 in both sexes (Rowland, 1995). An internet site for PD is available at www.apdaparkinson.com.

Etiology and Pathophysiology

Although the cause of PD remains unclear, the pathogenesis is well described. There is a marked loss of dopaminergic neurons (pigmented cells) in the substantia nigra as well as tyrosine hydroxylase, the rate-limiting enzyme for dopamine. Three theories are postulated for the etiology of PD: (1) altered dopamine metabolism from neural injury, (2) exposure to environmental neurotoxins, and (3) predisposition (Standaert and Stern, 1993).

The role of endogenous toxins from cellular oxidative reactions has emerged as one hypothesis, because aging has been associated with a loss of neurons containing dopamine and an increase in monoamine oxidase. Dopamine, when metabolized (enzymatic oxidation and auto-oxidation), produces endogenous toxins (hydrogen peroxide and free radicals), causing peroxidation of membrane lipids and cell death. In the presence of an inherited or acquired predisposition, severe oxidative injury can lead to substantial loss of dopaminergic neurons similar to that observed in PD (Standaert and Stern, 1993).

Several environmental factors have also been implicated in the etiology of PD and this theory of etiology has been strengthened considerably by the observation of intravenous drug users who self-administered an opiate substance, 1-methyl-4-phenyl-1,2,3,6-tetrahydropyridine (MPTP). This neurotoxin produces a rapidly progressive parkinsonian syndrome selectively destroying dopamine cells in the substantia nigra.

Dietary lipids and antioxidants are other environmental factors implicated in the etiology of PD. Recently, a case-controlled study found evidence linking high-fat intake from animal sources and PD (Logroscino et al., 1996). It has long been recognized that supplementing deficient subjects with vitamin E is an important preventive measure given the devastating peripheral neuropathy and ataxia that may result from vitamin E deficiency (Traber and Sies, 1996). Although serum levels of vitamin E were not significantly lower in patients with PD than in control subjects, researchers have concluded that a prolonged and severe vitamin E deficiency can result in loss of nigrostriatal nerve endings (Fernandez-Calle et al., 1996). These nutrient-related findings are biologically plausible and support the hypothesis that oxidative stress may contribute to the pathogenesis of PD.

The third environmental factor associated with the incidence of PD is geographic variation. There is a greater incidence of PD in industrialized countries and agrarian areas where toxins are more commonly used. Unfortunately, no one chemical toxin or heavy metal has been shown to definitely cause PD (Adams et al., 1997).

The genetic susceptibility for developing PD remains unclear. Twin studies are inclusive and most cases are sporadic, despite a family incidence rate of 5% (Adams et al., 1997).

Clinical Findings and Treatment

The "classic triad" of signs—tremor, rigidity, and bradykinesia—first described by James Parkinson in 1817 remains as accepted clinical criterion for diagnosis (Standaert and Stern, 1993). However, it was well over a century before an effective therapy, levodopa (L-dopa) was introduced for controlling symptoms. This remains the cornerstone of treatment. Because dopamine does not readily cross the blood–brain barrier, L-dopa is administered. L-Dopa, a precursor to dopamine, is subsequently converted to dopamine by dopa decarboxylase and it crosses the blood–brain barrier (Calne, 1993). To date, there are no primary preventive measures or curative treatments for PD. Additional pharmacotherapy agents as well as surgical interventions are adjunct therapies for treating PD along with physical therapy. Deprenyl (a monoamine oxidase inhibitor), but not vitamin E (2000 IU daily), was shown to delay the onset of disability associated with early otherwise untreated PD (Parkinson's Study Group, 1993). In older patients, drug-induced PD may occur as a side effect of neuroleptics or metoclopramide (see Chapter 18).

Nutritional Management

The primary nutritional intervention to consider when counseling patients with PD, especially with patients having refractory fluctuations of dyskinesias, should be to focus on drug–nutrient interactions; in particular, drug–nutrient interactions between dietary protein and L-dopa. Interactions between pyridoxine and aspartame should be considered as well. Large neutral amino acids are thought to compete for the transport mechanism in the gastrointestinal tract altering the rate of entry of L-dopa into circulation tract and uptake into the brain.

For some patients, symptoms may be reduced by eliminating (minimizing) dietary protein at breakfast and lunch and adding it to the evening meal. Several studies have claimed to reduce L-dopa fluctuations by restricting daytime protein to only 10 g and redistributing protein intake in the evening meal to meet the RDA protein requirement. Daytime mobility was improved, while rigidity occurred overnight (Karstaedt and Pincus, 1992; Pare et al., 1992). Table 42–13 presents a sample menu from this diet. Any benefit from this diet should be apparent within 1 week and a special effort should be made to ensure that the diet is not deficient in other nutrients such as calcium, iron, and B vitamins. However, another study found that regardless of the type of diet, L-dopa levels increased significantly and motor performance was maximized after a balanced 5:1 carbohydrate/protein intake at mealtime (Berry et al., 1991). Although the results of these studies are conflicting, dietary manipulation is harmless if the diet is nutritionally complete and it may be a significant adjunct to treating the symptoms of PD.

TABLE 42–13 PROTEIN REDISTRIBUTION IN L-DOPA THERAPY

Breakfast	**Amount of Protein (g)**
½ cup oatmeal	2
1 orange	0.5
1 cup Polyrich (nondairy creamer)	0.5
Egg Replacer (unlimited)	0
Low-protein bread, toasted	0
Margarine or butter (unlimited)	0
Jelly or jam (unlimited)	0
Sugar or sugar substitute (unlimited)	0
Coffee or tea (unlimited)	0
Lunch	
½ cup vegetable soup	2
1 cup tossed salad	1
Salad dressing (unlimited)	0
1 banana	1
Low-protein pasta (unlimited)	0
Margarine or butter (unlimited)	0
Low-protein cookies (unlimited)	0
Soda pop, coffee, tea, or water	0
Afternoon snack	
Gum drops or hard candy (unlimited)	0
Apple or cranberry juice (unlimited)	0
TOTAL	7
Dinner	
4 oz beef, pork, veal, chicken (at least)	28 or more
1 cup stuffing	4
Gravy	0
½ cup peas	2
1 cup pudding	8
1 cup milk	8
Evening Snack	
1 oz cheese	7
4 crackers	2
Soda pop	0
DAILY TOTAL	66 or more

Pyridoxine and aspartame have also been studied for their possible interaction with L-dopa. Decarboxylase, the enzyme required to convert L-dopa to dopamine, is dependent on pyridoxine. If excessive amounts of the vitamin are present, L-dopa may be metabolized in the periphery and not in the CNS where its therapeutic activity occurs. Therefore, vitamin preparations containing pyridoxine should not be taken with doses of L-dopa. Aspartame (NutraSweet), an artificial sweetener, is hydrolyzed in the stomach to phenylalanine, a large neutral amino acid, potentially competing with L-dopa for uptake across the blood–brain barrier. One study demonstrated that aspartame consumption in excess of 1200 mg/day, an intake considered to be more than what a heavy consumer would ingest, had no adverse effects. Although plasma phenylalanine increased, motor performance did not deteriorate (Karstaedt and Pincus, 1993).

Side effects of medications for PD include anorexia, nausea, reduced sense of smell, constipation, and dry mouth. To diminish the gastrointestinal side effects of L-dopa, it should be taken with meals. Additional foods, especially broad beans (fava beans), naturally contain L-dopa. A diet that substitutes these legumes for other protein foods may be useful in reducing fluctuations in response to L-dopa medication (Kempster and Wahlqvist, 1994).

As the disease progresses, rigidity of the extremities can interfere with the patient's ability to care for self, including self-feeding. Rigidity also interferes with the ability to control the position of the head and trunk, necessary for eating. Eating is slowed; mealtimes can take up to 1 hour. Simultaneous movements such as those required to handle both a knife and fork become difficult. Tremor in the arms and hands may make self-feeding of liquids impossible without spilling. Perception, including spatial organization, can become impaired (Burns and Carr-Davis, 1994). Dysphagia is a late complication but is not due to dopaminergic degeneration (Nilsson et al., 1996). A large number of patients may be silent aspirators, which affects nutritional status. One study identified a fourfold increase in weight loss greater than 10 lb in patients with PD than matched control patients (Beyer et al., 1995).

Neurotrauma

Head trauma refers to any of the following, alone or in combination: brain injury, skull fractures, extraparenchymal hemorrhage—epidural, subdural, subarachnoid—or hemorrhage into the brain tissue itself including intraparenchymal or intraventricular hemorrhage.

In the United States, trauma is the leading cause of death in persons up to 44 years of age, and more than one half of these deaths are due to head injuries (Adams et al., 1997). The annual incidence is estimated to be 200/100,000 people with a peak frequency between 15 and 24 years of age. Morbidity is also high, as estimated by the 74,000 newly disabled each year, yielding an incidence of 31 to 42/100,000 (Rowland, 1995). Motor vehicle collisions are the major source of injury.

Etiology and Pathophysiology

Brain injury can be subdivided into three types: concussion, contusion, and diffuse axonal injury. A *concussion* is described as a brief loss of consciousness (< 6 hours). No evidence of damage is found on computed tomography (CT) or magnetic resonance imaging (MRI) scans. Microscopic studies have failed to find any evidence of structural damage in areas of known concussion, though there is evidence of change in cellular metabolism. *Contusion* is similar to a bruise on the skin. It is characterized by damaged capillaries and swelling, followed by resolution of the damage. Note that large contusions may dramatically increase ICP and may lead to ischemia or herniation. Contusions can be detected by CT or MRI scans. **Diffuse axonal injury** results from the shearing of axons by a rotational acceleration of the brain inside the skull. Damaged areas are often found in the **corpus callosum** (the bridge between the two hemispheres) and the upper outer portion of the brain stem.

Skull fractures of the calvarium and the base are described in the same manner as other fractures. **Comminution** refers to splintering of bone into many fragments. Displacement refers to a condition where bones are displaced from their original apposition to each other. Open or closed describes whether a fracture is exposed to air. Open fractures dramatically increase the risk of infection (osteomyelitis) and open skull fractures in particular carry an increased risk for meningitis because the dura mater is often violated.

Epidural and **subdural hematomas** are often corrected by surgical intervention. The volume of these lesions often displaces the brain tissue and may cause diffuse axonal injury and swelling. When the lesion becomes large enough it may cause herniation of brain contents through various openings of the skull base. Consequent compression and ischemia of vital brain structures may rapidly lead to death.

Clinical Findings and Treatment

The body's response to stressors such as that seen in neurotrauma results in the production of cytokines such as interleukin 1, interleukin 6, interleukin 8, and tumor necrosis factor. These are elevated in the body after head injury and are associated with the hormonal milieu that negatively affects metabolism and organ function (see Chapter 33). Some of the metabolic events include fever, neutrophilia, muscle breakdown, altered amino acid metabolism, production of hepatic acute-phase reactants, increased endothelial permeability, and expression of endothelial adhesion molecules. It has also been proposed that specific cytokines cause organ demise. Specific tissue damage has been observed in the gut, liver, lung, and brain. Certain cytokines have also been found to cause brain cell death, increase blood–brain barrier permeability, and promote cerebral edema (Ott, 1994).

Clinical findings of brain injury often include a transient decrease in consciousness level. Headache and dizziness are relatively common and are less worrisome unless they become more intense or are accompanied by vomiting. Focal neurologic deficits, progressively decreasing level of consciousness, and penetrating brain injury are more ominous risk factors and demand prompt neurosurgical evaluation (Greenberg, 1997).

Skull fractures are suspected underneath lacerations, can often be felt as a "drop off" or discontinuity on the surface of the skull, and are readily identifiable by CT scan. Basilar skull fractures are manifested by **otorrhea, hemotympanum** (fluid or blood behind the eardrum or leaking from the ear) and rhinorrhea (salty fluid dripping from the nose or down the pharynx). Other signs include raccoon eyes and Battle's sign—blood behind the mastoid process. Basilar skull fractures may precipitate injuries to cranial nerves, which are essential for chewing, swallowing, taste, and smell. Epidural and subdural hematomas are neurosurgical emergencies because they may rapidly progress to herniation of brain contents through the skull base and to subsequent death. These lesions may present similarly, with decreased level of consciousness, contralateral hemiparesis, and pupillary dilation. Classically, the epidural hematoma presents with progressively decreasing consciousness after an interval of several hours in which the patient has been awake following a brief loss of consciousness. The subdural hematoma usually features progressively decreasing consciousness from the time of injury. These lesions damage brain tissue by gross displacement and traction. Sequelae most commonly include epilepsy and the *postconcussive syndrome,* a constellation of headache, vertigo, fatigue, and memory difficulties.

Treatment approaches for these patients can become highly complex, but the two goals of any therapeutic intervention are to maintain cerebral perfusion and to regulate ICP. Of possible interventions, perfusion and pressure control do have implications for nutritional therapy in the patient with a head injury.

Nutritional Management

The goal of nutritional management is to oppose the hypercatabolism and hypermetabolism associated with the inflammation. Hypercatabolism is manifested by protein degradation evidenced by profound urinary urea nitrogen excretion. Nitrogen catabolism in a fasting normal human is only 3 to 5 g N/day, whereas nitrogen excretion is 14 to 25 g N/day in the fasting patient with severe head injury. In the absence of nutritional intake, this degree of nitrogen loss can result in a 10% decrease in lean mass within 7 days. If this sequelae were to continue unabated, within 2 to 3 weeks a weight loss of 30% could impact mortality significantly (Brain Trauma Foundation, 1996) (see Chapter 33).

Hypermetabolism contributes to increased energy expenditure. Correlations between the severity of brain injury as measured by the Glascow Coma Scale and energy requirements have been shown. The mean resting metabolic rate in patients with head trauma is approximately 140% to 160% of the expected normal basal metabolic rate. In patients paralyzed with pancuronium bromide or barbiturates, metabolic expenditure may be decreased to 100% to 120% of basal metabolic rate. This decreased metabolic rate in pharmacologically paralyzed patients suggests that maintaining muscle tone is an important part of metabolic expenditure.

Nutriture of the neurologically critically ill patient is accomplished by administering either enteral or parenteral nutrition support. Nutritional replacement within the first week after injury has been shown to improve mortality (Rapp et al., 1983). Nutritional support is usually begun within 72 hours after injury and is necessary to achieve nutritional replacement by 7 days after injury. Both modes of therapy must be initiated at levels below actual requirements and increased gradually to meet nutritional requirements. For guidelines on estimating nutritional requirements in head trauma, refer to "*Clinical Insight:* Estimating Nutritional Requirements."

Spine Trauma

The term spine trauma encompasses many types of injuries ranging from stable fractures of the spinal column to catastrophic transsection of the spinal cord. Of nutritional significance is neurologic injury. A complete spinal cord injury (SCI) is defined as a lesion where there is no preservation of motor or sensory function more than three segments below the level of the injury (Greenberg, 1997). With an incomplete injury there is some degree of residual function, motor or sensory, more than three segments below the lesion.

Spinal cord injury is somewhat less common than head injury with an annual incidence of 40/1,000,000 people (Greenberg, 1997). SCI, like head injury, is most often seen in the young. Motor vehicle collisions account for one third to one half of SCIs with the balance caused by athletic injuries and domestic and industrial accidents.

Etiology and Pathophysiology

The spinal cord responds to insult in a manner similar to the brain. Bleeding, contusion, and shorn axons appear first, followed by a several-year remod-

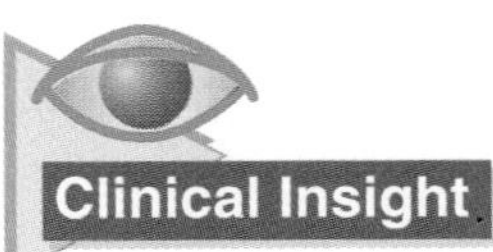

Estimating Nutritional Requirements

It is difficult to estimate nutritional requirements precisely, but they can be generalized as follows:

Ideally, caloric requirements should be measured by indirect calorimetry, but may be estimated from the Harris-Benedict equation if indirect calorimetry is not available.

140% to 160% of basal energy expenditure for severe head injuries
100% to 120% of basal energy expenditure in pharmacologically paralyzed patients

Protein requirements are accentuated in comparison to calorie requirements. Protein intake should be 15% to 20% of total calories and requirements should be measured using urinary urea nitrogen in an attempt to achieve positive nitrogen balance.

Initially, attenuation of negative nitrogen balance rather than achievement of positive nitrogen balance may be all that is possible. Other factors mediating protein requirements are hepatic and renal function. Renal function may be altered, especially in the head-injured patient due to dehydration therapy (Liebert, 1996; Schultz, 1994).

Free water should be given in accordance with the needs of either dehydration (increased ICP or hydrocephalus) or hypervolemic therapy (vasospasm risk). Concentrated enteral formulas providing 2 kcal/ml can be used to maintain adequate nutritional intake while providing minimal free water; about 2000 kcal can be provided in only 730 mL free water. Merely reducing the rate of infusion is not advised because this will contribute to nutritional deficits.

Nonprotein calories should be provided to prevent deleterious effects of excessive carbohydrate (hyperglycemia, hyperinsulinemia, gluconeogenesis, and hypercarbia) and fat (immunosuppression and hyperlipidemia) intake. Carbohydrate administration should range between 3 and 5 mg/kg/min/day with a minimum of about 150 g CHO/day to prevent gluconeogenesis. Lipids should not exceed 2 g/kg/day and should come from sources of ω-6 fatty acids.

Vitamin and mineral supplementation to meet the RDAs is important. Additional supplementation with calcium, phosphorus, and magnesium is often required when patients are on steroids, diuretics, or hypervolemic therapy.

eling process consisting of gliosis and fibrosis. Liquefactive necrosis may predispose to the formation of a syrinx, a fluid collection in the center of the spinal cord, whose mass effect may manifest as a slowly progressive neurologic deficit. Though SCI may strike at a single location, the significance of the injury lies more in the disruption of descending axons at that level, than in injury to the segment itself.

Traumatic extraparenchymal hematomas in the spine are unusual; however, SCIs are almost invariably associated with spinal column fractures and ligament instability. Such processes may be amenable to either surgical or nonsurgical reduction and stabilization.

Clinical Findings and Treatment

Spinal cord injuries have numerous clinical manifestations, depending on the level of the injury. Complete transsection results in complete loss of function below the level of the lesion, including the bladder and sphincters. Numerous incomplete cord syndromes have been described (Table 42–14).

After stabilizing the patient hemodynamically, the next step is to evaluate the degree of neurologic deficit. Patients with suspected SCI are usually immobilized promptly in the field. Complete radiographic evaluation of the spinal column is obligatory in multitrauma and unconscious patients. In the awake patient, clinical evidence of spine compromise is usually sufficient to determine the need for further workup. CT and MRI are used to more accurately delineate bony damage and spinal cord compromise. A dismal 3% of patients with complete spinal cord insults will recover some function after 24 hours. Failure to regain function after 24 hours predicts a 0% chance of reestablishment of function in the future. Incomplete spinal cord syndromes, described in Table 42–14, have variably improved outcomes.

An expeditiously implemented course of steroids is now an essential part of managing new SCIs (Bracken et al., 1990).

Nutritional Management

Morbidity and mortality rates associated with SCI have improved dramatically, particularly in the last two decades. Advances in acute-phase care have re-

TABLE 42–14 INCOMPLETE SPINAL CORD INJURY SYNDROMES

	RECOVERY (%)
Anterior cord: Paraplegia and heat/temperature loss. Fine sensation preserved.	10–20
Brown Sequard: Cord hemisection. Ipsilateral hemiparesis, fine sensation impaired. Contralateral pain and temperature sense loss.	90
Central cord: Upper extremities weaker than lower extremities. Bladder ileus. Variable sensory loss.	50
Posterior cord: Dysesthesias in neck, upper arms, and waist. Upper extremity hemiparesis.	Rare

(Adapted from Greenberg MS. Handbook of Neurosurgery, 4th ed. Lakeland, FL: Greenberg Graphics, 1997.)

The more common incomplete spinal cord injury syndromes. A course of steroids is strongly indicated for each of these.

duced early mortality and prevented complications frequently associated with early death, such as respiratory failure and pulmonary emboli (Barker, 1994; Ott et al., 1994). Fewer than 10% of patients with SCI die from the acute injury. Technological advances in enteral and parenteral feeding techniques and formulas have also played a role in maintaining nutritional status of these patients. Although the metabolic response to neurotrauma has been studied extensively, the acute metabolic response to SCI has not, but it is similar to that seen in neurotrauma during the acute phase. Initially, paralytic ileus may occur but may resolve within 72 hours after injury. See nutritional management for neurotrauma.

For those who survive the injury but are disabled for life there are significant alterations in life-style as well as the prevention of developing secondary complications that follow SCI. In general, the number and frequency of complications, constipation, pressure ulcers, obesity, and pain vary but are interrelated to nutrition. Figure 42–7 describes the rehabilitation potential based on the level of injury.

Constipation is a problem and can adversely affect appetite. Therapeutic diets consisting of high fiber and adequate water intake alone will not suffice for treatment of constipation. More than likely, a routine bowel preparation program is required. The individual with SCI is at risk for developing pressure ulcers, which, if left uncared for, can contribute to morbidity. Maintenance of nutritional health is one factor in preventing the development of pressure ulcers because poor nutrition is an underlying risk factor for infection. In one retrospective study, genitourinary infections accounted for 72.4% of all infections (Bhatt et al., 1987).

Loss of muscle tone due to skeletal muscle paralysis below the level of injury contributes to decreased metabolic activity, initial weight loss, and predisposition to osteoporosis. Acutely, the patient experiences some weight loss. Guidelines for accepted weights adjusted for paraplegia and quadriplegia are as follows: the paraplegic should weigh 10 to 15 lb less than ideal body weight (IBW); the quadriplegic should weigh 15 to 20 lb less than IBW (Blissett, 1990). The ability to maintain adequate weight is important for a number of reasons. Basal metabolic rates may be lower than predicted and significantly correlated with the level of the lesion. The higher the injury, the lower the metabolic rate.

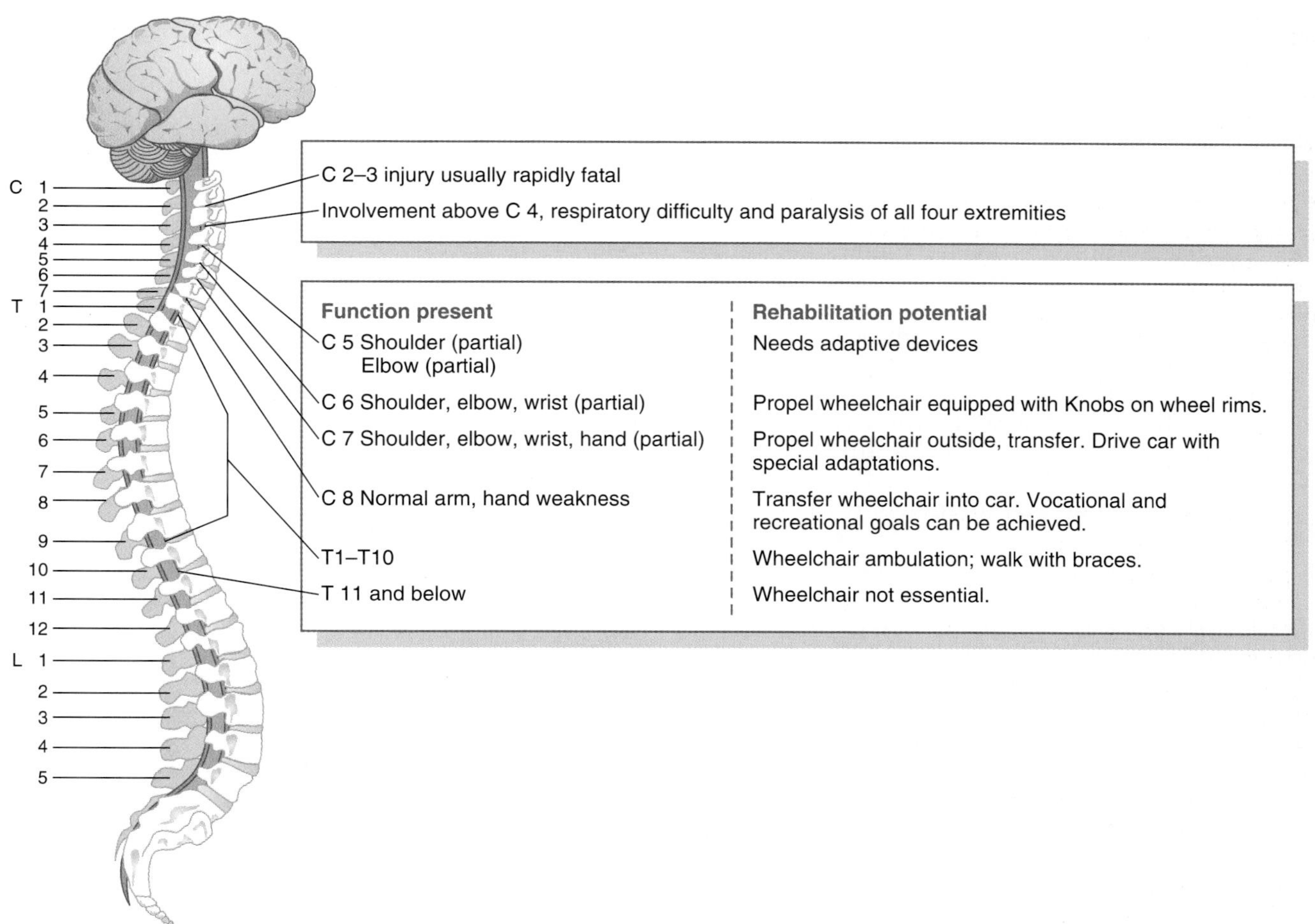

FIGURE 42–7 Sequelae of spinal cord injury and rehabilitation challenges.

CASE STUDY

Seizures

Clarence A., a hospitalized patient receiving enteral nutrition support is having mild seizure activity. Tube feedings have been infused via a PEG over 12 hours. Therapeutic serum level for phenytoin has not been achieved despite receiving a normal prescribed dose of phenytoin. The physicians would like input regarding the drug–nutrient interaction to achieve therapeutic serum phenytoin levels for control of the seizures.

1. As the clinician managing the nutritional care of this patient, what would be the most appropriate action based on the current enteral support regimen?
   a. Hold the feedings 2 hours before and after administering the phenytoin.
   b. Change the tube feeding regimen to gravity drip infusions of 480 mL four times per day.
   c. Change the tube feed formula to a blenderized formula.
   d. Suggest dosing phenytoin once per day via sustained-release capsule so that the tube feeding formula will not bind with the medication.
   e. Continue present enteral support regimen because answers a and c will not result in therapeutic phenytoin levels without increasing the dose of phenytoin.
2. Clarence's wife has suggested adding bolus feedings so the patient can walk with her more often. How would you design the feeding frequency and how will this affect the phenytoin administration?

Quadriplegic patients have lower metabolic rates than paraplegic patients and it is proportional to the amount of denervated muscle due in part to the loss of residual motor function.

In the rehabilitation phase, quadraplegics require 22.7 kcal/kg/day and paraplegics 27.9 kcal/kg/day which represents 45% to 90% of the recommended calories using conventional equations (Mollinger et al., 1985). Hence, these patients have the potential to become overweight. It has been proposed that obesity may actually influence the eventual rehabilitation process by limiting functional outcome. As a consequence of bone loss due to the loss of mineralization due to immobilization, SCI is associated with osteopenia and osteoporosis and the prevalence of long bone fractures is increased.

A diverse array of physical and psychosocial issues such as anemia, respiratory paralysis, pneumonia, ileus, pressure ulcers, hemorrhage, neurogenic bowel and bladder, depression, and social support all affect the patient's nutritional status (Blissitt, 1990). The nutritionist plays an important role.

CITED REFERENCES

Adams RD, et al. Principles of Neurology, 6th ed. New York: McGraw-Hill, Health Professions Division, 1997.

American Dietetic Association. The Handbook of Clinical Dietetics. New Haven, CT: Yale University Press, 1992.

Asbeck C, Burns BL. Nutritional management of amyotrophic lateral sclerosis. Diet Nutr Support 10(9):11, 1988.

Atkins D, et al. Cholesterol reduction and the risk for stroke in men. A meta-analysis of randomized controlled trials. Ann Intern Med 119:136, 1993.

Balaban DJ. Epidemiology and prevention of selected chronic diseases. The National Medical Series for Independent Study, Preventive Medicine and Public Health, 2nd ed. Baltimore: Harwal Publishing, 1992.

Barker E. Neuroscience Nursing. St. Louis: Mosby-Yearbook, 1994.

Barrett-Connor E, et al. Weight loss precedes dementia in community-dwelling older adults. J Am Geriatr Soc 44:1147, 1996.

Berry EM, et al. A balanced carbohydrate: Protein diet in the management of Parkinson's disease. Neurology 41(8):1295, 1991.

Berryman MS. The ketogenic diet revisited. J Am Diet Assoc 97:S192, 1997.

Beyer PL, et al. Weight change and body composition in patients with Parkinson's disease. J Am Diet Assoc 95:979, 1995.

Bhatt K, et al. Bacteremia in the spinal cord injury population. Journal of the American Paraplegia Society 10(1):11, 1987.

Blissitt PA. Nutrition in acute spinal cord injury. Crit Care Nurs Clin North Am 2:375, 1990.

Bracken MB, et al. A randomized controlled clinical trial of methylprednisolone or naloxone in the treatment of acute spinal cord injury. N Engl J Med 322:1405, 1990.

Brain Trauma Foundation. Nutritional support of brain-injured patients. J Neurotrauma 13(11):721, 1996.

Burns BL, Carr-Davis EM. Nutritional management of Parkinson's disease. In: Weiner WJ, Cohen A (eds.). Interdisciplinary Treatment of Parkinson's Disease. New York: Demos Publication, 1994.

Calne DB. Treatment of Parkinson's disease. N Engl J Med 329:1021, 1993.

Cecil RL, Underlie TE. Cecil Essentials of Medicine, 4th ed. Philadelphia: WB Saunders, 1997.

Cohen D. A primary care checklist for effective family management. Med Clin North Am 78(4):795, 1994.

Connor JR, Beard JL. Dietary iron supplements in the elderly: To use or not to use. Nutrition Today 32(3):102, 1997.

Curran JE. Nutritional considerations in dysphagia. In: Groher ME (ed.). Dysphagia: Diagnosis and Management, 3rd ed. Boston: Butterworth-Heinemann, 1997.

Davalos A, et al. Effect of malnutrition after acute stroke on clinical outcome. Stroke 27(6):1028, 1996.

De Girolami U, et al. The central nervous system. In: Cotran RS, et al. (eds.). Robbins Pathologic Basis of Disease, 5th ed. Philadelphia: WB Saunders, 1994.

Devanand DP, et al. Depressed mood and the incidence of Alzheimer's disease in the elderly living in the community. Arch Gen Psychiatry 53:175, 1996.

Diabetes Control and Complications Trial Research Group. Effect of intensive diabetes management on macrovascular events and risk factors in the Diabetes Control and Complications Trial. Am J Cardiol 75: 894,1995.

Fernandez-Calle P, et al. Serum levels of alpha-tocopherol (vitamin E) in Parkinson's disease. Neurology 42:1064, 1992.

Finley B. Nutritional needs of the person with Alzheimer's disease: Practical approaches to quality care. J Am Diet Assoc 97(10 suppl 2):S177, 1997.

Folstein M. Nutrition and Alzheimer's disease. Nutr Rev 55(1):23, 1996.

Freeman JM, et al. The Epilepsy Diet Treatment: An Introduction to the Ketogenic Diet, 2nd ed. New York: Demos Publication, 1996.

Frequin STFM, et al. Decreased vitamin B_{12} and folate levels in cerebrospinal fluid and serum of multiple sclerosis patients after high-dose intravenous methylprednisolone. J Neurol 240:305, 1993.

Friedman A, et al. Pyridostigmine brain penetration under stress enhances neural excitability and induces early immediate transcriptional response. Nat Med 2:1382, 1996.

Geula C, et al. Aging renders the brain vulnerable to amyloid B-protein neurotoxicity. Nat Med 4:827, 1998.

Gordis L. Epidemiology. Philadelphia: WB Saunders, 1996.

Greenberg MS. Handbook of Neurosurgery, 4th ed. Lakeland, FL: Greenberg Graphics, 1997.

Griffin JW. Neurological Disorders. In: Bennett JC, Plum F (eds.). Cecil Textbook of Medicine, 20th ed. Philadelphia: WB Saunders, 1996.

Hayes CE, et al. Vitamin D and multiple sclerosis (Review). Proc Soc Exp Biol Med 216(1):21, 1997.

Hillel AD, et al. ALS severity scale. J Neuroepidemiol 8:142, 1989.

Jacob RA, Milne DB. Biochemical assessment of vitamins and trace minerals. Clin Lab Med 13(2):371, 1993.

Karstaedt PJ, Pincus JH. Protein redistribution diet remains effective in patients with fluctuating parkinsonism. Arch Neurol 49(2):149, 1992.

Karstaedt PJ, Pincus JH. Aspartame use in Parkinson's disease. Neurology 43(3 Pt 1):611, 1993.

Kasarskis EJ, Neville HE. Management of ALS: Nutritional care. Neurology 47(4 suppl 2):S118, 1996.

Kasarskis EJ, et al. Nutritional status of patients with amyotrophic lateral sclerosis: Relation to the proximity of death. Am J Clin Nutr 63:130, 1996.

Kelly JH, Buchholz DW. Nutritional management of the patient with neurologic disorder. Ear Nose Throat J 75(5):293, 1996.
Kempster PA, Wahlqvist ML. Dietary factors in the management of Parkinson's disease. Nutr Rev 52(2 Pt 1): 51, 1994.
Kinsman SL, et al. Efficacy of the ketogenic diet for intractable seizure disorders: Review of 58 cases. Epilepsia 33:1132, 1992.
Kril JJ. Neuropathology of thiamine deficiency disorders. Metab Brain Dis 11(1):9, 1996.
Langlais PJ. Neuropathology of thiamine deficiency: An update on the comparative analysis of human disorders and experimental models. Metab Brain Dis 11(1):19, 1996.
LeBars PI, et al. A placebo-controlled, double-blind, randomized trial of an extract of ginkgo biloba for dementia. JAMA 278:1327, 1997.
Leira R, Rodriguez R. Diet and migraine: Review. Revista de Neurologia 24(129):534, 1996.
Liebert MA. Nutritional support of brain-injured patients. J Neurotrauma 13(11):721, 1996.
Logroscino G, et al. Dietary lipids and antioxidants in Parkinson's disease: A population-based, case-control study. Ann Neurol 39(1):89, 1996.
Mathus-Vliegen LM, et al. Percutaneous endoscopic gastrostomy in patients with amyotrophic lateral sclerosis and impaired pulmonary function. Gastrointest Endosc 40(4):463, 1994.
Mazzini L, et al. Percutaneous endoscopic gastrostomy and enteral nutrition in amyotrophic lateral sclerosis. J Neurol 242(10):695, 1995.
Miller RM. General treatment of neurologic swallowing disorders. In: Groher ME (ed.). Dysphagia: Diagnosis and Management, 3rd ed. Boston: Butterworth-Heinemann, 1997.
Mitsumoto H. Classification and clinical features of amyotrophic lateral sclerosis. In: Mitsumoto H, Norris FH (eds.). Amyotrophic Lateral Sclerosis: A Comprehensive Guide to Management. New York: Demos Publication, 1994.
Mollinger LA, et al. Daily energy expenditure and basal metabolic rates of patients with spinal cord injury. Arch Phys Med Rehabil 66(7):420, 1985.
Naidoo DP. Wernicke's encephalopathy and alcohol-related disease. Postgrad Med J 67:978, 1991.
Nilsson H, et al. Quantitative assessment of oral and pharyngeal function in Parkinson's disease. Dysphagia 11(4):274, 1996.
Ordunez-Garcia, et al. Cuban epidemic neuropathy, 1991 to 1994: History repeats itself a century after the "Amblyopia of the Blockade." Am J Public Health 86(5): 738, 1996.
Ott L, et al. Cytokines and metabolic dysfunction after severe head injury. J Neurotrauma 11(5): 447, 1994.
Ott L. Neurosurgery. In: Zalog G (ed.). Nutrition in Critical Care. St. Louis: Mosby-Yearbook, 1994.
Ozuna J, Friel P. Effects of enteral tube feeding on serum phenytoin levels. J Neurosurg Nurs 16:289, 1984.
Pare S, et al. Effect of daytime protein restriction on nutrient intakes of free-living Parkinson's disease patients. Am J Clin Nutr 55:701, 1992.
Parkinson's Study Group. Effects of tocopherol and deprenyl on the progression of disability in early Parkinson's disease. N Engl J Med 328:176, 1993.
Pinnock CB, et al. Relationship between milk intake and mucus production in adult volunteers challenged with rhinovirus-2. Am Rev Respir Dis 141:352, 1990.
Prospective Studies Collaboration. Cholesterol, diastolic blood pressure and stroke: 13,000 strokes in 450,000 people in 45 prospective cohorts. Lancet 341:1647, 1995.
Rapp RP, et al. The favorable effect of early parenteral feeding on survival in head injured patients. J Neurosurg 58:906, 1983.
Raskind MA, et al. Effect of tacrine on language, praxis and noncognitive behavioral problems in Alzheimer disease. Arch Neurol 54(7):838, 1997.
Rosen D, et al. Mutations in Cu/Zn superoxide dismutase gene are associated with familial amyotrophic lateral sclerosis. Nature 362:59, 1993.
Rothstein J, et al. Decreased glutamate transport of seasonal affective disorder. N Engl J Med 326:1464, 1992.
Roubenoff RA, et al. Hypermetabolism and hypercatabolism in Guillain-Barre syndrome. J Parenter Enteral Nutr 16(5):464, 1992.
Rowland LP. Merritt's Textbook of Neurology, 9th ed. Baltimore: Williams & Wilkins, 1995.
Sano M, et al. A controlled trial of selegitine, alpha-tocopherol or both as treatment for Alzheimer's disease. N Engl J Med 336:1216, 1997.
Schoenen J, et al. Effectiveness of high-dose riboflavin in migraine prophylaxis: A randomized controlled trial. Neurology 50:466, 1998.
Schultz P. Nutritional management in neurocritical care. In: Werner GT and Hacke W (eds.). NeuroCritical Care. New York: Springer-Verlag, 1994.
Smithard DG, et al. Complications and outcome after acute stroke. Does dysphagia matter? Stroke 27(7): 1200, 1996.
Standaert DG, Stern MB. Update on the management of Parkinson's disease. Med Clin North Am 77(1):169, 1993.
Strand EA, et al. Management of oral-pharyngeal dysphagia symptoms in amyotrophic lateral sclerosis. Dysphagia 11:129, 1996.
Swank RL, Dugan BB. Effect of low saturated fat diet in early and late cases of multiple sclerosis. Lancet 336:37, 1990.
Traber MG, Sies H. Vitamin E in humans: Demand and delivery (Review). Annu Rev Nutr 16:321, 1996.
Tufts University. Health and Nutrition Letter. February 1998, p. 7.
Warsama Jama J, et al. Dietary antioxidants and cognitive function in a population-based sample of older persons: The Rotterdam Study. Am J Epidemiol 144:275, 1996.
Wickelgren I. Estrogen stakes claim to cognition. Science 276:675, 1997.
Wozniak-Wowk CS. Nutrition intervention in the management of multiple sclerosis. Nutrition Today 28(6):12, 1993.
Yan SD, et al. An intracellular protein that binds amyloid-B peptide and mediates neurotoxicity in Alzheimer's disease. Nature 389:689, 1997.
Zubaran C, et al. Wernicke-Korsakoff syndrome. Postgrad Med J 73 (855):27, 1997.

ADDITIONAL REFERENCES

American Dietetic Association. Position of the American Dietetic Association: Legal and ethical issues in feeding permanently unconscious patients. J Am Diet Assoc 95:231, 1995.
Cantorna MT, et al. 1,25-Dihydroxyvitamin D_3 reversibly blocks the progression of relapsing encephalomyelitis, a model of multiple sclerosis. Proc Natl Acad Sci USA 93(15):7861, 1996.
Esparza ML, et al. Nutrition, latitude, and multiple sclerosis mortality: An ecologic study. Am J Epidemiol 142:733, 1995.
Franzoni S, et al. Good nutritional oral intake is associated with equal survival in demented and nondemented very old patients. J Am Geriatr Soc 44:1366, 1996.
Grap MJ, Munro CL. Ventilator-associated pneumonia: Clinical significance and implications for nursing. Heart Lung 26(6):419, 1997.
Guidry JR, et al. Phenytoin absorption in volunteers receiving selected enteral feedings. West J Med 15:659, 1989.
Homocysteine and Alzheimer's disease. Nutr Rev 57:126, 1999.
Keli S, et al. Dietary flavonoids, antioxidant vitamins and incidence of stroke: The Zutphen Study. Arch Intern Med 156: 637, 1996.
Lang AE, Lozano AM. Parkinson's disease, part I. N Engl J Med 339:1044, 1998.
Lang AE, Lozano AM. Parkinson's disease, part II. N Engl J Med 339:1130, 1998.
Lehman CA. Risk factors for pressure ulcers in the spinal cord injured in the community. Science Nursing 12(4):110, 1995.
Mann L, Wong K. Development of an objective method for assessing viscosity of formulated foods and beverages for the dysphagic diet. J Am Diet Assoc 96: 585, 1996.
Sano M, et al. A controlled trial of selegiline, alpha tocopherol, or both as treatment for Alzheimer's disease. N Engl J Med 336:1216, 1997.
Spindler A, et al. Nutritional status of patients with Alzheimer's disease: A 1-year study. J Am Diet Assoc 96:1013, 1996.
White H, et al. Weight change in Alzheimer's disease. J Am Geriatr Soc 44:265, 1996.

CHAPTER 43

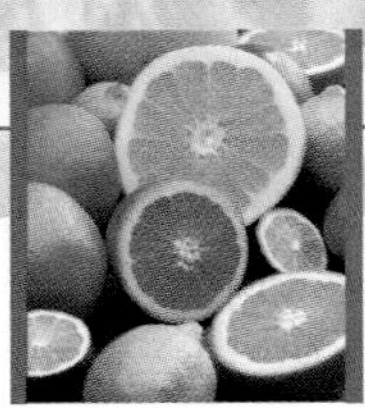

Medical Nutrition Therapy for Rheumatic Disorders

THERESE ANN FRANZESE, MS, RD, CD-N

Chapter Outline

- Rheumatic Diseases
- Osteoarthritis
- Rheumatoid Arthritis
- Gout
- Scleroderma
- Systemic Lupus Erythematosus
- Unproven Remedies for Rheumatic Disorders

Key Terms

ARACHIDONIC ACID—a fatty acid with four double bonds on the 5, 8, 11, and 14 carbon positions; a precursor for eicosanoid production

AUTOIMMUNE—having a specific type of humoral or cell-mediated immune response against constituents of the body's own tissues

CYTOKINES—small proteins, including lymphokines and monokines, that are produced by immunocytes, macrophages, and fibroblasts and that mediate or increase an inflammatory response

FIBROMYALGIA—generalized, widespread, nonarticular pain or inflammation

GOUT—a group of disorders of purine and pyrimidine metabolism characterized by hyperuricemia and deposition of uric acid crystals

JUVENILE RHEUMATOID ARTHRITIS—a chronic, autoimmune, multisystem condition occurring in children (mostly girls) that primarily affects the joints; characterized by changes in the synovial membranes and joint structures, atrophy, and osteopenia

OSTEOARTHRITIS—degenerative joint disease, also called the "wear-and-tear" disease, that occurs mainly in older persons; characterized by degeneration of the joint cartilage, hypertrophy of bone at the margins, and changes in the synovial membrane

PROSTAGLANDIN—any of a group of components derived from unsaturated 20-carbon fatty acids, primarily arachidonic acid, that are extremely potent mediators of a diverse group of physiologic processes; the series is designated with a subscript 1, 2, or 3, depending on the number of double bonds in the hydrocarbon skeleton and the fatty acid from which it was synthesized

PURINES—the nitrogenous bases adenine and guanine, which are constituents of nucleoproteins, the metabolic end-product of which is uric acid

RHEUMATIC DISEASES—more than 100 different manifestations of connective tissue and arthritic disease marked by degeneration, inflammation, pain, and swelling of the joints

RHEUMATOID ARTHRITIS—chronic inflammatory systemic disease, primarily involving the joints, which is characterized by changes in the synovial membranes, atrophy of joints, and osteopenia

RHEUMATOID FACTOR—abnormal circulating proteins found in the serum of individuals with rheumatoid arthritis; a group of immunoglobins that have been classified as antibodies

SCLERODERMA—progressive, systemic inflammation and hardening of the skin with deposition of fibrous connective tissue in the skin and visceral organs, including the gastrointestinal tract

SJÖGREN'S SYNDROME—a chronic inflammatory disorder characterized by diminished production of both tears in the eye and saliva

SYNOVIAL FLUID—transparent, alkaline fluid secreted by the synovial membrane and located in joints

SYSTEMIC LUPUS ERYTHEMATOSUS—a chronic, inflammatory, multisystem disorder of connective tissue, primarily affecting women, that involves the skin, joints, kidneys, and serosal membranes; of presumed immune mediated etiology

XEROPHTHALMIA—dryness of the cornea and conjunctiva of the eyes; manifestations include dry, sandy eyes with thick, white mucosa

XEROSTOMIA—dryness of the mouth secondary to reduced or absent saliva; consequences include an increased risk of dental decay, gingivitis, and difficulty chewing and swallowing

RHEUMATIC DISEASES

Rheumatic diseases include more than 100 different manifestations of connective tissue and arthritic disease marked by degeneration, inflammation, pain, and swelling of the joints. The most frequently affected tissues are the interstitial tissues, blood vessels, cartilage, bone, tendons, and ligaments, as well as the synovial membranes lining joint surfaces. In addition, some forms of arthritis can affect other organs, like the skin or blood vessels.

Arthritis and other rheumatic conditions are among the most prevalent chronic disease conditions in the United States, affecting an estimated 40 million persons (15% of the population or 1 of every 6 people) and projected to affect 60 million (more than 18% of the population) by 2020 (Lawrence et al., 1998). Recent increases are, to a large degree, a function of the marked aging of the U.S. population and, to a smaller degree, a function of changing sex and race distribution in the population.

According to The Arthritis Foundation (AF), arthritis is the leading cause of disability and is associated with total direct costs to the U.S. economy of $65 billion per year in medical care and lost wages. A useful internet website is www.nih.gov/niams.

Arthritis affects all population groups, including as many as 285,000 children (including juvenile rheumatoid arthritis) and two thirds of those diagnosed with arthritis are women. The most common forms of chronic arthritis in the United States are osteoarthritis (affecting 21 million), **fibromyalgia** (affecting 3.7 million people), gout (2.1 million), and rheumatoid arthritis (2.1 million) (Lawrence et al., 1998).

The major body changes associated with aging, including decreased body protein, body fluid, and bone density, as well as an increased proportion of total body fat, may all or partially contribute to the onset and progression of arthritis. Aging body mass causes changes in neuroendocrine regulators, immune regulators, and metabolism that affect the inflammation process (Roubenoff et al., 1997).

The etiology of most rheumatic conditions remains unknown. It is postulated that several types of arthritis are caused by either a virus or by constant stress (from obesity or inappropriate strenuous exercise) that initiates the inflammatory process. Other conditions, such as scleroderma and lupus erythematosus have also eluded scientific explanation.

Arthritis is usually chronic, but may present as acute episodes. An acute attack is of short duration, but may recur and develop into a chronic condition. Chronic arthritic conditions are associated with alternating periods of remission, or absence of symptoms, and flares, or worsening of symptoms, which often occur without any identifiable etiology.

Because there is usually no identifiable cause for the arthritic condition, disease flare, or remission, and very little public protection against fraud, individuals with arthritis often seek remedies from unorthodox sources. Chronic arthritic conditions have *no* known cure; pharmacotherapy, in addition to physical, occupational, and medical nutritional therapies, is the mainstay of management. Early detection, coupled with individualization and monitoring of treatment(s), is essential. Although various alternative diet theories have been proposed for the management of arthritis, these therapies are mostly based on anecdotal or nonscientific data, and could potentially cause additional damage. For these reasons, they are a continuing challenge for nutritionists.

Pathophysiology of Inflammation in Arthritic Disease

Inflammation, which is the predominant cause of pain, is the most debilitating component of arthritis. Pain reflects a neuroendocrine process associated with levels of corticotropin-releasing hormone (CRH), N-methyl-D-aspartate (NMDA), inflammatory mediators, unmyelinated C fibers sensitized to noradrenaline, and biologically active peptides (Harris, 1997).

The inflammatory process normally occurs to protect and repair tissue damaged by infections, sports injuries, toxicity, or wounds via accumulation of fluid and cells. Once the cause is resolved, however, the inflammation usually subsides. Whether inflammation is attributable to stress on the joints (osteoarthritis) or an **autoimmune** response (rheumatoid arthritis), in most forms of arthritis, the inflammatory reaction continues out of control, causing more damage than repair.

The complex inflammatory process is initiated by the production of histamine, **prostaglandins** (PGs), plasma proteases, and plasma activating factors. **Arachidonic acid** is a nonesterified fatty acid which, when released from cell membranes, is oxygenated to several classes of eicosanoids, including prostaglandin, thromboxanes, leukotrienes, and prostacyclin, which are proinflammatory.

Glucocorticoid therapy decreases the release of arachidonic acid from cell membrane phospholipids by binding to the receptor in the cell cytoplasm. This results in the development of a complex that moves into the nucleus as a transcription factor, interfering with expressions for the enzyme phospholipase (Harris, 1997).

Prostaglandins are produced by neutrophils, macrophages, and synovial fibroblasts in large quantities in synovial tissue as a response to specific activating protein hormones **(cytokines)** acting on oxygenated arachidonic acid. Examples of cytokines are tumor necrosis factors, interferons, and interleukins. Only a few years ago, little was known about the role of cytokines in rheumatic arthritis; now, tumor necrosis factor (TNF-α) has assumed particular importance (Firestein and Zvaifler,

1997). Prostaglandins have been shown to play a major role in the depletion of bone in rheumatoid arthritis (Harris, 1997).

There are many types of prostaglandins and other inflammatory mediators (i.e., PGE_1 and PGE_2) that are considered stable, induce inflammation, and potentiate the effects of histamine and other inflammatory mediators. For example, thromboxane activates platelet aggregation to initiate clotting and to release growth factors and proteases. Leukotrienes stimulate the attraction of neutrophils, macrophages, and fibroblasts into the circulating joint fluid. Prostacyclin (PGI_2), however, has the opposite effect of PGE_1 and PGE_2 (thromboxane and leukotrienes) by relaxing the smooth muscle and inhibiting platelet aggregation.

Many of the drugs used in treating rheumatic diseases affect the synthesis of prostaglandins, usually diminishing their production. Nonsteroidal anti-inflammatory drugs (NSAIDs) inhibit cyclo-oxygenase (COX), an enzyme which oxygenates arachidonic acid, leading to the formation of prostaglandins. Unfortunately, long-term use of NSAIDs and salicylates is often associated with renal failure, as well as gastrointestinal problems (Perneger, 1994). NSAIDs have been reported to be responsible for an estimated 7600 deaths and 76,000 hospitalizations per year (Tamblyn et al., 1997). Nevertheless, unless the risks are judged to be too great, NSAIDs are still favored in the management of arthritis, gout, and several other rheumatic disorders (Emmerson, 1996.)

Comparison of Osteoarthritis and Rheumatoid Arthritis

It is important to distinguish between osteoarthritis and rheumatoid arthritis. Generally speaking, osteoarthritis involves cartilage destruction with asymmetrical inflammation, whereas rheumatoid arthritis is a systemic autoimmune disorder that results in symmetrical joint inflammation.

OSTEOARTHRITIS

Pathophysiology

Osteoarthritis, formally known as degenerative arthritis or **degenerative joint disease** (DJD), is the most prevalent form of arthritis. Osteoarthritis is a steady, chronic process characterized by the softening of the articular (joint) cartilage and accompanied by reactive phenomena, such as vascular congestion and osteoblast activity in underlying bone, new growth of cartilage and bone (osteophytes) at the joint margins, and capsular fibrosis (Fig. 43–1). Although osteoarthritis occurs mostly in the aged, it is not necessarily age-related. Osteoarthritis is usually localized and has an arbitrary distribution in the body. It is thought that osteoarthritis results from past load impact injuries or from constant friction ("wear and tear"). Other diseases of the joints influenced by congenital and mechanical derangements of the joints may contribute to osteoarthritis. Inflammation occurs at times; however, it is not a primary symptom of this condition.

The joints most often affected in osteoarthritis are the distal interphalangeal joints, the thumb joint, and, in particular, the joints of the knees, hips, ankles, and spine, which bear the bulk of the body's weight. The elbow, wrist, and ankle are less often affected by osteoarthritis. The early stage of the disease is marked by stiffness, usually upon arising from a chair or after standing; this then progresses to generalized "soreness." One or more joints may be affected, and symptoms are usually confined to the afflicted parts.

Nutritional Care

A well-balanced diet that is consistent with established dietary guidelines and that promotes attainment and maintenance of a desirable body weight is an important part of medical nutrition therapy for osteoarthritis. The incidence of osteoarthritis among the obese is greater than among people of normal weight (Koopman, 1997). In fact, epidemiologic studies have shown that obesity and injury are the two greatest risk factors for osteoarthritis (Cooper et al., 1998). Excess weight puts an added burden on the weight-bearing joints; however, the benefits of weight reduction are not confined to these areas. For the patient with osteoarthritis, weight reduction seems to improve all joints (Hochberg et al., 1995). Obesity has been linked to osteoarthritis so convincingly that researchers are using the diagnosis of osteoarthritis as a risk factor for coronary heart disease (Philbin et al., 1996).

Intakes of calcium and vitamin D should be at levels specified in the new DRIs. Many patients with osteoarthritis do not consume enough dairy products and calcium, and low intake of vitamin D and low serum levels of vitamin D have been shown to be associated with progression of osteoarthritis (McAlindon et al., 1996). Although the study warrants confirmation, in 1996, McAlindon and colleagues, from Boston University Medical Center's Arthritis Center, demonstrated that high intakes of antioxidants, especially vitamin C, reduced the risk of progression of osteoarthritis, more so than thiamine, vitamin B_6, niacin, and folate. Vitamin C, E, and beta-carotene antioxidants, however, did not prevent the onset of osteoarthritis. Some experimental data have shown that vitamin B_6 deficiency may be responsible for the development of osteoarthritis-type lesions (Koopman, 1997). Comprehensive nutritional interviewing and counseling should include a determination of acceptable sources of *all* nutrients for the patient, as well as integration of sufficient amounts in the diet to achieve the recommended levels (van Weel, 1997).

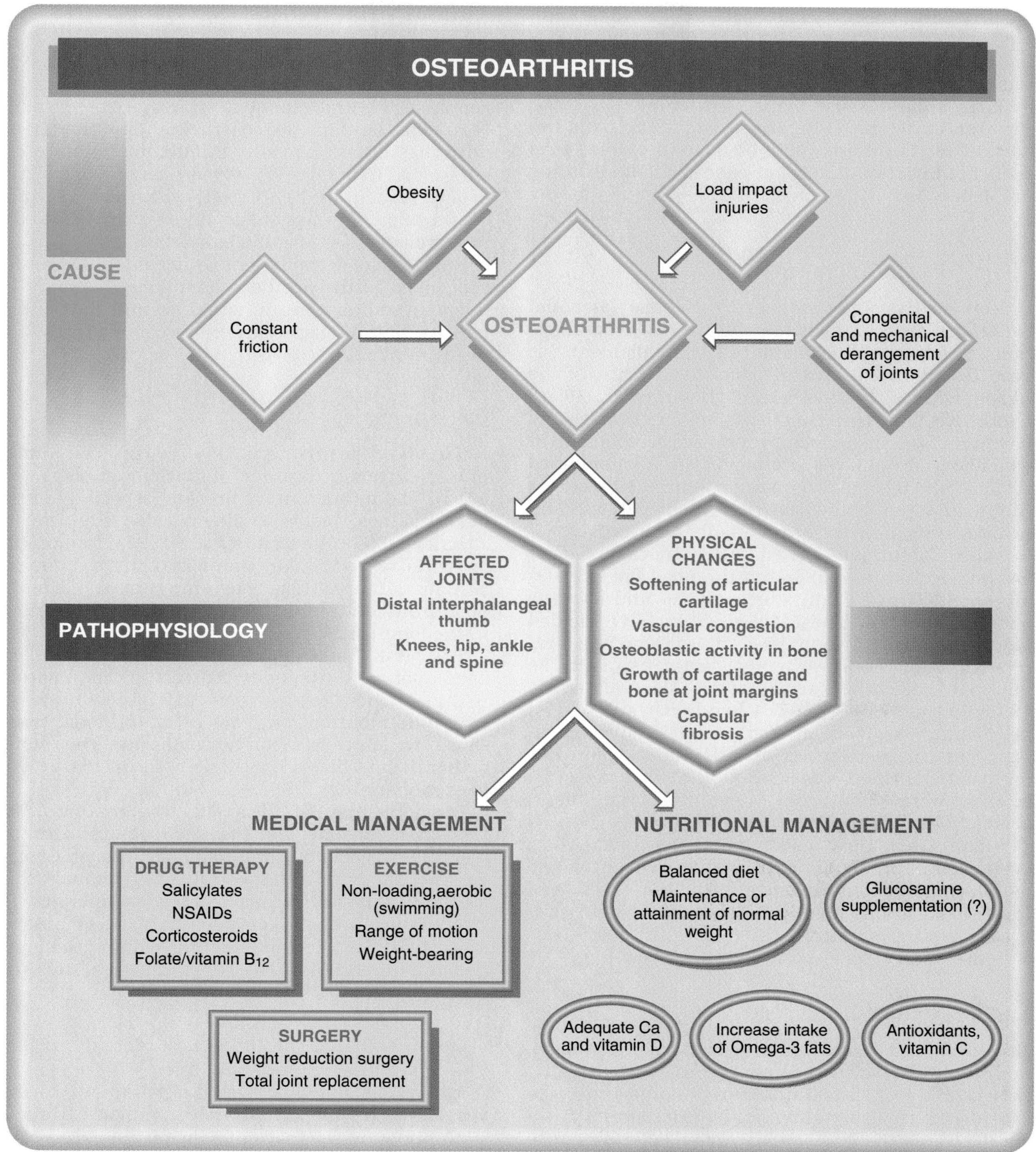

FIGURE 43–1 Pathophysiology algorithm—osteoarthritis. (Algorithm content developed by John Anderson, Ph.D., and Sanford C. Garner, Ph.D., 2000.)

Exercise

Sports or strenuous activities that subject joints to repetitive high impact and loading increase the risk of joint cartilage degeneration (Spector, 1996). Therefore, increased muscle tone and strength, correct form, general flexibility, and conditioning will help protect these joints in the habitual exerciser (Buckwalter and Lane, 1997). Weight reduction is challenging for individuals with osteoarthritis because the disease limits their ability to increase energy expenditure through exercise.

For treatment of osteoarthritis, nonloading aerobic (swimming), range-of-motion, and weight-bearing exercise have all been shown to reduce symptoms, increase mobility, and lessen continuing damage from osteoarthritis (Fisher et al., 1997; Fransen et al., 1997; Rejeski et al., 1998). It is important for the exercises to be done in correct form so as not to cause damage or exacerbate an existing problem.

Pharmacologic Therapy

Osteoarthritis can be managed with salicylates and NSAIDs. Corticosteroids may be given as local injections. A folate and cobalamin (B_{12}) supplement has been tested as a treatment for osteoarthritis of the hands, with fairly good results (Flynn et al., 1994.) Unlike NSAIDs, these nutrients are inexpensive and have minimal side effects when used for persons in whom low serum levels are identified. As mentioned earlier, NSAIDs have so many potential side effects (Bossingham and Hawkey, 1993), that patients and investigators alike are searching for alternatives.

Some alternative "investigative therapies" that are being used to help lessen the need for NSAIDs are chondroitin sulfate, glucosamine, and avocado and soybean oils. These alternatives have yielded favorable results when used in conjunction with conventional therapy for osteoarthritis, such as physical therapy and medications (Morreale et al., 1996; Blotman et al., 1997). Chondroitin sulfate and glucosamine are both molecules that produce cartilage, but the mechanism for eliminating pain has not been identified. Omega-3 fatty acids are just as likely to work as antagonists against prostaglandin production, the cause of much pain.

Weight reduction medications have sometimes been used in problematic cases of overweight. Close monitoring of potential side effects is essential, and these medications should not be used when risks are high (see Chapter 23).

Surgical Options

Because obesity contributes to continuous damage, and because exercise compliance in most arthritic patients is poor, intestinal bypass surgery may be considered. However, intestinal bypass surgery as a surgical treatment of obesity may actually cause bacterial overgrowth and formation of immune complexes in the joints that resemble arthritis (Bollet, 1994), and so should be used only as a last resort.

Surgical reconstruction (total joint replacement) may be considered for patients with osteoarthritis who are not responding to other medical therapies and who may be candidates for replacement surgery (Creamer et al., 1998). Surgical reconstruction has been quite successful, but should not be viewed as a replacement for overall good nutrition, maintenance of healthy body weight, and exercise.

RHEUMATOID ARTHRITIS

Rheumatoid arthritis is a debilitating and frequently crippling disease with overwhelming personal, social, and economic effects. Although much less common than osteoarthritis, the rheumatoid form may be more severe. Rheumatoid arthritis occurs more frequently in women than in men (ratio of approximately 3:1). Onset, which commonly occurs around 35 years of age, is generally followed by numerous remissions and exacerbations.

Epidemiologic studies have documented the fact that onset in the northern hemisphere is more frequent in winter than in summer, and that exacerbations of the disease are more common in winter (Kelly et al., 1997).

Pathophysiology

Rheumatoid arthritis (RA) is a chronic, autoimmune, systemic disorder of unclear etiology (Fig. 43–2). The inflammatory process, especially involving cytokines, seems to play a role (Firestein and Zvaifler, 1997; Moreland et al., 1997). Rheumatoid arthritis has articular manifestations that involve chronic inflammation, beginning in the synovial membrane and progressing to subsequent damage in the joint cartilage.

The term "angiogenesis-dependent disease" has been applied to rheumatoid arthritis. The inference is that, without extensive growth of new blood vessels, inflammation could not be maintained. In this sense, as in other arthritic conditions, rheumatoid arthritis acts like a cancer growth driven by antigens (Johanning, 1996).

Any joint may be affected by rheumatoid arthritis, but involvement of the small joints of the extremities, typically the proximal interphalangeal joints of the hands and feet, is most common. Pain, stiffness, and swelling are frequent complaints. The swelling or puffiness is caused by the accumulation of *synovial fluid* in the membrane lining the joints, and inflammation of the surrounding tissues (Fig. 43–3).

Nutritional Assessment

A comprehensive nutritional assessment of individuals with rheumatoid arthritis must include an evaluation of the patient's medical and surgical history, medication(s), disease sequelae, results of physical examination, weight history and anthropometric evaluation, laboratory data assessment, and a thorough diet history. The medical history should include a review of systems to determine the systemic impact of the disease process. A physical examination provides diagnostic information regarding signs and symptoms of nutrient deficits. Use of a "likelihood of malnutrition index" has been suggested for this population (Alarcon and Morgan, 1997) considering the number of medica-

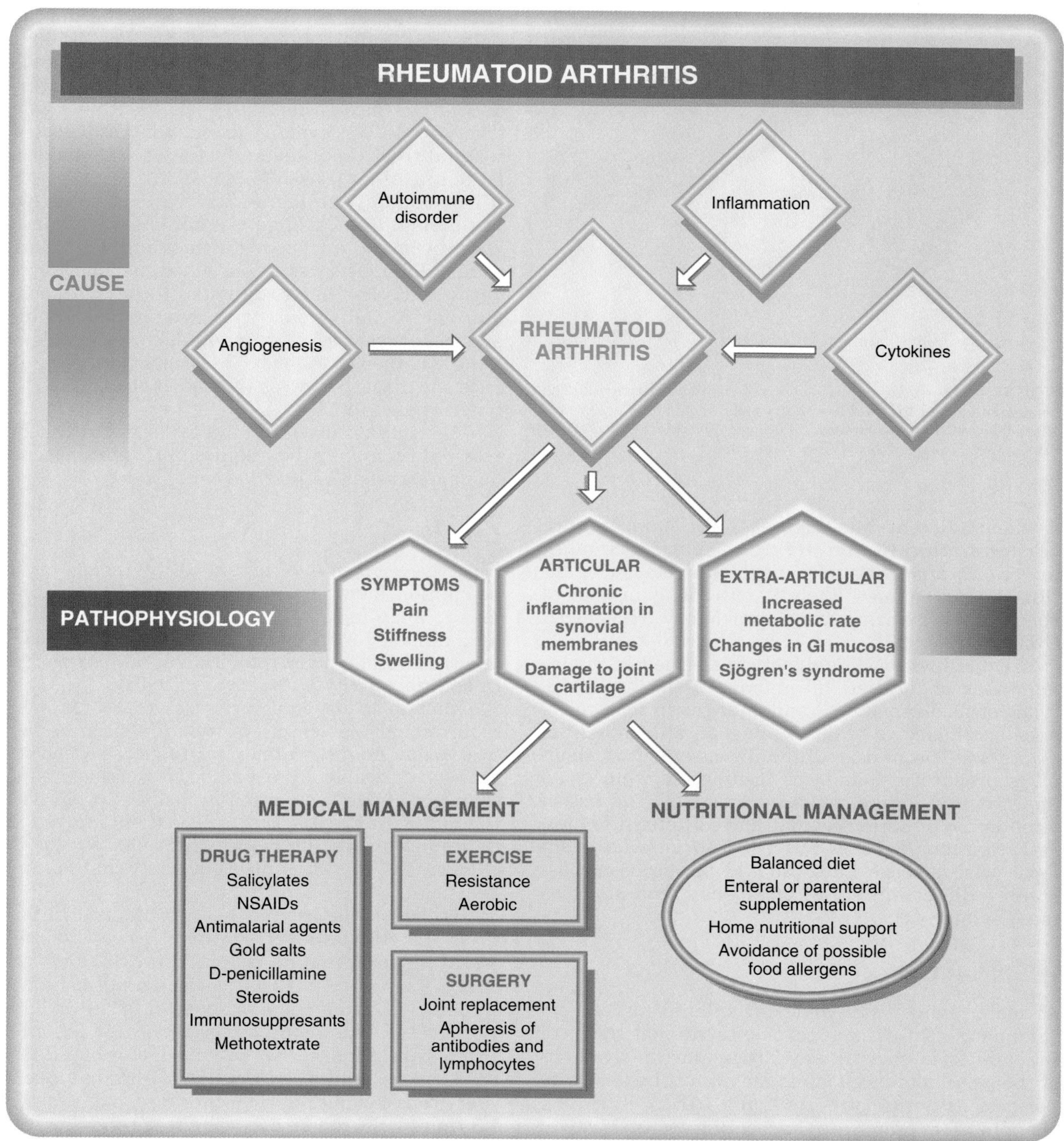

FIGURE 43–2 Pathophysiology algorithm—rheumatoid arthritis. (Algorithm content developed by John Anderson, Ph.D., and Sanford C. Garner, Ph.D., 2000.)

tions often used. A physical and occupational therapy evaluation helps to determine actual range of motion and activities that the individual can do independently.

Current weight and history of weight change over time are the least expensive, least invasive, and most reliable assessment tools to use with this population. Studies have demonstrated weight change as an important measure in individuals with rheumatoid arthritis. Increased cytokine production in rheumatoid arthritis may be associated with reduced body cell mass and altered energy intake and metabolism (Roubenoff et al, 1994).

Hematologic values should be assessed to determine the presence of anemia. Other laboratory values may be needed to evaluate other underlying

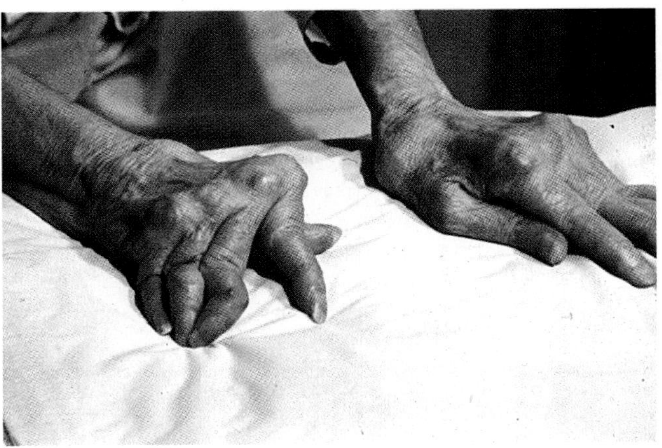

FIGURE 43–3 A patient with advanced rheumatoid arthritis. The twisted hands and the puffiness of the metacarpal joints are typical of the disease. (From Damjanov I. Pathology for the Health-Related Professions. Philadelphia: WB Saunders, 1996.)

problems. Recent data suggest that the appearance of **rheumatoid factor (RF),** an abnormal circulating protein that is an immunoglobulin-classified antibody, may be more likely to precede symptoms of rheumatoid arthritis than previously recognized (Kelly et al., 1997).

The diet history should include a review of the individual's usual diet, the impact of the handicap, types of food consumed, and changes in food tolerance secondary to oral, esophageal, and intestinal disorders. The impact of the disease on food shopping, preparation, and self-feeding, as well as on appetite and intake, must be assessed. The use of elimination or other diets purported to treat or cure arthritis should be evaluated. The association of foods with disease flares should be discussed, assuming the possibility of undetected food allergies (see Chapter 41).

Nutritional Care

Articular and extra-articular manifestations of rheumatoid arthritis affect the nutritional status of individuals in several ways. Articular involvement of the small and large joints may limit the ability to perform activities of daily living (ADL), including shopping for, preparing, and eating foods. Involvement of the temporomandibular joint can impact the ability to chew and swallow and may necessitate changes in diet consistency. Extra-articular manifestations include increased metabolic rate secondary to the inflammatory process, Sjögren's syndrome, and changes in the gastrointestinal mucosa.

The increase in metabolic rate secondary to the inflammatory process leads to increased nutrient needs, often in the face of a diminishing nutrient intake. Taste alterations secondary to **xerostomia** and dryness of the nasal mucosa, dysphagia secondary to pharyngeal and esophageal dryness, and anorexia secondary to medications, fatigue, and pain may reduce dietary intake. Changes in the gastrointestinal mucosa affect intake, digestion, and absorption. The impact of rheumatoid arthritis and of the medications used for treatment of the disease may be evident throughout the gastrointestinal tract, from the oral cavity to the small and large intestines (Bossingham, 1993).

In one study, patients with rheumatoid arthritis were found to be at high risk for obesity, abnormal vitamin levels, and poor nutrient intakes (Morgan et al., 1997). The use of uncooked, lactobacilli-rich, vegan diets has been suggested to have a positive outcome in individuals with rheumatoid arthritis; additional research is warranted, however, to determine whether changes in intestinal flora can influence the disease process (Nenonen et al., 1998; Peltonen et al., 1997).

When intakes are poor, enteral or parenteral supplementation may be required. In chronic cases, home nutritional support is beneficial.

Energy

Objective measures of actual energy needs for this population have not been determined. It is important to keep in mind that the actual impact of the inflammatory response on the metabolic rate is unknown, and may vary from individual to individual. In addition, activity levels vary greatly.

Although traditional measures to assess energy requirements can be used, weight should be monitored and energy intake modified as needed to achieve desirable or usual body weight. Reduced symptoms have been noted in fasting patients with rheumatoid arthritis, but most patients have experienced relapses after the reintroduction of food (Nenonen et al., 1998). It is not likely that fasting is beneficial.

Methods to determine energy requirements include the Harris-Benedict formula (see Chapter 2) and the Long equation (see Chapter 33) for resting energy expenditure (REE), with an additional factor for injury. During active disease, a factor of 1.14 to 1.35 times REE should be used to cover the effects of hypermetabolism. An activity factor of 1.2 times REE can be used for patients with limited mobility who are receiving physical therapy, and a factor of 1.3 times REE can be used for those receiving intensive daily physical therapy (Touger-Decker, 1988). For patients who are totally sedentary, calculations should be estimated at the REE and adjusted by weight changes that occur over time.

Protein

Well-nourished individuals require protein at levels comparable to the recommended dietary allowances (RDAs) for age and sex. One study revealed that patients with rheumatoid arthritis have increased whole body protein breakdown (regardless of age), which correlates with growth hormone factor, glu-

TABLE 43–1 PRODUCTION OF EICOSANOIDS FROM OMEGA-3 AND OMEGA-6 FATTY ACIDS

OMEGA-6: Linoleic acid 18:2~6 and Arachidonic acid 20:46~6
Thromboxane$_2$ (vasoconstrictor)—Platelet aggregation
Prostaglandin$_2$ (vasodilator)—Platelet antiaggregation
Leukotriene$_4$—Elongation
Desaturation—In platelets, blood vessels, leukocytes
OMEGA-3: Linolenic acid 18:3~3 and Eicosapentaenoic acid 20:5~3
Thromboxane$_3$ (vasoconstrictor)
Prostaglandin$_3$ (vasodilator)
Leukotriene$_5$

cagon, and tumor necrosis factor production (Rall et al., 1996b). Rall also concluded that strength training for patients receiving methotrexate yielded normal rates of protein catabolism (Rall et al., 1996a).

Requirements of patients who are poorly nourished or in an inflammatory phase of the disease increase to approximately 1.5 to 2 g/kg/day, with a nonprotein calorie:nitrogen ratio of 150:1 (Touger-Decker, 1988). To determine actual protein need objectively, a nitrogen balance study should be performed in each affected individual.

Lipids

German researchers have shown that low-fat diets (including utilization of low-fat substitutes) lead to low serum levels of vitamin A and E, and actually stimulate lipid peroxidation and eicosanoid production, aggravating rheumatoid arthritis (Adam et al., 1995). The typical emphasis on low-fat or fat-free dieting that has been the cornerstone of healthy eating in the United States may actually be counterproductive for patients susceptible to or afflicted by rheumatoid arthritis.

Rather than eliminating fat, it is probably more useful to change the type of fat in the diet. Omega-3 fatty acids, either in tablet form or as they occur in oils, have increased in popularity in the management of rheumatoid arthritis because of their role in inflammatory pathways (see Table 43–1 and "*Focus On:* Omega-3 Fatty Acids and the Inflammatory Process").

Although most studies (Ariza-Ariza et al., 1998; Hansen et al., 1998; James and Cleland, 1997) have demonstrated improvement in arthritic conditions and modulation of the inflammatory response with the administration of omega-3 and with lowered intake of omega-6 fatty acids, omega-3 oils should not replace conventional drug therapies. These oils should be used in conjunction with improved eating habits.

Research has also been conducted to determine whether the source of omega-3 fatty acids—that is, from a variety of whole food sources, like fish and oil-containing plants, rather than from pills—is significant. One study suggests that the pill form may enhance effectiveness of the food source (James and Cleland, 1997). Counselors should advise that fish oil supplements are not without their own side effects. Increased bleeding time, gastrointestinal distress, and fishy taste or odor may be associated with the ingestion of fish oil supplements.

Minerals and Vitamins

An observational study of 13 men and 35 women with rheumatoid arthritis showed that these patients had nutritional intakes below the RDA for calcium, folic acid, vitamin E, zinc, and selenium

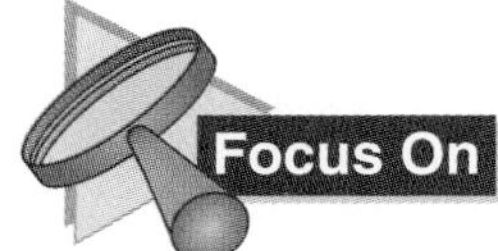

Omega-3 Fatty Acids and the Inflammatory Process

There are two classes of polyunsaturated omega fatty acids—Ω-6 and Ω-3—that are metabolized competitively, including conversion of their 20-carbon chain by oxygenase enzymes to form eicosanoids (eicosa meaning 20 in Greek). Prostaglandins, thromboxanes, leukotrienes, and prostacyclins are eicosanoids. Eicosapentaenoic acid (EPA) has a 20-carbon chain, and docosahexaenoic acid (DHA) has a 22-carbon chain; these are the Ω-3 polyunsaturated fatty acids that are abundant in fish, such as salmon, mackerel, herring, tuna, and some other fish oils. Alpha-linolenic acid (ALA) has an 18-carbon chain with an Ω-3 bond and is found in abundance in flaxseed, walnuts, and soy and canola (rapeseed) oils.

EPA, DHA, and ALA have all been shown to reduce the synthesis of aggressive inflammatory response cytokines by interfering with the conversion of arachidonic acid in various pathways. This process suppresses the activation of cytokines in the cell membrane. Cytokines are produced by antagonistic Ω-6 polyunsaturated acids that are mostly formed from linoleic acid, found in safflower and other oils (Grimble, 1998). The type of inflammatory mediator that is produced is determined by the composition of cellular membrane lipids, which in turn is influenced by the nature of the fatty acids in the diet.

Epidemiologic studies have supported the hypothesis that Ω-3 fatty acids may help prevent rheumatic arthritis (Shapiro, 1996). Diets that include supplemental doses (2.6 g) of Ω-3 fatty acids have been shown to improve the symptoms of rheumatic arthritis (Kremer et al., 1990) while allowing antiarthritic drug doses to be reduced (James and Cleloid, 1997). Overall, the effects on symptoms in individuals with rheumatoid arthritis have been beneficial (Kremer et al., 1995).

Additionally, Ω-3 fatty acids appear to inhibit tumor growth by limiting the production of prostaglandin E_2, which suppresses immune responses (Myrvik, 1994). Ω-3 and Ω-6 fatty acids that affect eicosanoids are listed in Table 43–1.

(Stone et al., 1997). Independent of drug-induced alterations in specific vitamin or mineral levels, there is mounting evidence that supports supplementation beyond the minimum levels for some nutrients.

There is preliminary evidence that indicates that vitamin therapy may complement conventional drug therapy, especially in the case of vitamin E (Edmonds et al., 1997), folic acid (Martin, 1998), selenium (Heinle et al., 1997), zinc (Naveh et al., 1997), and vitamin D (DeLuca and Zierold, 1998). There is also strong evidence that patients with rheumatoid arthritis are under pathophysiologic oxidative stress (Chiriac et al., 1996; Gambhir et al., 1997). Degradation of collagen and eicosanoid stimulation are associated with oxidative damage; therefore, increased intakes of supplemental antioxidants have been linked with beneficial effects in terms of both prevention and therapy for rheumatoid arthritis (Aaseth et al., 1998; Comstock et al., 1997; Hansen et al., 1998).

When metabolic bone disease is present, such as osteoporosis and osteomalacia, calcium and vitamin D supplementation are indicated (Gough et al., 1998). Animal studies have shown that vitamin D is beneficial because of its steroid-thyroid hormonal properties (DeLuca and Zierold, 1998).

Calcium and vitamin D malabsorption and bone demineralization are characteristic of advanced stages of the disease, which may lead to osteoporosis. Supplementation with calcium and vitamin D has been shown to help prevent and reduce these detrimental conditions (Buckley et al., 1996; Oelzner and Hein, 1997) (see Chapter 28).

Use of methotrexate in rheumatoid arthritis may be associated with elevated homocysteine levels caused by low folate levels. Thus, in patients with rheumatoid arthritis it makes good sense to pay special attention to adequate intakes of folate and vitamins B_6 and B_{12} (Morgan et al., 1998; Roubenoff et al., 1997).

Elevated levels of copper and ceruloplasmin in serum and joint fluid are seen in rheumatoid arthritis. Plasma copper levels correlate with the degree of joint inflammation, decreasing as the inflammation is diminished. Elevated plasma levels of ceruloplasmin may have a protective role, due to ceruloplasmin's antioxidant activity, against toxic oxygen radicals released during inflammation.

Variations in serum ferritin levels are less common in elderly persons than in young adults; this is true in rheumatoid arthritis as well (Lammi-Keefe et al., 1996). Plasma transferrin receptor levels are reliable for assessing iron status in this population. There does not appear to be any special requirement for iron supplementation in cases of rheumatoid arthritis.

Affected individuals should be cautioned to avoid falling prey to false claims of disease remission or cure using vitamins and minerals. It is important to remember that "nutrition only cures malnutrition;" the use of individual nutrients should be limited to situations in which the nutrient level or need is altered. The practice of megadosing should be addressed, especially in the case of vitamins A and D, and iron (Aaseth et al., 1998; Martin, 1998).

Disease Sequelae

Sjögren's Syndrome

Sjögren's syndrome, a chronic inflammatory disorder, is characterized by diminished production of tears and saliva resulting in *xerophthalmia*. The goal of dietary management in individuals with Sjögren's syndrome is relief of symptoms and eating comfort. Management of *xerostomia* should also include strategies for reducing the risk of dental decay (see Chapter 29), including frequent rinsing with water or brushing of teeth and the use of topical fluorides.

Because swallowing is a problem, ready-to-eat foods may be useful. Foods should all be moist, and extremes in temperature should be avoided. The tartness of artificially sweetened lemon drops may help stimulate salivary flow. Artificial saliva or products such as lemon glycerine may also be recommended by dental or dietetic professionals.

Temporomandibular Joint Syndrome

Severe temporomandibular joint (TMJ) syndrome, which may be associated with rheumatoid arthritis results in pain with eating. The goal of dietary management is to alter food consistency to reduce chewing pain. Diet consistency should be mechanical soft, and all foods should be cut into bite-size pieces to minimize the individual's need to chew.

Articular Manifestations

To facilitate self-feeding in individuals with rheumatoid arthritis, the dietitian or nurse should work closely with the occupational therapist to design a diet that maximizes independence in preparation and consumption and minimizes pain and frustration. Finger foods that do not fall apart easily when grasped may be helpful.

Pharmacologic Therapy

Pharmacologic therapy to control pain and inflammation is the mainstay of treatment for rheumatoid arthritis. The seven primary drug classifications used to treat rheumatoid arthritis are salicylates, NSAIDs, antimalarial agents, gold salts, D-penicillamine, steroids, and immunosuppressive agents. Unfortunately, it has been estimated that toxicity resulting from pharmacological treatments of rheumatoid arthritis contributes up to 60% of the total cost of treating affected patients in the United States (James and Cleland, 1997).

The goal of medication therapy is to control the inflammatory process. The choice of drug class and type is based on patient response to the medication, incidence and severity of adverse reactions, and patient compliance. Drug-nutrient side effects can occur with any of the drugs. Side effects of drug use may influence ingestion, digestion, and absorption, and, hence, nutritional status (see Table 43–2 and Chapter 18).

Salicylates are usually the first line of drug therapy. However, chronic aspirin ingestion is associated with gastric mucosal injury and bleeding, increased bleeding time, and increased urinary excretion of vitamin C. The gastrointestinal symptoms of gastritis are frequently alleviated by taking aspirin with milk, food, or an antacid. Vitamin C supplementation is prescribed when serum and platelet levels of ascorbic acid are abnormally low.

The second line of drug therapy involves the use of NSAIDs. The effectiveness of aspirin and NSAIDs lies in the inhibition of prostaglandin synthesis and immune modulation.

Corticosteroids, the most potent of the anti-inflammatory drugs used to treat rheumatoid arthritis, have extensive side effects. Their catabolic impact can result in negative nitrogen balance. Hypercalciuria and reduced calcium absorption can increase the risk of osteoporosis (see Chapter 28). Edema also occurs and may require diet modification, including a sodium-restricted diet and fluid restriction. Other side effects include Cushingoid changes in the body, gastrointestinal bleeding, diabetes mellitus, and osteoporosis.

One study has revealed that bone mineral loss, induced by prednisone at a mean daily dose of 5.5 mg, can be prevented with the daily addition of 1 g of calcium plus 500 IU of vitamin D (Canoso, 1997). Serum calcium levels greater than 11.0 mg/dL should be avoided (Harris, 1997). Despite these effects, oral glucocorticoids (such as prednisone) are widely used and have symptomatic benefits (Kirwan, 1995).

Gold salt therapy, antimalarials, and D-penicillamine are known as "remittive" agents and can cause a remission of rheumatoid arthritis. Proteinuria may occur with administration of gold and

TABLE 43–2 NUTRITIONAL SIDE EFFECTS OF ARTHRITIS MEDICATIONS

SIDE EFFECTS	SALICYLATES	NSAIDSs	ANTI-MALARIALS	D-PENICILLAMINE	CORTICO-STEROIDS	IMMUNOSUPPRESSIVE AGENTS	GOLD
Nutritional							
Anorexia			x	x		x	
Stomatitis		x		x		x	x
Nausea	x	x	x	x	x	x	
Vomiting	x	x	x	x			x
Gastritis	x						
Duodenal ulcer		x			x		
Peptic ulcer	x						
Constipation		x					
Gastrointestinal bleeding	x	x					
Diarrhea		x*	x	x		x	x
Altered taste				x		x	
Metabolic							
Glucose intolerance					x		
Proteinuria				x			x
Negative nitrogen balance					x		x
Altered serum K	x				x		
Edema		†			x		
Depressed total lymphocyte count (TLC)					x	x	
Anergy					x	x	
Increased BUN value		x					
Anemia	x	x		x			
Decreased Vitamin/Mineral							
Ascorbic acid	x						
Folate	x					x‡	
Zinc				x			
Copper				x			
Calcium					x	x	
Iron				x			

(Adapted from Touger-Decker R. Nutritional considerations in rheumatoid arthritis. J Am Diet Assoc 88:329, 1988.)

NSAIDs, nonsteroidal anti-inflammatory drugs.

*Meclomen only.

†May occur with preexisting edema.

‡Methotrexate only.

D-penicillamine. Toxicity from these drugs must be monitored continually.

Methotrexate is now commonly used to treat rheumatoid arthritis. Methotrexate toxicity is mostly related to its antifolate properties (Shirok, 1997). Folic acid supplementation (1 mg per day or 1 to 5 mg of folinic acid per week) is needed to offset the toxicity of this drug, for protection against gastrointestinal disturbances and maintenance of red blood cell production (Anderson et al., 1997; Morgan et al., 1997a, 1997b; Ortiz et al., 1998). It should be noted that folic acid supplementation does *not* decrease the efficacy of methotrexate therapy (Hunt et al., 1997). Although supplementation with folate in B_{12}-deficient patients will correct anemia, neurologic manifestations will continue to progress. Therefore, baseline B_{12} levels should be determined prior to vitamin therapy. Cyclosporine may be administered in combination with methotrexate, and it can produce other gastrointestinal side effects (Tugwell et al., 1995).

Other Treatments and Exercise

Surgery replaces irreversibly damaged joints, improves the functional capacity of damaged joints, and prevents damage to otherwise healthy joints. Circulating antibodies and lymphocytes are sometimes removed by a process called *apheresis.*

Regular resistance and aerobic activity in patients with rheumatoid arthritis increases their range of motion, improves strength and endurance, preserves bone mass, preserves lean body mass, prevents fatigue, decreases depression, and distributes the forces of muscle contraction more evenly over joint surfaces (Neuberger et al., 1997; Van den Ende et al., 1998). However, exercise does not appear to diminish inflammation or any other relevant inflammatory biochemical indices of rheumatoid arthritis (Rall et al., 1996a).

Recent research on the use of recombinant human tumor necrosis factor receptor (p75)-Fc protein has shown that it can diminish inflammatory symptoms of rheumatoid arthritis (Moreland et al., 1997). More studies are being conducted.

GOUT

Pathophysiology

Gout, one of the oldest diseases in recorded medical history, is a disorder of purine metabolism in which abnormally high levels of uric acid accumulate in the blood (hyperuricemia). As a consequence, sodium urates are formed and deposited as tophi in the small joints and surrounding tissues. Renal disease is common, and uric acid nephrolithiasis can occur. In chronic gout, a classic site is the helix of the ear (Fig. 43–4), but a more common site is the large toe or the elbow (Fig. 43–5). These urate deposits can destroy joint tissues, leading to chronic symptoms of arthritis (Fig. 43–6).

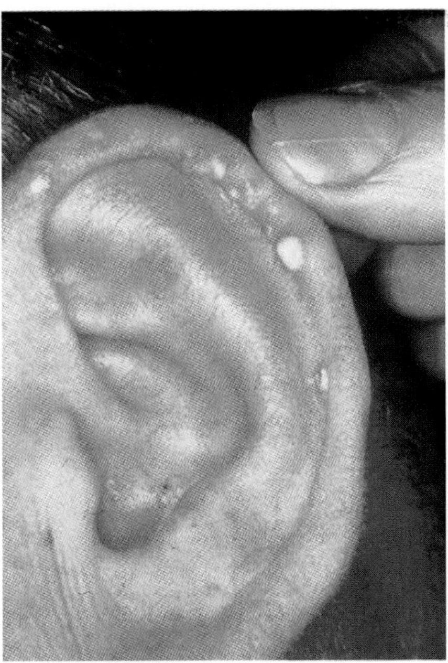

FIGURE 43–4 Tophi on the ear of a patient who has had gout for many years. (Courtesy of the American College of Rheumatology.)

The disease, which usually occurs after the age of 35 years and predominantly affects males, is characterized by the sudden and acute onset of localized arthritic pain that usually begins in the big toe and continues up the leg. As the disease advances, symptoms occur more frequently and are more prolonged. Trivial injury or unaccustomed exertion may precipitate the episodes, and attacks have been related to excessive eating, drinking, and exercise.

Obesity is commonly associated with a gouty condition. Ketosis associated with fasting or a low-carbohydrate diet can also precipitate an attack. Occasionally, the disturbance follows surgery.

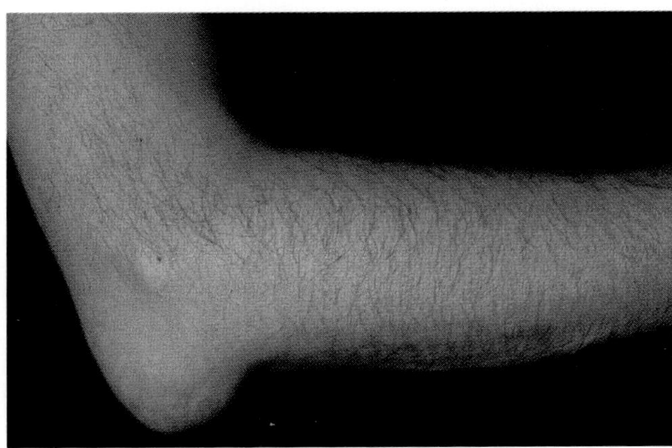

FIGURE 43–5 Gout. This markedly enlarged olecranon bursa is caused by gout. (Reprinted from the Clinical Slide Collection on the Rheumatic Diseases, copyright 1991, 1995, 1997. Used by permission of the American College of Rheumatology.)

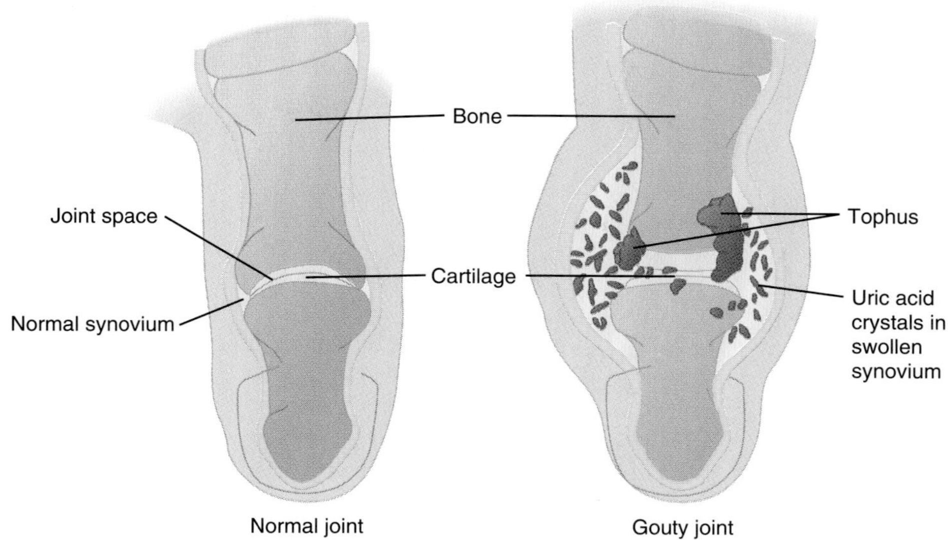

FIGURE 43–6 Comparison of a gouty joint and a normal joint. (From Black, JM et al. Medical Surgical Nursing, 5th ed. Philadelphia: WB Saunders, 1996.)

Nutritional Care

Role of Proteins and Purines

Uric acid is derived from the metabolism of **purines,** which constitute a part of **nucleoproteins.** Although gout has traditionally been treated with a low-purine diet, drugs have largely replaced the need for rigid restriction of dietary purines. Endogenous formation of uric acid from simple metabolites, as well as from purine breakdown, accounts for 85% of the urate formed, and is apparently influenced very little by dietary regulation. Even though limiting dietary purines is unlikely to decrease the uric acid pool significantly, individuals with gout should be encouraged to limit or avoid foods high in purines, to reduce metabolic stress (such as ketosis from excessive dieting), and to reduce medication use, if possible.

Traditionally, restriction of foods containing purines (see Table 43–3) has been recommended in the acute stage of gout in an attempt to avoid adding exogenous purines to the existing high uric acid load. Intake of fluids (3 L/day) should be encouraged to assist with the excretion of uric acid and to minimize the possibility of renal calculi formation. Because urate excretion tends to be reduced by fats and enhanced by carbohydrates, the diet should be relatively high in carbohydrate, moderate in protein, and low in fat. Dietary guidelines consistent with the food guide pyramid should be encouraged (see Chapter 15).

It has been suggested that tofu (bean curd) is a preferable source of protein in patients with gout. Tofu ingestion has been shown to alter plasma protein concentration and to increase uric acid clearance and excretion (Yamakita et al., 1998).

During the interval stage between attacks, dietary treatment for patients who are receiving maintenance medication for gout involves a normal adequate diet adjusted to achieve and maintain a desirable body weight and to avoid ketosis.

LOW-PURINE DIET. A typical diet contains 600 to 1000 mg of purines daily. Traditionally, in cases of severe or advanced gout, the purine content of the daily diet is restricted to approximately 100 to 150 mg. Other dietary guidelines to promote general health, including a high-carbohydrate (50% to 55% of calories), low-fat (30%), modified-cholesterol (<300 mg/day) diet, should be followed. The diet may be prescribed according to the groupings in Table 43–3, allowing for considerable individualization among patients. Table 43–4 summarizes the dietary guidelines for gout.

Alcohol

Ethanol does increase uric acid production, but does not always cause an attack of gout. The patient should be advised not to consume an excess of alcohol.

Pharmacotherapy

Gout is treated with drugs that inhibit or eliminate uric acid synthesis. Probenecid (Benemid) and sulfinpyrazone decrease the blood uric acid level by increasing elimination through the kidneys. Allopurinol inhibits uric acid production.

Both probenecid and sulfinpyrazone are frequently used in conjunction with colchicine, a drug that has no effect on uric acid metabolism but that has been shown to relieve the joint pain of gouty

TABLE 43–3 FOODS GROUPED ACCORDING TO PURINE CONTENT

Group 1: High Purine Content (100 to 1000 mg of Purine Nitrogen per 100 g of Food)

Anchovies	Mackerel
Bouillon	Meat extracts
Brains	Mincemeat
Broth	Mussels
Consommé	Partridge
Goose	Roe
Gravy	Sardines
Heart	Scallops
Herring	Sweetbreads
Kidney	Yeast (baker's and brewer's), taken as supplement

Foods in this list should be omitted from the diet of patients who have gout (acute and remission stages).

Group 2: Moderate Purine Content (9 to 100 mg of Purine Nitrogen per 100 g of Food)

Meat and Fish (except those listed in group 1):	*Vegetables*
Fish	Asparagus
Poultry	Beans, dried
Meat	Lentils
Shellfish	Mushrooms
	Peas, dried
	Spinach

One serving (2 to 3 oz) of meat, fish, or fowl or 1 serving (1/2 cup) of vegetables from this group is allowed daily (depending on condition) during remissions.

Group 3: Negligible Purine Content

Bread, white, and crackers	Fruit
Butter or margarine (in moderation)*	Gelatin desserts
Cake and cookies	Herbs
Carbonated beverages	Ice cream
Cereal beverage (e.g., Postum)	Milk
Cereals and cereal products	Macaroni products
Cheese	Noodles
Chocolate	Nuts
Coffee	Oil
Condiments	Olives
Cornbread	Pickles
Cream (in moderation)*	Popcorn
Custard	Puddings
Eggs	Relishes
Fats (in moderation)*	Rennet desserts
Vegetables (except those in group 2)	Rice
	Salt
	Sugar and sweets
	Tea
	Vinegar
	White sauce

Foods included in this group may be used daily.

*Recommended in moderation due to fat content.

arthritis. Colchicine is most valuable during the acute stage, but may be needed during symptom-free periods as a preventive measure. (For the nutritional effects of colchicine, see Chapter 18.)

Anti-inflammatory agents, such as indomethacin or phenylbutazone, are sometimes used in the acute stage of gout. NSAIDs are favored unless the side effects are too troublesome (Emmerson, 1996).

TABLE 43–4 SUMMARY OF NUTRITIONAL CARE FOR GOUT

1. Moderate intake of foods high in purines (see Table 43–3)
2. Moderate protein intake, with large proportion of protein coming from low-fat dairy products and soy
3. Liberal carbohydrate intake (at least 50% of total daily kilocalories)
4. Fat intake of about 30% of total kilocalories
5. Maintenance of, or gradual reduction to, ideal body weight
6. Restriction or elimination of alcohol
7. Liberal fluid intake to keep urine dilute
8. Management of side effects of NSAIDs, which are favored unless risks are too high

SCLERODERMA

Scleroderma is a progressive, systemic sclerosis characterized by deposition of fibrous connective tissue in the skin and visceral organs, including the gastrointestinal tract (Escott-Stump, 1998). Women tend to be afflicted three times more often then men (see internet site: www.Sjogren's.org/scl.htm). Raynaud's syndrome (ischemia or coldness in the small extremities, such as the fingers) can occur, causing difficulty in preparation and consumption of meals. Sjögren's syndrome is often also present. Weight loss, renal dysfunction, and multiple organ system dysfunction may result.

The disease is progressive, and there is no current treatment that produces a cure. Dysphagia may be one symptom that requires nutritional interventions (see Chapter 42). Malabsorption of lactose, vitamins, fatty acids, and minerals can cause further nutritional problems; supplementation may be required. A high-energy, high-protein supplement or enteral feeding may be effective in correcting or preventing weight loss, which is a common manifestation. Home enteral or parenteral nutritional support is often required when problems, such as chronic diarrhea, persist (see Chapter 22). Side effects of specific drug therapies, as prescribed for specific symptoms and organ involvement, are noted in Chapter 18.

SYSTEMIC LUPUS ERYTHEMATOSUS

Pathophysiology

Systemic lupus erythematosus (SLE) has an unclear etiology. A genetic predisposition (genetic marker HLA, or human leukocyte antigen), the presence of anti-DNA antibodies, and environmental factors, such as a viral infection, are thought to be involved. The condition is most prevalent in women of child-bearing age. About 25% of persons with SLE also develop Sjögren's syndrome.

SLE is considered to be an autoimmune disease that affects all organ systems. The disease itself, as well as the medications (e.g., steroids) that are commonly used to treat SLE, affects nutrient metabolism, needs, and excretion. Renal function is deranged, causing excessive excretion of protein and, often, renal failure.

Nutritional Care

There are no specific dietary guidelines for managing SLE. Rather, the diet needs to be tailored to the individual needs of the patient. Priorities include addressing the sequelae of the disease and the pharmacologic effects on organ function and nutrient metabolism (see Table 43–2). Protein requirements are altered as a result of disordered renal function, caused by the disease and steroid-induced side effects. Sodium and fluid intake are typically restricted for the same reasons. Although a diet low in saturated fats has been recommended, further studies are necessary to document its effectiveness.

Energy needs should be tailored to the individual's dry weight. In determining caloric requirements, the goal should be to attain and maintain usual body weight. Home enteral or parenteral nutritional support is often necessary (see Chapter 22).

The role of specific vitamins, minerals, and other nutrients, such as omega-3 fatty acids, is being studied. Although vitamin E may play a role in terminating the process of lipid peroxidation, this function has not been proven in connective tissue disorder therapy (Fairburn, 1992).

Pharmacotherapy

Corticosteroids cause alterations in protein, sodium, fluid, and calcium needs. Plaquenil, an antimalarial drug, appears to be effective in clearing up skin lesions for some individuals; side effects that must be managed include nausea, abdominal cramping, and diarrhea. Immunosupressants, such as azathioprine, may be used when there is brain or renal involvement, but gastrointestinal side effects may occur.

UNPROVEN REMEDIES FOR RHEUMATIC DISORDERS

Because modern medicine often has nothing to offer in the way of a cure or even relief of symptoms, many persons with rheumatic disorders understandably turn to folk medicine and even quackery for help. Surveys in the United States and other countries show that 50% to 94% of those affected try at least one self-help remedy, and usually more than one (Jarvis, 1990).

Favorable effects of self-help treatments are often reported anecdotally, but as a rule, no cause-and-effect relationships have been documented. Any amelioration can usually be attributed to the placebo effect or to characteristic cycles of worsening, followed by periods of improvement. When a home remedy coincides with a period of remission, the remedy is often continued indefinitely, even when it fails to perform through a later period of disease exacerbation (see "*Focus On:* Controversies in Rheumatic Disorders").

Some seemingly "natural" remedies have their roots in medicine, as in the case of willow bark and copper bracelets. Salicylate, derived from willow bark, has been around as a medicinal remedy for pain and inflammation since 1763, and some have even traced it back to ancient Egypt. Willow bark has the same gastrointestinal side effects as NSAIDs (Hedner & Everts, 1998). Although the folk remedy of wearing a copper bracelet to relieve arthritis pain has been suggested as a means of

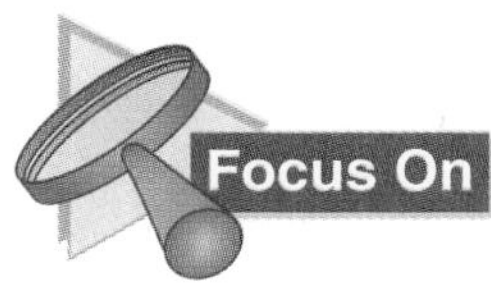

Controversies in Rheumatic Disorders: Chronic Fatigue Syndrome and Fibromyalgia

Disorders, such as chronic fatigue disorder syndrome (CFDS) and fibromyalgia, have rheumatic symptoms but no proven cure. In CFDS, chronic fatigue is the major symptom, lasting 6 months or longer and accompanied by a sore throat, multiple joint pain, headaches, postexertion lethargy, muscle pain, and impaired concentration. CFDS mimics autoimmune disorders, such as SLE or hypothyroidism. Graduated exercise programs, low-fat diets, antioxidant therapy, massive doses of vitamins, magnesium sulfate use, and costly intravenous immunoglobin therapy have been recommended, but their efficacy is as yet unconfirmed by controlled studies. When hypotension is identified medically, increases in sodium and fluid intakes have been suggested.

In **fibromyalgia,** nonarticular aches and fatigue cause disabling symptoms that are similar to those of rheumatoid arthritis. Muscle tenderness, sleep disturbances, fatigue, morning stiffness, numbness and tingling, chronic headaches, irritable bowel, and irritable bladder have all been reported to be associated with the "fibromyalgia syndrome." Several hypotheses have been proposed, including central pain derangement; central nervous system dysfunction; nutrient deficiencies of magnesium, malic acid, manganese, or thiamin; and other systemic abnormalities (www.sjogrens.org/fib.htm). Pain therapy, use of calcium channel blockers, physical reconditioning, psychological therapy, and alternative approaches have been recommended, but further studies are needed to evaluate their effectiveness.

promoting copper absorption through the skin (Bollet, 1994), no clinical studies have substantiated this claim.

Rhizoma smilacis glabrae, also known as glabrous green briar rhizome (china root), is an extract used in Chinese herbal medicine that has been shown to act as a therapeutic agent in rheumatoid arthritis and it is without side effects (Jiang et al., 1997). Initial studies suggest that china root extract acts through selective suppression of the cellular immune response involved in inflammation, as well as through a direct anti-inflammatory mechanism, including inhibition of PGE_2. This is not yet a proven remedy.

Megavitamin therapy and special foods and diets are among the most popular self-help remedies. Frequently, dietary variations are unusual, as evidenced by the "honey and apple cider vinegar" treatment or use of kombucha tea.

Shark cartilage is a popular remedy because it is a cheap source of chondroitin sulfate, but there have been no studies of the effect of shark cartilage on joint disease. Even with positive-effect evidence for cow trachea chondroitin sulfate and other promising "natural" remedies, some difficulties persist, including the following: (1) there is no regulation of such supplements in terms of dosage, purity, or claims; (2) using these nonregulated remedies is, in effect, self-medication without monitoring; and (3) there is no understanding of other drug interactions or long-term safety.

Animal studies have shown a positive response, in terms of reducing inflammation in arthritic paws of rats, from oral capsaicin (from red pepper) and curcumin (from turmeric) (Joe et al., 1997). One cannot assume, however, that studies in human subjects will yield the same results.

Few controlled trials of the effects of diet on the symptoms of arthritis are available. Among them are a few in which favorable results cannot be explained on the basis of the placebo effect. Underlying theories include exposing and eliminating unrecognized allergies or modifying the immune system response to inflammation.

Although much of the dietary experimentation is harmless (except for the cost of special foods or popular diet books), some self-treatment modalities can be harmful. Both comfrey and alfalfa are herbs that have been promoted as potential cures for arthritis, yet both have been deemed toxic by the scientific community. Rattlesnake meat has been touted as a remedy, but the risk of salmonella poisoning is high. Other unproven remedies involve the excessive use of supplements or other herbal remedies (see Chapter 19).

Rheumatic disorders may be disfiguring and painful. It would be ideal if nutritional therapies provided the answers, but the evidence is not clear that specific vitamins, minerals, fatty acids, amino acids, or carbohydrates make a difference in preventing or curing these disorders. Research in this field continues as a public health initiative to protect consumers from potentially harmful quackery and expensive fraud.

CASE STUDY

Sam T. is a 52-year-old white male who lives with his wife in a rural area. He is 5 feet 10 inches tall and weighs 230 lb. He has recently been diagnosed as having osteoarthritis. A nonsteroidal anti-inflammatory drug was prescribed for when he experiences severe flare-ups of the condition. Although the medication is generally effective, Sam now wants you to develop a special diet for him. He has heard that liver extract, bee pollen, and gold tablets will cure his condition. He brought you a bag full of various remedies, and has displayed them on your desk.

1. How will you tactfully advise him that these so-called remedies are not likely to be useful and may actually cause some harm?
2. He has read in the newspaper that vitamin E and other antioxidants are useful in alleviating his condition, but you have no scientific articles to prove this. How will you discuss this topic with Sam?
3. From his diet history, it appears that Sam eats little at breakfast and has a heavy, high-saturated-fat lunch. He eats no fish, few fruits and vegetables, and drinks a cocktail before dinner. What dietary changes would you suggest to improve his diet?
4. Sam does not mention his overweight. How would you bring up the subject, and what steps would you recommend for him?

CITED REFERENCES

Aaseth J, et al. Rheumatoid arthritis and metal compounds—Perspectives on the role of oxygen radical detoxification. Analyst 123:3, 1998.

Adam O, et al. Low-fat diet decreases alpha-tocopherol levels, and stimulates LDL oxidation and eicosanoid biosynthesis in man. Eur J Med Res 1:65, 1995.

Alarcon GS, Morgan SL. Guidelines for folate supplementation in rheumatoid arthritis patients treated with methotrexate: Comment on the guidelines for monitoring drug therapy. Arthritis Rheum 40:391, 1997.

Anderson LS, Hansen TM. Prospectively measured red cell folate levels in methotrexate treated patients with rheumatoid arthritis: Relation to withdrawal and side effects. J Rheumatol 25:830, 1997.

Ariza-Ariza R, et al. Omega-3 fatty acids in rheumatoid arthritis: An overview. Semin Arthritis Rheum 27:366, 1998.

Arthritis Foundation, 1330 West Peachtree Street, Atlanta, GA 30309. Available: www.arthritis.org. 1-800-283-7800.

Blotman F, et al. Efficacy and safety of avocado/soybean unsaponifiables in the treatment of symptomatic osteoarthritis of the knee and hip. A prospective, multicenter, three-month, randomized, doubleblind, placebo-controlled trial. Rev Rheum Engl Ed 64:825, 1997.

Bollet AJ. Nutrition and diet in rheumatic diseases. In: Shils ME, Olson JA, Shike M (eds.). Modern Nutrition in Health and Disease, 8th ed. Philadephia: Lea & Febiger, 1994.

Bossingham D, Hawkey CJ. Gastroenterology in the rheumatic diseases. Gastroenterol Rheum Dis 1:138, 1993.

Buckley LM, et al. Calcium and vitamin D_3 supplementation prevents bone loss in the spine secondary to low-dose corticosteroids in patients with rheumatoid arthritis. A randomized, double-blind, placebo-controlled trial. Ann Intern Med 125:961, 1996.

Buckwalter JA, Lane NE. Athletics and osteoarthritis. Am J Sport Med 25:873, 1997.

Canoso JJ. Rheumatology in Primary Care. Philadelphia: WB Saunders, 1997.

Chiriac R, et al. The antioxidant systems in rheumatoid polyarthritis. Rev Med Chir Soc Med Nat Iasi 100:79, 1996.

Comstock GW, et al. Serum concentrations of alpha-tocopherol, beta-carotene, and retinol preceding the diagnosis of rheumatoid arthritis and systemic lupus erythematosus. Ann Rheum Dis 56:323, 1997.

Cooper C, et al. Individual risk factors for hip osteoarthritis: Obesity, hip injury, and physical activity. Am J Epidemiol 147:516, 1998.

Creamer P, et al. Management of osteoarthritis in older adults. Clin Geriatr Med 14:435, 1998.
DeLuca HF, Zierold C. Mechanisms and functions of vitamin D. Nutr Rev 56:S4, 1998.
Edmonds SE, et al. Putative analgesic activity of repeated oral doses of vitamin E in the treatment of rheumatoid arthritis. Results of a prospective placebo controlled double blind trial. Ann Rheum Dis 56:649, 1997.
Emmerson B. The management of gout. N Engl J Med 334:445, 1996.
Escott-Stump S. Nutrition and Diagnosis-Related Care, 4th ed. Baltimore: Williams and Wilkins, 1998.
Fairburn K, et al. Alpha-tocopherol, lipids and lipoproteins in knee joint synovial fluid and serum from patients with inflammatory joint disease. Clin Sci 83:657, 1992.
Firestein G, Zvaifler N. Anticytokine therapy in rheumatoid arthritis. N Engl J Med 337:195, 1997.
Fisher NM, et al. Muscle function and gait in patients with knee osteoarthritis before and after muscle rehabilitation. Disabil Rehabil 19:47, 1997.
Flynn M, et al. The effect of folate and cobalamin on osteoarthritic hands. Am J Coll Nutr 13:351, 1994.
Fransen M, et al. A revised group exercise program for osteoarthritis of the knee. Physiother Res Int 2:30, 1997.
Gambhir JK, et al. Correlation between blood antioxidant levels and lipid peroxidation in rheumatoid arthritis. Clin Biochem 30:351, 1997.
Gough A, et al. Effect of vitamin D receptor gene alleles on bone loss in early rheumatoid arthritis. J Rheumatol 25:864, 1998.
Grimble RF, Tappia PS. Modulation of pro-inflammatory cytokine biology by unsaturated fatty acids. Z Ernahrungswiss 37:57, 1998.
Hansen G, et al. Nutritional status of Danish patients with rheumatoid arthritis and effects of a diet adjusted in energy intake, fish content and antioxidants. Ugeskr Laeger 160:3074, 1998.
Harris ED. Rheumatoid Arthritis. Philadelphia: WB Saunders, 1997.
Hedner T, Everts B. The early clinical history of salicylates in rheumatology and pain. Clin Rheumatol 17:17, 1998.
Heinle K, et al. Selenium concentration in erythrocytes of patients with rheumatoid arthritis. Clinical and laboratory chemistry infection markers during administration of selenium. Med Klin 92:29, 1997.
Heliovaara M, et al. Serum antioxidants and risk of rheumatoid arthritis. Ann Rheum Dis 53:51, 1994.
Hochberg MC, et al. Guidelines for the medical management of osteoarthritis. Arthritis Rheum 38:1535, 1995.
Hunt PG, et al. The effects of daily intake of folic acid on the efficacy of methotrexate therapy in children with juvenile rheumatoid arthritis. A controlled study. J Rheumatol 24:2230, 1997.
James MJ, Cleland LG. Dietary ω-3 fatty acids and therapy for rheumatoid arthritis. Semin Arthritis Rheum 27:85, 1997.
Jarvis WT. Arthritis: Folk remedies and quackery. Nutr Forum 7(1):1, 1990.
Jiang J, et al. Anti-inflammatory activity of the aqueous extract from rhizome smilacis glabrae. Pharmacol Res 36:309, 1997.
Joe B, et al. Presence of an acidic glycoprotein in the serum of arthritic rats: Modulation by capsaicin and curcumin. Mol Cell Biochem 169: 125, 1997.
Johanning GL. Modulation of breast cancer cell adhesion by unsaturated fatty acids. Nutrition 12:810, 1996.
Kelly WN, et al. Textbook of Rheumatology, vol. 2. Philadelphia: WB Saunders, 1997, p. 1383.
Kirwan J. The effect of glucocorticoids on joint destruction in rheumatoid arthritis. N Engl J Med 333:142, 1995.
Koopman WJ. Arthritis and Allied Conditions—A textbook of rheumatology, vol. 2. Baltimore, MD: Williams & Wilkins, 1997, p. 1970.
Kremer JM, et al. Effects of manipulation of dietary fatty acids on clinical manifestations of rheumatoid arthritis. Lancet 1:184, 1995.
Kremer J, et al. Dietary fish oil and olive oil supplementation in patients with rheumatoid arthritis. Arthritis Rheum 33:810, 1990.
Lammi-Keefe C, et al. Day-to-day variation in iron status indexes is similar for most measures in elderly women with and without rheumatoid arthritis. J Am Diet Assoc 96:247, 1996.
Lawrence RC, et al. Estimates of the prevalence of arthritis and selected musculoskeletal disorders in the United States. Arthritis Rheum 41:778, 1998.
Martin RH. The role of nutrition and diet in rheumatoid arthritis. Proc Nutr Soc 57:231, 1998.
McAlindon TE, et al. Relation of dietary intake and serum levels of vitamin D to progression of osteoarthritis of the knee among participants in the Framingham study. Ann Intern Med 125:353, 1996.
Moreland L, et al. Treatment of rheumatoid arthritis with a recombinant human tumor necrosis factor receptor (p75)-Fc protein. N Engl J Med 337:141, 1997.
Morgan S, et al. Nutrient intake patterns, body mass index, and vitamin levels in patients with rheumatoid arthritis. Arthritis Care Res 10(1):9, 1997a.
Morgan S, et al. Methotrexate in rheumatoid arthritis: Folate supplementation should always be given. BioDrugs 8(3):164, 1997b.
Morreale P, et al. Comparison of the anti-inflammatory efficacy of chondroitin sulfate and diclofenac sodium in patients with knee osteoarthritis. J Rheumatol 23:1385, 1996.
Myrvik QN. Immunology and nutrition. In: Shils ME, Olson JA, Shike M (eds.). Modern Nutrition in Health and Disease, 8th ed. Philadelphia: Lea & Febiger, 1994.
Naveh Y, et al. Zinc metabolism in rheumatoid arthritis: Plasma and urinary zinc and relationship to disease activity. J Rheumatol 24:643, 1997.
Nenonen T, et al. Uncooked, lactobacilli-rich, vegan food and rheumatoid arthritis. Br J Rheumatol 37:274, 1998.
Neuberger GB, et al. Effects of exercise on fatigue, aerobic fitness, and disease activity measures in persons with rheumatoid. Res Nurs Health 20:195, 1997.
Oelzner P, Hein G. Inflammation and bone metabolism in rheumatoid arthritis. Pathogenetic viewpoints and therapeutic possibilities. Med Klin 92:607, 1997.
Ortiz Z, et al. The efficacy of folic acid and folinic acid in reducing methotrexate gastrointestinal toxicity in rheumatoid arthritis. A meta-analysis of randomized controlled trials. J Rheumatol 25:36, 1998.
Peltonen R, et al. Faecal microbial flora and disease activity in rheumatoid arthritis during a vegan diet. Br J Rheumatol 36:64, 1997.
Perneger TV, et al. Risk of kidney failure associated with the use of acetaminophen, aspirin, and nonsteroidal anti-inflammatory drug. N Engl J Med 331:1675, 1994.
Philbin EF, et al. Osteoarthritis as a determinant of an adverse coronary heart disease risk profile. J Cardiovasc Risk 3:529, 1996.
Rall LC, et al. Effects of progressive resistance training on immune response in aging and chronic inflammation. Med Sci Sports Exerc 28:1356, 1996a.
Rall LC, et al. Protein metabolism in rheumatoid arthritis and aging—Effects of muscle strength training and tumor necrosis factor cc. Arthritis Rheum 39:1115, 1996b.
Rejeski WJ, et al. Treating disability in knee osteoarthritis with exercise therapy: A central role for self-efficacy and pain. Arthritis Care Res 11:94, 1998.
Roubenoff R, et al. Abnornal homocysteine metabolism in rheumatoid arthritis. Arthritis Rheum 40:718, 1997.
Roubenoff R, et al. Rheumatoid cachexia: Cytokine-driven hypermetabolism accompanying reduced body cell mass chronic inflammation. J Clin Invest 93:2379, 1994.
Shapiro JA. Diet and rheumatoid arthritis in women: A possible protective effect of fish consumption. Epidemiology 7:256, 1996.
Shiroky JB. The use of folates concomitantly with low-dose pulse methotrexate. Rheum Dis Clin North Am 23:969, 1997.
Spector TD, et al. Risk of osteoarthritis associated with long-term weight-bearing sports: A radiologic survey of the hips and knees in female ex-athletes and population controls. Arthritis Rheum 39:988, 1996.
Stone J, et al. Inadequate calcium, folic acid, vitamin E, zinc, and selenium intake in rheumatoid arthritis patients: Results of a dietary survey. Semin Arthritis Rheum 27:180, 1997.
Tamblyn R, et al. Unnecessary prescribing of NSAIDs and the management of NSAID-related gastropathy in medical practice. Am Coll Physicians 127:429, 1997.
Touger-Decker R. Nutritional considerations in rheumatoid arthritis. J Am Diet Assoc 88:327, 1988.
Tugwell P, et al. Combination therapy with cyclosporine and methotrexate in severe rheumatoid arthritis. N Engl J Med 333:137, 1995.
Van den Ende CH, et al. Dynamic exercise therapy in rheumatoid arthritis: A systematic review. Br J Rheumatol 37:677, 1998.
van Weel C. Morbidity in family medicine: The potential for individual nutritional counseling, an analysis from the Nijmegen continuous morbidity registration. Am J Clin Nutr 65:1928S, 1997.
Yamakita J, et al. Effect of tofu (bean curd) ingestion on uric acid metabolism in healthy and gouty subjects. Adv Exp Med Biol 431:839, 1998.

ADDITIONAL REFERENCES

Annelies E, et al. Methotrexate in rheumatoid arthritis: An update with focus on mechanisms involved in toxicity. Semin Arthritis Rheum 27:277, 1998.
Bautch JC, et al. Effects of exercise on knee joints with osteoarthritis: A pilot study of biologic markers. Arthritis Care Res 10:48, 1997.
Buckwalter JA. Maintaining and restoring mobility in middle and old age: The importance of the soft tissue. Instr Course Lect 46:459, 1997.
Chinn KS, et al. Modulation of adjuvant-induced arthritis by dietary arachidonic acid in essential fatty acid-deficient rats. Lipids 32:979, 1997.
Cleland LG, James MJ. Rheumatoid arthritis and the balance of dietary N-6 and N-3 essential fatty acids. Br J Rheumatol 36:514, 1997.
Hawkins CL, Davies MJ. Oxidative damage to collagen and related substrates by metal ion/hydrogen peroxide systems: Random attack or site-specific damage? Biochem Biophys Acta 1360:84, 1997.
Karsh J, Hetenyi G. An historical review of rheumatoid arthritis treatment: 1948 to 1952. Semin Arthritis Rheum 27:57, 1997.

Kyles AK, Ruslander D. Chronic pain: Osteoarthritis and cancer. Semin Vet Med Surg 12:122, 1997.

Martin RH. The role of nutrition and diet in rheumatoid arthritis. Proc Nutr Soc 57:231, 1998.

McAlindon TE, et al. Do antioxidant micronutrients protect against the development and progression of knee osteoarthritis? Arthritis Rheum 39:648, 1996.

Morgan S, et al. Folic acid supplementation prevents deficient blood folate levels and hyperhomocysteinemia during long-term, low dose methotrexate therapy for rheumatoid arthritis: Implications for cardiovascular disease prevention. J Rheumatol 25:441, 1998.

O'Relly S, et al. Effects of exercise on knee joints with osteoarthritis: A pilot study of biologic markers. Arthritis Care Res 10:48, 1997.

Pettersson T, et al. Serum homocysteine and methylmalonic acid in patients with rheumatoid arthritis and cobalaminopenia. J Rheumatol 25:859, 1998.

Ross C. A comparison of osteoarthritis and rheumatoid arthritis: Diagnosis and treatment. Nurse Pract 22:20, 1997.

Vijayalakshmi T, et al. Salubrious effect of semecarpus anacardium against lipid peroxidative changes in adjuvant arthritis studied in rats. Mol Cell Biochem 175:65, 1997.

White-O'Connor B, et al. Dietary habits, weight history, and vitamin supplement use in elderly osteoarthritis patients. J Am Diet Assoc 89:378, 1998.

Woolf K, Manore M. Nutrition, exercise, and rheumatoid arthritis. Top Clin Nutr 14(3):30, 1999.

CHAPTER 44

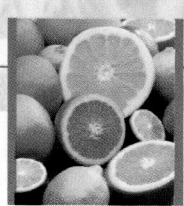

Medical Nutrition Therapy for Metabolic Disorders

CRISTINE M. TRAHMS, MS, RD

Chapter Outline

- Goals of Medical Nutrition Therapy
- Amino Acid Disorders
- Disorders of Carbohydrate Metabolism
- Disorders of Fatty Acid Oxidation
- Glycogen Storage Diseases
- Other Disorders
- Nutritional Care Management

Key Terms

ARGININOSUCCINIC ACIDURIA (ASA)—the presence of argininosuccinic acid in the blood and urine as a result of argininosuccinate lyase deficiency

AUTOSOMAL RECESSIVE—incapable of expression unless the responsible allele is carried by both members of a pair of homologous chromosomes that are not sex chromosomes

CARBAMYL-PHOSPHATE SYNTHETASE (CPS) DEFICIENCY—a defect in urea cycle metabolism that causes hyperammonemia and elevated plasma glycine

CARNITINE—a substance that functions as a carrier of fatty acids across the mitochondrial membranes

CITRULLINEMIA—elevated citrulline in the blood and urine secondary to a deficiency of argininosuccinic acid synthetase in the metabolism of citrulline to argininosuccinic acid

GALACTOSEMIA—a disturbance in the conversion of galactose to glucose because of the absence of the enzyme galactokinase or galactose-1-phosphate uridyl transferase

GLUCONEOGENESIS—the formation of glucose from noncarbohydrate molecules, such as glycerol, and the carbon skeletons of amino acids

GLYCOGEN STORAGE DISEASES—a group of inherited disorders of glycogen metabolism, such as glycogenosis, in which an enzyme deficiency causes glycogen to accumulate in abnormally large amounts in various parts of the body, especially the liver

GLYCOGENOLYSIS—the breakdown of glycogen to glucose

KETONE UTILIZATION DISORDER—possibly mitochondrial 2-methylacetoacetyl-CoA thiolase deficiency; a disorder of isoleucine and ketone body metabolism

LONG-CHAIN ACYL-CoA DEHYDROGENASE (LCAD) DEFICIENCY—a disorder of long-chain fatty acid oxidation

MAPLE SYRUP URINE DISEASE (MSUD) OR BRANCHED-CHAIN KETOACIDURIA—an autosomal recessive metabolic defect in decarboxylation that affects the metabolism of branched-chain amino acids

MEDIUM-CHAIN ACYL-CoA DEHYDROGENASE (MCAD) DEFICIENCY—a disorder of medium-chain fatty acid oxidation

METHYLMALONIC ACIDEMIA—an excess of methylmalonic acid in the blood and urine owing to a defect of methylmalonyl-CoA mutase or other similar enzyme

ORNITHINE TRANSCARBAMYLASE (OTC) DEFICIENCY—a sex-linked recessive disorder in the conversion of ornithine and carbamyl-phosphate to citrulline; usually lethal in males

PHENYLKETONURIA (PKU)—hyperphenylalaninemia in which phenylalanine is not metabolized to tyrosine because of a deficiency of phenylalanine hydroxylase

PROPIONIC ACIDEMIA—an excess of propionic acid in the blood secondary to defective propionyl-CoA reductase

Metabolic disorders are inherited traits that result in the absence or reduced activity of a specific enzyme or cofactor. Most metabolic disorders are inherited as **autosomal recessive** traits.

It is important to remember that not all biochemical disorders are diseases; some, such as histidinemia, may be normal variations in enzyme activity that are benign and do not require treatment (Snyderman et al., 1979). For many of the metabolic disorders, significant questions related to diagnosis and treatment still need to be answered.

Most inherited metabolic disorders are associated

with severe clinical illness, often appearing soon after birth. Mental retardation and severe neurologic involvement may be quickly apparent. Specific diagnosis may be difficult, and appropriate treatment measures may be uncertain. Prenatal diagnosis is available for many metabolic disorders, but it usually requires the identification of a family at risk, which can be done only after the birth of an affected child. However, the efficacy of newborn screening programs, as well as advanced diagnostic techniques and treatment modalities, has improved the outcome for many of these infants (see "*Focus On:* Time Line . . ."). Infants suspected of having a metabolic disorder should be afforded access to care offered by centers with expertise in treating these disorders. Infants who are afebrile but, for no apparent reason, are lethargic, vomiting, in respiratory distress, or having seizures should be evaluated for an undiagnosed metabolic disorder. The initial assessment should include blood gas measurements, electrolyte values, glucose and ammonia testing, and a urine test for ketones.

GOALS OF MEDICAL NUTRITION THERAPY

The goals of nutritional therapy are to maintain biochemical equilibrium for the affected pathway, provide adequate nutrients to support normal growth and development, and support social and emotional development.

Nutritional treatment is designed to circumvent the missing or inactive enzyme by (1) restricting the amount of substrate available, (2) supplementing the amount of product, (3) supplementing the enzymatic cofactor, or (4) combining any or all of these approaches.

AMINO ACID DISORDERS

Nutritional therapy for amino acid disorders most frequently consists of substrate restriction, which involves limiting one or more essential amino acids to the minimum requirement while providing adequate energy and nutrients to promote normal growth and development. However, care must be exercised because inadequate intake of an essential amino acid is often as detrimental as an excess. Dietary supplementation of the product of the reaction is usually required in nutritional therapy for amino acid disorders.

Requirements for individual amino acids are difficult to determine because normal growth and development can be achieved over a wide range of intake. The data of Holt and Snyderman (1967) are often used as the basis for prescribing amino acid therapy (Table 44–1). Careful and frequent monitoring is required to ensure the adequacy of the nutritional prescription (Acosta and Yannicelli, 1993). Although nitrogen studies would be the most precise, weight gain in infants is a sensitive and easily monitored index of well-being and nutritional adequacy.

Hyperphenylalaninemias

Of the amino acid disorders listed in Table 44–2, the hyperphenylalaninemias are the most frequent. These disorders provide a reasonable model for detailed discussion because (1) they occur relatively

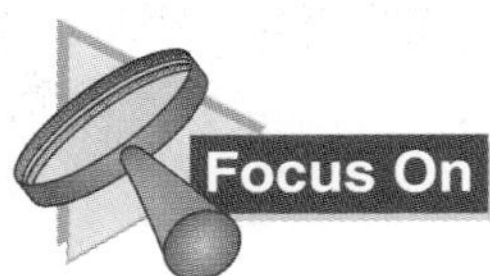

Time Line of Historical Events in the Diagnosis and Treatment of Phenylketonuria (PKU)

1934 A. Folling identifies phenylpyruvic acid in the urine of mentally retarded siblings in institutions. One percent of the institutionalized population was found to excrete phenylpyruvic acid.

1953 G. Jervis demonstrates a deficiency of phenylalanine oxidation in the liver tissue of an affected patient.

H. Bickel demonstrates that dietary phenylalanine restrictions lower the blood concentration of phenylalanine.

1961 R. Guthrie develops a bacterial inhibition assay for measuring blood phenylalanine levels.

Mid-1960s Semi-synthetic formulas restricted in phenylalanine content become commercially available.

1965–1970 States adopt newborn screening programs to detect phenylketonuria.

1967–1980 Collaborative Study of Children Treated for Phenylketonuria is conducted. Data from this study form the basis for treatment protocols for PKU clinics in the United States.

Late-1970s Detrimental effects of maternal phenylketonuria are recognized as a significant public health problem.

1983 The Maternal PKU Collaborative Study begins to study the effects of treatment on the pregnancy outcome of women with phenylketonuria.

1980s Lifelong restriction of phenylalanine intake becomes the standard of care for PKU clinics in the United States.

1987 Techniques for carrier detection and prenatal diagnosis of phenylketonuria are developed.

Late-1980s The gene for phenylalanine hydroxylase deficiency (MIM Number 261600) is located on chromosome 12q22-q24.1. DNA mutation analysis can be accomplished with peripheral leukocytes.

1990s Phenylalanine level of 2–6 mg/dL (60–360 μmol/L), lower than the previous level of less than 10 mg/dL, becomes the new standard of care for treatment of phenylketonuria.

TABLE 44–1 APPROXIMATE DAILY REQUIREMENTS FOR SELECTED NUTRIENTS AND AMINO ACIDS IN INFANCY AND CHILDHOOD*,†

AMINO ACID	UNIT	AGE			
		0 to 2 months	2 to 5 months	6 to 12 months	1 to 10 years
Phenylalanine					
Infants	mg/kg	47–900	47–900	25–470	—
Children	mg/day	—	—	—	200–500‡
Histidine	mg/kg	16–340	16–340	16–340	—
Tyrosine§	mg/kg	60–800	60–800	40–600	25–85
Leucine					
Infants	mg/kg	76–150	76–150	76–150	—
Children	mg/day	—	—	—	1000
Isoleucine					
Infants	mg/kg	79–110	79–110	50–750	—
Children	mg/day	—	—	—	1000
Valine					
Infants	mg/kg	65–105	65–105	50–800	—
Children	mg/day	—	—	—	400–600
Methionine‖					
Infants	mg/kg	20–450	20–450	20–450	—
Children	mg/day	—	—	—	400–800
Cyst(e)ine¶					
Infants	mg/kg	15–500	15–500	15–500	—
Children	mg/day	—	—	—	400–800
Lysine					
Infants	mg/kg	90–120	90–120	90–120	—
Children	mg/day	—	—	—	1200–1600
Threonine					
Infants	mg/kg	45–870	45–870	45–870	—
Children	mg/day	—	—	—	800–1000
Tryptophan					
Infants	mg/kg	13–220	13–220	13–220	—
Children	mg/day	—	—	—	60–120
Energy	kcal/kg	108	108	98	70–102
Water					
Infants	mL/kg	100	110	100	—
Children	mL/day	—	—	—	1100
Carbohydrate	g/day	→	kcal × 0.50	→	
Protein					
Infants	g/kg	2.2	2.2	1.6	—
Children	g/day	—	—	—	16–28
Fat	g/day	→	kcal × 0.35	→	

*Adapted from Committee on Nutrition, American Academy of Pediatrics. Special diets for infants with inborn errors of metabolism. Pediatrics 57:783, 1976; and Food and Nutrition Board, National Research Council, National Academy of Sciences. Recommended Dietary Allowances, 10th ed. Washington, DC: National Academy Press, 1989.

†Compiled from amino acid data of Holt and Snyderman. Information on amino acid requirements of infants and children at different ages is limited; the figures given here are in excess of minimum requirements. Consequently, this table should be used only as a guide and should not be regarded as an authoritative statement to which individual patients must conform.

‡More phenylalanine (>800 mg) is required in the absence of tyrosine.

§Total phenylalanine plus tyrosine should be considered in the prescription, as most phenylalanine is converted to tyrosine.

‖More methionine is required in the absence of cyst(e)ine.

¶More cyst(e)ine is required in the presence of a blocked trans-sulfuration outflow pathway for methionine metabolism.

frequently, and most neonates are screened for them; (2) they have a predictable course, with the greatest available documentation of "natural" and "intervention" history; (3) nutritional therapy is known to be successful; (4) the effects of various therapies, positive or negative, have been observed over time; and (5) the effect on the next generation can be observed.

Phenylketonuria (PKU) is the most common of the hyperphenylalaninemias. In this disorder, phenylalanine (Phe) is not metabolized to tyrosine (TYR) because of a deficiency or inactivity of *phenylalanine hydroxylase*, as shown in Figure 44–1. Nutritional treatment involves restricting the substrate (Phe) and supplementing the product (TYR) (Fig. 44–2). Approximately 97% of affected individuals exhibit phenylalanine hydroxylase deficiency; the remainder have a defect in associated pathways, either in the activity of *dihydropteridine reductase* (DHPR deficiency) or in the synthesis of biopterin (BH_4). Low-phenylalanine dietary therapy does not prevent the neurologic deterioration associated with these rare disorders (Early diagnosis . . . , 1980; New Varieties of PKU, 1979). How-

TABLE 44–2 METABOLIC DISORDERS THAT RESPOND TO DIETARY TREATMENT

DISORDER	ENZYME DEFECT	INCIDENCE	CLINICAL/BIOCHEMICAL FEATURES	DIETARY TREATMENT
Hyperphenylalaninemias				
Phenylketonuria	Phenylalanine hydroxylase	<1:10,000	Blood Phe > 20 mg/dL ↑ Phenylketones in urine Progressive severe MR, which can be prevented by early treatment	↓ Phe, ↑ tyrosine diet to maintain serum Phe at 2–6 mg/dL
Mild phenylketonuria	Phenylalanine hydroxylase	<1:13,000	Blood Phe > 6 mg/dL ↑ Phenylketones in urine	↓ Phe, ↑ tyrosine diet to maintain serum Phe at 2–6 mg/dL
Offspring of maternal phenylketonuria	None		Fetal brain damage	None
Dihydropteridine reductase deficiency	Dihydropteridine reductase	Rare	Blood Phe < 20 mg/dL Irritability, developmental delay, seizures	None; 5-hydroxytryptophan, 1-3,4-dihydroxyphenylalanine carbidopa may be useful in management
Tyrosinemias				
Tyrosinemia, type I	Fumaryl-acetoacetate hydroxylase	<1:120,000	Vomiting, acidosis, diarrhea, FTT, hepatomegaly, rickets; ↑ blood/ urine tyrosine, methionine; ↑ urine para-hydroxy derivatives of tyrosine; often fatal	NTBC; ↓ tyrosine, ↓ Phe diet; vitamin D for rickets
Tyrosinemia, type II	Tyrosine aminotransferase	Rare	Keratosis; MR; corneal dystrophy ↑ Blood/urine tyrosine levels; ↑ levels of urine parahydroxy derivatives of tyrosine	↓ Tyrosine, ↓ Phe diet
Transient neonatal tyrosinemia	?Parahydroxyphenyl-pyruvic acid oxidase (appears gradually during postnatal period)	Unknown	Initial lethargy; ?long-term effects ↑ Blood/urine tyrosine levels	Vitamin C, 100 mg/day may be beneficial; ↓ protein intake until tyrosine is cleared
Maple Syrup Urine Diseases (MSUD)				
MSUD	Keto acid decar-boxylase (<2% activity)	1:250,000	Early onset; seizures; acidosis; severe MR; often, death Plasma leucine, isoleucine, and valine levels 10 × normal	↓ Leucine, isoleucine, valine diet
Intermittent MSUD	Keto acid decar-boxylase (<20% activity between episodes)	Rare	Intermittent symptoms can cause death and some MR Plasma leucine, isoleucine, and valine levels 10 × normal during episodes	As for MSUD
Other Amino Acid Disorders				
Homocystinuria	Cystathionine synthase or similar enzyme	1:300,000	Arterial and venous thromboses; bony abnormalities; dislocated lens; fair hair and skin; mild to moderate MR, ↑ methionine; ↑ homocysteine	Trial of 500 mg of vitamin B_6/day for 1 month (if folate levels are normal) Low-protein, low-methionine diet with added L-cystine, betaine
Hyperlysinuria	Lysine ketoglutarate reductase, saccharopine oxidoreductase, saccharopine dehydrogenase	Rare	Probably benign ↑ Blood/urine lysine levels	None required
Histidinemia	Histidinase	1:18,000	Benign ↑ Blood/urine histidine levels	None required
Urea Cycle Disorders				
Carbamyl-phosphate synthetase deficiency	Carbamyl-phosphate synthetase	Rare	Vomiting; seizures; sometimes, coma → death Survivors usually have MR ↑ Plasma ammonia and glutamine levels	*Long-term treatment:* low-protein diet as tolerated and phenyl-butyrate *Acute treatment:* hemodialysis or peritoneal dialysis with energy and fluids

TABLE 44–2 METABOLIC DISORDERS THAT RESPOND TO DIETARY TREATMENT (continued)

DISORDER	ENZYME DEFECT	INCIDENCE	CLINICAL/BIOCHEMICAL FEATURES	DIETARY TREATMENT
Ornithine transcarbamylase deficiency	Ornithine transcarbamylase (X-linked)	Rare	Vomiting; seizures; coma → death as a newborn ↑ Plasma ammonia, glutamine, glutamic acid, and alanine levels	Low-protein diet and phenylbutyrate
Citrullinemia	Argininosuccinic acid synthetase	Rare	*Neonatal:* vomiting; seizures; coma → death *Infantile:* vomiting; seizures; progressive developmental delay ↑ Plasma citrulline, ammonia, and alanine levels	Low-protein diet; arginine supplements; phenylbutyrate
Argininosuccinic aciduria	Argininosuccinic acid lyase	Rare	*Neonatal:* hypotonia, seizures *Subacute:* vomiting, FTT, progressive developmental delay ↑ Plasma argininosuccinic acid, citrulline, and ammonia levels	Low-protein diet; arginine supplements; dialysis for crisis; phenylbutyrate
Argininemia	Arginase	Rare	Periodic vomiting; seizures; coma Progressive spastic diplegia and developmental delay ↑ Arginine and ↑ ammonia levels with protein intake	Low-protein diet
Organic Acidemias				
Methylmalonic acidemia	Methylmalonyl-CoA mutase or similar	Rare	Metabolic acidosis; vomiting; seizures; coma; often death Progressive developmental delay in survivors ↑ Organic acid and ammonia levels	*Long-term:* ↑ kcal, ↓ protein diet; ↓ isoleucine, methionine, threonine, valine, B_{12} supplements *Acute:* IV fluids, bicarbonate
Propionic acidemia	Propionyl-CoA carboxylase or similar	Rare	Metabolic acidosis; ↑ ammonia level; ↑ propionic acid in blood, ↑ methylcitric acid in urine	*Long-term:* ↑ kcal, ↓ protein diet *Acute:* IV fluids, bicarbonate
Isovaleric acidemia	Isovaleryl-CoA dehydrogenase	Rare	Poor feeding, lethargy, seizures, metabolic ketoacidosis, hyperammonemia	↓ Protein, leucine, glycine; supplement with L-carnitine
Ketone utilization disorder	2-methylacetoacetyl-CoA-thiolase or similar	Unknown	Vomiting, dehydration, metabolic ketoacidosis	↓ Protein intake; avoid fasting, provide complex carbohydrates, L-carinitine, and Bicitra (to buffer acid-base balance)
Carbohydrate Disorders				
Galactosemia	Galactose-1-phosphate uridyl transferase	<1:65,000	Vomiting, hepatomegaly, hypoglycemia, FTT, cataracts, MR, and often, early sepsis ↑ Urine/blood galactose levels	Low galactose- and lactose-free diet
Galactokinase deficiency	Galactokinase	1:40,000	Cataracts ↑ Blood/urine galactose levels after lactose feeding	Same as for galactosemia
Hereditary fructose intolerance	Fructose-1-phosphate aldolase	Rare	Vomiting, hepatomegaly, hypoglycemia, FTT, renal tubular defects after fructose introduction ↑ Blood/urine fructose levels after fructose feeding	Fructose-, sucrose-, and sorbitol-free diet
Fructose 1,6-diphosphatase deficiency	Fructose-1,6-diphosphatase	Rare	Hypoglycemia, hepatomegaly, hypotonia, metabolic acidosis upon fructose introduction No ↑ fructose level in blood or urine	Same as for hereditary fructose intolerance
Glycogen storage disease, type Ia	Glucose-6-phosphatase	1:60,000	Profound hypoglycemia, hepatomegaly	Exogenous glucose from uncooked cornstarch Avoidance of fructose, lactose ↑ Complex carbohydrate intake, ↓ fat intake

TABLE 44–2 METABOLIC DISORDERS THAT RESPOND TO DIETARY TREATMENT (continued)

DISORDER	ENZYME DEFECT	INCIDENCE	CLINICAL/BIOCHEMICAL FEATURES	DIETARY TREATMENT
Other Disorders				
Gyrate atrophy of the choroid and retina	Ornithine-keto-acid transferase	Rare	Progressive gyrate atrophy of choroid and retina with cataracts Possible FTT, hepatic cirrhosis, seizures, and MR ↑ Blood/urine ornithine levels ↓ Blood lysine levels	?Low-protein (low ornithine) diet with lysine supplements
Cystinuria	Defective proximal renal tubular transport of cystine and dibasic amino acids	1:13,000	Urinary tract calculi ↑ Cystine, ornithine, lysine, and arginine levels in urine	↑ Fluid intake Bicarbonate to alkalinize urine

Phe, phenylalanine; *MR,* mental retardation; *FTT,* failure to thrive; *NTBC,* 2-(2-nitro-4-trifluoro-methyl-benzoyl)-1,3-cyclohexanedione; *IV,* intravenous.

ever, certain therapies, including administration of tetrahydrofolate for DHPR deficiency and large amounts of BH_4 or neurotransmitter precursors in BH_4 deficiency, have been shown to be beneficial (Kaufman, 1986) (see Table 44–2).

Diagnosis and Outcome

Currently, most states have newborn screening programs for PKU and other metabolic disorders. The Guthrie bacterial inhibition assay (Guthrie and Susi, 1962), performed on blood, is the most frequently used screening test. The American Academy of Pediatrics has recommended that neonates with a positive screening result be tested again by both qualitative and quantitative methods (American Academy of Pediatrics, 1996).

Diagnostic criteria include blood concentrations of phenylalanine that consistently exceed 6 to 10 mg/dL (360 to 600 μmol/L), tyrosine levels of less than 3 mg/dL (165 μmol/L), and the presence of phenylpyruvic acid and o-hydroxyphenylacetic acid in the urine while consuming a normal diet (American Academy of Pediatrics, 1996). Confirmation of the diagnosis requires quantitative elevations of phenylalanine compounds in both blood and urine. A phenylalanine intake challenge is not performed.

Outcome, measured in terms of intelligence quotient (IQ) attainment or intellectual function, depends on the age at diagnosis, the age at the start of nutritional therapy, and biochemical control over time. The ages at diagnosis and at the start of nutritional therapy depend on the effectiveness of the screening program and an organized follow-up program, as infants with PKU do not manifest any clinical signs of abnormality in the immediate postnatal period. The advantage of rigorous nutritional

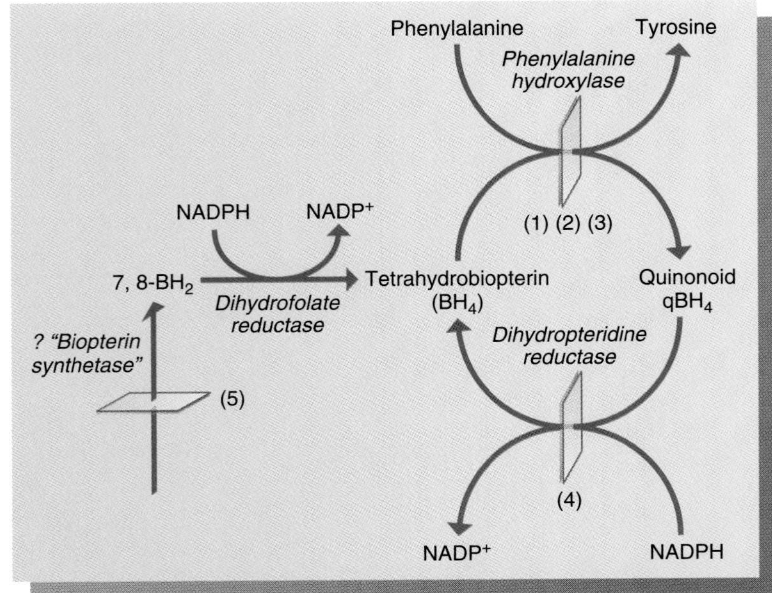

FIGURE 44–1 Hyperphenylalaninemias. (*1*) "Classic" phenylketonuria. (*2*) "Atypical" phenylketonuria. (*3*) Benign hyperphenylalaninemia. (*4*) Dihydropteridine reductase deficiency. (*5*) "Biopterin synthetase" deficiency. *NADPH,* nicotinamide-adenine dinucleotide phosphate; *NADP+,* nicotinamide-adenine dinucleotide phosphate (oxidized form).

therapy has been demonstrated by measurements of intellectual function. Individuals who do not receive diet therapy are severely mentally retarded (mean IQ of about 40), whereas individuals who are treated from birth have IQs in the normal range of intellectual function (Williamson et al., 1981; Legido et al., 1993).

Nutritional Care for Infants and Children

FORMULA

Restricted-phenylalanine dietary therapy is planned around the use of a formula or medical food with phenylalanine removed from the protein. The formulas or medical foods described in Table 44–3 provide a major portion of the daily protein and energy needs for affected infants, children, and adults. In general, the protein source in the formula or medical food is L-amino acids, with the critical amino acids being reduced or omitted. Carbohydrate sources are corn syrup solids, modified tapioca starch, sucrose, and hydrolyzed corn starch. Fat is provided by a variety of oils; however, some formulas contain no fat. The necessity for providing additional protein, carbohydrate, or fat is specific to the formula chosen for use. Most formulas or medical foods contain calcium, iron, and all other necessary vitamins and minerals, and are a reliable source of these nutrients.

Phenylalanine-free formula is supplemented with evaporated milk, regular infant formula, or breast milk during infancy and early childhood to provide high biologic value (HBV) protein, nonessential amino acids, and sufficient phenylalanine to meet the individualized requirements of the growing child. The phenylalanine-free formula and milk mixture should provide 90% of the protein and 80% of the energy needed by infants and toddlers. A method for calculating the appropriate quantities of a phenylalanine-free formula is shown in Table 44–4. It must be stressed that formula calculations should provide adequate but not excessive energy intake for infants, as well as appropriate fluid to maintain hydration. To support metabolic control effectively, formulas or medical foods must be consumed in three or four nearly equal portions throughout the day. Table 44–5 compares energy and protein intakes of affected and unaffected infants.

LOW-PHENYLALANINE FOODS

Foods of moderate- or low-phenylalanine content are used as a supplement to the formula mixture. These foods are offered at the appropriate ages to support developmental readiness and to meet energy needs. Puréed foods from a spoon might be introduced at 5 to 6 months of age, finger foods at 7 to 8 months, and the cup at 8 to 9 months, using the same timing and progression of texture recommended in Tables 8–7, 8–8, and 10–2 for children on free-choice food patterns. Table 44–6 lists phenylalanine and tyrosine values for selected food groups.

Low-protein pastas, breads, and baked goods made from wheat starch add variety to the food pattern and allow children to eat some foods "to appetite." Table 44–7 compares low-protein and regular food items. The relative protein and energy values indicate the advantage of the low-protein products in meeting energy needs. Sources for low-

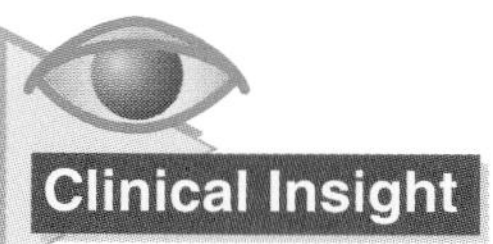

SOURCES OF LOW-PROTEIN FOODS

Low-protein products add energy, texture, and variety to restricted–amino acid and low-protein food patterns. A variety of low-protein pastas, rice, breads, rusks, crackers, cookies, egg replacers, and gelled dessert mixes is available. Wheat starch and a variety of low-protein baking mixes for breads, cakes, and cookies are also available.

SOURCES

Dietary Specialties
865 Centennial Ave.
Piscataway, NJ 08854
(1-888-MENU123)

Ener-G Foods, Inc.
5960 1st Ave., S.
P.O. Box 84487
Seattle, WA 98124-5787
(1-800-331-5222)

Med-Diet, Inc.
3600 Holly Lane, N., Suite 80
Plymouth, MN 55447
(1-800-633-3438)

SHS North America
P.O. Box 117
Gaithersburg, MD 20884
(1-800-365-7354)

TABLE 44–3 FORMULAS/MEDICAL FOODS FOR THE MANAGEMENT OF SELECTED INBORN ERRORS OF METABOLISM

DISORDER	PRODUCT	COMPOSITION*	MANUFACTURERS†	FORMULATED FOR		
				Infant	Child	Adult
Phenylketonuria	Lofenalac	g	MJ	X		
	Phenyl-free	a	MJ		X	X
	PKU 1	b	MJ	X		
	PKU 2	b	MJ		X	
	PKU 3	b	MJ			X
	XP	d	SHS	X		
	Analog XP	c	SHS		X	
	Maxamaid XP	c	SHS		X	X
	Periflex	e	SHS		X	
	Phenex 1	f	RL	X		
	Phenex 2	f	RL		X	X
Tyrosinemia	Low PHE/TYR diet powder	g	MJ	X	X	
	TYR 1	b	MJ	X		
	TYR 2	b	MJ		X	
	XPHEN, TYR Analog	d	SHS	X		
	XPHEN, TYR Maxamaid	c	SHS		X	
	Tyromex 1	f	RL	X		
	Tyrex 2	f	RL		X	X
MSUD	MSUD Diet Powder	a	MJ	X	X	
	MSUD 1	b	MJ	X		
	MSUD 2	b	MJ		X	
	MSUD Analog	d	SHS	X		
	MSUD Maxamaid	c	SHS		X	
	MSUD Maxamum	c	SHS		X	X
	Ketonex 1	f	RL	X		
	Ketonex 2	f	RL		X	X
Organic acid disorders	OS 1	b	MJ	X		
	OS 2	b	MJ		X	
	XMTVI Analog	d	SHS	X		
	XMTVI Maxamaid	c	SHS		X	
	Propimex 1	f	RL	X		
	Propimex 2	f	RL		X	X
Urea cycle disorders	UCD 1	b	MJ	X		
	UCD 2	b	MJ		X	
	Cyclinex 1	f	RL	X		
	Cyclinex 2	f	RL		X	X
Carbohydrate-free protein-free	RCF	j	RL	X		
	Protein-Free Diet Powder	h	MJ	X	X	
	Pro-Phree	i	RL	X	X	

*Formula contents as follows:

a—Free of critical amino acid(s); balanced mixture of other essential and nonessential L-amino acids; carbohydrate from sucrose/corn syrup solids/modified tapioca starch; fat from corn oil/coconut oil; minerals; trace elements added.

b—Free of critical amino acid(s); balanced mixture of other essential and nonessential L-amino acids; carbohydrate from sucrose; no fat; minerals; trace elements added.

c—Free of critical amino acid(s); balanced mixture of other essential and nonessential L-amino acids; carbohydrate from sucrose; trace of fat; minerals; trace elements added.

d—Free of critical amino acid(s); balanced mixture of other essential and nonessential L-amino acids; carbohydrate from corn syrup solids; fat from peanut oil/refined animal/coconut oil; minerals; trace elements added.

e—Free of critical amino acid(s); balanced mixture of other essential and nonessential L-amino acids; carbohydrate from corn syrup solids; fat from canola/safflower oil; minerals; trace elements added.

f—Free of critical amino acid(s); balanced mixture of other essential and nonessential L-amino acids; carbohydrate from hydrolyzed corn starch; fat from hydrogenated coconut/palm/soy oil; vitamins; minerals; trace elements added.

g—Protein supplied as enzymatic hydrolysate of casein processed to remove critical amino acid(s); carbohydrate from corn syrup solids, modified tapioca starch; fat from corn oil; vitamins; minerals; trace elements added.

h—Protein-free; carbohydrate supplied as corn syrup solids/modified tapioca starch; fat from corn oil; vitamins; minerals; trace elements added.

i—Protein-free; carbohydrate from hydrolyzed corn starch; fat from palm/hydrogenated coconut/soy oil; vitamins; minerals; trace elements added.

j—Protein from soy protein isolate; no carbohydrate; fat from soy/coconut oil; vitamins; minerals; trace elements added.

†Manufacturers: *MJ,* Mead Johnson & Company, Evansville, IN 47721; *SHS,* Scientific Hospital Supplies, Gaithersburg, MD 20884; *RL,* Ross Laboratories, Columbus, OH 43216.

TABLE 44–4 GUIDELINES FOR LOW-PROTEIN FOOD PATTERN CALCULATIONS

Case Study

M.S. is a 6-month-old infant with phenylketonuria. The information provided in Tables 44–1 and 44–6 can be used to plan a food and formula pattern for this child.

Baseline Data

Age	6 months
Sex	Male
Weight (kg)	7.7
Weight percentile	50th
Height (cm)	67.8
Height percentile	50th
Head circumference (cm)	43.3
General health	Good
Activity	Very active

Step 1. Calculate the child's requirement for phenylalanine, protein, and energy (kcal) using the information in Table 44–1.

A. Phenylalanine

7.7 kg body weight × 60* mg phenylalanine/kg/day = 462 mg phenylalanine/day

B. Protein

7.7 kg body weight × 3.3† g protein/kg/day = 25.4 g protein/day

C. Energy

7.7 kg body weight × 115† kcal/kg/day = 885 kcal/day

Step 2. Determine the amount of phenylalanine-free formula required per day. This information is determined from the infant's or child's protein requirement.

For example: 25.4 g protein/day × 90% of protein from phenylalanine-free formula powder (Phenex I) = 23 g protein = 145 g of formula powder per day.

Step 3. Determine the amount of evaporated milk or standard infant formula to be included in the food pattern.

Step 4. Determine the amount of water to mix with the phenylalanine-free formula. The consistency of the formula will vary according to the infant's age and fluid requirements.

For example: To prepare formula for the infant described in the case study, mix 145 g of Phenex I and 120 gm Enfamil powder with 4 oz of water to prevent lumps from forming. Then add water to make a total of 32 oz of formula. This provides 4 bottles of 8 oz each.

Step 5. Determine the amounts of phenylalanine, protein, and energy in the phenylalanine-free formula and evaporated milk, as shown in the examples below.

Formula	Phenylalanine (mg)	Protein (g)	Energy (kcal)
Phenex I powder (145 g)	0	21.6	695
Enfamil powder (120 g)	410	4.8	120
Total	410	26.4	815

Step 6. Determine the amount of phenylalanine, protein, and energy to be obtained from foods other than the formula mixture.

Total phenylalanine = 462 mg/day

Phenylalanine in formula = 410 mg/day

Phenylalanine from other foods = 52 mg/day

Total protein	25.4 g/day
Protein in formula	26.0 g/day
Protein from other foods	1.0–2.0 g/day
Total energy	885 kcal/day
Energy in formula	815 kcal/day
Energy from other foods	70 kcal/day

Step 7. Determine the amount of foods other than formula to be included in the dietary plan.‡ Use exchange lists in Table 44–6.

	PHENYLALANINE (mg)	PROTEIN (G)	Kcal
Baby rice cereal, 1 T	9	0.2	9
Green beans, strained, 1 T	9	0.2	4
Banana, mashed, 50 g	22	0.6	44
Carrots, strained, 3 T	9	0.3	12
Total	49	1.3	69

Step 8. Determine the actual amounts of phenylalanine, protein, and energy/kg of body weight by dividing the total available nutrients by the body weight (in kg).

Phenylalanine (mg)

460 mg phenylalanine ÷ 7.7 kg body weight = 60 mg phenylalanine/kg/day

Protein

27.7 g protein ÷ 7.7 kg body weight = 3.6 g protein/kg/day

Energy

869 kcal ÷ 7.7 kg body weight = 115 kcal/kg/day

*A phenylalanine intake of 60 mg/kg/day is chosen as a moderate intake level. The prescription for phenylalanine must be adapted to individual needs as judged by growth and blood levels.

†Although these intakes are higher than the RDA, they are the intakes found by the Collaborative Study to promote normal growth with consumption of protein hydrolysate–based formula. (Data from Acosta PB, et al. Nutrient intake of treated infants with phenylketonuria (PKU). Am J Clin Nutr 30:198, 1977.)

‡Total energy intake must be adjusted to meet individual needs, and an excess must be avoided.

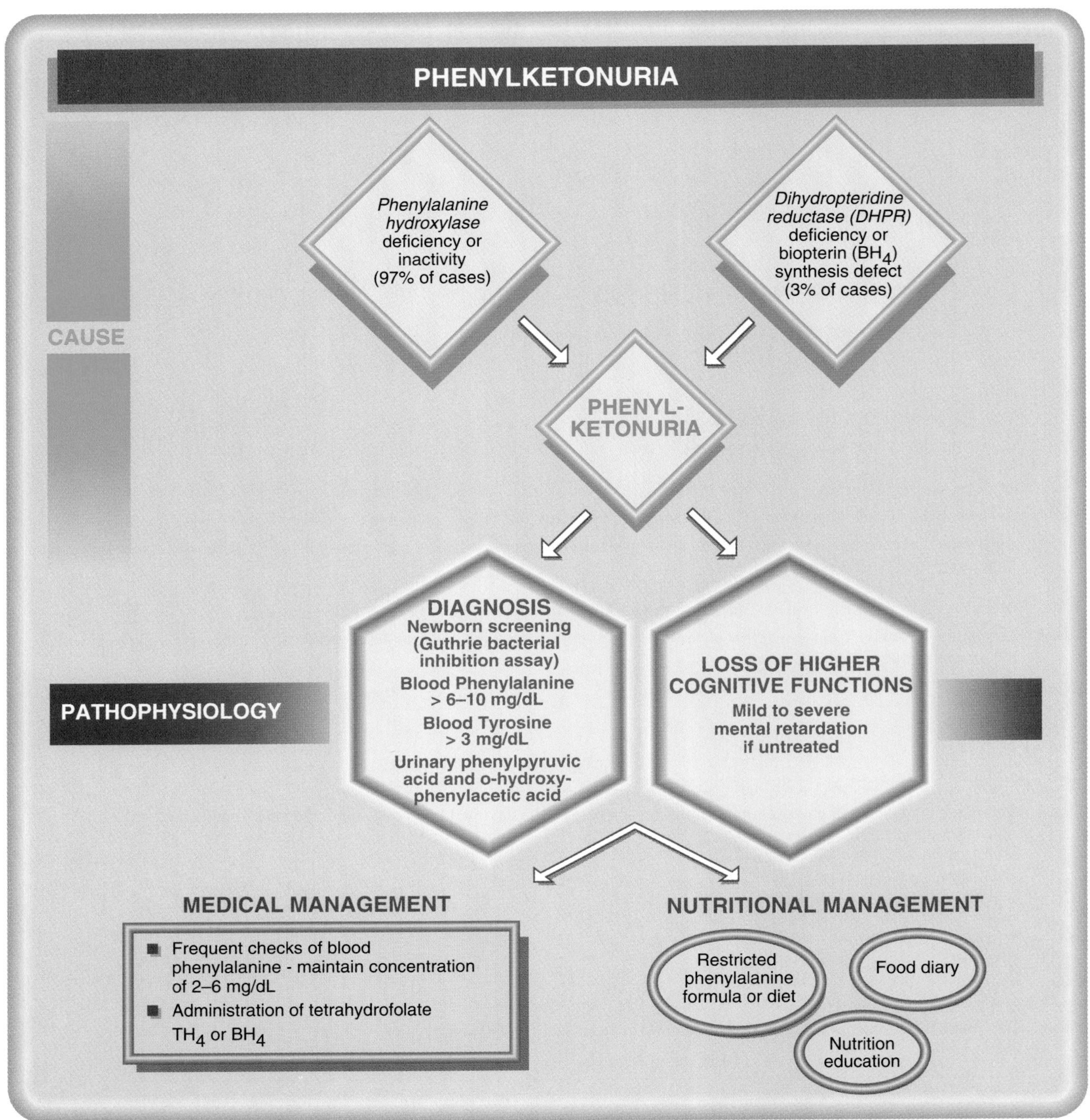

FIGURE 44–2 Pathophysiology algorithm—phenylketonuria. (Algorithm content developed by John Anderson, Ph.D., and Sanford C. Garner, Ph.D., 2000.)

protein products are given in *"Clinical Insight:* Sources of Low-Protein Foods." In many cases, parents create recipes or adapt family favorites to meet the needs of their children. These recipes offer the children a variety of textures and food choices, allowing them to participate in family meals. Families are also able to meet the energy and phenylalanine needs of their children without resorting to excessive intakes of sugars and concentrated sweets. The availability of aspartame (Nutrasweet), an artificial sweetener that contains phenylalanine, has made food choices more difficult, as it may not be labeled in many foods.

A formula that is free of phenylalanine and has a more appropriate amino acid, vitamin, and mineral composition for an older child is generally introduced in the toddler or preschool period. The criterion for introduction of the "next step" formula is that the child accept the food pattern and formula well and reliably consume a wide variety of foods

TABLE 44–5 COMPARISON OF DAILY INTAKES OF INFANTS WITH METABOLIC DISORDERS WHO ARE RECEIVING APPROPRIATE THERAPEUTIC FORMULAS AND ARE WELL MANAGED

	UNAFFECTED	PKU	MSUD	UREA CYCLE DISORDERS	ORGANIC ACID DISORDERS
Volume/day	24 oz	24 oz	24 oz	24 oz	24 oz
Dilution (kcal/oz)	20	20	20	20	20
Energy (kcal/kg)	110	110–120	110–120	110–120	120–140
Protein (g/kg)	2.7	2.0–2.5	1.5–2.0	1.0–2.0	1.0–2.0
Phenylalanine (mg/kg)	120	60	250	120	120
Tyrosine (mg/kg)	110	300	290	110	110
Isoleucine (mg/kg)	120	160	80	120	120
Leucine (mg/kg)	225	260	75	225	225
Valine (mg/kg)	130	180	65	130	130

PKU, phenylketonuria; *MSUD,* maple syrup urine disease.

from the low-phenylalanine food list. Successful management, with consistently low blood phenylalanine levels, is based on "habit," that is, the formula or medical food is offered and consumed without negotiation or threat. Children respond favorably to the regularity of the time of ingestion of the formula or medical food and the familiarity of its taste and presentation. Table 44–8 compares a food pattern using Phenyl-Free with a regular food pattern for a child.

BLOOD PHENYLALANINE CONTROL

The blood phenylalanine concentration must be checked frequently to be sure it remains within the range of 2 to 6 mg/dL, or 120 to 360 μmol/L (Medical Research Council, 1993a and 1993b). Phenylalanine-containing foods are offered as tolerated as long as the blood concentration level of phenylalanine remains in the range of good biochemical control. The child's rate of growth and mental development must be carefully monitored. Effective management requires a cohesive team in which the child, parents, dietitian, pediatrician, psychologist, social worker, and nurse work together to achieve and maintain biochemical control and provide an atmosphere for normal mental and emotional development.

An essential management tool for parents, children, and clinicians is the food diary, an example of which is shown in Figure 44–3. Daily record keeping supports compliance with treatment and builds self-management skills. An accurate record of food and formula intake for at least the 3 days before a laboratory specimen is obtained is mandatory for accurate interpretation of the results and subsequent adjustment of the amino acid prescription.

Elevations in blood phenylalanine concentration are generally caused by excessive phenylalanine intake or tissue catabolism. Intakes of phenylalanine in excess of the amount required for growth accumulate in the blood. Deficient energy intake, or the trauma of illness or infection, can result in protein breakdown and the release of amino acids, including phenylalanine, into the blood. In general, the anorexia of illness limits energy intake. It is essential to prevent tissue catabolism by maintaining the intake of formula as much as possible. Although it may occasionally be necessary to offer only clear liquids during an illness, the phenylalanine-free formula should be reintroduced as soon as it is feasible.

The necessity of continuing the restricted-phenylalanine dietary therapy beyond adolescence is a consideration in the management of children with

TABLE 44-6 SERVING LISTS FOR PHENYLALANINE-RESTRICTED DIETS: APPROXIMATE PHENYLALANINE (PHE), TYROSINE (TYR), PROTEIN, FAT, AND ENERGY CONTENT PER SERVING

	NUTRIENTS				
FOOD*	PHE (mg)	TYR (mg)	Protein (g)	FAT (g)	Energy (kcal)
Breads/cereals	30	20	0.6	0	30
Fats	5	4	0.1	5	60
Fruits	15	10	0.5	0	60
Vegetables	15	10	0.5	0	10
Free foods A[†]	5	4	0.1	0	65
Free foods B[‡]	0	0	0	Varies	55
Milk, whole (100 mL)	160	160	3.4	3.4	62

(From Acosta PB. Ross Metabolic Formula System Nutrition Support Protocols. Columbus, OH: Ross Laboratories, © 1993.)

*Only selected foods are allowed in each category, and these are usually simple foods so that the amino acid content can be estimated accurately.

[†]These foods contain small amounts of phenylalanine; this category includes low-protein pastas, breads, and some sweets.

[‡]These foods contain little or no phenylalanine; they include primarily sweet beverages and candies, and are used sparingly to satisfy appetite.

TABLE 44–7 COMPARISON OF PROTEIN AND ENERGY CONTENT OF FOODS USED IN LOW-PROTEIN DIETS

FOOD ITEM	ENERGY (kcal)	PROTEIN (g)
Pasta, ½ cup, cooked		
Low-protein	107	0.15
Regular	72	2.4
Bread, 1 slice		
Low-protein	135	0.2
Regular	74	2.4
Cereal, ½ cup, cooked		
Low-protein	45	0
Regular	80	1.0
Egg, 1		
Low-protein egg replacer	30	0
Regular	67	5.6

PKU. Progressively decreasing IQs, learning difficulties, poor attention span, and behavioral difficulties have been reported in some children who have discontinued the dietary regimen (Legido et al., 1993; Cabalska et al., 1977; Koch et al., 1982; Smith et al., 1978). As the cohort of children enrolled in the National Collaborative Study matures, those who maintain well-controlled blood phenylalanine levels are also seen to have comparatively higher intellectual achievement (Michals et al., 1988; Azen et al., 1991 and 1996). Good dietary control of blood phenylalanine concentrations by nutritional therapy is the best predictor of IQ, whereas "off-diet" blood phenylalanine concentrations of greater than 20 mg/dL (1200 μmol/L) are the best predictors of IQ loss (Waisbren et al., 1987). Subtle deficits in higher level cognitive function may persist even at blood phenylalanine levels of 6 to 10 mg/dL (Diamond, 1994); thus, some clinics are recommending treatment blood levels of 2 to 6 mg/dL. The current recommendation from most treatment centers is that restricted-phenylalanine therapy should be continued for life to maintain normal cognitive function (Ris et al., 1994).

EDUCATION ABOUT THERAPY MANAGEMENT

The energy needs and amino acid requirements of children with PKU do not differ appreciably from those of children in general. With proper management, normal growth can be expected. However, parents may tend to offer excessive energy as sweets because they feel the child is being deprived of food experiences. Health care providers and parents need to understand that children with PKU are well children who must make careful food choices for themselves, not chronically ill children who require food indulgences.

Appropriate clinical interaction with the family provides them with the information and skills to differentiate between food behaviors that are normal to the age and developmental level of the child and those related specifically to PKU (Trahms, 1986). To avoid power struggles and conflicts over food, it is advisable to involve the child in choosing appropriate foods at an early age. Two- and 3-year-old children can master the concept of appropriate choices when foods are categorized as YES foods and NO foods. The concept of an appropriate quantity of a food can be introduced to a 3- or 4-year-old child in terms of "how many" by counting crackers or raisins, and then in terms of "how much" by weighing or measuring foods, such as cereal or fruit (Heffernan and Trahms, 1981). The child then moves to more complex tasks (e.g., formula and food preparation) and planning of meals (e.g., breakfast or a packed lunch). Responsibility for planning a

TABLE 44–8 COMPARISON OF MENUS APPROPRIATE FOR CHILDREN WITH AND WITHOUT PHENYLKETONURIA

	PKU MENU	PHENYLALANINE (mg)	REGULAR MENU	PHENYLALANINE (mg)
Breakfast	Phenyl-Free	0	Milk	450
	Rice Krispies		Rice Krispies	
	Orange juice		Orange juice	
Lunch	Jelly sandwich with low-protein bread	18	Jelly sandwich with white bread	260
	Banana		Banana	
	Carrot and celery sticks		Carrot and celery sticks	
	Low-protein chocolate chip cookies	4	Chocolate chip cookies	60
	Juice		Juice	
Snack	Phenyl-Free	0	Milk	450
	Orange		Orange	
	Potato chips (small bag)		Potato chips	
Dinner	Phenyl-Free	0	Milk	450
	Salad		Salad	
	Low-protein spaghetti with tomato sauce	8	Spaghetti	240
			Spaghetti with meatballs	600
	Baskin-Robbins fruit ice	10	Ice cream	120
Estimated intake		400		2900

MY PKU FOOD RECORD

Name __________

Date __________

My formula is

______ gm (product)

______ oz water

My prescription is ______ mg PHE per day

NAME OF FOOD Was it fresh, canned, cooked?	HOW MUCH I ATE Use cups, tablespoons, pieces	PHENYLALANINE IN FOOD (use your list)

Today I drank ______ oz of formula

FIGURE 44–3 Sample phenylketonuria (PKU) food record. *PHE,* phenylalanine.

full day's menu by calculating the quantity of phenylalanine in portions of food and compiling the daily total is the ultimate goal. These age-related tasks are shown in Table 44–9.

Many young children are interested in participating in the school lunch program. School lunch personnel are often willing to provide extra foods or extra portions of allowed foods. If the parent reviews the published menu with the child and together they decide which foods can safely be eaten, the child has an opportunity for self-management decision making. If only one or two items are sanctioned for consumption, the child may wish to bring supplemental foods to school.

PSYCHOSOCIAL DEVELOPMENT

The necessity of carefully controlling food intake may prompt parents to overprotect their children and, perhaps, to restrict their social activities (Smith et al., 1988). The children, in turn, may react negatively to their parents and to their nutritional therapy. The ability of the family to respond to the stresses of PKU, as reflected by adaptability and cohesion scores, is demonstrated by improved blood phenylalanine concentrations and the positive coping behaviors of older children with PKU (Kazak et al., 1988; Nowak-Cooperman et al., 1987; Trahms et al., 1987). Thus, continuing nutritional therapy beyond early childhood requires that children become knowledgeable about and responsible for managing their own food choices. The health care team becomes responsible for working with families and children to provide strategies that enable children and adolescents to participate in social and school activities, interact with peers, and progress through the usual developmental stages with self-confidence and self-esteem (Rees and Trahms, 1987).

Children require parental and professional support as they begin to assume responsibility for their food management. Self-management of food choices avoids the risk of the child using dietary noncompliance as a wedge against parental restrictions. Nor-

TABLE 44–9 TASKS TO BE EXPECTED OF CHILDREN WITH PHENYLKETONURIA BY AGE LEVEL

AGE (yrs)	SCHOOL LEVEL	TASK
2–3	Preschool	Distinguishing between yes/no foods
3–4	Preschool	Counting: how many?
4–5	Preschool	Measuring: how much?
5–6	Kindergarten	Preparing own formula; using scale
6–7	Grade 1–2	Writing basic notes in food diary
7–8	Grade 2	Making some decisions on after-school snack
8–9	Grade 3	Preparing breakfast
9–10	Grade 4	Packing lunches
10–14	Middle school	Managing food choices with increasing independence
14–18	High school	Independently managing PKU

mal intellectual development is a laudable goal of management of PKU, but to be entirely successful, the children with PKU need to develop self-assurance and a strong self-image concomitantly. This can be achieved, in part, by fostering self-management, independence, and a normal life-style for these children.

Nutritional Care in Maternal Phenylketonuria

A pregnant woman with elevated blood phenylalanine concentrations endangers her fetus because of the amplified transport of amino acids across the placenta. The fetus is exposed to about twice the phenylalanine level contained in normal maternal blood. Babies whose mothers have elevated blood phenylalanine concentrations have an increased occurrence of cardiac defects, retarded growth, microcephaly, and mental retardation, as presented in Table 44–10. The fetus appears to be at risk of damage even with minor elevations in maternal blood phenylalanine levels, and the higher the level, the more severe the effect will be (Lenke and Levy, 1980; Rohr et al., 1987).

TABLE 44–10 FREQUENCY OF ABNORMALITIES IN CHILDREN BORN TO MOTHERS WITH PHENYLKETONURIA (PKU) (%)

	MATERNAL PHENYLALANINE LEVELS (mg/dL)				
COMPLICATION	20	16–19	11–15	3–10	Non-PKU Mother
Mental retardation	92	73	22	21	5.0
Microcephaly	73	68	35	24	4.8
Congenital heart disease	12	15	6	0	0.8
Low birth weight	40	52	56	13	9.6

(Adapted from Lenke RR, Levy HL. Maternal phenylketonuria and hyperphenylalaninemia: An international survey of the outcome of untreated and treated pregnancies. N Engl J Med 303:1202, 1980.)

The management of nutritional therapy during pregnancy for a women with hyperphenylalaninemia is complex. The changing physiology of pregnancy and changing nutritional needs are difficult to monitor with the precision required to maintain appropriately low blood phenylalanine concentrations. Even with meticulous attention to phenylalanine intake, blood concentrations, and the nutritional requirements of pregnancy, a woman cannot be assured of a normal infant. Prepregnancy management of blood phenylalanine concentrations may decrease the risk to the fetus, but success cannot be ensured. When prepregnancy management is not possible, restricted-phenylalanine therapy should be started as soon as possible after conception (Lenke and Levy, 1982). The risks of abnormal development of the fetus, even with therapeutic dietary management and maintenance of blood phenylalanine concentrations at 1 to 5 mg/dL (60 to 300 mmol/L), are an important consideration for young women with PKU considering pregnancy (Brenton et al., 1994; Brenton and Lilburn, 1996). The only risk-free choice is to avoid pregnancy (Lowitzer, 1987).

Nutritional management during pregnancy is difficult, even for women who have consistently followed a low-phenylalanine dietary regimen since infancy. Women who have discontinued treatment find that reinstituting medical food consumption and limitation of food choices is difficult, if not overwhelming. Compliance with nutritional therapy during pregnancy for even the well-motivated woman requires family and professional support, as well as frequent monitoring of biochemical and nutritional aspects of both pregnancy and phenylketonuria.

Nutritional Care for Adults with Phenylketonuria

Currently, most adults with PKU have had the benefits of early diagnosis and treatment and are less likely to be affected by neurologic damage. However, among those who have had some degree of mental retardation, hyperactivity and self-abuse are often major concerns. Not all patients have responded with improved behavioral or intellectual function. For the difficult-to-manage older patient, a trial of a low-phenylalanine food pattern is recommended. If successful, continued phenylalanine restriction therapy may facilitate behavioral management.

The current recommendation of most clinics is effective management of blood phenylalanine concentrations throughout one's lifetime. This recommendation is based on disturbing reports of declining intellectual capabilities (Smith et al., 1990), magnetic resonance imaging (MRI) studies that demonstrate white matter changes in the brain after prolonged, significant elevation of phenylalanine concentrations (Brismar et al., 1990; Shaw et al., 1991), and negative neuropathologic developments (Waisbren and Levy, 1991).

It is also clear that reinstituting a phenylalanine-restricted food pattern is difficult after the eating pattern has been liberalized (Schuett et al., 1985). However, the efficacy of continued treatment throughout adulthood has been documented by reports of improved current intellectual performance, especially in terms of response time (Krause et al., 1985), and improved problem-solving abilities (Ris et al., 1994) when blood phenylalanine concentrations are kept low.

Organic Acid Disorders

Organic acid disorders have been identified with increasing frequency because of an increased awareness of these disorders on the part of community-based physicians and because of improved laboratory technology. Treatment modalities, which continue to be refined, involve the increased or decreased intake of specific nutrients. L-Carnitine supplementation is currently recommended (Bartholomew et al., 1988).

Restricted protein intake is an essential component of the treatment of organic acid disorders. A daily protein intake of 1 to 1.5 g/Kg of body weight, supplied by standard infant formula that has been diluted to decrease the protein content, along with protein-free formula that has been added to meet nutrient needs, is often an effective treatment modality. Other specialized formulas (see Table 44–3) that limit isoleucine, methionine, threonine, and valine are used, as clinically indicated, to support an adequate protein intake.

Carnitine deficiency has recently been recognized as a metabolic disorder. Generally, it is a secondary deficiency that occurs as a result of an insufficiency of carnitine to meet metabolic requirements, as carnitine is provided primarily by animal products in the diet. Carnitine is a short-chain carboxylic acid containing nitrogen that facilitates the transport of long-chain fatty acids to the mitochondrial matrix. Generally, children with these disorders now receive supplements of L-carnitine. Levels of 50 to 300 mg/kg/day have been suggested (Ohtani et al., 1988; Roe et al., 1991). This level of supplementation appears to enhance metabolic function without notable side effects.

Propionic acidemia is a defect of propionyl-CoA carboxylase in the pathway of propionyl-CoA to methylmalonyl-CoA, as illustrated in Figure 44–4. The clinical course can be varied, but is generally marked by vomiting, lethargy, hypotonia, dehydration, seizures, and coma. Survivors often have permanent neurologic damage. Metabolic acidosis with a marked anion gap and hyperammonemia is characteristic. Long-chain ketonuria may also be present. Some patients with propionic acidemia may respond to pharmacologic doses of biotin. Long-term outcome in propionic acidemia is variable; hypotonia and cognitive delay may result even in children who are diagnosed early and who receive rigorous treatment (North et al., 1995).

At least five separate enzyme deficiencies have been identified that result in **methylmalonic acidemia.** The defect of methylmalonyl-CoA mutase apoenzyme is the most frequently identified (see Fig. 44–3). The clinical features are similar to those of propionic acidemia. Acidosis is common, and diagnosis is confirmed by the presence of large amounts of methylmalonic acid in blood and urine. Other findings include hypoglycemia, ketonuria, and elevation of plasma ammonia and lactate levels. Frank vitamin B_{12} deficiency must also be ruled out, as vitamin B_{12} yields two cofactors required to convert methylmalonate to succinate and homocysteine to methionine. The vitamin B_{12}–responsive patient may respond to pharmacologic doses of 1 to 2 mg/day (Walsher and Stewart, 1981). Progressive renal insufficiency is often a long-term outcome of methylmalonic acidemia (Molteni, 1991).

The goals of managing acute episodes of propionic acidemia and methylmalonic acidemia are to achieve and maintain normal nutrient intake and biochemical balance. Maintenance of energy and fluid intake is important to prevent tissue catabolism and dehydration. Electrolyte imbalances are corrected by the usual methods, and abnormal metabolites are removed through urinary excretion, promoted by a high fluid intake. Relapses of metabolic acidosis may result from excessive protein intake, infection, or unidentified factors. Parents become skilled at identifying early signs of illness. Treatment for these episodes must be rapid because coma and death can occur quickly.

Long-term nutritional therapy includes an appropriate balance of essential nutrients and a protein intake that is restricted to 1.0 to 1.5 g/kg/day for infants and toddlers. Requirements for the limited amino acids may vary widely. Growth rate, state of health, residual enzyme activity, and overall protein and energy intakes must be monitored carefully and correlated with plasma amino acid levels. A comparison of energy and protein intakes of affected and unaffected infants is shown in Table 44–5. An adequate fluid intake is required to normalize blood ammonia levels. Nutritional therapy may be complicated by food refusal and lack of appetite, which compromise medical management (Hyman et al., 1987). L-Carnitine supplementation at doses of 100 to 300 mg/kg/day is recommended (Acosta and Yannicelli, 1993).

Urea Cycle Defects

Diagnosis and treatment of defects in the urea cycle have also advanced (Ohtani et al., 1988). All such defects result in an accumulation of ammonia in the blood. The clinical signs of elevated ammonia are vomiting and lethargy, which may progress to seizures, coma, and ultimately, death. In infants, the adverse effects of elevated ammonia levels are rapid and devastating. In older children, symptoms of elevated ammonia may be preceded by hyperactivity and irritability. The severity and variation of

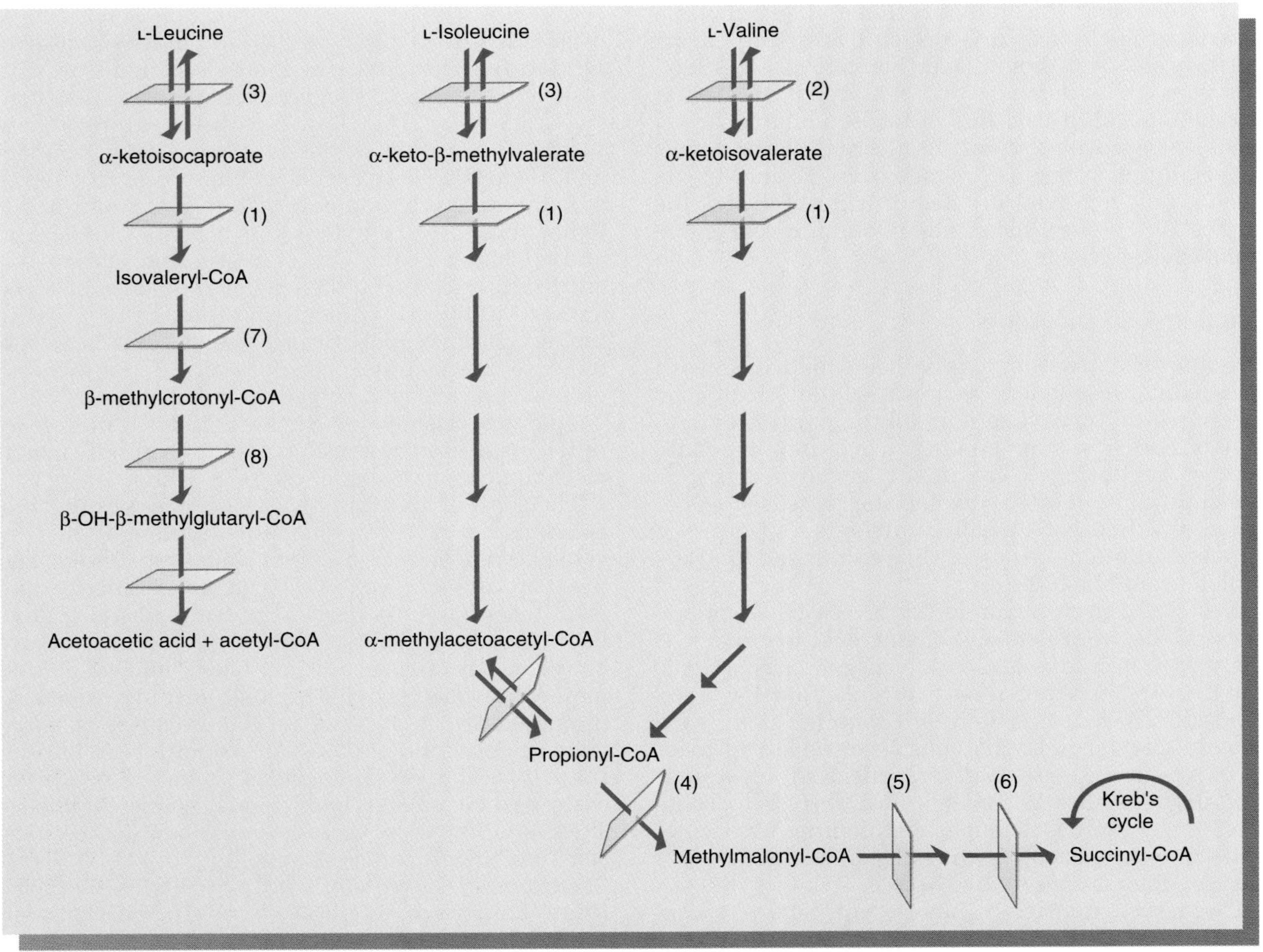

FIGURE 44–4 Organic acidemias and maple syrup urine disease (MSUD). (*1*) Branched-chain ketoacid decarboxylase (MSUD). (*2*) Valine aminotransferase. (*3*) Leucine-isoleucine aminotransferase. (*4*) Propionyl-CoA carboxylase (propionic acidemia). (*5*) Methylmalonyl-CoA racemase (methylmalonic aciduria). (*6*) Methylmalonyl-CoA mutase (methylmalonic aciduria). (*7*) Isovaleryl-CoA dehydrogenase (isovaleric acidemia). (*8*) Beta-methylcrotonyl-CoA carboxylase (biotin-responsive multiple carboxylase deficiency).

the clinical courses of all urea cycle defects may be related to the degree of residual enzyme activity. The common urea cycle defects are discussed in a progression that proceeds around the urea cycle, as shown in Figure 44–5. Treatment for all urea cycle disorders is similar: a low-protein food pattern. Frequently, a standard infant formula can be diluted to 1.0 to 1.5 g of protein per kilogram of body weight per day. Specialized formulas are often used to adjust protein composition in an effort to limit ammonia production. The energy, vitamin, and mineral concentrations can be brought up to recommended intake levels with the addition of a protein-free formula. L-arginine is supplemented based on individual needs, usually 400 to 700 mg/kg/day, except in the case of arginase deficiency (Brusilow and Howich, 1989). Phenylbutyrate or other compounds that enhance alternative metabolic pathways are usually required to normalize ammonia levels.

Ornithine transcarbamylase (OTC) deficiency is an X-linked recessive disorder marked by blockage in the conversion of ornithine and carbamyl phosphate to citrulline. OTC deficiency is identified by hyperammonemia and increased urinary orotic acid, with normal levels of citrulline, argininosuccinic acid, and arginine (Brubakk et al., 1982). OTC deficiency is usually lethal in male individuals, whereas heterozygous female subjects with various degrees of enzyme activity may not demonstrate symptoms until they are induced by stress, as from an infection, or a significant increase in protein intake.

Citrullinemia is the result of a deficiency of argininosuccinic acid synthetase in the metabolism of citrulline to argininosuccinic acid. Citrullinemia is identified by markedly elevated citrulline levels in the urine and blood. Argininosuccinic acid synthetase activity is absent or decreased in cultured skin fibroblasts. Symptoms may be present in the neonatal period, or they may develop gradually in

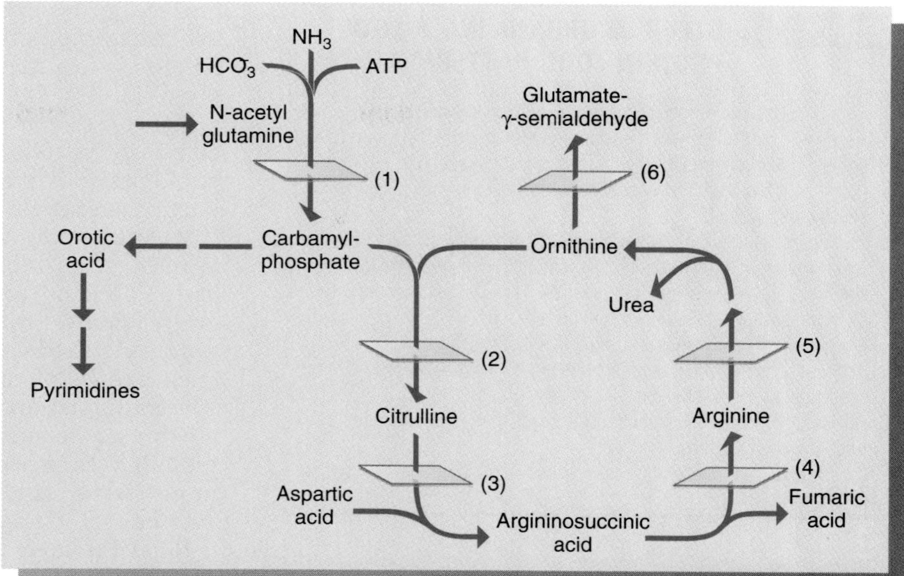

FIGURE 44–5 Urea cycle disorders. (*1*) Carbamyl-phosphate synthetase (CPS deficiency). (*2*) Ornithine carbamyl transferase (OTC deficiency). (*3*) Argininosuccinic acid synthetase (citrullinemia). (*4*) Argininosuccinic acid lyase (argininosuccinic aciduria). (*5*) Arginase (arginemia). *ATP,* adenosine triphosphate.

early infancy. They may include poor feeding and recurrent vomiting which, without immediate treatment, progress to seizures, neurologic abnormalities, and coma.

Argininosuccinic aciduria (ASA) is the result of a deficiency of argininosuccinate lyase, which is involved in the metabolism of argininosuccinic acid to arginine. ASA is identified by the presence of argininosuccinic acid in urine and blood. Citrulline levels may be moderately elevated in blood and urine. Argininosuccinate lyase activity is absent or decreased in cultured fibroblasts or red blood cells.

Citrullinemia and ASA have essentially the same clinical presentation. The aim of therapy for both of these defects is to prevent or decrease hyperammonemia and the detrimental neurologic consequences associated with high amino acid levels. Acute episodes of illness are managed by discontinuing protein intake and administering intravenous fluids and glucose to correct the dehydration and provide energy. If hyperammonemia is severe, peritoneal dialysis, hemodialysis, or exchange transfusion may be required. Intravenous arginine and sodium benzoate have also been beneficial in reducing the hyperammonemia.

Long-term therapy consists of restricting dietary protein to 1.0 to 2.0 g/kg/day, depending on individual tolerance. Table 44–5 compares energy and protein intakes for affected and unaffected infants. The food pattern should be supplemented with L-arginine (1 g/day for infants; 2 g/day for older children) to prevent arginine deficiency and assist in waste nitrogen excretion (Brusilow and Batshaw, 1979). Phenylbutyrate or other compounds are frequently prescribed to aid in ammonia excretion. Because of the effect of infection and illness on the urea cycle, infections should be treated aggressively.

Carbamyl-phosphate synthetase (CPS) deficiency is manifested in a very similar manner with hyperammonemic episodes. The onset is usually in the early neonatal period, with vomiting, irritability, hypothermia, respiratory distress, altered muscle tone, lethargy, and often, coma. Specific laboratory findings usually include elevated plasma glutamine levels and normal or low orotic acid levels in urine. Therapy for CPS deficiency is essentially the same as that described for citrullinemia and ASA, except that arginine in high doses is not indicated.

Neurologic outcome and intellectual development in those with urea cycle defects vary, with a range from normal IQ and motor function to severe mental retardation and cerebral palsy. Although information on long-term follow-up is limited, the use of alternative pathways for waste nitrogen excretion and a protein-restricted food pattern to control ammonia levels may improve the outcome.

Protein-Restricted Diets

Infants and children with metabolic disorders, such as urea cycle defects or organic acidemias, generally require restricted-protein intakes and specialized formulas. The most usual restrictions are for 1.0 g, 1.5 g, and 2.0 g of protein per kilogram of body weight. The appropriate prescription for protein level is based on the individual's tolerance or residual enzyme activity, age, and projected growth rate. The highest protein level tolerated should be given to ensure adequate growth and a margin of nutritional safety. The steps for effective planning of a low-protein food pattern are shown in Table 44–11.

In general, low-protein or restricted-protein food patterns can be formulated from readily available, lowered-protein infant, toddler, and table foods. Low-protein foods (see Table 44–7) can be used to

TABLE 44–11 STEPS IN ORGANIZING A LOW-PROTEIN FOOD PATTERN

1. Determine the protein tolerance of the individual based on (a) diagnosis, (b) age, and (c) growth. Consider the metabolic stability and total protein intake required for the infant's or child's weight.
2. Calculate the protein and energy needs of the individual based on age, activity, and weight.
3. Provide at least 70% of total protein as high biological value (HBV) protein—from formula for infants, and from milk or dairy foods for older children. Use a specialized formula if the infant or child cannot tolerate all of the protein intake from intact protein.
4. Provide energy and nutrient sources to meet basic needs.
5. Add water to meet fluid requirements and to maintain appropriate concentration of formula mixture.
6. For the older infant and child, provide foods to meet food variety, texture, and energy needs.
7. Provide adequate intake of calcium, iron, and all other vitamins and minerals for age.

provide energy, texture, and variety in the food pattern without appreciably increasing the protein load. Infant formula can be diluted with a protein-free formula product to meet the prescribed protein level. The resultant energy deficit is made up by supplementing carbohydrate and fat. Specialty modular formulas are also available (see Table 44–3). The appropriate choice depends on the level of protein restriction, age, and condition of the child. Formulas should contain 20 kcal/oz and should supply at least 100 kcal/kg of energy, depending on age. Osmolality of the formula must be considered; feedings of no more than 400 mOsm/L of solution have been recommended, although it must be noted that measurement of the osmolality of specific products is not always possible (Martin and Acosta, 1987). The usual recommendations for vitamins and minerals are appropriate for this population.

Maple Syrup Urine Disease

Classic **maple syrup urine disease (MSUD),** or **branched-chain ketoaciduria,** results from a defect in decarboxylation that affects the metabolism of the branched-chain amino acids (BCAAs) leucine, isoleucine, and valine (see Fig. 44–3). This rare autosomal recessive metabolic defect is estimated to occur in 1 in 225,000 neonates. Infants appear normal at birth, but by 4 or 5 days of age, they demonstrate poor feeding, vomiting, lethargy, and periodic hypertonia. A characteristic sweet, malty odor from the urine and perspiration can be noted toward the end of the first week of life. Failure to treat this condition leads to acidosis, neurologic deterioration, seizures, and coma, proceeding eventually to death. Because of the rapid onset of symptoms, results of newborn screening tests are often received too late to initiate treatment before symptom onset. Management of acute disease requires peritoneal dialysis and hydration. BCAAs are introduced gradually into the diet when plasma leucine concentrations are decreased to about 190 mmol/L.

The precise mechanism for the complete decarboxylase reaction and the resultant neurologic damage is not known. Neither is it understood why leucine metabolism is significantly more abnormal than that of the other two BCAAs. Clinical relapse is most often related to the degree of abnormality of the leucine concentrations, and these relapses are frequently related to infection. Acute infections represent medical emergencies in this population; most deaths of children receiving therapy have occurred during an episode of infection. If the plasma leucine concentration exceeds 20 mg/dL (1525 mmol/L), BCAAs should be removed from the diet immediately and intravenous therapy should be started.

Reports have indicated that early intervention and meticulous biochemical control can provide a more hopeful prognosis than was realized earlier. Reasonable growth and intellectual development in the normal to low-normal range have been described (Hilliges et al., 1993). Diagnosis before 7 days of age and long-term metabolic control are critical factors in long-term normalization of intellectual development (Kaplan et al., 1991; Nord et al., 1991). It is recommended that plasma leucine concentrations be maintained at between 2 and 5 mg/dL (150 to 380 μmol/L). Concentrations above 10 mg/dL (760 μmol/L) are often associated with alpha-ketoacidemia and neurologic symptoms.

Nutritional therapy requires very careful monitoring of blood concentrations (especially leucine, isoleucine, valine, and alloisoleucine), growth, and general nutritional adequacy. Several formulas specifically designed for the treatment of this disorder are now available to provide a reasonable amino acid and vitamin mixture (see Table 44–3). These are generally supplemented with a small quantity of standard infant formula or cow's milk to provide the BCAAs needed to support growth and development. The relative leucine, isoleucine, and valine values of the food groups are presented in Table 44–12.

Ketone utilization disorders (mitochondrial 2-methylacetoacetyl-CoA thiolase deficiency or similar enzyme defect) are disorders of isoleucine and ketone body metabolism. Affected individuals are usually older infants or toddlers who present with ketoacidosis, vomiting, and lethargy with secondary dehydration and, sometimes, coma. This event is frequently preceded by febrile illness or fasting (Slovik, 1993). The treatment is dietary protein restriction (usually 1.5 g of protein per kilogram of body weight per day), 100 to 300 mg of L-carnitine per kilogram of body weight per day; avoidance of fasting by providing small, frequent meals consisting primarily of carbohydrates; and the use of Bicitra to treat ketoacidosis.

TABLE 44–12 SERVING LISTS FOR BRANCHED-CHAIN AMINO ACID (BCAA)–RESTRICTED DIETS: AVERAGE ISOLEUCINE (ILE), LEUCINE (LEU), VALINE (VAL), PROTEIN, FAT, AND ENERGY CONTENT PER SERVING

FOOD*	ILE (mg)	LEU (mg)	VAL (mg)	PROTEIN (g)	FAT (g)	ENERGY (kcal)
Breads/cereals	18	35	25	0.5	0	30
Fats	7	10	7	0.1	8	70
Fruits	17	25	22	0.6	0	75
Vegetables	22	30	24	0.6	0	15
Free foods A†	3	5	4	0.1	Variable	50
Free foods B‡	0	0	0	0	Variable	55
Milk, whole (100 mL)	203	329	224	3.4	3.4	62

(From Acosta PB. Ross Metabolic Formula System Nutrition Support Protocols. Columbus, OH: Ross Laboratories, © 1993.)

*Only selected foods are allowed in each category, and these are usually simple foods so that the amino acid content can be estimated accurately.

†These foods contain small amounts of BCAAs; this category includes low-protein pastas, breads, and some sweets.

‡These foods contain little or no BCAAs; they are primarily sweet beverages and candies and are used sparingly to satisfy appetite.

DISORDERS OF CARBOHYDRATE METABOLISM

Disorders of carbohydrate metabolism are varied in presentation, clinical course, and clinical outcome. Some of the disorders present in the early newborn period with life-threatening seizures and sepsis, for example, galactosemia; others may present in mid-infancy at the time of introduction of solids which contain offending ingredients, such as hereditary fructose intolerance or at the time of spacing of feedings and subsequent hypoglycemia, for example, glycogen storage disease. All of these disorders require early and aggressive nutritional therapy.

Galactosemia

Galactosemia—a high level of plasma galactose-1-phosphate combined with galactosuria—is found in two autosomal recessive metabolic disorders, galactokinase deficiency and galactose-1-phosphate uridyl transferase deficiency, which is also called classic galactosemia.

Galactosemia results from a disturbance in the conversion of galactose to glucose because of the absence of one of the enzyme activities shown in Figure 44–6. The enzyme deficiency causes an accumulation of galactose, or galactose and galactose-1-phosphate, in body tissues. It is believed that galactose-1-phosphate in intercellular fluids causes the cellular disturbances in classic galactosemia.

If an infant has no galactose-1-phosphate uridyl transferase activity, illness generally occurs within the first 2 weeks of life. Symptoms are vomiting, diarrhea, lethargy, failure to thrive, jaundice, hepatomegaly, and cataracts. Infants with galactosemia may be hypoglycemic and are susceptible to infection from gram-negative organisms. If the condition is not treated, death frequently ensues secondary to septicemia. If diagnosis and therapy are delayed, mental retardation can result.

Diagnosis of transferase deficiency is accomplished in a stepwise fashion. Sick neonates are first screened for urinary non–glucose-reducing sugars, which are identified by a positive result from Benedict's test and a negative result from a glucose paper strip test. This is followed by the Beutler test for transferase enzyme activity and confirmation of diagnosis by specific enzyme tests.

Galactosemia is treated by lifelong galactose restriction. Although galactose is required for the production of galactolipids and cerebrosides, it can be produced by an alternative pathway if galactose is omitted from the diet. Galactose restriction mandates strict avoidance of all milk and milk products and lactose-containing foods because lactose is hydrolyzed into galactose and glucose. Infants are fed soy-based formula. Recent data suggest, in addition, the restriction of fruits and vegetables that contain significant amounts of galactose. Dates, papayas, bell peppers, persimmons, tomatoes, and watermelons all contain more than 10 mg of galactose

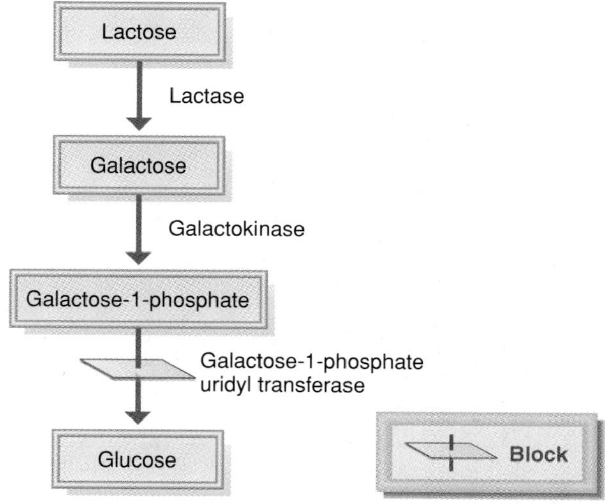

FIGURE 44–6 Schematic diagram of the metabolism of galactose in galactosemia.

per 100 g fresh weight of product (Gross and Acosta, 1991; Acosta and Gross, 1995). Effective galactose restriction requires careful reading of food product labels. Milk is added to many products, and lactose often appears in the coating of the tablet form of medications. Table 44–13 presents a low-galactose food pattern.

TABLE 44–13 FOOD LISTS FOR LOW-GALACTOSE FOOD PATTERN

ALLOWABLE FOODS	GALACTOSE-CONTAINING FOODS TO BE AVOIDED*
Milk and Milk Substitutes	
Isomil (Ross) Prosobee (Mead Johnson) Alsoy (Carnation) Gerber Soy (Gerber)	Breast milk All forms of animal milk Imitation or filled milk Cream, butter, some margarines Cottage cheese, cream cheese Hard cheeses Yogurt Ice cream, ice milk, sherbet
Fruits	
All fresh, frozen, canned, or dried fruits except those processed with unsafe ingredients†	Dates, papayas, bell peppers, persimmons, tomatoes, and watermelons, which contain > 10 mg galactose/100 g fresh weight Intake of fruits and vegetables containing galactose needs to be monitored carefully.
Vegetables	
All fresh, frozen, canned, or dried vegetables except those processed with unsafe ingredients,† seasoned with butter or margarine, breaded, or creamed	
Meat, Poultry, Fish, Eggs, Nuts	
Plain beef, lamb, veal, pork, ham, fish, turkey, chicken, game, fowl, Kosher frankfurters, eggs, nut butters, nuts	
Breads and Cereals	
Cooked and dry cereals, bread or crackers without milk or unsafe ingredients,† macaroni, spaghetti, noodles, rice, tortillas	
Fats	
All vegetable oils; all shortening, lard, margarines, and salad dressings except those made with unsafe ingredients;† mayonnaise; olives	

*NOTE: Lactose is often used as a pharmaceutical bulking agent, filler, or excipient; thus, tablets, tinctures, and vitamin and mineral mixtures should be evaluated carefully for galactose content. The *PDR (Physician's Desk Reference)* now lists active and inactive ingredients in medications, as well as manufacturers' telephone numbers.

†Unsafe ingredients include milk, buttermilk, cream, lactose, galactose, casein, caseinate, whey, dry milk solids, or curds. Labels should be checked regularly and carefully, as formulations of products change frequently.

With early diagnosis and treatment, physical and motor development should proceed normally. Mental development is generally slightly less than expected; patients often have an IQ of 85 to 100, and visual-perceptual and speech difficulties are common (Fischler et al., 1980).

A few women with galactosemia have become pregnant and given birth to healthy babies, although ovarian failure is a recognized problem in women affected with galactosemia (Kaufman et al., 1988 and 1995).

Galactokinase deficiency requires the same galactose-restricted regimen as galactosemia. Cataracts form, but the other sequelae of galactosemia have not been described.

DISORDERS OF FATTY ACID OXIDATION

Recent laboratory advancements in the identification of disorders involving fatty acid oxidation have enabled the treatment of **long-chain acyl-CoA dehydrogenase deficiency (LCAD)** and **medium-chain acyl-CoA dehydrogenase deficiency (MCAD).**

Children affected by LCAD or MCAD are generally identified during periods of fasting or clinical illness. These children present with symptoms of variable severity, including failure to thrive, episodic vomiting, and hypotonia. Children with LCAD become hypoglycemic and demonstrate abnormal liver function, reduced or absent ketones in the urine, and often, secondary carnitine deficiency. Children with MCAD have a similar presentation, in addition to mild metabolic acidosis (Bartlett et al., 1991).

The concept underlying effective treatment is simple: avoidance of fasting. This is accomplished by the regularly spaced intake of foods that provide an adequate energy intake and that are high in carbohydrates. A low-fat diet is advocated because fats are not effectively metabolized. Consumption of 15% to 20% of calories as fat has been recommended (Catzeflis et al., 1990). L-Carnitine supplementation is often required. Children often do very well with three meals and three snacks offered at regular intervals. Some children may require additional carbohydrate feedings during the night.

GLYCOGEN STORAGE DISEASES

Glycogen storage diseases, as a group, reflect an inability to metabolize glycogen to glucose in the liver. There are a number of possible enzyme defects along the pathway, including types I through IV. The most common of the disorders are types I and III. Their symptoms are poor physical growth, hypoglycemia, hepatomegaly, and abnormal biochemical parameters, especially for cholesterol and triglycerides. Advances in the treatment of glycogen storage diseases have improved the quality of life for affected children (Smit et al., 1990).

Glycogen storage disease type Ia (GSD Ia) is a defect in the enzyme glucose-1–6-phosphatase, which impairs **gluconeogenesis** and **glycogenolysis**. The affected person is unable to metabolize glycogen stored in the liver. Severe hypoglycemia can result, causing irreparable damage.

Currently, administration of raw cornstarch at regular intervals and a high-carbohydrate, low-fat dietary pattern are advocated to prevent hypoglycemia, which is the primary goal of treatment. Young infants may require administration of pancreatic enzyme before ingesting uncooked cornstarch, to increase its effectiveness (Goldberg and Slonin, 1993). Some infants and children do very well with oral cornstarch administration, whereas others require glucose polymers, administered via continuous-drip gastric feedings, to prevent hypoglycemic episodes during the night (Wolfsdorf and Crigler, 1997). The dose of cornstarch should be individualized; however, doses of 1.75 to 2.5 g/kg at 4- to 6-hour intervals have proved to be effective for young children (Lee et al., 1996). Overnight glucose delivery rates of 4 to 6 mg/kg/min have proved adequate (Goldberg and Slonin, 1993). Adolescents may be able to maintain plasma glucose concentrations with a single dose of cornstarch at bedtime (Wolfsdorf and Crigler, 1997). The glucose vehicle suggested is a lactose-free formula. Iron supplementation is required to maintain adequate hematologic status because cornstarch interferes with iron absorption. The rationale for intervention is to maintain plasma glucose in a safe range by providing a constant supply of exogenous glucose. The outcome of treatment has been good; the hazards of severe hypoglycemic episodes is diminished, physical growth is improved, and liver size is decreased. However, the risk of progressive renal dysfunction is not entirely eliminated by current treatment modalities (Wolfsdorf et al., 1997; Lee et al., 1996).

Amylo-1, 6-glucosidase deficiency (GSD III, or debrancher enzyme defect) prevents the glycogen breakdown beyond branch points. This disorder is similar to GSD I in that glycogenolysis is inefficient but gluconeogenesis is amplified to help maintain glucose production. The symptoms of GSD III are usually less severe, ranging from hepatomegaly to severe hypoglycemia (Gremse et al., 1990). Cornstarch therapy is sometimes efficacious when used in conjunction with a high-protein (25% of energy calories), moderate-fat (30% of energy calories) food pattern.

To some extent, treatment protocols for the glycogen storage diseases are still evolving. The protocols include various kinds of carbohydrates at various doses during the day and night. Individual tolerance, body weight, state of health, ambient temperature, and physical activity all play important roles in designing the specific pattern of carbohydrate administration. The goal for all of the protocols remains the same: normalization of blood glucose levels.

TABLE 44–14 INTERVENTION OBJECTIVES FOR THE NUTRITIONIST INVOLVED IN THE TREATMENT OF METABOLIC DISORDERS

In the clinic, the nutritionist has a major role in ongoing therapy and planning for each child. These responsibilities include gathering of objective food intake data from the family, assessing the adequacy of the child's intake, and working with the family to teach its members appropriate ways to monitor the restricted-food intake pattern.

The child with a metabolic disorder often presents a wide range of concerns, which may include unstable biochemical levels, failure to gain weight, excessive weight gain, difficulty adhering to diet, and behaviors that cause an adverse feeding situation. Thus, managing a child with a metabolic disorder requires input from the entire health care team. The nutritionist uses skills and a basic knowledge of foods as sources of nutrients, parent–child relationships, growth, development, and interviewing to obtain the necessary information for assessing and planning for the child with a metabolic disorder.

I. The nutritionist functions as an effective interdisciplinary team member by:
   A. Becoming familiar with the background and current status of the child through the medical record
   B. Recognizing and accepting the responsibility as the nutritionist by:
      1. Identifying appropriate intake of nutrients for growth, activity, and biochemical balance
      2. Identifying developmental stages of feeding behavior
      3. Understanding the concept of food as a support of developmental progress
      4. Identifying behavior as it affects nutrient intake
   C. Understanding, respecting, and utilizing the expertise of the team disciplines in providing care for the child with a metabolic disorder

II. The nutritionist provides adequate and supportive patient services by:
   A. Establishing a positive, cooperative working relationship with the parent and child
   B. Interviewing the parents about dietary intake and the feeding situation in a nonjudgmental manner
   C. Assessing the parent–child relationship as it relates to dietary management and control of the disorder
   D. Developing a plan for appropriate dietary management based on growth, biochemical levels, nutrient needs, and developmental progress
   E. Developing a plan that includes appropriate foods and recognizes the parents' skills in food preparation, as well as family routines
   F. Working with the parents to establish a method to deal effectively with negative feeding behaviors, if necessary
   G. Contacting the family after receiving laboratory results and calculating food records to make necessary and appropriate changes in diet prescription
   H. Supporting parents in their efforts at effective dietary and behavior management

III. The nutritionist develops a professional database by:
   A. Becoming familiar with the current literature on the treatment of metabolic disorders
   B. Understanding the genetic basis of metabolic disorders

IV. The nutritionist works with the team members to develop an understanding of long-term patient care and a written care plan for the patient.

OTHER DISORDERS

Table 44–2 outlines additional disorders by the enzymatic defects involved, distinctive clinical and biochemical features, and current approaches to dietary therapy.

NUTRITIONAL CARE MANAGEMENT

The role of the nutritionist in the treatment of inborn errors of metabolism is a complex one that requires expertise in medical nutrition therapy for the specific disorder, a family-centered counseling approach, feeding skill development and behavioral modification, as well as the support and counsel of a team of health care providers involved in the care of the patient. Nutritional intervention is often a lifelong consideration. Specific objectives of nutritional care are shown in Table 44–14.

CASE STUDY

Newborn Infant with Phenylketonuria

The 1-day newborn screening test result for phenylalanine (Guthrie method) for a 7-lb, 4-oz male child was 3 mg/dL. The infant was breast-fed with no supplemental formula. A repeat Guthrie sample was requested to further document the phenylalanine concentration. The result from this sample, collected on day 5 of life, was 24 mg/dL. To confirm the diagnosis for this child, who was considered to be "presumptive positive," a quantitative sample was obtained, and phenylalanine and tyrosine levels were measured. On day 9 of life, the serum phenylalanine concentration was 25.5 mg/dL and the tyrosine level was 1.1 mg/dL. The presence of urine phenylpyruvic and 0-hydroxyphenylacetic acids was documented.

To provide adequate protein and energy intake, and at the same time, decrease the serum phenylalanine concentration, a phenylalanine-free formula was introduced at standard dilution without a phenylalanine supplement. Within 24 hours, the infant's serum phenylalanine concentration had decreased to 16.5 mg/dL while being provided an intake of 16 oz of formula. Within 48 hours, the level was 8.8 mg/dL with an intake of 18 oz of formula. At this point, evaporated milk was added to bring the calculated phenylalanine concentration to about 60 mg/kg and to maintain a generous protein and energy intake for this 3.6-kg infant.

Phenylalanine concentrations were measured on alternate days for 4 days, and the levels were 7.6 mg/dL and 5.6 mg/dL, respectively. In subsequent weeks, growth and serum phenylalanine concentrations continued to be monitored carefully, and energy and phenylalanine intakes were adjusted as necessary to maintain blood phenylalanine concentrations between 2 and 6 mg/dL and to keep growth in appropriate channels.

1. What is the expected energy requirement for this infant with phenylketonuria?
2. What baseline formula would you use for this infant to provide phenylalanine at 60 mg/kg, formula at 20 kcal/oz, and protein and energy intakes at recommended levels?
3. What are the growth expectations for this infant?
4. What steps would you take if the plasma phenylalanine concentration exceeded 6 mg/dL on subsequent measurements?

CITED REFERENCES

Acosta PB, Gross KC. Hidden sources of galactose in the environment. Eur J Pediatr 154:S87, 1995.

Acosta PB, Yannicelli S. Nutrition support of inherited disorders of amino acid metabolism, Part I. Top Clin Nutr 9(1):65, 1993.

American Academy of Pediatrics, Committee on Genetics. Newborn screening fact sheets. Pediatrics 98:473, 1996.

Azen CG, et al. Intellectual development in 12-year-old children treated for phenylketonuria. Am J Dis Child 145:35, 1991.

Azen CG, et al. Summary of findings from the United States Collaborative Study of Children Treated for Phenylketonuria. Eur J Pediatr 155:S29, 1996.

Bartholomew DW, et al. Therapeutic approaches to cobalamin-C methylmalonic acidemia and homocystinuria. J Pediatr 112:32, 1988.

Bartlett K, et al. Inherited disorders of mitochondrial B-oxidation. In: Schaub J, Van Hoof F, Vis HL (eds.). Inborn Errors of Metabolism, Nestle Nutrition Workshop Series, Vol. 24. New York: Raven Press, 1991, p. 19.

Brenton DP, et al. Maternal phenylketonuria: Preconception dietary control and outcome. Int Pediatr 9(suppl 2):5, 1994.

Brenton DP, Lilburn M. Maternal phenylketonuria—A study from the United Kingdom. Eur J Pediatr 155:S177, 1996.

Brismar J, et al. Malignant hyperphenylalaninemia: CT and MRI of the brain. Am J Neurol Res 11:135, 1990.

Brubakk AM, et al. Successful treatment of severe OTC deficiency. J Pediatr 100:929, 1982.

Brusilow SW, Batshaw ML. Arginine therapy of arginine-succinase deficiency. Lancet 1:124, 1979.

Brusilow SW, Howich AL. Urea cycle enzymes. In: Scriver CR, Beaudet AL, Sly WS, Valle D (eds.). The Molecular and Metabolic Basis of Inherited Disease, 7th ed. New York: McGraw Hill, 1995.

Cabalska B, et al. Termination of dietary treatment in phenylketonuria. Eur J Pediatr 126:253, 1977.

Catzeflis C, et al. Early diagnosis and treatment of neonatal medium-chain acyl-CoA dehydrogenase deficiency: Report of two siblings. Eur J Pediatr 149:577, 1990.

Diamond A. Phenylalanine levels of 6–10 mg/dL may not be as benign as once thought. Acta Paediatr [Suppl] 407:89, 1994.

Diamond A, et al. Prefrontal cortex cognitive deficits in children treated early and continuously for phenylketonuria. Monog Soc Res Child Dev 62(4):1, 1997.

Early diagnosis of hyperphenylalaninemia due to tetrahydrobiopterin deficiency (malignant hyperphenylalaninemia). J Pediatr 96:854, 1980.

Fischler K, et al. Developmental aspects of galactosemia from infancy to childhood. Clin Pediatr 19:38, 1980.

Goldberg T, Slonin AE. Nutritional therapy for hepatic glycogen storage diseases. J Am Diet Assoc 93:1423, 1993.

Gremse DA, et al. Efficacy of cornstarch therapy in type III glycogen-storage disease. Am J Clin Nutr 52:671, 1990.

Gross KC, Acosta PB. Fruits and vegetables are a source of galactose: Implication in planning the diets of patients with galactosaemia. J Inherited Metab Dis 14:253, 1991.

Guthrie R, Susi A. A simple phenylalanine method for detecting phenylketonuria in large populations of newborn infants. Pediatrics 70:376, 1962.

Hanley WB, et al. Malnutrition with early treatment of phenylketonuria. Pediatr Res 4:318, 1970.

Heffernan JF, Trahms CM. A model preschool for patients with phenylketonuria. J Am Diet Assoc 79:306, 1981.

Hilliges C, et al. Intellectual performance of children with maple syrup urine disease. Eur J Pediatr 152:144, 1993.

Holt LE, Snyderman SE. The amino acid requirements of children. In: Nyhan WL (ed.). Amino Acid Metabolism and Genetic Variation. New York: McGraw-Hill, 1967, pp. 381–390.

Hyman SL, et al. Behavior management of feeding disturbances in urea cycle and organic acid disorders. J Pediatr 111:558, 1987.

Kaplan P, et al. Intellectual outcome in children with maple syrup urine disease. J Pediatr 119:46, 1991.

Kaufman FR, et al. Cognitive functioning, neurological status, and brain imaging in classical galactosemia. Eur J Pediatr 154:52, 1995.

Kaufman FR, et al. Correlation of ovarian function with galactose-1-phosphate uridyl transferase levels in galactosemia. J Pediatr 112:754, 1988.

Kaufman S. Unsolved problems in diagnosis and therapy of hyperphenylalaninemia caused by defects in tetrahydrobiopterin metabolism. J Pediatr 109:572, 1986.

Kazak AE, et al. Childhood chronic disease and family functioning: A study of phenylketonuria. Pediatrics 81:224, 1988.
Koch R, et al. Preliminary report on the effects of diet discontinuation on PKU. J Pediatr 100:870, 1982.
Krause W, et al. Biochemical and neuropsychological effects of elevated plasma phenylalanine in patients with treated phenylketonuria. J Clin Invest 75:40, 1985.
Lee PJ, Dixon MA, Leonard JV. Uncooked cornstarch—Efficacy in type 1 glucogenosis. Arch Dis Child 74:546, 1996.
Legido A, et al. Treatment variables and intellectual outcome in children with classic phenylketonuria. Clin Pediatr 32:417, 1993.
Lenke RR, Levy HL. Maternal phenylketonuria and hyperphenylalaninemia: An international survey of the outcome of untreated and treated pregnancies. N Engl J Med 303:1202, 1980.
Lenke RR, Levy HL. Maternal phenylketonuria: Results of dietary therapy. Am J Obstet Gynecol 142:548, 1982.
Lowitzer AC. Maternal phenylketonuria: Cause for concern among women with PKU. Res Dev Dis 8:1, 1987.
Martin SB, Acosta PB. Osmolalities of selected enteral products and carbohydrate modules used to treat inherited metabolic disorders. J Am Diet Assoc 87:48, 1987.
Medical Research Council Working Party on Phenylketonuria: Phenylketonuria due to phenylalanine hydroxylase deficiency: An unfolding story. Br Med J 306:115, 1993a.
Medical Research Council Working Party on Phenylketonuria: Recommendations on the dietary management of phenylketonuria. Arch Dis Child 68:426, 1993b.
Michals K, et al. Blood phenylalanine levels and intelligence of 10-year-old children with PKU in the National Collaborative Study. J Am Diet Assoc 88:1226, 1988.
Molteni KH, et al. Progressive renal insufficiency in methylmalonic acidemia. Pediatr Nephrol 5:323, 1991.
New varieties of PKU (editorial). Lancet 1:304, 1979.
Nord A, et al. Developmental profile of patients with maple syrup urine disease. J Inherited Metab Dis 14:881, 1991.
North KN, et al. Neonatal onset propionic acidemia: Neurologic and developmental profiles and implications for management. J Pediatr 126:916, 1995.
Nowak-Cooperman KM, et al. The impact of assertiveness, self-concept and coping behavior on self-management abilities in adolescents with phenylketonuria (abstract). J Adolesc Health Care 8:305, 1987.
Ohtani Y, et al. Secondary carnitine deficiency in hyperammonemic attacks of ornithine transcarbamylase deficiency. J Pediatr 112:409, 1988.
Rees JM, Trahms CM. The adolescent and phenylketonuria: Promoting self-management. Top Clin Nutr 2(3):35, 1987.
Ris MD, et al. Early-treated phenylketonuria: Adult neuropsychologic outcome. J Pediatr 124:388, 1994.
Roe CR, et al. Carnitine and the organic acidurias. In: Schaub J, Van Hoof F, Vis HL (eds.). Inborn Errors of Metabolism, Nestle Nutrition Workshop Series, Vol. 24. New York: Raven Press, 1991, p. 19.
Rohr FJ, et al. New England Maternal PKU Project: Prospective study of untreated and treated pregnancies and their outcomes. J Pediatr 110:391, 1987.
Schuett VE, et al. Reinstitution of diet therapy in PKU patients from twenty-two U.S. clinics. Am J Public Health 75:30, 1985.
Shaw DWW, et al. MR imaging of phenylketonuria. Am J Neurol Res 12:403, 1991.
Slovik O. Mitochondrial 2-methylacetoacetyl-CoA thiolase deficiency: An inborn error of isoleucine and ketone body metabolism. J Inherited Metab Dis 16:46, 1993.
Smit GPA, et al. The long-term outcome of patients with glycogen storage diseases. J Inherited Metab Dis 13:411, 1990.
Smith I, et al. Behavior disturbance in 8-year-old children with early treated phenylketonuria. J Pediatr 112:403, 1988.
Smith I, et al. Effect on intelligence of relaxing the low phenylalanine diet in phenylketonuria. Arch Dis Child 65:311, 1990.
Smith I, et al. Effect of stopping low-phenylalanine diet on intellectual progress of children with phenylketonuria. Br Med J 2:723, 1978.
Snyderman SE, et al. The nutritional therapy of histidinemia. J Pediatr 95:712, 1979.
Trahms CM. Long-term nutrition intervention model: The treatment of phenylketonuria. Top Clin Nutr 1(1):62, 1986.
Trahms CM. Low protein diets for children: Guidelines for treatment of common organic acidemias and urea cycle disorders. Top Clin Nutr 2(3):49, 1987.
Trahms CM, et al. Impact of patient attitudes and family function on compliance with treatment of phenylketonuria (abstract). J Adolesc Health Care 8:305, 1987.
Waisbren SE, Levy HL. Agoraphobia in phenylketonuria. J Inherited Metab Dis 14:755, 1991.
Waisbren SE, et al. Predictors of intelligence quotient and intelligence quotient change in persons treated for phenylketonuria early in life. Pediatrics 79:351, 1987.
Walsher M, Stewart PM. Organic acidemia and hyperammonaemia: A review. J Inherited Metab Dis 4:177, 1981.
Williamson MS, et al. Correlates of intelligence tests results in treated phenylketonuric children. Pediatrics 68:161, 1981.
Wolf B, et al. Propionic acidemia: A clinical update. J Pediatr 99:835, 1981.
Wolfsdorf JI, Crigler JF. Cornstarch regimens for nocturnal treatment of young adults with type I glycogen storage disease. Am J Clin Nutr 65:507, 1997.
Wolfsdorf JI, et al. Metabolic control and renal dysfunction in type I glycogen storage disease. J Inherited Metab Dis 20:559, 1997.

ADDITIONAL REFERENCES

Guides for Professionals

Acosta PB, Yannicelli S. A Practitioner's Guide to Selected Inborn Errors of Metabolism. Columbus, OH: Ross Laboratories, 1992.
Committee on Genetics, American Academy of Pediatrics. Newborn Screening Fact Sheets. Pediatrics 98:473, 1996.
de Freitas O, et al. New approaches to the treatment of phenylketonuria. Nutr Rev 57:65, 1999.
Dietary Management of Persons with Metabolic Disorders. Evansville, IN: Mead Johnson & Company, 1994.
Henderson RA, et al. Education of Students with Phenylketonuria (PKU): Information for Teachers, Administrators, and Other School Personnel. National Institutes of Health Publication No. 92-3318. Bethesda, MD: NIH, 1991.
Nutrition Support Protocols: The Ross Metabolic Formula System, 3rd ed. Columbus, OH: Ross Laboratories, 1997.
Scriver CR, et al. The Molecular and Metabolic Basis of Inherited Disease. New York: McGraw Hill, 1995.
Woolridge N (ed.). Quality Assurance Criteria for Pediatric Nutrition Conditions: A Model. V. Inborn Errors of Metabolism. Chicago: The Quality Assurance Committee, Dietitians in Pediatric Practice, The American Dietetic Association, 1988.

Selected Guides for Parents and Children

Dietary Specialties, 865 Centennial Ave., Piscataway, NJ 08854 (1-888-MENU123)—(1) Schuett VE. Low-Protein Bread Machine Baking for PKU, 1993; (2) Schuett VE. Low-Protein Food List for PKU, 1995.
Mead Johnson & Company, Evansville, IN 47721—Living with PKU, 1995.
PKU Clinic, CHDD, Box 357920, University of Washington, Seattle, WA 98195, or http://www.depts.u.washington.edu/pku—(1) New Parents' Guide to PKU; (2) Finger Foods Are Fun; (3) A Babysitter's Guide to PKU; (4) Games that Teach: Learning by Doing for Preschoolers with PKU; (5) Chef Lophe's Phe-nominal Cookbook; (6) The Essentials of PKU: An Informational Pamphlet for Young Adults with PKU and Their Significant Others; (7) Making the Change: From High Phe to Low Phe.
Ross Products Division, Abbott Laboratories, Columbus, OH 43215–1724A Guide for the Family of the CHild with (1) Galactosemia, (2) Phenyketonuria, (3) Maple Syrup Urine Disease, (4) Glutaric Acidemia Type I, (5) Homocystinuria, (6) Isoraleric Acidemia, (7) Tyrosenemia Type I, (8) Propionic Acidemia, 1998.
SHS North America, Gaithersburg, MD 20884, (1–800–365–7354)—Eat Right, Stay Bright: Guide for Hyperphenylalaninemia; (2) Denny the Dragon and His Magic Milk, 1995.
University of Wisconsin Biochemical Genetics Program, 1500 Highland Ave., Madison, WI 53705—Understanding Galactosemia: A Diet Guide, 1997.
University of Wisconsin Press, 114 N Murray Street, Madison, WI 53715—Schuett VE. Low-Protein Cookery for Phenylketonuria, 3rd ed., 1997.

Selected Newsletters and Family Support Groups:

Fatty Oxidation Disorder Communication Network at http://www.cinternet.net/FOD.
Glycogen Storage Disease (UK) at http://www.compulink.co.uk/~embra/agsdhome.html.
Maple Syrup Urine Disease Newsletter, 24806 SR 119, Goshen, IN 46526, or http://www.msud-support.org.
National PKU News, 6869 Woodlawn Ave NE, #116, Seattle, WA 98115, or http://pkunews.org.
Organic Acidemia Association Corporation, 14600 41st Ave. N., Plymouth, MN 55446, or OAANews@aol.com.
Parents of Galactosemic Children, Inc., 2871 Stage Coach Drive, Valley Springs, CA 95252.

Appendices

APPENDIX 1 GENERAL ABBREVIATIONS

ABGs	arterial blood gases	FX	fracture
ACTH	adrenocorticotropic hormone	GB	gallbladder
AD	Alzheimer's disease	GFR	glomerular filtration rate
ADH	antidiuretic hormone	GI	gastrointestinal
ADI	acceptable daily intake	GIP	gastric inhibitory polypeptide
ADL	activities of daily living	GTF	glucose tolerance factor
AI	adequate intake	GTT	glucose tolerance test
AIDS	acquired immunodeficiency syndrome	GVHD	graft-versus-host disease
ALS	amyotrophic lateral sclerosis	HA	hyperalimentation
AP	angina pectoris	HAV	hepatitis A virus
ARF	acute renal failure	Hgb	hemoglobin
ASHD	atherosclerotic heart disease	HBV	hepatitis B virus
ATP	adenosine triphosphate	HCT	hematocrit
BCAA	branched-chain amino acids	HDL	high-density lipoprotein
BEE	basal energy expenditure	HE	hepatic encephalopathy
BHA	butylated hydroxyanisole	HGB	hemoglobin
BHT	butylated hydroxytoluene	HIV	human immunodeficiency virus
BMR	basal metabolic rate	HPN	home parenteral nutrition
BMT	bone marrow transplantation	HSL	hormone-sensitive lipase
BPD	bronchopulmonary dysplasia	HTN	hypertension
BSA	body surface area	HX	history
BV	biologic value	IBD	inflammatory bowel disease
CA	cancer	IBS	irritable bowel syndrome
CAD	coronary artery disease	IBW	ideal body weight
CAPD	continuous ambulatory peritoneal dialysis	ICU	intensive care unit
CAVH	continuous arteriovenous hemofiltration	IDDM	insulin-dependent diabetes mellitus
CC	cardiac cachexia	IF	intrinsic factor
CCK	cholecystokinin	IgE	immunoglobulin E
CCU	coronary care unit	IGT	impaired glucose tolerance
CDC	Centers for Disease Control and Prevention	IL-2	interleukin-2
CHD	coronary heart disease	IM	intramuscular
CHF	congestive heart failure	INH	isonicotinic acid hydrazide
CHI	closed head injury	IV	intravenous
CNS	central nervous system	IVH	intravenous hyperalimentation
COPD	chronic obstructive pulmonary disease	J	joule
CPN	central parenteral nutrition	kcal (Cal)	kilocalorie
CSII	continuous subcutaneous insulin infusion	kJ	kilojoule
CSF	cerebrospinal fluid	KS	Kaposi's sarcoma
CVA	cerebrovascular accident	KUB	kidney, ureter, bladder
DCCT	Diabetes Control and Complications Trial	LBM	lean body mass
DHA	docosahexaenoic acid	LCT	long-chain triglyceride
DHEW	Department of Health, Education, and Welfare	LDL	low-density lipoprotein
DHHS	Department of Health and Human Services	LES	lower esophageal sphincter
DJD	degenerative joint disease	LFT	liver function tests
DKA	diabetic ketoacidosis	LNA	α-linolenic acid
DM	diabetes mellitus	LPL	lipoprotein lipase
DNA	deoxyribonucleic acid	MAOI	monoamine oxidase inhibitor
DRI	dietary reference intake	MCH	mean corpuscular hemoglobin
ECG/EKG	electrocardiogram	MCT	medium-chain triglyceride
EDTA	ethylenediaminotetraacetate	MCV	mean corpuscular volume
EFA	essential fatty acid	MET	metabolic equivalent
EPA	eicosapentaenoic acid	MFOS	mixed-function oxidase system
EPO	erythropoietin	MI	myocardial infarction
ERT	enzyme replacement therapy	MOM	milk of magnesia
ERT	estrogen replacement therapy	MSG	monosodium glutamate
ESR	erythrocyte sedimentation rate	MSUD	maple syrup urine disease
ESRD	end-stage renal disease	NANB	non-A, non-B hepatitis virus
FAD	flavin adenine dinucleotide	NCEP	National Cholesterol Education Program
FBG	fasting blood glucose	NCJ	needle catheter jejunostomy
FBS	fasting blood sugar	NG	nasogastric
FFA	free fatty acids	NI	nutritional index
FIGLU	formimino glutamic acid	NIDDM	non–insulin-dependent diabetes
FMN	flavin mononucleotide	NPO	nothing by mouth
FPG	fasting plasma glucose	NPU	net protein utilization
FTT	failure to thrive	NSAID	nonsteroidal anti-inflammatory drug

APPENDIX 1 GENERAL ABBREVIATIONS *(continued)*

NSP	nonstarch polysaccharides	ROS	review of systems
N & V	nausea and vomiting	RQ	respiratory quotient
OC	oral contraceptive	RS	resistant starches
OGTT	oral glucose tolerance test	RTA	renal tubular acidosis
OHA	oral hypoglycemic agent	SCA	sickle cell anemia
PAS	para-aminosalicylic acid	SCT	short-chain triglyceride
PBI	protein-bound iodine	SFA	saturated fatty acid
PCM	protein caloric malnutrition	SLE	systemic lupus erythematosus
PD	Parkinson's disease	SMBG	self-monitoring of blood glucose
PEG	percutaneous endoscopic gastrostomy	SOB	shortness of breath
PEM	protein energy malnutrition	TBSA	total body surface area
PER	protein efficiency ratio	TC	total cholesterol
PG	prostaglandin	TEE	total energy expenditure
PHE	phenylalanine	TEF	thermic effect of food
PKU	phenylketonuria	TG	triglyceride or triacylglycerol
PLP	pyridoxal phosphate	THFA	tetrahydrofolate
PPN	peripheral parenteral nutrition	TIA	transient ischemic attack
PT	patient	TIBC	total iron-binding capacity
PTA	prior to admission	TNF	tumor necrosis factor
PU	peptic ulcer	TPN	total parenteral nutrition
PUFA	polyunsaturated fatty acid	TS	transferrin saturation
RAST	radioallergosorbent test	UL	tolerable upper intake level
RBC	red blood cell	URI	upper respiratory infection
RDA	recommended dietary allowance	UTI	urinary tract infection
RDS	respiratory distress syndrome	VLCD	very-low-calorie diet
REE	resting energy expenditure	VLDL	very-low-density lipoprotein
RMR	resting metabolic rate	VOD	venous occlusive disease
RNA	ribonucleic acid	VS	vital signs
R/O	rule out	WNL	within normal limits

APPENDIX 2 UNIT ABBREVIATIONS

Along with the specialized vocabulary that is used in the medical, dietetic, and nursing fields, there are acceptable forms of abbreviations. Here is a list of abbreviations commonly used.

aa: Gr. *ana;* of each
ac: L. *ante cibum;* before meals
ad, add: L. *adde, addatus,* or *addantur;* add or added
ad lib: L. *ad libitum;* at pleasure, as desired
aq: L. *aqua;* water
aq dest: L. *aqua destillata;* distilled water
bid, bis in d: L. *bis in die;* twice a day
c: L. *cum;* with
c: cup
cc: cubic centimeter
Cent; cent; C: centrigrade, Celsius
cm: centimeter
dilut: L. *dilutus;* dilute
div: L. *divide;* divide
fac: make
g: gram
gr: L. *granum;* grain
gtt: L. *guttae;* drops
hs: L. *hora somni;* at hour of sleep
IU: international unit
kcal: kilocalorie
kg: kilogram
kJ: kilojoule
lb: pound
μg: microgram
mcg: microgram
μU: microunit
mEq: milliequivalent
mg: milligram
mil or mL: milliliter
mM: millimole
mOsm: milliosmole
oz: ounce
prn: L. *pro re nata:* may be repeated according to instructions
pt: pint
pulv: L. *pulvis;* powder
qd: L. *quaque die:* every day
QID, qid: L. *quater in die;* four times daily
q3h: every 3 hours
qs: L. *quantum satis;* a sufficient quantity
qt: quart
RE: retinol equivalent
s: L. *sine;* without
sol: solution
ss: L. *semis;* half
stat: L. *statim;* immediately
t, tsp: teaspoon
T, tbsp: tablespoon
tid. L. *ter in die:* three times a day

APPENDIX 3 POTENTIAL ICD-9-CM CODES FOR NUTRITION SERVICES

Carcinoma (Primary)

195.2 Carcinoma, abdomen
188 Carcinoma, bladder, ADR
170 Carcinoma, bone and articular cartilage, ADR
191 Carcinoma, brain, ADR
174 Carcinoma, breast (female), ADR
154.0 Carcinoma, colon
189.0 Carcinoma, kidney, except pelvis, NOS
155.0 Carcinoma, liver
145 Carcinoma, mouth, ADR
183.0 Carcinoma, ovary
157 Carcinoma, pancreas, ADR
185 Carcinoma, prostate
154.1 Carcinoma, rectum
173 Carcinoma, skin, ADR
151 Carcinoma, stomach, ADR
193 Carcinoma, thyroid
162 Carcinoma, trachea, lung and bronchus, ADR
182 Carcinoma, body of uterus, ADR

Cardiovascular

413.9 Angina pectoris, U, N
411.1 Angina, unstable
424.1 Aortic valve disorders, NOS
427.9 Arrythmia, NOS, U
785.9 Bruit, arterial, N
429.2 Cardiovascular disease, U, N
786.50 Chest pain, U, N
428.0 Congestive heart failure
414.01 Coronary atherosclerosis, of native coronary artery
401.1 Hypertension, essential, benign
401.1 Hypertension, essential, malignant
401.9 Hypertension, U, N
402.90 Hypertensive heart disease, U, w/o CHF
402.91 Hypertensive heart disease, U, w/CHF
403.00 Hypertensive renal disease, malignant, w/o renal failure
403.01 Hypertensive renal disease, malignant, w/renal failure
458.0 Hypotension, orthostatic
410.00 Myocardial infarction, of anterolateral wall, episode of care unspec., N
410.01 Myocardial infarction, acute, of other anterolateral wall, episode of care unspec., N
412 Myocardial infarction, status post
443.9 Peripheral vascular disease, U, N
416.0 Primary pulmonary hypertension
436 Stroke, acute but ill-defined, NOS
785.0 Tachycardia, U, N
435.9 Transient cerebral ischemia, U, N

Endocrine and Metabolic Disorders

790.2 Abnormal glucose tolerance test
255.4 Addison's disease, NOS
255.0 Cushing's syndrome
277.00 Cystic fibrosis, w/o meconium ileus
277.01 Cystic fibrosis, w/meconium ileus
253.5 Diabetes insipidus
250.0 Diabetes mellitus (DM), w/o mention of complications, ADR*
250.1 Diabetes w/ketoacidosis, ADR*
250.2 Diabetes w/hyperosmolar coma, ADR*
250.3 Diabetes w/other coma, ADR*
250.4 Diabetes w/renal manifestations, ADR*
250.5 Diabetes w/ophthalmic manifestations, ADR*
250.6 Diabetes w/neurological manifestations, ADR*
250.7 Diabetes w/peripheral circulatory disorders, ADR*
250.8 Diabetes w/other specified manifestations, ADR*
357.2 Diabetic polyneuropathy, NPD
271.1 Galactosemia
785.4 Gangrene, NOS
240.9 Goiter, U, N
242.00 Grave's disease, w/o thyrotoxic crisis or storm
242.01 Grave's disease, w/thyrotoxic crisis or storm
255.1 Hyperaldosteronism
275.4 Hypercalcemia
272.0 Hypercholesterolemia, pure
272.1 Hyperglyceridemia, pure
272.2 Hyperlipidemia, mixed
252.0 Hyperparathyroidism
242.9 Hyperthyroidism, NOS, N
251.2 Hypoglycemia, U, N
252.1 Hypoparathyroidism
244.0 Hypothyroidism, post surgical
244.9 Hypothyroidism, U, N, NOS
758.7 Klinefelter's syndrome
270.3 Maple syrup urine disease
278.00 Obesity, U, N, NOS
278.01 Obesity, morbid
270.1 Phenylketonuria

Gastrointestinal

571.2 Alcoholic cirrhosis of liver
571.0 Alcoholic fatty liver
535.30 Alcoholic gastritis, w/o hemorrhage
535.31 Alcoholic gastritis, w/hemorrhage
571.1 Alcoholic hepatitis, acute
571.3 Alcoholic liver damage, U, N
579.2 Blind loop syndrome
574.50 Calculus of bile duct w/o cholecystitis, w/o obstruction
574.51 Calculus of bile duct w/o cholecystitis, w/obstruction
579.0 Celiac disease
575.0 Cholecystitis, acute
575.10 Cholecystitis, chronic, U, N
571.5 Cirrhosis of liver, w/o mention of alcohol
749.10 Cleft lip, U, N
749.20 Cleft palate w/cleft lip, U, N
749.00 Cleft palate, U, N
558.2 Colitis and gastorenteritis, toxic
556.9 Colitis, ulcerative, U, N
564.0 Constipation
555.0 Crohn's disease, small intestine
555.1 Crohn's disease, large intestine
564.5 Diarrhea, functional
562.10 Diverticulosis
562.11 Diverticulitis
564.2 Dumping syndrome
536.8 Dyspepsia, other disorders of stomach, N
787.2 Dysphagia
787.3 Flatulence
575.9 Gallbladder, disorder, U
535.00 Gastritis, acute, w/o hemorrhage
535.01 Gastritis, acute, w/hemorrhage
558.9 Gastroenteritis, NOS, N
523.0 Gingivitis, acute
523.1 Gingivitis, chronic
529.0 Glossitis
787.1 Heartburn
578.0 Hematemesis
578.9 Hemorrhage of GI tract, U, N
573.3 Hepatitis, U, N
789.1 Hepatomegaly
271.2 Hereditary fructose intolerance
553.3 Hiatal hernia

APPENDIX 3 POTENTIAL ICD-9-CM CODES FOR NUTRITION SERVICES *(continued)*

536.2 Hyperemesis (not of pregnancy)
560.1 Ileus, paralytic
560.30 Impaction of colon, N
536.8 Indigestion
569.61 Infection, colostomy or enterostomy
564.1 Irritable colon (irritable bowel syndrome)
579.8 Steatorrhea, chronic, N
271.3 Malabsorption, glucose, lactose, sucrose
579.9 Malabsorption syndrome, NOS
578.1 Melena
787.01 Nausea with vomiting
787.02 Nausea alone
560.9 Obstruction, intestinal, U, N
577.9 Pancreas, unspec. disease of, N
577.0 Pancreatitis, acute
577.1 Pancreatitis, chronic
569.89 Pericolitis, intestine, N
528.9 Sore mouth, denture, N
528.0 Stomatitis
787.7 Stool, abnormal
525.1 Teeth loss
569.82 Ulceration, intestine
533.00 Ulcer, peptic, acute w/hemorrhage, w/obstruction
533.10 Ulcer, peptic, acute w/perforation, w/ obstruction
557.0 Vascular insufficiency of intestine, chronic
560.2 Volvulus
787.03 Vomiting alone
536.2 Vomiting, persistent

Genitourinary

626.0 Amenorrhea
753.10 Cystic kidney disease, U, N
595.9 Cystitis, U, N
625.3 Dysmenorrhea
403.9 Hypertensive renal disease, U, ADR
592.0 Kidney stones
627.2 Menopause symptoms
626.9 Menstrual disorders, U, N
626.0 Menstruation, absence
626.4 Menstruation, irregular
583.0 Nephritis, w/proliferative glomerulonephritis
583.9 Nephritis, NOS, N
583.81 Nephritis and nephropathy, NPD
626.1 Oligomenorrhea
625.4 Premenstrual tension syndromes
791.0 Proteinurea
590.80 Pyelonephritis, U, N
584.9 Renal failure, acute, U, N
585 Renal failure, chronic
592.9 Urinary calculus, U, N
599.0 Urinary tract infection, unspec. site, N

Hematology

285.9 Anemia, U, N
281.2 Anemia, folate deficiency
281.3 Anemia, folate & B_{12} deficiency
282.2 Anemia, G-6-PD deficiency
280.9 Anemia, iron deficiency, U, N
281.4 Anemia, protein deficiency
280.1 Anemia, secondary to lack of dietary iron intake
282.60 Anemia, sickle cell, U, N
281.9 Anemia, simple chronic
281.1 Anemia, vitamin B_{12} deficiency, U, N
276.9 Electrolyte and fluid disorders, NEC, N
275.4 Hypocalcemia
251.2 Hypoglycemia, U, N
276.8 Hypokalemia
282.5 Sickle-cell trait
282.4 Thalassemias

Infections

006.9 Ambebiasis, U, N
114.9 Coccidioidomycosis, U, N
078.5 Cytomegaloviral disease
008.00 *E. coli* infection, U, N
487.0 Flu w/pneumonia
008.8 Gastroenteritis, viral, N, NEC
007.1 Giardiasis
573.3 Hepatitis, U, N
070.1 Hepatitis A, viral, w/o hepatic coma
070.3 Hepatitis B, viral, w/o hepatic coma, acute, N
054 Herpes simplex, ADR
042 Human immunodeficiency virus (HIV) disease
075 Mononucleosis, infectious
136.3 Pneumocystosis
480.0 Pneumonia, due to adenovirus
481 Pneumonia, pneumococcal
486 Pneumonia, organism unspec., N
031.0 Pulmonary disease, mycobacterium infection
034.0 Streptococcal sore throat
112.0 Thrush, oral
463 Tonsillitis, acute
130.9 Toxoplasmosis, U, N
079.98 Viral and chlamydial infections, U, N

Musculoskeletal

714.0 Arthritis, rheumatoid
274.0 Arthropathy, gouty
724.5 Backache, U, N
727.3 Bursitis, NOS, N
724.2 Lumbago (low back pain)
340 Multiple sclerosis
729.1 Myalgia and myositis, U, N
268.2 Osteomalacia, U, N
730.00 Osteomyelitis, site unspec., N
733.00 Osteoporosis, U, N

Nervous System

305.00 Alcohol abuse, U, N
305.20 Cannabis abuse, U, N
343.9 Cerebral palsy, NOS, U
304.40 Drug dependence-amphetamines, U, N
304.10 Drug dependence-barbiturates, U, N
304.30 Drug dependence-cannabis, U, N
304.20 Drug dependence-cocaine, U, N
304.00 Drug dependence-opioid type, U, N
311 Depression disorder, NEC
300.4 Depression disorder, neurotic
345.0 Epilepsy, nonconvulsive, ADR
345.1 Epilepsy, convulsive, ADR
345.2 Epilepsy, Petit mal status
345.3 Epilepsy, Grand mal status
742.1 Microcephalus
346.9 Migraine, U, N, ADR
359.0 Muscular dystrophy, congenital hereditary
300.01 Panic disorder
780.50 Sleep disturbances, U, N
300.23 Social phobia, fear of eating in public
780.2 Syncope and collapse

Nutritional

790.6 Abnormal blood level, iron, zinc, N
783.1 Abnormal weight gain

APPENDIX 3 POTENTIAL ICD-9-CM CODES FOR NUTRITION SERVICES *(continued)*

Code	Description
783.2	Abnormal weight loss
783.0	Anorexia, loss of appetite (not nervosa)
307.1	Anorexia nervosa
263.2	Arrested development following protein-calorie malnutrition
265.0	Beriberi
307.51	Bulimia, nonorganic nature
267.0	Deficiency, ascorbic acid (Vit C)
264.7	Deficiency, vitamin A, xeropthalmia, N
266.9	Deficiency, vitamin B, U, N
265.1	Deficiency, vitamin B_1, U, N
266.0	Deficiency, vitamin B_2
266.1	Deficiency, vitamin B_6
266.2	Deficiency, B_{12} or folic acid
269.3	Deficiency, calcium
261	Deficiency, calorie (marasmus)
268.9	Deficiency, vitamin D, U, N
280.9	Deficiency, iron, anemia, U, N
271.3	Deficiency, lactose
265.2	Deficiency, niacin (pellagra)
269.9	Deficiency, nutritional, U
276.5	Dehydration, volume depletion
781.1	Disturbances of sensation of smell and taste
783.4	Failure to thrive
783.3	Feeding problem, elderly or infant
779.3	Feeding problem, newborn
005.9	Food poisoning, U, N
278.3	Hypercarotenemia
278.2	Hypervitaminosis A
278.4	Hypervitaminosis D
264.8	Keratosis, vitamin A deficiency, N
260	Kwashiorkor
579.3	Malnutrition, malabsorption, post gastro surgery, N
278.01	Obesity, morbid
307.52	Pica
263.9	Protein-calorie malnutrition, U, N
263.0	Protein-calorie malnutrition, moderate
783.6	Polyphagia
268.0	Rickets, active
783.4	Short stature

Perinatal

Code	Description
789.00	Abdominal pain, colic, unspec. site, N
758.0	Down syndrome
676.4	Lactation, failure, U, ADR
675.20	Mastitis, nonpurulent, U, ADR
775.1	Neonatal diabetes mellitus
760.70	Noxious substance, affecting fetus via placenta or breast milk, U, N
656.50	Poor fetal growth, unspec. as to care

Pregnancy

Code	Description
646.3	Aborter, habitual, ADR
648.8	Diabetes mellitus (gestational), U
V23.3	Grand multiparity
643.0	Hyperemesis gravidarum, ADR
646.8	Insufficient weight gain
V61.5	Multiparity
642.7	Pre-eclampsia or eclampsia superimposed on pre-existing hypertension, unspec. as to care
642.4	Pre-eclampsia, U or mild, ADR
643.9	Vomiting of pregnancy, U, N, ADR

Respiratory

Code	Description
786.09	Apnea, N
493.9	Asthma, U, N, ADR
466.0	Bronchitis, acute
491.0	Bronchitis, simple, chronic
491.1	Bronchitis, chronic, recurrent
492.8	Emphysema, NOS, N
780.53	Hypersomnia, w/sleep apnea
474.1	Hypertrophy of tonsils and adenoids
786.01	Hyperventilation
487.1	Influenza w/other respiratory manifestations, N
780.51	Insomnia, w/sleep apnea
482.9	Pneumonia, bacterial, U, N
480.9	Pneumonia, viral, U, N
472.0	Rhinitis, chronic (excludes allergic)
474.0	Tonsillitis, chronic

Signs & Symptoms

Code	Description
995.3	Allergy, excludes hayfever, dermatitis, allergic diarrhea, U, N
796.2	Blood pressure, elevated, w/o hypertension
782.3	Edema
780.7	Fatigue and malaise
780.6	Fever
784.0	Headache
789.1	Hepatomegaly
782.4	Jaundice, not of newborn, U
785.6	Lymph nodes, enlargement
789.2	Splenomegaly

Skin

Code	Description
682.9	Cellulitis and abscess, site unspec., N
707.0	Decubitus ulcer
708.9	Hives, NOS, N
696.1	Psoriasis, other, N
782.1	Rash and other nonspecific skin eruption, N
707.1	Ulcer of lower limbs, except decubitus

*The following fifth-digit is for use with category 250:
0 type II (non–insulin-dependent type) (NIDDM type) (adult-onset type) or unspecified type, not stated as uncontrolled
1 type I (insulin-dependent type) (IDDM) (juvenile type), not stated as uncontrolled
2 type II (non–insulin-dependent type) (NIDDM type) (adult-onset type) or unspecified type, uncontrolled
3 type I (insulin-dependent type) (IDDM) (juvenile type), uncontrolled

ADR = Additional digit required
N = Nonspecific code
NOS = Not otherwise specified
NEC = Not elsewhere classified
NPD = Not a primary diagnosis
U = Unspecified

Reference:
International Classification of Diseases, Clinical Modification 1997 (ICD-9-CM), Delaware: American Medical Association, 1996.

Each year, the ICD-9-CM is updated. Check the most recent publication year for accurate information, clarification and additional digits not listed here.
To obtain an ICD-9-CM book, contact the AMA at 800/621-8335 or visit website @ http://www.mcis.duke.edu/standards/termcode/codehome.htm/.
ICD-10 codes are the next generation of codes not yet implemented in the U.S.
From The American Dietetic Association, Reimbursement team. Chicago: The American Dietetic Association, 1998.

APPENDIX 4 MILLIEQUIVALENTS AND MILLIGRAMS OF ELECTROLYTES*

TO CONVERT MILLIGRAMS TO MILLIEQUIVALENTS

1. Divide milligrams by atomic weight and then multiply by the valence

$$\frac{\text{Milligrams}}{\text{Atomic weight}} \times \text{valence} = \text{milliequivalents}$$

MINERAL ELEMENT	CHEMICAL SYMBOL	ATOMIC WEIGHT	VALENCE
Calcium	Ca	40	2
Chlorine	Cl	35.4	1
Magnesium	Mg	24.3	2
Phosphorus	P	31	2
Potassium	K	39	1
Sodium	Na	23	1
Sulfate	SO_4	96	2
Sulfur	S	32	

TO CONVERT SPECIFIC WEIGHT OF SODIUM TO SODIUM CHLORIDE

1. Multiply by 2.54
   Example: 1,000 mg sodium = 1,000 × 2.54 = 2,540 mg sodium chloride (2.5 g)

TO CONVERT SPECIFIC WEIGHT OF SODIUM CHLORIDE TO SODIUM

1. Multiply by 0.393
   Example: 2.5 g sodium chloride = 2.5 × 0.393 = 1,000 mg sodium

MILLIGRAMS	SODIUM VALUES (MILLIEQUIVALENTS)	GRAMS OF SODIUM CHLORIDE
500	21.8	1.3
1,000	43.5	2.5
1,500	75.3	3.8
2,000	87.0	5.0

*Adapted from Nelson JK, Moxness KE, et al. *Mayo clinic diet manual,* 7th ed. St. Louis: Mosby-YearBook, 1994, p. 705.

APPENDIX 5 APPROXIMATE CONVERSIONS TO AND FROM METRIC MEASURES

APPROXIMATE CONVERSIONS TO METRIC MEASURES*†

When You Know	Multiply By	To Find
Length		
Inches	2.5	Centimeters
Feet	30	Centimeters
Yards	0.9	Meters
Miles	1.6	Kilometers
Area		
Square inches	6.5	Square centimeters
Square feet	9.09	Square meters
Square yards	0.8	Square meters
Square miles	2.6	Square kilometers
Acres	0.4	Hectares
Mass (weight)		
Ounces	28	Grams
Pounds	0.45	Kilograms
Short tons (2,000 lb)	0.9	Tonnes
Volume		
Teaspoons	5	Milliliters
Tablespoons	15	Milliliters
Fluid ounces	30	Milliliters
Cups	0.24	Liters
Pints	0.47	Liters
Quarts	0.95	Liters
Gallons	3.8	Liters
Cubic feet	0.03	Cubic meters
Cubic yards	0.76	Cubic meters
Temperature		
Fahrenheit	5/9 (after subtracting 32)	Celsius

APPROXIMATE CONVERSIONS FROM METRIC MEASURES*†

When You Know	Multiply By	To Find
Length		
Millimeters	0.04	Inches
Centimeters	0.4	Inches
Meters	3.3	Feet
Meters	1.1	Yards
Kilometers	0.6	Miles
Area		
Square centimeters	0.16	Square inches
Square meters	1.2	Square yards
Square kilometers	0.4	Square miles
Hectares (10,000 m^2)	2.5	Acres
Mass (weight)		
Grams	0.035	Ounces
Kilograms	2.2	Pounds
Tonnes (1,000 kg)	1.1	Short tons
Volume		
Milliliters	0.03	Fluid ounces
Liters	2.1	Pints
Liters	1.06	Quarts
Liters	0.26	Gallons
Cubic meters	35	Cubic feet
Cubic meters	1.3	Cubic yards
Temperature		
Celsius	9/5 (then add 32)	Fahrenheit

*Adapted from Nelson JK, Moxness KE, et al. *Mayo clinic diet manual,* 7th ed. St. Louis: Mosby-YearBook, 1994, p. 707.

†From U.S. Department of Commerce, National Bureau of Standards. Metric conversion card (NBS Special Publication 365). Washington, DC, Government Printing Office, 1972.

APPENDIX 6 BOYS: BIRTH TO 36 MONTHS; PHYSICAL GROWTH NCHS PERCENTILES

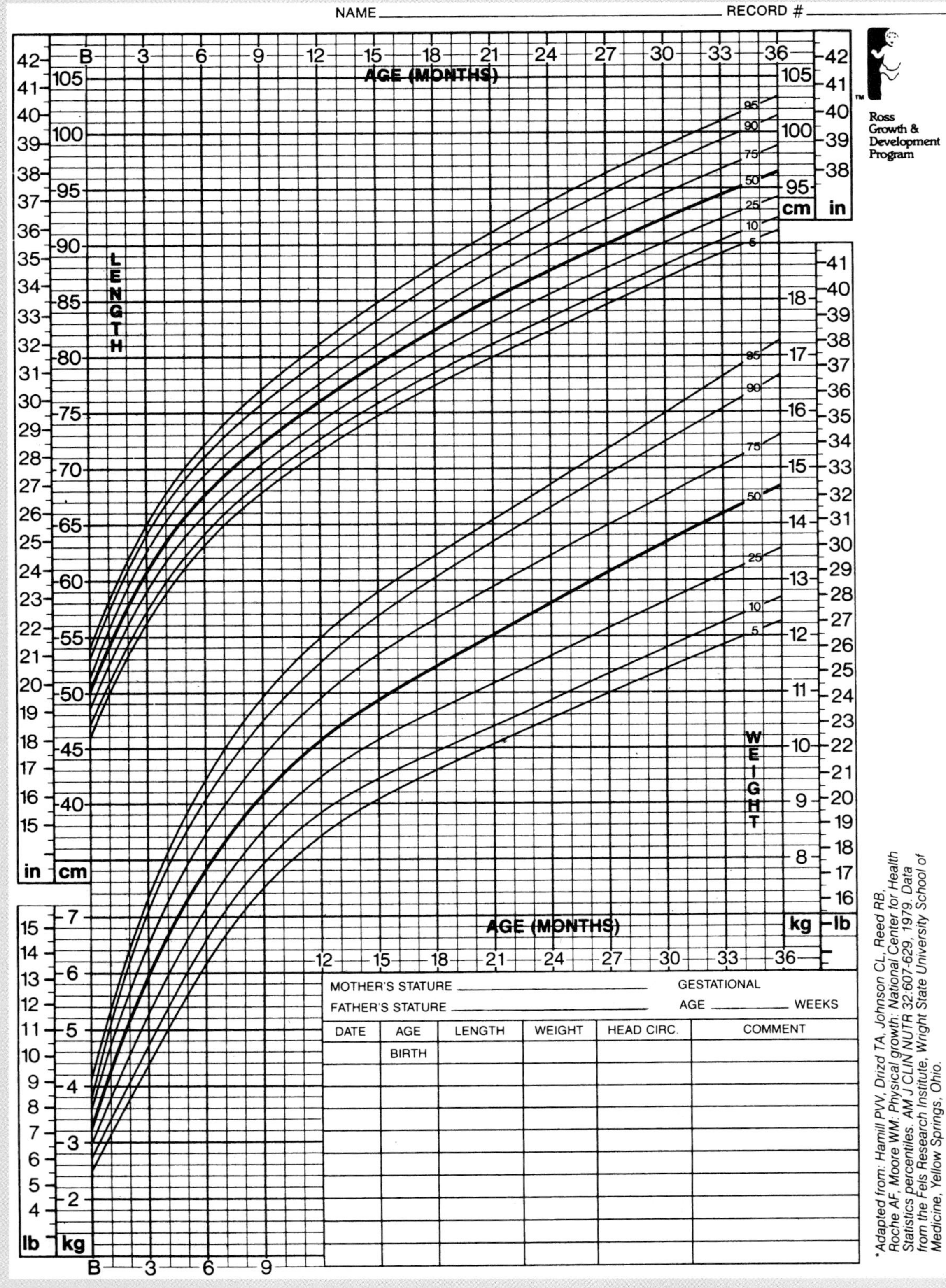

APPENDIX 7 BOYS: BIRTH TO 36 MONTHS; PHYSICAL GROWTH NCHS PERCENTILES*

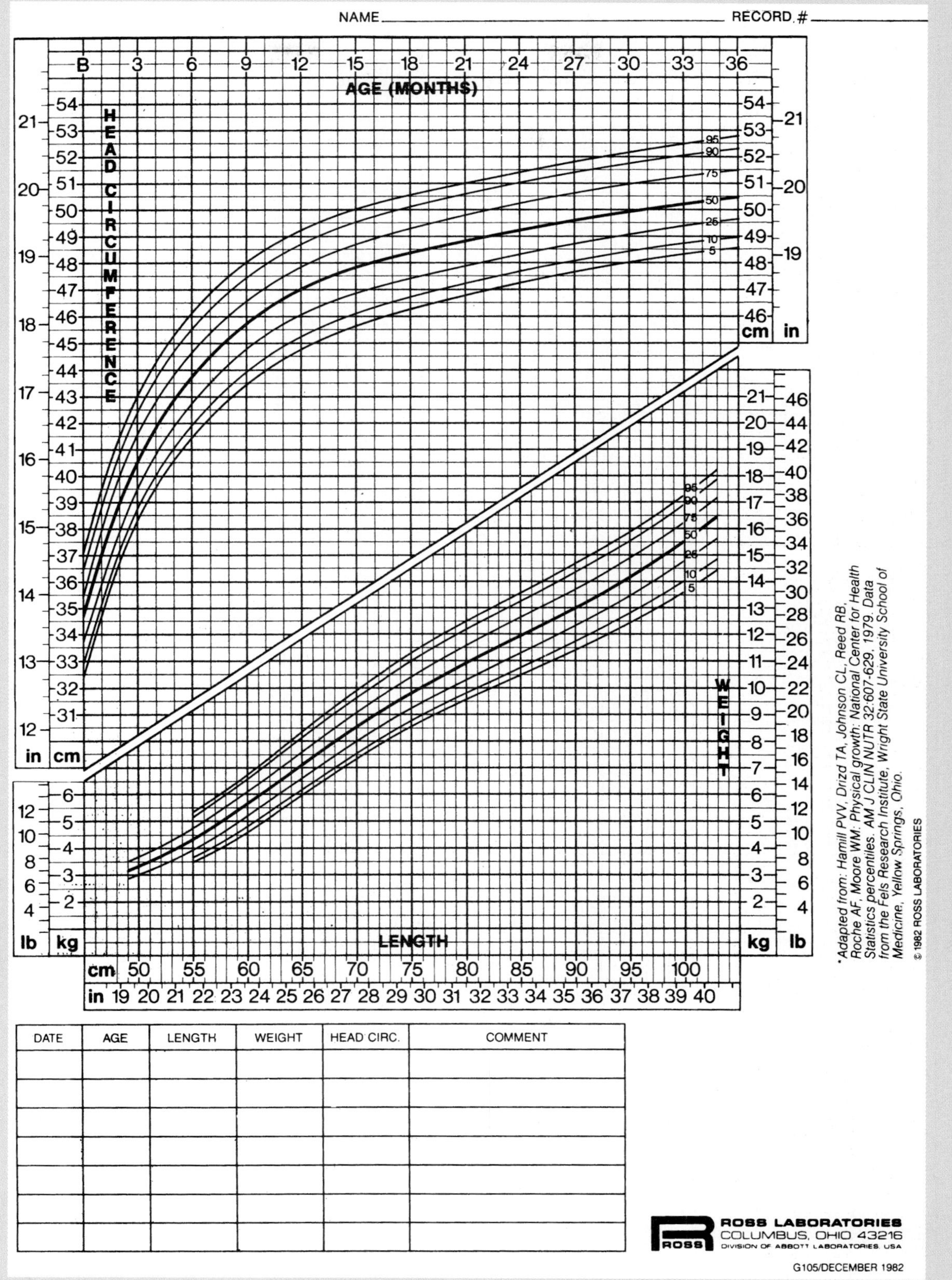

DATE	AGE	LENGTH	WEIGHT	HEAD CIRC.	COMMENT

APPENDIX 8 BOYS: 2 TO 18 YEARS; PHYSICAL GROWTH NCHS PERCENTILES*

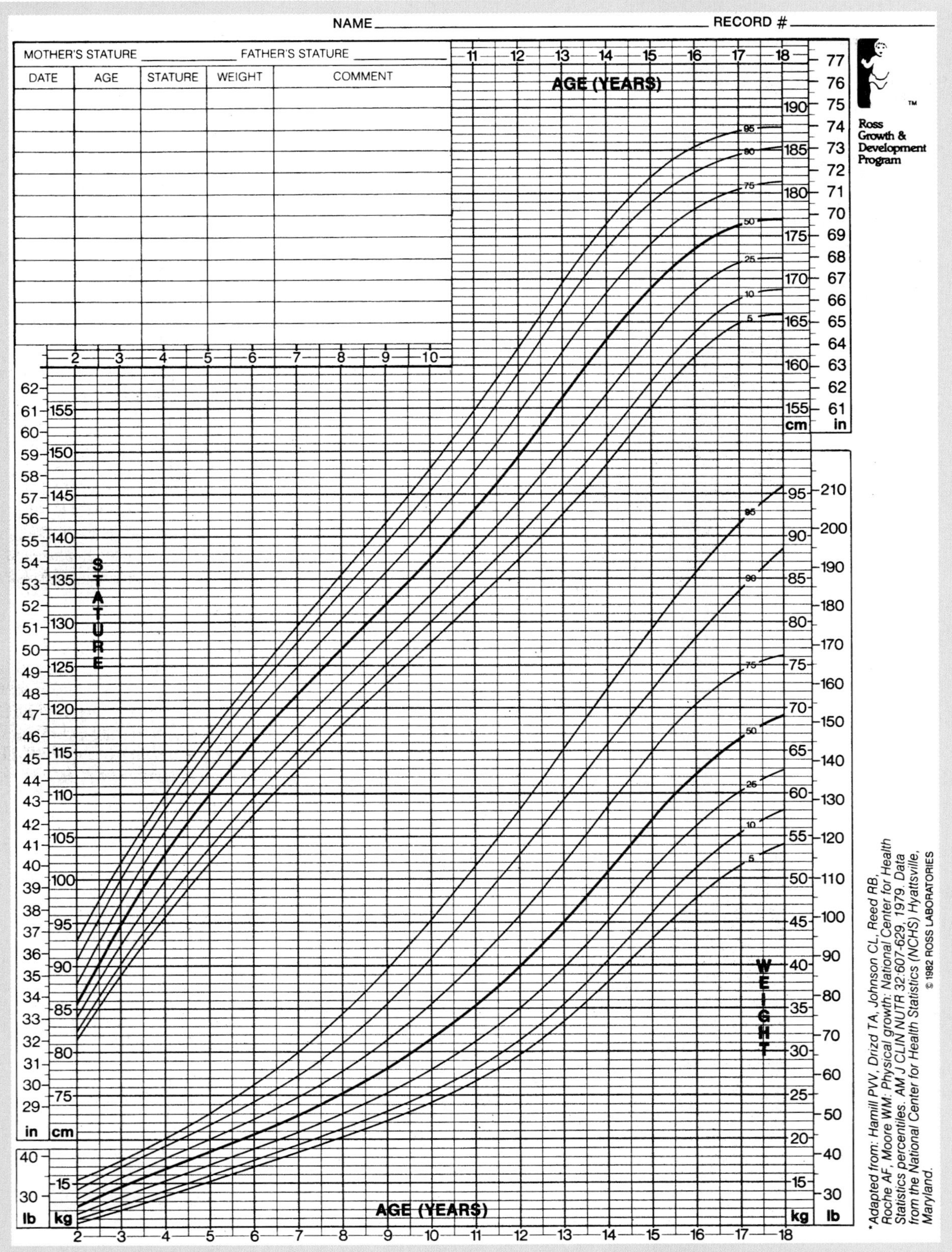

APPENDIX 9 BOYS: PREPUBESCENT; PHYSICAL GROWTH NCHS PERCENTILES*

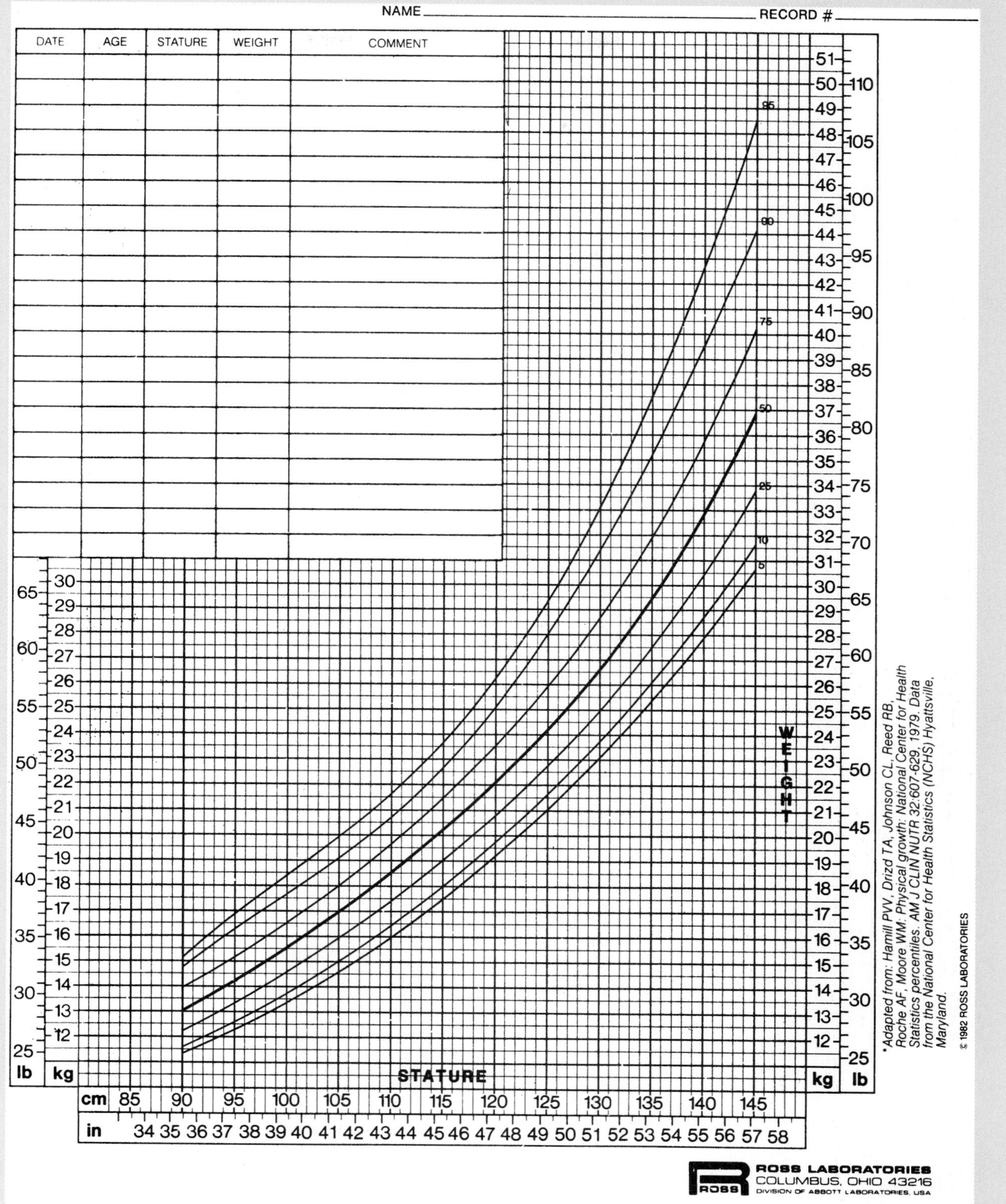

ROSS LABORATORIES
COLUMBUS, OHIO 43216
DIVISION OF ABBOTT LABORATORIES, USA

G107/DECEMBER 1982

APPENDIX 10 GIRLS: BIRTH TO 36 MONTHS; PHYSICAL GROWTH NCHS PERCENTILES*

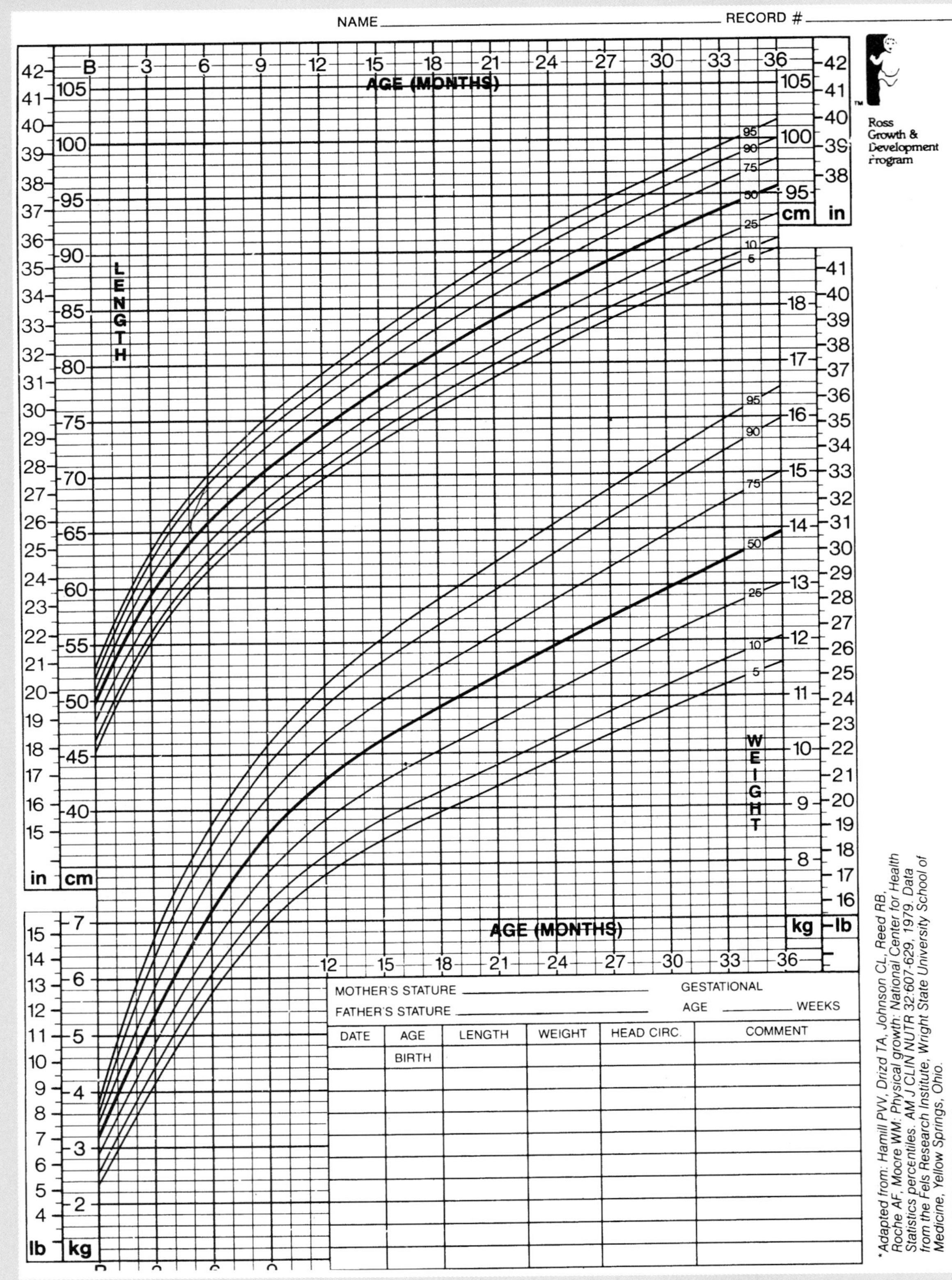

APPENDIX 11 GIRLS: BIRTH TO 36 MONTHS; PHYSICAL GROWTH NCHS PERCENTILES*

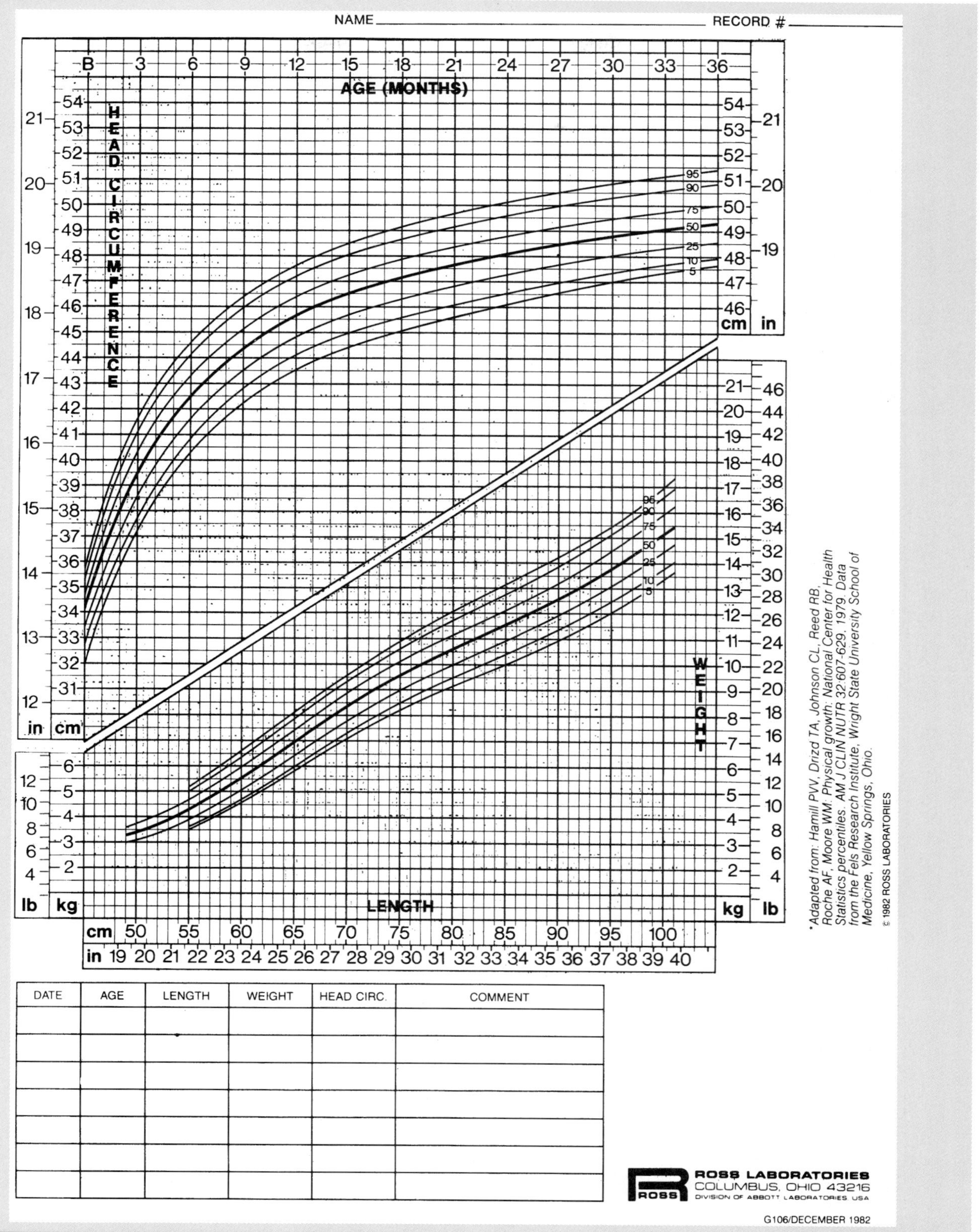

DATE	AGE	LENGTH	WEIGHT	HEAD CIRC.	COMMENT

APPENDIX 12 GIRLS: 2 TO 18 YEARS; PHYSICAL GROWTH NCHS PERCENTILES*

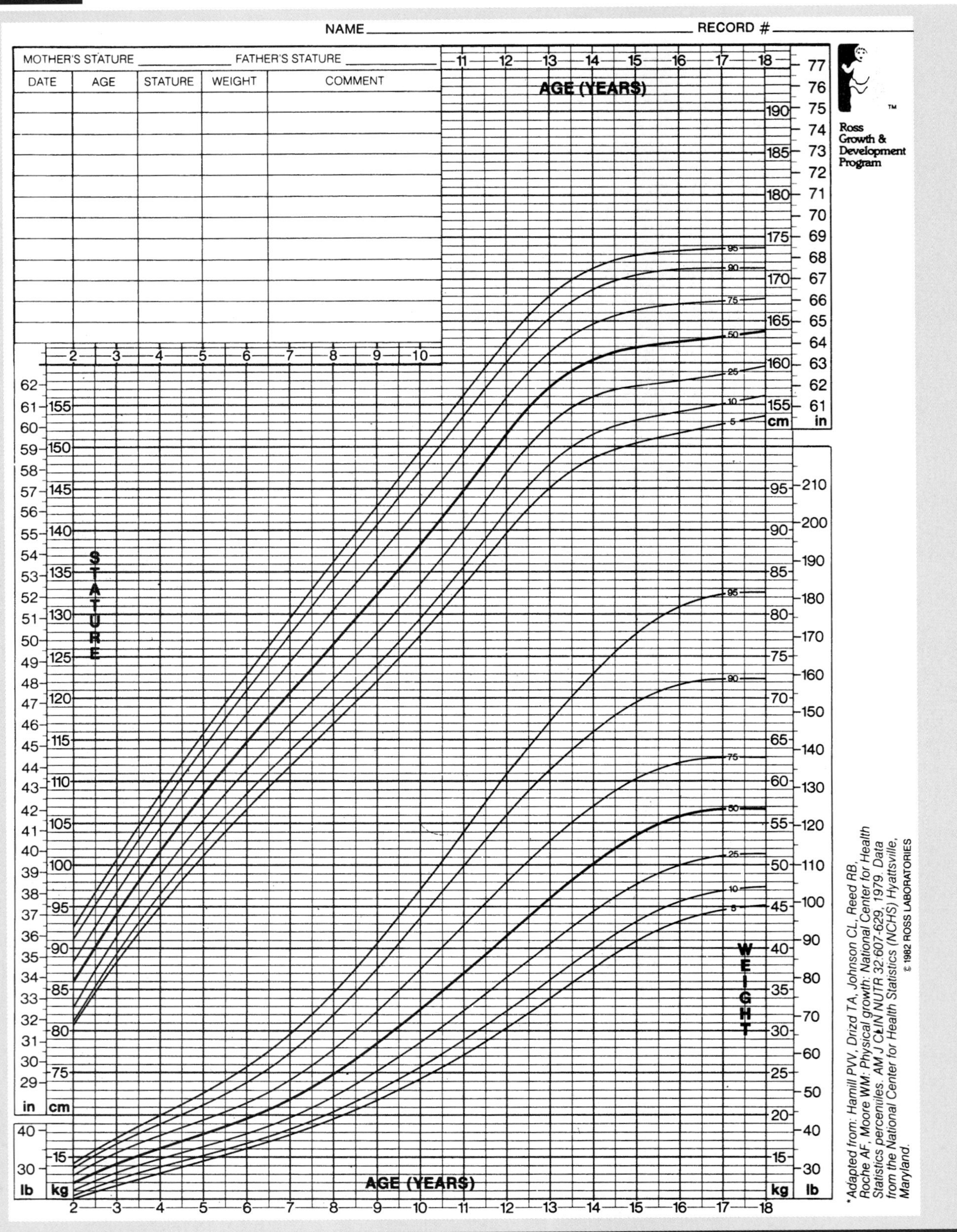

*Adapted from: Hamill PVV, Drizd TA, Johnson CL, Reed RB, Roche AF, Moore WM: Physical growth: National Center for Health Statistics percentiles. AM J CLIN NUTR 32:607-629, 1979. Data from the National Center for Health Statistics (NCHS) Hyattsville, Maryland.

APPENDIX 13 GIRLS: PREPUBESCENT; PHYSICAL GROWTH NCHS PERCENTILES*

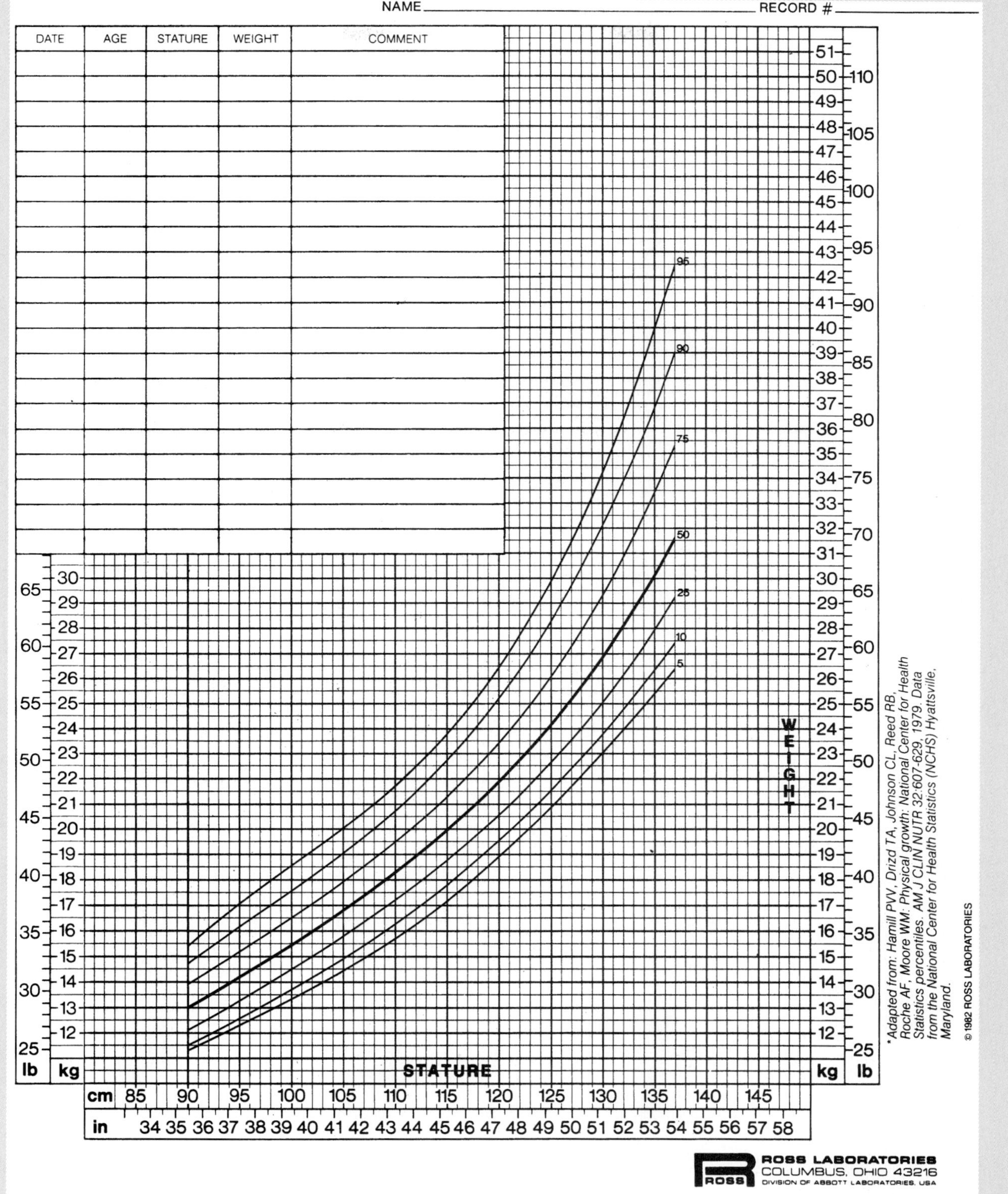

APPENDIX 14 STAGES OF ADOLESCENT DEVELOPMENT FOR FEMALES

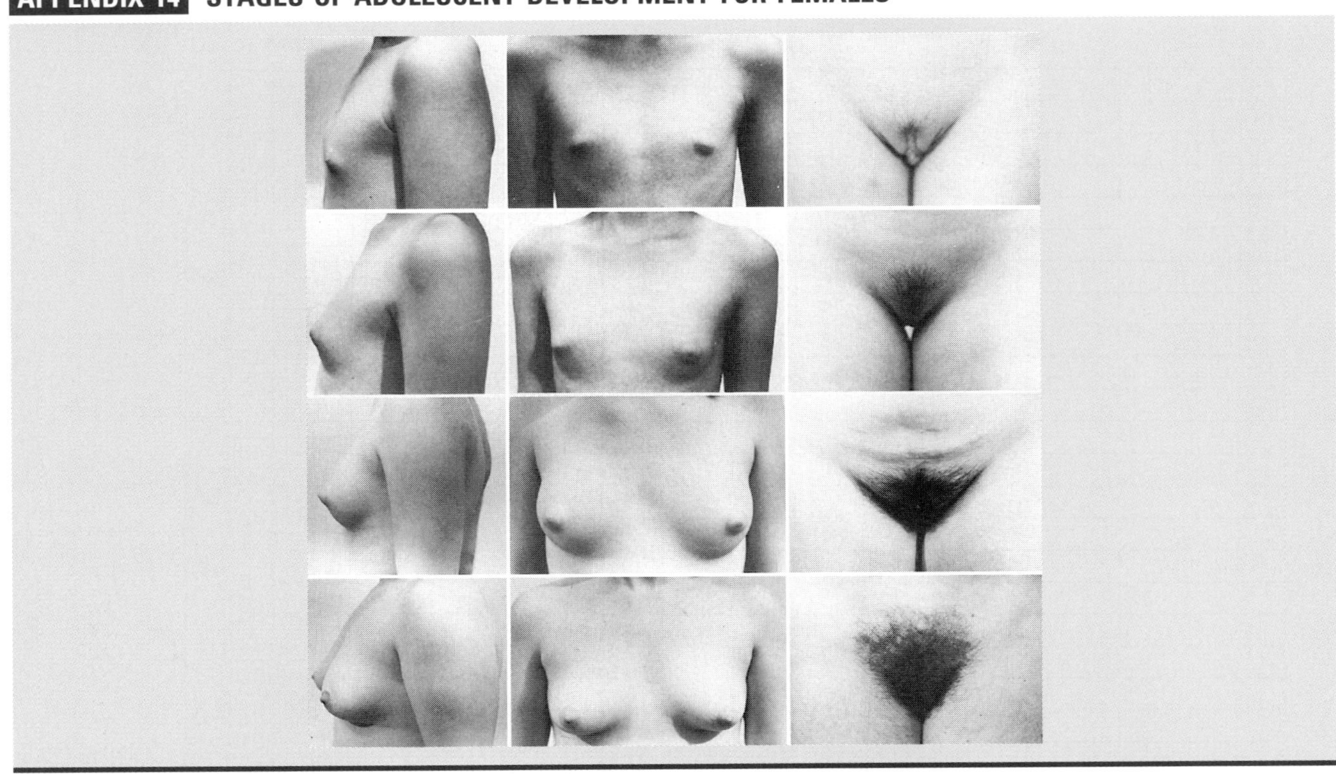

APPENDIX 15 STAGES OF ADOLESCENT DEVELOPMENT FOR MALES

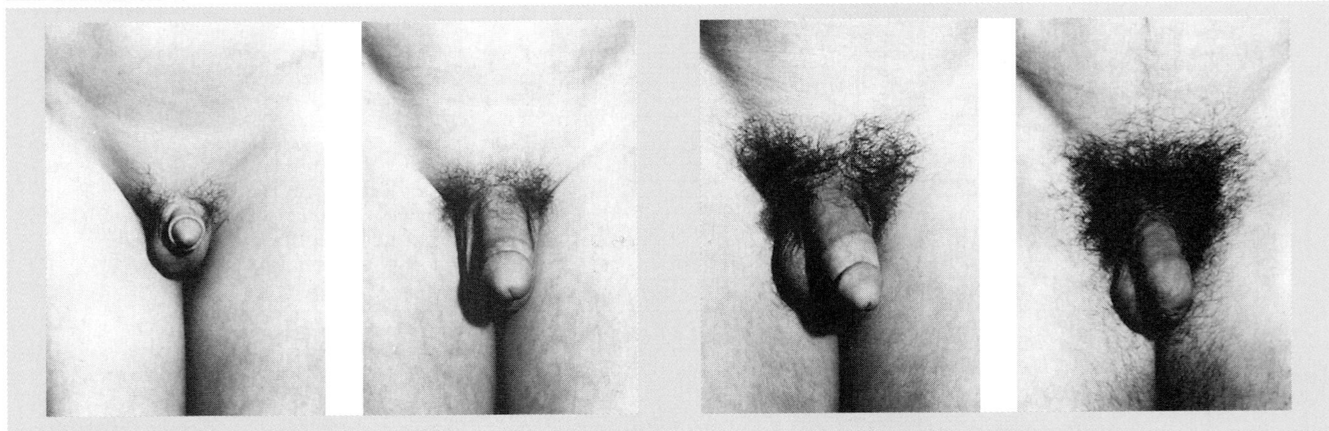

Chronological age is not always the best way to assess adolescent growth because of individual variations in beginning and completing the growth sequence. A more useful way of describing pubertal development, and thus the varying needs for nutrients throughout adolescence, is to divide growth into stages of breast and pubic hair development in girls (Appendix 14) and pubic hair and penis and testicle development in boys (Appendix 15). These are termed the Tanner Stages of Adolescent Development. Nutritional requirements vary depending upon the stage of development.

APPENDIX 16 DIRECT METHOD FOR MEASURING HEIGHT AND WEIGHT

Height

1. Height should be measured without shoes.
2. The individual's feet should be together, with the heels against the wall or measuring board.
3. The individual should stand erect, neither slumped nor stretching, looking straight ahead, without tipping the head up or down. The top of the ear and outer corner of the eye should be in a line parallel to the floor (the "Frankfort plane").
4. A horizontal bar, a rectangular block of wood, or the top of the statiometer should be lowered to rest flat on the top of the head.
5. Height should be read to the nearest ¼ inch or 0.5 cm.

Weight

1. Use a beam balance scale, not a spring scale, whenever possible.
2. Periodically calibrate the scale for accuracy, using known weights.
3. Weigh the subject in light clothing without shoes.
4. Record weight to the nearest ½ lb or 0.2 kg for adults, and ¼ lb or 0.1 kg for infants. Measurements above the 90th percentile or below the 10th percentile warrant further evaluation.

APPENDIX 17 INDIRECT METHODS FOR MEASURING HEIGHT

Measuring Arm Span

Steps:

1. The arms are extended straight out to the sides at a 90° angle from the body.
2. The distance from the longest fingertip of one hand to the longest finger of the other hand is measured.

Adult Recumbent

Steps:

1. Stand on right side of the body.
2. Align body so that the lower extremities, trunk, shoulders, and head are straight.
3. Place a mark at the top of the sheet in line with the crown of the head and one at the bottom of the sheet in line with the base of the heels.
4. Measure length between marks with measuring tape.

Knee Height*

Knee height measurement is highly correlated with upright height. It is useful in those who cannot stand and may have curvatures of the spine.

Steps:

1. Use the left leg for measurements.
2. Bend the left knee and the left ankle to 90° angles. A triangle may be used if available.
3. Using knee height calipers, open the caliper and place the fixed part under the heel. Place the sliding blade down against the thigh (approximately 2 inches behind the patella).
4. Measure from the heel to the anterior surface of thigh using a cloth measuring tape.
5. Obtain the measurement and convert it to centimeters by multiplying by 2.54.
6. Formulas to use to calculate estimated knee height:
   Men (ht in cm) = 64.19 – (0.04 × age) + (2.02 × knee height in cm)
   Women (ht in cm) = 84.8 – (0.24 × age) + (1.83 × knee height in cm)

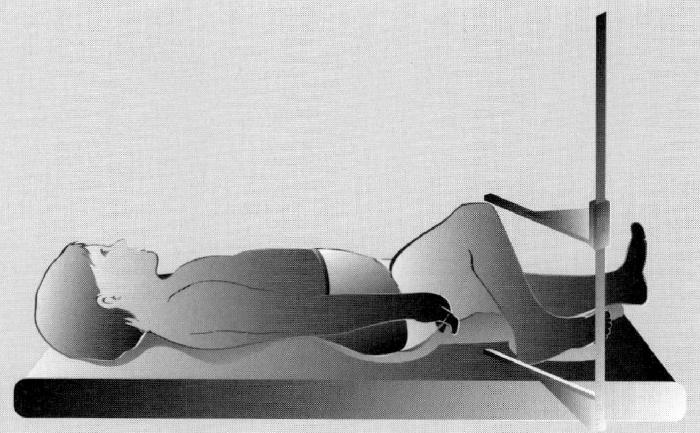

Recommended equations for predicting stature from knee height in adults (18 to 60 years of age) and children (6 to 18 years of age)

GROUP	EQUATION[a]
White men	Stature = 71.85 + (1.88 knee height) R^2 = .65; RMSE[a] = 3.97; SEI[b] = 3.97 cm; CV[c] = 2.28.
Black men	Stature = 73.42 + (1.79 knee height) R^2 = .69; RMSE = 3.60; SEI = 3.60 cm; CV = 2.08.
White women	Stature = 70.25 + (1.87 knee height) – (0.06 age) R^2 = .66; RMSE = 3.60; SEI = 3.60 cm; CV = 2.23.
Black women	Stature = 68.10 + (1.86 knee height) – (0.06 age) R^2 = .69; RMSE = 3.80; SEI = 3.80 cm; CV = 2.36.
White boys	Stature = 40.54 + (2.22 knee height) R^2 = .96; RMSE = 4.16; SEI = 4.21 cm; CV = 2.79.
Black boys	Stature = 39.60 + (2.18 knee height) R^2 = .95; RMSE = 4.44; SEI = 4.58 cm; CV = 2.99.
White girls	Stature = 43.21 + (2.15 knee height) R^2 = .95; RMSE = 3.84; SEI = 3.90 cm; CV = 2.63.
Black girls	Stature = 46.59 + (2.02 knee height) R^2 = .94; RMSE = 4.25; SEI = 4.39 cm; CV = 2.91.

[a]RMSE = root mean square error; [b]SEI = standard error for an individual; [c]CV = coefficient of variation.

*Chumlea WC, et al. Nutritional assessment of the elderly through anthropometry. Columbus, OH: Ross Laboratories, 1984.

APPENDIX 18 DETERMINATION OF FRAME SIZE

Method 1*

Height is recorded without shoes on.

Wrist circumference is measured just distal to the styloid process at the wrist crease on the right arm using a tape measure.

The following formula is used:

$$r = \frac{\text{Height (cm)}}{\text{Wrist circumference (cm)}}$$

Frame size can be determined as follows:

MALES	FEMALES
r > 10.4 small	r > 11.0 small
r = 9.6–10.4 medium	r = 10.1–11.0 medium
r < 9.6 small	r < 10.1 large

Method 2†

The patient's right arm is extended forward perpendicular to the body, with the arm bent so the angle at the elbow forms 90° with the fingers pointing up and the palm turned away from the body. The greatest breadth across the elbow joint is measured with a sliding caliper along the axis of the upper arm, on the two prominent bones on either side of the elbow. This is recorded as the elbow breadth. The following tables give the elbow breadth measurements for medium-framed men and women of various heights. Measurements lower than those listed indicate a small frame size; higher measurements indicate a large frame size.

MEN

Height in 1″ Heels	Elbow Breadth
5′2″–5′3″	2½″–2⅞″
5′4″–5′7″	2⅝″–2⅞″
5′8″–5′11″	2¾″–3″
6′0″–6′3″	2¾″–3⅛″
6′4″	2⅞″–3¼″

WOMEN

Height in 1″ Heels	Elbow Breadth
4′10″–4′11″	2¼″–2½″
5′0″–5′3″	2¼″–2½″
5′4″–5′7″	2⅜″–2⅝″
5′8″–5′11″	2⅜″–2⅝″
6′0″	2½″–2¾″

*From Grant JP. Handbook of total parenteral nutrition. Philadelphia: WB Saunders, 1980, p. 15.

† From Metropolitan Life Insurance Co., 1983.

APPENDIX 19 1983 METROPOLITAN HEIGHT AND WEIGHT TABLES*

MEN					WOMEN				
HEIGHT					HEIGHT				
FEET	INCHES	SMALL FRAME	MEDIUM FRAME	LARGE FRAME	FEET	INCHES	SMALL FRAME	MEDIUM FRAME	LARGE FRAME
5	2	128–134	131–141	138–150	4	10	102–111	109–121	118–131
5	3	130–136	133–143	140–153	4	11	103–113	111–123	120–134
5	4	132–138	135–145	142–156	5	0	104–115	113–126	122–137
5	5	134–140	137–148	144–160	5	1	106–118	115–129	125–140
5	6	136–142	139–151	146–164	5	2	108–121	118–132	128–143
5	7	138–145	142–154	149–168	5	3	111–124	121–135	131–147
5	8	140–148	145–157	152–172	5	4	114–127	124–138	134–151
5	9	142–151	148–160	155–176	5	5	117–130	127–141	137–155
5	10	144–154	151–163	158–180	5	6	120–133	130–144	140–159
5	11	146–157	154–166	161–184	5	7	123–136	133–147	143–163
6	0	149–160	157–170	164–188	5	8	126–139	136–150	146–167
6	1	152–164	160–174	168–192	5	9	129–142	139–153	149–170
6	2	155–168	164–178	172–197	5	10	132–145	142–156	152–173
6	3	158–172	167–182	176–202	5	11	135–148	145–159	155–176
6	4	162–176	171–187	181–207	6	0	138–151	148–162	158–179

*Source of basic data *1979 Build Study,* Society of Actuaries and Association of Life Insurance Medical Directors of America. Courtesy of the Metropolitan Life Insurance Co., 1983.

Weights for adults aged 25 to 59 years based on lowest mortality. For determination of frame size see Appendix 18. Weight in pounds according to frame size in indoor clothing (5 pounds for men and 3 pounds for women) wearing shoes with 1-inch heels.

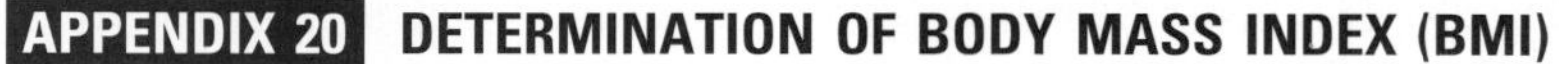

APPENDIX 20 DETERMINATION OF BODY MASS INDEX (BMI)

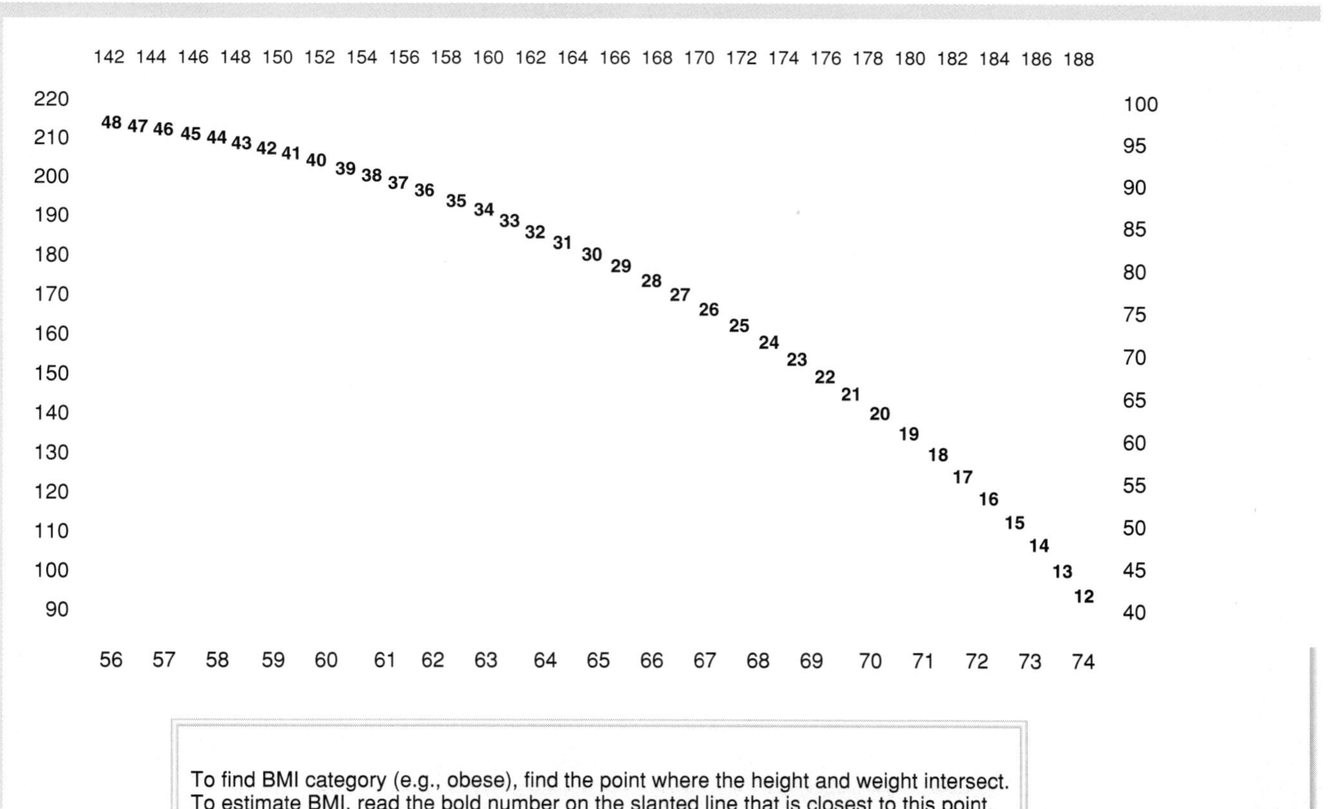

BMI charts are also available at this website: www.nhlbi.nih.gov/nhlbi/cardio/obes/prof/guidelns/bmi-tbl.htm

APPENDIX 21 ARM ANTHROPOMETRY FOR CHILDREN*

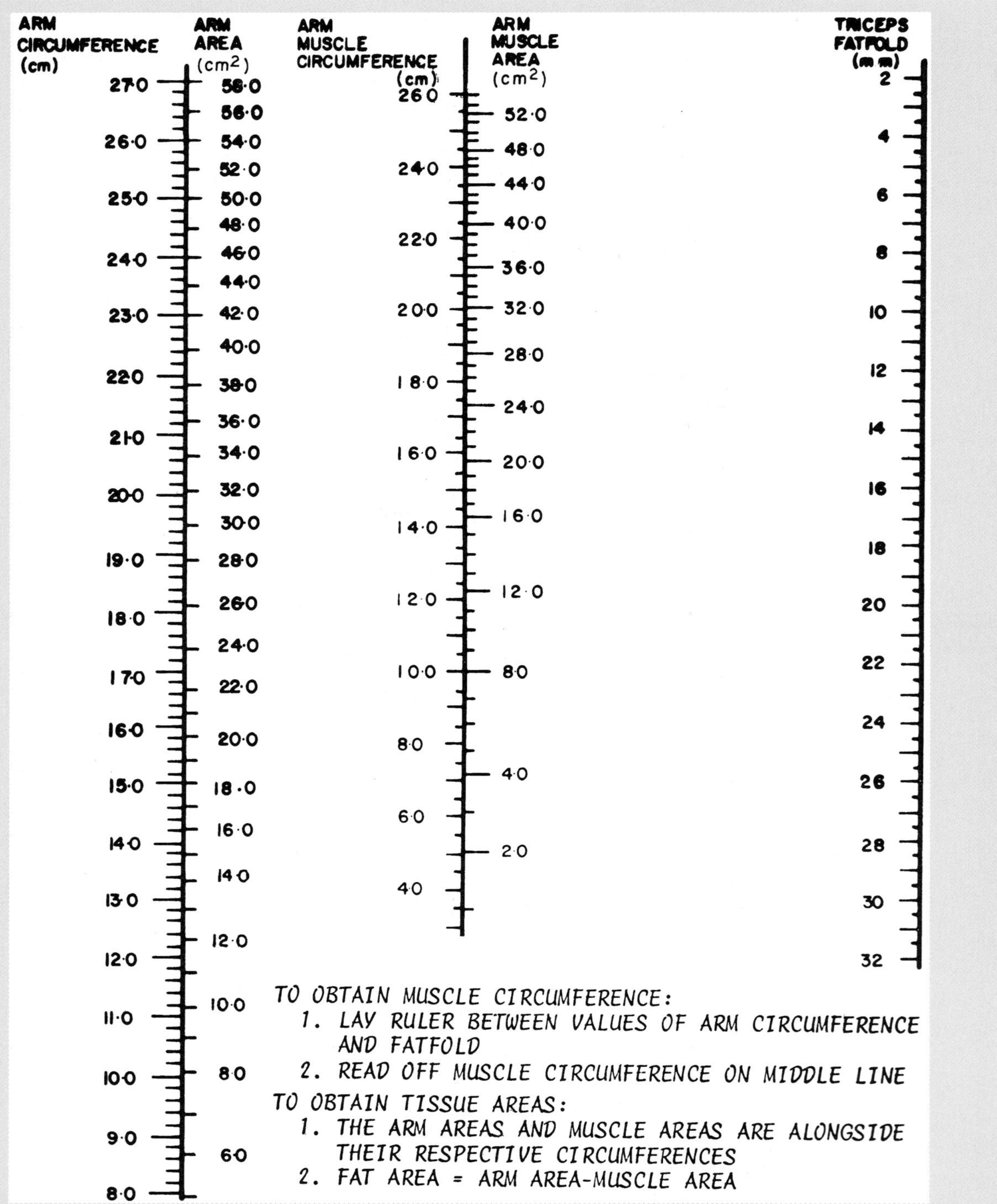

*From Gurney JM, Jelliffe DB. Arm anthropometry in nutritional assessment: Nomogram for rapid calculation of muscle circumference and cross-sectional muscle fat areas. Am J Clin Nutr 26:913, 1973.

APPENDIX 22 ARM ANTHROPOMETRY FOR ADULTS*

ARM CIRCUMFERENCE (cm): 40·0, 39·0, 38·0, 37·0, 36·0, 35·0, 34·0, 33·0, 32·0, 31·0, 30·0, 29·0, 28·0, 27·0, 26·0, 25·0, 24·0, 23·0

ARM AREA (cm²): 128·0, 124·0, 120·0, 116·0, 112·0, 108·0, 104·0, 100·0, 96·0, 92·0, 88·0, 86·0, 84·0, 82·0, 80·0, 78·0, 76·0, 74·0, 72·0, 70·0, 68·0, 66·0, 64·0, 62·0, 60·0, 58·0, 56·0, 54·0, 52·0, 50·0, 48·0, 46·0, 44·0, 42·0

ARM MUSCLE CIRCUMFERENCE (cm): 39·0, 38·0, 37·0, 36·0, 35·0, 34·0, 33·0, 32·0, 31·0, 30·0, 29·0, 28·0, 27·0, 26·0, 25·0, 24·0, 23·0, 22·0, 21·0, 20·0, 19·0, 18·0, 17·0, 16·0, 15·0, 14·0, 13·0, 12·0

ARM MUSCLE AREA (cm²): 120·0, 116·0, 112·0, 108·0, 104·0, 100·0, 96·0, 92·0, 88·0, 84·0, 80·0, 76·0, 72·0, 68·0, 64·0, 60·0, 56·0, 54·0, 48·0, 44·0, 40·0, 36·0, 32·0, 28·0, 24·0, 20·0, 16·0, 12·0

TRICEPS FAT FOLD (mm): 2, 4, 6, 8, 10, 12, 14, 16, 18, 20, 22, 24, 26, 28, 30, 32, 34, 36

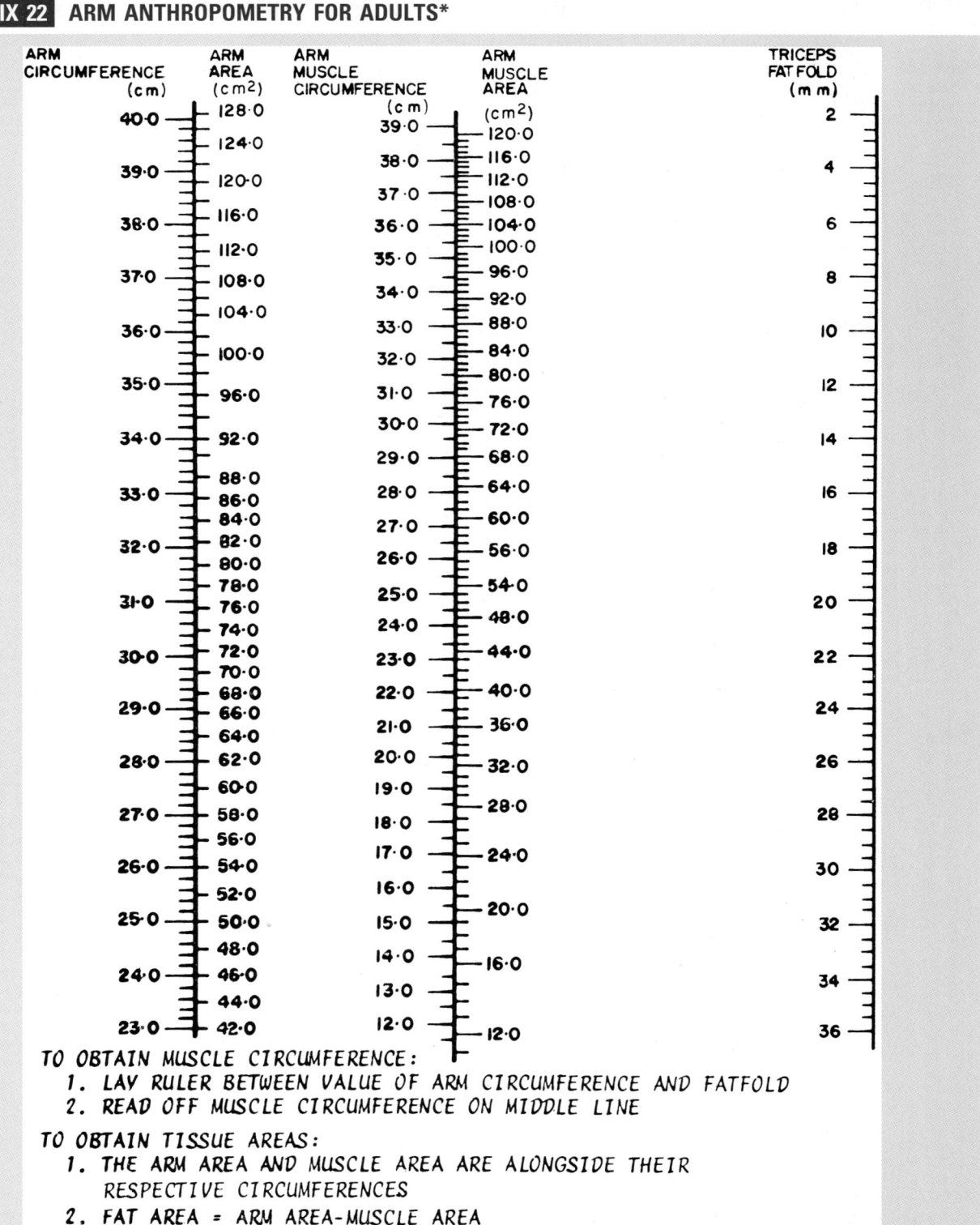

TO OBTAIN MUSCLE CIRCUMFERENCE:

1. *LAY RULER BETWEEN VALUE OF ARM CIRCUMFERENCE AND FATFOLD*
2. *READ OFF MUSCLE CIRCUMFERENCE ON MIDDLE LINE*

TO OBTAIN TISSUE AREAS:

1. *THE ARM AREA AND MUSCLE AREA ARE ALONGSIDE THEIR RESPECTIVE CIRCUMFERENCES*
2. *FAT AREA = ARM AREA-MUSCLE AREA*

*From Gurney JM, Jelliffe DB. Arm anthropometry in nutritional assessment: Nomogram for rapid calculation of muscle circumference and cross-sectional muscle fat areas. Am J Clin Nutr 26:913, 1973.

APPENDIX 23 TRICEPS SKINFOLD THICKNESS: YOUTH, 1–17 YEARS, UNITED STATES: 1971 TO 1974*

RACE AND AGE IN YEARS	NO. IN SAMPLE	ESTIMATED POPULATION IN THOUSANDS	MEAN	STANDARD DEVIATION	PERCENTILE								
					5th	10th	15th	25th	50th	75th	85th	90th	95th
					Triceps Skinfold in Millimeters								
Males													
White													
1	211	1,402	10.7	3.0	7.0	7.0	7.5	8.0	10.0	12.0	14.0	15.0	16.5
2	217	1,461	9.9	2.6	6.0	6.5	7.0	8.0	10.0	12.0	12.5	13.0	14.7
3	226	1,536	9.9	2.6	6.5	7.0	7.0	8.0	10.0	11.0	12.5	13.5	14.5
4	229	1,547	9.6	2.4	6.0	7.0	7.0	8.0	10.0	11.0	12.0	12.5	14.0
5	207	1,319	9.8	3.2	6.0	6.5	7.0	7.5	9.0	11.0	12.5	13.5	15.0
6	126	1,343	8.9	3.1	5.5	5.6	6.0	7.0	9.0	10.0	12.0	12.5	14.0
7	125	1,718	9.1	3.5	5.0	6.0	6.0	7.0	8.0	10.5	12.0	13.5	17.0
8	116	1,644	9.1	3.3	5.0	5.5	6.0	7.0	8.5	10.5	12.0	13.0	16.0
9	117	1,636	11.1	4.8	5.5	6.5	6.5	7.5	10.0	14.0	17.0	17.0	19.0
10	148	1,909	11.1	4.2	5.5	6.0	7.0	8.0	10.0	14.0	15.5	17.0	19.5
11	132	1,823	12.5	6.5	6.0	6.0	7.0	8.0	10.0	15.0	19.0	20.5	24.5
12	152	1,970	12.4	6.1	6.0	6.0	7.0	8.5	11.0	14.0	18.0	21.0	27.0
13	129	1,697	11.7	6.7	5.0	5.0	6.0	7.0	10.0	14.0	19.0	22.0	25.5
14	134	1,730	10.9	6.4	4.0	5.0	6.0	7.0	9.0	13.0	18.0	20.0	24.0
15	124	1,728	10.2	6.1	4.0	5.0	6.0	6.0	8.0	12.0	15.0	19.0	24.0
16	128	1,752	10.1	5.2	4.0	5.0	5.0	6.5	9.0	12.5	15.0	17.0	22.0
17	139	1,831	9.3	5.4	4.5	5.0	5.5	6.0	7.5	11.0	13.0	15.0	19.0
Black													
1	72	280	9.4	3.4	4.5	6.0	7.0	8.0	8.0	11.0	12.0	13.0	15.0
2	77	267	10.1	3.2	4.5	6.0	6.5	8.0	10.0	12.0	14.0	15.0	15.0
3	72	212	9.1	2.6	6.0	6.5	6.5	7.0	9.0	10.5	12.0	12.0	13.0
4	74	260	8.0	2.6	5.0	5.0	5.0	6.5	7.0	9.0	10.0	10.5	15.0
5	64	226	7.7	3.4	4.5	5.0	5.0	5.0	7.0	9.0	10.0	12.0	15.5
6	52	321	7.1	1.8	4.0	4.0	5.0	6.0	7.0	8.0	9.0	9.0	9.0
7	38	253	7.5	3.2	4.0	4.0	4.0	5.0	6.5	9.0	11.5	13.0	15.0
8	33	203	7.8	3.4	4.0	5.0	5.0	6.0	6.5	10.0	11.0	11.0	12.5
9	52	383	8.2	3.9	3.5	4.0	4.5	6.0	7.0	8.0	12.0	13.0	18.0
10	33	251	9.1	5.3	5.0	5.0	6.0	6.0	7.5	10.0	13.0	15.0	20.0
11	43	313	8.0	5.0	4.0	4.0	5.0	5.0	6.0	8.5	11.0	12.0	15.0
12	47	316	9.4	7.0	4.0	4.0	4.5	6.0	7.5	10.7	11.0	15.0	24.0
13	45	281	8.2	4.4	4.0	5.0	5.0	5.0	7.0	8.5	11.0	19.0	19.0
14	39	282	6.6	2.6	3.5	3.5	3.5	5.0	6.5	7.0	8.0	9.0	12.0
15	43	310	8.9	6.1	4.0	4.5	5.0	5.0	6.5	9.0	10.0	21.0	21.0
16	41	267	7.2	4.8	4.0	4.0	4.0	5.0	6.0	7.5	8.0	11.0	15.0
17	35	235	8.7	5.8	3.5	3.5	5.0	5.0	7.0	10.5	12.0	12.0	23.2

APPENDIX 23 TRICEPS SKINFOLD THICKNESS: YOUTH, 1–17 YEARS, UNITED STATES: 1971 TO 1974* *(continued)*

RACE AND AGE IN YEARS	NO. IN SAMPLE	ESTIMATED POPULATION IN THOUSANDS	MEAN	STANDARD DEVIATION	PERCENTILE								
					5th	10th	15th	25th	50th	75th	85th	90th	95th
					Triceps Skinfold in Millimeters								
					Females								
White													
1	189	1,328	10.2	2.8	6.0	7.0	7.0	8.0	10.0	12.0	13.0	13.5	15.5
2	203	1,434	10.6	2.6	7.0	7.5	8.0	9.0	10.0	12.0	13.5	14.0	15.0
3	211	1,438	11.1	2.6	7.0	8.0	8.5	9.0	11.0	13.0	13.5	14.0	15.0
4	204	1,339	10.8	2.6	7.5	8.0	8.0	9.0	10.5	12.0	13.0	14.5	16.0
5	224	1,416	10.7	3.7	6.0	7.0	8.0	8.5	10.0	12.0	13.0	15.0	17.5
6	125	1,445	10.6	3.3	6.5	7.0	7.5	8.0	10.5	12.0	13.0	14.0	16.0
7	122	1,507	10.9	4.2	4.0	6.0	7.0	8.0	11.0	12.0	15.0	15.5	17.5
8	117	1,507	12.4	4.7	7.0	8.0	8.0	9.0	11.5	15.0	16.5	18.0	22.0
9	129	1,751	13.6	4.6	7.5	8.0	9.0	10.0	13.0	16.0	18.0	20.0	22.0
10	148	1,855	13.4	4.8	7.5	8.0	8.5	10.0	12.5	15.5	19.0	20.0	23.0
11	122	1,569	14.9	6.1	8.0	8.5	9.0	10.0	13.0	17.5	20.5	24.5	28.5
12	128	1,506	15.2	5.6	8.0	9.0	10.0	11.0	14.0	18.5	20.0	23.0	26.0
13	153	1,886	16.2	6.8	7.0	8.0	10.0	11.5	15.0	20.0	24.0	25.0	28.5
14	132	1,731	17.8	7.3	9.0	9.5	10.5	13.0	16.7	21.0	24.0	28.5	33.0
15	125	1,752	17.7	6.7	9.0	10.5	11.0	13.0	17.0	21.0	24.0	25.0	28.5
16	141	1,933	18.2	6.6	10.0	10.5	12.5	14.0	17.0	21.0	24.0	26.0	32.1
17	117	1,549	19.8	8.0	10.0	12.0	12.5	13.5	19.0	24.0	26.5	29.5	35.0
Black													
1	73	257	10.0	3.0	5.5	5.5	7.0	8.0	10.0	12.0	13.0	14.0	15.0
2	66	261	10.0	2.3	7.0	8.0	8.0	8.0	10.0	11.0	12.0	14.0	15.5
3	78	245	9.7	2.9	6.0	7.0	7.0	8.0	10.0	11.0	12.0	13.0	14.0
4	73	246	8.8	2.7	5.0	6.0	7.0	7.0	8.0	10.5	12.0	13.0	14.0
5	88	265	9.4	3.9	5.0	5.0	6.5	7.0	8.0	10.0	12.0	13.5	17.0
6	50	336	9.0	3.1	5.5	6.0	6.0	8.0	8.0	10.0	11.5	12.0	13.0
7	46	241	10.1	4.0	5.0	6.0	7.0	7.5	9.0	11.0	17.5	18.0	18.0
8	35	293	11.5	5.1	5.0	6.5	7.0	8.0	10.0	13.5	18.0	18.0	23.0
9	41	247	10.2	5.1	5.5	6.0	6.0	6.5	8.0	12.0	18.0	18.0	20.0
10	48	303	11.7	5.6	6.5	6.5	7.0	7.5	10.0	16.0	18.0	19.0	24.0
11	42	315	12.7	6.4	4.0	5.0	6.5	7.5	10.0	18.0	22.0	23.0	23.0
12	47	284	13.6	7.6	5.5	6.0	6.0	7.5	12.0	17.0	22.0	25.0	30.0
13	44	287	16.1	7.0	7.0	8.5	10.0	11.0	14.0	18.0	24.0	24.0	33.5
14	50	265	15.9	6.7	8.0	8.0	9.0	10.5	14.0	20.5	24.0	24.5	24.5
15	46	411	14.0	7.6	6.5	6.5	8.0	10.0	12.5	16.0	16.5	20.0	32.8
16	33	203	18.9	8.0	8.0	8.0	10.0	12.0	19.0	24.0	24.5	33.0	33.1
17	39	239	16.9	6.6	7.5	9.0	11.0	12.0	14.5	20.0	24.0	28.0	31.0

*From the National Center for Health Statistics, Department of Health and Human Services. Health and Nutrition Examination Survey I, 1971–1974.

APPENDIX 24 TRICEPS SKINFOLD THICKNESS: ADULTS, UNITED STATES: 1971 TO 1974*

RACE AND AGE IN YEARS	NO. IN SAMPLE	ESTIMATED POPULATION IN THOUSANDS	MEAN	STANDARD DEVIATION	PERCENTILE								
					5th	10th	15th	25th	50th	75th	85th	90th	95th
					Triceps Skinfold in Millimeters								
Males													
White													
	4,344	54,694	12.2	5.8	5.0	6.0	6.5	8.0	11.0	15.0	18.0	20.0	23.0
18–19	203	3,206	11.3	5.9	5.0	5.5	6.0	7.0	9.0	15.0	18.0	20.0	23.0
20–24	423	7,094	11.5	6.0	4.0	5.0	6.0	7.0	10.0	15.0	18.0	21.0	23.0
25–34	672	11,594	12.7	6.2	5.0	6.0	6.5	8.0	12.0	16.0	18.5	21.0	24.0
35–44	569	9,516	12.6	5.4	5.0	6.0	7.0	9.0	12.0	15.5	17.5	20.0	23.0
45–54	628	10,039	12.6	5.9	5.5	6.5	7.0	8.5	11.0	15.0	18.0	20.0	26.0
55–64	505	8,275	11.7	5.0	5.0	6.0	7.0	8.0	11.0	14.0	16.5	18.0	21.0
65–74	1,344	4,970	12.0	5.4	5.0	6.0	7.0	8.0	11.0	15.0	17.0	19.0	22.0
Black													
	847	5,753	10.6	7.0	3.5	4.0	4.5	6.0	8.5	13.0	16.0	20.0	23.0
18–19	52	404	8.9	6.7	2.0	4.0	5.0	5.1	7.0	8.0	12.0	21.0	24.0
20–24	80	866	10.0	7.9	3.0	4.0	4.0	6.0	8.0	11.0	13.0	18.0	24.0
25–34	119	1,232	11.8	8.4	4.0	4.0	4.0	5.0	10.0	15.0	20.0	22.0	23.0
35–44	87	1,005	11.3	6.5	4.0	4.5	5.0	7.0	10.0	14.0	17.0	18.4	22.0
45–54	130	1,057	10.0	5.1	4.0	4.0	5.0	6.0	10.0	12.5	14.0	16.0	20.0
55–64	85	703	10.7	7.2	3.0	4.0	4.5	5.0	8.0	14.0	20.0	22.0	26.0
65–74	294	486	9.7	5.4	4.0	4.5	5.0	6.0	9.0	12.0	14.0	15.0	19.5
Females													
White													
	6,757	59,923	22.9	8.1	11.0	13.0	14.5	17.0	22.0	28.0	31.0	34.0	37.0
18–19	208	3,159	18.9	6.6	9.5	12.0	13.0	14.5	18.0	22.5	24.0	26.5	33.5
20–24	956	7,972	19.8	7.7	10.0	11.0	12.0	14.0	19.0	24.0	27.9	30.5	34.0
25–34	1,539	12,161	21.8	8.0	11.0	12.5	14.0	16.0	20.5	26.0	30.0	33.0	36.5
35–44	1,302	10,111	23.7	8.3	12.0	14.0	15.9	18.0	22.5	29.0	32.0	35.1	38.5
45–54	705	10,879	25.3	8.1	13.0	15.0	17.0	20.0	25.0	30.0	33.5	35.5	39.5
55–64	551	9,037	24.6	7.9	11.5	14.5	16.0	19.0	24.0	30.0	33.0	34.1	38.0
65–74	1,496	6,603	23.3	7.3	12.0	14.0	16.0	18.0	23.0	28.0	31.0	33.0	35.5
Black													
	1,557	7,302	23.7	10.3	9.0	11.0	12.0	15.5	23.0	30.5	34.0	36.6	41.0
18–19	70	504	16.2	7.3	8.0	9.0	9.0	11.5	14.0	20.0	25.0	29.0	32.0
20–24	259	1,073	19.3	8.7	9.0	10.0	11.5	12.5	17.0	24.5	28.6	32.0	36.0
25–34	335	1,646	22.5	9.6	8.5	10.0	12.0	14.0	22.0	30.0	32.6	34.1	40.0
35–44	334	1,318	25.8	9.2	11.5	13.0	16.0	20.0	25.5	32.0	35.0	36.5	41.0
45–54	126	1,237	26.8	9.8	12.0	14.0	17.0	20.0	26.0	34.0	37.1	40.0	42.2
55–64	115	871	28.2	12.9	10.0	11.0	13.0	19.0	28.0	34.0	40.0	45.0	51.5
65–74	318	652	23.8	9.0	7.5	11.5	15.0	17.5	24.0	30.0	32.2	35.5	40.0

*From the National Center for Health Statistics, Department of Health and Human Services, Health and Nutrition Examination Survey I, 1971–1974.

APPENDIX 25 PERCENTAGE OF BODY FAT BASED ON FOUR SKINFOLD MEASUREMENTS*†

SUM OF SKINFOLDS (mm)	MALES (AGE IN YEARS)				FEMALES (AGE IN YEARS)			
	17–29	30–39	40–49	50+	16–29	30–39	40–49	50+
15	4.8	—	—	—	10.5	—	—	—
20	8.1	12.2	12.2	12.6	14.1	17.0	19.8	21.4
25	10.5	14.2	15.0	15.6	16.8	19.4	22.2	24.0
30	12.9	16.2	17.7	18.6	19.5	21.8	24.5	26.6
35	14.7	17.7	19.6	20.8	21.5	23.7	26.4	28.5
40	16.4	19.2	21.4	22.9	23.4	25.5	28.2	30.3
45	17.7	20.4	23.0	24.7	25.0	26.9	29.6	31.9
50	19.0	21.5	24.6	26.5	26.5	28.2	31.0	33.4
55	20.1	22.5	25.9	27.9	27.8	29.4	32.1	34.6
60	21.2	23.5	27.1	29.2	29.1	30.6	33.2	35.7
65	22.2	24.3	28.2	30.4	30.2	31.6	34.1	36.7
70	23.1	25.1	29.3	31.6	31.2	32.5	35.0	37.7
75	24.0	25.9	30.3	32.7	32.2	33.4	35.9	38.7
80	24.8	26.6	31.2	33.8	33.1	34.3	36.7	39.6
85	25.5	27.2	32.1	34.8	34.0	35.1	37.5	40.4
90	26.2	27.8	33.0	35.8	34.8	35.8	38.3	41.2
95	26.9	28.4	33.7	36.6	35.6	36.5	39.0	41.9
100	27.6	29.0	34.4	37.4	36.4	37.2	39.7	42.6
105	28.2	29.6	35.1	38.2	37.1	37.9	40.4	43.3
110	28.8	30.1	35.8	39.0	37.8	38.6	41.0	43.9
115	29.4	30.6	36.4	39.7	38.4	39.1	41.5	44.5
120	30.0	31.1	37.0	40.4	39.0	39.6	42.0	45.1
125	30.5	31.5	37.6	41.1	39.6	40.1	42.5	45.7
130	31.0	31.9	38.2	41.8	40.2	40.6	43.0	46.2
135	31.5	32.3	38.7	42.4	40.8	41.1	43.5	46.7
140	32.0	32.7	39.2	43.0	41.3	41.6	44.0	47.2
145	32.5	33.1	39.7	43.6	41.8	42.1	44.5	47.7
150	32.9	33.5	40.2	44.1	42.3	42.6	45.0	48.2
155	33.3	33.9	40.7	44.6	42.8	43.1	45.4	48.7
160	33.7	34.3	41.2	45.1	43.3	43.6	45.8	49.2
165	34.1	34.6	41.6	45.6	43.7	44.0	46.2	49.6
170	34.5	34.8	42.0	46.1	44.1	44.4	46.6	50.0
175	34.9	—	—	—	—	44.8	47.0	50.4
180	35.3	—	—	—	—	45.2	47.4	50.8
185	35.6	—	—	—	—	45.6	47.8	51.2
190	35.9	—	—	—	—	45.9	48.2	51.6
195	—	—	—	—	—	46.2	48.5	52.0
200	—	—	—	—	—	46.5	48.8	52.4
205	—	—	—	—	—	—	49.1	52.7
210	—	—	—	—	—	—	49.4	53.0

*From Durnin JVGA, Wormersley J. Body fat assessed from total body density and its estimation from skinfold thickness: Measurements on 481 men and women aged from 16–72 years. Br J Nutr 32:77, 1974.

†Measurements made on the right side of the body, using biceps, triceps, subscapular, and suprailiac skinfolds.

APPENDIX 26 NOMOGRAM FOR DETERMINING ABDOMINAL/GLUTEAL CIRCUMFERENCE RATIO (WAIST/HIP RATIO)

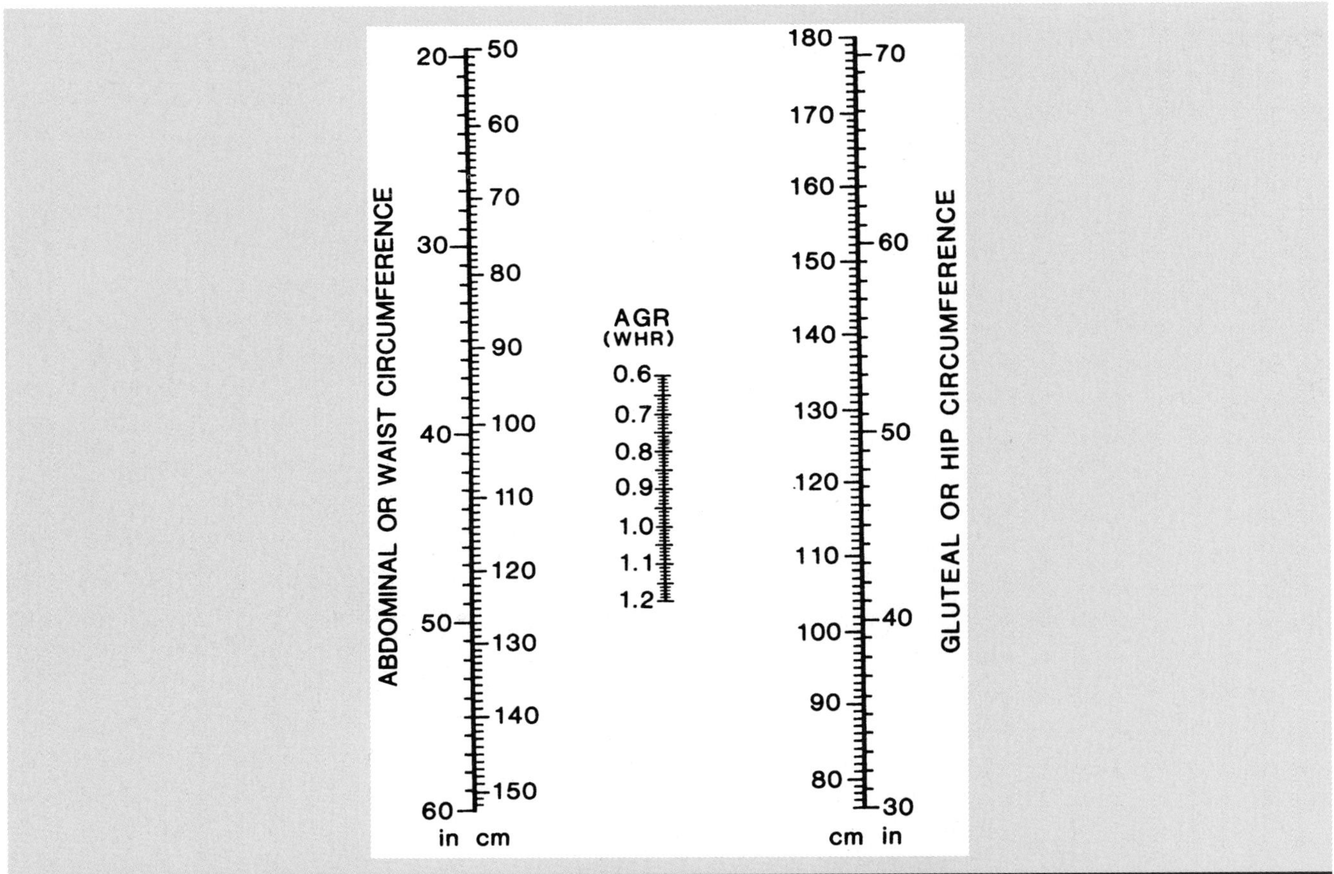

Nomogram for determining the ratio of abdominal (waist) circumference to gluteal (hips) circumference. Place a straight edge between the column for waist circumference and the column for hip circumference and read the ratio from the point where this straight edge crosses the AGR or WHR line. The waist or abdominal circumference is the smallest circumference below the rib cage and above the umbilicus, and the hips or gluteal circumference is taken as the largest circumference at the posterior extension of the buttocks. From Bray GA. Overweight is risking fate. Definition, classification, prevalence and risks. Ann N Y Acad Sci 249:14, 1987. (Copyright 1988, George A. Bray, M.D. Used with permission.)

APPENDIX 27 PERCENTILES FOR UPPER ARM CIRCUMFERENCE AND ESTIMATED UPPER ARM MUSCLE CIRCUMFERENCE OF WHITES IN THE UNITED STATES HEALTH AND NUTRITION EXAMINATION SURVEY I, 1971 TO 1974*†

	ARM CIRCUMFERENCE (mm)							ARM MUSCLE CIRCUMFERENCE (mm)						
AGE GROUP	5	10	25	50	75	90	95	5	10	25	50	75	90	95
Males														
1–1.9	142	146	150	159	170	176	183	110	113	119	127	135	144	147
2–2.9	141	145	153	162	170	178	185	111	114	122	130	140	146	150
3–3.9	150	153	160	167	175	184	190	117	123	131	137	143	148	153
4–4.9	149	154	162	171	180	186	192	123	126	133	141	148	156	159
5–5.9	153	160	167	175	185	195	204	128	133	140	147	154	162	169
6–6.9	155	159	167	179	188	209	228	131	135	142	151	161	170	177
7–7.9	162	167	177	187	201	223	230	137	139	151	160	168	177	190
8–8.9	162	170	177	190	202	220	245	140	145	154	162	170	182	187
9–9.9	175	178	187	200	217	249	257	151	154	161	170	183	196	202
10–10.9	181	184	196	210	231	262	274	156	160	166	180	191	209	221
11–11.9	186	190	202	223	244	261	280	159	165	173	183	195	205	230
12–12.9	193	200	214	232	254	282	303	167	171	182	195	210	223	241
13–13.9	194	211	228	247	263	286	301	172	179	196	211	226	238	245
14–14.9	220	226	237	253	283	303	322	189	199	212	223	240	260	264
15–15.9	222	229	244	264	284	311	320	199	204	218	237	254	266	272
16–16.9	244	248	262	278	303	324	343	213	225	234	249	269	287	296
17–17.9	246	253	267	285	308	336	347	224	231	245	258	273	294	312
18–18.9	245	260	276	297	321	353	379	226	237	252	264	283	298	324
19–24.9	262	272	288	308	331	355	372	238	245	257	273	289	309	321
25–34.9	271	282	300	319	342	362	375	243	250	264	279	298	314	326
35–44.9	278	287	305	326	345	363	374	247	255	269	286	302	318	327
45–54.9	267	281	301	322	342	362	376	239	249	265	281	300	315	326
55–64.9	258	273	296	317	336	355	369	236	245	260	278	295	310	320
65–74.9	248	263	285	307	325	344	355	223	235	251	268	284	298	306
Females														
1–1.9	138	142	148	156	164	172	177	105	111	117	124	132	139	143
2–2.9	142	145	152	160	167	176	184	111	114	119	126	133	142	147
3–3.9	143	150	158	167	175	183	189	113	119	124	132	140	146	152
4–4.9	149	154	160	169	177	184	191	115	121	128	136	144	152	157
5–5.9	153	157	165	175	185	203	211	125	128	134	142	151	159	165
6–6.9	156	162	170	176	187	204	211	130	133	138	145	154	166	171
7–7.9	164	167	174	183	199	216	231	129	135	142	151	160	171	176
8–8.9	168	172	183	195	214	247	261	138	140	151	160	171	183	194
9–9.9	178	182	194	211	224	251	260	147	150	158	167	180	194	198
10–10.9	174	182	193	210	228	251	265	148	150	159	170	180	190	197
11–11.9	185	194	208	224	248	276	303	150	158	171	181	196	217	223
12–12.9	194	203	216	237	256	282	294	162	166	180	191	201	214	220
13–13.9	202	211	223	243	271	301	338	169	175	183	198	211	226	240
14–14.9	214	223	237	252	272	304	322	174	179	190	201	216	232	247
15–15.9	208	221	239	254	279	300	322	175	178	189	202	215	228	244
16–16.9	218	224	241	258	283	318	334	170	180	190	202	216	234	249
17–17.9	220	227	241	264	295	324	350	175	183	194	205	221	239	257
18–18.9	222	227	241	258	281	312	325	174	179	191	202	215	237	245
19–24.9	221	230	247	265	290	319	345	179	185	195	207	221	236	249
25–34.9	233	240	256	277	304	342	368	183	188	199	212	228	246	264
35–44.9	241	251	267	290	317	356	378	186	192	205	218	236	257	272
45–54.9	242	256	274	299	328	362	384	187	193	206	220	238	260	274
55–64.9	243	257	280	303	335	367	385	187	196	209	225	244	266	280
65–74.9	240	252	274	299	326	356	373	185	195	208	225	244	264	279

*From Frisancho AR. New norms of upper limb fat and muscle areas for assessment of nutritional status. Am J Clin Nutr 34:2540, 1981.

†Percentiles are not yet available for the black population for upper arm circumference or arm muscle circumference.

APPENDIX 28 PERCENTILES FOR ESTIMATES OF UPPER ARM FAT AREA AND UPPER ARM MUSCLE AREA OF WHITES IN THE UNITED STATES HEALTH AND NUTRITION EXAMINATION SURVEY I, 1971 TO 1974*†

	ARM MUSCLE AREA PERCENTILES (mm²)							ARM FAT AREA PERCENTILES (mm²)						
AGE GROUP	5	10	25	50	75	90	95	5	10	25	50	75	90	95
Males														
1–1.9	956	1,014	1,133	1,278	1,447	1,644	1,720	452	486	590	741	895	1,036	1,176
2–2.9	973	1,040	1,190	1,345	1,557	1,690	1,787	434	504	578	737	871	1,044	1,148
3–3.9	1,095	1,201	1,357	1,484	1,618	1,750	1,853	464	519	590	736	868	1,071	1,151
4–4.9	1,207	1,264	1,408	1,579	1,747	1,926	2,008	428	494	598	722	859	989	1,085
5–5.9	1,298	1,411	1,550	1,720	1,884	2,089	2,285	446	488	582	713	914	1,176	1,299
6–6.9	1,360	1,447	1,605	1,815	2,056	2,297	2,493	371	446	539	678	896	1,115	1,519
7–7.9	1,497	1,548	1,808	2,027	2,246	2,494	2,886	423	473	574	758	1,011	1,393	1,511
8–8.9	1,550	1,664	1,895	2,089	2,296	2,628	2,788	410	460	588	725	1,003	1,248	1,558
9–9.9	1,811	1,884	2,067	2,228	2,657	3,053	3,257	485	527	635	859	1,252	1,864	2,081
10–10.9	1,930	2,027	2,182	2,575	2,903	3,486	3,882	523	543	738	982	1,376	1,906	2,609
11–11.9	2,016	2,156	2,382	2,670	3,022	3,359	4,226	536	595	754	1,148	1,710	2,348	2,574
12–12.9	2,216	2,339	2,649	3,022	3,496	3,968	4,640	554	650	874	1,172	1,558	2,536	3,580
13–13.9	2,363	2,546	3,044	3,553	4,081	4,502	4,794	475	570	812	1,096	1,702	2,744	3,322
14–14.9	2,830	3,147	3,586	3,963	4,575	5,368	5,530	453	563	786	1,082	1,608	2,746	3,508
15–15.9	3,138	3,317	3,788	4,481	5,134	5,631	5,900	521	595	690	931	1,423	2,434	3,100
16–16.9	3,625	4,044	4,352	4,951	5,753	6,576	6,980	542	593	844	1,078	1,746	2,280	3,041
17–17.9	3,998	4,252	4,777	5,286	5,950	6,886	7,726	598	698	827	1,096	1,636	2,407	2,888
18–18.9	4,070	4,481	5,066	5,552	6,374	7,067	8,355	560	665	860	1,264	1,947	3,302	3,928
19–24.9	4,508	4,777	5,274	5,913	6,660	7,606	8,200	594	743	963	1,406	2,231	3,098	3,652
25–34.9	4,694	4,963	5,541	6,214	7,067	7,847	8,436	675	831	1,174	1,752	2,459	3,246	3,786
35–44.9	4,844	5,181	5,740	6,490	7,265	8,034	8,488	703	851	1,310	1,792	2,463	3,098	3,624
45–54.9	4,546	4,946	5,589	6,297	7,142	7,918	8,458	749	922	1,254	1,741	2,359	3,245	3,928
55–64.9	4,422	4,783	5,381	6,144	6,919	7,670	8,149	658	839	1,166	1,645	2,236	2,976	3,466
65–74.9	3,973	4,411	5,031	5,716	6,432	7,074	7,453	573	753	1,122	1,621	2,199	2,876	3,327
Females														
1–1.9	885	973	1,084	1,221	1,378	1,535	1,621	401	466	578	706	847	1,022	1,140
2–2.9	973	1,029	1,119	1,269	1,405	1,595	1,727	469	526	642	747	894	1,061	1,173
3–3.9	1,014	1,133	1,227	1,396	1,563	1,690	1,846	473	529	656	822	967	1,106	1,158
4–4.9	1,058	1,171	1,313	1,475	1,644	1,832	1,958	490	541	654	766	907	1,109	1,236
5–5.9	1,238	1,301	1,423	1,598	1,825	2,012	2,159	470	529	647	812	991	1,330	1,536
6–6.9	1,354	1,414	1,513	1,683	1,877	2,182	2,323	464	508	638	827	1,009	1,263	1,436
7–7.9	1,330	1,441	1,602	1,815	2,045	2,332	2,469	491	560	706	920	1,135	1,407	1,644
8–8.9	1,513	1,566	1,808	2,034	2,327	2,657	2,996	527	634	769	1,042	1,383	1,872	2,482
9–9.9	1,723	1,788	1,976	2,227	2,571	2,987	3,112	642	690	933	1,219	1,584	2,171	2,524
10–10.9	1,740	1,784	2,019	2,296	2,583	2,873	3,093	616	702	842	1,141	1,608	2,500	3,005
11–11.9	1,784	1,987	2,316	2,612	3,071	3,739	3,953	707	802	1,015	1,301	1,942	2,730	3,690
12–12.9	2,092	2,182	2,579	2,904	3,225	3,655	3,847	782	854	1,090	1,511	2,056	2,666	3,369
13–13.9	2,269	2,426	2,657	3,130	3,529	4,081	4,568	726	838	1,219	1,625	2,374	3,272	4,150
14–14.9	2,418	2,562	2,874	3,220	3,704	4,294	4,850	981	1,043	1,423	1,818	2,403	3,250	3,765
15–15.9	2,426	2,518	2,847	3,248	3,689	4,123	4,756	839	1,126	1,396	1,886	2,544	3,093	4,195
16–16.9	2,308	2,567	2,865	3,248	3,718	4,353	4,946	1,126	1,351	1,663	2,006	2,598	3,374	4,236
17–17.9	2,442	2,674	2,996	3,336	3,883	4,552	5,251	1,042	1,267	1,463	2,104	2,977	3,864	5,159
18–18.9	2,398	2,538	2,917	3,243	3,694	4,461	4,767	1,003	1,230	1,616	2,104	2,617	3,508	3,733
19–24.9	2,538	2,728	3,026	3,406	3,877	4,439	4,940	1,046	1,198	1,596	2,166	2,959	4,050	4,896
25–34.9	2,661	2,826	3,148	3,573	4,138	4,806	5,541	1,173	1,399	1,841	2,548	3,512	4,690	5,560
35–44.9	2,750	2,948	3,359	3,783	4,428	5,240	5,877	1,336	1,619	2,158	2,898	3,932	5,093	5,847
45–54.9	2,784	2,956	3,378	3,858	4,520	5,375	5,964	1,459	1,803	2,447	3,244	4,229	5,416	6,140
55–64.9	2,784	3,063	3,477	4,045	4,750	5,632	6,247	1,345	1,879	2,520	3,369	4,360	5,276	6,152
65–74.9	2,737	3,018	3,444	4,019	4,739	5,566	6,214	1,363	1,681	2,266	3,063	3,943	4,914	5,530

*From Frisancho AR. New norms of upper limb fat and muscle areas for assessment of nutritional status. Am J Clin Nutr 35:2540, 1981.

†Percentiles are not yet available for the black population for upper arm fat and muscle areas.

APPENDIX 29 PERCENTILES FOR WEIGHT/STATURE RATIO IN THE ELDERLY

PERCENTILES FOR WEIGHT (IN KG) DIVIDED BY STATURE (IN CM) SQUARED × 10,000 (W/S^2)

MEN				WOMEN			
AGE (years)	95%	50%	5%	AGE (years)	95%	50%	5%
65	34.5	27.6	21.9	65	34.0	25.4	20.2
70	33.6	26.6	21.0	70	33.7	25.0	19.9
75	32.6	25.7	20.1	75	33.3	24.7	19.6
80	31.7	24.8	19.1	80	33.0	24.4	19.2
85	30.8	23.9	18.2	85	32.7	24.1	18.9
90	29.8	22.9	17.3	90	32.4	23.8	18.6

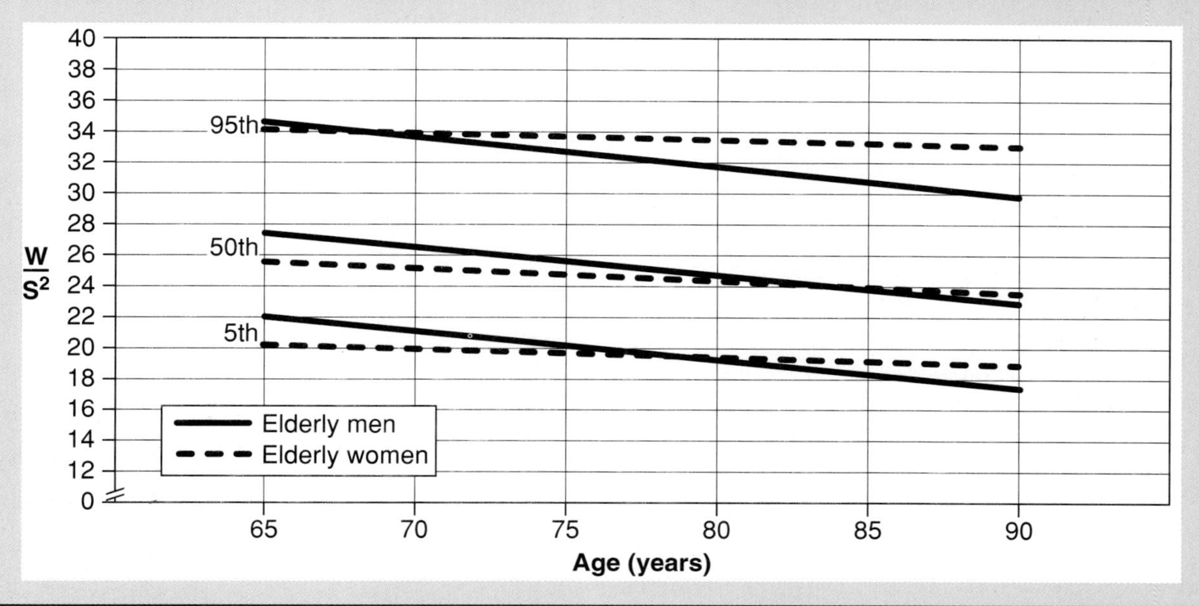

APPENDIX 30 PHYSICAL SIGNS AND NUTRITIONAL TERMS ASSOCIATED WITH MALNUTRITION*

GENERAL APPEARANCE

Apathy. Unreactive, unresponsive, disinterested, and inattentive to surroundings.

Clinical marasmus. Evidence of pronounced wasting of subcutaneous fat without edema. Significant apathy may be present. Frequently the face and eyes of the child may appear unusually bright due to the combination of wasting and prominence of the eyes. The child is usually considerably underdeveloped in relation to age, and there may or may not be associated hair changes such as dyspigmentation, thinness, ease in plucking, or signs of avitaminosis.

Irritability. Hyperresponsive; excessive or overreaction to minor stimuli, particularly manifest through crying or unusual indication of fear as a result of minor or relatively insignificant happenings.

Kwashiorkor. Pitting edema at least on the pretibial region; underweight, undersize, underdeveloped for age. Muscular wasting may be present but masked by edema. Apathy of some degree is present. Changes in the hair are usually noted, such as thinning, easily pluckable with dyspigmentation or "flag sign," and change in texture to silken, sparse hair. Dermatosis with desquamation of the so-called flaky-paint type, with or without hyperpigmentation. In severe cases the dermatosis may resemble a relatively severe burn but lacks erythema.

Pallor. Paleness and loss of color of skin, nail beds, mucosa, and lips.

Pre-kwashiorkor. An underweight, undersized, underdeveloped child, without the evident pronounced wasting present in marasmus. Child is thin and undersized but has relatively normal body proportions and rather poor muscle tone, and hair changes may be present. Not apathetic, although would not be described as alert.

HAIR

Dry staring. Dry, wirelike, unkempt, stiff hair, often brittle, sometimes may exhibit some bleaching of the normal color.

Dyspigmentation. Definite change from normal pigment of the hair, most usually evident distally and best seen by carefully combing hair strands upward and viewing the orderly array of hair in good light. Dyspigmentation includes both change of pigment (usually lightening of color) and depigmentation. Not to be confused with dyed or tinted hair. Dyspigmentation is often bandlike in character and usually is associated with some change in texture of hair in the depigmented band. In some ethnic groups, particularly among black groups, the pigment may be slightly red. In others, especially among straight black-haired peoples, the bandlike depigmentation ("flag sign") is common.

Easily pluckable. Easily pluckable hair is that in which the shafts are readily removed with minimum tug when a few strands are grasped between the finger and thumb and gently pulled. In such cases there is a lack of reaction of the child, indicating a lack of pain associated with removing of the hair.

SKIN

Crackled skin. Definite scales larger in size than those seen in xerosis. It is often congenital and is most prominent in cool weather. It is nonnutritional in origin.

Dependent edema. The presence of abnormally large amounts of fluid in the intercellular tissue spaces of the body; usually applied to demonstrate accumulation of excessive fluid in the subcutaneous tissues that is dependent on position and gravity.

SKIN *Continued*

Dermatitis with desquamation, or "crazy-pavement" type. Under this heading should be recorded those desquamating changes of the skin, usually with increased pigmentation, that occur on the extremities, especially legs, thighs, and buttocks, but may occur over the trunk in association with kwashiorkor. (These have been termed "flaky-paint" dermatoses.) Small, circumscribed bleblike lesions are sometimes seen in association with kwashiorkor and may occasionally precede the desquamation. In addition, any "crazy-pavement" type of lesions observed should be noted. These are characterized by a thin-appearing epithelium marked by striations usually resembling in outline the microscopic picture of epithelial cells. Not to be confused, however, with ichthyosis (scaly skin).

Follicular hyperkeratosis. This lesion has been likened to the "gooseflesh" that is seen on chilling, but it is not generalized and does not disappear with brisk rubbing of the skin. Readily felt, as it presents a "nutmeg grater" feel. Follicular hyperkeratosis is more readily detected by the sense of touch than by the eye. The skin is rough, with papillae formed by keratotic plugs that project from the hair follicles. The surrounding skin is dry and lacks the usual amount of moisture or oiliness. Differentiation from adolescent folliculosis can usually be made through recognition of the normal skin between the follicles in the adolescent disorder. It is distinguished from perifolliculosis by the ring of capillary congestion that occurs above each follicle in scorbutic perifolliculosis.

Pellagrous dermatitis. Symmetrical lesions typical of acute or chronic, mild or severe pellagra are observed; lesions are usually red, often swollen or blistered like sunburn, pigmented, scaly over exposed areas, clearly demarcated from normal skin.

Purpura or petechia. Small localized extravasations of blood, red or purplish in color, depending on time elapsed since formation. Usually distributed at sites of pressure, and may be perifollicular.

Xerosis. Xerosis is a clinical term used to describe a dry and crinkled skin that is accentuated by pushing the skin parallel to its surface. In more pronounced cases it is often mottled and pigmented and may appear as scaly or alligator-like pseudoplaques, usually not greater than 0.5 cm in diameter. Nutritional significance is not established. Different diagnoses must be made from changes due to dirt and exposure and ichthyosis.

SKELETAL

Bowleg. An outward curve of one or both legs at or below the knee (genu varum).

Costochondral beading. Palpable and visible enlargement of the costochondral junctions.

Cranial bossing. Abnormal prominence or protrusion of frontal or parietal areas.

Enlarged joints. When the more obvious ends of long bones are enlarged; that is, the wrist, ankles, knees.

Winged scapula. A scapula having a prominent vertebral border.

MUSCLE

Muscle wasting. Appearance indicates abnormal loss of muscle substance, as exhibited by unusual prominence of bony skeleton, undue degree of folding of the skin of the buttocks, or the abnormal flabby feel (sometimes described as jellylike) of the child with poor muscle tone.

APPENDIX 30 PHYSICAL SIGNS AND NUTRITIONAL TERMS ASSOCIATED WITH MALNUTRITION* *(continued)*

EYES

Bitot's spots. Bitot's spots are small, circumscribed grayish or yellowish gray, dull, dry, foamy superficial lesions of the conjunctiva. They most often occur on the lateral aspect of the bulbar conjunctiva in the interpalpebral area. Do not confuse with pterygium.

Blepharitis. Inflammation of eyelids.

Keratomalacia. Softening of the cornea.

Thickened opaque bulbar conjunctivae. All degrees of thickening may occur. The blueness of the sclera may disappear and the bulbar conjunctivae develop a wrinkled appearance with increase in vascularity. The thickened conjunctivae may result in a glazed, porcelain-like appearance, obscuring the vascularity.

Xerosis conjunctivae. The conjunctivae, on exposure by holding the lids open and having the subject rotate the eyes, appear dull and lusterless and exhibit a striated or roughened surface.

FACE

Angular lesions. Present bilaterally when mouth is held half open. May appear as pink or moist whitish macerated angular lesions that blur the mucocutaneous junction. Angular fissures are recorded when there is definite break in continuity of epithelium at the angles of the mouth.

Angular scars. Scars at the angles that, if recent, may be pink; if old, may appear blanched.

Cheilosis. Cheilosis is present when the lips are swollen, tense or puffy and, where it appears, the buccal mucosa extends out onto the lips. These lesions are also denuded. This category may be used to record vertical fissuring of the lips but not for lesions of the angles of the mouth only.

Nasolabial seborrhea. Definite greasy yellow scaling or filiform excrescences in the nasolabial area that become more pronounced on slight scratching with the fingernail or a tongue blade.

MOUTH

Filiform papillary atrophy. Filiform papillae exceedingly low or absent, giving the tongue a smooth appearance that remains after scraping slightly with an applicator stick. "Mild" involves less than one fourth of the tongue (tip and lateral margins only); "moderate" involves one fourth to three fourths of the tongue; "severe" involves over three fourths of the tongue.

Glossitis. Glossitis is any increase in redness, fissuring or swelling with color change (break in lingual mucosa), or diffuse involvement of mucosa. Geographic tongue has the typical irregularly shaped and distributed areas of atrophy with irregular white patches resembling leukoplakia. Glossitis is usually associated with some sensation of pain or burning, particularly upon eating.

Magenta color. The color of alkaline phenolphthalein.

Swollen gums. Swollen, red interdental papillae, with more than one papilla involved.

TEETH

Carious teeth. Molecular decay of a bone, in which it becomes friable, thinned, and dark and gradually breaks down, with the formation of pus.

Fluorosis. Opaque paper–white areas in the enamel of the tooth, ranging in size from a few flecks to entire enamel surface. In the latter case brown stain is a frequent accompaniment, as is attrition of opposing surfaces. The most severe forms of fluorosis include discrete or confluent pitting, with widespread brown staining and a general corroded appearance.

GLANDS

Parotid enlargement. Because of various types of facial configuration, parotid enlargement may be easily missed in certain populations. Check by palpation, moving the gland with fingers upward and backward toward the ear. Check if bilateral.

Thyroid enlargement. Thyroid enlargement occurs when a visually perceptible enlargement that is definitely palpable with or without swallowing is noted. It is preferable to examine the subject with his or her head slightly extended in order to detect thyroid enlargements.

ORGANS

Hepatomegaly. Liver edges more than 2 cm below the costal margin. (In children, the liver edge may normally be palpable.)

Splenomegaly. Spleen is palpable.

*From Christakis G (ed). Nutritional assessment in health programs. Washington, DC: American Public Health Association, 1973, pp. 26–27.

APPENDIX 31 FACTORS FOR PHYSICAL ACTIVITY LEVELS (PAL) BASED ON DOUBLY LABELED WATER (DLW) STUDIES

LIFE STYLE AND LEVEL OF ACTIVITY	FACTOR FOR PAL
Chair-bound or bed-bound	1.2
Seated work with no option of moving around and little or no strenuous leisure activity	1.4–1.5
Seated work with discretion and requirement to move around but little or no strenuous leisure activity	1.6–1.7
Standing work (e.g., housework, shop assistant)	1.8–1.9
Significant amounts of sport or strenuous leisure activity (30–60 min four to five times per week)	+0.3 (increment)
Strenuous work or highly active leisure activity	2.0–2.4

APPENDIX 32 A GUIDE TO THE USE OF LABORATORY DATA IN NUTRITIONAL ASSESSMENT AND MONITORING

I. Principles of Nutritional Laboratory Testing

By Timothy H. Carlson, Ph.D., R.D.

A. Purpose

Laboratory-based nutritional testing, used to estimate nutrient availability in biological fluids and tissues, is critical for assessment of both clinical and subclinical nutrient deficiencies. Laboratory data are the only objective data used in nutritional assessment that are "controlled." That is, the validity of the method of its measurement is checked each time a specimen is assayed by also assaying a sample with a known value. The known sample is called a control, and if the value obtained for the sample is outside the range of normal analytical variability, both the specimen and control are measured again.

The nutrition professional can use laboratory data to reduce the time required to gather subjective data and to eliminate the inevitable inconsistency associated with subjective judgment. Furthermore, because numeric values do not themselves connote personal judgment, this kind of data can often be passed on to a patient or client without implicit or perceived blame.

B. Specimen Types

Ideally, the specimen to be tested reflects the total body content of the nutrient to be assessed. Often, however, the best specimen is not readily available. The most common specimens for analysis are the following:

Whole blood—Must be collected with an anticoagulant if entire content of the blood is to be evaluated. The two common anticoagulants for whole blood analyses are ethylenediaminetetraacetic acid (EDTA, a calcium chelator used in hematologic analyses) and heparin (maintains the blood in its most natural state)[1]

Blood cells—Separated from anticoagulated whole blood for measurement of cellular analyte content.

Plasma—The uncoagulated fluid that bathes the formed elements (blood cells).

Serum—The fluid that remains after whole blood or plasma have coagulated. Coagulation proteins and related substances are missing or significantly reduced.

Urine—Contains a concentrate of excreted metabolites.

Feces—Important in nutritional analyses when nutrients are not absorbed and are, therefore, present in fecal material.

Hair—An easy to collect tissue; usually a poor indicator of actual body levels.

Other tissues—*Buccal cells* and *solid organ biopsy* specimens are rarely used in nutritional laboratory assessment.

C. Interpretation of Laboratory Data

As with all data, nutritional data may be quantitative (how much, how often, how fast, etc.), semi-quantitative (many, most, few, a lot, usually, majority, several, etc.), or qualitative (color, shape, species, etc.). The advantage of quantitative data is that it is less ambiguous or more objective than other types of observations. Although objective laboratory data are extremely important resources in nutrition assessment, one should be extremely cautious about using a single isolated laboratory test value to make an assessment. One value is often misleading, especially when taken out of the context of an individual's habitus, clinical status, and dietary and medical histories. The best data are obtained from analysis of changes in laboratory values.

When monitoring patients for changes in nutrition test values it is important to consider how much change is necessary to give confidence that a difference is significant. The change required for statistical significance has been called the *critical difference.* It is calculated from measurement of the variances calculated from repeated measurements of an analyte in 1) specimens that have been obtained, at several different times, from each of several healthy persons (intra-subject variation), and 2) separate samples from a large specimen pool (analytical variation).

The critical differences for some plasma proteins of nutritional significance are:[2]

Protein	Critical Difference
Albumin	8%
Transthyretin	32%
C-Reactive Protein	175%

The statistical probability that two consecutive albumin measurements are statistically different requires that the concentration change by 8% or more. Therefore, an albumin increase, for example, from 30.0 g/L to 32.4 g/L indicates a statistically significant change has occurred. For transthyretin (prealbumin), an increase from 30.0 mg/dL to 39.6 mg/dL would be significant, and for C-reactive protein, an increase from 3.0 mg/L to 8.2 mg/L would be significant. There are two reasons for the large discrepancy in the critical differences for these three proteins. The major reason is that albumin level is very stable in healthy persons, while transthyretin and C-reactive protein concentrations vary considerably. Also contributing to these differences is the fact that the currently available methods measure albumin more precisely than transthyretin or C-reactive protein.

In practice, assessments are not based on the measurement of a single analyte at one point in time. If you monitor, for example, transthyretin and C-reactive protein simultaneously, and both change so as to indicate a clinical improvement (opposite numerical directions), the amount of change required for significance decreases. The changes in laboratory data may precede changes in other nutritional indices, but generally, although not always, the data available should point to the same conclusion.

D. Reference Ranges

In order to determine if a particular laboratory value is abnormal, particularly when serial data are not available, the value is generally compared to a reference range. The reference range is constructed from a large number of test values (20 to > 1000). The average value and the standard deviation for these data are determined, and the reference range is calculated from the mean ±2 standard deviations.

APPENDIX 32 A GUIDE TO THE USE OF LABORATORY DATA IN NUTRITIONAL ASSESSMENT AND MONITORING *(continued)*

If the sample group is representative of the reference population, the reference range will include values reflecting those found in approximately 95% of the reference population. About 2.5% of this normal population will have values greater than the upper end of the reference range, and 2.5% will have values less than the lower end. This means that one normal individual in 20 would have a value below or above the reference range.

Reference ranges can be made for different populations. For example, reference ranges based on gender, age, race and so forth can be developed. In practice the differences between populations are often ignored because the importance of small differences in a nutrient analyte is not usually significant. However, when faced with borderline values, the possible influence differences between the population, which the patient is a member of, and the reference population may need to be taken into account. Often reference ranges are determined by obtaining blood from personnel working in or near the clinical laboratory. This population is often skewed toward younger persons, has few minorities, and is overrepresented by women.

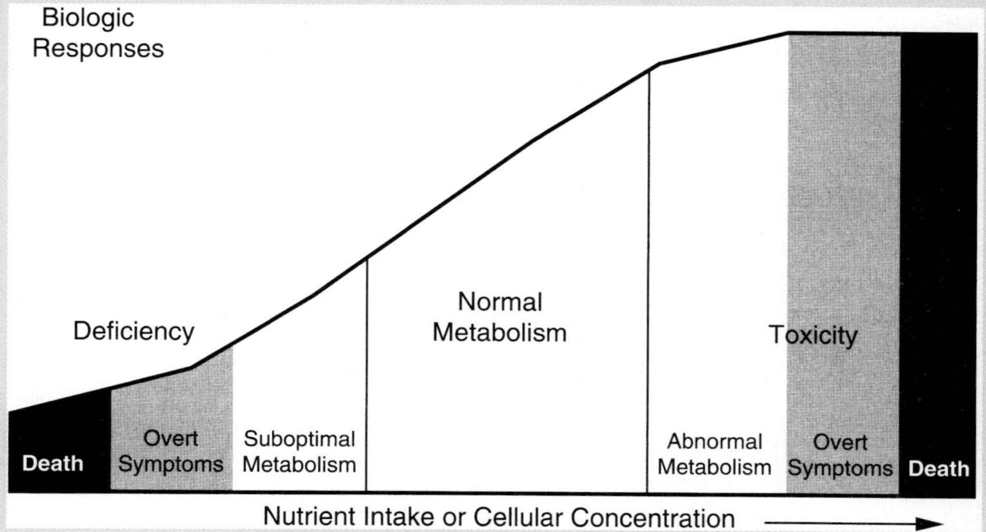

E. Units

Many types of units are used in reporting nutrient-dependent laboratory values. Two basic systems of units are in common use, the conventional system and the SI system (Système Internationale d'Unités).[3] The conventional system sometimes lacks convention, and so different laboratories adopt different units to report the same analyte! For example, the conventional report of an ionized calcium value could be 2.30 mEq/L, 46 mg/L, or 4.6 mg/dL. In the SI system, however, only 1.15 mmol/L is allowed.

F. Nature of Nutritional Testing and Types of Tests

Typically, laboratory tests are *static* assays, i.e., the concentration of an analyte is measured in a biological fluid (e.g., a fasting blood specimen) at a point in time. Assessment of nutrient status made by this approach is often inaccurate or distorted as explained in Chapter 17.

Some nutrients can be assessed by tests that are based on measurements that reflect the endogenous availability of a nutrient to a measurable biological function (e.g., biochemical, tissue, or organ). Most often, *functional* assessment of nutrient status may be done by measurement of a biochemical marker (i.e., a normal or abnormal metabolite) of function. The results of this type of testing can be reliably considered to reflect the adequacy of a nutrient pool. See Chapter 17.

As shown in the figure above, the size of a nutrient pool can vary continuously from frankly deficient, to adequate, to toxic. Most of these states can be assessed in the laboratory. This allows nutritional intervention before frank deficiency occurs. Furthermore, the response of the patient's body pool to nutritional intervention or change in patient behavior can be assessed before clinical or anthropometric changes take place.

[1]Samples obtained for blood coagulation tests are diluted with solutions containing sodium citrate (a calcium chelator). Because of the dilutional effect of the anticoagulant solutions, citrated samples are not suitable for measurement of the concentrations of analytes.

[2]Clark GH, and Fraser CG. Biological variation of acute phase proteins. Ann Clin Biochem 30:373, 1993.

[3]Monsen ER. The *Journal* adopts SI units for clinical laboratory values. J Am Diet Assoc, 37:356, 1987.

APPENDIX 32 A GUIDE TO THE USE OF LABORATORY DATA IN NUTRITIONAL ASSESSMENT AND MONITORING *(continued)*

II. A. Laboratory Measurement of Body Composition

TEST	PRINCIPLE AND REQUIREMENTS	INTERPRETATION	REFERENCE RANGE	LIMITATIONS
Creatinine-height ratio (CHR) and Creatinine-height index (CHI)	Creatinine is a continuously released by-product of energy metabolism in muscle; $CHR = \frac{\text{Urine Creatinine/24 h (mg)}}{\text{Height (cm)}}$ CHI = CHR (subject)/CHR (ideal)	Creatinine excretion related to muscle mass; tables of normal CHI values used to calculate percent deficit; % Deficit = 100 – CHI (%).	% Deficit 5–15 = mild 6–30 = moderate >30 = severe	Diet (creatinine in meat), and stress (infection, exercise, injury) ↑ creatinine excretion; age and renal insufficiency ↓ excretion; variability occurs during menstrual cycle.
3-Methyl histidine (3-MH)	3-MH, an amino acid found only in muscle, is measured by chromatographic analysis of 24-h urine collections.	3-MH excretion is related to muscle mass of adults; may be useful in monitoring or assessment for research purposes.	155–304 μmol/24h (young males; meat-free diet)	3-MH in meat; effects of age, hormone status not known; probably not useful in stressed patients or after intense muscular activity.
Hydroxyproline (HPro) index (HI)	HPro, an amino acid found in the collagen of connective tissue and bone, measured in random urine; HPro excretion related to tissue growth and repair.	$HI = \frac{\text{mg HPro per mL urine}}{\text{mg Creatinine per mL urine}}$. Can assess growth rate in children May monitor effect of nutrition support on wound healing.	Normal children: 0.7–4.7	HPro found in gelatin and other animal products; affected by age, sex, and presence of parasites, sprue, arthritis, and rheumatic fever.

II. B. Tests of Protein-Energy Status

TEST	PRINCIPLE AND REQUIREMENTS	INTERPRETATION	REFERENCE RANGE	LIMITATIONS
Urea urinary N (UUN)	The protein pool (visceral and somatic) N is catabolized to urea; urine urea represents ~80% of N catabolized; requires accurate estimate of protein intake, so usually used only for TPN or tube feeding patients.	UUN is compared to the actual N intake; $\text{N balance} = \frac{\text{protein (g)}}{6.25^*} - \text{UUN} + 4$; *factor = 5.95 for TPN; reflects severity of metabolic stress.	– = Catabolism 0 = Catabolism + = Anabolism (3–6 g/24 h = optimal utilization range)	Urine collection must be quantitative (complete); UUN not appropriate in renal insufficiency; does not account for wound leakage, cell losses, or diarrhea; inaccurate in metabolically stressed patients.
Total urinary N (TUN)	Some N is excreted as non-urea N (e.g., ammonia and creatinine); 24-h TUN reflects to protein catabolism, accounting for all sources of urinary N; as for UUN, requires accurate protein intake.	TUN is compared to the actual N intake; $\text{N balance} = \frac{\text{protein (g)}}{6.25^*} - \text{TUN} + 2$; *factor = 5.95 for TPN; reflects severity of metabolic stress; TUN gives the most accurate estimation of total protein catabolism.	– = Catabolism 0 = Catabolism + = Anabolism (3–6 g/24 h = optimal utilization range)	Urine collection must be quantitative; TUN not appropriate in renal insufficiency; not done in many institutions; does not account for wound leakage or cell losses, or diarrhea.
Urea kinetics	Formulas used to estimate protein catabolic rate (PCR) from changes in blood urea nitrogen (BUN) concentration in patients with impaired renal function.	Urinary urea (residual renal urea clearance—KrU) and BUN levels (urea generation rate—GU) are used to determine PCR; 1- to 3-day diet intake compared to PCR.	In protein balance, PRC = protein intake	Urea lost in dialysis must be accounted for in calculating urea nitrogen appearance. Dietary protein intake hard to estimate.
Visceral Proteins				
Total-protein (TP)	Protein concentration in serum is easily measured colorimetrically; largely reflects albumin (50–60% of TP).	TP levels parallel clinical signs of malnutrition; plasma TP is 0.4 g/dL greater than serum.	6.4–8.3 g/dL (64–83 g/L)	Does not reflect status during inflammatory (acute phase) response; conditions that affect individual protein affect TP.
Albumin	Easily and quickly measured colorimetrically; large body pool (3–5 g/kg body weight), ~60% is outside the plasma (in the extravascular pool); long half-life ≈3 weeks.	Decreased levels can occur following short-term protein and energy deficiency; often associated with other deficiencies, i.e., zinc, iron, and vitamin A.	3.5–5.0 g/dL (35–50 g/L)	Significance confounded by acute stress reaction, liver disease, protein-losing enteropathy, nephrotic syndrome, pregnancy, oral contraceptive use, strenuous exercise, and hemodilution.
Transferrin	Iron transport protein; smaller extravascular pool than albumin; measured by immuno-assay or calculated from TIBC (see below); half-life ≈8 d.	Levels increased during iron deficiency and decreased by protein-energy deficiency. Calculated values give inexact estimates of serum concentration.	200–400 mg/dL (2.0–4.0 g/L)	Significance confounded by acute stress reaction, liver disease, protein-losing enteropathy, nephrotic syndrome, pregnancy or estrogen administration, and hemodilution.

TEST	PRINCIPLE AND REQUIREMENTS	INTERPRETATION	REFERENCE RANGE	LIMITATIONS
Transthyretin	Transports thyroxin and acts as a carrier for retinol-binding protein; also called prealbumin and thyroxin-binding prealbumin; half-life ≈2 d. Soon will be available for routine laboratory measurement.	More sensitive protein-energy balance indicator than albumin or transferrin; responds rapidly to nutritional intervention; reportedly more sensitive to energy intake than to protein intake.	19–43 mg/dL (190–430 g/L) (Reference range varies considerably depending on methodology)	Very sensitive to stress response; also ↓ in liver disease, protein-losing enteropathy, nephrotic syndrome, and hemodilution.
Retinol-binding protein (RBP)	Transports retinol; because of low molecular weight, RBP is filtered by glomerulus and catabolized by the kidney tubule; half-life ≈0.5 d.	More sensitive protein-energy balance indicator than albumin or transferrin; responds rapidly to nutritional intervention; reportedly more sensitive to protein intake than to energy intake.	2.1–6.4 mg/dL (21–64 mg/L) (Children's values ~1/2 of adults until puberty)	Very sensitive to stress response; also ↓ in liver disease, protein-losing enteropathy, nephrotic syndrome, vitamin A, and zinc deficiencies, and hemodilution; ↑ in chronic renal disease.
Insulin-like growth factor-1 (IGF-1) (Somatomedin C)	The peptide mediator of growth-hormone activity produced by the liver; half-life of a few h; much less sensitive to stress response than other proteins.	Low in chronic undernutrition; increases rapidly during nutrition support when albumin, transferrin, transthyretin, and RBP are not affected.	95–395 ng/mL (95–395 μg/L)	Reduced levels seen in hypopituitarism, hypothyroidism, liver disease, and with estrogen use. Not generally available.
Metabolic Indicators				
Amino acid ratio	Serum ratio of nonessential to essential amino acids is an index of protein-energy status in kwashiorkor.	$\text{NEAA:EAA ratio} = \frac{\text{Gly + Ser + Gln + Tau}}{\text{Ile + Leu + Val + Met}}$ Decreased ratio in kwashiorkor, but not marasmus.	Risk — Ratio Low < 2.0 Medium 2.0–3.0 High >3.0	Not usually done because amino acid analysis is too expensive for this application.
Urea:creatinine ratio	Urinary urea to creatinine ratio (U:Cr) in fasting, first-void urine used to compare amino acid catabolism (BUN) with muscle mass (creatinine).	$\text{U:Cr} = \frac{\text{Urine urea (mg/dL)}}{\text{Urine creatinine (mg/dL)}}$ Can be used in uncomplicated protein-energy deficiency to approximate status.	Risk — Ratio Low >12.0 Medium 6.0–12.0 High < 6.0	Affected by recent protein intake, so not useful for estimating long-term status; ratio not used for accurate assessment or monitoring.

II. C. Immunological Tests

TEST	PRINCIPLE AND REQUIREMENTS	INTERPRETATION	REFERENCE RANGE	LIMITATIONS
Total lymphocyte count (TLC)	Calculated from the percentage of lymphocytes reported in the hemogram and the WBC count. Units = cells/μL or cells/mm^3	Decreased in protein-energy malnutrition and immunocompromised state.	Normal > 2700 Moderate depletion 900–1500 Severe depletion < 900	Decreased by viral infection, chemotherapy, radiation, and drugs (e.g., steroids, penicillin, sulfonamides, Lasix, phenylbutazone); increased by tissue necrosis and other types of infection.
Delayed cutaneous hypersensitivity	Anergy for antigens, such as mumps and *Candida;* occurs in malnutrition; antigens injected intradermally and redness (erythema) and hardness (induration) read 1, 2, or 3 d later.	Response affected by protein-energy status, and vitamin A, iron, zinc, and vitamin B_6 deficiencies.	Induration 1+ < 5 mm 2+ = 6–10 mm 3+ = 11–20 mm 4+ > 20 mm Erythema + or –	Usefulness in acute care limited by drugs, effect of aging and disease (metabolic, malignant and infectious diseases); difficult to administer and interpret results. Semiquantitative.

II. D. Prognostic Indices

TEST	PRINCIPLE AND REQUIREMENTS	INTERPRETATION	REFERENCE RANGE	LIMITATIONS
Albumin	↓ levels associated with increased incidence of medical or nutritional complications (morbidity), length of hospital stay, and mortality.	Levels <3.5 g/dL indicate need for further patient evaluation; <3.0 g/dL can be associated with edema; <2.5 g/dL implies extreme medical and nutritional risk.	See interpretation	Albumin responds slowly to treatment because of long $t_{1/2}$; markedly decreased during the metabolic response to injury.
Cholesterol	Low levels are associated with increased incidence of medical or nutritional complications and death.	Levels <150 indicate increased risk; concentration correlates with ↓ albumin, transthyretin, iron, zinc, and vitamins A and E.	See interpretation	Decreasing levels of total cholesterol may be more significant than absolute values.

APPENDIX 32 A GUIDE TO THE USE OF LABORATORY DATA IN NUTRITIONAL ASSESSMENT AND MONITORING *(continued)*

TEST	PRINCIPLE AND REQUIREMENTS	INTERPRETATION	REFERENCE RANGE	LIMITATIONS
Prognostic nutritional index (PNI)	PNI uses the following parameters to estimate nutritional risk: albumin (g/dL); transferrin (mg/dL); TSF = triceps skinfold (mm); DH = delayed hypersensitivity; (0-nonreactive; 1<5 mm; 2>5 mm)	PNI (%) = 158 – 16.6 [Alb] – 0.78 (TSF) – 0.2 [Tfn] – 5.8 (DH) Prospectively identifies patients who benefit from nutrition support.	PNI Low risk <40% Moderate 40–50% High risk >50%	Does not predict outcome in acute trauma; does not give specific information on nutritional deficiencies.

III. Tests of Carbohydrate Absorption

TEST	PRINCIPLE AND REQUIREMENTS	INTERPRETATION	REFERENCE RANGE	LIMITATIONS
Lactose Intolerance				
Breath hydrogen	Lactose loading (2 g/kg) in lactase deficiency allows bacterial metabolism of lactose with production of H_2 gas. Breath analyzed for H_2 by gas chromatography.	Breath H_2 measured fasting and 0.5 and 2 hr after dosing with lactose; a significant increase is associated with malabsorption.	Normal increase: <50 parts/million (i.e., <50 ppm)	Bacterial overgrowth can cause false positive results; consumption of soluble fiber or legumes and smoking are associated with H_2 production; false negative results caused by antibiotics.
Lactose tolerance test	Lactose loading (50 g) followed by blood sampling at 5, 10, 30, 60, 90, and 120 min after dose; glucose produced from lactose is assayed.	Lactase deficiency associated with <20 mg/dL increase in glucose.	Normal glucose increase ≥20 mg/dL	Test is not specific (many false positives) or sensitive (many false negatives).

IV. Tests of Lipid Status

TEST	PRINCIPLE AND REQUIREMENTS	INTERPRETATION	REFERENCE RANGE	LIMITATIONS
Fat Malabsorption				
Fecal fat screening	Microscopic inspection of fat-stained (Sudan stain) specimens for the presence of lipid droplets.	Trained observers are able to identify excessive fat in ~80% of persons with fat malabsorption.	Qualitative results	Patient must be consuming sufficient fat for analysis to reveal malabsorption. Semiquantitative.
Prothrombin time (PT)	Absorption of fat soluble vitamins, including vitamin K, decrease in fat malabsorption; vitamin K impairs coagulation causing an ↑ in PT.	A prolonged PT is a relatively sensitive but nonspecific indicator of fat malabsorption.	10.4–12.8 sec	Oral anticoagulant and other drugs, ↓ platelet count, acquired and hereditary bleeding diseases and liver disease ↑ PT.
Serum carotene (total serum carotenoids)	Carotenoids, fat soluble pigments in plant foods, are poorly absorbed in fat malabsorption; extracted by organic solvents for quantification.	A serum carotene level of less than 50 mg/dL is seen in ~85% of patients with fat malabsorption.	90–280 μg/dL (1.6–5.1 μmol/L)	Decreased serum carotenoid levels are also seen in low vegetable/fruit diets (e.g., in TPN or tube feeding), liver failure, and some lipoprotein disorders.
Quantitative fecal fat determination	Patient must consume 100 g fat/d (4 × 8 oz whole milk/d, or 2 Tbs vegetable oil/meal) during and for two days before collection.	Quantitative 72-hr stool collection required for accurate assessment; average daily discharge used for interpretation.	Normal: <5 g fat/24 h Malabsorption: ≥10 g/24 h	Failure to adhere to the diet invalidates the results.
Essential Fatty Acid Deficiency				
Fatty acid analysis	Levels of eicosapentaenoic acid (C20:3n9) and linoleic acid (C18:2n6) reflect essential fatty acid status; fatty acids in plasma or blood cell fractions assayed by gas chromatography.	Endogenous synthesis of C20:3n9 greatly increases during linoleic acid deficiency; plasma phospholipid C20:3n9/C18:2n6 ratio used to assess status.	C20:3n9/C18:2n6 ratio > 0.2 confirms deficiency	Test available only from laboratories specializing in nutritional or lipid analyses.

TEST	PRINCIPLE AND REQUIREMENTS	INTERPRETATION	REFERENCE RANGE	LIMITATIONS
Nonesterified Fatty Acids				
Serum-free fatty acids (FFA or NEFA)	Measured by a simple colorimetric procedure	↑ when medium chain fatty acids are administered.	8–25 mg/dL (0.28–0.89 mmol/L)	Many conditions ↑ FFA including hyperthryoidism, alcoholism, DM, acute MI; also ↑ in fasting and strenuous exercise.
V. Tests for Nutrition-influenced Risk Factors for Atherosclerotic Diseases				
Total serum or plasma cholesterol	Cholesterol is enzymatically released from cholesterol esters. Free cholesterol measured in automated enzyme assays.	Total cholesterol correlated with risk for cardiovascular diseases, but not as good an indicator as HDL-c and LDL-c. See National Cholesterol Education Program (NCEP) guidelines.	Desirable: <200 mg/dL (<5.2 μmol/L) Borderline: 200–239 mg/dL (5.2–6.2 μmol/L) High risk: ≥240 mg/dL (≥6.2 μmol/L)	Cholesterol measurements have considerable within-subject variability. May partly result from variability in specimen collection or handling.
HDL cholesterol (HDL-c)	LDL-c (and VLDL-c) are precipitated from the serum before measurement of residual HDL-c; direct measurement of HDL-c is now done in some laboratories.	HLD-c is called "good cholesterol" to indicate that it is a negative risk factor.	Desirable: >35 mg/dL (0.9 μmol/L)	Some precipitation methods cause underestimation of HDL. HDL can be divided into classes, HDL_1, HDL_2, and HDL_3; HDL_3 best correlates with risk of CHD.
LDL cholesterol (LDL-c)	LDL-c is estimated by the Friedewald formula, LDL-c = total cholesterol – HDL-c – TG/5, or by new direct assays.	LDL-c is called "bad cholesterol" to indicate that it is a positive risk factor. See NCEP guidelines.	Desirable: <130 mg/dL (<3.4 μmol/L) Borderline: 130–159 mg/dL (3.4–4.1 μmol/L) High risk: ≥160 mg/dL (≥4.1 μmol/L)	Calculation only valid when TG concentration is <400 mg/dL, so cannot be determined in nonfasting serum or plasma.
Triglycerides (TG)	Lipases release glycerol and fatty acids from TG; glycerol measured in automated enzyme assays.	The association of TG and CHD has been shown; may be a more important risk factor in women.[1]	<160 mg/dL (<1.80 mmol/L)	Fasting specimen is essential; alcohol ingestion can increase; some anticoagulants affect.
Lipoprotein (a) Lp(a)	Measured by a variety of immunoassay techniques.	Positive associations exists between CHD risk and serum Lp(a). Influence of diet is uncertain.		Results of different assay methods may not be comparable.
LDL subclass pattern and size	LDL particles of different sizes (densities) can be assessed by electrophoresis or other techniques.	Pattern B (small, dense LDL) is associated with ↑ risk of CHD and is responsive to diet. Pattern A (larger, buoyant LDL) is not associated with risk.		Measurements are generally inaccurate and imprecise. Only available from special laboratories.
Homocysteine (Hcy)	Total Hcy (oxidized + reduced forms) are measured by chromatography or by more rapid immunoassays that have recently become available.	Hcy level is an independent risk factor for CHD, venous thrombotic, and other diseases; folic acid and vitamins B_{12} and B_6 reduce plasma Hcy levels.	Normal: 3.8–18.6 μmol/L ♂ 0.2–20.1 μmol/L ♀ In CAD: 4.4–21.7 μmol/L ♂ 0–27.8 μmol/L ♀	Small Hcy differences between CAD and normal subjects; like LDL cholesterol, risk is increased even at slightly elevated levels.

VI. Tests of Micronutrient Status

TEST	PRINCIPLE AND REQUIREMENTS	INTERPRETATION	REFERENCE RANGE	LIMITATIONS
A. Vitamins				
Thiamin (B_1)[2]	Thiamin status is usually assessed by measuring the amount of thiamin pyrophosphate (TPP) needed to fully activate the RBC enzyme, transketolase.	The TPP needed to fully activate transketolase is inversely related to B_1 status; percent stimulation by TTP > 20% (index > 1.2) indicates deficiency.	% Stimulation >20% (index >1.2) indicates deficiency	Amount (and activity) of enzyme affected by drugs, iron, folate, or vitamin B_{12} status, malignant or GI diseases, and diabetes.

[1]See Austin MA, Hokanson JE. Epidemiology of triglycerides, small dense low-density lipoprotein, and lipoprotein(a) as risk factors for coronary heart disease. *Med Clin North Am,* 1994;78:99–115.

[2]Red blood cells are separated from plasma by centrifugation and washed with saline; after hemolyzing the cells the intracellular material is analyzed for vitamin availability.

APPENDIX 32 A GUIDE TO THE USE OF LABORATORY DATA IN NUTRITIONAL ASSESSMENT AND MONITORING *(continued)*

TEST	PRINCIPLE AND REQUIREMENTS	INTERPRETATION	REFERENCE RANGE	LIMITATIONS
Riboflavin (B_2)	Riboflavin status is assessed by measuring the amount of FAD needed to fully activate RBC enzyme, glutathione reductase (GR).	The FAD needed to fully activate GR is inversely related to B_2 status; percent stimulation.	% stimulation > 40% (index > 1.4) indicates deficiency	Amount and/or activity of enzyme may change with age, iron status, in liver disease, and glucose-6-phosphate dehydrogenase deficiency.
Niacin (B_3)[3]				
Pyridoxyl (PLP) compounds (B_6)[4]	1) RBC enzymes, ALT (GPT) or AST (GOT), are assayed for the presence of PLP as the enzymes' cofactor[5];	1) Difference between enzyme activities before and after addition of PLP is inversely related to B_6 status;	1) % ALT stimulation of >25% or AST activity of >50% in deficiency.	1) Disease and drugs which affect the liver and heart and pregnancy confound interpretation;
	2) Plasma PLP can be directly measured by chromatography;	2) PLP is the major transport form of B_6, so serum levels reflect body stores;	2) Normal: 0.50–3.0 μg/dL (20–120 nmol/L)	2) Deficiency may be seen clinically before plasma PLP levels ↓;
	3) Tryptophan load test, measures excretion of the PLP-dependent metabolite, xanthurenic acid (XA).	3) In this functional test, the levels of urinary XA should ↑ significantly when 2–5 g of Trp are ingested.	3) Marginal status: >50 mg/24 h	3) Steroid drugs and estrogen ↑ enzyme activity, some drugs cause analytical errors.
Folate[6]	1) Because of ↓ DNA synthesis large RBC are produced;	1) Deficiency leads to increase in MCV (mean cell volume);	1) Normal: MCV <100	1) Not sensitive or specific for folate;
	2) Shape of neutrophil nucleus affected by folate deficiency;	2) ↑ neutrophil lobe count seen in folate deficiency;	2) Normal: ≤ 4 lobes per neutrophil	2) Lobe count sensitive but not specific;
	3) Folate levels can be directly measured by radioimmunoassay;	3) Both red cell or serum folate are indicators of body stores;	3) 2–10 μg/L serum; 140–960 ng/L RBC (3.2–22 nmol/L)	3) Plasma from non-fasted subjects may reflect recent intake; RBC folate is not measured accurately;
	4) Functional folate status assayed by formiminoglutamic acid (FIGLU) in 24-h urine, or after oral histidine loading.	4) After 2–15 g loading dose, 10–50 mg of FIGLU should be excreted in 8 h.	4) Normal: <7.4 mg/24 h (<42.6 μmol/24 h) without loading	4) FIGLU affected by vitamin B_{12}, drugs, liver disease, cancer, TB, and pregnancy.
Cobalamin (B_{12})	1) Because of ↓ DNA synthesis large RBCs are produced;	1) Deficiency leads to increase in MCV (mean cell volume);	1) Normal: MCV <100	1) Not sensitive or specific for B_{12};
	2) Shape of neutrophil nucleus affected by B_{12} deficiency;	2) ↑ neutrophil lobe count in B_{12} deficiency;	2) Normal: ≤4 lobes per neutrophil	2) Lobe count sensitive but not specific;
	3) B_{12} can be directly measured by radioimmunoassay;	3) Levels <150 ng/L indicate deficiency (age affects level);	3) 200–1000 ng/L 150–750 pmol/L)	3) Marginal deficiency not correlated with level;
	4) Methylmalonic acid excretion reflects B_{12} available for branched-chain AA metabolism;	4) Methylmalonic acid excretion >300 mg/24 h in B_{12} deficiency;	4) Normal excretion: ≤9.0 mg/24 h (≤76 μmol/24 h)	4) Specific for B_{12}, but requires normal BCAA levels; done only in specialized laboratories;
	5) Schilling test for intrinsic factor and B_{12} absorption assesses radiolabeled B_{12} absorption as reflected by urinary excretion.	5) Abnormal B_{12} absorption indicated by excretion <3% of B_{12} radioactivity per 24 h.	5) Normal excretion: ≈8% of radioactivity per 24 h	5) Test must be repeated with oral administration of intrinsic factor (IF) to differentiate IF deficiency and malabsorption.
Ascorbic Acid (C)	Plasma or leukocyte C measured by 1) chromatography; 2) ascorbate oxidase; 3) spectrophotometrically by reaction with 2,4-dinitrophenylhydrazine.	Leukocyte C is less affected by recent intake, but well-fasted plasma levels parallel leukocyte levels; plasma preferred for acutely ill patients because leukocyte level is affected by infection, some drugs and hyperglycemia; < 0.2 mg/dL (<10 μg/10^8 WBC).	Plasma: 0.50–1.40 mg/dL (30–80 μmol/L) Leukocyte deficiency: 20–50 μg/10^8 WBC (1.1–3.0 fmol/cell)	Blood samples must by carefully prepared for assay to prevent C breakdown.Oxalate, glucose, and proteins interfere with some assays; recent intake can mask deficiency.

Fat-soluble Vitamins				
Retinols (A)	Serum retinol and retinol esters extracted by organic solvents and measured by chromatography; functional tests (e.g., dark adaptation) only detect severe deficiency.	Retinol levels <100 g/L indicate severe deficiency; retinol ester >5% of total retinols indicates hypervitaminosis A.	30–80 μg/dL (1.0–2.8 μmol/L)	Exposure of serum to bright light or oxygen destroys A; low retinol-binding protein level associated with low A (see protein-energy section).
Tocopherols (E)	Serum tocopherols measured by chromatography; α- and β-tocopherols serve different antioxidant functions.	Lower values found in infants; level associated with deficiency not determined.	0.5–1.8 mg/dL (12–42 μmol/L)	Plasma level dependent on recent intake and level of lipids, especially triglycerides, in blood.
Cholecalciferol (D_3) calcidiol calcitriol	1) Alkaline phosphatase activity reflects level of bone activity and, indirectly, D status;	1) Serum levels >190 units/L D deficiency; 30% is the form from bone;	1) Adult: 25–100 U/L 1–12 y < 350 U/L	1) Not specific, but a sensitive indicator; serum Ca and PO_4 should also be ↑;
Calciferol (D_2) ercalcidiol/ ercalcitriol	2) Calcidiol and ercalcidiol (25-OH-D) are assayed together by chromatography or radioimmunoassay;	2) <3 ng/mL (7.4 nmol/L) indicates deficiency; >200 ng/mL (500 nmol/L) indicates hyper-vitaminosis D;	2) 15–80 μg/L) summer (37–200 nmol/L) 14–42 μg/L winter (35–105 nmol/L)	2) Best indicator of status (liver stores), but marginal levels hard to interpret;
	3) Calcitriol [1,25-(OH)2-D_3] is assayed by chromatographic or immunoassay procedures.	3) Used to show that vitamin D metabolism is occurring normally.	3) 2.5–4.5 ng/dL (60–108 pmol/L) (little seasonal change)	3) Poor indicator of status because of tight control of synthesis independent of body stores.
Phyloquinone (K_1) and menadione (K_2)	Normal coagulation factor synthesis requires K; prothrombin (PT) assesses coagulation status.	In K deficiency, PT increases with increasing production of abnormal coagulation factors.[7]	10.4–12.8 s (varies significantly with method)	The level of vitamin K available for vitamin K–dependent bone proteins may not be reflected by the PT.
B. Minerals				
Electrolytes				
Sodium (Na^+)[8,9]	Serum electrolytes, including bicarbonate, are usually measured together by ion-specific electrodes in auto-analyzers; sometimes Na and K are measured by flame emission spectrophotometry.	↑ serum Na seen in water loss; ↓Na occurs in many conditions	135–145 mEq/L (1 mEq/L = mmol/L)	Electrolytes change rapidly in response to changes in physiology, e.g., hormonal stimulus, renal and other organ dysfunction, acid-base balance changes and drug action; serum electrolytes are minimally affected by diet.
Potassium (K^+)		↑ serum K seen in renal diseases and ↓ Na; ↓ K usually indicates ↓ intake or ↑ cellular uptake.	3.5–5.1 mEq/L (1 mEq/L = mmol/L)	
Chloride (Cl^-)		Chloride levels change with cation and osmotic changes in the body.	100–110 mEq/L (1 mEq/L = mmol/L)	
Bicarbonate or total CO_2		Bicarbonate levels reflect acid-base balance.	21–30 mEq/L (1 mEq/L = mmol/L)	
Major Minerals				
Calcium (Ca^{2+})	1) Total serum Ca^{2+} measured as chromogenic or fluorescent complexes, or by atomic absorption; 2) Ionized (free) Ca^{2+} measured by ion-specific electrodes.	Usually, slightly more than half of the serum Ca^{2+} is bound to albumin, or complexed with other molecules; the remaining C^{2+} is called ionized Ca (ICA); ICA is available physiologically.	1) 8.8–10 mg/dL (2.2–2.5 mmol/L) 2) 2.3–2.6 mEq/L (1.15–1.30 mmol/L)	Calcium status is related to many factors, including vitamin D, phosphate, parathyroid function and malignancy, and renal function.

[3]No biochemical tests have been developed to assess B_3 status; the fraction of whole blood niacin as NAD is a potentially useful test (see Jacobsen, EL. Niacin deficiency and cancer in women. *J Am Coll of Nutr* 1993;12:412–416).

[4]Several tests in addition to the ones described here have been used to assess B_6 status. For example, urinary B_6:creatinine ratios, urinary 4-pyridoxic acid excretion and the kynurenine load test are tests for B_6, but these are not usually available for clinical use.

[5]ALT (alanine aminotransferase) and GPT (glutamic-pyruvate transaminase) are the same enzyme; AST (aspartate aminotransferase) and GOT (glutamic-oxalacetic transaminase) are the same enzyme.

[6]Microbiological growth assays, the deoxyuridine suppression test and recently developed research tests for folate and vitamin B_{12} are not generally offered in the contemporary clinical laboratory.

[7]More sensitive procedures for measurement of vitamin K include serum chromatography and determination of the serum level of vitamin K–dependent bone protein called osteocalcin. Deficiency significantly increases the amount of abnormal forms of this protein. These tests are not yet widely available.

[8]These substances are measured by similar techniques when the concentration in urine or other body fluids is determined.

[9]These tests are combined with serum glucose, creatinine, and BUN on a test battery or panel. This set of tests are among the first and most frequently administered laboratory tests.

APPENDIX 32 A GUIDE TO THE USE OF LABORATORY DATA IN NUTRITIONAL ASSESSMENT AND MONITORING *(continued)*

TEST	PRINCIPLE AND REQUIREMENTS	INTERPRETATION	REFERENCE RANGE	LIMITATIONS
Phosphate (H_2PO^4, PO_4^2, and PO_4^{3-}) (Phosphorous)	Usually measured spectrophotometrically after reaction with ammonium phosphomolybdate.	Abnormal P level is most closely associated with disturbed intake, distribution, or renal function.	2.7–4.5 mg/dL (0.87–1.45 mmol/L) (higher in children)	Reported as phosphorous (P), not phosphate; hemolyzed blood cannot be used because of high RBC phosphate levels.
Magnesium (Mg^{2+})	1) Total serum Mg^{2+} measured after reaction to form chromogenic or fluorescent complexes, or by atomic absorption; 2) Ionized (free) Mg^{2+} measured by ion-specific electrodes.	Neuromuscular function (hyperirritability, tetany, convulsion, and electrocardiographic changes) affected when levels of total serum Mg^{2+} fall to <1.0 mEq/L.	1) 1.4–2.3 mEq/L (0.70–1.15 mmol/L) 2) 0.7–1.2 mEq/L (0.35–0.60 mmol/L)	Usually, about 45% of the serum Mg^{2+} is complexed with other molecules; the remaining Mg^{2+} is called ionized magnesium; serum levels remain constant until body stores are nearly depleted.
Trace Minerals				
Iron				
Complete blood count[10] (CBC) and red cell indices	HCT = % RBC in whole blood Hb = blood Hb concentration MCV = mean red blood cell volume	A CBC with red cell indices is one of the first set of tests that a patient receives; although CBC data are not specific for nutritional status, their universal and repeated presence in the patient's record make them very important.	42–52 (male) 37–47 (female)[12] 14–18 g/dL (male) 12–16 g/dL (female) 80–99 fl all except 96–108 in newborns.	These tests are affected only when iron stores are essentially depleted; HCT and Hb are sensitive to hydration status; low MCV also occurs in thalassemias and lead poisoning.
Serum iron (Fe);	Serum Fe^{3+} reduced to Fe^{2+} and then complexed with chromogen;	Slightly higher in males than premenopausal females; reflects recent Fe intake;	50–175 μg/dL (9–31 μmol/L)	Very insensitive index of total Fe stores; extremely variable (day-to-day and diurnal);
Total iron binding capacity (TIBC);	TIBC determined by saturating serum transferrin with Fe and then remeasuring serum Fe;	Reflects transferrin concentration;	250–450 μg/dL (45–81 μmol/L)	TIBC does not increase until Fe stores are essentially completely depleted.
Transferrin saturation (Tf-sat).	Tf-sat = Serum Fe/TIBC × 100	Used like TIBC in assessment of Fe deficiency; useful in diagnosis of iron toxicity or excess storage (hemochromatosis).	20–50% ♂ 15–50% ♀	↓ when Fe stores essentially depleted; ↑ in ↓ vitamin B_6 aplastic anemia.
Zinc protoprophyrin (ZPP)	1) ZPP:heme ratio measured by hematofluorometry; a single drop of blood required. 2) Free erythrocyte protoporphyrin (FEP) measures total red cell ZPP. These tests reflect substitution of zinc for iron during iron-deficient heme synthesis and erythropoiesis.	1) Because a ratio is measured, ZPP:H is insensitive to hemodilution; 2) Both ZPP:H and FEP also detect lead poisoning and hereditary tyrosinemia.	1) 30–80 μmol/mol 2) 17–77 μg/dL (cells) (0.27–1.23 μmol/L)	ZPP:heme ratio and FEP ↑ as iron availability ↓; both are excellent for screening and monitoring iron stores, but must be interpreted in light of possible lead poisoning and chronic inflammation.
Red cell distribution width (RDW)	Measurement of variation in RBC diameter (anisocytosis); reported to be helpful in distinguishing iron deficiency and anemia associated with chronic inflammation.	Very sensitive indicator of Fe status; normal RDW reportedly rules out anemia caused by chronic inflammatory diseases.[11]	Normal value < 16% (varies considerably with instrument used for measurement)	Specificity of RDW for Fe deficiency is relatively low; interpretation confounded by red cell transfusion; measurement usually not reported.
Ferritin	Intracellular Fe-storage protein; serum levels parallel iron stores; measured by immunoassays.	Best biochemical index of uncomplicated iron deficiency or overload (iron toxicity) and excess storage.	Males: 15–200 ng/mL (15–200 μg/L) Females: 12–150 ng/mL (12–150 μg/L)	Increases during metabolic response to injury, even when Fe stores are adequate; not useful in anemia of chronic disease.
Zinc (Zn)[13]	Serum levels measured by atomic absorption spectrophotometry.	Serum levels affected by diet and the inflammatory response. Zinc deficiency associated with many diseases and trauma.	0.7–1.5 mg/L (11–23 mmol/L)	Serum levels detect frank, but not marginal deficiency; blood must be collected in zinc free tubes.

Copper (Cu)	1) Serum levels measured by flame emission atomic absorption spectrophotometry;	1) Cu deficiency is associated with neutropenia, anemia, and scurvy-like bone disease;	1) 70–140 μg/dL ♂ (11–22 mmol/L) 80–155 μg/dL ♀ (13–24 μmol/L)	1) Serum levels detect frank, but not marginal deficiency; use of oral contraceptives ↑ serum Cu;
	2) Ceruloplasmin is the major Cu containing plasma protein; measured by immunoassay (e.g., nephelometry).	2) Ceruloplasmin is required for conversion of Fe^{3+} to Fe^{2+} during cellular Fe uptake; anemia can result from ↓ ceruloplasmin.	2) 150–600 mg/L	2) Ceruloplasmin not a useful marker of Cu status, but can be used to assess changes in status after supplementation.
Selenium (Se)	1) Serum levels measured by atomic absorption spectrophotometry; 2) Whole blood levels (measured by same methods) better reflect long-term status.	Margin between deficiency and toxicity is narrower for Se than any other trace element; important component of the antioxidant enzyme glutathione peroxidase.	1) 80–320 μg/L (1.0–4.0 μmol/L) 2) 60–340 μg/L (0.75–4.3 μmol/L)	Cutoff points for deficiency or toxicity are not well established.
Iodine (I)	Urinary excretion is best indicator of I status, either μg/24 h or μg/g creatinine; thyroid hormone level related to I status.	Excretion should be ≥ RDA for 24-h urine, or > 50 μg/g creatinine; thyroid hormone = T_3 or T_4	No urinary I reference range T_4 reference range: 5.0–12.0 μg/dL (65–155 nmol/L)	Thyroid hormone levels are affected by many factors beside iodine status.
Ultra-trace Minerals				
Chromium (Cr)	Urinary excretion usually tested by atomic absorption spectrophotometry.	Excretion should be ≥ ESADDI; deficiency reported in patients on long-term TPN; ↓ levels in DM.	10–200 ng/dL (1.9–38 nmol/L)	Test not available in most clinical laboratories; special handling required to prevent specimen contamination during collection.
Manganese (Mn)	Whole blood or serum assayed by atomic absorption spectrophotometry.	Mn is a cofactor for a variety of enzymes; ↑ in rheumatoid arthritis	Plasma: 0.7–1.2 μg/L (13–22 nmol/L) Whole Blood: 8.0–19 μg/L (150–340 nmol/L)	Test not available in most clinical laboratories; special handling required to prevent specimen contamination during collection.
Fluorine/Fluoride (Fl)	Serum assayed by gas chromatography	Levels >10–200 mμg/L are usually observed.	10–200 μg/L (0.5–10 μmol/L)	Not available in most clinical laboratories.

VII. Blood Gases and Water Status

TEST	PRINCIPLE AND REQUIREMENTS	INTERPRETATION	REFERENCE RANGE	LIMITATIONS
pH	pH = –log [H^+]; H^+ depends mainly on the CO_2 from respiration: $CO_2 + H_2O \Leftrightarrow H_2CO_3 \Leftrightarrow HCO_3 + H^+$; Measured by ion-selective electrodes (like those found in common pH meters).	In: Acidosis pH < 7.35 Alkalosis pH > 7.45 pH compatible with life 6.80–7.80.	Whole Blood: Arterial 7.35–7.45 Venous 7.32–7.42	Blood must not be exposed to air, before or during . measurement
pO_2 or PO_2 and O_2 saturation	Whole blood O_2 measured by oxygen electrode; PO_2 = "pressure" contributed by O_2 to the total "pressure" of all the gases dissolved in blood; $\text{saturation} = \frac{\text{content}}{\text{capacity}} (\times 100)$.	Affected by alveolar gas exchange, ventilation/ perfusion inequalities, generalized alveolar hypoventilation.	Arterial Blood: pO_2: 83–108 mm Hg <40 mm Hg = severe O_2 saturation: 0.95–0.98 (95–98%)	Blood must not be exposed to air, before or during . measurement

[10]The CBC includes the red cell count, the red cell indices, hemoglobin concentration (Hb), hematocrit (HCT), mean red blood cell volume (MCV), mean cell hemoglobin (MCH), mean cell hemoglobin concentration (MCHC), and white cell and platelet counts. Only HCT, Hb and MCV are dealt with here. See Savage RA. The red cell indices: Yesterday, today, and tomorrow. Clinics Lab Med 1993;13:773–785.

[11]See van Zeben D, Bieger R, van Wermeskerkan RK, Castel A, Herman J. Evaluation of microcytosis using serum ferritin and red cell distribution width. Eur J Haematol 1990;44:106–109.

[12]Ranges are for adult men and premenopausal women. Pregnant women, infants, and children have different reference ranges.

[13]Taste acuity tests can be used to supplement laboratory methods (see, e.g., Gibson RS, Smit-Vanderkooy PD, MacDonald AC, Goldman A, Ryan B and Berry M. A growth limiting mild zinc deficiency syndrome in some Southern Ontario boys with low growth percentiles. *Am J Clin Nutr* 1989;49:1266–1273).

APPENDIX 32 A GUIDE TO THE USE OF LABORATORY DATA IN NUTRITIONAL ASSESSMENT AND MONITORING *(continued)*

TEST	PRINCIPLE AND REQUIREMENTS	INTERPRETATION	REFERENCE RANGE	LIMITATIONS
pCO_2 or PCO_2	Measured by ion-selective electrode; "pressure" contributed by CO_2 to the total "pressure" of all the gases dissolved in blood.	↑ in respiratory acidosis (↑ CO_2 in inspired air or ↓ in alveolar ventilation), and ↓ in respiratory alkalosis [e.g., in hyperventilation from anxiety, mechanical ventilator, or closed head injury (damaged respiratory center)]	Whole Blood: Arterial 35–48 mm Hg ♂ 32–45 mm Hg ♀ Venous 6–7 mm Hg higher	Blood must not be exposed to air, before or during measurement.
Bicarbonate (HCO_3^-) and total CO_2 (tCO_2)	For whole blood [HCO_3^-] is calculated from the equation given in pH section.	↑ in compensated respiratory acidosis and in metabolic acidosis; ↓ in metabolic acidosis and in compensated respiratory alkalosis.	Whole Blood: Arterial 18–23 mEq/L (18–23 mmol/L)	Blood must not be exposed to air, before or during measurement.
Osmolality (osmol)	Osmol dependent on amount of particles (solutes) dissolved in a solution; measurement based on relationship between solute concentration and freezing point; serum osmo assesses hydration status and solute load.	Osmolality increases in dehydration, diabetic coma, diabetic ketoacidosis; also estimated from the formula: $mOsmol/L = 1.86\,[Na^+] + [Glucose]/18 + [BUN]/2.8$	282–300 mOsmol/kg (1 Osmol = 1 mol of solute particles; 1 kg serum ≈ 1 L)	Freezing point depression gives a more accurate estimate of osmolality than the calculated value (e.g., in ketoacidosis).

VIII. Tests of Antioxidant Status/Oxidative Stress

TEST	PRINCIPLE AND REQUIREMENTS	INTERPRETATION	REFERENCE RANGE	LIMITATIONS
Water soluble compounds	see Vitamin C			
Lipid soluble compounds: Vitamin E: See above Carotenoids Coenzyme Q10	The carotenoids: lutein, xanthein zeaxanthein, α- and β-carotene and lycopene; carotenoids and coenzyme Q10 (ubiquinone-10) are measured chromatographically.	Reference ranges for these compounds vary greatly, depending on the method used for their assay.	See reference for carotenoid range under fat malabsorption.	Tests for carotenoids and coenzyme Q are not yet available for routine clinical use.
Total antioxidant capacity: e.g., ORAC TEAC FRAP	ORAC: Oxygen radical absorbance capacity; TEAC: Trolox-equivalent antioxidant capacity FRAP: Ferric reducing ability of plasma.	These assays reflect the presence of all of plasma or serum antioxidants, including vitamins C and E, carotenoids, coenzyme Q10, glutathione, uric acid, bilirubin, superoxide dismutase, catalase, glutathione peroxidase, and albumin.		These assays are now commercially available, but are currently performed only in specialized laboratories.
Oxidative stress markers: e.g., *o*-tyrosine, nitro-tyrosine, 8-isoprostane, 4-hydroxynonenal, malondialdehyde	Free radical oxidation products of lipids (e.g., malondialdehyde, 8-isoprostane), proteins (e.g., *o*-tyrosine and nitro-tyrosine), or secondary oxidation products (e.g., 4-hydroxynonenal) can be measured chromatographically or by immunoassay.	8-Isoprostane (also called 8-epi-prostaglandin $F_{2\alpha}$) increases in plasma or urine of patients with lung disease, hypercholesterolemia, or DM.		8-Isoprostane assays are now commercially available. Markers of oxidative stress are currently assayed only in specialized laboratories.

IX. Tests for Monitoring Nutrition Support

TEST	PRINCIPLE AND REQUIREMENTS	INTERPRETATION	REFERENCE RANGE	LIMITATIONS
Chemistry panel with phosphate and Mg^{2+}	Panel includes electrolytes, glucose, creatinine, BUN and total CO_2 (bicarbonate); see above for additional test information.	Used to monitor carbohydrate tolerance, hydration status, and major organ system function.	See earlier	Very frequently ordered test panel.
Osmolality (see earlier)	Can be measured or calculated from chemistry-panel data.	Used to assess hydration status.	See earlier	Measured value accounts for substances in blood not accounted for by calculation.
Protein-energy Balance				
Serum proteins (see earlier)	Transthyretin, retinol binding protein, transferrin, albumin most often available.	These visceral proteins aid in assessing protein and energy balance.	See earlier	Stress reaction can markedly affect these and confound their interpretation as protein-energy indicators.
Nitrogen balance: UUN, TUN (see above)			Nitrogen balance in hospitalized patients ranges from −20 g to +6 g/d	UUN may greatly underestimate nitrogen excretion.
Minerals: Zn, Cu, Se, Cr (see above)			See earlier	Most trace minerals are measured only in long-term nutrition support patients.
Vitamins C and A (see above)	Because vitamin C and vitamin A are important in immune function and wound healing they should be assessed regularly.	Vitamin C levels can ↓ sharply in response to stress.	See earlier	Systematic, regular monitoring protocol should be followed.
Liver function tests (TPN only)	Bilirubin, alanine aminotransferase (ALT), gamma glutamyl transferase (GGT), and alkaline phosphatase (AlkP) assess liver function.	Excessive glucose or lipid administration, EFAD, impaired bile flow, or specific amino acid deficiency can ↑ liver enzymes and affect bilirubin.	ALT: 7–24 U/L GGT: 8–40 U/L AlkP: 20–90 U/L Bilirubin: 0.2–1.0 mg/dL (3.4–17.1 μmol/L)	Male values generally slightly higher than female; enzyme values are sensitive but not specific.
Triglycerides (TG) (see above)	Sepsis and stress can alter ability to metabolize fat, so TG should be regularly measured.	↑ TG indicates fat overload syndrome; measure TG before and after initial lipid infusion, and post-infusion weekly thereafter.	See earlier	Measurement only after lipid infusion may make interpretation impossible.
Vitamin K status (TPN only) (see above)	Contribution of the gut flora to vitamin K status is absent during TPN, and basic TPN formulas are devoid of it.	Prothrombin time (PT) is used to assess status.	See earlier	PT is affected by many other factors besides vitamin K status.

X. Tests for Metabolic Disease

TEST	PRINCIPLE AND REQUIREMENTS	INTERPRETATION	REFERENCE RANGE	LIMITATIONS
Amino acidurias	Dietary treatment is the major therapy for many of these genetic diseases; PKU, cystinuria, maple syrup urine disease, tyrosinemia, homocysteinuria, Hartnup disease are included.	Monitoring amino acid level in urine or serum is necessary to assess adequacy of treatment.	Examples: Phe 6–15 g/L (35–90 μmol/L) Cys 2–22 g/L (10–90 μmol/L) Val 17–37 g/L (145–315 μmol/L) Tyr 4–16 g/L (20–90 μmol/L)	There are several methods used to measure, e.g., phenylalaline; these usually do not have exactly equivalent reference ranges.

APPENDIX 32 A GUIDE TO THE USE OF LABORATORY DATA IN NUTRITIONAL ASSESSMENT AND MONITORING *(continued)*

TEST	PRINCIPLE AND REQUIREMENTS	INTERPRETATION	REFERENCE RANGE	LIMITATIONS
Diabetes mellitus			See Chapter 34.	
Diabetes diagnosis	1) Serum or whole blood glucose: After fasting 8–16 hr, or on a random blood sample;	1) ≥2 fasting levels >126 mg/dL is diagnostic; random level ≥200 followed by fasting level >126 is diagnostic. Fasting levels of 110 to 126 indicate impaired glucose tolerance (IGT);		1) Elevated glucose levels are normal in physiologic stress; whole blood gives slightly lower values;
	2) Glucose tolerance test (GGT); 75 g glucose (100 g during pregnancy) given after fasting; serum glucose measured by before and five times over 3 hr after oral dosing. Glucose measured by automated chemistry procedure.	2) Serum levels of >200 at 2 hr point is diagnostic; 2 hr level <140 and all 0–2 hr levels <200 is normal; 140–199 at 2 hr indicates IGT. Gestational diabetes: fasting >105, 1 hr GGT >190, 2 hr GGT >165, and 3 hr GGT >145.		2) Often used for confirmation; ambulatory patients only; bedrest or stress impairs GGT; inadequate carbohydrate consumption prior to test invalidates results.
Diabetes monitoring	1) Blood glucose—Monitoring requires that *the patient* monitor blood glucose level;	1) Tight diabetes control of requires frequent monitoring glucose levels;	1) 70–120 mg/dL (3.9–6.7 mmol/L);	A combination of glucose monitoring (by patient) and laboratory measurement of glycated proteins is needed to effectively monitor glucose control; fructosamine must be interpreted in light of plasma protein half-lives, and HbA_{1c} must be interpreted in light of red cell half-life.
	2) Serum fructosamine—assesses medium-term glucose control by measured glycated serum proteins; currently only tested in the laboratory;	2) Allows assessment of average glucose levels for previous 2–3 weeks.	2) Normal levels: 1–2% of total protein;	
	3) Serum glycated hemoglobin or HbA_{1c}—assesses longer-term glucose control; currently only tested in the laboratory.	3) Allows assessment of average glucose levels for previous 2–3 months and verification of patient's serum glucose log.	3) Normal levels: 5.0–7.5%	

APPENDIX 33 EFFECTS OF SOME DRUGS ON NUTRITIONAL STATUS

DRUG	POSSIBLE MECHANISM	NUTRITIONAL IMPLICATION
Analgesics		
Alcohol	Toxic effect on intestinal mucosa Excessive loss of magnesium in stool and urine	Decreased absorption of thiamin, folic acid, vitamin B_{12} Hypomagnesemic tetany
Colchicine	Decreases activity of intestinal disaccharidases Damages gastrointestinal mucosa by blocking mucosal cell replication	Decreased absorption of vitamin B_{12}, fat, carotene, sodium, potassium, lactose, xylose, protein Possible megaloblastic anemia
Antacids		
Aluminum hydroxide	Decreases absorption of phosphate	Phosphate depletion
Sodium bicarbonate	Alkalinization of proximal small intestine	Decreased folate absorption
Others	Basic environment inactivates thiamin and prevents formation of ferrous from ferric iron	Inadequate amount of thiamin Decreased absorption of iron
Anticoagulants		
Coumarins	Interference with regeneration of vitamin K from inactive form	Increased prothrombin time
Anticonvulsants		
Phenobarbital	Increases turnover of vitamin D, may block hydroxylation of vitamin D	Decreased serum levels of 24-hydroxyvitamin D_3 and calcium and magnesium
Phenytoin	May increase biliary excretion of vitamin D	Possible osteomalacia or rickets
Barbiturates	Accelerates inactivation of vitamin D Increases urinary excretion of vitamin C	Increased need for vitamin D with long-term use
Antidepressants		
Amitriptyline	Interference with riboflavin metabolism	
Imipramine	May increase appetite and craving for carbohydrate	Possible weight gain
Lithium carbonate	Causes change in sodium distribution and hyperexcretion	Altered blood glucose Hyponatremia Increased toxicity with low-sodium diet
Phenelzine and other MAOI drugs	MAO inhibitor Increases appetite and carbohydrate craving	Reactions with tyramine in foods Weight gain
Antifungals		
Amphotericin B	Nephrotoxicity Hepatotoxicity	Multiple side effects if kidney and liver damaged
Anti-Inflammatory Agents, Nonsteroidal		
Aspirin (salicylates)	Decreases leukocyte uptake of ascorbic acid and alters ascorbic acid distribution Damage to gastrointestinal tract; bleeding Malabsorption of vitamin B_{12}	Decreased plasma and platelet ascorbic acid levels Increased urinary loss of ascorbic acid Decreased absorption of glucose and vitamin B_{12}
Indomethacin	Gastrointestinal bleeding May cause fluid retention	Hyperkalemia Dyspepsia May cause anemia
Antimicrobials		
Cephalosporin	Inhibits prothrombin carboxylation	Increased prothrombin time Risk of vitamin K deficiency especially in elderly
Penicillins	Carry potassium with them into urine	Hypokalemia
Tetracyclines	Chelate divalent ions Decrease synthesis of vitamin K by intestinal bacteria	Net effect with minerals not clinically significant
Neomycin (Some of these changes also seen with kanamycin and paromomycin)	Causes mucosal injury resulting in decreased activity of disaccharidases and other enzymes	Decreased absorption of fat, medium-chain triglyceride, carbohydrate, protein, fat-soluble vitamins A, D, and K, vitamin B_{12}, calcium, and iron
Gentamicin	Nephrotoxicity	Increased urinary excretion of magnesium and potassium
Viomycin	Induces hyperaldosteronism	May cause hypomagnesemia, hypokalemia, hypocalcemia, alkalosis
Antineoplastics	Cytotoxic; damages intestinal mucosa	Extensive effects discussed in Chapter 36
Antipsychotics		
Chlorpromazine	Hepatotoxic May affect insulin release	Can reduce physical activity Possible weight gain
Molindone	Decreases appetite	Possible weight loss

APPENDIX 33 EFFECTS OF SOME DRUGS ON NUTRITIONAL STATUS *(continued)*

DRUG	POSSIBLE MECHANISM	NUTRITIONAL IMPLICATION
Antitubercular Agents		
Para-aminosalicylic acid	Causes intestinal injury	Decreased absorption of vitamin B_{12}, which may result in megaloblastic anemia
Isoniazid	Blocks conversion of tryptophan to niacin Inhibits pyridoxine-dependent enzymes Inhibits hydroxylation of vitamin D	Increased urinary excretion of pyridoxine Possible pyridoxine depletion May cause polyneuropathy, megaloblastic anemia Decreased serum folate
Cycloserine	Acts as a pyridoxine antagonist	May decrease serum folate, vitamin B_{12}, and pyridoxine
Antivitamins		
Methotrexate	Inhibits dihydrofolate reductase; decreases formation of active folate Causes gastrointestinal mucosal injury	Malabsorption of vitamin B_{12} and folate Weight loss, diarrhea, nausea, anorexia, vomiting, gingivitis, and stomatitis
Cardiac Drugs		
Propranolol	Suppresses normal sympathetic response to hypoglycemia	Masked signs of hypoglycemia
Digitalis glycosides	Inhibits glucose absorption	Diarrhea; cachexia; anorexia is early sign of toxicity Increased urinary excretion of potassium
Chelating Agents		
Penicillamine	Chelates with pyridoxine Chelates with zinc and copper	Increased urinary excretion of pyridoxine, zinc, and copper Peripheral neuritis, convulsions, mood changes Decreased taste acuity; unpleasant taste
CNS Stimulating Agents		
Methylphenidate	CNS effect on appetite	Decreased rate of growth in children due to decreased intake
Corticosteroids	Stimulate protein catabolism Depress protein synthesis Decrease calcium absorption	Decreased serum calcium Increased urinary excretion of potassium, zinc, and nitrogen Increased need for vitamin D Decreased bone formation
Diuretics		
Ethacrynic acid and furosemide	Anorexia and nausea	Decreased food intake Increased urinary excretion of calcium, magnesium, potassium Decreased serum magnesium and potassium
Spironolactone	Possible fluid and electrolyte imbalance May increase serum glucose	Decreased carbohydrate tolerance
Thiazides	May increase intestinal calcium absorption or increase bone resorption	Increased urinary excretion of potassium, magnesium, and sodium Possible potassium and magnesium depletion
Triamterene	Competitive inhibition of dihydrofolate reductase; reduces activation of folic acid	Decreased serum folate Possible increased calcium excretion Possible megaloblastic anemia
Hypocholesterolemics		
Cholestyramine	Binds bile salts and disrupts micelles Binds intrinsic factor at ileal pH Binds iron May bind calcium	Decreased absorption of cholesterol, vitamins A, D, K, and B_{12}, folate, fat, medium-chain triglycerides (MCTs), glucose, xylose, carotene, and iron Decreased calcium absorption Decreased serum calcium and vitamin B_{12} Increased urinary excretion of calcium
Clofibrate	May decrease activity of intestinal disaccharidases	Decreased taste acuity, unpleasant aftertaste Decreased absorption of carotene, glucose, iron, MCT, vitamin B_{12}, and electrolytes Possible anemia
Colestipol	Bile acid sequestrant	Reduced serum cholesterol Lowered plasma and serum levels of vitamins A and E

APPENDIX 33 EFFECTS OF SOME DRUGS ON NUTRITIONAL STATUS *(continued)*

DRUG	POSSIBLE MECHANISM	NUTRITIONAL IMPLICATION
Hypotensive Agents		
Hydralazine	Inactivates pyridoxine May chelate trace metals	Increased excretion of pyridoxine; pyridoxine depletion Possible peripheral neuritis
Diazoxide	Inhibits insulin release	Decreased tubular excretion of uric acid
Reserpine	Increases gastrointestinal motility and secretion	May cause weight gain May cause diarrhea
Laxatives		
Mineral oil (Petrolatum, liquid)	Dissolves fat-soluble vitamins Increases intestinal motility May decrease absorption of vitamins A, E, and K	Decreased absorption of carotene, vitamin D, and calcium and phosphate
Phenolphthalein	Can cause intestinal hyperperistalsis May irritate intestine	Can cause steatorrhea Can cause intestinal calcium and potassium loss
L-Dopa (levodopa)	Antagonizes pyridoxine Decreases absorption of some amino acids	Possible polyneuropathy related to pyridoxine depletion Risk of pyridoxine deficiency less with carbidopa/ievodopa preparation
Oral Contraceptives	May increase catabolism, decrease absorption or alter tissue uptake of vitamin C May inhibit folate conjugase May increase transport proteins for vitamin A Estrogens increase the rate of conversion of tryptophan to niacin	Altered tryptophan metabolism Decreased serum vitamin C levels Possibly decreased serum vitamin B_{12}, folate, pyridoxine, riboflavin, magnesium, and zinc Increased hemoglobin, hematocrit, serum levels of vitamins A and E, total lipids, triglycerides, iron, total iron-binding capacity (TIBC), and plasma copper Possible polyneuropathy, peripheral neuritis, and megaloblastic anemia Altered glucose tolerance
Oral Hypoglycemic Agents		
Metformin	Decreases activity of maltase, isomaltase, and sucrase in jejunum Competitive inhibition of B_{12} absorption	Decreased absorption of glucose, xylose, vitamin B_{12} Decreased serum folate, vitamin B_{12}
Phenoformin	May affect active transport mechanisms	Decreased rate of glucose absorption in human ileum Possible decreased absorption of vitamin B_{12}, fat, calcium, and amino acids
Potassium Supplements	Slow release of potassium chloride causes decrease of ileal pH (acidification)	Decreased absorption of vitamin B_{12}
Sedative-Hypnotics		
Glutethimide	Possibly increases inactivation of 25-hydroxy vitamin D_3	Increased vitamin D turnover Altered calcium need Increased bone resorption
Sulfonamides		
Salicylazosulfapyridine (Sulfasalazine)	Inhibits intestinal transport of folate Inhibits action of polyglutamyl folate conjugase	Decreased absorption of folate Decreased serum folate and serum iron Decreased response to folate supplement
Other sulfonamides	Decreased iron absorption	Possible anemia Peripheral neuritis Increased urinary excretion of ascorbic acid
Uricosuric Agents		
Probenecid	Alters renal excretion Decreases absorption of riboflavin and amino acids	Increased urinary excretion of riboflavin, calcium, magnesium, sodium, potassium, phosphate, and chloride Decreased urinary excretion of pantothenic acid
Urinary Germicides		
Nitrofurantoin	May inhibit intestinal folate conjugase	Decreased serum folate Possible megaloblastic anemia and peripheral neuritis

APPENDIX 34 MEDICATIONS WITH NUTRITION IMPLICATIONS

	SIDE EFFECTS								
MEDICATIONS	**Altered Taste**	**Anorexia**	**Hunger**	**Thirst**	**Diarrhea**	**Constipation**	**Nausea/ Vomiting**	**Flatulence**	**Dyspepsia**
Antacids									
Alka Seltzer						X	X		X
Aluminum carbonate (Basaljel)									
Aluminum hydroxide (Alterna Gel)		X			X	X	X		
Calcium carbonate (Tums)		X		X		X	X		
Gaviscon/aluminum hydroxide magnesium tristlicate		X							
Gelusil/magnesium hydroxide aluminum hydroxide smithecare					X	X			
Maalox/aluminum hydroxide magnesium hydroxide					X	X			
Riopan/Magaldrate					X				
Rolaids/dehydroxy aluminum sodium carbonate		X			X	X			
Sodium bicarbonate							X		
Antibiotics									
Amoxicillin (Amoxil, Larotid, Trimox)					X		X		
Amoxicillin, potassium Clawlanate (Augmenten)					X			X	
Amphotericin B		X			X		X		
Cefaclor (Ceclor)					X				
Cefazolin sodium (Ancef)		X			X		X		
Cefoxitin (Mefoxin)					X				
Ceftrioxone sodium (Rocephin)	X				X		X		
Cephalexin (Keflex)					X				
Chloramphenicol (Chloromycetin)	X				X		X		
Clindamycin HCl (Cleocin)		X		X	X			X	
Doxycycline (Doryx/Vibramycin)		X		X			X		
Erythromycin (Emycin, Ilosone)					X		X		
Imipenem & cilastatin (Primaxin)					X		X		
Metronidazole (Flagyl)		X			X	X	X		
Pediazole (Erythromycin)		X					X		
Tetracycline HCl (Sumycin)	X	X			X		X		
Trimethoprim with sulfamethoxazole (Bactrim)		X			X		X		
Anticoagulants									
Dicumarol					X	X	X		
Warfarin sodium (Coumadin)		X			X				
Antidiabetic Agents									
Acetohexamide (Dymelor)					X		X		X
Chlorpropamide (Diabinese)		X					X		
Glipizide (Glucotrol)	X				X	X	X		
Glyburide (DiaBeta/Micronase)					X	X	X		
Insulin									
Tolbutamide (Orinase)	X				X	X	X		
Antihypertensives									
Atenolol (Tenormin)		X			X		X		
Captopril (Capoten)	X	X			X		X		
Chlorothiazide (Diuril)		X			X	X	X		
Clonidine HCl (Catapres)		X				X	X		
Enalapril (Vasotec)					X		X		
Methyldopa (Aldomet)					X	X	X		

SIDE EFFECTS								
Abdominal Pain	**Wt Variances**	**Dry Mouth**	**Sore Tongue**	**Confusion**	**Headache**	**Fatigue/ Weakness**	**Glucose Variances**	**COMMENTS**
								w/8 oz water
								Suspension in H_2O, orange juice
								1–3 h after meals. Calcium and vitamin A deficiency
X		X						1–3 h after meals. Do not take with bran, dairy, or whole grain products
	X							1–3 h after meals
								1 h after meals
								1 h after meals & bedtime
								Empty stomach w/8 oz H_2O
X						X		1–3 h after meals
X								1–3 h after meals
								Anemia
								Take consistently with meal. Anemia and possible hypokalomia
X	X				X			
			X		X		X	Monitor diabetic, anemia, hypokalemia
X	X					X		Parenteral administration
								Parenteral administration
					X			Parenteral administration. Vitamin K deficiency (possible)
					X	X		
				X		X	X	Take on empty stomach. Monitor diabetes, anemia
X	X							
						X		Dysphagia, possible anemia
X								1–2 h before or after meal
X	X							Parenteral administration
		X			X	X		
X					X		X	Possible hypoglycemia, hepatitis
X					X			1 h before meals or 2 h after meals
					X		X	Caution with diabetes, jaundice, hepatitis
X							X	Limit foods with vitamin K. Caution with diabetic
X								Limit foods with vitamin K. Hepatitis and jaundice. Avoid proteolytic enzymes (Papain) and soybean oil.
						X		Before AM & PM meal. Anemia
						X		Anemia
					X	X		
						X		
							X	Parenteral. Monitor for hypo/hyperglycemia
X					X	X		Take in AM
	X	X		X		X	X	Caution with diabetics, may mask signs of hypoglycemia
	X	X			X			
		X						
	X	X			X	X		
					X			
	X	X			X			Edema, jaundice, depression

APPENDIX 34 MEDICATIONS WITH NUTRITION IMPLICATIONS *(continued)*

	SIDE EFFECTS								
MEDICATIONS	**Altered Taste**	**Anorexia**	**Hunger**	**Thirst**	**Diarrhea**	**Constipation**	**Nausea/ Vomiting**	**Flatulence**	**Dyspepsia**
Antiphypertensives *(continued)*									
Metoprolol tartrate (Lopressor)					X	X		X	
Minoxidil (Loniten)									
Prozosen HCl (Minipress)					X		X		
Spirinolactone (Aldactazide)		X			X				
Triamterene (Dyazide)		X		X	X		X		
Antiparkinsonian Agents									
Bromocriptine (Parlodel)		X			X	X	X		
Levodopa (Dopar/Larodopa)	X	X			X	X	X		
Levodopa Carbedopa (Sinemet)		X				X	X	X	
Selegiline (Eldepryl)	X	X			X	X	X		
Aspirin									
Aspirin, Ecotrin, Empirin		X					X		X
Barbiturates									
Phenobarbital					X	X	X		
Pentobarbital (Nembutal)						X	X		
Secobarbital (Seconal)						X	X		
Benzodiazepines									
Alprozolam (Xanax)		X			X	X	X		
Chlordiazepoxide (Librium)						X	X		
Diazepam (Valium) (Valrealse)			X						
Lorazepam (Ativan)		X			X	X			
Flurazepam (Dalmane)		X			X	X	X		
Clonazepam (Klonopin)		X							
Bronchodilator									
Theophyline preparations									
Theophyline (Bronkodyl)		X			X		X		
Elixophyllin Slo-Bid									
Slophyllin Theobid									
Theolair, Thea-24									
Diuretics									
Acetazolamide (Diamox)		X			X		X		
Bumetanide (Bumex)					X		X		
Furosemide (Lasix)		X		X			X		
Metolazone (Duilo/Zaroxolyn)		X			X	X	X		
Triamterene (Dypenium)					X		X		
Triamterene/Hydrochlorothiazide (Dyazide)					X		X		
Lithium Carbonate									
{Eskalith Lithane, Lithabid Lithonate & Lithotabs}				X	X		X		
Monoamine Oxidase (MAO) Inhibitors									
Phenelzine (Nardil)						X			
Tranylaypromine sulfate (Parnate)		X			X	X	X		
Penicillamine (Cuprimine, Depen)	X	X					X		
Sucralfate (Carafate)						X			
Thyroid Preparations									
Thyroglobulin (Proloid)					X		X		
Thyroid, Synthyroid									
Thyrolar, Liotrix									

Note: This is a partial list and is not inclusive of all medications.

SIDE EFFECTS								
Abdominal Pain	Wt Variances	Dry Mouth	Sore Tongue	Confusion	Headache	Fatigue/ Weakness	Glucose Variances	COMMENTS
X		X		X		X		
					X	X		Monitor fluid and electrolytes, edema
	X	X			X	X		
X		X		X	X		X	Monitor diabetic, bleeding
		X			X		X	Monitor diabetic and electrolytes (potassium)
X		X			X	X		
		X						
	X	X			X		X	Monitor diabetic, edema, anemia
X	X	X		X				
							X	Not for patient prone to vitamin K deficiency. Anemia. Caution with diabetics
	X			X	X		X	Caution with diabetes, low bone density, osteomalacia
	X							
				X	X			
		X		X	X			
				X				Edema, jaundice, blurred vision
	X	X		X		X		
	X	X						
		X		X				
	X	X			X	X		
			X			X		Caution with diabetics
	X			X			X	Monitor diabetic, anemia
X		X			X	X	X	Monitor diabetic and electrolytes
		X			X		X	Monitor diabetic and electrolytes (hypokalemia)
		X			X		X	Monitor diabetic and electrolytes
		X			X	X	X	Monitor diabetic and electrolytes
		X			X	X		
	X	X					X	Caution with diabetes and monitor electrolytes
					X	X		
	X	X			X		X	May result in hypertension. Monitor diabetics
X		X			X		X	Monitor diabetic and electrolytes. Limit caffeine
								Omit foods with Cu (chocolate, nuts, shellfish, mushrooms, liver, raisins, molasses, broccoli)
X		X			X			Empty stomach 1 h before meals
	X				X		X	Monitor diabetic

APPENDIX 35 MILK-BASED FORMULA, OR PRODUCTS DESIGNED TO BE MIXED WITH MILK*

PRODUCT	CARNATION INSTANT BREAKFAST	DIET CARNATION INSTANT BREAKFAST	COMPLEAT REGULAR	DELMARK INSTANT BREAKFAST	FORTA SHAKE	MERITENE POWDER	SUSTACAL POWDER	ULTRA SLIM FAST
Source	Nestlé	Nestlé	Novartis	Novartis	Ross	Novartis	Mead Johnson	Slim Fast Food Company
	Mixed as directed with 2% milk	Mixed as directed with 2% milk		Mixed as directed with whole milk	Mixed as directed with whole milk	Mixed as directed with whole milk	Mixed as directed with skim milk	Mixed as directed with skim milk
Form	Powder	Powder	Liquid	Powder	Powder	Powder	Powder	Powder
Kcal/mL	.93	.7	1.07	1.22	1.2	1.08	1.09	.74
Pro (%Kcal)	19	25	16	21	24	26	30	27
CHO (%Kcal)	63	51	48	51	51	45	68	66
Fat (%Kcal)	18	24	36	28	25	29	2	7
Pro (g/L)	51	68	43	62.4	71	69	79	50
CHO (g/L)	167	136	130	153.6	154	120	180	133
Fat (g/L)	21	28	43	37.2	33	34	4.6	6
Cal: N	130	99	156	120	107	96	88	93
Na^+ (mEq/L)	44.5	54.6	57	37.8	43	48	52.2	42
K^+ (mEq/L)	73	97	36	66	86	72	92.3	65
Osmol (mOsmol/kg)	661–747	467–485	450	796	808 (van)	690	950	NA
Vol to Meet RDI	1065	1065	1500	NA	948	1040	840	Not intended sole source of nutrition
Pro Source	Nonfat milk; fluid 2% milk used to mix	Nonfat milk, fluid 2% milk used to mix	Beef, nonfat milk	Nonfat dry milk, fluid whole milk used to mix	Nonfat dry milk, fluid whole milk for mixing	Nonfat milk, whole milk for mixing	Nonfat milk	Nonfat milk
CHO Source	Maltodextrin, sucrose, lactose	Maltodextrin	Maltodextrin, vegetables, fruit, nonfat milk	Dextrose, sugar, lactose	Sucrose, lactose	Lactose, sucrose, hydrolyzed starch	Sucrose, corn syrup solids, lactose	Lactose, sucrose
Fat Source	Butterfat from milk used to mix	Butterfat from milk used to mix	Corn oil, beef	Butterfat from milk used to mix	Butterfat from milk used to mix	Butterfat from milk used to mix	Milk fat	Vegetable oil
Flavors Available	Vanilla, chocolate, strawberry	Vanilla, chocolate	—	Vanilla, chocolate, strawberry	Vanilla, chocolate, eggnog, strawberry	Plain, chocolate, vanilla, eggnog, milk choc	Vanilla	Vanilla, chocolate, strawberry
Additional Comments		Contains aspartame	Benderized diet of traditional foods, 4.3 g dietary fiber/L	Vitamin & mineral fortified			Low fat	Contains 18.5 g fiber/L Low in fat
Ultratrace Mineral & Conditionally Essential Nutrient Fortified	No	No	Yes	No	No	No	No	Ultratrace minerals only

*Prepared by Marion Winkler and Susan Manchester.

APPENDIX 36A WHOLE PROTEIN, LACTOSE-FREE FORMULAS—.5 Kcal/mL*

PRODUCT	ENTRITION .5	INTRO-LYTE
Source	**Nestlé**	**Ross**
Form	Liquid	Liquid
Kcal/mL	.5	.53
Pro (%Kcal)	14	16.7
CHO (%Kcal)	54.5	53.3
Fat (%Kcal)	31.5	30.0
Pro (g/L)	17.5	22.2
CHO (g/L)	68	70.5
Fat (g/L)	17.5	18.4
Cal: N	179	150
Na^+ (mEq/L)	15.2	40.5
K^+ (mEq/L)	15.4	40.2
Osmol (mOsmol/kg)	120	220
Vol to meet RDI	4000	1321
Pro Source	Sodium-calcium caseinate	Soy protein isolate
CHO Source	Maltodextrin	Hydrolyzed corn starch
Fat Source	Corn oil	MCT, corn, soy oils
Flavors Available	Unflavored	Unflavored
Uses	Low osmo for initiating tube feedings	Introductory tube feed
Ultratrace Mineral & Conditionally Essential Nutrient Fortified	No	Ultratrace minerals only

*Prepared by Marion Winkler and Susan Manchester.

APPENDIX 36B WHOLE PROTEIN, LACTOSE-FREE FORMULAS—1 TO 1.2 Kcal/mL

PRODUCT	BENEFIT	BOOST	COMPLETE MODIFIED	ENSURE	ENSURE HIGH PROTEIN	ENSURE WITH FIBER	ENTRITION HN	FIBER SOURCE	FIBER SOURCE HN	ISOCAL
Company	**HMR**	**Mead Johnson**	**Novartis**	**Ross**	**Ross**	**Ross**	**Nestlé**	**Novartis**	**Novartis**	**Mead Johnson**
Form	Liquid	Liquid	Liquid	Liquid	Liquid	Liquid	Liquid	Liquid	Liquid	Liquid
Kcal/mL	1.04	1.0	1.07	1.06	.95	1.1	1.0	1.2	1.2	1.06
Pro (%Kcal)	22	17	16	14	21	14.5	17.6	14	18	13
CHO (%Kcal)	50	69	53	63.9	55	55	45.6	56	52	50
Fat (%Kcal)	29	14	31	22	24	30.5	36.8	30	30	37
Pro (g/L)	58	43	43	37.2	50	39.7	44	43	53	34
CHO (g/L)	137	171	140	169	128	162	114	170	160	135
Fat (g/L)	33	17	37	25.9	25	37.2	41	41	41	44
Cal:N	112	147	156	178	117	173	142	177	144	193
Na^+ (mEq/L)	41.6	23.7	43	36.8	52.4	36.8	36.7	48	48	23
K^+ (mEq/L)	47	43	36	40	53.3	43.4	40.5	46	46	34
Osmol (mOsmol/kg)	NA	590–620	300	555	610	480	300	390	390	270
Vol to meet RDI	1200	1180	1500	948	960	1390	1300	1500	1500	1890
Pro Source	Calcium caseinate, soy protein	Milk protein concentrate	Beef, calcium caseinate	Soy & calcium caseinates, soy protein isolate	Sodium & calcium caseinates, soy protein isolate	Sodium & calcium caseinates, soy protein isolate	Sodium & calcium caseinates, soy protein isolate	Sodium & calcium caseinates	Sodium & calcium caseinates	Sodium & calcium caseinates, soy protein isolate
CHO Source	Fructose, sucrose, dextrose	Sugar, corn syrup solids	Maltodextrin, vegetables, fruit	Corn syrup, maltodextrin	Sucrose, maltodextrin	Maltodextrin, sucrose	Maltodextrin	Hydrolyzed corn starch, soy fiber	Hydrolyzed corn starch, soy fiber	Maltodextrin
Fat Source	Corn oil	Canola, sunflower and corn oils	Canola oil, beef fat	Safflower, canola oils	Safflower, canola, soy oils	Corn oil	Corn oil	MCT, canola oils	MCT, canola oils	Soy, MCT oils
Flavors Available	Vanilla, choc	Vanilla, chocolate, chocolate mocha, strawberry	—	7 flavors available	Vanilla, choc, wildberry, banana	Vanilla, choc, butter pecan	Unflavored	Vanilla	Vanilla	Unflavored
Additional Comments	Powder form also available. 11 g dietary fiber/L (corn bran)	Natural milk taste but lactose-free	4.3 g dietary fiber/L. Blenderized diet of traditional foods	Powder form also available	Elevated levels vit E zinc, high protein	14.4 g dietary fiber/L (soy fiber)		10 g dietary fiber/L (soy fiber)	7 g dietary fiber/L (soy fiber)	
Ultratrace Mineral & Conditionally Essential Nutrient Fortified	Ultratrace minerals only	Ultratrace minerals only	Yes	Ultratrace minerals only	Ultratrace minerals only	Ultratrace minerals only	No	Ultratrace minerals only	Ultratrace minerals only	Ultratrace minerals only

*Prepared by Marion Winkler and Susan Manchester.

APPENDIX 36B WHOLE PROTEIN, LACTOSE-FREE FORMULAS—1 TO 1.2 Kcal/mL *(continued)*

PRODUCT	ISOCAL HN	ISOSOURCE	ISOSOURCE VHN	ISOTEIN HN	JEVITY	NUBASICS	NUBASICS VHP	NUTREN 1.0	OSMOLITE	OSMOLITE HN
Company	Mead Johnson	Novartis	Novartis	Novartis (Mixed @ Standard Dilution)	Ross	Nestlé	Nestlé	Nestlé	Ross	Ross
Form	Liquid	Liquid	Liquid	Powder	Liquid	Liquid	Liquid	Liquid	Liquid	Liquid
Kcal/mL	1.06	1.2	1.0	1.2	1.06	1.0	1.0	1.0	1.06	1.06
Pro (%Kcal)	17	14	25	23	16.7	14	25	16	14	16.7
CHO (%Kcal)	46	56	50	52	54.3	53	45	51	57	54.3
Fat (%Kcal)	37	30	25	25	29	33	30	33	29	29
Pro (g/L)	44	43	62	68	44.3	35	62.4	40	37.1	44.3
CHO (g/L)	123	170	130	160	154.4	132.4	112.8	127	151	143.9
Fat (g/L)	45	41	29	34	34.7	36.8	33.2	38	34.7	34.7
Cal:N	150	173	102	111	150	178	100	156	178	150
Na^+ (mEq/L)	40	52	57	27	40.5	38	38	38	27.8	40.5
K^+ (mEq/L)	41	43	41	28	40.2	32	32	32.1	26.1	40.2
Osmol (mOsmol/kg)	270	360	300	300	300	500–520	460	300–350	300	300
Vol to meet RDI	1180	1500	1250	1770	1320	2000	2000	1500	1887	1320
Pro Source	Sodium & calcium caseinates, soy protein isolate	Sodium & calcium caseinates, soy protein isolate	Sodium & calcium caseinates	Delactosed lactalbumin	Sodium & calcium caseinates	Calcium-potassium caseinate	Calcium-potassium caseinate	Casein	Sodium & calcium caseinates	Sodium & calcium caseinates, soy protein isolate
CHO Source	Maltodextrin	Hydrolyzed corn starch	Hydrolyzed corn starch, soy fiber	Hydrolyzed corn starch, fructose	Maltodextrin, corn syrup, soy fiber	Corn syrup solids, sucrose	Corn syrup solids, sucrose	Maltodextrin, corn syrup solids	Maltodextrin	Maltodextrin
Fat Source	Soy & MCT oils	MCT, canola oils	MCT, canola oils	Soybean, MCT oils	Safflower, canola, MCT oils	Canola, corn oils	Canola, corn oils	MCT, canola, corn oils	Safflower, canola, MCT oils	Safflower, canola, MCT oils
Flavors Available	Unflavored	Vanilla	Vanilla	Vanilla	Unflavored	Vanilla, chocolate, strawberry	Vanilla	Vanilla, unflavored also available with 14 g fiber/L	Unflavored	Unflavored
Additional Comments			10 g dietary fiber/L as soy		14.4 g dietary fiber/L as soy	Available with fiber (14 g/L)	High in protein			
Ultratrace Mineral & Conditionally Essential Nutrient Fortified	Yes	Ultratrace minerals only	Yes	Ultratrace minerals only	Yes	Yes	Yes	Yes	Yes	Yes

APPENDIX 36B WHOLE PROTEIN, LACTOSE-FREE FORMULAS—1 TO 1.2 Kcal/mL *(continued)*

PRODUCT	OSMOLITE HN PLUS	PROBALANCE	PROMOTE	PROTAIN XL	REPLETE	RESOURCE STANDARD	SUSTACAL	SUSTACAL WITH FIBER	ULTRACAL
Company	Ross	Nestlé	Ross	Mead Johnson	Nestlé	Sandoz	Mead Johnson	Mead Johnson	Mead Johnson
Form	Liquid	Liquid	Liquid	Liquid	Liquid	Liquid	Liquid	Liquid	Liquid
Kcal/mL	1.2	1.2	1.0	1.0	1.0	1.06	1.0	1.06	1.06
Pro (%Kcal)	18.5	18	25	25	25	14	24	17	17
CHO (%Kcal)	52.5	52	52	52	45	54	55	53	46
Fat (%Kcal)	29	30	23	26	30	32	21	30	37
Pro (g/L)	55.5	54	62.5	57	62.5	37.2	61	46	44
CHO (g/L)	157.5	156	130	129	113	140	139	139	123
Fat (g/L)	39.3	40.6	26	26	34	37.2	23	35	45
Cal:N	135	139	100	112	100	178	103	144	153
Na^+ (mEq/L)	61.7	32.8	43.5	40	38	39	40	31.2	40
K^+ (mEq/L)	49.7	40	50.6	45	39	41	54	36	41
Osmol (mOsmol/kg)	360	350–450	340	340	300–350	430	650–690	480	310
Vol to meet RDI	1000	1000	1000	1250	1000	1890	1060	1420	1180
Pro Source	Sodium caseinate	Calcium-potassium caseinate	Sodium & calcium caseinates, soy protein isolates	Sodium & calcium caseinates	Sodium & potassium caseinates	Sodium & calcium caseinates, soy protein isolates	Sodium & calcium caseinates, soy protein isolates	Sodium & calcium caseinates, soy protein isolate	Sodium & calcium caseinates
CHO Source	Maltodextrin	Maltodextrin, soy polysaccharides, gum arabic	Hydrolyzed corn starch, sucrose	Maltodextrin, soy fiber	Maltodextrin, corn syrup solids	Hydrolyzed corn starch, sugar	Sugar, corn syrup solids	Maltodextrin, sugar	Maltodextrin
Fat Source	Safflower, canola, MCT oils	Canola, MCT, corn oils	Safflower, canola, MCT oils	MCT, corn oils	Canola, MCT oils	Corn oil	Partially hydrogenated soy oil	Corn oil	Canola, MCT oils
Flavors Available	Unflavored	Vanilla & unflavored	Vanilla	Unflavored	Unflavored & vanilla	Vanilla, choc, strawberry	Vanilla, choc, eggnog, strawberry	Vanilla, choc, strawberry	Vanilla
Additional Comments	Contains β-carotene	For use in geriatric population; antioxidants & zinc 10 g dietary fiber/L	Added β-carotene, high protein Also available with fiber 14.4 g/L	Elevated levels zinc, vitamins C & A, 9 g dietary fiber/L from soy	Also available with fiber (14 g/L) enriched with vitamin C, zinc, β-carotene		High in protein, also available in powder form	11 g dietary fiber/L as soy fiber	14.2 g dietary fiber/L as soy fibers
Ultratrace Mineral & Conditionally Essential Nutrient Fortified	Yes	Yes	Yes	Ultratrace minerals only	Yes	No	Ultratrace minerals only	No	Yes

APPENDIX 36C WHOLE PROTEIN, LACTOSE-FREE HIGH-CALORIE FORMULAS

	1.5 Kcal/mL								2.0 Kcal/mL			
PRODUCT	**COMPLY**	**ENSURE PLUS**	**ENSURE PLUS HN**	**ISOSOURCE 1.5**	**NUBASICS PLUS**	**NUTREN 1.5**	**RESOURCE PLUS**	**SUSTACAL PLUS**	**DELIVER 2.0**	**NUBASICS 2.0 DRINK**	**NUTREN 2.0**	**TWO CAL HN**
Company	**Mead Johnson**	**Ross**	**Ross**	**Novartis**	**Nestlé**	**Nestlé**	**Novartis**	**Mead Johnson**	**Mead Johnson**	**Nestlé**	**Nestlé**	**Ross**
Form	Liquid	Liquid	Liquid	Liquid	Liquid	Liquid	Liquid	Liquid	Liquid	Liquid	Liquid	Liquid
Kcal/mL	1.5	1.5	1.5	1.5	1.5	1.5	1.5	1.52	2.0	2.0	2.0	2.0
Pro (%Kcal)	16	14.7	16.7	18	14	16	14	16	15	16	16	16.7
CHO (%Kcal)	48	53.3	53.3	44	47	45	58	50	40	39	39	43.2
Fat (%Kcal)	36	32	30	38	39	39	28	34	45	45	45	40.1
Pro (g/L)	60	54.9	62.6	68	52.4	60	55	61	75	80	80	83.7
CHO (g/L)	180	200	199.9	165	176.4	169.5	217	190	200	196	196	217.3
Fat (g/L)	60	53.3	50	63	64.8	67.5	46	57	102	106	106	90.9
Cal:N	160	171	150	138	179	156	173	160	167	156	160	150
Na^+ (mEq/L)	52	45.7	51.3	57	51	50.1	56	37	35	56.6	57	63.3
K^+ (mEq/L)	47	49.5	46.5	54	48	48.2	49	38	43	49.2	49	62.8
Osmol (mOsmol/kg)	460	690	650	650	620–650	430–530		630–670	640	750	720	690
Volume to meet RDI	830	1420	947	933	1330	1000	1400	1180	1000	750	750	947
Pro Source	Sodium & calcium caseinates	Sodium & calcium caseinates, soy protein isolate	Sodium & calcium caseinates, soy protein isolate	Sodium & calcium caseinates	Calcium-potassium caseinate	Calcium-potassium caseinates	Sodium & calcium caseinates, soy protein isolate	Sodium & calcium caseinates	Sodium & calcium caseinates	Calcium-potassium caseinate	Calcium-potassium caseinate	Sodium & calcium caseinates
CHO Source	Maltodextrin	Corn syrup, maltodextrin	Maltodextrin, sucrose	Hydrolyzed corn starch, sugar, soy fiber, guar gum	Corn syrup solids, sucrose	Maltodextrin	Corn syrup solids	Corn syrup solids, sugar	Corn syrup	Corn syrup solids, sugar	Corn syrup solids, sucrose	Maltodextrin, sucrose
Fat Source	Canola, MCT, corn oils	Corn oil	Corn oil	MCT, canola oils	Canola, corn oils	MCT, canola, corn oils	Sunflower, soy oils	Corn oil	Soy, MCT oils	MCT, canola oils	MCT, canola oils	Corn, MCT oils
Flavors Available	Unflavored	6 flavors available	Vanilla, chocolate	Vanilla	Vanilla, chocolate, strawberry	Unflavored, vanilla	Vanilla, chocolate, strawberry	Vanilla, chocolate, strawberry, eggnog	Vanilla	Vanilla	Vanilla	Vanilla
Additional Comments				3.8 g insol. fiber/L 4.2 g sol. fiber/L							—	
Ultratrace Mineral & Conditionally Essential Nutrient Fortified	Yes	Ultratrace minerals only	Yes	Yes	Yes	Yes	Ultratrace minerals only	Ultratrace minerals only	Ultratrace minerals only	Yes	Yes	Ultratrace minerals only

*Prepared by Marion Winkler and Susan Manchester.

APPENDIX 37 SPECIALLY DESIGNED FORMULA DIETS*

	Clear Liquid			*Fat Malabsorption*	
PRODUCT	**CITROTEIN**	**FORTA DRINK**	**RESOURCE FRUIT BEVERAGE**	**LIPISORB**	**TRAVASORB MCT**
Company	**Novartis**	**Ross**	**Novartis**	**Mead Johnson**	**Nestlé**
Form	Powder mixed at standard dilution	Powder mixed at standard dilution	Liquid	Liquid (also available in powder form)	Powder mixed at 1.0 KCal/mL
Kcal/mL	.67	.6	.76	1.35	1.0
Protein (% Calories)	25	24	20	17	20
Carbohydrate (% Calories)	73	71	80	48	50
Fat (% Calories)	2	6	0	35	30
Protein (g/L)	41	33.3	37	57	49.3
Carbohydrate (g/L)	120	100	150	161	122.8
Fat (g/L)	1.6	3.6	0	57	83
Cal: N	101	106	131	150	127
Na^+ (mEq/L)	29	20.3	6.5	59	15.2
K^+ (mEq/L)	14	12	1.1	43	26
Osmol (mOsmol/kg)	480–510	410–502	700	630	250
Volume to Meet RDI Vit/Min (mL)	Supplemental use only	1480	Supplemental use only	1180	2000
Protein Source	Pasteurized egg white solids	Whey protein concentrate	Whey protein concentrate	Sodium & calcium caseinates	Lactalbumin
Carbohydrate Source	Sucrose, maltodextrin	Sucrose, pineapple juice solids	Sugar, hydrolyzed corn starch	Maltodextrin, sugar	Corn syrup solids
Fat Source	Partially hydrogenated soy oil	Not available	—	MCT, soy oils	MCT, sunflower oils
Flavors Available	Orange, punch	Orange, fruit punch	Orange, peach, wild berry, iced tea	Vanilla	—
Use	Low-residue, low-fat, presurgery alternative to "milky" type supplements	Low-residue, low-fat, presurgery alternative to "milky" type supplements	Low-residue, low-fat, presurgery alternative to "milky" type supplements	Fat malabsorption (85% MCT oil)	Fat malabsorption (80% fat as MCT)
Special Features	—	—	Low electrolyte	—	—
Ultratrace Mineral & Conditionally Essential Nutrient Fortified	No	No	No	Yes	No

	Glucose Intolerance					*Hepatic*	
PRODUCT	**CHOICE DM**	**DIABETI-SOURCE**	**GLUCERNA**	**GLYTROL**	**RESOURCE DIABETIC**	**HEPATIC AID II**	**NUTRIHEP**
Company	**Mead Johnson**	**Novartis**	**Nestlé**	**Ross**	**Novartis**	**B/Braun**	**Nestlé**
Form		Liquid	Liquid	Liquid	Liquid	Powder mixed at standard dilution	Liquid
Kcal/mL	1.06	1.0	1.0	1.0	1.06	1.2	1.5
Protein (% Calories)	16.8	20	18	16.7	24	15	11
Carbohydrate (% Calories)	40	36	40	34.3	36	57	77
Fat (% Calories)	43	44	42	49	40	28	12
Protein (g/L)	45	50	45	41.8	63	45	40
Carbohydrate (g/L)	106	90	100	95.8	99	173	289
Fat (g/L)	53	49	47.5	54.4	47	37	21
Cal: N	150	100	142	150	106	174	234
Na^+ (mEq/L)	37	43	32.2	40.3	42	< 15	14
K^+ (mEq/L)	47	35.9	35.9	40.3	29	< 6	34
Osmol (mOsmol/kg)	440	360	380	355	450	560	690
Volume to Meet RDI Vit/Min (mL)	1000	1500	1400	1422	1890	Incomplete	1000
Protein Source	Milk protein concentrate, casein	Calcium caseinate, beef	Calcium-potassium caseinates	Sodium & calcium caseinates	Sodium & calcium caseinates	Free amino acids, 46% branched chain amino acids	L-Amino acids, whey protein (50% branched chain amino acids)
Carbohydrate Source	Maltodextrin, sucrose, soy fiber	Vegetables, fruits, maltodextrin, fructose	Maltodextrin, corn starch, fructose, gum arabic, pectin	Maltodextrin, soy fiber, fructose	Hydrolyzed corn starch, fructose	Maltodextrin, sucrose	Maltodextrin, modified corn starch (66%)

Fat Source	Canola, sunflower, corn, MCT oils	Sunflower, canola oils, beef fat	Canola, high-oleic safflower, MCT oils	Canola oil	Sunflower, soy bean oils	Soy oil	MCT, canola, corn, soy oils, lecithin
Flavors Available	Vanilla	—	Vanilla	Vanilla	Van, choc, strawberry	Eggnog, custard, chocolate	Vanilla & unflavored; flavored packets available
Use	—	Diabetes, stress	—	Patients with abnormal glucose tolerance	—	Liver disease	Liver disease
Special Features	—	10 g soy fiber/L	10 g soluble fiber/L 5 g insoluble fiber/L	14.4 g dietary fiber/L	13 g fiber/L	—	—
Ultratrace Mineral & Conditionally Essential Nutrient Fortified	—	Yes	Yes	Yes	Yes	No	Ultratrace minerals only

	Immune-Support				*Metabolic Stress*		
PRODUCT	**ADVERA**	**IMMUNE-AID**	**IMPACT**	**IMPACT 1.5**	**CRUCIAL**	**PERATIVE**	**TRAUMACAL**
Company	**Ross**	**B/Braun**	**Novartis**	**Novartis**	**Nestlé**	**Ross**	**Mead Johnson**
Form	Liquid	Powder mixed at standard dilution	Liquid	Liquid	Liquid	Liquid	Liquid
Kcal/mL	1.28	1.0	1.0	1.5	1.5	1.3	1.5
Protein (% Calories)	19	32	22	22	25	20	22
Carbohydrate (% Calories)	65	48	53	38	36	55	38
Fat16 (% Calories)	20	25	40	39	25	40	
Protein (g/L)	60	80	56	80	93.8	66.6	82
Carbohydrate (g/L)	215	120	132	140	135	177.2	142
Fat (g/L)	23	22	28	69	67.6	37.4	68
Cal: N	133	78	91	96	100	122	116
Na^+ (mEq/L)	45.9	25	48	56	50.8	45.2	51
K^+ (mEq/L)	72.5	27	36	43	48	44.2	36
Osmol (mOsmol/kg)	680	460	375	550	490	385	560
Volume to Meet RDI Vit/Min (mL)	1183	2000	1500	1250	1000	1155	2000
Protein Source	Soy protein hydrolysate, sodium caseinate	Lactalbumin, supplemental amino acids	Sodium & calcium caseinates, L-arginine	Sodium & calcium caseinates, L-arginine	Enzymatically hydrolyzed casein, L-arginine	Partially hydrolyzed sodium caseinate, lactalbumin hydrolysate	Sodium & calcium caseinates
Carbohydrate Source	Maltodextrin, sucrose, soy fiber	Maltodextrin	Hydrolyzed corn starch	Hydrolyzed corn starch	Maltodextrin, corn starch	Maltodextrin	Corn syrup, sugar
Fat Source	Canola, MCT, sardine oils	MCT, canola oils	Palm, sunflower, & menhaden oils	MCT, palm kernel, menhaden oils	MCT, marine, soy oils	Canola, MCT, corn oils	Soy, MCT oils
Flavors Available	Chocolate, vanilla	Custard	—	—	Unflavored	—	Vanilla
Use	HIV infection, AIDS	Stressed immune system surgery, burns, trauma	Sepsis, trauma, stressed immune system	Sepsis, trauma, burns, stressed immune system	Critical illness	Metabolically stressed patients	Hypermetabolic states
Special Features	8.7 g dietary fiber/L; fortified with β-carotene, vit E, C, B_6, B_{12} & folic acid	Enriched with arginine glutamine, and branched chain amino acids, nucleic acids	Enriched with arginine, dietary nucleotides, fish oils, structured lipids also available with 10 g fiber/L	Enriched with arginine, glutamine, branched chain amino acids, structured lipids	Peptide based, supplemented with arginine; high in n3 fatty acids	Supplemented with L-arginine, β-carotene; contains peptides and free amino acids	Increased amounts of MCT, B complex, E, copper, zinc
Ultratrace Mineral & Conditionally Essential Nutrient Fortified	Yes	Yes	Ultratrace minerals only	Yes	Yes	Yes	No

APPENDIX 37 SPECIALLY DESIGNED FORMULA DIETS* *(continued)*

Pulmonary					
PRODUCT	**NOVA-SOURCE PULMONARY**	**NUTRIVENT**	**OXEPA**	**PULMOCARE**	**RESPALOR**
Company	**Novartis**	**Nestlé**	**Ross**	**Ross**	**Mead Johnson**
Form	Liquid	Liquid	Liquid	Liquid	Liquid
Kcal/mL	1.5	1.5	1.5	1.5	1.52
Protein (% Calories)	20	18	16.7	16.7	20
Carbohydrate (% Calories)	40	27	28	28.2	39
Fat (% Calories)	40	55	55	55.1	41
Protein (g/L)	75	67.5	62	62.6	76
Carbohydrate (g/L)	146	100	104	105.7	148
Fat (g/L)	68	94	92	93.3	71
Cal: N	128	142	150	150	128
Na^+ (mEq/L)	56	51	56	57	55
K^+ (mEq/L)	63	48	50	44.2	37.9
Osmol (mOsmol/kg)	650	330–450	493	475	580
Volume to Meet RDI Vit/Min (mL)	NA	1000	947	947	1420
Protein Source	Sodium & calcium caseinates	Calcium-potassium caseinate	Sodium & calcium caseinates	Sodium & calcium caseinates	Sodium & calcium caseinates
Carbohydrate Source	Corn syrup, sugar, soy fiber	Maltodextrin	Sugar, maltodextrin	Sucrose, maltodextrin	Corn syrup, sugar
Fat Source	Canola, MCT oils	Canola, MCT, corn oils	MCT, canola, sardine, borage oils	Canola, MCT, corn, and safflower oils	Canola, MCT oils
Flavors Available	Vanilla	Vanilla & unflavored	Unflavored	Vanilla, strawberry	Vanilla
Use	Respiratory disease	Pulmonary patients	Patients at risk of acute respiratory distress syndrome	Pulmonary patients	Pulmonary patients
Special Features	8 g fiber/L; fortified with vit C, E & β-carotene	Elevated phosphorus low carbohydrate	Contains eicosapentaenoic acid, gamma-linolenic acid. Elevated levels of antioxidants	Includes vitamin E, β-carotene; low carbohydrate	Low carbohydrate
Ultratrace Mineral & Conditionally Essential Nutrient Fortified	Yes	Yes	Yes	Yes	Ultra-trace minerals only

Renal

PRODUCT	AMIN-AID	MAGNACAL RENAL	NEPRO	NOVASOURCE RENAL	RENALCAL	SUPLENA
Company	**R & D Labs**	**Mead Johnson**	**Ross**	**Novartis**	**Nestlé**	**Ross**
Form	Powder mixed at standard dilution	Liquid	Liquid	Liquid	Liquid	Liquid
Kcal/mL	2	2.0	2	2.0	2.0	2
Protein (% Calories)	4	15.3	14	15	6.9	6
Carbohydrate (% Calories)	75	40	43	40	58.1	51
Fat (% Calories)	21	45	43	45	35	43
Protein (g/L)	19.4	75	69.9	74	34.4	30
Carbohydrate (g/L)	365	200	215.2	200	290.4	256
Fat (g/L)	46	101	95.6	100	82.4	96
Cal: N	830	144	179	169	364	418
Na^+ (mEq/L)	<15	35	36	43	NA	34.2
K^+ (mEq/L)	<6	32	27	21	NA	28.6
Osmol (mOsmol/kg)	700	570	635	700	600	600
Volume to Meet RDI Vit/Min (mL)	Incomplete	1000	947	1000	1000	947
Protein Source	Essential amino acids, histidine	Sodium & calcium caseinates	Magnesium & sodium caseinates	Sodium & calcium caseinates, L-arginine	Essential L-amino acids, select non-essential amino acids, whey protein concentrate	Sodium & calcium caseinates
Carbohydrate Source	Maltodextrin, sugar	Maltodextrin, sugar	Corn syrup, sucrose	Corn syrup, fructose	Maltodextrin, modified corn starch	Maltodextrin, sucrose
Fat Source	Soy oil	Corn, canola, sunflower oils	High oleic safflower, soy oils	Sunflower, corn, MCT oils	MCT, canola, corn oils	Safflower, soy oils
Flavors Available	Lemon-lime, orange	Vanilla	Vanilla	Vanilla	Unflavored; flavor packets available	Vanilla
Use	Renal failure (protein restricted)	Dialyzed persons with renal failure	Dialyzed persons with renal failure	For dialyzed persons	Low protein	Renal failure (predialysis)
Special Features	—	—	Contains fructooligosaccharides	Added arginine	Negligible electrolytes	—
Ultratrace Mineral & Conditionally Essential Nutrient Fortified	No	NA	Yes	Yes	No	Yes

*Prepared by Marion Winkler and Susan Manchester.

APPENDIX 38 DEFINED FORMULAS*

PRODUCT	ALITRAQ	CRITICARE HN	L-EMENTAL	PEPTAMEN	PEPTAMEN VHP
Company	**Ross**	**Mead Johnson**	**Nutrition Medical**	**Nestlé**	**Nestlé**
Form	Powder mixed at standard dilution	Liquid	Powder mixed at standard dilution	Liquid	Liquid
KCal/mL	1.0	1.06	1.0	1.0	1.0
Protein (% Cal)	21	14	15	16	25
CHO (% Cal)	66	81.5	82	51	42
Fat (% Cal)	13	4.5	2.5	33	33
Pro (g/L)	52.5	38	38.2	40	62.5
CHO (g/L)	165	220	205	127	104
Fat (g/L)	15.5	5.3	3	39	39.2
Cal:N	120	174	164	156	100
Na^+ (mEq/L)	43.5	27	20	24.3	24
K^+ (mEq/L)	30.7	34	20	38.5	38.5
Osmol (mOsmol/kg)	575	650	630	270–380	300–430
Volume to meet RDI	1500	1890	2000	1500	1500
Pro Source	Soy & lactalbumin hydrolysates, whey, L-glutamine	Hydrolyzed casein, amino acids	L-amino acids	Enzymatically hydrolyzed whey	Enzymatically hydrolyzed whey
CHO Source	Maltodextrin, sucrose, fructose	Maltodextrin, modified corn starch	Maltodextrin, modified starch	Maltodextrin, corn starch	Maltodextrin, corn starch
Fat Source	MCT, safflower oils	Safflower oil, emulsifiers	Safflower oil	MCT, soybean oils	MCT, soybean oils
Flavors Available	Vanilla	—	—	Unflavored & vanilla	Unflavored & vanilla
Additional Features	Includes glutamine & arginine peptides and free amino acids	Elemental, low fat	100% free amino acids enriched with glutamine	Contains small peptides; 70% fat as MCT	Contains small peptides; elevated levels of beta carotene, vit C, zinc, & selenium
Ultratrace Minerals & Conditionally Essential Nutrient	Yes	No	Ultratrace minerals only	Yes	Yes

*Prepared by Marion Winkler and Susan Manchester.

REABILAN	REABILAN HN	SANDOSOURCE PEPTIDE	TOLEREX	VITAL HN	VIVONEX PLUS	VIVONEX TEN
Nestlé	**Nestlé**	**Novartis**	**Novartis**	**Ross**	**Novartis**	**Novartis**
Liquid	Liquid	Liquid	Powder mixed at standard dilution	Powder mixed at standard dilution	Powder mixed at standard dilution	Powder mixed at standard dilution
1.0	1.33	1.0	1.0	1.0	1.0	1.0
12.5	17.5	20	8	16.7	18	15
52.5	47.5	65	91	73.9	76	82
35	35	15	1	9.4	6	3
31.5	58.5	50	21	41.7	45	38
131.5	158	160	230	185	190	210
40.5	53.9	17	1.5	10.8	6.7	2.8
198	142	125	307	150	140	175
32.7	43.5	52	20	24.6	27	20
32.1	42.4	41	31	35.8	28	20
350	490	490	550	500	650	630
2000	1500	1750	3160	1500	1800	2000
Enzymatically hydrolyzed whey, casein	Enzymatically hydrolyzed casein and whey	Casein hydrolysate, free amino acids	Free amino acids	Partially hydrolyzed whey, meat, soy	100% free amino acids	100% free amino acids
Maltodextrin, corn starch	Maltodextrin, corn starch	Hydrolyzed corn starch	Maltodextrin	Hydrolyzed corn starch, sucrose	Maltodextrin	Maltodextrin
MCT, soy, canola oils	MCT, soy, & canola oils	MCT, soy oils	Safflower oil	Safflower, MCT oils	Soybean oil	Safflower oil
Unflavored	Unflavored	—	—	Vanilla	Flavor packets available	Flavor packets available
Small peptides; 50% fat as MCT	Small peptides; 50% fat as MCT, concentrated for fluid restriction	Semi-elemental low fat	100% free amino acids	Partially hydrolyzed diet	Enriched with glutamine and arginine	Enriched with glutamine
Yes	Yes	Yes	Ultratrace minerals only	Ultratrace minerals only	Yes	Ultratrace minerals only

APPENDIX 39 PEDIATRIC SPECIALIZED FORMULAS*

PRODUCT	COMPLEAT PEDIATRIC	KINDERCAL	PEDIASURE	PEDIASURE WITH FIBER	PEPTAMIN JR.	PORTAGEN	NUTREN JUNIOR	RESOURCE JUST FOR KIDS	VIVONEX PEDIATRICS
Company	**Novartis**	**Mead Johnson**	**Ross**	**Ross**	**Nestlé**	**Mead Johnson**	**Nestlé**	**Novartis**	**Novartis**
Form	Liquid	Liquid	Liquid	Liquid	Liquid	Powder diluted to 30 cal/fl oz	Liquid	Liquid	Powder mixed at standard dilution
KCal/mL	1.0	1.06	1.0	1.0	1.0	1.01	1.0	1.0	.8
Protein (% Cal)	15	13	12	12	12	14	12	12	12
CHO (% Cal)	50	50	43.9	43.9	55	46	51	44	63
Fat (% Cal)	35	37	44.1	44.1	33	40	37	44	25
Pro (g/L)	38	34	30	30	30	35.4	30	30	24
CHO (g/L)	50	135	109.7	114	137.5	116	127.5	110	130
Fat (g/L)	39	44	49.7	50	38.5	47.9	42	50	24
Cal:N	164	200	208	208	208	182	208	208	208
Na^+ (mEq/L)	30	14.8	16.5	16.5	20	23.5	20	17	17
K^+ (mEq/L)	38	33.6	33.5	33.5	33.8	32	33.8	33	31
Osmol (mOsmol/kg)	380	310	345	345	260–360	350	350	390	360
Volume to Meet RDI	900 (1–10 y)	950 mL (1–10 y)	1000 (1–6 y) 1300 (7–10 y)	1000 (1–6 y) 1000 (7–10 y)	1000 (1–10 y)	3800	1000 (1–10 y)	1000 (1–10 y)	1000 (1–6 y) 1170 (7–10 y)
Pro Source	Sodium & calcium caseinate, beef	Calcium & sodium caseinates, milk protein concentrate	Sodium caseinate, whey	Sodium caseinate, whey	Enzymatically hydrolyzed whey	Sodium caseinate	Isolated casein and whey proteins	Sodium & calcium caseinates	100% free amino acids
CHO Source	Hydrolyzed corn starch, apple juice, vegetables, fruit	Maltodextrins, sugar, soy fiber	Hydrolyzed corn starch, sucrose	Hydrolyzed corn starch, sucrose, soy fiber	Maltodextrin	Corn syrup solids, sucrose	Maltodextrin, sucrose	Hydrolyzed corn starch, sucrose	Maltodextrin, modified starch
Fat Source	Sunflower, soy, MCT oils	Canola, MCT, corn oils	High oleic safflower, soy, MCT oils	High oleic safflower, soy, MCT oils	MCT, soy, canola oils	MCT, corn oils	Soy, MCT, canola oils	Sunflower, soy, MCT oils	MCT, soybean oils
Flavors Available	Unflavored	Vanilla	Vanilla, chocolate, strawberry, banana cream	Vanilla	Unflavored available as oral product (vanilla) and flavor packets available in raspberry, grape, cherry, bubble gum, vanilla, chocolate	Unflavored	Vanilla	Choc, strawberry, vanilla	Flavor packets available
Additional Features	Blenderized from traditional foods	6.3 g dietary fiber/L	—	5 g dietary fiber/L	Elemental with peptides and MCT oil	MCT major source of fat for patients >2 y old with fat maldigestion/ malabsorption	Also available with 6 g/L fiber as soy polysaccharide	Contains m-inositol and beta carotene	Contains free glutamine
Ultratrace Mineral & Conditionally Essential Nutrient Fortified	Conditionally essential only	Yes	Yes	Yes	Yes	No	Yes	Yes	Yes

*Prepared by Marion Winkler and Susan Manchester.

APPENDIX 40A MODULAR COMPONENTS FOR ENTERAL FEEDINGS—PROTEIN*

PRODUCT	AMINESS TABLETS	CASEC	ELEMENTRA	PRO-MIX	PRO MOD	PURE GLUTAMINE POWDER
Company	**Nestlé**	**Mead Johnson**	**Nestlé**	**CORPAK**	**Ross**	**Cambridge Nutraceuticals**
Form	Tablets	Powder	Powder	Powder	Powder	Powder
Kcal/100 g powder	93/30 tablets	370	379	410	424	400
Protein (% Cal)	85	95	85	83	> 71	100
CHO (% Cal)	6	—	2.1	13	< 10	0
Fat (% Cal)	8	5	12.5	9	< 19	0
Pro (g/100 g powder)	20.7/30 tablets	90	79	75	75.8	100
CHO (g/100 g powder)	1.5/30 tablets	—	2	12.5	10.1	0
Fat (g/100 g powder)	.9/30 tablets	2	5	4	9	0
Cal:N	35	26	30	34	35	25
Na^+ (mEq/100 g powder)	Negligible	5.2	1.7	NA	9.8	0
K^+ (mEq/100 g powder)	Negligible	< 10	39	NA	25.1	0
Osmol (mOsmol/kg)	NA	No measurable increase in Osmol in a serving	Contributes minimally to Osmol of liquid	NA	NA	395
Volume to meet RDI	Incomplete	Incomplete	Incomplete	Incomplete	Incomplete	Incomplete
Pro Source	Free amino acids, essential and histidine	Calcium caseinate	Hydrolyzed whey (*Elemental protein module)	Whey protein	Whey protein concentrate	L-Glutamine
Carb Source	—	—	—	—	—	—
Fat Source	—	—	—	—	—	—

*Prepared by Marion Winkler and Susan Manchester.

APPENDIX 40B MODULAR COMPONENTS FOR ENTERAL FEEDINGS—CARBOHYDRATE

PRODUCT	KARO SYRUP	MODUCAL	POLYCOSE	POLYCOSE
Company	**Best Foods**	**Mead Johnson**	**Ross**	**Ross**
Form	Liquid	Powder	Powder	Liquid
Kcal/mL	4 cal/mL	380/100 g powder	380/100 g powder	2 cal/mL
Protein (% Cal)	—	—	—	—
Carbohydrate (% Cal)	100	100	100	100
Fat (% Cal)	—	—	—	—
Protein	—	—	—	—
Carbohydrate	100 g/L	95.09 g powder	94/100 g powder	200/100 mL
Fat	—	—	—	—
Cal:N	—	—	—	—
Na^+ (mEq/L)	50	3 mEq/100 g powder	4.8 mEq/100 g powder	3 mEq/100 mL
K^+ (mEq/L)	NA	< 1 mEq/100 g powder	< 1 mEq/100 g powder	< .15 mEq/100 mL
Osmol (mOsmol/kg)	NA	99 (30 g powder diluted in 250 mL distilled water)	Same osmol as liquid to which it is added	900
Volume to Meet RDI Vit/Min	Incomplete	Incomplete	Incomplete	Incomplete
Protein Source	—	—	—	—
Carbohydrate Source	Corn syrup, high fructose corn syrup	Maltodextrin	Glucose polymers	Glucose polymers

APPENDIX 40C MODULAR COMPONENTS FOR ENTERAL FEEDINGS—FAT

PRODUCT	VEGETABLE OIL	MCT OIL	MICROLIPID
Company	—	Mead Johnson	Mead Johnson
Form	Liquid	Liquid	Liquid
Kcal/mL	8	7.7	4.5
Protein (% Cal)	—	—	—
CHO (% Cal)	—	—	—
Fat (% Cal)	100	100	100
Pro (g/100 mL)	—	—	—
CHO (g/100 mL)	—	—	—
Fat (g/100 mL)	—	93	51
Cal:N	—	—	—
Na^+ (mEq/100 mL)	—	—	—
K^+ (mEq/100 mL)	—	—	—
Osmol (mOsmol/kg)	NA	NA	70
Volume to Meet RDI	Incomplete	Incomplete	Incomplete
Protein Source	—	—	—
Carb Source	—	—	—
Fat Source	Depends on selection	MCT oil	Safflower oil

APPENDIX 40D MODULAR COMPONENTS FOR ENTERAL FEEDINGS—MIXED

	SCANDI CAL	RESOURCE SELECT
Company	Scandipharm	Novartis
Form	Powder	Powder
Kcal/100g	538	406
Pro (% Cal)	0	25
CHO (% Cal)	46	45
Fat (% Cal)	64	30
Pro (g/100g)	0	22
CHO (g/100g)	62	45
Fat (g/100g)	38	15
Na^+ (mEq/100g)	6.7	15
K^+ (mEq/100g)	8.1	6.4
Osmol (mOsmol/kg)	NA	NA
Vol Meet RDA	Incomplete	Not intended for sole source of nutrition
Carb Source	Maltodextrin	Hydrolyzed corn starch
Fat Source	Coconut, soy oils	Soy, MCT oils
Pro Source	—	Whey protein isolate, glutamine, cystine
Additional comments		Contains 5 g fiber, enriched with vit C, E, selenium, zinc

APPENDIX 41 NUTRITIVE VALUE OF THE EDIBLE PART OF FOOD

Foods, Approximate Measures, Units, and Weight (weight of edible portion only)		Grams	Water (g)	Food Energy (Calories)	Protein (g)	Fat (g)	Fatty Acids: Saturated (g)	Fatty Acids: Monounsaturated (g)	Fatty Acids: Polyunsaturated (g)
Beverages									
Alcoholic									
Beer									
Regular	12 fl oz	360	92	150	1	0	0.0	0.0	0.0
Light	12 fl oz	355	95	95	1	0	0.0	0.0	0.0
Gin, rum, vodka, whiskey 80-proof	1½ fl oz	42	67	95	0	0	0.0	0.0	0.0
Table wine									
Red	3½ fl oz	102	88	75	tr	0	0.0	0.0	0.0
White	3½ fl oz	102	87	80	tr	0	0.0	0.0	0.0
Carbonated[2]									
Club soda	12 fl oz	355	100	0	0	0	0.0	0.0	0.0
Cola type									
Regular	12 fl oz	369	89	160	0	0	0.0	0.0	0.0
Diet, artificially sweetened	12 fl oz	355	100	tr	0	0	0.0	0.0	0.0
Ginger ale	12 fl oz	366	91	125	0	0	0.0	0.0	0.0
Coffee									
Brewed	6 fl oz	180	100	tr	tr	tr	tr	tr	tr
Instant, prepared (2 tsp powder plus 6 fl oz water)	6 fl oz	182	99	tr	tr	tr	tr	tr	tr
Fruit drinks, noncarbonated									
Canned									
Fruit punch drink	6 fl oz	190	88	85	tr	0	0.0	0.0	0.0
Tea									
Brewed	8 fl oz	240	100	tr	tr	tr	tr	tr	tr
Instant, powder, prepared:									
Unsweetened (1 tsp powder plus 8 fl oz water)	8 fl oz	241	100	tr	tr	tr	tr	tr	tr
Sweetened (3 tsp powder plus 8 fl oz water)	8 fl oz	262	91	85	tr	tr	tr	tr	tr
Dairy Products									
Butter. See Fats and Oils									
Cheese									
Natural									
Blue	1 oz	28	42	100	6	8	5.3	2.2	0.2
Camembert (3 wedges per 4-oz container)	1 wedge	38	52	115	8	9	5.8	2.7	0.3
Cheddar									
Cut pieces	1 oz	28	37	115	7	9	6.0	2.7	.03
	1 in³	17	37	70	4	6	3.6	1.6	0.2
Shredded	1 c	113	37	455	28	37	23.8	10.6	1.1

tr = nutrient present in trace amounts.
[1]Value not determined.
[2]Mineral content varies depending on water source.
(See also: Website http://www.nal.usda.gov/fnic/foodcomp/Data/index.html. Zinc and folic acid tables compiled in these tables by Elizabeth Summers, 1998.)

NUTRIENTS IN INDICATED QUANTITY

Cholesterol (mg)	Carbohydrate (g)	Calcium (mg)	Phosphorus (mg)	Iron (mg)	Potassium (mg)	Sodium (mg)	Zn (mg)	Vitamin A Value		Thiamin (mg)	Riboflavin (mg)	Niacin (mg)	Ascorbic acid (mg)	Folic acid (μg)
								IU	RE					
0	13	14	50	0.1	115	18	.07	0	0	0.02	0.09	1.8	0	21
0	5	14	43	0.1	64	11	.11	0	0	0.03	0.11	1.4	0	15
0	tr	tr	tr	tr	1	tr	tr	0	0	tr	tr	tr	0	.00
0	3	8	18	0.4	113	5	.09	([1])	([1])	0.00	0.03	0.1	0	2
0	3	9	14	0.3	83	5	.07	([1])	([1])	0.00	0.01	0.1	0	0
0	0	18	0	tr	0	78	.35	0	0	0.00	0.00	0.0	0	0
0	41	11	52	0.2	7	18	.04	0	0	0.00	0.00	0.0	0	0
0	tr	14	39	0.2	7	[3]32	.28	0	0	0.00	0.00	0.0	0	0
0	32	11	0	0.1	4	29	.18	0	0	0.00	0.00	0.0	0	0
0	tr	4	2	tr	124	2	.04	0	0	0.00	0.02	0.4	0	0
0	1	2	6	0.1	71	tr	NI	0	0	0.00	0.03	0.6	0	0
0	22	15	2	0.4	48	15	.22	20	2	0.03	0.04	tr	[4]61	2
0	tr	0	2	tr	36	1	NI	0	0	0.00	0.03	tr	0	12
0	1	1	4	tr	61	1	.00	0	0	0.00	0.02	0.1	0	1
0	22	1	3	tr	49	tr	.08	0	0	0.00	0.04	0.1	0	NI
21	1	150	110	0.1	73	396	.75	200	65	0.01	0.11	0.3	0	10
27	tr	147	132	0.1	71	320	.67	350	96	0.01	0.19	0.2	0	18
30	tr	204	145	0.2	28	176	.88	300	86	0.01	0.11	tr	0	5
18	tr	123	87	0.1	17	105	NI	180	52	tr	0.06	tr	0	NI
119	1	815	579	0.8	111	701	3.51	1,200	342	0.03	0.42	0.1	0	NI

NI = not indicated.
[3]Blend of aspartame and saccharin; if only sodium saccharin is used, sodium is 75 mg; if only aspartame is used, sodium is 23 mg.
[4]With added ascorbic acid.

APPENDIX 41 NUTRITIVE VALUE OF THE EDIBLE PART OF FOOD *(continued)*

Foods, Approximate Measures, Units, and Weight (weight of edible portion only)		Grams	Water (g)	Food Energy (Calories)	Protein (g)	Fat (g)	Fatty Acids: Saturated (g)	Fatty Acids: Monounsaturated (g)	Fatty Acids: Polyunsaturated (g)
Dairy Products (*cont.*)									
Cottage (curd not pressed down)									
Creamed (cottage cheese, 4% fat)									
Large curd	1 c	225	79	235	28	10	6.4	2.9	0.3
Small curd	1 c	210	79	215	26	9	6.0	2.7	0.3
With fruit	1 c	226	72	280	22	8	4.9	2.2	0.2
Low-fat (2%)	1 c	226	79	205	31	4	2.8	1.2	0.1
Uncreamed (cottage cheese dry curd, less than ½% fat)	1 c	145	80	125	25	1	0.4	0.2	tr
Cream	1 oz	28	54	100	2	10	6.2	2.8	0.4
Feta	1 oz	28	55	75	4	6	4.2	1.3	0.2
Mozzarella, made with									
Whole milk	1 oz	28	54	80	6	6	3.7	1.9	0.2
Part skim milk (low moisture)	1 oz	28	49	80	8	5	3.1	1.4	0.1
Muenster	1 oz	28	42	105	7	9	5.4	2.5	0.2
Parmesan, grated									
Cup, not pressed down	1 c	100	18	455	42	30	19.1	8.7	0.7
Tablespoon	1 tbsp	5	18	25	2	2	1.0	0.4	tr
Ounce	1 oz	28	18	130	12	9	5.4	2.5	0.2
Provolone	1 oz	28	41	100	7	8	4.8	2.1	0.2
Ricotta, made with									
Whole milk	1 c	246	72	430	28	32	20.4	8.9	0.9
Part skim milk	1 c	246	74	340	28	19	12.1	5.7	0.6
Swiss	1 oz	28	37	105	8	8	5.0	2.1	0.3
Pasteurized process cheese									
American	1 oz	28	39	105	6	9	5.6	2.5	0.3
Swiss	1 oz	28	42	95	7	7	4.5	2.0	0.2
Pasteurized process cheese food, American	1 oz	28	43	95	6	7	4.4	2.0	0.2
Pasteurized process cheese spread, American	1 oz	28	48	80	5	6	3.8	1.8	0.2
Cream, sweet									
Half-and-half (cream and milk)	1 c	242	81	315	7	28	17.3	8.0	1.0
	1 tbsp	15	81	20	tr	2	1.1	0.5	0.1
Light, coffee, or table	1 c	240	74	470	6	46	28.8	13.4	1.7
	1 tbsp	15	74	30	tr	3	1.8	0.8	0.1
Whipping, unwhipped (volume about double when whipped)									
Light	1 c	239	64	700	5	74	46.2	21.7	2.1
	1 tbsp	15	64	45	tr	5	2.9	1.4	0.1
Heavy	1 c	238	58	820	5	88	54.8	25.4	3.3
	1 tbsp	15	58	50	tr	6	3.5	1.6	0.2
Whipped topping (pressurized)	1 c	60	61	155	2	13	8.3	3.9	0.5
	1 tbsp	3	61	10	tr	1	0.4	0.2	tr
Cream, sour	1 c	230	71	495	7	48	30.0	13.9	1.8
	1 tbsp	12	71	25	tr	3	1.6	0.7	0.1

tr = nutrient present in trace amounts.

NUTRIENTS IN INDICATED QUANTITY

Cho-les-terol (mg)	Carbo-hydrate (g)	Calcium (mg)	Phos-phorus (mg)	Iron (mg)	Potas-sium (mg)	Sodium (mg)	Zn (mg)	Vitamin A Value IU	Vitamin A Value RE	Thiamin (mg)	Ribo-flavin (mg)	Niacin (mg)	Ascorbic acid (mg)	Folic acid (μg)
34	6	135	297	0.3	190	911	.80	370	108	0.05	0.37	0.3	tr	27
31	6	126	277	0.3	177	850	.80	340	101	0.04	0.34	0.3	tr	26
25	30	108	236	0.2	151	915	.66	280	81	0.04	0.29	0.2	tr	22
19	8	155	340	0.4	217	918	.95	160	45	0.05	0.42	0.3	tr	30
10	3	46	151	0.3	47	19	.68	40	12	0.04	0.21	0.2	0	NI
31	1	23	30	0.3	34	84	.32	400	124	tr	0.06	tr	0	4
25	1	140	96	0.2	18	316	.81	130	36	0.04	0.24	0.3	0	9
22	1	147	105	0.1	19	106	.90	220	68	tr	0.07	tr	0	2
15	1	207	149	0.1	27	150	.83	180	54	0.01	0.10	tr	0	3
27	tr	203	133	0.1	38	178	.84	320	90	tr	0.09	tr	0	3
79	4	1,376	807	1.0	107	1,861	NI	700	173	0.05	0.39	0.3	0	8
4	tr	69	40	tr	5	93	.16	40	9	tr	0.02	tr	0	0
22	1	390	229	0.3	30	528	1.00	200	49	0.01	0.11	0.1	0	2
20	1	214	141	0.1	39	248	.92	230	75	0.01	0.09	tr	0	3
124	7	509	389	0.9	257	207	2.85	1,210	330	0.03	0.48	0.3	0	30
76	13	669	449	1.1	307	307	3.29	1,060	278	0.05	0.46	0.2	0	14
26	1	272	171	tr	31	74	1.10	240	72	0.01	0.10	tr	0	2
27	tr	174	211	0.1	46	406	.93	340	82	0.01	0.10	tr	0	2
24	1	219	216	0.2	61	338	1.01	230	65	tr	0.08	tr	0	2
18	2	163	130	0.2	79	337	.85	260	62	0.01	0.13	tr	0	2
16	2	159	202	0.1	69	381	.78	220	54	0.01	0.12	tr	0	2
89	10	254	230	0.2	314	98	1.23	1,050	259	0.08	0.36	0.2	2	NI
6	1	16	14	tr	19	6	.08	70	16	0.01	0.02	tr	tr	2
159	9	231	192	0.1	292	95	.65	1,730	437	0.08	0.36	0.1	2	6
10	1	14	12	tr	18	6	.04	110	27	tr	0.02	tr	tr	NI
265	7	166	146	0.1	231	82	.60	2,690	705	0.06	0.30	0.1	1	1
17	tr	10	9	tr	15	5	.04	170	44	tr	0.02	tr	tr	1
326	7	154	149	0.1	179	89	.55	3,500	1,002	0.05	0.26	0.1	1	1
21	tr	10	9	tr	11	6	.03	220	63	tr	0.02	tr	tr	1
46	7	61	54	tr	88	78	.22	550	124	0.02	0.04	tr	0	1
2	tr	3	3	tr	4	4	.01	30	6	tr	tr	tr	0	0
102	10	268	195	0.1	331	123	.69	1,820	448	0.08	0.34	0.2	2	25
5	1	14	10	tr	17	6	.03	90	23	tr	0.02	tr	tr	1

NI = not indicated.

APPENDIX 41 NUTRITIVE VALUE OF THE EDIBLE PART OF FOOD *(continued)*

Foods, Approximate Measures, Units, and Weight (weight of edible portion only)		Grams	Water (g)	Food Energy (Calories)	Protein (g)	Fat (g)	Fatty Acids Saturated (g)	Fatty Acids Monounsaturated (g)	Fatty Acids Polyunsaturated (g)
Dairy Products (*cont.*)									
Milk									
Fluid									
Whole (3.3% fat)	1 c	244	88	150	8	8	5.1	2.4	0.3
Low-fat (2%)									
No milk solids added	1 c	244	89	120	8	5	2.9	1.4	0.2
Milk solids added, label claim less than 10 g of protein per cup	1 c	245	89	125	9	5	2.9	1.4	0.2
Low-fat (1%)									
No milk solids added	1 c	244	90	100	8	3	1.6	0.7	0.1
Milk solids added, label claim less than 10 g of protein per cup	1 c	245	90	105	9	2	1.5	0.7	0.1
Nonfat (skim)									
No milk solids added	1 c	245	91	85	8	tr	0.3	0.1	tr
Milk solids added, label claim less than 10 g of protein per cup	1 c	245	90	90	9	1	0.4	0.2	tr
Buttermilk	1 c	245	90	100	8	2	1.3	0.6	0.1
Milk desserts, frozen									
Ice cream, vanilla									
Regular (about 11% fat)									
Hardened	½ gal	1,064	61	2,155	38	115	71.3	33.1	4.3
	1 c	133	61	270	5	14	8.9	4.1	0.5
	3 fl oz	50	61	100	2	5	3.4	1.6	0.2
Soft serve (frozen custard)	1 c	173	60	375	7	23	13.5	6.7	1.0
Rich (about 16% fat), hardened	½ gal	1,188	59	2,805	33	190	118.3	54.9	7.1
	1 c	148	59	350	4	24	14.7	6.8	0.9
Ice milk, vanilla									
Hardened (about 4% fat)	½ gal	1,048	69	1,470	41	45	28.1	13.0	1.7
	1 c	131	69	185	5	6	3.5	1.6	0.2
Soft serve (about 3% fat)	1 c	175	70	225	8	5	2.9	1.3	0.2
Sherbet (about 2% fat)	½ gal	1,542	66	2,160	17	31	19.0	8.8	1.1
	1 c	193	66	270	2	4	2.4	1.1	0.1
Eggs									
Eggs, large (24 oz per dozen)									
Raw									
Whole, without shell	1 egg	50	75	80	6	6	1.7	2.2	0.7
White	1 white	33	88	15	3	tr	0.0	0.0	0.0
Yolk	1 yolk	17	49	65	3	6	1.7	2.2	0.7
Fat and Oils									
Butter (4 sticks per lb)									
Stick	½ c	113	16	810	1	92	57.1	26.4	3.4
Tablespoon (⅛ stick)	1 tbsp	14	16	100	tr	11	7.1	3.3	0.4
Pat (1 in square, ⅓-in high; 90 per lb)	1 pat	5	16	35	tr	4	2.5	1.2	0.2

tr = nutrient present in trace amounts.
[5]For salted butter; unsalted butter contains 12 mg sodium per stick, 2 mg per tbsp, or 1 mg per pat.

NUTRIENTS IN INDICATED QUANTITY

Cholesterol (mg)	Carbohydrate (g)	Calcium (mg)	Phosphorus (mg)	Iron (mg)	Potassium (mg)	Sodium (mg)	Zn (mg)	Vitamin A Value		Thiamin (mg)	Riboflavin (mg)	Niacin (mg)	Ascorbic acid (mg)	Folic acid (μg)
								IU	RE					
33	11	291	228	0.1	370	120	.93	310	76	0.09	0.40	0.2	2	12
18	12	297	232	0.1	377	122	.96	500	139	0.10	0.40	0.2	2	12
18	12	313	245	0.1	397	128	NI	500	140	0.10	0.42	0.2	2	NI
10	12	300	235	0.1	381	123	.96	500	144	0.10	0.41	0.2	2	12
10	12	313	245	0.1	397	128	NI	500	145	0.10	0.42	0.2	2	NI
4	12	302	247	0.1	406	126	.92	500	149	0.09	0.34	0.2	2	14
5	12	316	255	0.1	418	130	NI	500	149	0.10	0.43	0.2	2	NI
9	12	285	219	0.1	371	257	1.03	80	20	0.08	0.38	0.1	2	12
476	254	1,406	1,075	1.0	2,052	929	NI	4,340	1,064	0.42	2.63	1.1	6	NI
59	32	176	134	0.1	257	116	1.41	540	133	0.05	0.33	0.1	1	3
22	12	66	51	tr	96	44	NI	200	50	0.02	0.12	0.1	tr	NI
153	38	236	199	0.4	338	153	1.99	790	199	0.8	0.45	0.2	1	9
703	256	1,213	927	0.8	1,771	868	NI	7,200	1,758	0.36	2.27	0.9	5	NI
88	32	151	115	0.1	221	108	1.21	900	219	0.04	0.28	0.1	1	NI
146	232	1,409	1,035	1.5	2,117	836	NI	1,710	419	0.61	2.78	0.9	6	NI
18	29	176	129	0.2	265	105	.55	210	52	0.08	0.35	0.1	1	8
13	38	274	202	0.3	412	163	.86	175	44	0.12	0.54	0.2	1	5
113	469	827	594	2.5	1,585	706	NI	1,480	308	0.26	0.71	1.0	31	NI
14	59	103	74	0.3	198	88	1.33	190	39	0.03	0.09	0.1	4	4
274	1	28	90	1.0	65	69	.55	260	78	0.04	0.15	tr	0	24
0	tr	4	4	tr	45	50	0	0	0	tr	0.09	tr	0	1
272	tr	26	86	0.9	15	8	.54	310	94	0.04	0.07	tr	0	25
247	tr	27	26	0.2	29	[5]933	NI	[6]13,460	[6]852	0.01	0.04	tr	0	3.5
31	tr	3	3	tr	4	[5]116	.01	[6]430	[6]106	tr	tr	tr	0	0
11	tr	1	1	tr	1	[5]41	NI	[6]150	[6]38	tr	tr	tr	0	0

NI = not indicated.
[6]Values for vitamin A are year-round average.

APPENDIX 41 NUTRITIVE VALUE OF THE EDIBLE PART OF FOOD *(continued)*

Foods, Approximate Measures, Units, and Weight (weight of edible portion only)		Grams	Water (g)	Food Energy (Calories)	Protein (g)	Fat (g)	Fatty Acids: Saturated (g)	Fatty Acids: Monounsaturated (g)	Fatty Acids: Polyunsaturated (g)
Fats and Oils (*cont.*)									
Fats, cooking (vegetable shortenings)	1c	205	0	1,810	0	205	51.3	91.2	53.5
	1 tbsp	13	0	115	0	13	3.3	5.8	3.4
Lard	1 c	205	0	1,850	0	205	80.4	92.5	23.0
	1 tbsp	13	0	115	0	13	5.1	5.9	1.5
Oils, salad or cooking									
Corn	1 c	218	0	1,925	0	218	27.7	52.8	128.0
	1 tbsp	14	0	125	0	14	1.8	3.4	8.2
Olive	1 c	216	0	1,910	0	216	29.2	159.2	18.1
	1 tbsp	14	0	125	0	14	1.9	10.3	1.2
Peanut	1 c	216	0	1,910	0	216	36.5	99.8	69.1
	1 tbsp	14	0	125	0	14	2.4	6.5	4.5
Safflower	1 c	218	0	1,925	0	218	19.8	26.4	162.4
	1 tbsp	14	0	125	0	14	1.3	1.7	10.4
Soybean oil, hydrogenated (partially hardened)	1 c	218	0	1,925	0	218	32.5	93.7	82.0
	1 tbsp	14	0	125	0	14	2.1	6.0	5.3
Soybean-cottonseed oil blend, hydrogenated	1 c	218	0	1,925	0	218	39.2	64.3	104.9
	1 tbsp	14	0	125	0	14	2.5	4.1	6.7
Sunflower	1 c	218	0	1,925	0	218	22.5	42.5	143.2
	1 tbsp	14	0	125	0	14	1.4	2.7	9.2
Salad dressings									
Commercial									
Blue cheese	1 tbsp	15	32	75	1	8	1.5	1.8	4.2
French									
Regular	1 tbsp	16	35	85	tr	9	1.4	4.0	3.5
Low calorie	1 tbsp	16	75	25	tr	2	0.2	0.3	1.0
Italian									
Regular	1 tbsp	15	34	80	tr	9	1.3	3.7	3.2
Low calorie	1 tbsp	15	86	5	tr	tr	tr	tr	tr
Mayonnaise									
Regular	1 tbsp	14	15	100	tr	11	1.7	3.2	5.8
Imitation	1 tbsp	15	63	35	tr	3	0.5	0.7	1.6
Prepared from home recipe									
Cooked type[7]	1 tbsp	16	69	25	1	2	0.5	0.6	0.3
Vinegar and oil	1 tbsp	16	47	70	0	8	1.5	2.4	3.9
Fish and Shellfish									
Clams									
Raw, meat only	3 oz	85	82	65	11	1	0.3	0.3	0.3
Canned, drained solids	3 oz	85	77	85	13	2	0.5	0.5	0.4
Crabmeat, canned	1 c	135	77	135	23	3	0.5	0.8	1.4
Fish sticks, frozen, reheated (stick, 4 by 1 by ½ in)	1 fish stick	28	52	70	6	3	0.8	1.4	0.8

tr = nutrient present in trace amounts.

[7]Fatty acid values apply to product made with regular margarine.

NUTRIENTS IN INDICATED QUANTITY

Cholesterol (mg)	Carbohydrate (g)	Calcium (mg)	Phosphorus (mg)	Iron (mg)	Potassium (mg)	Sodium (mg)	Zn (mg)	Vitamin A Value		Thiamin (mg)	Riboflavin (mg)	Niacin (mg)	Ascorbic acid (mg)	Folic acid (μg)
								IU	RE					
0	0	0	0	0.0	0	0	NI	0	0	0.00	0.00	0.0	0	NI
0	0	0	0	0.0	0	0	NI	0	0	0.00	0.00	0.0	0	0
195	0	0	0	0.0	0	0	NI	0	0	0.00	0.00	0.0	0	0
12	0	0	0	0.0	0	0	.01	0	0	0.00	0.00	0.0	0	0
0	0	0	0	0.0	0	0	NI	0	0	0.00	0.00	0.0	0	0
0	0	0	0	0.0	0	0	.00	0	0	0.00	0.00	0.0	0	0
0	0	0	0	0.0	0	0	NI	0	0	0.00	0.00	0.0	0	0
0	0	0	0	0.0	0	0	.01	0	0	0.00	0.00	0.0	0	0
0	0	0	0	0.0	0	0	NI	0	0	0.00	0.00	0.0	0	0
0	0	0	0	0.0	0	0	.00	0	0	0.00	0.00	0.0	0	0
0	0	0	0	0.0	0	0	NI	0	0	0.00	0.00	0.0	0	0
0	0	0	0	0.0	0	0	.00	0	0	0.00	0.00	0.0	0	0
0	0	0	0	0.0	0	0	NI	0	0	0.00	0.00	0.0	0	0
0	0	0	0	0.0	0	0	.00	0	0	0.00	0.00	0.0	0	0
0	0	0	0	0.0	0	0	NI	0	0	0.00	0.00	0.0	0	0
0	0	0	0	0.0	0	0	.00	0	0	0.00	0.00	0.0	0	0
0	0	0	0	0.0	0	0	NI	0	0	0.00	0.00	0.0	0	0
0	0	0	0	0.0	0	0	.00	0	0	0.00	0.00	0.0	0	0
3	1	12	11	tr	6	164	.002	30	10	tr	0.02	tr	tr	1
0	1	2	1	tr	2	188	.01	tr	tr	tr	tr	tr	tr	1
0	2	6	5	tr	3	306	.03	tr	tr	tr	tr	tr	tr	0
0	1	1	1	tr	5	162	.02	30	3	tr	tr	tr	tr	1
0	2	1	1	tr	4	136	.02	tr	tr	tr	tr	tr	tr	0
8	tr	3	4	0.1	5	80	NI	40	12	0.00	0.00	tr	0	NI
4	2	tr	tr	0.0	2	75	.02	0	0	0.00	0.00	0.0	0	0
9	2	13	14	0.1	19	117	NI	70	20	0.01	0.02	tr	tr	NI
0	tr	0	0	0.0	1	tr	.00	0	0	0.00	0.00	0.0	0	0
43	2	59	138	2.6	154	102	1.17	90	26	0.09	0.15	1.1	9	14
54	2	47	116	3.5	119	102	2.32	90	26	0.01	0.09	0.9	3	24
135	1	61	246	1.1	149	1,350	5.42	50	14	0.11	0.11	2.6	0	22
26	4	11	58	0.3	94	53	.19	20	5	0.03	0.05	0.6	0	5

NI = not indicated.

APPENDIX 41 NUTRITIVE VALUE OF THE EDIBLE PART OF FOOD *(continued)*

Foods, Approximate Measures, Units, and Weight (weight of edible portion only)		Grams	Water (g)	Food Energy (Calories)	Protein (g)	Fat (g)	Fatty Acids: Saturated (g)	Fatty Acids: Monounsaturated (g)	Fatty Acids: Polyunsaturated (g)
Fish and Shellfish (*cont.*)									
Flounder or Sole, baked, with lemon juice									
With butter	3 oz	85	73	120	16	6	3.2	1.5	0.5
With margarine	3 oz	85	73	120	16	6	1.2	2.3	1.9
Without added fat	3 oz	85	78	80	17	1	0.3	0.2	0.4
Haddock, breaded, fried[8]	3 oz	85	61	175	17	9	2.4	3.9	2.4
Halibut, broiled, with butter and lemon juice	3 oz	85	67	140	20	6	3.3	1.6	0.7
Herring, pickled	3 oz	85	59	190	17	13	4.3	4.6	3.1
Ocean perch, breaded, fried[8]	1 fillet	85	59	185	16	11	2.6	4.6	2.8
Oysters									
Raw, meat only (13–19 medium Selects)	1 c	240	85	160	20	4	1.4	0.5	1.4
Breaded, fried[8]	1 oyster	45	65	90	5	5	1.4	2.1	1.4
Salmon									
Canned (pink), solids and liquid	3 oz	85	71	120	17	5	0.9	1.5	2.1
Baked (red)	3 oz	85	67	140	21	5	1.2	2.4	1.4
Smoked	3 oz	85	59	150	18	8	2.6	3.9	0.7
Sardines, Atlantic, canned in oil, drained solids	3 oz	85	62	175	20	9	2.1	3.7	2.9
Scallops, breaded, frozen, reheated	6 scallops	90	59	195	15	10	2.5	4.1	2.5
Shrimp									
Canned, drained solids	3 oz	85	70	100	21	1	0.2	0.2	0.4
French fried (medium)[10]	3 oz	85	55	200	16	10	2.5	4.1	2.6
Trout, broiled, with butter and lemon juice	3 oz	85	63	175	21	9	4.1	2.9	1.6
Tuna, canned, drained solids									
Oil pack, chunk light	3 oz	85	61	165	24	7	1.4	1.9	3.1
Water pack, solid white	3 oz	85	63	135	30	1	0.3	0.2	0.3
Tuna salad[11]	1 c	205	63	375	33	19	3.3	4.9	9.2
Fruits and Fruit Juices									
Apples									
Raw									
Unpeeled, without cores									
2¾-in diam. (about 3 per lb with cores)	1 apple	138	84	80	tr	tr	0.1	tr	0.1
3¼-in diam. (about 2 per lb with cores)	1 apple	212	84	125	tr	1	0.1	tr	0.2
Peeled, sliced	1 c	110	84	65	tr	tr	0.1	tr	0.1
Dried, sulfured	10 rings	64	32	155	1	tr	tr	tr	0.1
Apple juice, bottled or canned[13]	1 c	248	88	115	tr	tr	tr	tr	0.1
Applesauce, canned									
Sweetened	1 c	255	80	195	tr	tr	0.1	tr	0.1
Unsweetened	1 c	244	88	105	tr	tr	tr	tr	tr

tr = nutrient present in trace amounts.

[8]Dipped in egg, milk, and breadcrumbs; fried in vegetable shortening.

[9]If bones are discarded, value for calcium will be greatly reduced.

[10]Dipped in egg, breadcrumbs, and flour; fried in vegetable shortening.

NUTRIENTS IN INDICATED QUANTITY

Cholesterol (mg)	Carbohydrate (g)	Calcium (mg)	Phosphorus (mg)	Iron (mg)	Potassium (mg)	Sodium (mg)	Zn (mg)	Vitamin A Value		Thiamin (mg)	Riboflavin (mg)	Niacin (mg)	Ascorbic acid (mg)	Folic acid (μg)
								IU	RE					
68	tr	13	187	0.3	272	145	NI	210	54	0.05	0.08	1.6	1	10
55	tr	14	187	0.3	273	151	NI	230	69	0.05	0.08	1.6	1	10
59	tr	13	197	0.3	286	101	1.54	30	10	0.05	0.08	1.7	1	10
75	7	34	183	1.0	270	123	.85	70	20	0.06	0.10	2.9	0	14
62	tr	14	206	0.7	441	103	NI	610	174	0.06	0.07	7.7	1	8
85	0	29	128	0.9	85	850	.53	110	33	0.04	0.18	2.8	0	4
66	7	31	191	1.2	241	138	.410	70	20	0.10	0.11	2.0	0	6
120	8	226	343	15.6	290	175	152.56	740	223	0.34	0.43	6.0	24	25
35	5	49	73	3.0	64	70	12.35	150	44	0.07	0.10	1.3	4	NI
34	0	[9]167	243	0.7	307	443	4.19	60	18	0.03	0.15	6.8	0	13
60	0	26	269	0.5	305	55	NI	290	87	0.18	0.14	5.5	0	14
51	0	12	208	0.8	327	1,700	NI	260	77	0.17	0.17	6.8	0	1.6
85	0	[9]371	424	2.6	349	425	1.21	190	56	0.03	0.17	4.6	0	3
70	10	39	203	2.0	369	298	.99	70	21	0.11	0.11	1.6	0	11
128	1	98	224	1.4	104	1,955	1.07	50	15	0.01	0.03	1.5	0	2
168	11	61	154	2.0	189	384	1.24	90	26	0.06	0.09	2.8	0	7
71	tr	26	259	1.0	297	122	NI	230	60	0.07	0.07	2.3	1	20
55	0	7	199	1.6	298	303	.77	70	20	0.04	0.09	10.1	0	5
48	0	17	202	0.6	255	468	.41	110	32	0.03	0.10	13.4	0	2
80	19	31	281	2.5	531	877	2.30	230	53	0.06	0.14	13.3	6	30
0	21	10	10	0.2	159	tr	.050	70	7	0.02	0.02	0.1	8	4.0
0	32	15	15	0.4	244	tr	NI	110	11	0.04	0.03	0.2	12	NI
0	16	4	8	0.1	124	tr	NI	50	5	0.02	0.01	0.1	4	.5
0	42	9	24	0.9	288	[12]56	.13	0	0	0.00	0.10	0.6	2	0
0	29	17	17	0.9	295	7	.07	tr	tr	0.05	0.04	0.2	[14]2	0
0	51	10	18	0.9	156	8	.10	30	3	0.03	0.07	0.5	[14]4	2
0	28	7	17	0.3	183	5	.08	70	7	0.03	0.06	0.5	[14]3	2

NI = not indicated.
[11]Made with drained chunk light tuna, celery, onion, pickle relish, and mayonnaise-type salad dressing.
[12]Sodium bisulfite used to preserve color; unsulfited product would contain less sodium.
[13]Also applies to pasteurized apple cider.
[14]Without added ascorbic acid. For value with added ascorbic acid, refer to label.

APPENDIX 41 NUTRITIVE VALUE OF THE EDIBLE PART OF FOOD *(continued)*

Foods, Approximate Measures, Units, and Weight (weight of edible portion only)		Grams	Water (g)	Food Energy (Calories)	Protein (g)	Fat (g)	Fatty Acids: Saturated (g)	Fatty Acids: Monounsaturated (g)	Fatty Acids: Polyunsaturated (g)
Fruits and Fruit Juices (*cont.*)									
Apricots									
Raw, without pits (about 12 per lb with pits)	3 apricots	106	86	50	1	tr	tr	0.2	0.1
Canned (fruit and liquid)									
Heavy syrup pack	1 c	258	78	215	1	tr	tr	0.1	tr
	3 halves	85	78	70	tr	tr	tr	tr	tr
Juice pack	1 c	248	87	120	2	tr	tr	tr	tr
	3 halves	84	87	40	1	tr	tr	tr	tr
Dried									
Uncooked (28 large or 37 medium halves per cup)	1 c	130	31	310	5	1	tr	0.3	0.1
Cooked, unsweetened, fruit and liquid	1 c	250	76	210	3	tr	tr	0.2	0.1
Apricot nectar, canned	1 c	251	85	140	1	tr	tr	0.1	tr
Avocados, raw, whole, without skin and seed									
California (about 2 per lb with skin and seed)	1 avocado	173	73	305	4	30	4.5	19.4	3.5
Florida (about 1 per lb with skin and seed)	1 avocado	304	80	340	5	27	5.3	14.8	4.5
Bananas, raw, without peel									
Whole (about 2½ per lb with peel)	1 banana	114	74	105	1	1	0.2	tr	0.1
Sliced	1 c	150	74	140	2	1	0.3	0.1	0.1
Blackberries, raw	1 c	144	86	75	1	1	0.2	0.1	0.1
Blueberries									
Raw	1 c	145	85	80	1	1	tr	0.1	0.3
Frozen, sweetened	10-oz container	284	77	230	1	tr	tr	0.1	0.2
	1 c	230	77	185	1	tr	tr	tr	0.1
Cantaloupe. See Melons									
Cherries									
Sour, red, pitted, canned, water pack	1 c	244	90	90	2	tr	0.1	0.1	0.1
Sweet, raw, without pits and stems	10 cherries	68	81	50	1	1	0.1	0.2	0.2
Cranberry juice cocktail, bottled, sweetened	1 c	253	85	145	tr	tr	tr	tr	0.1
Cranberry sauce, sweetened, canned, strained	1 c	277	61	420	1	tr	tr	0.1	0.2
Dates									
Whole, without pits	10 dates	83	23	230	2	tr	0.1	0.1	tr
Chopped	1 c	178	23	490	4	1	0.3	0.2	tr
Figs, dried	10 figs	187	28	475	6	2	0.4	0.5	1.0

tr = nutrient present in trace amounts.
[14]Without added ascorbic acid. For value with added ascorbic acid, refer to label.

NUTRIENTS IN INDICATED QUANTITY

Choles-terol (mg)	Carbo-hydrate (g)	Calcium (mg)	Phos-phorus (mg)	Iron (mg)	Potas-sium (mg)	Sodium (mg)	Zn (mg)	Vitamin A Value		Thiamin (mg)	Ribo-flavin (mg)	Niacin (mg)	Ascorbic acid (mg)	Folic acid (μg)
								IU	RE					
0	12	15	20	0.6	314	1	.28	2,770	277	0.03	0.04	0.6	11	9
0	55	23	31	0.8	361	10	.27	3,170	317	0.05	0.06	1.0	8	4
0	18	8	10	0.3	119	3	.10	1,050	105	0.02	0.02	0.3	3	2
0	31	30	50	0.7	409	10	.27	4,190	419	0.04	0.05	0.9	12	5
0	10	10	17	0.3	139	3	.09	1,420	142	0.02	0.02	0.3	4	1
0	80	59	152	6.1	1,791	13	NI	9,410	941	0.01	0.20	3.9	3	4
0	55	40	103	4.2	1,222	8	NI	5,910	591	0.02	0.08	2.4	4	4
0	36	18	23	1.0	286	8	.23	3,300	330	0.02	0.04	0.7	[14]2	3
0	12	19	73	2.0	1,097	21	.73	1,060	106	0.19	0.21	3.3	14	113
0	27	33	119	1.6	1,484	15	1.28	1,860	186	0.33	0.37	5.8	24	162
0	27	7	23	0.4	451	1	.18	90	9	0.05	0.11	0.6	10	24
0	35	9	30	0.5	594	2	NI	120	12	0.07	0.15	0.8	14	NI
0	18	46	30	0.8	282	tr	.39	240	24	0.04	0.06	0.6	30	49
0	20	9	15	0.2	129	9	.16	150	15	0.07	0.07	0.5	19	9
0	62	17	20	1.1	170	3	NI	120	12	0.06	0.15	0.7	3	NI
0	50	14	16	0.9	138	2	.14	100	10	0.05	0.12	0.6	2	15
0	22	27	24	3.3	239	17	.18	1,840	184	0.04	0.10	0.4	5	20
0	11	10	13	0.3	152	tr	.04	150	15	0.03	0.04	0.3	5	8
0	38	8	3	0.4	61	10	.18	10	1	0.01	0.04	0.1	[15]108	NI
0	108	11	17	0.6	72	80	.14	60	6	0.04	0.06	0.3	6	2
0	61	27	33	1.0	541	2	.24	40	4	0.07	0.08	1.8	0	14
0	131	57	71	2.0	1,161	5	NI	90	9	0.16	0.18	3.9	0	NI
0	122	269	127	4.2	1,331	21	.94	250	25	0.13	0.16	1.3	1	16

NI = not indicated.
[15]With added ascorbic acid.

APPENDIX 41 NUTRITIVE VALUE OF THE EDIBLE PART OF FOOD *(continued)*

Foods, Approximate Measures, Units, and Weight (weight of edible portion only)		Grams	Water (g)	Food Energy (Calories)	Protein (g)	Fat (g)	Fatty Acids: Saturated (g)	Fatty Acids: Monounsaturated (g)	Fatty Acids: Polyunsaturated (g)
Fruits and Fruit Juices (*cont.*)									
Fruit cocktail, canned, fruit and liquid									
Heavy syrup pack	1 c	255	80	185	1	tr	tr	tr	0.1
Juice pack	1 c	248	87	115	1	tr	tr	tr	tr
Grapefruit									
Raw, without peel, membrane and seeds (3¾-in diam., 1 lb 1 oz, whole, with refuse)	½ grapefruit	120	91	40	1	tr	tr	tr	tr
Canned, sections with syrup	1 c	254	84	150	1	tr	tr	tr	0.1
Grapefruit juice									
Raw	1 c	247	90	95	1	tr	tr	tr	0.1
Canned									
Unsweetened	1 c	247	90	95	1	tr	tr	tr	0.1
Sweetened	1 c	250	87	115	1	tr	tr	tr	0.1
Frozen concentrate, unsweetened									
Undiluted	6-fl-oz can	207	62	300	4	1	0.1	0.1	0.2
Diluted with 3 parts water by volume	1 c	247	89	100	1	tr	tr	tr	0.1
Grapes, European type (adherent skin), raw									
Thompson Seedless	10 grapes	50	81	35	tr	tr	0.1	tr	0.1
Tokay and Emperor, seeded types	10 grapes	57	81	40	tr	tr	0.1	tr	0.1
Grape juice									
Canned or bottled	1 c	253	84	155	1	tr	0.1	tr	0.1
Frozen concentrate, sweetened									
Undiluted	6-fl-oz can	216	54	385	1	1	0.2	tr	0.2
Diluted with 3 parts water by volume	1 c	250	87	125	tr	tr	0.1	tr	0.1
Kiwifruit, raw, without skin (about 5 per lb with skin)	1 kiwifruit	76	83	45	1	tr	tr	0.1	0.1
Lemons, raw, without peel and seeds (about 4 per lb with peel and seeds)	1 lemon	58	89	15	1	tr	tr	tr	0.1
Lemon juice									
Raw	1 c	244	91	60	1	tr	tr	tr	tr
Canned or bottled, unsweetened	1 c	244	92	50	1	1	0.1	tr	0.2
	1 tbsp	15	92	5	tr	tr	tr	tr	tr
Frozen, single-strength, unsweetened	6-fl-oz can	244	92	55	1	1	0.1	tr	0.2
Lime juice									
Raw	1 c	246	90	65	1	tr	tr	tr	0.1
Canned, unsweetened	1 c	246	93	50	1	1	0.1	0.1	0.2
Mangos, raw, without skin and seed (about 1½ lb with skin and seed)	1 mango	207	82	135	1	1	0.1	0.2	0.1

tr = nutrient present in trace amounts.
[14]Without added ascorbic acid. For value with added ascorbic acid, refer to label.
[15]With added ascorbic acid.

NUTRIENTS IN INDICATED QUANTITY

Cholesterol (mg)	Carbohydrate (g)	Calcium (mg)	Phosphorus (mg)	Iron (mg)	Potassium (mg)	Sodium (mg)	Zn (mg)	Vitamin A Value		Thiamin (mg)	Riboflavin (mg)	Niacin (mg)	Ascorbic acid (mg)	Folic acid (μg)
								IU	RE					
0	48	15	28	0.7	224	15	.20	520	52	0.05	0.05	1.0	5	1.2
0	29	20	35	0.5	236	10	.22	760	76	0.03	0.04	1.0	7	1.5
0	10	14	10	0.1	167	tr	.09	[16]10	[16]1	0.04	0.02	0.3	41	13
0	39	36	25	1.0	328	5	.20	tr	tr	0.10	0.05	0.6	54	22
0	23	22	37	0.5	400	2	.12	20	2	0.10	0.05	0.5	94	52
0	22	17	27	0.5	378	2	.22	20	2	0.10	0.05	0.6	72	26
0	28	20	28	0.9	405	5	.15	20	2	0.10	0.06	0.8	67	26
0	72	56	101	1.0	1,002	6	.12	60	6	0.30	0.16	1.6	248	9
0	24	20	35	0.3	336	2	NI	20	2	0.10	0.05	0.5	83	9
0	9	6	7	0.1	93	1	.08	40	4	0.05	0.03	0.2	5	4
0	10	6	7	0.1	105	1	NI	40	4	0.05	0.03	0.2	6	4
0	38	23	28	0.6	334	8	.13	20	2	0.07	0.09	0.7	[14]tr	7
0	96	28	32	0.8	160	15	.10	60	6	0.11	0.20	0.9	[15]179	4
0	32	10	10	.03	53	5	NI	20	2	0.04	0.07	0.3	[15]60	4
0	11	20	30	0.3	252	4	.13	130	13	0.02	0.04	0.4	74	17
0	5	15	9	0.3	80	1	.03	20	2	0.02	0.01	0.1	31	6
0	21	17	15	0.1	303	2	.12	50	5	0.07	0.02	0.2	112	32
0	16	27	22	0.3	249	[17]51	NI	40	4	0.10	0.02	0.5	61	25
0	1	2	1	tr	15	[17]3	.01	tr	tr	0.01	tr	tr	4	2
0	16	20	20	0.3	217	2	NI	30	3	0.14	0.03	0.3	77	4
0	22	22	17	0.1	268	2	.15	20	2	0.05	0.02	0.2	72	21
0	16	30	25	0.6	185	[17]39	.15	40	4	0.08	0.01	0.4	16	20
0	35	21	23	0.3	323	4	.08	8,060	806	0.12	0.12	1.2	57	29

NI = not indicated.

[16]For white grapefruit; pink grapefruit have about 310 IU or 31 RE.

[17]Sodium benzoate and sodium bisulfite added as preservatives.

APPENDIX 41 NUTRITIVE VALUE OF THE EDIBLE PART OF FOOD *(continued)*

Foods, Approximate Measures, Units, and Weight (weight of edible portion only)		Grams	Water (g)	Food Energy (Calories)	Protein (g)	Fat (g)	Fatty Acids: Saturated (g)	Fatty Acids: Monounsaturated (g)	Fatty Acids: Polyunsaturated (g)
Fruits and Fruit Juices (*cont.*)									
Melons, raw, without rind and cavity contents									
Cantaloupe, orange-fleshed (5-in diam., 2⅓ lb, whole, with rind and cavity contents)	½ melon	267	90	95	2	1	0.1	0.1	0.3
Honeydew (6½-in diam., 5¼ lb, whole, with rind and cavity contents)	⅒ melon	129	90	45	1	tr	tr	tr	0.1
Nectarines, raw, without pits (about 3 per lb with pits)	1 nectarine	136	86	65	1	1	0.1	0.2	0.3
Oranges, raw	1 orange	131	87	60	1	tr	tr	tr	tr
Whole, without peel and seeds (2⅝-in diam., about 2½ per lb, with peel and seeds)									
Sections without membranes	1 c	180	87	85	2	tr	tr	tr	tr
Orange juice									
Raw, all varieties	1 c	248	88	110	2	tr	0.1	0.1	0.1
Canned, unsweetened	1 c	249	89	105	1	tr	tr	0.1	0.1
Chilled	1 c	249	88	110	2	1	0.1	0.1	0.2
Frozen concentrate									
Undiluted	6-fl-oz can	213	58	340	5	tr	0.1	0.1	0.1
Diluted with 3 parts water by volume	1 c	249	88	110	2	tr	tr	tr	tr
Orange and grapefruit juice, canned	1 c	247	89	105	1	tr	tr	tr	tr
Papayas, raw, ½-in cubes	1 c	140	86	65	1	tr	0.1	0.1	tr
Peaches									
Raw									
Whole, 2½-in diam., peeled, pitted (about 4 per lb with peels and pits)	1 peach	87	88	35	1	tr	tr	tr	tr
Sliced	1 c	170	88	75	1	tr	tr	0.1	0.1
Canned, fruit and liquid									
Heavy syrup pack	1 c	256	79	190	1	tr	tr	0.1	0.1
	1 half	81	79	60	tr	tr	tr	tr	tr
Juice pack	1 c	248	87	110	2	tr	tr	tr	tr
	1 half	77	87	35	tr	tr	tr	tr	tr
Dried									
Uncooked	1 c	160	32	380	6	1	0.1	0.4	0.6
Cooked, unsweetened, fruit and liquid	1 c	258	78	200	3	1	0.1	0.2	0.3
Frozen, sliced, sweetened	10-oz container	284	75	265	2	tr	tr	0.1	0.2
	1 c	250	75	235	2	tr	tr	0.1	0.2

tr = nutrient present in trace amounts.

NUTRIENTS IN INDICATED QUANTITY

Cholesterol (mg)	Carbohydrate (g)	Calcium (mg)	Phosphorus (mg)	Iron (mg)	Potassium (mg)	Sodium (mg)	Zn (mg)	Vitamin A Value		Thiamin (mg)	Riboflavin (mg)	Niacin (mg)	Ascorbic acid (mg)	Folic acid (μg)
								IU	RE					
0	22	29	45	0.6	825	24	NI	8,610	861	0.10	0.06	1.5	113	48
0	12	8	13	0.1	350	13	.12	50	5	0.10	0.02	0.8	32	10
0	16	7	22	0.2	288	tr	.12	1,000	100	0.02	0.06	1.3	7	5
0	15	52	18	0.1	237	tr	.09	270	27	0.11	0.05	0.4	70	44
0	21	72	25	0.2	326	tr	NI	370	37	0.16	0.07	0.5	96	NI
0	26	27	42	0.5	496	2	.12	500	50	0.22	0.07	1.0	124	109
0	25	20	35	1.1	436	5	.17	440	44	0.15	0.07	0.8	86	15
0	25	25	27	0.4	473	2	.13	190	19	0.28	0.05	0.7	82	45
0	81	68	121	0.7	1,436	6	.38	590	59	0.60	0.14	1.5	294	109
0	27	22	40	0.2	473	2	NI	190	19	0.20	0.04	0.5	97	109
0	25	20	35	1.1	390	7	.18	290	29	0.14	0.07	0.8	72	35
0	17	35	12	0.3	247	9	.21	400	40	0.04	0.04	0.5	92	48
0	10	4	10	0.1	171	tr	.12	470	47	0.01	0.04	0.9	6	3
0	19	9	20	0.2	335	tr	NI	910	91	0.03	0.07	1.7	11	6
0	51	8	28	0.7	236	15	.23	850	85	0.03	0.06	1.6	7	8
0	16	2	9	0.2	75	5	.07	270	27	0.01	0.02	0.5	2	2.6
0	29	15	42	0.7	317	10	.27	940	94	0.02	0.04	1.4	9	8
0	9	5	13	0.2	99	3	.09	290	29	0.01	0.01	0.4	3	2.6
0	98	45	190	6.5	1,594	11	NI	3,460	346	tr	0.34	7.0	8	0
0	51	23	98	3.4	826	5	NI	510	51	0.01	0.05	3.9	10	NI
0	68	9	31	1.1	369	17	NI	810	81	0.04	0.10	1.9	[15]268	NI
0	60	8	28	0.9	325	15	.13	710	71	0.03	0.09	1.6	[15]236	8

NI = not indicated.
[15]With added ascorbic acid.

Foods, Approximate Measures, Units, and Weight (weight of edible portion only)		Grams	Water (g)	Food Energy (Calories)	Protein (g)	Fat (g)	Fatty Acids Saturated (g)	Fatty Acids Monounsaturated (g)	Fatty Acids Polyunsaturated (g)
Fruits and Fruit Juices (*cont.*)									
Pears									
Raw, with skin, cored									
Bartlett, 2½-in diam. (about 2½ per lb with cores and stems)	1 pear	166	84	100	1	1	tr	0.1	0.2
Bosc, 2½-in diam. (about 3 per lb with cores and stems)	1 pear	141	84	85	1	1	tr	0.1	0.1
D'Anjou, 3-in diam. (about 2 per lb with cores and stems)	1 pear	200	84	120	1	1	tr	0.2	0.2
Canned, fruit and liquid									
Heavy syrup pack	1 c	255	80	190	1	tr	tr	0.1	0.1
	1 half	79	80	60	tr	tr	tr	tr	tr
Juice pack	1 c	248	86	125	1	tr	tr	tr	tr
	1 half	77	86	40	tr	tr	tr	tr	tr
Pineapple									
Raw, diced	1 c	155	87	55	1	1	tr	0.1	0.2
Canned, fruit and liquid									
Heavy syrup pack									
Crushed, chunks, tidbits	1 c	255	79	200	1	tr	tr	tr	0.1
Slices	1 slice	58	79	45	tr	tr	tr	tr	tr
Juice pack									
Chunks or tidbits	1 c	250	84	150	1	tr	tr	tr	0.1
Slices	1 slice	58	84	35	tr	tr	tr	tr	tr
Pineapple juice, unsweetened, canned	1 c	250	86	140	1	tr	tr	tr	0.1
Plantains, without peel									
Raw	1 plantain	179	65	220	2	1	0.3	0.1	0.1
Cooked, boiled, sliced	1 c	154	67	180	1	tr	0.1	tr	0.1
Plums, without pits									
Raw									
2⅛-in diam. (about 6½ per lb with pits)	1 plum	66	85	35	1	tr	tr	0.3	0.1
1½-in diam. (about 15 per lb with pits)	1 plum	28	85	15	tr	tr	tr	0.1	tr
Canned, purple, fruit and liquid									
Heavy syrup pack	1 c	258	76	230	1	tr	tr	0.2	0.1
	3 plums	133	76	120	tr	tr	tr	0.1	tr
Juice pack	1 c	252	84	145	1	tr	tr	tr	tr
	3 plums	95	84	55	tr	tr	tr	tr	tr
Prunes, dried									
Uncooked	4 extra large or 5 large prunes	49	32	115	1	tr	tr	0.2	0.1
Cooked, unsweetened, fruit and liquid	1 c	212	70	225	2	tr	tr	0.3	0.1
Prune juice, canned or bottled	1 c	256	81	180	2	tr	tr	0.1	tr
Raisins, seedless									
Cup, not pressed down	1 c	145	15	435	5	1	0.2	tr	0.2
Packet, ½ oz (1½ tbsp)	1 packet	14	15	40	tr	tr	tr	tr	tr

tr = nutrient present in trace amounts.

NUTRIENTS IN INDICATED QUANTITY

Cholesterol (mg)	Carbohydrate (g)	Calcium (mg)	Phosphorus (mg)	Iron (mg)	Potassium (mg)	Sodium (mg)	Zn (mg)	Vitamin A Value IU	RE	Thiamin (mg)	Riboflavin (mg)	Niacin (mg)	Ascorbic acid (mg)	Folic acid (μg)
0	25	18	18	0.4	208	tr	.20	30	3	0.03	0.07	0.2	7	12
0	21	16	16	0.4	176	tr	NI	30	3	0.03	0.06	0.1	6	NI
0	30	22	22	0.5	250	tr	NI	40	4	0.04	0.08	0.2	8	NI
0	49	13	18	0.6	166	13	.20	10	1	0.03	0.06	0.6	3	3
0	15	4	6	0.2	51	4	.06	tr	tr	0.01	0.02	0.2	1	.9
0	32	22	30	0.7	238	10	.22	10	1	0.03	0.03	0.5	4	3
0	10	7	9	0.2	74	3	.09	tr	tr	0.01	0.01	0.2	1	1.6
0	19	11	11	0.6	175	2	.12	40	4	0.14	0.06	0.7	24	16
0	52	36	18	1.0	265	3	.31	40	4	0.23	0.06	0.7	19	12
0	12	8	4	0.2	60	1	NI	10	1	0.05	0.01	0.2	4	NI
0	39	35	15	0.7	305	3	.25	100	10	0.24	0.05	0.7	24	12
0	9	8	3	0.2	71	1	NI	20	2	0.06	0.01	0.2	6	NI
0	34	43	20	0.7	335	3	.28	10	1	0.14	0.06	0.6	27	58
0	57	5	61	1.1	893	7	.27	2,020	202	0.09	0.10	1.2	33	33
0	48	3	43	0.9	716	8	.21	1,400	140	0.07	0.08	1.2	17	40
0	9	3	7	0.1	114	tr	.06	210	21	0.03	0.06	0.3	6	3
0	4	1	3	tr	48	tr	NI	90	9	0.01	0.03	0.1	3	NI
0	60	23	34	2.2	235	49	NI	670	67	0.04	0.10	0.8	1	NI
0	31	12	17	1.1	121	25	.08	340	34	0.02	0.05	0.4	1	2.8
0	38	25	38	0.9	388	3	NI	2,540	254	0.06	0.15	1.2	7	NI
0	14	10	14	0.3	146	1	.11	960	96	0.02	0.06	0.4	3	2.8
0	31	25	39	1.2	365	2	.22	970	97	0.04	0.08	1.0	2	1.5
0	60	49	74	2.4	708	4	.50	650	65	0.05	0.21	1.5	6	0
0	45	31	64	3.0	707	10	.54	10	1	0.04	0.18	2.0	10	1
0	115	71	141	3.0	1,089	17	.46	10	1	0.23	0.13	1.2	5	5
0	11	7	14	0.3	105	2	NI	tr	tr	0.02	0.01	0.1	tr	NI

NI = not indicated.

Foods, Approximate Measures, Units, and Weight (weight of edible portion only)		Grams	Water (g)	Food Energy (Calories)	Protein (g)	Fat (g)	Fatty Acids: Saturated (g)	Fatty Acids: Monounsaturated (g)	Fatty Acids: Polyunsaturated (g)
Fruits and Fruit Juices (*cont.*)									
Raspberries									
Raw	1 c	123	87	60	1	1	tr	0.1	0.4
Frozen, sweetened	10-oz container	284	73	295	2	tr	tr	tr	0.3
	1 c	250	73	255	2	tr	tr	tr	0.2
Rhubarb, cooked, added sugar	1 c	240	68	280	1	tr	tr	tr	0.1
Strawberries									
Raw, capped, whole	1 c	149	92	45	1	1	tr	0.1	0.3
Frozen, sweetened, sliced	10-oz container	284	73	275	2	tr	tr	0.1	0.2
	1 c	255	73	245	1	tr	tr	tr	0.2
Tangerines									
Raw, without peel and seeds (2⅜-in diam., about 4 per lb, with peel and seeds)	1 tangerine	84	88	35	1	tr	tr	tr	tr
Canned, light syrup, fruit and liquid	1 c	252	83	155	1	tr	tr	tr	0.1
Tangerine juice, canned, sweetened	1 c	249	87	125	1	tr	tr	tr	0.1
Watermelon, raw, without rind and seeds									
Piece (4 by 8 in wedge with rind and seeds; 1/16 of 32⅔-lb melon, 10 by 16 in)	1 piece	482	92	155	3	2	0.3	0.2	1.0
Diced	1 c	160	92	50	1	1	0.1	0.1	0.3
Grain Products									
Bagels, plain or water, enriched, 3½-in diam.[18]	1 bagel	68	29	200	7	2	0.3	0.5	0.7
Barley, pearled, light, uncooked	1 c	200	11	700	16	2	0.3	0.2	0.9
Biscuits, baking powder, 2-in diam. (enriched flour, vegetable shortening)									
From home recipe	1 biscuit	28	28	100	2	5	1.2	2.0	1.3
From mix	1 biscuit	28	29	95	2	3	0.8	1.4	0.9
From refrigerated dough	1 biscuit	20	30	65	1	2	0.6	0.9	0.6
Breadcrumbs, enriched									
Dry, grated	1 c	100	7	390	13	5	1.5	1.6	1.0
Soft. See White bread									
Breads									
Boston brown bread, canned, slice, 3¼ in by ½ in[19]	1 slice	45	45	95	2	1	0.3	0.1	0.1
Cracked-wheat bread (¾ enriched wheat flour, ¼ cracked wheat flour)[19]									
Loaf, 1 lb	1 loaf	454	35	1,190	42	16	3.1	4.3	5.7
Slice (18 per loaf)	1 slice	25	35	65	2	1	0.2	0.2	0.3
Toasted	1 slice	21	26	65	2	1	0.2	0.2	0.3

tr = nutrient present in trace amounts.

[18]Egg bagels have 44 mg cholesterol and 22 IU or 7 RE vitamin A per bagel.

NUTRIENTS IN INDICATED QUANTITY

Cholesterol (mg)	Carbohydrate (g)	Calcium (mg)	Phosphorus (mg)	Iron (mg)	Potassium (mg)	Sodium (mg)	Zn (mg)	Vitamin A Value IU	Vitamin A Value RE	Thiamin (mg)	Riboflavin (mg)	Niacin (mg)	Ascorbic acid (mg)	Folic acid (μg)
0	14	27	15	0.7	187	tr	.57	160	16	0.04	0.11	1.1	31	33
0	74	43	48	1.8	324	3	NI	170	17	0.05	0.13	0.7	47	NI
0	65	38	43	1.6	285	3	.45	150	15	0.05	0.11	0.6	41	65
0	75	348	19	0.5	230	2	.19	170	17	0.04	0.06	0.5	8	13
0	10	21	28	0.6	247	1	.19	40	4	0.03	0.10	0.3	84	28
0	74	31	37	1.7	278	9	NI	70	7	0.05	0.14	1.1	118	NI
0	66	28	33	1.5	250	8	.15	60	6	0.04	0.13	1.0	106	42
0	9	12	8	0.1	132	1	.38	770	77	0.09	0.02	0.1	26	17
0	41	18	25	0.9	197	15	NI	2,120	212	0.13	0.11	1.1	50	NI
0	30	45	35	0.5	443	2	.07	1,050	105	0.15	0.05	0.2	55	8
0	35	39	43	0.8	559	10	NI	1,760	176	0.39	0.10	1.0	46	NI
0	11	13	14	0.3	186	3	.11	590	59	0.13	0.03	0.3	15	4
0	38	29	46	1.8	50	245	.61	0	0	0.26	0.20	2.4	0	16
0	158	32	378	4.2	320	6	2.80	0	0	0.24	0.10	6.2	0	25
tr	13	47	36	0.7	32	195	.15	10	3	0.08	0.08	0.8	tr	7
tr	14	58	128	0.7	56	262	.18	20	4	0.12	0.11	0.8	tr	3
1	10	4	79	0.5	18	249	.09	0	0	0.08	0.05	0.7	0	1
5	73	122	141	4.1	152	736	1.32	0	0	0.35	0.35	4.8	0	27
3	21	41	72	0.9	131	113	.35	[20]0	[20]0	0.06	0.04	0.7	0	8
0	227	295	581	12.1	608	1,966	NI	tr	tr	1.73	1.73	15.3	tr	NI
0	12	16	32	0.7	34	106	.35	tr	tr	0.10	0.09	0.8	tr	12
0	12	16	32	0.7	34	106	.35	tr	tr	0.07	0.09	0.8	tr	12

NI = not indicated.

[19]Made with vegetable shortening.

[20]Made with white cornmeal. If made with yellow cornmeal, value is 32 IU or 3 RE.

APPENDIX 41 NUTRITIVE VALUE OF THE EDIBLE PART OF FOOD *(continued)*

Foods, Approximate Measures, Units, and Weight (weight of edible portion only)		Grams	Water (g)	Food Energy (Calories)	Protein (g)	Fat (g)	Fatty Acids Saturated (g)	Fatty Acids Monounsaturated (g)	Fatty Acids Polyunsaturated (g)
Grain Products (*cont.*)									
Breads (*cont.*)									
French or Vienna bread, enriched[19]									
Loaf, 1 lb	1 loaf	454	34	1,270	43	18	3.8	5.7	5.9
Slice									
French, 5 by 2½ by 1 in	1 slice	35	34	100	3	1	0.3	0.4	0.5
Vienna, 4¾ by 4 by ½ in	1 slice	25	34	70	2	1	0.2	0.3	0.3
Italian bread, enriched									
Loaf, 1 lb	1 loaf	454	32	1,255	41	4	0.6	0.3	1.6
Slice, 4½ by 3¼ by ¾ in	1 slice	30	32	85	3	tr	tr	tr	0.1
Mixed grain bread, enriched[19]									
Loaf, 1 lb	1 loaf	454	37	1,165	45	17	3.2	4.1	6.5
Slice (18 per loaf)	1 slice	25	37	65	2	1	0.2	0.2	0.4
Toasted	1 slice	23	27	65	2	1	0.2	0.2	0.4
Oatmeal bread, enriched[19]									
Loaf, 1 lb	1 loaf	454	37	1,145	38	20	3.7	7.1	8.2
Slice (18 per loaf)	1 slice	25	37	65	2	1	0.2	0.4	0.5
Toasted	1 slice	23	30	65	2	1	0.2	0.4	0.5
Pita bread, enriched, white, 6½-in diam.	1 pita	60	31	165	6	1	0.1	0.1	0.4
Pumpernickel (⅔ rye flour, ⅓ enriched wheat flour)[19]									
Loaf, 1 lb	1 loaf	454	37	1,160	42	16	2.6	3.6	6.4
Slice, 5 by 4 by ⅜-in	1 slice	32	37	80	3	1	0.2	0.3	0.5
Toasted	1 slice	29	28	80	3	1	0.2	0.3	0.5
Raisin bread, enriched[19]									
Loaf, 1 lb	1 loaf	454	33	1,260	37	18	4.1	6.5	6.7
Slice (18 per loaf)	1 slice	25	33	65	2	1	0.2	0.3	0.4
Toasted	1 slice	21	24	65	2	1	0.2	0.3	0.4
Rye bread, light (⅔ enriched wheat flour, ⅓ rye flour)[19]									
Loaf, 1 lb	1 loaf	454	37	1,190	38	17	3.3	5.2	5.5
Slice, 4¾ by 3¾ by 7⁄16 in	1 slice	25	37	65	2	1	0.2	0.3	0.3
Toasted	1 slice	22	28	65	2	1	0.2	0.3	0.3
Wheat bread, enriched[19]									
Loaf, 1 lb	1 loaf	454	37	1,160	43	19	3.9	7.3	4.5
Slice (18 per loaf)	1 slice	25	37	65	2	1	0.2	0.4	0.3
Toasted	1 slice	23	28	65	3	1	0.2	0.4	0.3
White bread, enriched[19]									
Loaf, 1 lb	1 loaf	454	37	1,210	38	18	5.6	6.5	4.2
Slice (18 per loaf)	1 slice	25	37	65	2	1	0.3	0.4	0.2
Toasted	1 slice	22	28	65	2	1	0.3	0.4	0.2
Slice (22 per loaf)	1 slice	20	37	55	2	1	0.2	0.3	0.2
Toasted	1 slice	17	28	55	2	1	0.2	0.3	0.2
Cubes	1 c	30	37	80	2	1	0.4	0.4	0.3
Crumbs, soft	1 c	45	37	120	4	2	0.6	0.6	0.4

tr = nutrient present in trace amounts.

NUTRIENTS IN INDICATED QUANTITY

Cholesterol (mg)	Carbohydrate (g)	Calcium (mg)	Phosphorus (mg)	Iron (mg)	Potassium (mg)	Sodium (mg)	Zn (mg)	Vitamin A Value		Thiamin (mg)	Riboflavin (mg)	Niacin (mg)	Ascorbic acid (mg)	Folic acid (μg)
								IU	RE					
0	230	499	386	14.0	409	2,633	NI	tr	tr	2.09	1.59	18.2	tr	NI
0	18	39	30	1.1	32	203	.22	tr	tr	0.16	0.12	1.4	tr	13
0	13	28	21	0.8	23	145	NI	tr	tr	0.12	0.09	1.0	tr	8
0	256	77	350	12.7	336	2,656	NI	0	0	1.80	1.10	15.0	0	NI
0	17	5	23	0.8	22	176	.26	0	0	0.12	0.07	1.0	0	9
0	212	472	962	14.8	990	1,870	NI	tr	tr	1.77	1.73	18.9	tr	NI
0	12	27	55	0.8	56	106	.30	tr	tr	0.10	0.10	1.1	tr	16
0	12	27	55	0.8	56	106	.30	tr	tr	0.08	0.10	1.1	tr	16
0	212	267	563	12.0	707	2,231	NI	0	0	2.09	1.20	15.4	0	NI
0	12	15	31	0.7	39	124	.28	0	0	0.12	0.07	0.9	0	8
0	12	15	31	0.7	39	124	.28	0	0	0.09	0.07	0.9	0	8
0	33	49	60	1.4	71	339	.50	0	0	0.27	0.12	2.2	0	12
0	218	322	990	12.4	1,966	2,461	NI	0	0	1.54	2.36	15.0	0	NI
0	16	23	71	0.9	141	177	.40	0	0	0.11	0.17	1.1	0	16
0	16	23	71	0.9	141	177	.40	0	0	0.09	0.17	1.1	0	16
0	239	463	395	14.1	1,058	1,657	NI	tr	tr	1.50	2.81	18.6	tr	NI
0	13	25	22	0.8	59	92	.16	tr	tr	0.08	0.15	1.0	tr	9
0	13	25	22	0.8	59	92	.16	tr	tr	0.06	0.15	1.0	tr	9
0	218	363	658	12.3	926	3,164	NI	0	0	1.86	1.45	15.0	0	NI
0	12	20	36	0.7	51	175	.38	0	0	0.10	0.08	0.8	0	10
0	12	20	36	0.7	51	175	.38	0	0	0.08	0.08	0.8	0	10
0	213	572	835	15.8	627	2,447	NI	tr	tr	2.09	1.45	20.5	tr	NI
0	12	32	47	0.9	35	138	.29	tr	tr	0.12	0.08	1.2	tr	13
0	12	32	47	0.9	35	138	.29	tr	tr	0.10	0.08	1.2	tr	13
0	222	572	490	12.9	508	2,334	NI	tr	tr	2.13	1.41	17.0	tr	NI
0	12	32	27	0.7	28	129	.15	tr	tr	0.12	0.08	0.9	tr	10
0	12	32	27	0.7	28	129	.15	tr	tr	0.09	0.08	0.9	tr	10
0	10	25	21	0.6	22	101	NI	tr	tr	0.09	0.06	0.7	tr	10
0	10	25	21	0.6	22	101	NI	tr	tr	0.07	0.06	0.7	tr	10
0	15	38	32	0.9	34	154	NI	tr	tr	0.14	0.09	1.1	tr	NI
0	22	57	49	1.3	50	231	NI	tr	tr	0.21	0.14	1.7	tr	NI

NI = not indicated.
[19]Made with vegetable shortening.

APPENDIX 41 NUTRITIVE VALUE OF THE EDIBLE PART OF FOOD *(continued)*

Foods, Approximate Measures, Units, and Weight (weight of edible portion only)		Grams	Water (g)	Food Energy (Calories)	Protein (g)	Fat (g)	Fatty Acids: Saturated (g)	Fatty Acids: Monounsaturated (g)	Fatty Acids: Polyunsaturated (g)
Grain Products (*cont.*)									
Breads (*cont.*)									
Whole-wheat bread[19]									
Loaf, 1 lb	1 loaf	454	38	1,110	44	20	5.8	6.8	5.2
Slice (16 per loaf)	1 slice	28	38	70	3	1	0.4	0.4	0.3
Toasted	1 slice	25	29	70	3	1	0.4	0.4	0.3
Bread stuffing (from enriched bread), prepared from mix									
Dry type	1 c	140	33	500	9	31	6.1	13.3	9.6
Moist type	1 c	203	61	420	9	26	5.3	11.3	8.0
Buckwheat flour, light, sifted	1 c	98	12	340	6	1	0.2	0.4	0.4
Bulgur, uncooked	1 c	170	10	600	19	3	1.2	0.3	1.2
Cakes prepared from cake mixes with enriched flour[21]									
Angel food									
Whole cake, 9¾-in diam. tube cake	1 cake	635	38	1,150	38	2	0.4	0.2	1.0
Piece, 1/12 of cake	1 piece	53	38	125	2	tr	tr	tr	0.1
Coffeecake, crumb									
Whole cake, 7¾ by 5⅝ by 1¼ in	1 cake	430	30	1,385	27	41	11.8	16.7	9.6
Piece, ⅙ of cake	1 piece	72	30	230	5	7	2.0	2.8	1.6
Devil's food with chocolate frosting									
Whole, 2-layer cake, 8- or 9-in diam.	1 cake	1,107	24	3,755	49	136	55.6	51.4	19.7
Piece, 1/16 of cake	1 piece	69	24	235	3	8	3.5	3.2	1.2
Cupcake, 2½-in diam.	1 cupcake	35	24	120	2	4	1.8	1.6	0.6
Gingerbread									
Whole cake, 8 in square	1 cake	570	37	1,575	18	39	9.6	16.4	10.5
Piece, ⅑ of cake	1 piece	63	37	175	2	4	1.1	1.8	1.2
Cheesecake									
Whole cake, 9-in diam.	1 cake	1,110	46	3,350	60	213	119.9	65.5	14.4
Piece, 1/12 of cake	1 piece	92	46	280	5	18	9.9	5.4	1.2
Cookies made with enriched flour									
Brownies with nuts									
Commercial, with frosting, 1½ by 1¾ by ⅞ in	1 brownie	25	13	100	1	4	1.6	2.0	0.6
From home recipe, 1¾ by 1¾ by ⅞ in[22]	1 brownie	20	10	95	1	6	1.4	2.8	1.2
Chocolate chip									
Commercial, 2¼-in diam., ⅜-in thick	4 cookies	42	4	180	2	9	2.9	3.1	2.6
Cornmeal									
Whole-ground, unbolted, dry form	1 c	122	12	435	11	5	0.5	1.1	2.5
Bolted (nearly whole-grain), dry form	1 c	122	12	440	11	4	0.5	0.9	2.2
Degermed, enriched									
Dry form	1 c	138	12	500	11	2	0.2	0.4	0.9
Cooked	1 c	240	88	120	3	tr	tr	0.1	0.2

tr = nutrient present in trace amounts; [20]Made with white cornmeal. If made with yellow cornmeal, value is 32 IU or 3 RE; [21]Excepting angel food cake, cakes were made from mixes containing vegetable shortening and frostings were made with margarine.

NUTRIENTS IN INDICATED QUANTITY

Cholesterol (mg)	Carbohydrate (g)	Calcium (mg)	Phosphorus (mg)	Iron (mg)	Potassium (mg)	Sodium (mg)	Zn (mg)	Vitamin A Value		Thiamin (mg)	Riboflavin (mg)	Niacin (mg)	Ascorbic acid (mg)	Folic acid (μg)
								IU	RE					
0	206	327	1,180	15.5	799	2,887	NI	tr	tr	1.59	0.95	17.4	tr	NI
0	13	20	74	1.0	50	180	.50	tr	tr	0.10	0.06	1.1	tr	16
0	13	20	74	1.0	50	180	.50	tr	tr	0.08	0.06	1.1	tr	16
0	50	92	136	2.2	126	1,254	.56	910	273	0.17	0.20	2.5	0	14
67	40	81	134	2.0	118	1,023	NI	850	256	0.10	0.18	1.6	0	22
0	78	11	86	1.0	314	2	2.56	0	0	0.08	0.04	0.4	0	100
0	129	49	575	9.5	389	7	1.04	0	0	0.48	0.24	7.7	0	33
0	342	527	1,086	2.7	845	3,226	NI	0	0	0.32	1.27	1.6	0	NI
0	29	44	91	0.2	71	269	.07	0	0	0.03	0.11	0.1	0	4
279	225	262	748	7.3	469	1,853	NI	690	194	0.82	0.90	7.7	1	NI
47	38	44	125	1.2	78	310	.62	120	32	0.14	0.15	1.3	tr	5
598	645	653	1,162	22.1	1,439	2,900	NI	1,660	498	1.11	1.66	10.0	1	NI
37	40	41	72	1.4	90	181	.35	100	31	0.07	0.10	0.6	tr	NI
19	20	21	37	0.7	46	92	NI	50	16	0.04	0.05	0.3	tr	NI
6	291	513	570	10.8	1,562	1,733	NI	0	0	0.86	1.03	7.4	1	NI
1	32	57	63	1.2	173	192	.610	0	0	0.09	0.11	0.8	tr	4
2,053	317	622	977	5.3	1,088	2,464	NI	2,820	833	0.33	1.44	5.1	56	NI
170	26	52	81	0.4	90	204	.39	230	69	0.03	0.12	0.4	5	17
14	16	13	26	0.6	50	59	NI	70	18	0.08	0.07	0.3	tr	7
18	11	9	26	0.4	35	51	NI	20	6	0.05	0.05	0.3	tr	4
5	28	13	41	0.8	68	140	.30	50	15	0.10	0.23	1.0	tr	4
0	90	24	312	2.2	346	1	NI	620	62	0.46	0.13	2.4	0	NI
0	91	21	272	2.2	303	1	2.44	590	59	0.37	0.10	2.3	0	70
0	108	8	137	5.9	166	1	.99	610	61	0.61	0.36	4.8	0	66
0	26	2	34	1.4	38	0	.99	140	14	0.14	0.10	1.2	0	66

NI = not indicated; [22]Made with vegetable oil.

APPENDIX 41 NUTRITIVE VALUE OF THE EDIBLE PART OF FOOD *(continued)*

Foods, Approximate Measures, Units, and Weight (weight of edible portion only)		Grams	Water (g)	Food Energy (Calories)	Protein (g)	Fat (g)	Fatty Acids: Saturated (g)	Fatty Acids: Monounsaturated (g)	Fatty Acids: Polyunsaturated (g)
Grain Products (*cont.*)									
Crackers[23]									
Cheese									
Plain, 1 in square	10 crackers	10	4	50	1	3	0.9	1.2	0.3
Sandwich type (peanut butter)	1 sandwich	8	3	40	1	2	0.4	0.8	0.3
Graham, plain, 2½ in square	2 crackers	14	5	60	1	1	0.4	0.6	0.4
Melba toast, plain	1 piece	5	4	20	1	tr	0.1	0.1	0.1
Rye wafers, whole-grain, 1⅞ by 3½ in	2 wafers	14	5	55	1	1	0.3	0.4	0.3
Saltines[24]	4 crackers	12	4	50	1	1	0.5	0.4	0.2
Snack-type, standard	1 round cracker	3	3	15	tr	1	0.2	0.4	0.1
Wheat, thin	4 crackers	8	3	35	1	1	0.5	0.5	0.4
Whole-wheat wafers	2 crackers	8	4	35	1	2	0.5	0.6	0.4
Croissants, made with enriched flour, 4½ by 4 by 1¾ in	1 croissant	57	22	235	5	12	3.5	6.7	1.4
Danish pastry, made with enriched flour									
Plain without fruit or nuts									
Packaged ring, 12 oz	1 ring	340	27	1,305	21	71	21.8	28.6	15.6
Round piece, about 4¼-in diam., 1 in high	1 pastry	57	27	220	4	12	3.6	4.8	2.6
Ounce	1 oz	28	27	110	2	6	1.8	2.4	1.3
Fruit, round piece	1 pastry	65	30	235	4	13	3.9	5.2	2.9
Doughnuts, made with enriched flour									
Cake type, plain, 3¼-in diam., 1 in high	1 doughnut	50	21	210	3	12	2.8	5.0	3.0
Yeast-leavened, glazed, 3¾-in diam., 1¼ in high	1 doughnut	60	27	235	4	13	5.2	5.5	0.9
English muffins, plain, enriched	1 muffin	57	42	140	5	1	0.3	0.2	0.3
Toasted	1 muffin	50	29	140	5	1	0.3	0.2	0.3
Pies, piecrust made with enriched flour, vegetable shortening, 9-in diam.									
Apple									
Whole	1 pie	945	48	2,420	21	105	27.4	44.4	26
Piece, ⅙ of pie	1 piece	158	48	405	3	18	4.6	7.4	4
Blueberry									
Whole	1 pie	945	51	2,285	23	102	25.5	44.4	27
Piece, ⅙ pie	1 piece	158	51	380	4	17	4.3	7.4	4
Cherry									
Whole	1 pie	945	47	2,465	25	107	28.4	46.3	27
Piece, ⅙ of pie	1 piece	158	47	410	4	18	4.7	7.7	4
Creme									
Whole	1 pie	910	43	2,710	20	139	90.1	23.7	6
Piece, ⅙ of pie	1 piece	152	43	455	3	23	15.0	4.0	1

tr = nutrient present in trace amounts.
[23]Crackers made with enriched flour except for rye wafers and whole-wheat wafers.

NUTRIENTS IN INDICATED QUANTITY

Cholesterol (mg)	Carbohydrate (g)	Calcium (mg)	Phosphorus (mg)	Iron (mg)	Potassium (mg)	Sodium (mg)	Zn (mg)	Vitamin A Value		Thiamin (mg)	Riboflavin (mg)	Niacin (mg)	Ascorbic acid (mg)	Folic acid (μg)
								IU	RE					
6	6	11	17	0.3	17	112	.16	20	5	0.05	0.04	0.4	0	3
1	5	7	25	0.3	17	90	.08	tr	tr	0.04	0.03	0.6	0	2
0	11	6	20	0.4	36	86	NI	0	0	0.02	0.03	0.6	0	2
0	4	6	10	0.1	11	44	.10	0	0	0.01	0.01	0.1	0	1
0	10	7	44	0.5	65	115	1.60	0	0	0.06	0.03	0.5	0	10
4	9	3	12	0.5	17	165	.08	0	0	0.06	0.05	0.6	0	4
0	2	3	6	0.1	4	30	NI	tr	tr	0.01	0.01	0.1	0	NI
0	5	3	15	0.3	17	69	.10	tr	tr	0.04	0.03	0.4	0	3
0	5	3	22	0.2	31	59	.23	0	0	0.02	0.03	0.4	0	2
13	27	20	64	2.1	68	452	.43	50	13	0.17	0.13	1.3	0	18
292	152	360	347	6.5	316	1,302	.48	360	99	0.95	1.02	8.5	tr	18
49	26	60	58	1.1	53	218	NI	60	17	0.16	0.17	1.4	tr	15
24	13	30	29	0.5	26	109	NI	30	8	0.08	0.09	0.7	tr	NI
56	28	17	80	1.3	57	233	.55	40	11	0.16	0.14	1.4	tr	11
20	24	22	111	1.0	58	192	.26	20	5	0.12	0.12	1.1	tr	4
21	26	17	55	1.4	64	222	.46	tr	tr	0.28	0.12	1.8	0	13
0	27	96	67	1.7	331	378	.40	0	0	0.26	0.19	2.2	0	18
0	27	96	67	1.7	331	378	.40	0	0	0.23	0.19	2.2	0	18
0	360	76	208	9.5	756	2,844	NI	280	28	1.04	0.76	9.5	9	NI
0	60	13	35	1.6	126	476	.27	50	5	0.17	0.13	1.6	2	8
0	330	104	217	12.3	945	2,533	NI	850	85	1.04	0.85	10.4	38	NI
0	55	17	36	2.1	158	423	.29	140	14	0.17	0.14	1.7	6	7
0	363	132	236	9.5	992	2,873	NI	4,160	416	1.13	0.85	9.5	0	NI
0	61	22	40	1.6	166	480	.36	700	70	0.19	0.14	1.6	0	13
46	351	273	919	6.8	796	2,207	NI	1,250	391	0.36	0.89	6.4	0	NI
8	59	46	154	1.1	133	369	.79	210	65	0.06	0.15	1.1	0	15

NI = not indicated.
[24]Made with lard.

APPENDIX 41 NUTRITIVE VALUE OF THE EDIBLE PART OF FOOD *(continued)*

Foods, Approximate Measures, Units, and Weight (weight of edible portion only)		Grams	Water (g)	Food Energy (Calories)	Protein (g)	Fat (g)	Fatty Acids: Saturated (g)	Fatty Acids: Monounsaturated (g)	Fatty Acids: Polyunsaturated (g)
Grain Products (*cont.*)									
Pies (*cont.*)									
Custard									
Whole	1 pie	910	58	1,985	56	101	33.7	40.0	19.1
Piece, ⅙ of pie	1 piece	152	58	330	9	17	5.6	6.7	3.2
Lemon meringue									
Whole	1 pie	840	47	2,140	31	86	26.0	34.4	17.6
Piece, ⅙ of pie	1 piece	140	47	355	5	14	4.3	5.7	2.9
Peach									
Whole	1 pie	945	48	2,410	24	101	24.6	43.5	26.5
Piece, ⅙ of pie	1 piece	158	48	405	4	17	4.1	7.3	4.4
Pecan									
Whole	1 pie	825	20	3,450	42	189	28.1	101.5	47.0
Piece, ⅙ of pie	1 piece	138	20	575	7	32	4.7	17.0	7.9
Pumpkin									
Whole	1 pie	910	59	1,920	36	102	38.2	40.0	18.2
Piece, ⅙ of pie	1 piece	152	59	320	6	17	6.4	6.7	3.0
Pies, fried									
Apple	1 pie	85	43	255	2	14	5.8	6.6	0.6
Cherry	1 pie	85	42	250	2	14	5.8	6.7	0.6
Popcorn, popped									
Air-popped, unsalted	1 c	8	4	30	1	tr	tr	0.1	0.2
Popped in vegetable oil, salted	1 c	11	3	55	1	3	0.5	1.4	1.2
Sugar syrup coated	1 c	35	4	135	2	1	0.1	0.3	0.6
Pretzels, made with enriched flour									
Stick, 2¼ in long	10 pretzels	3	3	10	tr	tr	tr	tr	tr
Twisted, dutch 2¾ by 2⅝ in	1 pretzel	16	3	65	2	1	0.1	0.2	0.2
Twisted, thin, 3¼ by 2¼ by ¼ in	10 pretzels	60	3	240	6	2	0.4	0.8	0.6
Rice									
Brown, cooked, served hot	1 c	195	70	230	5	1	0.3	0.3	0.4
White, enriched									
Commercial varieties, all types									
Raw	1 c	185	12	670	12	1	0.2	0.2	0.3
Cooked, served hot	1 c	205	73	225	4	tr	0.1	0.1	0.1
Wheat flours									
All-purpose or family flour, enriched									
Sifted, spooned	1 c	115	12	420	12	1	0.2	0.1	0.5
Unsifted, spooned	1 c	125	12	455	13	1	0.2	0.1	0.5
Cake or pastry flour, enriched, sifted, spooned	1 c	96	12	350	7	1	0.1	0.1	0.3
Self-rising, enriched, unsifted, spooned	1 c	125	12	440	12	1	0.2	0.1	0.5
Whole-wheat, from hard wheats, stirred	1 c	120	12	400	16	2	0.3	0.3	1.1

tr = nutrient present in trace amounts.

NUTRIENTS IN INDICATED QUANTITY

Cholesterol (mg)	Carbohydrate (g)	Calcium (mg)	Phosphorus (mg)	Iron (mg)	Potassium (mg)	Sodium (mg)	Zn (mg)	Vitamin A Value		Thiamin (mg)	Riboflavin (mg)	Niacin (mg)	Ascorbic acid (mg)	Folic acid (μg)
								IU	RE					
1,010	213	874	1,028	9.1	1,247	2,612	NI	2,090	573	0.82	1.91	5.5	0	NI
169	36	146	172	1.5	208	436	.79	350	96	0.14	0.32	0.9	0	21
857	317	118	412	8.4	420	2,369	NI	1,430	395	0.59	0.84	5.0	25	NI
143	53	20	69	1.4	70	395	.51	240	66	0.10	0.14	0.8	4	11
0	361	95	274	11.3	1,408	2,533	NI	6,900	690	1.04	0.95	14.2	28	NI
0	60	16	46	1.9	235	423	.35	1,150	115	0.17	0.16	2.4	5	5
569	423	388	850	27.2	1,015	1,823	NI	1,320	322	1.82	0.99	6.6	0	NI
95	71	65	142	4.6	170	305	1.47	220	54	.030	0.17	1.1	0	7
655	223	464	628	8.2	1,456	1,947	NI	22,480	2,493	0.82	1.27	7.3	0	NI
109	37	78	105	1.4	243	325	.99	3,750	416	0.14	0.21	1.2	0	17
14	31	12	34	0.9	42	326	.29	30	3	0.09	0.06	1.0	1	NI
13	32	11	41	0.7	61	371	.29	190	19	0.06	0.06	0.6	1	4
0	6	1	22	0.2	20	tr	NI	10	1	0.03	0.01	0.2	0	2
0	6	3	31	0.3	19	86	.31	20	2	0.01	0.02	0.1	0	3
0	30	2	47	0.5	90	tr	NI	30	3	0.13	0.02	0.4	0	NI
0	2	1	3	0.1	3	48	NI	0	0	0.01	0.01	0.1	0	10
0	13	4	15	0.3	16	258	.17	0	0	0.05	0.04	0.7	0	NI
0	48	16	55	1.2	61	966	.42	0	0	0.19	0.15	2.6	0	10
0	50	23	142	1.0	137	0	1.23	0	0	0.18	0.04	2.7	0	8
0	149	44	174	5.4	170	9	NI	0	0	0.31	0.06	6.5	0	6
0	50	21	57	1.8	57	0	.94	0	0	0.23	0.02	2.1	0	7
0	88	18	100	5.1	109	2	NI	0	0	0.73	0.46	6.1	0	NI
0	95	20	109	5.5	119	3	.88	0	0	0.80	0.50	6.6	0	32.5
0	76	16	70	4.2	91	2	.60	0	0	0.58	0.38	5.1	0	19
0	93	331	583	5.5	113	1,349	.78	0	0	0.80	0.50	6.6	0	NI
0	85	49	446	5.2	444	4	3.52	0	0	0.66	0.14	5.2	0	44

NI = not indicated.

APPENDIX 41 NUTRITIVE VALUE OF THE EDIBLE PART OF FOOD *(continued)*

Foods, Approximate Measures, Units, and Weight (weight of edible portion only)		Grams	Water (g)	Food Energy (Calories)	Protein (g)	Fat (g)	Fatty Acids: Saturated (g)	Fatty Acids: Monounsaturated (g)	Fatty Acids: Polyunsaturated (g)
Legumes, Nuts, and Seeds									
Almonds, shelled									
Slivered, packed	1 c	135	4	795	27	70	6.7	45.8	14.8
Whole	1 oz	28	4	165	6	15	1.4	9.6	3.1
Beans, dry									
Cooked, drained									
Black	1 c	171	66	225	15	1	0.1	0.1	0.5
Great Northern	1 c	180	69	210	14	1	0.1	0.1	0.6
Lima	1 c	190	64	260	16	1	0.2	0.1	0.5
Pea (navy)	1 c	190	69	225	15	1	0.1	0.1	0.7
Pinto	1 c	180	65	265	15	1	0.1	0.1	0.5
Canned, solids and liquid									
White with									
Frankfurters (sliced)	1 c	255	71	365	19	18	7.4	8.8	0.7
Pork and tomato sauce	1 c	255	71	310	16	7	2.4	2.7	0.7
Pork and sweet sauce	1 c	255	66	385	16	12	4.3	4.9	1.2
Red kidney	1 c	255	76	230	15	1	0.1	0.1	0.6
Black-eyed peas, dry, cooked (with residual cooking liquid)	1 c	250	80	190	13	1	0.2	tr	0.3
Brazil nuts, shelled	1 oz	28	3	185	4	19	4.6	6.5	6.8
Carob flour	1 c	140	3	255	6	tr	tr	0.1	0.1
Cashew nuts, salted									
Dry roasted	1 c	137	2	785	21	63	12.5	37.4	10.7
	1 oz	28	2	165	4	13	2.6	7.7	2.2
Roasted in oil	1 c	130	4	750	21	63	12.4	36.9	10.6
	1 oz	28	4	165	5	14	2.7	8.1	2.3
Chestnuts, European (Italian), roasted, shelled	1 c	143	40	350	5	3	0.6	1.1	1.2
Chickpeas, cooked, drained	1 c	163	60	270	15	4	0.4	0.9	1.9
Coconut									
Raw									
Piece, about 2 by 2 by ½ in	1 piece	45	47	160	1	15	13.4	0.6	0.2
Shredded or grated	1 c	80	47	285	3	27	23.8	1.1	0.3
Dried, sweetened, shredded	1 c	93	13	470	3	33	29.3	1.4	0.4
Filberts (hazelnuts), chopped	1 c	115	5	725	15	72	5.3	56.5	6.9
	1 oz	28	5	108	4	18	1.3	13.9	1.7
Lentils, dry, cooked	1 c	200	72	215	16	1	0.1	0.2	0.5
Macadamia nuts, roasted in oil, salted	1 c	134	2	960	10	103	15.4	80.9	1.8
	1 oz	28	2	205	2	22	3.2	17.1	0.4
Mixed nuts, with peanuts, salted									
Dry roasted	1 oz	28	2	170	5	15	2.0	8.9	3.1
Roasted in oil	1 oz	28	2	175	5	16	2.5	9.0	3.8
Peanuts, roasted in oil, salted	1 c	145	2	840	39	71	9.9	35.5	22.6
	1 oz	28	2	165	8	14	1.9	6.9	4.4

tr = nutrient present in trace amounts.

[25]Cashews without salt contain 21 mg sodium per cup or 4 mg per oz.

[26]Cashews without salt contain 22 mg sodium per cup or 5 mg per oz.

NUTRIENTS IN INDICATED QUANTITY

Cholesterol (mg)	Carbohydrate (g)	Calcium (mg)	Phosphorus (mg)	Iron (mg)	Potassium (mg)	Sodium (mg)	Zn (mg)	Vitamin A Value IU	Vitamin A Value RE	Thiamin (mg)	Riboflavin (mg)	Niacin (mg)	Ascorbic acid (mg)	Folic acid (μg)
0	28	359	702	4.9	988	15	NI	0	0	0.28	1.05	4.5	1	NI
0	6	75	147	1.0	208	3	4.15	0	0	0.06	0.22	1.0	tr	NI
0	41	47	239	2.9	608	1	1.92	tr	tr	0.43	0.05	0.9	0	256
0	38	90	266	4.9	749	13	1.55	0	0	0.25	0.13	1.3	0	181
0	49	55	293	5.9	1,163	4	1.34	0	0	0.25	0.11	1.3	0	86
0	40	95	281	5.1	790	13	1.93	0	0	0.27	0.13	1.3	0	255
0	49	86	296	5.4	882	3	1.85	tr	tr	0.33	0.16	0.7	0	294
30	32	94	303	4.8	668	1,374	4.79	330	33	0.18	0.15	3.3	tr	77
10	48	138	235	4.6	536	1,181	2.60	330	33	0.20	0.08	1.5	5	94
10	54	161	291	5.9	536	969	3.80	330	33	0.15	0.10	1.3	5	95
0	42	74	278	4.6	673	968	1.89	10	1	0.13	0.10	1.5	0	229
0	35	43	238	3.3	573	20	1.70	30	3	0.40	0.10	1.0	0	210
0	4	50	170	1.0	170	1	1.30	tr	tr	0.28	0.03	0.5	tr	1
0	126	390	102	5.7	1,275	24	.95	tr	tr	0.07	0.07	2.2	tr	30
0	45	62	671	8.2	774	[25]877	NI	0	0	0.27	0.27	1.9	0	95
0	9	13	139	1.7	160	[25]181	1.59	0	0	0.06	0.06	0.4	0	20
0	37	53	554	5.3	689	[26]814	6.18	0	0	0.55	0.23	2.3	0	88
0	8	12	121	1.2	150	[26]177	1.35	0	0	0.12	0.05	0.5	0	19
0	76	41	153	1.3	847	3	.82	30	3	0.35	0.25	1.9	37	100
0	45	80	273	4.9	475	11	2.51	tr	tr	0.18	0.09	0.9	0	282
0	7	6	51	1.1	160	9	.50	0	0	0.03	0.01	0.2	1	12
0	12	11	90	1.9	285	16	.88	0	0	0.05	0.02	0.4	3	21
0	44	14	99	1.8	313	244	1.69	0	0	0.03	0.02	0.4	1	8
0	18	216	359	3.8	512	3	3.24	80	8	0.58	0.13	1.3	1	97
0	4	53	88	0.9	126	1	NI	20	2	0.14	0.03	0.3	tr	NI
0	38	50	238	4.2	498	26	2.51	40	4	0.14	0.12	1.2	0	358
0	17	60	268	2.4	441	[27]348	1.47	10	1	0.29	0.15	2.7	0	91
0	4	13	57	0.5	93	[27]74	NI	tr	tr	0.06	0.03	0.6	0	5
0	7	20	123	1.0	169	[28]190	1.08	tr	tr	0.06	0.06	1.3	0	14
0	6	31	131	0.9	165	[28]185	1.44	10	1	0.14	0.06	1.4	tr	24
0	27	125	734	2.8	1,019	[29]626	9.60	0	0	0.42	0.15	21.5	0	181
0	5	24	143	0.5	199	[29]122	NI	0	0	0.08	0.03	4.2	0	36

NI = not indicated.

[27]Macadamia nuts without salt contain 9 mg sodium per cup or 2 mg per oz.

[28]Mixed nuts without salt contain 3 mg sodium per oz.

[29]Peanuts without salt contain 22 mg sodium per cup or 4 mg per oz.

Foods, Approximate Measures, Units, and Weight (weight of edible portion only)		Grams	Water (g)	Food Energy (Calories)	Protein (g)	Fat (g)	Fatty Acids Saturated (g)	Fatty Acids Monounsaturated (g)	Fatty Acids Polyunsaturated (g)
Legumes, Nuts, and Seeds (*cont.*)									
Peanut butter	1 tbsp	16	1	95	5	8	1.4	4.0	2.5
Peas, split, dry, cooked	1 c	200	70	230	16	1	0.1	0.1	0.3
Pecans, halves	1 c	108	5	720	8	73	5.9	45.5	18.1
	1 oz	28	5	190	2	19	1.5	12.0	4.7
Pine nuts (pinyons), shelled	1 oz	28	6	160	3	17	2.7	6.5	7.3
Pistachio nuts, dried, shelled	1 oz	28	4	165	6	14	1.7	9.3	2.1
Pumpkin and squash kernels, dry, hulled	1 oz	28	7	155	7	13	2.5	4.0	5.9
Refried beans, canned	1 c	290	72	295	18	3	0.4	0.6	1.4
Sesame seeds, dry, hulled	1 tbsp	8	5	45	2	4	0.6	1.7	1.9
Soybeans, dry, cooked, drained	1 c	180	71	235	20	10	1.3	1.9	5.3
Soy products									
Miso	1 c	276	53	470	29	13	1.8	2.6	7.3
Tofu, piece 2½ by 2¾ by 1 in	1 piece	120	85	85	9	5	0.7	1.0	2.9
Sunflower seeds, dry, hulled	1 oz	28	5	160	6	14	1.5	2.7	9.3
Tahini	1 tbsp	15	3	90	3	8	1.1	3.0	3.5
Walnuts									
Black, chopped	1 c	125	4	760	30	71	4.5	15.9	46.9
	1 oz	28	4	170	7	16	1.0	3.6	10.6
English or Persian, pieces or chips	1 c	120	4	770	17	74	6.7	17.0	47.0
	1 oz	28	4	180	4	18	1.6	4.0	11.1
Meat and Meat Products									
Beef, cooked[30]									
Cuts braised, simmered, or pot roasted									
Relatively fat, such as chuck blade									
Lean and fat, piece, 2½ by 2½ by ¾ in	3 oz	85	43	325	22	26	10.8	11.7	0.9
Lean only	2.2 oz	62	53	170	19	9	3.9	4.2	0.3
Relatively lean, such as bottom round									
Lean and fat, piece, 4⅛ by 2¼ by ½ in	3 oz	85	54	220	25	13	4.8	5.7	0.5
Lean only	2.8 oz	78	57	175	25	8	2.7	3.4	0.3
Ground beef, broiled, patty, 3 by ⅝ in									
Lean	3 oz	85	56	230	21	16	6.2	6.9	0.6
Regular	3 oz	85	54	245	20	18	6.9	7.7	0.7
Heart, lean, braised	3 oz	85	65	150	24	5	1.2	0.8	1.6
Liver, fried slice, 6½ by 2⅜ by ⅜ in[31]	3 oz	85	56	185	23	7	2.5	3.6	1.3
Roast, oven cooked, no liquid added									
Relatively fat, such as rib									
Lean and fat, 2 pieces, 4⅛ by 2¼ by ¼ in	3 oz	85	46	315	19	26	10.8	11.4	0.9
Lean only	2.2 oz	61	57	150	17	9	3.6	3.7	0.3

tr = nutrient present in trace amounts; [30]Outer layer of fat was removed to within approximately ½ in of the lean. Deposits of fat within the cut were not removed.

NUTRIENTS IN INDICATED QUANTITY

Cholesterol (mg)	Carbohydrate (g)	Calcium (mg)	Phosphorus (mg)	Iron (mg)	Potassium (mg)	Sodium (mg)	Zn (mg)	Vitamin A Value IU	Vitamin A Value RE	Thiamin (mg)	Riboflavin (mg)	Niacin (mg)	Ascorbic acid (mg)	Folic acid (μg)
0	3	5	60	0.3	110	75	.40	0	0	0.02	0.02	2.2	0	12
0	42	22	178	3.4	592	26	1.96	80	8	0.30	0.18	1.8	0	127
0	20	39	314	2.3	423	1	6.51	140	14	0.92	0.14	1.0	2	47
0	5	10	83	0.6	111	tr	NI	40	4	0.24	0.04	0.3	1	11
0	5	2	10	0.9	178	20	1.22	10	1	0.35	0.06	1.2	1	19
0	7	38	143	1.9	310	2	.38	70	7	0.23	0.05	0.3	tr	16
0	5	12	333	4.2	229	5	2.11	110	11	0.06	0.09	0.5	tr	16
0	51	141	245	5.1	1,141	1,228	2.96	0	0	0.14	0.16	1.4	17	150
0	1	11	62	0.6	33	3	.82	10	1	0.06	0.01	0.4	0	88
0	19	131	322	4.9	972	4	5.4	50	5	0.38	0.16	1.1	0	93
0	65	188	853	4.7	922	8,142	9.16	110	11	0.17	0.28	0.8	0	91
0	3	108	151	2.3	50	8	.83	0	0	0.07	0.04	0.1	0	16
0	5	33	200	1.9	195	1	1.42	10	1	0.65	0.07	1.3	tr	43
0	3	21	119	0.7	69	5	1.46	10	1	0.24	0.02	0.8	1	15
0	15	73	580	3.8	655	1	4.28	370	37	0.27	0.14	0.9	tr	83
0	3	16	132	0.9	149	tr	.97	80	8	0.06	0.03	0.2	tr	19
0	22	113	380	2.9	602	12	3.28	150	15	0.46	0.18	1.3	4	79
0	5	27	90	0.7	142	3	.77	40	4	0.11	0.04	0.3	1	19
87	0	11	163	2.5	163	53	6.66	tr	tr	0.06	0.19	2.0	0	5
66	0	8	146	2.3	163	44	NI	tr	tr	0.05	0.17	1.7	0	4
81	0	5	217	2.8	248	43	3.51	tr	tr	0.06	0.21	3.3	0	8
75	0	4	212	2.7	240	40	NI	tr	tr	0.06	0.20	3.3	0	9
74	0	9	134	1.8	256	65	4.44	tr	tr	0.04	0.18	4.4	0	7.7
76	0	9	144	2.1	248	70	4.29	tr	tr	0.03	0.16	4.9	0	7.7
164	0	5	213	6.4	198	54	2.66	tr	tr	0.12	1.31	3.4	5	NI
410	7	9	392	5.3	309	90	4.63	[32]30,690	[32]9,120	0.18	3.52	12.3	23	187
72	0	8	145	2.0	246	54	NI	tr	tr	0.06	0.16	3.1	0	6
49	0	5	127	1.7	218	45	NI	tr	tr	0.05	0.13	2.7	0	7

NI = not indicated; [31]Fried in vegetable shortening; [32]Value varies widely.

Foods, Approximate Measures, Units, and Weight (weight of edible portion only)		Grams	Water (g)	Food Energy (Calories)	Protein (g)	Fat (g)	Fatty Acids		
							Saturated (g)	Monounsaturated (g)	Polyunsaturated (g)
Meat and Meat Products (*cont.*)									
Beef, cooked (*cont.*)									
Relatively lean, such as eye of round									
Lean and fat, 2 pieces, 2½ by 2½ by ⅜ in	3 oz	85	57	205	23	12	4.9	5.4	0.5
Lean only	2.6 oz	75	63	135	22	5	1.9	2.1	0.2
Steak									
Sirloin, broiled									
Lean and fat, piece, 2½ by 2½ by ¾ in	3 oz	85	53	240	23	15	6.4	6.9	0.6
Lean only from item 587	2.5 oz	72	59	150	22	6	2.6	2.8	0.3
Beef, canned, corned	3 oz	85	59	185	22	10	4.2	4.9	0.4
Beef, dried, chipped	2.5 oz	72	48	145	24	4	1.8	2.0	0.2
Lamb, cooked									
Chops (3 per lb w/bone)									
Arm, braised									
Lean and fat	2.2 oz	63	44	220	20	15	6.9	6.0	0.9
Lean only	1.7 oz	48	49	135	17	7	2.9	2.6	0.4
Loin, broiled									
Lean and fat	2.8 oz	80	54	235	22	16	7.3	6.4	1.0
Lean only	2.3 oz	64	61	140	19	6	2.6	2.4	0.4
Leg, roasted									
Lean and fat, 2 pieces, 4⅛ by 2¼ by ¼ in	3 oz	85	59	205	22	13	5.6	4.9	0.8
Lean only	2.6 oz	73	64	140	20	6	2.4	2.2	0.4
Rib, roasted									
Lean and fat, 3 pieces, 2½ by 2½ by ¼ in	3 oz	85	47	315	18	26	12.1	10.6	1.5
Lean only	2 oz	57	60	130	15	7	3.2	3.0	0.5
Pork, cured, cooked									
Bacon									
Regular	3 medium slices	19	13	110	6	9	3.3	4.5	1.1
Canadian-style	2 slices	46	62	85	11	4	1.3	1.9	0.4
Ham, light cure, roasted									
Lean and fat, 2 pieces, 4⅛ by 2¼ by ¼ in	3 oz	85	58	205	18	14	5.1	6.7	1.5
Lean only	2.4 oz	68	66	105	17	4	1.3	1.7	0.4
Ham, canned, roasted, 2 pieces, 4⅛ by 2¼ by ¼ in	3 oz	85	67	140	18	7	2.4	3.5	0.8
Luncheon meat									
Canned, spiced or unspiced, slice, 3 by 2 by ½ in	2 slices	42	52	140	5	13	4.5	6.0	1.5
Chopped ham (8 slices per 6-oz pkg)	2 slices	42	64	95	7	7	2.4	3.4	0.9
Cooked ham (8 slices per 8-oz pkg)									
Regular	2 slices	57	65	105	10	6	1.9	2.8	0.7
Extra lean	2 slices	57	71	75	11	3	0.9	1.3	0.3

tr = nutrient present in trace amounts.

NUTRIENTS IN INDICATED QUANTITY

Cholesterol (mg)	Carbohydrate (g)	Calcium (mg)	Phosphorus (mg)	Iron (mg)	Potassium (mg)	Sodium (mg)	Zn (mg)	Vitamin A Value IU	Vitamin A Value RE	Thiamin (mg)	Riboflavin (mg)	Niacin (mg)	Ascorbic acid (mg)	Folic acid (μg)
62	0	5	177	1.6	308	50	NI	tr	tr	0.07	0.14	3.0	0	7
52	0	3	170	1.5	297	46	NI	tr	tr	0.07	0.13	2.8	0	7
77	0	9	186	2.6	306	53	3.91	tr	tr	0.10	0.23	3.3	0	6
64	0	8	176	2.4	290	48	4.44	tr	tr	0.09	0.22	3.1	0	7
80	0	17	90	3.7	51	802	3.03	tr	tr	0.02	0.20	2.9	0	5
46	0	14	287	2.3	142	3,053	2.75	tr	tr	0.05	0.23	2.7	0	6
77	0	16	132	1.5	195	46	4.28	tr	tr	0.04	0.16	4.4	0	13
59	0	12	111	1.3	162	36	3.98	tr	tr	0.03	0.13	3.0	0	12
78	0	16	162	1.4	272	62	2.22	tr	tr	0.09	0.21	5.5	0	12
60	0	12	145	1.3	241	54	1.91	tr	tr	0.08	0.18	4.4	0	11
78	0	8	162	1.7	273	57	3.74	tr	tr	0.09	0.24	5.5	0	17
65	0	6	150	1.5	247	50	4.20	tr	tr	0.08	0.20	4.6	0	20
77	0	19	139	1.4	224	60	2.96	tr	tr	0.08	0.18	5.5	0	15
50	0	12	111	1.0	179	46	3.80	tr	tr	0.05	0.13	3.5	0	22
16	tr	2	64	0.3	92	303	.62	0	0	0.13	0.05	1.4	6	1
27	1	5	136	0.4	179	711	.79	0	0	0.38	0.09	3.2	10	2
53	0	6	182	0.7	243	1,009	1.97	0	0	0.51	0.19	3.8	0	4
37	0	5	154	0.6	215	902	2.19	0	0	0.46	0.17	3.4	0	6
35	tr	6	188	0.9	298	908	1.97	0	0	0.82	0.21	4.3	[33]19	4
26	1	3	34	0.3	90	541	.62	0	0	0.15	0.08	1.3	tr	NI
21	0	3	65	0.3	134	576	.77	0	0	0.27	0.09	1.6	[33]8	NI
32	2	4	141	0.6	189	751	1.21	0	0	0.49	0.14	3.0	[33]16	0
27	1	4	124	0.4	200	815	1.09	0	0	0.53	0.13	2.8	[33]15	0

NI = not indicated; [33]Contains added sodium ascorbate. If sodium ascorbate is not added, ascorbic acid content is negligible.

APPENDIX 41 NUTRITIVE VALUE OF THE EDIBLE PART OF FOOD *(continued)*

Foods, Approximate Measures, Units, and Weight (weight of edible portion only)		Grams	Water (g)	Food Energy (Calories)	Protein (g)	Fat (g)	Fatty Acids		
							Saturated (g)	Monounsaturated (g)	Polyunsaturated (g)
Meat and Meat Products (*cont.*)									
Pork, fresh, cooked									
Chop, loin (cut 3 per lb with bone)									
Broiled									
Lean and fat	3.1 oz	87	50	275	24	19	7.0	8.8	2.2
Lean only	2.5 oz	72	57	165	23	8	2.6	3.4	0.9
Pan fried									
Lean and fat	3.1 oz	89	45	335	21	27	9.8	12.5	3.1
Lean only	2.4 oz	67	54	180	19	11	3.7	4.8	1.3
Ham (leg), roasted									
Lean and fat, piece, 2½ by 2½ by ¾ in	3 oz	85	53	250	21	18	6.4	8.1	2.0
Lean only	2.5 oz	72	60	160	20	8	2.7	3.6	1.0
Rib, roasted									
Lean and fat, piece, 2½ by ¾ in	3 oz	85	51	270	21	20	7.2	9.2	2.3
Lean only	2.5 oz	71	57	175	20	10	3.4	4.4	1.2
Shoulder cut, braised									
Lean and fat, 3 pieces, 2½ by 2½ by ¼ in	3 oz	85	47	295	23	22	7.9	10.0	2.4
Lean only	2.4 oz	67	54	165	22	8	2.8	3.7	1.0
Sausages (See also Luncheon meats)									
Bologna, slice (8 per 8-oz pkg)	2 slices	57	54	180	7	16	6.1	7.6	1.4
Braunschweiger, slice (6 per 6-oz pkg)	2 slices	57	48	205	8	18	6.2	8.5	2.1
Brown and serve (10–11 per 8-oz pkg), browned	1 link	13	45	50	2	5	1.7	2.2	0.5
Frankfurter (10 per 1-lb pkg), cooked (reheated)	1 frankfurter	45	54	145	5	13	4.8	6.2	1.2
Pork link (16 per 1-lb pkg), cooked[34]	1 link	13	45	50	3	4	1.4	1.8	0.5
Salami									
Cooked type, slice (8 per 8-oz pkg)	2 slices	57	60	145	8	11	4.6	5.2	1.2
Dry type, slice (12 per 4-oz pkg)	2 slices	20	35	85	5	7	2.4	3.4	0.6
Sandwich spread (pork, beef)	1 tbsp	15	60	35	1	3	0.9	1.1	0.4
Vienna sausage (7 per 4-oz can)	1 sausage	16	60	45	2	4	1.5	2.0	0.3
Veal, medium fat, cooked, bone removed									
Cutlet, 4⅛ by 2¼ by ½ in, braised or broiled	3 oz	85	60	185	23	9	4.1	4.1	0.6
Rib, 2 pieces, 4⅛ by 2¼ by ¼ in, roasted	3 oz	85	55	230	23	14	6.0	6.0	1.0

tr = nutrient present in trace amounts.

[33]Contains added sodium ascorbate. If sodium ascorbate is not added, ascorbic acid content is negligible.

NUTRIENTS IN INDICATED QUANTITY

Cholesterol (mg)	Carbohydrate (g)	Calcium (mg)	Phosphorus (mg)	Iron (mg)	Potassium (mg)	Sodium (mg)	Zn (mg)	Vitamin A Value IU	Vitamin A Value RE	Thiamin (mg)	Riboflavin (mg)	Niacin (mg)	Ascorbic acid (mg)	Folic acid (μg)
84	0	3	184	0.7	312	61	1.68	10	3	0.87	0.24	4.3	tr	4
71	0	4	176	0.7	302	56	1.61	10	1	0.83	0.22	4.0	tr	4
92	0	4	190	0.7	323	64	1.74	10	3	0.91	0.24	4.6	tr	4
72	0	3	178	0.7	305	57	1.61	10	1	0.84	0.22	4.0	tr	4
79	0	5	210	0.9	280	50	2.43	10	2	0.54	0.27	3.9	tr	10
68	0	5	202	0.8	269	46	2.77	10	1	0.50	0.25	3.6	tr	12
69	0	9	190	0.8	313	37	1.55	10	3	0.50	0.24	4.2	tr	6
56	0	8	182	0.7	300	33	1.47	10	2	0.45	0.22	3.8	tr	6
93	0	6	162	1.4	286	75	3.43	10	3	0.46	0.26	4.4	tr	5
76	0	5	151	1.3	271	68	3.33	10	1	0.40	0.24	4.0	tr	5
31	2	7	52	0.9	103	581	.92	0	0	0.10	0.08	1.5	[33]12	2
89	2	5	96	5.3	113	652	1.20	8,010	2,405	0.14	0.87	4.8	[33]6	16
9	tr	1	14	0.1	25	105	NI	0	0	0.05	0.02	0.4	0	NI
23	1	5	39	0.5	75	504	1.21	0	0	0.09	0.05	1.2	[33]12	2
11	tr	4	24	0.2	47	168	.33	0	0	0.10	0.03	0.6	tr	NI
37	1	7	66	1.5	113	607	.98	0	0	0.14	0.21	2.0	[33]7	0
16	1	2	28	0.3	76	372	1.28	0	0	0.12	0.06	1.0	[33]5	0
6	2	2	9	0.1	17	152	NI	10	1	0.03	0.02	0.3	0	NI
8	tr	2	8	0.1	16	152	.26	0	0	0.01	0.02	0.3	0	1
109	0	9	196	0.8	258	56	4.33	tr	tr	0.06	0.21	4.6	0	13
109	0	10	211	0.7	259	57	3.81	tr	tr	0.11	0.26	6.6	0	12

NI = not indicated.
[34]One patty (8 per pound) of bulk sausage is equivalent to 2 links.

Foods, Approximate Measures, Units, and Weight (weight of edible portion only)		Grams	Water (g)	Food Energy (Calories)	Protein (g)	Fat (g)	Fatty Acids		
							Saturated (g)	Monounsaturated (g)	Polyunsaturated (g)
Poultry and Poultry Products									
Chicken									
Fried, flesh, with skin[35]									
Batter dipped									
Breast, ½ breast (5.6 oz with bones)	4.9 oz	140	52	365	35	18	4.9	7.6	4.3
Drumstick (3.4 oz with bones)	2.5 oz	72	53	195	16	11	3.0	4.6	2.7
Flour coated									
Breast, ½ breast (4.2 oz with bones)	3.5 oz	98	57	220	31	9	2.4	3.4	1.9
Drumstick (2.6 oz with bones)	1.7 oz	49	57	120	13	7	1.8	2.7	1.6
Roasted, flesh only									
Breast, ½ breast (4.2 oz with bones and skin)	3.0 oz	86	65	140	27	3	0.9	1.1	0.7
Drumstick (2.9 oz with bones and skin)	1.6 oz	44	67	75	12	2	0.7	0.8	0.6
Stewed, flesh only, light and dark meat, chopped or diced	1 c	140	67	250	38	9	2.6	3.3	2.2
Chicken liver, cooked	1 liver	20	68	30	5	1	0.4	0.3	0.2
Duck, roasted, flesh only	½ duck	221	46	445	52	25	9.2	8.2	3.2
Turkey, roasted, flesh only									
Dark meat, piece, 2½ by 1⅝ by ¼ in	4 pieces	85	63	160	24	6	2.1	1.4	1.8
Light meat, piece, 4 by 2 by ¼ in	2 pieces	85	66	135	25	3	0.9	0.5	0.7
Light and dark meat									
Chopped or diced	1 c	140	65	240	41	7	2.3	1.4	2.0
Pieces (1 slice white meat, 4 by 2 by ¼ in and 2 slices dark meat, 2½ by 1⅝ by ¼ in)	3 pieces	85	65	145	25	4	1.4	0.9	1.2
Poultry food products									
Chicken									
Canned, boneless	5 oz	142	69	235	31	11	3.1	4.5	2.5
Frankfurter (10 per 1-lb pkg)	1 frankfurter	45	58	115	6	9	2.5	3.8	1.8
Roll, light (6 slices per 6 oz pkg)	2 slices	57	69	90	11	4	1.1	1.7	0.9
Turkey									
Gravy and turkey, frozen	5-oz package	142	85	95	8	4	1.2	1.4	0.7
Ham, cured turkey thigh meat (8 slices per 8-oz pkg)	2 slices	57	71	75	11	3	1.0	0.7	0.9
Loaf, breast meat (8 slices per 6-oz pkg)	2 slices	42	72	45	10	1	0.2	0.2	0.1
Patties, breaded, battered, fried (2.25 oz)	1 patty	64	50	180	9	12	3.0	4.8	3.0
Roast, boneless, frozen, seasoned, light and dark meat, cooked	3 oz	85	68	130	18	5	1.6	1.0	1.4

tr = nutrient present in trace amounts; [35]Fried in vegetable shortening; [36]If sodium ascorbate is used, product contains 11 mg ascorbic acid.

NUTRIENTS IN INDICATED QUANTITY

Cholesterol (mg)	Carbohydrate (g)	Calcium (mg)	Phosphorus (mg)	Iron (mg)	Potassium (mg)	Sodium (mg)	Zn (mg)	Vitamin A Value		Thiamin (mg)	Riboflavin (mg)	Niacin (mg)	Ascorbic acid (mg)	Folic acid (μg)
								IU	RE					
119	13	28	259	1.8	281	385	1.33	90	28	0.16	0.20	14.7	0	8
62	6	12	106	1.0	134	194	1.42	60	19	0.08	0.15	3.7	0	6
87	2	16	228	1.2	254	74	1.67	50	15	0.08	0.13	13.5	0	4
44	1	6	86	0.7	112	44	1.42	40	12	0.04	0.11	3.0	0	4
73	0	13	196	0.9	220	64	1.00	20	5	0.06	0.10	11.8	0	3
41	0	5	81	0.6	108	42	1.49	30	8	0.03	0.10	2.7	0	4
116	0	20	210	1.6	252	98	2.79	70	21	0.07	0.23	8.6	0	8
126	tr	3	62	1.7	28	10	.87	3,270	983	0.03	0.35	0.9	3	154
197	0	27	449	6.0	557	144	2.21	170	51	0.57	1.04	11.3	0	10
72	0	27	173	2.0	246	67	3.80	0	0	0.05	0.21	3.1	0	8
59	0	16	186	1.1	259	54	1.73	0	0	0.05	0.11	5.8	0	5
106	0	35	298	2.5	417	98	4.34	0	0	0.09	0.25	7.6	0	6
65	0	21	181	1.5	253	60	NI	0	0	0.05	0.15	4.6	0	NI
88	0	20	158	2.2	196	714	2.13	170	48	0.02	0.18	9.0	3	4
45	3	43	48	0.9	38	616	1.00	60	17	0.03	0.05	1.4	0	2
28	1	24	89	0.6	129	331	NI	50	14	0.04	0.07	3.0	0	NI
26	7	20	115	1.3	87	787	.99	60	18	0.03	0.18	2.6	0	NI
32	tr	6	108	1.6	184	565	NI	0	0	0.03	0.14	2.0	0	NI
17	0	3	97	0.2	118	608	NI	0	0	0.02	0.05	3.5	[36]0	NI
40	10	9	173	1.4	176	512	1.35	20	7	0.06	0.12	1.5	0	8
45	3	4	207	1.4	253	578	4.34	0	0	0.04	0.14	5.3	0	NI

NI = not indicated.

APPENDIX 41 NUTRITIVE VALUE OF THE EDIBLE PART OF FOOD *(continued)*

Foods, Approximate Measures, Units, and Weight (weight of edible portion only)		Grams	Water (g)	Food Energy (Calories)	Protein (g)	Fat (g)	Fatty Acids: Saturated (g)	Fatty Acids: Monounsaturated (g)	Fatty Acids: Polyunsaturated (g)
Sugars and Sweets									
Sugars									
Brown, pressed down	1 c	220	2	820	0	0	0.0	0.0	0.0
White									
Granulated	1 c	200	1	770	0	0	0.0	0.0	0.0
	1 tbsp	12	1	45	0	0	0.0	0.0	0.0
	1 packet	6	1	25	0	0	0.0	0.0	0.0
Powdered, sifted, spooned into cup	1 c	100	1	385	0	0	0.0	0.0	0.0
Syrups									
Chocolate-flavored syrup or topping									
Thin type	2 tbsp	38	37	85	1	tr	0.2	0.1	0.1
Fudge type	2 tbsp	38	25	125	2	5	3.1	1.7	0.2
Molasses, cane, blackstrap	2 tbsp	40	24	85	0	0	0.0	0.0	0.0
Table syrup (corn and maple)	2 tbsp	42	25	122	0	0	0.0	0.0	0.0
Vegetables and Vegetable Products									
Alfalfa seeds, sprouted, raw	1 c	33	91	10	1	tr	tr	tr	0.1
Artichokes, globe or French, cooked, drained	1 artichoke	120	87	55	3	tr	tr	tr	0.1
Asparagus, green									
Cooked, drained									
From raw									
Cuts and tips	1 c	180	92	45	5	1	0.1	tr	0.2
Spears, ½-in diam. at base	4 spears	60	92	15	2	tr	tr	tr	0.1
From frozen									
Cuts and tips	1 c	180	91	50	5	1	0.2	tr	0.3
Spears, ½-in diam. at base	4 spears	60	91	15	2	tr	0.1	tr	0.1
Canned, spears, ½-in diam. at base	4 spears	80	95	10	1	tr	tr	tr	0.1
Bamboo shoots, canned, drained	1 c	131	94	25	2	1	0.1	tr	0.2
Beans									
Lima, immature seeds, frozen, cooked, drained									
Thick-seeded types (Ford-hooks)	1 c	170	74	170	10	1	0.1	tr	0.3
Thin-seeded types (baby limas)	1 c	180	72	190	12	1	0.1	tr	0.3
Snap									
Cooked, drained									
From raw (cut and French style)	1 c	125	89	45	2	tr	0.1	tr	0.2
From frozen (cut)	1 c	135	92	35	2	tr	tr	tr	0.1
Canned, drained solids (cut)	1 c	135	93	25	2	tr	tr	tr	0.1

tr = nutrient present in trace amounts.
[37]For regular pack; special dietary pack contains 3 mg sodium.
[38]For green varieties; yellow varieties contain 101 IU or 10 RE.

NUTRIENTS IN INDICATED QUANTITY

Cholesterol (mg)	Carbohydrate (g)	Calcium (mg)	Phosphorus (mg)	Iron (mg)	Potassium (mg)	Sodium (mg)	Zn (mg)	Vitamin A Value		Thiamin (mg)	Riboflavin (mg)	Niacin (mg)	Ascorbic acid (mg)	Folic acid (μg)
								IU	RE					
0	212	187	56	4.8	757	97	.40	0	0	0.02	0.07	0.2	0	2
0	199	3	tr	0.1	7	5	.06	0	0	0.00	0.00	0.0	0	0
0	12	tr	tr	tr	tr	tr	.00	0	0	0.00	0.00	0.0	0	0
0	6	tr	tr	tr	tr	tr	.00	0	0	0.00	0.00	0.0	0	0
0	100	1	tr	tr	4	2	.04	0	0	0.00	0.00	0.0	0	0
0	22	6	49	0.8	85	36	.28	tr	tr	tr	0.02	0.1	0	2
0	21	38	60	0.5	82	42	NI	40	13	0.02	0.08	0.1	0	NI
0	22	274	34	10.1	1,171	38	.12	0	0	0.04	0.08	0.8	0	6
0	32	1	4	tr	7	19	1.66	0	0	0.00	0.00	0.0	0	0
0	1	11	23	0.3	26	2	.30	50	5	0.03	0.04	.02	3	12
0	12	47	72	1.6	316	79	.59	170	17	0.07	0.06	0.7	9	61
0	8	43	110	1.2	558	7	.86	1,490	149	0.18	0.22	1.9	49	176
0	3	14	37	0.4	186	2	NI	500	50	0.06	0.07	0.6	16	NI
0	9	41	99	1.2	392	7	1.01	1,470	147	0.12	0.19	1.9	44	176
0	3	14	33	0.4	131	2	NI	490	49	0.04	0.06	0.6	15	NI
0	2	11	30	0.5	122	[37]278	.48	380	38	0.04	0.07	0.7	13	104
0	4	10	33	0.4	105	9	.30	10	1	0.03	0.03	0.2	1	40
0	32	37	107	2.3	694	90	.74	320	32	0.13	0.10	1.8	22	18
0	35	50	202	3.5	740	52	1.00	300	30	0.13	0.10	1.4	10	14
0	10	58	49	1.6	374	4	.45	[38]830	[38]83	0.09	0.12	0.8	12	42
0	8	61	32	1.1	151	18	.84	[39]710	[39]71	0.06	0.10	0.6	11	42
0	6	35	26	1.2	147	[40]339	.39	[41]470	[41]47	0.02	0.08	0.3	6	43

NI = not indicated.
[39]For green varieties; yellow varieties contain 151 IU or 15 RE.
[40]For regular pack; special dietary pack contains 3 mg sodium.
[41]For green varieties; yellow varieties contain 142 IU or 14 RE.

APPENDIX 41 NUTRITIVE VALUE OF THE EDIBLE PART OF FOOD *(continued)*

Foods, Approximate Measures, Units, and Weight (weight of edible portion only)		Grams	Water (g)	Food Energy (Calories)	Protein (g)	Fat (g)	Fatty Acids: Saturated (g)	Fatty Acids: Monounsaturated (g)	Fatty Acids: Polyunsaturated (g)
Vegetables and Vegetable Products (*cont.*)									
Beans, mature. See Beans, dry and Black-eyed peas, dry									
Bean sprouts (mung)									
Raw	1 c	104	90	30	3	tr	tr	tr	0.1
Cooked, drained	1 c	124	93	25	3	tr	tr	tr	tr
Beets									
Cooked, drained									
Diced or sliced	1 c	170	91	55	2	tr	tr	tr	tr
Whole beets, 2-in diam.	2 beets	100	91	30	1	tr	tr	tr	tr
Canned, drained solids, diced or sliced	1 c	170	91	55	2	tr	tr	tr	0.1
Beet greens, leaves and stems, cooked, drained	1 c	144	89	40	4	tr	tr	0.1	0.1
Black-eyed peas, immature seeds, cooked and drained									
From raw	1 c	165	72	180	13	1	0.3	0.1	0.6
From frozen	1 c	170	66	225	14	1	0.3	0.1	0.5
Broccoli									
Raw	1 spear	151	91	40	4	1	0.1	tr	0.3
Cooked, drained									
From raw									
Spear, medium	1 spear	180	90	50	5	1	0.1	tr	0.2
Spears, cut into ½-in pieces	1 c	155	90	45	5	tr	0.1	tr	0.2
From frozen									
Piece, 4½ to 5 in long	1 piece	30	91	10	1	tr	tr	tr	tr
Chopped	1 c	185	91	50	6	tr	tr	tr	0.1
Brussels sprouts, cooked, drained									
From raw, 7–8 sprouts, 1¼- to 1½-in diam.	1 c	155	87	60	4	1	0.2	0.1	0.4
From frozen	1 c	155	87	65	6	1	0.1	tr	0.3
Cabbage, common varieties									
Raw, coarsely shredded or sliced	1 c	70	93	15	1	tr	tr	tr	0.1
Cooked, drained	1 c	150	94	30	1	tr	tr	tr	0.2
Cabbage, Chinese									
Pak-choi, cooked, drained	1 c	170	96	20	3	tr	tr	tr	0.1
Pe-tsai, raw, 1-in pieces	1 c	76	94	10	1	tr	tr	tr	0.1
Cabbage, red, raw, coarsely shredded or sliced	1 c	70	92	20	1	tr	tr	tr	0.1
Cabbage, savoy, raw, coarsely shredded or sliced	1 c	70	91	20	1	tr	tr	tr	tr
Carrots									
Raw, without crowns and tips, scraped									
Whole, 7½ by 1⅛ in, or strips, 2½ to 3 in long	1 carrot or 18 strips	72	88	30	1	tr	tr	tr	0.1
Grated	1 c	110	88	45	1	tr	tr	tr	0.1
Cooked, sliced, drained									
From raw	1 c	156	87	70	2	tr	0.1	tr	0.1
From frozen	1 c	146	90	55	2	tr	0.1	tr	0.1
Canned, sliced, drained solids	1 c	146	93	35	1	tr	0.1	tr	0.1

tr = nutrient present in trace amounts; [42]For regular pack; special dietary pack contains 78 mg sodium.

NUTRIENTS IN INDICATED QUANTITY

Cholesterol (mg)	Carbohydrate (g)	Calcium (mg)	Phosphorus (mg)	Iron (mg)	Potassium (mg)	Sodium (mg)	Zn (mg)	Vitamin A Value IU	Vitamin A Value RE	Thiamin (mg)	Riboflavin (mg)	Niacin (mg)	Ascorbic acid (mg)	Folic acid (μg)
0	6	14	56	0.9	155	6	.43	20	2	0.09	0.13	0.8	14	63
0	5	15	35	0.8	125	12	.58	20	2	0.06	0.13	1.0	14	35
0	11	19	53	1.1	530	83	.36	20	2	0.05	0.02	0.5	9	44
0	7	11	31	0.6	312	49	.25	10	1	0.03	0.01	0.3	6	86
0	12	26	29	3.1	252	[42]466	.28	20	2	0.02	0.07	0.3	7	NI
0	8	164	59	2.7	1,309	347	.72	7,340	734	0.17	0.42	0.7	36	47
0	30	46	196	2.4	693	7	1.7	1,050	105	0.11	0.18	1.8	3	210
0	40	39	207	3.6	638	9	2.4	130	13	0.44	0.11	1.2	4	120
0	8	72	100	1.3	491	41	NI	2,330	233	0.10	0.18	1.0	141	NI
0	10	205	86	2.1	293	20	NI	2,540	254	0.15	0.37	1.4	113	NI
0	9	177	74	1.8	253	17	.59	2,180	218	0.13	0.32	1.2	97	78
0	2	15	17	0.2	54	7	NI	570	57	0.02	0.02	0.1	12	NI
0	10	94	102	1.1	333	44	.56	3,500	350	1.10	0.15	0.8	74	55
0	13	56	87	1.9	491	33	.50	1,110	111	0.17	0.12	0.9	96	94
0	13	37	84	1.1	504	36	.55	910	91	0.16	0.18	0.8	71	157
0	4	33	16	0.4	172	13	.12	90	9	0.04	0.02	0.2	33	40
0	7	50	38	0.6	308	29	.24	130	13	0.09	0.08	0.3	36	31
0	3	158	49	1.8	631	58	.28	4,370	437	0.05	0.11	0.7	44	35
0	2	59	22	0.2	181	7	.17	910	91	0.03	0.04	0.3	21	60
0	4	36	29	0.3	144	8	.15	30	3	0.04	0.02	0.2	40	19
0	4	25	29	0.3	161	20	.26	700	70	0.05	0.02	0.2	22	32
0	7	19	32	0.4	233	25	.14	20,250	2,025	0.07	0.04	0.7	7	10
0	11	30	48	0.6	355	39	NI	30,940	3,094	0.11	0.06	1.0	10	16
0	16	48	47	1.0	354	103	.47	38,300	3,830	0.05	0.09	0.8	4	22
0	12	41	38	0.7	231	86	.35	25,850	2,585	0.04	0.05	0.6	4	16
0	8	37	35	0.9	261	[43]352	.38	20,110	2,011	0.03	0.04	0.8	4	14

NI = not indicated; [43]For regular pack; special dietary pack contains 61 mg sodium.

Foods, Approximate Measures, Units, and Weight (weight of edible portion only)		Grams	Water (g)	Food Energy (Calories)	Protein (g)	Fat (g)	Fatty Acids: Saturated (g)	Fatty Acids: Monounsaturated (g)	Fatty Acids: Polyunsaturated (g)
Vegetables and Vegetable Products (*cont.*)									
Cauliflower									
Raw (flowerets)	1 c	100	92	25	2	tr	tr	tr	0.1
Cooked, drained									
From raw (flowerets)	1 c	125	93	30	2	tr	tr	tr	0.1
From frozen (flowerets)	1 c	180	94	35	3	tr	0.1	tr	0.2
Celery, pascal type, raw									
Stalk, large outer, 8 by 1½ in (at root end)	1 stalk	40	95	5	tr	tr	tr	tr	tr
Pieces, diced	1 c	120	95	20	1	tr	tr	tr	0.1
Collards, cooked, drained									
From raw (leaves without stems)	1 c	190	96	25	2	tr	0.1	tr	0.2
From frozen (chopped)	1 c	170	88	60	5	1	0.1	0.1	0.4
Corn, sweet									
Cooked, drained									
From raw, ear 5 by 1¾ in	1 ear	77	70	85	3	1	0.2	0.3	0.5
From frozen									
Ear, trimmed to about 3½ in long	1 ear	63	73	60	2	tr	0.1	0.1	0.2
Kernels	1 c	165	76	135	5	tr	tr	tr	0.1
Canned									
Cream style	1 c	256	79	185	4	1	0.2	0.3	0.5
Whole kernel, vacuum pack	1 c	210	77	165	5	1	0.2	0.3	0.5
Cowpeas. See Black-eyed peas, immature, mature									
Cucumber, with peel, slices, ⅛ in thick (large, 2⅛-in diam.; small, 1¾-in diam.)	6 large or 8 small slices	28	96	5	tr	tr	tr	tr	tr
Dandelion greens, cooked, drained	1 c	105	90	35	2	1	0.1	tr	0.3
Eggplant, cooked, steamed	1 c	96	92	25	1	tr	tr	tr	0.1
Endive, curly (including escarole), raw, small pieces	1 c	50	94	10	1	tr	tr	tr	tr
Jerusalem artichoke, raw, sliced	1 c	150	78	115	3	tr	0.0	tr	tr
Kale, cooked, drained									
From raw, chopped	1 c	130	91	40	2	1	0.1	tr	0.3
From frozen, chopped	1 c	130	91	40	4	1	0.1	tr	0.3
Kohlrabi, thickened bulb-like stems, cooked, drained, diced	1 c	165	90	50	3	tr	tr	tr	0.1
Lettuce, raw									
Butterhead, as Boston types									
Head, 5-in diam.	1 head	163	96	20	2	tr	tr	tr	0.2
Leaves	1 outer or 2 inner leaves	15	96	tr	tr	tr	tr	tr	tr
Crisphead, as iceberg									
Head, 6-in diam.	1 head	539	96	70	5	1	0.1	tr	0.5
Wedge, ¼ of head	1 wedge	135	96	20	1	tr	tr	tr	0.1
Pieces, chopped or shredded	1 c	55	96	5	1	tr	tr	tr	0.1

tr = nutrient present in trace amounts; [44]For yellow varieties; white varieties contain only a trace of vitamin A.

NUTRIENTS IN INDICATED QUANTITY

Cholesterol (mg)	Carbohydrate (g)	Calcium (mg)	Phosphorus (mg)	Iron (mg)	Potassium (mg)	Sodium (mg)	Zn (mg)	Vitamin A Value IU	Vitamin A Value RE	Thiamin (mg)	Riboflavin (mg)	Niacin (mg)	Ascorbic acid (mg)	Folic acid (μg)
0	5	29	46	0.6	355	15	.18	20	2	0.08	0.06	0.6	72	66
0	6	34	44	0.5	404	8	.30	20	2	0.08	0.07	0.7	69	64
0	7	31	43	0.7	250	32	.23	40	4	0.07	0.10	0.6	56	74
0	1	14	10	0.2	144	35	.05	50	5	0.01	0.01	0.1	3	11
0	4	43	31	0.6	341	106	.21	150	15	0.04	0.04	0.4	8	NI
0	5	148	19	0.8	177	36	.14	4,220	422	0.03	0.08	0.4	19	8
0	12	357	46	1.9	427	85	.46	10,170	1,017	0.08	0.20	1.1	45	129
0	19	2	79	0.5	192	13	.87	[44]170	[44]17	0.17	0.06	1.2	5	49
0	14	2	47	0.4	158	3	.87	[46]130	[46]13	0.11	0.04	1.0	3	49
0	34	3	78	0.5	229	8	.79	[46]410	[46]41	0.11	0.12	2.1	4	38
0	46	8	131	1.0	343	[45]730	1.36	[46]250	[46]25	0.06	0.14	2.5	12	114
0	41	11	134	0.9	391	[46]571	.97	[46]510	[46]51	0.09	0.15	2.5	17	104
0	1	4	5	0.1	42	1	.69	10	1	0.01	0.01	0.1	1	4
0	7	147	44	1.9	244	46	.62	12,290	1,229	0.14	0.18	0.5	19	82
0	6	6	21	0.3	238	3	.24	60	6	0.07	0.02	0.6	1	23
0	2	26	14	0.4	157	11	.40	1,030	103	0.04	0.04	0.2	3	72
0	26	21	117	5.1	644	6	.18	30	3	0.03	0.09	2.0	6	15
0	7	94	36	1.2	296	30	.31	9,620	962	0.07	0.09	0.7	53	20
0	7	179	36	1.2	417	20	.23	8,260	826	0.06	0.15	0.9	33	30
0	11	41	74	0.7	561	35	.32	60	6	0.07	0.03	0.6	89	13
0	4	52	38	0.5	419	8	NI	1,580	158	0.10	0.10	0.5	13	NI
0	tr	5	3	tr	39	1	.03	150	15	0.01	0.01	tr	1	11
0	11	102	108	2.7	852	49	NI	1,780	178	0.25	0.16	1.0	21	NI
0	3	26	27	0.7	213	12	NI	450	45	0.06	0.04	0.3	5	11
0	1	10	11	0.3	87	5	.12	180	18	0.03	0.02	0.1	2	31

NI = not indicated; [45]For regular pack; special dietary pack contains 8 mg sodium; [46]For regular pack; special dietary pack contains 6 mg sodium.

APPENDIX 41 NUTRITIVE VALUE OF THE EDIBLE PART OF FOOD *(continued)*

Foods, Approximate Measures, Units, and Weight (weight of edible portion only)		Grams	Water (g)	Food Energy (Calories)	Protein (g)	Fat (g)	Fatty Acids: Saturated (g)	Fatty Acids: Monounsaturated (g)	Fatty Acids: Polyunsaturated (g)
Vegetables and Vegetable Products (*cont.*)									
Lettuce, raw (*cont.*)									
Looseleaf (bunching varieties including romaine or cos), chopped or shredded pieces	1 c	56	94	10	1	tr	tr	tr	0.1
Mushrooms									
Raw, sliced or chopped	1 c	70	92	20	1	tr	tr	tr	0.1
Cooked, drained	1 c	156	91	40	3	1	0.1	tr	0.3
Canned, drained solids	1 c	156	91	35	3	tr	0.1	tr	0.2
Mustard greens, without stems and midribs, cooked, drained	1 c	140	94	20	3	tr	tr	0.2	0.1
Okra pods, 3 by ⅝ in, cooked	8 pods	85	90	25	2	tr	tr	tr	tr
Onions									
Raw									
Chopped	1 c	160	91	55	2	tr	0.1	0.1	0.2
Sliced	1 c	115	91	40	1	tr	0.1	tr	0.1
Cooked (whole or sliced), drained	1 c	210	92	60	2	tr	0.1	tr	0.1
Onions, spring, raw, bulb (⅜-in diam.) and white portion of top	6 onions	30	92	10	1	tr	tr	tr	tr
Onion rings, breaded, pan-fried, frozen, prepared	2 rings	20	29	80	1	5	1.7	2.2	1.0
Parsley									
Raw	10 sprigs	10	88	5	tr	tr	tr	tr	tr
Freeze-dried	1 tbsp	0.4	2	tr	tr	tr	tr	tr	tr
Parsnips, cooked (diced or 2 in lengths), drained	1 c	156	78	125	2	tr	0.1	0.2	0.1
Peas, edible pod, cooked, drained	1 c	160	89	65	5	tr	0.1	tr	0.2
Peas, green									
Canned, drained solids	1 c	170	82	115	8	1	0.1	0.1	0.3
Frozen, cooked, drained	1 c	160	80	125	8	tr	0.1	tr	0.2
Peppers									
Hot chili, raw	1 pepper	45	88	20	1	tr	tr	tr	tr
Sweet (about 5 per lb, whole), stem and seeds removed									
Raw	1 pepper	74	93	20	1	tr	tr	tr	0.2
Cooked, drained	1 pepper	73	95	15	tr	tr	tr	tr	0.1
Potatoes, cooked									
Baked (about 2 per lb, raw)									
With skin	1 potato	202	71	220	5	tr	0.1	tr	0.1
Flesh only	1 potato	156	75	145	3	tr	tr	tr	0.1
Boiled (about 3 per lb, raw)									
Peeled after boiling	1 potato	136	77	120	3	tr	tr	tr	0.1
Peeled before boiling	1 potato	135	77	115	2	tr	tr	tr	0.1

tr = nutrient present in trace amounts.
[47]For regular pack; special dietary pack contains 3 mg sodium.
[48]For red peppers; green peppers contain 350 IU or 35 RE.
[49]For green peppers; red peppers contain 4,220 IU or 422 RE.

NUTRIENTS IN INDICATED QUANTITY

Cholesterol (mg)	Carbohydrate (g)	Calcium (mg)	Phosphorus (mg)	Iron (mg)	Potassium (mg)	Sodium (mg)	Zn (mg)	Vitamin A Value IU	Vitamin A Value RE	Thiamin (mg)	Riboflavin (mg)	Niacin (mg)	Ascorbic acid (mg)	Folic acid (μg)
0	2	38	14	0.8	148	5	.19	1,060	106	0.03	0.04	0.2	10	60
0	3	4	73	0.9	259	3	.60	0	0	0.07	0.31	2.9	2	14.8
0	8	9	136	2.7	555	3	.36	0	0	0.11	0.47	7.0	6	28
0	8	17	103	1.2	201	663	1.12	0	0	0.13	0.03	2.5	0	20
0	3	104	57	1.0	283	22	.30	4,240	424	0.06	0.09	0.6	35	20
0	6	54	48	0.4	274	4	.47	490	49	0.11	0.05	0.7	14	39
0	12	40	46	0.6	248	3	.30	0	0	0.10	0.02	0.2	13	30
0	8	29	33	0.4	178	2	.30	0	0	0.07	0.01	0.1	10	30
0	13	57	48	0.4	319	17	.44	0	0	0.09	0.02	0.2	12	16
0	2	18	10	0.6	77	1	.20	1,500	150	0.02	0.04	0.1	14	32
0	8	6	16	0.3	26	75	NI	50	5	0.06	0.03	0.7	tr	9
0	1	13	4	0.6	54	4	.22	520	52	0.01	0.01	0.1	9	55
0	tr	1	2	0.2	25	2	.09	250	25	tr	0.01	tr	1	NI
0	30	58	108	0.9	573	16	.40	0	0	0.13	0.08	1.1	20	91
0	11	67	88	3.2	384	6	.60	210	21	0.20	0.12	0.9	77	48
0	21	34	114	1.6	294	[47]372	.60	1,310	131	0.21	0.13	1.2	16	76
0	23	38	144	2.5	269	139	.75	1,070	107	0.45	0.16	2.4	16	94
0	4	8	21	0.5	153	3	.14	[48]4,840	[48]484	0.04	0.04	0.4	109	11
0	4	4	16	0.9	144	2	.32	[49]390	[49]39	0.06	0.04	0.4	[50]95	48
0	3	3	11	0.6	94	1	NI	[51]280	[51]28	0.04	0.03	0.3	[52]81	NI
0	51	20	115	2.7	844	16	.65	0	0	0.22	0.07	3.3	26	22
0	34	8	78	0.5	610	8	.45	0	0	0.16	0.03	2.2	20	14
0	27	7	60	0.4	515	5	.37	0	0	0.14	0.03	2.0	18	14
0	27	11	54	0.4	443	7	.41	0	0	0.13	0.03	1.8	10	12

NI = not indicated.

[50]For green peppers; red peppers contain 141 mg ascorbic acid.

[51]For green peppers; red peppers contain 2,740 IU or 274 RE.

[52]For green peppers; red peppers contain 121 mg ascorbic acid.

APPENDIX 41 NUTRITIVE VALUE OF THE EDIBLE PART OF FOOD *(continued)*

Foods, Approximate Measures, Units, and Weight (weight of edible portion only)		Grams	Water (g)	Food Energy (Calories)	Protein (g)	Fat (g)	Fatty Acids: Saturated (g)	Fatty Acids: Monounsaturated (g)	Fatty Acids: Polyunsaturated (g)
Vegetables and Vegetable Products (*cont.*)									
Potatoes, cooked (*cont.*)									
French fried, strip, 2 to 3½ in long, frozen									
Oven heated	10 strips	50	53	110	2	4	2.1	1.8	0.3
Fried in vegetable oil	10 strips	50	38	160	2	8	2.5	1.6	3.8
Potato products, prepared									
Au gratin									
From dry mix	1 c	245	79	230	6	10	6.3	2.9	0.3
From home recipe	1 c	245	74	325	12	19	11.6	5.3	0.7
Hashed brown, from frozen	1 c	156	56	340	5	18	7.0	8.0	2.1
Mashed									
From home recipe									
Milk added	1 c	210	78	160	4	1	0.7	0.3	0.1
Milk and margarine added	1 c	210	76	225	4	9	2.2	3.7	2.5
From dehydrated flakes (without milk), water, milk, butter, and salt added	1 c	210	76	235	4	12	7.2	3.3	0.5
Potato salad, made with mayonnaise	1 c	250	76	360	7	21	3.6	6.2	9.3
Scalloped									
From dry mix	1 c	245	79	230	5	11	6.5	3.0	0.5
From home recipe	1 c	245	81	210	7	9	5.5	2.5	0.4
Potato chips	10 chips	20	3	105	1	7	1.8	1.2	3.6
Pumpkin									
Cooked from raw, mashed	1 c	245	94	50	2	tr	0.1	tr	tr
Canned	1 c	245	90	85	3	1	0.4	0.1	tr
Radishes, raw, stem ends, rootlets cut off	4 radishes	18	95	5	tr	tr	tr	tr	tr
Sauerkraut, canned, solids and liquid	1 c	236	93	45	2	tr	0.1	tr	0.1
Seaweed									
Kelp, raw	1 oz	28	82	10	tr	tr	0.1	tr	tr
Spirulina, dried	1 oz	28	5	80	16	2	0.8	0.2	0.6
Southern peas. See Black-eyed peas, immature, mature									
Spinach									
Raw, chopped	1 c	55	92	10	2	tr	tr	tr	0.1
Cooked, drained									
From raw	1 c	180	91	40	5	tr	0.1	tr	0.2
From frozen (leaf)	1 c	190	90	55	6	tr	0.1	tr	0.2
Canned, drained solids	1 c	214	92	50	6	1	0.2	tr	0.4
Spinach souffle	1 c	136	74	220	11	18	7.1	6.8	3.1
Squash, cooked									
Summer (all varieties), sliced, drained	1 c	180	94	35	2	1	0.1	tr	0.2
Winter (all varieties), baked, cubes	1 c	205	89	80	2	1	0.3	0.1	0.5
Sunchoke. See Jerusalem-artichoke									

tr = nutrient present in trace amounts.

NUTRIENTS IN INDICATED QUANTITY

Cholesterol (mg)	Carbohydrate (g)	Calcium (mg)	Phosphorus (mg)	Iron (mg)	Potassium (mg)	Sodium (mg)	Zn (mg)	Vitamin A Value IU	Vitamin A Value RE	Thiamin (mg)	Riboflavin (mg)	Niacin (mg)	Ascorbic acid (mg)	Folic acid (μg)
0	17	5	43	0.7	229	16	.21	0	0	0.06	0.02	1.2	5	8
0	20	10	47	0.4	366	108	.19	0	0	0.09	0.01	1.6	5	15
12	31	203	233	0.8	537	1,076	.59	520	76	0.05	0.20	2.3	8	9
56	28	292	277	1.6	970	1,061	1.69	650	93	0.16	0.28	2.4	24	20
0	44	23	112	2.4	680	53	.50	0	0	0.17	0.03	3.8	10	26
4	37	55	101	0.6	628	636	.60	40	12	0.18	0.08	2.3	14	17
4	35	55	97	0.5	607	620	NI	360	42	0.18	0.08	2.3	13	NI
29	32	103	118	0.5	489	697	.51	380	44	0.23	0.11	1.4	20	15
170	28	48	130	1.6	635	1,323	.78	520	83	0.19	0.15	2.2	25	16
27	31	88	137	0.9	497	835	.61	360	51	0.05	0.14	2.5	8	13
29	26	140	154	1.4	926	821	.98	330	47	0.17	0.23	2.6	26	21
0	10	5	31	0.2	260	94	.29	0	0	0.03	tr	0.8	8	13
0	12	37	74	1.4	564	2	.45	2,650	265	0.08	0.19	1.0	12	33
0	20	64	86	3.4	505	12	.42	54,040	5,404	0.06	0.13	0.9	10	15
0	1	4	3	0.1	42	4	tr	tr	tr	tr	0.01	0.1	4	NI
0	10	71	47	3.5	401	1,560	.44	40	4	0.05	0.05	0.3	35	4
0	3	48	12	0.8	25	66	.35	30	3	0.01	0.04	0.1	(1)	51
0	7	34	33	8.1	386	297	2.00	160	16	0.67	1.04	3.6	3	94
0	2	54	27	1.5	307	43	.30	3,690	369	0.04	0.10	0.4	15	109
0	7	245	101	6.4	839	126	1.37	14,740	1,474	0.17	0.42	0.9	18	262
0	10	277	91	2.9	566	163	1.33	14,790	1,479	0.11	0.32	0.8	23	204
0	7	272	94	4.9	740	[53]683	.99	18,780	1,878	0.03	0.30	0.8	31	209
184	3	230	231	1.3	201	763	NI	3,460	675	0.09	0.30	0.5	3	NI
0	8	49	70	0.6	346	2	.70	520	52	0.08	0.07	0.9	10	36
0	18	29	41	0.7	896	2	.54	7,290	729	0.17	0.05	1.4	20	58

NI = not indicated.

[53]With added salt; if none is added, sodium content is 58 mg.

APPENDIX 41 NUTRITIVE VALUE OF THE EDIBLE PART OF FOOD *(continued)*

Foods, Approximate Measures, Units, and Weight (weight of edible portion only)		Grams	Water (g)	Food Energy (Calories)	Protein (g)	Fat (g)	Fatty Acids		
							Saturated (g)	Monounsaturated (g)	Polyunsaturated (g)
Vegetables and Vegetable Products (*cont.*)									
Sweet potatoes									
Cooked (raw, 5 by 2 in; about 2½ per lb)									
Baked in skin, peeled	1 potato	114	73	115	2	tr	tr	tr	0.1
Boiled, without skin	1 potato	151	73	160	2	tr	0.1	tr	0.2
Candied, 2½ by 2-in piece	1 piece	105	67	145	1	3	1.4	0.7	0.2
Canned									
Solid pack (mashed)	1 c	255	74	260	5	1	0.1	tr	0.2
Vacuum pack, piece 2¾ by 1 in	1 piece	40	76	35	1	tr	tr	tr	tr
Tomatoes									
Raw, 2⅗-in diam. (3 per 12 oz pkg.)	1 tomato	123	94	25	1	tr	tr	tr	0.1
Canned, solids and liquid	1 c	240	94	50	2	1	0.1	0.1	0.2
Tomato juice, canned	1 c	244	94	40	2	tr	tr	tr	0.1
Tomato products, canned									
Paste	1 c	262	74	220	10	2	0.3	0.4	0.9
Puree	1 c	250	87	105	4	tr	tr	tr	0.1
Sauce	1 c	245	89	75	3	tr	0.1	0.1	0.2
Turnips, cooked, diced	1 c	156	94	30	1	tr	tr	tr	0.1
Turnip greens, cooked, drained									
From raw (leaves and stems)	1 c	144	93	30	2	tr	0.1	tr	0.1
From frozen (chopped)	1 c	164	90	50	5	1	0.2	tr	0.3
Vegetable juice cocktail, canned	1 c	242	94	45	2	tr	tr	tr	0.1
Vegetables, mixed									
Canned, drained solids	1 c	163	87	75	4	tr	0.1	tr	0.2
Frozen, cooked, drained	1 c	182	83	105	5	tr	0.1	tr	0.1
Waterchestnuts, canned	1 c	140	86	70	1	tr	tr	tr	tr

[54]For regular pack; special dietary pack contains 31 mg sodium.
[55]With added salt; if none is added, sodium content is 24 mg.
[56]With no added salt; if salt is added, sodium content is 2,070 mg.

NUTRIENTS IN INDICATED QUANTITY

Cholesterol (mg)	Carbohydrate (g)	Calcium (mg)	Phosphorus (mg)	Iron (mg)	Potassium (mg)	Sodium (mg)	Zn (mg)	Vitamin A Value		Thiamin (mg)	Riboflavin (mg)	Niacin (mg)	Ascorbic acid (mg)	Folic acid (μg)
								IU	RE					
0	28	32	63	0.5	397	11	.33	24,880	2,488	0.08	0.14	0.7	28	26
0	37	32	41	0.8	278	20	.40	25,750	2,575	0.08	0.21	1.0	26	22
8	29	27	27	1.2	198	74	.16	4,400	440	0.02	0.04	0.4	7	12
0	59	77	133	3.4	536	191	.54	38,570	3,857	0.07	0.23	2.4	13	42
0	8	9	20	0.4	125	21	.46	3,190	319	0.01	0.02	0.3	11	NI
0	5	9	28	0.6	255	10	.11	1,390	139	0.07	0.06	0.7	22	19
0	10	62	46	1.5	530	[54]391	.38	1,450	145	0.11	0.07	1.8	36	35
0	10	22	46	1.4	537	[55]881	.34	1,360	136	0.11	0.08	1.6	45	49
0	49	92	207	7.8	2,442	[56]170	2.10	6,470	647	0.41	0.50	8.4	111	40
0	25	38	100	2.3	1,050	[57]50	.54	3,400	340	0.18	0.14	4.3	88	39
0	18	34	78	1.9	909	[58]1,482	.60	2,400	240	0.16	0.14	2.8	32	39
0	8	34	30	0.3	211	78	.17	0	0	0.04	0.04	0.5	18	14
0	6	197	42	1.2	292	42	.29	7,920	792	0.06	0.10	0.6	39	171
0	8	249	56	3.2	367	25	.68	13,080	1,308	0.09	0.12	0.8	36	64
0	11	27	41	1.0	467	883	.48	2,830	283	0.10	0.07	1.8	67	38
0	15	44	68	1.7	474	243	.67	18,990	1,899	0.08	0.08	0.9	8	39
0	24	46	93	1.5	308	64	.89	7,780	778	0.13	0.22	1.5	6	35
0	17	6	27	1.2	165	11	.54	10	1	0.02	0.03	0.5	2	16

NI = not indicated.
[57]With no added salt; if salt is added, sodium content is 998 mg.
[58]With salt added.
From Nutritive Value of Foods, U.S. Department of Agriculture, Home and Garden Bulletin No. 72.

APPENDIX 42 PROVISIONAL TABLE ON THE DIETARY FIBER CONTENT OF SELECTED FOODS (100 GRAMS EDIBLE PORTION)*

FOOD ITEM	MOISTURE	TOTAL DIETARY FIBER (AOAC)†
	g per 100 g edible portion	
Baked Products		
Bagels, plain	31.6	2.1
Biscuit mix:		
Dry	8.7	1.3
Baked	29.4	1.8
Biscuits, made from refrigerated dough, baked	28.7	1.5
Breads:		
Boston brown	47.2	4.7
Bran	37.7	8.5
Cornbread mix:		
Dry	6.0	6.5
Baked	34.4	2.6
Cracked-wheat	35.9	5.3
French	33.9	2.3
Hollywood-type, light	37.8	4.8
Italian	34.1	2.7
Mixed-grain	38.2	6.3
Oatmeal	36.7	3.9
Pita:		
White	32.1	1.6
Whole-wheat	30.6	7.4
Pumpernickel	38.3	5.9
Reduced-calorie, high-fiber:		
Wheat	43.7	11.3
White	41.8	7.9
Rye	37.0	6.2
Vienna		3.2
Wheat	37.0	3.5
Toasted		5.2
White	37.1	1.9
Toasted		2.5
Whole-wheat	38.3	7.4
Toasted		8.9
Bread crumbs, plain or seasoned	5.7	4.2
Bread stuffing, flavored, from dry mix	65.1	2.9
Cake mix:		
Chocolate:		
Dry	3.8	2.4
Prepared	33.3	2.2
Yellow:		
Dry	4.1	1.1
Prepared	40.0	0.8
Cakes:		
Boston cream pie	47.6	1.4
Coffeecake:		
Crumb topping	22.3	3.3
Fruit	31.7	2.5
Fruitcake, commercial	22.0	3.7
Baked Products *(continued)*		
Cakes (continued):		
Gingerbread, from dry mix	38.5	2.9
Cheesecake:		
Commercial	44.6	2.1
From no-bake mix	44.4	1.9
Cookies:		
Brownies	12.6	2.2
With nuts	12.6	2.6
Butter	4.7	2.4
Chocolate chip	4.0	2.7
Chocolate sandwich	2.2	2.9
Fig bars	16.7	4.6
Fortune	8.0	1.6
Oatmeal	5.7	2.9
Oatmeal, soft-type		2.7
Peanut butter	6.7	1.8
Shortbread with pecans	3.3	1.8
Vanilla sandwich	2.1	1.5
Crackers:		
Cheese, sandwich with peanut butter filling	4.0	1.1
Crisp bread, rye	6.1	16.2
Graham	4.1	3.2
Honey	4.1	1.7
Matzo:		
Plain	6.1	2.9
Egg/onion	8.0	5.0
Whole-wheat	3.0	11.8
Melba toast:		
Plain	5.6	6.3
Rye	6.7	7.9
Wheat	6.1	7.4
Rye	7.2	15.8
Saltines		2.6
Snack-type	4.2	1.2
Wheat	3.2	5.5
Whole-wheat	2.7	10.4
Croutons, plain or seasoned	5.6	4.7
Doughnuts:		
Cake	19.7	1.3
Yeast-leavened, glazed	26.7	2.2
English muffin, whole-wheat	45.7	6.7
French toast, commercial, ready-to-eat	48.1	3.1
Ice cream cones:		
Sugar, rolled type	3.0	4.6
Wafer-type	5.3	4.1
Baked Products *(continued)*		
Muffins, commercial:		
Blueberry	37.3	3.6
Oat bran	35.0	7.5
Pancake/waffle mix:		
Regular:		
Dry	8.7	2.7
Prepared	50.4	1.4
Buckwheat, dry	9.1	2.3
Pastry, danish:		
Plain	19.3	1.3
Fruit	27.6	1.9
Pies commercial:		
Apple	51.7	1.6
Cherry	46.2	0.8
Chocolate cream	43.5	2.0
Egg custard	46.5	1.6
Fruit and coconut		0.9
Lemon meringue	41.7	1.2
Pecan	19.8	3.5
Pumpkin	58.1	2.7
Rolls, dinner, egg	30.4	3.8
Taco shells	6.0	8.0
Toaster pastries	8.9	1.0
Tortillas:		
Corn	43.6	5.2
Flour, wheat	26.2	2.9
Waffles, commercial, frozen, ready-to-eat	45.0	2.4
Breakfast Cereals, Ready-to-Eat		
Bran, high fiber	2.9	35.3
Extra fiber		45.9
Bran flakes	2.9	18.8
Bran flakes with raisins	8.3	13.4
Corn flakes:		
Plain	2.8	2.0
Frosted or sugar-sparkled	1.9	2.2
Fiber cereal with fruit		14.8
Granola	3.3	10.5
Oat cereal	5.0	10.6
Oat flakes, fortified	3.1	3.0
Puffed wheat, sugar-coated	1.5	1.5
Rice, crispy	2.4	1.2
Wheat and malted barley:		
Flakes	3.4	6.8
Nuggets	3.2	6.5
With raisins		6.0
Wheat flakes	4.3	9.0
Cereal Grains		
Amaranth	9.8	15.2

APPENDIX 42 PROVISIONAL TABLE ON THE DIETARY FIBER CONTENT OF SELECTED FOODS (100 GRAMS EDIBLE PORTION)* *(continued)*

FOOD ITEM	MOISTURE	TOTAL DIETARY FIBER (AOAC)[†]
	g per 100 g edible portion	
Cereal Grains *(continued)*		
Amaranth flour, whole-grain	10.4	10.2
Arrowroot flour	11.4	3.4
Barley	9.4	17.3
Barley, pearled, raw	10.1	15.6
Bulgur, dry	8.0	18.3
Corn bran, crude	4.7	84.6
Corn flour, whole-grain	10.9	13.4
Cornmeal:		
Whole-grain	10.3	11.0
Degermed	11.6	5.2
Cornstarch	8.3	0.9
Farina, regular or instant:		
Dry	10.6	2.7
Cooked	85.8	1.4
Hominy, canned	79.8	2.5
Millet, hulled, raw		8.5
Oat bran, raw	6.6	15.9
Oat flour	7.8	9.6
Oats, rolled or oatmeal, dry	8.8	10.3
Rice, brown, long-grain:		
Raw	11.1	3.5
Cooked	73.1	1.7
Rice white:		
Glutinous, raw	10.0	2.8
Long-grain:		
Raw	11.6	1.0
Parboiled:		
Dry	10.5	1.8
Cooked		0.5
Precooked or instant:		
Dry	8.1	1.6
Cooked	76.4	0.8
Medium-grain, raw	12.9	1.4
Rice bran, crude	6.1	21.7
Rice flour:		
Brown	12.0	4.6
White	11.9	2.4
Rye flour, medium or light	9.4	14.6
Semolina	12.7	3.9
Tapioca, pearl, dry	12.0	1.1
Triticale	10.5	18.1
Triticale flour, whole-grain	10.0	14.6
Wheat bran, crude	9.9	42.4
Wheat flour:		
White, all purpose	11.8	2.7
Whole-grain	10.9	12.6
Cereal Grains *(continued)*		
Wheat germ:		
Crude	11.1	15.0
Toasted	2.9	12.9
Wild rice, raw	7.8	5.2
Fruits and Fruit Products		
Apples, raw:		
With skin	83.9	2.2
Without skin	84.5	1.9
Apple juice, unsweetened	87.9	0.1
Applesauce:		
Sweetened	79.6	1.2
Unsweetened	88.4	1.5
Apricots, dried	31.1	7.8
Apricot nectar	84.9	0.6
Bananas, raw	74.3	1.6
Blueberries, raw	84.6	2.3
Cantaloupe, raw	89.8	0.8
Figs, dried	28.4	9.3
Fruit cocktail, canned in heavy syrup, drained		1.5
Grapefruit, raw	90.9	0.6
Grapes, Thompson, seedless, raw	81.3	0.7
Kiwifruit, raw	83.0	3.4
Nectarines, raw	86.3	1.6
Olives:		
Green		2.6
Ripe		3.0
Oranges, raw	86.8	2.4
Orange juice, frozen concentrate:		
Undiluted	57.8	0.8
Prepared	88.1	0.2
Peaches:		
Raw	87.7	1.6
Canned in juice, drained		1.0
Dried	31.8	8.2
Pears, raw	83.8	2.6
Pineapple:		
Raw	86.5	1.2
Canned in heavy syrup, chunks, drained	79.0	1.1
Prunes:		
Dried	32.4	7.2
Stewed		6.6
Prune juice	81.2	1.0
Raisins	15.4	5.3
Strawberries	91.6	2.6
Watermelon	91.5	0.4
Legumes, Nuts, and Seeds		
Almonds, oil-roasted	3.3	11.2
Baked beans, canned:		
Barbecue-style		5.8
Sweet or tomato sauce:		
Plain	72.6	7.7
With franks	69.3	6.9
With pork	71.7	5.5
Beans, Great Northern:		
Raw	10.7	40.0
Canned, drained	69.9	5.4
Cashews, oil-roasted	5.4	6.0
Chickpeas, canned, drained	68.2	5.8
Coconut, raw	47.0	9.0
Cowpeas (black-eyed peas):		
Raw	12.0	27.0
Cooked, drained	70.0	9.6
Hazelnuts, oil-roasted	1.2	6.4
Lima beans:		
Raw	10.2	19.0
Cooked, drained	69.8	7.2
Miso	47.4	5.4
Mixed nuts, oil-roasted, with peanuts		9.0
Peanuts:		
Dry-roasted	1.6	8.0
Oil-roasted	2.0	8.8
Peanut butter:		
Chunky	1.1	6.6
Smooth	1.4	6.0
Pecans, dried	4.8	6.5
Pistachio nuts	3.9	10.8
Sunflower seeds, oil-roasted	2.6	6.8
Tahini	3.0	9.3
Tofu	84.6	1.2
Walnuts, dried:		
Black	4.4	5.0
English	3.6	4.8
Miscellaneous		
Beer, regular	92.3	.05
Candy:		
Caramels, vanilla	7.6	1.2
Chocolate, milk	0.8	2.8
Sugar-coated discs		3.1
Carob powder, unsweetened	1.2	32.8

APPENDIX 42 PROVISIONAL TABLE ON THE DIETARY FIBER CONTENT OF SELECTED FOODS (100 GRAMS EDIBLE PORTION)* *(continued)*

FOOD ITEM	MOISTURE	TOTAL DIETARY FIBER (AOAC)[†]
	g per 100 g edible portion	
Miscellaneous *(continued)*		
Chili powder	9.1	34.2
Chocolate, baking	0.7	15.4
Cocoa, baking	1.3	29.8
Cocoa mix, prepared	79.8	1.2
Curry powder	8.7	33.2
Gravy, beef, canned	89.1	0.4
Jelly apple	32.3	0.6
Milk, chocolate	82.3	1.5
Pepper, black	9.4	25.0
Pie filling:		
Apple	74.9	1.0
Cherry	69.7	0.6
Preserves:		
Peach	32.4	0.7
Strawberry	31.7	1.2
Soup, canned, condensed:		
Chicken with noodles or rice	86.5	0.6
Vegetable	84.9	1.3
Yeast active, dry	6.8	31.6
Pasta		
Macaroni (see spaghetti)		
Macaroni, protein-fortified, dry	10.2	4.3
Macaroni, tricolor, dry	9.8	4.3
Noodles, Chinese, chow mein	0.7	3.9
Noodles, egg, regular:		
Dry	9.7	2.7
Cooked	68.7	2.2
Noodles, Japanese, dry:		
Somen	9.2	4.3
Udon	8.7	5.4
Noodles, spinach, dry	8.5	6.8
Spaghetti and macaroni:		
Dry	10.5	2.4
Cooked	64.7	1.6
Spaghetti, dry:		
Spinach	8.7	10.6
Whole-wheat	7.1	11.8
Snacks		
Cheese-flavored, corn-based puffs or twists		1.0
Corn, toasted		6.9
Corn chips		4.4
Barbecue-flavored		5.2
Snacks *(continued)*		
Granola bars crunchy:		
Chocolate chip		4.4
Cinnamon		5.0
Popcorn:		
Air-popped		15.1
Oil-popped		10.0
Potato chips	2.5	4.8
Flavored		4.5
Potato chips, formulated	1.6	3.6
Pretzels		2.8
Tortilla chips		6.5
Flavored		6.2
Vegetables and Vegetable Products		
Artichokes, raw	84.4	5.2
Beans, snap:		
Raw	90.3	1.8
Canned:		
Drained solids	93.3	1.3
Solids and liquid	94.5	0.8
Beets, canned:		
Drained solids, sliced	91.0	1.7
Solids and liquid	91.3	1.1
Broccoli:		
Raw	90.7	2.8
Cooked	90.2	2.6
Brussels sprouts, boiled	87.3	4.3
Cabbage, Chinese:		
Raw	94.9	1.0
Cooked	95.4	1.6
Cabbage, red:		
Raw	91.6	2.0
Cooked	93.6	2.0
Cabbage, white, raw	91.5	2.4
Carrots:		
Raw	87.8	3.2
Canned, drained solids	93.0	1.5
Cauliflower:		
Raw	92.3	2.4
Cooked	92.5	2.2
Celery, raw	94.7	1.6
Chives	92.0	3.2
Corn, sweet:		
Raw	76.0	3.2
Cooked	69.6	3.7
Canned:		
Brine pack:		
Drained solids	76.9	1.4
Vegetables and Vegetable Products *(continued)*		
Canned Corn (continued):		
Brine pack: (continued)		
Solids and liquid	81.9	0.8
Cream-style	78.7	1.2
Cucumbers, raw	96.0	1.0
Pared		0.5
Lettuce:		
Butterhead or iceberg	95.7	1.0
Romaine	94.9	1.7
Mushrooms:		
Raw	91.8	1.3
Boiled	91.1	2.2
Onions, raw	90.1	1.6
Onions, spring, raw	91.9	2.4
Parsley, raw	88.3	4.4
Peas, edible-podded:		
Raw	88.9	2.6
Cooked	88.9	2.8
Peas, sweet, canned:		
Drained solids	81.7	3.4
Solids and liquid	86.5	2.0
Peppers, sweet, raw	92.8	1.6
Pickles:		
Dill	93.8	1.2
Sweet	68.9	1.1
Potatoes:		
Raw:		
Flesh and skin	80.0	1.8
Flesh	79.0	1.6
Baked:		
Flesh	75.4	1.5
Skin	47.3	4.0
Boiled	77.0	1.5
French-fried, home-prepared from frozen	52.9	4.2
Hashed brown	56.1	2.0
Spinach:		
Raw	91.6	2.6
Boiled	91.2	2.2
Squash:		
Summer:		
Raw	93.7	1.2
Cooked	93.7	1.4
Winter:		
Raw	88.7	1.8
Cooked	89.0	2.8
Sweet potatoes:		
Raw	72.8	3.0
Cooked	72.8	3.0
Canned, drained solids	72.5	1.8

APPENDIX 42 PROVISIONAL TABLE ON THE DIETARY FIBER CONTENT OF SELECTED FOODS (100 GRAMS EDIBLE PORTION)* *(continued)*

FOOD ITEM	MOISTURE	TOTAL DIETARY FIBER (AOAC)[†]	FOOD ITEM	MOISTURE	TOTAL DIETARY FIBER (AOAC)[†]	FOOD ITEM	MOISTURE	TOTAL DIETARY FIBER (AOAC)[†]
	g per 100 g edible portion			*g per 100 g edible portion*			*g per 100 g edible portion*	
Vegetables and Vegetable Products *(continued)*			**Vegetables and Vegetable Products** *(continued)*			**Vegetables and Vegetable Products** *(continued)*		
Tomatoes, raw	94.0	1.3	Turnip greens:			Vegetables, mixed,		
Tomato products:			Raw.	91.1	2.4	frozen, cooked. . . .	83.2	3.8
Catsup.		1.6	Boiled	93.2	3.1	Water chestnuts,		
Paste.	74.1	4.3	Turnips:			canned, drained		
Puree.	87.3	2.3	Raw.	91.9	1.8	solids.	87.9	2.2
Sauce	89.1	1.5	Boiled	93.6	2.0	Watercress	95.1	2.3

*From U.S. Department of Agriculture, Human Nutrition Information Service, HNIS/PT-106, Nutrient Data Research Branch, Nutrition Monitoring Division, September 1988.
[†]AOAC 5 accepted methods of dietary fiber analysis of the Association of Official Analytical Chemists.

APPENDIX 43 CAFFEINE CONTENT OF FOODS

CAFFEINE CONTENT	MG/SERVING
Coffee, 6-oz Cup	
Brewed, drip method	103
Brewed, percolator method	75
Instant, 1 rounded tsp	57
Decaffeinated	2
Flavored, regular and sugar-free	25–75
Tea	
3-minute brew, 6 oz cup	36
Instant, 1 rounded tsp in 8 oz of water	25–35
Decaffeinated, 5-minute brew, 6 oz cup	1
Cola Beverages, 12 oz	
Regular or diet	35–50
Decaffeinated	Trace
Cherry Colas, Dr. Pepper™, Mr. Pibb™, 12 oz	
Regular or diet	35–50
Decaffeinated	Trace
Mellow Yellow™, 12 oz	
Regular or diet	52
Mountain Dew™, 12 oz	
Regular or diet	54
Cocoa and Chocolate	
Cocoa beverage, 6 oz cup	4
Chocolate milk, 8 oz	8
Chocolate, sweet, semisweet, dark, milk, 1 oz	8–20
Chocolate, baking, unsweetened, 1 oz	58
Chocolate flavored, syrup, 1 oz	5
Chocolate pudding, ½ cup	4–8

Adapted from Pennington JAT. Bowes and Church's food values of portions used, 16th ed. Philadelphia: JB Lippincott, 1994.

APPENDIX 44 NUTRITIVE VALUES FOR ALCOHOLIC BEVERAGES AND MIXES

BEVERAGE	SERVING (oz)	ALCOHOL (g)	CARBOHYDRATE (g)	CALORIES	EXCHANGES FOR CALORIE CONTROL
Beer					
Regular	12	13	13	150	1 Starch, 2 Fat
Light	12	11	5	100	2 Fat
Near beer	12	1.5	12	60	1 Starch
Distilled spirits					
80-proof (gin, rum, vodka, whiskey, scotch)	1.5	14	Trace	100	2 Fat
Dry brandy, cognac	1	11	Trace	75	1.5 Fat
Table wine					
Dry white	4	11	Trace	80	2 Fat
Red or rosé	4	12	2	85	2 Fat
Sweet wine	4	12	5	105	⅓ Starch, 2 Fat
Light wine	4	6	1	50	1 Fat
Wine cooler	12	13	30	215	2 Fruit, 2 Fat
Dealcoholized wines	4	Trace	6–7	25–35	0.5 Fruit
Sparkling wines					
Champagne	4	12	4	100	2 Fat
Sweet kosher wine	4	12	12	132	1 Starch, 2 Fat
Appetizer/dessert wines					
Sherry	2	9	2	74	1.5 Fat
Sweet sherry, port, muscatel	2	9	7	90	0.5 Starch, 1.5 Fat
Cordials, liqueurs	1.5	13	18	160	1 Starch, 2 Fat
Vermouth					
Dry	3	13	4	105	2 Fat
Sweet	3	13	14	140	1 Starch, 2 Fat
Cocktails					
Bloody Mary	5	14	5	116	1 Vegetable, 2 Fat
Daiquiri	2	14	2	111	2 Fat
Manhattan	2	17	2	178	2.5 Fat
Martini	2.5	22	Trace	156	3.5 Fat
Old-fashioned	4	26	Trace	180	4 Fat
Tom Collins	7.5	16	3	120	2.5 Fat
Mixes					
Mineral water	Any	0	0	0	Free
Sugar-free tonic	Any	0	0	0	Free
Club soda	Any	0	0	0	Free
Diet soda	Any	0	0	0	Free
Tomato juice	4	0	5	25	1 Vegetable
Bloody Mary mix	4	0	5	25	1 Vegetable
Orange juice	4	0	15	60	1 Fruit
Grapefruit juice	4	0	15	60	1 Fruit
Pineapple juice	4	0	15	60	1 Fruit

With permission from: Franz MJ. Alcohol and diabetes: Its metabolism and guidelines for its occasional use. Part II Diabetes Spectrum 3(4):210–216, 1990.

CALORIC VALUE OF ALCOHOLIC BEVERAGES

The caloric contribution from alcohol of an alcoholic beverage can be estimated by multiplying the number of ounces by the proof and then again by the factor 0.8. For beers and wines, kilocalories from alcohol can be estimated by multiplying ounces by percentage of alcohol (by volume) and then by the factor 1.6.

APPENDIX 46 PROVISIONAL TABLE ON THE CONTENT OF OMEGA-3 FATTY ACIDS AND OTHER FAT COMPONENTS IN SELECTED FOODS (100 GRAMS EDIBLE PORTION) *(continued)*

		FATTY ACIDS						
FOOD ITEM	Total Fat (g)	Total Saturated (g)	Total Monounsaturated (g)	Total Polyunsaturated (g)	18:3 (g)	20:5 (g)	22:6 (g)	Cholesterol (mg)
Dairy and Egg Products								
Cheese, cheddar	33.1	21.1	9.0	0.9	0.4			105
Cheese, Roquefort	30.6	19.3	8.5	1.3	0.7			90
Cream, heavy whipping	37.0	23.0	10.7	1.4	0.5			137
Milk, whole	3.3	2.1	1.0	0.1	0.1			14
Egg yolk, chicken, raw	32.9	9.9	13.2	4.3	0.1			1,602
Fats and Oils								
Butter	81.1	50.5	23.4	3.0	1.2			219
Butter oil	99.5	61.9	28.7	3.7	1.5			256
Chicken fat	99.8	29.8	44.7	20.9	1.0			85
Duck fat	99.8	33.2	49.3	12.9	1.0			100
Lard	100	39.2	45.1	11.2	1.0			95
Linseed (flaxseed) oil	100	9.4	20.2	66.0	53.3			0
Margarine, hard, soybean	80.5	16.7	39.3	20.9	1.5			0
Margarine, hard, soybean, and soybean (hydrog.)	80.5	13.1	37.6	26.2	1.9			0
Margarine, hard, soybean (hydrog.), and palm	80.5	17.5	31.2	28.2	2.3			0
Margarine, hard, soybean (hydrog.), and cottonseed	80.5	15.6	36.1	25.3	2.8			0
Margarine, hard, soybean (hydrog.), and palm (hydrog.)	80.5	15.1	32.0	29.8	3.0			0
Margarine, liquid, soybean (hydrog.), soybean, and cottonseed	80.6	13.2	28.1	35.8	2.4			0
Margarine, soft, soybean (hydrog.), and cotton-seed	80.4	16.5	31.3	29.1	1.6			0
Margarine, soft, soybean (hydrog.), and palm	80.4	17.1	25.2	34.6	1.9			0
Margarine, soft, soybean, soybean (hydrog.), and cottonseed (hydrog.)	80.4	16.1	30.7	30.1	2.8			0
Mutton tallow	100	47.3	40.6	7.8	2.3			102
Rapeseed oil (Canola)	100	6.8	55.5	33.3	11.1			0
Rice bran oil	100	19.7	39.3	35.0	1.6			0
Salad dressing, comm., blue cheese, reg.	52.3	9.9	12.3	27.8	3.7			17
Salad dressing, comm., Italian, reg.	48.3	7.0	11.2	28.0	3.3			0
Salad dressing, comm., mayonnaise, imitation, soybean, w/o cholesterol	47.7	7.5	10.5	27.6	4.6			0
Salad dressing, comm., mayonnaise, safflower and soybean	79.4	8.6	13.0	55.0	3.0			59
Salad dressing, comm., mayonnaise, soybean	79.4	11.8	22.7	41.3	4.2			59
Salad dressing, comm., mayonnaise type	33.4	4.7	9.0	18.0	2.0			26
Salad dressing, comm., Thousand Island, reg.	35.7	6.0	8.3	19.8	2.5			0
Salad dressing, home recipe, French	70.2	12.6	20.7	33.7	1.9			0

APPENDIX 46 PROVISIONAL TABLE ON THE CONTENT OF OMEGA-3 FATTY ACIDS AND OTHER FAT COMPONENTS IN SELECTED FOODS (100 GRAMS EDIBLE PORTION) *(continued)*

		FATTY ACIDS						
FOOD ITEM	Total Fat (g)	Total Saturated (g)	Total Monounsaturated (g)	Total Polyunsaturated (g)	18:3 (g)	20:5 (g)	22:6 (g)	Cholesterol (mg)
Fats and Oils (Continued)								
Salad dressing, home recipe, vinegar, and soybean oil	50.1	9.1	14.8	24.1	1.4			0
Shortening, household, lard, and veg. oil	100	40.3	44.4	10.9	1.1			56
Shortening, household, soybean (hydrog.), and cottonseed (hydrog.)	100	25.0	44.5	26.1	1.6			0
Shortening, special-purpose, for bread, soy (hydrog.), and cottonseed	100	22.0	33.0	40.6	4.0			0
Shortening, special-purpose, for cake mixes, soybean (hydrog.), and cottonseed (hydrog.)	100	27.2	54.2	14.1	1.1			0
Shortening, special-purpose, heavy-duty, frying, soybean (hydrog.)	100	18.4	43.7	33.5	2.4			0
Soybean lecithin	100	15.3	10.9	45.1	5.1			0
Soybean oil	100	14.4	23.3	57.9	6.8			0
Soybean oil (hydrog.) and cottonseed oil	100	14.9	43.0	37.6	2.8			0
Soybean oil (partially hydrog.)	100	14.9	43.0	37.6	2.6			0
Spread, margarine-like, about 60% fat, soybean (hydrog.) and palm (hydrog.)	60.8	14.1	26.0	18.1	1.6			0
Spread, margarine-like, about 60% fat, soybean (hydrog.), palm (hydrog.), and palm	60.8	13.5	24.1	20.4	1.6			0
Tomatoseed oil	100	19.7	22.8	53.1	2.3			0
Walnut oil	100	9.1	22.8	63.3	10.4			0
Wheat germ oil	100	18.8	15.1	61.7	6.9			0
Fruits								
Avocados, California, raw	17.3	2.6	11.2	2.0	0.1			0
Raspberries, raw	0.6	Tr	Tr	0.3	0.1			0
Strawberries, raw	0.4	Tr	Tr	0.2	0.1			0
Lamb and Veal								
Lamb, leg, raw (83% lean, 17% fat)	17.6	8.1	7.1	1.0	0.3			71
Lamb, loin, raw (72% lean, 28% fat)	27.4	12.8	11.2	1.6	0.5			71
Veal, leg round with rump, raw (87% lean, 13% fat)	9.0	3.8	3.7	0.6	0.1			71
Legumes								
Beans, common, dry	1.5	0.2	0.1	0.9	0.6			0
Chickpeas, dry	5.0	0.5	1.1	2.3	0.1			0
Cowpeas, dry	1.9	0.6	0.1	0.8	0.3			0
Lentils, dry	1.2	0.2	0.2	0.5	0.1			0
Lima beans, dry	1.4	0.3	0.1	0.7	0.2			0
Peas, garden, dry	2.4	0.4	0.1	0.4	0.2			0
Soybeans, dry	21.3	3.1	4.4	12.3	1.6			0

APPENDIX 46 PROVISIONAL TABLE ON THE CONTENT OF OMEGA-3 FATTY ACIDS AND OTHER FAT COMPONENTS IN SELECTED FOODS (100 GRAMS EDIBLE PORTION) *(continued)*

		FATTY ACIDS						
FOOD ITEM	**Total Fat (g)**	**Total Saturated (g)**	**Total Monounsaturated (g)**	**Total Polyunsaturated (g)**	**18:3 (g)**	**20:5 (g)**	**22:6 (g)**	**Cholesterol (mg)**
Nuts and Seeds								
Beechnuts, dried	50.0	5.7	21.9	20.1	1.7			0
Butternuts, dried	57.0	1.3	10.4	42.7	8.7			0
Chia seeds, dried	26.3	10.5	7.3	7.3	3.9			0
Hickory nuts, dried	64.4	7.0	32.6	21.9	1.0			0
Soybean kernels, roasted, and toasted	24.0	3.2	5.6	12.7	1.5			0
Walnuts, black	56.6	3.6	12.7	37.5	3.3			0
Walnuts, English/Persian	61.9	5.6	14.2	39.1	6.8			0
Pork								
Pork, cured, bacon, raw	57.5	21.3	26.3	6.8	0.8			67
Pork, cured, breakfast strips, raw	37.1	12.9	16.9	5.6	0.9			69
Pork, cured salt pork, raw	80.5	29.4	38.0	9.4	0.7			86
Pork, fresh, ham, raw	20.8	7.5	9.7	2.2	0.2			74
Pork, fresh, jowl, raw	69.6	25.3	32.9	8.1	0.6			90
Pork, fresh, leaf fat, raw	94.2	45.2	37.2	7.3	0.9			110
Pork, fresh, separable fat, raw	76.7	27.9	35.7	8.2	0.7			93
Poultry								
Chicken, broiler fryers, flesh and skin, giblets, neck, raw†	14.8	4.2	6.1	3.2	0.1			90
Chicken, dark meat, w/o skin, raw†	4.3	1.1	1.3	1.0	Tr			80
Chicken, light meat, w/o skin, raw†	1.7	0.4	0.4	0.4	Tr			58
Chicken, skin only, raw†	32.4	9.1	13.5	6.8	0.3			109
Turkey, flesh, with skin, roasted†	9.7	2.8	3.2	2.5	0.1			82
Vegetables								
Beans, Navy, sprouted, cooked	0.8	Tr	Tr	0.5	0.3			0
Beans, pinto, sprouted, cooked	0.9	0.1	Tr	0.5	0.3			0
Broccoli, raw	0.4	Tr	Tr	0.2	0.1			0
Cauliflower, raw	0.2	Tr	Tr	Tr	0.1			0
Kale, raw	0.7	Tr	Tr	0.3	0.2			0
Leeks, freeze-dried, raw	2.1	0.3	Tr	1.2	0.7			0
Lettuce, butterhead, raw	0.2	Tr	Tr	0.1	0.1			0
Radish seeds, sprouted, raw	2.5	0.7	0.4	1.1	0.7			0
Seaweed, Spirulina, dried	7.7	2.6	0.7	2.0	0.8			0
Soybeans, green, raw	6.8	0.7	0.8	3.8	3.2			0
Soybeans, mature seeds, sprouted, cooked	4.5	0.5	0.5	2.5	2.1			0
Spinach, raw	0.4	Tr	Tr	0.1	0.1			0

Data from Human Nutrition Information Service, USDA. Provisional table on the content of omega-3 fatty acids and other fat components in selected foods, HNIS/PT-103, 1988.

†Contains trace amounts of 20:5, 22:5, and 22:6.

APPENDIX 47 CAROTENOID CONTENT OF FRUITS AND VEGETABLES

	β-CAROTENE[a,b]		α-CAROTENE[a,b]		LUTEIN + ZEAXANTHEIN		LYCOPENE		β-CRYPTOXANTHEIN
	Median	Conf code[c]	Median	Conf code	Median	Conf code	Median	Conf code	Median
	← μg/100g →		← μg/100g →		← μg/100g →		← μg/100g →		← μg/100g →
Apple, raw	26	C	0[d]	C	45	C	0	C	
Apricot, canned, drained	1,500[e]	B	0	C	2	C	65	C	
Apricot, dried	17,600[e]	C	...	...	0	C	864	C	
Apricot, raw	3,524	C	0	C	0	C	5	C	
Asparagus, raw	449	C	9	C	...	...	...	...	
Avocado, raw	34	C	...	...	320	C	...	...	
Banana, raw	0	C	0	B	0	C	0	C	
Basil, not dried	350	B	...	...	...	...	...	...	
Beet greens	2,560	B	3	B	...	...	...	...	
Beet, canned	1	C	0	C	4	C	0	C	
Bitter melon, raw	50	C	...	...	...	...	...	...	
Blueberries	...	...	0	C	...	...	...	...	
Bottle gourd, raw	4	C	...	...	...	...	...	...	
Broccoli, cooked	1,300	A	...	...	1,800	A	...	...	
Broccoli, raw	700	A	1[e]	B	1,900	C	0	C	
Brussels sprouts	480	A	6	C	1,300	A	0	C	
Cabbage, Chinese, bok choy, raw	62	C	1	C	40	C	0	C	
Cabbage, Chinese, wild	530	B	...	...	...	...	...	...	
Cabbage, red, raw	15	C	1	C	26	C	0	C	
Cabbage, white	80[e]	A	0	C	150	C	0	C	
Cantaloupe, raw	3,000[e]	A	35	C	0	C	0	C	
Carrot, cooked, canned, frozen	9,800	A	3,700	A	...	...	0	C	
Carrot, raw	7,900	A	3,600	A	260	C	0	C	
Carrot, A+ variety, raw	18,250	C	10,650	C	...	...	0	C	
Carrot, A+ variety, cooked	25,650	C	15,000	C	...	...	0	C	
Cashew apple, raw	155	C	14	C	...	...	...	..	
Cashew apple juice	80	C	...	...	...	...	...	...	
Cassava leaf	3,000	C	...	...	...	...	...	...	
Cauliflower	8[e]	B	0	B	33[e]	B	0	C	
Celeriac, raw	0	C	0	C	1	C	0	C	
Celery	710	B	0	C	3,600	C	0	C	
Chicory leaf, raw	3,430	C	...	...	...	...	...	...	
Coriander, not dried	2,000	C	...	...	...	...	...	...	
Corn, yellow	51	C	50	C	780	A	0	C	
Cranberries, raw	22	C	1	C	28	C	0	C	
Cress leaf, raw	4,150	C	...	...	...	...	...	...	

Cucumber, pickled	180	C	0	C	510	C	0	C	
Cucumber, raw	6[e]	C	0	C	240	C	0	C	
Currants, raw	62	C	0	C	240	C	0	C	
Dill, not dried	4,500	C	0	C	6,700	C	0	C	
Eggplant	35	B	...	...	...	...	...	...	
Endive	1,300	C	...	...	...	...	...	...	
Fennel leaves	4,440	C	...	...	...	...	...	...	
Grapefruit, pink, raw	1,310	C	0	C	0	C	3,362	C	
Grapefruit, white, raw	14[e]	B	1[e]	B	10	C	0	C	
Grapes, raw	33	C	1	C	72	C	0	C	
Green beans	630	A	44	C	740	B	0	C	
Greens, collard	5,400	B	...	...	...	...	...	...	
Greens, fiddlehead	1,950	B	280	B	...	...	...	...	
Greens, mustard	2,700	B	...	...	9,900	C	...	...	
Guava juice	270	C	...	...	...	...	3,340	C	
Guava, raw	812	C	...	...	...	...	5,400	C	
Jackfruit, raw	23	C	...	...	...	...	...	...	
Jellies, jams, preserves	16	C	1	C	6	C	0	C	
Kale	4,700	A	...	...	21,900	B	...	...	
Kale, Chinese	140	C	...	...	...	...	...	...	
Kiwi fruit, raw	43	C	0	C	180	C	0	C	
Leeks, raw	1,000	C	0	C	1,900	C	0	C	
Lemon, raw	3	C	0	C	12	C	0	C	
Lettuce, iceberg	480	C	4	C	...	...	...	...	
Lettuce, leaf	1,200	C	1	C	1,800	C	0	C	
Lettuce, romaine	1,900	B	...	...	...	...	...	...	
Lima beans, cooked	...	...	0	C	...	...	...	...	
Loofah fruit, raw	47	C	...	...	...	...	...	...	
Mango, raw	1,300	A	0	C	0	C	0	C	–54
Mint, not dried	730	C	...	...	...	...	...	...	
Mushroom	0	C	0	C	0	C	0	C	
Mushroom, chanterelle, raw	1,300	C	1	C	0	C	0	C	
Nectarine, raw	103	C	0	C	...	...	...	...	
Okra, raw	170	C	28	C	...	...	...	...	
Olive, green	280	C	0	C	510	C	0	C	–19
Onion, yellow, raw	160	C	0	C	16	C	0	C	
Orange juice	7	A	6	A	74	A	0	B	–24
Orange, raw	39[e]	B	20[e]	B	14	C	0	C	
Papaya, raw	99	C	0	C	...	...	0	C	–470
Parsley, not dried	5,300	C	0	C	10,200	C	0	C	
Peach, canned, drained	100	B	0	C	28	B	0	C	–47
Peach, dried	9,256	C	...	...	188	C	0	C	–251
Peach, raw	99	B	1	C	14	B	0	C	–42
Pear, raw	17	C	0	C	110	C	0	C	

APPENDIX 47 CAROTENOID CONTENT OF FRUITS AND VEGETABLES *(continued)*

	β-CAROTENE[a,b]		α-CAROTENE[a,b]		LUTEIN + ZEAXANTHEIN		LYCOPENE		β-CRYPTOXANTHEIN
	Median	Conf code[c]	Median	Conf code	Median	Conf code	Median	Conf code	Median
	← μg/100g →		← μg/100g →		← μg/100g →		← μg/100g →		← μg/100g →
Peas, green	350	A	16	C	1,700	A	0	C	
Pepper, green, raw	230	B	11	B	700	C	0	C	
Pepper, red	2,200	B	60	C	...	...	...	...	
Pepper, yellow, raw	150	C	92	C	770	C	0	C	
Pigeon peas	40	C	...	...	...	...	...	...	
Pineapple, canned, drained	18	C	1	C	2	C	...	...	
Plum, raw	430	C	...	...	240	C	0	C	
Potato salad	12	C	2	C	...	...	0	C	
Potato, white, cooked	0	C	0	C	0	C	0	C	
Potato, white, raw	6	C	0	C	36	C	0	C	
Prune, dried	140	C	31	C	120	C	0	C	
Pumpkin	3,100	A	3,800	A	1,500	C	0	B	
Radish, raw	9	C	0	C	12	C	0	C	
Raisins	0	C	0	C	1	C	C	C	
Raspberries, raw	6	C	6	C	76	C	0	C	
Rhubarb, raw	61	C	0	C	170	C	0	C	
Roquette, raw	3,460	C	...	...	...	...	...	...	
Rose hip, purée, canned	420	C	0	C	...	...	780	C	
Rutabaga, raw	1	C	0	C	0	C	0	C	
Scallion, raw	850	C	6	C	2,100	C	...	...	
Spinach, cooked, drained	5,500	A	...	...	12,600	A	...	...	
Spinach, raw	4,100	A	0	B	10,200	C	0	C	
Squash, summer	420	C	12	C	1,200	C	...	...	
Squash, winter, cooked	2,400	A	12[e]	B	38	C	...	...	
Squash, winter, raw	820[e]	A	12[e]	B	38	C	...	...	
Strawberries	9	C	2	C	31	C	0	C	
Sweet potato, cooked	8,800	A	0	C	...	...	0	C	
Sweet potato, raw	8,900	B	0	C	...	...	0	C	
Swiss chard, raw	3,647	C	45	C	...	...	...	...	
Tangerine, tangelo juice	8[e]	B	5	B	135	C	...	...	–214
Tangerine, raw	38	C	20	C	20	C	...	...	
Tomato catsup	5,000[f]	C	0[f]	C	210[f]	C	9,900[f]	...	

Tomato juice, canned	900	C	. . .	. . .	. . .	. . .	8,580	B
Tomato paste, canned	1,700	C	. . .	C	. . .	. . .	6,500	B
Tomato sauce, canned	1,000	C	. . .	. . .	. . .	. . .	. . .	. . .
Tomato, raw	520	A	. . .	. . .	100	C	3,100	A
Turnip, raw	72	C	1	C	1	C	0	C
Watermelon, raw	230	C	1	C	14	C	4,100	B
Yard-long beans, raw	44	C	. . .	. . .	. . .	. . .	. . .	. . .

[a]Missing values for minimum and maximum (min-max) alone indicate that only one acceptable analytic value was found for that carotenoid in that food.
[b]Missing value for median, minimum, maximum, and confidence code indicate that no acceptable analytic values were found for that carotenoid in that food. Refer below for imputed values.
[c]Conf code = Confidence code, see chart below.
[d]Zeroes represent values reported as not detected at a detection limit specified in the acceptable references.
[e]Mean for acceptable foods more than two times median.
[f]Values based only on data for Finnish catsup containing carrots.
See also: website www.nal.usda.gov/fnic/foodcomp/Data/car98/car98.html

A. The consensus of experts in carotenoid analysis is that this food does not contain detectable levels of this carotenoid. Impute the carotenoid level as 0.

B. Carotenoid present in similar food. For imputation purposes, cooked broccoli was used to estimate missing values for asparagus; guava for guava juice; white cabbage for iceberg lettuce; raw peach for raw nectarine; cucumber for okra; orange juice for oranges; green pepper for red pepper; tangerine juice for tangerines; tomato for tomato juice, tomato paste, and tomato sauce; and a mixture of greens (mustard greens, kale, parsley, raw spinach, and cooked spinach) for beet greens, chicory, cress leaf, endive, collard greens, romaine lettuce, and Swiss chard. Impute carotenoid using the ratio of the missing carotenoid to β-carotene in similar food multiplied by the β-carotene content of the food with missing carotenoid.

C. Impute using unpublished preliminary data for guava from Nutrient Composition Laboratory, Beltsville Human Nutrition Research Center, Agriculture Research Service, Beltsville, Md.

D. Impute value from similar food with highly similar levels of other carotenoids. For imputation purposes, carotenoid content of cloud berries (29) was used to replace missing values for blueberries, raw broccoli for cooked broccoli, and raw carrots for cooked carrots.

E. Impute based on unpublished preliminary data, 1988, for blueberries from Arthur D. Little, Inc., Cambridge, Mass.

Source: Adapted from Tables 3 and 4 in Mangels A et al. Carotenoid content of fruits and vegetables: An evaluation of the analytic data. J Am Diet Assoc 93:284, 1993.

APPENDIX 48 PROVISIONAL TABLE ON THE VITAMIN D CONTENT OF FOODS (100 GRAMS EDIBLE PORTION)

FOOD ITEM	VITAMIN D	
	µg	IU
Breakfast Cereals[1]		
All-Bran ®	3.5	140
Apple Jacks ®	3.5	140
Cap'n Crunch ®	*	140
Cheerios ®	3.5	140
Cinnamon Toast Crunch ®	3.5	140
Cocoa Pebbles ®	3.5	140
Corn Chex ®	*	140
Corn Pops ®	3.5	
Cracklin' Oat Bran ®	3.5	140
Crispix ®	3.5	140
Froot Loops ®	3.5	140
Frosted Flakes, Kellogg's ®	3.5	140
Frosted Mini-Wheats ®	*	
Fruity Pebbles ®	3.5	140
Golden Grahams ®	3.5	140
Grape-Nuts Brand Cereal ®	3.5	140
Honeycomb ®	3.5	140
Honey Nut Cherrios ®	3.5	140
Honey Smacks ®	3.5	140
Just Right ® with Fruit and Nuts	2.7	108
Kellogg's Bran Flakes ®	3.5	140
Kellogg's Corn Flakes ®	3.5	140
Kix ®	3.5	140
Life ®	*	
Lucky Charms ®	3.5	140
Nabisco Shredded Wheat ®	*	
Nabisco Shredded Wheat'n Bran ®	*	
Natural Bran Flakes ®	3.5	140
Natural Raisin Bran ®	3.8	152
Nut & Honey Crunch ®	3.5	140
Oatmeal Raisin Crisp ®	3.5	140
Product 19 ®	3.5	140
Raisin Bran, Kellogg's ®	2.5	100
Rice Chex ®	*	
Rice Krispies ®	3.5	140
Special K ®	3.5	140
Spoon-Size Shredded Wheat ®	*	
Super Golden Crisp ®	3.5	140
Total ®	3.5	140
Trix ®	3.5	140
Wheaties ®	3.5	140
Dairy and Egg Products		
Milk, cow, fortified[2]:		
Whole, 3.3% fat	1.0	40
Low-fat, 2% fat	1.0	40
Low-fat, 2% fat with nonfat milk solids added	1.0	40
Low-fat, 2% fat, protein fortified	1.0	40
Low-fat, 1% fat	1.0	40
Low-fat, 1% fat, with nonfat milk solids added	1.0	40
Low-fat, 1% fat, protein fortified	1.0	40
Skim	1.0	40
Skim, with nonfat milk solids added	1.0	40
Skim, protein fortified	1.0	40
Dry, whole	7.8	312
Dry, nonfat, regular	8.3	332
Dry, nonfat, instantized	11.0	440
Evaporated, skim	2.0	80
Chocolate, whole	1.0	40
Chocolate, low-fat, 2% fat	1.0	40
Chocolate, low-fat, 1% fat	1.0	40

FOOD ITEM	VITAMIN D	
	µg	IU
Dairy and Egg Products (continued)		
Milk, cow, fluid, whole, unfortified[3]:		
Summer	0.08	3
Winter	0.03	1
Season not specified	0.06	2
Milk, goat, whole, fluid	0.3	12
Milk, human, whole, fluid	0.09	4
Cheese:		
Camembert	0.3	12
Cheddar	0.3	12
Edam	0.9	36
Parmesan	0.7	28
Swiss	1.1	44
Cream, heavy whipping, fluid	1.3	52
Egg, chicken:		
Whole, fresh or frozen	1.3	52
Whole, dried	4.7	188
White, fresh	0	0
Yolk, fresh	3.7	148
Fast Foods		
Cheeseburger		
Regular	0.3	12
4-ounce	0.3	12
Eggs, scrambled	1.7	68
English muffin with egg, cheese, and bacon	0.8	32
Fish sandwich, regular, with cheese	0.5	20
Hamburger:		
Regular	0.3	12
Double meat and double-decker roll	0.4	16
4-ounce patty, regular roll	0.4	16
Ice cream cone	0.2	8
Shake:		
Chocolate	0.4	16
Strawberry	0.2	8
Vanilla	0.2	8
Sundae:		
Caramel	0.2	8
Hot Fudge	0.3	12
Strawberry	0.3	12
Fats		
Butter	1.4	56
Margarine, fortified[4]:		
Fleischmann's ®	1.5	60
Mazola ®	1.5	60
Promise ®	1.5	60
Margarine, unfortified	0	0
Fish oils:		
Cod liver:		
Medicinal, regular	417.5	16,700
Medicinal, high-potency	1,010.0	40,400
Low-potency	125.0	5,000
Commercial, refined	250.0	10,000
Dogfish liver	60.5	2,420
Halibut liver	9,200.0	368,000
Mackerel	3,250.0	130,000
Rockfish liver	2,445.0	97,800
Sardine, Atlantic or Pacific	8.3	332
Swordfish liver	17,325.0	693,000
Tuna liver	3,250.0	130,000
Fish oil, unspecified	5.0	200

APPENDIX 48 PROVISIONAL TABLE ON THE VITAMIN D CONTENT OF FOODS (100 GRAMS EDIBLE PORTION) *(continued)*

FOOD ITEM	VITAMIN D	
	μg	IU
Fish and Related Products		
Finfish, fillet, raw:		
Catfish, channel	12.5	500
Cod	1.1	44
Eel, European	5.0	200
Flounder	1.5	60
Garfish	8.5	340
Halibut, Greenland	15.0	600
Herring, Atlantic	40.7	1,628
Mackerel, Atlantic	9.0	360
Finfish roe, canned:		
Caviar, sturgeon	5.8	232
Cod	2.1	84
Herring:		
Pickled	17.0	680
Smoked	3.0	120
Mackerel, Atlantic:		
Canned in oil	5.7	228
Canned in tomato sauce	6.0	240
Mackerel, Pacific:		
Canned in oil	6.3	252
Salmon, canned:		
Chinook	8.1	324
Chum	5.6	224
Pink	15.6	624
Sardines:		
Atlantic, canned in oil	6.8	272
Pacific, canned in oil	8.3	332
Unspecified, canned in tomato sauce	12.0	480
Shellfish:		
Clam	0.1	4
Oyster	8.0	320
Shrimp	3.8	152
Sprat, smoked	3.0	120
Tuna, light meat, canned in oil, drained	5.9	236
Meat and Related Products		
Beef:		
Kidney	0.8	32
Lean cuts	0.3	12
Liver	0.4	16
Bologna:		
Beef	0.7	28
Meat and Related Products (continued)		
Bologna (continued):		
Beef and pork	1.1	44
Pork	1.4	56
Bratwurst, pork, smoked	1.1	44
Braunschweiger	1.2	48
Frankfurter:		
Beef	0.9	36
Beef and pork	0.9	36
Loaves:		
Beef, honeyroll	1.0	40
Pork:		
Ham and cheese	1.1	44
Luxury	0.7	28
Mother's loaf	1.0	40
Olive	1.1	44
Pickle and pimientc	1.1	44
Pork and beef:		
Barbecue	0.9	36
Honey	0.9	36
Old-fashioned	1.0	40
Peppered	0.8	32
Picnic	1.2	48
Salami:		
Beef:		
Beer	0.9	36
Cotto	1.2	48
Pork, beer	0.9	36
Sausage:		
Beef, summer	1.1	44
Beef and pork:		
Raw	1.1	44
Cooked	0.7	28
Pork	1.3	52
Vegetables		
Mushrooms:		
Chanterelle	2.1	84
Morel	3.1	124
Shitake, fresh	2.5	100
Shitake, dried	41.5	1,660
Yellow Boletus	3.1	124
Unspecified	1.9	76

μg = microgram.
IU = International Unit (1.0 μg = 40 IU).
[1]Values for breakfast cereals are based on label claim information.
*Level in unfortified cereals is negligible.
[2]Fortified so that one quart of milk contains 10 μg or 400 IU of vitamin D.
[3]Level of vitamin D varies with season.
[4]Values based on label claim information.

APPENDIX 49 VITAMIN E AS α-TOCOPHEROL (mg)*

Food	mg
Chips and Snacks	
Potato chips—1 oz (28 g)	1.20
Potato sticks—1 oz (28 g)	2.23
Eggs, Chicken	
Whole, fresh/frzn—1 large (50 g)	0.88
Yolk, fresh—yolk of large egg (17 g)	0.87
Entrées, Box Mix	
Pizza, cheese, from Contadina Pizzeria Kit	
Thick crust—¼ pizza (128 g)	0.14
Thin crust—¼ pizza (104 g)	0.14
Fats, Oils, and Shortenings	
Animal Fats	
Beef tallow, raw—1 T (13 g)	0.30
Pork fat (lard), raw—1 T (13 g)	0.20
Vegetable Oils	
Almond oil—1 T (14 g)	5.30
Coconut oil—1 T (14 g)	0.10
Corn oil—1 T (14 g)	1.90
Corn oil, Mazola—1 T (14 g)	3.00
Cottonseed oil—1 T (14 g)	4.80
Olive oil—1 T (14 g)	1.60
Palm oil—1 T (14 g)	2.60
Peanut oil—1 T (14 g)	1.60
Safflower oil—1 T (14 g)	4.60
Sesame oil—1 T (14 g)	0.20
Soybean oil—1 T (14 g)	1.50
Soybean oil, hydrogenated—1 T (14 g)	1.10
Sunflower oil—1 T (14 g)	6.10
Veg-oil spray, Mazola No Stick—2.5 sec spray (0.7 g)	0.51†
Wheat-germ oil—1 T (14 g)	20.30
Fruit and Vegetable Juices	
Apple jce, cnd/bottled—8 fl oz (248 g)	0.03
Grapefruit jce, cnd—8 fl oz (247 g)	0.10
Orange jce, fresh—8 fl oz (248 g)	0.10
Tomato jce—6 fl oz (182 g)	0.40
Fruits	
Apple	
Raw, w/skin—1 med (138 g)	0.81
Raw, w/o skin—1 med (128 g)	0.35
Apricots, cnd, in heavy syrup—4 halves (90 g)	0.80
Banana, raw—1 med (114 g)	0.31
Blackberries, raw—½ cup (72 g)	0.35
Cantaloupe, raw—1 cup pieces (160 g)	0.22
Cherries, sour, raw—½ cup (78 g)	0.10
Currants, European black, raw—½ cup (56 g)	0.56
Currants, red and white, raw—½ cup (56 g)	0.06
Gooseberries, raw—1 cup (150 g)	0.56
Grapefruit, raw, red and white—½ med (123 g)	0.30
Mango, raw—1 med (207 g)	2.32
Mixed fruit, frzn, in syrup, Bird's Eye—½ cup (142 g)	0.06
Orange, navel or valencia, raw—1 fruit (131 g)	0.30
Pear, raw—1 med (166 g)	0.83
Pineapple, raw—1 cup pieces (155 g)	0.16
Raspberries	
Raw—1 cup (123 g)	0.37
Frzn, in lite syrup, Bird's Eye—½ cup (142 g)	0.27
Strawberries	
Raw—1 cup (149 g)	0.18
Frzn, in lite syrup, Bird's Eye—½ cup (142 g)	0.13
Frzn, sweetened or unsweetened—1 cup (149 g)	0.31
Grain Products	
Pasta	
Macaroni, enr, ckd—1 cup (140 g)	1.03
Spaghetti, enr, ckd—1 cup (140 g)	1.03
Nuts, Nut Products, and Seeds	
Almonds	
Dried—1 oz (24 nuts) (28 g)	6.72
Oil roasted—1 oz (22 nuts) (28 g)	1.55
Toasted—1 oz (28 g)	1.41
Whole, Blue Diamond—1 oz (28 g)	1.66
Brazil nuts, dried—1 oz (8 med nuts) (28 g)	2.13
Cashews, dry roasted—1 oz (28 g)	0.16
Coconut, raw—1 piece (2″ × 2″ × ½″) (45 g)	0.33
Filberts (hazelnuts), dried—1 oz (28 g)	6.70
Peanut butter, creamy/smooth, Skippy—1 T (16 g)	3.00
Peanut butter, chunk style/crunchy, Skippy—1 T (16 g)	3.00
Peanuts	
Dried—1 oz (28 g)	2.56
Dry roasted—1 oz (28 g)	2.18
Oil roasted—1 oz (28 g)	2.07
Pecans, dried—1 oz (31 large nuts) (28 g)	0.87
Pistachio nuts, dried—1 oz (47 nuts) (28 g)	1.46
Sesame seeds, whole, dried—1T (9 oz)	0.20
Walnuts, English/Persian, dried—1 oz (14 halves) (28 g)	0.73
Spreads	
Butter—1 T (15 g)	0.20
Margarine by brand	
Mazola—1 T (14 g)	8.00
Mazola unsalted—1 T (14 g)	8.00
Margarine by form and type of oil	
Liquid, soybean and cottonseed—1 t (5 g)	0.20
Stick, safflower and soybean—1 t (5 g)	0.80
Stick soybean—1 t (5 g)	0.10
Stick, soybean and cottonseed—1 t (5 g)	0.30
Tub, corn—1 t (5 g)	0.50
Tub, safflower—1 t (5 g)	0.60
Tub, soybean—1 t (5 g)	0.10
Tub, soybean and cottonseed—1 t (5 g)	0.30
Margarine, imitation (diet) by brand	
Mazola diet—1 T (14 g)	3.00
Parkay, diet soft—1 T (14 g)	0.40
Margarine, imitation (diet) by form and type of oil	
Tub, soybean and cottonseed—1 t (5 g)	0.40
Mayonnaise	
Best Foods/Hellman's—1 T (14 g)	11.00
Soybean—1 T (14 g)	2.90
Miracle Whip, Kraft—1 T (14 g)	0.50
Miracle Whip, light, Kraft—1 T (14 g)	0.40
Sandwich spread, Best Foods/Hellmann's—1 T (15 g)	5.00
Vegetables	
Asparagus	
Cnd—½ cup (121 g)	0.46
Frzn, boiled—4 spears (60 g)	0.81
Raw—4 spears (58 g)	1.15
Avocado, raw, Calif—1 med (173 g)	2.32
Beet greens, raw—1 cup (38 g)	0.57
Beets, cnd, Harvard—½ cup slices (123 g)	0.04
Broccoli, raw—½ cup chopped (44 g)	0.20
Brussels sprouts	
Raw—½ cup chopped (44 g)	0.39
Boiled—½ cup (4 sprouts) (78 g)	0.66

APPENDIX 49 VITAMIN E AS α-TOCOPHEROL (mg)* *(continued)*

Food	α-Tocopherol (mg)
Vegetables (continued)	
Cabbage, Chinese (bok-choy), raw—½ cup shredded (35 g)	0.05
Cabbage, green, raw—½ cup shredded (35 g)	0.04
Carrots	
Raw—1 med (72 g)	0.32
Boiled—½ cup slices (78 g)	0.33
Cauliflower, raw—½ cup pieces (50 g)	0.02
Celery, raw—1 stalk (7.5″ long) (40 g)	0.14
Corn, sweet, yellow/white, cnd—½ cup (128 g)	0.05
Corn, sweet, yellow/white, frzn—½ cup (82 g)	0.02
Cucumber, raw—½ cup slices (⅙ cucumber) (52 g)	0.08
Dandelion greens, raw—½ cup chopped (28 g)	0.70
Eggplant, raw—½ cup pieces (41 g)	0.01
Garden cress, raw—½ cup (25 g)	0.18
Garlic, raw—3 cloves (9 g)	0.001
Green beans (snap beans)	
Raw—½ cup (55 g)	0.01
Cnd—½ cup (68 g)	0.03
Frzn—½ cup (62 g)	0.06
Frzn, boiled—½ cup (68 g)	0.09
Leeks, raw—¼ cup chopped (26 g)	0.24
Lettuce, iceberg, raw—¼ head (135 g)	0.54
Mushrooms, raw—½ cup pieces (35 g)	0.03
Mustard greens, raw—½ cup chopped (28 g)	0.56
Onion rings, frzn, heated—7 rings (70 g)	0.48
Vegetables (continued)	
Onions, raw—½ cup chopped (80 g)	0.25
Parsley, raw—½ cup chopped (30 g)	0.52
Parsnips, raw—½ cup (67 g)	0.67
Peas, green	
Raw—½ cup (78 g)	0.10
Frzn—½ cup (72 g)	0.09
Frzn, boiled—½ cup (80 g)	0.10
Peppers, sweet raw—½ cup chopped (50 g)	0.34
Potato	
Raw w/o skin—1 potato (112 g)	0.07
Baked w/o skin—1 potato (156 g)	0.05
Boiled w/o skin—1 potato (135 g)	0.05
French fried, frzn, heated—10 pieces (50 g)	0.10
Pumpkin, raw—½ cup (58 g)	0.58
Rutabaga, boiled—½ cup cubes (85 g)	0.13
Seaweed, kelp (kombu/tangle), raw—3.5 oz (100 g)	0.87
Spinach	
Raw—½ cup chopped (28 g)	0.53
Cnd—½ cup (107 g)	0.02
Squash, winter, all varieties, baked—½ cup cubes (102 g)	0.12
Sweet potato, raw—1 med (130 g)	5.93
Tomato, red, raw—1 tomato (123 g)	0.42
Turnip greens, raw—½ cup chopped (28 g)	0.63
Watercress, raw—½ cup chopped (17 g)	0.17

*From Pennington JAT. Bowes and Church's food values of portions commonly used, 17th ed. Philadelphia: JB Lippincott, 1989, pp. 284–285.

†Specified as tocopherols.

APPENDIX 50 PROVISIONAL TABLE ON THE VITAMIN K CONTENT OF FOODS (100 GRAMS EDIBLE PORTION)

FOOD ITEM	VITAMIN K
	μg/100 g
Apples, raw:	
Unpeeled	4
Peeled	0.46
Asparagus spears:	
Raw	39
Frozen	27
Bananas, raw	0.5
Beans, mung:	
Mature seeds, dry	170
Mature seeds, sprouted, raw	33
Beans, snap:	
Raw	28
Frozen	32
Beef, raw:	
Ground, regular	4
Ground, lean	0.6
Beef heart, raw	0
Beef kidney, raw	0
Beets, raw	5
Blueberries, canned	0.5
Broccoli, spears:	
Raw	154
Frozen	68
Cabbage, raw	149
Carrots, raw	13
Cauliflower, raw	191
Chicken breast, raw	0.01
Chickpeas:	
Mature seeds, dry	264
Mature seeds, sprouted, raw	48
Cola:	
Regular	0.01
Diet	0
Corn, sweet, yellow, raw	7
Cranberry juice	< 0.005
Cranberry sauce	1.4
Cucumbers, raw	5
Eggs:	
Whole	50
Yolk	147
White	0.02
Farina, dry	0.15
Fruit juice blend	< 0.005
Garlic powder	0.72
Ginger ale, regular	0.01
Grapefruit juice	0.02
Honey	0.02
Kale, raw	275
Lentils:	
Mature seeds, dry	264
Mature seeds, sprouted, raw	48
Lettuce, iceberg, raw	113
Lemonade	0.03
Liver, raw:	
Beef	104
Chicken	80
Lamb	0
Pork	88
Rabbit	35
Turkey	0
Veal	27
Milk, cow:	
Whole	4
Skim	4
Nonfat dry, regular	10
Milk, human	2
Mushrooms, raw	8
Mustard, dry	0.3
Nettle leaves, raw	372
Oats, rolled, dry	63
Oils:	
Almond	7
Canola	830
Coconut	10
Corn	5
Cottonseed	0
Olive	58
Palm	8
Peanut	2
Safflower	7
Sesame	12
Sunflower	10
Soybean	200
Walnut	16
Onions, mature, raw	0.52
Oranges, raw	1.35
Orange juice, fresh	0.04
Peaches, canned	3
Peanut butter	0.11
Pears, canned	0.46
Peas:	
Mature seeds, dry	81
Mature seeds, sprouted, raw	28
Pork, lean, raw	0.01
Potatoes, baked:	
Flesh and skin	0.53
Flesh	0.22
Pumpkin, canned	15
Rice flour:	
Brown, regular	0.04
White, regular	0.05
White, instant	0.01
Salt	0.01
Seaweed, raw:	
Dulse (*Rhocimeria palmenta*)	255
Rockweed (*Ascophyllum nodosum*)	255
Seagrass (*Enteromorpha clathrata*)	246
Sealettuce (*Ulva lactuca*)	68
Soybean, mature seeds, dry	190
Spinach:	
Raw	266
Frozen	138
Strawberries, raw	14
Sugar	0.01
Sweet potatoes, raw	4
Tea, black, brewed	0.05
Tea, black, decaffeinated, brewed	0.02
Tomatoes, raw:	
Green	47
Ripe	23
Vinegar	< 0.005
Wheat:	
Whole grain	20
Bran, crude	83
Germ, crude	39
Flour, all purpose	0.5
Flour, whole wheat	1.1
Starch	0.15
Wine, sherry	< 0.005

APPENDIX 51 MULTIPLE VITAMIN-MINERAL PREPARATIONS

	VITAMINS													MINERALS								
	A (IU)	D (IU)	E (IU)	K (μg)	C (mg)	FA (μg)	B_1 (mg)	B_2 (mg)	B_6 (mg)	Niacin (mg)	B_{12} (μg)	PA (mg)	Biotin (μg)	Fe (mg)	I (μg)	Zn (mg)	Cu (mg)	Mn (mg)	Cr (μg)	Se (μg)	Mo (μg)	Other
Adult MVI-12 Injection (10 mL, Armour)	3,300	200	10	—	100	400	3	3.6	4	40	5	15	60									
Peds IV MV's (5 mL, Armour)	2,300	400	7	200	80	140	1.2	1.4	1	17	1	5	20									
Centrum Liquid (15 mL, Lederle)	2,500	400	30	—	60	—	1.5	1.7	2	20	6	10	300	9	150	3	—	2.5	25	—	25	—
Theragran Liquid (5 mL, Squibb)	10,000	400	—	—	200	—	10	10	4.1	100	5	21.4	—	—	—	—	—	—	—	—	—	
Vi-Daylin Liquid (5 mL, Ross)	2,500	400	15	—	60	—	1.05	1.2	1.05	13.5	4.5	—	—	—	—	—	—	—	—	—	—	
Tri-Vi-Sol Drops (1 mL, Mead Johnson Nutritional)	1,500	400	—	—	35	—	—	—	—	—	—	—	—	10								
Poly-Vi-Sol Drops (1 mL, Mead Johnson Nutritional)	1,500	400	5	—	35	—	0.5	0.6	0.4	8	2	—	—									
Poly-Vi-Sol + Fe Drops (1 mL, Mead Johnson Nutritional)	1,500	400	5	—	35	—	0.5	0.6	0.4	8	—	—	—	10								
Vi-Daylin Drops (1 mL, Ross)	1,500	400	4.1	—	35	—	0.5	0.6	0.4	8	1.5	—	—									
Vi-Daylin + Fe Drops (1 mL, Ross)	1,500	400	4.1	—	35	—	0.5	0.6	0.4	8	—	—	—	10								
Flintstones (Chewable, Miles)	2,500	400	15	—	60	300	1.05	1.2	1.05	13.5	4.5	—	—									
Flintstones + Iron (Chewable, Miles)	2,500	400	15	—	60	300	1.05	1.2	1.05	13.5	4.5	—	—	15								
Poly-Vi-Sol (Chewable, Mead Johnson Nutritional)	2,500	400	15	—	60	300	1.05	1.2	1.05	13.5	4.5	—	—									
Poly-Vi-Sol + Iron (Chewable, Mead Johnson Nutritional)	2,500	400	15	—	60	300	1.05	1.2	1.05	13.5	4.5	—	—	12								

APPENDIX 51 MULTIPLE VITAMIN-MINERAL PREPARATIONS *(continued)*

	VITAMINS													MINERALS								
	A (IU)	D (IU)	E (IU)	K (µg)	C (mg)	FA (µg)	B_1 (mg)	B_2 (mg)	B_6 (mg)	Niacin (mg)	B_{12} (µg)	PA (mg)	Biotin (µg)	Fe (mg)	I (µg)	Zn (mg)	Cu (mg)	Mn (mg)	Cr (µg)	Se (µg)	Mo (µg)	Other
Theragran-M (Tablet, Squibb)	5,000	400	30	—	90	400	3	3.4	3	20	9	10	35	27	150	15	2	5	15	10	15	400 mg Ca 31 mg P
Centrum (Tablet, Lederle)	5,000	400	30	2.5	60	400	1.5	1.7	2	20	6	10	30	18	150	15	2	2.5	25	20	25	100 mg Mg 7.5 mg Cl 7.5 mg K 162 mg Ca 109 mg P 100 mg Mg 40 mg K 36 mg Cl 5 µg Ni 10 µg Tn 20 mg Si 10 µg V 150 µg B
One-A-Day Essential (Tablet, Miles)	5,000	400	30	—	60	400	1.5	1.7	2.0	20	6.0	10	—									—
Theragran (Tablet, Squibb)	5,000	400	30	—	90	400	3	3.4	3	30	9	10	35									1,250 IU β-carotene
Nephro Vite (Tablet, R and D Laboratories)	—	—	—	—	60	800	10	1.7	10	20	6	10	300	—	—	—	—	—	—	—	—	—
Materna (Tablet, Lederle)	5,000	400	30	—	100	1,000	3	3.4	10	20	12	10	30	60	150	25	2.0	5.0	25	—	25	250 mg Ca 25 mg Mg

APPENDIX 52 PROVISIONAL TABLE ON THE SELENIUM CONTENT OF FOODS (100 GRAMS EDIBLE PORTION)

FOOD ITEM	MEAN (μg)
Baked Products	
Bagels	32.0
Biscuits, refrigerated dough, baked	17.8
Bread:	
Cornbread mix	5.6
Prepared	9.9
Cracked-wheat	25.3
French or Vienna	31.5
Italian	27.2
Pita:	
White	27.1
Whole-wheat	44.0
Raisin	20.0
Rye	30.9
Wheat	30.9
White	28.2
Whole-wheat	36.6
Bread crumbs, dry, grated, plain	37.7
Bread stuffing, mix, dry	48.0
Cake:	
Chocolate, with chocolate frosting	3.3
Yellow:	
Prepared with chocolate frosting	3.4
Dry mix, pudding-type	2.4
Prepared with white frosting	3.3
Coffeecake	17.2
Cookies:	
Animal crackers	7.0
Chocolate chip	6.0
Chocolate sandwich with creme filling	5.0
Fig bars	3.3
Graham crackers	10.2
Oatmeal	9.8
Peanut butter:	
Regular	5.9
Soft	4.4
Refrigerated dough, baked	5.1
Peanut butter sandwich	7.7
Sugar	2.1
Vanilla wafers	11.3
Crackers:	
Cheese	8.6
Melba toast	34.8
Rye wafers	23.8
Saltines	11.7
Standard snack-type:	
Regular	6.6
Sandwich with peanut butter filling	4.8
Wheat	6.3
Whole-wheat	14.7
Danish pastry or sweet rolls	17.0
Doughnuts:	
Cake-type	9.3
Yeast-leavened	19.8
English muffins	20.1
Toasted	27.0
French toast, frozen	16.7
Ice cream cone	4.8
Muffins:	
Plain or blueberry	11.2
Corn	15.2
Baked Products (continued)	
Pancake mix	12.9
Prepared	9.8
Pie:	
Apple	1.0
Pumpkin	2.6
Rolls:	
Dinner	27.2
Hamburger or hot dog	26.5
Hard	39.1
Toaster pastries, fruit	4.4
Tortillas:	
Corn	5.5
Flour	23.4
Waffles, frozen, toasted	16.0
Beef Products	
Retail cuts:	
Chuck, separable lean:	
Raw	16.6
Cooked, braised	26.7
Cooked, roasted	24.0
Rib, whole, separable lean, raw	17.1
Round, full cut, separable lean, raw	20.8
Round, bottom round, separable lean, cooked, braised	28.1
T-bone, top loin, tenderloin, porterhouse: separable lean, raw	17.8
Top sirloin, separable lean:	
Raw	19.8
Cooked, broiled	32.9
Cooked, pan-cooked	23.6
Ground:	
Extra lean, raw	13.9
Lean:	
Raw	15.7
Cooked, broiled, medium	29.0
Regular:	
Raw	12.7
Cooked, baked	19.4
Variety meats:	
Kidneys, raw	148.8
Liver:	
Raw	41.3
Cooked, pan-fried	57.0
Beverages	
Beer	1.2
Cola, carbonated	.1
Chocolate-flavor mix, powder	2.6
Cocoa mix, prepared with water	.4
Coffee, brewed	.1
Coffee, instant powder	12.6
Fruit punch drink, canned	.0
Orange drink, canned	.0
Orange-flavor drink, powder, prepared with water	.1
Shake, fast-food, chocolate	1.7
Tea:	
Brewed	.0
Instant, unsweetened, powder	5.3
Thirst-quencher drink, bottled	.3
Wine, white	.2

APPENDIX 52 PROVISIONAL TABLE ON THE SELENIUM CONTENT OF FOODS (100 GRAMS EDIBLE PORTION) *(continued)*

FOOD ITEM	MEAN (μg)
Breakfast Cereals	
Cereals, ready-to-eat:	
All-Bran®	9.4
Bran Buds®	28.9
Bran Flakes, Kellogg's®	10.5
Cheerios®	37.5
Corn Chex®	3.5
Corn Flakes, Kellogg's®	5.1
Corn Pops®	6.5
Froot Loops®	7.3
Frosted Flakes, Kellogg's®	4.4
Frosted Mini-Wheats®	4.1
Golden Crisp®	48.6
Granola, commercial, plain	20.3
Grape-Nuts Brand Cereal®	9.6
Honey Nut Cheerios®	23.5
Life®	23.6
Lucky Charms®	19.8
Multi-Bran Chex®	9.0
100% Bran, Nabisco®	8.0
100% Natural Cereal®	17.3
Product 19®	12.0
Raisin Bran	7.0
Rice Chex®	3.9
Rice Krispies®	15.4
Rice, puffed	10.5
Special K®	54.9
Wheat germ, toasted	65.0
Wheat, puffed	123.1
Wheat, shredded	5.9
Wheaties®	4.7
Cereals, to-be-cooked:	
Corn grits, regular, quick and instant:	
Dry	17.0
Cooked	3.1
Cream of Wheat®:	
Regular, dry	20.0
Quick, cooked	12.8
Instant, cooked	11.4
Farina:	
Dry	23.5
Cooked	9.1
Oats, regular, quick, and instant:	
Dry	34.0
Cooked	8.1
Cereal Grains and Pasta	
Cereal grains:	
Bulgur, dry	2.3
Corn	15.5
Corn flour, masa	15.0
Cornmeal, degermed	7.8
Cornstarch	2.8
Oat bran	45.2
Rice, brown:	
Raw	23.4
Cooked	9.8
Rice, white:	
Regular:	
Raw	15.1
Cooked	7.5
Cereal Grains and Pasta (continued)	
Rice, white (continued):	
Parboiled:	
Dry	23.0
Cooked	8.2
Precooked or instant:	
Dry	46.9
Prepared	4.2
Rice bran	15.6
Rye flour	35.7
Wheat bran	77.6
Wheat germ	79.2
Wheat flour:	
Whole-grain	70.7
White:	
All-purpose	33.9
Bread	39.7
Cake	4.9
Wild rice, raw	2.8
Pasta:	
Macaroni or spaghetti:	
Dry	62.2
Cooked	21.3
Noodles, Chinese, chow mein	43.0
Noodles, egg:	
Dry	59.2
Cooked	21.7
Dairy and Egg Products	
Cheese:	
Cheddar	13.9
Cottage, creamed	9.0
Cream	2.4
Feta	15.0
Mozzarella, low-moisture, part-skim	16.3
Parmesan, grated	26.2
Pasteurized process, American:	
Cheese	14.4
Cheese food	16.1
Cheese spread	11.3
Swiss	12.7
Cream:	
Sour, cultured	2.2
Sweet, fluid:	
Half and half	1.8
Light, coffee or table	.6
Cream substitute, powdered	.6
Milk, cow:	
Fluid:	
Whole (3.3% fat)	2.0
Low fat, 2% fat	2.2
Skim	2.1
Buttermilk, cultured	2.0
Chocolate, low fat	1.9
Dry, nonfat	27.3
Evaporated, whole, canned	2.3
Milk, human, whole, mature, fluid	1.8
Yogurt, lowfat:	
Plain	3.3
Fruit-flavored	2.3

APPENDIX 52 PROVISIONAL TABLE ON THE SELENIUM CONTENT OF FOODS (100 GRAMS EDIBLE PORTION) *(continued)*

FOOD ITEM	MEAN (μg)
Dairy and Egg Products (continued)	
Eggs:	
Raw:	
Whole	30.8
White	17.6
Yolk	45.2
Cooked:	
Fried	26.9
Scrambled	22.5
Fast Food	
Chicken, breaded, fried, boneless pieces	16.3
Hamburger sandwich:	
Regular, single meat patty, with condiments	19.5
Large, single meat patty:	
Plain	19.8
With condiments and vegetables	15.4
Pizza:	
Cheese	21.4
Sausage	20.6
Fats and Oils	
Lard	.2
Salad dressings:	
Blue cheese	1.0
Mayonnaise	1.7
Thousand Island	2.1
Finfish and Shellfish	
Finfish:	
Catfish, channel, raw	12.6
Cod:	
Raw	33.1
Cooked	37.6
Fish portions and sticks, frozen, reheated	16.6
Flounder:	
Raw	32.7
Cooked	58.2
Haddock:	
Raw	30.2
Cooked	40.5
Mackerel, Atlantic:	
Raw	44.1
Cooked	51.6
Canned	52.8
Ocean perch, raw	43.3
Pollock, walleye, raw	21.9
Salmon, pink:	
Raw	44.6
Canned	33.2
Salmon, sockeye:	
Raw	33.7
Cooked	37.8
Canned, no bones or skin	38.6
Snapper, raw	38.2
Swordfish, raw	48.1
Tuna, canned, drained:	
Light meat:	
In oil	76.0
In water	80.4
White meat:	
In oil	60.1
In water	65.7
Finfish and Shellfish (continued)	
Finfish (continued):	
Whiting, raw	32.1
Shellfish:	
Crustaceans:	
Crab, blue:	
Canned	31.8
Cooked, moist heat	40.2
Shrimp:	
Raw	38.0
Breaded and fried	41.7
Canned, frozen or cooked	39.6
Mollusks:	
Clams, canned, drained	48.6
Oysters:	
Raw	63.7
Cooked	71.6
Scallops, mixed species, raw	22.2
Fruits and Fruit Juices	
Apples, raw	.3
Apple juice, bottled	.1
Applesauce, canned	.3
Avocados	.4
Bananas, raw	1.1
Fruit cocktail, canned, heavy syrup, drained	.5
Grapes, raw	.2
Melons, cantaloupe, raw	.4
Olives, ripe, canned	.9
Oranges, raw	.5
Orange juice, frozen concentrate, diluted with 3 parts water by volume	.1
Peaches, raw	.4
Peaches, canned, heavy syrup, drained	.3
Pears, raw	1.0
Pineapple, raw	.6
Pineapple, canned, drained	.4
Raisins, seedless	.7
Raisins, seeded	.6
Strawberries, frozen, sweetened	.7
Watermelon, raw	.1
Lamb and Veal	
Lamb, separable lean:	
Raw	23.4
Cooked	26.1
Lamb, chops, pan-cooked with added fat	22.9
Lamb kidney, raw	126.9
Lamb liver, raw	82.4
Veal, separable lean, cooked	13.0
Veal cutlet, breaded, pan-fried	13.5
Legumes	
Baked beans, canned	4.7
Beans, great northern:	
Raw	12.9
Cooked	4.1
Beans, kidney, cooked or canned	1.2
Beans, lima, large:	
Raw	7.2
Cooked	4.5

APPENDIX 52 PROVISIONAL TABLE ON THE SELENIUM CONTENT OF FOODS (100 GRAMS EDIBLE PORTION) *(continued)*

FOOD ITEM	MEAN (μg)
Legumes (continued)	
Beans, navy:	
Raw	11.0
Cooked	5.8
Beans, pinto:	
Raw	18.5
Cooked or canned	7.1
Cowpeas:	
Raw	9.0
Cooked	2.5
Canned	2.3
Peas, split, raw	1.6
Peanuts, roasted	7.5
Peanut butter	7.5
Soybeans, roasted	19.1
Soy sauce	.8
Tofu, raw	8.9
Nuts and Seeds	
Almonds	4.7
Brazil nuts	2,960.0
Cashew nuts, roasted	11.4
Coconut, dried, sweetened	16.1
Filberts or hazelnuts	4.0
Pecans	5.2
Sunflower seed kernels:	
Dried	59.5
Roasted	78.2
Walnuts, black	17.0
Walnuts, English	4.6
Pork Products	
Pork, fresh:	
Separable lean. (*See* individual cuts.)	
Separable fat:	
Raw	8.0
Cooked	16.3
Loin:	
Whole, separable, lean, roasted	35.1
Backribs, separable lean and fat:	
Raw	24.0
Roasted	39.3
Blade or country-style ribs, separate lean only:	
Raw	32.6
Roasted	42.3
Center loin (loin chops or roast), separable lean only:	
Raw	32.5
Broiled	47.3
Center rib (ribs or roasts), separable lean only:	
Raw	35.4
Roasted, bone-in or boneless	43.2
Broiled (*See* Center loin, broiled.)	
Sirloin, separable lean only:	
Raw	33.2
Broiled	51.6
Roasted	43.1
Tenderloin, separable lean only:	
Raw	28.9
Roasted	48.1
Toploin (loin chops, boneless), separable lean only:	
Raw (*See* Center loin, raw.)	
Broiled (*See* Center loin, broiled.)	
Roasted	48.2
Pork Products (continued)	
Pork, fresh (continued):	
Shoulder:	
Blade, Boston, separable lean only:	
Raw	28.9
Broiled	39.3
Ground:	
Raw	24.6
Cooked	35.4
Pork kidney, raw	190.0
Pork products, cured:	
Bacon:	
Raw	25.0
Cooked	24.7
Canadian-style bacon	25.0
Ham, canned	29.8
Ham, center slice, lean only, unheated	21.4
Ham, fully cooked, separable lean only, roasted	25.4
Poultry	
Chicken:	
Flesh and skin, cooked:	
Fried, flour-coated	21.7
Roasted	23.9
Livers:	
Raw	64.1
Cooked, broiled	70.9
Parts:	
Breast, meat only, roasted	27.6
Thigh, meat only, roasted	29.0
Turkey:	
Dark meat, without skin, roasted	40.9
Light meat, without skin, roasted	32.1
Sausages and Luncheon Meats	
Bologna, beef or beef and pork	11.3
Chicken roll	12.5
Frankfurters:	
Beef or beef and pork	13.8
Chicken	18.4
Ham, chopped	17.4
Ham, sliced	16.4
Kielbasa, Polish sausage	17.7
Liverwurst	58.0
Luncheon meat:	
Beef, sliced	28.2
Pork, canned	28.0
Pork sausage, fresh:	
Raw	11.5
Cooked	18.2
Salami, cooked	14.6
Turkey breast meat	30.8
Snacks and Sweets	
Snacks:	
Corn-based, extruded:	
Chips or tortilla chips	6.7
Puffs or twists, cheese-flavor	3.0
Popcorn, oil-popped	7.3
Potato chips	8.1
Pretzels, hard	5.8

APPENDIX 52 PROVISIONAL TABLE ON THE SELENIUM CONTENT OF FOODS (100 GRAMS EDIBLE PORTION) *(continued)*

FOOD ITEM	MEAN (μg)
Snacks and Sweets (continued)	
Sweets:	
Candies:	
Caramels	1.8
KIT KAT® Wafer Bar	4.7
Milk chocolate	3.9
SNICKERS® Bar	4.6
Cocoa, dry powder, unsweetened	14.3
Desserts:	
Egg custard, dry mix, prepared	14.1
Gelatins:	
Dry mix	6.7
Prepared with water	.3
Dry powder, unsweetened	39.5
Pudding, chocolate, dry mix, instant or regular, prepared	1.7
Frozen desserts:	
Ice cream, chocolate	2.5
Ice cream sandwich	3.2
Ice milk, vanilla	2.8
Honey	.8
Molasses	17.8
Sugars:	
Brown	1.2
Granulated	.6
Syrup, pancake	.7
Soups, Sauces, and Gravies	
Soups, canned:	
Bean with pork or bacon, condensed	6.4
Beef bouillon, prepared with water	.7
Beef noodle, condensed	5.9
Chicken broth, prepared with water	.0
Chicken noodle, condensed	9.8
Prepared with water	2.6
New England clam chowder, condensed	8.4
Mushroom, cream of, condensed	1.2
Tomato, condensed	.4
Prepared with milk	.9
Vegetarian vegetable, prepared with water	1.8
Vegetable beef, condensed	2.2
Prepared with water	1.8
Sauces:	
Barbecue, ready-to-serve	1.3
Cheese, dehydrated	13.6
Horseradish, prepared	2.8
Mustard, prepared	36.0
Sweet and sour, prepared	.4
Gravies:	
Beef	1.0
Chicken	.8
Vegetables	
Asparagus:	
Raw	2.3
Cooked; canned, drained; or frozen	1.7
Beans, lima, frozen	1.7
Beans, mung, mature seeds, sprouted, canned, drained	.6
Beans, snap:	
Raw	.6
Cooked; canned, drained; or frozen	.4

FOOD ITEM	MEAN (μg)
Vegetables (continued)	
Broccoli:	
Raw	3.0
Cooked or frozen	1.9
Cabbage:	
Raw	.9
Cooked	.6
Carrots:	
Raw	1.1
Cooked	.8
Cauliflower:	
Raw	.6
Frozen	.8
Celery, raw	.9
Collards, canned, drained; or frozen	1.4
Corn, sweet:	
Raw	.6
Cooked; canned, drained; or frozen	.7
Cowpeas, frozen, cooked	3.4
Eggplant:	
Raw	.3
Cooked	.4
Garlic, raw	14.2
Lettuce, raw	.2
Mushrooms:	
Raw	12.3
Cooked	11.9
Canned, drained	4.1
Mustard greens, canned, drained; or frozen	.7
Onions:	
Raw	.6
Canned, drained; frozen; cooked	.4
Onion rings, frozen, prepared	3.5
Peas, green:	
Canned, drained; or frozen	1.7
Frozen, cooked	1.0
Potatoes:	
Raw	.3
Baked	.8
Canned, drained	.9
Frozen, French-fried, heated in oven	.4
Potatoes, mashed, dehydrated:	
Dry	26.3
Prepared	1.4
Spinach:	
Raw	1.0
Cooked	1.5
Sweet potatoes:	
Raw	.6
Cooked or canned	.7
Tomatoes:	
Raw	.4
Canned	.7
Tomato juice or vegetable juice cocktail	.5
Tomato catsup	.8
Tomato sauce	.6
Turnips, raw	.7
Turnip greens, frozen	.9
Vegetables, mixed, canned, drained; or frozen, cooked	.3
Miscellaneous	
Yeast, baker's	8.1

APPENDIX 53 EXCHANGE LIST FOR MEAL PLANNING

MEAL PLAN

Meal Plan for: ______________________ Date: ______________

Dietitian: ______________________ Phone: ______________

	Grams	Percent
Carbohydrate	______	______
Protein	______	______
Fat	______	______
Calories	______	______

Time	Number of Exchanges/Choices	Menu Ideas	Menu Ideas
	______ Carbohydrate group ______ Starch ______ Fruit ______ Milk ______ ______ Meat group ______ ______ Fat group ______		
	______ ______ ______ ______		
	______ Carbohydrate group ______ Starch ______ Fruit ______ Milk ______ √ Vegetables ______ Meat group ______ Fat group		
	______ ______ ______ ______ ______ ______		
	______ Carbohydrate group ______ Starch ______ Fruit ______ Milk ______ √ Vegetables ______ Meat group ______ Fat group		
	______ ______ ______ ______ ______ ______		

Starch List

Cereals, grains, pasta, breads, crackers, snacks, starchy vegetables, and cooked dried beans, peas, and lentils are starches. In general, one starch is:

- ½ cup of cereal, grain, pasta, or starchy vegetable,
- 1 oz. of a bread product, such as 1 slice of bread,
- ¾ to 1 ounce of most snack foods. (Some snack foods may also have added fat.)

Nutrition Tips

1. Most starch choices are good sources of B vitamins.
2. Foods made from whole grains are good sources of fiber.
3. Dried beans and peas are a good source of protein and fiber.

Selection Tips

1. Choose starches made with little fat as often as you can.
2. Starchy vegetables prepared with fat count as one starch and one fat.
3. Bagels or muffins can be 2, 3, or 4 ounces in size, and can, therefore, count as 2, 3, or 4 starch choices. Check the size you eat.
4. Dried beans, peas, and lentils are also found on the Meat and Meat Substitutes list.
5. Regular potato chips and tortilla chips are found on the Other Carbohydrates list.
6. Most of the serving sizes are measured after cooking.
7. Always check Nutrition Facts on the food label.

APPENDIX 53 EXCHANGE LIST FOR MEAL PLANNING *(continued)*

ONE STARCH EXCHANGE EQUALS 15 GRAMS CARBOHYDRATE, 3 GRAMS PROTEIN, 0–1 GRAMS FAT, AND 80 CALORIES.

Bread

Food	Amount
Bagel	½ (1 oz)
Bread, reduced-calorie	2 slices (1½ oz)
Bread, white, whole-wheat, pumpernickel, rye	1 slice (1 oz)
Bread sticks, crisp, 4 in. long × ½ in.	2 (⅔ oz)
English muffin	½
Hot dog or hamburger bun	½ (1 oz)
Pita, 6 in. across	½
Roll, plain, small	1 (1 oz)
Raisin bread, unfrosted	1 slice (1 oz)
Tortilla, corn, 6 in. across	1
Tortilla, flour, 7–8 in. across	1
Waffle, 4½ in. square, reduced-fat	1

Cereals and Grains

Food	Amount
Bran cereals	½ cup
Bulgur	½ cup
Cereals	½ cup
Cereals, unsweetened, ready-to-eat	¾ cup
Cornmeal (dry)	3 Tbsp
Couscous	⅓ cup
Flour (dry)	3 Tbsp
Granola, low-fat	¼ cup
Grape-Nuts	¼ cup
Grits	½ cup
Kasha	½ cup
Millet	¼ cup
Muesli	¼ cup
Oats	½ cup
Pasta	½ cup
Puffed cereal	1½ cups
Rice milk	½ cup
Rice, white or brown	⅓ cup
Shredded Wheat	½ cup
Sugar-frosted cereal	½ cup
Wheat germ	3 Tbsp

Starchy Vegetables

Food	Amount
Baked beans	⅓ cup
Corn	½ cup
Corn on cob, medium	1 (5 oz)
Mixed vegetables with corn, peas, or pasta	1 cup
Peas, green	½ cup
Plantain	½ cup
Potato, baked or boiled	1 small (3 oz)
Potato, mashed	½ cup
Squash, winter (acorn, butternut)	1 cup
Yam, sweet potato, plain	½ cup

Crackers and Snacks

Food	Amount
Animal crackers	8
Graham crackers, 2½ in. square	3
Matzoh	¾ oz
Melba toast	4 slices

Crackers and Snacks (continued)

Food	Amount
Oyster crackers	24
Popcorn (popped, no fat added or low-fat microwave)	3 cups
Pretzels	¾ oz
Rice cakes, 4 in. across	2
Saltine-type crackers	6
Snack chips, fat-free (tortilla, potato)	15–20 (¾ oz)
Whole-wheat crackers, no fat added	2–5 (¾ oz)

Dried Beans, Peas, and Lentils
(Count as 1 starch exchange, plus 1 very lean meat exchange.)

Food	Amount
Beans and peas (garbanzo, pinto, kidney, white, split, black-eyed)	½ cup
Lima beans	⅔ cup
Lentils	½ cup
Miso*	3 Tbsp

Starchy Foods Prepared With Fat
(Count as 1 starch exchange, plus 1 fat exchange.)

Food	Amount
Biscuit, 2½ in. across	1
Chow mein noodles	½ cup
Corn bread, 2 in. cube	1 (2 oz)
Crackers, round butter type	6
Croutons	1 cup
French-fried potatoes	16–25 (3 oz)
Granola	¼ cup
Muffin, small	1 (1½ oz)
Pancake, 4 in. across	2
Popcorn, microwave	3 cups
Sandwich crackers, cheese or peanut butter filling	3
Taco shell, 6 in. across	2
Waffle, 4½ in. square	1
Whole-wheat crackers, fat added	4–6 (1 oz)

Some food you buy uncooked will weigh less after you cook it. Starches often swell in cooking, so a small amount of uncooked starch will become a much larger amount of cooked food. The following table shows some of the changes.

Food (Starch Group)	Uncooked	Cooked
Oatmeal	3 Tbsp	½ cup
Cream of Wheat	2 Tbsp	½ cup
Grits	3 Tbsp	½ cup
Rice	2 Tbsp	⅓ cup
Spaghetti	¼ cup	½ cup
Noodles	⅓ cup	½ cup
Macaroni	¼ cup	½ cup
Dried beans	¼ cup	½ cup
Dried peas	¼ cup	½ cup
Lentils	3 Tbsp	½ cup

Common Measurements

3 tsp = 1 Tbsp	4 ounces = ½ cup
4 Tbsp = ¼ cup	8 ounces = 1 cup
5⅓ Tbsp = ⅓ cup	1 cup = ½ pint

*400 mg or more of sodium per serving.

APPENDIX 53 EXCHANGE LIST FOR MEAL PLANNING *(continued)*

Fruit List

Fresh, frozen, canned, and dried fruits and fruit juices are on this list. In general, one fruit exchange is:

- 1 small to medium fresh fruit,
- ½ cup of canned or fresh fruit or fruit juice,
- ¼ cup of dried fruit.

Nutrition Tips

1. Fresh, frozen, and dried fruits have about 2 grams of fiber per choice. Fruit juices contain very little fiber.
2. Citrus fruits, berries, and melons are good sources of vitamin C.

Selection Tips

1. Count ½ cup cranberries or rhubarb sweetened with sugar substitutes as free foods.
2. Read the Nutrition Facts on the food label. If one serving has more than 15 grams of carbohydrate, you will need to adjust the size of the serving you eat or drink.
3. Portion sizes for canned fruits are for the fruit and a small amount of juice.
4. Whole fruit is more filling than fruit juice and may be a better choice.
5. Food labels for fruits may contain the words "no sugar added" or "unsweetened." This mans that no sucrose (table sugar) has been added.
6. Generally, fruit canned in extra light syrup has the same amount of carbohydrate per serving as the "no sugar added" or the juice pack. All canned fruits on the fruit list are based on one of these three types of pack.

ONE FRUIT EXCHANGE EQUALS 15 GRAMS CARBOHYDRATE AND 60 CALORIES.
THE WEIGHT INCLUDES SKIN, CORE, SEEDS, AND RIND.

Fruit

Apple, unpeeled, small	1 (4 oz)
Applesauce, unsweetened	½ cup
Apples, dried	4 rings
Apricots, fresh	4 whole (5½ oz)
Apricots, dried	8 halves
Apricots, canned	½ cup
Banana, small	1 (4 oz)
Blackberries	¾ cup
Blueberries	¾ cup
Cantaloupe, small	⅓ melon (11 oz) or 1 cup cubes
Cherries, sweet, fresh	12 (3 oz)
Cherries, sweet, canned	½ cup
Dates	3
Figs, fresh	1½ large or 2 medium (3½ oz)
Figs, dried	1½
Fruit cocktail	½ cup
Grapefruit, large	½ (11 oz)
Grapefruit sections, canned	¾ cup
Grapes, small	17 (3 oz)
Honeydew melon	1 slice (10 oz) or 1 cup cubes
Kiwi	1 (3½ oz)
Mandarin oranges, canned	¾ cup
Mango, small	½ fruit (5½ oz) or ½ cup
Nectarine, small	1 (5 oz)
Orange, small	1 (6½ oz)
Papaya	½ fruit (8 oz) or 1 cup cubes
Peach, medium, fresh	1 (6 oz)
Peaches, canned	½ cup
Pear, large, fresh	½ (4 oz)
Pears, canned	½ cup
Pineapple, fresh	¾ cup
Pineapple, canned	½ cup
Plums, small	2 (5 oz)
Plums, canned	½ cup
Prunes, dried	3
Raisins	2 Tbsp
Raspberries	1 cup
Strawberries	1¼ cup whole berries
Tangerines, small	2 (8 oz)
Watermelon	1 slice (13½ oz) or 1¼ cup cubes

Fruit Juice

Apple juice/cider	½ cup
Cranberry juice cocktail	⅓ cup
Cranberry juice cocktail, reduced-calorie	1 cup
Fruit juice blends, 100% juice	⅓ cup
Grape juice	⅓ cup
Grapefruit juice	½ cup
Orange juice	½ cup
Pineapple juice	½ cup
Prune juice	⅓ cup

Milk List

Different types of milk and milk products are on this list. Cheeses are on the Meat list and cream and other dairy fats are on the Fat list. Based on the amount of fat they contain, milks are divided into skim/very low-fat milk, low-fat milk, and whole milk. One choice of these includes:

	Carbohydrate (grams)	Protein (grams)	Fat (grams)	Calories
Skim/very low-fat	12	8	0–3	90
Low-fat	12	8	5	120
Whole	12	8	8	150

Nutrition Tips

1. Milk and yogurt are good sources of calcium and protein. Check the food label.
2. The higher the fat content of milk and yogurt, the greater the amount of saturated fat and cholesterol. Choose lower-fat varieties.
3. For those who are lactose intolerant, look for lactose-reduced or lactose-free varieties of milk.

Selection Tips

1. One cup equals 8 fluid ounces or ½ pint.
2. Look for chocolate milk, frozen yogurt, and ice cream on the Other Carbohydrates list.
3. Nondairy creamers are on the Free Foods list.
4. Look for rice milk on the Starch list.
5. Look for soy milk on the Medium-fat Meat list.

APPENDIX 53 EXCHANGE LIST FOR MEAL PLANNING *(continued)*

ONE MILK EXCHANGE EQUALS 12 GRAMS CARBOHYDRATE AND 8 GRAMS PROTEIN.

Skim and Very Low-fat Milk
(0–3 grams fat per serving)

Skim milk	1 cup
½% milk	1 cup
1% milk	1 cup
Nonfat or low-fat buttermilk	1 cup
Evaporated skim milk	½ cup
Nonfat dry milk	⅓ cup dry
Plain nonfat yogurt	¾ cup
Nonfat or low-fat fruit-flavored yogurt sweetened with aspartame or with a nonnutritive sweetener	1 cup

Low-fat
(5 grams fat per serving)

2% milk	1 cup
Plain low-fat yogurt	¾ cup
Sweet acidophilus milk	1 cup

Whole Milk
(8 grams fat per serving)

Whole milk	1 cup
Evaporated whole milk	½ cup
Goat's milk	1 cup
Kefir	1 cup

Other Carbohydrates List

You can substitute food choices from this list for a starch, fruit, or milk choice on your meal plan. Some choices will also count as one or more fat choices.

Nutrition Tips

1. These foods can be substituted in your meal plan, even though they contain added sugars or fat. However, they do not contain as many important vitamins and minerals as the choices on the Starch, Fruit, or Milk list.
2. When planning to include these foods in your meal, be sure to include foods from all the lists to eat a balanced meal.

Selection Tips

1. Because many of these foods are concentrated sources of carbohydrate and fat, the portion sizes are often very small.
2. Always check Nutrition Facts on the food label. It will be your most accurate source of information.
3. Many fat-free or reduced-fat products made with fat replacers contain carbohydrate. When eaten in large amounts, they may need to be counted. Talk with your dietitian to determine how to count these in your meal plan.
4. Look for fat-free salad dressings in smaller amounts on the Free Foods list.

ONE EXCHANGE EQUALS 15 GRAMS CARBOHYDRATE, OR 1 STARCH, OR 1 FRUIT, OR 1 MILK.

Food	Serving Size	Exchanges Per Serving
Angel food cake, unfrosted	1⁄12 cake	2 carbohydrates
Brownie, small, unfrosted	2 in. square	1 carbohydrate, 1 fat
Cake, unfrosted	2 in. square	1 carbohydrate, 1 fat
Cake, frosted	2 in. square	2 carbohydrates, 1 fat
Cookie, fat-free	2 small	1 carbohydrate
Cookie or sandwich cookie with creme filling	2 small	1 carbohydrate, 1 fat
Cupcake, frosted	1 small	2 carbohydrates, 1 fat
Cranberry sauce, jellied	¼ cup	2 carbohydrates
Doughnut, plain cake	1 medium (1½ oz)	1½ carbohydrates, 2 fats
Doughnut, glazed	3¾ in. across (2 oz)	2 carbohydrates, 2 fats
Fruit juice bars, frozen, 100% juice	1 bar (3 oz)	1 carbohydrate
Fruit snacks, chewy (pureed fruit concentrate)	1 roll (¾ oz)	1 carbohydrate
Fruit spreads, 100% fruit	1 Tbsp	1 carbohydrate
Gelatin, regular	½ cup	1 carbohydrate
Gingersnaps	3	1 carbohydrate
Granola bar	1 bar	1 carbohydrate, 1 fat
Granola bar, fat-free	1 bar	2 carbohydrates
Hummus	⅓ cup	1 carbohydrate, 1 fat
Ice cream	½ cup	1 carbohydrate, 2 fats
Ice cream, light	½ cup	1 carbohydrate, 1 fat
Ice cream, fat-free, no sugar added	½ cup	1 carbohydrate
Jam or jelly, regular	1 Tbsp	1 carbohydrate
Milk, chocolate, whole	1 cup	2 carbohydrates, 1 fat
Pie, fruit, 2 crusts	⅙ pie	3 carbohydrates, 2 fats
Pie, pumpkin or custard	⅛ pie	1 carbohydrate, 2 fats
Potato chips	12–18 (1 oz)	1 carbohydrate, 2 fats
Pudding, regular (made with low-fat milk)	½ cup	2 carbohydrates
Pudding, sugar-free (made with low-fat milk)	½ cup	1 carbohydrate
Salad dressing, fat-free	¼ cup	1 carbohydrate
Sherbet, sorbet	½ cup	2 carbohydrates
Spaghetti or pasta sauce, canned	½ cup	1 carbohydrate, 1 fat
Sweet roll or Danish	1 (2½ oz)	2½ carbohydrates, 2 fats
Syrup, light	2 Tbsp	1 carbohydrate
Syrup, regular	1Tbsp	1 carbohydrate
Syrup, regular	¼ cup	4 carbohydrates
Tortilla chips	6–12 (1 oz)	1 carbohydrate, 2 fats

APPENDIX 53 EXCHANGE LIST FOR MEAL PLANNING *(continued)*

ONE EXCHANGE EQUALS 15 GRAMS CARBOHYDRATE, OR 1 STARCH, OR 1 FRUIT, OR 1 MILK. ***(continued)***

Food	Serving Size	Exchanges Per Serving
Yogurt, frozen, low-fat, fat-free	⅓ cup	1 carbohydrate, 0–1 fat
Yogurt, frozen, fat-free, no sugar added	½ cup	1 carbohydrate
Yogurt, low-fat with fruit	1 cup	3 carbohydrates, 0–1 fat
Vanilla wafers	5	1 carbohydrate, 1 fat

Vegetable List

Vegetables that contain small amounts of carbohydrates and calories are on this list. Vegetables contain important nutrients. Try to eat at least 2 or 3 vegetable choices each day. In general, one vegetable exchange is:

- ½ cup of cooked vegetables or vegetable juice,
- 1 cup of raw vegetables.

If you eat 1 to 2 vegetable choices at a meal or snack, you do not have to count the calories or carbohydrates because they contain small amounts of these nutrients.

Nutrition Tips

1. Fresh and frozen vegetables have less added salt than canned vegetables. Drain and rinse canned vegetables if you want to remove some salt.
2. Choose more dark green and dark yellow vegetables, such as spinach, broccoli, romaine, carrots, chilies, and peppers.
3. Broccoli, brussels sprouts, cauliflower, greens, peppers, spinach, and tomatoes are good sources of vitamin C.
4. Vegetables contain 1 to 4 grams of fiber per serving.

Selection Tips

1. A 1-cup portion of broccoli is a portion about the size of a light bulb.
2. Tomato sauce is different from spaghetti sauce, which is on the Other Carbohydrates list.
3. Canned vegetables and juices are available without added salt.
4. If you eat more than 4 cups of raw vegetables or 2 cups of cooked vegetables at one meal, count them as 1 carbohydrate choice.
5. Starchy vegetables such as corn, peas, winter squash, and potatoes that contain larger amounts of calories and carbohydrates are on the Starch list.

ONE VEGETABLE EXCHANGE EQUALS 5 GRAMS CARBOHYDRATE, 2 GRAMS PROTEIN, 0 GRAMS FAT, AND 25 CALORIES.

Artichoke
Artichoke hearts
Asparagus
Beans (green, wax, Italian)
Bean sprouts
Beets
Broccoli
Brussels sprouts
Cabbage
Carrots
Cauliflower
Celery
Cucumber
Eggplant
Green onions or scallions
Greens (collard, kale, mustard, turnip)
Kohlrabi
Leeks
Mixed vegetables (without corn, peas, or pasta)
Mushrooms
Okra
Onions
Pea pods
Peppers (all varieties)
Radishes
Salad greens (endive, escarole, lettuce, romaine, spinach)
Sauerkraut*
Spinach
Summer squash
Tomato
Tomatoes, canned
Tomato sauce*
Tomato/vegetable juice*
Turnips
Water chestnuts
Watercress
Zucchini

Meat and Meat Substitutes List

Meat and meat substitutes that contain both protein and fat are on this list. In general, one meat exchange is:

- 1 oz meat, fish, poultry, or cheese,
- ½ cup dried beans.

Based on the amount of fat they contain, meats are divided into very lean, lean, medium-fat, and high-fat lists. This is done so you can see which ones contain the least amount of fat. One ounce (one exchange) of each of these includes:

	Carbohydrate (grams)	Protein (grams)	Fat (grams)	Calories
Very lean	0	7	0–1	35
Lean	0	7	3	55
Medium-fat	0	7	5	75
High-fat	0	7	8	100

Nutrition Tips

1. Choose very lean and lean meat choices whenever possible. Items from the high-fat group are high in saturated fat, cholesterol, and calories and can raise blood cholesterol levels.
2. Meats do not have any fiber.
3. Dried beans, peas, and lentils are good sources of fiber.
4. Some processed meats, seafood, and soy products may contain carbohydrate when consumed in large amounts. Check the Nutrition Facts on the label to see if the amount is close to 15 grams. If so, count it as a carbohydrate choice as well as a meat choice.

Selection Tips

1. Weigh meat after cooking and removing bones and fat. Four ounces of raw meat is equal to 3 ounces of cooked meat. Some examples of meat portions are:

- 1 oz cheese = 1 meat choice and is about the size of a 1-inch cube
- 2 oz meat = 2 meat choices, such as
  1 small chicken leg or thigh
  ½ cup cottage cheese or tuna
- 3 oz meat = 3 meat choices and is about the size of a deck of cards, such as
  1 medium pork chop
  1 small hamburger
  ½ of a whole chicken breast
  1 unbreaded fish fillet

* = 400 mg or more sodium per exchange.

APPENDIX 53 EXCHANGE LIST FOR MEAL PLANNING *(continued)*

Meat and Meat Substitutes List (continued)

2. Limit your choices from the high-fat group to three times per week or less.
3. Most grocery stores stock Select and Choice grades of meat. Select grades of meat are the leanest meats. Choice grades contain a moderate amount of fat, and Prime cuts of meat have the highest amount of fat. Restaurants usually serve Prime cuts of meat.
4. "Hamburger" may contain added seasoning and fat, but ground beef does not.
5. Read labels to find products that are low in fat and cholesterol (5 grams or less of fat per serving).
6. Dried beans, peas, and lentils are also found on the Starch list.
7. Peanut butter, in smaller amounts, is also found on the Fats list.
8. Bacon, in smaller amounts, is also found on the Fats list.

Meal Planning Tips

1. Bake, roast, broil, grill, poach, steam, or boil these foods rather than frying.
2. Place meat on a rack so the fat will drain off during cooking.
3. Use a nonstick spray and a nonstick pan to brown or fry foods.
4. Trim off visible fat before or after cooking.
5. If you add flour, bread crumbs, coating mixes, fat, or marinades when cooking, ask your dietitian how to count it in your meal plan.

Very Lean Meat and Substitutes List
One exchange equals 0 grams carbohydrate, 7 grams protein, 0–1 gram fat, and 35 calories.

One very lean meat exchange is equal to any one of the following items.

Poultry: Chicken or turkey (white meat, no skin), Cornish hen (no skin) . . . . . 1 oz
Fish: Fresh or frozen cod, flounder, haddock, halibut, trout; tuna fresh or canned in water . . . . . 1 oz
Shellfish: Clams, crab, lobster, scallops, shrimp, imitation shellfish . . . . . 1 oz
Game: Duck or pheasant (no skin), venison, buffalo, ostrich . . . . . 1 oz
Cheese with 1 gram or less fat per ounce:
- Nonfat or low-fat cottage cheese . . . . . ¼ cup
- Fat-free cheese . . . . . 1 oz

Other: Processed sandwich meats with 1 gram or less fat per ounce, such as deli thin, shaved meats, chipped beef,* turkey ham . . . . . 1 oz
- Egg whites 2
- Egg substitutes, plain . . . . . ¼ cup
- Hot dogs with 1 gram or less fat per ounce* . . . . . 1 oz
- Kidney (high in cholesterol) . . . . . 1 oz

Sausage with 1 gram or less fat per ounce . . . . . 1 oz

Count as one very lean meat and one starch exchange.

Dried beans, peas, lentils (cooked) . . . . . ½ cup

Lean Meat and Substitutes List
One exchange equals 0 grams carbohydrate, 7 grams protein, 3 grams fat, and 55 calories.

One lean meat exchange is equal to any one of the following items.

Beef: USDA Select or Choice grades of lean beef trimmed of fat, such as round, sirloin, and flank steak; tenderloin; roast (rib, chuck, rump); steak (T-bone, porterhouse, cubed), ground round . . . . . 1 oz
Pork: Lean pork, such as fresh ham; canned, cured, or boiled ham; Canadian bacon*; tenderloin, center loin chop . . . . . 1 oz
Lamb: Roast, chop, leg . . . . . 1 oz
Veal: Lean chop, roast . . . . . 1 oz
Poultry: Chicken, turkey (dark meat, no skin), chicken white meat with skin), domestic duck or goose (well-drained of fat, no skin) . . . . . 1 oz
Fish:
- Herring (uncreamed or smoked) . . . . . 1 oz
- Oysters . . . . . 6 medium
- Salmon (fresh or canned), catfish . . . . . 1 oz
- Sardines (canned) . . . . . 2 medium
- Tuna (canned in oil, drained) . . . . . 1 oz

Game: Goose (no skin), rabbit . . . . . 1 oz
Cheese:
- 4.5%-fat cottage cheese . . . . . ¼ cup
- Grated Parmesan . . . . . 2 Tbsp
- Cheeses with 3 grams or less fat per ounce . . . . . 1 oz

Other:
- Hot dogs with 3 grams or less fat per ounce* . . . . . 1½ oz
- Processed sandwich meat with 3 grams or less fat per ounce, such as turkey pastrami or kielbasa . . . . . 1 oz
- Liver, heart (high in cholesterol) . . . . . 1 oz

Medium-Fat and Meat Substitutes List
One exchange equals 0 grams carbohydrate, 7 grams protein, 5 grams fat, and 75 calories.

One medium-fat meat exchange is equal to any one of the following items.

Beef: Most beef products fall into this category (ground beef, meatloaf, corned beef, short ribs, Prime grades of meat trimmed of fat, such as prime rib) . . . . . 1 oz
Pork: Top loin, chop, Boston butt, cutlet . . . . . 1 oz
Lamb: Rib roast, ground . . . . . 1 oz
Veal: Cutlet (ground or cubed, unbreaded) . . . . . 1 oz
Poultry: Chicken dark meat (with skin), ground turkey or ground chicken, fried chicken (with skin) . . . . . 1 oz
Fish: Any fried fish product . . . . . 1 oz
Cheese: With 5 grams or less fat per ounce
- Feta . . . . . 1 oz
- Mozzarella . . . . . 1 oz
- Ricotta . . . . . ¼ cup (2 oz)

Other:
- Egg (high in cholesterol, limit to 3 per week) 1
- Sausage with 5 grams or less fat per ounce . . . . . 1 oz
- Soy milk . . . . . 1 cup
- Tempeh . . . . . ¼ cup
- Tofu . . . . . 4 oz or ½ cup

*1 gram or less fat per ounce = 400 mg or more sodium per exchange.

APPENDIX 53 EXCHANGE LIST FOR MEAL PLANNING *(continued)*

High-Fat Meat and Substitutes List
One exchange equals 0 grams carbohydrate, 7 grams protein, 8 grams fat, and 100 calories.

Remember these items are high in saturated fat, cholesterol, and calories and may raise blood cholesterol levels if eaten on a regular basis. One high-fat meat exchange is equal to any one of the following items.

Pork: Spareribs, ground pork, pork sausage . . . . . 1 oz
Cheese: All regular cheeses, such as American,* cheddar, Monterey Jack, Swiss . . . . . 1 oz
Other: Processed sandwich meats with 8 grams or less fat per ounce, such as bologna, pimento loaf, salami . . . . . 1 oz
Sausage, such as bratwurst, Italian, knockwurst, Polish, smoked . . . . . 1 oz
Hot dog (turkey or chicken)* 1 (10/lb)
Bacon . . . . . 3 slices (20 slices/lb)
Hot dogs with 1 gram or less fat per ounce* . . . . . 1 oz
Kidney (high in cholesterol) . . . . . 1 oz

Count as one high-fat meat plus one fat exchange.

Hot dog (beef, pork, or combination)* 1 (10/lb)
Peanut butter (contains unsaturated fat) . . . . . 2 Tbsp

Fat List

Fats are divided into three groups, based on the main type of fat they contain: monounsaturated, polyunsaturated, and saturated. Small amounts of monounsaturated and polyunsaturated fats in the foods we eat are linked with good health benefits. Saturated fats are linked with heart disease and cancer. In general, one fat exchange is:

- 1 teaspoon of regular margarine or vegetable oil
- 1 tablespoon of regular salad dressings.

Nutrition Tips

1. All fats are high in calories. Limit serving sizes for good nutrition and health.
2. Nuts and seeds contain small amounts of fiber, protein, and magnesium.
3. If blood pressure is a concern, choose fats in the unsalted form to help lower sodium intake, such as unsalted peanuts.

Selection Tips

1. Check the Nutrition Facts on food labels for serving sizes. One fat exchange is based on a serving size containing 5 grams of fat.
2. When selecting regular margarine, choose one with liquid vegetable oil as the first ingredient. Soft margarines are not as saturated as stick margarines. Soft margarines are healthier choices. Avoid those listing hydrogenated or partially hydrogenated fat as the first ingredient.
3. When selecting low-fat margarines, look for liquid vegetable oil as the second ingredient. Water is usually the first ingredient.
4. When used in smaller amounts, bacon and peanut butter are counted as fat choices. When used in larger amounts, they are counted as high-fat meat choices.
5. Fat-free salad dressings are on the Other Carbohydrates list and the Free Foods list.
6. See the Free Foods list for nondairy coffee creamers, whipped topping, and fat-free products, such as margarines, salad dressings, mayonnaise, sour cream, cream cheese, and nonstick cooking spray.

Monounsaturated Fats List
One fat exchange equals 5 grams fat and 45 calories.

Avocado, medium . . . . . ⅛ (1 oz)
Oil (canola, olive, peanut) . . . . . 1 tsp
Olives: ripe (black) . . . . . 8 large
green, stuffed* . . . . . 10 large
Nuts
almonds, cashews . . . . . 6 nuts
mixed (50% peanuts) . . . . . 6 nuts
peanuts . . . . . 10 nuts
pecans . . . . . 4 halves
Peanut butter, smooth or crunchy . . . . . 2 tsp
Sesame seeds . . . . . 1 Tbsp
Tahini paste . . . . . 2 tsp

Polyunsaturated Fats List
One fat exchange equals 5 grams fat and 45 calories.

Margarine: stick, tub, or squeeze . . . . . 1 tsp
lower-fat (30% to 50% vegetable oil) . . . . . 1 Tbsp
Mayonnaise: regular . . . . . 1 tsp
reduced-fat . . . . . 1 Tbsp
Nuts, walnuts, English . . . . . 4 halves
Oil (corn, safflower, soybean) . . . . . 1 tsp
Salad dressing: regular* . . . . . 1 Tbsp
reduced-fat . . . . . 2 Tbsp
Miracle Whip Salad Dressing®: regular . . . . . 2 tsp
reduced-fat . . . . . 1 Tbsp
Seeds: pumpkin, sunflower . . . . . 1 Tbsp

Saturated Fats List†
One fat exchange equals 5 grams fat, and 45 calories.

Bacon, cooked . . . . . 1 slice (20 slices/lb)
Bacon, grease . . . . . 1 tsp
Butter: stick . . . . . 1 tsp
whipped . . . . . 2 tsp
reduced-fat . . . . . 1 Tbsp
Chitterlings, boiled . . . . . 2 Tbsp (½ oz)
Coconut, sweetened, shredded . . . . . 2 Tbsp
Cream, half and half . . . . . 2 Tbsp
Cream cheese: regular . . . . . 1 Tbsp (½ oz)
reduced-fat . . . . . 2 Tbsp (1 oz)
Fatback or salt pork, see below‡
Shortening or lard . . . . . 1 tsp
Sour cream: regular . . . . . 2 Tbsp
reduced-fat . . . . . 3 Tbsp

*1 gram or less fat per ounce = 400 mg or more sodium per exchange.
†Saturated fats can raise blood cholesterol levels.
‡Use a piece 1 in. × 1 in. × ¼ in. if you plan to eat the fatback cooked with vegetables. Use a piece 2 in. × 1 in. × ½ in. when eating only the vegetables with the fatback removed.

APPENDIX 53 EXCHANGE LIST FOR MEAL PLANNING *(continued)*

Free Foods List

A *free food* is any food or drink that contains less than 20 calories or less than 5 grams of carbohydrate per serving. Foods with a serving size listed should be limited to three servings per day. Be sure to spread them out throughout the day. If you eat all three servings at one time, it could affect your blood glucose level. Foods listed without a serving size can be eaten as often as you like.

Fat-free or Reduced-fat Foods

Cream cheese, fat-free	1 Tbsp
Creamers, nondairy, liquid	1 Tbsp
Creamers, nondairy, powdered	2 tsp
Mayonnaise, fat-free	1 Tbsp
Mayonnaise, reduced-fat	1 tsp
Margarine, fat-free	4 Tbsp
Margarine, reduced-fat	1 tsp
Miracle Whip®, nonfat	1 Tbsp
Miracle Whip®, reduced-fat	1 tsp
Nonstick cooking spray	
Salad dressing, fat-free	1 Tbsp
Salad dressing, fat-free, Italian	2 Tbsp
Salsa	¼ cup
Sour cream, fat-free, reduced-fat	1 Tbsp
Whipped topping, regular or light	2 Tbsp

Sugar-free or Low-sugar Foods

Candy, hard, sugar-free	1 candy
Gelatin dessert, sugar-free	
Gelatin, unflavored	
Gum, sugar-free	
Jam or jelly, low-sugar or light	2 tsp
Sugar substitutes[§]	
Syrup, sugar-free	2 Tbsp

Drinks

Bouillon, broth, consommé[‖]	
Bouillon or broth, low-sodium	
Carbonated or mineral water	
Cocoa powder, unsweetened	1 Tbsp
Coffee	
Club soda	
Diet soft drinks, sugar-free	
Drink mixes, sugar-free	
Tea	
Tonic water, sugar-free	

Condiments

Catsup	1 Tbsp
Horseradish	
Lemon juice	
Lime juice	
Mustard	
Pickles, dill*	1½ large
Soy sauce, regular or light*	
Taco sauce	1 Tbsp
Vinegar	

Seasonings

Be careful with seasonings that contain sodium or are salts, such as garlic or celery salt, and lemon pepper.

- Flavoring extracts
- Garlic
- Herbs, fresh or dried
- Pimento
- Spices
- Tobasco® or hot pepper sauce
- Wine, used in cooking
- Worcestershire sauce

Combination Foods List

Many of the foods we eat are mixed together in various combinations. These combination foods do not fit into any one exchange list. Often it is hard to tell what is in a casserole dish or prepared food item. This is a list of exchanges for some typical combination foods. This list will help you fit these foods into your meal plan. Ask your dietitian for information about any other combination foods you would like to eat.

Food	Serving Size	Exchanges Per Serving
Entrees		
Tuna noodle casserole, lasagna, spaghetti with meatballs, chili with beans, macaroni and cheese[†]	1 cup (8 oz)	2 carbohydrates, 2 medium-fat meats
Chow mein (without noodles or rice)	2 cups (16 oz)	1 carbohydrate, 2 lean meats
Pizza, cheese, thin crust[†]	¼ of 10 in (5 oz)	2 carbohydrates, 2 medium-fat meats, 1 fat
Pizza, meat topping, thin crust[†]	¼ of 10 in (5 oz)	2 carbohydrates, 2 medium-fat meats, 2 fats
Pot pie[†]	1 (7 oz)	2 carbohydrates, 1 medium-fat meat, 4 fats
Frozen Entrees		
Salisbury steak with gravy, mashed potato[†]	1 (11 oz)	2 carbohydrates, 3 medium-fat meats, 3–4 fats
Turkey with gravy, mashed potato, dressing[†]	1 (11 oz)	2 carbohydrates, 2 medium-fat meals, 2 fats
Entree with less than 300 calories[†]	1 (8 oz)	2 carbohydrates, 3 lean meats

‖ = 400 mg or more sodium per exchange.

§Sugar substitutes, alternatives, or replacements that are approved by the Food and Drug Administration (FDA) are safe to use. Common brand names include: Equal® (aspartame), Sprinkle Sweet® (saccharin), Sweet One® (acesulfame K), Sweet-10® (saccharin), Sugar Twin® (saccharin), Sweet 'n Low® (saccharin).

* = 400 mg or more sodium per choice.

† = 400 mg or more sodium per exchange.

APPENDIX 53 EXCHANGE LIST FOR MEAL PLANNING *(continued)*

Combination Foods List (continued)

Food	Serving Size	Exchanges Per Serving
Soups		
Bean†	1 cup	1 carbohydrate, 1 very lean meat
Cream (made with water)†	1 cup (8 oz)	1 carbohydrate, 1 fat
Split pea (made with water)†	½ cup (4 oz)	1 carbohydrate
Tomato (made with water)†	1 cup (8 oz)	1 carbohydrate
Vegetable beef, chicken noodle, or other broth-type†	1 cup (8 oz)	1 carbohydrate

Fast Foods‡

Food	Serving Size	Exchanges Per Serving
Burritos with beef‡	2	4 carbohydrates, 2 medium-fat meats, 2 fats
Chicken nuggets‡	6	1 carbohydrate, 2 medium-fat meats, 1 fat
Chicken breast and wing, breaded and fried‡	1 each	1 carbohydrate, 4 medium-fat meats, 2 fats
Fish sandwich/tartar sauce‡	1	3 carbohydrates, 1 medium-fat meat, 3 fats
French fries, thin	20–25	2 carbohydrates, 2 fats
Hamburger, regular	1	2 carbohydrates, 2 medium-fat meats
Hamburger, large‡	1	2 carbohydrates, 3 medium-fat meats, 1 fat
Hot dog with bun‡	1	1 carbohydrate, 1 high-fat meat, 1 fat
Individual pan pizza‡	1	5 carbohydrates, 3 medium-fat meats, 3 fats
Soft-serve cone	1 medium	2 carbohydrates, 1 fat
Submarine sandwich†	1 sub (6 in.)	3 carbohydrates, 1 vegetable, 2 medium-fat meats, 1 fat
Taco, hard shell†	1 (6 oz)	2 carbohydrates, 2 medium-fat meats, 2 fats
Taco, soft shell†	1 (3 oz)	1 carbohydrate, 1 medium-fat meat, 1 fat

† = 400 mg or more sodium per exchange.

‡Ask at fast-food restaurant for nutrition information about favorite fast foods.

The Exchange Lists are the basis of a meal planning system designed by a committee of the American Diabetes Association and The American Dietetic Association. Although designed primarily for people with diabetes and others who must follow special diets, the Exchange Lists are based on principles of good nutrition that apply to everyone.

APPENDIX 54 THE GLYCEMIC INDICES OF FOODS

This table is a listing of the glycemic index (GI) for various foods. The GI values are based on more than 80 studies in the literature and summarized in the references. The GI value is based on the reference food, white bread having a GI of 100. To convert to the other standard often used, glucose, with it being 100, simply multiply the GI given here by 0.7.

FOOD	GLYCEMIC INDEX (GI) (WHITE BREAD = 100 = REFERENCE)
Bakery Products	
Cake, angel food	95
Cake, banana, made with sugar	67
Cake, banana, made without sugar	79
Cake, flan	93
Cake, pound	77
Cake, sponge	66
Croissant	96
Crumpet	98
Doughnut, cake type	108
Muffin	88
Pastry	84
Pizza, cheese	86
Waffle	109
Beverages	
Soy milk	43
Cordial, orange	94
Lucozade	136
Soft drink, Fanta	97
Breads	
Bagel, white	103
Barley kernel bread	57
Barley flour bread	95
Bread stuffing	106
Hamburger bun	87
Kaiser roll	104
Melba toast	100
Oat kernel bread	93
Oat bran bread	68
Rye kernel bread	66
Pumpernickel	71
Rye flour bread	92
Linseed rye bread	78
Wheat bread, white	100
French baguette	136
Wheat bread, high fiber	97
Wheat bread, Wonderwhite	112
Wheat bread, gluten free	129
Wheat bread, wholemeal flour	99
Whole-wheat snack bread	105
Pita bread, white	82
Semolina bread	92
Bulger bread	75
Mixed grain bread	64
Fruit loaf	67
Bürgen Oat Bran & Honey Loaf	43
Bürgen Soy Lin	27
Bürgen Fruit Loaf	62
Bürgen Mixed Grain	48
Holsom's	64
Breakfast Cereals	
All-bran	60
Bran Buds	75
Bran Chex	83
Breakfast bar	109
Cheerios	106
Cocoapops	110
Corn Bran	107

FOOD	GLYCEMIC INDEX (GI) (WHITE BREAD = 100 = REFERENCE)
Breakfast Cereals (continued)	
Corn Chex	118
Cornflakes	119
Cream of Wheat	100
Crispix	124
Golden Grahams	102
Grapenuts	96
Grapenuts Flakes	114
Life	94
Muesli	80
Nutri-grain	94
Oat Bran	78
Oatmeal	87
Pro Stars	102
Puffed Wheat	105
Red River Cereal	70
Rice Bran	27
Rice Bubbles	128
Rice Chex	127
Rice Krispies	117
Shredded Wheat	99
Special K	77
Sultana Bran	74
Sustain	97
Team	117
Total	109
Wheat Biscuit	100
Kellogg's All Bran Fruit 'n Oats	55
Kellogg's Guardian	59
Kellogg's Honey Smacks	78
Kellogg's Mini-Wheats (blackcurrant)	99
Kellogg's Mini-Wheats (whole wheat)	81
Kellogg's Just Right	84
Kellogg's Special K	77
Cereal Grains	
Barley, pearled	36
Barley, cracked	72
Barley, rolled	94
Buckwheat	78
Bulgur	68
Couscous	93
Cornmeal	97
Sweet corn	78
Taco shells	97
Millet	101
Rice, white	81
Rice, white, low amylose	126
Rice, white, high amylose, basmati	83
Rice, brown	79
Rice, Sunbrown Quick	114
Rice, Mahatma Premium	94
Rice	109
Rice, Calrose	124
Rice, instant, boiled 6 min	128
Rice, instant, boiled 1 min	65
Rice, parboiled	68
Rice, parboiled, high amylose	69
Rice, parboiled, low amylose	124

APPENDIX 54 THE GLYCEMIC INDICES OF FOODS *(continued)*

FOOD	GLYCEMIC INDEX (GI) (WHITE BREAD = 100 = REFERENCE)
Cereal Grains (continued)	
Rice, specialty	78
Rice, wild, Saskatchewan	81
Rye kernels	48
Tapioca, boiled with milk	115
Wheat kernels	59
Wheat, quick cooking	77
Cookies	
Digestives	84
Graham wafers	106
Arrowroot	95
Morning Coffee cookies	113
Oatmeal cookies	79
Rich Tea cookies	79
Shredded Wheatmeal	89
Shortbread	91
Vanilla wafers	110
Crackers	
Breton Wheat Crackers	96
Jatz	79
Puffed Crispbread	116
Rice Cakes	117
High Fibre Rye Crispread	93
Sao	100
Stoned Wheat Thins	96
Water Crackers	102
Dairy Foods	
Ice Cream	87
Ice cream, low-fat	71
Milk, full fat	39
Milk, skim	46
Milk, chocolate, sugar sweetened	49
Milk, chocolate, artificially sweetened	34
Milk + 30 g bran	38
Custard, milk + starch + sugar	61
Yakult (fermented milk)	64
Yogurt, low-fat, fruit, sugar sweetened	47
Yogurt, low-fat, artificially sweetened	20
Yogurt, unspecified	51
Fruit and Fruit Products	
Apple	52
Apple juice	58
Apricots, fresh	82
Apricots, canned, syrup	91
Apricots, dried	44
Banana	76
Cantaloupe	93
Cherries	32
Fruit cocktail	79
Grapefruit	36
Grapefruit juice, unsweetened	69
Grapes	62
Kiwifruit	75
Mango	80
Orange	62
Orange juice	74
Pawpaw	83
Peach, fresh	40
Peach, canned	79
Pear, fresh	51

FOOD	GLYCEMIC INDEX (GI) (WHITE BREAD = 100 = REFERENCE)
Fruit and Fruit Products (continued)	
Pear, canned	63
Pineapple	94
Pineapple juice	66
Plum	34
Raisins	91
Sultanas	80
Watermelon	103
Legumes	
Baked beans, canned	69
Beans, dried, not specified	40
Beans, dried, *P. vulgaris*	100
Black-eyed beans	59
Broad beans (fava beans)	113
Butter beans	44
Butter beans + 5 g sucrose	43
Butter beans + 10 g sucrose	44
Butter beans + 15 g sucrose	77
Chickpeas (garbanzo beans)	47
Chickpeas, canned	60
Chickpeas, curry, canned	58
Kidney beans	42
Kidney beans, autoclaved	49
Kidney beans, canned	74
Lentils, not specified	41
Lentils, green	42
Lentils, green, canned	74
Lentils, red	36
Lima beans, baby, frozen	46
Navy (haricot) beans	54
Pinto beans	55
Pinto beans, canned	64
Romano beans	65
Soya beans	25
Soya beans, canned	20
Split peas, yellow, boiled	45
Pasta	
Capellini	64
Fettuccine	46
Gnocchi	95
Instant noodles	67
Linguine, thick	65
Linguine, thin	78
Macaroni	64
Macaroni and cheese	92
Ravioli, durum, meat filled	56
Spaghetti, protein enriched	38
Spaghetti, white, boiled 15 min	59
Spaghetti, boiled 5 min	52
Spaghetti, durum	78
Spaghetti, wholemeal	53
Spirali, durum	61
Star pastina	54
Tortellini, cheese	71
Vermicelli	50
Rice pasta, brown	131
Root Vegetables	
Beets	91
Carrots	101
Parsnips	139

APPENDIX 54 THE GLYCEMIC INDICES OF FOODS *(continued)*

FOOD	GLYCEMIC INDEX (GI) (WHITE BREAD = 100 = REFERENCE)
Root Vegetables	
Potato, instant	118
Potato, baked	121
Potato, new	81
Potato, Pontiac, boiled	80
Potato, Prince Edward Island, boiled	90
Potato, boiled, mashed	104
Potato, canned	87
Potato, white, boiled	80
Potato mashed	100
Potato, steamed	93
Potato, microwaved	117
French fries	107
Sweet potato	77
Rutabaga	103
Yam	73
Snack Food and Confectionary	
Jelly beans	114
Life Savers	100
Chocolate	70
Muesli Bars	87
Popcorn	79
Corn chips	105
Potato crisps or chips	77
Peanuts	21
Pretzels	116
Mars Chocolate (Dove)	63
Mars M&Ms (peanut)	46
Mars Bar	91
Mars Skittles	98
Snack Food and Confectionary (continued)	
Mars Snickers Bar	57
Mars Twix Cookie Bars (caramel)	62
Mars Kudos Whole Grain Bars (choc chip)	87
Power Bar	81
VO_2 Max Energy Bar (chocolate; Mars)	69
Tofu frozen dessert, nondairy	164
Vitari, nondairy frozen fruit dessert	40
Soups	
Black bean soup	92
Green pea soup, canned	94
Lentil soup, canned	63
Split pea soup	86
Tomato soup	54
Sugars	
Honey	104
Fructose	32
Glucose	138
Glucose tablets	146
Maltose	150
Sucrose	92
Lactose	65
High fructose corn syrup	89
Maltodextrin	137
Vegetables	
Peas, dried	32
Peas, green	68
Pumpkin	107
Sweet corn	78

Adapted from Foster-Powell K, Brand Miller J. International tables of glycemic index. Am J Clin Nutr, 62:871s, 1995; Brand Miller J et al. In search of low glycaemic index foods. Proc Nutr Soc Aust, 19:177, 1995; Brand Miller JC, et al. The glycaemic index of more breads, breakfast cereals and snack products. Proc Nutr Soc Aust, 21:144, 1997; and Brand-Miller JC, et al. The glycaemic index of further Australian foods. Proc Nutr Soc Aust, 22:110, 1998.

Index

Note: Page numbers in italics indicate illustrations; page numbers followed by t indicate tables.